SIXTH EDITION

VOLUME I

# GLENN'S THORACIC AND CARDIOVASCULAR SURGERY

SIXTH EDITION
VOLUME I

# GLENN'S THORACIC AND CARDIOVASCULAR SURGERY


*Editor*

**Arthur E. Baue, MD**
Professor of Surgery
Saint Louis University School of Medicine
St. Louis, Missouri

*Coeditors*

**Alexander S. Geha, MD, MS**
Chief, Division of Cardiothoracic Surgery
University Hospitals of Cleveland
The Jay L. Ankeney Professor and Director
Division of Cardiothoracic Surgery
Case Western Reserve University School of Medicine
Cleveland, Ohio

**Graeme L. Hammond, MD**
Attending Surgeon
Yale-New Haven Hospital
Professor of Surgery
Yale University School of Medicine
New Haven, Connecticut

**Hillel Laks, MD**
Professor and Chief, Division of Cardiothoracic Surgery
University of California, Los Angeles School of Medicine
Los Angeles, California

**Keith S. Naunheim, MD**
Professor of Surgery
Saint Louis University School of Medicine
St. Louis, Missouri


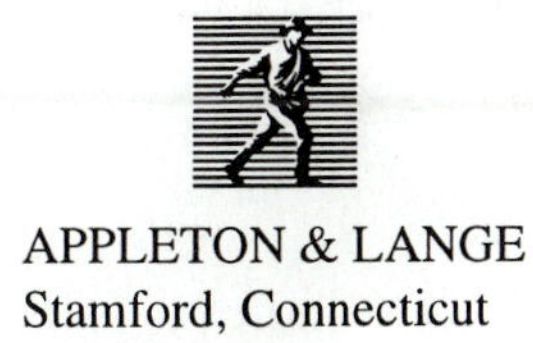


APPLETON & LANGE
Stamford, Connecticut

Notice: The authors and the publisher of this volume have taken care to make certain that the doses of drugs and schedules of treatment are correct and compatible with the standards generally accepted at the time of publication. Nevertheless, as new information becomes available, changes in treatment and in the use of drugs become necessary. The reader is advised to carefully consult the instruction and information material included in the package insert of each drug or therapeutic agent before administration. This advice is especially important when using new or infrequently used drugs. The publisher disclaims any liability, loss, injury, or damage incurred as a consequence, directly or indirectly, or the use and application of any of the contents of the volume.

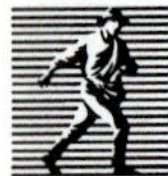



96 97 98 99 00 / 10 9 8 7 6 5 4 3 2 1

Prentice Hall International (UK) Limited, *London*
Prentice Hall of Australia Pty. Limited, *Sydney*
Prentice Hall Canada, Inc., *Toronto*
Prentice Hall Hispanoamericana, S.A., *Mexico*
Prentice Hall of India Private Limited, *New Delhi*
Prentice Hall of Japan, Inc., *Tokyo*
Simon & Schuster Asia Pte. Ltd., *Singapore*
Editora Prentice Hall do Brasil Ltda., *Rio de Janeiro*
Prentice Hall, *Englewood Cliffs, New Jersey*

**Library of Congress Cataloging-in-Publication Data**

Glenn's thoracic and cardiovascular surgery / [edited by] Arthur E. Baue . . . [et al.].—6th ed.
p. cm.
Includes bibliographical references and index.
ISBN 0–8385–3134–2 (set : casebound)
1. Chest—Surgery. 2. Cardiovascular system—Surgery. I. Glenn, William W. L. II. Baue, Arthur. III. Title: Thoracic and cardiovascular surgery.
[DNLM: 1. Thoracic Surgery. 2. Cardiovascular System—surgery. WF 980 G5581G558 1995]
RD536.G585 1995
617.5′4—dc20
DNLM/DLC
for Library of Congress 95–14257
CIP

Acquisitions Editor: Edward Wickland
Managing Editor, Development: Kathleen McCullough
Production Coordinator: Jean Finn
Production Service: Spectrum Publisher Services, Blair Woodcock
Production Supervisor: Karen Davis
Designer: Elizabeth Schmitz
Cover Designer: Janice Barsevich Bielawa

ISBN 0-8385-3134-2
90000
9 780838 531341

PRINTED IN THE UNITED STATES OF AMERICA

This book, the Sixth Edition, bears the name of
William W.L. Glenn, MD, who carried the tradition of the original
book by Gustav E. Lindskog, MD, and the late Averill A. Liebow, MD.
We remember them as we dedicate this edition to those who have
supported us in these endeavors—to Rosemary Baue, Diane Geha,
Janet Hammond, and Rosanne Naunheim.

Little do such men know the toil, the pains,
the daily, nightly racking of the brains
to arrange the thoughts, the matter to digest
to cull fit phrases, and reject the rest.

*Charles Churchill (1731–1764),*
*Gotham, Book II*

Surgery is in large part a handicraft with elaborate technics that may be grouped as Technology . . . if one be honest . . . he cannot fail to see that Surgery is seeded with ad hoc hypotheses, or, in more frank terms, empiricisms, and irrational beliefs.

*Edward D. Churchill*
*Ann Surg 126:381, 1947*

# Contents

# Contributors

**Michael A. Acker, MD**
Attending Staff, Surgical Director Cardiac Transplantation Program
Hospital of the University of Pennsylvania
Assistant Professor of Surgery
University of Pennsylvania School of Medicine
Philadelphia, Pennsylvania

**Lee P. Adler, MD**
Director Cardiovascular MR
University Hospital of Cleveland
Associate Professor of Radiology
Case Western Reserve University School of Medicine
Cleveland, Ohio

**Bradley S. Allen, MD**
Attending Cardiothoracic Surgeon
University of Illinois Hospital
Assistant Professor of Surgery
Division of Cardiothoracic Surgery
University of Illinois College of Medicine
Chicago, Illinois

**Mark S. Allen, MD**
Consultant in General Thoracic Surgery
Mayo Clinic
Assistant Professor of Surgery
Mayo Graduate School of Medicine
Rochester, Minnesota

**Nasser K. Altorki, MD**
Associate Attending Cardiovascular–Thoracic Surgeon
The New York Hospital
Associate Professor, Cardiothoracic Surgery
Cornell University Medical College
New York, New York

**Robert H. Anderson, BSc, MD, FRCPath**
Honorary Consultant
Royal Brompton Hospital NHS Trust
Joseph Levy Professor of Paediatric Cardiac Morphology
National Heart & Lung Institute
London, United Kingdom

**Joseph S. Auteri**
Attending Cardiothoracic Surgeon
Arizona Heart Institute
Health West Regional Medical Center
Phoenix, Arizona

**Carl L. Backer, MD**
Attending Cardiovascular–Thoracic Surgeon
The Children's Memorial Hospital
Assistant Professor of Surgery
Northwestern University Medical School
Chicago, Illinois

**Leonard L. Bailey, MD**
Attending Surgeon—Cardiothoracic
Loma Linda University Medical Center
Professor and Chairman, Department of Surgery
Loma Linda University School of Medicine
Loma Linda, California

**John C. Baldwin, MD**
Chief of Surgical Services
The Methodist Hospital
Surgeon-in-Chief
Ben Taub General Hospital
DeBakey Professor and Chairman, Department of Surgery
Baylor College of Medicine
Houston, Texas

**Paul G. Barash, MD**
Attending Anesthesiologist
Yale New Haven Medical Center
Professor of Anesthesiology
Yale University School of Medicine
New Haven, Connecticut

**Hendrick B. Barner, MD**
Christian Hospital NE
Professor of Surgery
Washington University School of Medicine
St. Louis, Missouri

**Arthur E. Baue, MD**
Professor of Surgery
Saint Louis University School of Medicine
St. Louis, Missouri

**Victor C. Baum, MD**
Attending Physician
Departments of Anesthesiology & Pediatrics
University of Virginia Medical Center
Associate Professor of Anesthesiology and Pediatrics
University of Virginia
Charlottesville, Virginia

**Carlos W.M. Bedrossian, MD**
Chief of Cytopathology
Detroit Medical Center
Professor of Pathology
Wayne State University School of Medicine
Detroit, Michigan

**Douglas M. Behrendt, MD**
Professor and Chairman
Division of Cardiothoracic Surgery
The University of Iowa
Iowa City, Iowa

**Ronald H.R. Belsey, MS, FRCS, FRCSI(Hon)**
Emeritus Professor of Cardiothoracic Surgery
Bristol University
Bath, United Kingdom

**John R. Benfield, MD**
Chief of the Division of Cardiothoracic Surgery
University of California, Davis Medical Center
Professor of Surgery
University of California, Davis School of Medicine
Sacramento, California

**Deborah A. Bishop, BS**
Research Associate
The Children's Hospital
University of Colorado Health Sciences Center
Denver, Colorado

**Edward L. Bove, MD**
Director, Pediatric Cardiovascular Surgery
C.S. Mott Children's Hospital
Professor of Surgery
University of Michigan School of Medicine
Ann Arbor, Michigan

**Carol M. Buchter, MD**
Director, Heart Failure Evaluation and Treatment Program
University Hospitals of Cleveland
Assistant Professor of Medicine
Case Western Reserve University School of Medicine
Cleveland, Ohio

**Gerald D. Buckberg, MD**
Attending Staff
University of California, Los Angeles Medical Center
Professor of Surgery
University of California, Los Angeles School of Medicine
Los Angeles, California

**Redmond P. Burke, MD**
Associate in Cardiac Surgery
Childrens Hospital, Boston
Instructor in Surgery
Harvard Medical School
Boston, Massachusetts

**Michael Burt, MD, PhD**
Attending Surgeon
Memorial Sloan-Kettering Cancer Center
Associate Professor of Surgery
Cornell University Medical College
New York, New York

**Alain Carpentier, MD, PhD**
Chairman, Cardiovascular Surgery Department
Hospital Broussais
Professor of Cardiac Surgery
University of Paris
France

**Bernard R. Chaitman, MD**
Chief of Cardiology
Saint Louis University Health Sciences Center
Professor of Medicine
Saint Louis University School of Medicine
St. Louis, Missouri

**Pauline W. Chen, MD**
Medical Staff Fellow
Surgery Branch
National Cancer Institute
National Institutes of Health
Bethesda, Maryland

**John S. Child, MD**
Co-Chief, Clinical Cardiology
Department of Medicine
Professor of Medicine
University of California, Los Angeles Medical School
Los Angeles, California

**Joseph M. Civetta, MD**
Director, Surgical Trauma Intensive Care Units
Jackson Memorial Hospital
Professor and Chief
Division of Surgical Critical Care
Department of Surgery
University of Miami School of Medicine
Miami, Florida

**David R. Clarke, MD**
Chief, Pediatric Cardiothoracic Surgery
The Children's Hospital
Professor of Surgery
University of Colorado
Denver, Colorado

**Brian L. Cmolik, MD**
Veterans Administration Medical Center/University Hospitals
Assistant Professor of Surgery
Case Western Reserve University School of Medicine
Cleveland, Ohio

**Lawrence H. Cohn, MD**
Chief of Cardiac Surgery
Brigham & Women's Hospital
Professor of Surgery
Harvard Medical School
Boston, Massachusetts

**Steven D. Colquhoun, MD**
Chief, Liver Transplantation
University of California, Davis Medical Center
Assistant Professor of Surgery
University of California, Davis School of Medicine
Sacramento, California

**John E. Connolly, MD**
Professor of Surgery
University of California, Irvine School of Medicine
Irvine, California

**Joseph S. Coselli, MD**
Attending Surgeon
The Methodist Hospital
Associate Professor of Surgery
Baylor College of Medicine
Houston, Texas

**John L. Cotton, MD**
Fellow, Division of Pediatric Cardiology
University of California, Los Angeles School of Medicine
Los Angeles, California

**James L. Cox, MD**
Chief, Division of Cardiothoracic Surgery
Washington University Medical Center/ Barnes Hospital
Evarts A. Graham Professor of Surgery
Washington University School of Medicine
St. Louis, Missouri

**Willard M. Daggett, Jr., MD**
Visiting Surgeon
Massachusetts General Hospital
Professor of Surgery
Harvard Medical School
Boston, Massachusetts

**Harry J. D'Agostino, Jr., MD**
Clinical Instructor
Division of Cardiothoracic Surgery
University of California, Los Angeles School of Medicine
Los Angeles, California

**Gordon K. Danielson, MD**
Consultant in Surgery
Mayo Medical Center
Roberts Professor of Surgery
Mayo Graduate School of Medicine Foundation
Rochester, Minnesota

**Robert Duane Davis, MD**
Surgical Director of Lung Transplantation
Duke University Medical Center
Assistant Professor of Surgery
Duke University School of Medicine
Durham, North Carolina

**Jacob G. Davtyan, MD**
Chief Resident, Cardiothoracic Surgery
Emory University School of Medicine
Atlanta, Georgia

**Malcolm M. DeCamp, Jr., MD**
Associate Thoracic Surgeon, Division of Thoracic Surgery
Brigham & Women's Hospital
Assistant Professor of Surgery
Harvard Medical School
Boston, Massachusetts

**Marc R. de Leval, MD, FRCS**
Consultant Cardiothoracic Surgeon
Great Ormond Street Hospital for Children NHS Trust
Institute of Child Health
London, United Kingdom

**Michael del Rio, MD**
Clinical Research Fellow in Cardiothoracic Pediatric Surgery
Loma Linda University Medical Center
Clinical Fellow
Division of Cardiothoracic Surgery, Department of Surgery
Loma Linda University School of Medicine
Loma Linda, California

**Tom R. DeMeester, MD**
Professor and Chairman
Department of Surgery
University of Southern California School of Medicine
Los Angeles, California

**Davis C. Drinkwater, Jr., MD**
Director, Pediatric Cardiac Transplant Program
University of California, Los Angeles Medical Center
Associate Professor of Surgery
University of California, Los Angeles School of Medicine
Los Angeles, California

**Jeffrey L. Duerk, Ph.D.**
Director, Physics Research
University Hospitals of Cleveland
Associate Professor, Radiology and Biomedical Engineering
Case Western Reserve University School of Medicine
Cleveland, Ohio

**André Duranceau, MD**
Professor of Surgery
University of Montreal
Division of Thoracic Surgery
Hôtel-Dieu de Montréal
Montreal, Quebec, Canada

**Cornelius M. Dyke, MD**
Fellow in Cardiothoracic Surgery
Medical College of Virginia/Virginia Commonwealth University
Richmond, Virginia

**L. Henry Edmunds, Jr., MD**
Active Staff, Division of Cardiothoracic Surgery
Hospital of the University of Pennsylvania
Julian Johnson Professor of Cardiothoracic Surgery
University of Pennsylvania School of Medicine
Philadelphia, Pennsylvania

**John A. Elefteriades, MD**
Attending Surgeon
Director of Adult Cardiac Procedures
Yale-New Haven Hospital
Professor of Surgery
Yale University Medical School
New Haven, Connecticut

**F. Henry Ellis, Jr., MD, PhD**
Chief Emeritus, Division of Cardiothoracic Surgery
Deaconess Hospital
Clinical Professor of Surgery Emeritus
Harvard Medical School
Boston, Massachusetts

**Richard P. Embrey, MD**
Director of Pediatric Cardiac Surgery
Medical College of Virginia Hospital
Assistant Professor of Surgery
Medical College of Virginia/Virginia Commonwealth University
Richmond, Virginia

**M. Arisan Ergin, MD**
Attending
Mount Sinai Hospital and Medical Center
Professor of Cardiac Surgery
Mount Sinai School of Medicine
New York, New York

**L. Penfield Faber, MD**
Director, Section General Thoracic Surgery
Presbyterian-St. Lukes Hospital
Professor of Surgery
Rush Medical College
Chicago, Illinois

**James I. Fann, MD**
Fellow, Cardiothoracic Surgery and Vascular Surgery
Stanford University Medical Center
Stanford, California

**Mark K. Ferguson, MD**
Chief, Section of Thoracic Surgery
University of Chicago Medical Center
Associate Professor of Surgery
University of Chicago Pritzker School of Medicine
Chicago, Illinois

**T. Bruce Ferguson, Jr., MD**
Associate Surgeon
Department of Surgery
Division of Cardiothoracic Surgery
Barnes Hospital
Associate Professor of Surgery
Washington University School of Medicine
St. Louis, Missouri

**Peter F. Ferson, MD**
University of Pittsburgh Medical Center and Veterans Administration Hospital
Professor of Surgery
University of Pittsburgh School of Medicine
Pittsburgh, Pennsylvania

**Andrew C. Fiore, MD**
Professor of Surgery
Saint Louis University School of Medicine
St. Louis, Missouri

**Eric W. Fonkalsrud, MD**
Professor of Surgery and Chief of Pediatric Surgery
University of California, Los Angeles School of Medicine
Los Angeles, California

**Gregory P. Fontana, MD**
Attending Cardiothoracic Surgeon
Cedars-Sinai Medical Center
Clinical Assistant Professor of Surgery
University of California, Los Angeles School of Medicine
Los Angeles, California

**Kenneth L. Franco, MD**
Yale-New Haven Hospital
Associate Professor of Surgery
Yale University School of Medicine
New Haven, Connecticut

**Robert W.M. Frater, MD**
Montefiore Medical Center
Jack D. Weiler Hospital of the Albert College of Medicine
Professor of Cardiothoracic Surgery
Albert Einstein College of Medicine
Bronx, New York

**Timothy J. Gardner, MD**
Chief, Division of Cardiothoracic Surgery
Hospital of the University of Pennsylvania
William M. Measey Professor of Surgery
University of Pennsylvania School of Medicine
Philadelphia, Pennsylvania

**Richard N. Gates, MD**
Congenital Heart Surgery/Transplant Fellow
University of California, Los Angeles Medical Center
University of California, Los Angeles School of Medicine
Los Angeles, California

**J. William Gaynor, MD**
Assistant Professor of Surgery
Duke University School of Medicine
Durham, North Carolina

**Alexander S. Geha, MD, MS**
Chief, Division of Cardiothoracic Surgery
University Hospitals of Cleveland
The Jay L. Ankeney Professor and Director
Division of Cardiothoracic Surgery
Case Western Reserve University School of Medicine
Cleveland, Ohio

**Barbara George, MD**
Associate Director, Cardiothoracic Intensive Care Unit
Center for the Health Sciences,
Associate Professor of Pediatrics
University of California, Los Angeles School of Medicine
Los Angeles, California

**Robert J. Ginsberg, MD**
Chief of Thoracic Service
Department of Surgery
Memorial Sloan-Kettering Cancer Center
Professor of Surgery
Cornell University Medical College
New York, New York

**Paul Gordon, MD**
Thoracic Surgery Resident
Southern Illinois University School of Medicine
Springfield, Illinois

**William J. Greeley, MD**
Division Chief, Division of Pediatric Cardiac Anesthesiology & Critical Care Medicine
Associate Professor of Anesthesiology & Pediatrics
Duke University School of Medicine
Durham, North Carolina

**Randall B. Griepp, MD**
Chairman, Department of Cardiothoracic Surgery
Mount Sinai Hospital
Professor of Cardiothoracic Surgery
Mount Sinai School of Medicine
New York, New York

**Bartley P. Griffith, MD**
Chief, Division of Cardiothoracic Surgery
Presbyterian University Hospital
Professor of Surgery
University of Pittsburgh
Pittsburgh, Pennsylvania

**Hermes C. Grillo, MD**
Visiting Surgeon, General Thoracic Surgery
Massachusetts General Hospital
Professor of Surgery
Harvard Medical School
Boston, Massachusetts

**Claude M. Grondin, MD**
Head, Division of Cardiothoracic Surgery
St. Luke's Hospital, Cleveland
Clinical Professor of Surgery
Case Western Reserve University School of Medicine
Cleveland, Ohio

**Gary Haas, MD**
Assistant Professor of Surgery and Pediatrics
University of California, San Francisco School of Medicine
San Francisco, California

**Alden W. Hall, BA**
Denver, Colorado

**Graeme L. Hammond, MD**
Attending Surgeon
Yale-New Haven Hospital
Professor of Surgery
Yale University School of Medicine
New Haven, Connecticut

**John R. Handy, MD**
Director of Lung Transplantation
Assistant Professor of Surgery
Assistant Professor of Clinical Services
Medical University of South Carolina
Charleston, South Carolina

**Frank L. Hanley, MD**
Chief, Division of Cardiothoracic Surgery
University of California, San Francisco Medical Center
Professor of Surgery
University of California, San Francisco
San Francisco, California

**Alden H. Harken, MD**
Professor and Chairman, Department of Surgery
University of Colorado
Denver, Colorado

**Lynn H. Harrison, Jr., MD**
Chief, Section of Cardiothoracic Surgery
University Hospital
Associate Professor of Surgery
Louisiana State University School of Medicine
New Orleans, Louisiana

**Stephen R. Hazelrigg, MD**
Chairman, Division of Cardiothoracic Surgery
Associate Professor
Southern Illinois University School of Medicine
Springfield, Illinois

**Richard F. Heitmiller, MD**
Chief, Division of General Thoracic Surgery
Johns Hopkins Hospital
Associate Professor of Surgery
Johns Hopkins University
Baltimore, Maryland

**John Hennecken, MD**
Director, Cardiac Cath Laboratories
Director Interventional Cardiology
Medical College of Georgia Hospital & Clinics
Augusta Veterans Affairs Medical Center
Associate Professor of Medicine
Medical College of Georgia
Augusta, Georgia

**Clement A. Hiebert, MD**
Chairman Emeritus
Department of Surgery
Maine Medical Center
Portland, Maine
Clinical Assistant in Surgery
Harvard Medical School
Boston, Massachusetts

**Alan D. Hilgenberg, MD**
Cardiac Surgeon
Massachusetts General Hospital
Associate Clinical Professor of Surgery
Harvard Medical School
Boston, Massachusetts

**Lucius D. Hill, MD**
Clinical Professor of Surgery
University of Washington School of Medicine
Seattle, Washington

**George T. Hodakowski, MD**
Resident in Cardiothoracic Surgery
The Emory University Hospital
Atlanta, Georgia

**E. Carmack Holmes, MD**
Chairman, Department of Surgery
University of California, Los Angeles Medical Center
Professor
University of California, Los Angeles School of Medicine
Los Angeles, California

**Thomas M. Hyers, MD**
Director, Division of Pulmonology & Pulmonary Occupational Medicine
Saint Louis University Health Sciences Center
James and Ethel Miller Professor of Internal Medicine
Saint Louis University School of Medicine
St. Louis, Missouri

**Michel N. Ilbawi, MD**
Director, Pediatric Cardiac Surgery
Heart Institute for Children
Associate Professor of Surgery
Northwestern University Medical School
Oak Lawn, Illinois

**Josephine B. Isabel-Jones, MD**
Professor of Pediatrics (Cardiology)
University of California, Los Angeles School of Medicine
Los Angeles, California

**Marshall L. Jacobs, MD**
Associate Cardiothoracic Surgeon
Children's Hospital of Philadelphia
Associate Professor of Surgery
University of Pennsylvania School of Medicine
Philadelphia, Pennsylvania

**Stuart W. Jamieson, MD, FRCS.**
Head of Cardiovascular and Thoracic Surgery
University of California, San Diego Medical Center
Professor of Surgery
University of California, San Diego School of Medicine
San Diego, California

**Adib D. Jatene, MD**
Director, Cardiovascular and Thoracic Surgery
Heart Institute
Professor of Surgery
University of Sao Paulo
Sao Paulo, Brazil

**Ellis L. Jones, MD**
Emory University Hospital
Professor of Cardiovascular Surgery
Emory University School of Medicine
Atlanta, Georgia

**M.J. Jurkiewicz, MD**
Attending Surgeon
Emory Affiliated Hospital
Professor of Surgery
Emory University School of Medicine
Atlanta, Georgia

**George C. Kaiser, MD**
Chief of Cardiothoracic Surgery
Saint Louis University Health Sciences Center
Professor of Surgery
Saint Louis University School of Medicine
St. Louis, Missouri

**Larry R. Kaiser, MD**
Chief, General Thoracic Surgery
Hospital of the University of Pennsylvania
Associate Professor of Surgery
University of Pennsylvania School of Medicine
Philadelphia, Pennsylvania

**Tom R. Karl, MS, MD**
Director, Cardiac Surgical Unit
Royal Children's Hospital
Melbourne, Australia

**Robert J. Keenan, MD, FRCSC**
Director, Lung Transplantation
University of Pittsburgh Medical Center
Assistant Professor of Surgery
University of Pittsburgh School of Medicine
Pittsburgh, Pennsylvania

**David P. Kelsen, MD**
Chief, Gastrointestinal Oncology Service
Memorial Sloan-Kettering Cancer Center
Professor of Medicine
Cornell University Medical College
New York, New York

**Frank H. Kern, MD**
Director, Pediatric Cardiac Anesthesia
and Associate Director
Pediatric Intensive Care Unit
Duke University Medical Center
Associate Professor of Anesthesiology & Pediatrics
Duke University School of Medicine
Durham, North Carolina

**Spencer B. King, III, MD**
Director Cardiovascular Labs
Emory University Hospital
Professor of Medicine
Emory University School of Medicine
Atlanta, Georgia

**Orlando C. Kirton, MD**
Assistant Director, Surgical Intensive Care Unit
University of Miami/Jackson Memorial Medical Center
Assistant Professor of Clinical Surgery
University of Miami School of Medicine
Miami, Florida

**Gary S. Kopf, MD**
Chief, Pediatric Cardiac Surgery
Yale-New Haven Hospital
Professor of Surgery
Yale University School of Medicine
New Haven, Connecticut

**Nicholas T. Kouchoukos, MD**
Surgeon and Cardiothoracic Surgeon-in-Chief
The Jewish Hospital of St. Louis
John M. Shoenberg Professor of Cardiovascular Surgery
Washington University School of Medicine
St. Louis, Missouri

**Jolene M. Kriett, MD**
Attending Surgeon
Division of Cardiothoracic Surgery
University of California, San Diego Medical Center
Associate Professor of Surgery
University of California, San Diego School of Medicine
San Diego, California

**Janine Krivokapich, MD**
Director, UCLA Adult Cardiac Non-Invasive Laboratories
Professor of Medicine
University of California, Los Angeles School of Medicine
Los Angeles, California

**Hillel Laks, MD**
Professor and Chief, Division of Cardiothoracic Surgery
University of California, Los Angeles School
of Medicine
Los Angeles, California

**John J. Lamberti, MD**
Chief of Cardiac Surgery
Children's Hospital—San Diego
Associate Clinical Professor
University of California, San Diego School
of Medicine
San Diego, California

**Rodney J. Landreneau, MD**
Head, Section of Thoracic Surgery
University of Pittsburgh Medical Center
Associate Professor
University of Pittsburgh School of Medicine
Pittsburgh, Pennsylvania

**Jai H. Lee, MD**
Attending Cardiothoracic Surgeon
University Hospitals of Cleveland
Assistant Professor of Surgery
Case Western Reserve University School of Medicine
Cleveland, Ohio

**K. Francis Lee, MD**
Fellow in Cardiothoracic Surgery
Medical College of Virginia/Virginia Commonwealth
University
Richmond, Virginia

**Toni Lerut, MD**
Chairman, Department of Thoracic
Surgery
Catholic University Hospitals Leuven
Professor in Surgery
Catholic University Leuven
Leuven, Belgium

**George V. Letsou, MD**
Attending Surgeon
The Methodist Hospital
Associate Professor of Surgery
Baylor College of Medicine
Houston, Texas

**James M. Lieberman, MD**
Staff Radiologist
University Hospitals of Cleveland
Associate Professor of Radiology
Case Western Reserve University School of Medicine
Cleveland, Ohio

**Wayne Lipson, MD**
Cardiac Surgery Fellow
Brigham & Women's Hospital
Harvard Medical School
Boston, Massachusetts

**Alex G. Little, MD**
Chief of Surgery
University Medical Center
Professor and Chairman
University of Nevada School of Medicine
Las Vegas, Nevada

**Joseph LoCicero, III, MD**
Chief, General Thoracic Surgery
New England Deaconess Hospital
New England Baptist Hospital,
Cambridge Hospital
Associate Professor
Harvard Medical School
Boston, Massachusetts

**Gary K. Lofland, MD**
Director, Congenital Heart Center
Columbia/HCA Henrico Doctors' Hospital
Clinical Professor of Surgery
Georgetown University School of Medicine
Richmond, Virginia

**Donald E. Low, MD, FRCS(C)**
Staff
Virginia Mason Clinic
Clinical Instructor
University of Washington School of Medicine
Seattle, Washington

**Michael J. Mack, MD**
Cardiothoracic Surgeon
Medical City Dallas Hospital
Clinical Assistant Professor of Thoracic Surgery
Southwestern Medical School
University of Texas
Dallas, Texas

**Judith A. Mackall, MD**
University Hospitals of Cleveland
Assistant Professor of Medicine
Case Western Reserve University School of Medicine
Cleveland, Ohio

**James W. Mackenzie, MD**
Chief of the Surgical Service
Robert Wood Johnson University Hospital
Professor and Chairman, Department of Surgery
University of Medicine & Dentistry of New Jersey
Robert Wood Johnson Medical School
New Brunswick, New Jersey

**Joren C. Madsen, MD, DPhil**
Assistant in Surgery
Massachusetts General Hospital
Assistant Professor of Surgery
Harvard Medical School
Boston, Massachusetts

**Mitchell J. Magee, MD**
Assistant Professor, Division of Cardiothoracic Surgery
Southern Illinois University School of Medicine
Springfield, Illinois

**James A. Magovern, MD**
Associate Attending Staff
Allegheny General Hospital
Associate Professor of Surgery
The Medical College of Pennsylvania
Pittsburgh, Pennsylvania

**Richard D. Mainwaring, MD**
Division of Cardiac Surgery
Children's Hospital—San Diego
San Diego, California

**James B.D. Mark, MD**
Head, Division of Thoracic Surgery
Stanford Medical Center
Johnson & Johnson Professor of Cardiothoracic Surgery
Stanford University School of Medicine
Stanford, California

**Nael Martini, MD**
Attending Thoracic Surgeon
Memorial Sloan-Kettering Cancer Center
Professor of Surgery
Cornell University Medical College
New York, New York

**Joseph P. Mathew, MD**
Attending Anesthesiologist
Yale New Haven Medical Center
Assistant Professor of Anesthesiology
Yale University School of Medicine
New Haven, Connecticut

**Douglas J. Mathisen, MD**
Visiting Surgeon and Chief,
General Thoracic Surgery
Massachusetts General Hospital
Associate Professor of Surgery
Harvard Medical School
Boston, Massachusetts

**Kenneth L. Mattox, MD**
Chief of Staff
Ben Taub General Hospital
Professor of Surgery
Baylor College of Medicine
Houston, Texas

**Constantine Mavroudis, MD**
Division Head and A.C. Buehler Professor
of Cardiovascular–Thoracic Surgery
The Children's Memorial Hospital
Professor of Surgery
Northwestern University Medical School
Chicago, Illinois

**Lawrence R. McBride, MD**
Director of Cardiac and Lung Transplantation
Saint Louis University Health Sciences Center
Professor of Surgery
Saint Louis University School of Medicine
St. Louis, Missouri

**Charles J. McCabe, MD**
Associate Chief, Emergency Services
Massachusetts General Hospital
Associate Professor of Surgery
Harvard Medical School
Boston, Massachusetts

**Patricia M. McCormack, MD**
Attending Surgeon, Thoracic Service,
Department of Surgery
Memorial Sloan-Kettering
Cancer Center
Associate Professor of Surgery
Cornell University Medical College
New York, New York

**Richard Burr McElvein, MD**
Chief, Thoracic Surgery
University Hospital and Birmingham Veterans
Administration Hospital
Professor of Surgery, Retired
University of Alabama at Birmingham
Birmingham, Alabama

**Joseph S. McLaughlin, MD**
Head, Division of Thoracic & Cardiovascular Surgery
University of Maryland Medical Center
Professor of Surgery
University of Maryland School of Medicine
Baltimore, Maryland

**D. Craig Miller, MD**
Professor of Cardiovascular Surgery
Stanford University School of Medicine
Stanford, California

**D. Douglas Miller, MD**
Director, Nuclear Cardiology
Director, Cardiovascular Biology
Saint Louis University Health Sciences Center
Associate Professor of Medicine
Saint Louis University School of Medicine
St. Louis, Missouri

**Joseph I. Miller, Jr., MD**
Professor, Department of Surgery, Division
of Cardiothoracic Surgery
The Emory Clinic
Emory University School of Medicine
Atlanta, Georgia

**Bruce D. Minsky, MD**
Associate Attending Physician
Memorial Sloan-Kettering Cancer Center
Associate Professor of Radiation Oncology
Cornell University Medical College
New York, New York

**Ralph S. Mosca, MD**
C.S. Mott Children's Hospital
Associate Professor of Surgery
University of Michigan School of Medicine
Ann Arbor, Michigan

**Keith S. Naunheim, MD**
Professor of Surgery
Saint Louis University School of Medicine
St. Louis, Missouri

**Scott H. Norwood, MD**
Director, Trauma Service
East Texas Medical Center
Tyler, Texas

**William I. Norwood**
Director, Division of Surgery
The Aldo Castañeda Institute
Clinique de Genolier
Genolier, Switzerland

**Mark F. O'Brien, FRCS, FRACS**
Cardiac Surgeon in Charge
Department of Cardiac Surgery
The Prince Charles Hospital
Brisbane, Australia

**James A. O'Neil, Jr., MD**
Surgeon-in-Chief
The Children's Hospital of Philadelphia
C. Everett Koop Professor of Pediatric Surgery
University of Pennsylvania School of Medicine
Philadelphia, Pennsylvania

**Mark B. Orringer, MD**
Professor and Head, Section of Thoracic Surgery
University of Michigan Medical Center
Ann Arbor, Michigan

**Walter E. Pae, Jr., MD**
Director of Cardiac Transplantation, Division of Cardiothoracic Surgery
University Hospital, The Milton S. Hershey Medical Center
Professor of Surgery
The Pennsylvania State University College of Medicine
Hershey, Pennsylvania

**K. Michael Pagliero, MB, BS, FRCS**
Consultant Thoracic Surgeon
Woodmill Hospital
Devon, United Kingdom

**Peter C. Pairolero, MD**
Chair, Department of Surgery
Mayo Medical Center
Professor of Surgery
Mayo Graduate School of Medicine
Rochester, Minnesota

**Christian E. Paletta, MD, FACS**
Associate Professor of Surgery
Division of Plastic and Reconstructive Surgery
Saint Louis University Health Sciences Center
Associate Professor of Surgery
Saint Louis University School of Medicine
St. Louis, Missouri

**Harvey I. Pass, MD**
Head, Thoracic Oncology Section
Senior Investigator, Surgery Branch
National Cancer Institute
National Institutes of Health
Bethesda, Maryland

**G.A. Patterson, MD**
Professor of Surgery
Washington University School of Medicine
St. Louis, Missouri

**Jeffrey M. Pearl, MD**
Chief Resident Cardiothoracic Surgery
University of California, Los Angeles School of Medicine
Los Angeles, California

**Carlos A. Pellegrini, MD**
Chairman, Department of Surgery
University of Washington Medical Center
Professor of Surgery
University School of Medicine
Seattle, Washington

**D. Glenn Pennington, MD**
Howard Holt Bradshaw Professor of Surgery and Chairman
Department of Cardiothoracic Surgery
Bowman Gray School of Medicine of Wake Forest University
Winston-Salem, North Carolina

**Lester C. Permut, MD**
Attending Surgeon
University of California, Los Angeles Medical Center
Assistant Professor of Surgery
University of California, Los Angeles School of Medicine
Los Angeles, California

**Richard M. Peters, MD**
Professor Emeritus Surgery
University of California at San Diego
Menlo Park, California

**William S. Pierce, MD**
Chief, Division of Cardiothoracic Surgery
University Hospital, The Pennsylvania State University
Professor, Cardiovascular & Thoracic Surgery
The Pennsylvania State University College of Medicine
Hershey, Pennsylvania

**Marvin Pomerantz, MD**
Professor of Surgery
Chief, Section of General Thoracic Surgery
University of Colorado
Denver, Colorado

**Thomas W. Prendergast, MD**
Fellow, Congenital Cardiothoracic Surgery
Children's Hospital of Los Angeles
University of California, Los Angeles School of Medicine
Los Angeles, California

**Francisco J. Puga, MD**
Chair, Division of Thoracic and Cardiovascular Surgery
Head, Section of Cardiovascular Surgery
Mayo Clinic
Professor of Surgery
Mayo Graduate School of Medicine
Rochester, Minnesota

**Jan M. Quaegebeur, MD**
Director of Pediatric Cardiac Surgery
Columbia Presbyterian Medical Center
Associate Professor of Surgery
Columbia University
New York, New York

**Marlene Rabinovitch, MD**
Staff Cardiologist, Department of Cardiology
Director, Cardiovascular Research
The Hospital For Sick Children
Professor of Pediatrics, Pathology and Medicine
University of Toronto
Toronto, Ontario, Canada

**Vadiyala Mohan Reddy, MD**
Fellow Pediatric Cardiac Surgery
University of California, San Francisco
Medical Center
San Francisco, California

**Carolyn E. Reed, MD**
Associate Professor of Surgery
Medical University of South Carolina
Charleston, South Carolina

**Michael S. Remetz, MD**
Director, Goodyer Cardiology FIRM
Yale-New Haven Medical Center
Associate Professor of Medicine
Yale University School of Medicine
New Haven, Connecticut

**Thomas W. Rice, MD**
Head of the Section
of General Thoracic Surgery
Department of Thoracic and Cardiovascular Surgery
The Cleveland Clinic Foundation
Cleveland, Ohio

**David J. Riley, MD**
Attending Staff
Robert Wood Johnson University Hospital
Professor of Medicine
University of Medicine & Dentistry of New Jersey
Robert Wood Johnson Medical School
New Brunswick, New Jersey

**Norman W. Rizk, MD**
Director of Clinical Services
Division of Pulmonary and Critical
Care Medicine
Stanford University Hospital
Associate Professor of Medicine
Stanford University School of Medicine
Stanford, California

**Eliot R. Rosenkranz, MD**
Chief, Cardiothoracic Surgery
Children's Hospital of Buffalo
Associate Professor of Surgery
State University of New York at Buffalo
Buffalo, New York

**Jack A. Roth, MD**
Professor and Chairman
Department of Thoracic and Cardiovascular Surgery
University of Texas M.D. Anderson Cancer Center
Professor of Tumor Biology
University of Texas School of Medicine
Houston, Texas

**Ehud Rudis, MD**
Visiting Assistant Professor
University of California, Los Angeles School of Medicine
Los Angeles, California

**Liisa A. Russell, MD**
Associate Clinical Professor of Pathology
University of California, Davis School of Medicine
Sacramento, California

**David H. Sachs, MD**
Director, Transplantation Biology Research Center
Massachusetts General Hospital
Paul S. Russell/Warner-Lambert Professor
of Surgery
Harvard Medical School
Boston, Massachusetts

**Robert M. Sade, MD**
Attending Surgeon
Medical University of South Carolina Medical Center
Professor of Surgery
Medical University of South Carolina
Charleston, South Carolina

**Susheela Sangwan, MD**
Assistant Clinical Professor of Anesthesiology
University of California, Los Angeles School
of Medicine
Los Angeles, California

**John S. Sapirstein, MD**
Research Fellow
Division of Cardiothoracic Surgery
The Pennsylvania State University
Hershey, Pennsylvania

**David S. Schrump, MD**
University of Texas M.D. Anderson Cancer Center
Assistant Professor of Surgery
Department of Thoracic and Cardiovascular
Surgery
University of Texas School of Medicine
Houston, Texas

**Stewart M. Scott, MD**
Chief, Surgical Service
Veterans Administration Medical Center
Consulting Professor of Surgery
Duke University Medical Center
Asheville, North Carolina

**Thomas W. Shields, MD**
Attending Surgeon Emeritus
Northwestern Memorial Hospital
Professor Emeritus of Surgery
Northwestern University
Medical School
Chicago, Illinois

**Dominique Shum-Tim, MD, MDCM, MSC, FRCS(C)**
Chief Resident
Cardiovascular and Thoracic Surgery
McGill University
Montreal Children's Hospital
Montreal, Quebec, Canada

**Mark L. Silen, MD**
Attending Surgeon
Cardinal Glennon Children's Hospital
Assistant Professor
Saint Louis University School of Medicine
St. Louis, Missouri

**Mika Sinanan, MD**
Attending Surgeon and Co-Director
IFDR Endoscopy Surgery Center
Department of Surgery
University of Washington Medical Center
Assistant Professor
University of Washington
Seattle, Washington

**David B. Skinner, MD**
Attending Surgeon
The New York Hospital
Cornell Medical Center
Professor of Surgery
Cornell University Medical College
New York, New York

**Philip C. Smith, MD, PhD**
Attending, Pediatric Cardiovascular Surgery
The Heart Institute for Children
Assistant Professor
University of Illinois at Chicago
Oak Lawn, Illinois

**Michael Sobel, MD**
Chief, Vascular Surgery
H.H. McGuire Veterans Medical Center
Associate Professor of Surgery
Medical College of Virginia/Virginia Commonwealth University
Richmond, Virginia

**Jonathan Somers, MD**
Attending Cardiovascular Surgeon
Rush–Presbyterian–St. Luke's Medical Center
Assistant Professor of Surgery
Rush Medical College
Chicago, Illinois

**Henry M. Spotnitz, MD**
Attending Cardiothoracic Surgeon
Columbia–Presbyterian Medical Center
George H. Humphreys, II, Professor of Surgery
Columbia University
New York, New York

**William D. Spotnitz, MD**
Director TCV Postoperative Unit
University of Virginia Health Sciences Center
Professor of Surgery
University of Virginia
Charlottesville, Virginia

**Thomas L. Spray, MD**
Division Chief, Cardiothoracic Surgery
The Children's Hospital of Philadelphia
Professor of Surgery
University of Pennsylvania School of Medicine
Philadelphia, Pennsylvania

**Jaroslav Stark, MD, FRCS**
Consultant Cardiothoracic Surgeon
Great Ormond Street Hospital for Children NHS Trust
London, United Kingdom

**Vaughn A. Starnes, MD**
Director, Cardiopulmonary Transplantation
University of California, Los Angeles Medical Center
Professor of Surgery, Department of Surgery
University of California, Los Angeles School of Medicine
Los Angeles, California

**David J. Sugarbaker, MD**
Chief, Division of Thoracic Surgery
Brigham & Women's Hospital
Associate Professor of Medicine
Harvard Medical School
Boston, Massachusetts

**R. Sudhir Sundaresan, MD**
Assistant Professor of Surgery
Washington University School of Medicine
St. Louis, Missouri

**Julie A. Swain, MD**
Chief, Cardiovascular Surgery
Professor of Surgery
University of Nevada School of Medicine
Las Vegas, Nevada

**Scott J. Swanson, MD**
Associate Thoracic Surgeon
Brigham & Women's Hospital
Instructor of Surgery
Harvard Medical School
Boston, Massachusetts

**Timothy Takaro, MD**
Formerly Chief of Staff
Veterans Administration Medical Center
Formerly Clinical Professor of Surgery
Duke University School of Medicine
Asheville, North Carolina

**Christo I. Tchervenkov, MD, FRCSC, FACS**
Director, Cardiovascular Surgery
The Montreal Children's Hospital
Associate Professor of Surgery
McGill University
Montreal, Quebec, Canada

**Marc D. Thames, MD**
Chief, Division of Cardiology
University Hospitals of Cleveland
Joseph T. Wearn University Professor in Medicine
Case Western Reserve University School of Medicine
Cleveland, Ohio

**Robert J. Touloukian, MD**
Chief, Pediatric Surgery
Children's Hospital of Yale-New Haven
Professor of Surgery and Pediatrics
Yale University School of Medicine
New Haven, Connecticut

**Thomas F. Tracy, Jr., MD**
Attending Surgeon
Cardinal Glennon Children's Hospital
Associate Professor
Saint Louis University School of Medicine
St. Louis, Missouri

**George A. Trusler, MD**
Professor Emeritus, Department of Surgery
University of Toronto
Senior Surgeon
Hospital For Sick Children
Toronto, Ontario, Canada

**Ross M. Ungerleider, MD**
Chief, Pediatric Cardiac Surgery
Duke University Medical Center
Professor of Surgery
Duke University
Durham, North Carolina

**Harold C. Urschel, Jr., MD**
Professor Thoracic and Cardiovascular Surgery
Baylor College of Medicine
Dallas, Texas

**Matthew Wall, Jr., MD**
Deputy Chief of Surgery
Ben Taub General Hospital
Assistant Professor of Surgery
Baylor College of Medicine
Houston, Texas

**Ralph L. Warren, MD**
Clinical Director, Trauma Service
Department of Surgery
Massachusetts General Hospital
Assistant Surgeon
Harvard Medical School
Boston, Massachusetts

**Paul F. Waters, MD**
Director, General Thoracic Surgery
Director, Lung Transplant Program
University of California, Los Angeles Medical Center
Professor of Surgery
University of California, Los Angeles School of Medicine
Los Angeles, California

**Thomas J. Watson, MD**
Clinical Fellow, Cardiothoracic Surgery
University of California, Los Angeles School of Medicine
Los Angeles, California

**Watts R. Webb, MD**
Chief, Cardiac Surgery
New Orleans Veterans Administration Hospital
Professor of Clinical Surgery
Louisiana State University School of Medicine
New Orleans, Louisiana

**Thomas R. Weber, MD**
Director, Division of Pediatric Surgery
Cardinal Glennon Children's Hospital
Professor of Surgery
Saint Louis University School of Medicine
St. Louis, Missouri

**Andrew S. Wechsler, MD**
Chairman, Department of Surgery
Head, Division of Thoracic Surgery
Medical College of Virginia Hospitals
Stuart McGuire Professor of Surgery and Physiology
Medical College of Virginia/Virginia Commonwealth University
Richmond, Virginia

**Debra E. Weese-Mayer, MD**
Associate Professor of Pediatrics
Rush Medical College
Chicago, Illinois

**Benson R. Wilcox, MD**
Professor of Surgery and Chief
Division of Cardiothoracic Surgery
University of North Carolina School of Medicine
Chapel Hill, North Carolina

**Roberta G. Williams, MD**
Chief, Pediatric Cardiology
University of California, Los Angeles Medical Center
Professor of Pediatrics
University of California, Los Angeles School of Medicine
Los Angeles, California

**Vallee L. Willman, MD**
C. Rollins Hanlon Professor and Chairman, Department of Surgery
Saint Louis University School of Medicine
St. Louis, Missouri

**Roger S. Wilson, MD**
Chairman
Department of Anesthesiology and Critical Care Medicine
Memorial Sloan-Kettering Cancer Center
Professor of Anesthesiology
Cornell University Medical College
New York, New York

**Michael K. Wolverson, MD**
Attending Radiologist
Saint Louis University Health Sciences Center
Professor of Radiology
Saint Louis University School of Medicine
St. Louis, Missouri

**James L. Zellner, MD**
Resident in Cardiothoracic Surgery
Medical University of South Carolina
Charleston, South Carolina

# Preface

The foundation for the sixth edition of *Glenn's Thoracic and Cardiovascular Surgery* was laid nearly 45 years ago by Drs. Gustav E. Lindskog, William H. Carmalt Professor of Surgery, and Averill A. Liebow, Professor of Pathology, both at the Yale University School of Medicine. They wrote a textbook entitled *Thoracic Surgery and Related Pathology* and included three contributing authors: Drs. Ralph D. Alley, William E. Bloomer, and Frederick C. Warring, Jr. Cardiovascular surgery was then in its infancy, and this subject was a very small part of the text.

Because of how well the first edition was received, a second edition was published in 1962. By that time, the fields of cardiac and vascular surgery had vastly expanded, and Dr. William W. Glenn, Professor of Surgery at Yale University School of Medicine, who had served as a consultant on the cardiovascular material in the first edition, was invited to be a coeditor and to write a section on cardiovascular surgery. The title of the book was expanded to *Thoracic and Cardiovascular Surgery with Related Pathology.* The three contributors to the first edition also participated in the second edition of the book.

In response to the favorable reception of the second edition of the book and the advances that had been made, especially in the surgical treatment of general thoracic and cardiovascular disease, a third edition was undertaken and published in 1975. The senior authors, who wrote portions of the text, were assisted by 11 contributing authors.

When the fourth edition was contemplated, it was evident that a simple revision would not suffice. The need was for a completely new book that involved a number of experts in the cardiothoracic field representing the basic sciences and clinical disciplines. Those of us who were at Yale University at that time joined Dr. Glenn as coeditors. The title was shortened to *Thoracic and Cardiovascular Surgery,* the text was completely rewritten, and there were 114 chapters contributed by 157 authors, more than 97% of whom were first-time contributors to the book. Broad-based expertise was emphasized. Approximately one third of the authors were from disciplines other than surgery.

The fifth edition of the book, now entitled *Glenn's Thoracic and Cardiovascular Surgery,* represented another complete revision. The general format of the three main divisions of the book was retained. This edition too was well accepted by the cardiothoracic community. In recent years, many requests have been made for a new edition, which brings us to the sixth edition.

Although this sixth edition of *Glenn's Thoracic and Cardiovascular Surgery* evolved from five previous editions of a venerable textbook on cardiovascular surgery, it is truly a new book in that most of the 140 chapters are either new (13 chapters) to this edition, reflecting the many exciting developments in the field in the last five years, or have been rewritten or drastically revised.

We welcome 110 new authors to this edition. They represent a whole new generation of cardiothoracic surgeons. We also welcome back more than 100 of the same authors who contributed to the fifth edition.

All of the revised chapters have been updated, and many have a new organization of material and expanded content, with new illustrations and current and comprehensive references. Results, statistics, and recommendations have all been derived for the most current information.

The chapter authors were not required to adhere to a totally uniform format, because it was thought that full freedom of expression would be a refreshing change in a textbook. Only complete coverage and strict adherence to an assigned subject were requirements. They all complied with these requirements admirably, which has provided continuity of thought throughout each section of the book with minimal duplication or overlap of material. Where applicable, cross references are made in certain chapters to other chapter(s) for details of diagnosis, therapy, and other information.

Each section and most chapters in this new edition present general information on a subject beginning with the historical background, surgical anatomy and pathophysiology, diagnosis with particular emphasis on the newest technical aids, perioperative care, anesthesia, and supportive medical therapy. Following the general considerations, specific diseases or deformities susceptible to surgical treatment are described along with diagnosis, operations, management of complications, and the results of operations. The sixth edition of this book is meant to be encyclopedic, and we therefore have tried to include all the information that is currently known about a subject or field. In addition, the authors have provided the reader with the evidence for the best methods of therapy presently known and the ones they currently use.

The book is divided into three major sections. In Section I, General Thoracic Surgery, topics include the technological advances in the use of video-assisted thoracoscopy and laparoscopy for diagnostic and therapeutic pulmonary procedures and for surgery of the esophagus and diaphragm. The molecular biology and immunology of thoracic neoplasms (lung and esophagus) are now included in this section. Several chapters from the previous edition have been incorporated in other chapters in this edition. For example, the chapter on vena caval syndrome was combined with the one on the mediastinum; the chapter on tracheotomy is now part of the one on reconstruction of the trachea; and the chapter on esophageal perforation has been combined with the one on chemical burns, foreign bodies, and bleeding. The chapters describing the three methods most commonly used for prevention of reflux esophagitis have been retained in this edition, and once again have been written by the experts in or developers of these procedures. In addition, other techniques for managing esophageal reflux are included in the chapter on the surgical treatment of hiatal hernia and gastroesophageal reflux.

In Section II, Surgery for Congenital Heart Disease, major advances in the care of congenital heart disease are described, Heart–lung transplantation in children is included, as are cardiac-assist devices in infants. Discussions of the use of nitric oxide gas in anesthesia and adenosine for the diagnosis and management of arrhythmias make this book current and comprehensive.

In Section III, Surgery for Acquired Heart Disease, the major developments in adult cardiac surgery are described. Angioplasty is compared with coronary bypass grafting for the treatment of coronary artery disease. The reader is given a better understanding of ventricular support, cardiopulmonary bypass, and other aspects of the management of adult heart disease. New chapters in this section are those on the clinical/biologic interface of the basic science of the myocardial muscle and the coronary circulation; transplantation immunology; mitral valve repair; homografts and autografts of cardiac valves; and indications for percutaneous (nonsurgical) coronary revascularization. The increasing importance of echocardiography is described, as is the use of intraoperative transesophageal echocardiography in both adults and infants.

New authors were selected on the basis of their contributions to the field of cardiothoracic surgery and their active involvement in operative surgery related to the subjects that they write about. In many instances, contributors who originally developed certain surgical operations or techniques and those who have popularized certain procedures continue their contributions in this edition. Thus, they know both the theoretical aspects of cardiothoracic surgery and what is practical in patients.

Indexing is a critical feature of a book such as this. Without an exhaustive index, vital information may not be readily apparent to the user of the book because it is buried within the text. We are very proud of the excellent and extensive index that has been compiled for this edition of the book.

The sixth edition of *Glenn's Thoracic and Cardiovascular Surgery* is truly international in scope in that it represents more than 100 medical schools worldwide. Therefore, it should serve as a reference source for practicing cardiothoracic surgeons and as a textbook and reference source for fellows in cardiothoracic surgery, particularly in preparation for the qualifying and certifying examinations of the American Board of Thoracic Surgery, and for students everywhere with an interest in cardiothoracic surgery. It should serve as the reference text of choice well into the twenty-first century.

A multiauthored textbook of this depth and breadth is not an easy undertaking for anyone involved in bringing it to fruition. Writing chapters for medical texts is a labor of love. Secretarial, medical illustration, and editorial costs must be borne in part or wholly by the departments or divisions of the institutions to which the participants belong. Authors have many other commitments for their time. They may be busy reporting the results of their work at national or international meetings, which require abstracts and manuscripts. Many others, because of their particular expertise, may be involved in the generation of material for several books at the same time. Acute and chronic overcommitment is characteristic of the capable surgeon. Thus, deadlines pass, chapters are not in, and months go by. As one of my senior colleagues once said, "There has been a certain amount of slippage in our editorial schedule." What he really meant was that the book was six months behind schedule. In spite of delays, the work eventually gets done. Overburdened authors come through and an excellent book such as this sixth edition of *Glenn's Thoracic and Cardiovascular Surgery* is produced. This book is the most comprehensive and complete work on cardiovascular surgery that I have ever seen.

We are grateful to many authors for their previous contributions and for helping to establish this textbook as a standard in the field. Many senior authors in previous editions, who have now retired, preferred not to continue as contributors in the sixth edition of the book. We are sad to report that two authors, Mr. Ian K. R. McMillan and Dr. E. Stanley Crawford, died in the years between the fifth and sixth editions.

We the editors are greatly indebted to all the contributors to this work for their participation and cooperation. It has been a most pleasant and stimulating experience to be associated with them in the vast effort to bring this sixth edition to publication.

I am particularly grateful to my coeditors, Drs. Keith S. Naunheim, Alexander S. Geha, Graeme L. Hammond, and Hillel Laks, and to their associates. Dr. Jai Lee has helped Dr. Geha with the work in Cleveland and has also contributed a chapter. Dr. Lester Permut has done yeoman service in developing Section II and helping to edit manuscripts and make suggestions for revisions and modifications.

I would also like to thank immensely those who have provided such excellent editorial assistance to us: My secretary Jean Finn, Delores Adams in Cleveland, Bambi Wojiechowski in Los Angeles, and Joan Batza in New Haven.

We would also like to acknowledge the fine photographic service and art work carried out in the divisions of medical illustrations from the many different universities from which contributors submitted original material for publication. We give special thanks to J. Anthony Stubblefield for his excellent medical illustrations prepared in the Department of Medical Illustrations at St. Louis University Health Sciences Center.

We greatly appreciate the help of Edward H. Wickland, Jr., Vice President and Publisher, and Kathleen McCullough, Managing Editor, Development, at Appleton & Lange.

We again salute Dr. William W. Glenn for his friendship, for his many contributions to this work, and for allowing us to continue this tradition in cardiothoracic education.

Finally, I want to again express my appreciation for the enormous effort put forth by the many people who contributed to this text. I am certain that the final product will be worthy of their trust in all of us who participated in the project.

*Arthur E. Baue*
*with*
*Alexander S. Geha*
*Graeme L. Hammond*
*Hillel Laks*
*Keith S. Naunheim*

SIXTH EDITION

VOLUME I

# GLENN'S THORACIC AND CARDIOVASCULAR SURGERY

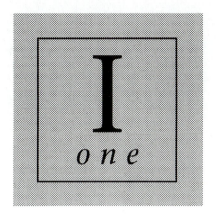


# GENERAL THORACIC SURGERY

CHAPTER

1

# Function of the Gas Exchange System and Its Evaluation

Richard M. Peters

The success of thoracic surgery during the last 60 years comes from increased understanding of the pathophysiology of cardiopulmonary function combined with innovative methods of support during operation and techniques to improve function and minimize loss due to ablative surgery. More than 70 years ago, when he wrote his extraordinary monograph on treatment of empyema, Evarts A. Graham set down much of the basis for the material presented in this chapter.[1,2] He discussed the effects of open chest wounds, decrease in lung compliance, ventilatory fatigue, and muscle condition. In 1932 this pioneer thoracic surgeon did the first successful pneumectomy, which started the modern era of general thoracic surgery.[3] The challenge required better understanding of surgical anatomy of the chest cage and its contents; function of the heart, lungs, and chest cage, and the effect of thoracotomy on the cardiopulmonary system. The development of cardiothoracic surgery has followed the model initiated by Dr. Graham. Alfred Blalock's studies of shock led to his collaboration with Helen Taussig to combine their physiologic knowledge with an imaginative procedure to increase circulation to the lungs.[4] John Gibbon was working on the development of methods of substituting artificial heart and lungs to permit cardiac surgery.[5] This chapter cannot begin to cover all the work of these pioneers. It attempts to bring together the basics of cardiopulmonary function with a focus on evaluating the amount of reserve and the effects of thoracotomy and pulmonary surgery on the cardiopulmonary systems.

The preoperative evaluation and perioperative care of a patient consists of three distinct parts: (1) diagnosis of the primary disease and decision whether an operative procedure is appropriate for its treatment, (2) determination of the patient's general condition and ability to tolerate the proposed procedure, and (3) the optimum preparation of the patient for surgery and the postoperative care required. Answers to these complex questions provide guides for predicting the particular problems that may be anticipated in the perioperative care of the patient.

Recovery from operative or accidental trauma requires an increase in metabolic rate and, therefore, more nearly approaches a state of continuous mild to moderate exercise than a state of rest. For short periods of time, most patients can sustain increases in functional demands. However, patients with compromised cardiopulmonary function have a limited ability to maintain high levels of function for prolonged periods. Fatigue develops resulting in decompensation. Preoperative evaluation needs to measure not only the immediate adequacy of function but also the amount of reserve capacity. The cardiopulmonary system's primary purpose is gas exchange that depends on (1) an adequate and intact circulation; (2) an adequate number of transport vehicles—the red cells in the blood containing properly functioning unique chemicals, hemoglobin, and carbonic anhydrase; (3) an adequate portion of the intact lung able to exchange gas effectively between air and the blood; and (4) a ventilatory pump able to ventilate the lungs adequately (Fig. 1–1).

The evaluation of pulmonary function requires some consideration of cardiac function, the oxygen-carrying red cells, the lungs, chest wall, and ventilatory muscular function. This chapter will emphasize the role of the lungs and ventilatory pump. It does not discuss methods for evaluation of cardiac function but does include discussion of the effects of compromised cardiac function on gas exchange, with emphasis on the interaction between pulmonary and cardiac dysfunction.

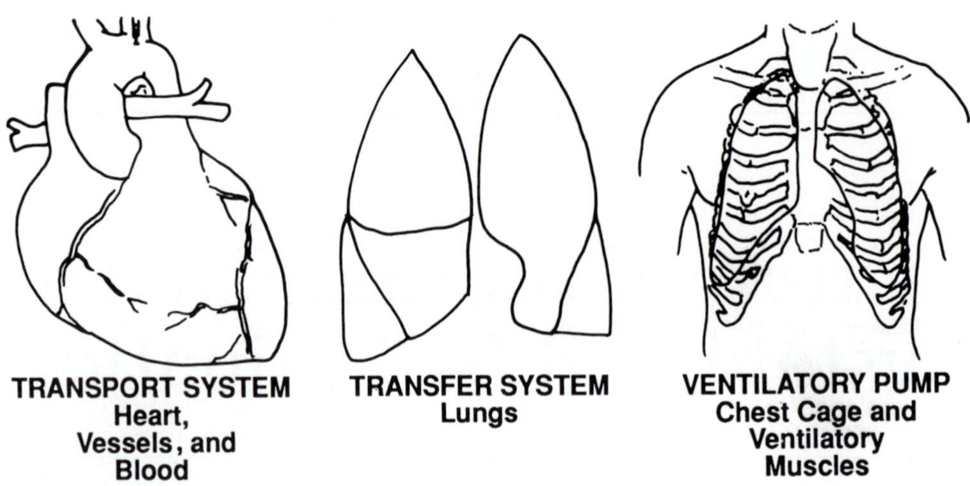


**Figure 1–1.** Three elements for gas exchange must be considered in assessing pulmonary function.

The lungs require a unique structure to efficiently exchange $O_2$ and $CO_2$ between the blood and ambient atmosphere. The vasculature of these relatively small organs, with a combined weight of 900–1100 g, must accommodate the entire cardiac output at a very low perfusion pressure. The lungs have about 300 million alveoli, with a surface area of 70–80 $m^2$ and as large a capillary surface area per gram of tissue as any organ in the body. For the lung to function, the richly perfused lumen of the alveolus must remain free of excess fluid. The large capillary bed in a small tissue volume and subject to high blood flow rates makes the lungs sensitive to even small changes in transcapillary filtration forces.

In essence, the lungs function as gas exchange membranes controlled by two pumps: (1) the right ventricular pump, which pumps blood through the lungs; and (2) the chest cage and diaphragms, which act as a reciprocating pump to stretch the lungs and pull air into them during inspiration. Inspiratory muscles relax during exhalation, and the elastic recoil of the lungs and chest wall provide the force to expel the inspired volume. Preexisting pulmonary disease, chest deformity, or cardiac disease can alter the mechanical and gas exchange efficiency of the lungs and chest cage, as can operative or accidental trauma.

One may divide the types of lung disease and dysfunction present in preoperative patients into five broad categories: (1) neoplastic or infectious processes that have destroyed or replaced a discrete portion of a lobe or lung, (2) diffuse multilobar fibrosis resulting from infectious disease or exposure to noxious gases, (3) degenerative disease of the lung or chronic obstructive pulmonary disease, (4) pulmonary consequences of cardiac dysfunction, and (5) acute lung dysfunction consequent to operative or traumatic injury.

In patients with neoplastic or infectious processes confined to a finite portion of the lung, a general assessment of function is essential prior to surgical removal of the diseased tissue. The surgeon now has a hierarchy of tests to provide objective measures of the functional reserve of a patient and predict the effect of lung resection or surgical correction of cardiac defects.

## CLINICAL EVALUATION

As in all clinical appraisals, the evaluation of pulmonary function depends on a pertinent and accurate history. To accommodate the marked increase in gas exchange required by vigorous exercise, the lungs have a large reserve capacity. Unfortunately, physicians evaluating lung function frequently fail to equate symptoms of dyspnea with activity level. No dyspnea and no exercise should not be reassuring but suggest that the patient may have dyspnea with activity. Dyspnea causes discomfort, and patients avoid levels of activity that result in dyspnea. At low levels of physical activity, even seriously compromised lungs can provide adequate function without symptoms. A sedentary individual without symptoms of dyspnea may have serious pulmonary disease. So it is imperative to include with a description of dyspnea the patient's level of physical activity. Postoperative recovery requires the patient to call on some of the gas exchange reserve. Assessing the limits that signifies a patient can tolerate a given procedure is difficult, because the range of normal reserve capacity and demands on reserve of operation are so large that no single clinical test of pulmonary function differentiates the patient with marginal from the patient with inadequate reserve capacity.[6–9]

With rare exceptions, patients with no symptoms during moderate exercise will have adequate functional reserve for a pneumonectomy (Fig. 1–2). However, even in patients who exercise, it is essential to inquire whether the patient has noticed any change in exercise capacity. If a change has occurred, objective testing is essential.

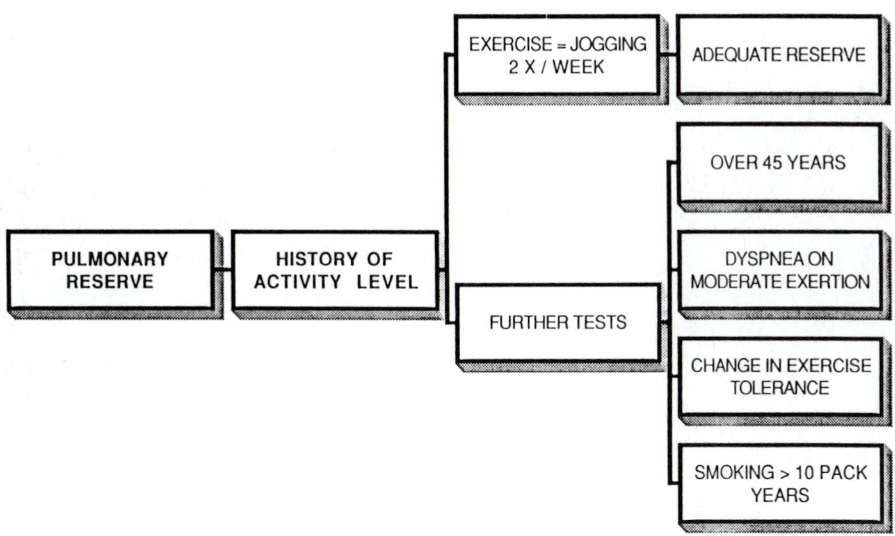


**Figure 1–2.** Patients with no symptoms with moderate exercise will have adequate functional reserve for a pneumonectomy. A tree for decision regarding ventilatory function tests.

## LUNG FUNCTION

The lungs have a complex structure of elastic and collagen fibers for supporting the bronchi and bronchioles. The elastic recoil of the lungs ejects gas, and the fibrous skeleton holds the small airways open. In a patient with normal lungs, only extreme exercise requires muscular effort for expiration. The inspiratory muscles expand the chest cage and lungs by stretching their elastic elements and overcoming the normally low airway resistance. Expiration is a passive process with force provided by the elastic recoil of the lungs and chest cage. Functional residual volume (FRV) is the volume of air in the lungs when all respiratory muscles are at rest. It is determined by a balance between the inward pull by the lungs on the chest cage, which has a large resting volume than lungs. If the lung becomes stiffer, FRV falls and, if the lung's fibroelastic skeleton is damaged compromising the lungs elastic properties, FRV increases. As a lung is emptied, airways decrease in diameter and, even in normal individuals below FRV, some airways are closed. The closed airways are those in the more dependent areas of the lungs. As airways close, the gas in the alveoli draining them is trapped.

After a careful history, the most useful tests of pulmonary function are a P-A and lateral x-ray of the chest cage and simple spirometry. Figure 1–3 shows a typical spirogram on a normal individual. The vital capacity is performed first by having the patient take a maximum deep inhalation followed by slow forced expiration, and a maximum inspiration followed forced expiration using maximum effort (FVC). Three sets of studies are usually done, and the best performance is recorded. Figure 1–4 shows a forced expiratory spirogram where the patient expired from full inspiration using maximal effort. The rate of flow of expired gas is estimated from the slope of the curve and reported as the first second forced expired volume ($FEV_1$). For interpretation of the spirogram, automatic analysis systems are used and provide a report of the values shown in

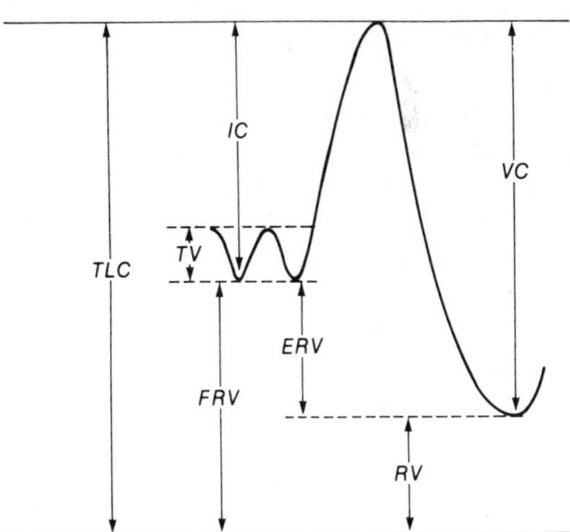


**Figure 1–3.** Spirogram tracing showing the subdivisions of the lung volume. The patient first breathes quietly at normal tidal volume (TV) and then, on command, takes in a maximum inspiration at the end of a normal expiration, using the full inspiratory capacity (IC). The patient then breathes out slowly the total vital capacity (VC) to residual volume (RV). ERV is expiratory reserve volume. FRV the functional reserve volume is the sum of ERV and RV. Since RV is the air left in the lungs at the end of maximum expiratory effort, it can only be measured indirectly with gas dilution or body box techniques. Total lung capacity (TLC) is the sum of RV and VC. *(From Peters RM et al: The Scientific Management of Surgical Patients, 1983. Courtesy of Little, Brown.)*

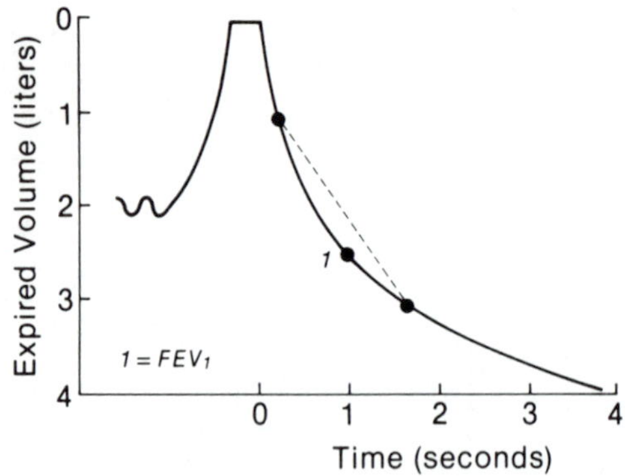


**Figure 1–4.** Tracing for forced vital capacity maneuver. The sequence is the same as for vital capacity measurements except that the patient is asked to expire as forcefully and fast as he or she can. The percent expired in the first second, $FEV_1$ is noted by the number 1. The dotted line is the slope of volume change between 25 and 75% of VC. From this forced expired flow, the $FEF_{25-75\%}$ can be derived. *(From Peters RM et al: The Scientific Management of Surgical Patients, 1983. Courtesy of Little, Brown.)*

Table 1–1. Standards or predicted levels for each age, sex, body weight, and height are also calculated by these systems. The norms were derived from nonsmoking Caucasians. These predictions are less accurate for other racial groups.

## RESTRICTIVE DISEASE

Spirometry (Fig. 1–3) permits characterization of ventilatory dysfunction due to restrictive disease and obstructive disease. In restrictive disease, the volume capacity of the lungs and/or chest cage is limited. Vital capacity and its subdivisions, inspiratory and expiratory reserves, are diminished. Restrictive disease can result from disease of the lung, the pleura, and the chest cage and its muscles or a combination of these three. The restrictive lung diseases include pulmonary congestions, atelectasis, pulmonary resection, pulmonary fibrosis following inhalation of toxic substances, acute respiratory distress syndrome (ARDS), and acute or chronic infection. Restrictive chest diseases are those that limit chest wall motion—kyphoscoliosis or muscular weakness or the capacity of the chest cavities—pleural effusion, pleural fibrosis.

With restrictive disease, the patient has limited capacity to expand the lungs but no difficulty emptying the lungs. *In patients with restrictive disease, the lungs are stiffer, the elastic recoil is greater, and FRV is decreased. These patients at FRV may not collapse their alveoli if the collagen elastic is intact. Because the lung disease is rarely uniformly distributed throughout the lungs, quantitative evaluation of regional function is essential in patients with moderate or severe restriction who need pulmonary resection.*

## OBSTRUCTIVE DISEASE

Obstructive disease is the more common and difficult problem for the modern thoracic surgeon. The major cause of obstructive disease is cigarette smoking, but it is also part of the aging process and a consequence of atmospheric pollution in an industrial society. Exposure to cigarettes fuels our lung cancer epidemic and is a major cause of diffuse injury to the lungs. The consequences of smoking disrupt the lungs' fibroelastic structure, which supports the bronchial tree and aleveoli. Lungs elastic recoil decreases, compromising the force for exhaling. The weakened alveoli become hyperexpanded, and alveolar septi lose their fibroelastic skeleton, causing them to coalesce into large alveoli. When alveolar septa are destroyed, their capillaries are destroyed and decrease the capillary bed and surface area for gas exchange. If compromise of the pulmonary capillary bed is extensive, the resistance to blood flow in the lung rises, leading to pulmonary hypertension. Smoking also damages the bronchi. They become inflamed, mucous glands hypertrophy, and secretions increase causing narrowing of the airway lumens. This combination of loss of elastic recoil and support of the bronchioles with resultant increase in airways resistance leads to expiratory obstruction of airways.

In a normal young person, no airways close at FRV. As they age, all people have some loss of elastic recoil, bronchial support, and lung surface area for the exchange of gas. The unsupported airways close at a higher lung volume so that despite an increase in FRV, small airways in the dependent area of lung close at FRV.[6,7,9] If a chronic obstructive lung disease (COLD) patient makes an active effort to push more air out of the lungs through unsupported airways, the airways collapse and trap the air in the lungs. Postoperative patients have a reduced FRV (see section on the ventilatory pump). In patients with obstructive lung disease, the postoperative decrease in lung volume results in closure of a significant portion of the airways in the dependent portions of the lungs. The areas of lung with closed airways are vulnerable to development of microatelectasis, an effect that is exaggerated if the patients are breathing gas with a high $FIO_2$. The elderly person who smokes, accelerates the process of aging, and becomes a victim of progressive obstructive pulmonary disease. FRV and closing volume of the lungs are important indicators of the vulnerability of the lungs to micro- and gross atelectasis.

The increase in FRV that results from the ravages of COLD affects the efficiency of the ventilatory muscles of the chest cage and diaphragms and the myocardium. Normal lungs at end expiration are stretched to greater than their unsupported volume, which produces a force that pulls the chest to a smaller volume than its nonstressed volume, a volume that provides an appropriate stretch for the inspiratory muscle fibers (see section on ventilatory pump).

In addition to the effect of loss of structural support for the airway in obstructive airways disease, there is also hy-

**TABLE 1–1A. EXAMPLE OF A REPORT OF A ROUTINE PULMONARY FUNCTION STUDY**

| | | | HT: 68.0 in | DATE: 03/18/94 |
|---|---|---|---|---|
| | AGE: 47 | SEX: F | WT: 190.0 lb | TIME: 13:49:32 |
| | | | OCC: | |
| | | DOB | | |
| DIAGNOSIS: | HAZARD: | | | PRED-COLLINS1 |
| PHYSICIAN: | TECH: | | | BP: 749TEMP: 24.0 |

| | | Predrug | | | | |
|---|---|---|---|---|---|---|
| **Spirometry** | **Predicted** | ***Actual*** | ***%Pred*** | **Actual** | **%Pred** | **%Change** |
| FVC (L) | 3.84 | 3.11 | 80 | | | |
| $FEV_1$ (L) | 2.94 | 2.25 | 76 | | | |
| $FEV_1/FVC$ (%) | 76 | 72 | 94 | | | |
| $FEV_3$ (L) | 3.73 | 2.80 | 75 | | | |
| $FEV_3/FVC$ (%) | 97 | 90 | 92 | | | |
| $FEF_{25-75\%}$ (L/S) | 3.22 | 1.61 | 50 | | | |
| FEFmax (L/S) | 6.50 | 5.76 | 88 | | | |
| $FEF_{25\%}$ (L/S) | 5.92 | 3.59 | 60 | | | |
| $FEF_{50\%}$ (L/S) | 4.55 | 2.18 | 47 | | | |
| $FEF_{75\%}$ (L/S) | 2.18 | 0.56 | 25 | | | |
| $FEF_{50\%}/FIF_{50\%}$ (%) | | 54 | | | | |

| | | Predrug | | | | |
|---|---|---|---|---|---|---|
| **Spirometry** | **Predicted** | ***Actual*** | ***%Pred*** | **Actual** | **%Pred** | **%Change** |
| MVV (L/Min) | 108.35 | 92.12 | 85 | | | |

| | | Predrug Avg | | | | |
|---|---|---|---|---|---|---|
| **Lung Volume** | **Predicted** | ***Actual*** | ***%Pred*** | **Actual** | **%Pred** | **%Change** |
| TLC (L) | 5.89 | 4.34 | 73 | | | |
| FRC (L) | 3.25 | 1.83 | 56 | | | |
| RV (L) | 2.05 | 1.41 | 68 | | | |
| VC (L) | 3.84 | 2.93 | 76 | | | |
| IC (L) | 2.64 | 2.51 | 94 | | | |
| ERV (L) | 1.20 | 0.42 | 35 | | | |
| RV/TLC (%) | 35 | 32 | 93 | | | |
| He Equil. (min) | | 2.00 | | | | |

| | | Predrug Avg | | | | |
|---|---|---|---|---|---|---|
| **Plethysmography** | **Predicted** | ***Actual*** | ***%Pred*** | **Actual** | **%Pred** | **%Change** |
| TLC (L) | 5.89 | 4.07 | 69 | | | |
| FRC (L) | 3.25 | 1.74 | 53 | | | |
| RV (L) | 2.05 | 1.41 | 68 | | | |
| VC (L) | 3.84 | 2.67 | 69 | | | |
| IC (L) | 2.64 | 2.34 | 88 | | | |
| ERV (L) | 1.20 | 0.33 | 27 | | | |
| RV/TLC (%) | 35 | 34 | 97 | | | |
| VTG (L) | | 1.96 | | | | |
| Raw (cm $H_2O$/L/S) | (0.20–2.50) | 6.27 | | | | |
| SGaw (L/S/cm $H_2O$) | (0.11–0.40) | 0.08 | | | | |

| | | Predrug Avg | | | | |
|---|---|---|---|---|---|---|
| **Diffusion** | **Predicted** | ***Actual*** | ***%Pred*** | **Actual** | **%Pred** | **%Change** |
| Dsb mL/min/mm Hg | 21.53 | 16.78 | 77 | | | |
| Dsb (adj) mL/min/mm Hg | 21.53 | 19.29 | 89 | | | |
| VA (sb) (L) | 5.89 | 4.55 | 77 | | | |
| D/VA | 3.65 | 3.69 | 101 | | | |

**TABLE 1–1B. EXAMPLE OF A REPORT OF A BLOOD GAS STUDY**

NAME: TEST DATE: 3/18/94

| Blood Gases | Predicted | Predrug (M) *Actual* | Predrug (M) *%Pred* | Actual | %Pred | %Change |
|---|---|---|---|---|---|---|
| $FIO_2$ (%) | | 21 | | | | |
| pH | (7.35–7.45) | 7.50 | | | | |
| $PaCO_2$ (mm Hg) | (35.00–45.00) | 31.00 | | | | |
| $PaO_2$ (mm Hg) | (80.00–100.00) | 112.00 | | | | |
| $HCO_3$ (mEq/L) | (22.00–26.00) | 24.10 | | | | |
| Base excess (mEq/L) | (–2.00–2.00) | 1.50 | | | | |
| Hb (g/100 mL) | | 11.30 | | | | |
| $SaO_2$ (%) | >95 | 96 | | | | |
| Hbco (%) | | 2.60 | | | | |
| HbMET (%) | | 0.40 | | | | |
| DLCO corrected for hemoglobin of 11.3 | | | | | | |

Spirometry: Forced vital capacity is normal. There is mild decrease in $FEV_1$ with normal $FEV_1$%. Lung volumes by helium dilution and body plethysmography show mild decrease in TLC. There is better vital capacity effort by helium dilution lung volumes. Diffusing capacity is normal when corrected for hemoglobin of 11. Arterial blood gases on room air are normal except for acute respiratory alkalosis.
Interpretation: There is no obstruction, and there is mild restriction.

pertrophy of the mucous glands with hypersecretion of a thick mucus that can cause plugging of bronchi. Dehydration can cause the mucus to become very thick and impacted, commonly resulting in segmental atelectasis. All of the described lung and chest mechanical problems of obstructive airways disease results in poor coordination of ventilation and perfusion (see section on ventilation perfusion coordination).

Destruction of the lung vascular bed as alveolar septa are destroyed leads to pulmonary hypertension, which can compromise cardiac function by increasing the right ventricular afterload and right ventricular work. The increased intraventricular pressure can also cause a shift in the ventricular septum to the left, which decreases left ventricular compliance and increases left heart filling pressure. The increased left heart filling pressure may cause an elevation in pulmonary capillary pressure and increase fluid filtration in the lungs. COLD creates a set of problems that amplify one another and result in progressive deterioration of gas exchange.

## THE VENTILATORY PUMP AND WORK OF BREATHING

Few clinicians include knowledge of the concepts of chest cage mechanics and the work of breathing in their clinical decision making. Lack of knowledge of these important concepts has led to failure to understand both bad and good outcomes of operative procedures carried out in the chest. The symptom dyspnea signals that the work required of the ventilatory muscles has reached a level that exceeds the comfortable capacity of the patient. Respiratory failure occurs when the $O_2$ demands of the gas exchange apparatus, the heart, and ventilatory pumps exceeds the capacity of the gas exchange to supply $O_2$ and remove $CO_2$.

The ventilatory pump, like the heart pump, gains its power from muscle function and works best if before contraction the muscle fibers have a proper preload—stretch and adequate supply of $O_2$ and nutrients.[10,11] The ventilatory pump is a suction pump that expands the chest cage to pull air into the lungs. The elastic recoil of the lungs and chest cage expel the air. Expiration is only assisted by active muscle force at extremes of exercise or if there is extraordinary airway obstruction. Design of a muscular suction pump requires that its muscles have optimum preload and stretch on the muscle fibers, when chest volume is small. In contrast to the heart that has optimum stretch on the muscle fibers when it is full, the inspiratory muscles are stretched at end expiration, when the chest cage and lungs have a low volume. In obstructive pulmonary disease, the combination of high airway resistance and low elastic recoil of the lungs (high compliance) prevent normal emptying during expiration. FRV is increased. A high lung volume at end expiration, typified by the flat diaphragms and increased A-P diameter of the chest, leaves the respiratory muscles unstretched and forced to function at a very inefficient position. These patients have both inefficient lungs and inefficient ventilatory pumps (Fig. 1–5).

Thoracotomy adds another type of insufficiency to the ventilatory pump and the lungs. Chest wall pain causes the patient to refuse to use the muscles that aggravate the pain. The effect is a region of noncontractile chest musculature that has the same effect as an infarct has on the heart. The tidal volume goes down, and the respiratory rate rises. To provide the same amount of alveolar ventilation, the minute ventilation must increase, because a greater portion of the

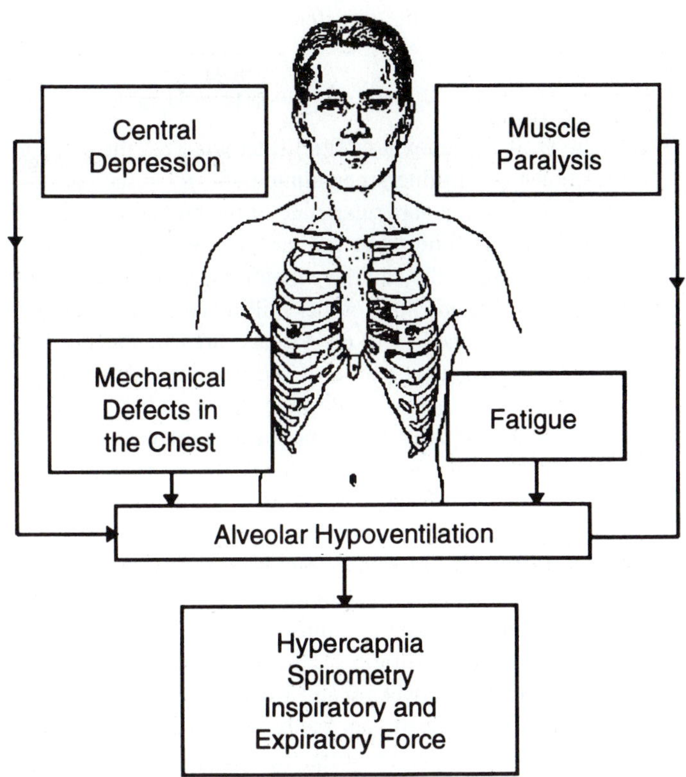


**Figure 1–5.** The ventilatory pump can fail from failure of the control system, central depression, or an increase in ventilatory work leading to muscle fatigue. Fatigue can result from lung disease, muscle weakness due to poor defects in the chest due to operative, or accidental injury.

tidal volume ventilates only the dead space. The region of the chest with muscle injury does not expand during inspiration, and FRV falls below normal. Low FRV increases the stretch on the muscle fibers, but it leads to deterioration in lung function. The number of airways and the number of alveoli at risk of having inadequate ventilation to keep them aerated increases at low FRV. The lack of ventilation of some alveoli leads to their collapse (microatelectasis), which makes the lung stiffer and increases the force required to expand the lungs. The combination of compromised ventilator pump and changing lung mechanics initiates a vicious cycle of progressive microatelectasis, ventilation perfusion abnormalities, and increasing ventilatory work (Fig. 1–6).

Mechanical injury to the muscle of the chest cage and distortion of the chest skeleton, which compromise the function and so the efficiency of the ventilatory pump, dictate the design of chest incisions to minimize the muscle injury and chest wall disruption. Minimal disruption of the chest cage, combined with effective control of postoperative pain, provide the strategy for preservation of ventilatory pump and lung efficiency. The sternal splitting incision that does not cut any muscles, combined with a sternal closure that minimizes motion across the split in the sternum, is the least disruptive thoracotomy incision. The most disruptive incision is a classical lateral thoracotomy, which divides large muscle groups and usually is combined with wide opening of the ribs. Muscle-sparing lateral thoracotomy incisions preserve a significant amount of chest wall function by avoiding muscle disruption and limiting opening of the rib spreader. The conservative incisions also reduce postoperative pain.

Following thoracotomy, ventilatory work increases because of stiffer lungs and less efficient gas exchange due to ventilation perfusion incoordination, lung dysfunction, and

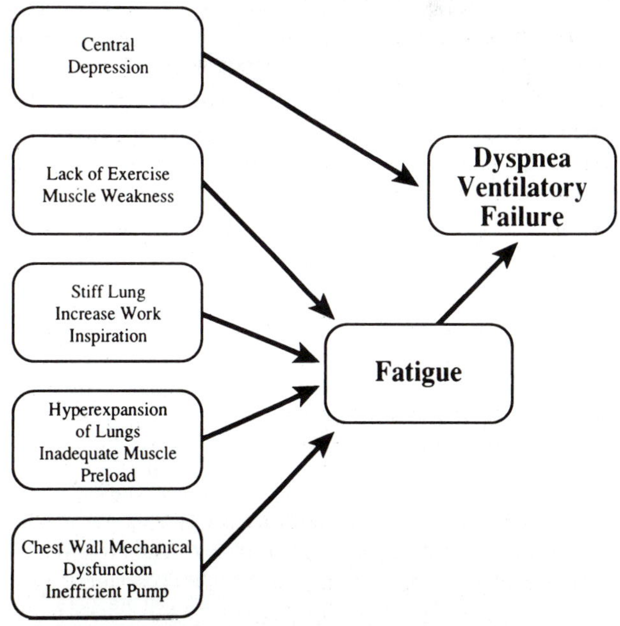


**Figure 1–6.** Increase in postoperative work of breathing is multifactorial. Shown are the relationships that lead to a cascade of factors that result from postoperative mechanical disruption and the effects of pain and muscle spasm.

increased dead space ventilation (Fig. 1–7). The interactions between chest dysfunction and lung dysfunction unfortunately usually aggravate rather than mitigate one another. Effective regional analgesia such as epidural narcotics prevents splinting and markedly reduces the limitation of chest cage motion. Patients can take deep breaths, cough effectively, and get up and move around. All of these measures preserve lung expansion and prevent microatelectasis.

The work capacity of muscles depends on the energy available to them and their strength. Like all other muscles, the work capacity of the ventilatory muscles increases with training and decreases with inactivity.[11,12] Bed rest for surprising short periods of time diminishes ventilatory reserve. Thoracic surgeons learned this lesson several decades ago when the treatment for tuberculosis included strict bed rest. Such patients had difficult intraoperative and postoperative courses unless they had a progressive exercise regimen to prepare them for surgery. A sedentary patient will tolerate a thoracotomy better if he or she is encouraged to start a modest exercise regime for even a week to 10 days prior to surgery.

## FLUID EXCHANGE AND LUNG WATER

The forces controlling the fluid filtration in the lungs are of paramount importance in determining the mechanical work required to ventilate the lungs and the gas exchange efficiency of the lungs. Accidental and operative trauma to the chest and cardiac and pulmonary disease all affect fluid transfer across the capillary surface. The interaction of forces controlling this transfer is defined by the Starling equation:

$$Q_f = K_f S\,[(P_c - P_t) - \phi(\Pi_c - \Pi_t)],$$

where $Q_f$ is the amount of fluid filtered across the capillary membrane in milliliters per minute and $K_f$ is the filtration coefficient for the particular state of the membrane with the dimensions milliliters per minute per millimeters of mercury. Damage to the capillary membranes increases $K_f$ and raises rate of fluid filtration per millimeter of transcapillary pressure difference. $S$ is the surface area of the capillary bed. A rise in surface area of the perfused alveolocapillary membrane increases filtration. Most authors include $S$ in $K_f$, but it is separated here, because an increase in the rate of blood flow through a lung opens larger portions of the alveolocapillary bed for perfusion. $P_c$ is microvascular or capillary hydrostatic pressure with the dimensions millimeters of mercury. A rise in $P_c$ increases fluid filtration. $P_t$ is tissue pressure around the capillary, perimicrovascular pressure with the dimensions millimeters of mercury. A rise in $P_t$ decreases fluid filtration. The coefficient $\phi$, is a dimensionless number between 0 and 1 that denotes the effectiveness of the alveolocapillary membrane in blocking the protein molecules from crossing the membrane. A fall in $\phi$ increases fluid filtration. $\Pi_c$ is colloidal osmotic pressure of plasma proteins in microvessels with the dimensions in millimeters of mercury. A fall in $\Pi_c$ increases fluid filtration. $\Pi_t$ is the colloidal osmotic pressure of proteins in the interstitial fluid with the dimensions in millimeters of mercury. A rise in $\Pi_t$ increases fluid filtration (Table 1–2).

Blood circulating through normal lung capillaries at normal rates and pressure causes a net fluid movement from

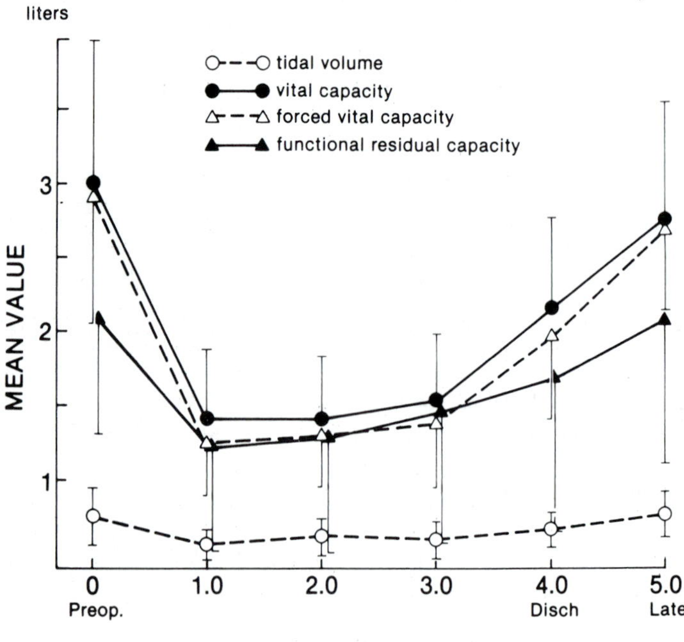


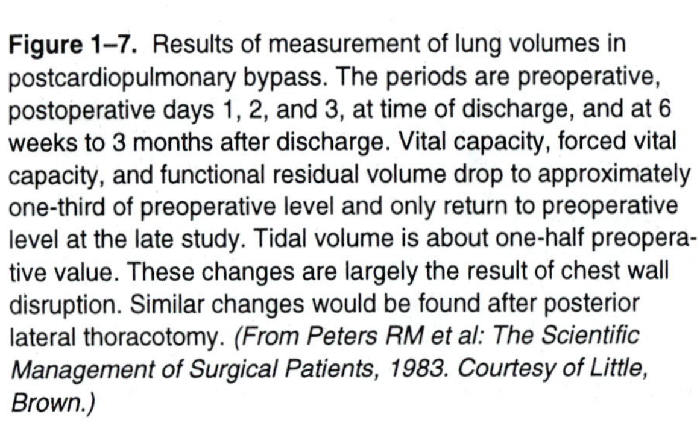

**Figure 1–7.** Results of measurement of lung volumes in postcardiopulmonary bypass. The periods are preoperative, postoperative days 1, 2, and 3, at time of discharge, and at 6 weeks to 3 months after discharge. Vital capacity, forced vital capacity, and functional residual volume drop to approximately one-third of preoperative level and only return to preoperative level at the late study. Tidal volume is about one-half preoperative value. These changes are largely the result of chest wall disruption. Similar changes would be found after posterior lateral thoracotomy. *(From Peters RM et al: The Scientific Management of Surgical Patients, 1983. Courtesy of Little, Brown.)*

**TABLE 1–2. FACTORS ALTERING FLUID FILTRATION IN THE LUNG**

| Filtration | | |
|---|---|---|
| ***Increase*** | | ***Decrease*** |
| Rise $K_f$ | Filtration coefficient | Fall in $K_f$ |
| Rise in $S$ | Capillary surface | Fall in $S$ |
| Rise in $P_c$ | Capillary pressure | Fall in $P_c$ |
| Fall in $P_t$ | Tissue pressure | Rise in $P_t$ |
| Fall in ∅ | Protein reflectance | Rise in ∅ |
| Rise in $\Pi_c$ | Serum protein | Rise in $\Pi_c$ |
| Rise in $\Pi_t$ | Interstitial protein | Fall in $\Pi_t$ |

the capillaries into the lung interstitium. The filtered fluid is picked up by lung lymphatics and returned to the circulation. Studies have shown that hemodilution with an electrolyte solution, which results in significant lowering of $\Pi_c$ and increased lung fluid filtration, does not cause pulmonary edema unless pulmonary capillary pressure is also elevated. The normal lung has a high interstitial protein content—$\Pi_t$. The low serum proteins do not cause pulmonary edema, because the interstitial protein ($\Pi_t$, concentration) is diluted by the increased filtered fluid and lymphatic removal of interstitial fluid is enhanced. The dilution of $\Pi_t$ and enhanced lymphatic removal of fluid neutralizes most of the drop in $\Pi_c$.[13–15]

In patients undergoing resection of major portions of the lung, particularly those requiring pneumonectomy, management of fluid therapy must take into account the multiple factors defined by the Starling equation that are altered by removal of portions of the lung.[16] See Figure 1–8. An uncomplicated postpulmonary resection patient has a cardiac output 1.5–2.0 times the resting level. Following pulmonary resection, the total cardiac output must flow through a pulmonary capillary bed reduced in proportion to the amount of lung resected. To accommodate the increased flow through the remaining lung, more of the capillary bed is actively perfused and at a higher pressure. Pulmonary resection results in an effectively increased surface area ($S$) open for filtration with a higher capillary hydrostatic pressure $P_c$. Fluid filtration per unit of perfused lung increases. The lymphatic pump capacity falls in proportion to the amount of lung resected. If a mediastinal node dissection removes additional lymphatic channels, this further compromises lymphatic pump capacity. The combination of factors, increasing filtration and decreasing lymphatic removal, makes it easy to put these patients into pulmonary edema, even if only modest excessive amounts of intraoperative or postoperative fluids are infused.[16] Monitoring the pulmonary capillary wedge pressure can be misleading following pneumectomy, when inflation of the balloon can obstruct enough of the remaining pulmonary circulation to increase the right ventricular afterload, lowering right heart output and giving a falsely low wedge pressure.[17]

Cardiopulmonary bypass, multiple transfusions, sepsis, and multiple trauma can cause injury to the capillary endothelium and the large capillary bed of the lungs, mak-

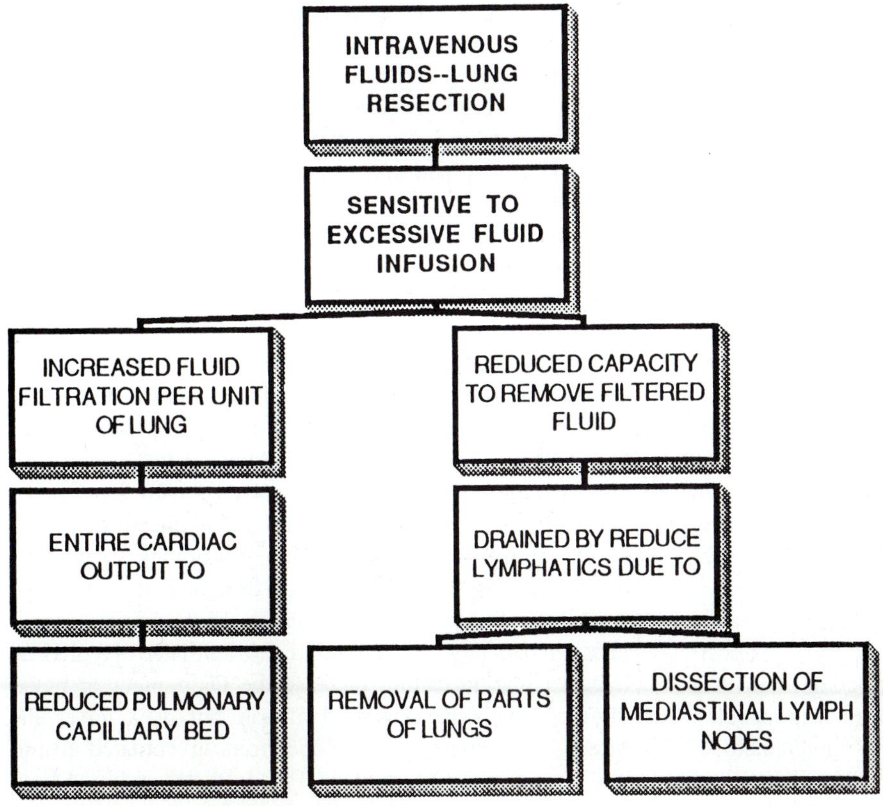


**Figure 1–8.** This figure depicts the effects of lung resection on rate of fluid filtration and accumulation in the lungs. On the left, fluid filtration is increased as remaining capillary bed must accommodate the entire cardiac output; on the right, the decrease in removal by lymphatics. *(From Peters RM: Matching pulmonary resection to patient function. J Jpn Assn Thorac Surg 5:674–684, 1988. Used with permission.)*

ing them a target after these injuries. Capillary injury results in an increase in filtration coefficient ($K_f$) and decrease in protein reflectance.[18] These patients develop high permeability pulmonary edema, a form of pulmonary edema that occurs without a rise in capillary pressure. Because the injured capillaries permit passage of protein and water, elevation of serum proteins has little effect on fluid filtration. On the other hand, such patients are extremely sensitive to an increase in capillary hydrostatic pressure. The dimensions of $K_f$ in milliliters per minute per millimeters of mercury dictate that when $K_f$ increased, the amount of fluid filtered for each millimeter rise in $P_c$ will be greater, regardless of whether the initiating cause of increased lung fluid filtration is a relatively larger surface area for filtration, a rise in pressure due to cardiac insufficiency, excessive fluid infusion, or increased capillary permeability. The most important therapeutic measure is to keep pulmonary capillary pressure at the lowest level compatible with adequate left heart filling. With normal capillary permeability, a rise in wedge pressure above 20, is likely to increase fluid filtration that will exceed the capacity of the lymphatic pump. If the volume of the capillary bed and lymphatic system has been restricted by pulmonary resection or disease, fluid filtration may exceed lymphatic pump capacity at lower wedge pressure.[16,17]

Consideration of pulmonary fluid exchange is an essential element of good preoperative assessment of a thoracic patient and volume restoration in the injured or bleeding patient. Inadequate fluid replacement resulting in a low cardiac output can reduce $O_2$ delivery to dangerous levels, particularly when pulmonary function is compromised. Indiscriminate fluid infusion can cause pulmonary edema.

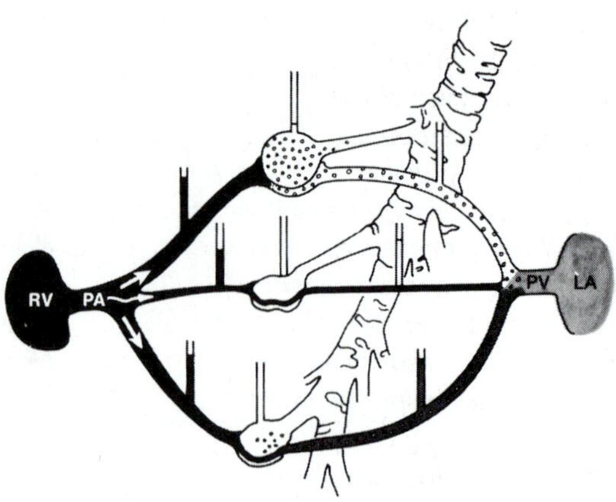


**Figure 1–9.** Three types of alveoli are depicted. The oxygen content of the mixed venous blood going to the three types of alveoli is the same. In the well-ventilated and well-perfused alveoli shown at the top, blood is fully oxygenated and carbon dioxide is removed. In the collapsed alveoli in the middle, no gas exchange takes place. In the poorly ventilated, perfused alveoli at bottom, the blood is only partially oxygenated and carbon dioxide is incompletely removed. Arterial blood is a mixture of blood from the three types of alveoli present. Low alveolar $Po_2$ increases pulmonary vascular resistance and limits flow to unventilated or poorly ventilated alveoli. In the acute respiratory distress syndrome, most alveoli are either well ventilated or collapsed. With chronic obstructive airways disease, many perfused, poorly ventilated alveoli are present. RV, right ventricle; PA, pulmonary artery; PV, pulmonary vein; LA, left atrium. *(From Peters RM. American Journal of Surgery 138:368, 1979. Used with permission.)*

## VENTILATION-PERFUSION INCOORDINATION

Most abnormalities of gas transfer in the lungs have as their basis disturbances in coordination of ventilation and perfusion. While the possible ratios of ventilation to perfusion are myriad, for our purposes we can consider three types (Fig. 1–9): (1) well-ventilated and well-perfused alveoli, (2) perfused unventilated alveoli, and (3) poorly ventilated but perfused alveoli. A fourth kind, ventilated unperfused alveoli, is seen following pulmonary emboli. Patients with normal lungs and ventilatory pump function before thoracotomy will have postoperatively a mixture of well-ventilated, well-perfused alveoli with varying fractions of unventilated but perfused alveoli, areas of diffuse patchy microatelectasis. These areas of microatelectasis result from the effects of splinting described earlier.

The microatelectasis develops over the first 48 hours after surgery. It is often worse on the second and third postoperative day as the effects of failure to cough and take deep breaths accumulate. Gross atelectasis can develop from improperly placed endotracheal tubes or retained secretions of blood and can be aggravated by splinting and failure to cough. Both gross and microatelectasis lead to an intrapulmonary shunt due to perfused but unventilated alveoli. Patients with obstructive lung disease have many regions of perfused but poorly ventilated alveoli. Airway obstruction and breakdown of the supporting structure result in uneven ventilation with major portions of lung poorly ventilated.

An abnormality of ventilation-perfusion coordination is the major cause of hypoxemia. Only as the discoordination becomes severe does hypercapnia develop. This discrepancy in response, hypoxemia preceding hypercapnia, provides essential information for the analysis of the preoperative and postoperative patient. The dissociation between $CO_2$ excretion and $O_2$ acquisition depends on the shape of $O_2$ and $CO_2$ dissociation curves. Above a $Pao_2$ of 95 mm Hg, hemoglobin is completely saturated with $O_2$. Further elevation of alveolar $Po_2$ will not increase the amount of $O_2$ in the blood. However, over the physiologic range, the amount of $CO_2$ in the blood has a straight-line relationship with $Pco_2$. In a patient with a shunt, the hypoxemia stimulates the patient to hyperventilate the ventilated alveoli. The hyperventilation cannot increase the $O_2$ content of blood draining the hyperventilated alveoli but does lower the blood's $CO_2$ content. The blood from unventilated alveoli will have a high $CO_2$ content (Fig. 1–9). When blood from these two sets of alveoli mix in the left heart, the result is a low $PaO_2$ and normal or low $PaCO_2$. In patients with a shunt, raising the $FIO_2$ has little effect, because the $O_2$ cannot reach unventilated alveoli.

During room air breathing in a patient with obstructive lung disease, the blood from regions of poorly ventilated but perfused alveoli will have a low $O_2$ and a high $CO_2$ content. When patients with obstructive airways disease breath air with increased $FIO_2$, the $PO_2$ in the gas of the poorly ventilated alveoli will rise, resulting in a matched rise in $PaO_2$. Since inspired air $CO_2$ is near zero, there is no way to adjust the inspired air to reduce $CO_2$. In patients with COLD, breathing air with an elevated $FIO_2$ corrects the low $PaO_2$, and the hypoxic ventilatory drive is suppressed, but alveolar ventilation can fall resulting in a rise of $PaCO_2$. The $FIO_2$ must be adjusted to only partially correct the depressed $PaO_2$. *The implications of these simple analyses to the evaluation of the pre- and postoperative patients are profound. The arterial $PaCO_2$ is an indicator of the adequacy of alveolar ventilation. $PaO_2$ is not an indicator of the adequacy of alveolar ventilation, because shunt and $FIO_2$ influence $PaO_2$ independent of the adequacy of alveolar ventilation. If $PaCO_2$ is normal, a low $PaO_2$ is an indicator of the degree of ventilation perfusion incoordination.*

What are some of the causes of incoordination of ventilation and perfusion? One of these is described earlier, a fall in FRV, which places part of the lung below closing volume during all or a portion of the ventilatory cycle. The portions of lung below closing volume develop diffuse alveolar collapse. In the supine posture, the abdominal contents push up on the diaphragms, lowering FRV. In addition, more lung is lower than the left atrium. The combination of these two factors puts more lung below closing volume due to lowering of FRV and increasing interstitial lung fluid (see "Fluid Exchange and Lung Water" earlier in this chapter). Aging results in degeneration of the lungs' elastic and collagen structure, which supports and holds airways open. The airways will close at higher lung volume. The normal progression of aging is accelerated and complicated by bronchitis in smokers. In elderly patients who smoke, the fall in FRV that occurs following thoracotomy places more unstable airways below closing volume than in a patient with normal lungs. An increased number of closed airways increases the amount of microatelectasis.

## SHUNT FRACTION

The physiologic evaluation of the extent of ventilation-perfusion incoordination is determined by measuring the shunt fraction, the fraction of the blood ejected by the left ventricle that has no gas exchange in the lungs (Fig. 1–10). Shunt is spoken of as true shunt—the amount of blood with no gas exchange—or physiologic shunt—the amount of blood that

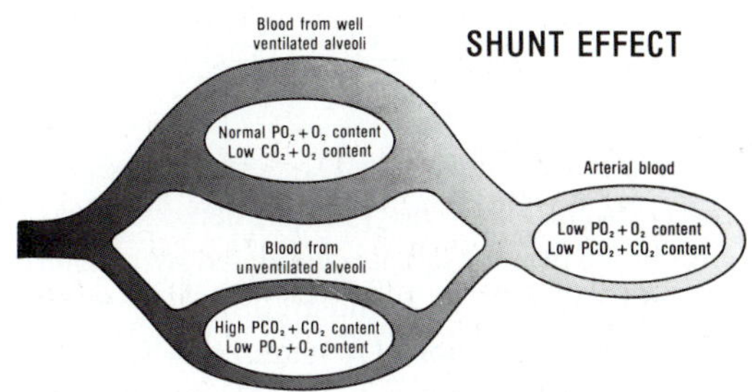


**Figure 1–10.** Effect on the arterial blood gas partial pressure and contents of alveoli of mixing blood from unventilated and well-ventilated alveoli. The ventilated alveoli are hyperventilated because of central stimulus from the depressed arterial $PO_2$. The hyperventilation lowers $PCO_2$ and $CO_2$ content of the perfusing blood. Because of the shape of the oxygen dissociation curve, the perfusing blood has only a normal $O_2$ content. Blood perfusing the unventilated alveoli has low $O_2$ and high $CO_2$ partial pressure and content. In this illustration, 25% blood is perfusing unventilated alveoli. Arterial blood, a mixture of blood from ventilated and unventilated alveoli, has low $PO_2$—a mixture of normal oxygen content and low oxygen content—and low $PCO_2$—a mixture of more low $CO_2$ content than high. This is the mechanism that results in the combination of hypoxemia and hypocapnia. *(From Peters RM et al: The Scientific Management of Surgical Patients, 1983. Courtesy of Little, Brown.)*

would be shunted to give the measured arterial $O_2$ content. The latter includes the effects of perfusion of poorly ventilated as well as unventilated alveoli. Theoretically, one can separate the hypoxemia due to perfusion of hypoventilated alveoli from that due to perfusion of unventilated alveoli by having the patient breathe 100% $O_2$ for 10 minutes. The high inspired $O_2$ provides enough $O_2$ to well- and poorly ventilated alveoli to eliminate hypoxemia caused by under ventilation. Unfortunately, washing out all the stabilizing gas (nitrogen) from the alveoli can lead to absorption of alveolar gas and collapse of the low-ventilation alveoli. Breathing high concentrations of $O_2$ can of itself increase the intrapulmonary shunt. Because the effect on the patient's gas exchange is essentially the same whether a group of alveoli is not ventilated or a large group is markedly hypoventilated, it is better to estimate the physiologic shunt without raising the $FIO_2$. Estimation of the physiologic shunt requires measurement of arterial and mixed venous $PO_2$, $PCO_2$, and pH, and the hemoglobin or hematocrit. The assumption is made that blood coming from ventilated alveoli has the same $PO_2$ as alveolar air. The alveolar $PO_2$ can be estimated from the inspired $O_2$ concentration by indirect calculation or by measuring end-expired $O_2$ concentration. The following calculations permit estimations of the elements needed to calculate the shunt fraction. To estimate alveolar $PO_2$ ($PaO_2$), $FIO_2 \times$ barometric pressure = inspired $PO_2$ ($PIO_2$). $PaO_2 = PIO_2 - PH_2O - PaCO_2$, where $PH_2O$ is the water vapor pressure of fully saturated gas at the patient's temperature and $PaCO_2$ is the measured end-expired $CO_2$ that is usually equal to the arterial $PCO_2$ ($PaCO_2$). The formula for calculating the fraction of cardiac output that goes to unventilated lungs is:

$$Q_s / Q_t = \frac{CAO_2 - CaO_2}{CAO_2 - CVO_2}$$

$CAO_2$ has two components—the $O_2$-carrying capacity of hemoglobin (1.34 mL of $O_2$ per gram of hemoglobin) and $O_2$ in solution in the blood. $CaO_2$ is calculated by measuring arterial $O_2$ saturation ($SaO_2$) and multiplying $SaO_2$ times (1.34 × Hgb). Mixed venous $O_2$ saturation ($SvO_2$) is calculated by measured $SvO_2$ times (1.34 × Hgb). Arteriovenous $O_2$ content difference ($avDO_2 = CaO_2 - CvO_2$). In this information age, a programmed calculator or the intensive care unit computer system should provide the physician with calculations to assess whether a fall in $CaO_2$ and $PaO_2$ is the result of increase in shunt fraction or fall in cardiac output.

It is apparent that the numerator of the equation (and so the calculated shunt) will become larger as the systemic arterial $O_2$ content decreases. Often neglected is the fact that the shunt can be unchanged while the $PaO_2$ can fall significantly as a result of a fall in venous $O_2$ content ($CvO_2$). This is more apparent when the equation is solved for arterial content: $CaO_2 = CAO_2 - Qs/Qt\ (CAO_2 - CvO_2)$. As $CvO_2$ becomes smaller, the expression $Q_s/Q_t(CAO_2 - CvO_2)$ becomes larger and $CaO_2$ smaller. If arterial blood is a mixture of blood from ventilated and unventilated alveoli, both a rise in the proportion of blood going to unventilated alveoli and a fall in the $O_2$ content of the venous blood can widen the $avDO_2$ and lower $PaO_2$ (Fig. 1–11). A patient with atelectasis will have a lower $PaO_2$ if there is a low cardiac output that causes a large $avDO_2$ than will a patient with atelectasis who has an adequate or high cardiac output and a small $avDO_2$. Because sampling of mixed venous blood requires introducing a Swan-Ganz catheter, certain criteria must be met to determine the necessity of this procedure. In a study on 41 patients with depressed $PaCO_2$, we found that to assume an $avDO_2$ of 4.5 vol% produced good shunt estimates if the shunt fraction did not exceed 20%. The $avDO_2$ must be measured when the estimated shunt exceeds 20%. When the calculated size of shunt exceeds 20%, a low $PaCO_2$ can result from a fall in mixed venous $O_2$ content due to a low cardiac output, an increase in shunt fraction, or both.

Patients with incoordination of ventilation and perfusion and a shunt fraction of greater than 0.15 to 0.20 are critically vulnerable to a low cardiac output. $O_2$ extraction from the blood increases, and $CvO_2$ falls. There is admixture of venous blood with less $O_2$ causing a fall in $PaCO_2$. The analysis of the shunt equation provides another important factor for estimate of gas exchange reserve. Patients with ventilation-perfusion incoordination require hyperventilation to remove $CO_2$ and an increase in cardiac output to compensate for the low blood $O_2$ content. Unless cardiac output increases, tissue $O_2$ delivery will fall further, lowering $PaO_2$. The effect of a fall in $CvO_2$ in a patient with an intrapulmonary shunt provides an excellent example of the importance of cardiac reserve on the gas exchange systems.

A Swan-Ganz catheter should be inserted to measure wedge pressure, control cardiac preload and optimize cardiac output with any of the following:

1. An intrapulmonary shunt greater than 0.2 calculated by assuming an arteriovenous $O_2$ content difference ($avDO_2$) of 4.5 mL $O_2$/100 mL of blood. In such a cir-

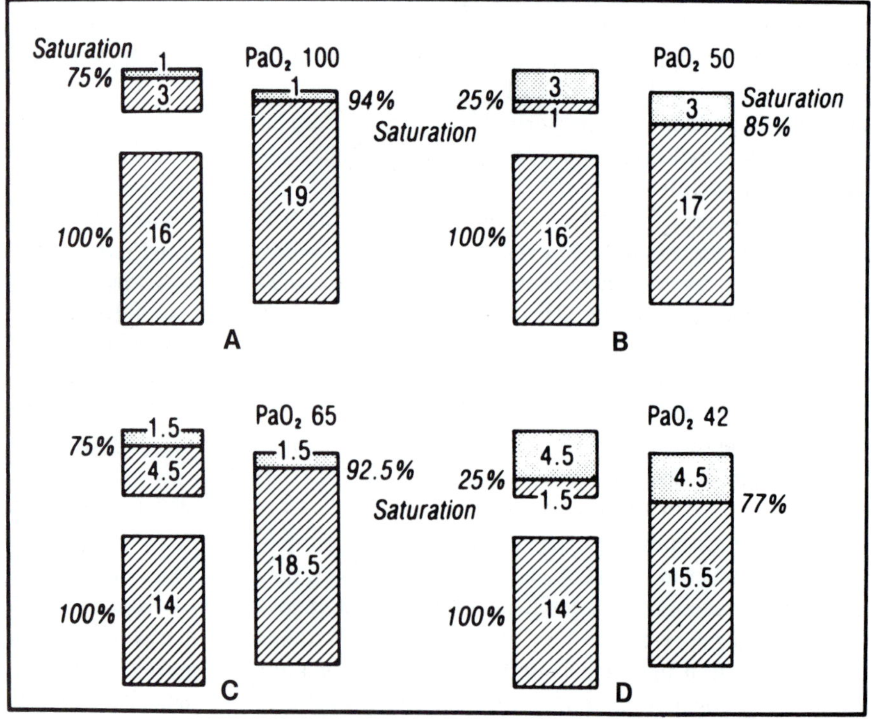


**Figure 1–11.** The effect of change in venous oxygen content on arterial $Po_2$ and oxygen saturation. **A.** At a 20% shunt with normal venous oxygen, the saturation level of 20% of arterial blood is 75%; that of the remaining 80% is 100%. When the two sets of blood are mixed (second bar), the result is normal or near normal $Po_2$ and oxygen saturation. **B.** If venous saturation falls to 25% due to decrease in cardiac output or increased oxygen utilization, the low venous oxygen making up 20% of the arterial blood causes the $PaO_2$ to drop to 50 mm Hg and the saturation to 85% (right upper bars). **C, D.** If shunt is raised to 30%, the effects of fall in venous oxygen are exaggerated. *(From Peters RM et al: The Scientific Management of Surgical Patients, 1983. Courtesy of Little, Brown.)*

cumstance, it is imperative to measure mixed venous $O_2$ to determine avD$O_2$ for an accurate shunt fraction calculation.[19,20]

2. Multiple trauma
3. Compromised cardiac function

### One-Lung Anesthesia

Over the last 10 years, use of a double lumen endotracheal tube to separate the ventilation to the two lungs has become the anesthesia methodology of choice for pulmonary resection. The advent of videothoracoscopy has further increased the need for this form of ventilation, because the lung must be collapsed. The surgeon must understand the unique physiologic disturbances created during one-lung anesthesia.[21]

The unventilated lung is perfused and is a source of an intrapulmonary shunt that can lead to a fall in $PaO_2$. A patient on one-lung anesthesia is ventilated with an $FIO_2$ of 1.0 for two reasons. The high $FIO_2$ in the unventilated lung leads to rapid collapse when ventilation is stopped and allows the surgeon to proceed as soon as the ventilation to the lung is stopped. Alveolar hypoxemia induces vasoconstriction and increases vascular resistance to the unventilated lung, and lung collapse enhances the increased resistance. This protective reflex improves oxygenation by increasing vascular resistance and decreasing the flow to the unventilated lung and the intrapulmonary shunt. The high $FIO_2$ to the unventilated lung provides an increase of 1.5 to 2.0 vol% of $O_2$ in blood draining the collapsed lung. The combination of high venous $O_2$ from the ventilated lung and decreased perfusion to the unventilated lung prevents dangerous systemic hypoxemia. To maintain normal $PaCO_2$, the patient must be hyperventilated to lower the $PaCO_2$ of blood from the ventilated lung enough to dilute the high $PaCO_2$ of the blood perfusing the unventilated lung. If the ventilated lung is normal, the $PaO_2$ should remain above the critical 60–65 mm Hg the shoulder of the oxyhemoglobin dissociation curve and hyperventilation should maintain a normal $PaCO_2$.

Careful placement of the tube is critical. An improperly positioned bronchial tube can obstruct exhalation and raise the intra-alveolar pressure in the collapsed lung. The increased alveolar pressure compresses the capillaries, increases resistance, and cuts down the portion of cardiac output going to the dependent lung, increasing the shunt fraction.[21] The surgeon should expect the mediastinum to move with each inflation of the lung. A still mediastinum is a sign that the patient is not getting good ventilation to the ventilated lung. Partial inflation of the unventilated lung with a low level of continuous positive airway pressure (CPAP) with $O_2$ is another method of preventing a fall in $PaO_2$. The venous blood perfusing the inflated but unventilated lung pulls $O_2$ from the alveoli to transport $O_2$ to the blood. The partial inflation of the unventilated lung with $O_2$ does not remove $CO_2$. Most patients requiring one-lung ventilation do not have normal lungs, and many have severely compromised lungs. Patients with emphysema are at risk of developing dangerous hypoxemia with one-lung ventilation, often requiring temporary interruption of the procedure to ventilate the lung on the operated side for some time. In others, the procedure may need to be abandoned.

A great deal of effort to develop an artificial blood substitute has resulted in the development of perfluorocarbons for supplementing $O_2$-carrying capacity of blood. These compounds have only a 2-hour half-life in the patient, but they have a unique potential for patients on one-lung anesthesia. Their $O_2$ dissociation curve is a straight line similar to the blood $CO_2$ dissociation curve. An infusion of these compounds at the time of initiation of one-lung ventilation would increase the amount of $O_2$ in the blood, draining the lung ventilated with $FIO_2$ of 1. This compensates for the lack of $O_2$ pickup in the unventilated lung. In patients with severe lung disease that need one-lung ventilation such as single-lung transplant or pneumectomy as described by Cooper et al,[22] these compounds may provide another safety factor to aid the skillful anesthesiologist. They will not substitute for a surgeon who understands the deranged physiology of single-lung ventilation and aids the anesthesiologist in tailoring the operative procedure to the need to preserve oxygenation.

## FUNCTIONAL RESIDUAL VOLUME AND SHUNT FRACTION

Measurements of delta increase in shunt fraction and delta decrease in FRV show that they are almost linearly correlated. In patients with an intrapulmonary shunt caused by pulmonary congestion, positive end-expiratory pressure (PEEP) opposes the increased elastic recoil of the congested lungs and increases FRV. Increasing FRV with PEEP or CPAP can increase pulmonary vascular resistance, because the high alveolar pressure in the ventilated alveoli compresses the capillary sheet between opposing alveolar surfaces. The compression of the capillaries raises pulmonary vascular resistance in the ventilated alveoli and may lower right heart output and shunt blood away from ventilated to unventilated alveoli, resulting in a fall in cardiac output and $PaO_2$. This combination decreases $O_2$ delivery. Hypovolemic patients are particularly at risk for this adverse effect of increasing airway pressures.

### Interaction of Lungs and the Ventilatory Pump

Patients can tolerate considerable dysfunction of either the chest cage or the lung, but the combination of chest cage and lung dysfunction leads to fatigue and respiratory failure. A rise or fall in FRV above or below normal compromises both the lung and chest wall function. A fall in FRV puts areas of the lungs below closing volume and leads to alveolar collapse, fall in lung compliance, and intrapulmonary shunt. Airways disease and lack of elastic recoil of the lung lead to an increase in FRV in patients with obstructive disease. An increase in FRV makes the preload of the inspiratory muscles inadequate and the ventilatory pump inefficient. The flat diaphragms and the barrel chest of patients with obstructive airways disease indicate that the inspiratory muscles are not stretched at end expiration and must start inspiratory work when already partially shortened.

Loss of alveolocapillary bed volume resulting from destructive effects of infection, resection of lung, or degenerative lung disease can compromise pulmonary circulation. Patients with obstructive airways disease and breakdown of alveolar septa lose significant portions of the alveolocapillary bed. Hypoventilation leading to low alveolar $Po_2$ initiates reflex precapillary vessel constriction. In advanced disease, destruction of capillary bed and vasoconstriction lead to pulmonary hypertension.

Interstitial and alveolar congestion change the dynamics about the precapillary and postcapillary vessels and raise pulmonary vascular resistance (PVR). Atelectasis with a fall in lung volume allows vessels to collapse and increases vascular resistance. In patients with COLD, elevation of PVR is an indicator of the extent of alveolar wall and capillary breakdown. Measurement of PVR can provide useful criteria for predicting lung reserve in borderline cases.

### Pneumectomy (Volume Reduction)

Pneumectomy is a term coined by Cooper et al[22] to describe an operation to reduce the size of the lungs in patients with emphysema. Patients with the late stages of obstructive airways disease characterized by bullae of varying size or just hyperinflated diffuse emphysematous changes have frustrated pulmonologists and thoracic surgeons. Such patients have hyperinflated lungs with flat diaphragms and intercostal spaces that are widened, even at end expiration. It was not known what would happen to these large chests if a normal-sized lung was used for transplantation. Cooper et al reported that after transplantation, the chest cage immediately adapted to the transplanted lung sized to fit a normal patient of comparable size.[12] The chest volume was not determined by chest wall function but by the lung. Brantigan et al[23] operated on a series of patients with diffuse emphysematous changes and resected portions of the lung to lower the lung volume. The patients were greatly improved symptomatically, but the operative mortality was 20%. Brantigan et al were not able to get support for continuing this series, because they had no objective measures of increases in lung function. Cooper et al independently reasoned from their experience with chest cage adaption in lung transplantation and stimulated perhaps by frustration with the large number of patients with emphysema waiting for donor lungs, that reducing the volume of the lungs in these patients might improve their function. In a carefully selected group of eight patients, they have developed a method of using a median sternotomy approach for bilateral stapling and excision of the periphery of the lungs to diminish their volume (bullous and nonbullous areas). Initially there were problems with prolonged air leaks. This has been reduced by overlying each of the stapling devices with a strip of bovine pericardium. Postoperatively, the patients had significant improvement in symptoms and in $FEV_1$. Postoperative sophisticated dynamic magnetic resonance imaging scans demonstrated that diaphragmatic motion was greatly improved. The reduction in the lung and chest cage volumes at end expiration increases the efficiency of the ventilatory pump by increasing the stretch (preload) on the muscle fibers of the diaphragm and chest. The lung tissue removed from the periphery was the most hyperexpanded and provided little surface for gas exchange. To palliate these patients, they sacrificed poorly ventilated lung to improve chest cage function and relieve the symptom of severe dyspnea.

If, as seems likely, Cooper et al's early results justify the continued use of pneumectomy, surgeons and pulmonologists must understand the pathophysiology of the disease and the therapeutic effects of reducing lung volume. Tests are needed to indicate those patients who are candidates for the procedure and document the functional improvement. For decades, pulmonologists and surgeons have concentrated on ways to identify patients with bullae compressing surrounding good lung.[24] These were the individuals in whom surgical resection of bullae seemed indicated. There are a few such patients. However, most patients with emphysema have diffuse disease. It is now apparent that the earlier studies were misdirected. Dyspnea presages ventilatory failure as an indicator that the effort to breathe is reaching the limits of the individual's reserve. Concentration on the disintegrating lungs in emphysema and ignoring the associated compromise of the ventilatory pump led to severe criticism of Brantigan et al and the abandonment of a procedure that with better methods of patient management and better understanding of the mechanism of ventilatory compromise, might have increased the quality of life of many patients. One need only try to breathe at increased lung volume or look at the hyperdeveloped chest cage muscle of the asthmatic child to recognize that when lungs are hyperinflated, the chest cage mechanics are compromised. Cooper et al's studies of change in diaphragmatic function and position suggest simpler studies evaluating the indication for pneumectomy and measuring postoperative improvement in function such as mean, end-expired, and delta pleural pressures. Noncompliant lungs do not exert the normal pull on the chest, so the mean end-expired pressures are less subatmospheric, the force across the lung and pulling the chest cage in is lower. The delta pressure oscillations are smaller, the lung is easy to stretch, and the chest muscle is at a mechanical disadvantage. Unstretched ventilatory muscles cannot generate force to provide a normal inspiratory fall in pleural pressure. A less subatmospheric peak inspiratory pressure provides another good indication of the mechanical disadvantage of the hyper-expanded chest cage.

The high pleural pressure also compromises the filling of the heart. The heart is in the chest cavity, so its actual transmural filling pressure is the difference between the venous or capillary wedge pressure and the intrapleural pressure. Normal pleural pressures are subatmospheric through the resting breathing cycle and become more subatmospheric as depth of breathing increases. Increased activity calls first on the inspiratory reserve of the patients, making pleural pressure more subatmospheric. As the intrapleural pressure falls, the heart filling pressure increases, causing an increase in ventricular volume and cardiac output. The restoration of negative pleural pressure in the pneumectomy patients increases heart filling pressure. It is likely that a decrease in dyspnea postoperatively is associated with increased cardiac function. Discussion of this procedure is included in this chapter on function, because it illustrates so clearly the importance of including the efficiency of the chest cage in evaluation of gas exchange.

### Summary of Evaluation of Gas Exchange Function

The background facts for assessing pulmonary function are the following: (1) There is a very large reserve of pulmonary function in normal, healthy individuals. (2) The condition of muscles of respiration depends on the exercise habits of the individual, just as in all other muscles.[11,12] (3) As lung volume falls, airways in dependent areas of the lung close. (4) With aging and in smokers, airways close at higher lung volumes. (5) When airways close, alveolar collapse may lead to ventilation-perfusion incoordination. (6) Ventilation-perfusion incoordination requires increased alveolar ventilation to maintain the same level of gas exchange as with a normal *V/Q* ratio. (7) Spirometry measures the volumes of lung and the ability to move air. (8) The level of $Paco_2$ is the indicator of adequacy of alveolar ventilation. (9) The level of $Pao_2$ is the indicator of adequacy of oxygenation. (10) Depression of $Pao_2$ in patients breathing room air at sea level is an indicator of ventilation-perfusion incoordination.

## ASSESSING PREOPERATIVE PULMONARY FUNCTION

The first steps in evaluation of patients preoperatively are an accurate history, physical examination, and chest x-ray. If the patient has no symptoms with vigorous exercise, chest wall motion is symmetrical and normal in range, and a chest x-ray shows disease limited to one lobe or less, clinical judgment will rarely be wrong in assuming that function is adequate. However, in my opinion, this assumption is not appropriate for a preoperative evaluation of a patient scheduled for cardiothoracic surgery. As part of the preoperative work-up, patients should all have complete blood counts, urine examination, a chemistry panel, an ECG, and assessment of blood coagulation. Many of these studies are more expensive than useful. All patients should have screening spirometry, a 10-minute test that should cost no more than \$50 to \$100. This simple test will avoid mistakes and provide an excellent reference for later clinical decisions. The simplest test for evaluating obstructive lung disease is to measure the $FEV_1$.[9] A normal individual can expel 80% of vital capacity in 1 second. Forced expired volume less than 35% of the total inspired volume in the first second puts a patient in the high-risk group for pulmonary surgery. Another frequently used test is the forced expired flow between 25% and 75% of expired vital capacity (FEF25–75%).[25] An FEF25–75% less than 1 L/s denotes severe obstructive disease. The maximum voluntary ventilation (MVV) measured for 15 seconds is also a useful predictor. AMVV of less than 28 L/min denotes severe decrease in function. Spirometry is effort-dependent, and so patients must be able to cooperate to make a maximum effort.[6,7,9] The lung volumes measured at spirometry are reported as absolute values in liters and also as percent of predicted for the patient's age and body size. Figure 1–12 shows the predicted normal volumes for a 70-kg, 165-cm

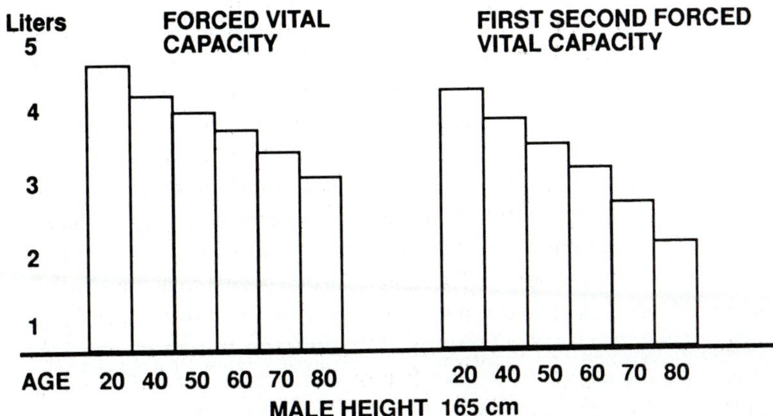


**Figure 1–12.** This figure shows the effect of age on predicted lung volumes. With aging, the amount of ventilatory reserve needed following lung resection does not decrease. Therefore, we suggest use of value at age 50 as norm for lung resection. *(From Peters RM: Matching pulmonary resection to patient function. J Jpn Assn Thorac Surg 5:674–684, 1988. Used with permission.)*

patient with the FRV and $FEV_1$ corrected for age. Note that with aging, normal values decrease. The use of predicted lung volumes to select patients for operation implies that an elderly patient needs less reserve for an operation than does a younger patient. This is obviously a ridiculous conclusion. To avoid this error, I prefer to use the age 50 norms for patients above age 50 (Fig. 1–12). If the patients' spirometry results place them in the low-risk category as shown in Table 1–3, no other studies are needed. If they function below this level, further studies are needed.[26] If vital capacity is down but $FEV_1$ is above 70%, the patient has restrictive disease. For patients being studied to evaluate tolerance to lung resection, we need to know the predicted postoperative lung volumes. Interpretation of spirometry with review of the x-ray identifies a patient with obstructive atelectasis of a lobe for whom resection of the affected lobe does not remove functional lung. Quantitative radioisotopic ventilation-perfusion scanning, with calculation of regional distributions of ventilation and perfusion, provides the most precise method for predicting postoperative function.[25,27,28]

Estimation of the proportion of total function ascribed to the region to be resected allows one to calculate what will remain after resection. Some studies have shown a good correlation between predicted postoperative function and measured postoperative function using the percent of normal lung volume for each lobe or lung for the calculations.[28] To define as a limit for resection a minimal for postoperative activity compatible with self-care, many clinicians use a predicted postoperative $FEV_1$ of 800 mL as their low limit.[7,9,26,27,29] This assumption, like all attempts to produce absolute values, has proven wrong. A predicted function at this level certainly places the patient in a marginal group that requires careful evaluation. Any patient who has predicted postoperative $FEV_1$ less than 1200 mL needs further evaluation.

Arterial blood drawn at rest and exercise for measurement of pH and blood gas partial pressures is the next step. The pH and $Paco_2$ indicate whether alveolar ventilation is adequate. If the $Paco_2$ is elevated above 45 mm Hg at rest or rises above this level with exercise, the patient has clear evidence of a marginal level of alveolar ventilation. Such a patient is not a candidate for pulmonary resection unless a medical regimen improves gas exchange, usually by improving the obstructive airways disease component. In all marginal patients, an effective regimen of bronchopulmonary toilet, bronchodilators, cessation of smoking and appropriate antibiotics, if infection is present, is essential to good preoperative preparation. The regimen must be tailored to the patient but usually includes oral bronchodilators and bronchopulmonary toilet. Corticosteroids may be required but should be avoided if possible. All patients who are candidates for a thoracotomy should cease smoking to eliminate a major cause of bronchopulmonary dysfunction. Measurement of blood carbon monoxide level provides a monitor of patient compliance to a nonsmoking agreement. Cooper et al have shown that a graded exercise regimen, even in candidates who are candidates for lung transplantation or pneumectomy, can increase their preoperative functional capacity and enhance their postoperative recovery.[12,22] If, despite such an optimal regimen, $Paco_2$ remains above 45 mm Hg, there is a high risk of postresection respiratory insufficiency.

If $Pao_2$ is depressed below 65 mm Hg, the shoulder of the oxyhemoglobin dissociation curve, a further fall in $Pao_2$ will cause a sharp drop in $O_2$ saturation. If the $Paco_2$ is low and $Paco_2$ is not elevated, the decrease in $Pao_2$ is due to ventilation perfusion mismatch. Correlation of spirometry with chest x-ray and ventilation-perfusion lung scans can indicate whether the physiologic shunt will be improved by resection of an area of unventilated lung. There is no single or combination of findings that provides absolute criteria to deny a resection for a patient.[9,26,27,29–31]

## The Marginal Patient

The difficult problems in evaluating patients for surgery are not those with excellent function or those with persistent elevation of $Paco_2$ and predicted $FEV_1$ less than 800 mL, but

**TABLE 1–3. GUIDELINES FOR INTERPRETING PULMONARY FUNCTION STUDIES**

| | High Risk | Pneumonectomy | Lobectomy | Wedge |
|---|---|---|---|---|
| Preoperative $FEV_1$ liters | <2.01 <60% | >2.01 | >1.01 | >0.61 |
| Predicted postop $FEV_1$ liters | | >0.81 | >0.81 | |
| Preoperative FVC liters | <2.01 <60% | | | |
| Predicted FVC liters | | >0.81 | >0.81 | >0.61 |
| pH | <7.25 | >7.40 | >7.40 | >7.40 |
| $Po_2$ mm Hg | <55 | >60[a] | >60[a] | >60[a] |
| $Pco_2$ mm Hg | >45 | | | |
| $Mvo_2$ mL/kg/min | >20 | >10 | >10 | >10 |

Prediction values should be based on age 50. Tolerance to decrease pulmonary reserve does not improve with age. For the borderline patient, the age factor in the prediction of normal makes the patient over 50 appear a better risk than they actually are.

[a] If pulmonary resection will remove perfused unventilated lung and thus decrease shunt, a low $Po_2$ is less of a risk factor.

rather marginal patients with a low FVC or $FEV_1$ that invite errors of both commission and omission. Among the reasons for inaccurate decisions regarding pulmonary resection for patients with compromised reserve care are the following: (1) Failure to match the type of resection to the patient's functional level. All surgeons doing pulmonary resections for carcinoma should read Churchill et al's article[32] on lobectomy vs. pneumectomy and its discussion. The issue of how much lung to remove to treat cancer of the lung persists, but now the issue is wedge resection vs. lobectomy.[8,33] A recent report by Martini et al[34] documents the fact that local recurrences are more common after wedge resection. The balance of preservation of lung tissue vs. wide margin for removal of cancer remains. The dilemma is magnified by the high incidence of a second carcinoma. The surgeon must recognize the consequences of removal of more lung than is necessary for the first cancer may preclude removal of a second cancer,[33] (2) failure to design a postoperative regimen suited to the patient's needs for postoperative pain control with epidural analgesia,[35,36] (3) inadequate control of fluids and early ambulation,[30,31] and (4) refusing a patient for resection who could tolerate removal of the necessary lung. We do not know how many patients are denied surgery who had adequate pulmonary reserve to tolerate complete removal of their lung carcinoma. *Unfortunately*, none of the simple function tests gives a firm answer about prognosis for pulmonary resection,[5,7,9,26–30,37] A number of investigators have attempted multifactorial analyses to improve predictability.[32,33] While such analyses improve statistical predictability of outcome, their standard errors are large, and they cannot provide guidelines to completely replace clinical judgment. Table 1–3 gives the rough indications of risk identified by commonly used pulmonary function tests. There are useful criteria only for broad grouping to appropriate risk, and prediction of outcome is limited.[9,26,28]

The classic criterion of requiring a predicted postoperative $FEV_1$ of 800 to 1000 can result in both pulmonary resections that produce ventilator dependence and in denial of resection to patients who could tolerate it.[26] Efforts to improve outcome prediction by a more complete analysis of the interrelating systems that control gas exchange do not prevent all postoperative pulmonary failure.[28] A number of authors have advocated the use of exercise-induced maximum $O_2$ consumption ($MVO_2$) to access the integrated function of the three systems—circulation, pulmonary function, and ventilatory pump function. Bechard and Wetstein[31] concluded that an $MVO_2$ of 10 mL/kg defined the lower limit for safe lung resection. More recent studies have questioned whether $MVO_2$ is any more predictive than multifactorial analysis of clinical, spirometric, and blood gas measurements.[28] Ferguson et al[38] found that the best single predictor of morbidity and mortality after lung resection was the predicted postoperative diffusing capacity for carbon monoxide (PPODLCO %). This was calculated by the percentage of unresected lung segments multiplied by the percent of predicted preoperative DLCO. A value of 40% or less was associated with a mortality of 20% and morbidity of 56%.

Clinical assessment must supplement function tests. An important negative clinical factor is obesity.[28] Obese patients have restricted motion of the chest cage and diaphragms. They must do greatly increased amounts of ventilatory muscle work to displace the fat to move the chest cage. The weight of the fat presses on the chest cage and diaphragms and requires extra effort to displace the chest wall on inspiration and to move about postoperatively. Obesity decreased FVC, $FEV_1$, FRV, and total lung volume.

Very muscular individuals also suffer some of the same disadvantages as the obese. The large muscle mass adds weight to the chest cage to lift with each inspiration. If pain is controlled, the muscular individual's superior physical condition compensates for the extra work without difficulty, but without adequate pain control, chest immobilization due to muscle spasm is exaggerated. Cooper et al have shown that in patients with severe pulmonary disease, carefully planned, preoperative, progressive exercise protocols result in a significant increase in performance on spirometry.[12,22] If two patients have the same degree of lung dysfunction, the one who has maintained physical activity is a far better risk.

In the earlier discussion of pulmonary function, the importance of a rise in cardiac output to compensate for a fall in efficiency of ventilation was emphasized. A patient with compromised cardiac function and borderline pulmonary function is a poor candidate for resection.

## TAILORING RESECTION TO FUNCTION

The type of pulmonary resection or other operative procedure is an important consideration in preoperative evaluation. The resection can and should be tailored to the patient's functional capacity. Removal of a lobe that is not involved with cancer does not improve survival. It increases operative mortality and morbidity, however, and may preclude a subsequent resection for the all-too-frequent second carcinoma.[32–34] Patients with seriously compromised function should have a careful preoperative regimen to clear up bronchial infection and bronchospasm, combined with insistence that they stop smoking. If they have not been physically active, they need a supervised, graded exercise regimen. A patient unwilling to cooperate in such preoperative preparation will most likely be his own worst enemy in the postoperative period.

The preoperative preparation should include plans for a postoperative regimen to meet the peculiar needs of the patient with compromised pulmonary function. The goals are to maintain the condition of the respiratory muscles by forcing patients to do their own respiratory work, enable coughing and deep breathing, and encourage mobilization. A great asset that is seldom available in the United States is a skilled team of physical therapists interested in pulmonary function. They can teach the patient breathing exercises and how to turn and sit up with minimal postoperative pain.

The surgeon and anesthesiologist can improve the patient's chances by a plan to use local analgesia to control pain instead of narcotics, which depress respiration. An example of the effectiveness of such regimens is the general acceptance of epidural analgesia to control pain in patients with flail chest due to trauma.[35,36] Early effective pain control enables patients to cough, keep lungs clear, and hyperventilate to compensate for flail chest wall. Seventy percent of patients with flail chest do not need ventilator support early, if effective regional analgesia is achieved.[39] Similarly, aggressive use of regional anesthesia (particularly epidural anesthesia) is extremely helpful in patients with obstructive airways disease. If these pain control measures are not planned preoperatively and initiated immediately, lung collapse and retained secretions result in atelectasis and failure to re-expand the remaining lung in the operative chest.

The exact equating of type of resection to a given set of preoperative criteria is not and will not be feasible. The interaction of various predictors—the surgeon's evaluation of the required extent of resection, its technical difficulty, function of chest cage, physical conditioning of the patient, and the amount of pleural disease—must all be entered into the complex decision-making process. Often, the deciding element is careful appraisal of the patient's clinical, physiologic state. This is a fancy term for the indefinable art of clinical judgment, and this type of clinical acumen comes only with careful practice. It cannot be acquired without time for critical evaluation of all data in a thorough manner. The need for judgment continues into the operating room, where the preoperative suppositions about the type of resection needed are tested and finally fit to the patient's respiratory reserve. Solutions to these problems do not come from looking at numbers. They require the synthesis of a complexity of information, clinical and laboratory, to make a wise judgment. Judgments require review of available laboratory studies in relation to an evaluation of the type of operation proposed and the other indicators of the patient's general health.

## REFERENCES


1. Graham EA: Some fundamental considerations in the treatment of empyema thoracis. St. Louis, Mosby, 1925
2. Peters RM: Empyema thoracis: Historical perspective. *Ann Thorac Surg* **49:**306-308, 1989
3. Graham EA, Singer JJ: Successful removal of entire lung for carcinoma of the bronchus. *JAMA* **101:**1371-1374, 1933
4. Blalock A: Reminiscence: Shock after thirty-four years. In Ravitch M (ed): *The Papers of Alfred Blalock*, Vol 1. Baltimore, The Johns Hopkins Press, 1966, p 16–19
5. Gibbon JH: Development of the artificial heart and lung extracorporeal blood circuit. *JAMA* **206:**1983–1986, 1968
6. Tisi GM: Preoperative evaluation of pulmonary function. Validity, indications and benefits. *Am Rev Respir Dis* **119:**293, 1979
7. Tisi GM: Preoperative identification and evaluation of the patient with lung disease. *Med Clin North Am* **71:**399, 1987
8. Peters RM: How big and when? *Ann Thorac Surg* **44:**338–339, 1987
9. Clausen J: Assessment of pulmonary function. In Peters RM, Toledo J (eds): *Current Topics in General Thoracic Surgery, an International Series*, Vol 2, *Perioperative Care*. Amsterdam, Elsevier, 1992, pp 3–27
10. Peters RM: The lung. In Peters RM, Peacock EE Jr, Benfield JR (eds): The *Scientific Management of Surgical Patients*. Boston, Little-Brown, 1983, p 349
11. Braun NMT, Faulkner J, Hughes RL, et al: Clinical conference in pulmonary disease. When should respiratory muscles be exercised? *Chest* **84:**76–84, 1983
12. Patterson GA, Grossman R, Maurer J, et al: Toronto lung transplant group. Double lung transplant for advanced chronic obstructive lung disease. *Am Rev Respir Dis* **139:**303–307, 1989
13. Taylor AE, Grimbert F, Rutilli G, et al: Pulmonary edema: Changes in Starling forces and lymph flow. In Hargens AR (ed): *Tissue Fluid Pressure and Composition*. Baltimore, Williams & Wilkins, 1981
14. Peters RM, Hargens A: Protein versus electrolytes and all of the Starling forces. *Arch Surg* **116:**1293, 1981
15. Peters RM: Pulmonary physiologic studies of the perioperative period. *Chest* **76:**576–584, 1979
16. Zeldin RA, Normandin D, Landtwing D, et al: Postpneumonectomy pulmonary edema. *J Thorac Cardiovasc Surg* **87:**359–365, 1984
17. Wittnich C, Trudel J, Sidulka A, Chui RC: Misleading "pulmonary wedge pressure" after pneumonectomy: Its importance in postoperative fluid therapy. *Ann Thorac Surg* **42:**192–196, 1986
18. Gosling P, Path MRC, Sanghera K, Dickson G: Generalized vascular permeability and pulmonary function in patients following serious trauma. *J Trauma* **36:**477–481, 1994
19. Shapiro AR, Virgilio RW, Peters RM: Interpretation of alveolar-arterial oxygen tension difference. *Surg Gynecol Obstet* **144:**547–552, 1977
20. Hennein HA, Swain JA: Preoperative cardiac assessment. In Peters RM, Toledo J (eds): *Current Topic in General Thoracic Surgery, an International Series*, Vol 2, *Perioperative Care*. Amsterdam, Elsevier, 1992, pp 39–61
21. Benumof JL: Anesthesia-specific problems for pulmonary resection. In Peters RM, Toledo J (eds): *Current Topics in General Thoracic Surgery, an International Series*. Vol 2, *Perioperative Care*. Amsterdam, Elsevier, 1992, pp 253–287
22. Cooper JD, Trulock EP, Patterson GA, et al: Bilateral pneumectomy (volume reduction) for chronic obstructive pulmonary disease. *J Thorac Cardiovasc Surg* **109:**106–119, 1995
23. Brantigan OE, Muller E, Dress MO: A surgical approach to bullous emphysema. *Am Rev Resp Dis* **80:**194–204, 1959
24. Gaensler EA, Gaensler EHL: Surgical treatment of bullous emphysema. In Baue AE, et al, (eds): *Glenn's Thoracic and Cardiovascular Surgery*, 5th Ed. Norwalk, CT, 1990, Chap 14, p 193
25. Kristersson S, Lindell SE, Svanberg L: Prediction of pulmonary function loss due to pneumonectomy using "Xe-radiospirometry." *Chest* **62:**694–698, 1972
26. Dunn WF, Scanlon PD: Preoperative pulmonary function testing for patients with lung cancer. *Mayo Clin Proc* **68d:**371–377, 1993
27. Keagy BA, Schorlemmer GR, Murray GF, et al: Correlation of preoperative pulmonary function testing with clinical course in patients after pneumonectomy. *Ann Thorac Surg* **36:**253–257, 1983
28. Nakahara K, Ohano K, Hashimoto J, et al: Prediction of postoperative respiratory failure in patients undergoing lung resection for cancer. *Ann Thorac Surg* **46:**549–552, 1988
29. Epstein SK, Faling J, Benedict DTD, Batrolome RC: Predicting complications after resection—preoperative exercise testing vs a multifactorial cardiopulmonary risk index. *Chest* **104:**694–700, 1993
30. Miller JI, Grossman GD, Hatcher C: Pulmonary function criteria for

operability and pulmonary resection. *Surg Gynecol Obstet* **153:** 893–895, 1981

31. Bechard D, Wetstein L: Assessment of exercise oxygen consumption as preoperative criterion for lung resection. *Ann Thorac Surg* **44:**344–349, 1987
32. Churchill ED, Sweet RH, Soutter L, Scannell JG: The surgical management of carcinoma of the lung. *J Thorac Surg* **20:**349–365, 1950
33. Peters RM: The role of limited resection in cancer of the lung. *Am J Surg* **143:**706–710, 1982
34. Martini N, Manfit SM, Burt ME, et al: Incidence of local recurrence and secondary primary tumors in resected stage 1 lung cancer. *J Thorac Cardiovasc Surg* **109:**120–129, 1995
35. Lomessy A, Magnin C, Viale J, et al: Clinical advantages of fentanyl given epidurally for postoperative analgesia. *Anesthesiology* **61:** 466–469, 1984
36. Benumof JL: Analgesia following thoracotomy. In Peters RM, Toledo J (eds). *Current Topics in General Thoracic Surgery, an International Series,* Vol 2, *Perioperative Care.* Amsterdam, Elsevier, 1992, pp 343–353
37. Goldman L, Caldera D, Nussbaum SR, et al: Multifactorial index of cardiac risk in noncardiac surgical procedures. *N Engl J Med* **297:**845–850, 1977
38. Ferguson MK, Reeder LB, Mick R: Optimizing selection of patients for major lung resection. *J Thorac Cardiovasc Surg* 1994
39. Shackford SR, Virgilio RW, Peters RM: Selective use of ventilatory therapy in flail chest injury. *J Thorac Cardiovasc Surg* **81:**194–201, 1981

CHAPTER

2

# Anesthesia for Thoracic Surgery

Roger S. Wilson

## INTRODUCTION

Management of the thoracic surgical patient has improved in many ways in recent years.[1] Improved diagnostic techniques and approaches have been developed to evaluate preoperative pulmonary function.[2] There has also been a better understanding of the complex changes in cardiac and pulmonary physiology during the perioperative period,[3] and approaches to anesthetic care have paralleled these changes. Anesthetic management of patients scheduled for noncardiac thoracic surgical procedures requires an approach that, in many ways, is unique to this surgical population. Noticeable differences include the need for a heightened awareness of preoperative pulmonary impairment and the specific delineation of any preexisting multisystem disease. Anesthetic management during the intraoperative period is potentially more complicated when compared with many other major surgical procedures, since the manipulation of lung and other intrathoracic organs may interfere, albeit temporarily, with gas exchange, cardiovascular function, and the delivery of volatile anesthetic agents. Finally, the technique of lung isolation or "one-lung" anesthesia is frequently utilized for a variety of reasons during these surgical procedures. Inherent in this practice is the need for the anesthesia and surgical teams to understand the application and design of isolation techniques, the safe and appropriate placement of these devices, and the altered pulmonary physiology produced when a significant portion of lung is temporarily unused during the intraoperative period.

This chapter will consider selected aspects of anesthetic management. It will focus on the role of the anesthesiologist during the preoperative period, the specifics of one-lung anesthetic techniques, and relevant aspects of altered cardiopulmonary physiology occurring with the resection of benign and malignant lesions of the lung, esophagus, and the major airways.

## PREANESTHETIC EVALUATION

The preoperative evaluation of the thoracic patient differs in several ways from the approach used for many other surgical candidates. One notable difference is the need to focus specific attention on the physiologic sequela of preexisting neoplastic, bronchospastic, and infectious pulmonary pathology. The potential impact of age and cardiovascular disease must be carefully considered to the extent that they can contribute to postoperative multiple organ system dysfunction. Patients with preexisting cardiopulmonary pathology, especially coronary artery disease complicated by ischemia and ventricular dysfunction, can be expected to experience significant perioperative morbidity. Intraoperative cardiovascular instability can result from postural changes, the lateral decubitus position with upper torso and lower extremities in the dependent position. This is often compounded by systemic effects of intraoperative manipulation and compression of pulmonary parenchyma and intrathoracic vascular structures. These and other acute physiologic derangements including hypoxemia, hypercarbia, and acidosis, especially when combined with the pharmacologic effects of anesthetic agents, can compromise both cardiac and pulmonary function. When superimposed on preexisting disease, this can produce immediate life-threatening situations during surgery. Preoperative evaluation must define the nature and extent of any existing cardiac and pulmonary disease. Several excellent studies have considered the specific approach to the preoperative evaluation in these surgical patients.[4–7]

The presence of preoperative cardiac disease requires special consideration. Of importance is any history of atrial or ventricular arrhythmias, valvular pathology, and evidence of coronary artery disease, especially with existing ventricular dysfunction. Arrhythmias are of special concern, since it is well documented that supraventricular dysrhythmias are common and potentially life-threatening during the postoperative period in this group of patients.[8,9] Any preexisting condition that would potentially increase the occurrence and severity of such rhythm disturbances should be carefully evaluated. Special consideration must be given to either prophylactic or early therapy whenever warranted. The manifestations of organic heart disease, although well tolerated in the preoperative period, may become more serious and life-threatening as a result of inadequate gas exchange and resulting hypoxemia and hypercarbia occurring in the perioperative period.

Detailed evaluation of pulmonary function is important to the anesthesiologist for several reasons. This patient population frequently presents with a significant history of cigarette smoking. Important are the inherent complications of chronic bronchitis with excessive sputum production and reactive airways. The presence of preoperative infection involving airways or pulmonary parenchyma could increase postoperative morbidity. Postoperative limitation of secretions clearance due to an ineffective cough increase the potential for pulmonary complications. Pulmonary disease that produces significant restrictive or obstructive patterns will further compromise postoperative pulmonary function. This is complicated by reduction in function associated with loss of lung occurring with pulmonary resection.

It is important to select an anesthetic technique that does not further impair respiratory function, gas exchange, and pulmonary toilet during the immediate postoperative period. Also, specific consideration must be given to adequacy of pain control in the attempt to maximize these functions while respiratory depression is limited.

## PREOPERATIVE MEDICATION

The choice of preanesthetic medication is dictated by need, the proposed surgical procedure, and coexisting disease. Selection from drug groups including tranquilizers, barbiturates, narcotics, and antisialagogues is often modified for the thoracic patient. Specific objectives of premedication differ little from other surgical patients with the exception that specific side effects, especially those adversely affecting pulmonary function, must be avoided or minimized. Central nervous system depression with barbiturates, tranquilizers, and narcotics can promote retention of secretions and decreased efficiency of gas exchange prior to anesthesia and surgery. Drying agents, including atropine and scopolamine, although they do not increase secretion viscosity, can adversely effect secretion clearance. Since they are not necessary with the use of contemporary inhalation agents, they are generally not used.

## MONITORING

The selection of specific monitoring techniques used during thoracic procedures is based on a variety of factors. Although there are published guidelines concerning monitoring, there is no universally accepted "minimal" standard.[10] A contemporary approach would always include use of noninvasive measurement of blood pressure, oxygen saturation, expired carbon dioxide, and body temperature and a continuous recording of cardiac rate and rhythm. Use of supplementary monitoring techniques are generally determined by availability, presence of preexisting disease, and the likelihood of adverse alteration in cardiopulmonary function from anesthetic technique or surgical manipulation. Other basic noninvasive approaches would also include the use of a precordial or esophageal stethoscope to monitor heart and breath sounds and on-line analysis of inspired and expired concentration of respiratory gases and anesthetic agents.

The use of invasive arterial and venous pressure monitoring is governed by standard indications. This would include significant preoperative impairment in cardiopulmonary function and anticipated adverse hemodynamic effects of anesthesia and surgery. Use of peripheral arterial cannulation is determined by the need for direct and continuous blood pressure monitoring and frequent sampling of arterial blood for gas analysis. The decision to use an arterial line is based on the presence of preexisting cardiopulmonary disease, anesthetic approach, and the complexity of the surgical procedure. The radial artery is most commonly used for cannulation. Advantages of this site include its accessibility, the presence of collateral circulation, and compatibility with good patient care in the postoperative setting, since it does little to limit patient mobility. Other sites, less frequently used, include femoral, axillary, and dorsalis pedis arteries. Controversy exists as to the suitability of the brachial artery, in part due to its potential for producing peripheral ischemia with vascular injury and thrombosis and also with difficulty in maintaining immobility. Complications of cannulation include thrombosis, hematoma formation, laceration of the arterial wall, and infection.

Objective assessment of hemodynamic function is accomplished using central venous pressure (CVP) or pulmonary artery (PA) monitoring during intraoperative and postoperative period. The decision to place a catheter in the central circulation is determined in part by need for vascular monitoring and also by need for vascular access for drug therapy when these are not suitable for administration via the peripheral route. Specific decisions as to use of a CVP vs. a PA catheter are based on individual preference, preexisting cardiac and/or pulmonary disease, the complexity of operation, and requirements in the postoperative period. Since its introduction in 1970, the merits and risks of PA catheters have been extensively debated.[11,12] A CVP clearly provides useful information regarding venous return and right heart function and, thus, adequacy of volume replacement. Significant blood loss is generally not a factor during most thoracic (noncardiac) operations and thus the need for CVP use on a regular basis can be debated. Central access to provide a safe route of administration for a variety of vasoactive drugs does justify its use. Potential benefits of

PA catheters during anesthesia and surgery have recently been described by the American Society of Anesthesiologists in published practice guidelines.[13] Benefits include the direct measurement pressures in the PA, right atrial and right ventricle, and indirect measure of left atrial pressure. In addition, the sampling of mixed venous blood, measurement of cardiac output, and determination of venous saturation are also possible with this approach. The inability to monitor biventricular function with a CVP in the presence of pulmonary disease does influence the decision to use PA monitoring. It is also possible that PA pressure monitoring provides more specific and useful information in the immediate postoperative period. This is especially important in the presence of multisystem disease. Randomized controlled trials generally fail to show any difference in variables such as intraoperative mortality, duration of postoperative hospital stay, or postoperative mortality in surgical patients when either monitored by PA catheter or CVP or when compared with surgical populations without central monitoring.[13] Complications with use of any central venous catheters include those occurring during placement, passage, and the period of use (Table 2–1). Factors such as the site of entry, insertion technique, and experience of the operator will likely determine the frequency and the complexity of complications.[14] Arterial puncture is a recognized complication with both internal jugular and subclavian venous approaches. The morbidity associated with this complication is minimized with the use of small gauge "finder" needles, recognition of arterial cannulation, and the appropriate control of bleeding. Complications such as pneumothorax and hemothorax may pose serious threats to life in situations where there is preexisting cardiopulmonary compromise, especially in circumstances when the complication is not properly recognized and treated. Complications relating to catheter passage are more frequent with PA lines when compared with CVP.[15] Although CVP can cause cardiac arrhythmias secondary to stimulation of the atrium, this is more likely to occur with the passage of a PA catheter. Well-described atrial and ventricular arrhythmias are produced with passage of PA catheter through right heart chambers and also pose the potential for bundle branch or complete heart block. Again, recognition and appropriate management generally limit significant morbidity with such complications. Complications relating to the presence of the catheter include thrombosis; infection; and, with use of PA monitoring, the potential for pulmonary artery rupture. The incidence, prevention, and management of all of these complications have been clearly defined.[13]

**TABLE 2–1. COMPLICATIONS OF CENTRAL VENOUS CANNULATION**

| |
|---|
| Vascular (venous/arterial) injury |
| Hematoma/Hemorrhage |
| Pneumothorax |
| Nerve injury |
| Cardiac arrhythmias |
| Air embolization |
| Thrombosis |
| Infection |

A special consideration is the technique used to place a PA catheter in the thoracic surgical patient. It is advisable to position the catheter in the dependent, nonsurgical lung in order to minimize interference of measurement produced by direct compression within the surgical field and also to ensure that the catheter tip does not reside in a segment or lobe of the lung that will be resected. One approach, although not the most cost-effective, is to position the catheter electively into the nonoperative lung using fluoroscopy. Limitations of the approach include the need for coordination of radiology, surgical, and anesthesiology teams and also the well-recognized possibility that, even in a short time, PA catheters may move in position, and relocate the lung opposite to the original one cannulated.

Specific design modifications of PA catheters provide for (1) measurement of mixed venous saturation (using oximetry), (2) ability to measure right ventricular ejection fraction, and (3) use as a temporary cardiac pacing catheter. Questions concerning the accuracy and also the utility of mixed venous saturation and right ventricle ejection fraction measurement must be weighed against the benefit of use of such catheters. Indications for the use of pacing catheters is determined by the presence of preexisting cardiac disease and the ability to use alternative approaches. As recently described, transcutaneous pacing is a viable alternative during the intraoperative period in the thoracic surgical population.[16]

Measurement of urine output is not mandatory in less complex and shorter procedures. Included are pulmonary resections and major airway surgery where there is minimal blood loss and the duration of operation is limited to a few hours. In more complex operations such as esophagectomy, adequacy of fluid replacement is effectively monitored, in part, with serial measurement of urine output.

Other more specific monitoring techniques including continuous measurement of inspired and expired anesthetic and respiratory gas concentrations are not universally used and are of limited value under most clinical circumstances. Use of transesophageal echocardiography during the perioperative period is dictated by availability and the need to monitor specific cardiac function.

## ANESTHETIC AGENTS

Many techniques including local, regional, and general anesthesia, alone or in combination, are suitable for management of thoracic surgical patients. The choice of a specific technique is influenced by the nature of the procedure and the specific objectives that must be met during the intraoperative and immediate postoperative period. The presence of coexisting disease, the complexity of the procedure, and the experience of surgeon and anesthetist are all important factors. The most common approach uses general anesthesia with one of several inhalation agents (Table 2–2) preceded by an induction with a suitable intravenous agent (Table 2–3). Endotracheal intubation is facilitated with use of muscle relaxant. Supplemental analgesia is provided with short- or long-acting narcotics such as demerol, morphine, fentanyl, sufentanil, and alfentanil. Narcotics and local anesthetic agents, placed in either the epidural or subarachnoid space, are used frequently for postoperative pain relief and will be discussed later in this chapter.

It is well recognized that major surgery, including thoracotomy, evokes a major endocrine stress response characterized by an increase in markers such as serum cortisol, plasma epinephrine, and norepinephrine and a variety of cytokines.[17–19] The combined use of epidural anesthesia with a "light" general anesthesia has been shown to be of potential benefit with decreasing postoperative morbidity in nonthoracic[20] and thoracic surgical patients.[21] Additional studies are necessary to delineate clearly the importance of such an approach in the thoracic surgical population.

A wide variety of intravenous and inhalation agents are suitable for use to produce general anesthesia.[22] There are few specific advantages to guide their individual selection. Use of one of several potent inhalation anesthetics listed in Table 2–2, is generally a matter of personal preference. These halogenated compounds differ in the way they alter function of the cardiovascular, respiratory, and central nervous systems. Central nervous system depression is produced in dose-related fashion with all of these agents. There is an overall reduction in cortical function with increased cerebral blood flow with all agents (halothane > enflurane > isoflorane), and this effect is attenuated by use of hyperventilation. This situation could prove problematic when thoracotomy is necessary with a concomitant head injury, especially where there are limitations in the ability to control the level of carbon dioxide.

Cardiovascular effects are prominent with all agents. Although agent specific, the circulatory effects are related to (1) myocardial contractility, (2) peripheral vascular resistance, and (3) autonomic nervous system function. All agents will produce a dose-dependent decrease in blood pressure. This mechanism is agent specific but in general is determined by the net sum of effects on contractility, heart rate, and peripheral vascular resistance. All decrease contractility in a dose-dependent manner. Increase in heart rate, relative to preinduction values, occurred with enflurane, isoflurane, and desflurane. Decrease in systemic vascular resistance is most notable with isoflurane and desflurane. Volatile agents differ to the extent to which they increase the potential for ventricular arrhythmias during conditions of increased levels of epinephrine. The potential for epinephrine to evoke premature ventricular beats is greatest with halothane and least with enflurane.

**TABLE 2–2. INHALATION AGENTS**

Halothane
(Fluothane, $F_3CHBrCl$)
Enflurane
(Ethrane, $CFHCl\text{-}CF_3\text{-}0\text{-}CHF_2$)
Isoflurane
(Forane, $CF_3\text{-}CHCl\text{-}0\text{-}CHF_2$)
Desflurane
(Suprane, $CF_3\text{-}CFH\text{-}0\text{-}CHF_2$)
Sevoflurane
(I-653, $(CF_3)_2\text{-}CH\text{-}0\text{-}CH_2F$)
(Not presently available in United States)

**TABLE 2–3. INDUCTION AGENTS**

| Drug | Comments |
|---|---|
| Barbiturates | |
| Thiopental<br>Thiamyal<br>Methohexital | Rapid onset and ultra short-acting. Minor differences exist for individual agents |
| Ketamine | A congener of phencyclidine administered via IV or IM route. Sympathomimetic effect is useful in specific patients |
| Benzodiazipines | |
| Midazolam<br>Diazepam<br>Lorazepam | Used for sedative effects and as adjuncts for general anesthesia. Agents produce anxiolysis and amnesia |
| Etomidate | An imidazole-containing hypnotic. Rapid onset with minimal circulatory effects |
| Propofol | 2,6-diisopropylphenal used for sedation, induction, and maintenance anesthesia (bolus or continuous infusion). No analgesic properties and rapid awakening |

Respiratory depression occurs with all agents in a dose-related manner. This effect is accentuated by use of narcotics, tranquilizers, and other drugs influencing the nervous system. Irritation of the airway, especially during light levels of anesthesia, exists with all agents, with isoflorane causing somewhat more irritation than enflurane, which in turn causes more irritation than halothane. Of the newer agents, desflurane is very pungent, while sevoflurane is much like halothane. All agents appear to cause bronchodilatation and obtund airway reflex activity at deep levels of anesthesia.

The pharmacokinetic activity of these drugs differs considerably. The extent to which they are metabolized differs considerably. Approximately 20% of the administered dose of halothane is eliminated as degradation products of metabolism. In comparison, biotransformation for enflurane is approximately 2% and isoflurane about 0.2%. Biotransformation and production of metabolites, especially with halothane, raise the question of potential for the organ system impairment. This is of concern with prolonged or repeated use of these agents. Halothane, by virtue of many properties, is a superior inhalation agent for airway and thoracic procedures; however, concern for its potential role in producing postoperative liver dysfunction, although controversial, has tended to minimize the frequency of use in most elective thoracic cases. Use of desflurane and sevoflurane for thoracotomy is limited due to their recent induction into clinical practice.

An IV technique, which uses one of several potent short-acting narcotic agents with supplemental nitrous oxide, is suitable provided that care is taken to avoid undesirable postoperative respiratory depression. This approach is most applicable for short procedures including all types of endoscopy and other superficial operations.

Muscle relaxation, although not absolutely necessary for many thoracic procedures provided that sufficiently deep levels of general anesthesia are utilized, is indicated during specific circumstances. Included are procedures such as rigid bronchoscopy and, when necessary, to minimize the potential for coughing and bucking. The latter is likely to occur during periods of airway and lung manipulation and may produce iatrogenic complications including bleeding and barotrauma. Many agents are available to produce relaxation of skeletal muscle. In general relaxants fall into two categories: depolarizing and nondepolarizing agents. Succinylcholine is the classic example of the depolarizing relaxants. This agent mimics the action of acetylcholine on both nicotinate and muscarinic receptors. It usually is the drug of choice for intubation due to its rapid onset of action providing optimal conditions within 1 minute. Muscle pain, ganglionic stimulation with increased heart rate and blood pressure in adults and bradycardia in children, hyperkalemia, and increases in intragastric and intraocular pressure are all undesirable side effects of this agent. Numerous nondepolarizing muscle relaxants are available for use both for induction and as maintenance agents during the procedure. They differ with respect to onset and duration of action, their route of metabolism and their effect on cardiovascular function by way of histamine release, ganglionic stimulation, and their ability to block or stimulate phagolytic and sympathetic activity. Choice of these agents is based on the nature and extent of operation, the need to minimize specific side effects in a given patient, and an approach that is consistent with no residual effects in the immediate postoperative period if spontaneous respiration and extubation of the airway are planned. A variety of approaches is used to monitor the extent of residual neuromuscular function and to assess the efficacy of chemical reversal with a number of specific agents such as edrophonium, neostigmine, and pyridostigmine.

## SPECIFIC ANESTHETIC APPROACHES

### Bronchoscopy

Laryngoscopy and bronchoscopy with flexible fiberoptic or rigid techniques often require some form of anesthesia. The anesthetic approach, including regional, local, or general, is dictated by the bronchoscopic technique utilized; the level of anticipated patient cooperation; and the nature, extent, and location of the surgical pathology. The specific objectives to be met include the ability to provide analgesia or anesthesia to the airway, adequacy of gas exchange during the procedure itself, and the need to depress or eliminate reflex airway activity. The latter is important to reduce probability of coughing, straining, and bucking. It is often necessary to attenuate or totally prevent the untoward side effects of the airway stimulation including tachycardia, hypertension, and the potential for inducing cardiac arrhythmias in patients with significant cardiovascular disease.

Fiberoptic bronchoscopy is easily accomplished in most patients with topical anesthesia of the nasal or oral pharynx, larynx, and trachea. It is often necessary to supplement this with judicious and careful use of IV narcotics and a variety of sedatives and tranquilizers. Several anesthetic agents and techniques are utilized to provide profound anesthesia throughout the airway. Local infiltration and selective nerve blocks, such as the superior laryngeal nerve, may be used to augment the use of topical anesthesia when necessary.[23] When bronchoscopy is performed in conjunction with mediastinoscopy or done immediately prior to thoracotomy, a general anesthetic technique is usually preferred. This is also the case when managing uncooperative patients or when patients are deemed medically unsuitable for the potential hazards of an uncontrolled local or sedative technique.

Several approaches are used to provide for control ventilation during rigid and fiberoptic bronchoscopy. During fiberoptic bronchoscopy with endotracheal intubation, positive pressure ventilation with appropriate airway adaptor is the standard of care. Use of a rigid endoscope provides a greater challenge. Suitable jet or venturi techniques using a variety of adapters with high-pressure gas flow to provide tidal ventilation has been well described.[24]

### Mediastinoscopy

Mediastinoscopy is generally accomplished with a general anesthetic technique. In virtually all circumstances, endotracheal intubation is done to guarantee airway control. Again, a variety of approaches are suitable including potent inhalation agents, narcotics, and sedatives. These are generally preceded by a barbiturate or propofol induction. Specific sequela of surgical stimulation including coughing, bucking, tachycardia, and hypertension. This is frequently associated with digital exploration of the pretracheal space. Increased intrathoracic pressure with bucking and coughing can produce engorged venous plexuses within the mediastinum with potential for an increased risk of venous bleeding. Muscle relaxation is frequently used to reduce the untoward consequences of motion during surgical manipulation and, thus, to decrease incidence of iatrogenic complications in this setting. The objectives of general anesthesia would include (1) sufficient depth of anesthesia to reduce reflex activity during periods of intense surgical stimulation, (2) minimal intraoperative cardiovascular depression, and (3) minimal respiratory depression at the conclusion of the procedure. This is even more important when such surgical procedures are carried out in an outpatient facility, where it is incumbent upon the anesthesiologist to select a technique consistent with safe and early discharge.

## LUNG ISOLATION TECHNIQUES

One anesthetic technique commonly used during thoracotomy and thoracoscopy deals with selected isolation of a portion of the airway and pulmonary parenchyma. Such isolation, commonly known as "one-lung" anesthesia, is indicated in a variety of circumstances (Table 2–4). An absolute indication for using isolation is pulmonary resection in the presence of lung abscess. A similar case could be made for thoracotomy and lung manipulation in the presence of significant bronchiectasis. Under such circumstances isolation should be considered in an attempt to avoid interoperative spillage of infected materials into the dependent, nonsurgical lung. Isolation techniques are also utilized to facilitate management of acute and chronic bronchopleural or complex bronchopleural-cutaneous fistulas. This is especially true in the setting of large air leaks, which could result in inadequate gas exchange with positive pressure ventilation prior to surgical correction. In appropriate circumstances one-lung anesthesia can prove to be beneficial in the management of acute penetrating thoracic wounds. A relative but similar indication for isolation technique is use during pulmonary resection involving lobectomy with a sleeve resection.[25] A common indication is the need to improve operating conditions by producing complete collapse of the operative lung during pulmonary and nonpulmonary resection. Other indications from the anesthesiologists' perspective would include the use of these techniques on an elective basis for the purposes of teaching residents and routine use to maintain technical skills. This is most essential to ensure that one is proficient when the method is clearly indicated especially if required in an emergent setting. One indication that is controversial is use during thoracotomy for acute hemoptysis. The hazard during such application would include the potential for occlusion of the smaller diameter endotracheal or endobronchial tubes necessitated with this approach. This issue will be specifically considered when isolation techniques are described.

**TABLE 2–4. INDICATIONS FOR ONE-LUNG ANESTHESIA**

1. Control of secretions
   a. Abscess
   b. Bronchiectasis
2. Airway control
   a. Bronchopleural fistula
   b. "Sleeve" resection
   c. Lung cyst/bullous disease
3. "Quiet" lung
   a. Pulmonary resection
   b. Exposure for nonpulmonary structures
4. Teaching
5. ?Hemoptysis

Three approaches have been used to facilitate isolation during thoracic surgery. These methods, although not used with similar frequency, include (1) endobronchial blockers,[26,27] (2) single-lumen endobronchial tubes,[28] and (3) double-lumen endobronchial tubes.[29,30] A brief description and applications of each of these techniques will be given. Factors governing the selection of any of these techniques include the surgical procedure, anatomic considerations, availability of equipment, and experience of the anesthesiologist.[31] Each technique must be considered based on specific advantages and disadvantages that are offered for a given surgical procedure.

### *Endobronchial Blockers*

Endobronchial isolation blockers, first described in the 1930s, have a limited role in contemporary thoracic surgery. This approach, however, is utilized when there is need to isolate a limited portion rather than the entire lung or due to the location of the lesion. Endobronchial occlusion is also useful when anatomic abnormalities, often due to prior pulmonary resection, may obviate endobronchial intubation, and when anatomic or oral pharyngeal pathology limit ability to use large-bore single and double-lumen endobronchial tubes. Finally, bronchial blockers used with a large-bore endotracheal tube are effective and practical during the operative management of hemoptysis.[32] The blocker, as described, will afford isolation of the lung with the active bleeding site and allow for a large-bore standard endotracheal tube. This approach decreases the potential for tube occlusion when there are excessive quantities of blood in the airway, a situation that is problematic during use of endobronchial tubes with limited cross-sectional area.

The original technique incorporating a latex (McGill) catheter with an inflatable distal balloon is of historical interest only. The contemporary approach is to use a Fogarty (venous occlusion) catheter (#8–14 with 10-cc balloon), which is available in most operating suites where major vascular surgery is performed. The Fogarty catheter is positioned with use of fiberoptic bronchoscopy. With this technique both the endotracheal tube and catheter are passed into the larynx under direct visualization using standard laryngoscopy. The Fogarty catheter is best placed through the vocal cords, external to the endotracheal tube. It is then advanced alongside the tube into the distal airway. Localization and appropriate placement of the catheter into optimal position in the distal airway is accomplished visually using a flexible fiberoptic scope passed through the endotracheal tube. Inflation of the balloon is confirmed with both visual inspection and chest auscultation to assure absence of breath sounds in the area of lung distal to the site of catheter balloon occlusion.

The catheter can also be placed into the lumen of the endotracheal tube, especially when intubation was done at a prior time. A disadvantage of this approach is movement of the distal portion of the Fogarty catheter with any movement of the endotracheal tube common during change in posture and with head motion during the operative procedure. The disadvantage of blocker techniques is the distinct possibility of dislodgement of the balloon tip during surgery. Common causes of this include use of positive pressure ventilation, unanticipated coughing and bucking, and surgical manipulation of lung. Bronchoscopic confirmation of catheter and balloon position is frequently necessary during the course of surgical procedure when this technique is used. An additional problem is the lack of inability to remove secretions and other foreign material situated distal to the catheter balloon. Although this is not problematic during the period of lung collapse, there is potential for contamination when the catheter is removed at the termination of the procedure and a cause for persistent atelectasis due to secretion retention within distal airways. Lung collapse during the surgical procedure is dependent almost entirely on reabsorption of trapped alveolar gas into the blood that continues to perfuse through this isolated lung. This process often requires several minutes or longer to give complete atelectasis and so must be considered well in advance of surgical need.

The Univent (Fuji Systems Corp, Tokyo, Japan) is a single-lumen tube equipped with a small channel on the anterior wall that contains a cuffed hollow catheter (Fig. 2–1).[33,34] This tube is available in several sizes from 6 through 9 mm I.D. in 0.5-mm increments. Once the tube is placed into the trachea with standard laryngoscopy, the blocker is advanced into the appropriate mainstem bronchus "blindly" or under direct vision using a fiberoptic bronchoscope. There are multiple applications for this airway device.[35,36] Special circumstances that lend themselves to use of this device include procedures where postoperative ventilation is desired, and, thus, use of this tube eliminates the need to convert a double-lumen to a single-lumen tube at the end of the case. Another specific application would be in the setting of hemoptysis where the larger or internal diameter potentially reduces the risk of tube occlusion with clotted blood and facilitates fiberoptic bronchoscopy for diagnostic or therapeutic purposes.

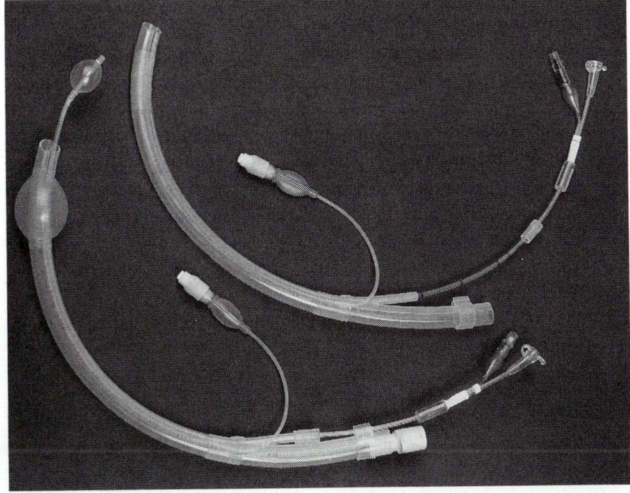

**Figure 2–1.** Univent tube shown on top with the blocker withdrawn and in the lower with blocker extended and balloon inflated.

### *Single-Lumen Endobronchial Tubes*

Single-lumen endobronchial tubes, although utilized for several decades, are infrequently used in current practice.[37] There are several limitations with this technique including the inability to suction secretions in the nonintubated (surgical lung) and the difficulty in providing adequate, retrograde gas flow from the intubated nonsurgical bronchus into the operative (nonintubated) lung. Two existing designs of single-lumen endobronchial tubes are fashioned for the left or right mainstem bronchi. These are still manufactured in nondisposable red rubber configurations. The MacIntosh-Leatherdale (left) endobronchial tube is designed for intubation of the left mainstem bronchus.[26] This tube is fitted with both tracheal and endobronchial cuffs. The terminal endobronchial portion of the tube is angled approximately 45 degrees off the midline to facilitate intubation of the left mainstem bronchus using standard direct laryngoscopy, oral intubation, and blind placement of the tube into the appropriate distal position. Confirmation of proper position is accomplished with intermittent inflation and deflation of the endobronchial cuff (tracheal cuff in an inflated position) to ensure respective presence and absence of breath sounds in the operative side when the cuff is inflated in the nonoperative lung.

A right-sided version, the Gordon-Green tube, is designed for left thoracotomy.[28] This tube includes a carinal spur on the body of the tube to facilitate placement at the carina. It differs significantly from the MacIntosh-Leatherdale, since the distal end is angled at approximately 30 degrees from the midline, and the endobronchial cuff incorporates a slitlike orifice in the lateral wall for ventilation of the right upper lobe bronchus. Appropriate positioning of this slit to assure ventilation and patency of the bronchus through the operative procedure is difficult to ascertain with auscultatory technique. Exact cuff placement would require use of flexible fiberoptic bronchoscopy.

Disadvantages of single-lumen endobronchial tubes include the inability to clear material from the operative lung and the potential for limited ventilation to the nonintubated surgical lung. Intraoperative difficulties with inflation of the operative lung secondary to inadequate gas flow and the presence of secretions often create problems in lung reexpansion once isolation is no longer necessary.

### *Double-Lumen Endobronchial Tubes*

Double-lumen endobronchial tubes are by far the most common method used for isolation during thoracic surgical

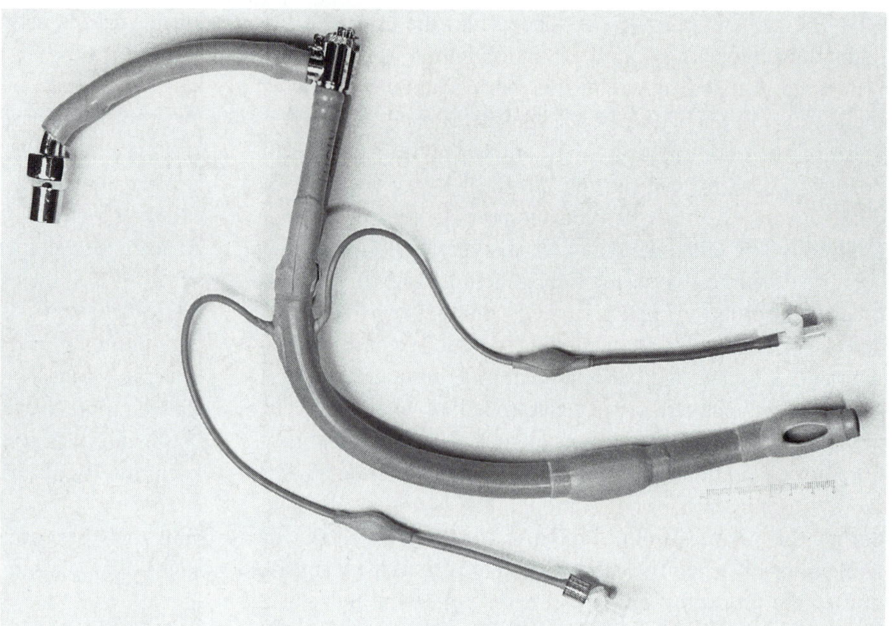

**Figure 2–2.** Right-sided Robertshaw double-lumen endotracheal tube shown from the side.

procedures.[31,37] Although this approach has been utilized since 1949, when first described for bronchospirometry, tube designs have undergone multiple transformations to improve their utility and function. Several types are currently available, all designed in the left- and right-sided versions for appropriate operative procedures. The oldest of techniques, the Carlens[38] (left) and the White[30] (right), although once the mainstay of double-lumen endobronchial tubes, have given way to the use of either Robertshaw design (red rubber) nondisposable tubes or the more conventional polyvinylchloride (PVC) design, which are manufactured by several companies. The Robertshaw and PVC types offer specific design and advantages when compared with preexisting tubes.[39,40] Included are larger internal cross-sectional diameter for a given external tube size and the absence of the carinal spur, although the carinal spur is available from one manufacturer of PVC double-lumen tubes. Due to design features, it is less problematic than the original Carlens design during passage through the larynx.

The Robertshaw double-lumen tube (Fig. 2–2) is a nondisposable red rubber design that incorporates a D-shaped internal lumen. This provides a reasonably low resistance to gas flow (approximately 10 cm $H_2O$/L/s). The tubes are manufactured in three sizes: small, medium, and large. Thus, they are suitable for use in adolescents to a large male adult patient. The right-sided endobronchial tube has a well-designed slit in the endobronchial cuff (Fig. 2–3) to facilitate a right upper lobe ventilation with minimal opportunity for occlusion.

The disposable PVC tube (Fig. 2–4) has continued to gain in popularity since introduction several years ago. These tubes are generally available in French sizes 28, 35, 37, 39, and 41. Depending on the manufacturer, they are available in right- and left-sided designs. The right-sided cuff design incorporates several features to accommodate ventilation through the right upper lobe bronchus. This cuff is somewhat more complex in design when compared with that of the Robertshaw tube (Fig. 2–5). There is potential for a significant incidence of upper lobe collapse when right-sided tubes are utilized. A practice in many centers is to use the left-sided endobronchial tube for operative procedures carried out either in the right and left hemithorax. This practice, although accepted by many, must consider the potential for dislodgement of the endobronchial limb when it is placed in the surgical lung and also the potential for obstruction to ventilation of the dependent, nonsurgical lung that occurs through the lateral (tracheal) port located in the distal airway. All isolation techniques carry the poten-

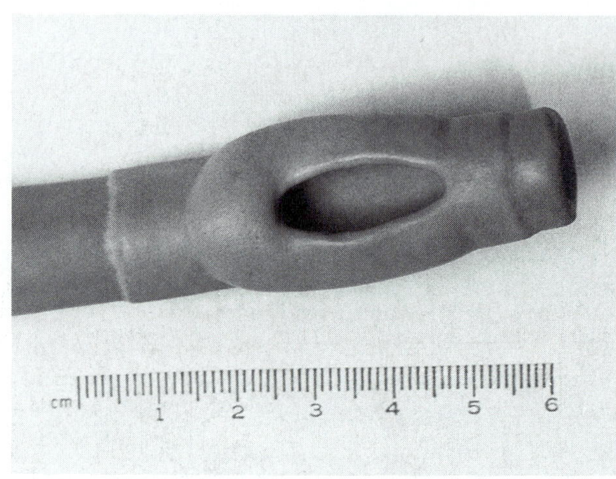


**Figure 2–3.** Enlarged view of slotted distal cuff on the Robertshaw tube.

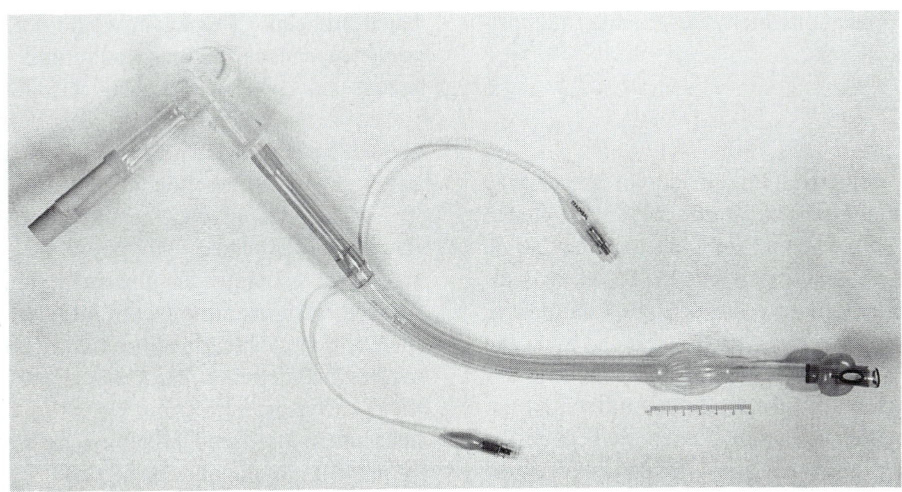

**Figure 2–4.** Right-sided polyvinylchloride double-lumen endobronchial tube shown from the side.

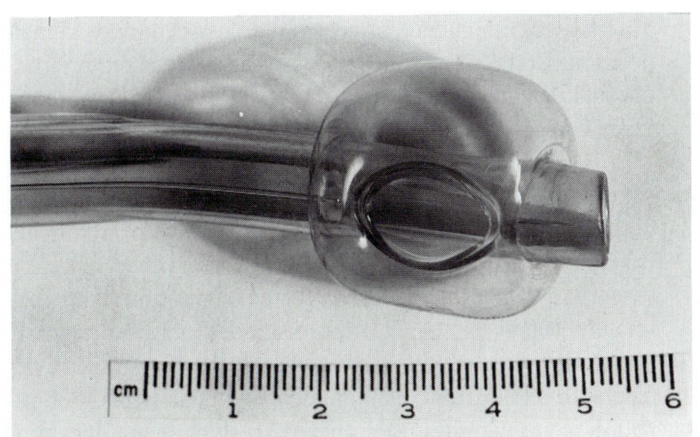


A

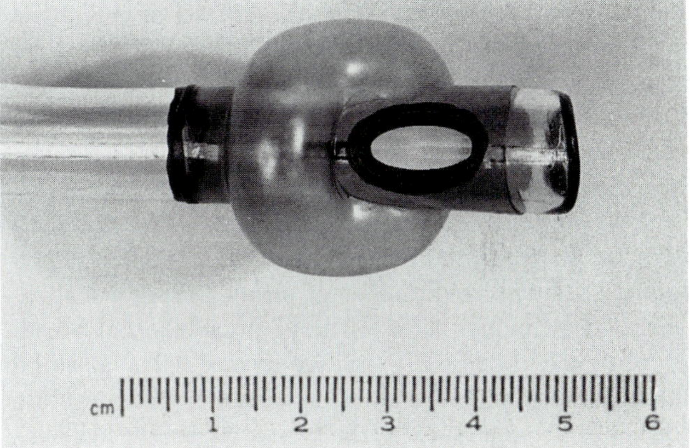


B

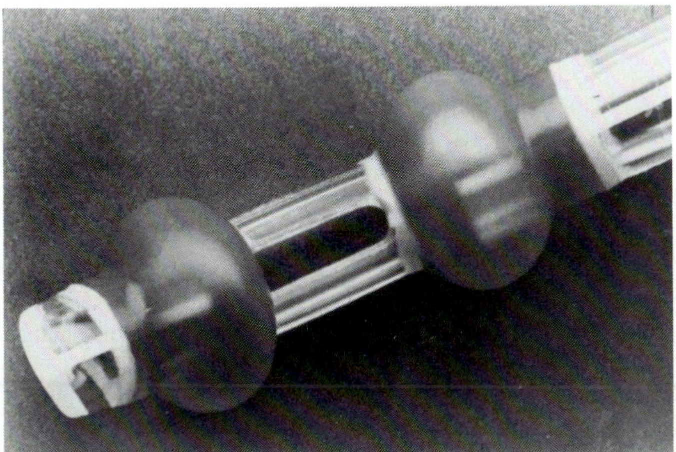

C

**Figure 2–5.** Cuff designs on the polyvinylchloride right-sided tubes: (**A**) conventional, (**B**) S-shaped, (**C**) double cuff.

tial for specific complications including trauma, malposition, and hypoxemia.

## Complications

Trauma can occur throughout the length of the airway under a variety of circumstances. Single- and double-lumen endobronchial tubes, due to their size, bulk, and angulation, are potentially more difficult to pass into the larynx with direct visualization. Hence, during the period of intubation, there is potential for dental and soft tissue injury with the oral and posterior pharynx. In addition, laryngeal injury owing to the large external diameter of these tubes is possible. Tracheobronchial rupture, a rare but reported complication, has occurred with standard single-lumen tubes as well as double-lumen devices.[41–43] The location of such trauma is generally confined to the posterior membranous wall of the distal trachea and proximal mainstem bronchi. When reported, injury has been noted during thoracotomy as evidenced by air within mediastinal tissue, the presence of the endobronchial cuff or endobronchial limb protruding through the bronchial wall into the surgical field, or loss of pressure and volume in the anesthetic circuit. The true incidence of this complication cannot be ascertained. Selected case reports would indicate that once detected, immediate surgical repair is generally consistent with survival. Trauma to the bronchial wall can occur secondarily to cuff inflation, especially with high-pressure, low-volume cuffs. Although theoretically an issue, such trauma has not been reported with significant frequency.

Malposition of double-lumen tubes within the airway is an obvious source of complications.[44,45] The true incidence of malposition is not ascertainable. Careful attention to placement and confirmation of position using visualization of chest motion with inflation, auscultation of breath sounds, and fiberoptic visualization of tube position through endobronchial and endotracheal lumen reduce the likelihood of occurrence.[46] The most common type of malposition results from advancement of the endobronchial limb too distally into the airway. This creates potential for isolation of the upper lobe on the nonoperative side and resulting lobar atelectasis. In this position the tracheal lumen opening enters into the bronchus rather than being positioned in the distal trachea. This would obviate ventilation to the nonintubated lung. A potential for such placement is increased with inadvertent selection of a "smaller-than-necessary" size tube that is easily advanced too far into the bronchus. A second type of malposition would be placement of the tube in a position that is too proximal in the airway. With such, the endobronchial limb does not adequately pass into the desired bronchus. Under such circumstances there is gas flow to both lungs with inability to isolate the surgical lung in the absence of endobronchial intubation. A variation of this type of malposition would include location of the endobronchial cuff just proximal to the carina, producing partial or total occlusion of the nonintubated bronchus. This again would not interrupt ventilation to the dependent lung but would limit ventilation to the operative side with occlusion of gas flow from the tracheal lumen to the operative lung. This particular complication should be detected with careful auscultation of the chest and with use of fiberoptic techniques.

As a general rule, the incidence of tube malposition should be minimized with careful attention to selection of tube size, technique for placement, and with confirmation of tube position during cuff inflation. When question of malposition exists, fiberoptic techniques are clearly advantageous in defining the exact problem and affording a means of visual correction. Use of elective fiberoptic bronchoscopy to position all double-lumen tubes is controversial at present. Smith and associates[47] used fiberoptic bronchoscopy to confirm the position of double-lumen (PVC) tubes placed "blindly" in 23 patients. In only 52% of the cases did they find the position to be optimal by their criteria. In 26% of the cases they found that the endobronchial limb had been advanced too far beyond the carina. Variables include right- vs. left-sided tubes and tube type. Burton and co-workers[48] found a 4% incidence of complications, such as malposition, with PVC tubes when compared with a 28% incidence with conventional red rubber types. Anatomic differences on the right side are likely to predispose a higher incidence of complications secondary to malposition. Complex cuff design with these tubes requires additional accuracy with respect to placement. Fiberoptic visualization is the most accurate technique to assure this.

Hypoxemia is the most serious of all potential complications with use of one-lung anesthesia. Unfortunately, as described in numerous studies, it occurs with significant frequency in patients undergoing noncardiac thoracic surgery in spite of inspired oxygen concentration of approximately 100%.[49,50] As will be discussed, its occurrence is not always predictable prior to surgery, and in general, occurs with all isolation techniques.[51] Fortunately, $CO_2$ elimination is not compromised during one-lung techniques providing an adequate minute ventilation is delivered and there are no mechanical problems such as air leak or tube kinking.

The incidence of hypoxemia ($Pa_{O_2} < 60$ torr) is variable as reported in several clinical studies.[51,52] In general, factors such as age, preexisting cardiopulmonary disease, and intraoperative management will dictate the frequency and the level of impairment.

It is important to consider the physiologic mechanisms that can produce increased inefficiency of gas exchange during one-lung anesthesia.[53,54] Several factors, working alone or in conjunction, have been identified. These include (1) the distribution of blood flow (percent of cardiac output) to the operative (nondependent) and nonoperative (dependent) lung, (2) the presence of air space collapse (atelectasis) and/or the existence of vascular disease in the dependent lung, (3) the inspired oxygen concentration, and (4) cardiac output. Although this is not an all-inclusive list, it represents those factors that are most likely responsible for the increased shunt fraction during one-lung techniques, and defines the issues that can be addressed with respect to therapy. Optimal arterial oxygenation should occur when there is minimal blood flow distributed to the nondependent, and collapsed, surgical lung.

In addition, optimal alveolar recruitment or expansion in the nonsurgical dependent lung, where maximal distribution of blood flow exists, is equally important. Any factor that influences the distribution of blood flow from the dependent to the nondependent lung, or is responsible for alveolar collapse in the dependent lung, will undoubtedly decrease the efficiency of oxygenation. Factors that can alter distribution of blood flow would include the hydrostatic pressure in the pulmonary artery, in part determined by the cardiac output, and the pulmonary vascular resistance in both lungs. High cardiac output, with increased pulmonary artery pressure, could result in distribution of flow into the surgical lung. In addition, preexisting vascular disease, especially in the dependent lung, would again favor redistribution of flow to the operative lung where it is not desired.

Factors that govern the integrity of air space include simple problems such as inadequate tidal volume being delivered to the dependent and potentially less compliant lung; the presence of alveolar or air space disease, including pneumonia and edema in the dependent lung; and direct compression of the dependent lung secondary to the weight of mediastinal and abdominal contents. Thus, the presence of acute or chronic pulmonary disease can influence these factors in adverse fashion during the time of surgery. As described by Hurford and associates,[55] one potentially predictive variable would be knowledge concerning the distribution of pulmonary blood flow in the preoperative setting as determined by radioactive perfusion scans. The greater the distribution of blood flow to the operative (collapsed) lung, the lower is arterial oxygen tension during one-lung anesthesia.

A variety of therapies is used to minimize the potential for hypoxemia during one-lung anesthesia.[51,56,57] A major objective is to maintain alveolar expansion in the dependent lung. This is accomplished with a large (12–15 mL/kg body weight) total volume delivered to the dependent lung during one-lung ventilation. Positive end-expired pressure (generally less then 10 cm $H_2O$) is added to the large tidal volume when $PaO_2$ is inadequate. In addition, the use of continuous positive airway pressure (CPAP) in the operative, nondependent lung causes partial reinflation without ventilation of the lung. This improves oxygenation, since it supplies oxygen to any blood flow that continues to perfuse through the operative lung during the procedure. As recently described by Slinger et al,[58] application of CPAP to a partially inflated lung is more beneficial than when applied after total collapse. A similar approach is to instill small aliquots of oxygen (approximately 4–5 mL/kg body weight) into the surgical lung with subsequent clamping of that limb of the double-lumen tube. This "residual volume" of oxygen is then allowed to reabsorb over the course of the next 10–20 minutes. This technique requires repeated instillation during the course of lung isolation but serves to maintain a quiet surgical field with a minimal lung inflation. An alternative is intermittent reinflation with large (tidal) volume ventilator on a periodic (q5–10 min) basis.[59]

Factors that govern the distribution of blood flow, including hypoxic pulmonary vasoconstriction (HPV), are clinically of limited importance, since there are few techniques to influence this variable. It appears that inhalation anesthetic agents and/or barbiturates and narcotic techniques have a similar influence on the HPV (or lack of HPV) during one-lung anesthesia.[60–62] The ultimate therapy for life-threatening hypoxemia during one-lung techniques (without returning to two-lung ventilation) is temporary occlusion of the pulmonary artery supplying the surgical lung. During pneumonectomy, early ligation of the pulmonary artery inevitably results in improved gas exchange. In cases where total lung resection is not anticipated, a decision has to be made as to whether the risk of dissecting and clamping the main pulmonary artery outweighs the potential complications of vascular damage. Arterial oxygen tension generally returns to control levels within minutes once two-lung ventilation is reinstituted.

The safe time course for continued elective lung collapse and the potential for complications occurring within pulmonary parenchyma are not well described. It appears, based on a number of anecdotal reports, that continued lung collapse can be carried out for several hours without need for reinflation. This practice fails to show evidence of postoperative complications due to change in compliance characteristics or gas exchange in the surgical lung. There is no evidence to support need for repeated lung (surgical) inflations during the operative procedure. The occurrence of postinflation pulmonary edema is rare.

## Major Airway Reconstruction

A complete discussion of the anesthetic approach to surgical resection and reconstruction of the trachea is not warranted due to the existence of several previous publications detailing these.[63–65] In addition, there is limited exposure to this procedure for most anesthesiologists and surgeons.

Complete preoperative evaluation, when clinically feasible, is necessary to define the extent and nature of the tracheal pathology, the presence of cardiac disease, and other conditions that could adversely affect the intraoperative and postoperative course. It is essential that the anesthesiologist have a complete understanding of the pathology and the plan for surgical correction to allow an optimal approach to premedication, monitoring, induction, airway management, and postoperative care. Standard methods for preoperative diagnosis of tracheal pathology encompass pulmonary function testing, radiologic evaluation, and endoscopy.

Premedication is selected using a conservative approach. This is done to minimize complications resulting from respiratory depression and airway obstruction and to ensure minimal residual postoperative effect. Monitoring techniques are similar to those previously described for other thoracic procedures, dictated in part by the presence and nature of preexisting cardiac and pulmonary disease.

Induction of anesthesia must be done with caution, especially with critical limitations of airflow, to ensure continued spontaneous respiratory effort and minimal compromise to the upper airway resulting from soft-tissue obstruction. Except in cases demonstrating little to no airway compromise, induction is accomplished using high inspired oxygen concentration, potent inhalation agents (halothane is optimal), and careful use of intravenous barbiturate. The latter is dictated by need; it is commonly used to reduce the "excitement phase" of induction. Bronchoscopy, generally using a rigid approach, is accomplished using "deep" general anesthesia, often supplemented with topical anesthesia to the airway. Once the extent of the tracheal pathology is determined and estimation of airway diameter at the level of the lesion is achieved, endotracheal intubation is performed.

The size and type of tube is determined by the location of pathology and the anticipated surgical approach. With surgical approach to the upper one-half of the trachea using a cervical (collar) incision, an uncut, standard red-rubber endotracheal tube is most suitable. A size 26 or 28 Fr is optimal for gas exchange, suctioning of secretions, and surgical exposure. It offers minimal limitation to intraoperative airway manipulation. When the airway diameter is less than 5 to 6 mm, endoscopic dilatation—provided that it can be safely accomplished—is performed to allow the endotracheal tube to be passed into the trachea distal to the lesion. This will maximize gas exchange and ensure an unobstructed airway during initial surgical dissection. Pathology involving the distal trachea, carina, or bronchi, especially utilizing a right thoracotomy, requires special consideration and use of modified endotracheal tubes. This description is beyond the scope of this discussion. Anesthesia is maintained with an inhalation technique usually with maximal inspired oxygen concentration.

Airway management during tracheal resection and placement of sutures is accomplished with a sterile flexible wire-reinforced endotracheal tube. This is inserted into the distal tracheal lumen via the surgical field and connected to the anesthesia machine with sterile anesthesia tubes and Y-piece. Following the placement of all sutures, the trachea is approximated. The "field tube" is removed, and the translaryngeal endotracheal tube is advanced through the anastomosis as the sutures are tied in a circumferential fashion.

In most cases, extubation is accomplished in the operating room. This is done either at a "deep" level of anesthesia or with the patient awake. The approach, considering the advantages and disadvantages of each, is determined by the anticipated need for immediate reintubation, usually optimal in anesthetized patients, and minimal soft-tissue obstruction to airflow and protection from aspiration existing in awake patients. The approach to optimal anesthetic management is designed to result in a comfortable, cooperative, awake patient with adequate spontaneous respiration in the immediate postoperative period.

## POSTOPERATIVE PAIN MANAGEMENT

Control of surgical pain in the postthoracotomy patient has been accomplished using a variety of techniques. In addition to the conventional approach using parenteral and orally administered analgesics, specialty techniques such as intercostal nerve block, transcutaneous electrical nerve stimulation (TENS), and cryotherapy have been proven to be of benefit.[66–68] In the past several years a number of potentially more effective approaches to pain management have been described in the literature including patient controlled analgesia (PCA), use of intrapleural local anesthetics, and intraspinal opioids and/or local anesthetics.[69,70]

PCA provides a continuum of intravenous or subcutaneous narcotic with administration that is self-regulated by the patient. Fixed doses of a variety of narcotics may be infused intravenously in a preprogrammed manner, by patient activation of a "control button." With this technique it is possible to establish both dose limitation and the time periods between doses (lockout interval) with appropriate pump programming. In addition, systems can be designed to provide a continuous background infusion that is then supplemented by the demand dose system. This technique has been used following a variety of surgical procedures and affords a number of advantages over standard intermittent intermuscular or intravenous drug administration.[71]

Intrathecal and epidural administration of opioids has gained acceptance during the past decade as a technique for control of chronic and acute postsurgical pain. Use of this mode has been the subject of numerous recent studies and several comprehensive reviews.[72,73] Small doses of a variety of opioids will produce effective and frequently prolonged analgesia in the postoperative patient when administered either directly into the epidural or intrathecal space. Administration may be done with single-dose technique or with multiple-dose methods, usually with a catheter placed into the appropriate space. The latter method is favored with epidural administration, while single-dose technique is reserved generally for the intrathecal approach. In the case of postthoracotomy pain where analgesia is often desirable for periods of several days, narcotic administration is often accomplished with intermittent injection or continuous infusion through a lumbar or thoracic epidural catheter.[74–76] The approach is generally dictated by the choice of agent; longer-acting narcotics such as morphine are suitable for intermittent injection while lipid soluble agents such as fentanyl are conveniently given by continuous infusion.[77,78]

Clinical studies have confirmed not only effectiveness of pain relief but, unfortunately, a number of untoward side effects.[74,78] Delayed respiratory depression, although the most serious and life-threatening complication, is uncommon. More frequent complications of intrathecal and epidural opioids include nausea and vomiting, pruritus, urinary retention, and drowsiness. Although the incidence of such side effects has varied considerably in studies to date, it is evident that several factors, including drug type, route, and dosage, and factors inherent in given patients, are important.[79,80] It is likely that with additional pharmacokinetic and pharmacodynamic studies and further clinical experience, there will follow improved prevention and treatment of these undesirable side effects.

Thus, it is evident that the anesthetic management of thoracic surgical patients offers several unique challenges to the anesthesiologist. The overall approach must consider the nature of the surgical pathology and must focus on the presence of associated organ system dysfunction with its potential to alter intraoperative and postoperative morbidity.

## REFERENCES


1. Grillo HC, Austen WG, Wilkins EW, Mathisen DJ, et al (eds): *Current Therapy in Cardiothoracic Surgery.* Toronto, Decker, 1989
2. Tisi GM: Preoperative evaluation of pulmonary function. *Am Rev Respir Dis* **119:**293–310, 1979
3. Marshall BE, Marshall C: Anesthesia and the pulmonary circulation. In: Covino BG, Fozzard HA, Rehder K, Strichartz GS (eds): *Effects of Anesthesia Clinical Physiology Series.* Bethesda, American Physiological Society, 1985, pp 121–136
4. Miller JI, Grossman GD, Hatcher CR: Pulmonary function test criteria for operability and pulmonary resection. *Surg Gynecol Obstet* **153:**893, 1981
5. Epstein SK, Faling LJ, Benedict DT, et al: Predicting complications after pulmonary resection: Preoperative exercise testing vs a multifactorial cardiopulmonary risk index. *Chest* **104:**694–700, 1993
6. Zibrak JD, O'Donnell CR, Marton K: Indications for pulmonary function testing. *Ann Int Med* **112:**763–771, 1990
7. Fishman RS, Systrom DM: Preoperative cardiopulmonary exercise testing: Determining the limit to exercise and predicting outcome after thoracotomy. *J Cardiothor Vasc Anesth* **5:**614–626, 1991
8. von Knorring J, Lepantalo M, Lindgren L, Lindfors O: Cardiac arrhythmias and myocardial ischemia after thoracotomy for lung cancer. *Ann Thorac Surg* **53:**642–647, 1992
9. Krowka MJ, Pairolero PC, Trastek VF, et al: Cardiac dysrhythmia following pneumonectomy: Clinical correlates and prognostic significance. *Chest* **4:**490–495, 1991
10. Eichhorn JH, Cooper JB, Cullen DJ, et al: Standards for patient monitoring during anesthesia at Harvard Medical School. *JAMA* **256:** 1017–1020, 1986
11. Ganz W, Donoso R, Marcus H, et al: A new technique for measurement of cardiac output by thermodilution in man. *Am J Cardiol* **27:**392–396, 1971
12. Vender JS: Pulmonary artery catheter monitoring. In Barash PG (ed): *Cardiac Monitoring.* Philadelphia: Saunders, 1988, pp 743–767
13. American Society of Anesthesiologists: Task Force on Pulmonary Artery Catheterization. Practice guidelines for pulmonary artery catheterization. *Anesthesiology* **78:**380–391, 1993
14. Murray IP: Complications of invasive monitoring. *Med Instrum* **15:**85–89, 1981
15. Sprung CL, Poen RG, Rozanski JJ, et al: Advanced ventricular arrhythmias during Swan-Ganz catheterization of the critically ill. *Am J Med* **72:**203–208, 1982
16. Amar D, Gross JN, Burt M, et al: Transcutaneous cardiac pacing during thoracic surgery: Feasibility and hemodynamic evaluation by transesophageal echocardiography. *Anesthesiology* **79:**715–723, 1993
17. Toft P, Svendsen P, Tonnesen E, et al: Redistribution of lymphocytes after major surgical stress. *Acta Anaesth Scand* **37:**245–249, 1993
18. Tonnesen E, Wanscher M, Hohndorf K, et al: Effect of methylprednisolone on the cytokine response in patients undergoing lung surgery. *Acta Anaesth Scand* **37:**410–414, 1993
19. Tonnesen E, Hohndorf K, Lerbjerg G, et al: Immunological and hormonal responses to lung surgery during one-lung ventilation. *Eur J Anaesth* **10:**189–195, 1993
20. Yeager MP, Glass DD, Neff RK: Epidural anesthesia and analgesia in high-risk surgical patients. *Anesthesiology* **66:**729–736, 1987
21. Temeck BK, Schafer PW, Park WY, Harmon JW: Epidural anesthesia in patients undergoing thoracic surgery. *Arch Surg* **124:**415–418, 1989
22. Eger EI II: New Inhaled anesthetics. *Anesthesiology* **80:**906–922, 1994
23. Gotta AW, Sullivan CA: Anesthesia of the upper airway using topical anesthetic and superior laryngeal nerve block. *Br J Anaesth* **53:** 1055–1058, 1981
24. Seki S, Gotta K, Kondo T, et al: Gas exchange and facilitation of high-frequency ventilation in intrathoracic surgery. *Ann Thorac Surg* **37:**491–496, 1984
25. Newton JR, Grillo HC, Mathisen DJ: Main bronchial sleeve resection with pulmonary conservation. *Ann Thorac Surg* **52:**1272–1280, 1991
26. Macintosh R, Leatherdale RAL: Bronchus tube and bronchus blocker. *Br J Anaesth* **27:**556–557, 1955
27. Ginsberg RJ: New technique for one-lung anesthesia using an endobronchial blocker. *J Thorac Cardiovasc Surg* **82:**542–546, 1981
28. Green R, Gordon W: Right lung anesthesia. Anesthesia for left lung surgery using a new right endobronchial tube. *Anesthesia* **12:**86–87, 1957
29. Robertshaw FL: Low resistance double-lumen endobronchial tubes. *Br J Anaesth* **34:**576–579, 1962
30. White GMJ: A new double-lumen tube. *Br J Anaesth* **32:**232–234, 1960
31. Edwards EM, Hatch DJ: Experiences with double-lumen tubes. *Anaesthesia* **20:**461–467, 1965
32. Gottlieb LS, Hillberg R: Endobronchial tamponade therapy for intractable hemoptysis. *Chest* **67:**482–483, 1975
33. Inoue H, Shohtsu A, Ogawa J, et al: New device for one-lung anesthesia: Endotracheal tube with movable blocker. *J Thorac Cardiovasc Surg* **83:**940–941, 1982
34. Inoue H, Shohtsu A, Ogawa J, et al: Endotracheal tube with movable blocker to prevent aspiration of intratracheal bleeding. *Ann Thorac Surg* **37:**497–499, 1984
35. Benumof JL, Gaughan S, Ozaki GT: Operative lung constant positive airway pressure with the Univent bronchial blocker tube. *Anesth Analg* **74:**406–410, 1992
36. MacGillivray RG: Evaluation of a new tracheal tube with a movable bronchus blocker. *Anaesthesia* **43:**687–689, 1988
37. Pappin JC: The current practice of endobronchial intubation. *Anesthesia* **34:**57–64, 1979
38. Carlens E: A new flexible double-lumen catheter for bronchospirometry. *J Thorac Cardiovasc Surg* **18:**742–746, 1949
39. Zeitlin GL, Short DH, Rider GH: An assessment of the Robertshaw double-lumen tube. *Br J Anaesth* **37:**858–860, 1965
40. Nelson AB, Watson DC, Brodsky JB, Mark JBD: Advantages of a new polyvinyl chloride double-lumen tube in thoracic surgery. *Ann Thorac Surg* **36:**78–84, 1983
41. Guernelli N, Bragaglia RB, Briccoli A, et al: Tracheobronchial ruptures due to cuffed Carlens tubes. *Ann Thorac Surg* **28:**66–68, 1979
42. Heiser M, Steinberg JJ, Macvaugh H, et al: Bronchial rupture, a complication of use of the Robertshaw double-lumen tube. *Anaesthesia* **51:**88, 1979

43. Burton NA, Fall SM, Lyons T, Graeber M: Rupture of the left mainstem bronchus with a polyvinylchloride double-lumen tube. *Chest* **83:**928–929, 1983
44. Black AMS, Harrison GA: Difficulties with positioning Robertshaw double-lumen tubes. *Anesth Intens Care* **3:**299–304, 1975
45. Brodsky JB, Shulman MS, Mark JBD: Malposition of left-sided double-lumen endobronchial tubes. *Anesthesiology* **62:**667–669, 1985
46. Shulman MS, Brodsky JB, Levesque PR: Fiberoptic bronchoscopy for tracheal and endobronchial intubation with a double-lumen tube. *Can J Anaesth* **34:**172–173, 1987
47. Smith G, Hirsch N, Ehrenwerth J: Placement of double-lumen endobronchial tubes. *Br J Anaesth* **58:**1317–1320, 1986
48. Burton NA, Watson DC, Brodsky JB, et al: Advantages of a new polyvinylchloride double-lumen tube in thoracic surgery. *Ann Thorac Surg* **36:**78–84, 1981
49. Torda TA, McCulloch CH, O'Brien HD, et al: Pulmonary venous admixture during one-lung anaesthesia. *Anaesthesia* **29:**272–279, 1974
50. Kerr JH, Crampton Smith A, Prys-Robert C, et al: Observations during endobronchial anesthesia II oxygenation. *Br J Anaesth* **46:**84–92, 1974
51. Capan LM, Turndorf H, Patel C, et al: Optimization of arterial oxygenation during one-lung anesthesia. *Anesth Analg* **59:**847–851, 1980
52. Slinger P, Suissa S, Adam J, Triolet W: Predicting arterial oxygenation during one-lung ventilation with continuous positive airway pressure to the nonventilated lung. *J Cardiothor Anesth* **4:**436–440, 1990
53. Marshall BE, Marshall C: Continuity of response to hypoxic pulmonary vasoconstriction. *J Appl Physiol* **59:**189–196, 1980
54. Benumof JL: One-lung ventilation and hypoxic pulmonary vasoconstriction: Implication for anesthetic management. *Anesth Analg* **64:**821–833, 1985
55. Hurford WE, Kolker AC, Strauss HW: The use of ventilation/perfusion lung scans to predict oxygenation during one-lung anesthesia. *Anesthesiology* **67:**841–844, 1987
56. Katz JA, Laverne RG, Fairley HB, et al: Pulmonary oxygen exchange during endobronchial anesthesia: Effect of tidal volume and PEEP. *Anesthesiology* **56:**164–171, 1982
57. El-Baz NM, Kittle CF, Faber LP, et al: High frequency ventilation with an uncuffed endobronchial tube. A new technique for one-lung anesthesia. *J Thorac Cardiovasc Surg* **84:**823–828, 1982
58. Slinger P, Triolet W, Wilson J: Improving arterial oxygenation during one-lung ventilation. *Anesthesiology* **68:**291–295, 1988
59. Malmkvist G: Maintenance of oxygenation during one-lung ventilation: effect of intermittent reinflation of the collapsed lung with oxygen. *Anesth Analg* **68:**763–766, 1989
60. Rogers SN, Benumof JL: Halothane and isoflurane do not decrease $PaO_2$ during one-lung ventilation in intravenously anesthetized patients. *Anesth Analg* **64:**946–954, 1985
61. Benumof JL: Isoflurane anesthesia and arterial oxygenation during one-lung ventilation. *Anesthesiology* **64:**419–422, 1986
62. Benumof JL, Augustine SD, Gibbons JA: Halothane and isoflurane only slightly impair arterial oxygenation during one-lung ventilation in patients undergoing thoracotomy. *Anesthesiology* **67:**910–915, 1987
63. Grillo HC: Primary reconstruction of airway after resection of subglottic laryngeal and upper tracheal stenosis. *Ann Thorac Surg* **33:**3–8, 1982
64. Geffin B, Bland J, Grillo HC: Anesthetic management of tracheal resection and reconstruction. *Anesth Analg* **48:**884–894, 1969
65. Wilson RS: Tracheostomy and tracheal reconstruction. In Kaplan J (ed): *Thoracic Anesthesia.* New York, Churchill Livingstone, 1983, pp 421–445
66. Galway JE, Caves PK, Dundee JW: Effect of intercostal nerve blockade during operation on lung function and the relief of pain following thoracotomy. *Br J Anaesth* **47:**730–735, 1975
67. Rooney SM, Jain S, McCormack P, et al: A comparison of pulmonary function tests for post-thoracotomy pain using cryoanalgesia and transcutaneous nerve stimulation. *Ann Thorac Surg* **41:**204–207, 1986
68. Warfield CA, Stein JM, Frank HA: The effect of transcutaneous electrical nerve stimulation on pain after thoracotomy. *Ann Thorac Surg* **39:**462–465, 1985
69. McKenzie R: Patient-controlled analgesia. *Anesthesiology* **69:** 1027, 1988
70. Ferrante FM, Chan VW, Arthur GR, et al: Interpleural analgesia after thoracotomy. *Anesth Analg* **72:**105–109, 1991
71. Church JJ: Continuous narcotic infusions for relief of postoperative pain. *Br Med J* **1:**977–979, 1979
72. Cousins MJ, Mather LE: Intrathecal and epidural administration of opioids. *Anesthesiology* **61:**276–310, 1984
73. Morgan M: Epidural and intrathecal opioids. *Anaesth Intens Care* **15:**60–67, 1987
74. James EC, Kolberg HL, Iwen GW, et al: Epidural analgesia for postthoracotomy patients. *J Thorac Cardiovasc Surg* **82:**898–903, 1981
75. Shulman M, Sandler AN, Bradley JW, et al: Postthoracotomy pain and pulmonary function following epidural and systemic morphine. *Anesthesiology* **61:**569–575, 1984
76. El-Baz NM, Faber LP, Jensik RJ: Continuous epidural infusion of morphine for treatment of pain after thoracic surgery: A new technique. *Anesth Analg* **63:**757–764, 1984
77. Gray JR, Fromme GA, Nauss LA, et al: Intrathecal morphine for postthoracotomy pain. *Anesth Analg* **65:**873–876, 1986
78. Logas WG, El-Baz N, El-Ganzouri A, et al: Continuous thoracic epidural analgesia for postoperative pain relief following thoracotomy: A randomized prospective study. *Anesthesiology* **67:**787–791, 1987
79. Shulman MS, Brebner J, Sandler A: The effect of epidural morphine on post-operative pain relief and pulmonary function in thoracotomy patients. *Anesthesiology* **59:**A192, 1983
80. Salomaki TE, Laitinen JO, Nuutinen LS: A randomized double-blind comparison of epidural versus intravenous fentanyl infusion for analgesia after thoracotomy. *Anesthesiology* **75:**790–795, 1991

CHAPTER

# 3

# Postoperative Care and Complications in the Thoracic Surgery Patient

Mark S. Allen and Peter C. Pairolero

## PREOPERATIVE EVALUATION

The number of patients who can safely undergo thoracotomy has increased greatly in recent years. Better understanding of cardiopulmonary physiology and expanded knowledge in clinical pharmacology have contributed to this increase. There can be no doubt, however, that some of the increase is also due to greater attention to preoperative preparation and improved intraoperative and postoperative management. Recent economic pressures, forcing same-day admissions for major thoracic surgical procedures and early hospital discharge, stress the need for preoperative assessment of risks and careful postoperative management.

A recent development in postoperative management has been the use of critical pathways. These predetermined guidelines are an attempt to reduce costs by reducing variability in postoperative care without compromising quality. Critical pathways are a tool of total quality management, initially developed by the business community.[1,2] These pathways have been initially applied to operative procedures such as coronary artery bypass grafting and total hip replacement with good success. For these techniques to reduce costs, surgeons must be involved in each aspect of development and implementation.

The patient at high risk for developing postoperative complications can often be identified by history and physical, roentgenographic, and routine laboratory examination. The importance of a careful respiratory history cannot be overemphasized. The patient's smoking habits, present and past, should be documented. Information regarding occupational and other possible exposure to pulmonary irritants should also be obtained. The presence of underlying lung disease and a positive smoking history are definite risk factors, and the patient at greatest risk is the one in whom existing lung disease is not recognized preoperatively. Information regarding the presence and extent of dyspnea, cough, sputum, and wheeze should also be obtained.

Routine pulmonary function testing should be performed in all patients undergoing pulmonary surgery. Spirometry is obtained early, and measurements of vital capacity, forced expiratory volume in 1 second ($FEV_1$), and maximum voluntary ventilation (MVV) should be done. MVV is an extremely valuable test. Although the results are influenced by a variety of nonspecific factors such as muscle strength, physical condition, and lack of cooperation. MVV is indicative of excellent overall pulmonary function and a low risk for pulmonary complication if normal. In contrast, MVV less than 50% of predicted normal is associated with an increased operative risk, especially if pneumonectomy is contemplated. If abnormal pulmonary function is found, several days of preoperative pulmonary preparation as described in the section on early postoperative management may be of help. In general, this preparation should include cessation of smoking; bronchodilator therapy; measures to minimize sputum production, including antibiotic administration if there is any evidence of infection; and adequate hydration.

Nonpulmonary risk factors are equally important in the preoperative evaluation. Significant cardiac disease carries a high risk. Since postoperative myocardial infarction is associated with a high mortality, some groups routinely screen all patients with an exercise treadmill test or thallium-201 imaging.[3] Heart failure, recent myocardial infarction, and unstable angina are usually contraindications to operation. Systemic diseases such as diabetes mellitus, hypertension, atherosclerosis, and renal insufficiency are especially common, and all may affect the postoperative course. Although patients over the age of 70 tend to have greater morbidity and mortality, age itself is relatively unimportant if the patient is otherwise in good health.

## POSTOPERATIVE MANAGEMENT

Successful postoperative management of patients undergoing general thoracic surgical procedures is dependent on an early recognition of physiologic alterations that may be developing so that early corrective measures may be instituted. Observation by experienced personnel, assisted by information gathered from various monitoring devices, combined with a free and open communication among the nurse, resident, intensivist, and surgeon, are essential to effective management.

Postoperative care of a thoracic surgical patient begins in the operating room. A catheter is positioned in the radial artery for monitoring of arterial blood pressure and blood gas analysis. Oxygen saturation monitors and end tidal $CO_2$ mass spectrometry are used to monitor pulmonary function. Large central venous lines also are placed for the instillation of fluids and for monitoring of right heart pressures. If there is a history of cardiac or pulmonary disease, a catheter should be positioned in the pulmonary artery for monitoring of pulmonary capillary wedge pressure.

After completion of the intrathoracic operative procedure, large (28° to 32°F) pleural drainage tubes are inserted into the thorax. These tubes should have multiple fenestrations over the distal 20 cm, which will allow for suction and drainage from several different areas within the pleural cavity. The most proximal opening should be well within the pleural space to prevent slippage of the opening to outside the chest. Two tubes are generally required; one should be directed toward the apex of the thorax, especially after upper lobe resections to help obliterate the air space, and one directed posteriorly to drain fluid or blood. For lateral thoracotomy incisions, the tubes should be inserted through separate stab wounds in the skin located in the anterolateral aspect of the thorax caudal to the incision. This skin position allows the patient to be supine without compression and occlusion of the tubes. The tubes are tunneled subcutaneously to an intercostal space several centimeters cephalad, where they are passed through the intercostal space. When the tube is removed, the subcutaneous tunnel prevents a direct communication between the pleural space and the skin. Drainage tubes should be carefully fixed in position by skin sutures.

For mediastinal procedures performed through a median sternotomy, drainage can be accomplished by a single tube placed in the mediastinum through a stab wound just below the xiphoid process. If one or both pleural cavities are entered, a single tube can be inserted in each thorax from the same subxiphoid position.

The pleural space should not be drained routinely following pneumonectomy. Intrapleural pressure, however, should be regulated to approximately –4 to –10 cm of water to prevent shifting of the mediastinum. This can be done by an intercostal catheter connected to a manometric system or a needle simply inserted through the skin into the pleural cavity, after completion of the procedure. The tube or needle is removed once the intended pressure is achieved with the patient in the supine position.

After a pneumonectomy, suction should not be applied to chest tubes, since the mediastinum may shift too far. Placing the tube to water seal creates a slight negative intrapleural pressure (–4 to –10 cm of $H_2O$). The tube can be removed in the operating room after the patient is placed supine, during a full inspiration, or it can be left to water seal overnight to monitor the amount of intrapleural drainage.

Following closure of the thoracic wound, postoperative care can be divided into immediate, early, and late management. The discussion in this chapter will be devoted to the overall care of a patient following general thoracic operation. Postoperative management of specific operative procedures will be discussed in the chapters relative to these subjects.

### Management in the Immediate Postoperative Period

Immediate postoperative care is also performed in the operating room, and the principal considerations are protection of the wound, connection of the pleural drainage tubes to an underwater seal, maintenance of an adequate airway, and transportation of the patient.

#### *Wound*

A light dressing is applied to the wound, supported by elastic adhesive tape. The adjacent skin is first rescrubbed with an antiseptic agent followed by an application of tincture of benzoin that, when allowed to dry, makes a sticky surface to which the elastic adhesive easily adheres without undue skin traction. This type of dressing avoids restriction of motion in the thoracic cage and allows coughing and deep breathing in the immediate postoperative period. It is usually removed the day after operation, exposing the closed incision to the air.

#### *Underwater Suction*

The drainage tubes are connected to a commercially available sealed sterile suction unit that is available from various vendors. These units all have the advantage that they are single and disposable. All of these commercially available drainage units are similar and consist of the classical three-bottle suction system (Fig. 3–1). The first bottle is for collection and measurement of fluid drained from the chest. Aspiration of air back into the pleural space is prevented by an underwater seal in the second bottle. The tip of the seal usually is not more than 2.5 cm below the surface of the water, and positive intrapleural pressure is required to displace the fluid column before air can escape from the thorax. Negative intrapleural pressure is maintained by the third bottle, which has a water column for regulating the amount of suction applied to the pleural space according to the depth of the tube beneath the level of the water.

### *Respiration*

Most patients can be extubated at the end of anesthesia and do not require mechanical ventilation. Indications for prolonged endotracheal intubation and mechanical ventilation include central nervous system depression due to anesthetic agents, hypoxemia for any reason, the possibility of continuing bleeding, and inadequacy of cardiac performance. If the endotracheal tube has been left in place in the operating room, usually it can be removed within the following 12–48 hours. It should not be removed until spontaneous respirations have been well established. If there is any question of secretions in the tracheobronchial tree, the trachea should be aspirated. After the patient has been breathing spontaneously a humidified inspiratory gas mixture containing 70% oxygen through a T-piece attached to the endotracheal tube, the measurements of tidal volume and blood gas analysis are used to evaluate the adequacy of ventilation. Generally, the endotracheal tube may be removed after 20 minutes of spontaneous respiration if the vital capacity is greater than 10 mL/kg, the respiratory rate is below 30 breaths/per minute, and the blood gas determinations are normal ($PaO_2 > 60$ torr, $PaCO_2 < 50$ torr) (Chapter 4). As the endotracheal tube is removed, a suction catheter is inserted through it until the catheter protrudes just beyond the tube's distal opening. Secretions that have accumulated in the upper part of the trachea and larynx are thus aspirated as the tube is removed. Upon extubation, the pharynx likewise is thoroughly aspirated if the patient is not fully awake. Increased concentrations of humidified oxygen are provided by mask for at least 48 hours.

### *Transportation*

Following most thoracic operations, the patient is transferred to a recovery room or an intensive care unit. Oxygen is administered by a face mask if the patient is extubated. If the patient cannot be extubated, ventilation must be assisted by using an anesthesia bag and a portable oxygen delivery system. Chest tubes should *not* be clamped during transport but connected to an underwater seal. This is especially true if assisted ventilation is required. Even a minimal air leak combined with assisted ventilation, or a spontaneous cough if the patient is extubated, can produce a tension pneumothorax with possible cardiopulmonary collapse if air cannot be vented from the pleural space.

## Early Postoperative Management

Following arrival of the patient in the recovery room or the intensive care unit, arterial blood pressure, electrocardiogram, and oxygen saturation should be monitored continuously. This permits the immediate recognition of problems. Heart and respiratory rates should be recorded every 15 minutes until the patient is stable and at hourly intervals thereafter. Urinary output, chest tube drainage, central venous pressure, and temperature are measured hourly. Body weight is recorded daily. Chest roentgenograms are obtained the evening of surgery and every morning thereafter until the day following chest tube removal.

### *Pulmonary Care*

Many patients who undergo thoracic operations have abnormal pulmonary function due to chronic obstructive lung disease. In these patients, preoperative pulmonary preparation—including chest physical therapy, aerosolized bronchodilators, mist, hydration, antibiotics, and the avoidance of bronchial irritants—has been shown to decrease significantly the frequency of postoperative pulmonary complications.[4] Operative trauma, incisional pain, and sedation are

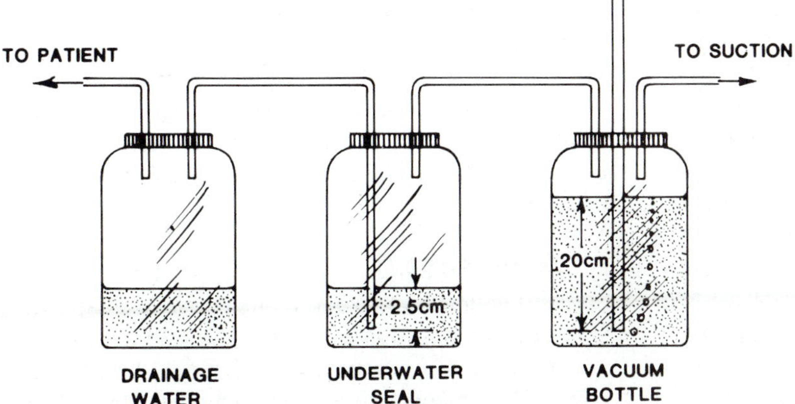


**Figure 3–1.** Three-bottle system for underwater seal suction.

additional factors that lead to retention of secretions, atelectasis, and arteriovenous shunting within the lung.

As consciousness is regained in the early postoperative period, the patient should be encouraged to breathe deeply and cough vigorously. Placing a pillow against the incision helps to support the chest wall, which decreases the pain of coughing and gives the patient a sense of assurance. The patient should be encouraged to cough every hour or two. If rales are present, the patient should be encouraged to cough until the rales are clear.

Chest physical therapy should be a major part of the postoperative respiratory care program.[5] When postoperative convalescence proceeds normally, treatments are administered twice daily and timed to follow the usual administration of analgesics by 30 minutes. If the patient has copious secretions, treatment may be given as often as every 2 hours. A treatment begins with 20 minutes of mist inhalation to wet down the upper airways and liquefy secretions. Then 10–15 minutes of aerosolized inhalation of a bronchodilator decongestant, or occasionally a mucolytic agent, is given. This is followed by 20 minutes of postural drainage, chest percussion and vibration, and vigorous coughing. If the patient can be instructed preoperatively in breathing exercises and the use of the respiratory therapy equipment, the patient will be more cooperative and receive greater benefit from the treatments postoperatively.

The position of the patient should be changed at regular intervals. Maintaining the patient in one position tends to promote the retention of bronchial secretions in the dependent portion of the lung. Most patients can breathe more comfortably and with less effort when they are in the semierect position. For coughing, it is also best to have the patient sit up because this aids in taking a deep breath. Patients who are mechanically ventilated should be turned from side to side hourly.

Atelectasis and intrapulmonary shunting can be reduced by the production of a large pressure gradient between the airway and the pleura. This transpulmonary gradient can be increased by intermittent positive pressure breathing (IPPB), which expands the lungs under pressure during inspiration, opening some airways that otherwise would remain closed. As a result, ventilation matches perfusion, and intrapulmonary shunting decreases. Removal of secretions is also facilitated by IPPB. Once the expiratory cycle is initiated from a high intraalveolar pressure following IPPB, an increased endobronchial velocity develops, moving secretions from the alveolus to the trachea. IPPB, however, carries a significant risk of insufflation of the gastrointestinal tract. Incentive spirometry, which requires the patient to inspire deeply (thereby increasing transpulmonary pressure by decreasing intrapleural pressure), is equally effective and carries less risk of gaseous abdominal distention. We favor incentive spirometry because it is inexpensive and easily performed. It can be instituted the day following operation, utilized every 2–3 hours, and continued up to hospital dismissal.

If, following vigorous coughing, chest physical therapy, and incentive spirometry, tracheal secretions cannot be cleared, nasotracheal aspirations should be performed (Fig. 3–2). With the patient in an upright position, the tongue, covered with a gauze sponge, is grasped between the thumb and forefinger and drawn forward. A sterile catheter is handled with sterile precautions. The catheter is passed through the nose until it reaches the pharynx, where a gagging reflex is usually produced. The patient is then instructed to breathe slowly and deeply. At the beginning of a deep inspiration, the catheter is rapidly advanced through the vocal cords and into the trachea. The catheter is then attached to low suction and moved proximally and distally while it is being rotated. The catheter can usually be inserted into each mainstem bronchus by turning the head and neck of the patient in the opposite direction. Finger closure of an open port on the suction tube easily controls the duration of suction. Suction should not be applied for more than 5–10 seconds. Longer periods of suctioning lead to hypoxemia and vagal stimulation, which may produce cardiac arrhythmias and even cardiac arrest.[6] Prior to suction and between periods of aspiration, the patient should breathe a humidified, oxygen-enriched atmosphere. Instillation of 5–10 mL of sterile physiologic saline dilutes tenacious secretions that can be aspirated more easily through the catheter. Because nasotracheal suctioning contributes to bacterial contamination of the lower airway by carrying organisms from the nasopharynx into the trachea on the catheter, it should not be used routinely. Probably as important as the aspiration of secretions is the stimulus to cough provoked by the catheter. Patients can also be stimulated to cough by the instillation of several milliliters of saline inserted by way of a small needle through the cricothyroid membrane or even a percutaneous endotracheal catheter.[7] This usually can be accomplished aseptically at the bedside under local anesthesia. When nasotracheal aspiration is anticipated to be required frequently, placement of a "mini-tracheostomy" is often helpful. This device, which can be placed at the bed-

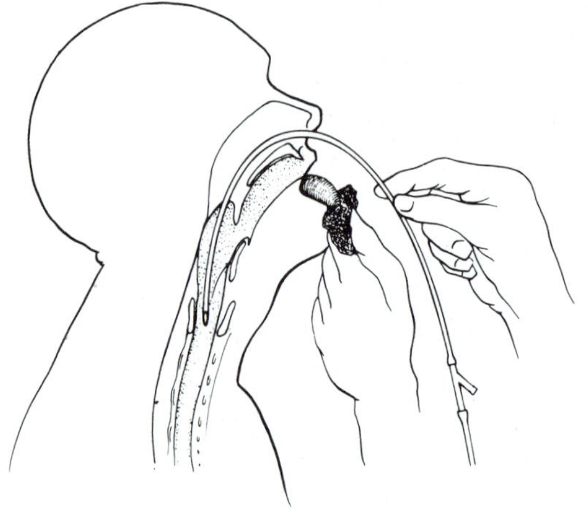

**Figure 3–2.** Passage of catheter for nasotracheal aspiration.

side with local anesthesia, allows a 10 F suction catheter to aspirate secretions from the trachea. Unlike nasotracheal aspiration, it is easy to suction secretions through, more comfortable, and less morbid. A mini-tracheostomy is generally well tolerated but is not a substitution for a formal tracheostomy or endotracheal intubation[8] (Fig. 3–3).

When the secretions become so tenacious or copious that nasotracheal aspiration fails to clear the tracheobronchial tree, fiber-optic bronchoscopy is indicated. This is generally performed at the bedside under topical anesthesia. To prevent hypoxemia, it is important to ventilate the patient with humidified oxygen for several minutes prior to and throughout the procedure and to employ short, intermittent periods of aspiration. If bronchoscopy is unsuccessful in opening the airway, reinsertion of an endotracheal tube may be required and the patient mechanically ventilated. Frequent tracheal aspirations are performed through the endotracheal tube, using sterile techniques. Instillation of 5–10 mL aliquots of saline into the trachea, followed by hyperinflation of the lungs with oxygen by compression of an anesthesia bag, tends to loosen secretions prior to suctioning. Bronchoscopy can also be performed through a port attached to the endotracheal tube, thereby allowing continued ventilation. For patients with prolonged need of tracheal aspiration, tracheostomy should be performed.

The secretions obtained during tracheal aspiration or bronchoscopy should be collected aseptically, cultured, and examined microscopically by Gram stain. If pathogenic organisms are present, appropriate antibiotics should be administered.

Breathing humidified air is very important in the postoperative care. This is especially true in the care of infants and children. A highly humid atmosphere helps to avoid dry, tenacious bronchial secretions, which are difficult for the patient to expectorate. Humidity is easily provided by a device attached to an oxygen supply line. The concentration of oxygen in the atmosphere should be carefully regulated, since prolonged use of high levels ($FIO_2 > 50\%$) can produce pulmonary parenchymal damage.

### *Fluids and Electrolytes*

The patient, upon leaving the operating room, is usually normovolemic with electrolytes in balance if fluid administration and blood replacements have been given properly. Intravenous fluid therapy consists of the administration of daily maintenance fluids plus replacement of any losses. Administration of 1000 mL of 5% dextrose and 0.2% sodium chloride per square meter of body surface area during the first 24 postoperative hours, and 1500 mL/m$^2$ for each subsequent 24-hour period, is usually adequate to maintain fluid balance. Included in these figures are all additional fluids given with intravenous medication and flushing of the arterial and venous lines. Potassium is given as necessary according to serum electrolyte determinations. When large amounts of potassium are needed, up to 40 mEq of potassium chloride may be placed in 200 mL of 5% dextrose and infused into the patient.

A urinary catheter is generally required, since epidural anesthesia frequently is utilized postoperatively, making monitoring of urinary output difficult. An adult with normal renal function should excrete at least 25–30 mL urine/h. Decreased urinary output frequently is due to hypovolemia. Measurement of central venous pressure should be taken,

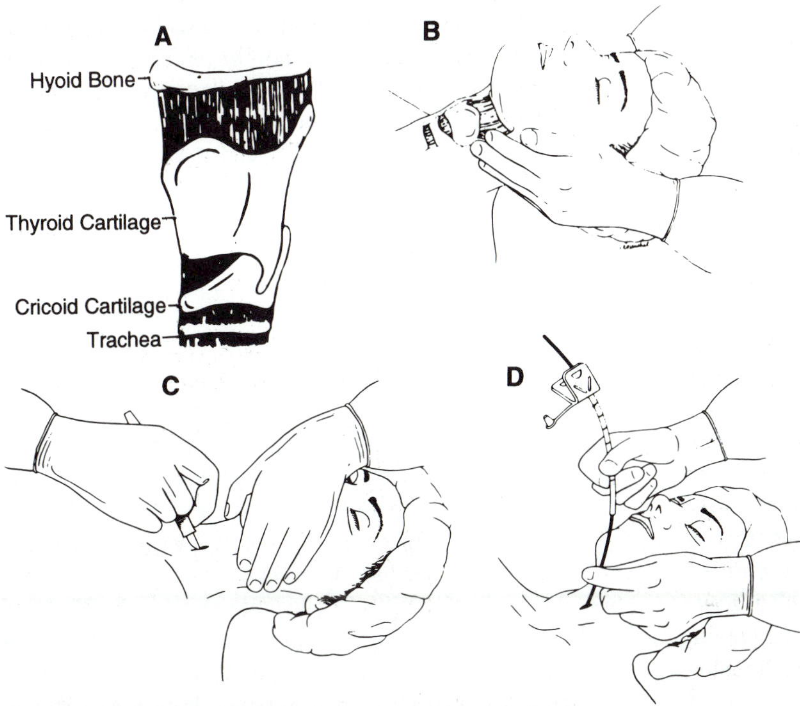


**Figure 3–3.** Mini-tracheostomy insertion technique. **A.** Anatomy of the upper airway. The cannula (outer diameter, 5.4 mm) is inserted through a vertical incision in the cricothyroid membrane. **B.** The head is positioned with the neck in extension, and the thyroid notch, cricoid cartilage, and cricothyroid membrane are identified. **C.** After instillation of local anesthetic, a vertical incision in the cricothyroid membrane is made with the bevel of the knife directed caudally. Egress of air should be identified with successful incision into the subglottic space. **D.** The obturator is passed through the incision; its curvature directs it distally into the trachea. Resistance should be minimal. The cannula is guided over it into the trachea. After removal of the obturator, intratracheal placement of the minitracheostomy is confirmed by respiration through the cannula, aspiration of airway secretions, and elicitation of cough by direct stimulation of the carina.

and if it is low, additional fluids or blood should be administered.

If the abdominal cavity has not been entered, oral intake may be started as soon as the patient desires. The patient should be encouraged to ingest at least 1500–2000 mL of fluid daily.

### *Pleural Space*

Pleural drainage tubes must be examined frequently to make certain they remain patent. When the tubes are patent, fluids within the tubes fluctuate with respiration. To prevent clotted blood from occluding them, the tubes should be milked throughout their length at frequent intervals. If this does not restore patency, the tube should be irrigated with 30 mL of sterile saline. The amount of pleural drainage should be recorded at hourly intervals. Blood loss should be replaced with equal amounts of blood administered intravenously. In adult patients, drainage is generally not replaced unless it exceeds 600 mL/24h. Continued steady loss of blood greater than 200 mL/h over a 4- to 6-hour period in the absence of any coagulation defect requires reexploration of the thorax to achieve hemostasis.

Drainage from the pleural tubes should decrease progressively during the first 12 hours. The tubes may be removed when there is no leakage of air and when drainage has ceased or is less than 75 mL per 8-hour period. Daily chest roentgenograms provide valuable confirmatory evidence of the effective elimination of air and fluid from the pleural space. The tube is clamped during removal, and the patient is instructed to perform a Valsalva maneuver. This increases the intrapleural pressure above that of the atmosphere. The tube is rapidly withdrawn, and the stab wound is covered by petroleum gauze reinforced by an elastic compression dressing. This dressing may be removed in 48 hours.

### *Medications*

Following operation intermittent epidural administration of either local anesthetics, such as 5 mL of 0.5% bupivacaine, or narcotics, such as morphine (5 mg/injection), effectively relieves pain, improves pulmonary function, and allows early ambulation.[9,10] Despite these advantages, however, intermittent epidural anesthesia for postoperative control of pain has been limited because of associated problems and side effects. The short duration of pain control requires constant participation of an anesthesiologist in postoperative management. Local anesthetics tend to be associated with motor and sensory blockade of the upper thoracic and lower cervical spine nerves, which can produce severe anxiety in many patients. Sympathetic blockade resulting in hypotension also occurs. Morphine administration, in contrast, can cause central depression of consciousness and respiratory depression. Morphine has also been associated with pruritus and urinary retention, requiring bladder catheterization. More recently, fentanyl given as a continuous infusion seems to be better tolerated than intermittent infusions of either local anesthetics or morphine. The analgesic effect of fentanyl is similar to morphine, but respiratory depression is less. Urinary retention also is reduced, and very few patients complain of pruritus. It has been our practice to place a small polyvinyl catheter in the second lumbar interspace immediately following thoracotomy. Fentanyl is then administered as a bolus, 1μg/kg, followed by a continuous infusion of 1.0–2.0 μg/kg per hour. Respiratory depression and somnolence are constantly evaluated to determine infusion rate. Epidural anesthesia has been given up to 96 hours without encountering any difficulties.

Following discontinuance of epidural anesthesia all patients are given supplemental medication to relieve pain. The severity of the pain depends on the type of incision and the reaction of the patient to the painful stimuli. Commercial patient controlled anesthesia (PCA) pumps are available that allow the patient to self-administer a predetermined dose of parenteral medication. Morphine sulfate, 0.5–1.5 mg, or meperidine hydrochloride, 5–15 mg, are usually administered intravenously. Parameters can be set to prevent overdose. Lockout periods during which time the drug cannot be self-administered are usually 10–15 minutes. Total 4-hour dosage (morphine sulfate 10–20 mg, meperidine hydrochloride 100–200 mg) can also be preset. Oral medications such as aspirin 600 mg (acetaminophen, 2 tablets, if the patient has peptic ulcer disease) or codeine, 30 mg every 3–4 hours, are usually sufficient to keep the patient comfortable in the late postoperative period. Division of the intercostal nerves in our experience has not been successful in preventing postoperative pain. However, intercostal nerve blocks have provided some relief of acute pain as well as improved forced vital capacity.

Fever is deleterious because the metabolic requirements of the patient with fever are increased. Acetaminophen, 1 g administered rectally, should be given if the body temperature rises above 101°F (38.3°C). If the temperature is above 103°F (39.4°C), a hypothermic mattress should be used. If hypothermia is present, the patient should be covered with a warm blanket and placed on a heating mattress.

### *Prophylactic Antibiotics*

Controversy exists regarding the need of prophylactic antibiotics during thoracic surgery. Those who oppose antibiotic prophylaxis warn of possible allergic side effects and the development of resistance. Others claim that because infectious respiratory complications significantly compromise ventilatory capacity postoperatively, prophylactic antibiotics are justified. Since common pathogens in bronchial secretions are *Hemophilus influenzae* and *Staphylococcus aureus,* antibiotics that are effective against these common bacteria may reduce the incidence of postoperative infection. In 1977, Kvale and colleagues,[11] in a double-blind control study, demonstrated that cefazolin prophylaxis significantly reduced postoperative infections compared with the placebo group. Other investigators, however, were unable to substantiate their findings.[12] In 1982 penicillin prophylaxis was reported to show a reduction in wound infections in patients undergoing elective pulmonary surgery, although penicillin did not have any effect on the incidence of pulmonary infection.[13] Similarly, short-term cephalothin prophylaxis has also been demonstrated to decrease infection in the operative sites in patients undergoing a variety of thoracic procedures.[14]

Only in a few control studies has the reduction in the rate of postoperative pulmonary infections been found.[11,15] The decrease in the incidence of postoperative wound infections is well documented in studies utilizing penicillin G, cephazolin, cephalothin, or cefuroxime as the prophylactic agent.[11,13,15] More recently, in a prospective randomized study utilizing either tetracycline or cephalosporin, Tarkka and associates[16] demonstrated that cephalosporin was slightly more effective in reducing infection than tetracyclines. This difference, however, was not statistically significant.

Although frequently used, the value of prophylactic antibiotic continues to be uncertain. Nonetheless, certain guidelines have emerged. The antibiotic should have a broad spectrum (tetracycline or cephalosporin) and should be administered for only a short duration (24–48 hours). The first dose should be given IV on call or in the operating room before the incision is made.

### *Gastric Distention*

Mechanical ventilation by mask or mouthpiece frequently forces air and anesthetic gases into the stomach. Patients with endotracheal tubes in place often swallow a great deal of air. Even in the absence of these mechanisms, anesthetic gases may diffuse into the gastrointestinal tract. It is advisable to position a nasogastric tube into the stomach to evacuate the gases. This maneuver is especially important after a right pneumonectomy, where a distended stomach may interfere with movement of the left hemidiaphragm.

### Late Postoperative Management

By this time, bronchial secretions are less of a problem, since coughing is no longer as painful. Chest physical therapy can generally be discontinued. The support provided by the elastic dressing to the wound is also no longer necessary, and the dressing can be removed. The wound can then either be not covered at all or covered with a light gauze dressing. If the wound is left open, care must be taken to avoid its irritation by rubbing against bedsheets. This is especially important with a posterior thoracotomy wound, where the patient may frequently lie on the wound. Irritation can be reduced by a frequent change of position and placement of the patient on a sheepskin cover.

The patient should be up and out of bed as much as possible. Generally, this can be started, even if only for short periods, the day after operation if the patient is hemodynamically stable and not being mechanically ventilated. Even with drainage tubes in place, the patient can stand to cough and deep breathe and walk. Male patients should stand to void. After drainage tubes have been removed, the patient should be encouraged to walk when out of bed and to lie down again when tired. Prolonged sitting, especially with legs crossed, should be avoided to prevent venous stasis. The patient should be encouraged to eat his meals sitting in a chair and not in bed. By the third postoperative day, the patient should be on a general diet. Patients are encouraged to take frequent warm showers after the drainage tubes are removed. Gentle bathing of the wound has a mild analgesic effect and provides relaxation.

Prophylactic antibiotics usually are discontinued when the pleural drainage tubes have been removed. Skin stitches may be removed on the seventh or eighth postoperative day but should remain in place longer if the patient is chronically debilitated. The use of absorbable subcuticular sutures greatly facilitates wound care postoperatively.

Patients generally are ready for hospital dismissal when they are ambulatory and are able to care for themselves. The medication doses should be stable, and there should be no complications. An exercise program should be outlined that will prepare these patients for resumption of normal life activity and return them to their previous occupations without producing excessive fatigue or undue stress upon the operative wounds. Strenuous physical activity or lifting objects heavier than 10 lbs is prohibited for 6 weeks, but patients are encouraged to walk or perform light exercise immediately upon discharge.

Oral narcotic analgesics are usually required at discharge. Requirements for narcotics gradually reduces with time, and by 1 month after discharge, most patients only require analgesics at bedtime. Long-term pain occurs in about 1% of patients and is referred to as "postthoracotomy pain syndrome." It is usually from intercostal nerve irritation and is effectively treated by local injection. If unsuccessful, transcutaneous electrical nerve stimulation (TENS) is helpful. Reoperation is rarely indicated.

## POSTOPERATIVE COMPLICATIONS

The complications common to most general thoracic surgical procedures are discussed in this section. Complications peculiar to a specific type of thoracic operation are discussed in the chapters relative to these procedures.

### *Bleeding*

Inadequate hemostasis at the time of initial thoracotomy is the most common cause of postoperative bleeding in patients undergoing general thoracic surgery. Bleeding due to an abnormality in the coagulation mechanism is unusual, and most are secondary to massive (greater than 10 U) transfusions of stored blood. Other causes include liver failure or a previously abnormal clotting mechanism, such as occurs in patients with hemophilia or von Willebrand's disease.

Signs and symptoms of hemorrhage are dependent on the amount of blood loss. Although hypotension, tachycardia, and pallor are classic findings, their absence does not exclude the possibility of significant bleeding. Continued pleural drainage in excess of 200 mL of blood per hour over a 4- to 6-hour period is an indication for reexploration of the thorax to control the source of bleeding.

Once intrathoracic bleeding is suspected, coagulation studies and a chest roentgenogram should be obtained. If coagulation studies demonstrate an abnormal clotting mechanism, appropriate treatment should be instituted. Most bleeding coagulopathies are corrected with the administration of fresh frozen plasma or cryoprecipitate. The presence of significant thrombocytopenia should be corrected by the transfusion of fresh platelet concentrates. If the chest roentgenogram demonstrates accumulation of blood in the pleural cavity, an estimate of the pooled amount must be added to that already drained for adequate volume replacement. If the clot cannot be evacuated or if the estimated blood loss exceeds 1000 mL, reexploration is generally indicated to control bleeding and to remove the clot in order to prevent late entrapment of the lung in a collapsed position.

### Pulmonary Embolism

Pulmonary embolism is an infrequent but lethal postoperative complication. Diagnosis is difficult because of preexisting conditions such as chronic obstructive pulmonary disease (COPD) and postoperative changes in the lung. Therefore, a high index of suspicion is necessary to diagnose a postoperative pulmonary embolism. Usually, ventilation and perfusion scanning will be indeterminate because of preexisting pulmonary disease, and a pulmonary angiogram will be required for diagnosis. Long-term treatment based on an empiric diagnosis is not recommended, since these patients are at high risk to develop complications of therapy. Treatment is usually systemic anticoagulation that can be cautiously administered in the postoperative period with careful monitoring. Occasionally, caval interruption or embolectomy is indicated. Prophylaxis is recommended in almost all patients and should begin prior to the operation. Intermittent pneumatic compression cuffs and subcutaneous heparin administration (5000 U q12h) are the two most common means of prophylaxis.

### Hypotension

Hypotension in the early postoperative period is most commonly due to hypovolemia secondary to unrecognized blood loss. Other causes include myocardial infarction with low cardiac output and cardiac tamponade. When hypotension does occur, the effective circulating blood volume must be assessed by measurement of central venous pressure. Central venous pressure reflects the filling pressure of the right ventricle, and if it is low, blood or fluid should be administered until it is normal. If systemic arterial blood pressure does not return to normal with elevation of the central venous pressure, left ventricle end diastolic pressure should be assessed by measuring the pulmonary capillary wedge pressure. Even though the central venous pressure may be normal, pulmonary capillary wedge pressure may be low, particularly in patients with pulmonary vascular obstructive disease. Pulmonary capillary wedge pressure can be measured by insertion of a Swan Ganz catheter.[17,18] The balloon-tip catheter is inserted into a peripheral vein, usually the jugular or subclavian vein, and advanced through the superior vena cava into the right atrium. The balloon is then inflated, which permits the tip of the catheter to float through the right ventricle and into the pulmonary artery as the catheter is advanced. The position of the catheter can be determined by measurement of the pressure at its tip. When the pulmonary arterial pressure curve is observed, the catheter is slowly advanced until it is wedged in a segmental pulmonary artery, and a wedge pressure is recorded.[19] The balloon is then deflated. If the left atrial pressure is low, blood and fluid replacement should be continued until the wedge pressure returns to normal (14–16 mm Hg).

Hypotension accompanied by an elevated central venous pressure and an elevated capillary wedge pressure usually implies heart failure. Treatment should be directed toward improving ventricular contractility and decreasing peripheral vascular resistance. If the patient is not receiving digitalis, rapid digitalization may be helpful. An estimate of the digitalizing dose by the parenteral route is made on the basis of 0.9 mg of digoxin per square meter of body surface area, with half being administered initially intravenously. Subsequently, one eighth to one quarter of the total calculated dose is provided at 1- to 2-hour intervals under close electrocardiographic control until the total dose is administered. When digitalis appears ineffectual or is contraindicated, or more commonly, when treatment is required more urgently, another inotropic agent is employed. We prefer dopamine administered at a rate of 5–10 μg/kg per minute. Dopamine has a potent inotropic effect on the myocardium, with fewer chronotropic and arrhythmic effects. It also dilates renal arterial vessels, and both renal blood flow and glomerular filtration are improved.[20] If the heart rate is slow, isoproterenol administered as a dilute IV drip improves myocardial contractility, increases heart rate, and reduces vascular resistance. With dilation of the peripheral vessels, additional blood or fluid may be necessary to maintain an adequate effective circulating blood volume.

### Cardiac Tamponade

Cardiac tamponade must be considered whenever hypotension is accompanied by elevated central venous pressure following operations in which the pericardium has been opened. The increased intrapericardial pressure results in an increase of ventricular end-diastolic pressure, mean atrial pressure, and mean venous pressure. As a result, ventricular filling is reduced, leading to a reduced stroke volume and cardiac output.

In rapidly developing cardiac tamponade the patient is cyanotic and has dyspnea, dizziness, diaphoresis, anxiety, and hypotension. Eventually, hemodynamic collapse occurs. The late sign of tamponade are characterized by a decreasing blood pressure and a small quiet heart. Pericardial rubs are often present. Pulsus paradoxus is present, and the neck veins are distended. Chest roentgenograms demonstrate a widened pericardium. Electrocardiogram demonstrates reduction in the amplitude of both the T-waves and QRS complex with normal P-wave voltage. Often the T-wave is flat or shows minor inversion. Echocardiography is diagnostic. When pericardial tamponade is suspected in the early postoperative patient, the patient should be immediately returned to the operating room, the wound should be reopened, the pericardium inspected, and bleeding controlled. Echocardiographic decompression is generally inadequate in the patient who has active postoperative bleeding within the pericardium.

### Pulmonary Edema

Pulmonary edema generally presents as acute respiratory failure with tachypnea, cyanosis, and restlessness. The basic pathophysiology is the accumulation of fluid from the pulmonary capillaries into the interstitial space, with eventual flooding of the alveoli.[21] Blood gas exchange is impaired, and hypotension develops. Under normal conditions, the hydrostatic pressure of the pulmonary capillary bed is approximately 7 mm Hg, and the plasma oncotic pressure is approximately 27 mm Hg. The net effect is a 20 mm Hg pressure gradient from the interstitial space into the capillaries, which favors movement of fluid into the capillaries, thereby keeping the alveoli dry under normal conditions. Pulmonary edema develops when this gradient is reversed or when capillary permeability is increased. As fluid accumulates in the interstitial space, the distance between the alveoli and the capillary increases, and diffusion of gases becomes impaired. Eventually, the alveoli become congested, which further decreases diffusion and inactivates surfactant, leading to alveolar collapse. Blood now flowing through the capillaries adjacent to nonventilated alveoli passes without an exchange of oxygen, and a right-to-left intrapulmonary shunt is produced.

The most common cause of pulmonary edema in the postoperative thoracic patient is hypervolemia secondary to overinfusion of fluids. Myocardial infarction with acute left heart failure may result in elevation of the pulmonary capillary pressure. Decreased serum protein concentration may contribute to the severity of edema by lowering plasma oncotic pressure. Pulmonary capillary injury from sepsis or prolonged inspiration of a high oxygen concentration can lead to increased capillary permeability.

Treatment is directed toward removal of fluid from the interstitial space and improvement of blood gas exchange.[22] Excess circulating volume should be eliminated by diuresis, rotating tourniquets, and, if necessary, phlebotomy. Heart failure is treated by the administration of digitalis and other appropriate inotropic agents. Administration of morphine sulfate reduces anxiety and peripheral resistance. Mild hypoxemia can be improved by the administration of oxygen with a close-fitting face mask. If the edema is severe, and particularly if there is severe hypoxemia with hypercarbia, endotracheal intubation with positive pressure ventilation is indicated. The positive pressure generated during inspiration with mechanical ventilation is important to treatment and favors a shift of fluid into the capillary. Positive end-expiratory pressure (PEEP) of 5–10 cm $H_2O$ is also effective in decreasing pulmonary edema and at this level generally does not impair cardiac output. If acute heart failure secondary to cardiac dysrhythmia occurs, correction of the dysrhythmia is most important.

### Atelectasis and Pneumonitis

Retained bronchial secretions from ineffective coughing are the most common cause of atelectasis following thoracic operations. The lung distal to the obstructed bronchus collapses as air is absorbed. If the obstruction is partial and unrelieved, infection is superimposed on the atelectasis. Treatment is directed toward removal of secretions, maintenance of oxygenation, and institution of appropriate antibiotic coverage.

Aspiration of liquid gastric contents into the lung may also produce pneumonitis. Aspiration of low pH gastric juice in sufficient volume produces a distinct clinical syndrome, with dyspnea, cyanosis, bronchospasm, and shock.[23] Once this condition is suspected, prompt and vigorous therapy is necessary. The airway must be cleared by suction, and if the aspirate was particulate, bronchoscopy should be performed. Tracheal lavage with saline, bicarbonate, or steroids is of no benefit and may produce additional areas of involvement. Severe hypoxemia should be aggressively treated with increased concentrations of oxygen, IV injection of aminophyllin, and mechanical ventilation. Hypotension is usually a result of hypovolemia, and appropriate volume replacement is indicated. Corticosteroids administered intravenously in large doses (1–2 g hydrocortisone) are recommended.[23] Broad-spectrum antibiotic coverage is also indicated to prevent secondary bacterial infection.

### Respiratory Insufficiency

Respiratory insufficiency may develop in any postoperative thoracic patient but is more common in patients with reduced pulmonary reserve secondary to chronic obstructive lung disease who develop such complications as atelectasis and pneumonitis. Despite a well-executed preventive program of supportive respiratory care, some patients who have been extubated after operation develop progressive respiratory difficulties. The interval from extubation to the onset of distress varies, but it tends to be between 36 to 48 hours. The cause is not always clear. However, the inability to clear bronchial secretions, which leads to increased airway resistance, and the accumulation of water in the pulmonary interstitium, which leads to a decrease in lung compliance, often seem to be significant contributing factors. Both add to the work of breathing and, when severe or protracted, may produce acute respiratory failure.

It may be difficult to distinguish respiratory failure from cardiac failure, and often they occur concomitantly. The patient is dyspneic, tachypneic, and often exhausted. Tachycardia and ventricular dysrhythmias may result from hypoxemia and hypercarbia, as well as from myocardial failure.

Blood gas analysis may demonstrate early hypoxemia and hypercarbia while the patient's clinical condition still remains satisfactory. A low $PaO_2$ (less than 50 torr) in spite of increasing concentration of inspired oxygen may indicate the need for mechanical ventilation. Another indication is an elevated arterial $PCO_2$ (greater than 50 torr).

Initial treatment is establishment of a patent airway and ventilation of the lungs with 100% oxygen. Intubation with a soft-cuffed endotracheal tube follows. Oral endotracheal tubes are used for resuscitation and in other emergency situations. In most other circumstances, nasal endotracheal tubes are employed because they are better tolerated. However, because of their smaller internal diameter and greater length, they offer more resistance to breathing. Consequently, suctioning of the patient and assessment of the adequacy of spontaneous ventilation are also more difficult. Either tube may be left in place for 6–7 days or, in some instances, for up to 2 weeks. The incidence of complications, however, rises significantly with time. When required, morphine sulfate in doses of 1–2 mg administered intravenously every 2–3 hours improves the tolerance of endotracheal tubes. We prefer morphine sulfate to diazepam unless seizure disorders are present.

We use volume preset ventilators, since there is often a need for peak inspiratory pressures greater than 35 cm $H_2O$ or controlled mechanical ventilation with PEEP. When indicated, PEEP is applied by immersing the expiratory limb of the ventilatory circuit to an appropriate depth in a column of water. Generally, PEEP is started at 2.5–5.0 cm $H_2O$ and gradually increased. Each increase is followed by continuous hemodynamic monitoring and by blood gas analysis after 15–30 minutes. Close observation both clinically and radiographically for the appearance of subcutaneous or mediastinal air and pneumothorax is also required. With 10 cm or more of PEEP, it may be necessary to reduce tidal volume and increase respiratory frequency in order to lower peak inspiratory pressures and lessen the risk of barotrauma. PEEP is contraindicated in patients with known bullous disease and in patients with a possible air leak following pulmonary resection who do not have a pleural drainage tube in place. Once initiated, PEEP is maintained until the $FIO_2$ can be reduced to $< 0.5$. After patients can maintain acceptable blood gas exchange on mechanical ventilation with zero end-expiratory pressure and with an $FIO_2$ of 0.4 or less, spontaneous ventilation through a T-piece is started, and the procedure leading to extubation is followed as described in the "Respiration" section near the start of the chapter.

A decision regarding tracheostomy is usually made 7–10 days after endotracheal intubation. The optimal time to proceed with tracheostomy is often difficult to decide. Factors in favor of early tracheostomy are salvageability of the patient, difficulty in clearing secretions via an endotracheal tube, and expectations of a long period of mechanical ventilation. Factors tending to delay tracheostomy include a hopeless prognosis, childhood, drug overdose, and the likelihood that only another 24–48 hours of mechanical ventilation will be necessary.

### *Subcutaneous Emphysema*

After operations that involve the lungs, tracheobronchial tree, or esophagus, air trapped within the pleural cavity is evacuated by pleural drainage tubes. Should entrapped air not be removed, as may occur when drainage tubes become occluded or when a large air leak develops, the normal mechanics of respiration may force air through the intercostal incision into the soft tissues of the chest wall. Since muscle is too dense for air to dissect and the skin prevents egress of the air, most air spreads through the subcutaneous tissue planes. If the subcutaneous emphysema is excessive, it will extend up into the face from the tissues of the neck, sometimes inflating the eyelids until the eyelids are forced closed. It may extend down the abdomen into the scrotum, where it is generally prevented from extending into the thighs by the attachments of the inguinal ligament.

If subcutaneous emphysema does develop, the drainage tubes should be checked to determine if they are patent. If they are occluded and patency cannot be restored, they should be removed and replaced with new tubes. If the tubes are patent and the emphysema progresses, an additional tube should be inserted into the pleural space. The sudden appearance of a large air leak may indicate the development of a bronchopleural fistula. A large fistula that develops during the first new postoperative days should be closed by reoperation. The use of cervical incisions to release the air, unless necessary for tracheostomy, has little merit. On rare occasions, upper airway obstruction may occur, necessitating endotracheal intubation or tracheostomy for management.

### *Cardiac Dysrhythmia*

Cardiac dysrhythmias are common after general thoracic surgical procedures, with the frequency being reported to range from 3% to 50%.[24] Dysrhythmias are most common in patients with preexisting cardiovascular disease who are over 50 years of age and who undergo either pneumonectomy or esophageal surgery.[25,26] The dysrhythmias most commonly observed are sinus tachycardia, premature atrial and ventricular contraction, atrial fibrillation, and atrial flutter. In our series of 236 recent pneumonectomies, dysrhythmias occurred in 22% of patients.[27] Nearly all occurred within the first postoperative week and did not correlate with preoperative pulmonary function. Dysrhythmias occurred more frequently following intrapericardial dissection and in patients who developed postoperative interstitial pulmonary edema. Cardiac dysrhythmias are associated with significant morbidity and mortality. In our series, 25% of patients who developed cardiac dysrhythmias died within 30 days following pneumonectomy. Careful electrocardiographic monitoring, with prompt recognition of the dysrhythmia, is essential for successful management.

Sinus tachycardia is the most frequent dysrhythmia observed in the postoperative period and is the result of increased sympathetic or decreased vagal tone. The most common precipitating factors are pain, anxiety, hypoxemia, hypercarbia, and hypovolemia. Other causes include fever, drugs, congestive heart failure, and myocardial infarction. The appearance of sinus tachycardia necessitates careful evaluation of the patient to rule out a serious etiology. Therapy should be directed toward the abnormal clinical state and not the tachycardia itself.

The most common significant dysrhythmia after general thoracic surgery is atrial fibrillation or atrial flutter. Paroxysmal atrial trachycardia can also occur alone, or it can precede an episode of atrial fibrillation. These dysrhythmias present with rapid ventricular rates and inadequate ventricular filling due to a loss of atrial contraction and decreased filling time. Consequently, they are frequently associated with a reduction in cardiac output, leading to ischemia of the brain, heart, and kidneys. Transient ischemia may be tolerated in an otherwise healthy individual, but in elderly patients, transient ischemia may lead to stroke, myocardial infarction, or renal failure. Adenosine is useful to control the ventricular rate in atrial flutter or other supraventricular tachycardia. The first dose is usually 6 mg IV. The dose can be doubled on the second dose. It functions by inducing a pharmacologic block of the atrioventricular node. The ventricular rate in atrial fibrillation, atrial flutter, and paroxysmal atrial tachycardia can also be controlled by the rapid administration of intravenous digitalis (see p. 44). Frequently, conversion to a normal sinus rhythm spontaneously follows slowing of the ventricular rate to normal limits in atrial fibrillation. Verapamil is also effective in the management of supraventricular dysrhythmias. Verapamil is administrated intravenously in a dosage of 0.075 mg/kg (approximately 5 mg) given over 1 or 2 minutes. If this dosage is ineffective in terminating the supraventricular dysrhythmia or in slowing the ventricular response, a second dose of 0.15 mg/kg (approximately 10 mg) can be administered 20 minutes after the initial dose. If successful, oral therapy is then instituted starting with 80 mg every 8 hours and increasing to 120 mg three or four times a day if needed. The primary side effect is vasodilation and cardiac depression; therefore, blood pressure should be monitored closely. Cardioversion with synchronized countershock is also effective in the majority of patients with supraventricular tachycardia, and it may be preferred over drug therapy. This is particularly true in atrial flutter, especially if the situation is urgent. Digitalis should be discontinued for 24 hours prior to cardioversion.

Ventricular tachycardia requires prompt attention, since ventricular fibrillation may develop. Lidocaine hydrochloride in a bolus of 50–100 mg administered IV followed by countershock is the treatment of choice. Once the dysrhythmia is controlled, a continuous lidocaine drip (1–3 mg/min) should be administered intravenously. Premature ventricular contractions often occur in normal individuals and may be of little significance if they have occurred preoperatively. When they occur postoperatively in a patient who did not have them preoperatively, they can lead to ventricular tachycardia or ventricular fibrillation. Generally, premature ventricular contractions can be controlled with a bolus of lidocaine followed by a lidocaine infusion.

Isolated premature atrial contractions are also common and generally are of little significance. Usually, no treatment is indicated. When they are frequent, atrial contractions can be a sign of congestive heart failure or digitalis intoxication and can lead to atrial fibrillation. If they are due to digitalis intoxication, digitalis should be withheld. Otherwise, they can be controlled with small doses of digitalis.

Prophylactic digitalization of all patients undergoing thoracic operations has been widely debated in the literature.[24,28,29] Most authors concur that prophylactic digitalization reduces the incidence of postoperative dysrhythmias in older individuals. Arguments against prophylactic digitalization are the potential toxic effect of the drug and the difficulty in assessing adequate digitalization in patients without cardiac failure. It has been our practice not to routinely digitalize patients preoperatively but rather to monitor them closely electrocardiographically postoperatively. If there is any evidence of any cardiac dysrhythmia, the patient is then rapidly digitalized with a short-acting digitalis preparation (digoxin).

### *Wound Dehiscence and Infection*

Dehiscence of a lateral thoracotomy wound is rare. When it occurs in the early postoperative period, respirations, even if the skin closure remains intact, may become ineffective. Complete dehiscence interferes with the negative pressure cycle necessary for ventilation and may be associated with shifting of the mediastinum. Cough also may become ineffective, which leads to accumulation of secretions. Early dehiscence generally requires immediate reclosure of the wound. If dehiscence develops in the late postoperative period, as may occur with wound infections, chest wall mechanics are less likely to be interfered with. In this situation, reclosure of the wound can be delayed until after adequate local debridement and pleural drainage have been performed.

Lateral thoracotomy wound infections are uncommon. Most are confined to the subcutaneous tissues and can usually be detected by erythema, swelling, and tenderness in the wound. Frequently, the patient is febrile and has a leukocytosis. Once an infection is suspected, the wound should be opened and drained, and cultures should be obtained. Following thorough irrigation, necrotic tissue should be debrided. If cellulitis surrounds the wound, appropriate antibiotics should be instituted. Wet dressings of 5% Betadine are applied several times a day, or more frequently if drainage is excessive. After a few days and if the patient's condition permits, further cleaning of the wound can be accomplished by placing the patient in a whirlpool tank once a day. When uniform healthy granulation tissue is present, the patient may be brought back to the operating room and the wound closed secondarily.

Median sternotomy wound infections can be life-threatening. Early diagnosis requires a high incidence of suspicion. Purulent drainage is an obvious sign of infection. More common but less specific signs and symptoms include fever, chest pain, serosanguinous wound drainage, sternal instability, and leukocytosis. Wound cultures demonstrate no growth in approximately one fifth of patients; when positive, however, staphylococcal species is encountered nearly half the time. These wounds must be thoroughly debrided. At times the entire sternum and associated costal arches need to be resected. The wound is then dressed with gauze moistened with saline solution and changed every 4–6 hours in the patient's room.[30,31] Open irrigation with a pulsatile water jet, such as a Water Pik, is routinely used and greatly facilitates cleaning. If at all possible, the patient also showers, since drainage is considerably better in the upright position. If at any time there is evidence of new or persistent necrotic tissue, the patient is returned to the operating room for further debridement.

Closure of the wound is performed when there is no evidence of drainage; when there is no gray or green perichondrium, bone, or cartilage; and when the edges of the debrided sternum or ribs are clean. Quantitative bacterial counts have not been helpful. In many of these patients there is a persistent mediastinal space following debridement, and simple closure of the skin and subcutaneous tissues is inadequate.

We prefer to obliterate the mediastinal space with the pectoralis major muscle transposed on a dominant proximal thoraco-acromial neurovascular leash. Most commonly both pectoralis muscles are mobilized. The humeral attachments are divided as needed to permit the degree of rotation and advancement required. One muscle is transposed into the mediastinal dead space.[31] The overlying skin and subcutaneous tissue are usually then closed with direct suture.

### Residual Pleural Space

Following pulmonary resection, the pleural space is normally obliterated by several mechanisms. These include expansion of the remaining lung parenchyma, shifting of the mediastinum toward the ipsilateral side, elevation of the ipsilateral diaphragm, and narrowing of the intercostal spaces on the ipsilateral side. If a residual pleural space can be anticipated at the time of initial operation, as may occur when there is marked fibrosis of the remaining ipsilateral lung, several operative maneuvers can be used to reduce the size of the pleural cavity. In the past, apical thoracoplasties had been performed.[32] Alternative but less satisfactory procedures have included development of a pleural tent[33] and transplantation of the diaphragm to a higher level.[34,35] Another method has been to fill the residual pleural space with healthy, viable muscle. We currently favor this latter technique and transplant either the pectoralis major or the latissimus dorsi muscle into the apex of the chest.[36] Both of these muscles when mobilized have adequate length and volume, which, when rotated on their neurovascular leash, reach and fill the pleural cavity (see Chapter 31).

### Persistent Air Leak

Air leak in the immediate postoperative period following pulmonary resection occurs in most patients and usually is secondary to leakage from areas where incomplete fissures were divided. Most air leaks cease by the second or third postoperative day. Leakage beyond this time, however, does occasionally occur. If the postoperative chest roentgenogram demonstrates that the remaining lung parenchyma completely fills the pleural cavity, most leaks will eventually stop. Persistent air leaks are generally associated with a small residual pleural space. If the air leak continues beyond 7 days, we generally lower intrapleural negative pressure and add a sclerosing agent intrapleurally. If the pleural space does not increase in size, intrapleural suction is discontinued, leaving the patient connected only to an underwater seal. Most persistent air leaks cease with this method of management between the second and third postoperative weeks. However, if the air leak continues beyond this time or suddenly increases, strong consideration should be given to the possibility of reoperation and control of the leak.

### Bronchopleural Fistula

When a bronchopleural fistula develops following pulmonary resection, early thoracotomy with reclosure of the bronchial stump is usually indicated. The diagnosis can be suspected by the sudden appearance of postoperative hemoptysis, fever, and a persistent air leak. If a pneumonectomy has been previously performed, there is usually aspiration of large quantities of serosanguineous fluid. Bronchoscopy should be done, and if the fistula is not readily apparent, 3–5 mL of propyliodone in the region of the bronchial stump should be injected. Extravasation of contrast material into the pleural cavity confirms the diagnosis.

Another method to demonstrate an occult bronchopleural fistula is to perform a ventilation scan. If radioactivity is detected in the pleural space, a fistula is present. For a small fistula (i.e., <2 mm), occlusion with fibrin glue, placed through a bronchoscope, may be attempted; however, a larger fistula usually requires operative intervention.

The goals of reoperation include closure of the bronchial stump and obliteration of any associated empyema cavity. Reamputation of the stump, if possible, should be done. Occasionally, completion pneumonectomy may be required. The stump should be reinforced with transposition of viable tissue. Although intercostal muscle and diaphragmatic flaps have been used previously with success, we prefer transposition of either the serratus anterior, latissimus dorsi, or pectoralis major muscle[36,37] (see the section on postpneumonectomy empyema that follows). These muscles all have a sufficient arc of rotation that allows them to reach most areas of the pleural cavity. They also have significant mass that obliteration of most residual pleura spaces is possible.

### Empyema

Postoperative empyema is uncommon following pulmonary resection. It is most likely to occur if the pleural space is not completely obliterated and serosanguineous fluid is allowed to accumulate. Adequate preoperative preparation to control pulmonary infection, careful intraoperative technique, and good postoperative management with adequate pleural drainage should prevent the development of an empyema. However, if it should develop, pleural tube drainage must be maintained and parenteral antibiotics administered. Obliteration of the pleural space with adequate pleural drainage and systemic antibiotics is usually sufficient to manage most patients with acute empyema. If the empyema becomes chronic, thoracotomy with decortication is required. If a bronchopleural fistula is present, it must be closed as described above. If, following decortication, the remaining lung does not expand to completely fill the pleural space, the cavity must be obliterated by one of the methods discussed above.

The incidence of empyema following pneumonectomy is approximately 5%.[38–40] Signs and symptoms of postpneumonectomy empyema vary and may not appear until months later. This possibility should always be suspected in any patient with signs of infection following pneumonectomy, no matter how far in the past the patient underwent the procedure. Fever of unknown origin, expectoration of serosanguineous fluid, or an air–fluid level visualized on chest roentgenogram should immediately arouse suspicion of an infected pleural space.

In the past, management consisted of drainage and thoracoplasty. Clagett and Geraci, in 1963,[41] described an alternative method of management that we have continued to use with modifications. Following control of the infection by closed pleural drainage, open drainage in the most dependent portion of the thorax is performed. Cultures are obtained, and the pleural cavity is thoroughly debrided. If a bronchopleural fistula is present, this must be closed and then reinforced with viable tissue. We prefer the intrathoracic transposition of extrathoracic skeletal muscle such as the serratus anterior or latissimus dorsi.[42] All extrathoracic muscles require a route of entry when transposed into the thorax. Generally a 5-cm segment of one rib, usually the anterior portion of the second, needs to be resected to provide an adequate chest wall entrance. The location of this opening is best determined by the transposed muscle's blood supply, and the opening should be selected to avoid kinking of the neurovascular leash and subsequent muscle necrosis. The purpose of the muscle transposition is to reinforce the closed bronchial stump. Wet dressings of dilute antibiotic solution (gentamicin 20 mg/L adjusted to a pH of 7.4) are then packed into the thorax and changed four times daily, more frequently if drainage is excessive.[43] A dental Water Pik to mechanically debride the wound at the time of dressing change is also a value in cleaning the wound. Further debridement can be accomplished by placing the patient in a whirlpool tank after several days if his condition permits. When pink, healthy granulation tissue is present, the pleural cavity is closed following instillation of DABS antibiotic solution to obliterate the pleural space. DABS solution consists of 80 mg of gentamicin, 1,000,000 units of polymixin, and 500 mg of neomycin mixed into 1 L of normal saline. Alternatively, the pleural space could be obliterated by further intrathoracic transposition of both extrathoracic skeletal muscle (latissimus dorsi, pectoralis major, rectus abdominis) and omentum as suggested by Miller and associates,[44] but in our experience this has not been necessary.

### Indications

Indications for thoracoplasty today are rare and, in general, include the obliteration of an empyema cavity or a noninfected residual pleural space. A still acceptable, though even more rare, indication is a patient who required surgery to supplement chemotherapy for tuberculosis but who clearly cannot tolerate pulmonary resection because of severely limited pulmonary reserve.

### Extrapleural Paravertebral Thoracoplasty

Extrapleural paravertebral thoracoplasty is the classic procedure described by Alexander for control of tuberculosis.[45] It consists of extrapleural subperiosteal resections of ribs 1–7 and associated transverse processes. It is generally performed in two stages, with the first stage consisting of resection of the first through third ribs. Two weeks later, the second stage is performed, in which the remaining ribs are resected. Excision of the inferior angle of the scapula is also performed at this time to permit maximal collapse and to prevent dysfunction of the shoulder girdle and pain caused by impingement of the scapular angle on the remaining intact ribs.

### Schede Thoracoplasty

The thoracoplasty described by Schede in 1890 for obliteration of a chronic empyema cavity is rarely performed today. This procedure consisted of unroofing an empyema cavity by resecting the overlying ribs, intercostal muscle bundles, and adjacent parietal pleura. The soft tissue and skin were closed over gauze packing, which was then removed several days later. This procedure has been modified to resemble paravertebral thoracoplasty, where only the ribs are resected, allowing the intercostal muscle bundles to collapse against the visceral pleura.

### Plombage Thoracoplasty

The most important variation of the classic thoracoplasty is the plombage thoracoplasty. In this procedure, the periosteum and intercostal muscle bundles are separated from the ribs, allowing the parietal pleura to collapse against the lung. The subperiosteal space is then filled with a foreign material, which has included fat, oil, paraffin, polyethylene spheres, and plastics.[47, 48] This procedure has the advantage of being performed in one stage, is cosmetically acceptable, and does not result in as much impairment of pulmonary function.

## REFERENCES


1. Critical paths: A pre-existing tool ready-made for TQM implementation. *QI/TOM* **2:**2–4, 1992
2. Hofmann PA: Critical path method: An important tool for coordinating clinical care. *J Comm Qual Improv* **19:**235–146, 1993
3. Miller JI: Preoperative evaluation, complications of pulmonary surgery. *Chest Surg Clin North Am* **2:** 701–711, 1992
4. Tarhan S. Moffitt EA, Sessler AD, et al: Risk of anesthesia and surgery in patients with chronic bronchitis and chronic obstructive pulmonary disease. *Surgery* **74:**720, 1973
5. Muldoon SM, Rehder K, Didier EP, et al: Respiratory care of patients undergoing intrathoracic surgery. *Surg Clin North Am* **53:**843, 1973
6. Shim C, Fine N, Fernandez R, Williams MH Jr: Cardiac arrhythmias resulting from tracheal suctioning. *Ann Intern Med* **71:**1149, 1969
7. Sizer JS, Frederick PL, Osborne, MP: The prevention of postoperative pulmonary complications by percutaneous endotracheal catheterization. *Surg Gynecol Obstet* **123:**336, 1966
8. Wain JC, Mathisen DJ, Wilson D: Clinical experience with minitracheostomy. *Ann Thorac Surg* **49:**881–886, 1990
9. El-Baz NM, Faber LP, Jerrik RJ: Continuous epidural infusion of morphine for treatment of pain after thoracic surgery: A new technique. *Anesth Analg* **63:**757–764, 1984
10. Lamessy A, Magnin C, Viale JP, et al: Clinical advantages of fentanyl given epidurally for postoperative analgesia. *Anesthesiology* **61:**466–469, 1984
11. Kvale PA, Ranga V, Kopacz M: Pulmonary resection. *South Med J* **70:**64, 1977
12. Truesdale R, D'Alessanderi R, Manuel V, et al: Antimicrobial vs placebo prophylaxis in noncardiac surgery. *JAMA* **241:**1254, 1979
13. Frumodt-Moller N, Ostri P, Pedersen IBK, et al: Antibiotic prophylaxis in pulmonary surgery. *Ann Surg* **195:**444, 1982
14. Ilves R, Cooper JD, Todd TRJ, et al: Prospective randomized double blind studies using prophylactic cephalothin for major elective general thoracic operations. *J Thorac Cardiovasc Surg* **81:**813, 1981
15. Walker WS, Faichney A, Raychandhury T, et al: Wound prophylaxis in thoracic surgery. A new approach. *Thorax* **39:**121, 1984
16. Tarkka M, Polela R, Lepojarvi M, Nissinen J, Karkola P: Infection prophylaxis in pulmonary surgery: A randomized prospective study. *Ann Thorac Surg* **44:**508–513, 1987
17. Gooding JM, Kirby RR: Comparison of central venous and pulmonary capillary wedge pressure in critically ill patients with and without ischemic heart disease. *Crit Care Med* **6:**92, 1978
18. Luchsinger PC, Seipp HW, Patel DJ: Relationship of pulmonary artery wedge pressure to left atrial pressure in man. *Circ Res* **10:**315, 1962
19. Swan HJC, Ganz W: Guidelines for use of balloon-tipped catheter. *Am J Cardiol* **34:**119, 1974
20. Goldberg LI: Cardiovascular and renal action of dopamine: Potential clinical applications. *Pharmacology* **24:**1, 1972
21. Levine OR, Mellins RB, Senior RM, Fishman AP: The application of Starling's law of capillary exchange to the lungs. *J Clin Invest* **46:**934, 1967
22. Giodano JM, Joseph WL, Klingenmaier CH, Adkins PC: The management of interstitial pulmonary edema. *J Thorac Cardiovasc Surg* **64:**739, 1972
23. Tinstman TC, Dines DE, Arms RA: Postoperative aspiration pneumonia. *Surg Clin North Am* **53:**859, 1973
24. Shields TW, Ujiki GT: Digitalization for prevention of arrythmias following pulmonary surgery. *Surg Gynecol Obstet* **126:**743, 1968
25. Ghosh B, Pakreshi BC: Cardiac dysrhythmias after thoracotomy. *Br Heart J* **34:**374, 1972
26. Mowry FM, Reynolds EW Jr: Cardiac rhythm disturbances complicating resectional surgery of the lung. *Ann Intern Med* **61:**688, 1964
27. Krowka, MJ, Pairolero PC, Trastek VF, et al: Cardiac dysrhythmia following pneumonectomy. Clinical correlates and prognostic significance. *Chest* **91:**490–495, 1987
28. Wheat MW Jr, Burford TH: Digitalization in surgery: Extension of classical indications. *J Thorac Cardiovasc Surg* **41:**162, 1961
29. Burman SO: The prophylactic use of digitalis before thoracotomy. *Ann Thorac Surg* **14:**359, 1972
30. Arnold PG, Pairolero PC: Use of pectoralis major muscle flaps to repair defects of anterior chest wall. *Plast Reconstr Surg* **63:**205, 1979
31. Pairolero PC, Arnold PG, Harris JB: Long-term results of pectoralis major muscle transposition for infected sternotomy wounds. *Ann Surg* **213:**583–590, 1991
32. Bjork VO: Thoracoplasty. A new osteoplastic technique. *J Thorac Surg* **28:**194, 1954
33. Brewer LA III: Pleural partition procedure: A technique for management of large intrapleural dead space following lobectomy. *Bull Soc Int Chir* **17:**305, 1958
34. Burdette WJ: Transplantation of the diaphragm for obliteration of dead space following pulmonary resection. *J Thorac Surg* **33:**803, 1957
35. Brewer LA III, Gazzaniga AB: Phrenoplasty: A new operation for the management of dead pleural space following pulmonary resection. *Ann Thorac Surg* **6:**119, 1968
36. Pairolero PC, Arnold PG: Bronchopleural fistula: Treatment by transposition of pectoralis major muscle. *J Thorac Cardiovasc Surg* **79:**142, 1980
37. Pairolero PC, Arnold PG: Bronchopleural fistula: Management with muscle transposition. In Grillo HC, Eschapasse H (eds): *International Trends in General Thoracic Surgery,* vol 2. *Major Challenges.* Philadelphia, Saunders, 1987
38. Ruckdeschel JC, Codish SD, Stranahan A, McKneally MF: Postoperative empyema improves survival in lung cancer. *N Engl J Med* **287:**1013, 1972
39. LeRoux BT: Empyema thoracis. *Br J Surg* **52:**89, 1965
40. Karkola P, Kairalvoma MI, Larmi TK: Postpneumonectomy empyema in pulmonary carcinoma patients: treatment with antibiotic irrigation and closed chest drainage. *J Thorac Cardiovasc Surg* **72:**319, 1976
41. Clagett OT, Geraci JE: A procedure for the management of post-pneumonectomy empyema. *J Thorac Cardiovasc Surg* **45:**141, 1963
42. Pairolero PC, Arnold PG, Piehler JM: Intrathoracic transposition of extrathoracic skeletal muscle. *J Thorac Cardiovasc Surg* **86:**809–817, 1983
43. Stafford EG, Clagett OT: Post-pneumonectomy empyema: neomycin insulation and definitive closure. *J Thorac Cardiovasc Surg* **63:**771, 1972

44. Miller JI, Mansour KA, Nahai F: Single-stage complete muscle flap closure of the postpneumonectomy empyema space: A new method and possible solution to a disturbing complication. *Ann Thorac Surg* **38:**227–231, 1984.
45. Alexander J: *The Surgery of Pulmonary Tuberculosis.* New York, Lea & Febiger, 1927
46. Schede M: Die Behandlung der Empyema. *Verh Kongr inn Med Wiesbaden* **9:**41, 1890
47. O'Neill TJE, Ramirez HPR, Trout RG: Experimental and clinical studies of collapse therapy using fiberglass wool and fabric. *J Thorac Surg* **18:**181, 1949
48. Wilson D: Extrapleural pneumonolysis with lucite plombage. *J Thorac Surg* **17:**111, 1948

CHAPTER

# 4

# Ventilatory Assistance and Support

Orlando C. Kirton, Scott H. Norwood, and Joseph M. Civetta

## INTRODUCTION

Modern ventilatory techniques have become more varied and complex, providing physicians with multiple modes from which to choose. Therefore, it is important to define those patients who require ventilatory assistance; become familiar with the various modes of support available; understand guidelines important to the initiation, optimization, and termination of therapy; and, finally, identify what special conditions may require alternative vs. conventional therapy. Understanding the indications, benefits, limitations, and potential complications will permit appropriate individualization of ventilator support to meet each patient's needs.

## HISTORICAL PERSPECTIVE

Negative pressure systems were the first used. By the mid-1930s, these negative pressure "iron lungs" had numerous limitations including cumbersome size and restrictions on mobilization and concomitant medical procedures. These difficulties were responsible in part for the development of devices that delivered positive pressure ventilation. By the mid-1940s, pressure-limited ventilators were available; however, inconsistent delivery of tidal volumes and minute ventilation resulted in atelectasis, hypoxemia, and hypercarbia. By the 1960s, volume preset ventilators delivered relatively constant tidal volumes to most patients with respiratory failure that, at that time, was associated with reduced compliance, hypoxemia, and hypercarbia. Unfortunate therapeutic complications were barotrauma and impairment of cardiac performance. In the 1970s, intermittent mandatory ventilation (IMV) was introduced. For the first time, ventilatory support supplemented rather than substituted for the patient's efforts. IMV also reduced intrathoracic pressure compared with previous forms of positive pressure ventilation because of decreased ventilator cycle-time. Improved distribution of inspired gases, less sedation requirements, decreased adverse effects on renal blood flow, and preservation of ventilatory muscle conditioning and coordination are also positive effects of IMV. In the 1980s, microprocessor ventilators were introduced. These permitted modifications in the modes of ventilation, control over parameters such as inspiratory flow patterns, and they had improved monitoring and measuring characteristics. Conceptually, ventilatory support has shifted from total takeover of the patient's work of breathing to supplementation and treatment of the underlying disease process with eventual decrementation of this support.

### Intubation

The decision to intubate is usually based on the need to manage hypoxemic and/or hypercapnic respiratory insufficiency, decrease the patient's work of breathing, assure airway patency, or facilitate pulmonary toilet (Table 4–1). Difficult intubation is anticipated in patients with (1) difficulties in positioning the neck due to cervical arthritis, trauma, or previous surgery; (2) anatomic variations such as a small mouth, "bull neck," receding lower jaw, prominent maxillary dentition, high arched palate, and marked obesity; (3) limitations of mouth opening due to trismus, mandibular trauma, lingual or submandibular pathology, ankylosis of

**TABLE 4–1. INDICATIONS FOR MECHANICAL VENTILATORY AND POSITIVE AIRWAY PRESSURE SUPPORT**

| Oxygenation | Ventilation |
|---|---|
| $Pao_2$ < 65 torr on supplemental $O_2$ | Respiratory rate > 38/min[a] |
| $Pao_2$ < 55 torr on room air[a] | Vital capacity < 15 mL/kg |
| A–a gradient > 450 after 10 min 100% $O_2$ | Negative inspiratory force < –20 cm $H_2O$ |
| $\dot{Q}_{sp}/\dot{Q}_T$ > 25%[a] | Minute ventilation > 10 L/min |
| | $V_D/V_T$ > 0.6 |

[a]Authors' preferred indications.

the temporal-mandibular joint or perioral contractions of the soft tissue, and "jaw clenching" in head-injured patients; (4) upper airway inflammation due to epiglottitis or laryngeal infections or burns; (5) trauma to the larynx or trachea; and (6) congenital malformation of the face, head, or neck.1 Procedures available for difficult intubations include (1) fiberoptic laryngoscopy, (2) retrograde intubation, (3) blind nasal intubation, (4) dual-lumen airway devices, (5) laryngeal mask airway, and (6) minitracheostomy or cricothyroidotomy.[1–3]

### Complications of Intubation

Early complications include trauma to the tissues of the oro/nasopharynx and larynx, oro-esophageal intubation, endobronchial intubation, or obstruction of the endotracheal tube from blood and mucus. Prolonged intubation can sequentially produce mucosal edema, ulceration, fibrous scarring, and stenosis of the larynx or trachea. Injury is now less frequent with high-volume, low-pressure cuffed tubes unless the cuff is overinflated. Mucosal injury is less likely if cuff pressure is < 25 mm Hg.[4] However, higher pressures may be necessary to achieve adequate alveolar ventilation and oxygenation in severe cases of adult respiratory distress syndrome (ARDS). In patients requiring prolonged mechanical ventilatory support, the incidence of laryngeal complications tends to plateau with the duration of endotracheal intubation; therefore, early tracheostomy is usually not indicated and may create stoma-related problems.[5,6]

Late complications include laryngeal or tracheal stenosis. This rare but serious complication may develop weeks or months after extubation as a consequence of scar formation in healing mucosal lesions.[1] Persistent chronic hoarseness or stridor should be evaluated by an otolaryngologist for traumatic lesions of the vocal cords and their attachments, polyp formation, or injury to the recurrent laryngeal nerves.[7]

### Oral Tracheal Intubation

**Indications.** Orotracheal intubation is the most rapid method of airway control and, under most clinical circumstances, the method of choice. Exceptions are massive facial or neck trauma requiring an emergency surgical airway and acute trauma situations where cervical spine injury precludes uncontrolled manipulation of the neck. Initial management in unconscious trauma victims and victims with head injury must assume the presence of a cervical spine injury, and the method of airway control (orotracheal with inline cervical traction, nasotracheal, or surgical cricothyroidotomy) is determined by the individual physician's level of expertise with each method.

General guidelines for selection of tube size are: adult males 9.0 mm, adult females 8.0 mm, premature infants uncuffed 2.5 mm, newborns uncuffed 3.5 mm, older children age in years + 16 divided by 4.

### Nasotracheal Intubation

Nasotracheal intubation is used in situations where orotracheal intubation is difficult or contraindicated, including suspected cervical spine injury, maxillofacial anomalies, and during maxillofacial surgical procedures. Nasotracheal intubation cannot be safely performed if the patient is apneic or has very shallow breaths.

Nasal intubation has a number of significant complications including: epistaxis, trauma to the posterior pharyngeal wall, creation of false passages, bacteremia, necrosis of the external nares, and increased resistance to air flow during spontaneous ventilation.

While nasal vs. oral intubation has long been a popular controversy, the smaller tube size usually required using the nasal route increases the imposed work of breathing[8] and may make suctioning and adequate pulmonary toilet more difficult. Studies have documented an increased rate of maxillary sinusitis,[9] and the alleged increase in patient comfort and tolerance is not documented. Thus, orotracheal intubation has become the preferred route for long-term mechanical ventilation (> 4 days).

### Tracheostomy

The optimum time to perform a tracheostomy remains controversial, and some techniques may be accompanied by significant morbidity. Endotracheal intubation can safely be employed for 3–6 weeks under most circumstances, and it is associated with a low risk for subglottic stenosis.[3] The inflammatory injuries and mucosal necrosis as a result of translaryngeal intubation reaches the maximum threshold early, i.e., within the first 7 days.[5,6] Because early tracheostomy adds tracheal complications to laryngeal problems already present, tracheostomy *before* 3 weeks should only be considered when the advantage of a more secure airway could permit discharge from the intensive care unit (ICU) in cases of predicted long recovery, such as severe head injury. Since most patients are extubated before 3 weeks, only a few patients remain to be considered for late tracheostomy. Tracheostomy may offer advantages to some patients in terms of comfort and ability to eat and communicate; however, there is no good evidence that tracheostomy facilitates weaning or improves pulmonary toilet compared to orotracheal tubes.

In trauma situations where surgical cricothyroidotomy is necessary, early conversion to formal tracheostomy is sometimes recommended to prevent subglottic stenosis. Others believe that prolonged use of cricothyroidotomy has no more complications than formal tracheostomy. Stoma site stenosis occurs following tracheostomy as the stoma heals with the formation of scar tissue. Scar formation can be limited by dividing the tracheal rings longitudinally rather than forming a "trapdoor" or excising a portion of the anterior tracheal wall.[10] Stomal stenosis and the other risks of tracheostomy may be easier to treat than subglottic laryngeal stenosis.[10]

Percutaneous dilatational tracheostomy has become an increasingly popular alternative to formal surgical tracheostomy.[11] However, this form of airway control is contraindicated in emergency situations.

## Physiologic Basis of Disease, Support, and Monitoring

### *Pulmonary Pathophysiology*

In the presence of decreased lung-thorax compliance, compensatory mechanisms to overcome the increased intrathoracic pressure required for respiration include diminished tidal volumes and increased respiratory frequency so that the total work of breathing is minimized (the so-called minimal work concept).[12] However, this compensation, in turn, increases oxygen utilization due to the increased breathing frequency and associated increased pressure changes. These evolved mechanisms are no longer ontogenically appropriate for individual patients. Our evolved mechanisms, from the caveman, were only capable of attaining short-term survival, there being no intensive care support for failing organ systems until recovery could occur. To understand how to design and monitor ventilatory support, we must first explore the expression of this evolved response during the imposed prolonged critical care support of today.

**Systemic Mechanisms Leading to Pulmonary Pathophysiology.** The most advanced clinical situation, ARDS, is not a single disease process but represents a final common pathway for a variety of lung insults. The common expression is increased capillary permeability and inflammatory edema with damage and destruction to the alveolar/capillary interface. The increased permeability leads to pulmonary edema, decreased compliance, and a large right to left intrapulmonary shunt, due to ventilation/perfusion ($\dot{V}/\dot{Q}$) abnormalities in the earliest stages and eventually alveolar flooding. The resulting respiratory failure is rarely the ultimate cause of death but rather the subsequent multiple-organ system failure. The underlying disease, sepsis, or trauma that leads to ARDS is the predominant determinant of outcome. The goals of therapy are early recognition, elimination of predisposing conditions, and aggressive patient support. Positive end-expiratory pressure (PEEP) has become the mainstay for managing oxygenation deficits in patients with ARDS, whether its application is specified explicitly by the practitioner or achieved indirectly (i.e., auto-PEEP) by the ventilatory method used.[13]

The polymorphonuclear leukocyte (neutrophils) is the principal inflammatory cell involved in ARDS. Neutrophils are activated by potent chemotactic factors (e.g., Interleukin-1, [IL-1], IL-8, the complement peptide C5a, and leukotrienes [e.g., LTB4]).[14] The neutrophils marginate in pulmonary capillaries and release free oxygen radicals that in turn damage the capillary endothelium and increase their permeability. The neutrophils also release proteases, particularly elastase, that further damage the interstitium. Proinflammatory cytokines (IL-1, IL-6, IL-8, TNF, IFNα) may participate in the local organ injury that leads to ARDS, and there is evidence that an imbalance between the proinflammatory cytokines and the endogenous cytokine inhibitors may be necessary for ARDS to develop following injury.[15] Several clinical and experimental studies have demonstrated normal or moderately elevated systemic plasma levels of TNF, IL-1, and IFNα compared with those levels in the lung (via bronchoalveolar lavage).[16,17] This has been confirmed both in the early and the most severe disease stages, implying that the lung cytokine response rather than the systemic cytokine environment may be responsible for the end-organ injury. This also indicates that early local organ mediator production may regulate this injury independent of the systemic (global) cytokine production. Understanding how the pulmonary cytokine response impacts and modulates the pulmonary air spaces and immunologic function is an active focus of investigation. Once understood, it may be possible to attenuate or block cytokine production, yielding targeted and clinically relevant therapies.[18]

Work of breathing, which relates to the product of the change in pressure and volume, is a measure of the process of overcoming the elastic and frictional forces of the lung and chest wall.[19] The work of breathing ($WOB_{Pt}$)in the critically ill patient who requires ventilatory support can be divided into three sections: the normal physiologic work ($WOB_{Phys}$); the work to overcome the pathophysiologic changes in the lung and chest wall ($WOB_{Dis}$); and imposed work of breathing ($WOB_{Imp}$), created by the endotracheal tube, breathing circuit, and ventilator. The sum is total work. Physiologic work of breathing consists of three elements: elastic work of breathing, flow resistive work, and inertial work.[20] Elastic work is the work necessary to overcome the elastic forces of the lung and is inversely proportional to the compliance of the lung. If compliance becomes diminished, the work of breathing increases dramatically. The second element of physiologic work is flow resistive work, or the work that is needed to overcome the resistance of the airways and parenchymal tissues. This may increase the pressure change necessary to inhale the same tidal volume, but it also adds another component of work during expiration, that necessary to expel the gas from the lungs through the narrow airways. The third component of physiologic work is the inertial work to overcome the tendency of gas volume to remain at rest. This element is negligible when compared with the elastic and flow resistive work elements. In addition to the normal physiologic work, patients with respiratory failure must overcome the increased work of breathing caused by superimposed disease ($WOB_{Dis}$). This is clinically manifested as a change from relatively large tidal volumes at a slow respiratory rate to small tidal volumes at a rapid rate. Finally, the patient must do additional work to breathe spontaneously against the breathing apparatus. This imposed work of breathing ($WOB_{Imp}$) is the work performed by the patient to breathe through the breathing apparatus (i.e., the endotracheal tube, the breathing circuit, the humidifier and ventilator demand valves, and flow system). Imposed work is an additional flow resistive work load superimposed on the patient's physiologic work of breathing. Banner et al[8] showed that the endotracheal tube acts as a resistor in series in the breathing apparatus thereby causing an increase in work of breathing. Imposed work has been shown to exceed physiologic work of breathing by a factor of 6 under conditions of spontaneous breathing through a narrow internal diameter endotracheal tube at a high inspiratory flow rate demand during continuous positive airway pressure. Poor demand system sensitivity, ventilator dyssynchrony, malfunctioning demand valves, inadequate inspiratory flow, and especially small endotracheal tubes are contributing factors.[21] The goal of ventilatory support is to titrate carefully the ventilator's contribution to minute ventilation so that the patient's effort remains a nonfatiguing work load. Failure to do so by supplying either too much or too little ventilatory support may result in unsuccessful weaning trials and increase the duration of mechanical ventilation. Normal range for $WOB_{pt}$ is 0.3–0.6 J/L.

**Therapy-Induced Pathologic Pulmonary Changes.** Pulmonary barotrauma, alveolar edema, hyaline membrane formation, and vascular injury are all attributed to the use of positive pressure ventilatory techniques (Table 4–2). Until recently, the elevation of airway pressure (PAW) consequent to positive pressure ventilation was generally considered the cause. However, in most studies, elevation of PAW was achieved by increasing the tidal volume to 10 times the normal level or even more (65 mL/kg and to over 100 mL/kg).[22] Dreyfuss et al,[23] using an experimental rat model to study airway pressure and tidal volume independently, found that lung structure was normal in the control animals as well as in those of the low-volume, high-pressure group. That is, large cyclic changes in airway pressure with tidal volumes between 13 and 19 mL/kg (still two to three times normal) had no demonstrable effect on pulmonary microstructure. In contrast, pulmonary edema and structural lung injuries, similar to that seen in ARDS, were observed in the high-volume group administered both by positive and negative pressure ventilation. Thus, large lung volume and not high airway pressures produced pulmonary pathology in their model. Also, adding PEEP ameliorated the damage produced by the high volumes. Zapol[24] has suggested that this therapy-induced damage be called volutrauma rather than barotrauma, a nomenclature that accents the role of hyperinflation in the genesis of secondary lung injury.

**TABLE 4–2. COMPLICATIONS OF MECHANICAL VENTILATION**

1. Related to positive intrathoracic pressure
   - Pulmonary barotrauma
   - Decreased venous return and cardiac output
   - Hypotension
   - Increased pulmonary artery pressure and right ventricular afterload
   - Decreased extrathoracic organ blood flow
2. Related to length of time on the ventilator
   - Mucous plugging and atelectasis
   - Nosocomial pneumonia and sepsis
   - Thromboembolism
   - Technical complications of intubation and ventilation
   - Respiratory muscle atrophy and deconditioning

### *Monitoring During Therapy*

**Measurement of Lung Mechanics.** Several lung volume measurements are useful for monitoring ventilatory function (Table 4–3). These include tidal volume, vital capacity, minute ventilation, and dead space ventilation. Tidal volume (expressed in liters) can be measured both during inspiration and expiration. Tidal volume is monitored during mechanical ventilation to determine if alveolar ventilation is adequate. A small spontaneous tidal volume may be an indicator of respiratory fatigue. If tidal volume is diminished, both oxygenation and ventilation may be impaired. A 25% difference between inspired and expired tidal volume may indicate obstruction, system leaks, or air trapping. In order to obtain accurate measurements, tidal volume must be measured between the ventilator Y piece and the endotracheal tube.[25] If measurements are made at the expiratory valve of the breathing circuit, the entire tidal volume delivered by a ventilator, rather than the volume received by the patient, is measured. Under conditions of decreased lung compliance or increased airway resistance, the high peak inspiratory pressure (PIP) can result in an increase of gas volume compressed in the breathing circuit, with correspondingly less delivered to the patient. The product of PIP (centimeters of water) times 5 mL/cm water provides an estimation of the compression volume in commonly used disposable ventilator circuits. This must be subtracted from the machine-measured tidal volume to calculate the actual tidal volume received by the patient. Vital capacity is the total amount of air exhaled in one breath. Vital capacity reflects the patient's ability to breathe deeply and to cough. The vital capacity is reduced in diseases involving the respiratory muscles or the neurologic pathways, in obstructive and restrictive disease, and in patients who fail to cooperate

**TABLE 4–3. MEASURED AND DERIVED RESPIRATORY AND BLOOD GAS PARAMETERS**

| Parameter | Normal Range | Indication for Weaning |
|---|---|---|
| **Lung mechanics** | | |
| Dead space/Tidal volume ratio $V_D/V_T$ | 0.3–0.45 | <.5 |
| Respiratory rate (**f**) | 10–30 breaths/min | <35 breaths/min |
| Tidal volume ($V_T$) | 7–10 mL/kg | >5 mL/kg (ideally) |
| Vital capacity (VC) | 10–15 mL/kg | >15 mL/kg (ideally) |
| Resting minute ventilation (VE) | 5–10 LPM | <10 LPM (ideally) |
| Lung compliance dynamic ($C_{Dyn}$) | 100–200 mL/cm $H_2O$ | >30 mL/cm $H_2O$ |
| Lung compliance static ($C_{Static}$) | 50–100 mL/cm $H_2O$ | >25 mL/cm $H_2O$ |
| Airway resistance (RAW) | 2–5 cm $H_2O$/1/s | <15 cm $H_2O$/1/s |
| Auto PEEP ($PEEP_a$) | <3 cm $H_2O$ | <3 cm $H_2O$ |
| Forced expiratory volume ($FEV_1$) | 5–10 mL/kg | >10 mL/kg |
| **Respiratory muscle strength** | | |
| Maximum inspiratory pressure (MIP) | –30 Low effort<br>–140 High effort | >(–)30 cm $H_2O$ |
| Change in esophageal pressure ($\Delta P_{ES}$) | (–)5–(–)10 cm $H_2O$ | <(–)15 cm $H_2O$ |
| Respiratory drive ($P_{0.1}$) | 2–4 cm $H_2O$ | <6 cm $H_2O$ |
| **Respiratory muscle endurance** | | |
| Pressure time product (PIP) | 200–300 cm $H_2O$–s/min | <300 cm $H_2O$–s/min |
| Pressure time index (PTI) | 0.05–0.12 | <0.15 |
| Rapid shallow breathing index ($^f/V_T$) | 60–90 | <105 |
| Maximum voluntary ventilation (MVV) | 10–20 LPM | >20 LPM (ideally) |
| Patient work of breathing (pWOB) | 0.3–0.6 Js/L | <.80 J/L (ideally) |
| Respiratory time fraction ($T_I/T_{TOT}$) | 0.3–0.4 | Increase <0.1 |
| **Arterial blood gases** | | |
| $PaO_2$ | 75–105 mm Hg with $FIO_2$ 0.21 | $PaO_2$ > 60 mm Hg on $FIO_2$ <0.40 |
| $PaCO_2$ | 35–40 mm Hg | <45 in a previous eucapneic patient |
| pH | 7.35–7.45 | >7.3 or <7.45 |

fully. Vital capacity is normally 65–75 mL/kg, and a value of 10 mL/kg or greater is commonly considered a favorable predictor in weaning. However, this value is quite dependent upon patient cooperation and its power to predict successful weaning is poor. Minute ventilation is the product of respiratory rate and tidal volume. A resting minute ventilation of less than 10 L/min and the ability to double the respiratory ventilation on command have been associated with successful weaning from mechanical ventilation. The dead space ($V_D$) is the proportion of tidal volume that does not participate in gas exchange and can be calculated from the Enghoff equation (modified from the Bohr equation) as follows:

$$V_D = \frac{PaCO_2 - P\bar{E}CO_2}{PaCO_2}\ \dot{V}_E,$$

where $P\bar{E}CO_2$ is the mean partial pressure of exhaled $CO_2$ in the total exhaled volume of gas after thorough mixing (collected in a bag reservoir) over 3 minutes. This is divided into two components: the volume of gas occupying the conducting airways (the anatomic dead space, approximately 150 cc in the 70-kg adult) and the volume of gas within unperfused alveoli (the physiologic dead space). The ratio of dead space to tidal volume provides a useful expression of the efficiency of ventilation. The normal ratio is between 0.3 and 0.45. The $V_D/V_T$ ratio is increased in a number of diseased states associated with high ventilation–low perfusion ratios, such as adult respiratory distress syndrome, emphysema, pulmonary embolism, and shock with low cardiac output. It may also be elevated during positive pressure ventilation with high tidal volume and positive end expiratory pressure. Patients whose $V_D/V_T$ exceeds .60 cannot usually be weaned from ventilatory support. By multiplying minute ventilation by the $V_D/V_T$ ratio, the alveolar ventilation can be calculated. Respiratory rate (**f**) is the number of respirations per minute. An elevated respiratory rate may be a compensating mechanism for a decreased tidal volume, which in turn is compensating for an increased pressure work load. A low respiratory rate may result in hypoventilation and respiratory acidosis.

The Shallow Breathing Index of Yang and Tobin ($^f/V_T$)[26] and the Weaning Index of Jabour et al[27] identified target values ($^f/V_T < 105$ and WI < 4 $min^{-1}$, respectively), to discriminate between successful and unsuccessful outcome during weaning. They were found to have high positive predictive value (0.78:Yang/0.95:Jabour) and negative predictive values (0.95:Yang and Jabour). Unfortunately, additional trials of these indices have not validated the results nor confirmed the inferred relationship to total work of breathing ($r^2$ 0.275: WOB vs. $^f/V_T$, 0.355 WOB vs. **f**).[28–30]

**Newly Available Measurements.** Portable microprocessor-based respiratory monitors such as the CP-100 (Bicore Monitoring Systems, Inc., Irvine, CA) measure many mechanical ventilation and respiratory muscle parameters, including compliance, airway resistance, strength and endurance, and both patient and ventilator work of breathing. (Table 4–3). Physiologic data are accrued from a miniature pneumotachograph and airway pressure sensor positioned between the "Y" piece of the breathing circuit tubing and the endotracheal tube. A catheter with a distally annealed balloon is positioned in the distal esophagus to measure changes in intraesophageal pressure as an estimate of changes in intrathoracic pressure.

Esophageal pressure changes are used to distinguish lung mechanical properties from those of the chest wall; assess inspiratory effort; and calculate airway resistance, compliance, and elasticity. During a patient-initiated breath, there is a negative deflection of the esophageal pressure. During ventilator-supplied or -assisted breaths, positive airway pressure may be transmitted across the pleural space causing a rise in esophageal pressure. An esophageal pressure change of less than 15 cm $H_2O$ indicates adequate ventilatory reserve. The normal range for a nonmechanically ventilated patient is (–)2 to (–)10 cm $H_2O$.

Maximal inspiratory pressures, thoracic, static, and dynamic compliance can also be monitored. Compliance is the quotient of change in gas volume divided by change in driving pressure. Thoracic compliance is an indicator of lung and chest wall elasticity. Dynamic compliance ($C_{Dyn}$) represents the elastic properties of the lung. $C_{Dyn}$ (normal range 100–200 mL/cm $H_2O$) has been proven to be an indicator for successful weaning if greater than 30 mL/cm water. Static compliance ($C_{Static}$) includes all the forces applied across the lung and chest wall. $C_{Static}$ normal values are reported to be 50–100 mL/cm $H_2O$. A value of >25 cm/$H_2O$ predicts successful weaning.[31,32] In patients receiving mechanical ventilation, a rough measure of total thoracic compliance (both the lungs and chest wall) can be obtained by dividing the delivered tidal volume by the inflation pressure displayed on the ventilator gauge during conditions of zero gas flow, preferably using a 1-L inflation in a passively ventilated patient. It can be estimated by employing an inspiratory hold during mechanical ventilation. The peak airway pressure falls to a plateau, PEEP is subtracted and the exhaled (at the endotracheal tube) tidal volume is divided by the change in pressure. Decreased values are observed with disorders of the thoracic cage or reduction in the number of functioning lung units (resection, bronchial intubation, pneumothorax, pneumonia, atelectasis, or pulmonary edema). The dynamic characteristic is calculated by dividing the volume delivered by the peak (rather than the plateau) airway pressure minus the PEEP. It is not correct to call this value dynamic compliance because it includes both compliance and resistive components. (The dynamic characteristic is normally about 50–80 mL/cm $H_2O$). This component may be decreased by disorders of the airway, lung parenchyma, or chest wall. A reduced dynamic component relative to static compliance suggests an increase in airway resistance, i.e., bronchospasm, mucus plugging, kinking of the endotracheal tube, or an excessive flow rate. Airway resistance is a measure of the frictional resistance to air flow created by the entire system of air passages in the respiratory system. Maximal inspiratory pressure (MIP) is the maximal pressure below atmospheric that a patient can exert against an occluded airway. MIP corresponds reasonably well with the ability to cough and reflects ventilatory muscle pump strength. An MIP value of more than –20 to –25 cm $H_2O$ has been used to confirm recovery from neuromuscular blockade after general anesthesia. MIP at values more negative than –30 cm $H_2O$ have been used to predict successful weaning from short-term (<3–4 days) mechanical ventilation.[33] MIP is less useful after prolonged mechanical ventilation because it assesses the instantaneous strength of the respiratory muscle pump and not endurance function, which is the more important determinant of successful weaning. Respiratory drive ($P_{0.1}$) is a measurement that directly relates to the patient's ability to breathe spontaneously. $P_{0.1}$ measures the neurologic stimulus to create the force of diaphragmatic contraction. It is defined as the decrease in airway pressure during the first 100 ms after airway closure. It is measured as the decrease in esophageal pressure before the onset of ventilator flow. A high value increases work expenditure during a patient-initiated ventilator breath and may indicate a problem in the sensitivity setting of the ventilator or a sticking demand valve. A low value of $P_{0.1}$ may indicate blunting of respiratory drive. It is also a good indicator of strength for predicting successful weaning. Pressure time product (PTP), reflecting the patient's effort to overcome both mechanical and isometric forces, is an estimate of the oxygen consumption of the respiratory muscles.[34] Intubated patients normally will exert between 200 and 300 cm $H_2O$ – s/min when capable of sustaining successful weaning.[35] Nonintubated patients should average between 60–80 cm $H_2O$ – s/min values.

The respiratory time fraction, $T_I/T_{Tot}$, is defined as the ratio of inspired time to total time in the respiratory cycle and is an inference of endurance. As the respiratory muscles are fatiguing, the fraction of the breathing cycle spent in inspiration tends to increase. Excessive work of breathing is the most common cause for an elevated inspiratory time fraction. Issues such as imposed ventilatory work, dyssynchrony, increased expiratory airway resistance, auto PEEP, and malnutrition must be explored.

Pressure time index (PTI) is a measure of strength and endurance combined into one value. It combines the strength measure of MIP with the endurance value of $T_I/T_{Tot}$. The PTI correlates directly with oxygen consumption and inversely with respiratory muscle fatigue. PTI may predict the onset of respiratory muscle fatigue.[36]

### Methods of Assessing Gas Exchange

***Intermittent.*** Arterial blood gas analysis for oxygen, carbon dioxide, and acid base balance remains an important monitoring method (Table 4–3). Derived indices such as the alveolar—arterial oxygen partial pressure difference ($PAO_2 - PaO_2$) and the arterial to alveoli oxygen tension ratio ($PaO_2/PAO_2$) have been suggested for evaluating the efficiency of gas exchange.[37] However, they are not always accurate, because the relationship between physiologic shunt and the oxygen tension indices is nonlinear and substantially influenced by changes in the inspired oxygen concentration and arterial venous oxygen content difference.

### *Capnography*

Capnography is the display of $CO_2$ concentration as a wave form. Currently available systems for $CO_2$ analysis include infrared spectroscopy, mass spectrometry, and Raman scattering.[38] In addition, disposable noninvasive and inexpensive calorimetric devices are available. In the majority of stand alone capnographs, the $CO_2$ concentration is measured by infrared spectroscopy. End tidal $CO_2$ measurement ($E_TCO_2$) is the most reliable means of determining proper endotracheal tube placement short of direct laryngoscopy.[39] Proper endotracheal tube position produces discernible $CO_2$ wave forms, while esophageal intubation causes ET $CO_2$ to rapidly decrease to zero after a few breaths. In the ICU, end tidal $CO_2$ can also be utilized as a ventilator disconnect alarm and to indicate ventilator malfunction. Measurement of end tidal $CO_2$ has been proposed as a substitute for arterial blood gas sampling during adjustment of mechanical ventilation and to guide weaning in critically ill patients.[40] However, end tidal $CO_2$ is often misleading since arterial and end tidal $CO_2$ values do not change in unison or even in the same direction in diseases characterized by $\dot{V}/\dot{Q}$ abnormalities.

### *Pulse Oximetry*

Pulse oximetry provides a reliable, real-time estimation of functional arterial hemoglobin oxygen saturation ($SpO_2$). Pulse oximeters measure the absorbance of light at two wave lengths: 660 nm (red) and 940 nm (infrared) to distinguish between oxyhemoglobin and deoxyhemoglobin. Continuous display of $SpO_2$ provides safety since desaturation is immediately detected. Continuous $SpO_2$ may also guide therapy during titration of PEEP and $FIO_2$.[38] Pulse oximetry provides continuous data at a lower cost since blood gas testing is reduced. Hemoglobin species other than oxyhemoglobin and deoxyhemoglobin are not detected by pulse oximetry. However, if carboxyhemoglobin and metahemoglobin are suspected, laboratory co-oximetry will reveal their concentrations.

### *Criteria for the Institution of Ventilatory Support*

Mechanical ventilatory support is initiated to (1) improve gas exchange, (2) decrease patient work of breathing, and (3) secure airway patency.[41] A clinical classification includes prophylaxis, early intervention to abort or ameliorate progression, and support for advanced pulmonary parenchymal disease.

**Type of Support Considered.** The patient who can not ventilate adequately should be treated with mechanical ventilation to achieve adequate alveolar ventilation. If hypoxemia alone is present, then continuous positive airway pressure (CPAP) or biphasic positive airway pressure (Bi-PAP), which do not require intubation, may be sufficient to increase functional residual capacity, decrease intrapulmonary shunt, and improve oxygenation. Prophylactic ventilatory support is indicated in patients who have received long-acting narcotics or muscle relaxants and/or who have no pulmonary disease. Prophylaxis need only be maintained until the patient is fully awake, responsive, cooperative, and able to ventilate adequately. If there are no other reasons to continue ventilation, an alternative would be to reverse the muscle relaxants or narcotics to permit early extubation. Early intervention includes ventilatory support in patients with mild reversible disease (i.e., pulmonary contusion, viral pneumonia, aspiration) and in patients with preexisting pulmonary disease such as chronic obstructive pulmonary disease (COPD), bronchitis, or asthma, if combined with other factors such as pulmonary edema or upper respiratory tract infection. Other factors would include a history of smoking, obesity, and lengthy operations (>4–6 hours). In both prophylactic support and early intervention, the time of extubation is based on the clinician's preference since reasonably normal pulmonary function has been maintained. Ordinarily this process should require no more than 4–6 hours. Measured criteria such as a spontaneous vital capacity of >15 mL/kg and a negative inspiratory force in excess of 20 cm $H_2O$ are usually easily met; weaning, strictly speaking is not necessary.

Postoperative atelectasis associated with elevated diaphragms and decreased expiratory lung volumes may complicate prophylaxis. If abnormalities such as hypoxemia or hypercarbia are present, ventilatory support should be considered therapeutic. Requirement for prolonged ventilatory support (i.e., ≥72 hours) can be anticipated in patients with acute major reversible disease (i.e., ARDS secondary to trauma or sepsis), and in patients with preexisting chronic disease (COPD), especially if there is a superimposed acute problem, such as pneumonia or lengthy operation.

Despite the myriad of pulmonary function studies used, there are no clear-cut methods to determine which patients will develop respiratory complications postoperatively or require ventilatory support. However, patients who have an $FEV_1$ of less than 50%, a maximum ventilatory volume of less than 50%, and an elevated arterial carbon dioxide level at rest usually will require ventilatory support in the postoperative period.

### *Achievement of Adequate Ventilatory Support*

Prolonged mechanical ventilation is both expensive and associated with many complications, chiefly pneumonia. Thus, it is advantageous to reduce support (wean) and extubate patients as soon as possible. Ventilatory muscle fatigue or use dystrophy can be caused by increased muscle loading from breathing through a highly resistant breathing apparatus.[42–44] Muscle atrophy and deconditioning can result from totally unloading the ventilatory muscle pump for too long by using controlled mechanical ventilation (CMV), high-rate (>10) intermittent mandatory ventilation (IMV), or high levels of pressure support ventilation (PSV); all prolong ventilatory support. As the disease process improves, ventilatory support must be reduced to reload the ventilatory muscle pump, thereby preventing detraining of the respiratory musculature. When the disease process has resolved, no further weaning is required because the patient is performing the normal physiologic work, and the ventilator only offsets the imposed work of the breathing. Once adequate gas exchange is demonstrated, the patient can be extubated. We have coined the term "fast-track weaning" to describe ventilatory support titrated to preserve respiratory muscle pump strength and endurance while avoiding use dystrophy or disuse atrophy.[12] Adequate ventilatory support now means ensuring that the patient does the normal physiologic work, neutralizing imposed work and decrementing support as disease improves. Measurement of imposed, physiologic, and ventilator-provided works of breathing provides objective information to set the ventilator to prevent fatigue or atrophy.

## Modes of Mechanical Ventilation

### *Assist Control Ventilation (A/C)*

This is a mode of ventilation in which every patient breath is supported by the ventilator. With assist control (A/C) ventilation, the ventilator delivers a breath, either when triggered by the patient's inspiratory effort or independently, if such an effort does not occur within a preselected period. Volume-cycled and pressure-limited or pressure-targeted modes are available (Fig. 4–1B).

***Setup Parameters.*** With the use of volume-targeted A/C ventilation, the tidal volume, inspiratory flow rate, flow wave form, sensitivity, and mandatory ventilatory rate are set. With pressure-limited or pressure-targeted A/C modes, pressure level, $T_I$, mandatory ventilatory rate and sensitivity are set.

***Suggested Initial Settings.*** Set back-up rate: 6–8 breaths per minute; flow rate (60–80 L/min) commensurate with patient's spontaneous inspiratory flow demand or to achieve I:E ratio of at least 1:2 to avoid auto PEEP; tidal volume: 8–10 mL/kg; high-pressure limit 20% > peak inspiratory pressure; trigger: 1 cm $H_2O$, or more to avoid auto cycling.

***Advantages.*** Assist control ventilation combines the security of controlled ventilation with the possibility of synchronizing the breathing rhythm of patient and ventilator, and it ensures ventilatory support during each breath.

***Risks.*** Excessive patient work occurs in cases of inadequate peak flow or inspiratory sensitivity setting, especially if the patient's respiratory drive is excessive. Volume-targeted A/C may be poorly tolerated in awake nonsedated patients and may require sedation to ensure synchrony of patient and machine cycle lengths. This mode of ventilatory support can be associated with respiratory alkalosis and may potentially lead to stacking of breaths, air trapping, and barotrauma. Pressure-targeted A/C may result in inadequate minute ventilation during changes in lung impedance, patient-ventilatory drive, or patient-ventilatory dyssynchrony.[45]

### *Intermittent Mandatory Ventilation (IMV)*

IMV is a mode of ventilation that combines a preset number of ventilator-delivered mandatory breaths of predetermined tidal volume and patient-generated spontaneous breaths (Fig. 4–1C). Minute ventilation combines patient-initiated (high-pressure–low-volume) breaths with ventilator (high-volume–high-pressure) breaths. Several ventilators offer pressure-targeted breaths instead of volume-targeted breaths during mandatory cycles. If the mandatory breaths are patient-triggered, the technique is termed synchronized (SIMV).

***Setup Parameters.*** Parameters include tidal volume, flow rate and/or inspiratory time, frequency of controlled breath, and sensitivity. When pressure-targeted breaths are used, pressure level and inspiratory time must be set.

***Suggested Initial Settings.*** Set tidal volume: 10–12 mL/kg; inspiratory time: 1.5–2 s, or flow rate adjusted to provide this inspiratory time with the set tidal volume; initial IMV rate (postop) 4 breaths per minute if awake to 8 breaths per minute if still anesthetized or paralyzed; trigger effort: 1 cm $H_2O$ or more to prevent auto cycling (SIMV); $FIO_2$: .4 (unless hypoxic in OR); PEEP or CPAP: 5 cm $H_2O$; high-pressure limit approximately 25% above peak inspiratory pressure.

***Advantages.*** The patient performs a variable amount of respiratory work, yet there is a security because of the preset mandatory ventilation. IMV or SIMV allow varying support from continuous mechanical ventilation (IMV rates > 10/min) to spontaneous breathing (IMV rate = 0) and thus can be used as a weaning tool.

***Risks.*** With IMV, the machine-delivered volume may be delivered at the peak of a spontaneous breath. The total is little more than most programmed "sighs" and has not been a problem clinically. Excessive work of breathing due to the presence of a poorly responsive demand valve, suboptimal ventilator circuit, or inappropriate flow delivery can occur. The patient's breaths in ARDS are unphysiologic—high pressure and low volume. In each case, excess work is im-

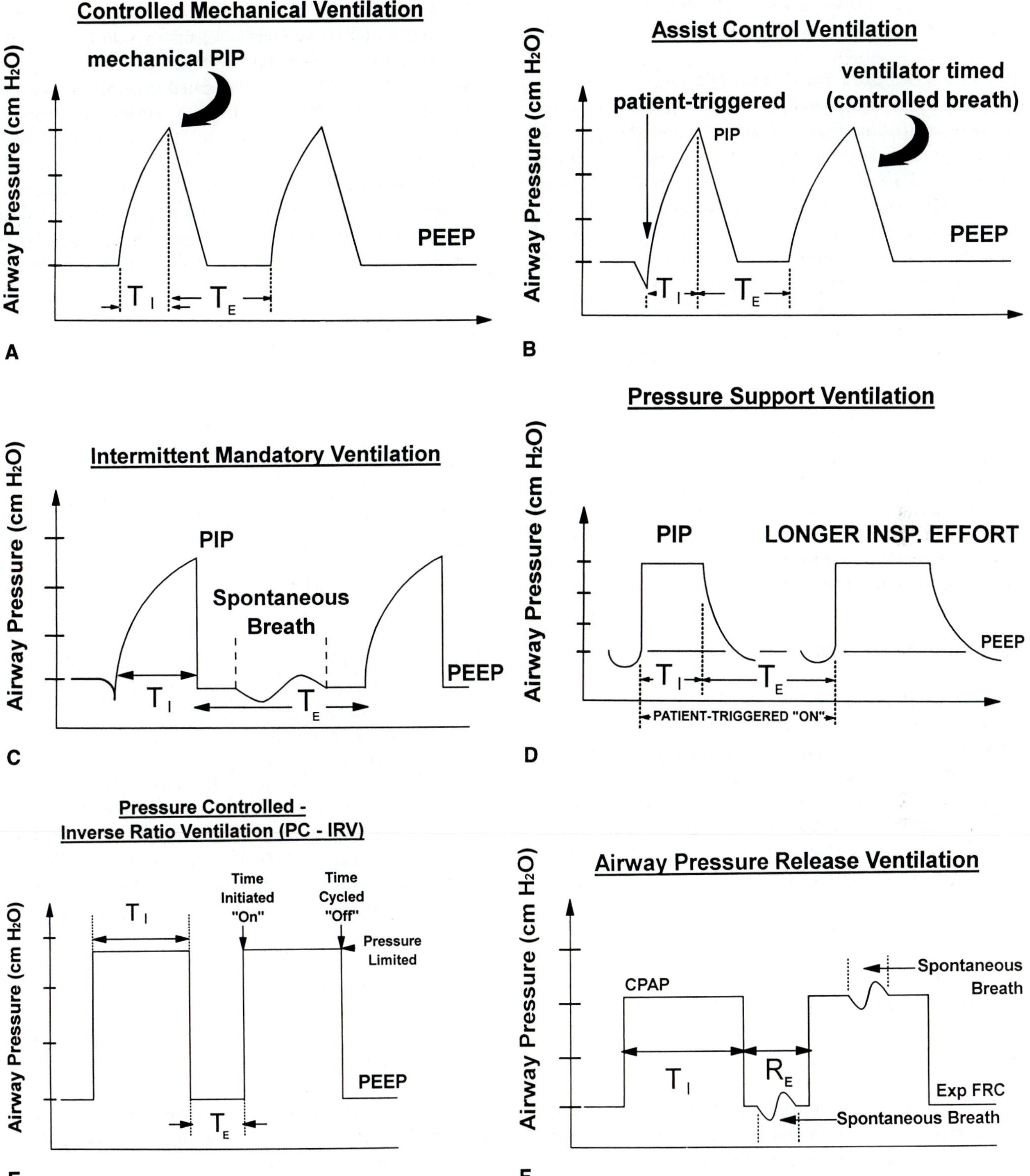


**Figure 4–1.** (**A**) Controlled mechanical ventilation, (**B**) assist-control ventilation, (**C**) intermittent mandatory ventilation, (**D**) pressure support ventilation, (**E**) pressure controlled-inverse ratio ventilation, (**F**) airway pressure release ventilation. Spontaneous breaths are shown, PIP indicates peak Inflation pressure; PEEP, positive end-expiratory pressure; CPAP, continuous positive airway pressure; $T_I$, inspiratory time; and $T_E$, expiratory time; $R_E$, release (expiratory) time; exp FRC, end-expiratory functional residual capacity.

posed on the respiratory muscle pump. Worsening dynamic hyperinflation has been described with patients in COPD.[22]

### *Pressure Support Ventilation (PSV)*

PSV is a pressure-triggered, pressure-targeted flow-cycled mode of ventilation (Fig. 4–1D). It is used both as a mode of ventilation during stable ventilatory support periods and in weaning. PSV is used to unload the ventilatory muscles and decrease work of breathing.[46] It augments spontaneous breaths and offsets the work imposed by the endotracheal tube and breathing apparatus. Since PSV is designed to assist spontaneous breathing, the patient should have an intact respiratory drive if it is to be used during weaning. At initiation of inspiration, the pressure rises rapidly to the preselected positive pressure plateau that is maintained for the remainder of inspiration. Gas flow from the ventilator cycles off, when the patient's inspiratory flow rate decreases to a predetermined percentage of the initial inspiratory flow rate, usually 25%. The patient and the ventilator work in synchrony to achieve the total work required for each breath.

***Setup Parameters.*** Parameters include pressure level and sensitivity, and no mandatory PSV rate is set. In some ventilators, it is possible to adjust the rate of rise in the pressure at the beginning of inspiration or to adjust the flow threshold for cycling from inspiration to expiration. Many ventilators incorporate volume-targeted backup modes in the event of apnea.

***Suggested Initial Settings.*** Set trigger level: 1 cm $H_2O$, or more to prevent auto cycling; flow triggering: set (as instructed by device manufacturer's recommendation) so that minimal inspiratory effort (1–2 cm $H_2O$) will initiate breath; initiation level corresponding to one half the PIP-PEEP, adjust as necessary to provide initial tidal volume 7–8 mL/kg; optional SIMV rate of 1 breath at a tidal volume 10–12 mL/kg (sigh breath to prevent atelectasis); tidal volume to be delivered in 1.5–2.0 s.

***Advantages.*** Improved patient ventilator synchrony and comfort have been identified in studies and in practice. The patient interacts with the pressure-assisted breaths but retains control over inspiratory time and flow rate, expiratory time, frequency, tidal volume, and minute ventilation. Peak airway pressures are lower than IMV or CMV. PSV should also be used to compensate for the imposed work produced by the endotracheal tube, the demand valve system, and breathing circuit. It permits variation from nearly total ventilatory support to essentially spontaneous breathing. PSV may be useful in patients who are difficult to wean.

***Risks.*** Tidal volume is not controlled and will vary with compliance, cycling frequency, and synchrony between the patient and ventilator. Backup mandatory ventilation is recommended for unstable patients. One or two volume-cycled breaths (10–12 mL/kg) per minute prevents atelectasis. PSV may be poorly tolerated in patients with high airway resistance because of the preset high initial flow and terminal respiratory flow algorithms. Adjustment of initial flow rates, possible in newer systems, may ameliorate this problem.

### *Inverse Ratio Ventilation (IRV)*

Inverse ratio ventilation uses inspiratory times greater than exhalation, thus reversing the normal ratio of inhalation to exhalation of 1:2 (Fig. 4–1C). It may be created by pressure-controlled or volume-cycled modes. Pressure-controlled IRV with a rapidly decelerating inspiratory flow pattern is more widely used than volume-cycled IRV in patients with ARDS. At present there is a lack of convincing data to support any outcome superiority of IRV over conventional ventilation, although it is quite popular because it limits peak inspiratory pressures.[47] Because high volume, rather than high pressure, has been identified as causing pulmonary damage, limiting peak inspiratory pressure has no proven advantage. In addition, inversion of conventional I/E ratios produces no significant improvement in the overall cardiorespiratory profile. Its proposed clinical utility is in advanced ARDS with refractory hypoxemia or hypercapnea.[48]

***Setup Parameters.*** Choose the pressure limit desired. Increase time of inspiration or inspiratory hold incrementally until oxygen and $CO_2$ elimination are in the desired range. Deep sedation is required in most patients under IRV to avoid dyssynchrony with the ventilator. Careful monitoring of peak airway pressure and end inspiratory plateau pressure are required during volume control IRV. The high-pressure alarm should be set at 10 cm of water above intended peak airway pressure. Careful monitoring of minute ventilation is required during pressure control IRV; tidal volume is markedly dependent on the patient's respiratory mechanics. Auto PEEP level may develop as the I:E ratio increases and should be regularly measured. Because auto PEEP and increased mean airway pressure associated with IRV may compromise cardiac function, hemodynamic status should be assessed using a Swan-Ganz catheter when IRV is implemented.

***Suggested Initial Settings.*** Set pressure limit arbitrarily at half the prior peak inspiratory pressure; I:E ratio 1.5:1 to 2:1 with either inspiratory time control or flow rate control; trigger effort: usually not synchronized to patient's inspiratory effort; high-pressure alarm: 10% above pressure limit; adjust PEEP and $FIO_2$ (<50%) to maintain $PaO_2 \geq 65$ mm Hg.

***Advantages.*** Peak airway (alveolar) pressures are minimized while maintaining mean airway pressure relatively high. Prolongation of inspiration allows recruitment of lung units with long time constants.

***Risks.*** Excessive gas trapping can cause auto PEEP and barotrauma. Cardiac output and tissue oxygen delivery may fall as mean airway pressure, and auto PEEP increases although several studies report no significant alteration in oxygen transport.[49,50] Tidal volume may vary with changing respiratory mechanics; therefore, minute ventilation must be monitored carefully. With pressure-controlled IRV, progressive atelectasis can occur in the presence of poor lung compliance. Deep sedation and/or paralysis are nearly always required with the potential for atrophy and detraining of the respiratory musculature.

### *Airway Pressure Release Ventilation (APRV)*

Airway pressure release ventilation (APRV) is another technique that minimizes lung expansion. APRV is a pressure-controlled, time-triggered, pressure-limited, time-cycled ventilation that allows spontaneous breathing throughout the ventilator cycle (Fig. 4–1F). In this mode, CPAP (usually 10–20 cm $H_2O$) is maintained until the timed release valve opens, allowing the pressure in the system to fall to a lower preset level, usually the functional residual capacity or a lower preset end expiratory pressure (EEP). When the release valve closes again, insufflation rapidly restores the original airway inflation pressure. This form of mechanical ventilation is the opposite of the intermittent positive pressure ventilation methods in terms of the direction of lung volume change. In conventional and spontaneous ventilation, inspiration increases lung volume to eliminate $CO_2$; APRV achieves this goal by decreasing lung volume and eliminates large volume changes above the optimal resting lung volume. The goal of APRV is to limit peak airway pressures, thereby minimizing barotrauma and cardiac compromise. There are two types of pressure release ventilation: APRV, during which pressure release time is preset, and intermittent mandatory pressure release ventilation (IMPRV),[51] which is integrated into the ventilator circuit, providing end-expirated pressure change according to the patient's spontaneous breathing activity. Oxygenation is improved by increasing CPAP, lengthening inspiratory time, or increasing $FIO_2$ while $CO_2$ elimination is effected by increasing the APRV rate and the airway pressure change (i.e., release pressure). When compared with conventional intermittent positive-pressure ventilation plus PEEP, APRV was shown to produce comparable oxygenation and hemodynamic effects at lower peak and end expiratory pressures but similar mean airway pressures in patients with acute respiratory failure.[52]

***Setup Parameters.*** Respiratory monitoring and alarms are available. During APRV, the following respiratory parameters are preset: upper and lower airway pressure levels (i.e., CPAP and EEP), inspiratory time, frequency of pressure release, and pressure release time (expiratory time). During IMPRV, the following respiratory parameters are preset: upper and lower PEEP levels, frequency of PEEP changes, and sensitivity of the trigger. Ventilatory assistance is progressively decremented by decreasing the spacing of PEEP/CPAP changes (positive airway pressure released every 2, 3, 4, 5, 6 ventilatory cycles, etc. to spontaneous expiration).

***Suggested Initial Settings.*** Set $FIO_2$ to maintain $PaO_2 \geq$ 65 mm Hg; CPAP initially at 20 cm $H_2O$; EEP 0 (FRC) to −10 cm $H_2O$); release pressure; expiratory time fixed at 1.5 s to ≥ three times expiratory time constant of patient ($R_{AW} \times C_L$) to avoid auto PEEP; set APRV rate: 4–8 breaths per minute depending on level of sedation. Inspiratory time (seconds) ($T_I$) = 60 (seconds)/frequency (breaths per minute) − expiratory time ($T_E$:seconds).

***Advantages.*** APRV allows spontaneous breathing. The potential for alveolar hyperinflation and iatrogenic lung injury is minimized. Also, there is improved matching of ventilation and perfusion at lower peak and end-expired pressures, and theoretically, less hemodynamic compromise.

***Risks.*** This technique has not been evaluated in patients with poor compliance. It is not applicable in patients with severe airflow obstruction. Minute ventilation must be carefully monitored. Excessive auto PEEP may develop if the respiratory frequency increases above 30 breaths per minute.

### *High Frequency Ventilation (HFV)*

High frequency ventilation uses small tidal volumes (1–3 mL/kg) at high frequencies (100–300 breaths per minute) (Fig. 4–2). The mechanism of gas transfer changes from conventional bulk flow to other types when $V_T < V_D$. Proposed mechanisms include coaxial flow, Taylor dispersion,

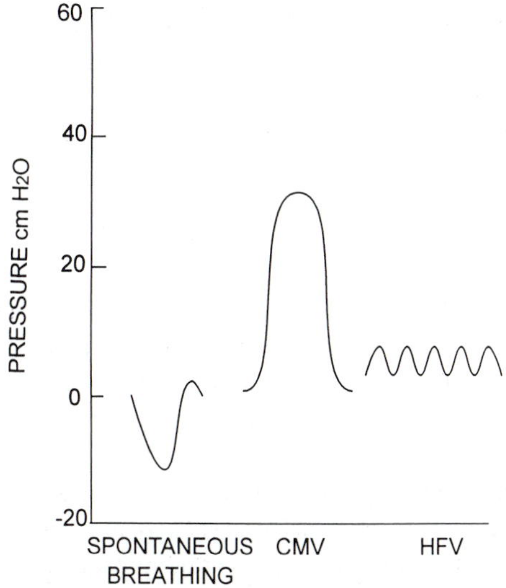


**Figure 4–2.** Pressure changes during spontaneous breathing, conventional mechanical ventilation, and high-frequency positive pressure ventilation. Gas exchange can be maintained with lower mean airway pressure using HFV rather than CMV or high levels of IMV.

pendelluft, and augmented molecular diffusion. The tidal volume and frequency product is usually much higher than during conventional mechanical ventilation. Alveolar ventilation appears to be influenced more by tidal volume than frequency. There are a number of different types of high-frequency ventilation: The three most common are high-frequency oscillation, high-frequency positive-pressure ventilation that is used in anesthesia, and high-frequency jet ventilation that is used in both anesthesia and in the critically ill patient with acute respiratory failure.[53]

***Setup Parameters.*** The clinician sets the driving pressure, inspiratory time, respiratory rate, $FIO_2$ and PEEP. Adequate humidification of delivered gases is mandatory if high-frequency jet ventilation is to be administered for periods longer than 8 hours. Mean airway pressure, which approximates alveolar pressure, should be continuously monitored with an endotracheal catheter located at least 5 cm from the injection site. $PaO_2$ is affected by altering the $FIO_2$ and PEEP. Increase in the I:E ratio and the driving pressure increase tidal volume and decrease $PaCO_2$. Increasing respiratory frequency, decreasing the driving pressure, and decreasing inspiratory time decrease tidal volume and increase $PaCO_2$. FRC can also be increased by increasing the I:E ratio, driving pressure, and respiratory frequency.

***Suggested Initial Settings.*** Follow manufacturer's device specific algorithms or recommendations since settings vary with type of high-frequency ventilator and type of circuit utilized; HFV: $T_I$ – 0.3, ventilatory frequency 80–100/min, drive pressure: 30–40 PSI, titrate to achieve acceptable low mean airway pressure and adequate alveolar ventilation; adjust PEEP and $FIO_2$ (< 50%) to maintain $PaO_2 \geq 65$ mm Hg.

***Advantages.*** High-frequency ventilation is useful during laryngoscopy, bronchoscopy, tracheal surgery, bronchopleural fistula, and tracheoesophageal fistula. A prospective randomized study comparing high-frequency jet ventilation with conventional ventilation performed in a nonhomogeneous population of cancer patients with ARDS did not demonstrate any significant advantage over conventional methods.[46] Ultrahigh frequency ventilation (up to rates of 900 breaths per minute) has improved oxygenation and the elimination of $CO_2$ at lower airway pressures, but no clinical trials have shown superior outcome. A subset of patients with hypovolemia may be more likely to tolerate high-frequency jet ventilation compared with CMV.

***Risks.*** Outflow obstruction can rapidly lead to increases in lung volume that can cause hemodynamic compromise and barotrauma. Air trapping is especially of concern in patients with compliant lungs and airway obstruction. It can be assessed by measuring airway opening pressure under static conditions after airway occlusion by monitoring esophageal pressure, or by measurements of lung volume obtained at the chest wall (e.g., inductive plethysmography). Inadequate humidification can induce severe necrotizing tracheobronchitis. Long-term jet ventilation can result in squamous metaplasia with submucosal inflammatory cell infiltration.

### *Continuous Positive Airway Pressure (CPAP)*

Continuous positive airway pressure elevates airway pressure above atmospheric pressure throughout spontaneous inspiration and exhalation. It increases lung volume and improves oxygenation by elevating functional residual volume above the closing volume, thereby preventing airway closure and alveolar collapse (Figs. 4–3, 4–4). Continuous positive airway pressure is also used to reduce the pressure gradient between the mouth and the alveoli in patients with air trapping. Since it only assists spontaneous breathing, it requires an intact respiratory drive and adequate alveolar ventilation.

***Setup Parameters.*** These include pressure level, flow rate, sensitivity, and amount of inspiratory pressure descent (demand valves or flow-triggered system) or flow rate (continuous-flow system).

***Suggested Initial Settings.*** Demand-flow systems require minimal triggering effort (approximately 1 cm $H_2O$ or more) to avoid auto cycling; flow rate adjusted to avoid deflection of more than 2–4 cm $H_2O$ below baseline during peak inspiration; set continuous-flow system to 2.5–3 times minute volume and titrate to produce 2–4 cm $H_2O$ pressure drop during inspiration; the larger the deflection during inspiration, the greater the work for the patient.

***Advantages.*** CPAP offers the benefit of PEEP to spontaneously breathing patients. It will improve oxygenation if hypoxemia is caused by decreased lung volume. It may help reduce the work of breathing in patients with dynamic hyperinflation and auto PEEP. Recent data suggest that the

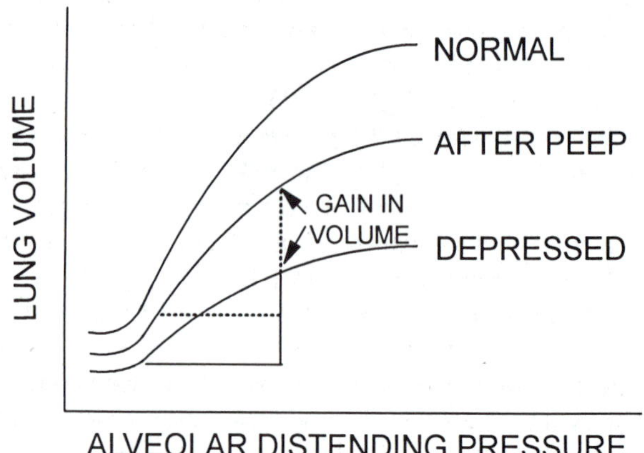


**Figure 4–3.** Representation of an additional effect of PEEP. When compliance is reduced, PEEP can shift the curve toward normal. This will permit delivery of tidal volume at lower transpulmonary pressure gradients.

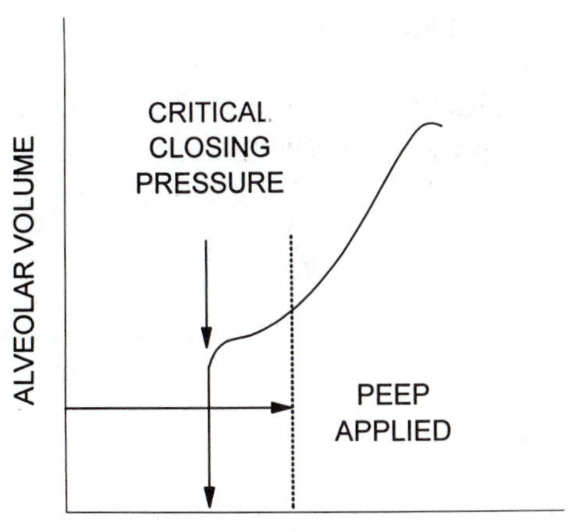


**Figure 4–4.** Representation of the effect of PEEP. If transpulmonary pressure returned to ambient pressure, the critical closing pressure would be reached, and the alveolus would lose all remaining volume i.e., would collapse. An artificial positive airway pressure is added during expiration in order to prevent critical closing and maintaining alveolar volume.

work of breathing is reduced with systems incorporating a continuous flow system in comparison to demand flow systems.[8]

***Risks.*** Hyperinflation and excessive expiratory work may result if excessive CPAP levels are used. High-flow resistance or inadequate inspiratory flow rates may increase inspiratory work of breathing.

### *Minimal Excursionary Ventilation (MEV)*

If alveolar hyperinflation is the primary etiologic factor causing the structural lung injury associated with positive pressure ventilation, a reduction in cyclical volume expansion during mechanical ventilation should be expected to be beneficial. This approach has been called minimal excursionary ventilation; several approaches are available:

(1) *Permissive hypercapnia:* The simplest method of minimal excursionary ventilation is permissive hypercapnia or controlled hypoventilation. In this approach, total minute ventilation is reduced, and the consequent rise in $Paco_2$ is accepted, provided the pH is >7.2. $Paco_2$ as high as 90 mm Hg has been reported[54]; if bicarbonate is conserved, pH will increase just as in the metabolic compensation for the respiratory acidosis associated with COPD.

(2) *Extracorporeal $CO_2$ with venovenous bypass using a membrane oxygenator:* $CO_2$ is removed by a membrane oxygenator, while arterial oxygenation by the native lung is enhanced by CPAP. Mechanical tidal volumes are limited to 45 cm $H_2O$ peak inflation pressure. The reduction in lung volume excursions during ventilatory support result in less injury visualized at pathologic examination. This technique, first described by Gattinoni et al,[55] has not been found superior to conventional mechanical ventilation in prospective controlled trials.[56] Also, extracorporeal $CO_2$ removal is expensive, effort-intensive, and not without complications, especially related to the systemic heparinization.

(3) *IVOX (intravascular oxygenator):* This technique of extrapulmonary gas exchange does not require an extracorporeal circuit. The intravascular oxygenator is a device made up of several hundred gas-permeable hollow fibers that are inserted into the vena cava by femoral cut down. Flow of gas through each fiber adds $O_2$ and removes $CO_2$ from the bloodstream. Insertion of the IVOX was found to decrease cardiac index and systemic oxygen delivery despite maximum fluid and inotropic support in a study by Gentilello.[57] Mortality was 80%. Although some gas exchange occurred, the device did not allow significant reduction in the level of mechanical ventilatory support and adversely affected systemic oxygen transport. It is unclear what role IVOX may eventually play in the treatment of severe respiratory failure, although the concept is exciting because it does not require extracorporeal circulation.

## Decision to Terminate Ventilatory Support

### *The New Approach to Weaning*

The process of weaning the patient from mechanical ventilation now begins as soon as the patient can begin spontaneous breathing. The primary goal of the clinical team is to determine when mechanical ventilatory support is no longer needed. Although the patient's respiratory status is considered the most important factor, nonrespiratory variables such as nutritional status, cardiac function, sepsis, and mental status have varying influences. The mental processing leading up to the decision must combine art with science. Newer monitoring techniques may transform much of the art into the arena of science, benefiting the patient by providing increased safety while reducing the number of days of ventilation.

Criteria have been designed to address alveolar ventilation and oxygenation (Table 4–1) on a short-term basis, though total elimination of ventilatory support is an endurance-related phenomenon. Many weaning parameters (e.g., vital capacity, negative inspiratory pressure, minute ventilation) that address respiratory muscle pump strength, lack specificity and negative predictive value.[58–60] In addition, the weaning method chosen (e.g., abrupt discontinuation, T-piece, IMV, PSV) has not been shown to influence weaning outcome.[61] Both of these statements reflect the large number of patients who received ventilatory support for a short time without significant disease. Thus, success reflects the underlying ability of the patient to ventilate adequately rather than the precision of the test or mode of weaning. In patients requiring prolonged ventilatory support (> 72 hours), work of breathing may be a reliable parameter because it directly assesses endurance rather than using indirect inferences such as respiratory rate or frequency (f) even when combined with tidal volume ($V_T$). Extubation should be based upon (1) the resolution of initial indications for ventilatory support, (2) satisfactory overall clinical status, (3) no need for airway control (or tracheostomy present), (4) appropriate mental status and, (5) acceptable breathing pattern.

### *Weaning with IMV*

The concept of IMV supposes that the patient's spontaneous breathing efforts plus mechanical ventilations result in a clinically acceptable breathing pattern and adequate alveolar ventilation. The three most common criteria used in this assessment are arterial pH > 7.35, $PaCO_2 \leq 45$ torr (in previously eucapneic patient), and a spontaneous respiratory rate < 30 breaths per minute. The IMV rate is reduced 2 breaths per minute at the clinician's discretion, perhaps every 1–2 hours as long as the above criteria are satisfied. If not, mechanical ventilation is increased until a satisfactory ventilatory status is obtained. After the rate has been reduced to 2, final weaning (extubation) proceeds when desired. Also, satisfactory oxygenation at 5 cm $H_2O$ PEEP or CPAP must precede extubation. This is still a simple and effective way to wean patients who are prophylactically ventilated or after early intervention.

### *Weaning with Pressure Support Ventilation*

Pressure support ventilation supplements the patient's efforts and results in lower peak airway pressures, coordination, a full range of respiratory muscle excursion, and greater patient comfort. The ventilator-added pressure enables the patient to perform high-volume, low-pressure work, associated with endurance, even though compliance is reduced. MacIntyre and Leatherman[44] advocate beginning with PSV maximum, usually 10 mL/kg tidal volume. However, at this level of PSV the patient does little if any work of breathing. At tidal volumes of 7–8 mL/kg, most patients perform 0.3–0.6 J/L, a normal workload. Pressure support is decremented by 2–3 cm $H_2O$. In short-term ventilation, blood gases and clinical assessment are sufficient to assess weaning. Low levels of PSV (5 cm or less) may cause increased inspiratory muscle loading as the patient's inspiratory flow demand exceeds the flow capacity of the ventilator (Fig. 4–5). The resulting tachypnea may be interpreted as ventilatory failure and ventilatory support augmented inappropriately. In actuality, extubation is all that is required. PSV may be used in long-term ventilation. Work of breathing measurements may help select appropriate support levels more accurately than respiratory rate alone.

### *PEEP/CPAP Auto PEEP*

Auto PEEP is persistent positive alveolar pressure at the end of the exhalation cycle during mechanical ventilation. It is also termed occult PEEP or intrinsic PEEP and will artificially increase central venous pressure and pulmonary capillary wedge pressure readings, limit the accuracy of monitored respiratory mechanical variables, and especially increase inspiratory work of breathing.[62] The patient exhales through the combined resistances of the endotracheal tube and exhalation (positive pressure) valve, increasing the expiratory time constant. If inspiration begins before the prior exhalation has been completed, alveolar pressure will not have returned to baseline airway pressure nor will inspired tidal volume have exited completely. This is termed air trapping or dynamic hyperinflation. Factors leading to dynamic hyperinflation include a prolonged time constant (resistance × compliance), shortened expiratory time, and increased tidal volume. Finally, to initiate gas flow for the next breath, the patient must decrease airway pressure sufficiently to activate the ventilator (sensitivity).

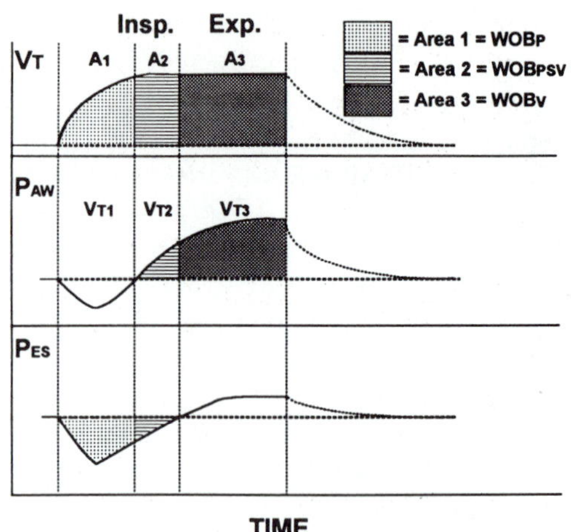


**Figure 4–5.** Work of breathing during pressure support and assist control ventilation. Patient work of breathing ($WOB_P$) is the amount of work done by the respiratory muscles to move a given volume of gas during spontaneous breathing or in a ventilator-assisted breath. Ventilator work of breathing ($WOB_V$) is the physical force required by the ventilator to move a given volume of gas into the lung with a relaxed chest wall.

A greater change in intrapleural pressure is required in the presence of auto PEEP as the change in intrapleural pressure must first overcome the elevation above baseline and then activate the demand valve. Thus, the patient must perform more work, the product of the change in pressure and change in volume. A number of adverse effects may occur, including hypoxemia and hypercarbia, and chief among these is a decrease in the elastic force generated by the inspiratory muscles because of the unfavorable position on the length tension curve, again resulting in an increase in inspiratory work of breathing. Auto PEEP can be displayed on most respiratory monitors.[63] When present, it may be decreased by lengthening expiratory time or decreasing tidal volume. Treating bronchospasm if present might also decrease auto PEEP.

### *Weaning from PEEP or CPAP*

Patients who have adequate ventilatory ability and can maintain normal $PaCO_2$ while breathing spontaneously but are hypoxemic can be treated with PEEP or CPAP to increase functional residual capacity (FRC) which will improve arterial $Po_2$. The term PEEP is often used to indicate end-expiratory pressure (EEP) added during mechanical ventilation, while CPAP refers to continuous positive EEP during spontaneous breathing or IMV when flows are adjusted to maintain inspiratory airway pressure above 0 during the entire cycle. The level of EEP is not the only determinant of the overall effects of PEEP or CPAP on the lungs or cardiovascular system. Mean airway pressure is higher during positive pressure ventilation with PEEP, whereas the mean airway pressure is slightly lower than EEP during CPAP breathing. High airway pressures may cause a redistribution of blood flow in the lungs. In addition to increasing FRC and decreasing intrapulmonary shunt, PEEP increases ventilation to lung units with low ventilation perfusion ($\dot{V}/\dot{Q}$) ratios. We use EEP when $Pao_2$ is < 65 mm Hg or $Fio_2$ is > 0.40. High levels of inspired oxygen depress mucocilliary motion, enhance mediator-induced pulmonary damage, and worsen the already abnormally low $\dot{V}/\dot{Q}$ ratios. Because PEEP may reduce venous return and cardiac output, fluid status should be monitored and hypovolemia corrected as PEEP is increased, usually in 2–3 cm $H_2O$ increments. Individuals and institutions differ in their conception of the best or optimal PEEP. Our preferences reflect fear of the detrimental aspects of $Fio_2$, which definitely may occur at levels > 0.6 and possibly as low as $Fio_2$ = 0.4. Though it had been common practice to use pulmonary artery catheters routinely at PEEP > 15 cm $H_2O$, having recognized the importance of adequate fluid resuscitation, we now selectively use catheters only when cardiac compromise is suspected or high levels of PEEP (e.g., > 25 cm $H_2O$) are used. Weaning is the same process in reverse: 2–3 cm $H_2O$ decrements in PEEP and decrease in $Fio_2$ as long as $Pao_2$ > 65 or $Spo_2$ > 0.90. "Minimal support" is reached when PEEP = 5 cm $H_2O$ and $Fio_2$ = 0.3.

### *Final Weaning Process*

A CPAP room-air trial (15 minutes, CPAP = 5 cm $H_2O$ PEEP, $Fio_2$ = 0.21) serves as an adequate test for 80–90% of patients, especially those ventilated for a short time. Using these criteria, we have achieved a 92% successful extubation rate.[64] If the results of the CPAP room air trial are $Pao_2$ > 55 mm Hg, pH > 7.35 and $Paco_2$ < 45 mm Hg (prior eucapnea) with a respiratory rate of < 30 breaths per minute, the patient is extubated. Following extubation, pulse oximetry is used to follow oxygenation continuously, and blood gases at $Fio_2$ = 0.21 are determined periodically.

Increased but undetected imposed work of breathing ($WOB_{Imp}$) may be interpreted as a patient's physiologic failure (e.g., tachypnea, accessory muscle use, etc.) and weaning attempts halted, prolonging intubation, even if blood gas criteria were satisfied. For these patients, the additional imposed work of breathing of the breathing apparatus causes the failure to successfully complete the final weaning test. If the clinician erroneously concludes that the cause of the failure is physiologic and decides that the patient should remain intubated, the opportunity to extubate the patient safely is missed and intubation and ventilation prolonged. If tachypnea develops during the CPAP room air trial, we believe that the work of breathing should be measured: If total work is low (< 0.8 J/L), the patient is extubated. If total work is high (> 0.8 J/L), the $WOB_{Imp}$ is determined and $WOB_{Phys}$ calculated. If the $WOB_{Phys}$ is < 0.8, the patient can be extubated safely.

## Monitoring During Therapy

### *Invasive Cardiovascular Monitoring*

Functional cardiovascular compromise, often present in patients undergoing cardiovascular and thoracic surgery, can be detected and treated by invasive cardiovascular monitoring. Therapy to improve respiratory function may compromise cardiovascular function and arterial hypoxemia may be produced by both cardiac and pulmonary components. Arterial catheterization provides direct monitoring of arterial blood pressure and ready access for arterial blood specimens. In stable patients, pulse oximetry for measuring arterial oxygen saturation may suffice. A pulmonary artery catheter measures left ventricular and right ventricular filling pressures, pulmonary artery pressures, mixed venous oxygen saturation and cardiac output. The basic information from blood gases and arterial and pulmonary artery catheters can be used to calculate many derived variables. The necessary data bases to quantitate both cardiac and respiratory function are listed in Tables 4–4 and 4–5. Invasive cardiovascular monitoring provides precise information to dispel the uncertainty of clinical judgment.[65]

### *Continuous Mixed Venous Oximetry ($S\bar{v}o_2$)*

($S\bar{v}o_2$) is helpful in the assessment of oxygen supply/demand relationship in critically ill patients. The normal range for $S\bar{v}o_2$ in healthy subjects is 0.65–0.80 with an average of .75 corresponding to a $P\bar{v}o_2$ of 40 mm Hg at a normal pH of 7.4. A rapid or prolonged fall from the normal range suggests significant deterioration, but it cannot distinguish among decreased cardiac output, increased oxygen consumption, or change in oxygen content. It is a signal that further data are needed. However, Astiz and colleagues[66] were unable to identify the critical levels of $S\bar{v}o_2$ associated with lactic acidosis in patients with sepsis or acute myocardial infarction. Potential cost savings lie in decreased use of other intermittent tools, i.e., cardiac output measurements and venous blood gas analysis. Continuous $S\bar{v}o_2$ monitoring serves three major functions. First, it serves as an indicator of adequacy of the oxygen supply/demand balance of perfused tissue. Second, continuous measure of $S\bar{v}o_2$ may function as an early warning signal of cardiopulmonary deterioration. Third, continuous monitoring $S\bar{v}o_2$ may improve the efficacy of the delivery of critical care by providing immediate feedback as to the effectiveness of

**TABLE 4–4. MEASURED AND DERIVED HEMODYNAMIC PARAMETERS**

| Parameter (Abbreviation) | Measurements/Calculations | Normal Range |
|---|---|---|
| Systolic blood pressure (SBP) | Direct measurement | 100–140 mm Hg |
| Diastolic blood pressure (DBP) | Direct measurement | 60–90 mm Hg |
| Pulmonary artery systolic pressure (PASP) | Direct measurement | 15–30 mm Hg |
| Pulmonary artery diastolic pressure (PADP) | Direct measurement | 4–12 mm Hg |
| Mean pulmonary artery pressure (MPAP) | Direct measurement | 9–16 mm Hg |
| Right ventricular systolic pressure (RVSP) | Direct measurement | 15–30 mm Hg |
| Right ventricular end-diastolic pressure (RVEDP) | Direct measurement | 0–8 mm Hg |
| Central venous pressure (CVP) | Direct measurement | 0–8 mm Hg |
| Pulmonary artery occlusion pressure (PAOP) | Direct measurement | 2–12 mm Hg |
| Cardiac output (CO) | Direct measurement | 4–6 L/min[a] |
| Mean arterial blood pressure (MAP)[a] | $MAP = DBP + \frac{(SBP - DBP)}{3}$ | 70–105 mm Hg |
| Cardiac index (CI) | $CI = \frac{CO}{BSA}$ | 2.8–4.2 L/min/m$^2$ |
| Stroke volume (SV) | $SV = \frac{CO}{HR}$ | 60–80 mL/beat[a] |
| Stroke index (SI) | $SI = \frac{SV}{BSA}$ | 30–65 mL/beat/m$^2$ |
| Left ventricular stroke-work index (LVSWI) | $LVSWI = \frac{SV \times (MAP - PAOP)}{BSA} \times 0.0136$ | 43–61 g × m/m$^2$ |
| Right ventricular stroke-work index (RVSWI) | $RVSWI = \frac{SV \times (MPAP - CVP)}{BSA} \times 0.0136$ | 7–12 g × m/m$^2$ |
| Systemic vascular resistance (SVR) | $SVR = \frac{MAP - CVP}{CO} \times 80$ | 900–1400 dyne × s × cm$^{-5}$ |
| Pulmonary vascular resistance (PVR) | $PVR = \frac{MPAP - PAOP}{CO} \times 80$ | 150–250 dyne × s × cm$^{-5}$ |
| Coronary perfusion pressure (CCP) | CPP = DBP − PAOP | 60–90 mm Hg |

BSA = body surface area; HR = heart rate.
[a] Varies with size.
[b] Can also be measured directly.

**TABLE 4–5. PARAMETERS DERIVED FROM BLOOD GAS ANALYSIS**

| Parameter (Abbreviation) | Measurements/Calculations | Normal Range |
|---|---|---|
| Arterial blood $O_2$ tension ($PaO_2$) | Direct measurement | 70–100 mm Hg |
| Arterial hemoglobin $O_2$ saturation ($SaO_2$) | Direct measurement | >0.92 (fraction) |
| Mixed venous blood $O_2$ tension ($P\bar{v}O_2$) | Direct measurement | 35–45 mm Hg |
| Mixed venous hemoglobin $O_2$ saturation ($S\bar{v}O_2$) | Direct measurement | 0.65–0.80 (fraction) |
| Arterial blood $O_2$ content ($CAO_2$) | $CaO_2 = (Hb \times SaO_2 \times 1.39) + (0.0031 \times PaO_2)$ | 16–22 mL $O_2$/dL blood |
| Mixed venous $O_2$ content $C\bar{v}O_2$ | $C\bar{v}O_2 = (Hb \times S\bar{v}O_2 \times 1.39) + (0.0031 \times P\bar{v}O_2)$ | 12–17 mL $O_2$/dL blood |
| Arterial-venous $O_2$ content difference ($C(a - \bar{v})O_2$) | $C(a - \bar{v})O_2 = CaO_2 - C\bar{v}O_2$ | 3.5–5.5 mL $O_2$/dL blood |
| $O_2$ delivery ($\dot{D}O_2$) | $\dot{D}O_2 = CaO_2 \times CO \times 10$ | 700–1400 mL/min |
| $O_2$ consumption ($\dot{V}O_2$) (Fick) | $\dot{V}O_2 = C(a - \bar{v})O_2 \times CO \times 10$ | 180–280 mL/min |
| $O_2$ utilization coefficient ($O_2UC$) | $O_2UC = \frac{\dot{V}O_2}{\dot{D}O_2} = \frac{C(a - \bar{v})O_2 \times CO}{CaO_2 \times CO} = \frac{C(a - \bar{v})O_2}{CaO_2}$ | 0.23–0.32 (fraction) |
| Physiologic shunt (venous admixture) ($\dot{Q}_{sp}/\dot{Q}_t$) | $\dot{Q}_{sp}/\dot{Q}_t = \frac{Cc'O_2 - CaO_2}{Cc'O_2 - C\bar{v}O_2}$ | 0.03–0.05 (fraction) |
| Pulmonary end-capillary $O_2$ content ($Cc'O_2$) | $Cc'O_2 = (Hb \times 1.39)^a + (0.0031 \times PAO_2)$ | [b] mL $O_2$/dL blood |
| Alveolar $O_2$ tension ($PAO_2$) | $PAO_2 = FIO_2 (P_B - P_{H_2O}) - \frac{PaCO_2}{RQ}$ | [b] mm Hg |

Hb = hemoglobin concentration; CO = cardiac output; $FIO_2$ = inspired $O_2$ fraction: $P_B$ = barometric pressure; $P_{H_2O}$ = partial pressure of water vapor (47 mm Hg at 37°C); $PaCO_2$ = arterial blood $CO_2$ tension; RQ = respiratory quotient ($CO_2$ production/$O_2$ consumption).
[a]Assumes 100% Hb saturation.
[b]Varies with $FIO_2$.

therapeutic interventions aimed at improving oxygen transport balance.

### Cardiorespiratory Interactions

Should ventilatory support improve arterial oxygenation and yet compromise cardiac output and lower total oxygen delivery, the patient would not be well served.

Arterial oxygenation is determined by inspired oxygen tension, alveolar oxygen tension, pH, temperature, mixed venous oxygen content, diffusion of oxygen, the $\dot{V}/\dot{Q}$ abnormalities, and the intrapulmonary shunting. The influence of venous oxygen content upon arterial oxygenation is often not appreciated. Increased intrapulmonary shunt and decreased venous oxygen content both lower arterial oxygen tension. An increased shunt will add a greater volume of poorly oxygenated blood, and a decreased venous oxygen content will have an increased dilutional effect. If cardiac output is decreased, and if oxygen consumption must be maintained, more oxygen will be extracted from the arterial blood. This results in a diminished venous oxygen content, producing an increase in the arterial-venous oxygen content difference. This mixed venous blood, when shunted through the lungs, will then result in diminished arterial oxygen tension. For instance (Fig. 4–6), a patient with a 20% intrapulmonary shunt and normal cardiovascular function (cardiac output = 5 L/min) would have an arterial oxygen tension of 250 torr at an inspired oxygen tension ($FIO_2$) of 1.0 (100% oxygen). *Without altering pulmonary function*, decreasing cardiac output to 2.5 L/min would result in an arterial oxygen tension of 90 torr (Fig. 4–7). This decrease in oxygen tension from 250 to 90 torr occurs because the cardiac output is decreased. Because this effect is so important and can only be recognized by proper testing, ventilatory support must include cardiovascular monitoring to quantify its effects upon arterial oxygen tension.

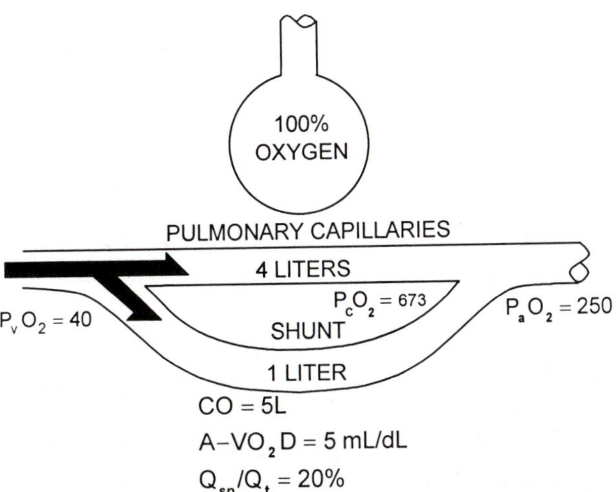


**Figure 4–6.** Relationship between cardiac and pulmonary effect upon arterial oxygen tension. Note normal cardiac output (5 L/min) and $A - VO_2$ difference (5 mL/dL). With $FIO_2 = 1.0$, a 20% shunt results in an arterial $PO_2$ of 250 torr.

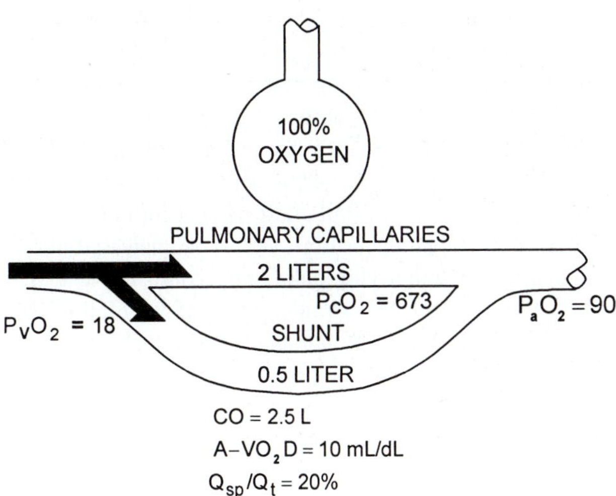


**Figure 4–7.** Cardiac output falls to 2.5 L/min, $A-VO_2$ difference increases to 10 mL/dL to maintain oxygen consumption. Intrapulmonary shunt remains unchanged, but shunting highly desaturated mixed venous blood lowers arterial $PO_2$ to 90 torr.

### Gastric Tonometry

The gastric intramucosal $pH_i$ is a measure of tissue pH; normal $pH_i$ is 7.38 ± 0.03 and is unrelated to the pH of gastric juice, normally pH 1–7. The measurement provides clinicians with a specific index of the adequacy of tissue oxygenation. A normal $pH_i$ is indicative of a normoxic tissue, a low $pH_i$ of a dysoxic tissue. The gut has been called the "canary" of the body[67] because of the selective impact of endogenous vasoconstrictors and a high demand for oxygen, making gastric mucosa a desirable site to detect inadequate tissue oxygenation. $pH_i$ seems to be a good prognostic indicator of outcome, especially major morbidity and organ system failure, and suggests the need for more aggressive resuscitation in cardiac surgical patients. It may also reduce ICU costs and ICU stay. ICU mortality and multiple organ system failure have been confined in large part to those who seem hemodynamically compensated, yet still have a low $pH_i$.[68] Resuscitative efforts aimed at reversing the inadequacy of mucosal oxygenation may prevent multiple system failure and improve survival.

## Special Situations

### Flail Chest

Flail chest is encountered primarily after direct thoracic injury, whether induced by an automobile accident or after cardiopulmonary resuscitation. Flail chest can be divided into orthopedic and pulmonary components. In order to create a "flail" segment—one that moves paradoxically inward with inspiration—it is necessary to have fractures of the ribs and/or sternum in two separate places so that a segment of chest wall is no longer fixed during inspiration and expiration. However, this paradoxical motion rarely results in hypoventilation. The flailing motion initially attracted the attention of clinicians to stabilize the segment, first with external traction and thereafter using "internal stabilization" by supplying continuous mechanical ventilation.[69] However, most patients with flail chest present initially with arterial hypoxemia and hypocarbia, signifying increased minute ventilation. The underlying pulmonary contusion and associated hypoxia seem to stimulate minute ventilation. The principle that increased minute ventilation does not require mechanical ventilatory support suggests that treatment should be directed to reversing hypoxemia through the restoration of functional residual capacity.[70] Thus, the techniques of IMV or PSV plus PEEP or CPAP seem appropriate. In many cases, mechanical support can be diminished rapidly utilizing CPAP to improve oxygenation; minute ventilation and respiratory rate then return to normal.

### *Unilateral Pulmonary Disease*

Physiologic principles governing ventilation–perfusion relationships can sometimes be utilized to improve oxygenation in patients with unilateral pulmonary disease. Major disease in one lung, such as lobar pneumonia, unilateral aspiration during thoracotomy in lateral position, or as a direct result of unilateral thoracic injury, occurs with some frequency and usually responds to conventional therapy as outlined above. However, in rare instances, this therapeutic approach worsens the already abnormal $\dot{V}/\dot{Q}$ ratios, and two alternatives may be considered.

With "positional" therapy, the diseased lung is positioned superiorly so that blood flow and ventilation increase to the dependent undamaged lung. This results in improvement of $\dot{V}/\dot{Q}$ matching and may improve arterial oxygen tension.[71,72] Rotational beds, providing lateral rotation to angles up to 70 degrees, can effect the necessary position changes. Rapid resolution of unilateral pulmonary contusion has been achieved in this manner.

Independent lung ventilation can also be used so that different tidal volume and PEEP can be delivered to each lung. This requires insertion of a Carlen's type endobronchial tube so that ventilation to each lung can be maintained independently. Selective CPAP and synchronous or nonsynchronous ventilation with one or two ventilators have been successfully utilized.

### *Bronchopleural Cutaneous Fistulas*

Patients, who have had pulmonary resection or pleurodesis, or who have suffered traumatic and iatrogenic pneumothorax, often develop bronchopleural cutaneous fistulas. Inspired gas always takes the path of least resistance, immediate egress of a large portion of the tidal volume through the bronchopleural cutaneous fistula. This loss is increased if suction is increased to the chest tube. In many instances, an increased tidal volume or ventilator rate can compensate for this volume loss. However, in rare circumstances, the increased total ventilatory support may depress cardiovascular function, produce further pulmonary barotrauma, or be unable to provide sufficient alveolar ventilation.

High-frequency, positive-pressure ventilation is presently the treatment of choice for massive bronchopleural fistulae, since adequate oxygenation and ventilation can be achieved at much lower airway pressures. By minimizing airway pressure changes during inspiration and expiration, high-frequency ventilation diminishes air loss through bronchopleural fistula. Similar results may be achievable with other pressure-limited mechanical ventilatory modes (i.e., APRV, PSV).[54] Simultaneous independent lung ventilation has also been used to direct the tidal volume to the lung that has not been afflicted by the bronchopleural cutaneous fistula. Obviously, this technique is only applicable if unilateral involvement is present.[72] Nonventilatory treatment approaches include use of fibrin and tissue glue adhesives, endobronchial occlusion coils, video thoracoscopy, and open thoracotomy with pedicle flap closure.[73,74]

### *Weaning the Long-Term Ventilator-Dependent Patient*

In the critically ill, hypermetabolic, ventilator-dependent, ICU patient, near total ventilatory support may cause atrophy of the respiratory muscles. If too little support had been provided, fatigue and use dystrophy would result.[12] The failure to wean or maintain spontaneous ventilation is often due to inadequate endurance, not inadequate strength of the respiratory muscle pump.[75] In the case of either disuse atrophy or use dystrophy, a period of ventilatory muscle training may help reestablish the patient's maximal ventilatory capacity, which in turn enables the patient to perform the normal physiologic work of breathing, weaning, and extubation. We use PSV and increase the afterload on the ventilatory muscles by placing external weights (four 1-L IV bags taped together) over the lower thorax and upper abdomen to increase the elastic work of breathing. We found a 50% reduction in PSV days in patients who had multiple weaning failures (e.g., tachypnea, abnormal blood gases, or required reintubation).[76] External chest weights seem to be a method to regain strength and endurance lost during long-term ventilatory support. In-line inspiratory resistive loading using either a nonlinear resistor device or a threshold breathing device are other methods that can also be employed with pressure support ventilation to achieve or recapture lost strength.[77,78] The noninvasive pulmonary monitor is used to titrate muscle afterload and inspiratory resistance to guide retraining and reconditioning.

## SUMMARY

Recent advances in our knowledge of the pathophysiology of acute and chronic respiratory failure have significantly revised our strategies for ventilatory support. Furthermore, technologic innovations have enabled the clinician to monitor the patient–ventilator interaction and variables previously available only in the laboratory. This combination has resulted in a variety of techniques so that individual problems can be specifically addressed.

## REFERENCES


1. Mulvey DA, Mallett SV, Browne DRG: Endotracheal intubation. *Intensive Care World* **10:**122, 1993
2. Heath ML: Endotracheal intubation through the laryngeal mask—helpful when laryngoscopy is difficult or dangerous. *Eur J Anaesthesiol* **14:**41, 1991
3. Heffner JE: Medical indications for tracheostomy. *Chest* **96:**186, 1989
4. Black AMS, Seegobin RD: Pressures on endotracheal tube cuffs. *Anesthesia* **36:**498, 1981
5. Bishop MJ: Mechanisms of laryngotracheal injury following prolonged tracheal intubation. *Chest* **96:**185, 1989
6. Marsh HM, Gillespie DJ, Baumgartner AE: Timing of tracheostomy in the critically ill patient. *Chest* **96:**190, 1989
7. MacKenzie CF, Shin B, McAslan TC, et al: Severe stridor after prolonged endotracheal intubation using high-volume cuffs. *Anesthesiology* **50:**235, 1979
8. Banner MJ, Blanch PB, Kirby RR: Imposed work of breathing and methods of triggering a demand-flow continuous positive airway pressure system. *Crit Care Med* **21:**183, 1993
9. Areus JF, LeJeune FE, Webre DR: Maxillary sinusitis, a complication of nasotracheal intubation. *Anesthesiology* **40:**415, 1974
10. Streitz JM, Shapshay SM: Airway injury after tracheotomy and endotracheal intubation. *Surg Clin North Am* **71:**1211, 1991
11. Friedman Y, Mayer AD: Bedside percutaneous tracheostomy in critically ill patients. *Chest* **104:**532, 1993
12. Civetta JM: Nosocomial respiratory failure or iatrogenic ventilator dependency. *Crit Care Med* **21:**171, 1993
13. Stoller JK, Kacmarek RM: Ventilatory strategies in the management of the adult respiratory distress syndrome. *Clin Chest Med* **11:**755, 1990
14. Windsor AC, Mullen PG, Fowler AA, et al: Role of the neutrophil in adult respiratory distress syndrome. *Br J Surg* **80:**10, 1993
15. Rodriguez JL: Hospital-acquired gram-negative pneumonia in critically ill injured patients. *Am J Surg* **165:**34S, 1993
16. Hyers TM, Tricomi SM, Dettenmeier PA, et al: Tumor necrosis factor levels in serum and bronchoalveolar lavage fluid of patients with the adult respiratory distress syndrome. *Am Rev Respir Dis* **144:**268, 1991
17. Sutter PM, Sutter S, Girardin E, et al: High bronchoalveolar levels of tumor necrosis factor and its inhibitors, interleukin-1, interferon, and elastase in patients with adult respiratory distress syndrome after trauma shock or sepsis. *Am Rev Respir Dis* **145:**1016, 1992
18. St. John RC, Dorinsky PM: Immunologic therapy for ARDS, septic shock and multiple-organ failure. *Chest* **103:**932, 1993
19. Hubmayr RD, Abel MD, Rehder K: Physiologic approach to mechanical ventilation. *Crit Care Med* **18:**103, 1990
20. Banner MJ, Jaeger MJ, Kirby RR: Components of the work of breathing and implications for monitoring ventilator dependent patients. *Crit Care Med* **22:**515, 1994
21. Kirton OC, Banner MJ, Axelrad A, et al: Detection of unsuspected imposed work of breathing: Case reports. *Crit Care Med* **21:**790, 1993
22. Kolobow T, Moretti MP, Fumagalli R, et al: Severe impairment in lung function induced by high peak airway pressure during mechanical ventilation—an experimental study. *Am Rev Respir Dis* **135:**312, 1987
23. Dreyfuss D, Soler P, Bassett G, et al: High inflation pressure pulmonary edema—respective effects of high airway pressure, high tidal volume, and positive end-expiratory pressure. *Am Rev Respir Dis* **137:**1159, 1988
24. Zapol W: Volutrauma and the intravenous oxygenator in patients with adult respiratory distress syndrome *(editorial). Anesthesiology* **77:**847, 1992
25. Banner MJ, Kirby RR, Blanch PB: Site of pressure measurement during spontaneous breathing with continuous positive airway pressure: Effect on calculating imposed work of breathing. *Crit Care Med* **20:**528, 1992
26. Yang KL, Tobin MJ: A prospective study of indexes predicting the outcome of trials of weaning from mechanical ventilation. *N Engl J Med* **324:**1445, 1991
27. Jabour ER, Rabil DM, Truwit JD, et al: Evaluation of a new weaving index based on ventilatory endurance and the efficiency of gas exchange. *Am Rev Respir Dis* **144:**531, 1991
28. Kirton OC, Banner M, DeHaven CB, et al: Respiratory rate and related assessments are poor inferences of patient work of breathing. *Crit Care Med* **21:**5242, 1993
29. Shikora SA, Benotti PN, Johannigman JA: The oxygen cost of breathing may predict weaning from mechanical ventilation better than the respiratory rate to tidal volume ratio. *Arch Surg* **129:**269, 1994
30. Lee KH, Hui KP, Chan TB, et al: Rapid shallow breathing (frequency-tidal volume ratio) did not predict extubation outcome. *Chest* **105:**540, 1994
31. Bone RC: Compliance and dynamic characteristics curve in acute respiratory failure. *Crit Care Med* **4:**173, 1976
32. Ross A, Gottfried SB, Zocchi L, et al: Measurement of static compliance of the total respiratory system in patients with acute respiratory failure during mechanical ventilation. *Am Rev Respir Dis* **131:**672, 1985
33. Boysen PG: Respiratory muscle function and weaning from mechanical ventilation. *Respir Care* **32:**572, 1987
34. Marini JJ: Monitoring during mechanical ventilation. *Clin Chest Med* **9:**73, 1988
35. Collett PW, Perry C, Engle LA: Pressure time product, flow and oxygen cost of resistive breathing in human. *J Appl Physiol* **58:**1263, 1985
36. Grassino A, Macklem P: Respiratory muscle fatigue and ventilator failure. *Ann Rev Med* **35:**625, 1984
37. Matthay MA: The adult respiratory distress syndrome—definition and prognosis. *Clin Chest Med* **11:**575, 1990
38. Weingarteen M: Respiratory monitoring of carbon dioxide and oxygen: A ten year perspective. *J Clin Monit* **6:**217, 1990
39. Varon AJ, Morrina J, Civetta JM: Clinical utility of a calorimetric end-tidal $CO_2$ detector in cardiopulmonary resuscitation and emergency intubation. *J Clin Monit* **7:**289, 1991
40. Hoffman RA, Krieger BPL: End tidal carbon dioxide in critically ill patients during changes in mechanical ventilation. *Am Rev Respir Dis* **140:**1265, 1989
41. Tobin MJ: Mechanical ventilation. *N Engl J Med* **330:**1056, 1994
42. Kirton OC, DeHaven BC, Morgan J, et al: Endotracheal tube flow resistance and elevated imposed work of breathing masquerading as ventilator weaning intolerance. *Chest* **104:**1335, 1993
43. Banner MJ, Kirby RR, Blanch PB, et al: Decreased imposed work of the breathing apparatus to zero using pressure support ventilation. *Crit Care Med* **21:**1333, 1993
44. MacIntyre NR, Leatherman NE: Ventilatory muscle loads and the frequency-tidal volume pattern during inspiratory pressure-assisted (pressure-support) ventilation. *Am Rev Respir Dis* **141:**327, 1990
45. Slutsky AS: ACCP consensus conference mechanical ventilation. *Respir Care* **38:**1389, 1993
46. Tokioka H, Saito S, Kosaka F: Comparison of pressure support venti-

lation and assist control ventilation in patients with acute respiratory failure. *Intens Care Med* **15**:364, 1989
47. Marcy TW, Marini JJ: Inverse ratio ventilation in ARDS—rationale and implementation. *Chest* **100**:494, 1991
48. Chan K, Abraham E: Effects of inverse ratio ventilation on cardiorespiratory parameters in severe respiratory failure. *Chest* **102**:1556, 1992
49. Abraham E, Yoshihara G: Cardiorespiratory effects of pressure controlled inverse ratio ventilation in severe respiratory failure. *Chest* **96**:1356, 1989
50. Mercat A, Graini L, Teboul JL, et al: Cardiorespiratory effects of pressure controlled ventilation with and without inverse ratio in the adult respiratory distress syndrome. *Chest* **104**:871, 1993
51. Rouby JJ, Ameur MB, Jawish D, et al: Continuous positive airway pressure (CPAP) vs intermittent mandatory pressure release ventilation (IMPRV) in patients with acute respiratory failure. *Intens Care Med* **18**:69, 1992
52. Räsänen J, Cane RD, Downs JB, et al: Airway pressure release ventilation during acute lung injury: A prospective multi-center trial. *Crit Care Med* **19**:1234, 1991
53. Standiford TJ, Morganroth ML: High-frequency ventilation. *Chest* **96**:1380, 1989
54. Bray JG, Cane RD: Mechanical ventilatory support and pulmonary parenchymal injury: positive airway pressure or alveolar hyperinflation. *Intens Crit Care Digest* **12**:33, 1993
55. Gattinoni L, Kolobow T, Tomlinson T, et al: Low frequency positive pressure ventilation with extra corporeal $CO_2$ removal in severe acute respiratory failure. *JAMA* **256**:881, 1986
56. Pesenti A, Gattinoni L, Bombino M: Long term extracorporeal respiratory support: 20 years of progress. *Intens Crit Care Digest* **12**:15, 1993
57. Gentilello LM, Jurkovich GJ, Gubler KD, et al: The intravascular oxygenator (IVOX): preliminary results of a new means of performing extra pulmonary gas exchange. *J Trauma* **35**:399, 1993
58. Fiastro JF, Habib MP, Shon BY, et al: Comparison of standard weaning parameters and the mechanical work of breathing in mechanically ventilated patients. *Chest* **94**:232, 1988
59. DeHaven CB, Hurst JM, Branson RD: Evaluation of two different extubation criteria: attributes contributing to success. *Crit Care Med* **14**:92, 1986
60. Jounieavx V, Duran A, Levi-Valensi P: Synchronized intermittent mandatory ventilation with and without pressure support ventilation in weaning patients with COPD from mechanical ventilation. *Chest* **105**:1204, 1994
61. Tomlinson JR, Miller KS, Lorch DG, et al: A prospective comparison of IMV and T-piece weaning from mechanical ventilation. *Chest* **96**:348, 1989
62. Brown DG, Pierson D: Auto-PEEP is common in mechanically ventilated patients: A study of incidence, severity and detection. *Respir Care* **31**:1069, 1986
63. Haluska J, Chartrand DA, Grassino AE, et al: Intrinsic PEEP and arterial $PCO_2$ in stable patients with chronic obstructive pulmonary disease. *Am Rev Respir Dis* **141**:1194, 1990
64. Dagostino DW, DeHaven B, Kirton OC, et al: Elective extubation failures in a surgical ICU using a room air-CPAP trial criteria: Frequency and cause. *Chest* **104**:1445, 1993
65. Swan HJC: Monitoring the seriously ill patient with heart disease (including use of Swan-Ganz catheter). In JW Hurst (ed). *The Heart*, 7th ed, chap 120. McGraw-Hill, New York, 1990
66. Astiz ME, Rackow EC, Kaufman B: Relationship of oxygen delivery and mixed venous oxygenation to lactic acidosis in patients with sepsis and acute myocardial infraction. *Crit Care Med* **16**:655, 1988
67. Dantzker DR: Adequacy of tissue oxygenation. *Crit Care Med* **21**:S40, 1993
68. Mythen MG, Webb AR: Intra-operative gut mucosal hypoperfusion is associated with increased post-operative complications and cost. *Intens Care Med* **20**:99, 1994
69. Freedland M, Wilson RF, Bender JS, et al: The management of flail chest injury: factors affecting outcome. *J Trauma* **30**:1460, 1990
70. Zimmerman T, Muhrer KH, Padberg W, et al: Closure of acute bronchial stump insufficiency with a musculus latissimus dorsi flap. *Thorac Cardiovasc Surg* **56**:644, 1993
71. Marcum RF, Norwood SH: Trendelenburg positioning to correcy hypoxemia from chest trauma. *Chest* **85**:716, 1984
72. Crim G, Candiani A, Conti G, et al: Clinical application of independent lung ventilation with unilateral high-frequency jet ventilation (ILV-UHFJV). *Intens Care Med* **12**:90, 1986
73. Ferguson MK: Thoracoscopy for empyema, bronchopleural fistula, andchylothorax (review). *Ann Thoracic Surg* **56**:644, 1993
74. Litmanovitch M, Joynt GM, Cooper PJ, et al: Persistent bronchopleural fistula in a patient with adult respiratory distress syndrome, treatment with pressure-controlled ventilation. *Chest* **104**:1901, 1993
75. Tobin MJ: Respiratory muscles in disease. *Clin Chest Med* **9**:263, 1988
76. Kirton OC, Civetta JM, Murtha M. et al: Respiratory muscle conditioning may improve outcome of pressure support weaning. *Chest* **104**:494, 1993
77. Larson JL, Kim MJ, Sharp JT, et al: Inspiratory muscle training with a pressure threshold breathing device in patients with chronic obstructive pulmonary disease. *Am Rev Respir Dis* **138**:689, 1988
78. Harver A, Mahler DA, Daubenspeck JA: Targeted inspiratory muscle training improves respiratory muscle function and reduces dyspnea in patients with chronic obstructive pulmonary disease. *Ann Intern Med* **111**:117, 1989

CHAPTER

# 5

# Thoracic Incisions

Richard F. Heitmiller

## INTRODUCTION

The reason why a chapter on thoracic incisions is included in thoracic surgery texts is that thoracic anatomy, by virtue of its large-volume intrathoracic space; separate pleural spaces; and rigid, ribbed chest wall, makes specific incision selection crucial to the ease and safety of a given thoracic procedure. The development and evolution of thoracic surgical incisions has been closely related to developments in thoracic surgery. Prior to the introduction of methods allowing safe open pleural space procedures, thoracic incisions were used predominantly to drain localized infectious pulmonary and pleural space complications, or they were ingenious techniques employing extrapleural approaches to lower thoracic structures.[1] With the advent of general endotracheal anesthesia, major open thoracic procedures became possible. Wide-exposure thoracotomy incisions were stressed. Subsequently, the emphasis shifted to more conservative thoracotomy techniques including rib and muscle sparing, and skin incisions that were more cosmetically appealing. The evolution of cardiac surgery has made the median sternotomy one of the most widely used thoracic incisions. Currently, video-thoracoscopic surgery has introduced a whole new array of incision options.

## PRINCIPLES

Regardless of the specific incision used, there are certain principles shared by all approaches to optimize the likelihood of a successful outcome. A thoracic incision must *provide adequate exposure.* If a small incision with limited exposure is planned, the incision must be placed directly over the underlying lesion. Preoperative radiographic localization is often helpful.[2] For major open procedures, the incision should give adequate exposure to the area of greatest expected operative difficulty. Options for achieving wider exposure, if necessary, such as extending the original incision, counterincisions, or perpendicular "T-off" incisions, should be considered in advance. Creation of excess skin flaps are best avoided.

After adequate exposure to permit a safe operative procedure, the next priority is to *preserve chest wall function and appearance.* Examples of this principle include muscle sparing techniques, rib preservation, protection of the neurovascular bundles, and avoiding excessive rib or sternal retraction. Skin incisions are ideally placed along Langer's lines or otherwise positioned to minimize visibility as with a low vertical median sternotomy incision, and with use of axillary thoracotomy techniques.

For closure, *rigid chest wall reapproximation* and strict *layered closure* are the rule. Excess rib or sternal motion decrease the efficiency of chest wall mechanics and increase the work of breathing. Therefore, as with a flail segment, there is an increased likelihood for retained secretions and respiratory failure. Chest wall motion also contributes to postoperative incisional pain and may increase the chance of wound complications. Strict layered closure means that all divided tissues should be reapproximated even if the tissue seems insignificant. In doing so, divided individual chest wall muscles are not pexed to deeper layers or other muscles that may delay their recovery or range of motion. As well, a layered closure *isolates* the wound layers. Therefore, if a superficial infection develops, it remains superficial, without deeper extension to form a more serious infectious problem such as mediastinitis or empyema.

### Median Sternotomy

#### *Indications*

The median sternotomy incision, by virtue of its anterior, midline, vertical configuration, provides a broad range of lower cervical and intrathoracic exposure. Median sternotomy, partial or complete, has been advocated for lower cervical procedures including tracheal resection and reconstruction,[3] excision of thyroid masses or parathyroid adenomas, lower cervical lymph node dissection,[4] and resection of cervical esophageal tumors.[5,6] Within the chest, all mediastinal tumors and cysts bilaterally are potentially accessible using this incision. Exposure of mediastinal structures decreases from anterior to middle to posterior mediastinum. The excellent exposure of the heart and great vessels has made median sternotomy the gold standard incision for most cardiac surgical procedures, especially those requiring cardiopulmonary bypass. Finally, median sternotomy allows access to the lungs, their hila, and pleural spaces bilaterally. Urschel and Razzuk[7] and Cooper et al[8] have stressed the utility and technical aspects of using median sternotomy for pulmonary resection. Numerous reports advocate using median sternotomy to perform bilateral pulmonary metastasectomy.[9–13] In patients who have previously undergone thoracotomy, who now require redo pulmonary resection, especially pneumonectomy, this incision provides a relatively adhesion-free approach to the pulmonary hilum.

### Advantages

The advantages of this incision are that it is quick to perform and yields excellent exposure of the heart, proximal great vessels, and anterior mediastinum. As a midline incision, it permits exposure of both lungs, their hila, and pleural spaces. The median sternotomy incision is safe; heals quickly (especially true for partial sternal split); and, compared with a thoracotomy, produces less incisional pain.

### Disadvantages

Many find the vertical skin incision unsightly. Median sternotomy gives limited exposure of the lower chest and posterior mediastinum bilaterally. Depending on a patient's size, and the shape of the chest, there is often variability in the exposure obtained. Disadvantages also include postoperative complications, most notably unstable sternum, sternal osteomyelitis, and mediastinitis.

### Technique

**Standard Sternotomy.** The technique of median sternotomy has been well described previously and has not significantly changed. The standard approach uses a vertical midline incision beginning at or below the sternal notch, extending to at least the xiphoid tip and often several centimeters below. The dissection is then carried down in the midline with the electrocautery to the anterior table of the sternum. The superior end of the skin incision is then retracted cephalad in order to delineate the superior edge of the manubrium. A crossing anterior jugular vein within the suprasternal space of Burns should be sought and controlled. The dissection is continued for a short distance retrosternally either digitally or with a short-tipped, right-angled clamp. Inferiorly, the xiphoid process is dissected out, split in the midline with heavy straight scissors, and the inferior, retrosternal space entered. The sternum is then vertically divided, in the midline, using an oscillating saw, or less commonly, a Lebsche knife or Gigli saw. Hemostasis is obtained using the electrocautery to control bleeding vessels from the cut periosteal edges. Some also use bone wax to control marrow bleeding. Specially designed sternal retractors, with blades designed to distribute evenly the retraction tension along the cut sternal edges, minimize the chance of injury to the sternum and are preferable to standard rib spreaders. The sternal retractor should not be placed too high along the sternum to avoid the risk of injury to the innominate vein or brachial plexus.

Following appropriate drainage of the mediastinum or pleural space, the sternal edges are rigidly reapproximated. Numerous reports have been published on how to rejoin optimally the sternal edges using parasternal sutures, mersilene ribbon,[14] or stainless steel bands[15] or wire. The use of absorbable sutures has been shown to be safe and effective in both adults[16] and children.[17] Increasingly, the effectiveness of a figure of eight suture technique to reapproximate the sternum is being appreciated. DiMarco et al[18] stressed two crucial technical factors common to successful sternal closure. The first is the use of a figure of eight suture technique, which avoids direct perpendicular sternal wire shear, and the second is some method to reinforce the lateral table of the sternum, which allows for tighter sternal closure. The authors advocate an interlocking figure of eight sternal wire closure technique that simply accomplishes these goals (Fig. 5–1). For those patients in whom the sternum is fractured or osteoporotic, Robicsek et al[19] described a sternal wire weave technique that reenforces the sternal edges for secure closure. After sternal closure, the remainder of the wound is closed in layers.

Some have found the vertical skin incision, especially at its upper end, cosmetically unappealing, and have therefore advocated a low vertical,[20] a Y-shaped or champagne glass, or a submammary incision.[21,22] The advocates of each approach stress the superior cosmetic appearance, and that exposure is not compromised.

**Open Sternotomy.** Furnary et al[23] reported leaving an open sternotomy as adjunctive therapy of the severely impaired heart in 1.8% of adults undergoing open cardiac procedures. The indications for prolonged open sternotomy was hemodynamic instability (37%), myocardial edema (17%), intractable bleeding (22%), arrythmia (8%), and implantation of ventricular assist device (16%). In their series, 67% of patients who underwent delayed sternal closure survived and were discharged home. Predictors of mortality in patients with prolonged open sternotomy were renal insufficiency and serious ventricular arrhythmias.

**Reoperative Sternotomy.** Reoperative median sternotomy for cardiac procedures carries an increased mortality over initial sternotomy. The increased mortality is directly re-

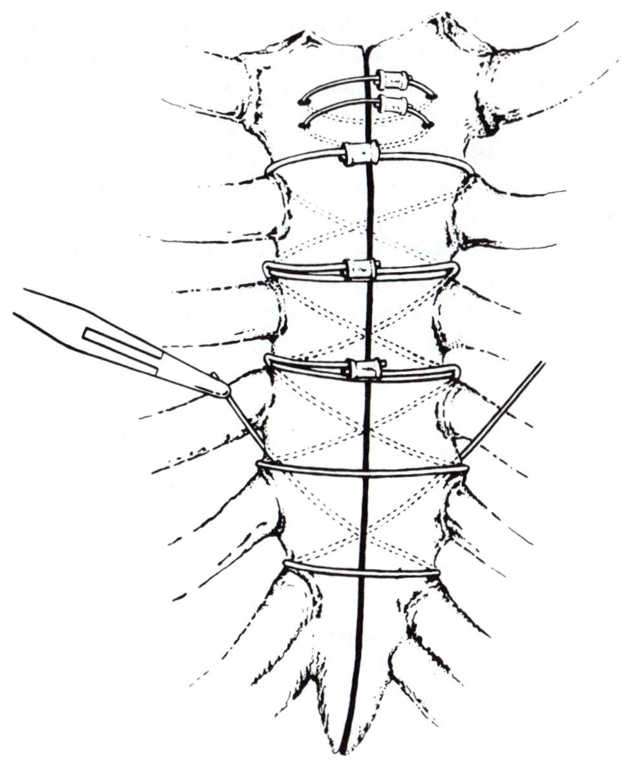

**Figure 5–1.** An interlocking wire suture technique for sternal closure is illustrated which provides lateral sternal reenforcement, and uses a figure of eight suture technique which reduces perpendicular wire shear.[18] *(From DiMarco RF Jr. et al: Interlocking figure-of-eight closure of the sternum. Ann Thorac Surg 47:927–929, 1989. Courtesy of Elsevier Science, Inc.)*

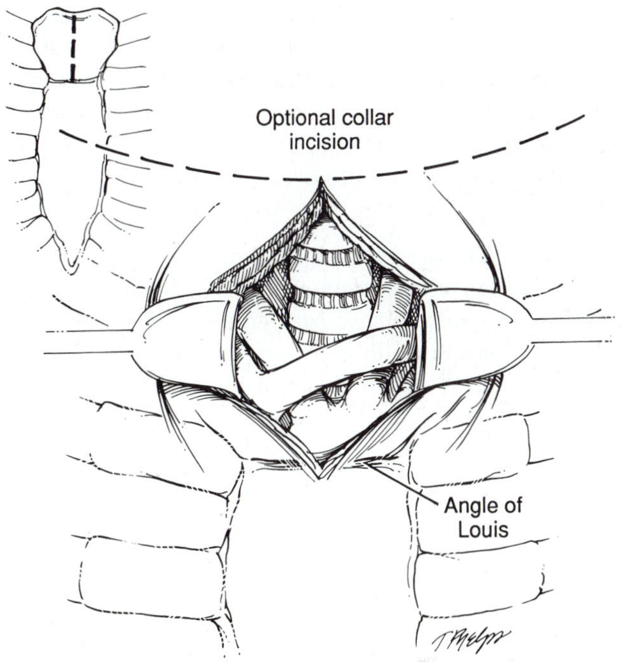


**Figure 5–2.** A partial sternal split which divides only the manubrium sternum, gives excellent exposure of the anterior superior mediastinum. An optional collar incision for cervicomediastinal exposure is shown.

lated to the increased operative mortality in performing the repeat sternotomy. There is general consensus that use of an oscillating saw facilitates sternal reopening. Garrett and Matthews[24] described a technique of reoperative median sternotomy in which the previous sternal wires are used to provide upward retraction of the sternum and limit the depth of penetration of the oscillating saw.

**Partial Sternal Split.** A useful variation of the median sternotomy incision is the partial sternal split (Fig. 5–2). A vertical skin incision is used extending from the sternal notch superiorly, to the angle of Louis inferiorly. The dissection is carried down to the anterior table of the manubrium. The suprasternal rim is mobilized as for a standard sternotomy. The manubrium sternum is divided in the midline, from above down, to the angle of Louis, using the Lebsche knife or sternal saw. A Tuffier, or pediatric rib spreader retracts the divided manubrium. This incision results in exposure of the anterior superior mediastinum and may be combined with a collar neck incision to provide wide cervicomediastinal exposure. For closure the substernal space is drained with closed suction drainage, the manubrium reapproximated with sternal wires or sutures, and the remainder of the incision closed in layers.

### Complications

Mediastinitis is the most serious of the complications following median sternotomy. The reported incidence of mediastinitis after coronary artery bypass surgery is 0.6–5%, with an associated mortality of 0–36%.[25–28] In their experience, Kutsal et al[25] reported *Staphylococcus aureus* as the responsible pathogen in 31% of patients, *Escherichia coli* in 3%, and enterococcus in 2%; no positive cultures were obtained in 64% of patients. Demmy et al[27] reported that chronic obstructive pulmonary disease, prolonged intensive care unit stay, respiratory failure, connective tissue disease, and male sex were all associated with a higher incidence of sternal wound complications. Hazelrigg et al[29] reported that the probability of wound complication after median sternotomy with single or bilateral internal mammary artery grafting was increased three to five times respectively that of saphenous vein grafting. Francel et al[30] described the perfusion distribution of the internal mammary artery and made recommendations to minimize wound complication after internal mammary artery harvesting.

Sternal osteomyelitis is an infrequent postoperative complication. Treatment principles include IV antibiotics, operative debridement of involved sternum, and either delayed primary closure or closure after transposition of muscle flaps or omentum.[31]

The reported incidence of brachial plexus injury after median sternotomy for cardiac surgery is 1.4–6.5%.[32,33] The most important factors responsible for this injury are the extent of sternal spread and the height of placement of the sternal spreader. Cannulation of the left internal jugular vein with hematoma formation is also thought to be a contributing factor.[33]

## Thoracotomy

### *Standard Thoracotomy Incisions*

Anterior, anterolateral, lateral, posterolateral, and posterior thoracotomy incisions have been grouped together for discussion. Although all thoracic surgeons are familiar with these incisions, it is difficult to find a specific written definition for each. For the purposes of this chapter, standard thoracotomy incisions are defined according to their relationship to the latissimus dorsi muscle, which arbitrarily is considered lateral (Fig. 5–3). A standard thoracotomy incision that only divides the latissimus dorsi muscle, or a part of it, is considered a *lateral* thoracotomy. Standard incisions that divide the latissimus and extend anteriorly are called *anterolateral,* and, similarly, an incision that extends posteriorly is defined as *posterolateral.* Those standard incisions that are entirely anterior or posterior to the latissimus dorsi muscle are called *anterior* and *posterior* thoracotomies, respectively.

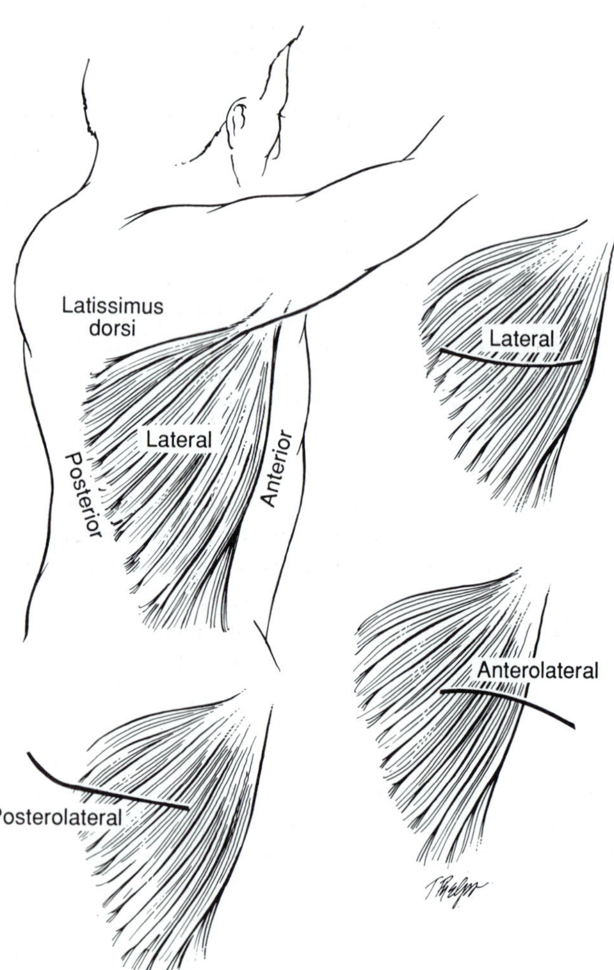


**Figure 5–3.** The nomenclature for standard thoracotomy incision is arbitrarily based on the latissimus dorsi muscle which is defined as lateral.

#### *Indications*

Standard thoracotomy incisions can be used for a wide range of surgical procedures involving the heart, esophagus, mediastinum, and ipsilateral lung.

#### *Advantages*

The flexibility, wide range of intrathoracic exposure, and proven experience with these incisions, has made them the "standard" thoracic incisional approach.

#### *Disadvantages*

The disadvantages of these incisions include the potential for poor exposure if the wrong interspace is chosen, unilateral hemithorax exposure, incisional pain, disability related to division of the chest wall muscles, documented detrimental effect on pulmonary function, a prominent incision, and often the need for single-lung anesthesia in order to achieve the desired exposure.

#### *Technique*

**Posterolateral Thoracotomy.** Following the adequate induction of single- or double-lumen general anesthesia, appropriate monitoring, including placement of a urinary catheter, the patient is positioned in the lateral decubitus position oriented with the operating table flex point at the level of the iliac crest. Either soft rolls or a bean bag may be used to secure the patient in position on the table. The lower leg is flexed at the hip and the knee, and the upper leg is straight with pillows in between. The arms are extended with the upper arm supported with pillows or a padded arm rest. An axillary roll may be used to minimize the risk of "downside" brachial plexus injury. The operating table is flexed to widen the ipsilateral intercostal spaces, and wide adhesive tape placed across the hip to prevent rotation. The patient is widely prepped and draped to accommodate the skin incision and chest tube drainage sites. The skin incision used is in the form of a crescent or "lazy-S." The incision shape is designed to permit upward retraction of the scapula. Some prefer to have the incision follow the rib angle, while others prefer to have the incision flat along its lateral portion. The incision begins anteriorly near the anterior border of the latissimus dorsi muscle, passes 2–3 cm below the scapular tip, and extends posteriorly, turning cephalad, along a line midway between the posterior scapular border and the spine. The dissection is carried sharply down through the subcutaneous tissue, the anterior border of the latissimus dorsi muscle is identified, and the latissimus divided using the electrocautery, coagulating or ligating the individual muscular vessels. The serratus anterior muscle is divided low, close to its muscular attachment, to minimize the length of denervated distal segment, and the auscultory triangle is opened posteriorly. A portion of the trapezius and rhomboid muscles may be divided as needed for additional exposure. The hand is then passed superiorly along the lateral edge of the erector spinae muscle to identify the first rib. Various scapular retractors may help with this maneuver. By counting from above down, an appropriate interspace is selected depending on the operative procedure planned. For most pulmonary resections, the fifth intercostal is preferred.

There are four options for entering the pleural space (Fig. 5–4). The first is an intercostal approach. The intercostal muscle is incised, by using the electrocautery, along the superior rib border in order to avoid injury to the adjacent intercostal neurovascular bundle. Alternatively, the periosteum over the rib is scored with the electrocautery, the periosteum is raised off the superior rib border, and the intercostal space is opened through the periosteal bed. After the pleural space is opened in one point to ensure a free space, the lung is gently retracted away from the chest wall, and the intercostal opening is widened to encompass the length of the incision. To facilitate rib retraction without rib fracture, the superior rib border is mobilized further, from within the pleural space, posteriorly to the costotransverse process articulation preserving the sympathetic chain, and anteriorly preserving the internal mammary vessels. A rib spreader is introduced, and the ribs are slowly retracted. The second approach is to utilize an intercostal incision but to divide one or more ribs, usually by resecting a short segment of rib posteriorly, in order to achieve a wider rib opening. The third approach is to resect a rib and to enter the pleural space through its periosteal bed.

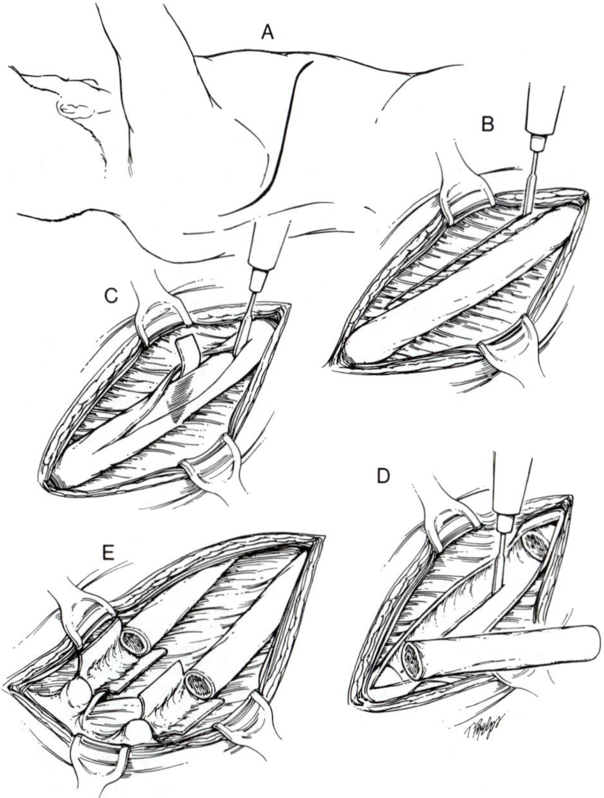


**Figure 5–4.** The options for entering the pleural space after posterolateral thoracotomy (**A**), include dividing the intercostal muscle from the superior rib edge with the electrocautery (**B**), reflecting the periosteum off the superior rib edge, and entering through the periosteal bed without rib resection (**C**), subperiosteal rib resection (**D**), and an intercostal approach with short segment rib resection posteriorly (**E**).

There continues to be some controversy as to which is the optimal thoracotomy technique. Advocates in favor of rib resection argue that this approach results in wider exposure reducing the risk of adjacent rib fracture from retraction. For this reason, Sweet[34] preferred rib resection for patients over 30 years of age. Opponents of rib resection point out that the technique is time-consuming to open and close; increases the likelihood of intercostal neuralgia[35]; increases postoperative pain and, therefore, the incidence of respiratory complications; and results in developmental chest wall structural abnormalities in children. Weinberg and Kraus[36] stressed the ease, exposure, and low incidence of intercostal neuralgia with the intercostal thoracotomy technique. More recently Kittle[37,38] has stated that there is little justification for rib resection unless the rib is needed as a graft. Therefore, whereas rib resection is an acceptable thoracotomy technique, it should no longer be considered the "standard" approach.

Before closure, adequate pleural space drainage is instituted. There is some variation on the technique of chest wall closure depending on whether or not a rib resection was performed. For an intercostal space approach, with or without rib division, paracostal sutures are employed using heavy absorbable sutures taking care not to injure the neurovascular bundle superior or inferior to the interspace opening. A figure of eight suture technique provides rigid rib reapproximation, and, by pulling up on the figure of eight stitches, the ribs are easily approximated without the need for a Bailey rib reapproximator. If rib is resected, then the chest wall is closed either by wide paracostal sutures around the remaining superior and inferior ribs, or by use of interrupted sutures to approximate the opposing intercostal muscles. The muscular layers, and auscultory triangle soft tissue, are closed in layers using heavy absorbable sutures. The latissimus dorsi is ideally closed in two layers, separately reapproximating the anterior and posterior fascial layers, to minimize muscular bunching, which is cosmetically unappealing. The remainder of the incision is closed in layers as per surgical preference.

**Anterior and Anterolateral Thoracotomy.** The anterior and anterolateral thoracotomy incision have seen greater use historically, when many used it as the preferred approach to pulmonary and cardiac operations. Currently, although this incision may be used for pulmonary resection, cardiac procedures, or management of mediastinal masses or esophageal pathology, the incision is much less frequently used than a posterolateral approach. The anesthetic and monitoring considerations are the same as for a posterolateral thoracotomy. The patient is positioned in the supine position with the chest elevated at 30–45 degrees by means of soft rolls or a bean bag. The ipsilateral arm is either positioned at the patient's side or flexed and suspended to the ether screen so that the arm is extended away from the chest wall. A gentle curved submammary skin incision is used (Fig. 5–5). Laterally, the incision may either be curved upwards toward the axilla (as with a pure anterior thoracotomy) or extended horizontally more laterally (anterolateral). The dissection is carried down to the chest wall with the electrocautery dividing the pectoralis major, minor, and medial aspect of the serratus anterior muscles. Rib counting is performed by identifying the angle of Louis and, therefore, the second rib, and counting up or down as needed. To expose the higher ribs, the divided chest wall musculature is dissected up off the chest wall, controlling the anterior perforating arterial branches to the pectoralis muscles. The options for opening the chest wall are the same with a posterolateral incision, except if an intercostal incision and rib division is performed, the rib is divided anteriorly through its cartilaginous portion. Further exposure may be obtained medially by ligating and dividing the internal mammary vessels, and by extending the incision transsternally. Laterally the serratus anterior muscle may be divided, and the anterior rim of the latissimus retracted posteriorly or divided. Closure proceeds after appropriate drainage of the hemithorax in the same fashion as described for a posterolateral incision. Anteriorly, it is difficult to achieve close rib to rib reapposition, and, therefore, extra care is necessary to ensure secure, multiple layered muscular and soft tissue closure to prevent local wound dehiscence.

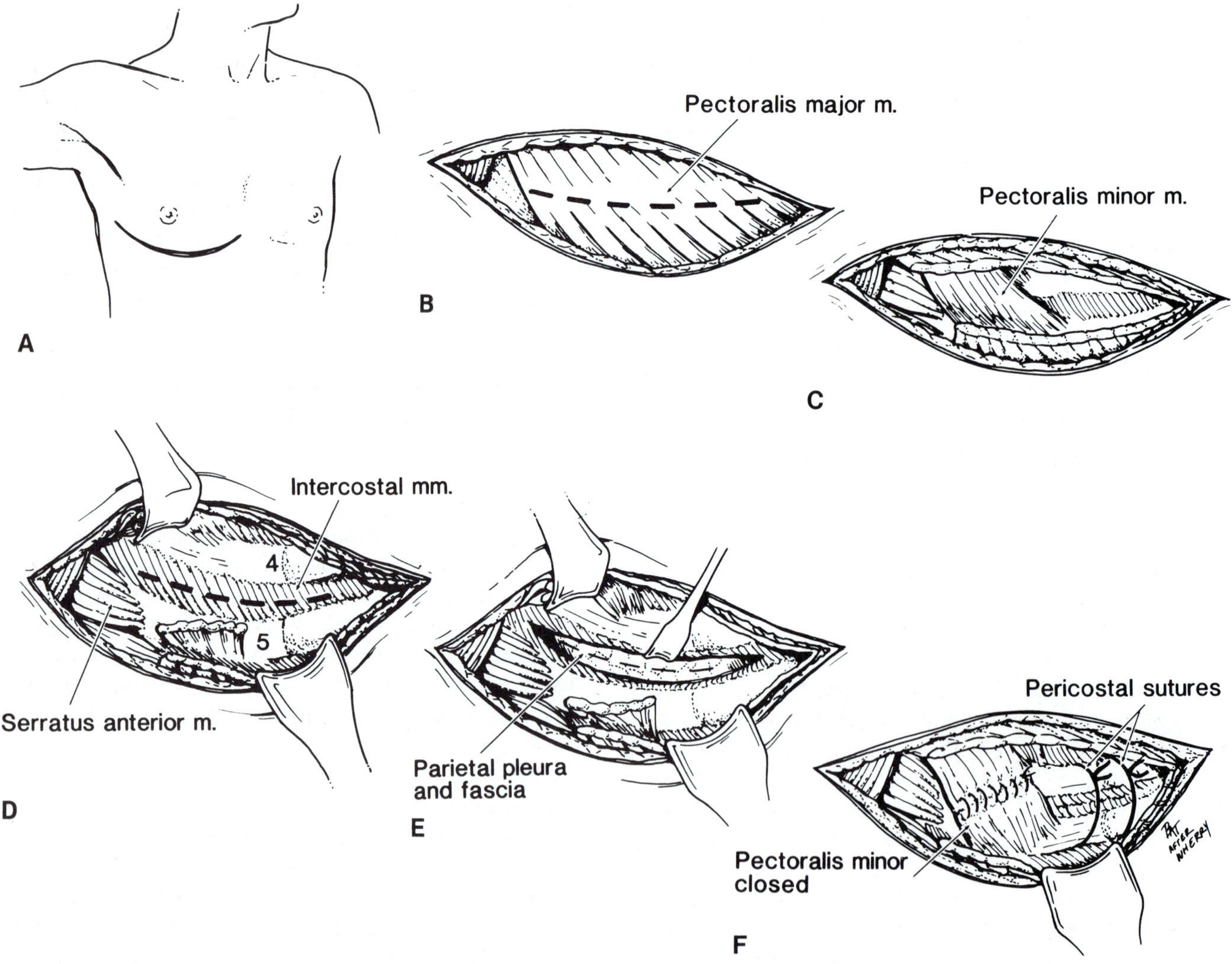


**Figure 5–5.** Anterolateral thoracotomy showing position of patient and anatomy encountered in fourth intercostal incision. Incision is identified by the solid line; the sternum is indicated by a dotted line. *(From Foster ED, Dobell ARC: Thoracic incisions. In Goldsmith HS, Ellis FH Jr [eds]: Thoracic Surgery. Philadelphia, Harper and Row, 1985, p 25, with permission.)*

**Lateral Thoracotomy.** Many use the term *lateral thoracotomy* to refer to a muscle-sparing thoracotomy technique. However, as defined in this chapter, a lateral thoracotomy is an incision within the confines of the latissimus dorsi muscle. This incision is ideal for limited lateral, or inferior exposure is required. The incision is quick to open and close, can easily be extended to a standard posterolateral incision, and divides only one muscle. The incision provides limited exposure of the upper hemithorax. Patients are positioned as for a posterolateral incision. A transverse skin incision is used oriented horizontally, or parallel to the underlying rib. The incision is located 1–2 cm inferior to the scapular tip, or over any inferior rib, as dictated by the specific intrathoracic pathology. All or frequently only a portion of the latissimus muscle is divided with the electrocautery. The serratus is not divided, and the chest wall is exposed, opened, and later closed in the same fashion as described for a posterolateral incision.

### Complications

The excellent exposure and safety of the standard thoracotomy incisions have been demonstrated for a wide variety of applications over many years of use. The most bothersome complication is postthoracotomy incisional pain, which will be discussed later in this chapter. Wound infection, or dehiscence, is uncommon. Tedder et al[39] reported bronchopleural fistula in 8.8% and empyema in 2.2% but no wound infections following bronchoplastic procedures for malignancies. Naunheim et al[40] reported a wound infection rate of only 2% in the octogenarian patient, and Lozac'h et al[41] noted a 1% thoracic wound dehiscence rate in patients undergoing Ivor Lewis esophagectomy for squamous cell carcinoma. In patients with superior sulcus tumors who receive preoperative radiation therapy, the incidence of superficial wound infection does not appear to be increased, further attesting to the safety of these incisions.[42,43]

## Muscle-Sparing Thoracotomy

### Indications

The muscle-sparing techniques included in this section are variations of the standard incisions described in the preceding section. Much of the enthusiasm created by the initial reports of muscle-sparing techniques have now been eclipsed by the introduction of thoracoscopic surgery. Nonetheless, muscle-sparing variants of standard thoracotomy incisions have become well established, and many now use at least one of these approaches as their standard open thoracotomy incision. Although it is generally accepted that muscle-sparing results in less postoperative pain, and improved postoperative cough and mobility, this has been difficult to prove. Lemmer et al[44] reported that use of a "limited lateral" muscle-sparing technique resulted in less early postoperative reduction in $FEV_1$ and FVC compared with use of a standard thoracotomy incision. The authors noted no difference; however, in other postoperative pulmonary function parameters, narcotic use, complications, or length of hospital stay. In their series, Hazelrigg et al[45] demonstrated less postoperative pain, less narcotic use in the first 24 hours, lower visual analog scales for the first week, and increased shoulder girdle strength at 1 week postoperatively when a muscle-sparing approach was used instead of a standard posterolateral incision. No difference was noted in postoperative morbidity, mortality, pulmonary function, shoulder range of motion, or length of hospital stay. Shoulder girdle strength had equalized and returned to baseline in both the muscle-sparing and non–muscle-sparing groups by the end of the first month. Ponn et al[46] reported a comparison of late pulmonary function after posterolateral and muscle-sparing thoracotomy and concluded that the differences in late pulmonary function were small and of no apparent clinical significance. In neonates, infants, and children,[47–49] the impact of muscle-sparing techniques may be greater than in adults.

### Advantages

There is some evidence to show that by preserving major muscle groups, muscle-sparing variations of the standard thoracotomy result in less early postoperative pain and greater shoulder girdle strength. Most result in quick closure as the muscle groups do not have to be reapproximated. Chest wall muscles are saved for later use as muscle flaps if needed. In the pediatric age group, there is evidence to suggest that muscle-sparing techniques may prevent chest wall deformity with growth following thoracotomy.[48]

### Disadvantages

Disadvantages include limited exposure compared with standard thoracotomy, and an increased incidence of postoperative wound seroma.

### Technique

There has been confusion regarding the terminology that should be used to describe muscle-sparing variants of the standard thoracotomy. For simplicity, in this chapter the terminology used to describe standard incisions, based on the incision's relationship to the latissimus dorsi muscle, has been adopted. Muscle sparing incisions can be divided into three groups: (1) anterolateral, (2) vertical axillary, and (3) posterolateral.

**Anterolateral.** Numerous anterolateral muscle sparing techniques have been reported under various names including limited lateral,[50] simplified lateral,[51] muscle-sparing posterolateral,[52] extensive lateral,[55] axillary thoracotomy,[54] and the French incision.[55] Although there is some variation in the specifics of the skin incision used, all are otherwise similar. In general (Fig. 5–6), superior and inferior skin flaps are raised, the medial border of the latissimus dorsi is delineated and retracted laterally, and the ser-

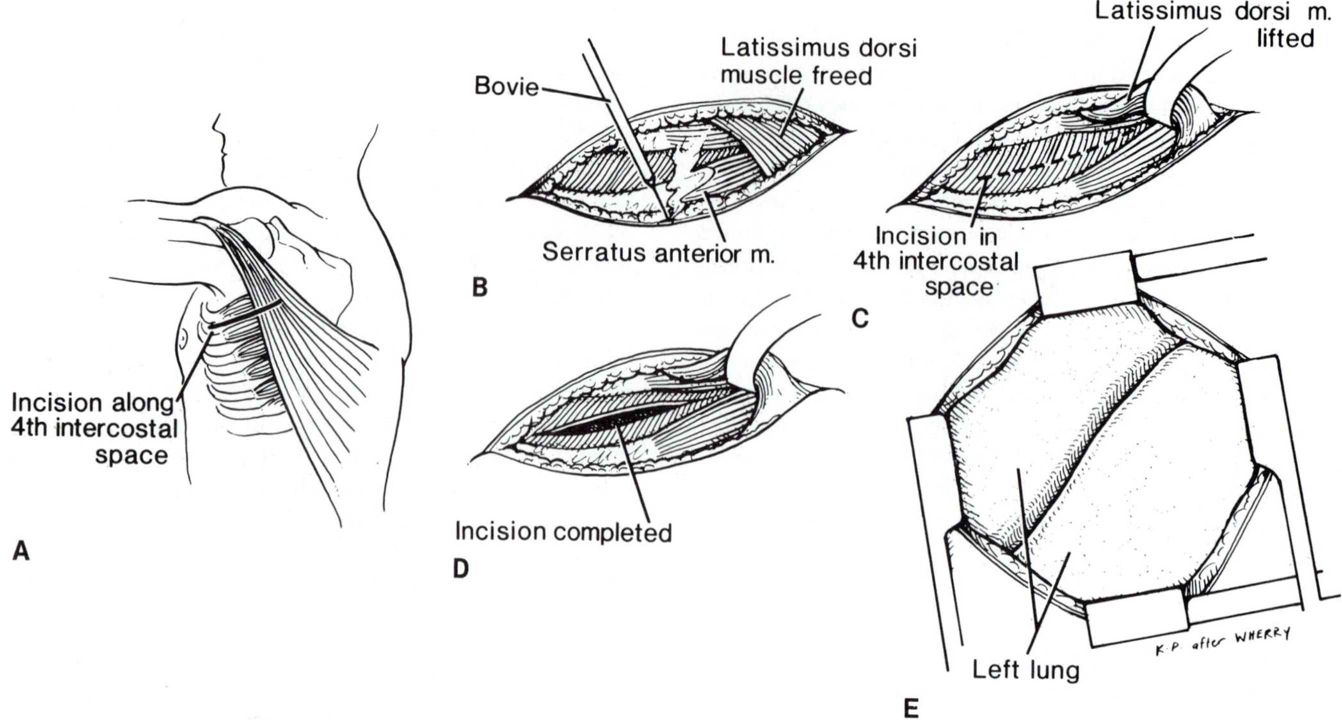


**Figure 5–6.** The technique of muscle sparing anterolateral thoracotomy incision is illustrated. The positions of the patient and incision are shown. The anterior edge of the latissimus dorsi muscle is retracted laterally to expose the chest wall.[51] *(From Mitchell R, Angell W, Wuerflein R, Dor. Simplified lateral chest incision for most thoracotomies other than sternotomy. Ann Thorac Surg 22:284–286, 1976.)*

ratus anterior muscle is either partially split or laterally retracted as well. After an appropriate interspace is chosen, the chest wall is opened as with a standard thoracotomy incision. Frequently two rib retractors are used for exposure resulting in a square or rectangular chest wall opening. Closure is simply performed. After appropriate chest drainage, the ribs are reapproximated as with a standard incision, the retracted muscles are released, the deep soft tissue anterior to the serratus is closed with a running absorbable suture, and then the subcutaneous tissue and skin are closed as per the surgeon's routine. Frequently, a subcutaneous closed suction drain is used.

**Vertical Axillary.** Baeza and Foster[56] described a muscle-sparing thoracotomy technique using a midaxillary vertical skin incision in which anterior and posterior skin flaps are raised, the latissimus is retracted posteriorly, and the serratus is split vertically, to expose the chest wall (Fig. 5–7). Siegel and Steiger[57] reported a similar technique that they called an axillary thoracotomy. Ginsberg[58] reported on his use of a vertical axillary thoracotomy in which the same skin incision is used, no skin flaps are raised, the latissimus is retracted posteriorly, and the serratus is elevated from the chest wall, by detaching its rib insertions, until the appropriate interspace is exposed. In most instances, the fourth interspace proved optimal. Regardless of the specific technique, the vertical incision is closed by rib approximation, closure, or reattachment of the serratus, followed by subcutaneous and skin closures. Given the cosmetic result, full postoperative shoulder girdle motion, and decreased incisional pain, Ginsberg preferred the approach for most routine thoracotomies. It was not recommended if difficult hilar dissections were anticipated.

**Posterolateral.** Ashour[59] reported a modified muscle-sparing posterolateral thoracotomy. A standard posterolateral skin incision is used, and extensive skin flaps are raised over the latissimus and posteriorly over the trapezius muscle. The latissimus and trapezius muscles are separated, the latissimus is detached posteriorly by a 6–7-cm incision in the thoracolumbar fascia, the serratus anterior is detached inferiorly from its rib insertion, and both are retracted anteriorly to expose the chest wall, which is opened in the standard fashion. Closure includes reattachment of the serratus, and latissimus muscles with running absorbable suture, followed by subcutaneous and skin closure. Heitmiller[60] reported on a modified posterolateral incision in which the latissimus is divided per routine; however, the serratus anterior muscle is preserved and retracted medially by means of a penrose sling (Fig. 5–8).

### *Complications*

The reported incidence of wound seroma using an anterolateral muscle sparing incision is 0–23%.[44,45,51] Mitchell[50] reported a 2.9% overall morbidity using an anterolateral muscle-sparing technique in a large number of patients

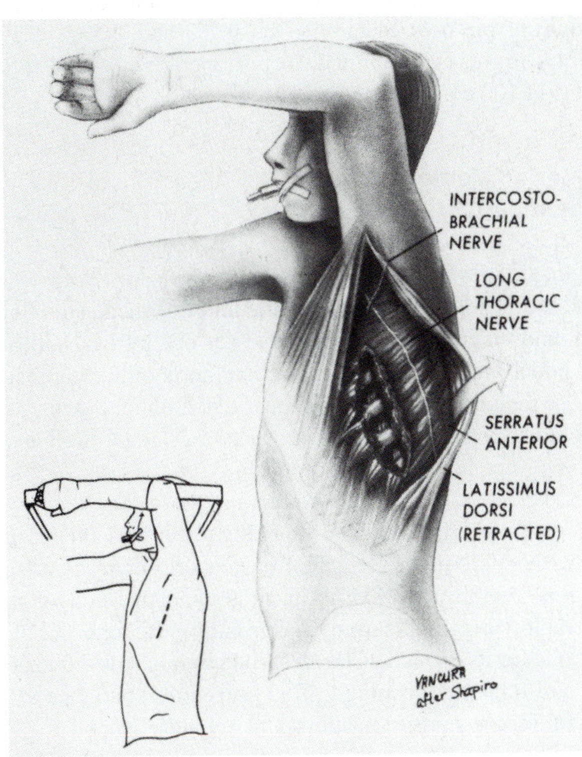


**Figure 5–7.** Patient positioning and incision for a vertical axillary incisions are shown. The latissimus dorsi muscle is retracted laterally and the serratus anterior muscle split along it muscle fibers to expose the chest wall.[56] *(From Baeza OR, Foster ED: Vertical axillary thoracotomy: A functional and cosmetically appealing incision. Ann Thorac Surg 22:287–288, 1976. Courtesy of Elsevier Science, Inc.)*

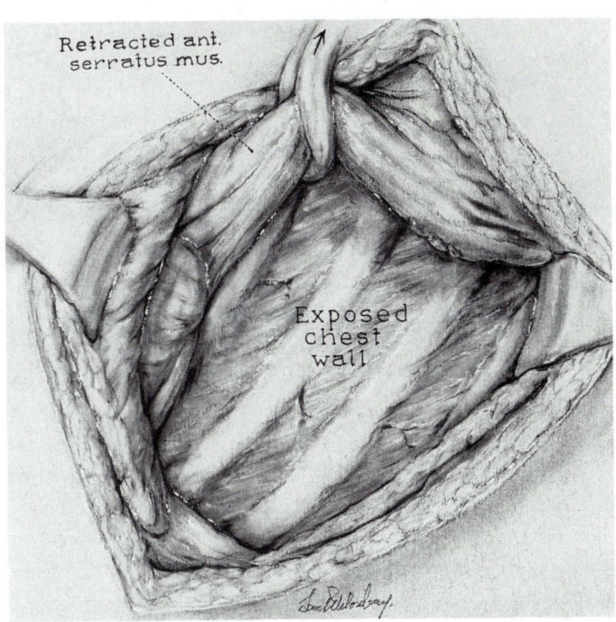


**Figure 5–8.** A simple, modified posterolateral incision spares the serratus anterior muscle by encircling it with a penrose sling.[60] *(From Heitmiller RF: The serratus sling: A simplified serratus-sparing technique. Ann Thorac Surg 48:867–868, 1989. Courtesy of Elsevier Science, Inc.)*

for a wide range of intrathoracic procedures. In that series, there was a 0.4% incidence of wound infection, and a 0.4% incidence of wound dehiscence.

Ginsberg[58] reported that wound seromas occurred occasionally with the vertical axillary thoracotomy, but that none required treatment. Siegel and Steiger[57] reported a 1.8% incidence of wound infection after vertical axillary thoracotomy.

Ashour,[59] using a muscle-sparing posterolateral thoracotomy for a wide range of thoracic procedures, noted that exposure was inadequate in only 4% of cases. In those instances, the muscle-sparing incision was converted to a standard approach. Wound seroma occurred in 2% and wound infection in 2% of patients.

## Axillary Thoracotomy

### *Indications*

The indications for this incision are first rib resection, apical bleb disease, management of spontaneous pneumothorax with apical pleurectomy or pleurodesis, staging of lung cancer, and sympathectomy. Fry et al[54] described an extended axillary thoracotomy technique that has broadened the indications for its use to include anatomic lung resection, including pneumonectomy. Many of the procedures performed through an axillary approach, such as management of bleb disease, pleural scarification, staging of lung cancer, and wedge resection, are now routinely performed thoracoscopically.

### *Advantages*

The axillary thoracotomy is a small incision, which is quickly performed, muscle-sparing, and cosmetically appealing since it is largely hidden under the arm. Its limited size and muscle-sparing characteristics make it an ideal approach for use in patients with poor pulmonary function. The incision is easily extended anteriorly if further exposure is needed.

### *Disadvantages*

The main disadvantage for use of this incision is its exposure, which is primarily limited to the upper half of the chest. Other disadvantages include intercostobrachial nerve injury, and proximal long thoracic nerve injury.

### *Technique*

The patient is positioned in the lateral decubitus position with the ipsilateral arm generously padded, flexed at the elbow, and rotated superiorly where it is secured to a stand or an ether screen. The patient is widely prepped and draped to permit anterior extension of the incision if necessary (Fig. 5–9). A curvilinear incision is made at the base of the hairline. Care must be taken not to position the incision too far posteriorly. The dissection is carried down to the chest wall retracting the pectoralis and serratus muscles posteriorly, and the pectoralis major muscle anteriorly. The chest is usually entered through the third intercostal space. The second interspace is easily identified by the intercosto-brachial nerve, which emanates from it. Closure is quickly performed, reapproximating the ribs, subcutaneous, and skin layers.[61]

Fry et al[54] describe an axillary thoracotomy approach in which the incision is lower (fourth or fifth interspace) and extended anteriorly. The muscle layers are managed as with a muscle-sparing anterolateral technique by retracting the latissimus posteriorly, splitting the serratus in the direction of its muscle fibers, and preserving the long thoracic nerve. The chest is entered through the fourth or fifth intercostal space with two rib retractors placed at 90 degrees for exposure. Closure is performed as with an anterolateral approach.

### *Complications*

In general this incision is simple, safe, and with few complications. In their series, Deslauriers et al[62] reported the incidence of wound infection and limited shoulder mobility requiring physical therapy to be 0.7% and 0.5%, respectively. Fry et al[54] reported no postoperative wound infections in 100 consecutive patients.

## Anterior Mediastinotomy (Chamberlain Procedure)

### *Indications*

The indications for the use of the anterior mediastinotomy continue to be the same as those set out by McNeill and Chamberlain[63] in their original description of the technique. These include cases of lung cancer that are thought to be inoperable by virtue of mediastinal lymph nodal metastasis, or by direct mediastinal invasion, and biopsy of mediastinal masses. As stated in their report, this procedure ". . . was designed to fill the gap in our diagnostic armamentarium between such minor surgical procedures as endoscopic and scalene lymph node biopsy and the extensive undertaking of exploratory thoracotomy." Currently, although the indications for its use have been lessened by improved diagnostic and imaging techniques, this procedure continues to be useful for the same indications as originally intended.

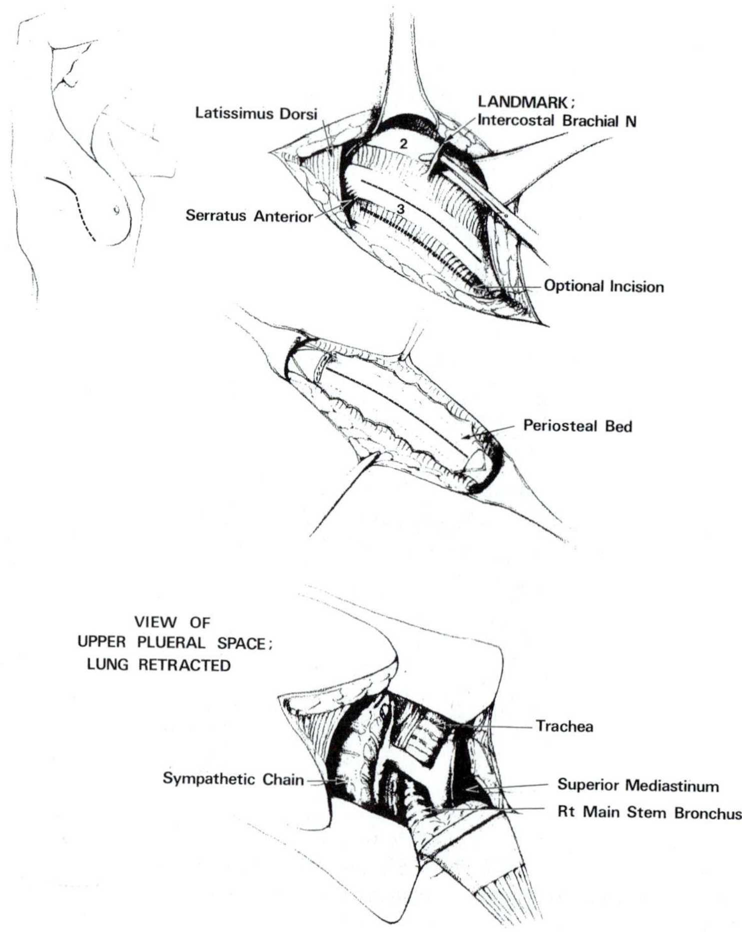


**Figure 5–9.** The technique of axillary thoracotomy is shown including the anterior extension of the incision if necessary. Posterior extension of this incision risks injury to the long thoracic nerve. *(From Becker RM, Munro DD: Transaxillary minithoractomy: The optimal approach for certain pulmonary and mediastinal lesions. Ann Thorac Surg 22:254–259, 1976. Courtesy of Elsevier Science, Inc.)*

### *Advantages*

The advantages include quick easy access to the anterior, superior lung hilar structures bilaterally, and the mediastinum. The incision may be extended as an anterior thoracotomy if needed.

### *Disadvantages*

Disadvantages include limited exposure, inability to visualize the posterior hilar region, the need to sacrifice the internal mammary vessels, and wound-healing problems related to the limited anterior soft tissue for closure.

### *Technique*

The procedure is performed under general anesthesia, although in the original report[63] it is stated that local anesthesia is an option. The patient is placed in the supine position with the head of the bed elevated so that the sternum lies flat. A 6-cm transverse incision is positioned over the cartilaginous portion of the left or right second or third costal cartilage (Fig. 5–10). The entire costal cartilage is excised from its perichondrial bed. The internal mammary vessels are identified, ligated, and divided. The mediastinal space is entered sweeping the ipsilateral pleura laterally (Fig. 5–11). An alternative technique uses an intercostal incision, preserving the costal cartilage. If necessary, the pleural space is opened for exposure. Other technical factors that help with deep mediastinal exposure are a deep, narrow retractor; a Carlens mediastinoscope; and headlight illumination.

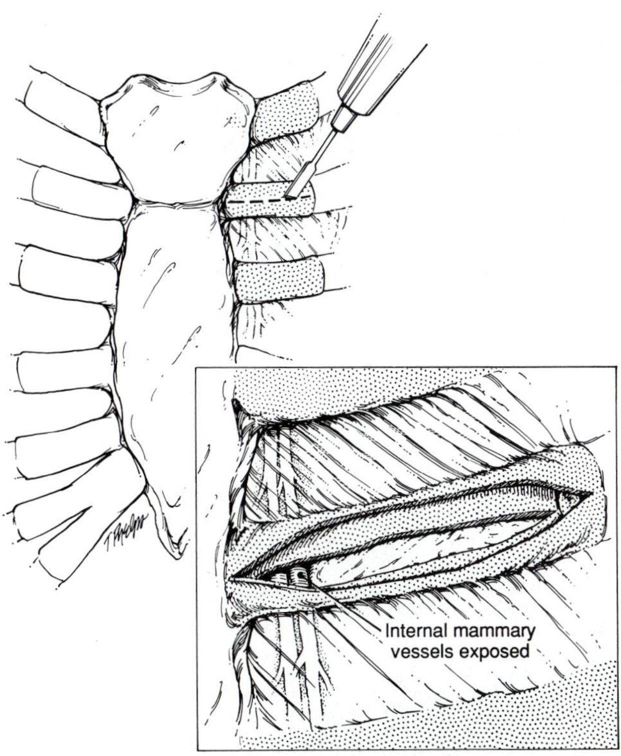


**Figure 5–10.** Anterior mediastinotomy employs a transverse incision over the cartilaginous portion of the second or third rib. The rib cartilage is removed from its perichondrial bed to enter the mediastinum. The medially located internal mammary vessels (insert) are shown.

For closure, the wound is closed in multiple layers with running absorbable suture. If the pleural space is opened and no prolonged airleak is anticipated, the wound is closed around a small drainage catheter placed to suction, which is withdrawn after wound closure. Otherwise, a standard pleural drain is placed through a separate stab incision.

### *Complications*

Complications are infrequent and include wound infection, pneumothorax, hemorrhage, and injury to exposed mediastinal structures. McNeill and Chamberlain[63] reported an incidence of pneumothorax and wound infection of 2% and 4%, respectively.

## Left Thoracoabdominal Incision

### *Indications*

The left thoracoabdominal incision provides excellent exposure for operative procedures involving the spleen, stomach, left hemidiaphragm, aorta, and lower esophagus.

### *Advantages*

The incision provides excellent, wide exposure of the abdominal left upper quadrant and left lower hemithorax. It provides single-incision exposure of the thoracoabdominal aorta, and it maximizes reconstructive options in patients with esophageal tumors at or near the gastroesophageal junction.

### *Disadvantages*

The wide thoracoabdominal exposure from this incision results from the size of the incision, division of the costal margin, and diaphragm. Despite these factors, the incision is remarkably well tolerated. Disadvantages of this incision include postoperative complications including incisional pain, wound infection, costal margin instability, and transdiaphragmatic herniation of abdominal contents.

### *Technique*

Following the induction of general, left-sided general anesthesia, the patient is placed in the right lateral decubitus position with the hips rotated back to a 45-degree angle to increase abdominal exposure (Fig. 5–12). The left arm and neck are included in the field if a cervical esophageal anastamosis is anticipated. The incision extends in a straight line from one finger 2 cm below the scapular tip to a point midway between the umbilicus and the xiphoid process. In the case of a malignant process, the abdominal portion of the incision may be made first to assess operability. The latissimus dorsi muscle is divided with the electrocautery. The serratus anterior is divided close to its rib insertion site to

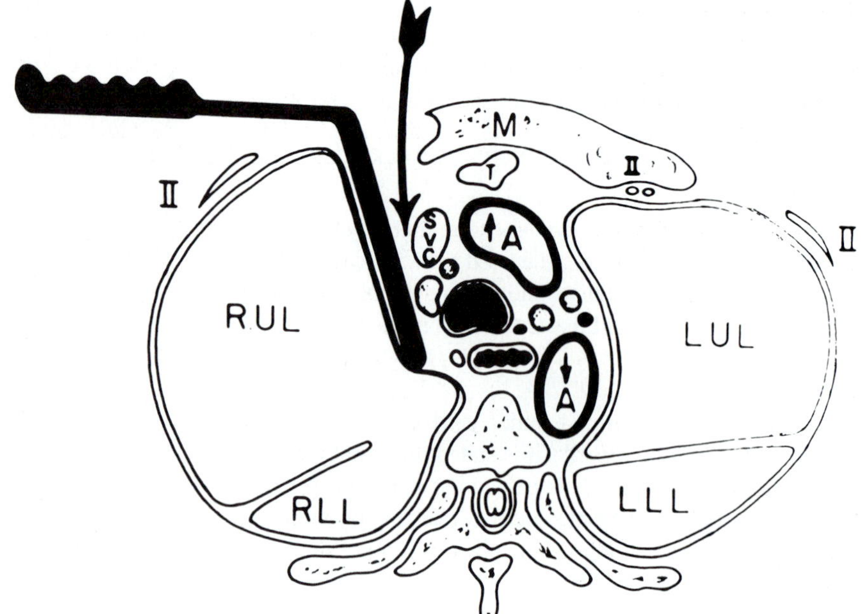


**Figure 5–11.** Diagram to illustrate anatomy encountered in a right-sided anterior mediastinotomy. *(From McNeill TM, Chamberlain JM: Ann Thorac Surg 2:532–539, 1966. Reprinted with permission from The Society of Thoracic Surgeons.)*

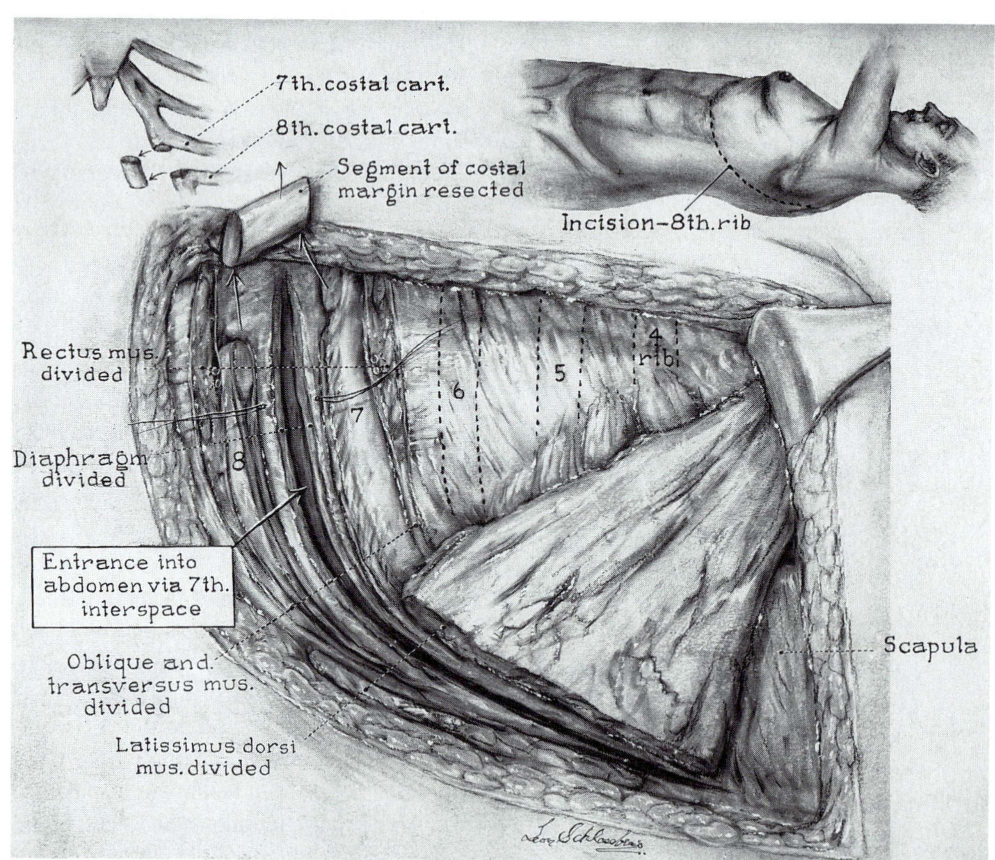


**Figure 5–12.** Patient positioning for a seventh interspace left thoracoabdominal incision is illustrated. Resection of a short segment of costal cartilage allows for closer rib reapproximation with closure.[1] *(From Heitmiller RF: The left thoracoabdominal incision. Ann Thorac Surg 46:250–253, 1988. Courtesy of Elsevier Science, Inc.)*

expose the chest wall. The level for chest wall opening is identified by counting ribs from above (as with a standard thoracotomy) and is determined by the specific operative procedure. A seventh interspace approach is most commonly employed. The chest wall is opened without rib resection. The costal margin is opened, and a short segment of costal cartilage removed to facilitate later rib and costal margin reapproximation with closure. The abdomen is opened in layers using the electrocautery. The left hemidiaphragm is divided radially protecting the phrenic nerve branches (Fig. 5–13), and chest and abdominal wound retractors placed. The chest incision may be extended posteriorly as with a standard posterolateral thoracotomy. The abdominal incision may be extended by carrying the incision across the midline or by turning the incision inferiorly in the abdominal midline.

For closure, the chest is drained per routine. The diaphragm is reconstructed with interrupted, nonabsorbable sutures. The ribs are reapproximated with absorbable figure-of-eight paracostal sutures. The costal margin is closed by a single, heavy absorbable figure-of-eight suture that incorporates the upper edge of the diaphragm to prevent herniation of abdominal contents into the chest. The remainder of the chest and abdominal closure proceed in layers as per routine.[1]

### *Complications*

Respiratory complications are most common. A high incidence of postoperative atelectasis, usually involving the left lower lobe, is generally reported. When used as an approach for esophagogastrectomy, the incidence of pneumonia is 0–24%, atrial fibrillation occurs in up to 10%, and the incidence of wound infection is 1.5–5.2%. Both empyema and subphrenic abscess are uncommon complications in the absence of an esophageal leak.[64]

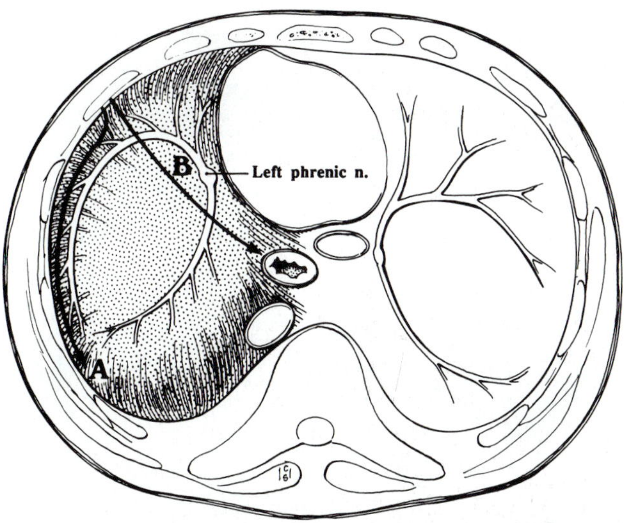


**Figure 5–13.** When using a left thoraco-abdominal incision, the left hemic diaphragm may be divided circumferentially (**A**) preserving the anterior branch of the left phrenic nerve, or radially (**B**).[64] *(From Heitmiller RF: Results of standard left thoracoabdominal esophagogastrectomy. In Loop FD, Mathisen DJ (eds): Seminars in Thoracic and Cardiovascular Surgery, vol. 4, Philadelphia, Saunders, 1992, pp 314–319, with permission.)*

## Bilateral Trans-Sternal Thoracotomy (Clam-Shell Incision)

### *Indications*

This incision has been referred to by several different names including bilateral trans-sternal thoracotomy, "clamshell," and "cross bow" incision. The incision results in exposure of both lungs and their hila, pleural spaces, the mediastinum, and great vessels. The incision has demonstrated its greatest utility for exposure during bilateral sequential lung transplantation,[65,66] but it has also been described for use in bilateral pulmonary metastasectomy.[67] More recently, Bains et al[68] have reported their experience with this incision for bilateral pulmonary or combined pulmonary and mediastinal disease.

### *Advantages*

The incision provides wide exposure of both lungs, their hila, the mediastinum, and proximal great vessels. For bilateral sequential lung transplantation, the pleural spaces can be opened sequentially, which optimizes intraoperative ventilation.

### *Disadvantages*

The incision takes time to perform and close and results in a significant impact on early postoperative respiratory function. Patients frequently require postoperative ventilatory support, and there is significant early postoperative pain.

### *Technique*

General double lumen endotracheal anesthesia is instituted. The patient is placed in the supine position with both arms padded, extended upward over the face, the elbows flexed, and secured to a stand or ether screen. Bilateral anterior thoracotomies are performed (Fig. 5–14), the internal mammary vessels are ligated and divided, and the two thoracotomies are joined by a transverse sternotomy. Usually a fourth or fifth intercostal space approach is selected. When bilateral sequential lung transplantation is performed, the pleural spaces are opened sequentially to optimize intraoperative ventilation.

After appropriate intrathoracic drainage, the divided sternum is closed with interrupted or figure-of-eight heavy-gauge wire sutures, and then the bilateral anterior thoracotomies are closed in layers as previously described.

### *Complications*

Kaiser et al[66] reported an incidence of early sternal instability and wound infection of 11% and 7%, respectively, in pa-

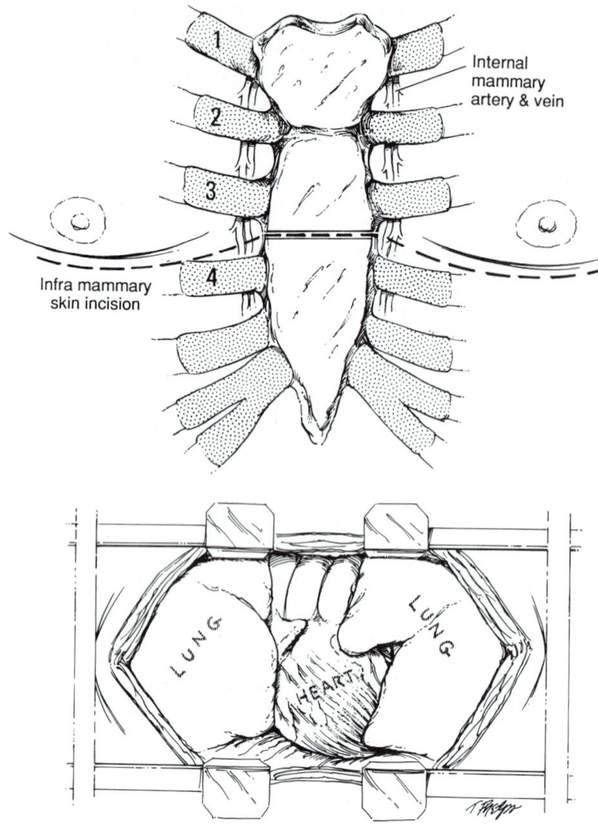


**Figure 5–14.** A "clamshell" incision uses bilateral anterior thoracotomy incisions that are joined by transternal division. The excellent bilateral lung, pleural space, and mediastinal exposure in shown.

tients undergoing bilateral lung transplantation. Shimizu et al,[67] using the trans-sternal incision for pulmonary metastasectomy, reported that only 30% of patients could be extubated at the conclusion of the operation. For those left intubated, the average time to extubation was 2.7 days. The main cause of prolonged intubation was reported to be incisional pain.

## Extrathoracic Approaches to the Thorax

Three extrathoracic approaches—transcervical, subxiphoid, and transdiaphragmatic—are discussed. All three techniques share avoidance of a chest wall incision and limited intrathoracic exposure as their advantage and disadvantage, respectively.

The transcervical approach may be used for "closed" chest thymectomy, resection of a mediastinal parathyroid adenoma,[69] or substernal goiter. Patients are positioned in the supine position with the neck extended and a standard collar incision employed. The substernal space is bluntly developed, and the manubrium sternum retracted upward with a right-angled, self-retaining retractor to expose the anterior, superior mediastinum. Headlight illumination helps. The neck wound is closed in layers.

The subxiphoid approach is used as an alternative method of accessing the pericardial space and has been used for management of pericardial effusions and placement of AICD patch electrodes.[70]

Thirlby et al[71] reported a transdiaphragmatic approach to the lower esophagus and the posterior mediastinum (Fig. 5–15). Patients are positioned supine, a midline abdominal incision is employed, and the diaphragm is incised using a semicircular incision in the central tendinous portion.

## Postthoracotomy Pain

Postoperative incisional pain has been a well-recognized, and often criticized, sequela following thoracotomy. Pain may result from division of skin, soft tissue, and muscle or irritation of the parietal pleura and diaphragm. However, most significant pain is derived from the bony chest wall as a consequence of rib retraction, including injury to rib articulation joints, ligamentous strain, rib fractures, and intercostal nerve injury. Limited, muscle-sparing, and conservative rib retraction techniques have been developed to reduce postoperative pain and respiratory depression, and there is some evidence to suggest they do so. Analgesic strategies that have been devised to treat postthoracotomy pain are systemic medications, local or regional techniques, and combination analgesic methods. More recently, there is evidence that analgesic administration before the onset of pain, or "preemptive analgesia," is more effective than pain management after the onset of pain.[72–74]

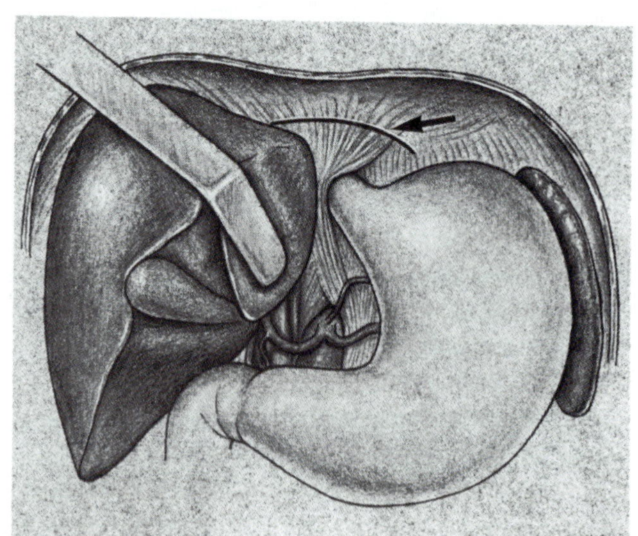

**Figure 5–15.** An unusual approach to the lower esophagus and lower posterior mediastinum involves transabdominal and transdiaphragmatic (arrow) incisions as shown. *(From Thirlby RC, Kraemer SJ, Hill LD: Transdiaphragmatic approach to the posterior mediastinum and thoracic esophagus. Arch Surg 128:897–901, 1993. Courtesy of American Medical Association.)*

### Systemic Medications

Oral or parenteral narcotics are limited in their effectiveness by the side effects including sedation, respiratory depression, diminished gastrointestinal motility, nausea, and urinary retention. Continuous IV administration using patient-controlled systems minimizes "break-through" pain inherent with bolus techniques; however, side effects are not reduced. *Nonsteroidal anti-inflammatory drugs (NSAIDs)* are generally not effective acutely when used alone; however, they do provide enhanced pain control when used in conjunction with other analgesic methods. NSAIDs produce little respiratory depression, and their long dosing interval minimizes the chance of break-through pain. Complications of NSAID use are gastritis, peptic ulceration, and decreased renal function.

### Local or Regional Techniques

*Epidural morphine* is considered by many to be the gold standard in postthoracotomy pain relief because it provides excellent pain control with a low incidence of narcotics-related side effects.[75,76] Patients receiving epidural morphine require monitoring in an intensive care or a special nursing unit in the event of hypotension or respiratory depression. The development of respiratory depression is unpredictable of delayed onset and is reported to occur in 0.25–13.5%[77–79] of patients. Other complications include urinary retention and nausea. Inability to place an epidural catheter is reported to occur in up to 10.9% of patients.[80] *Intrathecal morphine* has uniformly been demonstrated to be effective at reducing postthoracotomy pain with minimal respiratory depression.[81,82] The duration of relief is limited, and, therefore, this approach is mainly used in an adjuvant setting. *Intercostal nerve blocks* reduce pain with some authors showing an associated benefit in terms of respiratory function,[83] and others do not.[84] As with intrathecal morphine, the duration of pain relief is limited, although a continuous infusion technique has been described.[85] Cryoprobe intercostal nerve blocks have been reported to provide effective postthoracotomy pain relief; however, the technique is associated with neuralgia symptoms in up to 20% of patients.[86] *Continuous extrapleural nerve blockade,* also known as a paravertebral block, is an approach that blocks both the intercostal and sympathetic nerves, and it has been shown to provide effective pain control with a minimum of analgesic-related side effects.[87,88] The extrapleural catheters may be placed preoperatively or intraoperatively. Although some report the variable effectiveness with *intrapleural analgesia,*[89] others have shown no benefit with its use.[90] In patients without chest tube drainage, there is a risk of pneumothorax.[91]

**Combined Analgesia.** Eng and Sabanathan[74] have recently advocated a "balanced analgesia" approach to postthoracotomy pain that includes premedication with narcotics and NSAIDs, preincision local nerve blocks, and postoperative continuous regional block plus systemic NSAIDs. In their experience, such an approach has resulted in superior pain relief with little respiratory depression.

### REFERENCES


1. Heitmiller RF: The left thoracoabdominal incision. *Ann Thorac Surg* **46:**250–253, 1988
2. Daly BD, Faling LJ, Diehl JT, et al: Computed tomography-guided minithoracotomy for the resection of small peripheral pulmonary nodules. *Ann Thorac Surg* **51:**465–469, 1991
3. Grillo HC: Surgical treatment of postintubation tracheal injuries. *J Thorac Surg* **78:**860–875, 1979
4. Sugenoya A, Asanuma K, Shingu K, et al:. Clinical evaluation of upper mediastinal dissection for differentiated thyroid carcinoma. *Surgery* **113:**541–544, 1993
5. Fujita H, Kakegawa T, Inoue Y, et al: Upper esophagectomy with pharyngolaryngectomy for esophageal carcinoma at the cervicothoracic junction. *Jpn J Surg* **21:**650–654, 1991
6. Orringer MB: partial median sternotomy: Anterior approach to the upper thoracic esophagus. *J Thorac Cardiovasc Surg* **87:**124–129, 1984
7. Urschel H, Razzuk M: Median sternotomy as the standard approach for pulmonary resection. *Ann Thorac Surg* **41:**130–134, 1986
8. Cooper JD, Nelems JF, Pearson FG: Extended indications for median sternotomy in patients requiring pulmonary resection. *Ann Thorac Surg* **26:**413–420, 1978
9. Swoboda L, Ioomes H: Results of surgical treatment for pulmonary metastasis. *Thorac Cardiovasc Surg* **34:**149–152, 1986
10. Pogrebniak HW, Pass HI: Initial and reoperative pulmonary metastasectomy: indications, technique, and results. *Semin Surg Oncol* **9:**142–149, 1993
11. Ueda I, Uchida A, Kodama K, et al: Aggressive pulmonary metastasectomy for soft tissue sarcomas. *Cancer* **72:**1919–1925, 1993
12. McAfee MK, Allen MS, Trastek VF, et al: Colorectal lung metastasis: results of surgical excision. *Ann Thorac Surg* **53:**780–785, 1992
13. Stewart JR, Carey JA, Merrill WH, et al: Twenty years' experience with pulmonary metastasectomy. *Am Surg* **58:**100–103, 1992
14. Sirivella S, Zikria EA, Ford WB, et al: Improved technique for closure of median sternotomy incision. Mersilene tapes versus standard wire closure. *J Thorac Cardiovasc Surg* **94:**591–595, 1987
15. Kalush SL, Bonchek LI: Peristernal closure of median sternotomy using stainless steel bands. *Ann Thorac Surg* **21:**172, 1976
16. Zieren HU, Muller JM, Zieren J, Pichlmaier H: Closure of partial median sternotomy with absorbable sutures: A practical and safe option. *Am Surg* **59:**596–597, 1993
17. Kreitmann B, Riberi A, Metras D: Evaluation of an absorbable suture for sternal closure in pediatric cardiac surgery. *J Card Surg* **7:**254–256, 1992
18. DiMarco RF Jr, Lee MW, Bekoe S, et al: Interlocking figure-of-eight closure of the sternum. *Ann Thorac Surg* **47:**927–929, 1989
19. Robicsek F, Daugherty HK, Cook JW: The prevention and treatment of sternum separation following open-heart surgery. *J Thorac Cardiovasc Surg* **73:**267–268, 1977
20. Tatebe S, Eguchi S, Miyamura H, et al: Limited vertical skin incision for median sternotomy. *Ann Thorac Surg* **54:**787–788, 1992
21. Deutinger M, Deutinger J: Breast feeding after aesthetic mammary operations and cardiac operations through horizontal submammary skin incision. *Surg Gynecol Obstet* **176:**267–270, 1993
22. Martinez-Sanz R, Fleitas MG, de la Llana R, et al: Submammary median sternotomy. *J Cardiovasc Surg* **31:**578–580, 1990
23. Furnary AP, Magovern JA, Simpson KA, Magovern GJ: Prolonged open sternotomy and delayed sternal closure after cardiac operations. *Ann Thorac Surg* **54:**233–239, 1992
24. Garrett HE Jr, Matthews J: Reoperative median sternotomy. *Ann Thorac Surg* **48:**305, 1989

24. Garrett HE Jr, Matthews J: Reoperative median sternotomy. *Ann Thorac Surg* **48:**305, 1989
25. Kutsal A, Ibrisim E, Catav Z, Tasdemir O, Bayazit K: Mediastinitis after open heart surgery. Analysis of risk factors and management. *J Cardiovasc Surg* **32:**38–41, 1991
26. Belcher P, McLean N, Breach N, Paneth M: Omental transfer in acute and chronic sternal wound breakdown. *Thorac Cardiovasc Surg* **38:**186–191, 1990
27. Demmy TL, Park SB, Liebler GA, et al: Recent experience with major sternal wound complications. *Ann Thorac Surg* **49:**458–462, 1990
28. Lovich SF, Iverson LI, Young JN, et al: Omental pedicle grafting in the treatment of postcardiotomy sternotomy infection. *Arch Surg* **124:**1192–1194, 1989
29. Hazelrigg SR, Wellons HA Jr, Schneider JA, Kolm P: Wound complications after median sternotomy. Relationship to internal mammary grafting. *J Thorac Cardiovasc Surg* **98:**1096–1099, 1989
30. Francel TJ, Dufresne CR, Baumgartner WA, O'Kelley J: Anatomic and clinical considerations of an internal mammary artery harvest. *Arch Surg* **127:**1107–1111, 1992
31. Iacobucci JJ, Stevenson TR, Hall JD, Deeb GM: Sternal osteomyelitis: treatment with rectus abdominous muscle. *Br J Plast Surg* **42:**452–459, 1989
32. Stangl R, Altendorf-Hofmann A, von der Emde J: Brachial plexus lesions following median sternotomy in cardiac surgery. *Thorac Cardiovasc Surg* **39:**360–364, 1991
33. Rieke H, Benecke R, DeVivie ER, et al: Brachial plexus lesions following cardiac surgery with median sternotomy and cannulation of the internal jugular vein. *J Cardiothorac Anesth* **3:**286–289, 1989
34. Sweet RH: Thoracic incisions. In Sweet RH (ed): *Thoracic Surgery,* 1st ed. Philadelphia, Saunders, 1950, pp 59–80
35. Grimson KS: Complications of thoracotomy observed during operations upon sympathetic and vagus nerves. *Surg Clin North Am* **26:**1108–1123, 1946
36. Weinberg JA, Kraus AR: Intercostal incisions in transpleural operations. *J Thorac Surg* **19:**769–778, 1950
37. Kittle CF: Thoracic incisions. In Baue AE, Geha AS, Hammond GL, et al (eds): *Thoracic and Cardiovascular Surgery,* 5th ed. East Norwalk, CT, 1991, pp 67–82
38. Kittle CF: Which way in? The thoracotomy incision. *Ann Thorac Surg* **45:**234, 1988
39. Tedder M, Anstadt MP, Tedder SD, Lowe JE: Current morbidity, mortality, and survival after bronchoplastic procedures for malignancy. *Ann Thorac Surg* **54:**387–391, 1992
40. Naunheim KS, Kesler KA, D'Orazio SA, et al: Thoracotomy in the octogenarian. *Ann Thorac Surg* **51:**547–551, 1991
41. Lozac'h P, Topart P, Etienne J, Charles JF: Ivor Lewis operation for epidermoid carcinoma of the esophagus. *Ann Thorac Surg* **52:**1154–1157, 1991
42. Shaw RR, Paulson DL, Kee JL: The treatment of the superior sulcus tumor by irradiation followed by resection. *Ann Surg* **154:**29–40, 1961
43. Wright CD, Moncure AC, Shepard JO, et al. Superior sulcus lung tumors. *J Thorac Cardiovasc Surg* **94:**69–74, 1987
44. Lemmer JH, Gomez MN, Symreng T, et al: Limited lateral thoracotomy. *Arch Surg* **125:**873–877, 1990
45. Hazelrigg SR, Landreneau RJ, Boley TM, et al: The effect of muscle-sparing versus standard posterolateral thoracotomy on pulmonary function, muscle strength, and postoperative pain. *J Thorac Cardiovasc Surg* **101:**394–400, 1991
46. Ponn RB, Ferneini A, D'Angostino RS, et al: Comparison of late pulmonary function after posterolateral and muscle-sparing thoracotomy. *Ann Thorac Surg* **53:**675–679, 1992
47. Brereton RJ, Goh DW: Muscle-sparing thoracotomy has much to recommend it in neonates. *J Pediatr Surg* **27:**1257–1258, 1992
48. Soucy P, Bass J, Evans M: The muscle-sparing thoracotomy in infants and children. *J Pediatr Surg* **26:**1323–1325, 1991
49. Karwanda SV, Rowles JR: Simplified muscle-sparing thoracotomy for patent ductus arteriosus ligation in neonates. *Ann Thorac Surg* **54:**164–165, 1992
50. Mitchell RL: The lateral limited thoracotomy incision: Standard for pulmonary operations. *J Thorac Cardiovasc Surg* **99:**590–596, 1990
51. Mitchell R, Angell W, Wuerflein R, Dor V: Simplified lateral chest incision for most thoracotomies other than sternotomy. *Ann Thorac Surg* **22:**284–286, 1976
52. Bethencourt DM, Holmes EC: Muscle-sparing posterolateral thoracotomy. *Ann Thorac Surg* **45:**337–339, 1988
53. Noirclerc M, Dor V, Chavin et al: Extensive lateral thoracotomy without muscle section. *Ann Chir Thorac Cardiovasc* **12:**181–183, 1973
54. Fry WA, Kehoe TJ, McGee JP: Axillary thoracotomy. *Am Surg* **56:**460–462, 1990
55. Heitmiller RF, Mathisen DJ: French incision. In Grillo HC, Austen WG, Wilkins EW Jr, et al (eds): *Current Therapy in Cardiothoracic Surgery,* B.C. Decker Inc, 1989, pp 268–269
56. Baeza OR, Foster ED: Vertical axillary thoracotomy: A functional and cosmetically appealing incision. *Ann Thorac Surg* **22:**287–288, 1976
57. Siegel T, Steiger Z: Axillary thoracotomy. *Surg Gynecol Obst* **155:**725–727, 1982
58. Ginsberg RJ: Alternative (muscle-sparing) incisions in Thoracic surgery. *Ann Thorac Surg* **56:**752–754, 1993
59. Ashour M: Modified muscle sparing posterolateral thoracotomy. *Thorax* **45:**935–938, 1990
60. Heitmiller RF: The serratus sling: A simplified serratus-sparing technique. *Ann Thorac Surg* **48:**867–868, 1989
61. Becker RM, Munro DD: Transaxillary minithoracotomy: The optimal approach for certain pulmonary and mediastinal lesions. *Ann Thorac Surg* **22:**254–259, 1976
62. Deslauriers J, Beaulieu M, Despres JP, et al: Transaxillary pleurectomy for treatment of spontaneous pneumothorax. *Ann Thorac Surg* **30:**569–574, 1980
63. McNeill TM, Chamberlain JM: Diagnostic anterior mediastinotomy. *Ann Thorac Surg* **2:**532–539, 1966
64. Heitmiller RF: Results of standard left thoracoabdominal esophagogastrectomy. In Loop FD, Mathisen DJ (eds): *Seminars in Thoracic and Cardiovascular Surgery,* vol. 4. Philadelphia, Saunders, 1992, pp 314–319
65. Pasque MK, Cooper JD, Kaiser LR, et al: Improved technique for bilateral lung transplantation: Rationale and initial clinical experience. *Ann Thorac Surg* **49:**785–791, 1990
66. Kaiser LR, Pasque MK, Trulock EP, et al: Bilateral sequential lung transplantation: The procedure of choice for double-lung replacement. *Ann Thorac Surg* **52:**438–446, 1991
67. Shimizu N, Ando A, Matsutani T, et al: Transternal thoracotomy for bilateral pulmonary metastasis. *J Surg Oncol* **50:**105–109, 1992
68. Bains MS, Ginsberg RJ, Jones WG II, et al: The clamshell incision: An improved approach to bilateral pulmonary and mediastinal tumors. Abstract presented at the 30th meeting of the Society of Thoracic Surgeons, New Orleans, January 1994
69. Wells SA, Cooper JD: Closed mediastinal exploration in patients with persistent hyperparathyroidism. *Ann Surg* **214:**555–561, 1991
70. Marrin CA, Canver CC, Greenberg M, et al: Subxiphoid approach for insertion of ICDs after previous median sternotomy. *Ann Thorac Surg* **56:**312–315, 1993
71. Thirlby RC, Kraemer SJ, Hill LD: Transdiaphragmatic approach to the posterior mediastinum and thoracic esophagus. *Arch Surg* **128:**897–901, 1993
72. Wolf CJ: Recent advances in the pathophysiology of acute pain. *Br J Anaesth* **63:**139–146, 1989
73. Wall PD: The prevention of postoperative pain. *Pain* **33:**289–290, 1988
74. Eng J, Sabanathan S: Post-thoracotomy analgesia. *J R Coll Surg Edinb* **38:**62–68, 1993

75. El-Baz NMI, Faber LP, Jensik RJ: Continuous epidural infusion of morphine for treatment of pain after thoracic surgery: A new technique. *Anesth Analg* **63:**757–764, 766, 1984
76. Pflug AE, Murphy TM, Butler SH, Tucker GT: The effects of postoperative peridural analgesia on pulmonary therapy and pulmonary complications. *Anesthesiology* **41:**8–17, 1974
77. Faber LP: Epidural analgesia: different strokes for different folks. *Ann Thorac Surg* **50:**862–863, 1990
78. Gustafsson LL, Schildt B, Jacobson K: Adverse effects of extradural and intrathecal opiates: report of a nationwide survey in Sweden. *Br J Anaesth* **54:**479–486, 1982
79. Stenseth R, Sellevold O, Breivik H: Epidural morphine for postoperative pain: experience with 1085 patients. *Acta Anaesthesiol Scand* **29:**148–156, 1985
80. James EC, Kolberg HL, Iwen GW, Gellaatly TA: Epidural analgesia for post-thoracotomy patients. *J Thorac Cardiovasc Surg* **82:**898–903, 1981
81. Neustein SM, Cohen E: Intrathecal morphine during thoracotomy, part II: Effect on post-operative meperidine requirements and pulmonary function tests. *J Cardiovasc Vasc Anesth* **7:**157–159, 1993
82. Gray JR, Fromme GA, Nauss LA, Wang JK: Intrathecal morphine for post-thoracotomy pain. *Anesth Analg* **6:**873–876, 1986
83. Kaplan J, Miller ED Jr, Gallagher EG Jr: Post-operative analgesia for thoracotomy patients. *Anesth Analg* **54:**773–777, 1975
84. de la Rocha AG, Chambers K: Pain amelioration after thoracotomy: A prospective randomized study. *Ann Thorac Surg* **37:**239–242, 1989
85. Eng J, Sabanathan S: Site of action of continuous extrapleural intercostal nerve block. *Ann Thorac Surg* **51:**387–389, 1991
86. Muller LC, Salzer GM, Ransmayr G, Neiss A: Intraoperative cryoanalgesia for postthoracotomy pain relief. *Ann Thorac Surg* **48:**15–18, 1989
87. Kirvela O, Antila H: Thoracic paravertebral block in chronic postoperative pain. *Reg Anaesth* **17:**348–350, 1992
88. Eng J, Sabanathan S: Continuous extrapleural intercostal nerve block and post-thoracotomy pulmonary complications. *Scand J Thorac Cardiovasc Surg* **26:**219–223, 1992
89. Inderbitzi R, Flueckiger K, Ris HB: Pain relief and respiratory mechanics during continuous intrapleural bupivacaine administration after thoracotomy. *Thorac Cardiovasc Surg* **40:**87–89, 1992
90. Schneider RF, Villamena PC, Harvey J, et al: Lack of efficacy of intrapleural bupivicaine for postoperative analgesia following thoracotomy. *Chest* **103:**414–416, 1993
91. Stromskag KE, Minor B, Steen PA: Side effects and complications related to intrapleural analgesia: an update. *Acta Anaesthesiol Scand* **34:**473–477, 1990

# CHAPTER 6

# Thoracic Trauma

Kenneth L. Mattox and Matthew Wall, Jr.

## HISTORIC PERSPECTIVES

Until the 19th century, references to chest injury were either descriptions of internal injuries found at autopsy or treatment schemas for chest wall injuries. Of the 58 cases cited in the Edmund Smith Surgical Papyrus, two involved injury to the chest, one involved injury to the sternum, and another involved fractured ribs.[1] By the second century, Galen[2] had described successful drainage of a posttraumatic sternal infection that required a pericardiectomy. By the 16th century, debates concerning closure of an open chest wound were published by Ambrose Paré.[3] In 1535, while wandering through Texas to Mexico, the Spanish explorer Cabeza de Vaca recorded in his diary the first documented operation in North America: removal of an arrowhead from the sternum and pericardium of an Indian. The patient's recovery resulted in "Doctor" de Vaca's ongoing sustenance, allowing him to return to Spain.[4] In 1814, Larrey[5] commented on injuries of the thoracic outlet, particularly the subclavian artery. Since the time of Homer, all cardiac wounds have been considered fatal. Although Tourby,[6] in 1642, discovered a spontaneously healed heart in a man who had been stabbed with a sword, Rehn[7] in 1897 was the first to report successful suturing of a cardiac wound 4 years earlier. Although successful repair of cardiac wounds was sporadically reported, by the mid-20th century, conservative thought still dictated repeated pericardiocentesis for treating these injuries.[8]

Injuries to the great vessels were recognized as early as 1557, when Vesalius described a blunt thoracic aortic injury.[9] Successful treatment of great vessel injuries did not occur until the 20th century, with the advent of endotracheal anesthesia and a better understanding of chest physiology. Dshanelidze[10] in 1922 repaired a puncture wound of the ascending aorta. By the 1950s and 1960s, several significant series of injuries to the great vessels and heart appeared in the literature. Although Alexis St. Martin (William Beaumont's patient) is best known for his gastric fistula, he actually had an injury to the sixth rib, the left lung, and diaphragm.[11] The herniated lung was reduced, and the chest wound was closed. During World Wars I and II, knowledge of proper timing for drainage of posttraumatic and postinfectious empyema resulted in treatises on both open and closed drainage.[12,13]

The treatment of thoracic injuries has been simplified during the last 25 years with tracheostomy for flail chest, positive pressure ventilators, broad-spectrum and specific antibiotics, resuscitative thoracotomy in the emergency room (ER), autotransfusion and cardiopulmonary bypass, sophisticated radiologic techniques, and surgical intensive care units (ICU).

Prior to the 20th century, the mortality rate for penetrating wounds of the chest exceeded 50%. There were no civilian experiences. One must look to military campaigns for mortality rates. The mortality for chest injury in the Crimean War was 91.6% for the French, and 79.3% for the British; other rates were as follow: Italian War of 1859, 61%; American Civil War, 33.4%; Franco-Prussian War, 55.8%. The mortality rate was 7.7% in World War I and 12% in World War II.[14–18] In the later half of the 20th century, thoracic trauma gained medico-political attention. Texas Governor John Connally in 1963 sustained a near fatal and highly publicized gunshot wound to the right chest from the same gun that resulted in President John Kennedy's death.[19] President Ronald Reagan also sustained a near fatal gunshot wound to the left chest in 1981. Each of these events was photographed, each victim was taken to a trauma center, and two patients survived.

## SPECIFIC ANATOMIC CONSIDERATIONS

The chest is a truncated, dynamic structure with upper and lower boundaries that vary with respiration and patient position. The general surgeon considers the thoracic outlet to be zone 1 of the neck. Some articles define both the subclavian and axillary vessels to be part of the thoracic outlet, and others describe these vessels as belonging to the upper extremity. The cupola of the lung may rise into supraclavicular spaces of the neck. With respiration, especially in the supine position, the dome of the diaphragm may rise as high as the fourth interspace. When the patient is standing and lungs are fully expanded, the dome of the diaphragm may be as low as the 10th interspace. These variable anatomic considerations are important when determining associated neck and abdominal injuries in a patient with a major thoracic injury.

Pericardial reflections are so positioned that portions of the ascending aorta, the main pulmonary artery, portions of the right and left pulmonary arteries, and portions of the pulmonary veins, as well as portions of the superior and inferior vena cava are intrapericardial. Even trivial injuries to these vessels as well as cardiac injuries may produce pericardial tamponade with major physiologic derangement with relatively small volumes of blood loss.

The visceral and parietal pleura are normally separated by a thin film of plasma. The pleural space is only a potential space, developing if injury to the lung or chest wall occurs. The visceral and parietal pleura are attached at the hilum but not attached peripherally to allow free movement of the lung within the confines of the pleural space. However, in up to 25% of individuals, isolated or significant areas of pleural symphysis are secondary to old injury or inflammation. The muscular chest wall supports the upper extremities and provides aid in respiration. Laterally, at the midaxillary line at approximately the fifth intercostal space, the auscultatory triangle is most devoid of muscle. Insertion of a chest tube in this location for a hemo- or pneumothorax is not only most expeditious, but also least painful.

The blood supply to the spinal cord is of specific interest to the thoracic surgeon. Approximately nine paired segmental arteries branch from the descending thoracic aorta, with the highest pairs to the first few intercostal spaces branching from either the highest intercostal artery or directly off of the subclavian or innominate artery.[20] The segmental arteries divide into the intercostal and radicular arteries (Fig. 6–1). The radicular artery further branches to supply a single anterior spinal artery and paired posterior spinal arteries. The anterior spinal artery is extremely variable and rudimentary. It may be continuous throughout the entire length of the spinal cord, or it may be interrupted repeatedly. The size of the radicular arteries supplying the anterior spinal artery varies. This variability in the blood supply to the anterior part of the spinal cord is the most important factor in the occurrence of posttraumatic paraplegia when operations must be performed on the thoracic aorta.

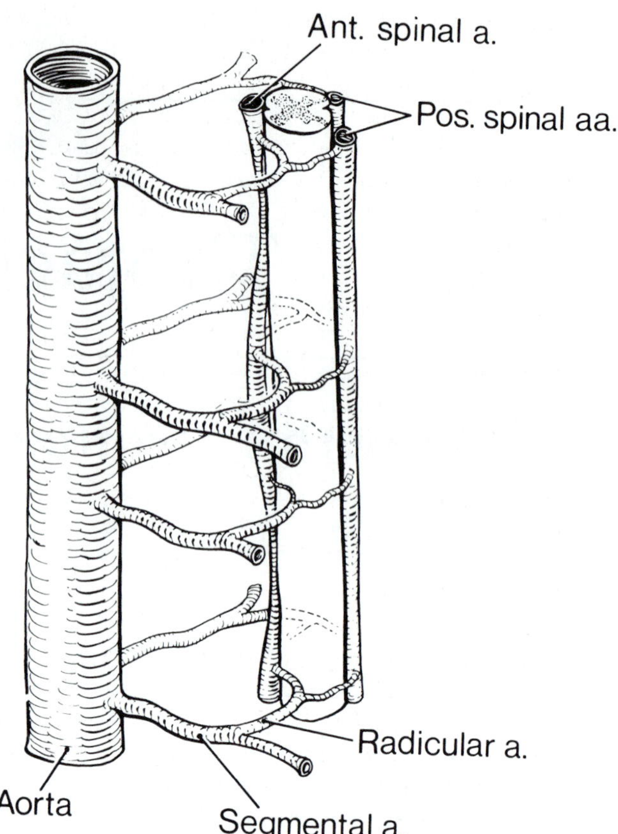


**Figure 6–1.** Drawing of thoracic segmental arteries depicting the variability of radicular and anterior spinal arteries.

## ETIOLOGY, PATHOGENESIS, AND NATURAL HISTORY

Injury to the chest and its structures may be due to (1) penetrating trauma; (2) blunt trauma, including blast injuries; (3) pulmonary injury secondary to aspiration or infection; (4) pulmonary, vascular, and cardiac alterations secondary to hormonal, immunologic, and cell mediator responses; and (5) iatrogenic injuries.[21–32] Penetrating wounds may be produced by a knife, a portion of an automobile, or a gunshot wound. Blunt trauma, most commonly produced by motor vehicle accidents, causes deceleration injuries. Blunt injuries include those produced by blasts, falls, and other impacts. Iatrogenic injuries may be secondary to both diagnostic and therapeutic interventions resulting in injury to the esophagus or tracheobronchial tree during endoscopy, to the lungs or heart during catheterization and percutaneous biopsies, to the heart or even the great vessels during cardiopulmonary resuscitation, and in other injuries during various procedures.

Although not usually reported with chest injuries, numerous iatrogenic injuries to the chest occur. Chest tubes containing trocars have perforated the lung, heart, aorta, esophagus and all of the upper abdominal organs, including liver, spleen, colon, kidney, stomach, pancreas, and small bowel. The use of trocar chest tubes is not recommended. Penetration of the lung during thoracentesis may occur, with subsequent development of pneumothorax. Barotrauma during positive pressure ventilation may result in pneumothorax and massive air leak. Long IV catheters, especially those that are relatively stiff, may perforate the subclavian or innominate veins and the heart.[25,33] A tracheostomy tube may produce a fistula from the innominate artery to the trachea, resulting in exsanguinating hemorrhage.[32,34] During mediastinoscopy, thoracoscopy, insertion of trocar chest tubes, and even percutaneous biopsy of lung masses, arterial, venous, and pleural structures may be injured.

Of patients dying from trauma, 25% die as a direct result of the chest injury. In an additional 25%, the chest injury contributes to their demise.[35] There are approximately 12 thoracic injuries per day per 1 million population. Of these 12, 4 will require hospitalization, with 1 being severe.[36] In the United States, of 50,000 injuries in the major outcome study, 15,000 patients had chest injuries.[37] Of these, 70% were secondary to blunt trauma and 30% from penetrating trauma. From 1962 to 1970, 60% of thoracic injuries were from motor vehicle accidents, 14% occurring at work, 10% at home, and 18% resulting in death.[36] Of these, 71% involved the chest wall, 41% produced a pneumothorax or hemothorax, 7% involved the heart, and 7% involved the diaphragm (Table 6–1). About 4% of patients will have injury to a great vessel, with less than 5% having injury to the tracheobronchial tree or esophagus. Blunt and penetrating thoracic injury may involve the liver, kidney, and spleen. The many organs involved and problems produced by penetrating thoracic trauma are listed in Table 6–2.

**TABLE 6–1. PERCENTAGE OF ORGAN INJURY FOLLOWING BLUNT THORACIC TRAUMA**

| Organ | Kemmerer[18] (%) | Besson[36] (%) |
|---|---|---|
| **Chest wall** | | |
| Rib fracture | 39 | 47 |
| Sternal fracture | 5 | 22 |
| **Pleural "space"** | | |
| Hemothorax | 28 | 24 |
| Lung laceration | 10 | 21 |
| Lung contusion | 6 | 12 |
| **Mediastinum** | | |
| Great vessel | 10 | 4 |
| Myocardial | 6 | 7 |
| Trachea | 1 | 5 |
| **Diaphragm** | 5 | 7 |

## PREHOSPITAL ISSUES

With the development of trauma systems came emergency medical services (EMS), trauma centers, and the concepts and devices to assist in the care of patients with chest injury.[38–40] Triage criteria established by the American College of Surgeons require all patients with significant thoracic trauma to be directed by the EMS to a designated trauma center.[41] The use of air ambulance for patients with truncal trauma being transported less than 35 miles is discouraged. Ground ambulances for these distances are quicker, more expeditious, and more cost-effective.[42,43] Prehospital external cardiac compression for more than 4 minutes for patients with truncal trauma is usually unsuccessful.[44] The pneumatic antishock garment (MAST) has not improved survival in patients with thoracic injuries and may actually slightly decrease survival, especially in patients with cardiac tamponade.[45] Inserting chest tubes in the field has no effect on survival in the urban setting. Currently in the urban setting, the value of prehospital administration of IV fluids for the patient in shock from penetrating trauma has not been demonstrated and may actually be detrimental.[46,47]

Endotracheal intubation is one of the few prehospital interventions demonstrated with proven efficacy. In patients with truncal trauma requiring prehospital cardiopulmonary resuscitation (CPR), survival is extremely rare after 5 minutes in the unintubated patient and after 10 minutes in the intubated patient.[48]

## EMERGENCY CENTER EVALUATION AND TREATMENT

In the emergency area of the trauma center, resuscitation and treatment algorithms are always under the direction of a surgeon.[49] The initial survey is a quick overview to assess major physiologic derangements as well as provide immediate life-saving maneuvers. The basics of these assessments cannot be overemphasized and include assess and secure the airway, control and treat hemorrhage, replace volume when appropriate, splint fractures, and perform surgery as part of resuscitation—not as a sequela to it. Specific assessments include status of neck veins, presence of consolidation of one hemothorax or the other, hyperresonance to percussion, presence or absence of breath sounds, presence of a deviated trachea, and systemic blood pressure. Arterial blood gases and an initial chest x-ray provide additional immediate information. Patients with injuries close to the trachea or esophagus should undergo endoscopy, and patients with radiologic clues suggestive of great vessel injury should undergo arteriography. For clinical findings of a

**TABLE 6–2. PERCENTAGE OF ORGAN INJURY FOLLOWING PENETRATING THORACIC TRAUMA**

| | Stab Wound | | Gunshot Wound | |
|---|---|---|---|---|
| Organ or Symptom | *Incidence (%)* | *Mortality (%)* | *Incidence (%)* | *Mortality (%)* |
| Pneumothorax | 49 | 0 | 30 | 17 |
| Hemothorax | 47 | 19 | 54 | 19 |
| Lung | 24 | 0 | 54 | 12 |
| Abdominal viscus | 16 | 14[a] | 35 | 18 |
| Thoracic great vessel | 16 | 14[a] | 6 | 60[a] |
| Diaphragm | 9 | 25[a] | 31 | 20 |
| Heart | 7 | 67 | 13 | 40 |
| Pericardium | 7 | 67[a] | 19 | 20 |
| Chylothorax | 4 | 0 | — | — |
| Esophagus | — | — | 6 | 60[a] |
| Trachea | — | — | 1 | 100[a] |

[a]Less than ten cases.
*(From Besson A, Saegesser F: Color Atlas of Chest Trauma and Associated Injuries. Oradell, New Jersey, Medical Economics Books, 1983, with permission.)*

significant hemopneumothorax and/or radiologic confirmation of such, tube thoracostomy with a nontrocar chest tube of 32F or greater is indicated.[50,51] Chest tubes are inserted in the fourth or fifth midaxillary line and directed posteriorly for all hemopneumothoraces (Fig. 6–2). A limited digital exploration of the chest is done prior to insertion of the chest tube. The diaphragm, lung, and pericardium can be palpated, at times ascertaining the presence of a tense pericardium, a hole in the pericardium, or a hole in the diaphragm. The subcutaneous tissue and intercostal muscles may be divided by a sharp instrument, but the pleura should be entered only with the finger, since 25% of the population will have pleural symphysis.

A patient with a thoracic injury may rapidly deteriorate, on entering the emergency center or shortly thereafter. Patients with chest injury, especially to the heart, may benefit from emergency center thoracotomy.[52–55] This procedure should not be performed if (1) a surgeon is not available to assist other emergency center personnel, (2) if the patient is obviously dead, or (3) if hospital policy dictates against this procedure. Emergency center thoracotomy for extrathoracic injury or blunt trauma to the chest has a very low yield for successful resuscitation.[56,57] In male patients, emergency center thoracotomy is usually performed through a fourth intercostal anterolateral incision and through the inframammary fold in women, lifting the breast up to enter the fourth intercostal space (Fig. 6–3). In hypovolemic patients, the descending thoracic aorta may be crossclamped to preserve coronary and cerebral perfusion during resuscitation. The pericardium is entered anterior to the phrenic nerve and the heart massaged preparatory to cardiorrhaphy.

Patients who are hypotensive without arrest but with signs of pericardial tamponade may, on rare occasion, benefit from pericardiocentesis. Clotted blood is frequently present, and a minimal amount may be removed. During the late 1980s, subxiphoid pericardiotomy (sometimes under local anesthesia) performed in the emergency center and/or the operating room (OR) was proposed by some as an alternate to pericardiocentesis.[58,59] Subxiphoid pericardiotomy has greatest value if tamponade is *not* present and as such "rules out" a heart injury. Should there be a significant heart injury, this procedure may convert the emergency situation from tamponade to exsanguination through a "peek hole" incision.

Eighty-five percent of patients with chest injury may be managed by simple techniques, either tube thoracostomy or endotracheal intubation with simple techniques, or either tube thoracostomy or endotracheal intubation with respiratory support. Only for specific indications should a thoracotomy be performed in the emergency center or operating room (OR).

## Airway

In the ER, evaluation of the airway is of primary importance. It may be compromised by an obstructing hematoma, deviation of the trachea, obstruction by a foreign body, obstruction by a relaxed mandible or tongue, direct injury to the air passages, or injury to the neuromuscular structures that control respiration.

## Hemothorax/Pneumothorax

A variety of specific injuries produces relatively few clinical symptoms and signs. Hemothorax, pneumothorax, and hemopneumothorax are variants of the same process: loss of integrity of the pleural space. They may be the result of external penetration with disruption of the parietal pleura, disruption of the visceral pleura secondary to lung injury caused by external trauma or barotrauma, or disruption of the mediastinal pleura secondary to injury of the esophagus

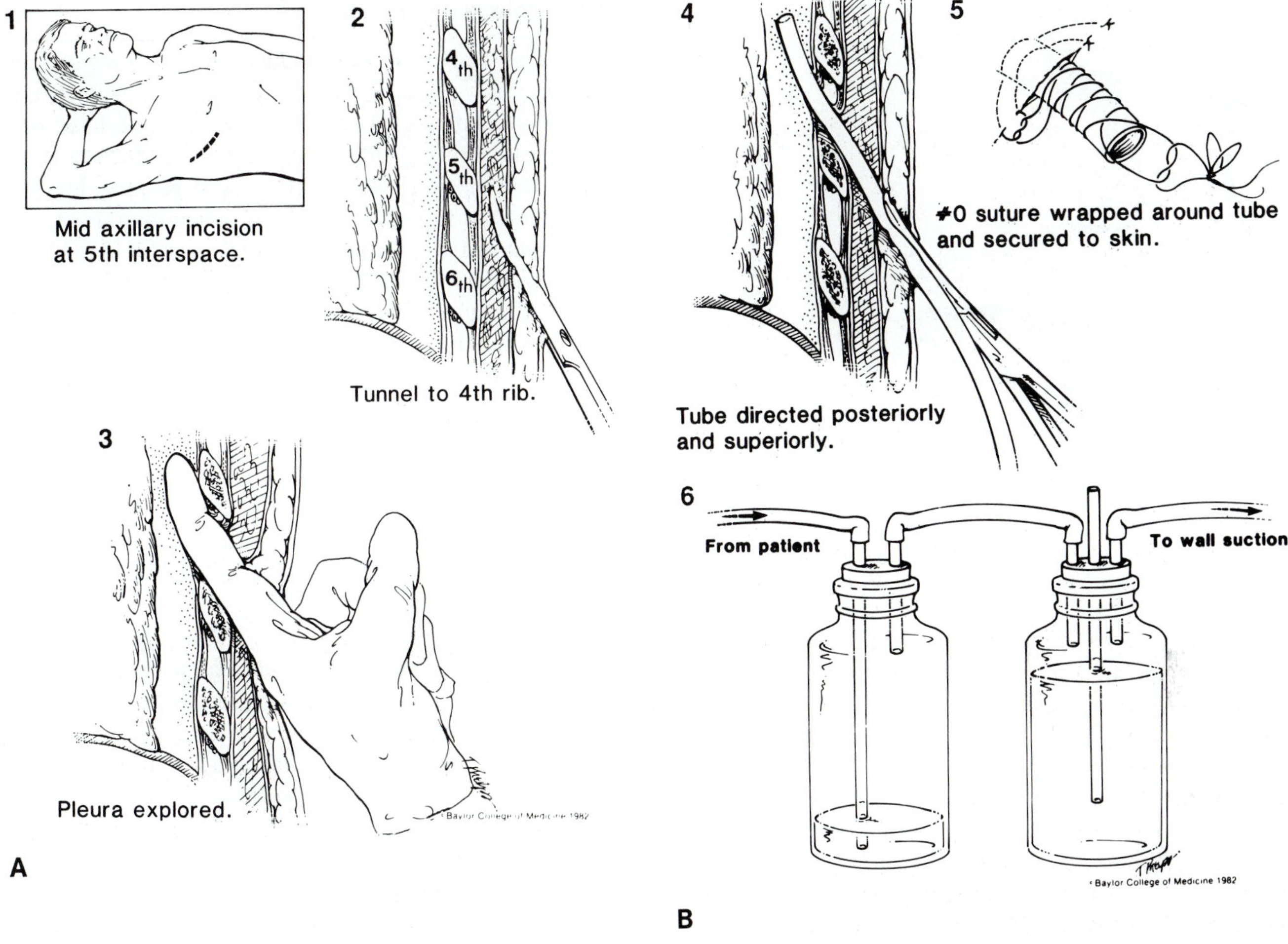


**Figure 6–2. A.** Technique of chest tube insertion. Note that the gloved finger is the instrument used to penetrate and explore the pleural space. **B.** Insertion of chest tube and connection to "two-bottle" controlled negative pressure collection device.

or tracheobronchial tree. Hemopneumothorax is the most common variant. If the injury to a visceral organ is large or involves a large vessel, hemothorax predominates. Because 25% of patients may have pleural symphysis, the hemopneumothorax may be loculated or limited. Four or more liters of fluid may accumulate in the pleural space. Because the mediastinum usually is not "fixed," clamping of a chest tube through which a large volume of blood is flowing should not be done to achieve "tamponade" of bleeding unless it is preparatory to autotransfusion.

## Pneumomediastinum and Subcutaneous Emphysema

Pneumomediastinum and subcutaneous emphysema may occur from the same mechanisms that produce hemopneumothorax, especially in patients with injury in an area of pleural symphysis. Subcutaneous emphysema is common with soft tissue injury from blunt trauma, especially with multiple rib fractures. If a tension pneumothorax is present, subcutaneous emphysema may quickly become exaggerated, especially if the patient is on positive pressure ventilation. Injury to the trachea, main stem bronchus, or the esophagus may produce isolated pneumomediastinum. A pneumomediastinum may be present without subcutaneous emphysema or a pneumothorax in patients with barotrauma secondary to a blast or Valsalva maneuver. Pneumopericardium is rare after injury. It implies loss of pericardial integrity. Rarely in the adult, tension pneumopericardium may occur.[60–63]

## Tension Pneumothorax

Tension pneumothorax is a special form of pneumothorax that occurs when an injury to the lung results in a ball valve mechanism with air from the lung entering the pleural space and accumulating (Fig. 6–4). With each breath, particularly with Valsalva maneuvers and positive pressure ventilation, pressure in the pleural space increases, and the mediastinum is deviated to the opposite side, causing kinking of the vena cavae and decreased venous return to the heart. The diaphragm on the affected side is depressed, and the trachea is deviated in the neck to the opposite side. Hyperresonance to percussion and distant breath sounds are present. The

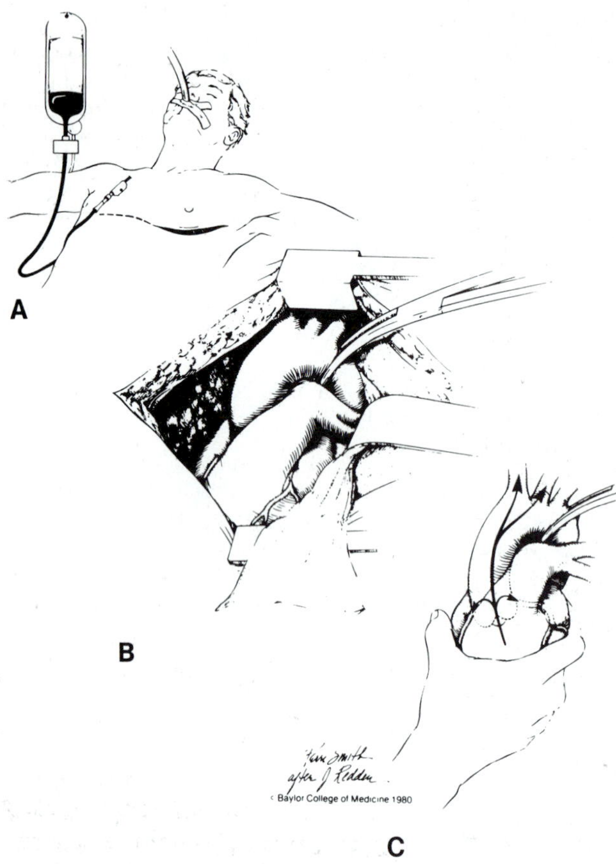


**Figure 6–3.** Technique of fourth interspace resuscitative anterolateral thoracotomy for cross clamping of the descending thoracic aorta and/or internal cardiac massage. Note that patient is intubated and incision may be carried across the sternum if necessary.

clinical pictures of tension pneumothorax and cardiac tamponade are very similar. In both conditions, hypotension and distended neck veins are present.

### Pulmonary Hematoma and Pulmonary Contusion

Pulmonary contusion and/or hematoma may occur from both blunt and penetrating trauma. Blood within the substance of the lung usually resolves in about 2 weeks. Occasionally, a hematoma may cavitate if it becomes infected. Rarely do such hematomas require surgery. Pulmonary contusion is secondary to direct blunt trauma, blast injury, or indirect forces from a bullet. A contusion is a diffuse infiltration of all blood elements, especially albumin, without marked derangement of the basic pulmonary architecture. A pulmonary contusion will contribute to pulmonary A–V shunting. The contused lung is more amenable than the normal lung to sequestration of fluid and contributes to the adult respiratory distress syndrome (ARDS).[64]

### Pericardial Tamponade

Pericardial tamponade may be the result of a seemingly innocuous injury (such as internal mammary artery injury), or may be secondary to a severe injury (ruptured heart or a penetrating aortic or pulmonary artery wound). Any structures within the pericardial sac may cause bleeding that prevents the heart from passive filling during diastole. As the pericardial and venous pressures rise, systolic blood pressure may remain normal until a venous pressure of 20–25 cm $H_2O$, at which time systemic blood pressure may fall precipitously. Just before the drop in blood pressure, the pulse pressure is narrowed. With increased intrathoracic pressure from a Valsalva maneuver, the pulse may be completely lost (see Chapter 139).

### Myocardial Depression

Myocardial depression may be due to direct cardiac injury (myocardial contusion) or frank tears with a ventricular septal defect or valvular insufficiency. The patient in shock with low perfusion rapidly becomes acidotic with release of numerous cellular mediators, many of which depress the myocardium. Prolonged hypotension, acidosis, hyperkalemia, and hypothermia all contribute to myocardial depression, possibly by way of these cell mediators.

## DECISION TO OPERATE

Decisions to perform various procedures in the chest follow an orderly and logical sequence. Each procedure will be discussed separately.

### Tube Thoracostomy

Tube thoracostomy is a very useful procedure in thoracic trauma.[51] Repeated thoracentesis or a small catheter connected to a plastic needle and to underwater seal may alleviate a small pneumothorax in some patients. For patients with significant chest trauma, a formal tube thoracostomy, as described previously, may not only be life-saving but also provides a valuable monitoring technique for continued blood loss. Tube thoracostomy is indicated for a wide variety of conditions including iatrogenic pneumothorax after subclavian catheter insertion, hemothorax, pneumothorax, and/or tension pneumothorax. A patient with a penetrating wound below the nipples and without hemopneumothorax, for whom an exploratory laparotomy is planned should have a prophylactic tube thoracostomy performed on the side of the penetrating injury. Patients with ARDS who require high levels of positive end-expiratory pressure (PEEP) benefit from a prophylactic tube thoracostomy, as do patients with extensive subcutaneous emphysema. The subcutaneous emphysema may be the result of a tear in the

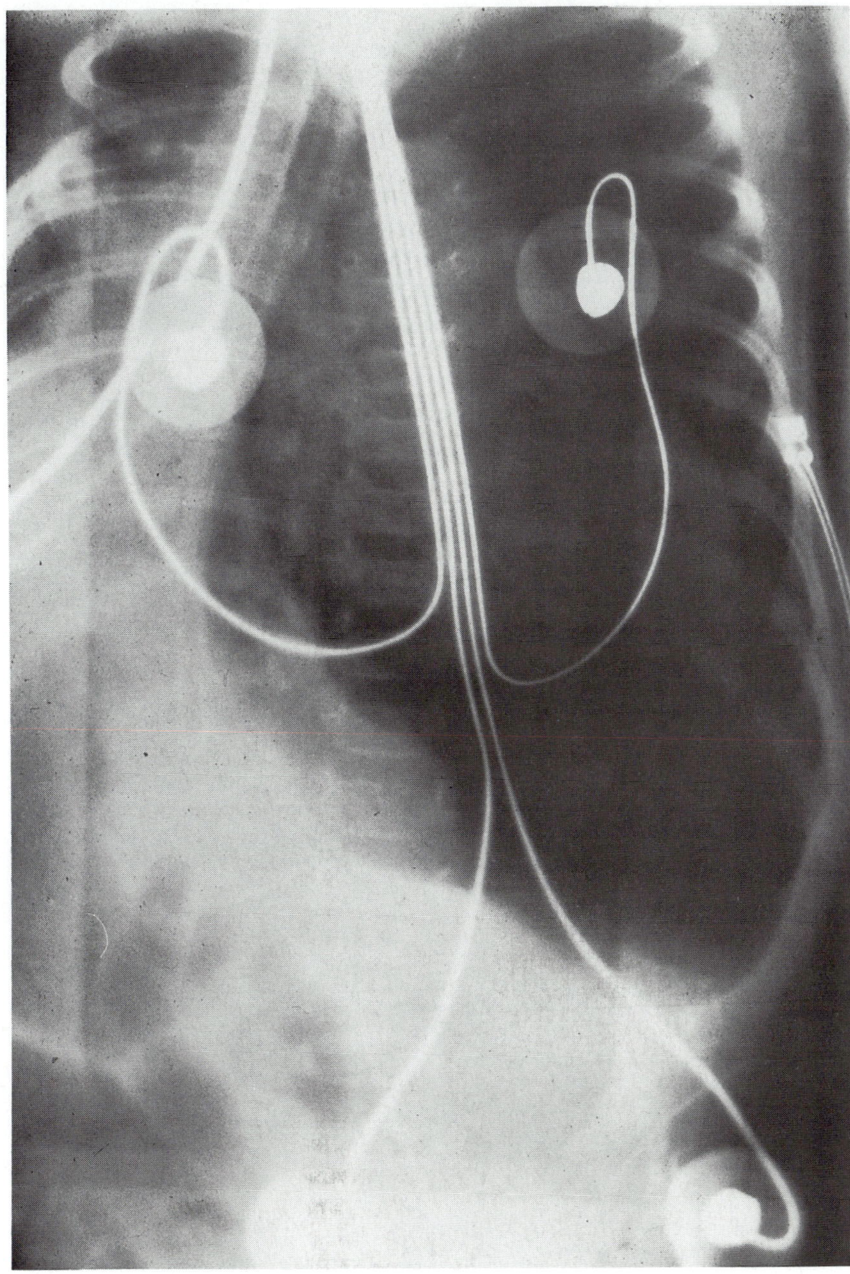

**Figure 6–4.** Chest x-ray (of a child) demonstrating a severe tension pneumothorax. Note the marked deviation of the mediastinum and depressed hemidiaphragm.

lung in an area of pleura symphysis or secondary to mediastinal dissection of an injury along the peribronchial septal planes. Because air breaking into the pleural space is common, a tube thoracostomy is beneficial.

## Decision for a Surgical Airway

Tracheostomy or cricothyroidotomy may be necessary in patients with chest injury. For the patient with a cervical fracture in whom the anesthesiologist has difficulty performing an oral or nasotracheal intubation, a cricothyroidotomy may be life-saving. Jet ventilation through a catheter placed in the trachea or cricothyroid membrane may be used until a definitive airway is obtained. A patient with a fractured larynx or transection of the trachea secondary to "clothesline" tear of the trachea may require an airway in the emergency center. An endotracheal tube inserted through an anterior wound is preferable to a tracheostomy. A formal tracheostomy in the emergency center may be difficult and lead to complications. For a patient with multisystem trauma (especially a head injury) who will require intubation for more than a week, early tracheostomy is advised. A patient with a flail chest and/or ARDS who requires intubation for periods in excess of 7–10 days is usually easier to manage with fewer pulmonary infections with a tracheostomy rather than orotracheal or nasotracheal intubation (see Chapter 4). A tracheostomy should be done at a high level through the second tracheal ring, so the tube will not ride low on the innominate artery, producing the dreaded complication of innominate artery-tracheal fistula. Should such occur, ligation of the innominate artery near the arch of the aorta and near the origin of the subclavian artery is the procedure of choice.[34]

## Indication for Thoracotomy

The decision to perform a thoracotomy is made on an urgent, emergent, or elective basis. An urgent thoracotomy is performed in the emergency center, ICU, or OR on a patient who is rapidly deteriorating because of exsanguinating hemorrhage or cardiac tamponade. Thoracotomy is required for cardiac resuscitation with cross-clamping of the descending thoracic aorta, cross-clamping of the hilum of the lung, or other techniques to control life-threatening hemorrhage or airway compromise. The procedure is most frequently performed in the emergency center.[48–53] An emergency thoracotomy may be performed in the OR for cardiac tamponade, loss of chest wall substance, penetrating injury to zone I of the neck (thoracic outlet), air embolism, and bronchial rupture.

An elective thoracotomy may be required for traumatic diaphragmatic rupture. A traumatic diaphragmatic hernia is usually approached through a laparotomy.[65] Delayed posttraumatic sequelae of penetrating cardiac injury, such as valvular or septal defects, posttraumatic false aneurysms, stenosis of the trachea or main stem bronchus, constrictive pericarditis, chronic emphysema, and evacuation of a clotted hemothorax may require an elective thoracotomy.

On rare occasions, cardiopulmonary bypass or extracorporeal circulatory support devices may be indicated for postmyocardial depression secondary to severe intramyocardial hemorrhage (usually from blunt trauma), systemic hypothermia secondary to exposure, acute aortic valve insufficiency, acute massive left-to-right shunt through a ventricular septal defect, tears of the ascending aorta or aortic arch, complex injuries involving the posterior left atrium or pulmonary hilum, and posttraumatic pulmonary embolism.[66–73] Rarely, proximal coronary artery injuries or myocardial depression secondary to fluid overload, cardiac distension, and electrolyte imbalance may require cardiopulmonary bypass (Fig. 6–5).[73–76]

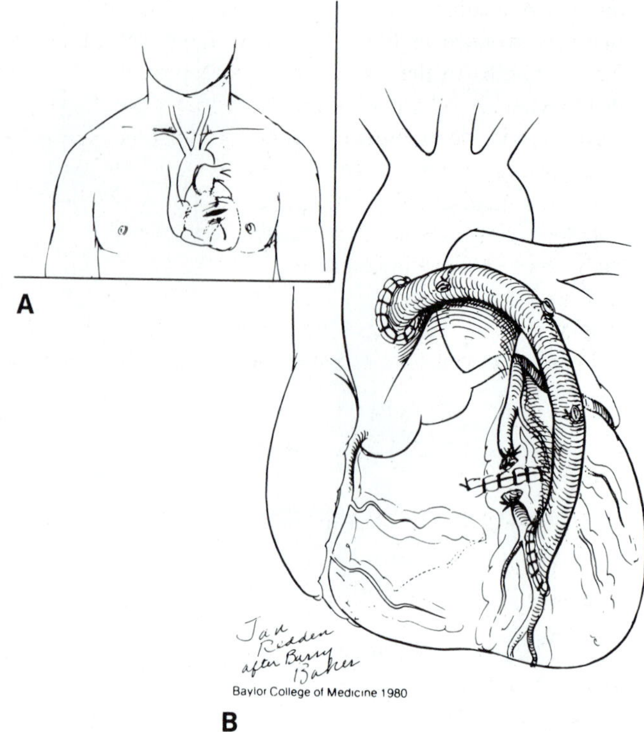


**Figure 6–5.** Acute emergency coronary artery bypass for stab wound to the left anterior descending coronary artery, with proximal ligation of injured artery. Patient was placed on battery-operated portable cardiopulmonary bypass in emergency room.

## Incisions

One of several incisions may be used: anterolateral, bilateral anterolateral with or without transsternal extension, median sternotomy, "book" or "trap door" incision, and posterolateral thoracotomy (Fig. 6–6). The anterolateral incision is used principally for resuscitation and for cross-clamping the aorta while anterior repairs are performed. A bilateral anterolateral thoracotomy is used for extensive bilateral injuries, including traversal of the mediastinum by a

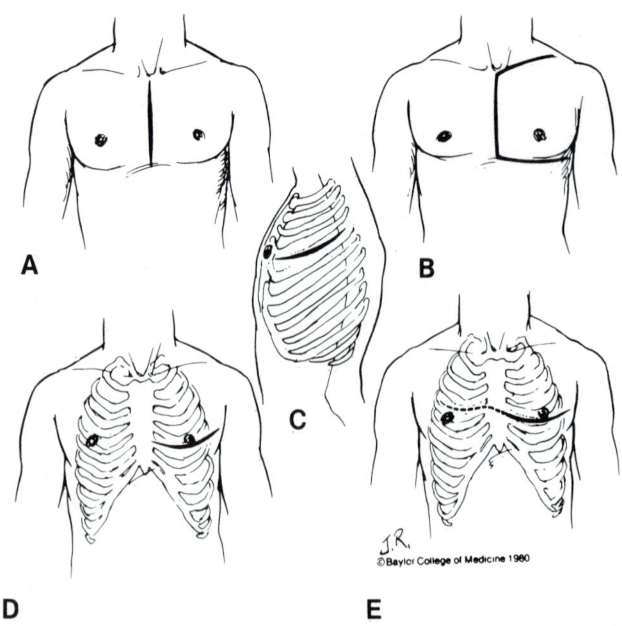


**Figure 6–6.** The variety of incisions available for exposure of thoracic injuries.

missile. A median sternotomy may be performed for anterior stab wounds and for thoracic outlet great vessel injuries. Injuries to the trachea may be approached through this incision. A subxiphoid pericardiotomy should never be performed in the emergency center. A subxiphoid pericardiotomy has no advantage over an anterolateral thoracotomy for a mediastinal or intrapericardial injury. A book or trap door incision is utilized primarily for injuries of the intrathoracic left subclavian artery. The posterolateral incision is used for injuries to the descending thoracic aorta, the esophagus, the diaphragm, posterior aspects of the lung, right and left main stem bronchus, and trachea in the area of the carina.

## DESCRIPTION OF INJURIES

### Chest Wall

Injuries to the chest wall are the most common thoracic trauma and often are treated on an outpatient basis. They range from minor lacerations and muscle strain, to perforation of the subcutaneous tissue and muscle alone, to fracture of the bony skeleton, to complete disruption of the chest wall with flail chest and its underlying visceral injury.

Fracture of the sternum is relatively uncommon.[77,78] The 5–15% mortality rate associated with a fractured sternum is more a function of associated injury to the heart and great vessels rather than the sternal fracture itself. A fractured sternum usually occurs with deceleration injuries and/or direct blows to the sternum. The fracture is usually linear in the midportion of the body of the sternum. It is frequently painful, with overlapping edges. The step deformity can be confirmed by lateral or oblique x-rays (Fig. 6–7). Sternal fractures are frequently self-limiting and do not cause any significant morbidity except for the deformity. A small percentage of patients will have respiratory insufficiency and cannot be extubated until operative fixation of the sternum has been performed. This procedure is done under general anesthesia and requires reduction and fixation with stainless steel wire.[77,78]

The flail chest syndrome is associated with fracture of the ribs anterior/posterior on the same side, at the costochondral junction on both sides, or a combination of several fractures that result in paradoxical movement of the chest wall with respiration. Contusion of the underlying lung leads to mild to severe respiratory insufficiency. Patients with flail chest frequently do not have evidence of paradoxical movement immediately in the ER. The contused underlying lung responds to vigorous fluid resuscitation by filling the interstitial spaces and alveoli with proteinaceous and cellular material. Arteriovenous shunting occurs. The work of breathing increases, and blood gases deteriorate. The flail segment only then manifests itself. With judicious management of fluid replacement, especially crystalloids, patients with flail chest may not develop respiratory insufficiency.[64,79] In the prehospital and emergency center periods, crystalloid resuscitation of these patients should be limited to <1000 mL. If volume expansion is required, blood or other colloids should be used. In the patient with a flail chest, decisions of when to observe or when to intubate may not be easy. The underlying pulmonary contusion and accumulated interstitial fluid with a ventilation/perfusion imbalance are more important than the degree of flailing. Although there are no clear cut guidelines, presence of the following in a patient prompts strong consideration of intubation:

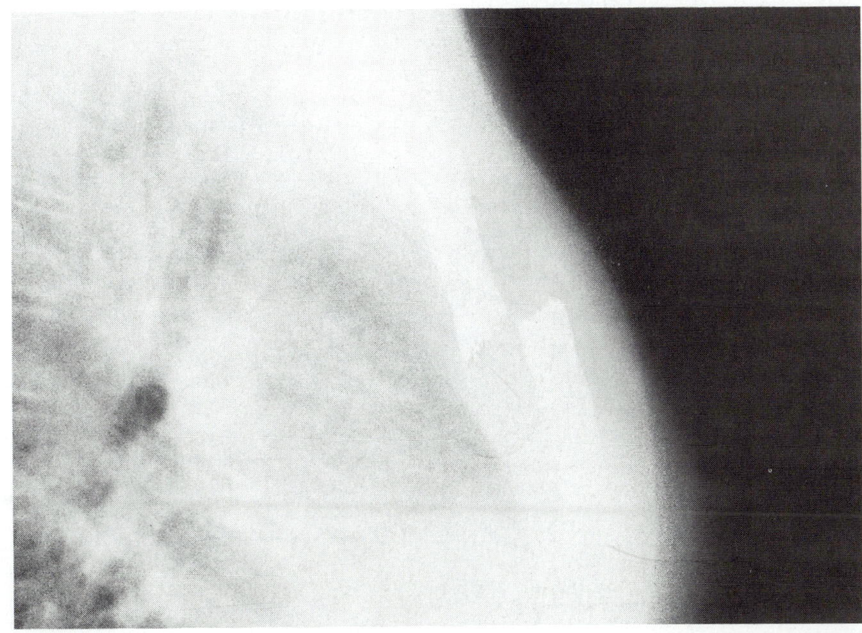

**Figure 6–7.** Lateral chest x-ray focusing on the sternum and demonstrating a sternal fracture. Note overriding of the lower segment and underriding of the upper segment. Fracture graphically enhanced by author.

- Combined severe head injury and flail chest
- Respiratory rate of 35–40/min
- Arterial $Po_2$ of 60 torr or less
- Arterial $Pco_2$ of 50 torr or more
- Vital capacity of less than 12 mL/kg
- Right-to-left pulmonary shunt >15%
- Maximum inspiratory force of <25 cm $H_2O$
- Injury severity score of >50
- Patients >50 years of age
- Poor nutrition or loss of immunocompetence

Assisted ventilation should be continued until the chest x-ray and ventilation status indicate weaning from controlled respiration. The use of intermittent mandatory ventilation (IMV) with pressure support or other alterations in positive pressure-assisted ventilation will decrease the total time intubation is required. IMV with pressure support is especially helpful for patients who have had prolonged intubation, since it helps to "retrain" the patient to breathe spontaneously. Ventilatory support serves as a form of internal stabilization for the flail chest and allows the underlying lung injury to heal. When the lung is healed, the patient may be extubatable, even if flailing persists.

Intubation is indicated if excessive fluids are required for associated injuries or prolonged operation, or if respiratory insufficiency develops with $Po_2$ of <60 and $Pco_2$ of <50. The use of colloids to maintain a satisfactory colloidal osmotic pressure as well as steroid and loop diuretics has been postulated, but the value of these agents is questionable. Operative fixation of the flail segments was popular in the past but is not believed to be necessary now. Rib fracture fixation is currently being studied by a few centers to determine its potential for reducing the long-term incidence of pain and respiratory insufficiency.[80] At least one third of patients with flail chest will have significant complaints later of decreased respiratory reserve, chronic pain, and respiratory insufficiency, among other problems.[81,82]

The finding of chest wall injuries alerts the clinician to potential underlying injury. Lower rib fractures are associated with injury to the liver and spleen. Fracture of the first and/or second rib has a high association with thoracic great vessel injuries, particularly the aorta and innominate and subclavian arteries.[83–85] Fracture of the scapula indicates severe injury and is associated with injury to the brachial plexus and intrathoracic great vessel injury (Fig. 6–8).

## Blunt Cardiac Injury

Because of variations in definitions of cardiac contusion, the incidence of blunt cardiac injury is unknown. The spectrum of blunt cardiac injury ranges from hemorrhage into the cardiac muscle secondary to cardiac contusion, myocardial depression secondary to cardiac contusion, septal or cardiac valve tears, to rupture of the heart. Tests to determine cardiac injury include CPK-MB, isoenzymes, radioisotope scans, electrocardiographic monitoring, echocardiography, and cardiac catheterization.[86–88] In general, cardiac contusion (cardiac concussion) has been overdiagnosed. Admission to an ICU should be individualized, treating identifiable problems, such as blunt chest trauma with severe cardiac arrhythmias or blunt chest trauma with valvular disruption.[88–89] The patient with valvular or septal pathology or a ruptured heart has obvious physiologic derangement manifest by either cardiac tamponade or congestive heart failure. This patient can be quickly evaluated and have appropriate repair. The most common site of rupture is the right atrium, although other chambers of the heart have been reported to rupture. Septal and aortic and mitral valve injuries have also been reviewed.[72,73,90–92] For patients surviving initial injury, the results of surgery are excellent.

The diagnosis and treatment of cardiac contusion are much more complex. Perhaps the term cardiac contusion should be eliminated. Cardiac enzymes have a very low diagnostic yield and may be positive in patients with no phys-

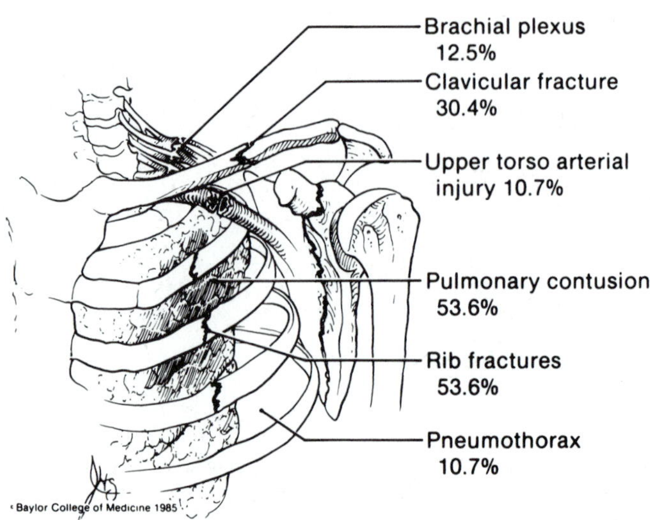


**Figure 6–8.** Ipsilateral upper torso injuries associated with fracture of the scapula.

iologically identifiable lesion. Although electrocardiographic changes of bundle branch block, premature ventricular contractions, ST segment depression, and T-wave abnormalities have all been described in association with myocardial contusion, these changes occur in patients with no myocardial pathology. Thus, the significance of EKG abnormalities is unclear. Radioisotope scanning of the heart may show septal or cardiac wall abnormalities. Moderate to severe derangement of such scans has been present in patients with little physiologic derangements, who recover uneventfully. The role of such scans as a guide to therapy remains unclear. Echocardiography may show pericardial effusion, septal wall abnormalities, alterations in valvular function, intracardiac shunts, and abnormal sounds.[93] Transesophageal echocardiography (TEE) may demonstrate intimal flaps and tears of the descending thoracic aorta.[93,94,95] The continuous monitored electrocardiogram is best.

## Penetrating Cardiac Injury

Penetrating cardiac wounds have been successfully managed since the late 19th century, and now numerous reports of large series from civilian trauma centers are available.[96–98] Although injuries to all chambers of the heart have been reported, the anterior surface is most frequently injured (Fig. 6–9).[98,99] The coronary arteries are seldom injured. On rare occasions, emergency coronary artery bypass utilizing extracorporeal support is required (Fig. 6–6). With stab wounds of the heart, a large rent in the pericardium may result in hemothorax without pericardial tamponade. With a missile and some stab wounds, the hole in the pericardium may not allow egress of blood, and pericardial tamponade results. Some patients who arrive at the hospital alive may benefit from pericardiocentesis.[99,100] Although subxiphoid pericardiotomy in the ER or OR has been suggested, such a small incision is beneficial only if no injury to the heart is present. If a cardiac injury is present, this small incision results in extensive blood loss during the time that either a median sternotomy or anterolateral thoracotomy is performed to expose the injury. If a cardiac wound is suspected, the incision of choice is one that allows repair. For missile and stab wounds lateral to the midclavicular line, an anterolateral incision is preferred. For stab wounds to the pericardium, a median sternotomy may be better.

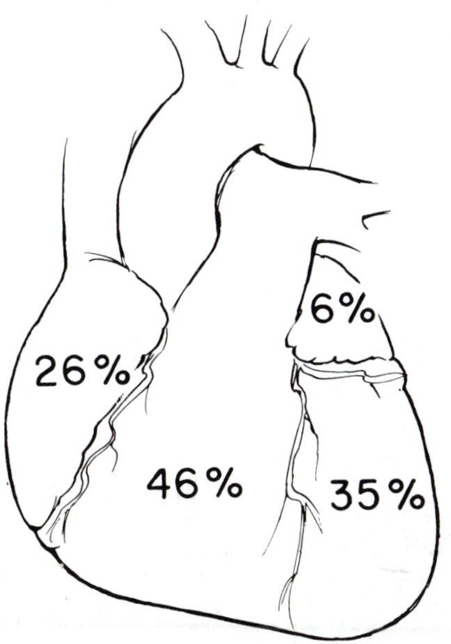


**Figure 6–9.** Baylor College of Medicine experience with heart injuries and the chambers injured. Note that 11% had multichamber injury.

Repair can be done by cardiorrhaphy using a 3-0 or 4-0 polypropylene suture.[31] Supportive pledgets are required in approximately 5–10% of patients in whom distension of the cardiac chamber is present. Injury to the coronary arteries is rare, and injuries on either side of the coronary arteries may require a mattress suture on a double-ended needle placed around the cardiac wound so that it does not occlude the coronary artery. On rare occasions, a Foley catheter balloon placed through the injury into the heart, inflated and pulled back against the wall, may achieve hemostasis and allow time for resuscitation and proper placement of sutures. Posterior cardiac wounds occasionally may require cardiopulmonary bypass for repair. Care should be taken not to overhydrate the patient or to give pressor drugs that unnecessarily increase cardiac contractility, since both of these techniques may cause the sutures to pull out of friable cardiac muscle. Postoperatively, patients having cardiorrhaphy should undergo cardiography to rule out an internal cardiac wound that occurs in approximately 6–10% of patients (Fig. 6–10).[93]

Patients who reach the hospital alive with cardiac wounds and a blood pressure of >90 mm Hg have >90% chance of survival. Cardiac injury patients who undergo external cardiac massage for less than 5 minutes prehospital and who have electrical activity when they reach the ER benefit from emergency center cardiorrhaphy.[44,55] Endotracheal intubation in the field may extend this time to 10 minutes.[48] With aggressive ER thoracotomy in selected patients, successful resuscitation may occur in up to 30% of patients with heart wounds when the resuscitation is directed by surgical personnel.[56] Emergency center thoracotomy and cardiorraphy are rarely successful in patients who undergo more than 10 minutes' prehospital cardiopulmonary resuscitation, who have no electrical activity, or who are victims of blunt chest trauma.[44]

## Lung Injury

After the chest wall, the lung is the most commonly injured intrathoracic organ.[36,101–103] Manifestations of lung injury are pneumothorax, hemothorax, pulmonary contusion, pulmonary hematoma, systemic air emboli, and ARDS. Most

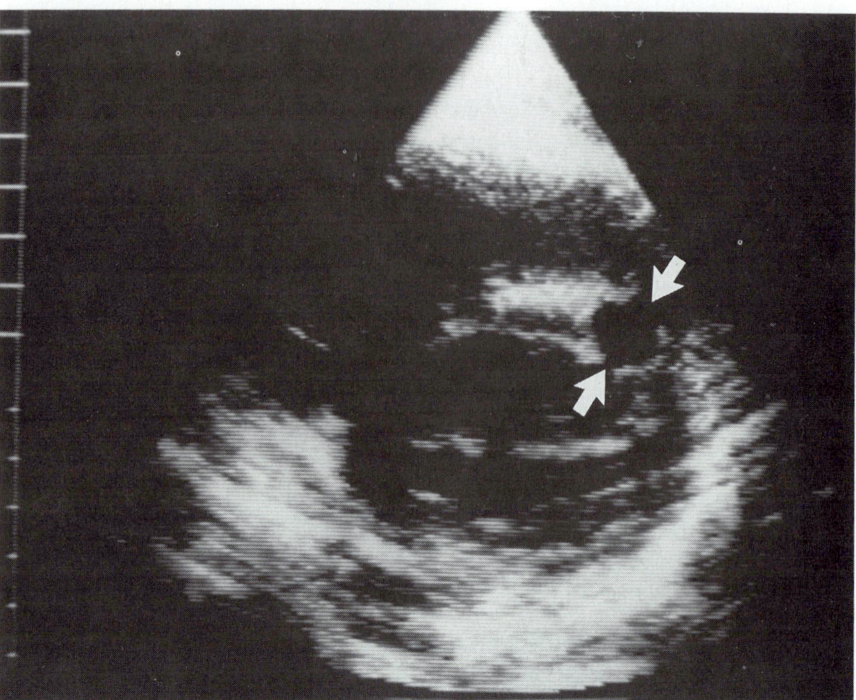

**Figure 6–10.** Two-dimensional echocardiogram of patient 3 months after stab wound of the heart and demonstrating (between arrows) a traumatic intraventricular septal defect.

patients with injured lung have only the above manifestations of injury and do not require thoracotomy. Tube thoracostomy and/or ventilatory support allow most lung injuries to heal. Continued hemothorax of more than 1500 mL, massive air leak, development of a nonhealing lung abscess, pulmonary necrosis, and other complications may prompt thoracotomy, at which time a large lung injury is found. Most peripheral lung injuries may be handled by simple pneumorrhaphy, suturing, or stapling. A large injury through the substance of the lung that will not respond to simple pneumorrhaphy will require unroofing of the lung, with specific ligation of deep vasculature and oversewing of the pulmonary parenchyma. In "filleting open" the lung (not necessarily via lobar anatomy) along the route of the coagulation, devices such as the Argon Beam Coagulator (Bard Electro Medical Systems, Englewood, Colorado) may aid in control of bleeding from the lung surface. On rare occasions, especially if associated hilar, major tracheobronchial, or major vascular injury is present, lobectomy or pneumonectomy may be required. With penetrating injuries of the lung, especially when entrance and exit sites have been oversewn and either marked Valsalva maneuver by the patient (such as coughing or straining) or positive pressure ventilation in excess of 60 torr occurs, systemic air emboli can be created from a bronchiolar-alveolar to pulmonary venous fistula (Fig. 6–11).[104,105] Manifestations of this condition include seizure activity, confusion, and cardiac arrest. Once the syndrome is recognized, immediate thoracotomy, cross-clamping of the hilum, removal of air from the left ventricle and ascending aorta, and cardiac resuscitation are necessary for successful resuscitation. Success in reversing this process is rare. To prevent such complications, positive-pressure ventilation in excess of 60 torr should be avoided.[104,105] Avoiding oversewing both open ends of a missile tract that traverses the lung may help prevent the problem.

Formal pulmonary resection for lung injury was required in only 1.1% of stab wounds and 2.3% of the gunshot wounds in 1168 patients with lung injury. In 666 other patients, 91 (13.6%) required thoracotomy, with only 8 (1.2%) requiring resection, and 6 of these were segmental.[103] Repair of other intrathoracic structures (heart, aorta, trachea, etc.) was more common than formal pulmonary resection in both series.

### Ascending Aorta/Main Pulmonary Artery

Injuries to the ascending aorta or main pulmonary artery usually result in pericardial tamponade and death prior to arrival at the emergency center. Among those patients who arrive alive, virtually all will have gunshot wounds and manifestations of cardiac tamponade, with thoracotomy revealing an injury to an intrapericardial great vessel. On a rare occasion, blunt injury to the ascending aorta occurs in a patient with a widened mediastinum. Cardiopulmonary bypass with reconstruction is then possible (Fig. 6–12).[106]

### Aortic Arch and Thoracic Outlet Vascular Injury

The innominate artery at the aortic arch is the second most common site of blunt injury to the thoracic aorta in patients who arrive at a hospital alive. Injuries to the distal innominate artery and/or innominate vein are the most common thoracic outlet injuries (Figs 6–13 and 6–14). There are few

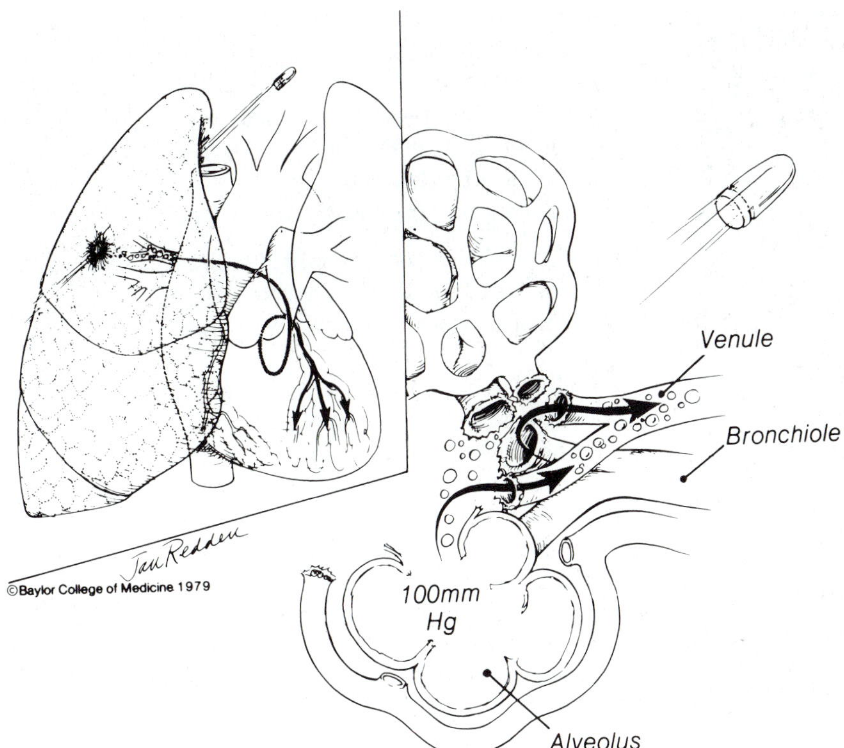


**Figure 6–11.** Drawing of isolated gunshot wound to the lung and demonstrating the mechanism of alveolar to pulmonary venous fistula and producing systemic air embolism.

series of thoracic outlet great vessel injuries. Management is by simple bypass grafting without systemic heparinization, hypothermia, to intraluminal shunts of cardiopulmonary bypass (Figs. 6–15 and 6–16).[107–112] The left innominate vein may be ligated. Complex injuries of the aortic arch, like those of the ascending aorta, require cardiopulmonary bypass for repair (Fig. 6–17).

A subclavian vascular injury is a thoracic outlet injury. Numerous incisions have been described for exposure and control of such injuries.[111–115] The most conservative incision is one that provides maximum exposure and proximal and distal control prior to entering the hematoma. This is frequently an anterior chest incision for proximal control combined with either an upper sternotomy with a supraclavicular extension or a separate supraclavicular incision. At times, the clavicle must be removed separately for exposure. Because of friability of the subclavian artery and inability to mobilize it, an interposition prosthesis of knitted Dacron or saphenous vein is indicated rather than end-to-end anastomosis.

## Descending Thoracic Aorta

Injury to the descending thoracic aorta may be produced by either penetrating or blunt trauma. Penetrating injuries to the descending thoracic aorta carry a mortality rate of approximately 50%, primarily due to exsanguinating hemorrhage prior to arrival at the hospital. Penetrating injuries are usually repaired by lateral aortorrhaphy (Fig. 6–18).[116–120]

Blunt injury to the descending thoracic aorta occurs in over 8000 patients per year in the United States. Its incidence world wide is unknown. Eight-five percent of patients with this injury die before reaching a hospital.[119,120] Of those who arrive alive, the 48-hour in-hospital mortality without treatment is 50%. Half of these patients will have no external sign of trauma. Clues obtained from information relative to the accident and suggestive of descending thoracic aortic injury include severe deceleration injury, death of another occupant in the same accident, and marked deformity of the passenger area of the vehicle.

Clues that should prompt suspicion of injury to the descending thoracic aorta include an intrascapular murmur; pulse or blood pressure discrepancy between upper and lower extremities; palpable fractures of clavicle or sternum; presence of lower extremity pulse deficit, paresis or paralysis; and presence of steering wheel imprint on the anterior chest wall.

Radiologic clues (Figs. 6–19, 6–20)[121] on an original chest x-ray that should suggest the need for a confirmatory arteriogram include:

- widening of the mediastinum >8 cm.
- depression of the left main stem bronchus >140 degrees.
- presence of a hematoma in the left apical area (apical cap).
- fracture of the first and/or second rib.
- fracture of the sternum and/or clavicle.
- massive left hemothorax.
- multiple fractured ribs on the left side.
- fracture dislocation of the thoracic spine.
- loss of the aortopulmonary window.

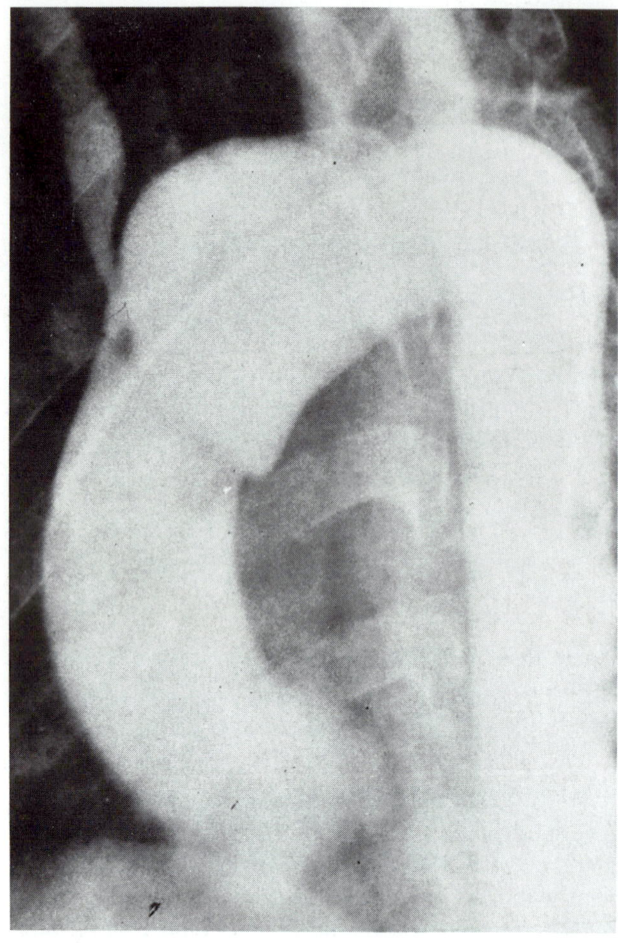

**Figure 6–12.** Ascending aortogram demonstrating blunt injury of ascending aorta to include origin of the innominate artery, requiring cardiopulmonary bypass for graft reconstruction.

- anterior displacement of the trachea on lateral chest x-ray.
- deviation to the right of the nasogastric tube in the esophagus.
- deviation of the trachea to the right.
- calcium layering in the aorta.
- loss of the aortic knob contour.
- loss of the paraspinal pleural stripe.

None of these signs are diagnostic but should alert the clinician to the need for the arteriography.[109]

When arteriography confirms an injury to the descending thoracic aorta, the patient is taken to the OR as soon as possible. Although traditional treatment has been early operation, in the patient with multisystem trauma and a known contained, stable hematoma from aortic injury, delay in thoracic operation has been suggested.[122,123] During arteriography, use of afterload reduction agents such as beta blockers might be helpful to alter the DP/DT. MRI and CT scanning may show a mediastinal hematoma but do not show the specific area of aortic injury and are not the best imaging techniques for specific diagnosis.[124–129]

Transeophageal echocardiogram (TEE) has been advocated to demonstrate intimal flaps and tears of the descending thoracic aorta.[94,95] This technique might be especially adaptable in the OR when one is performing an urgent laparotomy for hemoperitoneum in a patient with a widened mediastinum but without time to have obtained an aortogram. Similarly, in the ICU, TEE may have some utility.

A double-lumen endotracheal tube and a right arm intra-arterial line for monitoring blood pressure are of assistance during surgery. Use of the Swan-Ganz catheter and sophisticated monitoring techniques for assessing somatosensory evoked potentials, spinal fluid pressure, and other factors should be left to the discretion of the anesthe-

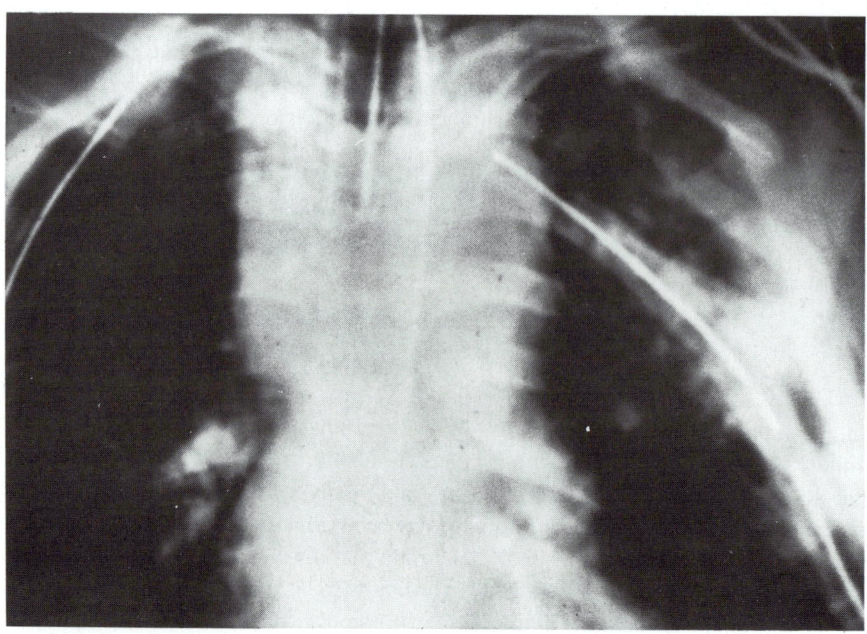

**Figure 6–13.** Chest x-ray demonstrating a widened superior mediastinum in patient injured in motorcycle accident. Note that trachea is midline, and descending aorta at isthmus is not widened.

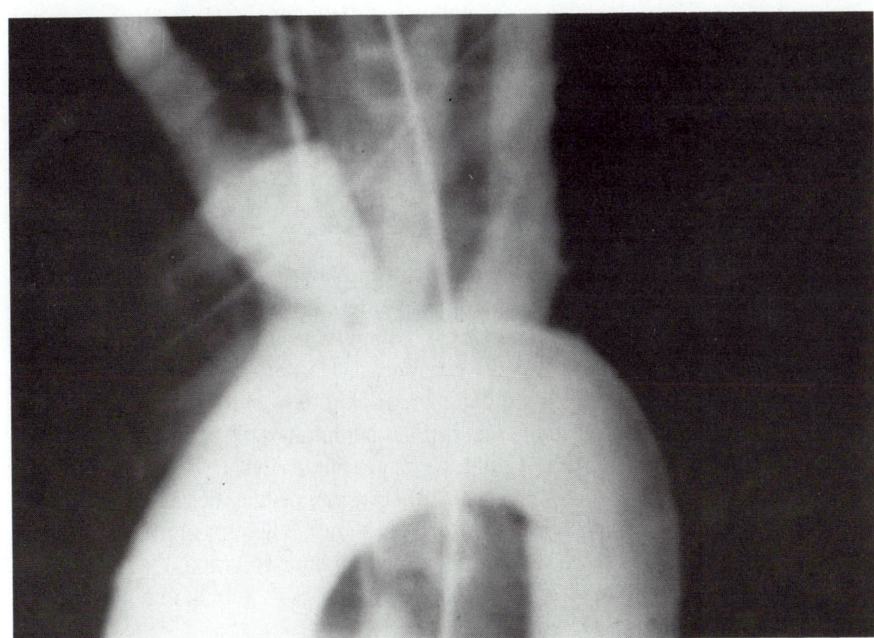

**Figure 6–14.** Arch aortogram of patient depicted in Figure 6–13. Note that there is injury of the aortic arch involving proximal innominate artery.

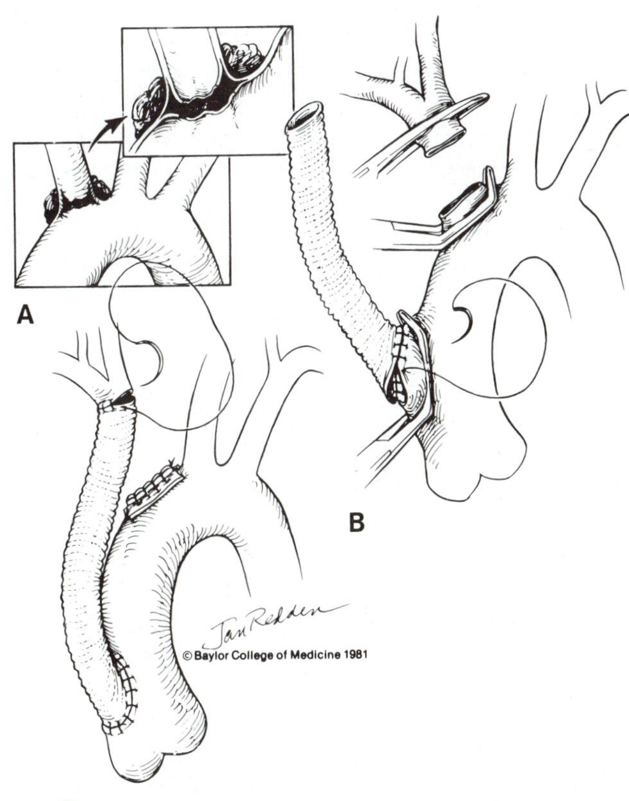


**Figure 6–15.** Technique for reconstruction of patient with an innominate artery injury, not requiring systemic heparinization, internal shunts, hypothermia, temporary bypass shunt, or pump bypass. Note that the hematoma is entered only after proximal end of graft has been attached to ascending aorta.

siologist and surgeon.[130–132] Debate exists as to the protective role of cardiopulmonary bypass, temporary bypass, shunts (centrifugal pump without systemic heparinization, Gott shunt, etc.), or clamp repair with pharmacologic control to prevent the dread complications of paraplegia and renal failure (Fig. 6–21).[133–140] Analysis of the large series in the literature indicates that no technique completely eliminates paraplegia, and some techniques have a higher mortality rate.[140] The paraplegia rate is approximately 7%, and the mortality rate approximately 15% for patients who arrive alive at a trauma center.[141] In a recent series using

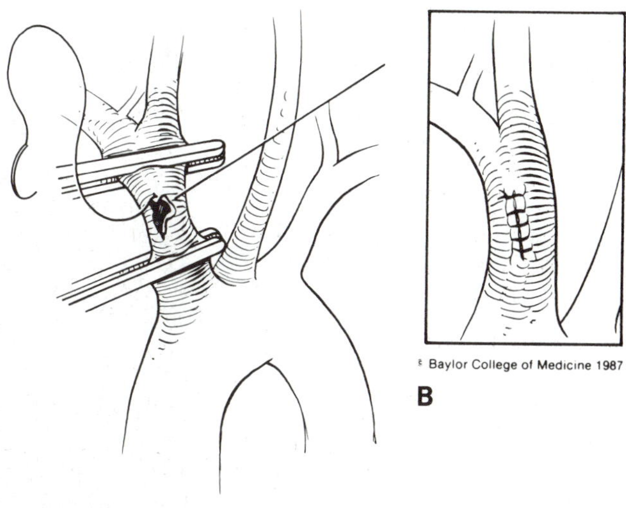


**Figure 6–16.** Lateral arteriorrhaphy for penetrating injury of innominate artery.

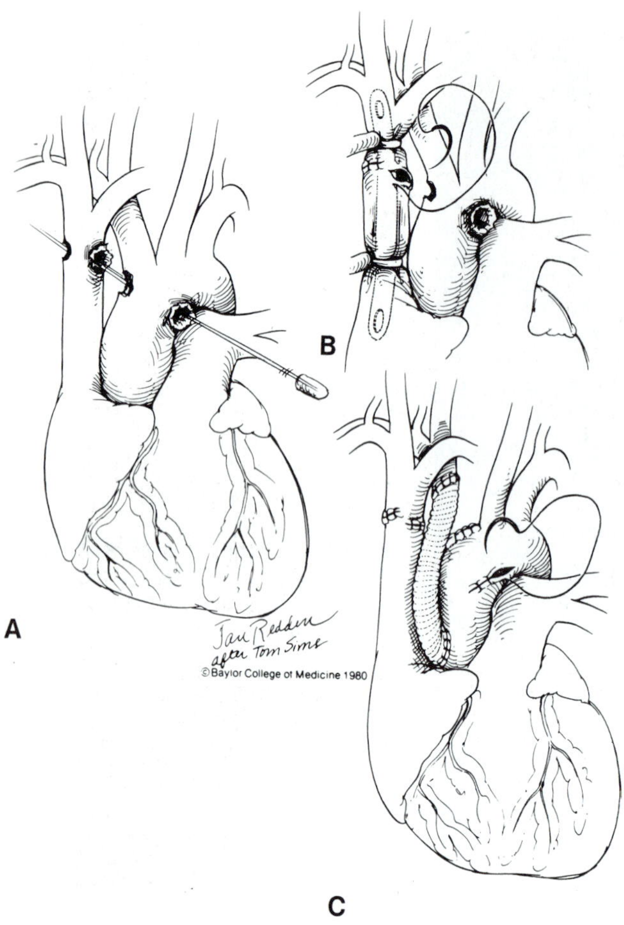


Figure 6–17. Techniques of bypass grafting for a complex injury of the thoracic outlet in a 68-year-old man: (A) lateral arch aortorrhaphy, (B) internal temporary shunting of the superior vena cava, and (C) lateral vena cavorrhaphy.

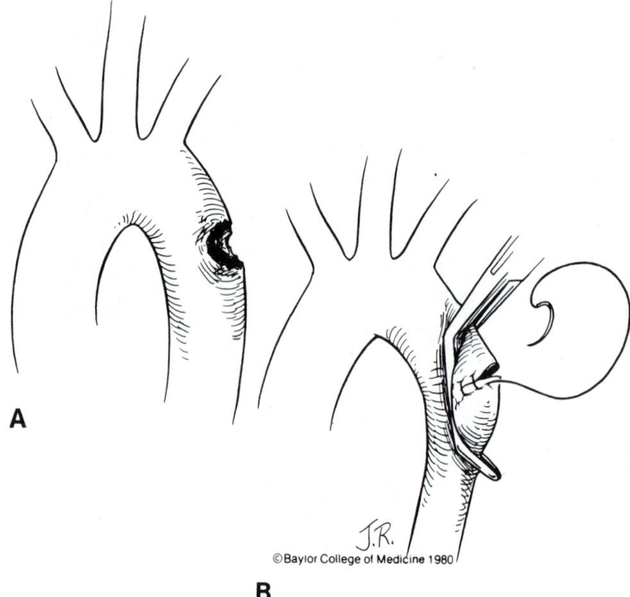


Figure 6–18. Lateral descending aortorrhaphy for patient with a penetrating injury. For larger defects, a patch graft aortoplasty or tube graft interposition could be used.

each of the techniques (clamp/repair, Gott shunt, and cardiopulmonary bypass), no cases of paraplegia were reported.[83,136–146] Thus, none of these techniques should be championed or condemned. The choice of technique is less important than the anatomy of the patient. In patients with unfavorable anatomy, any area between the aortic clamps is at risk regardless of the perioperative adjunctive techniques (see Chapter 137).

Intraoperatively, following proximal and distal control, the hematoma is entered and the aortic tear repaired. Approximately 15% of patients can have primary repair, but the majority require a Dacron graft interposition. For the unstable patient with multisystem injury and an apparently stable mediastinal hematoma, the abdominal injury, in general, should be approached first.[122,123] Patients with chronic traumatic aneurysms of the descending thoracic aorta have perioperative paraplegia, and mortality rates are at least one third the rate for acute injuries.[144]

## Tracheobronchial Injury

Injury to the trachea and/or bronchi may be secondary to penetrating, blunt, or iatrogenic trauma.[147–153] Penetrating trauma may produce injury at any location but most often injures the cervical trachea. Blunt trauma usually occurs within 1 cm of the carina, most often in the right or left main stem bronchus. Iatrogenic tracheobronchial trauma may occur during intubation, tracheostomy, or bronchoscopy. Tracheobronchial injury is manifest by pneumothorax, pneumomediastinum, atelectasis, and/or subcutaneous emphysema. Patients with penetrating injuries usually develop symptoms immediately, whereas those with blunt injuries may have a delay of up to 1 week before atelectasis and pneumonia prompt a detailed evaluation such as bronchography or bronchoscopy. A number of clinical clues suggestive of a bronchial injury include:

- unusually large and persistent air leak.
- need for a second (or third) chest tube.
- incomplete expansion of a pneumothorax despite functioning chest tubes and pleural collection devices.
- inability to keep lung expanded.
- refractory and recurrent lobar or whole lung atelectasis.
- chest x-ray showing a pneumothorax with downward displacement of the hilum of the lung.

With suspicion of bronchial injury, bronchoscopy and/or bronchography will confirm the diagnosis. On bronchoscopy, the initial clue may be inability to discern the usual tracheal and endobronchial landmarks, even by an experienced bronchoscopist.

Control and repair are aided by a double-lumen endotracheal tube. Injury to the intrathoracic trachea and the bronchi is approached by a posterolateral thoracostomy. The bronchus is mobilized following anastomosis using in-

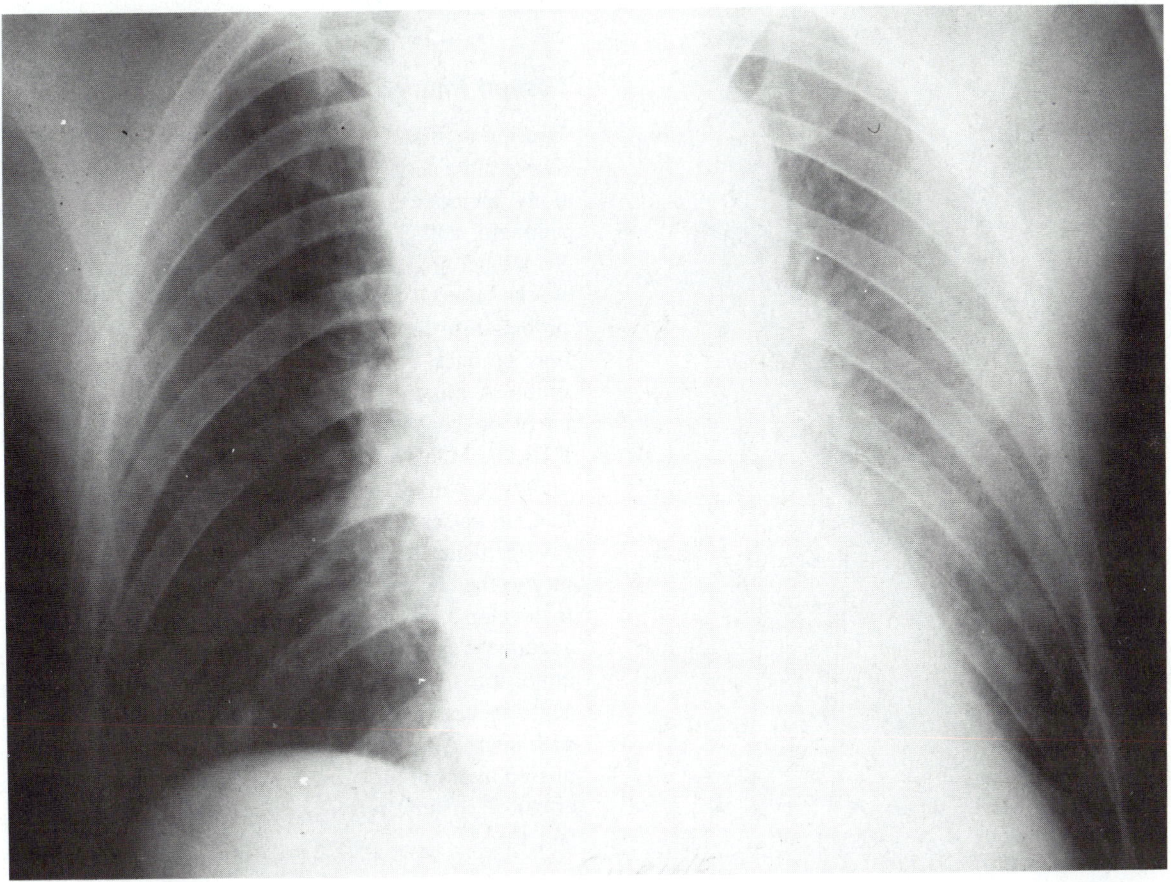

**Figure 6–19.** Chest x-ray of patient with blunt injury of descending thoracic aorta. Note widened mediastinum, loss of aortic knob contour, and left hemothorax. Confirmatory aortography is indicated.

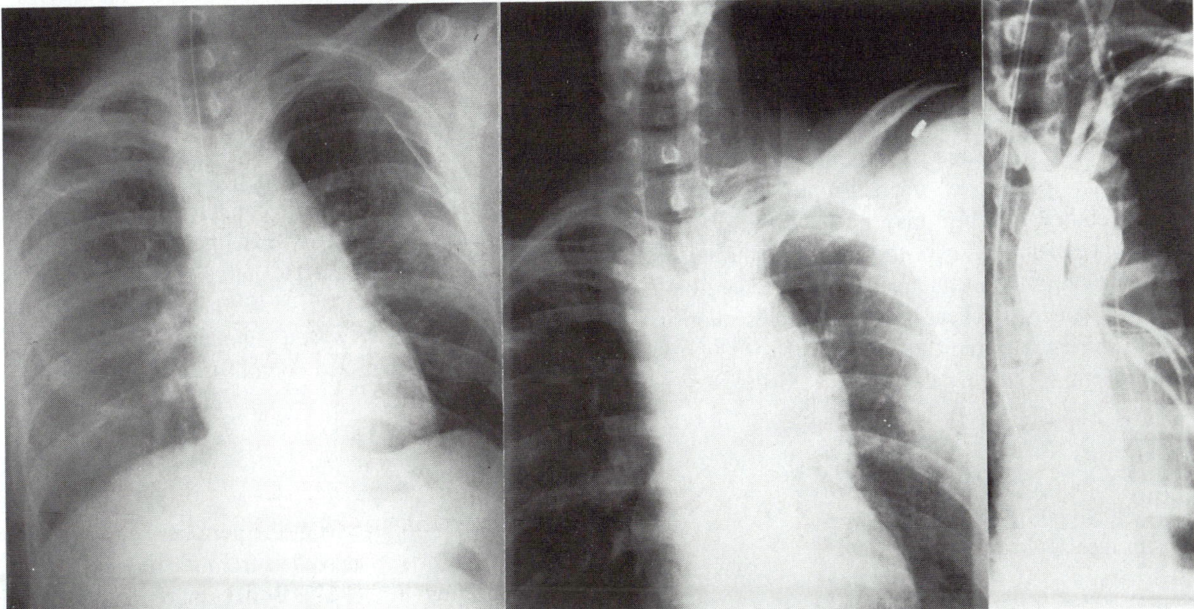

**Figure 6–20.** Chest x-rays and aortography of patient with blunt injury to the descending thoracic aorta. Note depression of the left mainstem bronchus, loss of aortic knob contour, and left apical hematoma cap.

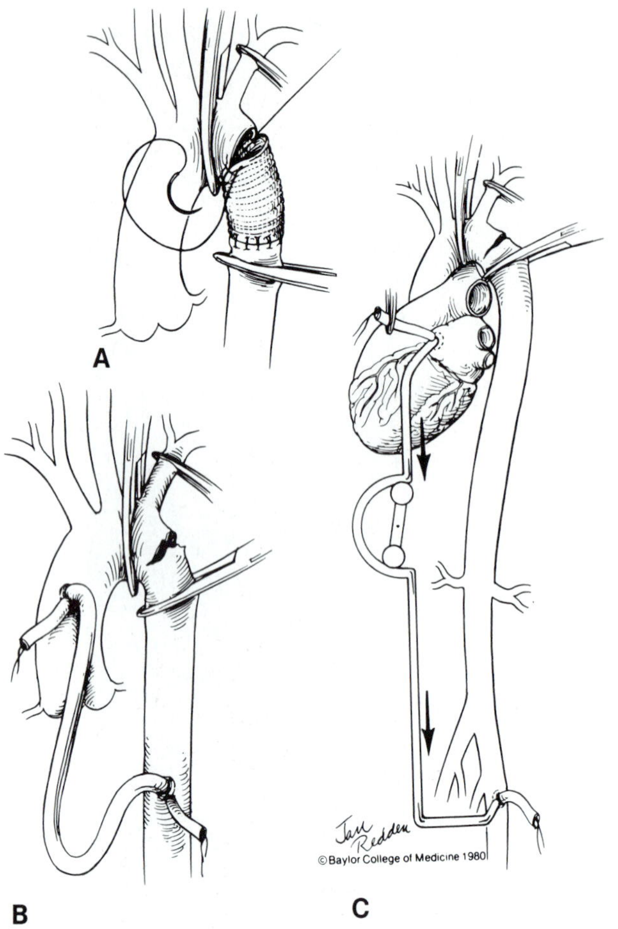


Figure 6–21. Current techniques used to control and repair blunt injuries of descending thoracic aorta. A new variation of pump bypass (B) is to incorporate a centrifugal pump not requiring heparinization. Unfortunately, this technique has not reduced the incidence of paraplegia.

terrupted 000 Vicryl.[148,149] With isolated injuries, a protective proximal tracheostomy is not required. With complex injuries involving thoracic outlet vasculature or the esophagus, a proximal protective tracheostomy is recommended.[150] A chronic stricture may occur with a missed tracheal or bronchial injury or in the trachea subjected to the balloon of a long-term endotracheal or tracheostomy tube. In such instances, tracheal or broncheal resection in the area of the stricture is indicated, and reconstruction is accomplished using techniques described by Grillo[153] (see Chapter 38).

### Esophagus

For injuries of the esophagus, see Chapter 41.

### Diaphragm

For injuries to the diaphragm, see Chapter 35.

## COMPLICATIONS

### Missed Injuries

Injuries to thoracic organs may not be detected initially. Those most susceptible to missed injury and late complications include the tracheobronchial tree, esophagus, diaphragm, and descending thoracic aorta. Blunt injuries to the tracheobronchial tree may not be detected for 1 or more weeks after injury. Atelectasis and pneumonia should prompt bronchoscopy. A missed injury to the esophagus may produce a chronic or fulminant empyema or mediastinitis. A missed injury to the esophagus or breakdown of an esophageal tear may have a mortality rate as high as 50%.[147] Many patients with diaphragmatic hernia, secondary to blunt or penetrating trauma have chest x-rays that, in retrospect, should have prompted the diagnosis. Five percent of patients arriving at a hospital alive with injury to the descending thoracic aorta may live long enough to develop a chronic traumatic false aneurysm. Similar false aneurysms may occur in other intrathoracic vessels but are quite rare. Chronic aneurysms may be treated the same as acute aneurysms: precise diagnosis, proximal distal control, with interposition grafting or primary repair. Occasionally a missed injury to the heart may result in a chronic pericardial effusion, constrictive pericarditis, or a late intracardiac defect.[72,73,91]

### Paraplegia

The tragic complication of paraplegia may be secondary to the injury or may accompany operations on the descending thoracic aorta. Numerous factors affect this complication, including spinal cord compartment syndrome, variant anatomy, ischemic times, reperfusion injury, spinal cord pressure, reaction to various medications, and unknown factors. Operative and monitoring techniques have been suggested to minimize paraplegia.[129,130,134,154–156] Despite all of these techniques, the complication continues. It seems to be more a function of the contributory factors than any specific surgical or protective technique. Patient and family must be made cognizant (with witnesses) of the potential for this complication and the lethality of the injury. The record must reflect that this information is understood by the patient and family with a completed informed consent. Paraplegia is a recognized complication of thoracic trauma and not malpractice.[157]

### Embolism

Missiles may embolize from the periphery to the heart and the pulmonary artery, as well as from the heart and the aorta to distal arteries (Fig. 6–22). Bullet emboli to the chest present confusing pictures on original chest x-ray and require a high index of suspicion (Fig. 6–23).[158] With bullet emboli, the area of injury in the cardiovascular system should be

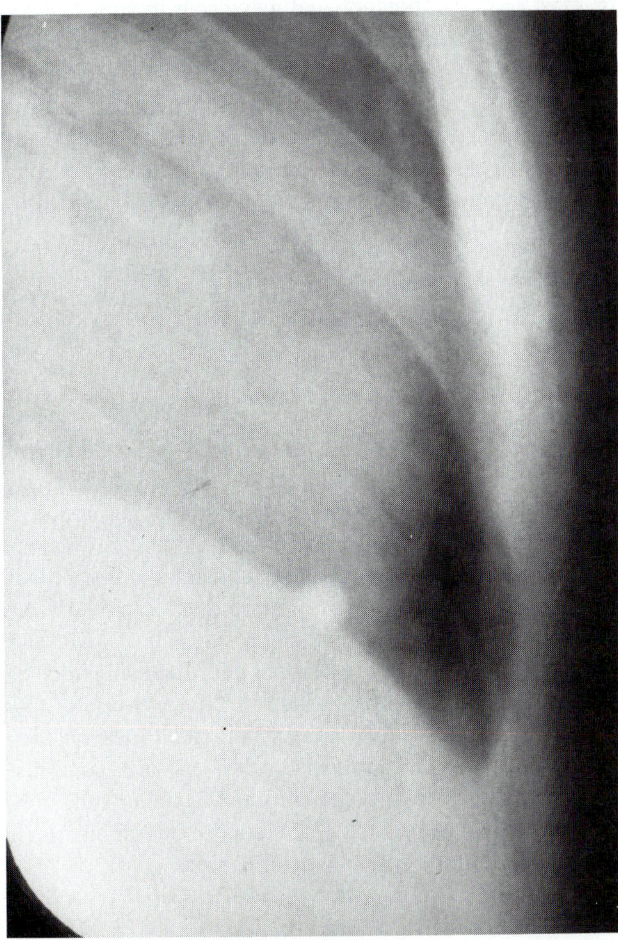

Figure 6–22. Lateral chest x-ray demonstrating ribs in focus and missile (which had embolized to the heart from entry in left iliac vein) out of focus over cardiac silhouette.

controlled first and the distal embolus removed secondarily. A bullet embolus to the heart is usually removed using cardiopulmonary bypass, although direct removal is sometimes possible.[159]

## Adult Respiratory Distress Syndrome (ARDS)

The term ARDS is used to describe a constellation of clinical conditions manifest by pulmonary consolidation on chest x-ray, progressive hypoxemia, increasing hypercarbia, pulmonary arteriovenous shunting, and typical pathologic findings on lung tissue at biopsy or autopsy. The term ARDS evolved because the posttraumatic and postseptic findings in the lungs of adults closely resembled those seen in the infant respiratory distress syndrome and in soldiers exposed to phosgene gas during World War I. This syndrome is secondary to numerous factors, including fat emboli, shock lung, pulmonary contusion, fluid overload, hypoxemia, inhalation, central nervous system injury, hepatic injury, pancreatitis, remote infection, and many more.[160,161] ARDS occurs in the trauma patient either early after the injury (2–3 days) or 2 weeks to 2 months after. Early manifestations are pulmonary injury and/or fluid imbalance. Late-appearing ARDS is clearly secondary to complications of trauma, such as multiple organ failure, sepsis, and loss of immunocompetence, among others. ARDS is now felt to be a regional manifestation of a systemic inflammatory response syndrome (SIRS). Many cell mediators have been postulated to either contribute or be present in patients with ARDS; however, none have been found singularly or in combination to be the major causal factor. Attempts to block such cell mediators by pharmacologic

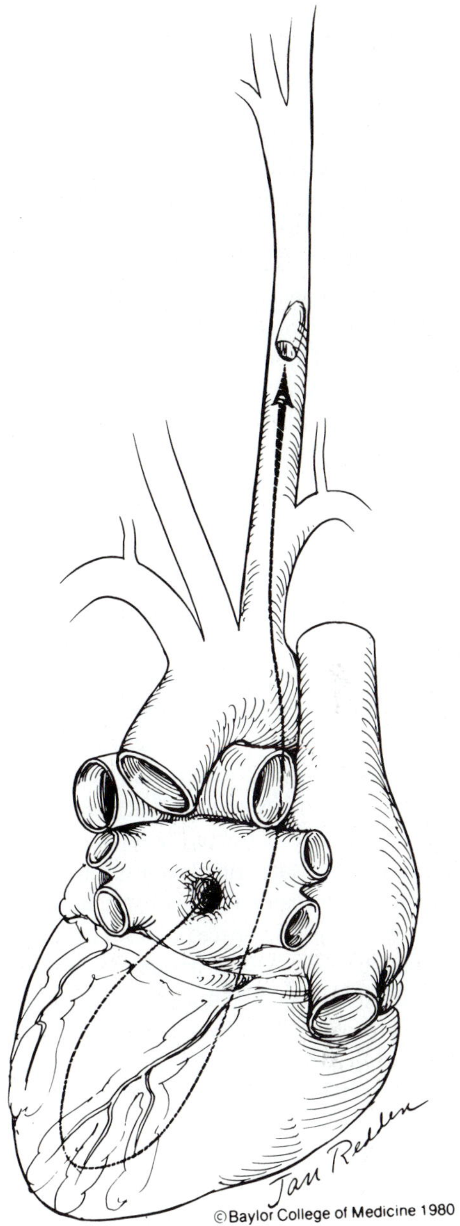


Figure 6–23. Drawing demonstrating patient who had a gunshot wound to the heart (left atrium). The bullet embolized to the left carotid artery, resulting in an acute cerebrovascular accident that ultimately caused this patient's death.

means have been successful in some experimental animals but have yet to reach clinical significance for the patients.

Initial therapy of the patient in shock is 3 cc of crystalloids for every 1 cc of blood lost. For a patient with a significant injury, large volumes of both crystalloid, banked blood, fresh frozen plasma, and, at times, colloid, are needed to maintain, not only blood pressure but also urinary output. The patient who has had a preoperative blood pressure of less than 90 mm Hg and pulmonary contusion is susceptible to pulmonary capillary leak and the development of ARDS. Treatment involves the early use of PEEP and judicious use of fluid management.[162–166] In a patient who does not have irreversible metabolic acidosis and has functioning kidneys, this early form of ARDS usually clears within 2–3 days. The use of diuretics, colloidal osmotic agents, and micropore filters as a means of treating, monitoring, or altering ARDS is currently being studied.[161–167]

The late-appearing form of ARDS, which presents similarly clinically and radiologically to early ARDS, is extremely complex and difficult to treat. It is a manifestation of the multiorgan failure syndrome and also may be a manifestation of an unrecognized abscess or systemic sepsis. Such patients frequently have marginal renal function, may have lost immunocompetence, and have evidence of altered gastrointestinal and hepatic function as well. Thus, the pulmonary insult is a manifestation of a total body response. The clinician must be extremely aggressive in seeking a treatable cause of this late complication. Causes include venous line sepsis, intra-abdominal abscess, acalculous cholecystitis, empyema, pelvic abscess, and pancreatitis, among others. Late-appearing ARDS frequently develops rapidly into a fulminant pneumonia from resistant organisms and requires progressively higher levels of PEEP and $FIO_2$. Death is often secondary to overwhelming sepsis, pneumonia, renal failure, hepatic insufficiency, or a combination.

### Infections

Incomplete evacuation of a clotted hemothorax by an intercostal tube occurred frequently in the past. This was due to long periods of time before treatment of the hemothorax, use of small chest tubes, or repeated thoracentesis as primary treatment. Empyema and fibrothorax were further complications of clotted hemothoraces. The reduced complication rate and cost with early evacuation of a clotted hemothorax is well established. This can be done with a limited thoracotomy or by thoracoscopy.[102,168,169]

If a clotted hemothorax is not evacuated, a noninfectious fever may occur, but often an empyema develops. Empyema is especially common when upper abdominal enteric injury is present.

Other posttraumatic infectious complications include pneumonia, sternal wound infections, costochondral infections, subcutaneous wound infections, line sepsis, and colonization of the tracheobronchial tree. Many such infections are due to prolonged stays in the ICU. Pneumonia is by far the most common infection and may occur in very sick patients despite the most fastidious pulmonary toilet. Infections in bony or cartilaginous tissue may be resistant to the most active local wound care and may require resection and/or coverage by transposed viable muscle flaps. Line sepsis requires removing the offending catheter, culturing the line tip and replacing it at a second site if still needed.

## MISCELLANEOUS CONSIDERATION

### Long-term Disability

Most patients with thoracic injury do not have long-term disability and require very little rehabilitation. Up to 30% of patients with flail chest, however, have some long-term disability,[81,170] including chest pain and chronic respiratory insufficiency with measured alterations in pulmonary function. A patient with a "book" or "trap door" type thoracotomy may have chronic pain in the skin, chest wall, and upper extremity. This chronic pain and the availability of alternate approaches have resulted in decreased use of this incision. A patient with a thoracoabdominal incision may have chronic costochondral pain or even chronic chondritis. With infection in the cartilage or a chronic sternal infection, a myocutaneous flap from the rectus or latissimus dorsi with or without resection may be of benefit.

### Autotransfusion

Autotransfusion is valuable in the ER, OR, and ICU for patients with trauma.[76] In the ER, hemothorax blood can be collected and immediately reinfused using a nonprocessing type autotransfusion device. In the OR, patients with thoracic outlet or other great vessel injury are ideal candidates for use of an intraoperative processing autotransfusion device such as the Baylor Rapid Autologous Transfuser (BRAT) (COBE Laboratories, Cardiovascular Division, Arvada, CO). For patients with hypothermic and dilutional associated coagulopathy, continued autotransfusion in the ICU allows time for rewarming and replacement of clotting factors.

### Substitute Vascular Conduits

Extensive experience has accumulated with the use of substitute vascular conduits in the innominate, subclavian, and thoracic aortic locations. Because of the size of these vessels, autogenous vascular transposed conduits are not acceptable. Infection around these synthetic conduits is rare. Knitted Dacron appears to be the most useful in these locations. Experimentally and clinically, the acceptability of synthetic grafts over transposed scavenged autologous tissue has been repeatedly demonstrated.[171–174]

## Nutrition

The thoracic injured patient has the same nutritional requirements as any postsurgery or nonthoracic injured patient. Fortunately, the majority of patients undergoing surgery or admitted to the hospital for thoracic injury do not require supplemental nutrition. Most will be taking oral feedings, even regular diets, within a day or two of their injury. Some who are given large doses of opiate analgesia may have ileus. For those with sedation, concomitant head injury, or severe injuries, a nasogastric or nasointestinal tube provides the better route for nutrition. For patients with a concomitant abdominal injury, a jejunostomy tube placed at the time of the laparotomy allows enteral nutrition supplements by the second hospital day. Few patients will require IV "hyperalimentation." Complications of line sepsis, acalculous cholecystitis, fatty acid deficiencies, and possible increase in ARDS should be kept in mind when IV nutrition is necessary for the patient with chest injury.

## Pain

Patients with simple rib fractures may have considerable pain. Puncture of the underlying lung, heart, spleen, or other abdominal viscera is always a possibility in a patient with rib fractures. Patients with rib fractures do not breathe deeply and can develop atelectasis and ultimately pneumonia. Pain can be relieved by either intercostal nerve block or continuous epidural anesthesia. In patients with multiple rib fractures, such as with the flail chest syndrome, continuous epidural anesthesia is gaining popularity.[82] Circumferential binders to produce a rigid chest wall limit chest wall excursion as well as the ability to cough and, especially in older individuals, increase the chances of atelectasis and pneumonia.

## Postoperative Care

For most patients with thoracic injury, postoperative care is straightforward. For the patient requiring a stay in the ICU, there are several special considerations: who writes orders and who supervises patient care, monitoring, and airway.

Trauma is a surgical disease, and thoracic trauma is no exception. Despite the recent trend for added certification in "critical care" by at least three specialties within the American Board of Medical Specialists, the thoracic, general, or trauma surgeon is still the best suited to care for the patient with thoracic injury. Only one physician (or team) should write orders, place/remove tubes, and determine priorities. Appropriate consultants should be requested and integrated into the patient's care as the surgeon sees fit, based on the surgeon's special understanding of the complexities of the trauma patient.

ICU monitoring capabilities continue to evolve. Many devices and monitors are very useful, others are merely expensive fads or trends that produce confusing information and may ultimately be dangerous. The thoracic surgeon should be slow to adopt an expensive and "trendy" gadget that does not provide any new, useful information. Furthermore, it is axiomatic that one should not lose sight of the patient in the midst of a room full of machinery. For the trauma patient, much of the monitoring discussed in the recent literature could still be described as experimental, an example being somatosensory evoked potentials for prediction of spinal ischemia in acute aortic traumatic tears.

Intra-arterial blood pressure monitoring also allows for blood sampling as indicated. Transcutaneous oximetry is useful for monitoring. Abnormal readings require arterial blood gases and a reason for change. Oximetric measurements can also be made with transducers coupled with a pulmonary artery catheter; though somewhat expensive, they provide helpful information when surgeons are familiar with their use. The Swan-Ganz catheter is widely used and produces many direct and indirect physiologic measurements including readouts of cardiac function. Trend analysis provides a guide to respiratory settings, inotropic drugs, insertion of cardiac assist devices, or decreasing support tactics. A chest x-ray taken at least daily in the ICU (and more often if indicated) is a valuable monitoring technique along with physical examination. Other monitoring techniques include central venous pressure, electrocardiogram, blood chemistry, myocardial enzyme determinations, ventilation-perfusion radioisotope scanning, ventilator pressure and lung compartment measurements, end-tidal $CO_2$ measurements, and echocardiography.

Maintenance of a clear airway is an active process that combines mucocilliary clearance and all coughing in the noninjured person. In the postoperative patient, pulmonary toilet includes any or all of the following: coughing and deep breathing exercises, incentive spirometry, chest physiotherapy including "clapping" if necessary, postural drainage, endotracheal suctioning, fiberoptic bronchoscopy, and rigid bronchoscopy. Each of these is aided by appropriate respiratory therapy support. Oxygen delivered without adequate humidification becomes desiccant, especially in a mouth-breathing patient. Excessive doses and prolonged use of opiate analgesia depress respiration, producing atelectasis, pneumonia, and prolonged hospitalization. Early ambulation and activity reduces postoperative pulmonary problems, even including pulmonary emboli.

## Antibiotics

Antibiotics administered for chest tube prophylaxis or as an initial therapeutic dosage should not be continued beyond 48 hours unless there is specific indication. Antibiotics are administered immediately prior to surgery for penetrating or blunt injury of the chest and abdomen. Multiple agent or broad-spectrum single agents are used and discontinued within 48 hours after operation. Currently, patients with tube thoracostomy are kept on antibiotics in most centers of the country.[26,120,175] Controversy exists as to the efficacy of antibiotics with a thoracostomy. Because the incidence of tube thoracostomy empyema is so low, it would take an extremely large multicenter study with thousands of randomized patients to achieve significance and answer the questions of efficacy. For established infections, such as empyema, endocarditis, and others, specific organism-directed antibiotics are indicated.

## ACKNOWLEDGMENTS

The authors wish to gratefully acknowledge the superb secretarial and editorial assistance of Ms. Mary K. Allen and the excellent artwork of the Medical Illustration and Audiovisual Education Department at Baylor College of Medicine.

## REFERENCES

1. Breasted JH: *The Edwin Smith Surgical Papyrus,* vol. 1. Chicago, University of Chicago Press, 1930
2. Hewson W: *The Works of William Hewson, FRS,* George Gulliver (ed). London, Sydenham Society, 1986
3. Paré A: *The Works of Ambrose Pare,* Johnson T (transl). London, Richard Cotes and Willie DeGaud (printers), 1678
4. Sparkman RS, Nixon PI, Crosthwait RW, et al: *The Texas Surgical Society, The First Fifty Years.* Dallas, Texas Surgical Society, 1965, pp 5–7
5. Larrey DJ: *Memoirs of a Military Surgeon,* Willmott R (transl). Birmingham, Alabama, Joseph Cushing, special edition by Classics of Surgery Library, 1814
6. Meade RH: *A History of Thoracic Surgery.* Thomas, Springfield, Illinois, 1961
7. Rehn L: Ueber Penetrirende Herzwunden und Herznagt. *Arch Klin Chir* **55**:315, 1897
8. Blalock A, Ravitch M: A consideration of the nonoperative treatment of cardiac tamponade resulting from wounds of the heart. *Surgery* **14**:157–162, 1943
9. Glinz W: *Chest Trauma. Diagnosis and Treatment.* West Berlin, Springer-Verlag, 1981
10. Dshanelidze II: Manuscript, Petrograd, 1922; cited by Lilienthal H: *Thoracic Surgery: The Surgical Treatment of Thoracic Diseases.* Philadelphia, Saunders, 1926, p 489
11. Beaumont W: *Experiments and Observations on the Gastric Juice and the Physiology of Digestion.* Pittsburg, New York, F.P. Allen, 1833
12. Brewer LA: Wounds of the chest in war and peace. *Ann Thor Surg* **7**:387–408, 1969
13. Burford T, Parker EF, Samson PC: Early pulmonary decortication in the treatment of posttraumatic empyema. *Ann Surg* **122**:163, 1945
14. Blaisdell FW: Initial assessment. In Blaisdell FW, Trunkey DD (eds): *Trauma Management,* vol 3, *Cervicothoracic Trauma.* New York, Thieme, 1986, pp 1–11
15. Billings JS: *War of the Rebellion. Medical and Surgical History.* Washington, DC, U.S. Government Printing Office, 1870
16. Carter BN, De Bakey ME: Current observations on war wounds of the chest. *J Thorac Surg* **13**:271, 1944
17. Duval P: *War Wounds of the Lungs. Notes on Their Surgical Treatment at the Front.* Bristol, England, John Wright, 1918
18. Kemmerer WT: Patterns of thoracic injuries in fatal traffic accidents. *J Trauma* **1**:595, 1961
19. President's Commission on the Assassination of President Kennedy: *The Warren Report,* The Associated Press, 1964
20. Djindjian R, Huth M, Houdart M, et al: Arterial supply of the spinal cord. In: *Angiography of the Spinal Cord.* Baltimore, University Park Press, 1970
21. Adkins RB, Whiteneck JM, Woltering EA: Penetrating chest wall and thoracic injuries. *Am Surg* **51**:140–148, 1985
22. Beall AC Jr, Bricker DL, Crawford HW, Noon GP, DeBakey ME: Considerations in the management of penetrating thoracic trauma. *J Trauma* **8**:408–414, 1968
23. Beall AC Jr, Crosthwait RW, Crawford ES, DeBakey ME: Gunshot wounds of the chest: A plea for individualization. *J Trauma* **4**:382–389, 1964
24. Blass DZ, James EC, Reed RJ, et al: Penetrating wounds of the neck and upper thorax. *J Trauma* **18**:2–7, 1979
25. Feliciano DV, Mattox KL, Graham JM, et al: Major complications of percutaneous subclavian catheters. *Am J Surg* **138**:969–974, 1979
26. Kish G, Kozloff J, Joseph WL, et al: Indications for early thoracotomy in the management of chest trauma. *Ann Thorac Surg* **22**:623–628, 1976
27. Mattox KL: Thoracic injury requiring surgery. *World J Surg* **7**:47–55, 1982
28. Mattox KL, Allen MK: Systematic approach to pneumothorax, haemothorax, pneumomediastinium and subcutaneous emphysema. *Injury* **17**:309–312, 1986
29. Mattox KL, Allen MK: Penetrating wounds of the thorax. *Injury* **17**:313–317, 1986
30. Mattox KL, Pickard LR, Allen MK: Emergency thoracotomy for injury. *Injury* **17**:327–331,1986
31. Oparah SS, Mandal AK: Operative management of penetrating wounds of the chest in civilian practice: Review of indications in 125 consecutive patients. *J Thorac Cardiovasc Surg* **77**:162–168, 1979
32. Reul GJ, Jr, Mattox KL, Beall AC Jr, Jordan GL Jr: Recent advances in the operative management of massive chest trauma. *Ann Thorac Surg* **16**:521–662, 1973
33. Kappes S, Towne J, Adams M, et al: Perforation of the superior vena cava, a complication of subclavian dialysis. *JAMA* **249**:2232–2233, 1983
34. Cooper JD: Trachea-innominate artery fistula: Successful management of three consecutive patients. *Ann Thorac Surg* **24**:439, 1977
35. Wilson RF, Murray C, Antonenko DR: Nonpenetrating thoracic injuries. *Surg Clin North Am* **57**:17–36, 1977
36. Besson A, Saegesser F: *Color Atlas of Chest Trauma and Associated Injuries.* Oradell, New Jersey, Medical Economics Books, 1983
37. LoCicero J: Epidemiology of thoracic trauma. *Surg Clin North Am* **69**:15–20, 1988
38. Trunkey D: Trauma. *Sci Am* **249**:28–35, 1983
39. McSwain NE: Medical control of prehospital care. *J Trauma* **24**:172, 1984
40. Jacobs LM, Sinclair A, Beiser A: Prehospital advanced life support: Benefits in trauma. *J Trauma* **24**:8–13, 1984
41. American College of Surgeons Committee on Trauma: *Hospital and Prehospital Resources for Optimal Care of the Injured Patient and Appendices A-J.* Chicago, American College of Surgeons, 1987
42. Schiller WR, Knox R, Zinnicker H, et al: Effect of helicopter transport of trauma victims on survival in an urban trauma center. *J Trauma* **28**:1127, 1988
43. Baxt WG, Moody P: The impact of rotocraft aeromedical emergency care service on trauma mortality. *JAMA* **249**:3047–3051, 1983
44. Mattox KL, Feliciano DV: Role of external cardiac compression in truncal trauma. *J Trauma* **22**:934–935, 1982
45. Mattox KL, Bickell WH, Pepe PE, et al: Prospective randomized evaluation of antishock MAST in posttraumatic hypotension. *J Trauma* **26**:779–786, 1986
46. Lewis FR: Prehospital intravenous fluid therapy: Physiologic computer modeling. *J Trauma* **26**:804–811, 1986

47. Martin RR, Bickell W, Mattox KL, et al: Prospective evaluation of preoperative fluid resuscitation in hypotensive patients with penetrating truncal injury: A preliminary report. *J Trauma* **33**:354–362, 1992
48. Durham LA, Richardson RJ, Wall MJ, et al: Emergency center thoracotomy: Impact of prehospital resuscitation. *J Trauma* **32**:775–779, 1992
49. Thompson CT: Trauma center development. *Am Emerg Med* **10**:662–665, 1981
50. Bricker DS, Mattox KL: About chest tubes. *Curr Concepts Trauma Care* **2**:16–19, 1979
51. Miller KS, Sahn FA: Chest tubes, indication, technique, management and complications. *Chest* **91**:258, 1987
52. Moore EE, Moore JB, Galloway AC, et al. Post-injury thoracotomy in the emergency department: A critical evaluation. *Surgery* **86**:590–598, 1979
53. Baker CC, Thomas AN, Trunkey DD: The role of emergency room thoracotomy in trauma. *J Trauma* **20**:848–855, 1980
54. Harnar TJ, Oreskovich MR, Copass MK, et al: Role of emergency thoracotomy in the resuscitation of moribund trauma victims: 100 consecutive cases. *Am J Surg* **142**:96–99, 1981
55. Mattox KL, Beall AC Jr, Jordan GL Jr, DeBakey ME: Cardiorrhaphy in the emergency center. *J Thorac Cardiovasc Surg* **68**:886–895, 1974
56. Mattox KL, Espada R, Beall AC Jr: Performing thoracotomy in the emergency center. *JACEP* **3**:13–17, 1974
57. Bodai BI, Smith JP, Ward RE, et al: Emergency thoracotomy in the management of trauma. *JAMA* **249**:1891–1896, 1983
58. Mayor-Davis JA, Britz RS: Subxiphoid pericardial windows—helpful in selected cases. *Trauma* **30**:1399–1401, 1990
59. Trinkle JK, Marcos J, Gover FL, Cuello LM. Management of the wounded heart. *Ann Thorac Surg* **17**:230–236, 1974
60. Cummings RG, Wesly RLR, Adams DH: Pneumopericardium resulting in cardiac tamponade. *Ann Thorac Surg* **37**:511, 1984
61. Spotnitz AJ, Kaufman JL: Tension pneumopericardium following penetrating chest injury. *J Trauma* **27**: 806–808, 1987
62. Shorr RM, Mirvis SE, Indeck MC: Tension pneumopericardium in blunt chest trauma. *J Trauma* **27**:1078–1082, 1987
63. Westaby S: Pneumopericardium and tension pneumopericardium after closed chest injury. *Thorax* **32**:91–97, 1977
64. Trinkle JK, Richardson JD, Franz JL, et al: Management of flail chest without mechanical ventilation. *Ann Thorac Surg* **19**:355, 1975
65. Strug B, Noon GP, Beall AC Jr: Traumatic diaphragmatic hernia. *Ann Thorac Surg* **17**:444–449, 1974
66. Snow N, Lucas AE, Richardson JD: Intra-aortic balloon counterpulsation for cardiogenic shock from cardiac contusion. *J Trauma* **22**:426–429, 1982
67. Saunders CR, Doty DB: Myocardial contusion: Effect of intra-aortic balloon counterpulsation of cardiac output. *J Trauma* **18**:706–708, 1978
68. Beall AC Jr, Morris GC Jr, Cooley DA: Temporary cardiopulmonary bypass in the management of penetrating wounds of the heart. *Surgery* **52**:330–337, 1962
69. Gewertz B, O'Brien C, Kirsh MM: Use of the intraaortic balloon support for refractory low cardiac output in myocardial contusion. *J Trauma* **17**:325–327, 1977
70. Mattox KL, Beall AC Jr: Application of portable cardiopulmonary bypass to emergency instrumentation. *Med Instrumentation* **11**:347–349, 1977
71. Orlando R, Drezner D: Intra-aortic balloon counterpulsation in blunt cardiac injury. *J Trauma* **23**:424–427, 1983
72. Pickard LR, Mattox KL, Beall AC Jr: Ventricular septal defect from blunt chest injury. *J Trauma* **20**:329–331, 1980
73. Reyes LH, Mattox KL, Gaasch WH, et al: Traumatic coronary artery-right heart fistula. *J Thorac Cardiovasc Surg* **70**:52–56, 1975
74. Espada R, Whisennand H, Beall AC Jr, Mattox KL: Surgical management of penetrating injuries of the coronary arteries. *J Cardiovasc Surg* **17**:97, 1976
75. Espada R, Whisennand HH, Mattox KL, Beall AC Jr: Surgical management of penetrating injuries to the coronary arteries. *Surgery* **78**:755–760, 1975
76. Von Koch L, Defore WW, Mattox KL: A practical method of autotransfusion in the emergency center. *Am J Surg* **133**:770–772, 1977
77. Foley NT, Mattox KL: Fracture of the sternum. *Curr Concepts Trauma Care* **8**:9–11, 1985
78. Harley DP, Mena I: Cardiac and vascular sequelae of sternal fractures. *J Trauma* **26**:553–555, 1986
79. Clark GC, Schecter WP, Trunkey DD: Variables affecting outcome in blunt chest trauma: Flail chest vs pulmonary contusion. *J Trauma* **28**:298–304, 1988
80. Moore BP: Operative stabilization of nonpenetrating chest injuries. *J Thorac Cardiovasc Surg* **70**:619, 1975
81. Landercasper J, Cogbill TH, Lindesmith LA: Long-term disability after flail chest. *J Trauma* **24**:414, 1984
82. Moss G, Regal ME, Lichtig L: Reducing postoperative pain, narcotics and length of hospitalization. *Surgery* **99**:206–210, 1986
83. Stiles QR, Cohimia GS, Smith JH, et al: Management of injuries of the thoracic and abdominal aorta. *Am J Surg* **150**:132–140, 1985
84. Kirshner R, Seltzer S, D'Orsi C, et al: Upper rib fractures and mediastinal widening; Indications for aortography. *Ann Thorac Surg* **35**:450, 1983
85. Woodring JH, Fried AM, Hatfield DR, et al: Fractures of first and second ribs: Predictive value for arterial and bronchial injury. *AJR* **138**:211–215, 1982
86. Waxman K, Soliman MH, Braunstein P, et al: Diagnosis of traumatic cardiac contusion. *Arch Surg* **121**:689–692, 1986
87. Frazee RC, Mucha P, Farnell MB, et al: Objective evaluation of blunt cardiac trauma. *J Trauma* **26**:510–520, 1986
88. Mattox KL, Flint LM, Carrico CJ, Grover F, et al: Blunt cardiac injury. *J Trauma* **33**:649–650, 1992. Editorial.
89. Fabian TC, Mangiante EC, Patterson CR, et al: Myocardial contusion in blunt trauma: Clinical characteristics, means of diagnosis and implications for patient management. *J Trauma* **28**:50–57, 1988
90. Noon GP, Boulafendis D, Beall AC Jr: Rupture of the heart secondary to blunt trauma. *J Trauma* **11**:122–128, 1971
91. Whisennand HH, Van Pelt SA, Beall AC Jr, et al: Surgical management of traumatic intracardiac injuries. *Ann Thorac Surg* **28**:530–536, 1979
92. Beall AC Jr, Shirkey AL: Successful surgical correction of traumatic aortic valve regurgitation. *JAMA* **187**:507–510, 1964
93. Mattox KL, Limacher MC, Feliciano DV, et al: Cardiac evaluation following heart injury. *J Trauma* **25**:758–765, 1985
94. Brooks SW, Young JC, Cmolik B, et al: The use of transesophageal echocardiography in the evaluation of chest trauma. *J Trauma* **32**:761–766, 1992
95. Kearney PA, Smith DW, Johnson SB, et al: Use of transesophageal echocardiography in the evaluation of traumatic aortic injury. *J Trauma* **34**:696–703, 1993
96. Beall AC Jr, Gasior RM, Bricker DL: Gunshot wounds of the heart: Changing patterns of surgical management. *Ann Thorac Surg* **11**:523–531, 1971
97. DeGennaro VA, Bonfils-Robert EA, Ching N, et al: Aggressive management of potential penetrating cardiac injuries. *J Thorac Cardiovasc Surg* **79**:883–887, 1980
98. Beall AC Jr, Patrick TA, Okies JE, et al: Penetrating wounds of the heart: Changing patterns of surgical management. *J Trauma* **12**:468–473, 1972
99. Mattox KL, Von Koch L, Beall AC Jr, et al: Logistic and technical considerations in the treatment of the wounded heart. *Circulation* **51**:210–214, 1975
100. Breaux ED, DuPont JB, Albert HM, et al: Cardiac tamponade following penetrating mediastinal injuries: Improved survival with early pericardiocentesis. *J Trauma* **19**:461–466, 1979

101. Robinson PD, Harman DL, Trinkle JK, et al: Management of penetrating lung injuries in civilian practice. *J Thorac Cardiovasc Surg* **95:**184–190, 1988
102. Beall AC Jr, Crawford HW, DeBakey ME: Considerations in the management of acute traumatic hemothorax. *J Thorac Cardiovasc Surg* **52:**351–360, 1966
103. Graham JM, Mattox KL, Beall AC Jr: Penetrating trauma of the lung. *J Trauma* **19:**665–669, 1979
104. Graham JM, Beall AC Jr, Mattox KL, Vaughn GD: Systemic air embolism following penetrating trauma to the lung. *Chest* **72:**449–454, 1977
105. Graham JM, Mattox KL, Feliciano DV, Beall AC Jr: Air embolism following penetrating thoracic trauma. *Curr Concepts Trauma Care* fall:7–9, 1979
106. Reyes LH, Rubio PA, Korompai FL, Guinn GL: Successful treatment of transection of aortic arch and innominate artery. *Ann Thorac Surg* **19:**468–471, 1975
107. Graham JM, Feliciano DV, Mattox KL, et al: Innominate vascular injury. *J Trauma* **22:**647–655, 1982
108. Carlsson E, Silander T: Rupture of the subclavian and innominate artery due to nonpenetrating trauma to the chest. *Acta Chir Scand* **125:**294, 1963
109. Fisher RG, Hadlock F, Ben-Menachem Y: Laceration of the thoracic and brachiocephalic arteries by blunt trauma. *Radiol Clin North Am* **19:**91,1981
110. Beall AC Jr, Roof WR, DeBakey ME: Successful surgical management of through and through stab wound of the aortic arch. *Ann Surg* **156:**823–826, 1962
111. Richardson JD, Smith JM, Grover FL, et al: Management of subclavian and innominate artery injuries. *Am J Surgery* **134:**780, 1977
112. Bricker DL, Noon GP, Beall AC Jr, DeBakey ME: Vascular injuries of the thoracic outlet. *J Trauma* **10:**1–15, 1970
113. Wyatt DA, Kellum CD, Joob AW, et al: Isolated injury of the proximal vertebral artery associated with blunt chest trauma. *J Vasc Surg* **4:**196, 1986
114. Graham JM, Feliciano DV, Mattox KL, et al: Management of subclavian vascular injuries. *J Trauma* **20:**537–544, 1980
115. Scaff HV, Brawley RK: The operative management of penetrating vascular injuries of the thoracic outlet. *Surgery* **82:**182, 1977.
116. Allen TW, Reul GJ, Morton JR, Beall AC Jr: Surgical management of aortic trauma. *J Trauma* **12:**862–868, 1972
117. Reul GJ Jr, Beall AC Jr, Jordan GL Jr, Mattox KL: The early operative management of injuries to the great vessels. *Surgery* **74:**862–873, 1973
118. Reul GJ, Rubio PA, Beall AC Jr: The surgical management of acute injury to the thoracic aorta. *J Thorac Cardiovasc Surg* **67:**272–281, 1974
119. Parmley LF, Mattingly TW, Marion WC, et al: Non-penetrating traumatic injury to the aorta. *Circulation* **17:**1086, 1958
120. Mattox KL: Invited commentary on blunt injury to the descending thoracic aorta. *World J Surg* **4:**551, 1980
121. Seltzer SE, D'Orsi C, Kirshner R, et al: Traumatic aortic rupture: Plain radiographic findings. *AJR* **137:**1011, 1981
122. Akins CW, Buckley MJ, Daggett W, et al: Acute traumatic disruption of the thoracic aorta: A ten-year experience. *Ann Thorac Surg* **31:**305, 1980
123. Borman KR, Aurbakken CM, Weigelt JA: Treatment priorities in combined blunt abdominal and aortic trauma. *Am J Surg* **144:**728–732, 1982
124. Akins EW, Carmichael MJ, Hill JA, et al: Preoperative evaluation of the thoracic aorta using MRI and angiography. *Ann Thorac Surg* **44:**499–507, 1987
125. Egan TJ, Neiman HL, Herman RJ, et al: Computed tomography in the diagnosis of aortic aneurysm dissection of traumatic injury. *Radiology* **136:**141–146, 1980
126. Heiberg E, Wolverson MK, Sundaram M, et al: CT in aortic trauma. *AJR* **140:**1119–1124, 1983
127. Moore EH, Webb WR, Verrier ED, et al: MRI of chronic posttraumatic aneurysms of the thoracic aorta. *AJR* **143:**1195–1196, 1984
128. Oudkerk M, Overbosch E, Dee P: CT recognition of acute aortic dissection. *AJR* **141:**671–676, 1983
129. Sherck JP, Oakes DD, Baker LW: Computed tomography in the management of thoracic, abdominal and pelvic trauma. *Infections in Surgery,* July:505, 1985
130. Blaisdell FW, Cooley DA: The mechanism of paraplegia after temporary thoracic aortic occlusion and its relationship to spinal fluid pressure. *Surgery* **51:**51, 1962
131. Crawford ES, Fenstermacher JM, Richardson W, et al: Reappraisal of adjuncts to avoid ischemia in treatment of thoracic aortic aneurysms. *Surgery* **67:**182, 1970
132. Cunningham JN, Laschinger JC, Merkin HA, et al: Measurement of spinal cord ischemia during operations on the thoracic aorta. *Ann Surg* **196:**285, 1982
133. Read RA, Moore EE, Moore J, Haenel JB. Partial left heart bypass for thoracic aorta repair. *Arch Surg* **128:**746–752, 1993
134. Stavens B, Hashim SW, Hammond GL, et al: Optimal methods of repair of descending thoracic aortic transections and aneurysms. *Am J Surg* **145:**508, 1983
135. Svensson LG, Von Ritater CM, Groeneveld HT, et al: Cross-clamping of the thoracic aorta: Influence of aortic shunts, laminectomy, papaverine, calcium channel blocker, allopurinol, etc., on blood flow and paraplegia. *Ann Surg* **204:**38–47, 1986
136. Mattox KL, Holzman M, Pickard LR, Beall AC Jr, Debakey ME: Clamp/repair: A safe technique for treatment of blunt injury to the descending thoracic aorta. *Ann Thorac Surg* **40:**456–463, 1985
137. Antunes MJ: Acute traumatic rupture of the aorta: Repair by simple aortic cross-clamping. *Ann Thorac Surg* **44:**257–259, 1987
138. Garcia-Rinaldi R, Defore WW, Mattox KL, Beall AC Jr: Unimpaired renal myocardial and neurologic function after cross clamping of the thoracic aorta. *Surg Gynecol Obstet* **143:**249–252, 1976
139. Livesay JJ, Cooley DA, Ventemiglia RA, et al: Surgical experience in descending thoracic aneurysmectomy with and without adjuncts to avoid ischemia. *Ann Thorac Surg* **39:**37, 1985
140. Mattox KL: Reply to Mayo Clinic letter to editor re Clamp/repair of traumatic transection of descending aorta. *Ann Thorac Surg* **43:**351–352, 1987
141. Olivier HF Jr, Maher TD, Liebler GA, et al: Use of the BioMedicus centrifugal pump in traumatic tears of the thoracic aorta. *Ann Thorac Surg* **38:**586–591, 1984
142. Verdant A, Cossette R, Dontigny L, et al: Acute and chronic traumatic aneurysms of the descending thoracic aorta: A 10 year experience with a single method of aortic shunting. *J Trauma* **25:**601–607, 1985
143. Heberer G, Becker HM, Stelter WJ: Vascular injuries in polytrauma. *World J Surg* **7:**68–79, 1983
144. McCollum CH, Graham JM, Noon GP, DeBakey ME: Chronic thoracic aneurysm of the thoracic aorta: An analysis of 50 patients. *J Trauma* **19:**248, 1979
145. Pate JW: Traumatic rupture of the aorta: Emergency operation. *Ann Thorac Surg* **39:**531–537, 1985
146. Williams TE, Vasko JS, Kakos GS, et al: Treatment of acute and chronic traumatic rupture of the descending thoracic aorta. *World J Surg* **4:**545, 1980
147. Sulek M, Miller RH, Mattox KL: The management of gunshot and stab injuries of the trachea. *Arch Otolaryngol* **109:**56–59, 1983
148. Deslauriers J, Beaulieu M, Archambault G, et al: Diagnosis and long term follow-up of major bronchial disruptions due to nonpenetrating trauma. *Ann Thorac Surg* **33:**32, 1982
149. Jones WS, Mavroudis C, Richardson D, et al: Management of tracheo-bronchial disruption resulting from blunt trauma. *Surgery* **95:**319, 1984
150. Grover FL, Ellestad C, Arom KV, et al: Diagnosis and management of major tracheobronchial injuries. *Ann Thorac Surg* **28:**384, 1979

151. Feliciano DV, Bitondo CG, Mattox KL, et al: Combined tracheoesophageal injuries. *Am J Surg* **150**:710–715, 1985
152. Antkowiak JG, Cohen ML, Kyllnen AS: Tracheoesophageal fistula following blunt trauma. *Arch Surg* **109**:529, 1974
153. Grillo HC, Surgery of the trachea. In *Current Problems in Surgery*. Chicago, Year Book, 1970
154. Defore WW, Mattox KL, Hansen HA, et al: Surgical management of penetrating injuries of the esophagus. *Am J Surg* **134**:734–738, 1977
155. McCullough JL, Hollier LH, Nugent M: Paraplegia after thoracic aortic occlusion: Influence of cerebrospinal fluid drainage—Experimental and early clinical results. *J Vasc Surg* **7**:153–160, 1987
156. Cunningham JN Jr: Discussion of clamp repair: A safe technique for treatment of blunt injury to the descending thoracic aorta. *Ann Thorac Surg* **40**:462, 1985
157. Weigel CJ: Medicolegal aspects of trauma. In Mattox KL, Moore EE, Feliciano DV (eds): *Trauma*. Norwalk, Connecticut, Appleton and Lange, 1988, pp 53–60
158. Mattox KL, Beall AC, Ennix CL, DeBakey ME: Intravascular migratory bullets. *Am J Surg* **137**:192–195, 1979
159. Graham JM, Mattox KL: Right ventricular bullet embolectomy without cardiopulmonary bypass. *J Thorac Cardiovasc Surg* **82**:310–313, 1981
160. Pepe PE: The clinical entity of adult respiratory distress syndrome. *Crit Care Clin* **2**:377–403, 1986
161. Weigelt JA: Current concepts in the management of adult respiratory distress syndrome. *World J Surg* **11**:161–166, 1987
162. Pepe PE, Hudson LD, Carrico CJ: Early application of positive end-expiratory pressure in patients at risk for the adult respiratory distress syndrome. *N Engl J Med* **311**:281–286, 1984
163. Johnson KD, Cadambi A, Seibert GB: Incidence of adult respiratory distress syndrome in patients with multiple musculoskeletal injuries: Effects of early operative stabilization of fractures. *J Trauma* **25**:375–384, 1985
164. Fein AM, Lippman M, Holtzman H, et al: The risk factors, incidence and prognosis of ARDS following septicemia. *Chest* **83**:40–42, 1983
165. Pepe PE, Potkin RT, Reus DH, et al: Clinical predictors of the adult respiratory distress syndrome. *Am J Surg* **144**:124–130, 1982
166. Weigelt JA, Snyder WH, Mitchell RA: Early identification of patients prone to develop adult respiratory distress syndrome. *Am J Surg* **142**:687–691, 1981
167. Reul GJ Jr, Greenberg SD, Lefrak EA, et al: Prevention of post-traumatic pulmonary insufficiency: Fine-screen filtration of blood. *Arch Surg* **106**:386–394, 1973
168. Milfeld DJ, Mattox KL, Beall AC Jr: Early evacuation of clotted hemothorax. *Am J Surg* **136**:686–692, 1978
169. Coselli JS, Mattox KL, Beall AC Jr: Reevaluation of early evacuation of clotted hemothorax. *Am J Surg* **148**:786–790, 1984
170. Mulder DS, Greenwood FAH, Brooks CE: Posttraumatic thoracic outlet syndrome. *J Trauma* **13**:706–715, 1973
171. Knott LH, Crawford FA Jr, Grogan JB: Comparison of autogenous vein, Dacron, and Gore-Tex in infected wounds. *J Surg Research* **24**:288, 1978
172. Stone KS, Walshaw R, Sugiyama GT, et al: Polytetrafluoroethylene versus autogenous vein grafts for vascular reconstruction in contaminated wounds. *Am J Surg* **147**:692, 1984
173. Weiss JP, Lorenzo FV, Campbell CD, et al: The behavior of infected arterial prostheses of expanded polytetrafluoroethylene (Gore-Tex). *J Thorac Cardiovasc Surg* **73**:630, 1977
174. Schramel RJ, Creech O Jr: Effects of infection and exposure on synthetic arterial prostheses. *Arch Surg* **78**:271, 1959
175. LoCurto JJ, Tischler CD, Swan KG, et al: Tube thoracostomy and trauma-antibiotics or not? *J Trauma* **26**:1067–1072, 1986

CHAPTER

7

# Pulmonary Resection

## *Anatomy and Techniques*

Larry R. Kaiser

### INTRODUCTION

Pulmonary resection is a routine part of the work of a thoracic surgeon, but the techniques are barely 60 years old. Until the mid-1930s, pulmonary resection was rarely employed and had an almost prohibitive mortality. The techniques of pulmonary resection form the basis of modern thoracic surgery and often are the introduction to the specialty for the general surgery resident and thoracic surgical trainee. To safely perform pulmonary resections, the surgeon must have an intimate understanding of pulmonary anatomy that is more complex, because the thoracic surgeon works from both anterior and posterior aspects of the pulmonary hilum, unlike procedures in the abdomen, where the surgeon works only from an anterior approach. Anatomic relationships from both aspects are particularly important to safely and expeditiously perform pulmonary resections.

Modern thoracic surgery began in World War I, when a large number of chest wounds forced surgeons to operate in the open chest and, thus, directed many toward surgical problems of the chest when they returned to civilian life.[1] The specialty is a creation of the 20th century in that it took numerous developments in anesthetic techniques as well as a general appreciation of the physiology of respiration before chest operations could be undertaken. During the first 20 years of this century, the major problem was the control of pneumothorax in operations of the open chest. Developments in fluid replacement, blood transfusion, and antibiotics along with positive pressure ventilation ultimately made it feasible to operate in the chest.

### HISTORICAL ASPECTS

The most pressing problem in the development of chest surgery was the control of pneumothorax with an open chest. Sauerbruch[2] devised a negative pressure chamber into which both the patient's body and the operating surgeon were placed. This device proved extremely impractical. Matas,[3] in 1900, developed intralaryngeal insufflation to maintain artificial respiration in surgery of the chest. Finally, Meltzer and Auer[4] introduced a simple practical method for control of intrapleural pressure by peroral intubation in 1909. The technique of positive pressure ventilation with an endotracheal tube initially was not widely accepted, and considerable skepticism remained even as late as 1918.

The physiologic principles of the open pneumothorax were finally elucidated by Graham and Bell[5] as part of the work of the Empyema Commission. Graham[6] recognized that avoidance of an open pneumothorax before the mediastinum was stabilized could significantly decrease the mortality from empyema. This observation and others made by Graham resulted in a giant leap forward in the management of thoracic pathology. He also noted that an open pneumothorax on one side exerted a deleterious effect on both lungs, depending on the fixation of the mediastinum.

In 1922, Lilienthal[7] reported a series of lung resections for suppurative infections with a high mortality. There was a 42% mortality when the process involved one lobe and a 70% mortality when the infective process involved more than one lobe. In 1923, Graham[8] described his technique for pneumonectomy with cautery, a multiple-stage procedure using a soldering iron to remove portions of diseased lung tissue. If, at the time of the first procedure, the lung was adherent to the pleura, a red hot iron was used to make an excavation into the lung tissue. If pleural symphysis was not present, Iodoform gauze was used to create pleural symphysis as a prelude to a second stage when cautery destruction would be undertaken. It was necessary to remove all diseased tissue, and this often required multiple stages.

Before 1929, essentially all attempts at excising lung tissue utilized Graham's operation or an operation described by Whitmore, in which the diseased lobe was exteriorized and the base of the lobe secured to the chest wall.[1] The lobe was then allowed to slough or could be removed in stages. In 1929, Brunn[9] described six one-stage lobectomies carried out for bronchiectasis with only one death. This astounding accomplishment served to stimulate renewed interest in pulmonary resection. Most of these early one-stage lobectomies utilized tourniquet techniques with mass ligation of the hilum, followed by sloughing of the lung tissue. It took several more years before precise hilar anatomy became of practical importance as individual ligation techniques of hilar structures eventually were developed and first attempted in carcinoma of the lung by Churchill in 1932.[10]

The concept of anatomic dissection of the pulmonary hilum with individual ligation was proposed by several investigators in animals in the early 1920s.[11] However, these same surgeons continued to perform mass hilar ligation. In retrospect, the "dissection lobectomy" for tumor performed by Morriston Davies in 1912 was an historic yet little recognized achievement, probably because the patient died 8 days following the operation.[12]

In 1931, Nissen[13] of Berlin performed the first pneumonectomy by excising the left lung of a 12-year-old girl using mass ligation of the hilum with subsequent slough of the lung. Soon after, Haight[14] performed the second successful pneumonectomy using a similar technique. In 1933, Graham and Singer[15] described the first successful pneumonectomy for cancer performed in one stage accompanied by a partial thoracoplasty to deal with the resultant space. Reinhoff,[16] in Baltimore, subsequently described and successfully accomplished an elegant technique for individual ligation of hilar structures. Despite these rapid developments, the early mortality from pulmonary resection was quite high, mainly because of bronchial dehiscence with resultant empyema. The reduction in mortality achieved today for pulmonary resection resulted from improved techniques, instruments, antibiotics, and anesthesia.

## ANATOMY AND GENERAL CONSIDERATIONS

The gross anatomic features of each lung and its surface projection as well as the basic relationships of the major hilar structures can be found in any standard textbook of anatomy. The bronchopulmonary segment is the anatomic, surgical, and pathologic unit of the lung that is most important. Aspects of hilar and lobar anatomy of importance to the surgeon will be described within the sections dealing with specific pulmonary resections. The concept of bronchopulmonary segments developed in response to clinical need. During the early development of thoracic surgery, suppurative infections, specifically bronchiectasis, were a major problem, and lung conservation was key. Segmental resections were feasible to resect infected areas of the lung and conserve normal lung tissue. It was often necessary to perform multiple segmental resections. Boyden[17] described segmental anatomy in all its complexity in his classic *Segmental Anatomy of the Lungs,* published in 1955. The bronchopulmonary segments are detailed in Figures 7–1 and 7–2 and listed in Table 7–1. It is important to have a knowledge of segmental anatomy, especially when one is looking at a chest radiograph, since it is the common language of the physician and surgeon dealing with chest disorders. The numerical nomenclature is more confusing than helpful for clinical purposes. We distinguish the three segments of the upper lobe on each side, whereas the lower lobes can be conceptualized as "two segments": the superior segment and the "unit" of basilar segments. From the standpoint of resection, this classification summarizes what is relevant. Now, segmental resection plays a small role in the management of chest pathology. The major anatomic unit for resection is the lobe. This is because malignant disease is the major reason for pulmonary resection, not suppurative disease, and the standard operation for malignant disease is lobectomy.

Since thoracic incisions are dealt with in Chapter 5, we will only mention them briefly here. The standard thoracotomy incision is a posterolateral one that divides the latissimus dorsi and serratus anterior muscle. Variations on this include muscle-sparing incisions. Morbidity from a thoracic incision is due mainly to rib spreading, and it is incumbent on the surgeon to avoid breaking ribs if possible. Removal of a rib, usually the fifth rib, often facilitates entry into the chest. It allows use of a rib spreader without breaking ribs. Alternatively, a small portion of the posterior sixth rib can be removed in a subperiosteal fashion, allowing the sixth rib to move more readily and avoid breaking the ribs. I prefer to enter the chest through the bed of the resected fifth rib or in the fifth intercostal space for all pulmonary resections. Others prefer to enter through the sixth intercostal space for lower lobe resections, but the major extent of dissection is at the hilum, which is fixed in its location no matter where the pathology is located.

For most procedures, the patient is positioned in the lateral decubitus position so that a posterolateral incision may be carried out. There are times, however, that a posterolateral thoracotomy is not the appropriate incision. The median sternotomy incision has engendered renewed enthusiasm for pulmonary resection in patients with compromised pulmonary function.[18] There is seemingly less post-

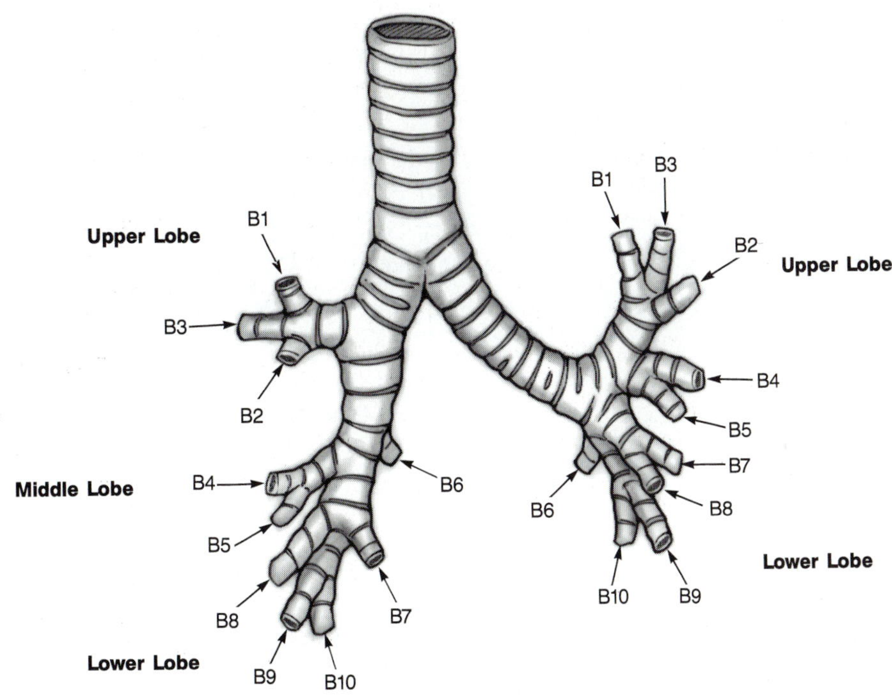


**Figure 7–1.** Segmental anatomy of the bronchial tree. Segmental numbering corresponds to Table 7–1.

operative pain with the sternotomy incision, and, for most resections, this incision is adequate. It is more difficult to accomplish a left lower lobectomy through a sternotomy because of the heart. A left lower lobectomy is rarely performed through this incision. Entry to both hemithoraces can also be gained by a bilateral thoracosternotomy incision, an anterolateral thoracotomy on each side with transverse division of the sternum.[19] This incision is useful in bilateral sequential lung transplantation but has also been utilized for complex resections of mediastinal lesions as well as for some pulmonary resections. A posterior thoracotomy, with the patient in the prone position, was often used in the early days of thoracic surgery, when infection was the major indication for operation, but currently is of historical interest only.

In perhaps no other surgical procedure is one working in as deep a space, and a headlight provides optimal illumination and should be employed for pulmonary resections. Vascular instruments should be available, since it is often necessary to take portions of vessels for complex resections. Mechanical staplers have greatly advanced pulmonary surgery and are used for both bronchial closure and division of pulmonary vessels by most thoracic surgeons. For video-assisted thoracic operations, stapling devices are even more important. The ability to place a linear cutting stapler through a small incision has allowed the performance of pulmonary resections using this video-assisted approach (see Chapter 12B). The principles that apply to resection via the open chest also apply for resection by a video-assisted approach.

Placement of a double-lumen, endobronchial tube is key to visualization of hilar structures, especially for complex resections of central lesions. To be able to work in a field with the lung collapsed and easily maneuverable is far preferable to fighting an inflated lung or working during short periods of apnea. The double-lumen tube was initially introduced to protect the side opposite the pathology from being soiled with pus, but this problem is encountered far less now. Accurate placement of the tube is crucial, and the surgeon must occasionally assist the anesthesiologist in this regard.

Postoperative pain management is particularly important. I strongly recommend preoperative placement of a thoracic epidural catheter for continuous infusion of a narcotic and/or local anesthetic postoperatively. It is important for the patient to take deep breaths and cough productively to prevent atelectasis and pneumonia in the early postoperative period. Preoperative teaching of the postoperative coughing and use of an incentive spirometer helps minimize postoperative morbidity.

## SPECIFIC PULMONARY RESECTIONS

The surgeon must have intimate familiarity with the anatomy of the pulmonary hilum. Resectability must be distinguished from operability. A patient may have an otherwise resectable lesion yet be inoperable because of disseminated disease. On the other hand, a patient may be operable, with disease limited to the chest, yet be found to be unresectable at the time of operation because of mediastinal invasion. We use the chest radiograph as well as the com-

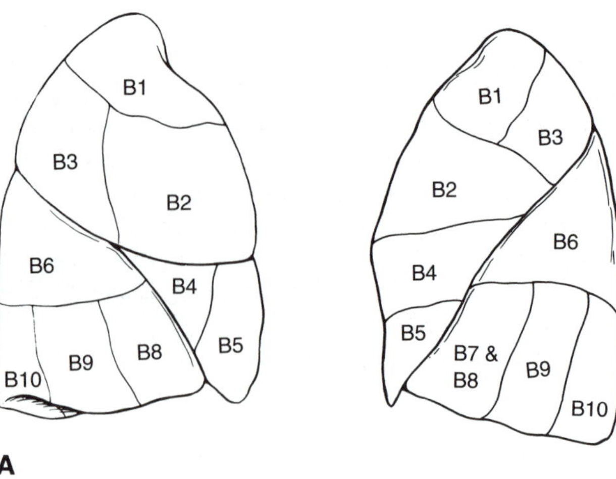


**Figure 7–2. A.** Lateral view of the bronchopulmonary segments for both the right and left lung. The key for the numbering system appears in Table 7–1. **B.** Medial view of the bronchopulmonary segments of the right and left lung with the hilar structures labeled. Note the relationships at the hilum of the bronchovascular structures.

puted tomographic (CT) scan to help determine resectability. Unfortunately, magnetic resonance imaging (MRI) scan does not increase our ability to determine resectability, especially in delineating whether a lesion directly invades adjacent structures in the mediastinum. Neither CT nor MRI is accurate for distinguishing between invasion and abutment when a lung cancer is contiguous with the mediastinum or

**TABLE 7–1. BRONCHOPULMONARY SEGMENTS**

| | |
|---|---|
| **Right Upper Lobe** | **Left Upper Lobe** |
| 1. Apical | 1 and 3. Apicoposterioı |
| 2. Anterior | 2. Anterior |
| 3. Posterior | 4. Superior lingular |
| **Right Middle Lobe** | 5. Inferior lingular |
| 4. Lateral | **Left Lower Lobe** |
| 5. Medial | 6. Superior |
| **Right Lower Lobe** | 7 and 8. Anteromedial |
| 6. Superior | 9. Lateral basal |
| 7. Medial basal | 10. Posterior basal |
| 8. Anterior basal | |
| 9. Lateral basal | |
| 10. Posterior basal | |

chest wall. Although resecting a lobe in continuity with chest wall is a well-accepted procedure, removing mediastinal structures invaded by tumor is only rarely warranted.

Although many patients will have had bronchoscopy performed by the referring pulmonologist, we feel it is important for the operating surgeon to repeat the bronchoscopy prior to thoracotomy. The location of an endobronchial lesion is important in planning the resection, and unsuspected findings may be noted. The possibility of a sleeve resection or another bronchoplastic procedure may become evident to the surgeon by observation of the endobronchial pathology.

Following bronchoscopy, the standard endotracheal tube is removed, and a double-lumen endobronchial tube is placed. For most resections, including those on the left, a left-sided tube, which is easier to place, is acceptable. However, when a left endobronchial lesion is present, and the possibility exists that a left pneumonectomy or a bronchoplastic procedure may be required, a right-sided endobronchial tube is preferable. The right-sided tube is more difficult to place in the correct location and requires aligning the side hole of the tube at the right upper lobe orifice.

The patient is positioned in the appropriate lateral decubitus position and secured in place. Care is taken to pad pressure sensitive areas, and the position of the upper extremities is also particularly important. After the incision is made and the pleura is seen, the lung moving within indicates at least a partially free pleural space. The pleura is incised and adhesions, if present, are divided sharply, using electrocautery for bleeding points on the chest wall. The lung is allowed to collapse. The entire lung is mobilized in the pleural space. Beginning medially, at the mediastinum, may expedite the dissection, as the adhesions tend to be less dense in this location or may be absent when adhesions elsewhere are quite dense. If one encounters difficulty in one area, moving to another less difficult area is often helpful. Care is taken at the apex to avoid the brachiocephalic vessels. Dissection of adhesions along the diaphragm may be difficult, since the correct plane may be difficult to discern.

The entire visceral and parietal pleura surface is inspected for metastatic disease. The lung is then thoroughly palpated to locate the lesion and rule out additional disease. Palpation of the hilum is particularly important to note enlarged or likely metastatic lymph node involvement. The location of the primary tumor and its proximity to the hilum is important in assessing resectability. Potential invasion of contiguous structures in the mediastinum is evaluated as is the need to resect these structures. Palpation of the superior mediastinum and subcarinal space is performed. If unsuspected mediastinal nodal disease is found, a determination must be made as to whether it is resectable. Discrete, enlarged mediastinal lymph nodes (intranodal disease) should be removed with the resected lobe and consideration given to postoperative treatment. We prefer performing a resection, if possible, even if unsuspected mediastinal nodal metastatic disease is found.

Several factors determine resectability. Not the least of these is the experience of the operating surgeon. What is resectable for one surgeon may not be resectable for another, but certain key maneuvers are necessary in order to assess fully the possibility of resection. It is often helpful to open the pericardium to assess fully the extent of involvement of a lesion occurring in a central location where the pulmonary veins or left atrium may be involved. Palpation of the lesion through the opened pericardium gives a better idea of its location and proximity to the central vascular structures. It is important to note whether the confluence of the veins is free of disease and, if it is not, whether there is enough atrium to place a clamp proximal in order to complete a resection. Once the initial decision for resection is made, it is critically important to dissect all structures prior to "burning any bridges." It would not be desirable to have divided the main pulmonary artery, only to find that one cannot get a clamp proximal enough on the atrium to complete a resection. All bronchovascular structures should be dissected or their dissection deemed feasible prior to dividing any structures. Occasionally, this may prove quite difficult.

## Right-Sided Resections

Key anatomic features on the right side are the superior vena cava and the azygos vein. Access to the pulmonary hilum on the right is best gained through the fifth intercostal space or the bed of the resected fifth rib. The location of the phrenic nerve as it courses along the superior vena cava must be noted and care taken to avoid injuring this nerve (Fig. 7–3).

## Right Upper Lobectomy

A right upper lobectomy is the most common lobectomy performed and is, perhaps, the easiest resection for the novice surgeon. The anatomic considerations are usually quite straightforward and easily seen. The dissection is undertaken with the operator standing at the posterior aspect of the patient placed in the lateral decubitus position, but the resection may be more easily accomplished with the operating surgeon standing anterior to the patient. The dissection is begun by incising the anterior and superior aspects of the hilar pleura. Again, the location of the phrenic nerve must be kept in mind. As the hilar pleura is incised, the superior pulmonary vein is usually the first structure to be seen. It commonly has two trunks as can be seen in Figure 7–3. Variations of venous anatomy are many, and there may be more than two trunks, depending upon where the vessel branches. Often, a third trunk is easily seen. The middle

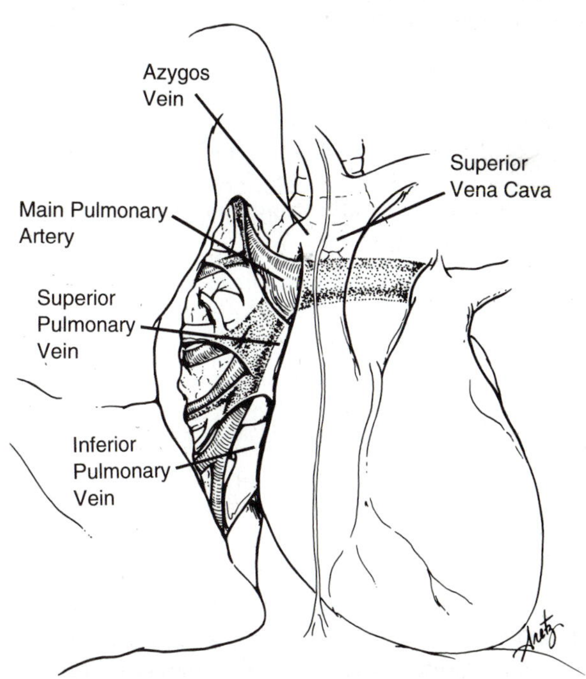


**Figure 7–3.** The hilum of the right lung viewed from the anterior aspect. Note the position of the main pulmonary artery in relation to the superior vena cava, the location of the phrenic nerve as it courses along the vena cava, and the relationships of the pulmonary veins to the arterial branches.

lobe vein most commonly arises from the superior pulmonary vein. The main trunk of the superior pulmonary veins is seen, and the dissection is carried down onto the cleavage plane, where the pericardial reflection may be reflected medially to expose a longer segment of extrapericardial vein. The pulmonary artery lies superior and posterior to the superior pulmonary vein (Fig. 7–3). As one carries the dissection superiorly, there is a wedge of areolar tissue containing mostly lymphatics and few, if any, small vessels. The electrocautery is used to coagulate the small vessels. Dissecting slightly more superior, one encounters the "truncus anterior" of the pulmonary artery, which includes the apical and anterior segmental arteries.

The right main pulmonary artery courses posterior to the vena cava just inferior to the junction of the azygos vein and the superior vena cava. It is rarely necessary to divide the azygos vein in order to adequately expose the pulmonary artery, but, depending upon the location of the tumor, this may be necessary. The right main pulmonary artery is relatively long, and adequate length of the artery can be obtained as the artery courses posterior to the vena cava.

Great care is taken in exposing and surrounding the pulmonary artery. The artery is quite fragile, having no muscular layer, and may be easily damaged or torn, especially if the tumor is close. Often, lymph nodes are densely adherent to the pulmonary artery and may, in fact, invade the wall of the artery. If the surgeon suspects the upper lobe arterial branches are adherent to lymph nodes or the primary tumor, then proximal control of the main pulmonary artery is advisable. The main artery is then circumferentially dissected in the adventitial plane. The final (deep) portion of the dissection can be accomplished with the thumb and forefinger. It is far safer to complete the last portion of the dissection digitally than it is to try to encircle the artery with a clamp. Once the artery is encircled, a blunt clamp, guided by the finger, is placed and an umbilical tape passed. A Rumel tourniquet is then placed so that proximal control may now be rapidly established, if necessary. Dissection is then carried distally and the truncus anterior and the bifurcation of the apical and anterior branches exposed. The apical segmental branch of the superior pulmonary vein may obscure the bifurcation of the truncus anterior, and it may be easiest to divide this segmental branch of the vein to facilitate dissection of the artery. The arterial dissection is then carried distally along the inferior division of the artery posterior to the superior pulmonary vein. The superior pulmonary vein is circumferentially dissected and encircled. Using the thumb and forefinger for safety, a loose ligature is placed around it. Care is taken not to include the middle lobe branch when encircling the vein. The hilar pleura is then incised further superiorly and then posteriorly. The truncus anterior is then freed with its branches and loose ligatures placed around them. The azygos vein, at this point, is well visualized and delineates the tracheobronchial angle. Just inferior to the azygos is the takeoff of the upper lobe bronchus, seen best from the posterior view (Fig. 7–4). The hilar pleura is incised posteriorly to the level of the bifurcation between the upper lobe bronchus and bronchus intermedius. This is a significant anatomic feature of a right upper lobectomy. The "crotch" between the upper lobe bronchus and bronchus intermedius provides the key to completing an upper lobectomy. Bronchial arterial branches are present in this location and require either clipping or electrocautery, depending upon the size. The "crotch" is palpated but usually can be easily seen. Dissection is begun just at the bifurcation and carried along the bronchus intermedius and inferior wall of the upper lobe bronchus. The pulmonary artery lies just medial at this location and is visualized as the dissection is carried down to it. This is a common location for lymph node involvement, and the dissection to remove the lymph node is accomplished by dissecting the plane between the lymph node and the bronchus. Once this area has been dissected, it is then possible to encircle the bronchus, having previously dissected the truncus anterior artery away from the bronchus anteriorly.

Attention is then directed to the fissure. Not uncommonly, the major or oblique fissure is well developed, and the distal pulmonary artery is easily visualized. However, this may not be the case, and it may be necessary to dissect into the fissure in order to see the artery. This move is facilitated once the bifurcation between the upper-lobe bronchus

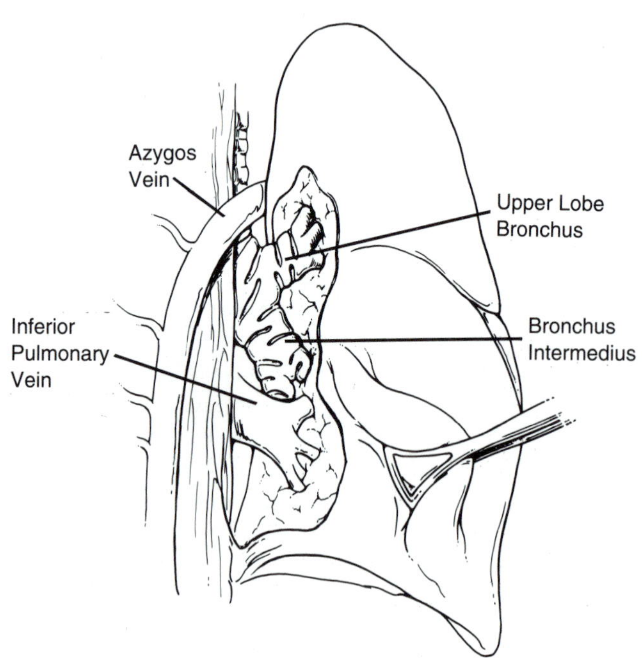


**Figure 7–4.** The right hilum as seen from the posterior aspect. Note particularly the position of the azygos vein in relation to the mainstem bronchus and the takeoff of the right upper-lobe bronchus. The bifurcation formed by the right upper-lobe takeoff and the bronchus intermedius is the key anatomic feature of this aspect of the hilum. The location of the inferior pulmonary vein in relation to the lower-lobe bronchus should also be noted.

and bronchus intermedius has been dissected. If the branch of the pulmonary artery to the superior segment of the lower lobe has been visualized from behind, it is often quite easy to dissect the most medial aspect of the oblique fissure with the thumb and forefinger. The posterior fissure can then be divided safely with a linear stapler, since there are no vascular structures posterior to the takeoff of the superior segmented artery (Fig. 7–5). Once the artery has been identified in the fissure, an additional arterial branch to the upper lobe, the so-called recurrent branch, is sought. This is actually a posterior segmental branch and is easily seen in the fissure. The dissection is directed superiorly along the artery until this branch is identified (Fig. 7–4). The minor fissure is rarely well developed, and care must be taken to avoid injuring the middle-lobe artery when dividing this fissure. Once the pulmonary artery is identified in the fissure, however, proceeding along the artery will identify the takeoff of the middle-lobe arterial branch, which usually occurs just opposite the superior segmental branch. The minor fissure is safely divided, once the middle-lobe artery or arteries have been identified, or it may be divided, once all other bronchovascular structures have been divided.

Once all the bronchovascular structures to the upper lobe have been exposed, they may then be divided. There is no particular importance to the order in which the structures are divided. Classically, the arterial branches have been divided first, followed by the venous branches and, finally, the bronchus. It is important to remember that whichever structure is the easiest should be taken on first. Depending upon the location of the primary tumor or of the lymph node involvement, it is sometimes easiest to divide the superior pulmonary vein prior to dividing the arterial branches.

Adequate length must be gained on an arterial branch prior to dividing it. Once a proximal tie is placed, dissection to gain length on an arterial branch should be done with extreme care, if at all. We prefer to do all the dissection of an arterial branch prior to placing a ligature on the proximal artery. The vessels may be divided in several different ways. For the arterial branches, we prefer to ligate with silk ligatures, usually doubly ligating proximally. We do not use metal clips on proximal arterial branches. Care must be taken when tying a pulmonary artery not to exert traction on the ties. The artery is susceptible to cracking, usually at the origin of the branch from the arterial trunk. The ligatures must be tied securely but not so tight as to crush the vessel. Some prefer a 2-0 silk suture ligature on the proximal vessel. This is placed distal to the proximal ligature. The vessel distal to the point of division should be secured by a ligature or clip. Loss of control of the distal vessel leads to bothersome back bleeding. The main trunk of the superior pulmonary vein may be handled in several ways. We prefer to use a vascular stapler for ligation of the venous trunk; however, acceptable alternatives include suture ligation or clamping with division and oversewing the divided vein.

Once the pulmonary vessels have been divided, the lobar bronchus is divided as close to its origin as possible. We prefer to close the bronchus with a mechanical stapler (TA-30, U.S. Surgical Corp., Norwalk, CT) that provides an excellent closure, with two layers of titanium staples. Following division, the bronchial stump is checked to assure that it is airtight. This is done by inflating the remain-

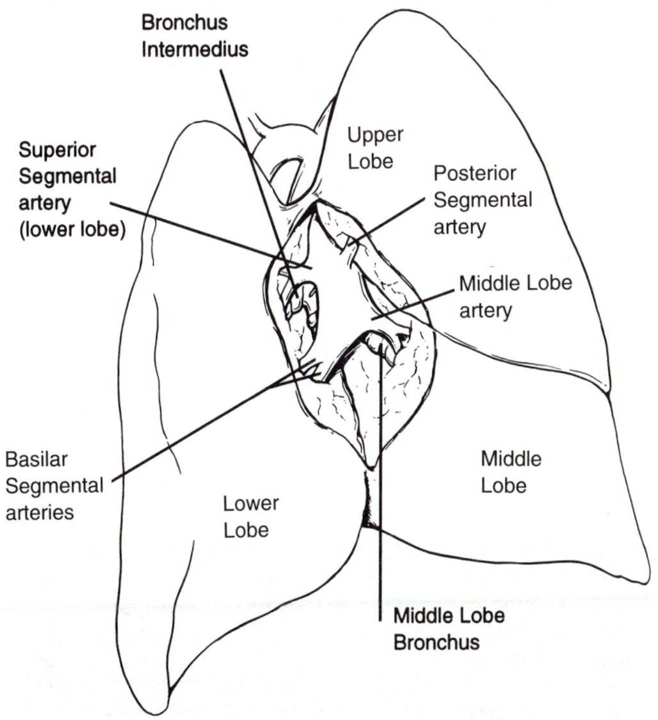


**Figure 7–5.** View of the right pulmonary artery in the fissure in relation to the location of the bronchus. Note the position of the middle-lobe artery relative to the superior segment arterial branch. The relationship between the artery to the superior segment and the basilar arterial trunk determines how one divides the arterial supply to the lower lobe. Care must be taken to avoid injury to the middle-lobe artery and vein during performance of a lower lobectomy.

ing lung to 20–30 cm $H_2O$ with the stump under water. Before the advent of mechanical staplers, the divided bronchus was sutured. Suture closure may still be performed and is carried out after dividing the bronchus as close as possible to its origin. The bronchus is closed by placing fine, interrupted absorbable sutures to approximate the cartilaginous to the membranous bronchus. The initial suture is placed in the center of the closure, and sutures are placed approximately 1–2 mm apart. The sutures are tied after all have been placed, and the bronchial closure is checked to assure that it is airtight. A flap of pleura or intercostal muscle may be used to reinforce the bronchial closure but probably is unnecessary, especially with a stapled closure.

Usually by the time the bronchus is transected, the oblique fissure has been divided and all that remains is the division of the minor fissure. We use a linear stapler (GIA, U.S. Surgical Corp., Norwalk, CT) to divide the minor fissure. The stapler is placed so as not to injure the middle-lobe artery or vein but should be inferior to the distal stumps of the previously divided venous branches.

For staging, it is important to know the status of the mediastinal lymph nodes. If a mediastinoscopy has been performed, the status of the mediastinal lymph node samples is known. During thoracotomy, further evaluation of node regions should be done. The mediastinal pleura is incised at the level of the azygos vein and is carried superiorly to the level of the subclavian vein. The contents of the superior mediastinum are dissected from the trachea posteriorly, the superior vena cava anteriorly, the subclavian vein superiorly, and the azygos vein inferiorly. Small vessels in the mediastinal areolar tissue are controlled with clips. Dissection is also carried out in the subcarinal space after incising the overlying mediastinal pleura. Lymph nodes also are sampled in the periesophageal region as well as in the inferior pulmonary ligament. Following such a procedure, the status of the mediastinal lymph nodes is known definitively. Although it is controversial whether or not mediastinal lymph node dissection is therapeutic, it is certainly of great value from a prognostic standpoint. Finally, the inferior pulmonary ligament is divided up to the inferior pulmonary vein. This allows the remaining lower lobe to rise in the pleural space and fill the apex of the chest. A problem after upper lobectomy is a residual airspace at the apex, if the lung does not expand to fill it.

### Right Middle Lobectomy

The relationship of the middle-lobe artery to the posterior segmental arterial branch to the upper lobe and the superior segmental branch to the lower lobe have been described as shown in Figure 7–5. If the major fissure is nearly complete and dissection proceeds easily, the artery can be identified in the fissure as the initial maneuver. Often, there are two middle-lobe arterial branches. The middle-lobe bronchus is posterior and slightly inferior to the middle-lobe arterial branch. The bronchus is easily seen following division of the artery. The middle-lobe vein most commonly drains into the superior pulmonary vein. Occasionally, it drains directly into the left atrium or may be part of the inferior pulmonary vein. The vein is the key structure in the dissection of the middle lobe, since middle lobectomy often may be accomplished more easily by first dividing the vein. This is certainly true when dissection in the fissure proves difficult. Following division of the middle-lobe vein, the middle-lobe bronchus is seen and divided. This allows the middle-lobe artery to be seen and divided. Once the bronchovascular structures are divided, the minor fissure may be divided with a stapler. The major fissure is usually complete, and the middle lobe is removed, followed by mediastinal lymph node dissection or sampling.

### Right Lower Lobectomy

Because of the relationship of the middle-lobe bronchus to the lower-lobe bronchus, a lower lobectomy can at times be quite difficult. As seen in Figure 7–5, note the relationship of the superior segmental arterial branch to the basilar arterial trunk. Here the length of the basilar arterial trunk appears quite long, but it actually may be significantly shorter, depending on the location of the superior segmental branch. It is sometimes possible to ligate the entire lower lobe arterial supply, including the superior segmental branch, with one ligature, but just as often it is necessary to divide the superior segmental branch and the basilar segmental trunk separately. Dissection usually is begun in the major fissure, and, if this proceeds easily, the artery may be identified and divided. The basilar arterial trunk is of a size that it should be either doubly ligated or suture ligated. Alternatively, a vascular stapler may be used to divide this arterial trunk. Once the pulmonary artery to the lower lobe is divided, the bronchus is readily seen immediately posterior (Fig. 7–4). The location of the middle-lobe bronchus must be noted so that division of the lower-lobe bronchus does not damage or compromise it. The position of the superior segmental bronchus must also be considered, since this may have to be divided separately from the basilar segmental bronchus. Usually, a stapler can be placed obliquely across the lower-lobe bronchus, approximating the membranous to the cartilaginous portion of the entire bronchus, including the superior segmental bronchus.

The inferior pulmonary vein is located inferiorly and posterior to the superior pulmonary vein as seen in Figure 7–4. Incising the hilar pleura over the vein readily reveals the entire vein. The inferior pulmonary ligament, that band of tissue tethering the lower lobe medially, should be divided prior to dividing the inferior pulmonary vein. The relationship of the vein to the lobar bronchus is seen in Figure 7–3. The lower lobectomy is completed by dividing what remains of the major fissure with a linear stapler.

Depending upon the location of the tumor in the lower lobe and the relationship of any nodal disease to middle-lobe structures, occasionally it may be necessary to perform a bilobectomy, removing both the middle and lower lobes. The bronchial division occurs at the level of the bronchus intermedius, just distal to the right upper-lobe takeoff (Fig. 7–4). The inferior pulmonary vein along with the middle-lobe vein must be divided, as would the appropriate arterial branches.

### Right Pneumonectomy

For centrally located tumors, it is often necessary to remove the entire lung. Indications for pneumonectomy include involvement of the proximal pulmonary artery to such an extent that it is not possible to isolate lobar branches, or involvement of the confluence of the pulmonary veins. An entire lung should not be removed without histologic confirmation of malignancy. It should be kept in mind that a bronchoplastic procedure (see Chapter 26) should always be considered a possibility, so that pulmonary parenchyma might be preserved. Even in the current era, mortality following pneumonectomy still approaches 5–10%, and complete removal of the lung should be performed only when absolutely necessary. The presence of tumor in the main stem bronchus is not necessarily an indication for pneumonectomy, if the surgeon is familiar with bronchoplastic techniques. If lobar vessels to the middle and lower lobe are able to be isolated, it may be possible to perform an upper lobectomy, with resection of the main stem bronchus and reanastomosis of the bronchus intermedius to the most proximal portion of the main stem bronchus or distal trachea.

If the surgeon determines that pneumonectomy is necessary, dissection begins by incising the hilar pleura. The inferior and superior pulmonary veins are encircled (Fig. 7–3, 7–4). The right main pulmonary artery is also dissected as it courses posterior to the superior vena cava in its extrapericardial location. Occasionally, it may be necessary to open the pericardium and isolate the vessels within the pericardium and perform an intrapericardial pneumonectomy. This becomes necessary when tumor involves most of the extrapericardial length of the pulmonary artery, and additional length is needed for a safe division. Once the artery has been encircled, it is then possible to encircle the right main stem bronchus as it courses posterior to the azygos vein (Fig. 7–4).

Depending upon the location of the tumor and the length of the pulmonary artery available, division of the vascular structures is begun. It is often safer to divide the veins prior to dividing the artery, since this may allow for more length and a safer division of the artery. Sometimes it is necessary to divide the main stem bronchus prior to taking the artery, since, again, this may make arterial division safer. We prefer to divide the veins with a vascular stapler, but they may also be suture ligated or clamped, divided, and sutured. The pulmonary artery may also be clamped, divided, and sutured or taken with a vascular stapler. It is not sufficient to simply place a ligature on the main pulmonary artery or on a pulmonary vein. An additional suture ligature, however, is satisfactory. The hilar pleura must be incised circumferentially, and the main stem bronchus should be divided as close to the carina as possible. This may be accomplished with either a mechanical stapler or divided and closed with interrupted sutures. The bronchial stump must be buttressed with either a flap of pleura or intercostal muscle. The incidence of bronchial stump problems is highest after a right pneumonectomy. This is because of its exposed location. Thus, the bronchial stump should be protected. Dividing the bronchus as close as possible to the carina obviates leaving a long segment of relatively ischemic bronchus.

If an intrapericardial dissection has been performed, it often is advisable to replace the pericardial defect with prosthetic material to prevent the heart from herniating out of the pericardial sac. This is necessary only when a large pericardial defect has been made. Division of the phrenic nerve should be avoided, if possible, since the function of the contralateral hemidiaphragm may be hindered by dysfunction of the diaphragm on the surgical side. Complete removal of the lung is not an indication for division of the phrenic nerve. It is sometimes necessary, however, because of tumor involvement, to take the phrenic nerve.

Despite the best intentions of the operating surgeon, problems occasionally occur. It is far better to avoid problems in the chest rather than try to manage them, so that one should always be thinking safety and how to stay out of trouble. Encircling the main pulmonary artery to gain proximal control prior to beginning dissection is one way to prevent a catastrophe, should there be a problem in dissecting the distal artery. At least on the right side, because of the length of the main pulmonary artery, even a problem with the artery in a proximal location can usually be managed, although at times it may be necessary to gain intrapericardial control. Care should also be taken when working in the fissure to prevent injury to an artery or a bronchial structure that one does not wish to remove. In particular, injury to the middle-lobe bronchus when one is dividing the lower-lobe bronchus can be prevented by visualizing the middle-lobe bronchial takeoff prior to dividing the lower-lobe bronchus and only dividing the bronchus from within the fissure. The lower-lobe bronchus should not be divided from the posterior approach, since the middle-lobe bronchus cannot easily be seen.

Following a lobectomy, the hemithorax should be drained, with tubes placed to control suction. After a pneumonectomy, a tube may also be left in place, but a balanced drainage system should be employed that is not placed on suction. Many surgeons do not put in a chest tube after a pneumonectomy. After the incision is closed and a dressing applied, the patient is turned to a supine position. At that time, the location of the trachea and heart are observed to be sure that the trachea and mediastinum are in the midline. The opposite lung is not overexpanded or compressed. This can be adjusted by a needle and syringe to remove or inject air into the empty hemithorax. During the operative procedure, air leaks should be minimized by using mechanical staplers to divide fissures and avoiding dissection through parenchyma when possible. Anatomic segmental resections will be discussed in a separate chapter, but it should be mentioned in the context of pulmonary resections that segmental resection, as a way of conserving lung tissue, may be performed for smaller lesions or in the occasional patient with limited bronchiectasis. Excision of the superior segment of the right lower lobe is the easiest and most common segmentectomy performed on the right side. The superior segmental bronchus is a discrete structure, readily located and usually accompanied by a single arterial branch and a separate superior segmental pulmonary vein. Because of this favorable anatomic arrangement, the basilar segments also may be taken as a block, leaving the superior segment (Fig. 7–5). Rarely is segmentectomy done in the middle lobe. Segmental resections are possible in the upper lobe, especially excision of the posterior segment or a combination anterior-apical segmentectomy. Segmental resections can be quite challenging from a technical standpoint, and it is safe to say that they are performed infrequently by most surgeons.

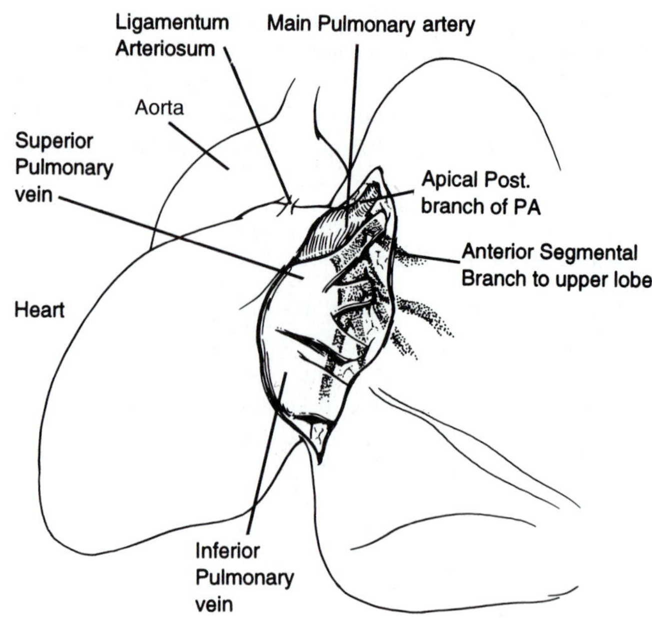


**Figure 7–6.** The left pulmonary hilum as viewed from the anterior aspect. Note the position of the left main pulmonary artery in relation to the aortic arch and the location of the ligamentum arteriosum. The apical-posterior branch of the pulmonary artery is short and broad and is the most proximal branch. The inferior pulmonary vein lies inferior and posterior to the superior vein.

### Left-Side Resection

The location of the aortic arch and its relationship to the left main pulmonary artery are the major anatomic landmarks in the left chest. The left main pulmonary artery is significantly shorter than the right artery, and the ligamentum arteriosum tethers the proximal left main pulmonary artery proximally under the arch (Fig. 7–6). Although there are only two lobes on the left, the lingula is analogous to the middle lobe from an anatomic stand point.

### Left Upper Lobectomy

As on the right side, the patient is positioned in the lateral decubitus position, and the chest is entered most commonly through the fifth intercostal space or the bed of the resected fifth rib. Entry through this space provides excellent access to the hilum. The hilar pleura overlying the pulmonary artery and superior pulmonary vein is incised. At the most superior aspect of the hilum, one encounters the left main pulmonary artery (Fig. 7–6). Great care must be taken not to exert too much traction on the left upper lobe, since it is very easy to tear or avulse the apical-posterior trunk of the pulmonary artery, the most proximal branch of the left main pulmonary artery and a branch that is usually short and broad (Fig. 7–5). A centrally located tumor close to this branch makes dissection of the artery extremely difficult, and proximal control of the left main pulmonary artery should be obtained. Occasionally, it is necessary to divide the ligamentum arteriosum, taking care to avoid the recurrent laryngeal nerve that courses around the arch of the aorta medially to the ligamentum arteriosum. Dividing the ligamentum provides additional useable length of the left main pulmonary artery, facilitating further dissection. The lingular venous branch drains into the superior pulmonary vein in most circumstances (Fig. 7–6). The apical segmental branch of the superior pulmonary vein may obscure the apical posterior branch of the pulmonary artery and may be divided in order to adequately see the arterial branch. The hilar pleura is incised superiorly and posteriorly, and the artery is dissected posteriorly toward the fissure. An anterior segmental branch comes into view as this dissection continues (Fig. 7–7). Continued distal dissection on the artery reveals the superior segmental arterial branch to the lower lobe (Fig. 7–6). Once this branch is visualized, the posterior portion of the major fissures may be divided, with a linear stapler, although this portion of the fissure is often quite attenuated. Further dissection along the pulmonary artery in the fissure reveals one and often two lingular branches as seen in Fig. 7–8. Note the relationship of the bronchus to the pulmonary artery, which we describe as "epibronchial," that is positioned slightly superior to the bronchus.

To complete the upper lobectomy, the arterial branches are divided, followed by division of the superior pulmonary vein, including the lingular branch, although the order of division is unimportant. The left main bronchus is quite long in comparison with the right main bronchus, and it is necessary to see the bifurcation of the bronchus in order to safely divide only the left upper bronchus (Fig. 7–6). Once the arterial branches have been divided, it is usually quite easy to see the bronchial bifurcation and use either a mechanical stapler or to divide the bronchus and suture it

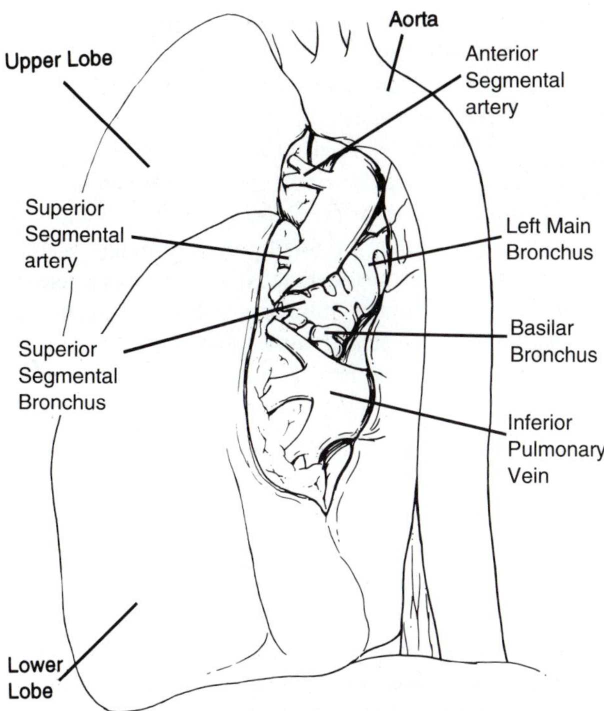


**Figure 7–7.** View of the left hilum from the posterior aspect showing the epibronchial location of the pulmonary artery and the location of the inferior pulmonary vein relative to the left main bronchus. The left pulmonary hilum is tethered by the aortic arch.

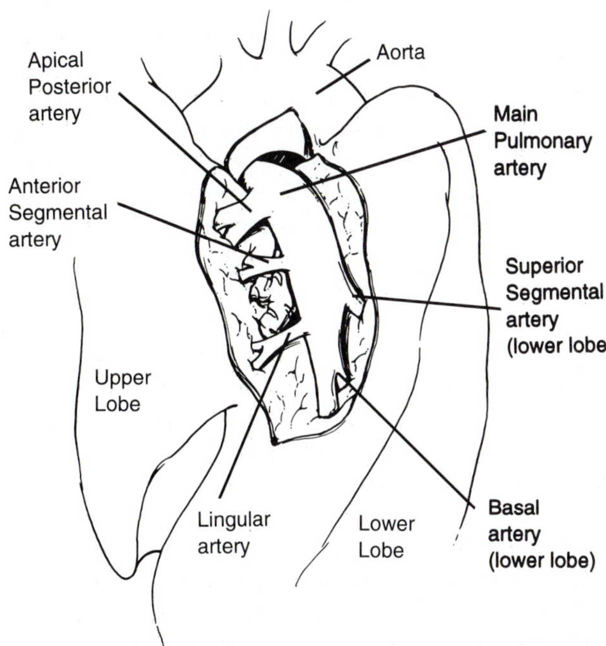


**Figure 7–8.** The left pulmonary artery in the fissure showing the location of the lingular branch in relation to the superior segmental branch. Note the location of the lingular branch relative to the superior segmental branch and how these relate to the length of the basilar arterial trunk.

closed. It is necessary to see the upper-lobe bronchus at its origin, in order to include the lingular bronchus in the division. The remaining fissure is divided with a linear stapler, once the bronchovascular structures have been divided.

From the anterior aspect of the hilum, the bronchus may be seen between the anterior segmental venous branch and the pulmonary artery. Often, it is necessary to mobilize lobar lymph nodes distally to include them with the resected specimen in order to completely encircle the bronchus. The bronchus should ideally be divided from within the fissure, in order to avoid damage to the lower-lobe bronchus, although following division of the superior pulmonary vein, the bifurcation of the bronchus may be seen anteriorly.

It is not possible to perform a formal lymph node dissection as elegantly on the left as on the right because of absence of a well-defined superior mediastinal compartment. However, for complete staging, it is necessary to remove the nodes from the aortopulmonary window, the area lateral to the ligamentum arteriosum between the aortic arch and main pulmonary artery (Fig. 7–6). Nodes located at the level of or slightly superior to the aortic arch should also be removed. The subcarinal space may be entered and dissected, although it is slightly more difficult to gain access to this space from the left side because of the location of the aortic arch. Because of the difficulty in gaining access to the left paratracheal region, obscured by the aortic arch, we routinely perform preoperative mediastinoscopy for left-sided lesions to facilitate sampling of the lymph nodes in this location. Again, the inferior pulmonary ligament is divided up to the inferior pulmonary vein to sample lymph nodes and to allow the lower lobe to rise to the apex of the pleural space.

Depending upon the location of the tumor, left upper lobectomy may be a technically challenging operation. This is especially true because of the short apical posterior arterial branch that comes off the artery quite proximally. It is for this reason that proximal control of the pulmonary artery should be obtained whenever there appears to be any difficulty in dissection.

## Left Lower Lobectomy

If one had to pick the easiest lobectomy, one would have to choose either the left lower lobe or right lower lobe. If the fissure is complete, dissection may begin within the fissure to identify the pulmonary artery (Fig. 7–7). If the fissure is incomplete, dissection begins at the hilar level on the main pulmonary artery, proceeding down into the fissure until the superior segmental arterial branch is seen (Fig. 7–6). Once this arterial branch is identified, the posterior portion of the fissure is divided with a linear stapler. The location of the superior segmental arterial branch relative to the upper lobe anterior segmental branch and the lingular branches should be noted. Usually, the superior segmental branch comes off just opposite the lingular branches, and there is a length of basilar segmental trunk (Fig. 7–7). The dissection is carried along the artery, mobilizing the basilar arterial trunk. As on the right side, it is occasionally necessary to divide the superior segmental branch distinct from the basilar trunk.

The inferior pulmonary ligament is divided and the inferior pulmonary vein exposed. It is inferior and posterior, relative to the superior pulmonary vein. The inferior vein is readily identified from the posterior aspect of the hilum (Fig. 7–6). From the anterior aspect, the lower-lobe bronchus may be seen just posterior to the inferior pulmonary vein. It is most readily identified following division of the vein.

Once all pertinent structures have been identified, the arterial trunk frequently may be divided, since a single branch with a suture ligature or superior segmental branch and basilar trunk can be divided separately. The inferior pulmonary vein is divided, revealing the bronchus. The main bronchial bifurcation should be identified, and the lower-lobe bronchus is divided with a stapler or sewn according to individual preference.

Adhesions of the left lower lobe are most commonly associated with contralateral mediastinal lymph node spread, and, therefore, mediastinoscopy should be performed if there is any suspicion on the CT scan (nodes 1.0–1.5) of mediastinal nodal disease. Right-sided lymph nodes cannot be reached from a left thoracotomy approach, although the converse is true. It is difficult to dissect lymph nodes in the left paratracheal region because of the aortic arch. Access to these nodes may be gained by dividing the ligamentum arteriosum to open the left tracheobronchial angle. Damage to the left recurrent laryngeal nerve must be avoided.

### Left Pneumonectomy

Pneumonectomy should only be undertaken when there are no other options. One should always consider the possibility of a sleeve resection or other bronchoplastic procedure. If, based on the location of the primary tumor or lymph node involvement, it is felt that a pneumonectomy is necessary, the left main pulmonary artery is identified and encircled. It may be necessary to approach the artery from within the pericardium. It may be necessary to divide the ligamentum arteriosum in order to get adequate length of the left main pulmonary artery in order to divide it (Fig. 7–6).

The superior and inferior pulmonary veins are identified and encircled (Fig. 7–5). Once the artery has been dissected, the left main bronchus is mobilized. Bronchial vessels are identified as they course along the left main stem bronchus and are clipped or cauterized, depending upon their size. It is necessary to dissect as far proximal as possible on the bronchus, recognizing that this dissection is more difficult because of the tethering of the left main stem bronchus by the aortic arch. However, with some persistence, it is possible to dissect back to the carina. Lateral (or distal) traction is applied to the left main stem bronchus to facilitate proximal dissection.

The pulmonary artery is clamped, divided and sutured, or divided with a mechanical vascular stapler (TA-30V, U.S. Surgical Corp., Norwalk, CT). The pulmonary veins are then divided, usually with the vascular stapler. The bronchus is divided as far proximally as possible, with care taken not to leave a long length of bronchial stump. We prefer to staple the bronchus, but, again, it may be divided and closed using interrupted sutures accurately placed. The bronchial closure is patched with a flap of pleura or intercostal muscle. The bronchial stump readily disappears under the arch of the aorta following proximal bronchial division.

### Segmental Resections

On the left side it is feasible to perform a segmental resection of the superior segment of the left lower lobe as well as a segmental resection of the lingula. Both of these are done "anatomically," taking the arterial supply, the segmental bronchus, and veins. It is also possible to leave the superior segment and take the basilar segments as a unit. For the upper lobe, a lingulectomy is the easiest and most commonly performed segmentectomy. It is also feasible to take the apical and posterior segment as a block or perform an anterior segmentectomy.

### Problems Unique to the Left Chest

The location of the left main pulmonary artery in relation to the aortic arch provides a potential problem. Lymph nodes in this area may make the dissection extremely difficult and occasionally may lead to a situation where a lesion is found to be unresectable. Involvement of lymph nodes or primary tumor in the aortopulmonary window may extend to the left recurrent laryngeal nerve, and the patient presents with hoarseness. Involvement of the left recurrent laryngeal nerve usually indicates unresectability. Lymph nodes in the aortopulmonary window are not accessible by routine cervical mediastinoscopy. Classically, a parasternal mediastinotomy, or Chamberlain procedure, was utilized to sample these lymph nodes, but newer video thoracoscopic techniques allow excellent visualization of the subaortic window, facilitating lymph node sampling.

The location and nature of the apical posterior arterial branch makes it vulnerable to injury if excess force is applied when retracting the left upper lobe. If this arterial branch is injured, it may force a pneumonectomy in order to control the problem. Great care should be taken when performing a left upper lobectomy to avoid injury to this arterial branch.

The location of the left main stem bronchus in relation to the aortic arch makes it difficult to approach the proximal portion of the bronchus. Despite this, the bronchus must be taken as close as possible to the carina when one is performing a pneumonectomy.

## CONCLUSIONS

As a well-known thoracic surgeon once said, "Thoracic surgery is either terribly simple or simply terrible." Perhaps in no other field of surgery is this quite as true. It is far better to avoid problems in the chest than to try to manage them, no matter how expert one may be in getting out of trouble. Bleeding from the pulmonary artery is notoriously difficult to control, especially if proximal control of the artery has not been obtained. In the chest, we work in a hole with limited space, and it is difficult to manually control bleeding while trying to obtain proximal control. Bleeding may be torrential, and the patient may deteriorate rapidly. It should be recognized that, in the chest, unlike working in the abdomen, one has to be familiar with anatomical relationships from both anterior and posterior aspects. For the experienced surgeon, this is an advantage in that it leads to expeditious pulmonary resections. For an inexperienced operator, this may present problems. The surgeon operating in the chest must know various approaches to each individual resection, so that if there are problems at one location, an easier approach can be done. Pulmonary resection may be an elegant operative procedure, if care is taken to anticipate problems.

## REFERENCES


1. Blades B: Intrathoracic surgery, 1905–1955. Lung, heart, and great vessels: Surgical management of diseases of the esophagus. In Loyal Davis (ed): *Fifty Years of Surgical Progress.* Chicago, The Franklin H. Martin Memorial Foundation, 1955, pp 163–174
2. Nissen R, Wilson RHL: *Pages in the History of Chest Surgery.* Springfield, Illinois, Charles C Thomas, 1960, pp 10–13
3. Matas R: Intralaryngeal insufflation. For the relief of acute surgical pneumothorax. Its history and methods with a description of the latest devices for this purpose. *JAMA* **34:**1371, 1900
4. Meltzer SJ, Auer J: Continuous respiration without respiratory movements. *J Exp Med* **11:**622, 1909
5. Graham EA, Bell RD: Open pneumothorax: Its relation to the treatment of empyema. *Am J Med Sci* **156:**839, 1918
6. Graham EA: *Some Fundamental Considerations in the Treatment of Empyema Thoracis.* St. Louis, Mosby, 1925
7. Lilienthal H: Surgical diseases of the lung. In: *Thoracic Surgery.* Philadelphia, Saunders, 1922, pp 134–218
8. Graham EA: Pneumonectomy with the cautery. *JAMA* **81:**1010, 1923
9. Brunn H: Surgical principles underlying one-stage lobectomy. *Arch Surg* **18:**490, 1929
10. Churchill ED: The surgical treatment of carcinoma of the lung. *J Thorac Surg* **2:**254, 1932
11. Naef AP, Hugh Morriston Davies: First dissection lobectomy in 1912. *Ann Thorac Surg* **56:**988, 1993
12. David, HM: Recent advances in the surgery of the lung and pleura. *Br J Surg* **1:**228, 1913
13. Nissen R: Exstirpation eines ganzen lungenflugels. *Zentralbl Chir* **58:**3003, 1931
14. Haight C: Total removal of left lung for bronchiectasis. *Surg Gynecol Obstet* **58:**768, 1934
15. Graham EA, Singer JJ: Successful removal of an entire lung for carcinoma of the bronchus. *JAMA* **100:**1371, 1933
16. Rienhoff WF: Pneumonectomy. A preliminary report of the operative technique in two successful cases. *Bull Johns Hopkins Hosp* **53:**590, 1933
17. Boyden EA: *Segmental Anatomy of the Lungs.* New York, McGraw-Hill, 1955
18. Cooper JD, Nelems JF, Pearson FG: Extended indications for median sternotomy in patients requiring pulmonary resection. *Ann Thorac Surg* **26:**413, 1978
19. Pasque MK, Cooper JD, Kaiser LR, et al: Improved technique for bilateral lung transplantation: rationale and initial clinical experience. *Ann Thorac Surg* **49:**785–791, 1990

CHAPTER

# 8

# Thoracic Imaging

Michael K. Wolverson

## HISTORICAL PERSPECTIVE

Application of x-rays to medical diagnosis occurred rapidly following their discovery by Roentgen in 1895.[1] The first x-ray department in a U.S. institution was established at the Boston City Hospital in 1896. In the period up to 1920 many advances were made in radiographic and fluoroscopic systems, including the hot cathode x-ray tube, antiscatter movable grids, the motor-driven tilting x-ray table, double-coated x-ray film, intensifying screens, and lead protective devices. During the 1920s combined radiographic and fluoroscopic units were introduced, and the rotating anode x-ray tube was developed. The latter allowed electrical power exposures hundreds of times greater than with a stationary anode tube and without damage to the tube's focal spot. This also contributed to the later development of rapid filming techniques. Research and development of contrast materials also began during this period. The 1930s saw the introduction of three-phase electrical generators providing better quality radiographs because much shorter exposure times were possible. Tomographic techniques and portable equipment also came into use. Chest x-ray surveys were begun during this period using photofluorography, which was installed in traveling vans. Their use impacted the control of tuberculosis and continued for the next 20 years. In the 1940s, phototiming devices for x-ray exposures were developed and eventually led to automatic exposure systems. The most significant advance in this period, however, was the early development of the image intensifier, which increased the brightness of the fluoroscopic image over 1000 times, greatly improving fluoroscopic capability in diagnosis and monitoring of procedures. In the 1950s, high-kilovolt chest radiography was introduced that overcame the problem with chest x-rays of masking of the heart and lung fields by bony structures. Rapid film changers were developed and corresponded in time with the earliest performance of angiographic and cardiac procedures. Motion picture images of image intensifier output became possible with the development of cineradiography. The development of the Seldinger technique for the percutaneous introduction of vascular catheters was another important event in the 1950s. The 1960s saw further technical improvements in conventional radiographic and fluoroscopic techniques, but it was in the 1970s that the most dramatic breakthrough occurred since the discovery of x-rays. Computed tomography (CT) revolutionized imaging techniques and contributed significantly to the development later in the decade of magnetic resonance imaging (MRI) and gray scale ultrasound imaging (US). Digital or computerized fluoroscopic apparatus was also introduced during this period that provided digital radiographic images and digital subtraction angiography. These new modalities most impacted chest radiology in the 1980s due to technical improvements and their application in clinical diagnoses.

## CURRENT DEVELOPMENTS IN IMAGING TECHNOLOGY

### Computed Radiography[2]

Nonfilm imaging technology for conventional radiography is now practicable and will be more widely available in the near future. Images are processed and archived on an optical disk and can be sent to a laser printer for hard and soft copy use. Multiple copies or displays of the images are easily obtained and can be transmitted between departments or hospitals in seconds. The major advantage of the technique is its tolerance of a wide latitude of x-ray exposure compared with conventional film. This is especially valuable for portable imaging where exposures can vary greatly. Thus, consistent film densities are available for viewing, enabling the detection of subtle pathologic changes on sequential images. The capability of postprocessing image manipulation also enables evaluation of the lung fields and mediastinum with separate adjustments from one image exposure.

Reduced radiation exposure is theoretically possible with this technique but has to date been realized only in pediatric radiology where the small size of the patient permits a 30–70% x-ray exposure reduction.

### Helical Computed Tomography[3]

In conventional CT a series of single scans is obtained during suspended respiration. In helical CT, rotation of the x-ray source around the patient and patient movement through the machine occur simultaneously. This offers three main advantages. First, scanning time is greatly reduced so that groups of images can be obtained in a single breath-hold. Examinations can be completed much more rapidly and multiple images obtained during peak vascular enhancement with contrast material. Second, since the imaging data is acquired continuously, the location of the slice reconstruction can be shifted retrospectively. Collimation is set before acquisition, but the acquired raw data can be reconstructed and shifted by any distance up to that of the thickness of the slice collimation. Thus, overlapping slices may be obtained that can be of value for applications such as better visualization of small lesions or three dimensional (3D) imaging.

Readily obtained high-quality multiplanar images and 3D imaging is the third advantage of helical CT and does not entail the acquisition of additional scans and radiation exposure.

### Fast Magnetic Resonance Imaging[4]

Until recently, cardiac and respiratory motion have limited application of MRI in the thorax because of motion artifacts related to the prolonged imaging times. Also, lung parenchyma is difficult to image by MRI because of magnetic susceptibility artifacts related to the air interfaces in the lung. Its usefulness is enhanced, however, by its ability to demonstrate flow without contrast material, its multiplanar image capability, and high tissue differentiation. Recent technical advances have permitted more rapid image acquisition. These include newer pulsing sequences that enable imaging to be completed in a single breath-hold with most current equipment installations. In addition, ultrafast imaging is now possible with special purpose machines, including those that employ the echoplanar technique. In this method all the data for formation of a complete image can be obtained following a single radio frequency excitation. An image can be obtained in as little as 30 ms, and imaging as rapidly as 20 images/s is possible. This permits freezing of cardiac and vascular motion and enables high-quality dynamic cardiac and pulmonary vascular imaging. These capabilities have resulted in MRI being the preferred imaging modality to evaluate initially a variety of cardiovascular lesions and to define the relationship of masses to vascular structures. It is also well suited to evaluate processes located near the lung apex, those involving mediastinal structures and lesions located at or near the thoracoabdominal junction. Its ability to differentiate tissue assists in the distinction between tumor and fibrosis that is of importance in the monitoring of treatment for various malignancies.

### Positron Emission Tomography (PET Scanning)[5]

This was developed in the 1970s but has only recently begun to impact clinical practice. PET is capable of depicting a variety of physiologic processes in vivo, especially those involving glucose metabolism. The data can then be displayed in a way that permits viewing of physiologic processes tomographically. The positron-emitting isotopes, such as $^{11}C$, $^{15}O$, $^{18}F$, and $^{13}N$ provide the basis for labeling almost any organic compound and the possibility to study a wide variety of physiologic and pathologic processes. PET is used mainly as a complementary imaging modality to more structurally oriented methods such as CT and MRI. Its value in chest diagnosis, to date, has centered on its ability to exploit the biochemical differences between benign and malignant cells in the diagnosis of malignant disease. Scanning with $^{18}F$-2-fluoro-2 deoxyglucose (FDG) takes advantage of the high glucose metabolism of neoplastic cells. Studies have shown consistently increased uptake of FDG by all lung cancer cell types and PET has shown promise in the accurate characterization of pulmonary nodules.[6] It may also be used to identify residual or recurrent neoplasms following treatment.[5]

### Endoscopic Ultrasound

This technique involves combining the advantages of direct endoscopic visualization of the wall of the gastrointestinal tract with high-frequency sonography to visualize individual layers of the bowel wall and the immediately surrounding spaces.[7] Direct contact of the transducer with the bowel wall via a water-filled balloon in the lumen overcomes the problem air presents in being impenetrable to ultrasound. This approach has proved useful in the preoperative diagnosis and staging of esophageal cancer, by using relatively high-frequency transducers (7–12.5 MHz).[8] More recently transducers have been developed that can be passed through the biopsy channel of a flexible endoscope. Most recently, flexible, ultrasound transducer-containing catheters (4.8–9F), originally designed for intravascular ultrasound application, have become available, and their use overcomes many of the limitations of earlier instruments.[9] They can be used without an endoscope by being passed through a simple nasogastric tube. Ease and accuracy of placement of the transducer is facilitated by its passage over a guidewire under fluoroscopic control. Ultrasound frequencies as high as 20 MHz can be achieved and provide exquisite detail of the esophageal wall in which seven distinct layers may be identified in normal subjects. These devices have a potential role in the diagnosis and evaluation of many esophageal disorders including tumors, mucosal and submucosal lesions, motility disorders, and esophageal and periesophageal varices. Transesophageal echocardiography is also now an established method for the diagnosis of aortic dissection.[10]

## Solitary Pulmonary Nodule

The solitary pulmonary nodule is often an incidental finding on a chest film. The discovery immediately raises the following questions: Is it real? Is it truly solitary? Where is it? What is it?

Often the abnormality can be seen on only one view. Physical examination may reveal a skin lesion such as a mole or commonly a nipple superimposing the area in question. Repeat film with markers may answer. With most examinations performed at high kilovoltage, detection of calcification may be difficult. Fluoroscopy with a low (50–60) kilovolt spot film may establish the presence of calcification within the lesion. Old chest films should be obtained and reviewed. A lesion seen on only one of several chest films and on only one view may indeed be real. Rarely can the single-vs.-multiple-lesion issue be resolved by this means. Calcification may be obvious in a lesion that is completely calcified or that has concentric ring calcifications, but otherwise may not be appreciated.

CT (Fig. 8–1) is the most sensitive method of demonstrating nodules; their position within the lung can be precisely determined, and calcifications may be shown when not evident on conventional radiographs. The nature of the nodule, benign or malignant, cannot be ascertained except for calcification. If the nodule's calcification is complete, a concentric ring or a small central nidus defines the probability that the lesion is benign is very high. Siegelman and associates[11] showed that the CT density of an indeterminate lesion could, if high, also define benignancy. Their results are translatable to all types of CT equipment by means of a chest phantom.[12] A recent report has shown promise in the use of iodinated contrast enhancement of lung nodules at CT as a means of distinguishing benign from malignant nodules.[13] Encouraging results have also been obtained with PET scanning for this clinical problem[5] (Fig. 8–2).

In CT the most significant pitfall in diagnosis of nodules is the possibility of missing them because of misregistration due to respiratory or other patient movement during the examination. Helical CT enhances nodule detection by overcoming this, especially for smaller nodules in the lung periphery.[14,15] It also improves evaluation of nodule morphology, vascularity, and relationship to airways due to the increased number of available contiguous images. Helical CT is of particular value in improving CT densitometry of nodules because images reconstructed retrospectively can be obtained precisely at the center of lesions. Detailed assessment of pulmonary arteriovenous malformations is also possible with helical CT, especially following IV contrast injection. Also, the detailed evaluation of lesions related to the diaphragm is facilitated by use of helical CT because of avoidance of misregistration from diaphragmatic movement and high-quality multiplanar image reconstruction. The relationship of the lesion to the diaphragm is thus readily shown in sagittal and coronal planes.

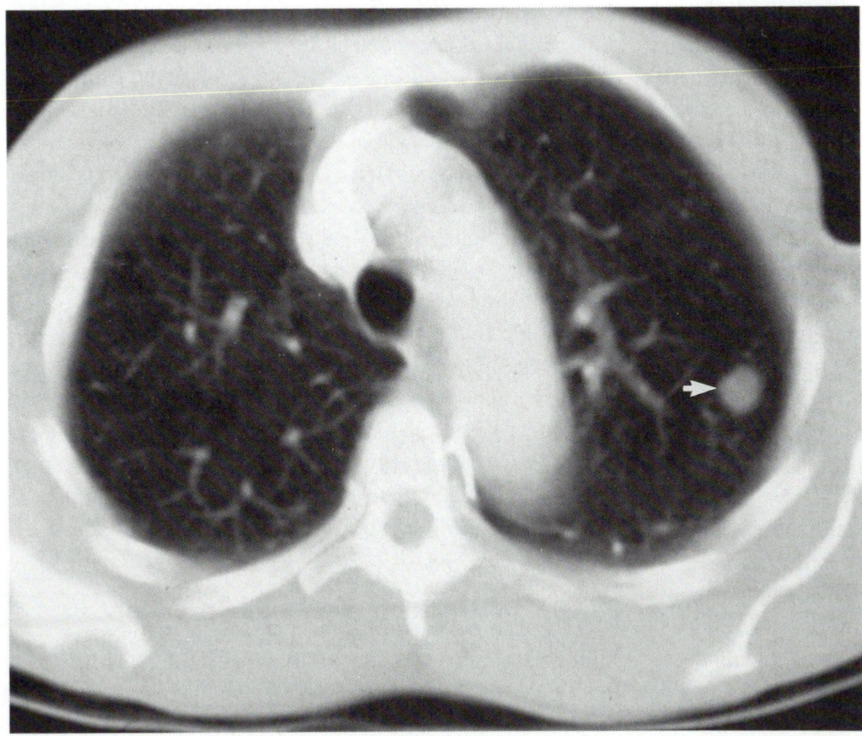

**Figure 8–1.** A nodule, 1 cm in diameter, is shown in the left upper lobe (arrow). Its CT attenuation is identical to that of the soft tissues of the chest wall indicating absence of calcification.

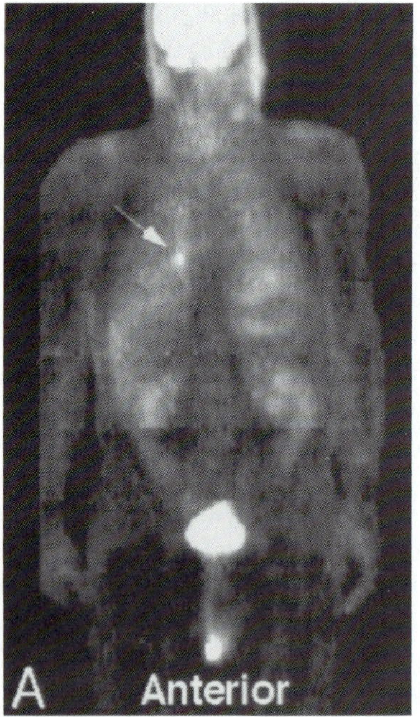


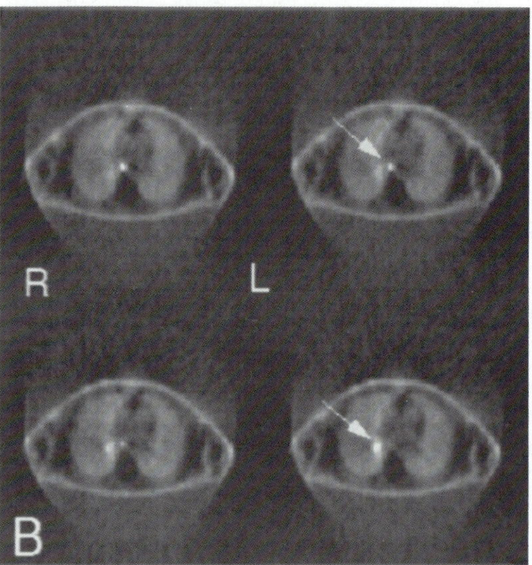


**Figure 8–2. A.** Whole body $^{18}$F-FDG image. Solitary pulmonary nodule in right infra-hilar region shows increased tracer uptake (arrow, see also bottom arrow in **B**). **B.** Serial 3.0-mm transverse slices from apex to base through the nodule reveal a second area of $^{18}$F-FDG uptake (top arrow) that was unsuspected by CT. Both lesions had SUV values >2.5 and were malignant by surgical pathology.

## BIOPSY PROCEDURES

### Percutaneous Biopsy of Chest Lesions

Improved cytology, imaging techniques, and needle design have resulted in percutaneous needle biopsy (PNB) becoming a definitive, safe procedure for the diagnosis of many pulmonary, hila, and mediastinal lesions.[16–19] Relative contraindications include severely compromised lung function, coagulopathy, and severe pulmonary hypertension.

### Technique of Lung Biopsy

If the lesion is visible at fluoroscopy, its use is preferable to CT, especially in the lower lung fields. CT is of value for lesions that cannot be well localized on chest films or that are close to the heart, major vessels, or hilum of the lung[20,21] (Fig. 8–3). It is also of value in identifying the optimal location for open-lung biopsy in patients with parenchymal lung disease in whom the changes are asymmetric in distribution. Premedication for percutaneous lung biopsy is rarely required. Twenty and twenty-two gauge needles are popular, but their use is not associated with a lower risk of pneumothorax than with larger needles. This complication is more related to the number of times the pleura is punctured by the needle. Aspirated tissue fragments may be used to make histologic preparations that are processed differently from cytologic material.

The lesion to be biopsied is localized under fluoroscopy and the needle inserted vertically through an intercostal space under fluoroscopy. The needle is advanced until resistance is felt at the edge of the lesion. If no resistance to the needle can be felt, lateral radiographs or biplane fluoroscopy may be needed to localize its tip. For CT- guided procedures, the mass is first localized while the patient suspends breathing at end expiration. A single- or a double-needle technique may be used. For the latter a guidance cannula is advanced to the edge of the lesion; a 22–23-gauge biopsy needle is then passed through the cannula into the mass. Maximum suction through an attached syringe is applied, and the needle is moved briskly to and fro and rotated within the lesion. It is then withdrawn slowly during continued suction. Aspirates are spread on glass slides and fixed immediately in 95% alcohol. Flushings of the syringe and needle are centrifuged for further pathologic examination, and aliquots may be placed in culture medium for microbiologic studies.

Successful biopsy depends upon the expertise of the cytologist and the handling of specimens in close cooperation with the radiologist.[22] Immediate processing of specimens for cytologic study in, or close to, the biopsy room ensures that adequate material has been obtained for diagnosis before the procedure is terminated.

### Patient Observation and Complications

Minor hemoptysis occurs in about 10% of patients, pneumothorax in 25%, and pneumothorax requiring treatment in

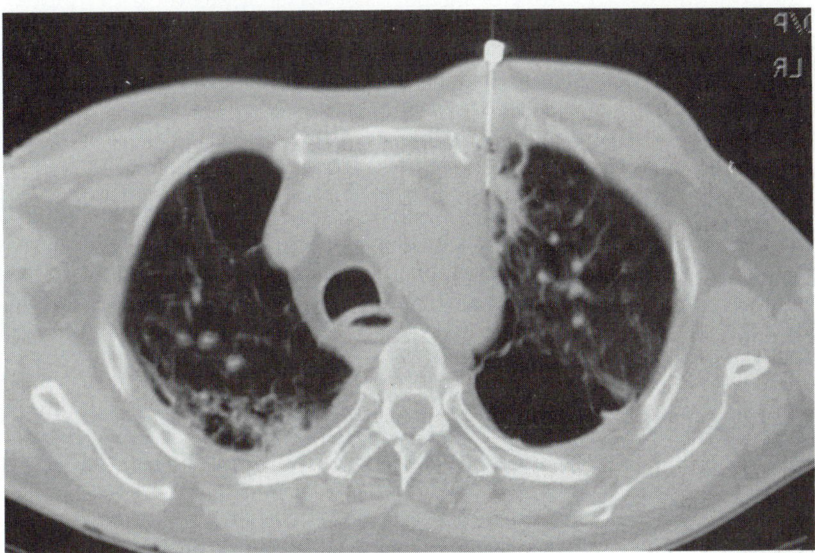

A

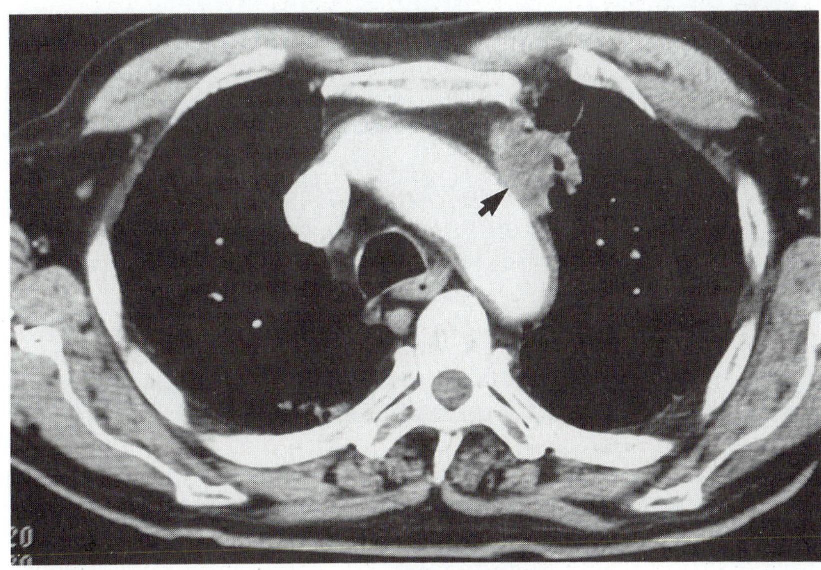

B

**Figure 8–3.** CT guided biopsy of intrathoracic mass: **A.** At window settings to demonstrate lung detail, the tip of the fine needle of a co-axial needle set is shown in a mass contiguous to the anterior mediastinum. **B.** The same scan, at window settings to demonstrate soft tissue detail, shows the relationship of the mass (arrow) to the anterior mediastinum and aortic arch. Cytologic examination of the needle aspirate showed bronchogenic carcinoma.

10%. Air embolism is a rare but potentially fatal complication. Following biopsy, an upright chest radiograph is performed, and, if no pneumothorax is found, the patient is observed for dyspnea for 24 hours. If a pneumothorax is found, and the patient is symptomatic, a chest tube is inserted without delay.

Outpatients who have PNB are discharged after 2–3 hours if a 2-hour chest radiograph shows no pneumothorax. Hemoptysis is managed by turning the patient on the side biopsied, and oxygen is administered.

## Needle Biopsy of Mediastinal and Hilar Lesions

CT is preferred for guidance of biopsies of hilar and mediastinal masses (Fig. 8–3). CT shows the lesions in relation of the heart and great vessels, and an approach is selected that avoids their injury.[20]

## Biopsy Results

Malignant pulmonary lesions are correctly diagnosed by PNB in more than 95% of cases and hila or mediastinal lesions in more than 90% of cases. The success of the procedure increases with the number of needle passes made in the attempt to obtain tissue for histology. The accuracy of PNB is much lower for lymphomatous lesions compared with epithelial lesions.

In some patients with biopsies negative for malignancy, a specific benign diagnosis may be possible.[23–25] Such lesions include granulomas, hamartomas, infarcts, abscesses, or specific infections such as tuberculosis.

## STAGING OF BRONCHOGENIC CARCINOMA

### Primary Tumor

The trend toward more aggressive surgery has increased the importance of accurate primary tumor staging by CT. Its most important role is to assess whether a T4 classification is justifiable based on the reliable demonstration of mediastinal soft-tissue invasion or involvement of major mediastinal structures such as the heart, great vessels, trachea, esophagus, and vertebral bodies. Also, demonstration of malignant pleural disease and a malignant effusion constitute a T4 lesion.[26]

Interpretation of tumor invasion can be difficult, however, especially when the lesion makes only limited contact with surrounding structures because desmoplastic reactions and inflammation may mimic invasion. Also, microscopic invasion may be missed. Signs likely to be associated with resectable disease include less than 3 cm of tumor contact with the mediastinum, less than 90 degrees circumferential contact with the aorta, and the presence of fat between the lesion and mediastinum.[27] Thin-section helical CT with

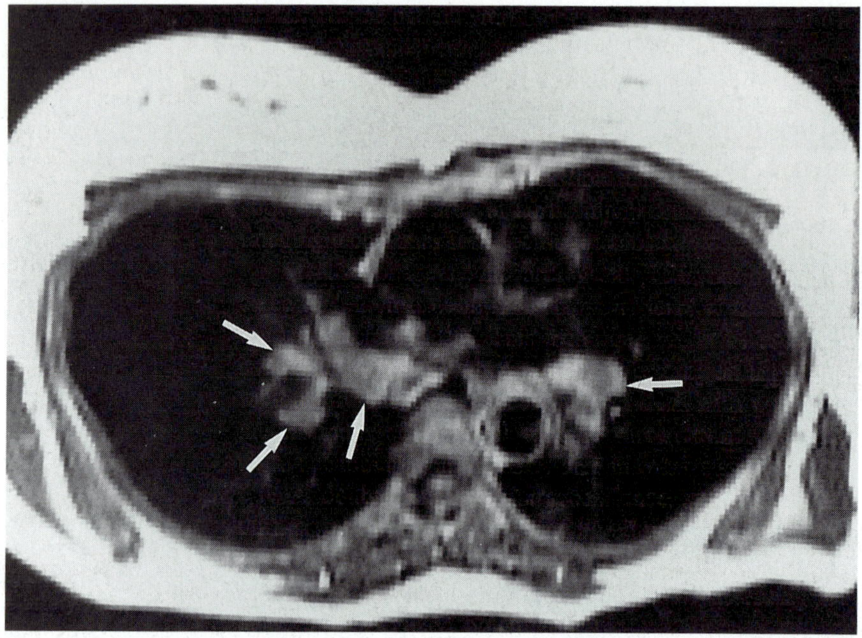

A

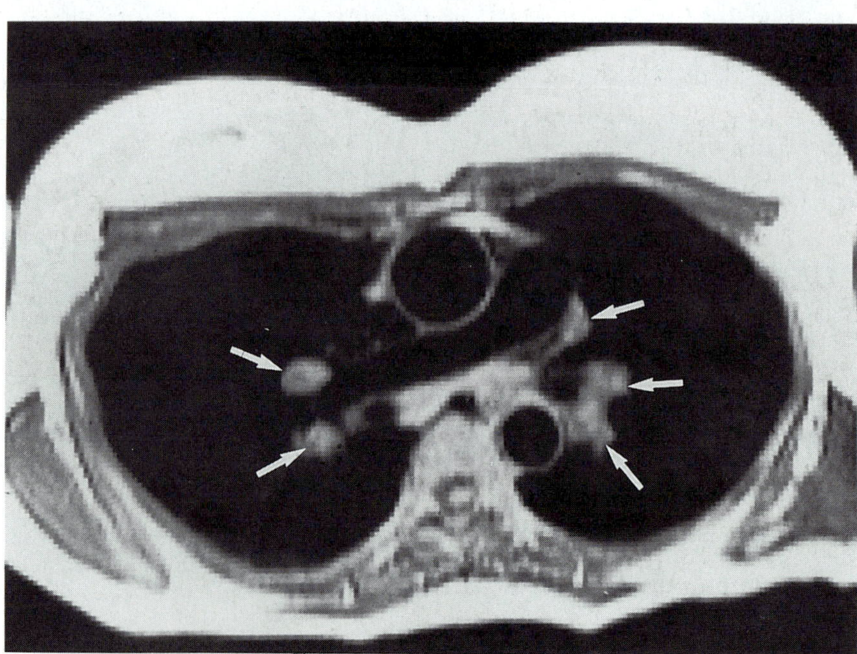

B

**Figure 8–4.** MRI of hilar adenopathy. **A, B.** Axial scans at two levels through the hila show masses of intermediate signal intensity corresponding to enlarged lymph nodes.

multiple contiguous image reconstructions often assist in the evaluation, and contrast enhancement is critical where the relationship of tumor to major vessels is in question.

### The Hilum

Hilar metastases are shown on radiographs in 50–75% of patients. Contrast-enhanced dynamic CT is the method of choice in depiction of metastases.[28–30] Sources of error include nodal micrometastases and contiguous parenchymal disease that obliterates hila contours. MRI also shows neoplastic tissue[31] (Fig. 8–4), and coronal views are useful after lung resection, especially if surgical clips preclude satisfactory CT. CT is better for evaluation of bronchi, but MRI appears superior in differentiating proximal tumor from distal collapse and consolidation. Disadvantages of MRI are poorer spatial resolution, longer scan times, thicker image slices, and inability to detect calcifications.

### Mediastinum

CT depicts normal and abnormal mediastinal nodes[32–34] (Figs. 8–5, 8–6). One centimeter is the upper limit of normal for the short axis of a node on axial CT.[35] By using this criterion, it has been reported that a patient with a normal mediastinum by CT may not need a staging mediastinoscopy but can proceed to thoracotomy with an 88–94% expectation of finding no mediastinal metastases.[36–37] More recent reports, however, have indicated a lower sensitivity for detection of nodal metastases by CT.[38] Twenty to thirty per cent of patients with enlarged nodes on CT have no tumor in lymph nodes at surgery. This lack of specificity is due to reactive hyperplasia owing to infection or previous granulomatous disease. Such patients must undergo biopsy confirmation of metastases prior to surgery, and CT serves as a road map for guiding the biopsy procedure. Mediastinal extension may be shown by MRI and, in some cases, may be more helpful than CT in distinguishing tumor from vessels and in detection of invasion of vessels by neoplasm[39–40] (Fig. 8–7).

### Evaluation of Pleura and Chest Wall

Rib destruction shown on radiographs is evidence of chest wall invasion by neoplasm. The same is true on CT, but CT evaluation of pleural invasion is difficult.[41,42] MRI has been shown to be more accurate than CT in showing chest wall invasion and also extrathoracic spread in apical neoplasms. MRI is also better able to define the structures of the brachial plexus.

Pleural fluid shown on CT may be due to infection and not be an indication of disseminated disease. Pleural involvement by tumor must be confirmed by biopsy or cytology of pleural fluid.

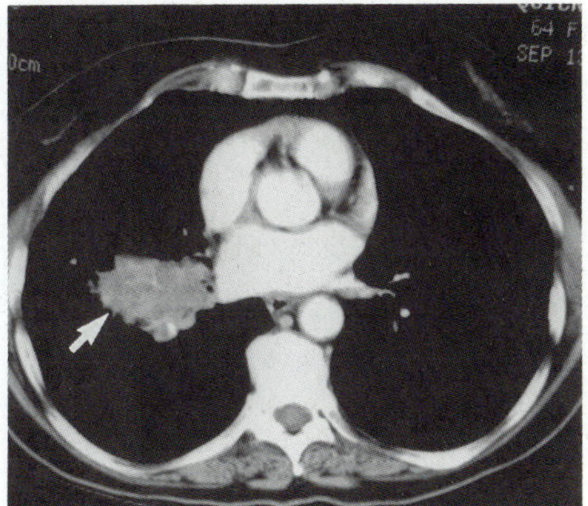

**A**

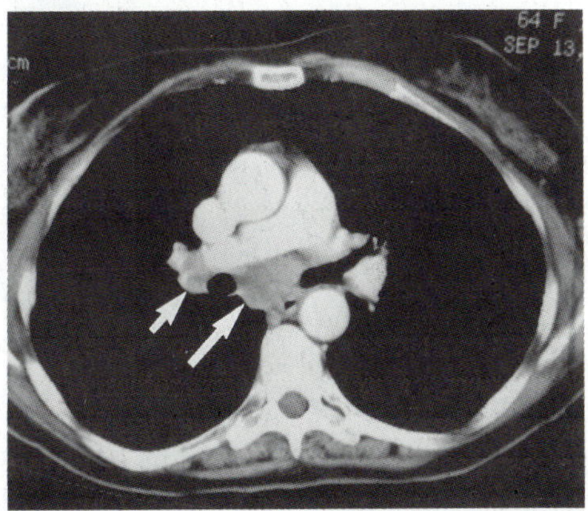

**B**

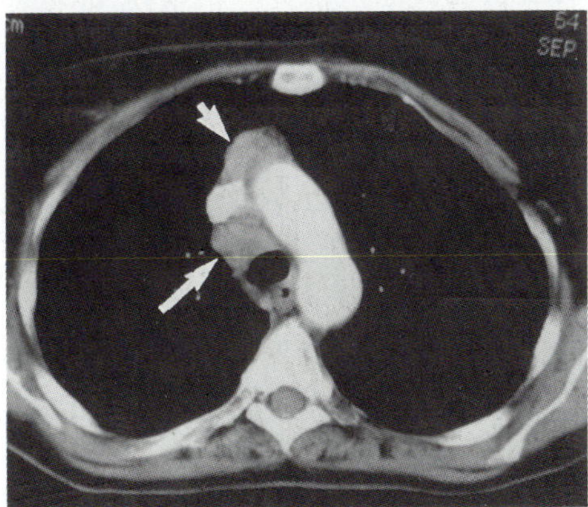

**C**

**Figure 8–5.** Bronchogenic carcinoma and metastatic mediastinal lymphadenopathy: **A.** A large mass (arrow) is shown involving the lower portion of the right lung hilum. **B.** Enlarged lymph nodes are seen in the upper portion of the right hilum (short arrow) and in the subcarinal region (long arrow). The lesions stand out in sharp contrast to vascular structures densely opacified by intravenously injected contrast material. **C.** Metastatic nodal masses anterolateral to the lower trachea (large arrow) and in the anterior mediastinum (short arrow).

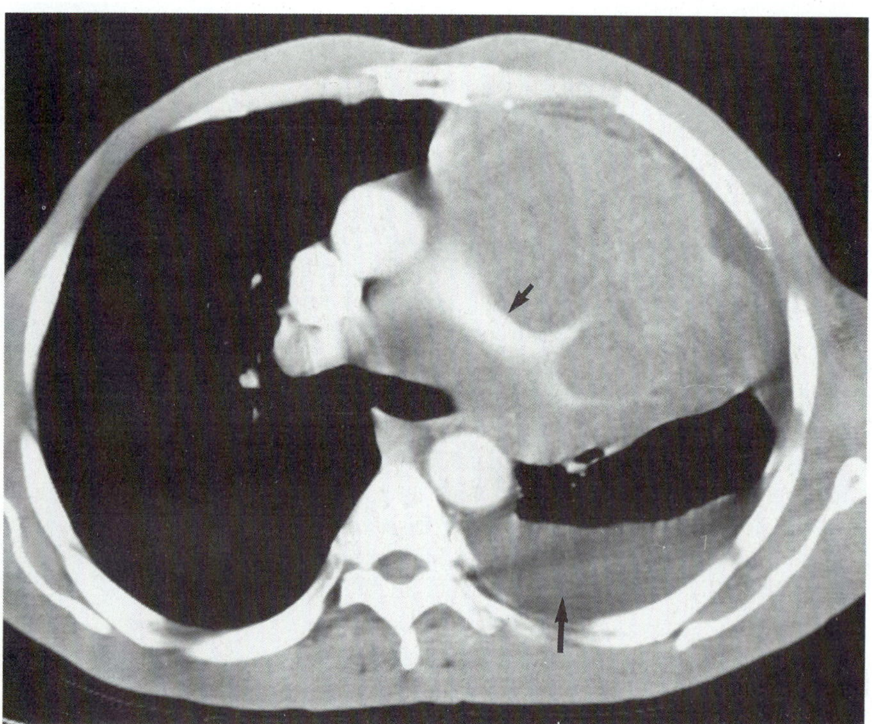

**Figure 8–6.** CT of lung cancer. A large mass in the left upper lobe is invading the mediastinum and encasing the left main pulmonary artery (short arrow). Fluid is present in the left pleural cavity (long arrow).

### Extrapulmonary Disease

The upper abdomen, included in chest CT for staging, may show liver and adrenal metastases. Biopsy confirmation is important to exclude benign hepatic and adrenal lesions. Radionuclide bone scanning is the screening examination of choice for suspected bone metastases. Positive findings on bone scan are not specific and should be correlated with conventional radiographs of the bone(s) in question. Benign lesions, such as degenerative changes and Paget's disease, may account for the findings, and only instances of radiographically normal bones require further evaluation which, in the spine at least, should be by MRI. Areas of obvious bone destruction may be biopsied by needle aspiration with CT guidance.

## PLEURAL DISEASE

### Conventional Radiography

Pleural and extrapleural lesions cast a sharp margin with lung where projected tangential to the x-ray beam and will often be elongated in vertical dimension. Obtuse angles with the chest wall are usual compared with peripheral lung lesions that usually show acute angles of interface. Pleural lesions may project across a fissure and, if solid and arising in visceral pleura, may move with the lung on respiration. A pedunculated parietal or visceral pleural lesion moves independently. Fluid may change its shape with breathing or with a change in patient position. Rib destruction, if present, distinguishes extrapleural from pleural lesions. Rib notching and intervertebral foramen enlargement point to an extrapleural lesion associated with a neurogenic tumor.

A shift of pleural shadowing on a decubitus radiograph is characteristic of mobile fluid and pneumothorax. Small effusions and pneumothoraces may thus be shown. Oblique films and fluoroscopy may help distinguish pleural and lung lesions by placing a pleural lesion tangential to the x-ray beam.

### Ultrasound

The distinction between solid masses and fluid can often be made. A sonolucent collection that changes shape with respiration is typical of pleural fluid.[43,44] Exudates are distinguishable from transudates when septations or other echogenic material is seen in the fluid or the fluid is associated with pleural thickening or lung lesions. The lower chest and upper abdomen may be viewed at once when a subdiaphragmatic abscess or fluid collection is suspected. The diaphragm is easily identified and its relationship to collections shown. Movement of the diaphragm with respiration, paralysis, or eventration are readily documented. A major advantage of ultrasound is that it can be performed at the bedside of a sick patient.

### Computed Tomography

CT provides the means to examine the entire pleural margin and associated disease elsewhere in the chest[45] (Fig. 8–8). It provides reliable evidence of chest wall disease only

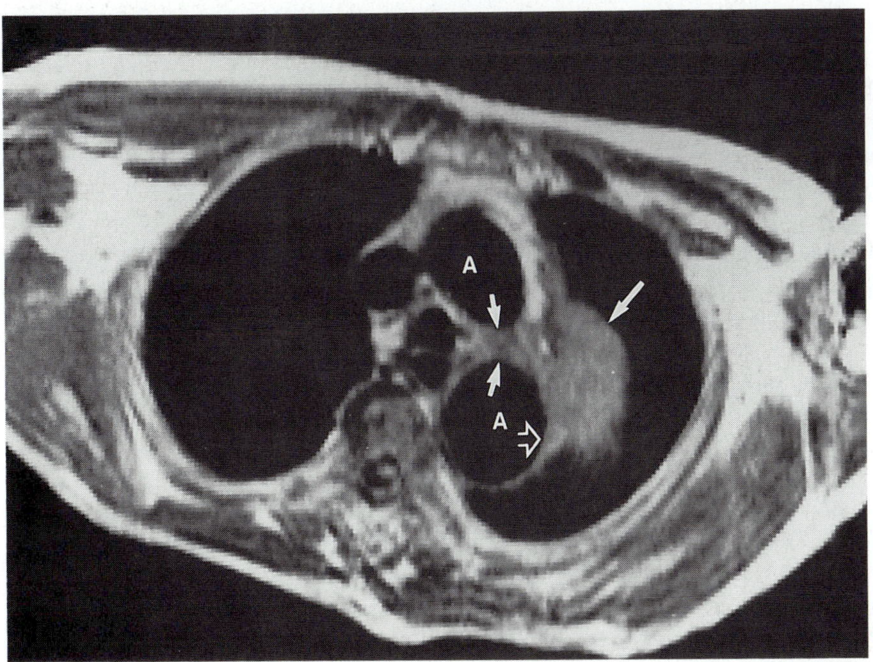


**A**

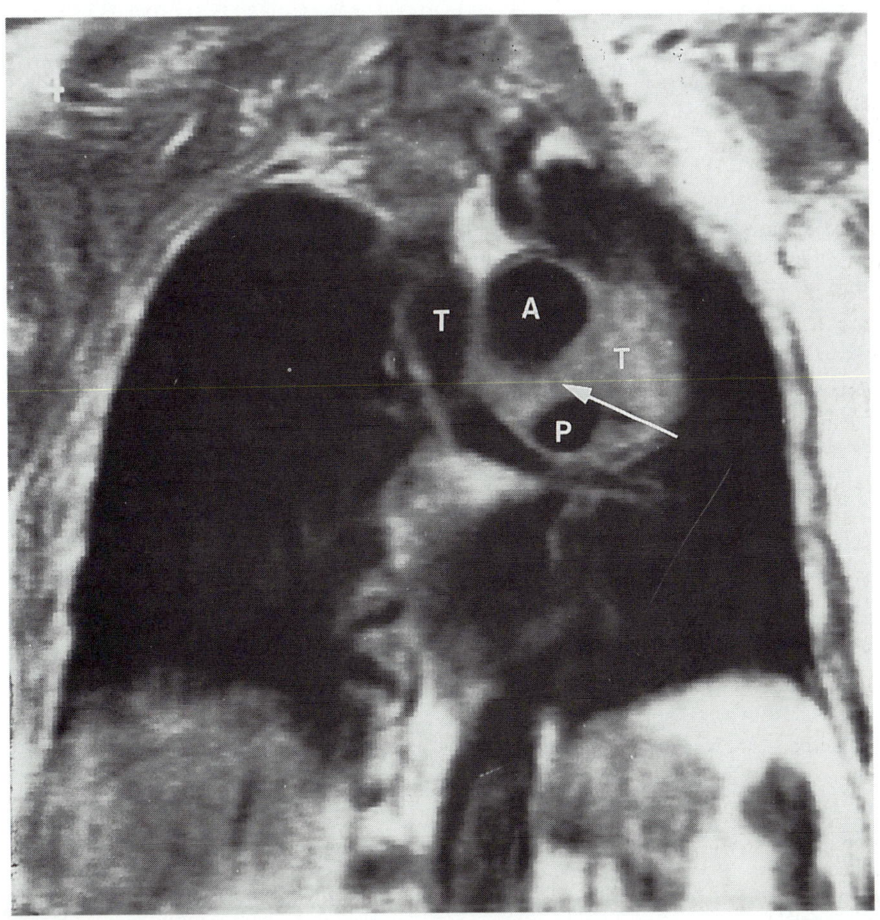


**B**

**Figure 8–7.** MRI of lung cancer. **A.** Axial scan through the aortic arch shows a mass in the left lung (long arrow) infiltrating the aortic wall (open arrow) and extending into the mediastinum below the aortic arch (short closed arrows). (A = aorta, T = trachea, P = pulmonary artery.) **B.** Coronal scan of the chest at the level of the trachea better demonstrates extension of neoplasm into the aortopulmonary window (arrow).

when there is rib destruction or marked distortion of extrathoracic tissues.

CT is superior to chest films in the detection of pleural calcification, thickening, and plaques (Fig. 8–9). CT attenuation values of pleural collections range from levels in the range of fat with chylous effusions to levels in excess of those of soft tissues in acute hemothorax. Transudates or exudates have intermediate readings (Fig. 8–10). The distinction between pleural and pulmonary lesions is easily made. It is also usually possible to characterize round atelectasis of the lung that results from a rolling-up of the lung edge in association with pleural thickening and may simulate neoplasm. The crowding of curvilinear vessels into the mass resembles a comet tail (Fig. 8–11). Empyema and peripheral lung abscess may also be distinguished on CT[46] (Figs. 8–12, 8–13). A lung abscess usually shows an irregular contour with walls of varying thickness, whereas an empyema has a regular shape with walls of uniform thickness and a smooth inner margin. Typical of empyema is a fluid collection between thickened visceral and parietal pleura. Pneumonia and air bronchograms accompany lung abscesses, whereas empyemas compress lung and displace bronchi and pulmonary vessels around their periphery.

CT helps in the investigation of unexplained pleural effusion if aspiration of fluid is not diagnostic. Associated lung disease, pleural masses, and lymph node enlargement at the hilum or mediastinum may direct subsequent diagnostic procedures.

Primary neoplasms of the pleura are well shown by CT, but pleural thickening may be indistinguishable from mesothelioma unless obvious nodular or irregular thickening is shown with associated invasion of the chest wall or mediastinum. CT may be of value in directing biopsy of a dominant pleural mass in these circumstances.[47]

## THE TRACHEOBRONCHIAL TREE

Volume acquisition of imaging data by helical CT enables 95% of normal segmental bronchial divisions to be identified. This includes the lingular bronchi, which are often difficult to show on conventional CT.[48] Screening for bronchiectasis is readily and accurately conducted with spiral CT in patients with hemoptysis,[49] (Fig. 8–14) and it is superior to conventional CT in the demonstration of tumor obstruction of segmental bronchi. Easily obtained axial and coronal reformatted images are useful in the assessment of tumors of the trachea and major bronchi for local infiltration, mediastinal invasion, and tumor extent. Multiplanar reconstructions are also of value in the demonstration of bronchopleural fistulae, in surgical planning for tracheal reconstruction, in the detection of complications at sites of tracheal or bronchial anastomoses after lung transplantation, in showing the size and form of bronchial stenoses, and in the localization of intrabronchial stents.

At the present time MRI is less good for demonstration of lesions of the bronchial tree than helical CT.

## PULMONARY EMBOLUS

There is no simple, accurate means for diagnosis of pulmonary embolus. Were an ideal means of diagnosis available, it possibly would be to no avail due to low clinical suspicion despite postmortem studies of hospitalized patients showing its frequent occurrence.[50]

Most patients at risk for pulmonary embolism are ill. Consequently, the chest film most often is abnormal and may show pulmonary vascular congestion, pleural effusions, pulmonary infiltrates, atelectasis from bronchial plugs, or hypostatic pneumonia. Occasionally the film will

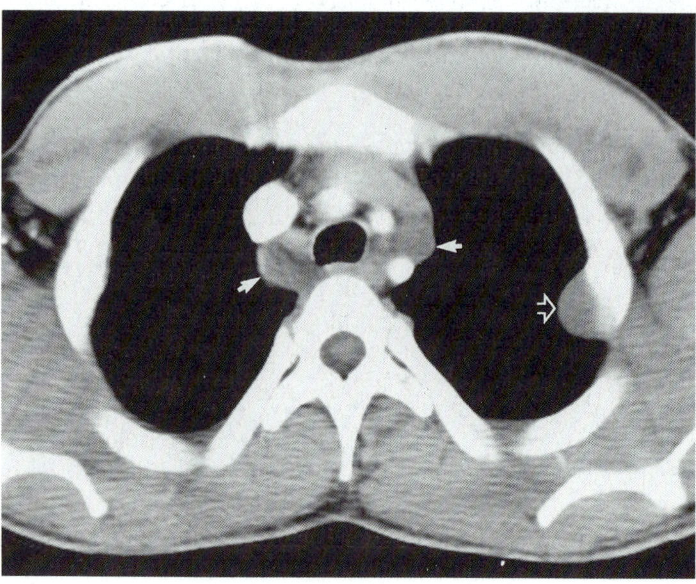

**Figure 8–8.** CT of pleural-based mass. A pleural-based lesion (open arrow) is seen arising from the upper left lateral chest wall. Its margins form obtuse angles with the adjacent normal pleura. This was a neurofibroma of an intercostal nerve in a patient with neurofibromatosis. Additional lesions (closed arrows) are seen to both sides of the superior mediastinum.

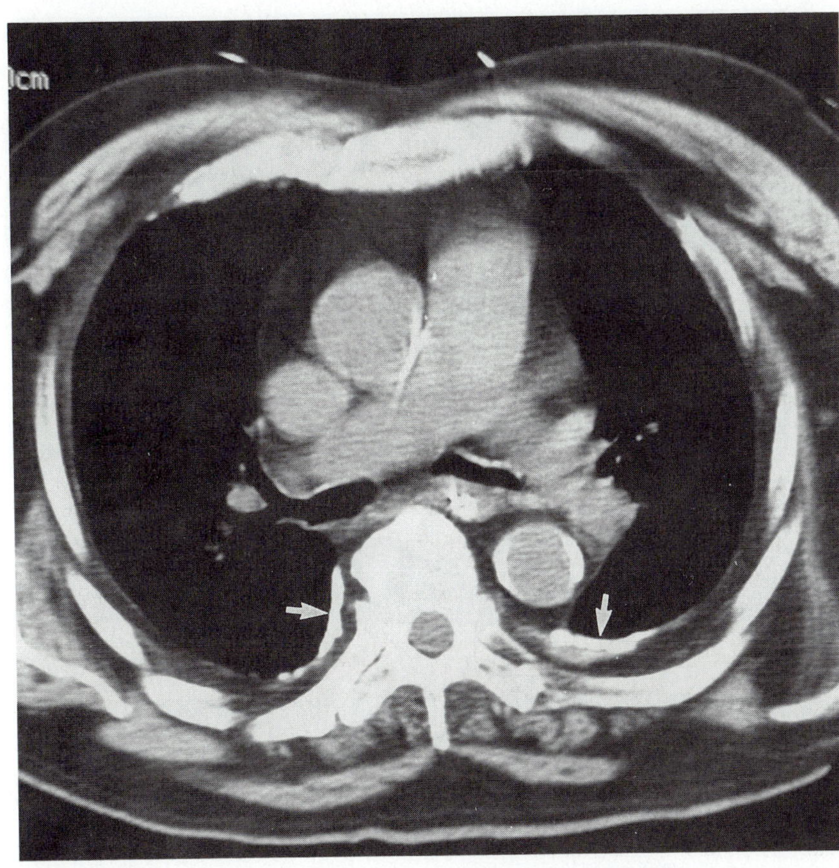

**Figure 8–9.** CT of pleural calcification. Calcified pleural plaques (arrows) are shown in the posterior aspect of the chest on each side in this subject with a history of asbestos exposure.

suggest the possibility of a pulmonary embolus, but most often not and specific signs are infrequent. Nevertheless, a chest film is an important step in the evaluation of suspected pulmonary embolus both for guidance and interpretation of scintigraphy (if chosen) and to evaluate possible other causes of the patient's signs and symptoms.

Perfusion and ventilation scintigraphy is a noninvasive means of evaluation for suspected pulmonary embolism.[51,52] Interpretation of the combined scans are reported as normal, low probability, indeterminate, and high probability. These have been further refined but, if one uses pulmonary arteriography as the standard, some patients

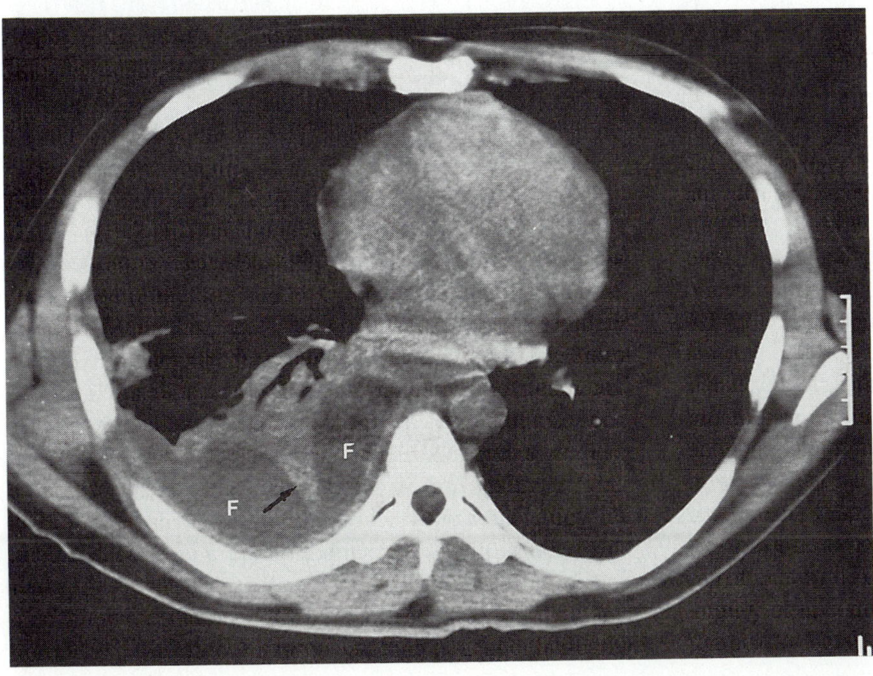


**Figure 8–10.** CT of loculated pleural effusion. Scan obtained through the lower chest shows a loculated pleural fluid collection. The underlying collapsed and consolidated lung is tethered to the posterior pleural surface (arrow).(F = fluid.)

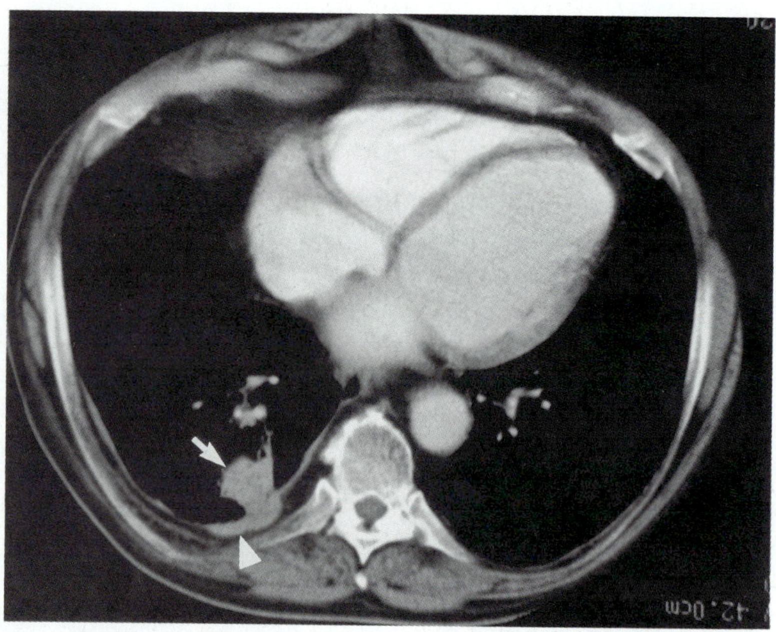

A

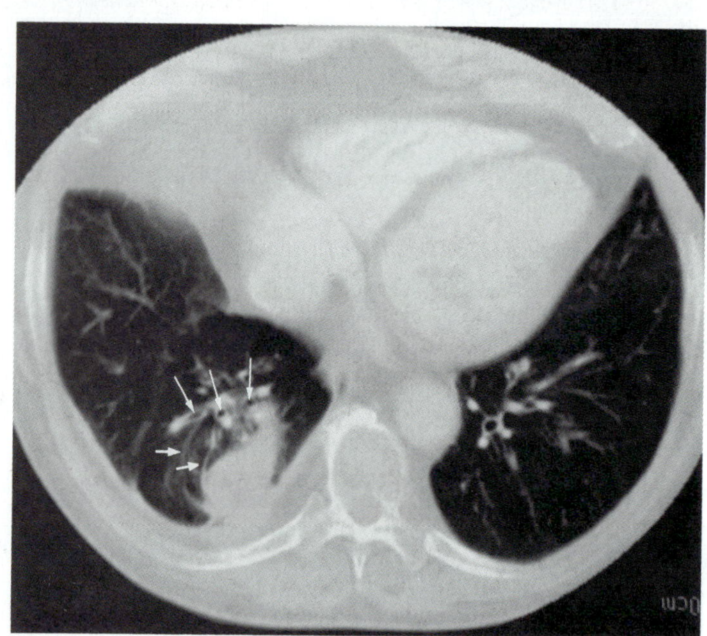

B

**Figure 8–11.** CT of round atelectasis of the lung: **A.** At window settings to demonstrate soft tissue detail, an angular-shaped mass (arrow) is seen in the posterior aspect of the right lower lobe and is associated with a region of pleural thickening (arrowhead). **B.** At window settings to optimize lung detail, bronchi (long arrows) and curvilinear vessels (short arrows) converge toward the mass. This is the so-called comet-tail sign.

with low-probability combined scan do have emboli, some patients with a high-probability scan do not, and the patient with the indeterminate scan has embolus about half the time. Thus, a more definitive study is needed.

Pulmonary arteriography is an invasive study with some (although low) risk, requiring moderate expertise and sophisticated, expensive equipment. The injection of opaque medium should be into each main pulmonary artery and at least two views obtained. Selective magnification arteriography should be done if lesser studies are indeterminate. The only unequivocal diagnostic finding is an intraluminal filling defect due to thrombus. The accuracy of pulmonary arteriography is open to question as is any study requiring human perception. A study comparing interobserver concordance revealed high concordance in the diagnosis of larger emboli in vessels up to the fourth order. The concordance for more distal vessels and for selective studies was poor.[53] It is hard to lend credence then to accuracy of interpretation of abnormalities in these smaller vessels and to selective studies.

Fast MRI and helical CT have made it possible to image the pulmonary vascular tree and accurately identify large central pulmonary emboli as intraluminal filling defects. Small peripheral emboli may be missed, however, so that neither technique can replace pulmonary angiography.[54]

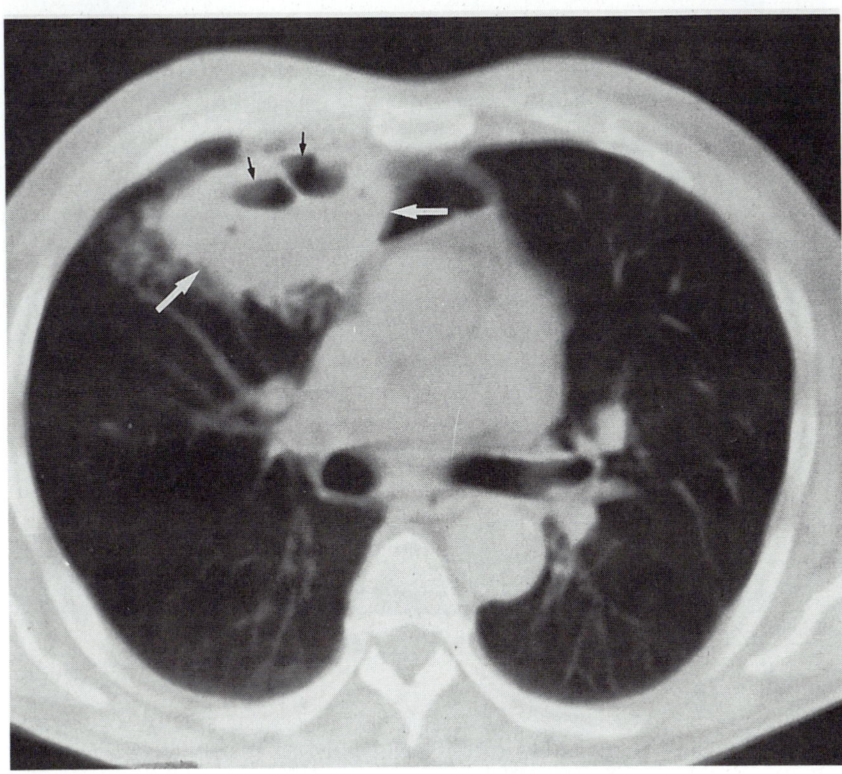

**Figure 8–12.** CT of lung abscess. Scan obtained just below the carina shows an area of confluent consolidation in the right anterior lung field abutting the pleural surface. Areas of cavitation are present within the lesion.

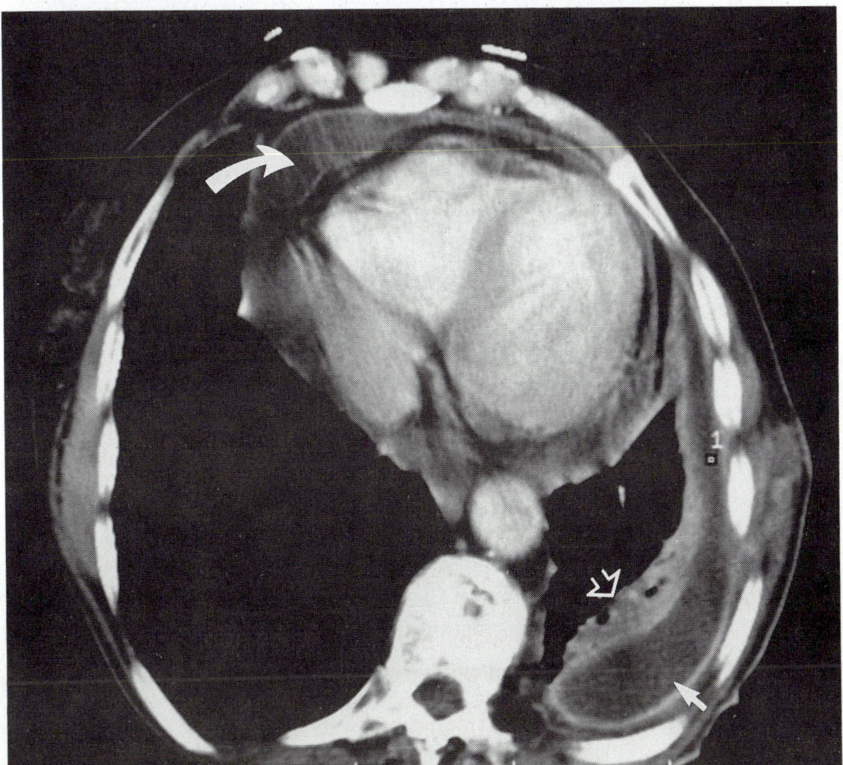

**Figure 8–13.** CT of empyema. A loculated fluid collection is seen in the left posterior pleural space (arrow). The surrounding pleura is thickened and is enhanced by intravenously administered contrast material. The underlying lung (open arrow) is compressed. A pericardial effusion is also present (curved arrow).

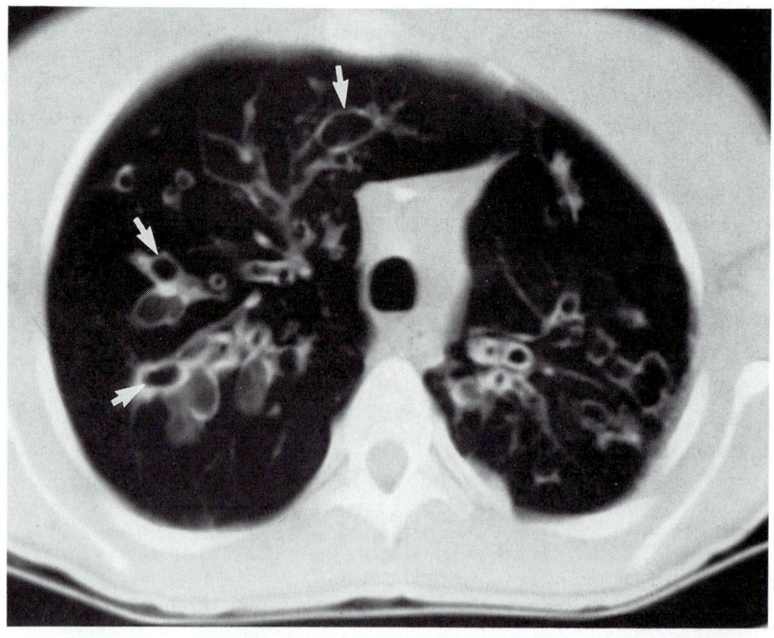

A

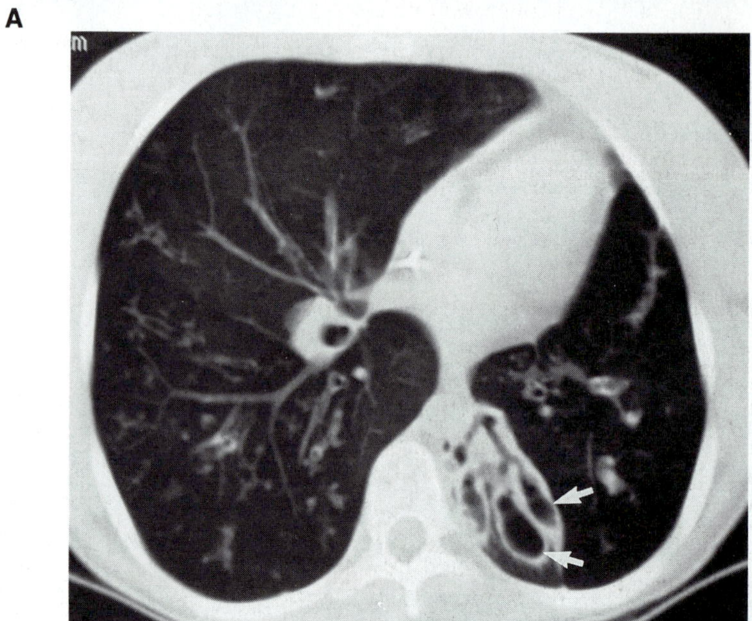

B

**Figure 8–14.** CT showing bronchiectasis in a young adult with cystic fibrosis: **A.** Scan through the upper lobes shows multiple, contiguous dilated bronchi (arrows) in both lung fields. **B.** Scan through the lung bases show bronchiectasis in association with a collapsed left lower lobe (arrows).

We believe that in all but the most critical clinical circumstance (in that case, pulmonary arteriography following heparinization) an appropriate approach to diagnosis would be:

1. heparinization.
2. a chest x-ray to rule out other causes of symptoms and for comparison to ventilation-perfusion scans, particularly if the chest x-ray is normal.
3. evaluation of the lower extremity for thrombosis by venography, duplex sonography, or impedance plethysmography. If the leg study reveals thrombosis, treatment should be started inasmuch as it is the same for embolus as for venous thrombosis. No further study is justified.
4. if the lower extremity is nonrevealing, and suspicion remains, then pulmonary arteriography should be performed.

The above suggestions do not include pulmonary scintigraphy. If the patient has few if any contraindications to anticoagulation, if the chest film is quite normal, then pulmonary scintigraphy would be a reasonable approach. A normal scan, for practical purposes, rules out pulmonary embolus. A high-probability scan under the circumstance might well be sufficient information to institute anticoagulation. However, for the further therapy, such as caval interruption or thrombolysis, pulmonary arteriography would still be a necessity, and perhaps the step of pulmonary scintigraphy could be avoided.

The roles of fast MRI and helical CT in the diagnosis of pulmonary embolism are being actively investigated. Possible uses at present might be for suspicion of acute central pulmonary embolism in very sick patients, in patients at high risk for pulmonary angiography, and the identification of candidates for thromboendarterectomy related to chronic embolic disease.[48]

## MEDIASTINAL MASSES

### Conventional Radiography

Most mediastinal masses are detected on chest radiographs performed routinely or for symptoms related to a mediastinal lesion. A mass is often well defined by the deformed mediastinal pleura, although malignant lesions may be ill defined if there is pleural invasion. An obtuse angle formed by the mass at its point of contact with the mediastinum is usual and differs from the acute angle formed by a lung mass in contiguity with the mediastinum. The location of the mass is indicated by its relationship to the pleural reflection and interfaces. Density differences related to gas, fat, or calcification may help characterize the lesion as may an associated abnormality such as a mass in the lung or at the hilum.

The esophagram is helpful in the evaluation of a suspected esophageal abnormality and may demonstrate a mediastinal mass by showing displacement due to extrinsic compression.

Fluoroscopy may confirm the presence of a lesion before more specific diagnostic methods are used. A pulsatile mass suggests a vascular lesion, although one in contact with a major vessel may also appear to pulsate. Variation in size with the Valsalva maneuver may also indicate the vascular nature of an abnormality. Angiography is still used for detailed evaluation of specific vascular lesions, such as aortic dissection, but contrast CT and MRI (Fig. 8–15). are sensitive screening studies in distinguishing vascular from nonvascular lesions.

### Computed Tomography

CT can correctly distinguish among four categories of pathology—soft tissue masses, fatty lesions, vascular lesions, and fluid-filled cysts.[55] Bronchogenic cysts may be a source of confusion because the density of their fluid may be relatively high due to high protein concentration (Fig. 8–16). CT is indicated in the evaluation of an abnormal mediastinum on chest radiographs and a specific diagnosis may be possible (Figs. 8–17, 8–18). The distinction between atelectasis, with collapsed lung against the medi-

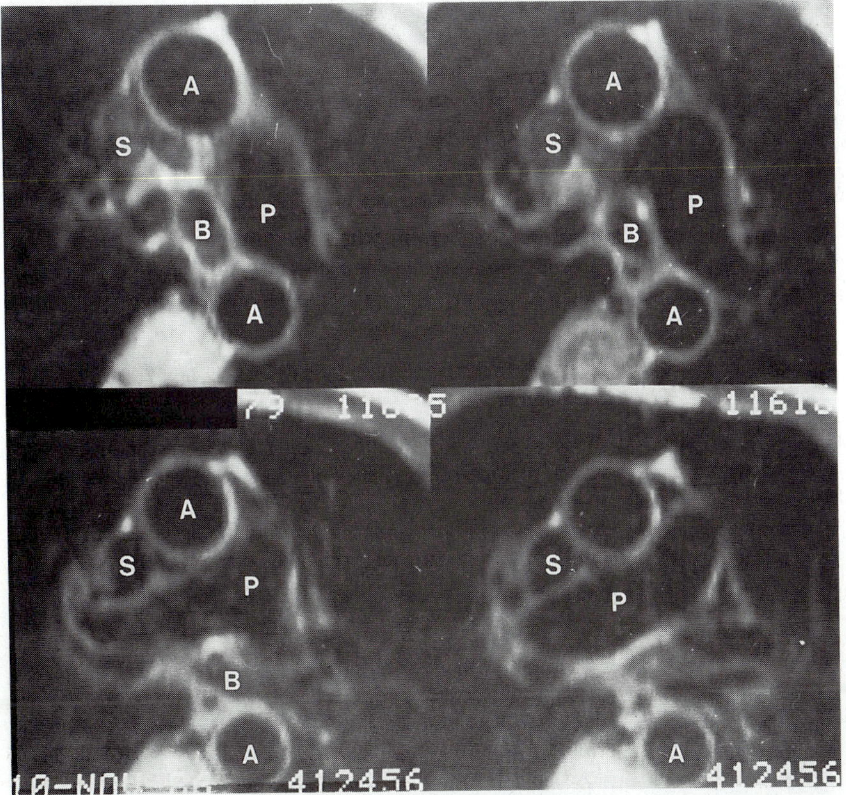


**Figure 8–15.** MRI of normal mediastinal major vessels and bronchi. Four scans at slightly different levels show the lumina and walls of the aortic arch, pulmonary artery and its main branches and the proximal main stem bronchi. (A = aorta, P = pulmonary artery, B = bronchus, S = superior vena cava.)

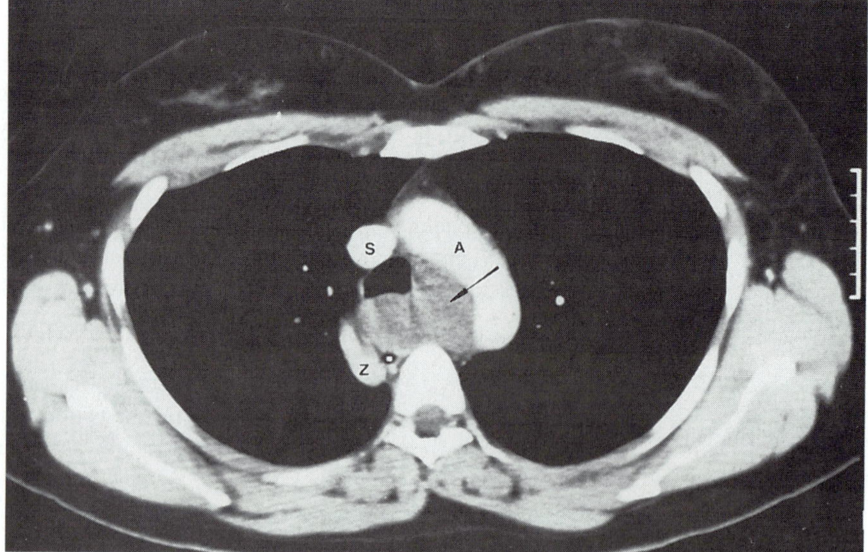


**Figure 8–16.** CT scan of a mediastinal bronchogenic cyst. Scan obtained at the level of the aortic arch shows the contrast opacified aorta, superior vena cava, and azygos arch at the periphery of a large central mediastinal mass (arrow) due to a surgically proven bronchogenic cyst. Although this is a cystic lesion, the density of the mass is intermediate between that of fluid and soft tissue due to a high protein concentration in the cyst fluid. (A = aorta, S = superior vena cava, Z = azygos arch.)

astinum, and a mediastinal lesion is readily made. Similarly, CT can distinguish pleural masses and fluid collections from mediastinal lesions. Contrast studies are essential to accurately identify vascular lesions such as aneurysms, which may simulate soft tissue tumors. In patients with malignancy, CT may detect direct invasion of the mediastinum or tumor involvement of mediastinal lymph nodes. It also has an important application in the planning and localization of treatment fields used in radiation therapy of mediastinal neoplasm.

CT may permit the diagnosis of specific conditions in certain clinical situations such as thymoma associated with myasthenia gravis or parathyroid adenoma in hyperparathyroidism.[56] It is helpful in directing the biopsy of a mediastinal mass by fine-needle aspiration, and aspiration and catheter drainage of mediastinal abscesses.

## Magnetic Resonance Imaging

Because flowing blood is devoid of signal on MRI, vascular lesions and the relationship of masses to vessels are clearly shown without contrast injection. The margins of lesions

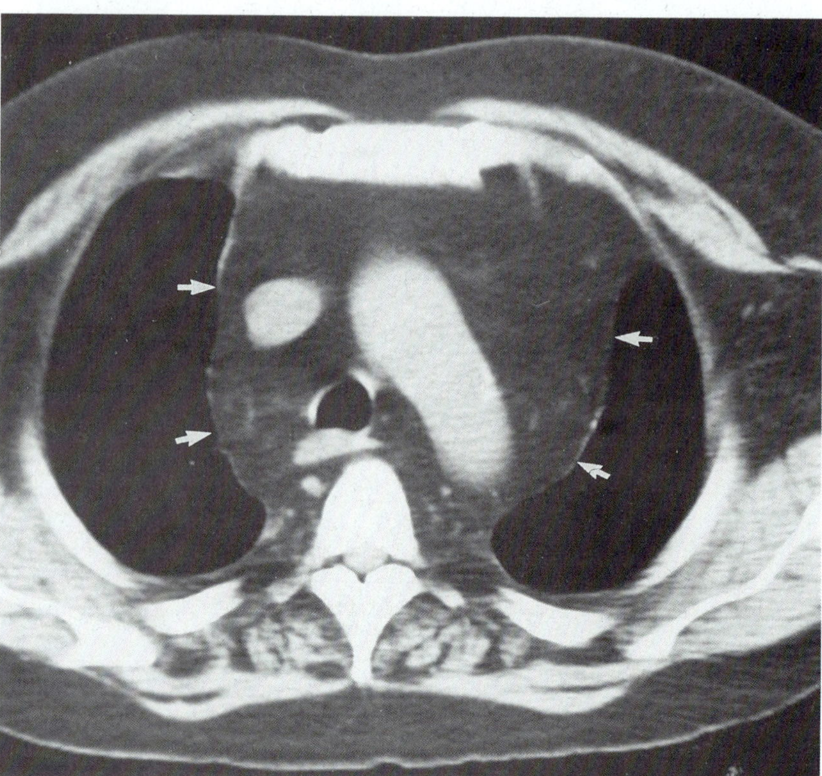

**Figure 8–17.** CT of mediastinal enlargement. A scan at the level of the aortic arch shows mediastinal enlargement due to adipose tissue (arrows).

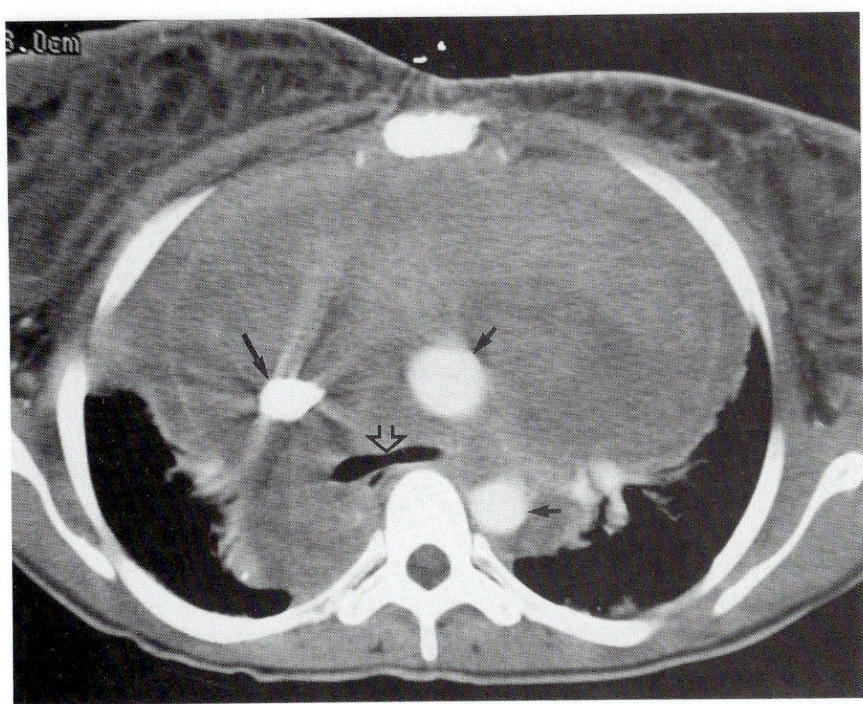

**Figure 8–18.** CT of mediastinal Hodgkins disease. A huge anterior mediastinal mass encroaches into both lung fields. It encases, displaces, and separates the ascending and descending thoracic aorta (short arrows), superior mediastinum (long arrow), and carina (open arrow).

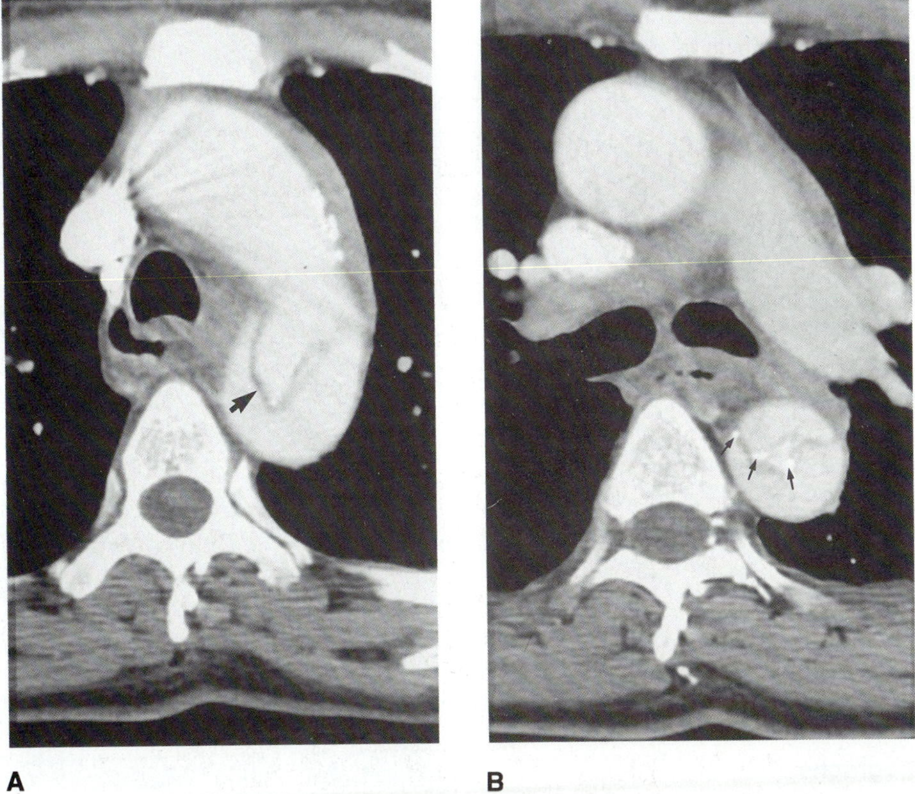


**Figure 8–19.** Aortic dissection: **A.** A curvilinear intimal flap (arrow) is shown in the opacified distal aortic arch. **B.** A scan at a lower level in the chest, a little below the carina, also shows a curvilinear intimal flap. Calcified and displaced atheromatous lesions (arrows) are seen in association with the intimal flap.

may not be as well defined as on CT, however, due to poorer spatial resolution (see Fig. 8–15).[57,58] Differentiation of benign from malignant lesions is not possible although fluid-filled and necrotic lesions can be characterized. Imaging in sagittal and coronal planes permits structures such as the trachea, aorta, and spine to be imaged in their long axes. Failure to identify calcification handicaps MRI studies with regard to characterization of lymph node masses, goiters, and some thrombosed aortic dissections.

### Endoscopic Ultrasound

The accuracy of preoperative staging of esophageal cancer has been improved by the introduction of endoscopic US, which enables evaluation of the true extent of tumor invasion of the esophageal wall and its immediate vicinity. CT is more accurate in staging distant metastases and the highest correspondence with surgical and pathologic findings in overall stage occurs with combined use of endoscopic ultrasound and dynamic CT.

## DRAINAGE OF PLEURAL COLLECTIONS, LUNG, AND MEDIASTINAL ABSCESSES

This is requested when fluid cannot be localized by physical examination, is loculated, or requires to be drained completely. The fluid is localized by ultrasound with the patient sitting and leaning over the back of a chair or a bed table.[59]

Infected pleural collections should be drained, in the first instance, by percutaneous means under imaging guidance using a soft pigtail, or gently curved tip, catheter with numerous side holes.[60] It is introduced by the trochar or Seldinger technique. The method is preferable to chest tube placement because it is less traumatic, the tube tip is accurately placed in the dependent portion of the collection, and most collections are easily drained through catheters of this size. More than one catheter may be used for loculated pockets, and very thick material is removed by rinsing with sterile saline. The integrity of the catheter is monitored daily and kept patent by frequent irrigation with a few cubic centimeters of sterile saline. The catheter is only removed when the cavity has collapsed and drainage has ceased. This may take several weeks.

Lung and mediastinal abscesses are drained in a similar fashion if they abut the chest wall and if medical treatment is ineffective.[61]

## THE THORACIC AORTA

### Conventional Radiographs

Chest films, including oblique views obtained after swallowing barium, are of value as initial studies in suspected aortic disease. An aneurysm may bulge the mediastinum in some portion of the course of the aorta. The mass usually has sharply curved borders. Calcification is common, is often curvilinear, and parallels the aortic contour. Lesions of the right sinus of Valsalva may project to the right at the level of the inferior pulmonary veins. This appearance differs from that of other mediastinal masses at this site in that no posterior border is discernable on lateral radiographs. Aneurysms of the left sinus of Valsalva do not bulge the mediastinum but may increase mediastinal density and simulate a subcarinal bronchogenic cyst or enlarged left atrium.

Aneurysms of the ascending aorta fill the lower retrosternal space on the lateral radiograph and project to the right on frontal views. It is difficult to distinguish fusiform aneurysms at this location from tortuosity and aortography or CT is needed for diagnosis.

Aneurysms at the aortic arch more often bulge to the

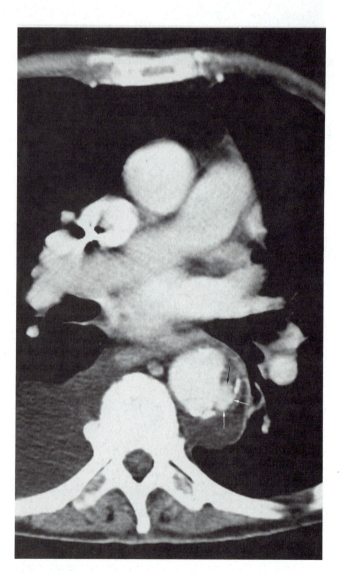

**Figure 8–20.** CT of penetrating ulcer of the distal aortic arch. An ulcer, 1 cm in antero-posterior diameter, is seen arising from the lateral aspect of the aortic lumen in the distal aortic arch.

left than to the right of the mediastinum. An esophagram helps in distinction of aneurysm from a mass at this site, since a mass displaces the esophagus to the same side as the aorta, whereas an aneurysm displaces it to the opposite side. Traumatic pseudoaneurysms of the aorta usually involve the isthmus distal to the left subclavian artery. A localized bulge of the aortic contour may be seen on chest x-ray. Associated hemorrhage from small vessels widens the mediastinum in 40–50% of cases, and the trachea may be displaced to the right. Extrapleural extension of hemorrhage may result in an "apical cap" or displacement of the paravertebral pleural–pulmonary interface. Pleural effusion from hemorrhage may also occur.

Aneurysms of the descending aorta project within the heart on frontal radiographs and bulge into the left lung field. Distinguishing aneurysm from dissection may not be possible on plain chest films. Findings suggestive of dissection are widening of the mediastinum at the level of the aortic arch with progressive increase in width on sequential films. A localized bulge of the distal aortic arch may be seen. Separation of intimal calcification from the aortic contour is a characteristic but infrequent sign of dissection. It is valid when seen in the descending aorta, but not on frontal views of the aortic arch due to foreshortening.

## Computed Tomography

This should be the next procedure in the nonurgent evaluation of aortic aneurysm or dissection and is usually definitive. The ease of performance of the studies has improved

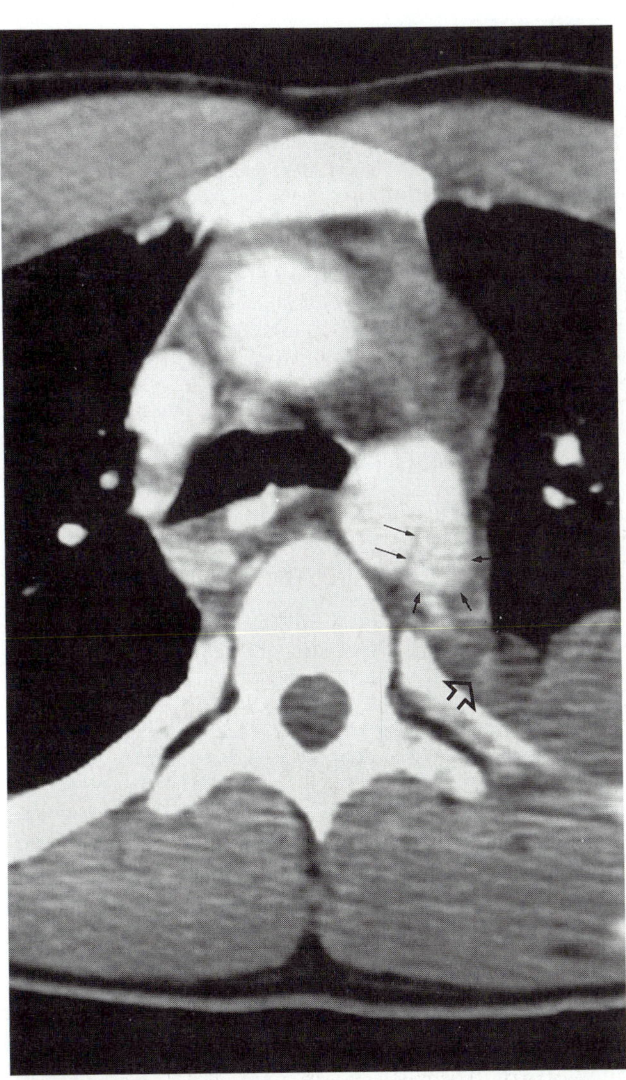

A

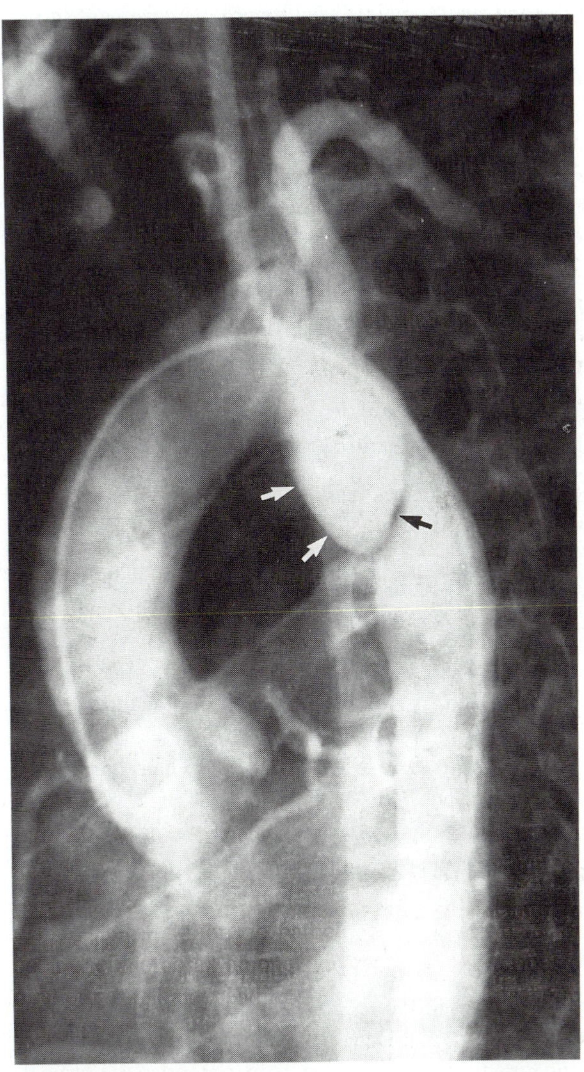

B

**Figure 8–21.** Aortic trauma: **A.** CT image through the aortic arch and descending thoracic aorta. An intimal flap is seen within the lumen of the distal aortic arch (long arrows) and forms the medial margin of a traumatic false aneurysm (short arrows). Blood is shown in the contiguous pleural space (open arrow). **B.** Arteriogram of the thoracic aorta shows the intimal flap (black arrow) and false aneurysm (white arrows) shown in A.

and the consistency in obtaining high-quality examinations has increased with helical CT.[62] It shows aortic dilatation, mural calcification, intraluminal thrombus, and effects on surrounding structures such as tracheal displacement and bone erosion. In aortic dissection, dynamic scanning shows the intimal flap and patency of true and false lumens[63,64] (Fig. 8–19). Distinction between Type A and Type B dissections is accurately made, and extension into the abdomen can be identified. CT may document rupture of a dissection into the pericardium or pleura and is of value in follow-up whether treatment is medical or surgical. A limitation of CT is that associated aortic regurgitation and coronary disease cannot be assessed.

Penetrating ulceration of the descending aorta can usually be distinguished from classic dissection on dynamic contrast CT[65] (Fig. 8–20). A focal ulcer is shown with an adjacent subintimal hematoma most often in the middle or distal third of the thoracic aorta. Inward displacement of intimal calcifications may be seen, and there is often associated thickening and contrast enhancement of the aortic wall. In classic dissection, a smoothly spiralling flap begins in the proximal aorta. Calcification of the displaced flap is seen less frequently because atherosclerosis does not predispose to classic dissection.

CT may demonstrate acute aortic injuries, but there is difficulty in its use for this application[66] (Fig. 8–21).

### Ultrasound

Transthoracic and transesophageal echocardiography are effective in the evaluation of the aorta for suspected aneurysms and aortic dissection.[10,67,68] The transthoracic approach is most successful in evaluating the ascending aorta and the transesophageal approach the aortic arch and descending aorta. As with other modalities, the diagnosis of dissection depends on demonstration of two lumina separated by an intimal flap. The method is noninvasive and can be performed at the bedside. It is, however, highly dependent on the operator's skill and experience in evaluating the aorta. In most cases sedation is required, and esophageal perforation is a potential complication when the transesophageal approach is used. Its ability to identify lesions of the ascending aorta is useful in determining which patients with dissection require urgent surgery.

### Angiography

Suspected trauma to the thoracic aorta calls for urgent angiography (Fig. 8–21). Deceleration injury, chest pain, and a widened mediastinum on chest x-ray comprise the typical clinical picture. A false aneurysm just below the aortic isthmus is the usual finding, but more than one tear may be present in 15–20% of cases.

Suspected acute aortic dissection is also often an indication for urgent angiography. Diagnosis depends on demonstration of two channels separated by an intimal flap. If the false channel is thrombosed, then diagnosis may be based on the appearance of a compressed true channel and aortic wall thickening. The status of the aortic valve and coronary vessels can be determined.

### Magnetic Resonance

Imaging of major thoracic blood vessels is an excellent use for MRI.[31] Good resolution, especially with electrocardiogram-gated images, permits detailed evaluation of congenital vascular malformations, aneurysms, and aortic dissections. For congenital lesions, it is superior to CT and has comparable accuracy in evaluation of dissections and aneurysms.

### REFERENCES


1. Krohmer JS: Radiography and fluoroscopy, 1920 to the present. Monograph. *Radiographics* **9:**1129–1153, 1989
2. Wandtke JC: Bedside chest radiography. *Radiology* **190:**1–10, 1994
3. Heiken JP, Brink JA, Vannier MW: Spiral (helical) CT. *Radiology* **189:**647–656, 1993
4. Stark DD, Bradley WG: *Magnetic Resonance Imaging.* 2nd ed. St. Louis, Mosby, 1992
5. Hoffman JM, Hanson MY, Coleman RE: Clinical positron emission tomography imaging. *Radiol Clin North Am* **314:**935–959, 1993
6. Patz EF, Lowe VJ, Hoffman JM, et al: Focal pulmonary abnormalities: Evaluation with F-18 fluorodeoxyglucose PET scanning. *Radiology* **188:**487–490, 1993
7. Botet JF, Lightdale C: Endoscopic sonography of the upper gastrointestinal tract. *AJR* **156:**63–68, 1992
8. Botet JF, Lightdale CL, Zauber AG, et al: Preoperative staging of esophageal cancer: Comparison of endoscopic US and dynamic CT. *Radiology* **181:**419–425, 1991
9. Liu J, Miller LS, Goldberg BB, Feld RI, et al. Transnasal US of the esophagus: Preliminary morphologic and function studies. *Radiology* **184:**721–727, 1992
10. Erbel R, Daniel W, Visser C, et al. Echocardiography in diagnosis of aortic dissection. *Lancet* **4:**457–460, 1989
11. Siegelman SS, Zerhouni EA, Leo FP, et al: CT of the solitary pulmonary nodule. *AJR* **135:**1, 1980
12. Zerhouni EA, Boukadoum M, Siddiky MA, et al: A standard phantom for quantitative CT analysis of pulmonary nodules. *Radiology* **149:**767, 1983
13. Swensen SJ, Morin RL, Schueler BA, et al: Solitary pulmonary nodule: CT evaluation with iodinated contrast material—A preliminary report. *Radiology* **182:**343–347, 1992
14. Vock P, Soueck M, Daepp M, Kalender WA: Lung: Spiral volumetric CT with single-breath-hold technique. *Radiology* **176:**864–867, 1990
15. Costello P, Anderson W, Blume D: Pulmonary nodule: Evaluation with spiral volumetric CT. *Radiology* **179:**875–876, 1991
16. Greene R: Transthoracic needle aspiration biopsy. In Athanasoulis CA (ed): *Interventional Radiology.* Philadelphia, Saunders, 1982, pp 587–634
17. Westcott JL: Percutaneous needle biopsy of hilar and mediastinal masses. *Radiology* **141:**323, 1981
18. Westcott JL: Direct percutaneous needle aspiration of localized pulmonary lesions: Results in 422 patients. *Radiology* **137:**31, 1980
19. Adler OB, Rosenberger A, Peleg H: Fine-needle aspiration biopsy of mediastinal masses: Evaluation of 136 experiences. *AJR* **140:**893, 1983

20. Fink I, Gamsu G, Harter LP: CT-guided aspiration biopsy of the thorax. *J Comput Assist Tomogr* **6:**958, 1982
21. Gobien RP, Skucas J, Paris BS: CT-assisted fluoroscopically guided aspiration biopsy of central hilar and mediastinal masses. *Radiology* **131:**443, 1981
22. Austin JHM, Cohen MB: Value of having a cytopathologist present during percutaneous fine-needle aspiration biopsy of lung: Report of 55 cancer patients and metaanalysis of the literature. *AJR* **160:**175, 1993
23. Gobien RP, Valicent JF, Paris BS, Danielli C: Thin needle aspiration biopsy: Methods of increasing the accuracy of a negative prediction. *Radiology* **145:**603, 1982
24. Khouri NF, Stitik FP, Erozan YS, et al: Transthoracic needle aspiration biopsy of benign and malignant lung lesions. *AJR* **144:**281, 1985
25. Sinner WN: Fine needle biopsy of hamartomas of the lung. *AJR* **138:**65, 1982
26. Naidich DP, Zerhouni EA, Siegelman SS: Lung cancer in computed tomography and magnetic resonance of the thorax. In: *Computed Tomography and Magnetic Resonance of the Thorax.* Raven, New York, 1991: pp 275–302
27. Glazer HS, Duncan-Meyer J, Aronberg DJ, et al: Pleural and chest wall invasion in bronchogenic carcinoma: CT evaluation. *Radiology* **157:**191–194, 1985
28. Glazer GM, Francis IR, Shirazi KK et al: Evaluation of the pulmonary hilum: Comparison of conventional radiography, 55° posterior oblique tomography, and dynamic computed tomography. *J Comput Assist Tomogr* **7:**983, 1983
29. Webb WR, Glazer G, Gamsu G: Computed tomography of the normal pulmonary hilum. *J Comput Assist Tomogr* **5:**476, 1981
30. Webb WR, Gamsu G, Speckman JM: Computed tomography of the pulmonary hilum in patients with bronchogenic carcinoma. *J Comput Assist Tomogr* **7:**219, 1983
31. Gamsu G, Webb WR, Sheldon P, et al: Nuclear magnetic resonance imaging of the thorax. *Radiology* **147:**473, 1983
32. Daly BDT Jr, Faling LJ, Pugatch et al: Computed tomography: An effective technique for mediastinal staging in lung cancer. *J Thorac Cardiovasc Surg* **88:**486, 1984
33. Clinical staging of primary lung cancer: American Thoracic Society node mapping scheme. *Am Rev Respir Dis* **127:**659, 1983
34. Baron RL, Levitt RG, Sagel SS et al: Computed tomography in the preoperative evaluation of bronchogenic carcinoma. *Radiology* **145:**727, 1982
35. Glazer GM, Gross BH, Quint LE, et al: Normal mediastinal lymph nodes: Number and size according to American Thoracic Society node mapping. *Am Rev Respir Dis* **144:**261, 1983
36. Faling LJ, Pugatch RD, Jung-Legg Y: Computed tomography scanning of the mediastinum in the staging of bronchogenic carcinoma. *Am Rev Respir Dis* **124:**690–695, 1981
37. Osborne DR, Korobkin M, Ravin CE, et al: Comparison of plain radiography, conventional tomography, and computed tomography in detecting lymph node metastasis from lung carcinoma. *Radiology* **142:**157–161, 1982
38. McLoud TC, Bourgouin PM, Greenberg RW, et al. Bronchogenic carcinoma: Analysis of staging in the mediastinum with CT by correlative lymph node mapping and sampling. *Radiology* **183:**319–323, 1992
39. Webb WR, Jensen BG, Sollitto R, et al. Bronchogenic carcinoma: Staging with MR compared with staging with CT and surgery. *Radiology* **156:**117, 1985
40. Cohen AM, Creviston S, LiPuma JP, et al. NMR evaluation of hilar and mediastinal lymphadenopathy. *Radiology* **148:**739, 1982
41. Pennes DR, Glazer GM, Wimbish KJ, et al: Chest wall invasion by lung cancer: Limitations of CT evaluation. *AJR* **144:**507, 1985
42. O'Connell RS, McLoud TC, Wilkins EW: Superior sulcus tumor: Radiographic diagnosis and workup. *AJR* **140:**25, 1983
43. Hirsch JH, Rogers JV, Mack LA: Real-time sonography of pleural opacities. *AJR* **136:**297, 1981
44. Marks WM, Filly RA, Callen PW: Real-time evaluation of pleural lesions: New observations regarding the probability of obtaining free fluid. *Radiology* **142:**163, 1982
45. Williford ME, Hidalgo H, Putman CE, et al: Computed tomography of pleural disease. *AJR* **140:**909, 1983
46. Stark DD, Federle MP, Goodman PC, et al: Differentiating lung abscess and empyema: Radiography and computed tomography. *AJR* **141:**163, 1983
47. Grant DC, Seltzer SE, Antman KH, et al: Computed tomography of malignant pleural sothelioma. *J Comput Assist Tomogr* **7:**626, 1983
48. Costello P: Finding thoracic hernias in breath-hold intervals. *Diagn Imaging* 1993;Nov(suppl): 25–29, 1993
49. Phillips MS, Williams MP, Flower CDR: How useful is computed tomography in the diagnosis and assessment of bronchiectasis? *Clin Radiol* **37:**321, 1986
50. Consensus Conference, Medical Applications of Research, National Institutes of Health: Prevention of venous thrombosis and pulmonary embolism. *JAMA* **256:**744, 1986
51. Biello DR, Mattar AG, McKnight RC, Siegel BA: Interpretation of ventilation-perfusion studies in patients with suspected pulmonary embolism. *AJR* **133:**1033, 1979
52. Hull R, Hirsh J, Carter C, et al: Diagnostic value of ventilation-perfusion lung scanning in patients with suspected pulmonary embolism. *Chest* **88:**819, 1985
53. Quinn MF, Lundell CJ, Klotz TA, et al: Reliability of selective pulmonary arteriography in the diagnosis of pulmonary embolism. *AJR* **149:**469, 1987
54. Getter WB, Krishann BG, Holland G: MR and CT enhance the diagnosis of thromboemboli. *Diagn Imaging* Aug:80–85, 1993
55. Paguatch RD, Faling LJ, Robbins AH, et al: CT diagnosis of benign mediastinal abnormalities. *AJR* **134:**685, 1980
56. Krudy AG, Koppman JL, Brennan MF, et al: The detection of mediastinal parathyroid glands by computed tomography, selective arteriography, and venous sampling: An analysis of 17 cases. *Radiology* **140:**739, 1981
57. Gamsu G, Stark DD, Webb WR, et al: Magnetic resonance imaging of benign mediastinal masses. *Radiology* **151:**709, 1984
58. Cohen AM, Creviston S, LiPuma JP, et al: NMR imaging of the mediastinum and hila: Early impressions of its efficacy. *AJR* **141:**1163, 1983
59. Harnsberger HR, Lee TG, Mukuno DH: Rapid, inexpensive real-time directed thoracentesis. *Radiology* **146:**545, 1983
60. Westcott JL: Percutaneous catheter drainage of pleural effusion and emphysema. *AJR* **144:**1189, 1985
61. Gobien RP, Stanley JH, Gobien BS, et al: Percutaneous catheter aspiration and drainage of suspected mediastinal abscesses. *Radiology* **151:**69, 1984
62. Costello P, Ecker CP, Tello R, et al: Assessment of the thoracic aorta by spiral CT. *AJR* **158:**1127, 1992
63. Heiberg E, Wolverson MK, et al: CT findings in thoracic aortic dissection. *AJR* **136:**13, 1981
64. Vasile N, Mathieu D, Keita K, et al: Computed tomography of thoracic aortic dissection: accuracy and pitfalls. *J Comput Assist Tomogr* **9:**78, 1985
65. Kazerooni EA, Bree RL, Williams DM: Penetrating atheroclerotic ulcers of the descending thoracic aorta: Evaluation with CT and distinction from aortic dissection. *Radiology* **183:**759, 1992
66. Heiberg E, Wolverson MK, Sundaram M, et al: CT in aortic trauma. *AJR* **160:**1119, 1983
67. Mathew T, Nanda NC: Two-dimensional and Doppler echocardiographic evaluation of aortic aneurysm and dissection. *Am J Cardiol* **54:**379–385, 1984
68. Hashimoto S, Kumada T, Osakada G, et al: Assessment of transesophageal Doppler echography in dissecting aortic aneurysm. *J Am Coll Cardiol* **14:**1253–1262, 1989

CHAPTER

# 9

# Esophagoscopy and Endoscopic Esophageal Ultrasonography

Thomas W. Rice

## INTRODUCTION

Although esophagoscopy has been practiced for more than 100 years, it was not until the introduction of the flexible fiberoptic endoscope in the 1970s that esophagoscopy became a routine and practical investigation. Refinements in optics and instrumentation have further increased the diagnostic capabilities of esophagoscopy. Today, flexible fiberoptic esophagoscopy has nearly eliminated the need for rigid esophagoscopy. Flexible esophagoscopy allows evaluation of symptoms, planning of therapy, and assessment of treatment. This is accomplished by the luminal examination of the esophagus with direct evaluation of the mucosa and indirect appraisal of extramucosal structures. The development of endoscopic esophageal ultrasonography has extended this useful examination beyond the esophageal mucosa into the esophageal wall and the paraesophageal tissue. These two instruments are most powerful tools for the diagnosis of esophageal diseases. Although therapeutic esophagoscopy has evolved at a slower rate, it is increasingly possible to treat selected esophageal diseases via a flexible fiberoptic endoscope.

## INSTRUMENTS

### Flexible Fiberoptic Endoscope

A flexible fiberoptic endoscope has four components: the control section, the insertion tube, the bending section, and the distal tip (Fig. 9–1). The control section, which houses the controls for deflection of the bending section and the suction and air insufflation/water irrigation valves, is approximately 0.3 m long. The control section is either fitted with an eyepiece for direct viewing of the upper gastrointestinal (GI) tract or a miniature video camera for remote display of the image. The insertion tube, the bending section, and the distal tip, which are inserted into the patient, have an overall working length of approximately 1 m. These sections house the optic bundles and the instrument/suction and air/water channels. The optic bundles are of two types: the light guide (LG) and the optic guide (OG) bundles. The LG bundles are incapable of producing an image and are designed for maximum light transmission. Adequate illumination is provided by endoscopes with one LG bundle. However, a second LG bundle in specialized endoscopes produces a sharper, brighter image and minimizes instrument shadowing. The OG bundle transmits the image; its design characteristics determine the resolution of the endoscope.

The diameter of the insertion tube, the bending section, and the distal tip are determined by the size of the optic bundles and the channels. The outside diameter (OD) of the insertion tube of a pediatric endoscope is as little as 5.3 mm. In these units the inside diameter (ID) of the instrument channel is usually 2 mm, and this channel must be used for air, water, suction, and instrumentation. The OD of adult endoscopes range from 9 to 11 mm, and the ID of the instrument/suction channel is 2.2–2.8 mm. Generally there is a separate channel for air and water. For therapeutic procedures endoscopes of 12.8 mm, OD with two instrument channels of 2.8-mm and 3.7-mm ID are available.

For esophagoscopy forward-viewing endoscopes that provide a 120-degree field of view are used. The depth of field is 3–100 mm; objects closer than 3 mm to the distal tip are not in view, and objects further than 100 mm from the

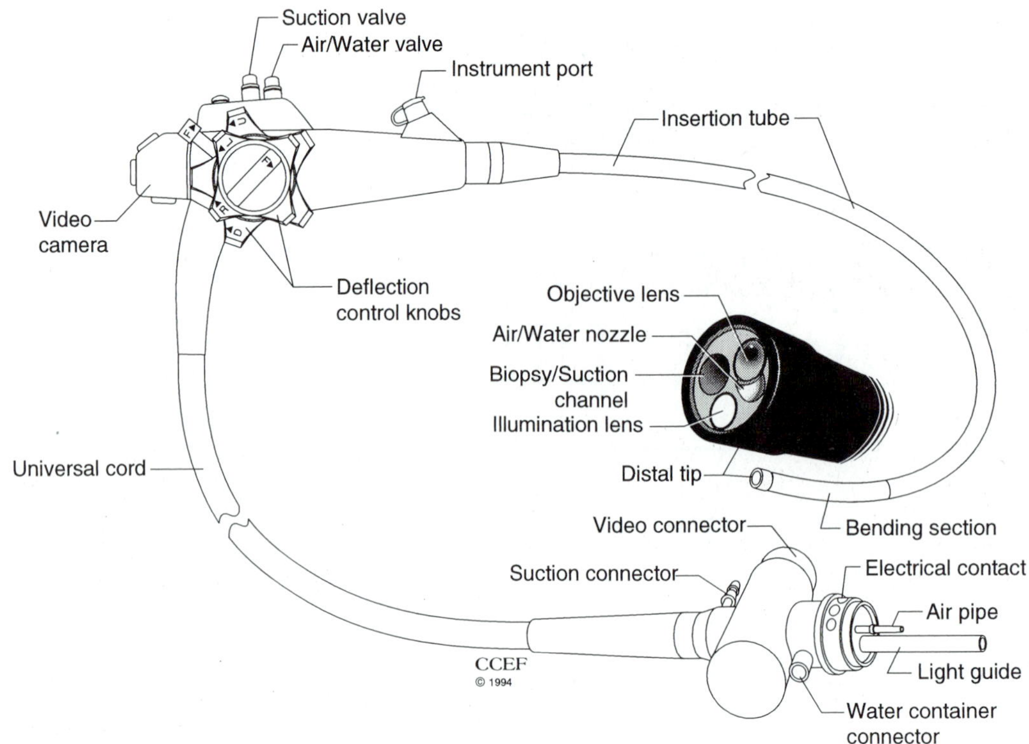


**Figure 9–1.** The flexible fiberoptic video endoscope.

distal top are not in focus. The bending section is capable of being deflected through 210 degrees in an upward direction, 90 degrees in a downward direction, and 100 degrees to the right or left. The direction of the distal tip deflection is with respect to the control section of the endoscope when the insertion tube is straight.

Illumination is provided by a light source. Low output halogen sources (150 W) are adequate for nonvideo systems. However, high-output xenon systems (300 W) are required for optimum examinations with today's video endoscopes. The light source also contains an air pump for pressurization of the water irrigation and air insufflation systems. The universal cord connects the endoscope to the light source.

There is an ever increasing number of endoscopic instruments designed for use through the instrument channel of these endoscopes. An abbreviated list includes biopsy forceps, cytology brushes, aspiration needles, curettes, retrival forceps, magnetic extractors, polypectomy snares, coagulation electrodes, injection needles, guide wires, balloon catheters, suture cutters, scissors, and knives. A wide variety of dilators and pulsion prosthesis is available for management of esophageal strictures.

## Ultrasound Endoscope

The ultrasound endoscope allows a limited visual examination of the esophagus, as well as ultrasonography of the esophagus, stomach, duodenum, and adjacent tissue (Fig. 9–2). The ultrasound transducer, which is housed in the tip of the endoscope, continuously rotates at a speed of seven revolutions per minute. Since the transducer is endoscopically placed immediately adjacent to the tissues to be examined, higher frequencies than those employed in extracorporeal ultrasound examinations can be used. In recent ultrasound endoscopes two frequencies are available, 7.5 and 12 MHz. The 7.5-MHz transducer allows adequate study to a depth of 4–5 cm, while the 12-MHz transducer allows study to a depth of 1–2 cm. An acoustic interface between the transducer and the tissue being examined must be obtained to assure good-quality ultrasound images. This is accomplished by covering the ultrasound tip of the endoscope with a latex balloon, which can be filled with water to provide an excellent acoustic interface. A less commonly employed technique is the rapid insufflation of the esophageal lumen with water. This provides an excellent, but transient, acoustic interface without the tissue compression that can occur with the latex balloon technique.

Located behind the ultrasound transducer is the distal tip of the fiberoptic endoscope. This positioning results in a limited field of view, 80 degrees at a 45-degree forward oblique angle. This depth of field is 3–100 mm. A 2-mm ID suction channel is oriented at this oblique 45-degree angle. The OD of the distal endoscope tip is 13.2 mm, while the OD of the insertion tube is 11.7 mm. Deflection of the bending section is 130 degrees up and down and 100 degrees right and left.

The control section contains the deflection controls

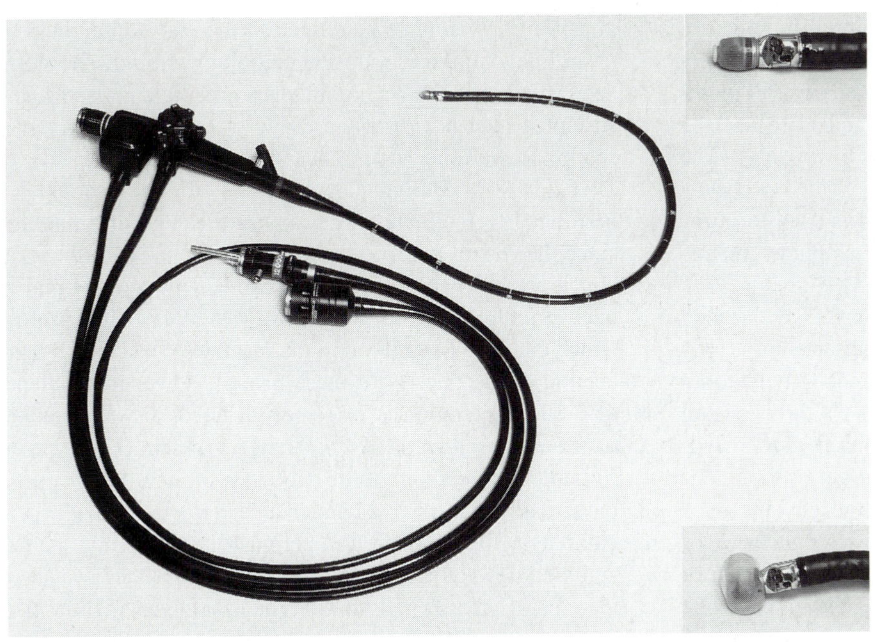

**Figure 9–2.** An Olympus UM20 ultrasound endoscope. Right upper inset: the distal tip contains the ultrasound transducer and the endoscopic tip. Right lower inset: inflation of the latex balloon covering the ultrasound transducer provides an excellent acoustic interface between the transducer and the esophageal wall.

and air/water and suction valves similar to those of a standard endoscope. A water inflation/deflation system for the balloon is incorporated into the air/water and suction valve mechanisms. A DC motor and drive mechanism, which rotate the ultrasound transducer, are housed in the control section.

The instrument is used in conjunction with an image processor. The controls of the image processor allow adjustment of gain, contrast, and sensitivity time control, which regulates the strength of the returning echo at different depths of penetration. On-screen calibration and labeling can be done with the image processor. The image may be displayed on a TV monitor, imaged on Polaroid film, or stored in a computer or on videotape. The image processor has been refined and miniaturized with successive generations of endoscopic ultrasound equipment. The current models are rack mounted and weigh about 80 lb.

## TECHNIQUES OF EXAMINATION

Esophagoscopy and endoscopic esophageal ultrasonography should be performed in an endoscopy suite designed for these investigations and the preparation and postprocedural care of the endoscopy patient. The majority of endoscopic esophageal examinations may be conducted in the outpatient setting with a conscious, sedated patient. Preparation is crucial to assure good outcome. The patient is instructed to take a light dinner the night prior to the procedure and remain NPO after midnight if the examination is scheduled before noon. If an afternoon examination is planned, then a fluid breakfast may be taken early in the morning, after which the patient should remain NPO. Patients with achalasia should be placed on clear fluids 24–48 hours before the procedure, and those with significant emptying abnormalities may require esophageal lavage prior to a clear fluid restriction. Complex examinations should be performed early in the day, allowing adequate observation time; should complications arise, further investigations and management may then be performed optimally. An appropriate history and review of pertinent investigations must be done by the endoscopist prior to esophagoscopy. The patient should then receive detailed instructions, to ensure full cooperation during the procedure. Prior to the examination a peripheral IV catheter is inserted. Prophylactic antibiotics should be administered by this route prior to the examination of patients with valvular heart disease or implanted prosthetic material. IV medication using a narcotic analgesic and a minor tranquilizer (Meperidine 25–75 mg and Midazolam 1–3 mg IV) provides sufficient sedation so that the patient is comfortable and cooperative but not stuporous and combative.[1,2] The indwelling IV cannula allows additional medication to be given if the initial dose is inadequate or a prolonged procedure requires further medication. IV access is crucial for the immediate administration of Naloxone (0.4 mg) and Flumazenil (0.5 mg) if rapid reversal of sedation is required.[3] Uncommonly these examinations may be performed without sedation. Topical anesthesia (4% viscous xylocaine gargle or 1% topical spray) is optional. Continuous monitoring of oxygen saturation (percutaneous), blood pressure (noninvasive), and ECG is mandatory in all patients.[4,5] Supplemental oxygen should be delivered by nasal prongs.

A right-handed endoscopist holds the endoscope in the left hand; the junction of the universal cord and the control section hangs in the web space between the thumb and index finger. The left thumb is used to manipulate the up and down control knob. Right and left deflection is accomplished by flexion and extension of the left wrist, rotation of the elbow, and raising or lower the left shoulder; the right/left control knob is infrequently required for this deflection. The left index finger controls the upper valve (suction). Although the left index finger may also be used to operate the lower valve (air/water), it is practical to use the left middle finger to separately control this lower valve. The ring and little fingers of the left hand support the lower portion of the control section. The right hand is used to introduce and advance the endoscope and manipulate instruments within the instrument channel.

Upper gastrointestinal (GI) endoscopy is performed with the patient in the left lateral decubitus position. It is best to introduce the endoscope under direct visualization. Use of the video endoscope further enhances direct vision passage of the endoscope. Blind passage has distinct disadvantages and is more likely to result in injury to the endoscopist (bite injuries) and the patient. Blind passage does not allow examination of the oropharynx, hypopharynx, or upper esophagus. With the patient's head flexed, the endoscope is placed on the posterior portion of the tongue. The endoscope is then visually guided into the posterior portion of the oropharynx, and the epiglottis is visualized. The endoscope is passed over the epiglottis and larynx, and the pyriform sinuses come in to view. The vocal cords should be inspected routinely and their mobility noted. The endoscope is kept on the posterior pharyngeal wall and as close to the midline as possible, and the patient is asked to swallow. This will open the cricopharyngeus, and the endoscope can be advanced through this rosette of tissue into the upper esophagus. If the endoscope fails to pass into the esophagus, it is usually because the endoscope has been deflected into the left pyriform sinus. The endoscope may be withdrawn into the hypopharynx and this maneuver attempted again, or the endoscope tip may be manipulated out of the pyriform sinus into the esophagus. This is accomplished by rotating the endoscope tip to the midline (to the right), dislodging it from the pyriform sinus. If the patient is asked to swallow during this process, the endoscope can usually be advanced into the upper esophagus. The cricopharyngeus and upper esophagus are the most difficult areas to examine, and a careful viewing on removal of the endoscope will add to the initial observations at endoscope insertion. The examination of the esophagus is carried out with air insufflation, sufficient to distend the esophagus but not excessive so as to cause patient discomfort, retching, or vomiting. Complete examination of the stomach, with retroflexed inspection of the gastric cardia, and the duodenum should be included with every esophagoscopy.

Since the ultrasound endoscope provides an inadequate endoscopic inspection of the upper GI tract, every ultrasound study should be preceded by a standard flexible endoscopic upper GI examination. This provides precise location, mucosal definition, and biopsy of the esophageal lesion and guides the ultrasound examination. The ultrasound endoscope is generally passed blindly through the oropharynx and hypopharynx. Care must be taken, since the distal end containing the ultrasound transducer and endoscope tip is rigid. For complete examination the endoscope must be passed beyond the esophageal pathology and into the stomach. This is not always possible since malignant esophageal strictures may not permit passage of the ultrasound endoscope. In various series, this has occurred at a rate of 12–62.5%.[6–11] Malignant esophageal strictures should not be dilated to facilitate endoscopic ultrasound examination, since the risk of perforation with dilation and ultrasonography is unacceptably high.[11] Ultrasound imaging of malignant strictures can be conducted with small thin probes, which can be passed through the channel of a standard therapeutic endoscope. With these probes, however, the depth of tissue penetration is extremely limited, and the maintenance of consistent tissue contact is a problem. Thus, the information gained with these probes is limited. If it is possible to pass the ultrasound endoscope beyond the esophageal pathology, the stomach and perigastric tissues may be examined with water distension of the stomach. However, if the area of interest is limited to the esophagus or if the purpose of transgastric scanning is only to image areas such as the celiac axis, water distension of the stomach is not necessary.

The patient should recover in a monitored setting. Once the sedation has worn off, the patient should be questioned concerning odynophagia, dysphagia, and chest pain. If these are present, or if they occur within the next 24–48 hours, the physician who performed the procedure should be immediately contacted. The patient should not drive and must be accompanied home by a companion.

## ANATOMY

### Endoscopic Anatomy

The esophagus begins at the cricopharyngeus and ends at the esophagogastric junction, and in the adult it is approximately 25–30 cm long. Since the normal esophagus is a relatively straight mucosal lined muscular tube, it possess no intrinsic markings, and there are few extrinsic landmarks. For recording purposes, endoscopic findings are measured as a distance in centimeters from the incisor teeth. The cricopharyngeus is encountered at 15–18 cm from the incisor teeth. The esophagus passes into the mediastinum at 18–20 cm. The next landmark seen is the indentation of the anterior and left lateral wall of the esophagus produced by the aortic arch. This physiologic narrowing and the transmitted aortic pulsation are usually seen approximately 25 cm from the incisors. The left pulmonary hilum, which lies below the aortic arch, does not generally cause any recognizable extrinsic compression of the esophagus. Approximately 30–35 cm from the incisors, the pulsations of the left atrium are transmitted to the anterior esophageal wall. At 40–45 cm the diaphragmatic hiatus is encountered. The position can be confirmed by asking the patient to sniff or perform a Valsalva maneuver causing the esophagus to be pinched by the contracting diaphragm. The intraabdominal portion of the esophagus is 1–2 cm long. It is typically not appreciated endoscopically, and, immediately after passing through the diaphragm, the stomach is entered. The lower esophageal sphincter is not identifiable at esophagoscopy.

The esophageal lumen can be distended to 2 cm in AP diameter and 3 cm in lateral diameter. An undistensible or redundant dilated esophagus are signs of esophageal pathology. Esophageal distension is crucial to esophagoscopy and allows assessment of the mucosa. The esophageal mucosa is a pearly gray homogenous color, with a pale, dull appearance. Submucosal vessels can be seen to course longitudinally in the esophageal wall. These vessels are absent in the distal 2–3 cm of the esophagus. In the lower third of the esophagus, longitudinal folds can sometimes be seen. The abrupt transition from the squamous epithelium of the esophagus to the shiny, velvety, salmon pink-orange mucosa of the stomach marks the squamocolumnar junction. Recognition of this transition and documenting its location is essential in the diagnosis of Barrett's esophagus. Islands of gastric mucosa may be seen throughout the esophageal body and must be distinguished from the normal squamocolumnar junction.

Inspection of the esophagus includes evaluation of peristalsis. If the patient is asked to swallow when the endoscope is positioned in the proximal esophagus, primary esophageal waves can be seen to traverse the length of the esophagus. The endoscope, especially with insufflation, will stimulate secondary waves, which can be observed to be transmitted from the point of stimulation to the distal esophagus. Tertiary nonpropulsive waves can be seen at esophagoscopy in certain motility disorders.

## Ultrasound Anatomy

The normal esophagus is usually viewed as five discrete layers at endoscopic esophageal ultrasonography (Fig. 9–3). These layers are seen as alternating hyperechoic (white) and hypoechoic (black) rings. The five layers correspond to the balloon/mucosa interface, the mucosa deep to this interface, the submucosa and the acoustic interface between the submucosa and the muscularis propria, the muscularis propria minus the acoustic interface between the submucosa and the muscularis propria, and the periesophageal tissue.[12,13] For clinical purposes these layers represent the superficial mucosa, the deep mucosa, the submucosa, the muscularis propria, and the periesophageal tissue. In the upper esophagus or with overdistention of the examining balloon, only three layers of the esophageal wall may be apparent on the ultrasound image: the superficial mucosa, deep mucosa, and submucosa are compressed into one hyperechoic layer (Fig. 9–3). The thickness of each ultrasound band is approximately equal and represents the time it takes the ultrasound wave to traverse this tissue layer, and not the thickness of the tissue.

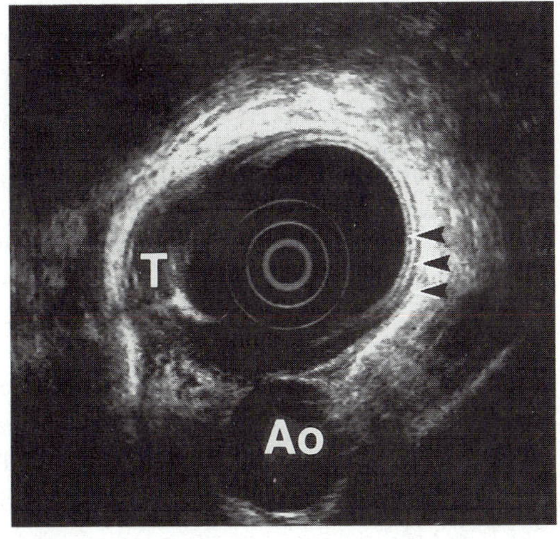


A

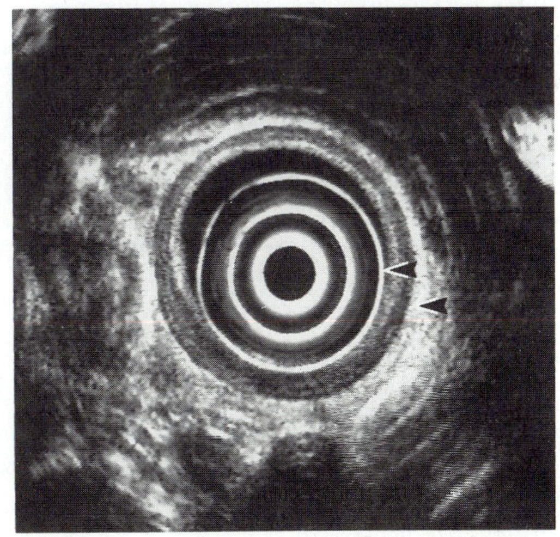

B

**Figure 9–3.** The esophageal ultrasonography image of the esophageal wall. **A.** Five layers—the first layer (upper arrow) is hyperechoic (white) and represents the superficial mucosa. The second layer is hypoechoic (black) and represents the deep mucosa. The third layer (middle arrow) is hyperechoic (white) and represents the submucosa. The fourth layer is hypoechoic (black) and represents the muscularis propria. The fifth layer (lower arrow) is hyperechoic (white) and represents the periesophageal tissue. Ao is the aorta. T is a hypoechoic tumor. **B.** Three layers—the first layer (upper arrow) is hyperechoic (white) and represents the mucosa and submucosa. The second layer is hypoechoic (black) and represents the muscularis propria. The third layer (lower arrow) is hyperechoic (white) and represents the periesophageal tissue. *(From Rice TW, Boyce GA, Sivak MV Jr: Esophageal ultrasound and the preoperative staging of carcinoma of the esophagus. J Thorac Cardiovasc Surg 101:536, 1991, with permission.)*

## INDICATIONS

Esophagoscopy is indicated in the evaluation of dysphagia, odynophagia, heartburn, regurgitation, atypical chest pain, and upper GI bleeding. Esophagoscopy is useful in the definition of abnormalities seen on barium esophagram and chest roentgenogram.[14] Strictures, diverticula of the esophageal body, ulcers, tumors, intramural masses, varices, hiatal hernias, and aspiration pneumonia may all require further evaluation at esophagoscopy. Established esophageal diseases such as esophagitis, chemical injuries, infections, achalasia, scleroderma, diffuse esophageal spasm, and esophageal neoplasms may require esophagoscopy during the management of these disorders. Esophagoscopy is the best means of surveillance of patients at risk for esophageal malignancies. Patients with Barrett's esophagus and treated esophageal malignancies should undergo routine endoscopy and biopsy. Esophagoscopy is also indicated in the postoperative evaluation of patients who have had resection or repair of esophageal disorders.

Therapeutic esophagoscopy is indicated for the dilatation of strictures, coagulation of upper GI bleeding sites, laser ablation of esophageal malignancies, placement of esophageal stents, removal of foreign bodies, and sclerosis of esophageal varices.

Endoscopic esophageal ultrasonography is primarily indicated for the clinical staging of esophageal malignancies and the restaging of treated esophageal carcinomas. It is extremely useful in the investigation of intramural esophageal lesions and extra-esophageal lesions that are adjacent to the esophageal wall. Endoscopic esophageal ultrasonography may be used to direct transesophageal fine-needle aspiration of extramucosal structures.

Endoscopy is contraindicated in uncooperative or moribund patients, patients with severe cardiac or pulmonary compromise, and patients with certain cervical vertebral diseases.[15] Age is not a contraindication to esophagoscopy.[16] If an experienced endoscopist or appropriate equipment is not available, the examination should be postponed.

## ESOPHAGEAL DISORDERS

### Esophageal Carcinoma

Flexible esophagoscopy is the procedure of choice for the diagnosis of esophageal carcinoma (Fig. 9–4, 9–5, see Color Plates following page 608). Modern endoscopy equipment provides excellent visualization of all areas of the upper GI tract, including the cervical esophagus, esophagogastric junction, and gastric cardia. In addition, flexible endoscopy permits assessment of the GI tract distal to obstructing esophageal carcinomas in approximately 80% of patients.[17] Inspection of the mucosa distant from the primary tumor site allows detection of intramural metastases, which are associated with advanced tumor stage and decreased survival. Intramural metastases have been reported to occur in 11.9% of patients with squamous cell carcinoma of the esophagus.[18]

The clinical diagnosis of esophageal carcinoma requires tissue confirmation prior to treatment. Improved equipment and techniques have increased the diagnostic capabilities of fiberoptic endoscopic biopsy from 70–80% to nearly 100%.[19–22] The number of biopsy specimens obtained increases the diagnostic yield from 93% for one specimen to 98–100% with six or seven specimens. Lusink and colleagues[23] reported flexible endoscopy to be unreliable in the diagnosis of adenocarcinoma of the lower esophagus due to inflammation of the mucosa and tumor infiltration of the submucosa. Recent work reports that neither site nor type of malignancy adversely affects diagnostic yield.[22] The area biopsied within an esophageal lesion has not been reported to influence diagnostic accuracy. However, if an esophageal ulcer is encountered, experience with gastric ulcers shows the combination of biopsies from the rim of the ulcer, and the ulcer crater provides a diagnostic accuracy of 95%.[24]

Endoscopic cytology brushings of esophageal lesions are easily obtained and should be considered for all lesions. Brush cytology has a reported accuracy of 80–97% and a false positive rate of 0.3–2.0%.[19,20,25–27] O'Donoghue and colleagues[27] analyzed both endoscopic brush cytology and biopsy and reported a sensitivity of 81% and 87%, specificity of 98% and 99%, and positive predictive value of 92% and 96%, respectively, in the diagnosis of esophageal malignancies. Brush cytology is particularly helpful when adequate biopsies are difficult to obtain, such as with small, superficial cancers or strictures. It has been reported that when obstructing lesions preclude biopsy, cytology may provide a diagnosis in 75% of patients.[28] The diagnostic yield of endoscopic biopsy is increased with the addition of brush cytology by as much as 20.8%.[28] Cytology specimens should be obtained before biopsies. The accuracy of brush cytology is reduced from 93.5% to 82.6% if done after biopsy.[29] The accuracy of endoscopic biopsy is not altered by preceding brush cytology. Brush cytology is complementary to biopsy and may be used to improve diagnostic yield.

Endoscopic fine-needle aspiration may be helpful in the diagnosis of mucosal and submucosal esophageal lesions. This procedure should be reserved for deeper lesions and those that remain undiagnosed by both biopsy and brush cytology.[30,31]

Rigid esophagoscopy allows large biopsy specimens to be obtained and may permit assessment of fixation of an esophageal carcinoma. Without insufflation and magnification, the esophageal assessment may be difficult and incomplete. However, examination of the entire esophagus with rigid esophagoscopy was possible in 79% of patients with esophageal carcinoma.[32] It has been reported that the passage of the rigid scope through a tumor increases the risk of perforation from negligible levels to 1.13%.[33] Although rigid esophagoscopy may be as likely as flexible esophagoscopy to allow passage of the instrument through the carcinoma, examination of the esophagogastric junction is inferior, and examination of the stomach and duodenum is not possible with rigid esophagoscopy. General anesthesia is usually required for this examination. Since flexible endoscopy provides more information, is easier and safer to perform, and is better tolerated than rigid esophagoscopy, rigid esophagoscopy should be reserved for failure of flexible fiberoptic esophagoscopy.

Endoscopic esophageal ultrasound is the most accurate modality for the determination of depth of tumor invasion prior to treatment.[10,34–38] This is a result of the definition of the esophageal wall and the periesophageal tissue afforded by esophageal ultrasonography. Although five ultrasound layers are seen in the examination of the esophagus and periesophageal tissues, it is the fourth ultrasound layer, which represents the muscularis propria, that must be examined carefully to differentiate T1, T2, and T3 tumors (Fig. 9–6, 9–7, and 9–8). The same definition of the esophageal wall is not offered by computed tomography (CT). The thickened esophageal wall, the principal CT finding in esophageal carcinoma, is not specific for esophageal carcinoma and lacks the definition required to distinguish T1, T2, and T3 tumors.[39]

In the differentiation of T3 and T4 tumors, esophageal ultrasonography is superior to CT (Fig. 9–9). The evaluation of fat planes is used to define local invasion at CT examination. The obliteration or lack of fat planes is not sensitive in the prediction of local invasion; however, the preservation of these planes is specific for the absence of T4 disease.[40–46] In the evaluation of aortic invasion, obliteration of the smooth contour of a quarter or more of the circumference of the aorta and an angle of contact between the tumor and the aorta greater than 45 degrees are the CT criteria for aortic invasion. Compared with CT, esophageal ultrasonography provides a more sensitive and reliable determination of vascular involvement.[47]

Despite its superiority, there are shortcomings of endoscopic esophageal ultrasonography in the determination of depth of tumor invasion. There is a learning curve for ultrasonography. Improved technical and interpretative skills have increased the accuracy of determination of depth of tumor invasion from 59% to 81% at our institution.[48,49] Loss of definition of the first three ultrasound layers and their merging into one layer makes the identification of early stage carcinoma difficult, and may lead to the overstaging of these tumors.[48] The inability to pass the ultrasound probe through a malignant stricture occurs in a significant number of patients. Attempts at staging the tumor in the region above the stenosis is inaccurate.[11,50] Despite this incomplete examination, the inability to advance the ultrasound probe through the malignant stricture is a finding that is highly predictive of advanced disease. Ninety-one percent of patients in whom the malignant stricture was severe enough to prevent passage of the ultrasound probe had stage III or IV tumors.[11]

In the assessment of regional lymph nodes, CT relies solely on lymph node size to predict metastatic disease. Studies of mediastinal lymph nodes of normal patients show that N0 nodes are usually < 1.0 cm and not > 1.6 cm in largest dimension.[51,52] Regional lymph nodes > 1.5 cm are considered suspicious for N1 disease. As well as size, esophageal ultrasonography evaluates nodal shape, border,

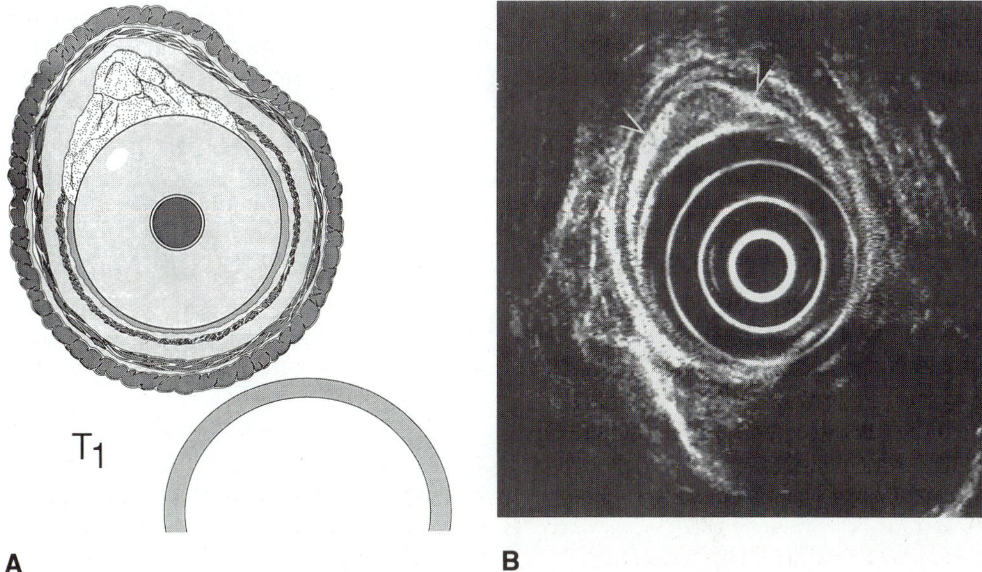


**Figure 9–6. A.** A T1 tumor invades but does not breach the submucosa. **B.** A T1 tumor as seen at esophageal ultrasonography. The hypoechoic (black) tumor invades the hyperechoic (white) third ultrasound layer (submucosa) but does not breach the boundary between the third and fourth layers (arrows). *(From Rice TW, Boyce GA, Sivak MV Jr: Esophageal ultrasound and the preoperative staging of carcinoma of the esophagus. J Thorac Cardiovasc Surg 101:536, 1991, with permission.)*

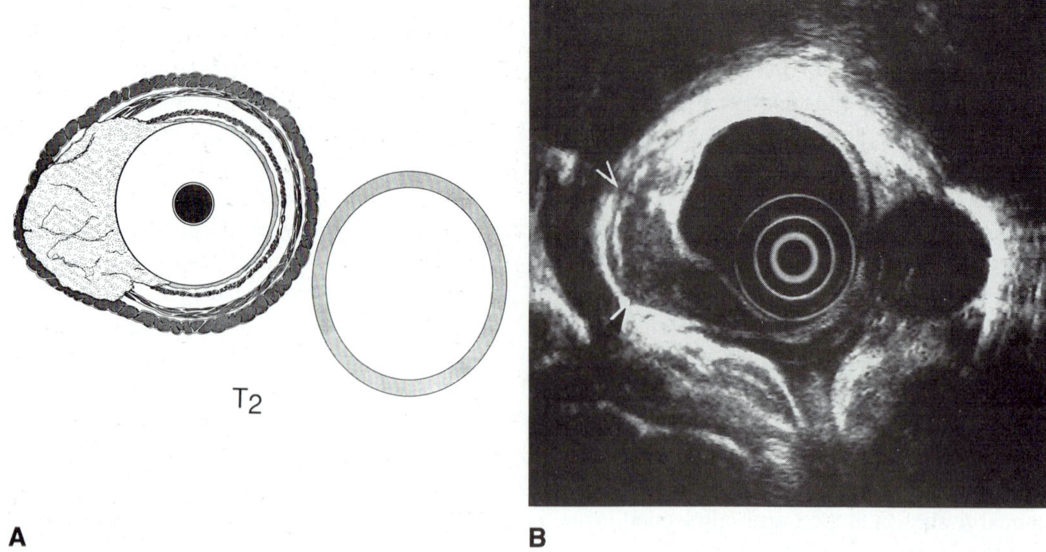


**Figure 9–7.** **A.** A T2 tumor invades but does not breach the muscularis propria. **B.** A T2 tumor as seen at esophageal ultrasonography. The hypoechoic (black) tumor invades the hypoechoic (black) fourth ultrasound layer but does not breach the boundary between the fourth and fifth layers (arrows). *(From Rice TW, Boyce GA, Sivak MV Jr: Esophageal ultrasound and the preoperative staging of carcinoma of the esophagus. J Thorac Cardiovasc Surg 101:536, 1991, with permission.)*

and internal echo characteristics in regional lymph node assessment (Fig. 9–10). These additional factors account for the superiority of endoscopic esophageal ultrasonography in the determination of regional lymph node status.[10,34,36–38] The major shortcomings of esophageal ultrasonography in the determination of N are the inability to detect micrometastases, which may not display detectable ultrasonographic changes, and to differentiate large inflammatory nodes from nodal metastases, which sometimes share the same esophageal ultrasonography findings. These problems may be overcome by endoscopic esophageal ultrasonography-directed, fine-needle aspiration of indeterminate nodes.[53] The prediction of regional lymph node metastases may be extrapolated from the ultrasonographic determination of depth of tumor invasion. The incidence of lymph node metastases increases with increasing depth of

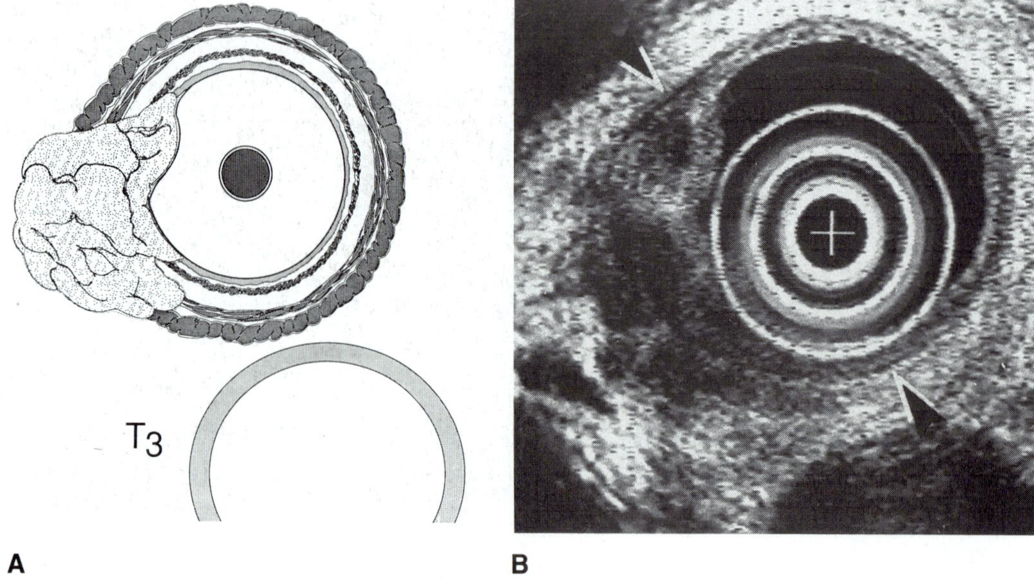


**Figure 9–8.** **A.** A T3 tumor invades the periesophageal tissue but does not involve adjacent structures. **B.** A T3 tumor as seen at esophageal ultrasonography. The hypoechoic (black) tumor breaches the boundary between the fourth and fifth ultrasound layers (arrows) and invades the hyperechoic (white) fifth ultrasound layer (periesophageal tissue). *(From Rice TW, Boyce GA, Sivak MV Jr: Esophageal ultrasound and the preoperative staging of carcinoma of the esophagus. J Thorac Cardiovasc Surg 101:536, 1991, with permission.)*

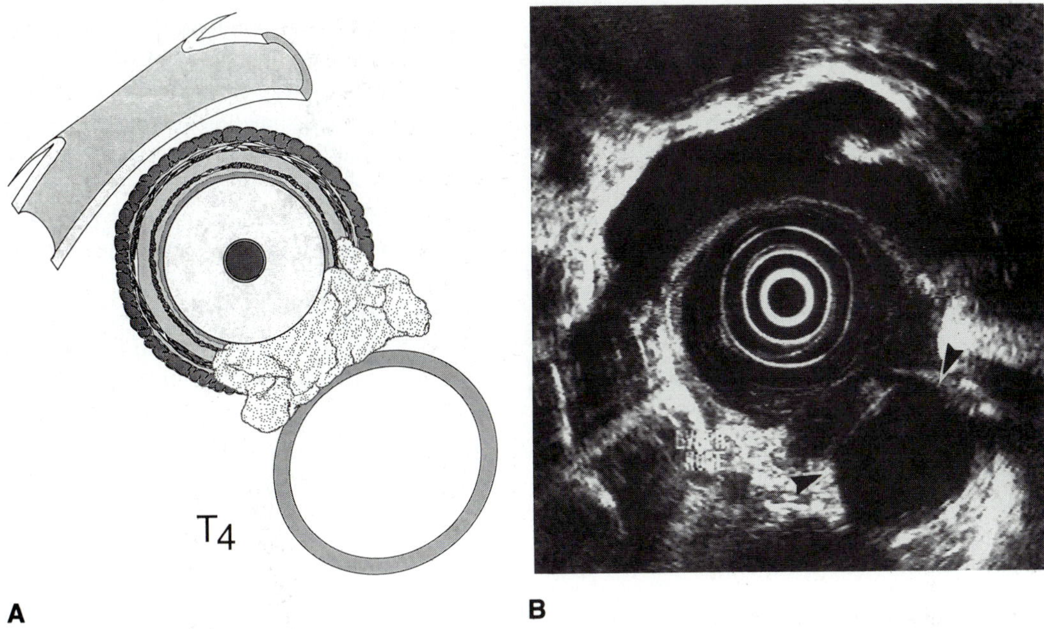


**Figure 9–9. A.** A T4 tumor invades the aorta. **B.** A T4 tumor as seen at esophageal ultrasonography. The hypoechoic (black) tumor invades the aorta. The tumor breaches the boundary between the periesophageal tissue and the aorta (arrows). *(From Rice TW, Boyce GA, Sivak MV Jr: Esophageal ultrasound and the preoperative staging of carcinoma of the esophagus. J Thorac Cardiovasc Surg 101:536, 1991, with permission.)*

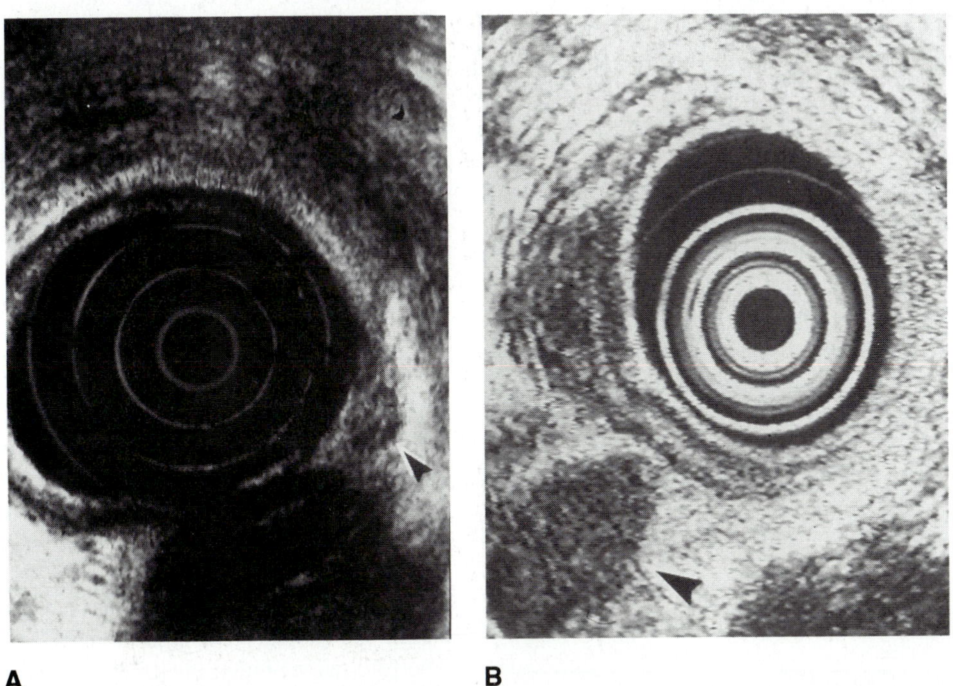


**Figure 9–10. A.** A N0 node (arrow) as seen at esophageal ultrasonography. The node is 5 mm in diameter and has an ill-defined border and a hyperechoic (white) internal structure. **B.** An N1 node (arrow) as seen at esophageal ultrasonography. The large node, 12 mm in diameter, has a sharply demarcated border. The internal structure is hypoechoic (black) and is similar to that of the primary tumor (T). *(From Rice TW, Boyce GA, Sivak MV Jr: Esophageal ultrasound and the preoperative staging of carcinoma of the esophagus. J Thorac Cardiovasc Surg 101:536, 1991, with permission.)*

tumor invasion.[34,54] This association of T with N may be one of the most sensitive indicators of regional lymph node metastases (Table 9–1).[55,56]

Endoscopic esophageal ultrasonography is of limited value in the assessment of sites of distant metastases. Esophageal ultrasonography is only useful if the distant organ is in direct contact with the upper GI tract (Fig. 9–11). The celiac axis and left lateral segment of the liver are two such sites.

Endoscopic esophageal ultrasonography has been used in the assessment of induction therapy prior to resection and in the evaluation of palliative therapy in patients who are inoperable and therefore will not undergo pathologic staging.[57,58] In these situations, restaging may prove difficult. After treatment it may not be possible to differentiate fibrosis and tumor necrosis from viable tumor.[59] Esophageal ultrasonography has been useful in the diagnosis and restaging of patients with anastomotic recurrences that are not endoscopically visible.[60]

## Intramural Tumors

At esophagoscopy, an intramural tumor appears as an extramucosal mass bulging into the lumen with no involvement of the esophageal mucosa (Fig. 9–12, see Color Plates following page 608). These tumors are usually mobile, and the endoscope can generally pass without any evidence of obstruction. It is difficult to differentiate these uncommon tumors at esophagoscopy. There are few features or locations that are pathognomonic for any tumor. If a hemangioma lies superficially in the submucosa, it will appear as a bluish mass that will blanch with pressure exerted by the tip of the endoscope. If the overlying mucosa is normal, biopsy is contraindicated, for it may complicate enucleation.

The detailed examination of the esophageal wall provided by endoscopic esophageal ultrasonography has improved the diagnosis of benign esophageal tumors. The identification of intramural masses relies on both the ultrasound characteristics of the tumor and the layer from which the tumor arises. Leiomyomas of the esophagus originate in the fourth layer of the esophagus as local thickening and are typically sharply defined hypoechoic tumors (Fig. 9–13). It may be difficult to differentiate a leiomyoma from a leiomyosarcoma. The probability of malignancy is greater for lesions >4 cm in diameter. Heterogeneous internal echoes, large internal blood vessels, ulceration, and visualization of regional lymph nodes are all suggestive of malignancy.[61] Cysts and lipomas arise from the third ultrasound layer (submucosa) of the esophageal wall.[62] Cysts are echo-free, rounded, and sometimes septated. Lipomas are homogeneous, intensely hyperechoic lesions. Lipomas can often be recognized by endoscopy alone, since they frequently have a yellow tint and are soft and pliable when probed. Granular cell tumors also arise in the submucosa. These tumors have hypoechoic ultrasound characteristics and are very well demarcated.[63] Endoscopically guided fine-needle aspiration or biopsy may increase the diagnostic accuracy of endoscopic ultrasound in the evaluation of submucosal tumors.[64,65]

**TABLE 9–1. ASSOCIATION OF TUMORS AND REGIONAL LYMPH NODES**

| | Percentage of Tumors with N1 Disease | | | | |
|---|---|---|---|---|---|
| | *Tis* | *T1* | *T2* | *T3* | *T4* |
| Catalano[55] | 0 | 14.3 | 33.3 | 73.3 | 85.7 |
| Dittler[56] | — | 4 | 52 | 82 | 91 |

## Esophageal Varices

Esophageal varices have variable appearances at esophagoscopy depending upon their complexity and previous treatment. They can lie deep in the muscular wall or entirely extraluminal and may not be visible at esophagoscopy. In a patient with known varices, a complete upper GI endoscopy is required during each bleeding episode to exclude other common sources of upper GI bleeding. Sclerotherapy is an effective means of bleeding control. No one sclerosing agent has been demonstrated to be superior.[66] Variceal sclerotherapy may be complicated by fever, chest pain, dysphagia, ulcers, and perforation. Complications have been reported to be less frequent with rubber band ligation.[67]

Esophageal varices have the typical appearance of blood vessels at endoscopic esophageal ultrasonography. They appear as tubular, round, or serpiginous echo-free structures. They may be visualized within the submucosal layer of the esophageal wall or in tissues adjacent to the esophagus. These ultrasonographic patterns change following sclerosis.[68] Intravariceal sclerosis fills the varix with echogenic material, representing thrombus. Paravariceal injection leads to obliteration of the varix with hypoechoic extravariceal thickening.

## Gastroesophageal Reflux Disease (GERD)

Hiatal hernia, reflux esophagitis, Schatzki's ring, peptic stricture, and Barrett's esophagus are part of the spectrum of endoscopic findings seen at esophagoscopy in patients with GERD. An understanding of the esophagogastric junction (EGJ) and its anatomic landmarks is critical to the endoscopist in defining a hiatal hernia and diagnosing the complications of GERD. EGJ can be defined as the point at which the tubular esophagus joins the saccular stomach. The EGJ can be either muscular or mucosal. The muscular EGJ is defined manometrically as the distal most portion of the lower esophageal sphincter (LES). LES is a 2–4-cm zone of increased resting pressure that is higher than the pressure in the stomach or esophageal body. Although LES can be defined physiologically, no distinct anatomic struc-

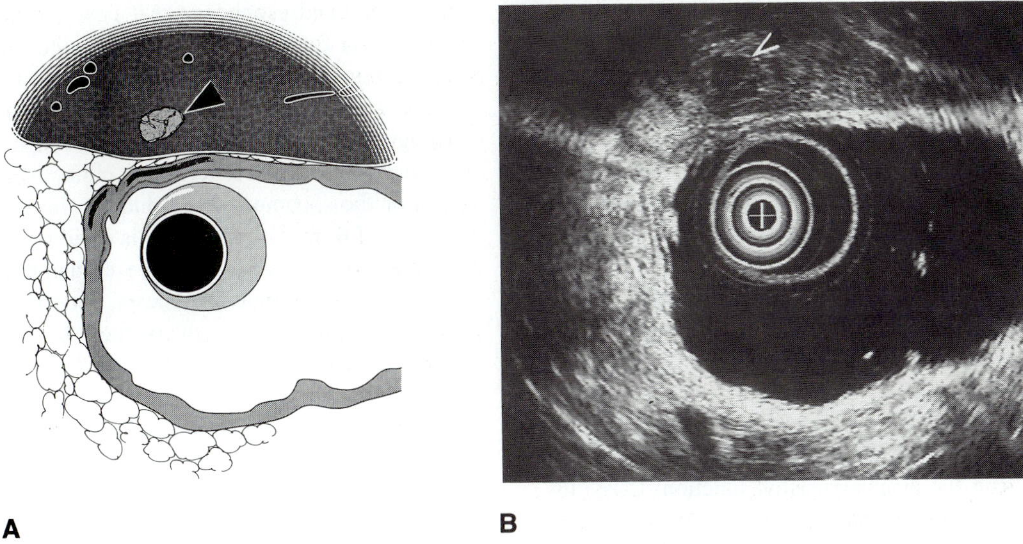


**Figure 9–11. A.** A hepatic metastasis (arrow) in the left lateral segment of the liver. The ultrasound probe is seen in the gastric cardia. **B.** The hepatic metastasis (arrow) as seen from the gastric cardia by ultrasonography; the metastasis was imaged only by esophageal ultrasonography. *(From Rice TW, Boyce GA, Sivak MV, et al: Esophageal carcinoma: Esophageal ultrasound assessment of preoperative chemotherapy. Ann Thorac Surg 53:972, 1992.)*

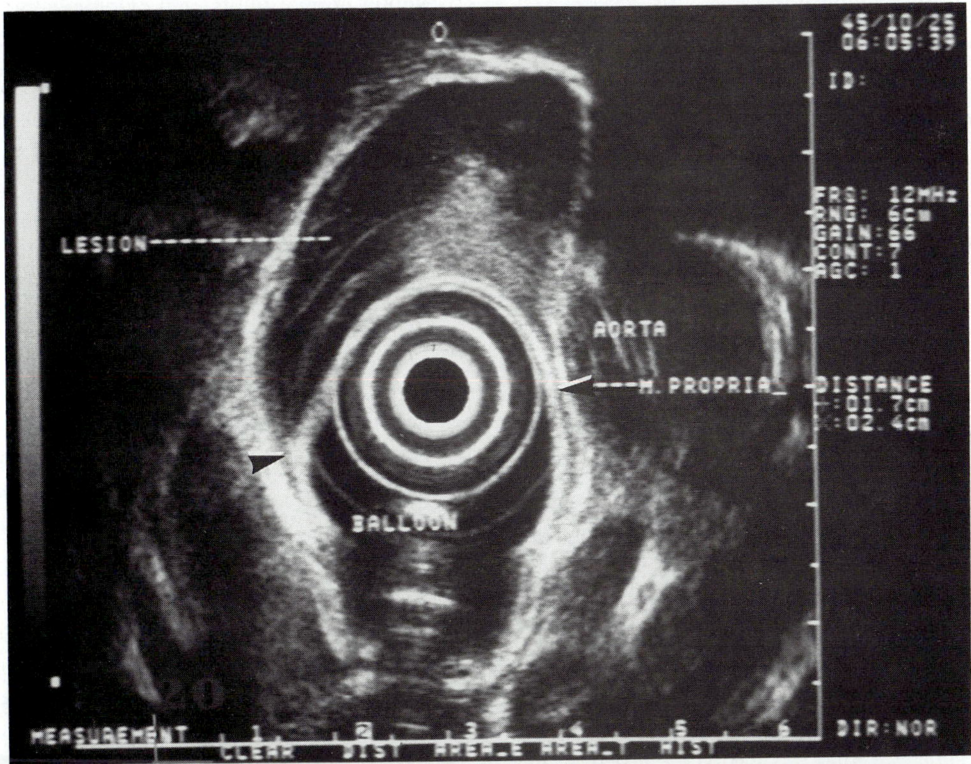


**Figure 9–13.** An esophageal leiomyoma as seen at esophageal ultrasonography hypoechoic. The leiomyoma (lesion) can be seen arising from the hypoechoic, fourth ultrasound layer (arrows). This intramural mass in confined to this layer with no invasion of adjacent layers; there is a hyperechoic portion that suggests necrosis.

ture has been identified. Endoscopically, the proximal margin of the gastric folds has been shown to approximate closely the muscular EGJ.[69] The mucosal EGJ, which normally lies within LES, does not correspond to the muscular EGJ and is usually 1–2 cm above the muscular junction. If the muscular EGJ is used to define the limits of the esophagus, the distal 1–2 cm of the esophagus is lined by columnar epithelium that is either gastric cardiac or fundic in type. It is for this reason, that in the absence of intestinal metaplasia, many physicians require at least 3 cm of columnar epithelium above the EGJ before the diagnosis of Barrett's esophagus is accepted.

The diagnosis of a type I hiatal hernia requires the esophagogastric junction to be displaced above the diaphragm. Generally the squamocolumnar junction is used to identify grossly the esophagogastric junction. Large hiatal hernias are easily appreciated, since the squamocolumnar junction is seen well above the diaphragm and the diaphragmatic impression is located about the intrathoracic portion of the stomach. Smaller hiatal hernias are sometimes easier to verify with the retroflexed endoscopy placed in the stomach (Fig. 9–14, see Color Plates following page 608). Type II hiatal hernias may be more easily appreciated with a retroflexed view from the gastric body (Fig. 9–15, see Color Plates following page 608).

Reflux esophagitis can be visually graded. The classification of Sonnenberg and colleagues is a simple scheme[70]:

- Grade 1: (mild) isolated linear or round erosions
- Grade 2: (severe) confluence of erosions involving the total luminal circumference
- Grade 3: (complicated) grade 1 or 2 erosions associated with deep ulcers, strictures, or Barrett's esophagus

Esophagitis should be confirmed by biopsy in all cases of suspected reflux esophagitis.

A Schatzki's ring, which is located at the squamocolumnar junction, is a benign disorder presenting with dysphagia. Histologically the ring is the result of fibrosis in lamina propria, muscularis propria, or submucosa. Endoscopically a Schatzki's ring appears as a circumferential constriction at the squamocolumnar junction with maximal esophageal distension. There is always an associated hiatal hernia and rarely reflux esophagitis.

Esophagoscopy is the crucial invasive investigation in the diagnosis of peptic esophageal strictures. A diagnosis can be obtained at endoscopy in 90–95% of patients.[71,72] Cytologic brushing of the stricture must be added to random biopsy to reach this level of diagnostic accuracy. Endoscopy, biopsy, and dilatation can be safely performed at one sitting.[73] After dilatation, careful endoscopic examination of the stricture and the distal GI tract is required.

Barrett's esophagus may be easily identified if the squamocolumnar junction has retreated well above the gastroesophageal junction (Fig. 9–16, see Color Plates following page 608). Short-segment Barrett's esophagus, which is a columnar lined esophagus that is < 3 cm in length, requires biopsy for diagnosis. Biopsy is indicated in all suspected cases of Barrett's esophagus to confirm the diagnosis and to assess dysplasia. If a biopsy specimen from the esophagus shows specialized epithelium with goblet cells or columnar epithelium overlying either the submucosal glands or the squamous-lined duct of these glands, then a diagnosis of Barrett's esophagus is established. However, if either cardiac-type or fundic-type epithelium is present in the absence of intestinal metaplasia, underlying submucosal glands, or squamous-lined ducts, then the changes are consistent with Barrett's esophagus only if the specimen comes from an area above LES.

A metaplasia-dysplasia-carcinoma sequence, similar to that described in the colon, has been to be hypothesized present in Barrett's esophagus.[74] Dysplasia is unequivocally neoplastic epithelium that is confined within the basement membrane of the glands from which it arose. Once a diagnosis of Barrett's esophagus is established, patients should be placed into a cancer surveillance program, with the identification of epithelial dysplasia as the surveillance goal. Histologically, a diagnosis of dysplasia is based on both architectural and cytologic changes that suggest a neoplastic transformation. A dysplasia classification, which is a modification of the classification for dysplasia in inflammatory bowel disease,[75] has been applied to Barrett's esophagus, and is as follows:

- *Negative for dysplasia*: The mucosal architecture is within normal limits, and cytologically there is little nuclear hyperchromatism or pleomorphism.
- *Indefinite for dysplasia*: In areas adjacent to erosions or ulcerations, inflammatory reactive changes may be difficult to differentiate from low-grade dysplasia. In general, true dysplasia is characterized by more prominent nuclear enlargement and hyperchromasia as well as more irregular nuclear contours and nuclear crowding than is seen in inflammatory repair. However, since it is often difficult to differentiate between these two, the term *indefinite for dysplasia* is acceptable.
- *Positive for dysplasia*: These biopsies show both cytologic and architectural abnormalities that suggest neoplastic transformation. Both low- and high-grade dysplasia are recognized depending upon the severity of the changes.
- *Intramucosal carcinoma*: This is a carcinoma that has penetrated through the glandular basement membrane and into the lamina propria, but there is no transgression of the muscularis mucosae.

Despite these criteria, there is still considerable interobserver variation in the diagnosis of dysplasia. In a consensus conference, intramucosal carcinoma and high-grade dysplasia had the best interobserver agreement in this histologic classification, with 85% and 87% agreement in successive reviews of selected cases.[76] In this study, "negative for dysplasia" had only 71% and 72% agreement among experienced GI pathologists.

Endoscopic esophageal ultrasonography has not been helpful in the surveillance of patients with Barrett's esophagus. The mucosal definition provided by esophageal ultrasonography cannot differentiate dysplasia from intramucosal carcinoma.[77]

### Motility Disorders

Endoscopy is indicated in achalasia to exclude the mucosal complications of esophagitis and squamous cell carcinoma (Fig. 9–17, see Color Plates following page 608). A careful inspection of the stomach with a retroflexed examination of EGJ is necessary to rule out an obstructing carcinoma of the cardia masquerading as achalasia. Endoscopy is indicated in diffuse esophageal spasm (DES) to exclude other disorders that may be misdiagnosed as DES. The endoscopic finding of scleroderma are those seen complicating gastroesophageal reflux. The lack of peristalsis and monilial esophagitis in advanced cases may be recognized at endoscopy.

The endoscopic ultrasonographic findings in achalasia are controversial. Some authors have reported thickened esophageal wall in most patients examined.[78,79] However, this excessive thickening may be artifactual. In a dilated and convoluted esophagus, the ultrasound transducer may orient at an angle oblique to the esophageal wall, giving a false appearance of wall.[80] The main role of ultrasonography in achalasia is to exclude other mural abnormalities.[81,82]

### Diverticula

A Zenker's diverticulum is a relative contraindication to esophagoscopy. If endoscopic inspection is required to investigate a mass lesion complicating a Zenker's diverticulum or to study associated upper GI pathology, passage of the endoscope under direct vision is compulsory. The endoscopic evaluation of an epiphrenic diverticulum (Fig. 9–18, see Color Plates following page 608) is mandated by the associated motility disorder, hiatal hernia, or stricture.

### Paraesophageal Diseases

Endoscopic esophageal ultrasonography has been used to examine mediastinal lymph nodes in patients with bronchogenic carcinoma.[83,84] In this setting, esophageal sonography has a reported positive value of 77%, a negative predictive value of 93%, and an overall accuracy of 92%, by using criteria similar to that used for regional lymph node evaluation in esophageal carcinoma.[84] However, anatomic constraints limit its usefulness for evaluation of lymph nodes in proximity to the airway.

Endoscopic esophageal ultrasonography has proven useful in the diagnosis of foregut cysts.[85,86] These cysts are generally hypoechoic and located outside the esophageal wall. They may occasionally be found within the esophageal wall. If foregut cysts contain proteinaceous material, they may have a hyperechoic or an inhomogeneous (hyper/hypoechoic) ultrasound appearance. Extrinsic esophageal compression may also be characterized with endosonography.[87] However, examination of structures distant from the esophagus is best performed with transducers of lower frequencies. Transesophageal cardiac ultrasound provides better definition of these structures using probes with frequencies of 3–5 MHz.

## COMPLICATIONS

Flexible fiberoptic esophagoscopy is an extremely safe procedure. The overall complication rate for upper GI endoscopy is in the range of 0.1%, and the mortality rate is <0.005%.[88] Cardiopulmonary complications are the most frequent complications. Careful monitoring and oxygen supplementation during the procedure may minimize these problems.

Esophageal perforation is the most feared complication of esophagoscopy. Replacement of rigid endoscopy with flexible fiberoptic endoscopy has significantly reduced perforations (from 0.11% or more to 0.03%) but has not eliminated them. Perforations are more likely to occur during complex examinations, therapeutic esophagoscopy, or when there is significant esophageal pathology. Prompt recognition and treatment will minimize further morbidity and mortality. It should be suspected in a patient who complains of excessive and prolonged pain following esophagoscopy. Subcutaneous emphysema and a pneumothorax may be detected on physical examination. An urgent chest roentgenogram will demonstrate a hydropneumothorax and possibly mediastinal and subcutaneous emphysema. Early surgical intervention is required with lavage and debridement of the mediastinum and pleural cavity, repair of the perforation, and surgical management of the underlying pathology. Rarely, there may be a contained leak with free, preferential drainage into the esophagus, which may be managed nonsurgically.

Other less frequent complications of esophagoscopy include bacteremia, cerebral abscess, septic arthritis, bacterial endocarditis, bleeding, and equipment failure.[88,89]

## REFERENCES


1. Bianchi Porro G, Baroni S, Parente F, et al: Midazolam versus diazepam as premedication for upper gastrointestinal endoscopy: A randomized, double-blind, crossover study. *Gastrointest Endosc* **34:**252, 1988
2. Carrougher JG, Kadakia S, Shaffer RT, et al: Venous complications of midazolam versus diazepam. *Gastrointest Endosc* **39:**396, 1993
3. Birkenfeld S, Federico C, Dermansky-Avni Y, et al: Double-blind controlled trial of flumazenil in patients who underwent upper gastrointestinal endoscopy. *Gastrointest Endosc* **35:**519, 1989
4. Hayward SR, Sugawa C, Wilson RF: Changes in oxygenation and pulse rate during endoscopy. *Am Surg* **55:**198, 1989
5. Dark DS, Campbell DR, Wesselium LJ: Arterial oxygen desaturation

during gastrointestinal endoscopy. *Am J Gastroenterol* **85:**1317, 1990

6. Dancygier H, Classen M: Endoscopic ultrasonography in esophageal disease. *Gastrointest Endosc* **35:**220, 1989
7. Heyder N, Lux G: Malignant lesions of the upper gastrointestinal tract. *Scand J Gastroenterol* **123:**47, 1986
8. Takemoto T, Ito T, Aibe T, et al: Endoscopic ultrasonography in the diagnosis of esophageal carcinoma with particular regard to staging it for operability. *Endoscopy* **3:**22, 1986.
9. Tio TL, Schouwink MH, Cikot RJ, et al: Preoperative TNM classification of gastric carcinoma by endosonography in comparison with the pathological TNM system: A prospective study of 72 cases. *Hepato-Gastroenterol* **36:**51, 1989.
10. Vilgrain V, Mompoint D, Palazzo L, et al: Staging of esophageal carcinoma: Comparison of results with endoscopic sonography and CT. *AJR* **155:**277, 1990
11. Van Dam J, Rice TW, Catalano MF, et al: High-grade malignant stricture is predictive of esophageal tumor stage. Risks of endosonographic evaluation. *Cancer* **71:**2910, 1993
12. Bolondi L, Casanova P, Santi V, et al: The sonographic appearance of the normal gastric wall: An in vitro study. *Ultrasound Med Biol* **12:**991, 1986
13. Kimmey MB, Martin RW, Hagitt RC, et al: Histologic correlates of gastrointestinal ultrasound images. *Gastroenterology* **96:**433, 1989
14. Tabibian N: Endoscopy versus x-ray studies of the gastrointestinal tract: future health care implications. *South Med J* **84:**219, 1991
15. Welsh LW, Welsh JJ, Chinnici JC: Endoscopic problems due to cervical vertebral diseases. *Ann Otol Rhinol Laryngol* **98:**597, 1989
16. Brussaard CC, Vandewoude MF: A prospective analysis of elective upper gastrointestinal endoscopy in the elderly. *Gastrointest Endosc* **34:**118, 1988
17. Cheung HC, Siu KF, Wong J: A comparison of flexible and rigid endoscopy in evaluating esophageal cancer patients for surgery. *World J Surg* **12:**117, 1988
18. Takubo K, Sasajima K, Yamashita K, et al: Prognostic significance of intramural metastasis in patients with esophageal carcinoma. *Cancer* **65:**1816, 1990
19. Prolla JC, Reilly W, Kirsner JB, et al: Direct-vision endoscopic cytology and biopsy in the diagnosis of esophageal and gastric tumors: current experience. *Acta Cytol* **21:**399, 1977
20. Witzel L, Halter F, Gretillat PA, et al: Evaluation of specific value of endoscopic biopsies and brush cytology for malignancies of the esophagus and stomach. *Gut* 17:375,1976
21. Graham DY, Schwartz JT, Cain GD, et al: Prospective evaluation of biopsy number in the diagnosis of esophageal and gastric carcinoma. *Gastroenterology* **82:**228, 1982
22. Lal N, Bhasin DK, Malik AK, et al: Optimal number of biopsy specimens in the diagnosis of carcinoma of the oesophagus. *Gut* **33:**724, 1992
23. Lusink C, Sali A, Chou ST: Diagnostic accuracy of flexible endoscopic biopsy in carcinoma of the oesophagus and cardia. *Aust N Z J Surg* **53:**545, 1983
24. Hatfield AR, Slavin G, Segal AW, et al: Importance of the site of endoscopic gastric biopsy in ulcerating lesions of the stomach. *Gut* **16:**884, 1975
25. Kasugai T, Kobayashi S, Kuno N: Endoscopic cytology of the esophagus, stomach, and pancreas. *Acta Cytol* **22:**327, 1978
26. Chambers LA, Clark WE 2nd: The endoscopic diagnosis of gastroesophageal malignancy. A cytologic review. *Acta Cytol* **30:**110, 1986
27. O'Donoghue J, Waldron R, Gough D, et al: An analysis of the diagnostic accuracy of endoscopic biopsy and cytology in the detection of oesophageal malignancy. *Eur J Surg Oncol* **18:**332, 1992
28. Cusso X, Monés-Xiol J, Vilardell F: Endoscopic cytology of cancer of the esophagus and cardia: a long-term evaluation. *Gastrointest Endosc* **35:**321, 1989
29. Zargar SA, Khuroo MS, Jan GM, et al: Prospective comparison of the value of brushings before and after biopsy in the endoscopic diagnosis of gastroesophageal malignancy. *Acta Cytol* **35:**549, 1991
30. Graham DY, Tabibian N, Michaletz PA, et al: Endoscopic needle biopsy: a comparative study of forceps biopsy, two different types of needles, and salvage cytology in gastrointestinal cancer. *Gastrointest Endosc* **35:**207, 1989
31. Layfield LJ, Reichman A, Weinstein WM: Endoscopically directed fine needle aspiration biopsy of gastric and esophageal lesions. *Acta Cytol* **36:**69, 1992
32. Bacon CK, Hendrix RA: Open tube versus flexible esophagoscopy in adult head and neck endoscopy. *Ann Otol Rhinol Laryngol* **101:**147, 1992
33. Ritchie AJ, McManus K, McGuigan J, et al: The role of rigid oesophagoscopy in oesophageal carcinoma. *Postgrad Med J* **68:**892, 1992
34. Tio TL, Cohen P, Coene PP, et al: Endosonography and computed tomography of esophageal carcinoma. Preoperative classification compared to the new (1987) TNM system. *Gastroenterology* **96:**1478, 1989
35. Date H, Miyashita M, Sasajima K, et al: Assessment of adventitial involvement of esophageal carcinoma by endoscopic ultrasonography. *Surg Endosc* **4:**195, 1990
36. Botet JF, Lightdale CJ, Zauber AG, et al: Preoperative staging of esophageal cancer: comparison of endoscopic US and dynamic CT. *Radiology* **181:**426, 1991
37. Heintz A, Hohne U, Schweden F, et al: Preoperative detection of intrathoracic tumor spread of esophageal cancer: endosonography versus computer tomography. *Surg Endosc* **5:**75, 1991
38. Ziegler K, Sanft C, Zeitz M, et al: Evaluation of endosonography in TN staging of oesophageal cancer. *Gut* **32:**16, 1991
39. Reinig JW, Stanley JH, Schabel SI: CT evaluation of thickened esophageal walls. *AJR* **140:**931, 1983
40. Duignan JP, McEntee GP, O'Connell DJ, et al: The role of CT in the management of carcinoma of the oesophagus and cardia. *Ann R Coll Surg Engl* **69:**286, 1987
41. Ruol A, Rossi M, Ruffatto A, et al: Reevaluation of computed tomography in preoperative staging of esophageal and cardial cancers: a prospective study. In Siewert JR, Hölscher AH (eds): *Diseases of the Esophagus*, 1st ed. Berlin, Springer-Verlag 1988, pp 194–197
42. Kasbarian M, Fuentes P, Brichon PY, et al: Usefulness of commuted tomography in assessing the extension of carcinoma of the esophagus and gastroesophageal junction. In Siewart JR, Hölscher AH (eds): *Diseases of the Esophagus*, 1st ed. Berlin, Springer-Verlag, 1988, pp 185-188
43. Markland CG, Manhire A, Davies P, et al: The role of computed tomography in assessing the operability of oesophageal carcinoma. *Eur J Cardio-thorac Surg* **3:**33, 1989
44. Kirk SJ, Moorehead RJ, McIlrath E, et al: Does preoperative computed tomography scanning aid assessment of oesophageal carcinoma? *Postgrad Med J* **66:**191, 1990
45. Søndenaa K, Skaane P, Nygaard K, et al: Value of computed tomography in preoperative evaluation of resectability and staging of oesophageal carcinoma. *Eur J Surg* **158:**537, 1992
46. Consigliere D, Chua CL, Hui F, et al: Computed tomography for oesophageal carcinoma: its value to the surgeon. *J R Coll Surg Edinb* **37:**113, 1992
47. Ginsberg GG, Al-Kawas FH, Nguyen CC, et al: Endoscopic ultrasound evaluation of vascular involvement in esophageal cancer: a comparison with computed tomography. *Gastrointest Endosc* **39:**276, 1993
48. Rice TW, Boyce GA, Sivak MV Jr: Esophageal ultrasound and the preoperative staging of carcinoma of the esophagus. *J Thorac Cardiovasc Surg* **101:**536, 1991
49. Rice TW, Sivak MV Jr, Kirby TJ: Ultrasound staging of esophageal carcinoma. *Can J Surg* **34:**399, 1991
50. Hordijk ML, Zander H, van Blankenstein M, et al: Influence of tumor

stenosis on the accuracy of endosonography in preoperative T staging of esophageal cancer. *Endoscopy* **25:**171, 1993

51. Genereux GP, Howie JL: Normal mediastinal lymph node size and number: CT and anatomic study. *AJR* **142:**1095, 1984
52. Glazer GM, Gross BH, Quint LE, et al: Normal mediastinal lymph nodes: number and size according to American Thoracic Society mapping. *AJR* **144:**261, 1985
53. Wiersema MJ, Kochman ML, Chak A, et al: Real-time endoscopic ultrasound-guided fine-needle aspiration of a mediastinal lymph node. *Gastrointest Endosc* **39:**429, 1993
54. Tio TL, Coene PP, Luiken GJ, et al: Endosonography in the clinical staging of esophagogastric carcinoma. *Gastrointest Endosc* **36:**S2, 1990
55. Catalano MF, Sivak MV Jr, Rice TW, et al: Depth of tumor invasion of esophageal carcinoma (ECA) is predictive of lymph node metastasis: Role of endoscopic ultrasonography (EUS). *Am J Gastroenterol* **87:**1245A, 1992.
56. Dittler HJ, Rosch T, Lorenz R, et al: Failure of endoscopic ultrasonography to differentiate malignant from benign nodes in esophageal cancer. *Gastrointest Endosc* **38:**240A, 1992
57. Rice TW, Boyce GA, Sivak MV, et al: Esophageal carcinoma: esophageal ultrasound assessment of preoperative chemotherapy. *Ann Thorac Surg* **53:**972, 1992
58. Nousbaum JB, Robaszkiewicz M, Cauvin JM, et al: Endosonography can detect residual tumor infiltration after medical treatment of oesophageal cancer in the absence of endoscopic lesions. *Gut* **33:**1459, 1992
59. Souquet JC, Napoleon B, Pujol P, et al: Endosonography-guided treatment of esophageal carcinoma. *Endoscopy* **1:**324, 1992
60. Lightdale CJ, Botet JF, Kelsen DP, et al: Diagnosis of recurrent upper gastrointestinal cancer at the surgical anastomosis by endoscopic ultrasound. *Gastrointest Endosc* **35:**407, 1989
61. Tio TL, Tytgat GN, den Hartog Jager FC: Endoscopic ultrasonography for the evaluation of smooth muscle tumors in the upper gastrointestinal tract: An experience with 42 cases. *Gastrointest Endosc* **36:**342, 1990
62. Yasuda K, Nakajima M, and Kawai K: Endoscopic ultrasonographic imaging of submucosal lesions of the upper gastrointestinal tract. *Gastrointest Endosc Clin North Am* **2:**615, 1992
63. Tada S, Iida M, Yao T, et al: Granular cell tumor of the esophagus: endoscopic ultrasonographic demonstration and endoscopic removal. *Am J Gastroenterol* **85:**1507, 1990
64. Caletti GC, Brocchi E, Ferrari A, et al: Guillotine needle biopsy as a supplement of endosonography in the diagnosis of gastric submucosal tumors. *Endoscopy* **23:**251, 1991
65. Wiersema MJ, Hawes RH, Tao LC, et al: Endoscopic ultrasonography as an adjunct to fine needle aspiration cytology of the upper and lower gastrointestinal tract. *Gastrointest Endosc* **38:**35, 1992
66. Kochhar R, Goenka MK, Mehta S, et al: A comparative evaluation of sclerosants for esophageal varices: a prospective randomized controlled study. *Gastrointest Endosc* **36:**127, 1990
67. Steigmann GV, Goff JS, Michaletz-Onody PA, et al: Endoscopic sclerotherapy as compared with endoscopic ligation for bleeding esophageal varices. *N Engl J Med* **326:**1527, 1992
68. Yasuda K, Cho E, Nakajima M, et al: Diagnosis of submucosal lesions of the upper gastrointestinal tract by endoscopic ultrasonography. *Gastrointest Endosc* **36:**S17, 1990
69. McClave SA, Boyce HW Jr, Gottfried MR: Early diagnosis of columnar-lined esophagus: A new endoscopic criterion. *Gastrointest Endosc* **33:**413, 1987
70. Sonnenberg A, Lepsien G, Muller-Lisner SA, et al: When is esophagitis healed? esophageal endoscopy, histology, and function before and after cimetidine treatment. *Dig Dis Sci* **27:**297, 1982
71. Eastman MC, Gear MW, Nicol A: An assessment of the accuracy of modern endoscopic diagnosis of oesophageal stricture. *Br J Surg* **65:**182, 1978
72. Webb WA, McDaniel L, Jones L: The use of endoscopy in assessment and treatment of peptic strictures of the esophagus. *Am Surg* **50:**476, 1984
73. Barkin JS, Taub S, Rogers AI: The safety of combined endoscopy, biopsy and dilation in esophageal strictures. *Am J Gastroenterol* **76:**23, 1981
74. Hamilton SR, Smith RR: The relationship between columnar epithelial dysplasia and invasive adenocarcinoma arising in Barrett's esophagus. *Am J Clin Pathol* **87:**301, 1987
75. Riddell RH, Goldman H, Ransohoff DF, et al: Dysplasia in inflammatory bowel disease: standardized classification with provisional clinical applications. *Hum Pathol* **14:**931, 1983
76. Reid BJ, Haggitt RC, Rubin CE, et al: Observer variation in the diagnosis of dysplasia in Barrett's esophagus. *Hum Pathol* **19:**166, 1988
77. Falk GW, Catalano MF, Sivak MV Jr, et al: Endosonography in the evaluation of patients with Barrett's esophagus and high-grade dysplasia. *Gastrointest Endosc* **40:**207, 1994
78. Deviere J, Dunham F, Rickaert F, et al: Endoscopic ultrasonography in achalasia. *Gastroenterology* **96:**1210, 1989
79. Bergami GL, Fruhwith R, Di Mario M, et al: Contribution of ultrasonography in the diagnosis of achalasia. *J Pediatr Gastroenterol Nutr* **14:**92, 1992
80. Falk GW, Van Dam J, Sivak MV, et al: Endoscopic ultrasonography (EUS) in achalasia. *Gastrointest Endosc* **37:**241, 1991
81. Ziegler K, Sanft C, Friedrich M, et al: Endosonographic appearance of the esophagus in achalasia. *Endoscopy* **22:**1, 1990
82. Ponsot P, Chaussade S, Palazzo L, et al: Endoscopic ultrasonography in achalasia. *Gastroenterology* **98:**253, 1990
83. Kobayashi H, Danabara T, Sugama Y, et al: Observation of lymph nodes and great vessels in the mediastinum by endoscopic ultrasonography. *Jpn J Med* **26:**353, 1987
84. Kondo D, Imaizumi M, Abe T, et al: Endoscopic ultrasound examination for mediastinal lymph node metastases of lung cancer. *Chest* **98:**586, 1990
85. Rice TW: Benign neoplasms and cysts of the mediastinum. *Sem Thorac Cardiovasc Surg* **4:**25, 1992
86. Van Dam J, Rice TW, Sivak MV Jr: Endoscopic ultrasonography and endoscopically guided needle aspiration for the diagnosis of upper gastrointestinal tract foregut cysts. *Am J Gastroenterol* **87:**762, 1992
87. Silva SA, Kouzu T, Ogino Y, et al: Endoscopic ultrasonography of esophageal tumors and compressions. *J Clin Ultrasound* **16:**149, 1988
88. Pasricha PJ, Fleischer DE, Kalloo AN: Endoscopic perforations of the upper GI tract: A review of their pathogenesis, prevention, and management. *Gastroenterology* **106:**787, 1994
89. Katz D: Morbidity and mortality in standard and flexible gastrointestinal endoscopy. *Gastrointest Endosc* **14:**143, 1967

CHAPTER

# 10

# Bronchoscopy

## *Transbronchial Biopsy and Bronchoalveolar Lavage*

Richard Burr McElvein

### INTRODUCTION

The ability to carefully inspect the tracheobronchial tree with a variety of instruments for both diagnostic and therapeutic purposes is the hallmark of the compleat thoracic surgeon. The bronchoscope is an indispensable instrument for dealing with a wide variety of respiratory tract diseases such as infection and cancer. This chapter will discuss the many facets of bronchoscopy and the use of this instrument in a wide variety of patients and diseases.

### HISTORY

From a candle and a disk of polished metal at the end of a rod to inspect the oropharynx, we have progressed to the point where we have a sophisticated array of devices that allow minute inspection of the airways for diagnosis and treatment.

The first reported endoscopy was in 1895 by Kilian, who was successful in removing a piece a bone from the right main stem bronchus of a patient.[1] Coolidge in 1898 used a urethroscope to remove a displaced portion of a tracheal cannula from the airway. Einhorn in 1902 used an auxiliary light tube for distal illumination. Jackson in 1904 started his large series of foreign body extractions, and his teachings had a profound effect on many who made notable contributions to endoscopy including Moersch, Vinson, Broyles, and Hollinger. The era of flexible instrumentation began in 1930 when Lamm noted the passage of light through a flexible glass fiber. Hopkins in 1954 developed a rigid lens light fiber system that was a major improvement in optics. Hirschowitz in 1957 solved the problem of flexible fiber orientation in intestinal endoscopes, and Ikeda in 1968 reported the use of the flexible fiberoptic bronchoscope. Today we have a wide variety of rigid instruments and forceps, light sources, flexible instruments in varying diameters, and good optical systems for visualization of the airway directly or by video screening.[1]

### INDICATIONS

#### Diagnostic

The diagnostic indications for bronchoscopy can be grouped into three categories. First are a set of symptoms. Second are radiographic findings, and third are clinical settings that indicate a bronchoscopy should be performed.

A persistent unexplained cough is ominous and needs to be investigated even in the absence of other physical findings or chest x-ray abnormalities. Hemoptysis either persistent or massive is an obvious indication unless a single episode in a patient with no physical findings, a normal chest x-ray, a nonsmoker, and a preceding respiratory tract infection. Bronchoscopy need not be delayed even if bleeding is massive, since the rigid instrument permits clearing of the airway, identification of the anatomic site of bleeding, and establishment of the diagnosis. Control of bleeding can be accomplished in some by tamponade with pledgets or balloons, and irrigation with iced saline or epinephrine 1:10,000 applied topically. A wheeze, not a component of known bronchospastic disease and especially if unilateral, is an indication for bronchoscopy.[2–4]

Multiple radiographic findings occur and individually or collectively indicate a bronchoscopy should be performed. A local persistent infiltrate or diffuse bilateral infiltrates are common problems. Deviation of the trachea or bronchi, atelectasis, a hilar mass, a peripheral circular lesion, and a lung abscess all require a bronchoscopy. An unexplained pleural effusion and elevation of a hemi-diaphragm also require bronchoscopic investigation.

The presence of a recurrent or unresolved pneumonia, history of foreign body aspiration, a positive sputum cytology, vocal cord paralysis, and suspected airway stricture require investigation. Thoracic trauma especially with mediastinal air, subcutaneous emphysema, or a persistent pneumothorax despite thoracostomy tube drainage is a further indication.

The bronchoscope is indispensable in diagnosis and staging of pulmonary carcinoma. The presence of a superior vena caval syndrome or esophageal carcinoma in the upper and middle thirds where the lesion is in juxtaposition with the airway dictate the need for bronchoscopy. Bronchoscopy is useful in lung transplantation both for diagnosis and postoperative surveillance.

The immunocomprised patient with respiratory symptoms or a radiographic abnormality needs investigation. Steroids are widely used for a variety of diseases. Chemotherapy induces immunosuppression. Increasingly there are patients who have been the recipients of organ transplants, and by necessity they are immunosuppressed. Finally, the rapid worldwide dissemination of the human immunodeficiency virus (HIV) has rendered thousands to be at risk for immunosuppression, and their numbers continue to increase (Table 10–1).

### Therapeutic

Atelectasis secondary to retained pulmonary secretions, usually postoperative or posttraumatic, can be resolved readily by bronchoscopy if other measures fail. Aspiration of a foreign body, vomitus, or blood requires bronchoscopic inspection. A refractory lung abscess may be drained internally by bronchoscopy.[2]

Physical modalities for malignant respiratory tract obstruction such as lasers, electrocautery, and cryotherapy are all administered through the bronchoscope. The bronchoscope is necessary to insert laser probes to activate hematoporphyrin derivatives (HpD) and to place radiation sources in the airway. A difficult intubation can be accomplished with a bronchoscope. It is helpful for accurate placement of a bilumen tube. Placement of an airway stent is performed with a bronchoscope. Evaluation of airway injury in cases of prolonged intubation can be readily accomplished. Closure of a bronchopleural fistula with fibrin glue and coils inserted through a bronchoscope has been reported[5] (Table 10–1).

**TABLE 10–1. PRINCIPLE INDICATIONS FOR BRONCHOSCOPY**

| Diagnostic | Therapeutic |
|---|---|
| **Symptoms** | Atelectasis |
| Cough | Foreign body removal |
| Hemoptysis | Lung abscess |
| Wheezing | Laser therapy |
| **Radiographic findings** | Brachy therapy |
| Persistent infiltrate | HpD activation |
| Diffuse bilateral infiltrates | Intubation |
| Deviation of trachea/main stem bronchi | Stent placement |
| Hilar mass | Bronchopleural fistula |
| Peripheral circular lesion | |
| Lung abscess | |
| Pleural effusion, unexplained | |
| Elevation of hemidiaphragm | |
| **Clinical setting** | |
| Pneumonia, persistent or recurrent | |
| History of aspiration | |
| Positive sputum cytology | |
| Vocal cord paralysis | |
| Suspected airway stricture | |
| Thoracic trauma | |
| SVC syndrome | |
| Staging of pulmonary carcinoma | |

## CONTRAINDICATIONS

Most reported contraindications to bronchoscopy have proven to be relative rather than absolute and do not preclude a careful bronchoscopy if the need for diagnosis and subsequent therapy outweigh the risk involved. Patients with intracranial lesions whether tumor or stroke can be safely bronchoscoped.[6] A recent myocardial infarction increases the risk but not prohibitively. Bleeding disorders are vexing whether from planned anticoagulation, deficient platelets, uremia, or other factors. Usually they can be corrected transiently to permit a safe examination.[7] Patients on ventilators can be bronchoscoped with only transient depression of oxygenation and no demonstrable long-term deficit.[8] The presence of tracheal obstruction while worrisome should not deter the bronchoscopist providing adequate ventilation can be attained and maintained. Severe cervical arthritis or kyphoscoliosis are not a deterrent with the availability of flexible instruments.

Active tuberculosis is not a contraindication but does present a hazard to the bronchoscopist and personnel. Due care can be exercised and minimal risk encountered. The same is true for patients who have hepatitis or are infected with HIV. Terminal, adequate sterilization of the instruments is mandatory.[9]

There are a few absolute contraindications that are obvious. Lack of informed consent, inexperience, improper facilities, and the inability to oxygenate the patient for any reason are cause for not proceeding with a bronchoscopy.

## COMPLICATIONS

Bronchoscopy is generally a safe procedure, and the complications that can occur are usually minor with mortality an uncommon event. Careful attention to premedication drugs and dosages, the conduct of anesthesia, and the procedure itself can reduce the incidence of both major and minor complications to a minimum. One large series reported by Credle involved 24,251 fiberoptic bronchoscopies with an incidence of 0.08% of major complications, defined as respiratory compromise, syncope, bradycardia, and ventricular tachycardia; with a mortality of 0.01%. This author considered most of these complications preventable.[10]

Another series detailed by Lukomsky included 4595 bronchoscopies, 1146 fiberoptic done with local anesthesia, and 3449 rigid done with general anesthesia. He reported a rate of complications of 5.1% of which 1.1% were categorized as major. He observed the complications with fiberoptic bronchoscopy to be more likely secondary to premedication and topical anesthesia, while the complications with rigid bronchoscopy were more likely to be the result of instrument manipulation.[11] Cordasco addressed the issue of bronchoscopically induced bleeding. In a series of 6969 bronchoscopies, he identified 58 (0.5%) cases of bleeding. No deaths occurred. Risk factors included immunosuppression and malignancy.[12]

Premedication if doses are excessive can result in respiratory depression, hypotension, and syncope. The topical anesthetic agents can induce laryngospasm and bronchospasm as well as hypoxia and arrhythmias. The procedure itself can induce bleeding, hypoxia, and arrhythmia. If transbronchial biopsy is performed at the periphery, a pneumothorax can be induced. Postbronchoscopy infiltrates have been noted after biopsy and segmental bronchoalveolar lavage, but they appear to be of little consequence.[2]

Even thrombocytopenic patients can be bronchoscoped safely. Weiss et al[7] reported 47 such patients who underwent 66 separate bronchoscopies with bronchoalveolar lavage. The procedure was diagnostic in 22 patients, 47%. Only one major episode of bleeding, epistaxis, was encountered in a patient with a history of previous epistaxis.

The bronchoscope probably does not propagate infection. Prakash[9] after review of his experience and that of others could find no consistent evidence that oropharyngeal bacteria are transmitted to the lower respiratory tract and produce an infection. The possibility of spread of a preexisting infection to other portions of the lung is suggested but not proven. Hematogenous spread to other sites has rarely occurred. It is possible to spread infection from one patient to another with an improperly cleaned instrument, but this can be avoided by using adequate cleaning and sterilization procedures. Because the risk of infection is so low, there is no indication for the use of prophylactic antibiotics except for those patients with a history of endocarditis, a prosthetic valve, shunt, or conduit where their use would be prudent (Table 10–2).

**TABLE 10–2. COMPLICATIONS OF BRONCHOSCOPY**

| |
|---|
| Premedication |
| Respiratory depression |
| Hypotension/syncope |
| Anesthesia |
| Laryngospasm |
| Bronchospasm |
| Hypoxia |
| Arrhythmia |
| Procedure |
| Pneumothorax |
| Hemorrhage |
| Pneumonia |

## INSTRUMENTS

### Rigid

A wide variety of rigid instruments are manufactured. They are available in varying lengths and diameters to accommodate the anatomy of the patient. The contour of the interior channel varies from circular to oval with the available working space dependent upon the interior placement of other conduits for a light source, aspiration, or oxygen administration. A light source may be incandescent or halogen and is connected to the instrument with a flexible fiberoptic cable (Fig. 10–1).

Telescopes with excellent optics have varying viewing angles from straight ahead to right angle. Combinations of telescopes and forceps have proven very useful.

Many different types of forceps have been produced that can perform special functions such as grasping safety pins and marbles.

The rigid instrument is preferred for removal of foreign bodies and investigation of massive hemoptysis. It is also the instrument of choice for infants[13] (Table 10–3).

Airway obstruction can be dealt with much more easily with a rigid than a flexible instrument, since the latter by its design partially occludes the airway. Insertion of airway stents is accomplished with a rigid bronchoscope.

Despite its many virtues, there is a limited range of vision of the rigid instrument when it is used alone. Insertion of a flexible instrument through the rigid scope obviates this deficiency. Patient comfort under local anesthesia is much less with the rigid instrument.

### Flexible

The flexible bronchoscope has been developed into a utilitarian instrument that has expanded the role of bronchoscopy. The instruments are available in several lengths

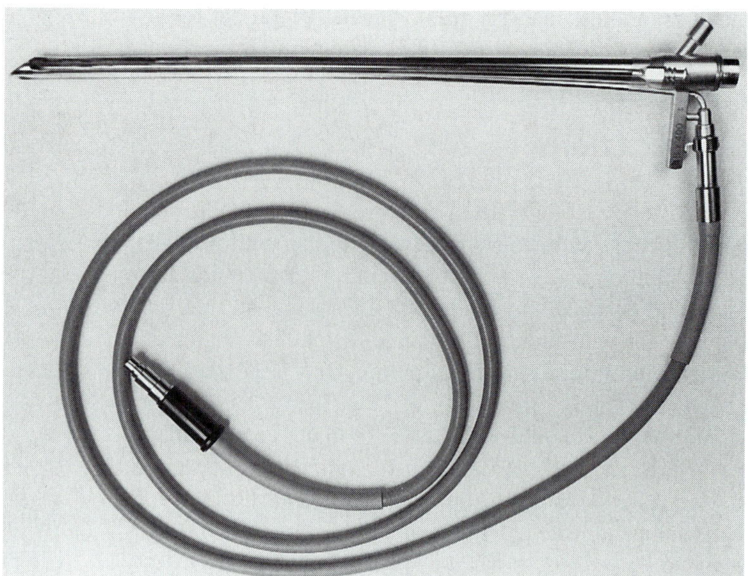

**Figure 10–1.** Rigid bronchoscope with flexible fiber-optic light cable and sidearm for ventilation.

and have outer diameters ranging from 3.6 to 6.1 mm. The number of fiberoptic bundles for transmission of light and images and the number and size of auxiliary channels determine the diameter of an instrument. A light source is attached to the flexible light cable of the bronchoscope. The field of vision is usually about 80 degrees, and the angle of deflection is variable up to 180 degrees (Fig. 10–2).

Video cameras can be affixed to the proximal end of the bronchoscope for large-screen display. Some instruments now include the camera as a built-in feature.

Great improvements have been made in construction so they may be totally immersed in liquids for greater ease and safety in cleaning and sterilization (Table 10–4).

## PREOPERATIVE EVALUATION

The preparation of a patient for a bronchoscopy begins with a history, followed by a physical examination and chest x-ray. Pulmonary function studies, while desirable for evaluating the underlying disease, are not a prerequisite to bronchoscopy. Some have advocated the routine performance of a complete blood count, bleeding time, coagulation time, and prothrombin time. However, unless indicated by the history and physical, they have no predictive value. Similarly, the routine ECG is not necessary unless the history and physical provide some information to indicate the test would be worthwhile and would alter the conduct of a bronchoscopy. Flow-volume loops are performed only if they are a part of airway evaluation.[14]

Renal failure predisposes to bleeding and might deter biopsy. Steroids are commonly used for so many reasons, and caution should be exercised to obtain this history. Cervical arthritis and congenital maxillo-facial deformities are self evident.

Several considerations are prerequisites. First, the bronchoscopy should be indicated. Second, the patient should be informed fully about the procedure with a discus-

**TABLE 10–3. INSTRUMENT SIZE RELATED TO AGE**

| | Millimeters |
|---|---|
| Adult | 8 × 40 |
| Adolescent | 7 × 40 |
| 6–12 y | 6 × 35 |
| 12–24 mo | 4 × 30 |
| 6–12 mo | 3.5 × 15 |
| <6 mo | 3 × 25 |

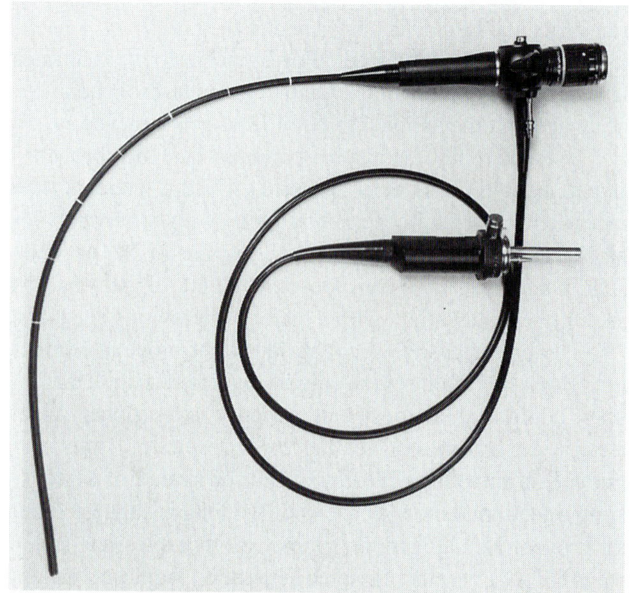

**Figure 10–2.** Flexible fiber-optic bronchoscope with light cable.

**TABLE 10–4. RIGID V. FLEXIBLE BRONCHOSCOPES**

| Advantages | Disadvantages |
|---|---|
| Rigid bronchoscope | |
| Large biopsies | Peripheral biopsy difficult |
| Improved airway | Segment visualization poor |
| Greater ease of aspiration and retrieval | Patient discomfort |
| Flexible bronchoscope | |
| Patient comfort | Small biopsies |
| Segment visualization good | Small lumen for aspiration |
| Distal biopsies easier | Maintenance |
| Bronchoscopy on ventilator | |

sion of the risks and possible complications such as post-bronchoscopy intubation pneumothorax and tracheostomy. Finally, these discussions are written in the records and verified by a signed consent form.

## ANESTHESIA

### Topical

A wide variety of anesthetic agents is available, and it is not possible to describe all with exact doses. The drugs and agents used should be those with which the endoscopist is familiar both in method of administration and duration of action and recovery, along with a knowledge of toxicity dosages and idiosyncrasies.

The patient who is to undergo bronchoscopy should be NPO for 12 hours and all dentures removed. Premedication is desirable and should include a sedative agent, a drying compound, and an antitussive drug. Examples of sedatives are the barbiturates, valium, or a benzodiazipine given orally. Atropine and glycopyrrolate are both excellent drying agents. Codeine is an excellent cough suppressant as are morphine derivatives.[15]

The three commonest topical agents in use are cocaine 4 and 10%; tetracaine 0.5, 1.0, and 2.0%; and lidocaine 2%. The toxic levels of these compounds are 300 mg for cocaine, 80 mg for tetracaine, and 40 mg for lidocaine. The anesthetic agent can be applied to the nasal, oral, and laryngeal mucosa by atomizer, gargle, nose drops, and pledgets applied with a curved forcep. The larynx is anesthetized by using a syringe and malleable curved cannula. Additional anesthetic agent can be instilled through the bronchoscope as it is introduced into the posterior pharynx or after placement into the airway.

A laryngeal block is preferred by some. The superior laryngeal nerve is numbed by applying an anesthetic soaked pledget into the pyriform sinuses. Alternately, percutaneous injection of the nerve at the cornu of the hyoid bone can be used. Finally, direct injection of the agent percutaneously into the trachea provides rapid effective distribution of the drug in the airway.

Monitoring of a patient having a bronchoscopy using local anesthesia should include IV access, an electrocardiograph, and a pulse oximeter to determine requirements for supplemental oxygen.[16] Postprocedure the patient should be observed in a suitable recovery area until the effects of sedation and anesthesia have worn off. The patient should not eat or drink until full recovery from the topical anesthesia to avoid aspiration.

### General

Flexible bronchoscopy is performed by passing the instrument through a right-angle connector and an endotracheal tube (Fig. 10–3).

If a rigid bronchoscope is used, ventilation can be maintained using the side arm of the bronchoscope connected to an anesthesia machine with high gas flow, which is inefficient, or by using a bronchoscope with a proximal covering port, which has the disadvantage of requiring removal for insertion of suction devices or instruments. A

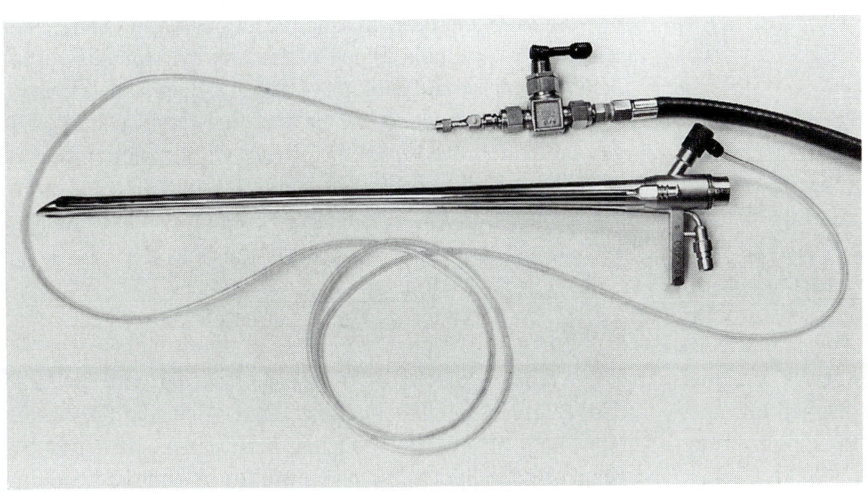

**Figure 10–3.** Right angle connector joining the anesthesia circuit and endotracheal tube with port for passage of flexible bronchoscope.

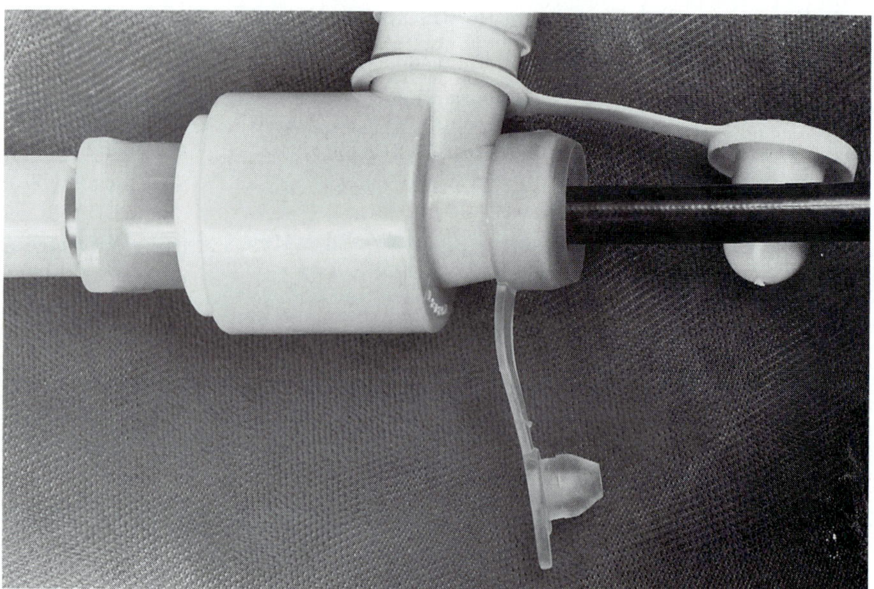

**Figure 10–4.** Rigid bronchoscope with Sanders attachment on sidearm with flow control valve for use with general anesthesia.

preferable technique is to use a Sanders ventilation device, which can be placed either at the proximal end of the bronchoscope or bent to fit the side arm (Fig. 10–4).

If lasers or cautery are to be used, the airway gases must contain oxygen in a concentration approximating room air, to reduce the risk of fire. If a Sanders system is used, this is easily accomplished by using two tanks, one of oxygen and another of compressed air. At the time of laser use, switching to air results in a prompt reduction of oxygen concentration in the airway, and the laser can be used, with reversion to oxygen when the laser is no longer in use. Monitoring for general anesthesia should include IV access, electrocardiograph, and pulse oximeter with end-tidal oxygen measurement if air is used for ventilation during laser use.

As with a local anesthetic, the patient must be observed in a suitable area until the effects of the anesthetic agents have dissipated and the patient can return to hospital or home environment.

## TECHNIQUE

### Flexible

There is considerable variety in the position of the patient and the operator when a flexible instrument is used. The patient may be supine, semi-sitting, or even in the upright sitting position. The operator can be at the head of the patient or can be face to face, laterally depending on handedness of the operator and placement of equipment. The trans-nasal technique is common. The instrument is passed directly posterior and is flexed over the soft palate. The epiglottis is seen, the instrument is passed behind the epiglottis bringing the cords into view, and the instrument is inserted into the airway. At this point it may be necessary to administer an additional dose of topical anesthesia.

If the nares are small or the operator cannot advance the scope easily, or if the patient has a history of severe epistaxis or nasal deformity, then the oral route is chosen. To accomplish this, the tongue is pulled forward, and the instrument is inserted to the back of the pharynx and flexed; the cords will come into view. A bite block is used to prevent inadvertent damage to the instrument. A common error in introducing the instrument is to pass it posteriorly into the postlaryngeal area, missing the epiglottis and cords and entering the valleculae, pyriform sinuses, or esophagus.

Once the flexible instrument is in place, it can be advanced or withdrawn, rotated or flexed to achieve access to the bronchial tree. The bronchoscopist should have a plan of investigation in mind so that a thorough evaluation is accomplished.

If the bronchoscope is to be used through an endotracheal tube, it is prudent to make sure it will pass easily through the lumen and still provide a space for ventilation. For example, a 5- or 5.5-mm scope mandates an 8.5 endotracheal tube. If there is doubt, it should be tried beforehand.

The flexible bronchoscope is an occluding device that reduces the available lumen of the airway, which, in a patient with marginal ventilatory capacity, may be deleterious. Not usually appreciated is the fact that large quantities of gas can be removed from the airway via the suction port of an instrument. Depending on aspirating port size and negative pressure of the suction system, it is possible to remove 14 L of gas per minute from the airway.

### Rigid

The patient is placed in the supine position with the head extended. No special table is required. A standard operating table with a movable head rest suffices. A small pad beneath the shoulders may be helpful to extend the head and neck. The operator stands at the head of the table and grasps the maxilla with padded fingers. The head of the patient is turned slightly to the left, and the instrument is passed in a vertical direction through the side of the mouth. The fulcrum of the bronchoscope is the thumb of the operator to prevent injury to the teeth and gums. The proximal end of the bronchoscope is depressed pivoting on the operator's thumb. At this point it is convenient for the operator to sit on a movable stool adjusted to a comfortable height. The tip of the epiglottis is elevated with the beveled tip of the bronchoscope exposing the cords. The bronchoscope is rotated 90 degrees to the right and is pointed at the left vocal cord and advanced. Because of the bevel, the bronchoscope will pass easily into the trachea. The bronchoscope is straightened, and additional topical anesthesia is given if necessary.

By rotating the head to the left, it is easy to pass into the right main stem bronchus and view the right upper lobe tangentially or with a telescope. By advancing further the middle lobe and superior dorsal orifices come into view with the basilar segmental bronchi in the distance.

With the instrument in the trachea and the patient's head turned to the right, the bronchoscope can be passed into the left main stem bronchus, where the left upper lobe and lingula can be viewed followed by the lower lobe bronchi, once again with the use of, as necessary, telescopes.

Insertion of a rigid bronchoscope initially that gives control of the airway and then passage of a flexible instrument through the rigid instrument permits complete inspection of the airway. Errors in passing the instrument are incomplete anesthesia, poor cooperation of the patient, and inserting the instrument too deep, thus bypassing the laryngeal apparatus.

The reader is referred to Stradling,[17] who has produced a work depicting not only the normal anatomy of the tracheobronchial tree but also examples of most of the endobronchial lesions encountered.

## SPECIMENS

### Procurement

Tissue and fluids obtained at bronchoscopy must be collected and accurately labeled to be useful. The cost of procuring such specimens is significant, and all efforts should be made to ensure they are appropriately obtained and processed.

Specimens fall into three categories: washings, brushings, and biopsies. Washings are obtained by installation of saline into the bronchial tree and catching the aspirate in a trap receptacle such as a Lukens tube inserted in the suction line. Brushings are obtained by rubbing the brush on the surface of a lesion or in an area of a parenchymal lesion and then wiping the brush on a slide that is then fixed promptly by spray or immersed in a liquid fixative such as alcohol to avoid a drying artifact that distorts cellular anatomy. Biopsies are performed with either rigid forceps passed through a rigid instrument or with flexible instruments passed through a flexible instrument. The larger the size of the biopsy forcep, the more tissue is retrieved and the better the chance is of establishing an accurate diagnosis[18] (Fig. 10–5).

A biopsy through a rigid instrument is straightforward. With a flexible instrument, the location of the tip of the biopsy forcep may not be visible unless fluoroscopy is used. The biopsy forcep should be advanced to the lesion; then the jaws should be separated and the forcep advanced following by closure of the forcep and withdrawal. The instru-

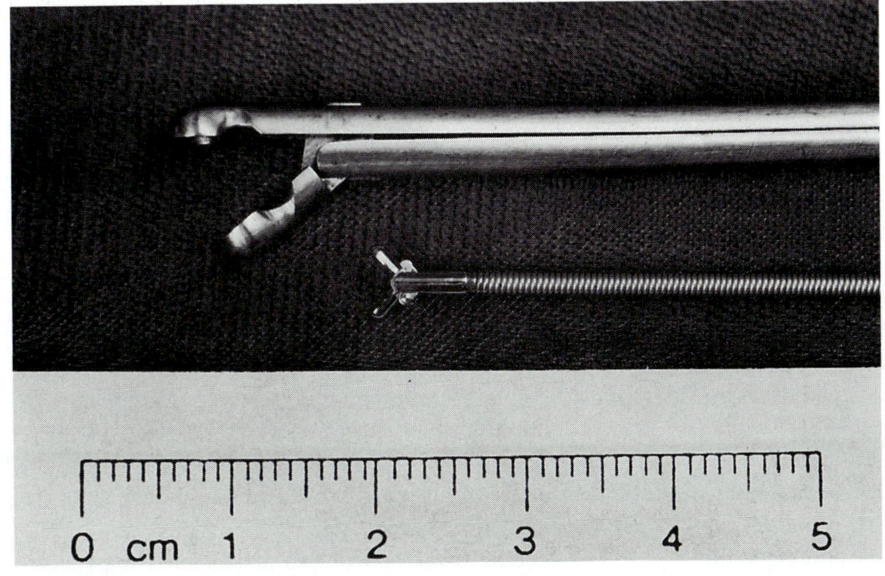


**Figure 10–5.** Relative size of rigid and flexible biopsy forceps.

ment should be retained in position so that in the case of bleeding, it can be controlled with tamponade or irrigation with epinephrine solution.

Needle biopsy of peripheral lesions is possible by using the flexible instrument and fluoroscopy.[19] Para-tracheal and para-bronchial lesions noted radiographically are biopsied using a Wang-type needle. The needle, commonly 18 gauge, is placed in position and then advanced to penetrate the wall of the airway. Aspiration confirms that a blood vessel has not been penetrated. Sampling through the needle is aided by injection of small amounts of saline.[20]

Fluoroscopy is not necessary when diffuse disease is present or there is an obvious central radiographic lesion.

### Handling

Bronchial washings should be sent in a fresh state without preservative to the laboratory for cytologic processing that includes centrifugation and Papanicolaou staining. Similarly specimens destined for culture are also sent fresh without preservative to the bacteriology laboratory with specifications whether standard techniques, acid-fast, fungal, or viral cultures are to be used.

Brushings are wiped on a slide and immediately fixed for cytology. A protected specimen brush is used for accurate bacteriology studies.[21]

Biopsies are placed in formalin for standard processing. If electron microscopy is contemplated, then a portion should be placed in glutaraldehyde. If a frozen section is deemed necessary, then the specimen should be placed in saline and given to the pathologist.

Needle aspirates should be expelled on a slide, perhaps with the aid of a little saline, and immediately fixed. If enough tissue is obtained or a large-bore needle has been used to obtain a core of tissue, then it is expelled into saline and processed as with other tissue. Rapid on-site evaluation by a pathologist of brush and biopsy specimens is of help to determine if a diagnosis has been established or if additional specimens are needed.

## AIRWAY OBSTRUCTION

### Dilatation and Extraction

Obstruction of the airway can be either benign or malignant. The diagnosis is usually not difficult, but the management can be troublesome. A complete array of instruments must be available including rigid and flexible bronchoscopes of various sizes plus dilators, balloons and forceps. General anesthesia is preferred, and a skilled anesthesiologist who is capable of assisting the bronchoscopist is essential. The operator must possess skill and confidence that the airway will be improved at the conclusion of the procedure. The patient must be informed as to the goals of the procedure and the possibility that tracheostomy or prolonged intubation and ventilator support may ensue.

The simplest method is to pass a small-bore rigid bronchoscope and follow this with instruments of increasing diameter, aided by dilators, until the obstruction is relieved. This works well for benign strictures. If the obstruction is secondary to malignancy, then the rigid bronchoscope can be used to core out fragments of tissue and extract these with forceps.[22] Balloons may also be used for dilatation. The procedure may have to be repeated if the obstruction recurs. The role of steroid injection for benign strictures is not settled. The idea is attractive, but the results are not well documented.

### Lasers

The use of lasers for airway obstruction has now become commonplace. A number of different types of lasers are available but the two most widely used are the $CO_2$ laser operating in the 10.6-μm range and the Neodymium aluminum garnet laser (YAG), which operates at the 1.06-μm wavelength.

Laser is an acronym for *l*ight *a*mplification by *s*timulated *e*mission of *r*adiation, first described by Einstein in 1917. A laser beam delivers a high level of energy with great precision, ensuring destruction of tissue with minimal adjacent tissue effects.

A laser is a coherent beam of monochromatic light generated from different substrates that are stimulated either by electricity or light. Raising the molecules of the substrate to a high level, transiently and repetitively, produces photons that form the laser beam. This beam is then directed either by an articulated arm and mirrors in the case of the $CO_2$ laser or by a flexible fiber-optic wave guide in the case of the YAG laser.

The $CO_2$ laser beam is formed by electrical stimulation of a gas mixture, and its use is restricted to the rigid bronchoscope. No flexible wave guild is available. The energy is absorbed by tissues containing water. The destructive action is superficial. The beam can be focused into a small spot size and seals lymphatic and vascular channels.

The YAG laser is formed by flash lamp excitation of a compound crystal and can be passed through a flexible guide. It has a deeper depth of penetration, is a better coagulation device, and has a rapid thermal drop-off like the $CO_2$ laser.

The results using a laser and dilatation in benign strictures are good.[23] In malignant disease the use of lasers provides an improved airway with amelioration of symptoms and increased longevity.[24] The issue of rigid vs. flexible bronchoscopy for a YAG laser is not settled. The combination of a rigid bronchoscope to obtain control of the airway with a flexible bronchoscope for accurate manipulation of the fiber appears optimum.[25]

The advantages of laser treatment are the immediate ablation of tissue with an improved airway and the ability to repeat the process as necessary.

Protection of the patient and personnel is imperative. A laser beam may be deflected, and eye protection is mandatory. Fire is a constant hazard and can be reduced if airway gases are nonflammable. This can be accomplished by transiently using air as a ventilating gas. Plastic and rubber endotracheal tubes can be ignited with a laser beam and should be foil wrapped. Adjacent drapes and coverings can also be ignited.

## Brachytherapy

The application of radiation sources to areas of malignancy in the airway has a long history. Insertion of seeds or pellets of radioactive 125 I, 198 Au, 192 IR, and radon has been accomplished through the bronchoscope. They have the disadvantage of radiation hazard to personnel during placement and subsequently until the radiation source decays.

Low-dose internal radiation has been accomplished by placement of a catheter in the airway with indwelling radioactive materials. The catheter was left in place for 24–36 hours depending on the source and calculated amount of radiation. The disadvantages were the lack of assurance that the catheter would remain in position and the fact that the patient had to be kept in radioactive isolation.

Currently high-dose intraluminal radiation therapy is available. A catheter is placed under visual and fluoroscopic guidance following which a radioactive source, iridium, is passed into the catheter. A computer calculates isodose curves and determines the time interval at each position to provide the exact radiation dose. Treatment time ranges from 2 to 6 minutes depending on the age of the source. Treatments are repeated, usually two to three times, at weekly intervals until the calculated total dose is administered. The advantages are precise placement and short treatment time. The patient does not require posttreatment isolation.

The results of the high-dose brachytherapy are generally good. The quality of life is improved, and the quantity of life is extended.[26,27] The complications of necrosis, hemorrhage, and esophageal fistula are uncommon but catastrophic and dose-dependent.[28]

Brachytherapy can be combined with laser therapy. The latter provides immediate relief of obstruction, while the radiation provides a more lasting benefit. The combination treatment is an improvement over either method alone.[29,30]

## Electrocautery

The use of electrocautery to eradicate malignant disease has been used for many years. Both rigid and flexible instruments may be used. Ball and needle electrodes are available. Occasionally the lesion is amenable to the use of a snare. Fulgurated tissue is removed with forceps and suction. There are no large reported series to indicate the results, but from a methodologic standpoint the technique is applicable.[31]

## Cryotherapy

The application of cold probes to malignant tissue for destruction has been used in many parts of the body. In the airway the cryotherapy probe has been inserted through a rigid bronchoscope under general anesthesia. The probe, fueled by liquid nitrogen operates at a temperature of −89.5°C, produces almost instant freezing of tissue that is removed by forceps. Repeat bronchoscopy is necessary to remove the tissue slough that occurs subsequent to freezing.[32]

## Photodynamic Therapy (HpD)

Hematoporphyrin derivatives are substances injected into the body that are absorbed by all tissues, then excreted but preferentially retained in malignant tissue. Activation of HpD by light results in the development of singlet oxygen that destroys the malignant cell but not adjacent normal cells. This material has been in use for years, and the methodology has recently been standardized. A calculated dose of purified HpD obtained from bovine blood altered with a mixture of acids is injected into a patient. Bronchoscopy is performed 48 hours later and the tissue illuminated with an argon pumped dye laser in the 630-μm range. The activated HpD produces malignant tissue death. Subsequent bronchoscopies are necessary to rid the airway of slough. The advantage is precise tumor cell death with good palliation.[33] The disadvantages are the difficulty of getting the light to deeper parts of the tumor, photosensitivity of the patient for several weeks, and the expense of the equipment.

Photodynamic therapy has proven successful as an alternative to surgery for a group of patients with early superficial squamous cell carcinoma.[34]

## Stents

Once the airway has been enlarged, it may be necessary to insert a stent to retain the diameter of the lumen and its patency. A number of materials have been used but at the present silastic seems to be the must useful. The tubes are formulated by manufacturers in a number of configurations. Simple straight tubes of varying lengths and diameters are available for the bronchi or trachea. They may have flanges or knobs to help maintain position. "T" tubes are available to provide access through a tracheostomy site and aid in removal of secretions. The "T" tube has had "Y" arms connected to provide stenting of both the trachea and main stem bronchi. Plain "Y" tubes are also available.[35,36]

A new development is the use of expandable wire stents that are inserted in a collapsed state and, when released, expand to provide a suitable airway.[37,38]

The results of stenting are good for benign airway obstruction. Survival of patients with malignancy depends on the extent of the disease. Stents are not easy to insert in all cases, and the endoscopist must be skilled in all phases of bronchoscopy. They may migrate and require extraction and replacement.

## FOREIGN BODIES

The presence of a foreign body in the airway can usually be detected by a combination of history, respiratory tract symptoms, usually wheezing and cough, and x-ray findings of either an opaque foreign body or perhaps an infiltrate or atelectasis. Segments of the population susceptible include infants and children, the mentally retarded, the physically handicapped, epileptics, and alcoholics.

Foreign bodies are categorized into organic and inorganic. The organic foreign bodies have a tendency to absorb water, swell, and produce obstruction or infection even leading to abscess if not extracted. Inorganic foreign bodies, while they produce symptoms may not obstruct a lobar bronchus completely, and there is less urgency in their removal. The location of a foreign body in the respiratory tree is a function of the geometry of the foreign body, the anatomy of the bronchial tree, and the position of the patient. More commonly, foreign bodies come to rest in the right bronchial tree since this is a more direct path than angulating into the left main stem bronchus.

The removal of a foreign body is best done under general anesthesia. The rigid bronchoscope is preferred. A wide variety of special forceps has been developed such as cups and spoon to remove spherical objects and pointed tips to allow grasping the millage of a coin (Fig. 10–6). Some organic material may have degenerated and require multiple bites of the material followed by irrigation and aspiration. On occasion, passing a balloon catheter distally may dislodge a foreign body and aid in extraction. If the foreign body is fenestrated, it may be possible to pass a forcep or balloon through the fenestration and then open the forcep or expand the balloon and withdraw the object.

Several precautions should be taken. If the object is known, practice with a forcep and a replacement object will aid in grasping and removal. If a foreign body is too large to pass through the lumen of the bronchoscope, keep a firm grip with the forcep, impinge the object in the tip of the bronchoscope, and withdraw the instrument, forcep, and foreign body as a unit, relaxing your grip only after the foreign body is completely clear of the patient so as not to drop the object in the posterior pharynx. Once a foreign body has been removed, reinsert the instrument and look again. Foreign bodies can be multiple. Fragments of organic material may have been dislodged and still remain.

## BRONCHOALVEOLAR LAVAGE (BAL)

### Diagnostic

The technique of bronchoalveolar lavage is an extension of simple bronchial washing. It provides a larger volume of cellular and noncellular material from distal airways. There is great variability in the technique of BAL from one institution to another. Comparison data is difficult to analyze. A common method is described.

A flexible bronchoscope of approximately 5.2 mm is gently wedged into a third- or fourth-generation bronchial segment. If disease is local, the appropriate bronchus is chosen. If diffuse disease is present, the middle lobe or lingula is used.

Sterile buffered or unbuffered saline is instilled in increments of 30–60 mL and aspirated into a trap using a gentle suction to avoid trauma to the airway.

A total aspirate of 150–200 mL is sought. Each sample is kept separate and numbered in sequence. The initial specimen contains mostly airway cells, while later specimens sample the alveoli. Whether to pool specimens or not is

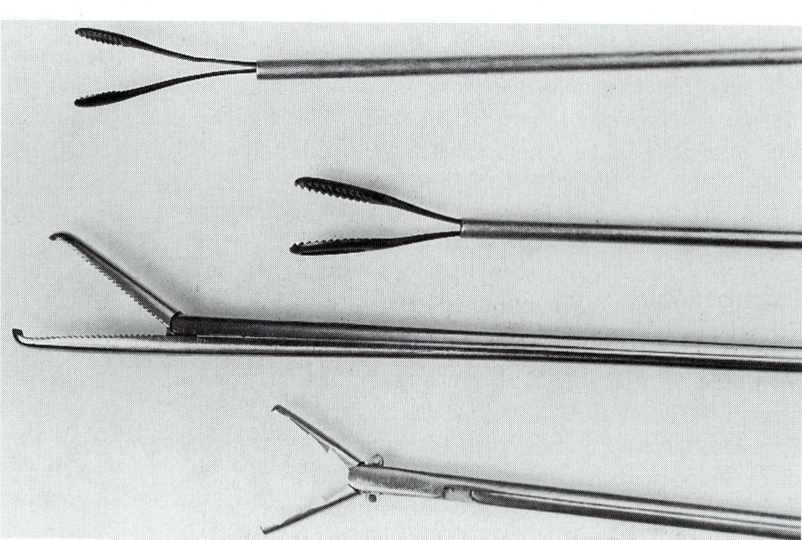

**Figure 10–6.** Types of foreign body forceps.

controversial. The lavage fluids are transported, iced, to the laboratory.

Differential cell counts on cytocentrifuge preparations is performed along with protein analysis of the supernatant fluid.[39] Cultures are carried out.

BAL is a safe procedure with only minor complications including fever, pneumonitis, bleeding, and bronchospasm. None of these usually require treatment. Patients on ventilators can have a BAL without undue risk.[40]

BAL is diagnostic for many infectious diseases including *Pneumocystis carinii, Mycobacterium tuberculosis,* histoplasmosis, and mycoplasma. It is helpful but not necessarily diagnostic for herpes simplex, cytomegalovirus, aspergillus, and others.

BAL is diagnostic for alveolar proteinosis, eosinophilic granuloma, and cancer. The role of BAL in the diagnosis of sarcoidosis is debatable but probably is reliable to establish the diagnosis.[41]

Many other diseases are being investigated with BAL and as experience is gained more diseases will probably be identified with certainty.[39]

### Therapeutic

Whole lung lavage has been performed for several abnormalities most notably pulmonary alveolar proteinosis, a disease of unknown cause characterized by the accumulation of amorphous material in the bronchial tree with resultant decrease in the forced vital capacity (FVC) and total lung capacity (TLC).

The procedure is performed one lung at a time with a 2–3-day interval. Under general anesthesia a bilumen tube is inserted. It is imperative this be in accurate position to ensure complete isolation of the lungs. Through a "Y" connector attached to one arm of the bilumen tube, saline warmed to body temperature is instilled into the lung from a height of 1 m. As this is done, carefully listen with a stethoscope to ensure the fluid is entering only the desired lung and not spilling into the opposite side, which is to be used for ventilation. Most adult patients will accept 1 L without difficulty. Gravity drainage of the effluent is then accomplished with subsequent instillation of additional liters of fluid. The volume of the first exchange recovered will be small, since the functional residual capacity (FRC) has been filled and is not recovered. A running tally is kept to document the fluid load absorbed by the patient, usually under 1 L. Percussion of the thorax with both installation and drainage aides in removal of the debris. An aliquot of each effluent is taken. The end point is when the effluent is clear enough so news type can be read through a test tube of perfusate. Addition of heparin and acetyl cystic acid has not shown any improvement over plain saline. After clearing of the effluent, flexible bronchoscopy with a small-bore instrument is performed through the bilumen tube. This is replaced with a single lumen tube, and repeat bronchoscopy is performed to remove any residual saline and debris. Generally it will take 20–25 L of saline to reach the end point.[42]

A few patients have been critically ill and have required additional support while lavage has been performed. This has taken the form of hyperbaric oxygenation and the use of extracorporeal circulation.

## BRONCHOSCOPY SITE AND EQUIPMENT

The area where bronchoscopy is performed should be of sufficient size to accommodate all of the equipment and have adequate electrical power.

A standard operating room table is sufficient. There should be space for storage and cleaning of all instruments. Complete anesthesia and resuscitation equipment must be at hand including anesthetic agents and drugs. If lasers are to be used, entrance to the area needs to be restricted, and eye protection is mandatory. The potential for fire exists when lasers are in use; fire extinguishers are necessary.

On occasions it is necessary to perform a bronchoscopy in a special care unit. This is best accomplished if a mobile cart is stocked with the necessary items including light sources and power cables. Personnel experienced with the instruments and techniques should accompany the bronchoscopist to ensure proper distribution of specimens and appropriate cleaning of contaminated instruments.

## EDUCATION AND TRAINING

A thoracic surgeon should be trained in both rigid and flexible bronchoscopy and be facile in the use of all the equipment used for diagnosis and treatment of airway and pulmonary disease. To accomplish this residents must see patients with a variety of disorders that require the use of all bronchoscopic techniques and modalities. There are some who have proscribed specific numbers of each type of procedure to become proficient. Absolute numbers are less important than learning with a teacher who will demonstrate the proper way to perform the procedures and to ensure the safety and comfort of the patient. A few good bronchoscopic teaching sessions are superior to many unsupervised insertions of instruments into the bronchial tree. If a training program does not have sufficient patient volume to achieve this goal, then provision should be made for training in other settings.

## SUMMARY

The development of the bronchoscope and its accessories has resulted in a versatile system for use in the diagnosis and treatment of patients with a wide variety of diseases. Many lives have been saved, and others have had an improvement in their quality life as well as an extension of their life spans.

Perfection has not been achieved. Further developments in instrumentation—such as a flexible wave guide for the $CO_2$ laser, a miniaturized camera to be applied to the tip of the bronchoscope, and the development of smaller ultrasonic probes for investigation of lymph nodes adjacent to the airway to predict malignant involvement—are awaited.

Tumor-specific compounds with identification systems will be developed. Tissue sensitizers and activators will expand the scope of treatment using a bronchoscope. Finally, advancements in molecular biology will allow accurate analysis of tissue obtained at bronchoscopy to determine specific tumor identification as a determinant for therapy.

## REFERENCES


1. Sackner MA: Bronchofiberoscopy. *Am Rev Respir Dis* **111:**62, 1975
2. Miller MB, Kvale PA: Diagnostic bronchoscopy. *Chest Surg Clin North Am* **2:**599, 1992
3. Knott-Craig CJ, Oostuizen JG, Russouw G, et al: Management and prognosis of massive hemoptysis. *J Thorac Cardiovasc Surg* **105:**394, 1993
4. Prakash UBS, Offord KP, Stubbs SE: Bronchoscopy in North America. The ACCP Survey. *Chest* **100:**1668, 1991
5. Ponn RB, D'Agostino RS, Stern H, Westcott JL: Treatment of peripheral bronchopleural fistulas with endobronchial occlusion coils. *Ann Thorac Surg* **56:**1343, 1993
6. Bajwa NK, Henein S, Kamholz SL: Fiberoptic bronchoscopy in the presence of space occupying intracranial lesions. *Chest* **104:**101, 1993
7. Weiss SM, Hert RC, Gianola FJ, et al: Complications of fiberoptic bronchoscopy in thrombocytopenic patients. *Chest* **104:**1025, 1993
8. Montravers P, Gauzit R, Dombret MC, et al: Cardiopulmonary effects of bronchoalveolar lavage in critically ill patients. *Chest* **104:**1541, 1993
9. Prakash UBS: Does the bronchoscope propagate infection? *Chest* **104:**552, 1993
10. Credle WF Jr, Smiddy JF, Elliott RC: Complications of fiberoptic bronchoscopy. *Am Rev Respir Dis* **109:**67, 1974
11. Lukomsky GI, Ovchinnikov AA, Bilal A: Complications of bronchoscopy. *Chest* **79:**316, 1981
12. Cordasco EM Jr, Mehta AC, Ahmad M: Bronchoscopically induced bleeding. *Chest* **100:**1141, 1991
13. Rodgers BM, McGahren ED: Endoscopy in children. *Chest Surg Clin North Am* **3:**405, 1993
14. Prakash UBS, Stubbs SE: The bronchoscopy survey, some reflections. *Chest* **100:**1660, 1991
15. Reed AP: Preparation of the patient for awake flexible fiberoptic bronchoscopy. *Chest* **101:**244, 1992
16. Council on Scientific Affairs, American Medical Association: The use of pulse oximetry during conscious sedation. *JAMA* **270:**1463, 1993
17. Stradling P: *Diagnostic Bronchoscopy*, 4th ed. New York, Churchill Livingstone, 1981
18. Loube DI, Johnson JE, Wiener D, et al: The effect of forceps size on the adequacy of specimens obtained by transbronchial biopsy. *Am Rev Resp Dis* **148:**1411, 1993
19. Harrow EM, Oldenburg FA Jr, Lingenfelter MS, Smith AM Jr: Transbronchial Needle aspiration in clinical practice. *Chest* **96:**1268, 1989
20. Shure D: Transbronchial biopsy and transbronchial-transtracheal needle aspiration. *Chest Surg Clin North Am* **2:**617, 1992
21. Lorch DG Jr, John JF Jr, Tomlinson JR, et al: Protected transbronchial needle aspiration and protected specimen brush in the diagnosis of pneumonia. *Am Rev Respir Dis* **136:**565, 1987
22. Mathisen DJ, Grillo HC: Endoscopic relief of malignant airway obstruction. *Ann Thorac Surg* **48:**469, 1989
23. Mehta AC, Lee FYW, Cordasco EM, et al: Concentric tracheal and subgottic stenosis. *Chest* **104:**673, 1993
24. Cavaliere S, Fuccoli P, Farina PL: Nd: Yag laser bronchoscopy: a five year experience with 1,396 applications in 1,000 patients. *Chest* **94:**15, 1988
25. Chan AL, Tharratt RS, Siefkin AD, et al: Nd: Yag laser bronchoscopy rigid or fiberoptic mode. *Chest* **98:**271, 1990
26. Nori D, Allison R, Kaplan B, et al: High dose-rate intraluminal irradiation in bronchogenic carcinoma. *Chest* **104:**1006, 1993
27. Pisch J, Villamena PC, Harvey JC, et al: High dose-rate endobronchial irradiation in malignant airway obstruction. *Chest* **104:**721, 1993
28. Khanavkar B, Stern P, Alberti W, Nakhosteen JA: Complications associated with brachytherapy alone or with laser in lung cancer. *Chest* **99:**1062, 1991
29. Miller JI Jr, Phillips TW: Neodymium: Yag laser and brachytherapy in the management of inoperable bronchogenic carcinoma. *Ann Thorac Surg* **50:**190, 1990
30. Shea JM, Allen RP, Tharratt RS, et al: Survival of patients undergoing Nd:Yag laser therapy compared with Nd:Yag laser therapy and brachytherapy for malignant airway disease. *Chest* **103:**1028, 1993
31. Hooper RG, Jackson FN: Endobronchial electrocautery. *Chest* **94:**595, 1988
32. Marasso A, Gallo E, Massaglia GM, et al: Cryosurgery in bronchoscopic treatment of tracheobronchial stenosis. *Chest* **103:**472, 1993
33. Lo Cicero J III, Metzdorff M, Almgren C: Photodynamic therapy in the palliation of late stage obstructing non-small cell lung cancer. *Chest* **98:**97, 1990
34. Edell ES, Cortese DA: Photodynamic therapy in the management of early superficial squamous cell carcinoma as an alternative to surgical resection. *Chest* **102:**1319, 1992
35. Orlowski TM: Palliative intubation of the tracheobronchial tree. *J Thorac Cardiovasc Surg* **94:**343, 1987
36. Bolliger CT, Probst R, Tschopp K, et al: Silicone stents in the management of inoperable tracheobronchial stenoses. *Chest* **104:**1653, 1993
37. Nomori H, Kobayashi R, Kodera K, et al: Indications for an expandable metallic stent for tracheobronchial stenosis. *Ann Thorac Surg* **56:**1324, 1993
38. Tsang V, Williams AM, Goldstraw P: Sequential silastic and expandable metal stenting for tracheobronchial strictures. *Ann Thorac Surg* **53:**856, 1992
39. American Thoracic Society: Clinical role of bronchoalveolar lavage in adults with pulmonary disease. *Am Rev Resp Dis* **142:**481, 1990
40. Steinberg KP, Mitchell DR, Maunder RJ, et al: Safety of bronchoalveolar lavage in patients with adult respiratory distress syndrome. *Am Rev Resp Dis* **148:**556, 1993
41. Winterbauer RH, Lammert J, Selland M, et al: Bronchoalveolar lavage cell populations in the diagnosis of sarcoidosis. *Chest* **104:**352, 1993
42. Selecky PA, Wasserman K, Benfield JR, Lippman M: The clinical and physiological effect of whole-lung lavage in pulmonary alveolar proteinosis: A ten-year experience. *Ann Thorac Surg* **24:**451, 1977

CHAPTER

11

# Diagnostic and Staging Procedures

## *Mediastinal Evaluation, Scalene Lymph Node Biopsy, Mediastinoscopy, and Mediastinotomy*

James W. Mackenzie and David J. Riley

### INTRODUCTION

The diagnostic and staging procedures discussed in this chapter have decreased the unnecessary thoracotomies from approximately 50% in the 1940s to approximately 10% at the present time.[1] The first of these procedures was that suggested by Daniels[2] in 1949 whereby the lymph nodes of the scalene fat pad were excised. It seemed reasonable then and does now that patients in whom the cancer had spread to the scalene area would not benefit from thoracotomy. Approximately 10 years later, Carlens described the technique of mediastinoscopy.[3] This technique has largely replaced scalene node biopsy in the evaluation of patients with nonpalpable nodes because of the increased yield with this procedure.[4,5] As will be discussed later, there are theoretical objections to the use of standard cervical mediastinoscopy in evaluation of patients with lesions of the left upper lobe, in that the anterior mediastinal nodes and the aortopulmonary nodes (stations 5 and 6) are not accessible through this approach. Accordingly, Stemmer et al[6] in 1965 and McNeil and Chamberlain[7] in 1966 described techniques of anterior mediastinoscopy or mediastinotomy for evaluation of these lesions. Several authors have addressed the problem of access to other regions of the mediastinum in other ways. Extended mediastinoscopy was described by Kirschner[8] in 1971 and Specht[9] in 1965 to approach the prevascular (retrosternal) space. In 1987, Ginsberg et al[10] extended this technique to provide access to the aorto-pulmonary nodes (station 5) as well. When combined with standard cervical mediastinoscopy, extended mediastinoscopy provides an appropriate method for full preoperative evaluation of left upper lobe lesions through one incision. Arom and associates[11] in 1977 described a subxiphoid approach to the substernal area that is occasionally useful. In 1976, Deslauriers and co-workers[12] advocated mediastinal pleuroscopy at the time of mediastinoscopy to permit lung biopsy and pleural evaluation. These modifications of the standard cervical mediastinoscopy may well be replaced, at least in part, by thoracoscopic techniques.[13]

### PULMONARY LYMPHATIC DRAINAGE

Understanding of the lymph drainage pathways from the lung is complicated by changing terminology for the various mediastinal lymph node groups. Fortunately, the terminology of the regional lymph nodes are standardized by the American Joint Committee for Cancer Staging and End-Results Reporting (AJC) and is shown in Figure 11–1.[14] Subsequently, the terminology was slightly modified by the

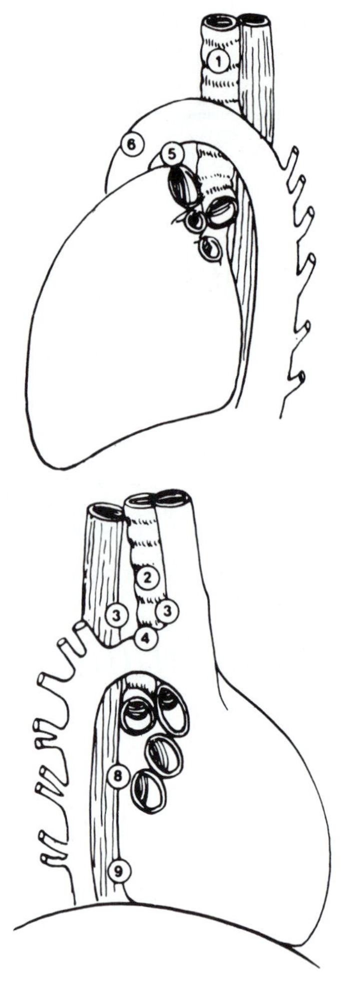

**N2 Nodes**

**Superior mediastinal nodes**

1. Highest mediastinal
2. Upper paratracheal
3. Pre- and retrotracheal
4. Lower paratracheal (including azygos nodes)

**Aortic nodes**

5. Subaortic (aortic window)
6. Para-aortic (ascending aorta or phrenic)

**Inferior mediastinal nodes**

7. Subcarinal
8. Paraesophageal (below carina)
9. Pulmonary ligament

**N1 Nodes**

10. Hilar
11. Interlobar
12. Lobar
13. Segmental

**Figure 11–1.** AJC terminology. *(From Beahrs OH, Meyers MH (eds): American Joint Committee on Cancer Manual for Staging of Cancer, 2nd ed. Philadelphia, Lippincott, 1983, with permission.)*

American Thoracic Society (ATS) based upon anatomic structures identifiable at mediastinoscopy.[15] A comparison of these nodal group classifications is given in Table 11–1. However, there are differences as determined by anatomists using dye injection methods, and the findings of nodal involvement in metastatic carcinoma of the lung.[16] Further, even among anatomists, there is no unanimity of opinion.[17–19] In general, anatomists agree that lymphatic drainage from the right upper lobe is to the lower and then to the higher paratracheal nodes on the right and from there into the neck. The lymphatic drainage from the middle lobe and from part of the lower portion of the upper lobe is to the subcarinal nodes and from there to the right paratracheal chain. The lymph flow from the right lower lobe is primarily to the subcarinal nodes and from there into the right paratracheal chain.

Normally, drainage from the upper left lobe is primarily to the aortopulmonary (subaortic) (Botallo's) node(s) and from there into the anterior mediastinal nodes or to the left paratracheal nodes. Drainage from the left lower lobe is primarily to the subcarinal nodes and from there along the right paratracheal chain.

It should be noted that although major emphasis is placed on the ascending drainage pattern, anatomists have described drainage through the diaphragm from the basal portions of the lung.

The findings of nodal involvement at the time of operation often do not follow the pathways described by the anatomists. Blockage of lymphatic channels may well provide explanation for unexpected nodal involvement. As described by Nohl-Oser,[16] nodal involvement from lesions of the left upper lobe, is *contralateral*, i.e., to the right side, as frequently as it is to the left. These findings are not those expected from the anatomical studies. In lesions of the left lower lobe, there is the expected finding of more contralateral spread than of ipsilateral or left-sided spread.

These considerations are of importance in planning biopsy procedures. The frequency of right-sided spread even with left upper lobe lesions makes conventional mediastinoscopy a reasonable first approach, even though nodes in the anterior mediastinum and in the subaortic (aortopulmonary) region cannot be reached by conventional mediastinoscopy.

**TABLE 11–1. COMPATIBILITY OF AJC AND ATS NODAL CLASSIFICATIONS**

| Nodal Station | AJC | ATS |
|---|---|---|
| 1. | Highest mediastinal | Included in station 2. |
| 2. | Upper paratracheal | Essentially unchanged. |
| 3. | Pre- and retrotracheal | If pretracheal, included in regions 2, 4, or 6 depending on anatomic location; if retrotracheal, included in region 8. |
| 4.[a] | Lower paratracheal | Boundaries of this *critical* station are defined. |
| 5. | Subaortic | Renamed aortopulmonary to include nodes along the lateral surfaces of the aorta and left or main pulmonary artery as well as those along the aortopulmonary window. |
| 6. | Paraortic | Renamed anterior mediastinal nodes; includes some pretracheal and preaortic nodes. |
| 7. | Subcarinal | Unchanged. |
| 8. | Paraesophageal | Unchanged. |
| 9. | Pulmonary ligament | Unchanged. |
| 10.[a] | Hilar | Designation of "hilar" dropped because of ambiguity of the radiologic use of this term; renamed peribronchial on the left and tracheobronchial on the right; this station is now outside the pleural reflection. |
| 11. | Interlobar | Reclassified as intrapulmonary. |
| 12. | Lobar | Included in station 11. |
| 13. | Segmental | Included in station 11. |

[a]The critical modifications that are being suggested.
*(From American Thoracic Society,[2] with permission of the American Lung Association.)*

## SCALENE NODE BIOPSY

In 1949, Daniels[2] suggested excision of lymph nodes of the scalene fat pad to diagnose intrathoracic disease. This operation was widely adopted, particularly for patients suspected of having bronchogenic carcinoma, sarcoidosis, or metastatic disease from other sites. Most authorities agree that palpable scalene nodes warrant biopsy in patients with intrathoracic disease. Controversy exists regarding the use of scalene biopsy for *nonpalpable* nodes.

In patients with suspected *carcinoma of the lung*, the use of scalene node biopsy in initial staging has decreased.[20–22] Although scalene node biopsy is usually done under local anesthesia and mediastinoscopy under general anesthesia, the reported mortality rates are not significantly different.[4,22] The choice of operation is based, therefore, on the anticipated yield from scalene node biopsy as compared with that from mediastinoscopy. Most authors report a yield of approximately 10% from scalene node biopsy in patients with nonpalpable node and no other indications of inoperability.[21,22] The anticipated yield from mediastinoscopy in this group of patients appears to be between 20% and 30%.[23] Therefore, we, like most other thoracic surgeons, prefer cervical mediastinoscopy in patients without palpable anterior cervical nodes if an invasive staging procedure is done before thoracotomy. Other authors, however, reporting positive findings as high as 23% from scalene node biopsy in patients with carcinoma who have nonpalpable nodes, believe that scalene node biopsy does have a place in initial staging procedures.[24,25] In the rare case where one is considering thoracotomy in spite of histologic evidence of mediastinal metastases, scalene node biopsy certainly would seem worthwhile, particularly when ultrasound or CT scan documents significant nodal involvement there.[26]

In patients with sarcoidosis, fiberoptic bronchoscopy with transbronchial biopsy is the diagnostic procedure of choice (Chap. 10). If further procedures are needed, mediastinoscopy is a better choice than scalene node biopsy because, again, the yield is higher with mediastinoscopy (98% vs. 75–85%).[27,28] If, however, the patient's condition makes general anesthesia hazardous, scalene node biopsy is a better choice.

## TECHNIQUE

This operation is performed under local anesthesia unless it is combined with other procedures. The incision is made on the side of palpable nodes. If nodes are not palpable, the incision is made on the right side for all lesions of the lung and mediastinum except those that appear to be confined to the left upper lobe. In the latter case and if disease metastatic from sites other than the thorax is under consideration, the left side is chosen. The incision, approximately 6 cm long, is made about 2 cm above the clavicle in the skin crease and usually extends about 2–3 cm over the lateral border of the sternocleidomastoid muscle (Fig. 11–2). This incision is deepened through the subcutaneous tissues and platysma, and the sternocleidomastoid muscle is retracted medially. In obese or muscular patients, it may be necessary to divide a portion of the clavicular head of this muscle or to carry the incision between its two heads. The omohyoid muscle is then identified and its fascia incised, after which the muscle is retracted superiorly and laterally. The fat pad containing the scalene lymph nodes is then excised from the

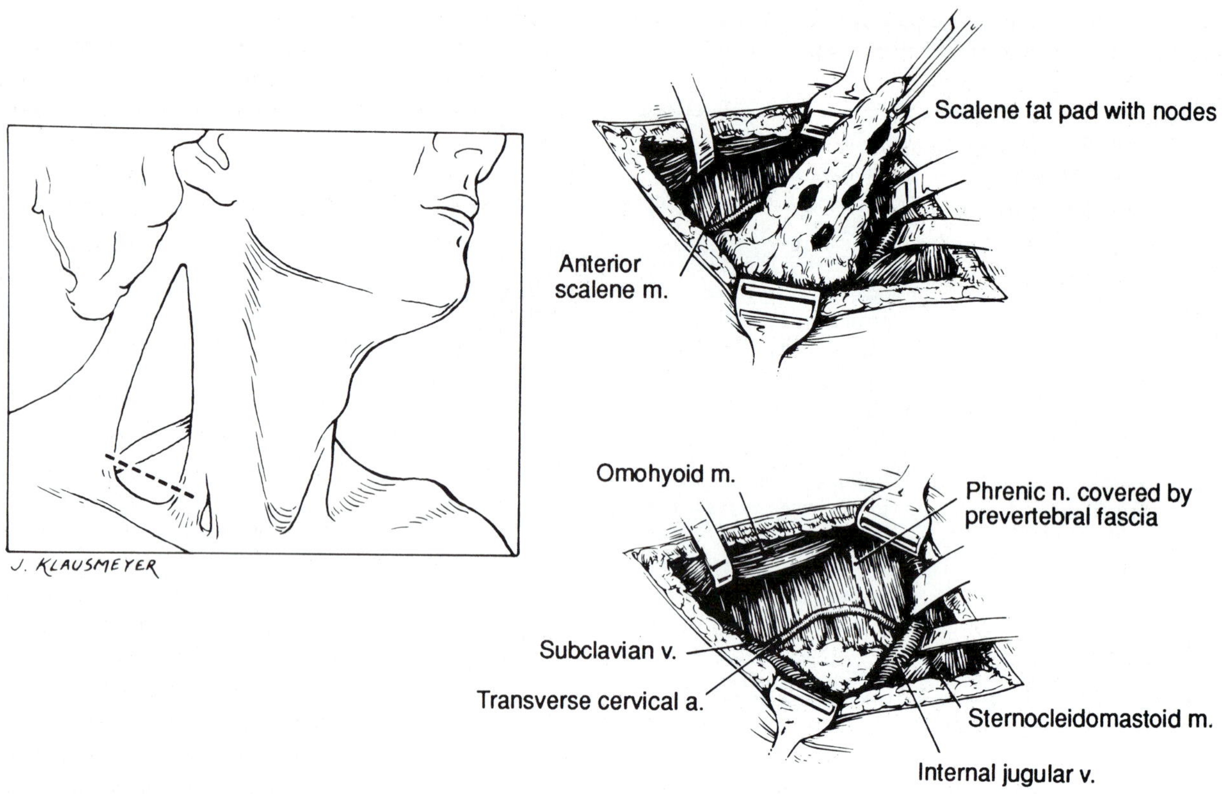


**Figure 11–2.** Scalene node biopsy.

anterior surface of the anterior scalene muscle. The dissection is carried to the internal jugular vein medially and to the omohyoid superiorly and laterally. The inferior border of the dissection is the subclavian vein, but frequently this is not clearly identified. If grossly abnormal nodes are present, the entire pad need not be excised.[28] The transverse cervical artery may require ligation and division. The phrenic nerve runs from a lateral to a medial position immediately on the anterior scalene muscle, but it is protected by a fascial sheath so that it need not be injured. On the left side the thoracic duct must be avoided; if it is severed, it should be ligated with nonabsorbable sutures. The platysma muscle is closed with interrupted 4-0 suture and the skin closed with subcuticular stitches as well and a pressure dressing applied until the next morning. The specimen should not only be sent for histologic examination, but a portion of it should be preserved for special stains and cultures to rule out granulomatous disease such as tuberculosis, histoplasmosis, and brucellosis. Potential complications include pneumothorax, chylous fistula, and, rarely, injury to the phrenic nerve. Serious complications are extremely infrequent, and the mortality from the procedure is a small fraction of 1% in experienced hands.[24]

## MEDIASTINOSCOPY

Since the description by Carlens[3] in 1959, this procedure has slowly gained wide acceptance. In most clinics, mediastinoscopy has replaced scalene node biopsy for invasive preoperative evaluation of patients with *suspected carcinoma of the lung*, unless there are palpable cervical nodes. As noted previously, this reasoning is based on the negligible mortality from either procedure and the increase in positive nodes from approximately 10–15% in scalene node biopsy to approximately 30–35% in mediastinoscopy.[4,5] Even patients who have had prior cervical mediastinoscopy or who have severe vena caval obstruction may safely undergo operation if reasonable care is exercised.[29–33]

There are currently two unresolved questions regarding this procedure in patients with bronchogenic carcinoma: (1) Which patients with suspected carcinoma of the lung, otherwise operable, should undergo this procedure? (2) What is the significance of positive mediastinal metastases (N2 disease) in such patients? Obviously, these two questions are interrelated. If one does not believe that positive mediastinal lymph nodes are a contraindication to thoracotomy, there is little reason for the liberal use of this procedure.

A strong case is made for preoperative mediastinoscopy in all patients by Maassen.[5] In his experience of 1921 cases of central tumors in stages I and II, 23% were positive and of the peripheral tumors in stage I and II, 19% were positive. Even exclusion from preoperative mediastinoscopy of peripheral tumors with a diameter of < 3 cm would lead to mediastinal metastases being missed in 11% of cases. Many authors, however, have advocated mediastinoscopy only in cases of central lesions, hilar involvement, or obvious mediastinal nodal involvement on standard radiographic examinations, or in those cases with positive gallium 67 scans of mediastinal nodes.[34–38]

The development of computed tomography (CT) has heightened this controversy. Several papers have reported significant numbers of patients who were presumably resectable and had been evaluated by preoperative CT scans and the findings correlated with mediastinoscopy and thoracotomy. Data from five such studies are summarized in Table 11–2.[40–43]

Histologic confirmation of a positive scan is clearly indicated. Whether or not patients should be excluded from mediastinoscopy on the basis of a negative CT scan is controversial. Data from the largest of these series have a negative predictive index (NPI) of 93%, and the authors, therefore, suggest that most patients with normal CT by their criteria can proceed directly to thoracotomy. However, in 1990, Dales and co-workers[44] published a meta-analysis of the literature regarding the ability of computed tomography to detect mediastinal lymph node metastases from non–small-cell bronchogenic carcinoma. The result of this analysis convinced them that CT scanning of the mediastinum results in approximately 21% false-positive and 20% false-negative results. They were unconvinced that a negative CT exam even with a peripheral lung lesion was adequate reason to exclude mediastinoscopy. Further, in 1992 Kerr et al[45] published a careful examination of mediastinal lymph nodes taken from patients who underwent thoracotomy. They found metastatic disease in 15% of lymph nodes <10 mm in diameter and believe this finding called into question the confidence that could be placed in a so-called negative computed tomographic examination.

In summary, all positive CT reports should be confirmed by histologic or cytologic study. Even negative CT reports have an unacceptable margin of error if one accepts the importance of positive mediastinal nodes in excluding most patients from resection.

The significance of metastatic disease in mediastinal lymph nodes (N2) still causes debate among surgeons. Questions regarding the significance of mediastinal metastases were generated by the reports of Kirsh et al,[46] Martini et al,[47] and others[48,49] of reasonable survival following resection in patients with known positive mediastinal nodal involvement. In discussions of the benefits of resections in patients with known N2 disease, one must recall the work of Paulson and Urschel[50] in which they found a 5-year survival rate of 3% following exploratory thoracotomy and 1% in patients with primary inoperable tumors.

Therefore, one must be careful in evaluating results of resection in patients with known N2 disease that the reported survival (including operative mortality) is greater than that of the natural history of the disease. There are certain subsets of patients, however, that may well benefit from resection of N2 disease. Selected patients in whom there is limited involvement of the aortopulmonary nodes but not involvement of the anterior mediastinal nodes and those patients with non–small-cell cancer in whom there is limited ipsilateral tracheobronchial intranodal involvement may fall into this category.[51,52] We continue to believe that except for patients in these latter two categories, patients with N2 disease discovered preoperatively should not be subjected to resection in spite of reports advocating a contrary view.[53,54] Obviously, if nodal involvement is discovered at the time of resection, and a nodal dissection can be carried out without leaving gross tumor behind, resection is indicated.[55,56] Confirmation of the accuracy of frozen section diagnosis and the ability to perform mediastinoscopy in the outpatient setting contribute to the attractiveness of this procedure.[57,58]

On the Robert Wood Johnson Thoracic Surgical Service (formerly Rutgers Thoracic Surgical Service), we have performed over 3650 mediastinoscopies with one mortality. The mortality in over 11,000 mediastinoscopies collected by Specht[59] was about 0.15%. Therefore, the negligible mortality and doubt concerning the reliability of CT scan even for peripheral lesions causes us to continue to recom-

**TABLE 11–2. CT LUNG CANCER (Mediastinal Nodes)**

| | | | | Percent | |
|---|---|---|---|---|---|
| **Author** | **Year** | **No. Patients** | **Criterion Positivity** | ***Negative Predictive Index***[a] | ***Positive Predictive Index***[b] |
| Brion | 1985 | 153 | >5 mm | 88 | 48 |
| Redina | 1987 | 171 | >10 mm | 97 | 82 |
| Daly | 1987 | 345 | 15 mm or larger | 93 | 68 |
| Staples | 1988 | 151 | >10 mm | 80 | 83 |
| McLoud | 1991 | 143 | >10 mm | 79 | 44 |

[a]Negative predictive value:

$$\frac{\text{No. of True Negative}}{\text{No. of True Negative + No. False Negative}} \times 100.$$

[b]Positive predictive value:

$$\frac{\text{No. of True Negative}}{\text{No. of True Negative + No. False Negative}} \times 100.$$

mend mediastinoscopy for most patients. Patients with peripheral lesions less than 2 cm in diameter and no risk factor with a negative mediastinal CT scan are an occasional exception to this policy, but the newest data described above make even this exception questionable.

## TECHNIQUE

CT scans are carefully reviewed prior to operation. The operation is done under general anesthesia with the opening table adjusted to decrease obvious venous distention but not enough to increase the possibility of air embolism. The patient's neck should be slightly extended; hyperextension decreases the space between the sternum and the trachea and increases the possibility of compression of the innominate artery. Although continuous recording or palpation of the right radial artery pulse has been advocated, we find this unnecessary if excessive anterior compression is avoided. The transverse incision is made approximately 1 cm above the sternal ends of the clavicles and deepened through the platysma muscle (Fig. 11–3). The strap muscles are divided vertically in the midline, principally by spreading of a small hemostat; the thyroid isthmus is retracted superiorly and the pretracheal fascia incised. With finger dissection, a tunnel is created within the pretracheal fascia anterior to the trachea and beneath the innominate artery as it is palpated slightly to the right of the midportion of the trachea and beneath the aortic arch as it curves over the left main bronchus. Approaching the lower portion of this dissection, the envelope of pretracheal fascia is opened to expose the paratracheal and tracheobronchial lymph nodes. Careful palpation often reveals enlarged nodes, and these findings are correlated, if possible, with CT scan.

The finger is withdrawn and the mediastinoscope is inserted with the aid of an Allyce forcep on the inferior flap of the tracheal fascia. Nodes previously identified by palpation are biopsied; if there is any question as to whether this structure is a lymph node or a blood vessel, aspiration is done prior to biopsy. A combination insulated sucker and coagulating device is helpful. If no palpable nodes are present, biopsy of the paratracheal nodes and of the tracheobronchial nodes is carried out. Subcarinal nodes are ordinarily not biopsied unless they are abnormal to palpation with the finger or sucker or they are abnormally enlarged on CT scan. Hemostasis is obtained by coagulation, clipping, and packing. Should significant bleeding occur, the mediastinoscope is left in place and the area packed with gauze for at least 10 minutes. Packing is then removed, and, if the bleeding is still significant, the packing is reapplied and preparation made for thoracotomy.

If one assumes that hemostasis is satisfactory, the wound is thoroughly irrigated and strap muscles closed

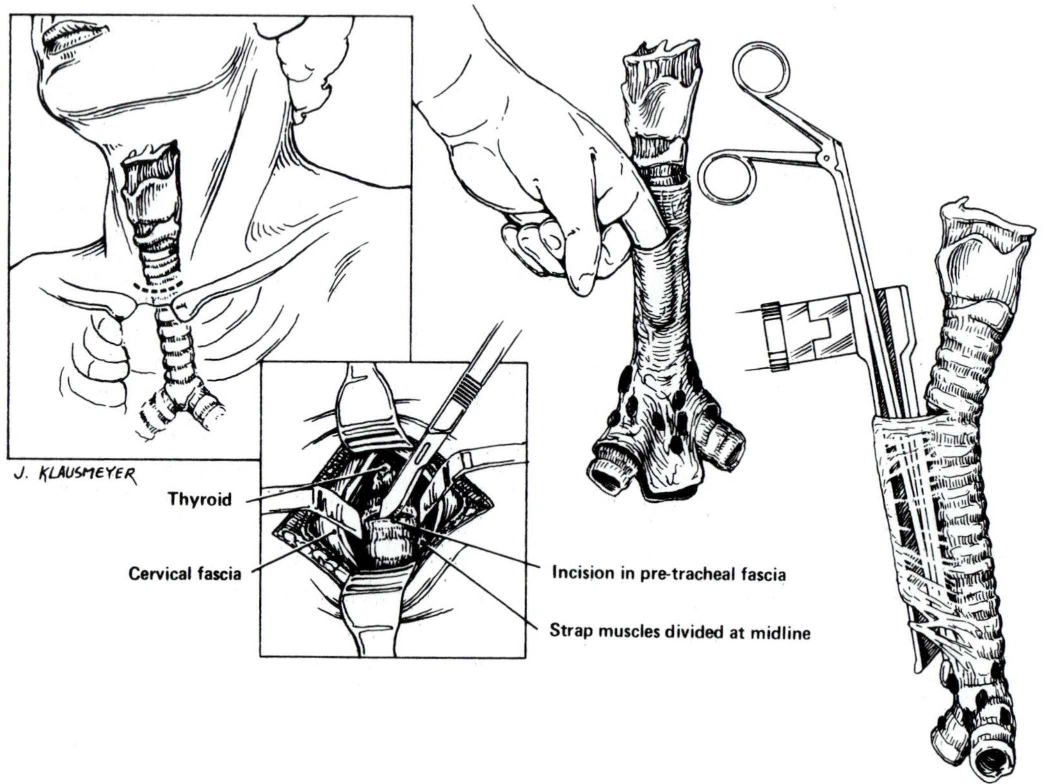


**Figure 11–3.** Mediastinoscopy.

with interrupted 3-0 silk suture. An interrupted 3-0 polyglactin (Vicryl) (Trademark—Ethicon) suture is used to close the subcutaneous tissue and subcuticular stitch of 4-0 polyglactin (Vicryl) applied.

The incidence of serious bleeding is between 0.1 and 0.2%[59]; the complications of vocal cord paralysis and pneumothorax occur slightly more frequently. Extremely rare complications include damage to the esophagus, thoracic duct, bronchus and trachea, cardiac arrhythmias, and wound seeding.[60–62]

## MODIFIED MEDIASTINOSCOPY

Particularly in evaluation of lesions of the left upper lobe and in the evaluation of some lymphomas or benign mediastinal tumors, standard cervical mediastinoscopy does not provide appropriate access. Percutaneous needle biopsy may be helpful in these cases. If necessary, entry into what has been termed the prevascular or retrosternal zone, may be reached through the same skin incision used for standard mediastinoscopy.[8,9]

Although lesions from the left upper lobe do spread to the right side as often as to the left, standard cervical mediastinoscopy does not provide appropriate access to other early sites of metastasis (stations 5 and 6).[16] Ginsberg et al's[10] extended mediastinoscopy does provide staging appropriate for left upper lobe lesions through a single incision (Fig. 11–4). Other authors have utilized this technique, and recently Ginsberg[63] has updated his experience to report 300 personal cases with a negligible morbidity and no mortality.[64] Nevertheless, extended mediastinoscopy does have a significant learning curve, and, as noted previously, the recent availability of video-assisted thoracoscopic exploration of the thorax may make extended mediastinoscopy less attractive.

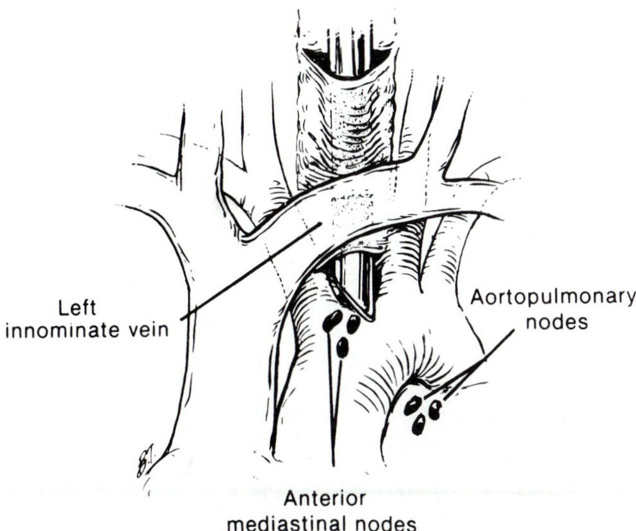


**Figure 11–4.** Transcervical biopsy of anterior mediastinal and subaortic nodes.

## ANTERIOR MEDIASTINOTOMY

As discussed in the preceding section, the theoretical drainage from lesions of the left upper lobe is to areas not accessible by standard cervical mediastinoscopy. For this reason, a number of authors have advocated anterior mediastinotomy as the initial procedure of choice for these lesions.[65,66] Since paratracheal metastases from left upper lobe lesions are a clear-cut contraindication to pulmonary resection in the opinion of most surgeons, we have preferred cervical mediastinoscopy as the initial procedure for all lesions, including those of the left upper lobe. Anterior mediastinoscopy does result in chest wall discomfort that may interfere with coughing; it may delay radiation therapy if it is indicated, and advances in transcutaneous needle biopsy and transtracheal biopsy have also decreased the need for anterior mediastinotomy.[67–69] Finally, videoscopic techniques will probably contribute still further to the decreased utilization of anterior mediastinotomy or mediastinoscopy.

## TECHNIQUE

The original report by Stemmer et al[6] described an approach through a vertical incision after subperichondrial resection of the second and third cartilages. The more popular modification described by McNeil and Chamberlain[7] advocated an incision over the second costal cartilage with removal of the costal cartilage subperichondrially. We have found the use of a second interspace incision without removing the cartilage satisfactory for most patients. Occasionally, a portion or all of the cartilage must be removed in patients with a narrow intercostal space (Fig. 11–5).

The internal mammary artery and vein are usually ligated, preferably individually. The mediastinum is entered after lateral mobilization of the pleura. The anterior mediastinal and the aortopulmonary nodes are evaluated. Fine-needle aspiration may make the operation easier and safer. The pericardium may be entered to evaluate extensive central involvement. Appropriate samples are obtained. If the pleural cavity is entered, it is drained with an intercostal tube attached to underwater seal.

Certainly, firmly matted nodes in the aortopulmonary window or spread to the anterior mediastinal nodes preclude thoracotomy as does extensive central involvement. Nodes restricted to the aortopulmonary window that are easily resectable as judged by palpation should not preclude thoracotomy. A 5-year survival rate of 28% has been reported in such cases.[52]

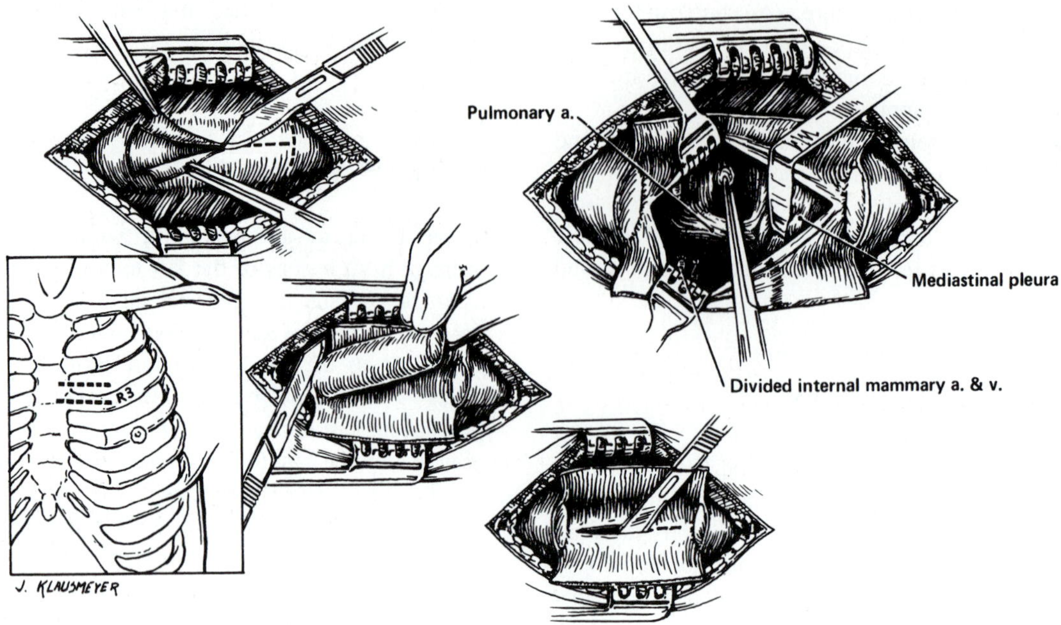


**Figure 11–5.** Anterior mediastinotomy.

## SUMMARY

The importance of staging in patients with bronchogenic carcinoma is increasingly appreciated. Not only does proper staging avoid unnecessary operations, but it allows accurate comparisons on various treatments including the use of adjuvant therapy. Only with accurate staging can valid comparisons be made.

## REFERENCES


1. Pearson FG: Staging of the mediastinum. Role of mediastinoscopy and computed tomography. *Chest* **103:**346S, 1993
2. Daniels AC: A method of biopsy useful in diagnosing certain intrathoracic diseases. *Dis Chest* **16:**360, 1949
3. Carlens E: Mediastinoscopy: A method for inspection and tissue biopsy in the superior mediastinum. *Dis Chest* **36:**343, 1959
4. Luke WP, Pearson FG, Todd TRJ, et al: Prospective evaluation of mediastinoscopy for assessment of carcinoma of the lung. *J Thorac Cardiovasc Surg* **91:**53, 1986
5. Maassen W: The staging issue—problems: Accuracy of mediastinoscopy. In Delarue NC, Eschapasse H (eds): *International Trends in General Thoracic Surgery. Lung Cancer*, vol. 1. Philadelphia, Saunders, 1985, Chapter 3, pp 42–53
6. Stemmer EA, Calvin JW, Chandor SB, et al: Mediastinal biopsy for indeterminate pulmonary and mediastinal lesions. *J Thorac Cardiovasc Surg* 405, 1965
7. McNeill TM, Chamberlain JM: Diagnostic anterior mediastinotomy. *Ann Thorac Surg* **2:**532, 1966
8. Kirschner PA: "Extended" mediastinoscopy. In Jespen O, Sorensen HR (eds): *Mediastinoscopy*. Denmark, Odense University Press, 1971, 131
9. Specht G: Erweiterte mediastinoskopie. *Thoraxchir Vask Chir* **13:**401, 1965
10. Ginsberg RJ, Rice TW, Goldberg M, et al: Extended cervical mediastinoscopy. A single staging procedure for bronchogenic carcinoma of the left upper lobe. *J Thorac Cardiovasc Surg* **94:**673, 1987
11. Arom KV, Franz JL, Grover FL, Trinkle JK: Subxiphoid anterior mediastinal exploration. *Ann Thorac Surg* **24:**289, 1977
12. Deslauriers J, Beaulieu M, Dufour C, et al: Mediastinopleuroscopy: A new approach to the diagnosis of intrathoracic diseases. *Ann Thorac Surg* **22:**265, 1976
13. Landreneau RJ, Hazelrigg SR, Mack MJ, et al: Thoracoscopic mediastinal lymph node sampling: Useful for mediastinal lymph node stations inaccessible by cervical mediastinoscopy. *J Thorac Cardiovasc Surg* **106:**554, 1993
14. Beahrs OH, Myers MH: Lung. In Beahrs O, Myers M (eds): *Manual for Staging of Cancer, American Joint Committee on Cancer*, 2nd ed. Philadelphia, Lippincott, 1983, pp 99–105
15. American Thoracic Society, Medical Section of the American Lung Association: Clinical staging of primary lung cancer. *Am Rev Resp Dis* **127:**659, 1983
16. Nohl-Oser HC: An investigation of the anatomy of the lymphatic drainage of the lungs. *Ann R Coll Surg Engl* **51:**157, 1972
17. Rouviere H: Lymphatics of the lungs. In Rouviere H (ed): *Anatomy of the Human Lymphatic System*. Ann Arbor, Michigan, Edwards Brothers Inc, 1938, pp 113–118
18. Shimazaki H: Lymphatic system. In Nagaishi C (ed): *Functional Anatomy and Histology of the Lung*, Baltimore, University Park Press, 1972, pp 149–150
19. Oka H: Lymphatic system. In Nagaishi C (ed): *Functional Anatomy and Histology of the Lung*, Baltimore, University Park Press, 1972, pp 150
20. Leckie WJ, McCormack RJM, Walbaum PR: The case against routine scalene node biopsy in bronchial carcinoma. *Lancet* **1:**853, 1963
21. Shields TW, Shocket E: Preoperative evaluation of patients with clinically resectable bronchogenic carcinoma. *Arch Surg* **76:**707, 1958
22. Skinner DB: Scalene lymph node biopsy. Reappraisal of risks and indications. *N Engl J Med* **268:**1324, 1963
23. Ashraf MH, Milsom PL, Walesby RK: Selection by mediastinoscopy and long-term survival in bronchial carcinoma. *Ann Thorac Surg* **30:**208, 1980
24. Brantigan JW, Brantigan CO, Brantigan OC: Biopsy of nonpalpable

scalene lymph nodes in carcinoma of the lung. *Am Rev Resp Dis* **107:**962, 1973

25. Brousseau JD, Reinecke ME, Banerjee TK, et al: The continuing importance of scalene node biopsy in lung cancer patients. *Wis Med J* **76:**97, 1977
26. van Overhagen H, Lameris JS, Berger MY, et al: Supraclavicular lymph node metastases in carcinoma of the esophagus and gastroesophageal junction: Assessment with CT, US, and Us-guided fine-needle aspiration biopsy. *Radiology* **179:**155, 1991
27. Greschuchna D, Maassen W: Results of mediastinoscopy and other biopsies in sarcoidosis and silicosis. In Jespen O, Sorensen HR (eds): *Mediastinoscopy*. Denmark, Odense University Press, 1971, pp 79–82.
28. Truedson H, Stjernberg N, Thunell M: Scalene lymph node biopsy. A diagnostic method in sarcoidosis. *Acta Chir Scan* **151:**121, 1985
29. Kirschner PA: Mediastinoscopy in superior vena cava obstruction. In Jespen O, Sorensen HR (eds): *Mediastinoscopy*. Denmark, Odense University Press, 1971, pp 40–42.
30. Lewis RJ, Sisler GE, Mackenzie JW: Mediastinoscopy in advanced superior vena cava obstruction. *Ann Thorac Surg* **32:**458, 1981
31. Lewis RJ, Sisler GE, Mackenzie JW: Repeat mediastinoscopy. *Ann Thorac Surg* **37:**147, 1984
32. Jahangiri M, Taggart DP, Goldstraw P: Role of mediastinoscopy in superior vena cava obstruction. *Cancer* **71:**3006, 1993
33. Meersschaut D, Vermassen F, de la Riviere AB, et al: Repeat mediastinoscopy in the assessment of new and recurrent lung neoplasm. *Ann Thorac Surg* **53:**120, 1992
34. Acosta JL, Manfredi F: Selective mediastinoscopy. *Chest* **71:**150, 1977
35. DeMeester TR, Bekerman C, Joseph JG, et al: Gallium-67 scanning for carcinoma of the lung. *J Thorac Cardiovasc Surg* **72:**699, 1976
36. Hutchinson CM, Mills NL: The selection of patients with bronchogenic carcinoma for mediastinoscopy. *J Thorac Cardiovasc Surg* **71:**768, 1976
37. Whitcomb ME, Barham E, Goldman AL, Green DC: Indications for mediastinoscopy in bronchogenic carcinoma. *Am Rev Resp Dis* **113:**189, 1976
38. Baker RR, Lillemoe KD, Tockman MS: The indications for transcervical mediastinoscopy in patients with small peripheral bronchial carcinoma. *Surg Gynecol Obstet* **148:**860, 1979
39. Brion JP, Depauw L, Kuhn G, et al: Role of computed tomography and mediastinoscopy in preoperative staging of lung carcinoma. *J Comput Assist Tomogr* **9:**480, 1985
40. Daly BDT Jr, Faling LJ, Bite G, et al: Mediastinal lymph node evaluation by computed tomography in lung cancer. An analysis of 345 patients grouped by TNM staging, tumor size, and tumor location. *J Thorac Cardiovasc Surg* **94:**664, 1987
41. Redina EA, Bognola DA, Mineo TC, et al: Computed tomography for the evaluation of intrathoracic invasion by lung cancer. *J Thorac Cardiovasc Surg* **94:**57, 1987
42. McLoud TC, Bourgouin PM, Greenberg RW, et al: Bronchogenic carcinoma: Analysis of staging in the mediastinum with CT by correlative lymph node mapping and sampling. *Radiology* **182:**319, 1992
43. Staples CA, Muller NL, Miller RR, et al: Mediastinal nodes in bronchogenic carcinoma: Comparison between CT and mediastinoscopy. *Radiology* **167:**367, 1988
44. Dales RE, Stark RM, Raman S: Computed tomography to stage lung cancer. Approaching a controversy using meta-analysis. *Am Rev Respir Dis* **141:**1096, 1990
45. Kerr KM, Lamb D, Wathen CG, et al: Pathological assessment of mediastinal lymph nodes in lung cancer: implications for non-invasive mediastinal staging. *Thorax* **47:**337, 1992
46. Kirsch MM, Kahn DR, Gaggo O, et al: Treatment of bronchogenic carcinoma with mediastinal metastases. *Ann Thorac Surg* **12:**11, 1971
47. Martini N, Flehinger BJ, Zaman MB, Beattie EJ: Prospective study of 445 lung carcinomas with mediastinal lymph node metastases. *J Thorac Cardiovasc Surg* **80:**390, 1980
48. Rubinstein I, Baum GL, Kalter Y, et al: Resectional surgery in the treatment of primary carcinoma of the lung with mediastinal lymph node metastases. *Thorax* **34:**33, 1979
49. Pearson FG, DeLarue NC, Ilves R, et al: Significance of positive superior mediastinal nodes identified at mediastinoscopy in patients with resectable cancer of the lung. *J Thorac Cardiovasc Surg* **83:**1, 1982
50. Paulson DL, Urschel HC Jr: Selectivity in the surgical treatment of bronchogenic carcinoma. *J Thorac Cardiovasc Surg* **62:**554, 1971
51. Shields TS: The significance of ipsilateral mediastinal lymph node metastasis (N2 disease) in non-small cell carcinoma of the lung. *J Thorac Cardiovasc Surg* **99:**48, 1990
52. Patterson GA, Piazza D, Pearson FG, et al: Significance of metastatic disease in subaortic lymph nodes. *Ann Thorac Surg* **43:**155, 1987
53. Watanabe Y, Shimizu J, Oda M, et al: Aggressive surgical intervention in N2 non-small cell cancer of the lung. *Ann Thorac Surg* **41:**253, 1991
54. Naruke T, Goya T, Tsuchiya R, Suemasu K: The importance of surgery to non-small cell carcinoma of lung with mediastinal lymph node metastasis. *Ann Thorac Surg* **46:**603, 1988
55. Goldstraw P, Mannam GC, Kaplan DK, Michail P: Surgical management of non-small-cell lung cancer with ipsilateral mediastinal node metastasis (N2 disease). *J Thorac Cardiovasc Surg* **107:**19, 1994
56. van Klaveren RJ, Festen J, Otten HJAM, Cox AL, et al: Prognosis of unsuspected but completely resectable N2 non-small cell lung cancer. *Ann Thorac Surg* **56:**300, 1993
57. Gephardt GN, Rice TW: Utility of frozen-section evaluation of lymph nodes in the staging of bronchogenic carcinoma at mediastinoscopy and thoracotomy. *J Thorac Cardiovasc Surg* **100:**853, 1990
58. Vallieres E, Page A, Verdant A: Ambulatory mediastinoscopy and anterior mediastinotomy. *Ann Thorac Surg* **52:**1122, 1991
59. Specht G: Discussion by Carlens. In Jespen O, Sorenson HR (eds): *Mediastinoscopy*. Denmark, Odense University Press, 1971, 130
60. Hoyer ER, Leonard CE, Hazuka MB, Wechsler-Jentzsch K: Mediastinoscopy incisional metastasis. A radiotherapeutic approach. *Cancer* **70:**1612, 1992
61. Basca S, Czako Z, Vezendi S: The complications of mediastinoscopy. *Panminerva Med* **16:**402, 1974
62. Foster ED, Munro DD, Dobell ARC: Mediastinoscopy. A review of anatomical relationship and complications. *Ann Thorac Surg* **13:**273, 1972
63. Ginsberg RJ: The role of preoperative surgical staging in left upper lobe tumors. *Ann Thorac Surg* **57:**526, 1994
64. Lopez L, Varela A, Freixinet J, et al: Extended cervical mediastinoscopy: Prospective study of fifty cases. *Ann Thor Surg* **57:**555, 1994
65. Bowen TE, Zajtchuk R, Green DC, Brott WH: Value of anterior mediastinotomy in bronchogenic carcinoma of the left upper lobe. *J Thorac Cardiovasc Surg* **76:**269, 1978
66. Jolly PC, Li W, Anderson RP: Anterior and cervical mediastinoscopy for determining operability and predicting resectability in lung cancer. *J Thorac Cardiovasc Surg* **79:**366, 1980
67. Cheung DK, Stibal D, Weinberg S, Poleksic S: Needle aspiration biopsy as an adjunct to mediastinoscopy. *South Med J* **79:**1067, 1986
68. Wang KP, Brower R, Haponik EF: Flexible transbronchial needle aspiration for staging of bronchogenic carcinoma. *Chest* **84:**571, 1983
69. Callol L, Garcia-Perez C, Sevillano A, et al: Letter to the editor. *Resp Med* **84:**177, 1990

CHAPTER

# 12A

# Thoracoscopy

## *General Principles and Diagnostic Procedures*

Peter F. Ferson, Rodney J. Landreneau, and Robert J. Keenan

### INTRODUCTION

Minimally invasive surgery has been widely accepted in gynecology, abdominal surgery, and orthopedic surgery. The concept of performing standard surgical procedures through limited incisions has the advantages of decreasing pain, accelerating recovery, and potentially decreasing operative risk and morbidity. Development of video optic systems and design of new instruments overcomes the limitations of visibility and access.

The keystone of minimally invasive surgery is the introduction of a video camera through a small incision for intracavitary visualization. In thoracic surgical procedures this requires a chest tube-sized interspace incision through which a 10–12-mm-diameter cylindrical port is inserted to allow introduction of the video camera (the thoracoscope). Similar incisions may be placed at strategic locations to insert instruments designed to function through the small access ports. Alternatively, a limited intercostal incision can be performed, without a rib-spreading retractor, and standard instruments can be used to perform the procedure while one observes through the video system. This latter method has spawned the term *video-assisted thoracic surgery* (VATS) (Figs. 12A–1, 12A–2).

### HISTORY

Hans Jacobaeus[1,2] proposed thoracoscopy in 1910 and performed the first procedure in 1913. He introduced a cystoscope into the pleural cavity to lyse adhesions to enhance pneumothorax therapy of tuberculosis. Thoracoscopic techniques for the next 30 years were mostly applied to the management of tuberculosis.[3]

Interest in thoracoscopy for investigation of pleural diseases or diagnosis of intrathoracic malignancies persisted.[4,5] A few isolated series reported biopsy of the lung parenchyma.[6,7] With the development of instruments initially for laparoscopic gynecologic procedures and advanced video systems for laparoscopy and orthopedic arthroscopy, further efforts rapidly followed in thoracic surgery.

The use of lasers and development of endoscopic staplers permitted direct therapy for bullous disease,[8] wedge resection of the lung for parenchymal biopsy, and resection of pulmonary masses.[9,10]

### GENERAL PRINCIPLES AND STRATEGIES

#### Patient Selection

As experience with VATS has developed, the selection of patients has become a patient-related factor. With small accessory interspace incisions, it is possible to perform nearly all intrathoracic procedures videoscopically. All major anatomic lung resections can be safely performed in this fashion,[11–13] as can resection of mediastinal tumors[14] and mobilization of the esophagus.[15,16] The decision to proceed

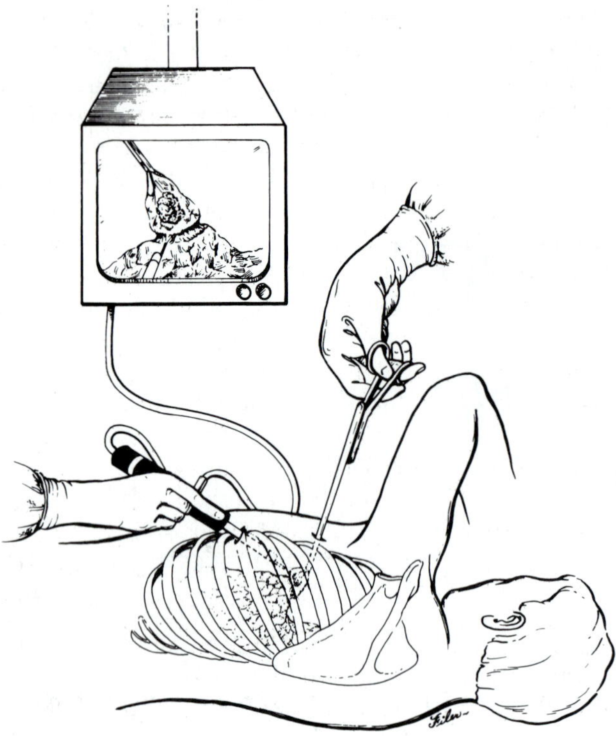

**Figure 12A–1.** Illustration of video-assisted approach to intrathoracic manipulation. Both the thoracoscope and the working instruments are introduced through intercostal cannulae. *(From Dowling RD, Landreneau RJ, Wachs ME, Ferson PF. Thoracoscopic Nd:YAG laser resection of a solitary pulmonary nodule. Chest 102:1903–1905, 1992 with permission.)*

with a video-assisted procedure is no longer dependent on the procedure to be performed but rather on the presence or absence of adhesions, the completeness of fissure development, or the ability to control ventilation.

Patients with previous thoracotomies or with a history of extensive pleural disease are not good candidates for video-assisted procedures, since a complete pneumothorax with good visibility is difficult to obtain. This is not an absolute contraindication, since often the adhesions can be dealt with and complete mobilization of the lung achieved.

Inability to tolerate one-lung anesthesia is rare. Even patients with end-stage interstitial lung disease who are oxygen dependent will usually tolerate single-lung ventilation with 100% oxygen.[17] Patients who are intubated, on high concentrations of oxygen, with positive end-expiratory pressure (PEEP) and elevated peak airway pressures (such as candidates for lung biopsy in the clinical setting of sepsis and respiratory distress syndrome) will not be considered for video-assisted procedures.

Nearly all lung resections with a free pleural space can be initially approached thoracoscopically. This will allow initial evaluation of the structures, localization of the site of abnormality, assessment of the mediastinal and hilar lymph nodes, and observation of the fissures. If the impression is favorable for the VATS approach to pulmonary resection, then further progress can be made with an accessory incision if necessary. If visibility becomes inadequate, or if the dissection becomes difficult, the accessory incision can easily be extended to an open thoracotomy.

## Anesthetic Management

Anesthesia for video-assisted thoracic procedures is similar to that for open thoracotomies. For most major procedures,

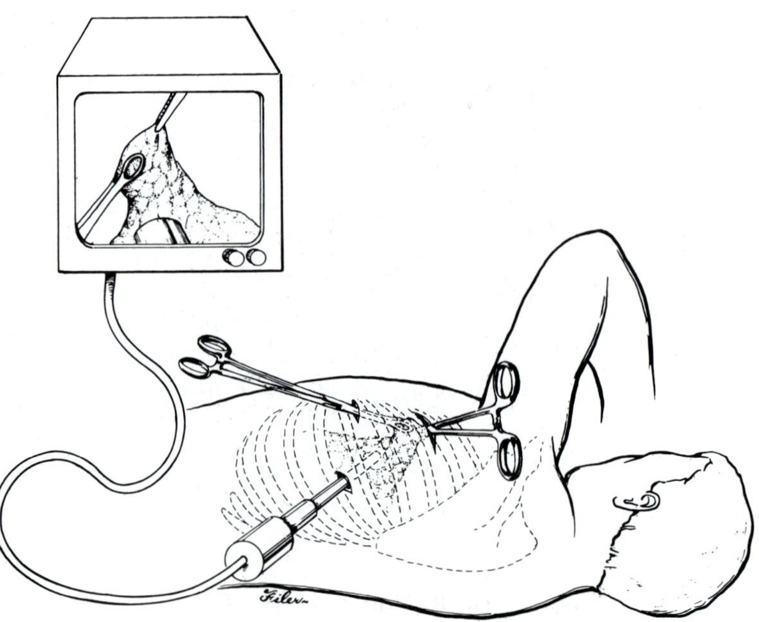

**Figure 12A–2.** VATS using an accessory incision to permit introduction of standard instruments.

an arterial monitoring catheter is inserted. Pulse oximetry and end-tidal $CO_2$ determinations are useful for continuous assessment of the adequacy of ventilation.

Since ipsilateral lung collapse with resulting pneumothorax is necessary, single-lung ventilation is essential. This can be achieved with the use of a "bronchus blocker" system. Such systems have been built into a standard endotracheal tube, but alternatively one can place a balloon catheter alongside the endotracheal tube and into the desired bronchus to achieve ipsilateral collapse of the lung. This bronchus blocker mechanism provides very slow emptying of the lung, and the balloon can be easily dislodged, resulting in loss of pulmonary collapse. This is particularly a problem when collapse of the right lung is desired. A double-lumen endotracheal tube with left mainstem intubation provides more reliable control of ventilation with greater ability to suction and empty the collapsed lung when appropriate. The left-sided endobronchial tube works equally well to exclude either lung. Conversely, right-sided endobronchial tubes are difficult to place and to maintain in a stable position.

Since collapse of the lung is necessary for thoracoscopy, it is important to recognize the potential airway circumstances resulting in inadequate atelectasis. Retained secretions can obstruct airways with delayed emptying of the lung. These can usually be removed with suctioning. Inadequate seal of the bronchus around the endobronchial balloon can allow crossed ventilation. This is uncommon if the endotracheal tube lumen to the isolated lung is left open to air and is free to empty. The most common technical problem is positioning of the left bronchial extension of the endotracheal tube, which is easily identified and corrected.

Initial misplacement of the double-lumen tube will usually result in the left endobronchial limb being inserted into the bronchus intermedius. This can often be recognized by auscultation; however, bronchoscopic assessment is the essential evaluation.

A properly placed double-lumen catheter may shift position during a procedure. This is most likely to occur with lateral positioning of the patient or when the pulmonary parenchyma and hilum are manipulated. This will present distinct and easily recognizable problems. Proximal displacement of the endotracheal tube will cause herniation of the endobronchial cuff over the carina and will obstruct the right bronchus. The right lung will not ventilate when left-lung collapse is desired or will not collapse for right-sided procedures. Distal displacement of the tube will cause the left endobronchial limb to impact in the left lower lobe, causing inadequate ventilation when one is ventilating the left lung or inadequate collapse when performing a left-sided procedure. When these problems develop, the surgical and anesthesia team must reexamine the position of the endotracheal tube bronchoscopically. Minor adjustments in tube position will usually correct the problem.

Carbon dioxide insufflation is used routinely during VATS. It may help expeditious induction of pneumothorax and collapse of emphysematous lung. Once a pneumothorax has been produced, a closed system needed for $CO_2$ pressurization is a disadvantage.

## Video Equipment

The difference between "video-assisted" procedures and "open" procedures is the method of viewing. The difference in visualization from direct vision to video-reproduced images on a monitor introduces a fundamental change in perception and motor orientation. The surgeon and assistant must become familiar with camera orientation, magnification, and change of depth perception. The inability to easily change viewing angle decreases three-dimensional perception; therefore, knowledge of intrathoracic relationships is vital.

Our standard camera and thoracoscope system is a rigid lens thoracoscope with light fibers and an operating channel (Karl Storz Corp., Culver City, California) (Fig. 12A–3A,B). The camera is attached to the eyepiece of the thoracoscope and transmits a video image to a camera converter and video monitor. The quality of the image produced depends on many factors such as the size of the light-

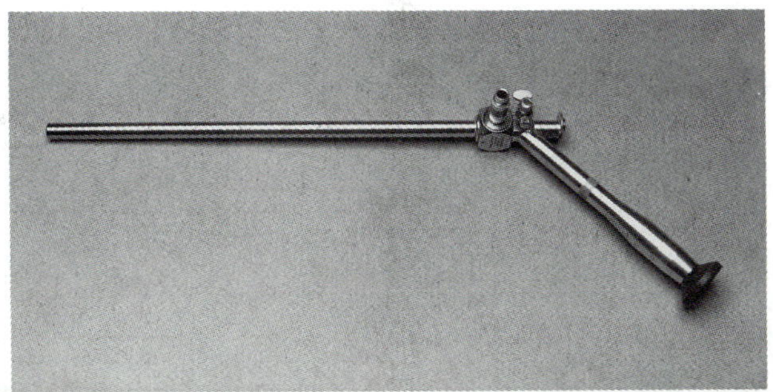

A

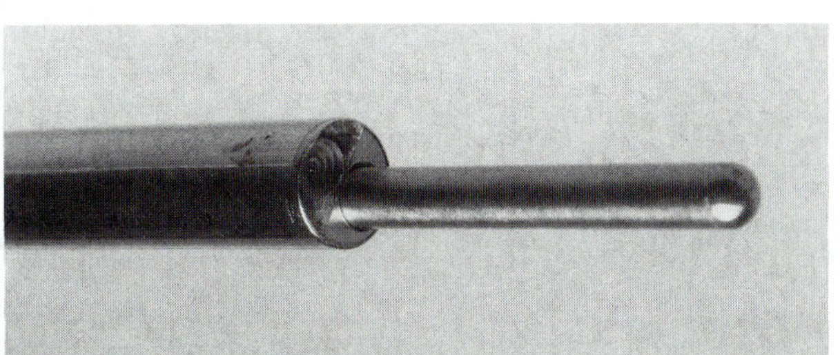

B

**Figure 12A–3. A.** A standard thoracoscope with an offset viewing lens. **B.** A 5-mm working channel allows introduction of instruments. (A blunt probe is demonstrated.)

carrying bundles within the thoracoscope, the resolution and light sensitivity of the camera, the resolution of the video monitor, and the field of view of the thoracoscope. A wide-angle field of view is helpful for orientation. The light-carrying needs of a thoracoscope are greater than for laparoscopes, since the empty chest is a larger cavity to be illuminated, and viewing intrathoracic structures is often from a greater distance than in the peritoneal cavity. The apparent intensity of the light also depends on other factors such as the presence of blood in the pleural space. Light is absorbed by intrapleural blood, and frequent suctioning of free blood will increase the overall intrathoracic illumination.

A straight viewing telescope is easiest to manipulate and to maintain in proper vertical and horizontal orientation, but angled viewing thoracoscopes are available for specific needs. Flexible fiberoptic thoracoscopes are also being developed to allow viewing around structures and along the internal aspect of the chest wall (Olympus, Strongville, Ohio). In our practice, we have found little need for angled or flexible thoracoscopes. Strategic placement of intercostal access sites allows for periodic change for the site of thoracoscope insertion. Such changes in perspective allow for complete visualization of the thoracic cavity.

The video system consists of the television camera mounted on the thoracoscope. The signal is carried to an image converter and then to the monitor. The video recorder may be easily attached to the visual system, and provides the ability to document procedures and record technical details for later review. Printing equipment for still reproductions is also available (Sony, Montvale, New Jersey). We use two separate video monitors for VATS interventions. One monitor is positioned behind the shoulder of the assistant for the surgeon to observe. Similarly, a monitor for the assistant is placed behind the shoulder of the surgeon. This allows each person to stand in a neutral position and to work with instruments in a direct line with his perceived vision (Fig. 12A–4).

## Operating Equipment

Currently available operating instruments attempt to duplicate the function of traditional instruments with extended handle length, and a shaft that can be inserted through a trocar. Success at accomplishing this objective has been variable. Grasping forceps, scissors with or without cautery, separate cautery tips, hemoclip appliers, and retractors are available (Fig. 12A–5A,B). These tools have been adapted to be introduced through endosurgical intercostal ports.

An advantage of the "operating" thoracoscope is that it allows us to do simple diagnostic procedures through a single intercostal site. This thoracoscope also provides direct line of sight suctioning and a Nd:YAG laser during more complex procedures. Special 45-cm-long instruments are necessary to work through the biopsy channel with an "operating" thoracoscope with a channel of at least 5 mm in diameter so that these instruments can be introduced (Fig. 12–3B).

Many VATS interventions can be accomplished by using one or more small intercostal incisions and trocar access sites. However, small accessory intercostal incision, usually about 5 cm in length, will often facilitate the VATS intervention. This incision allows for introduction of stan-

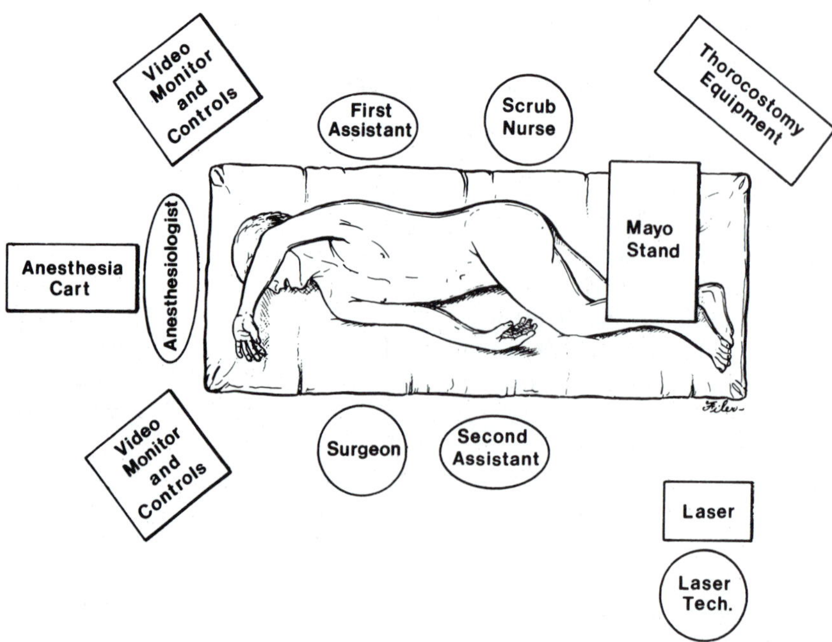


**Figure 12A–4.** Orientation of operating room with video monitors and equipment tables.

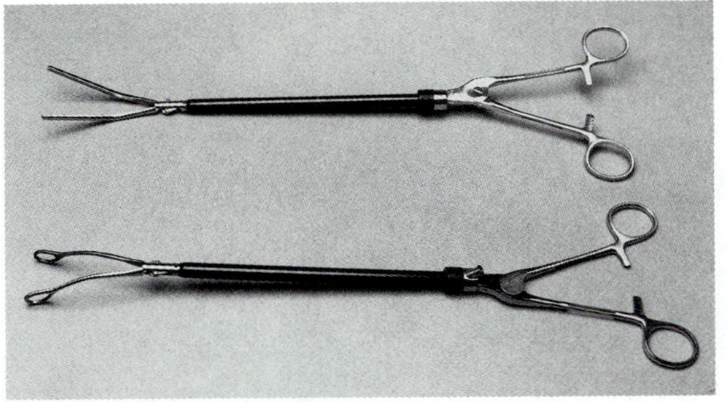

A

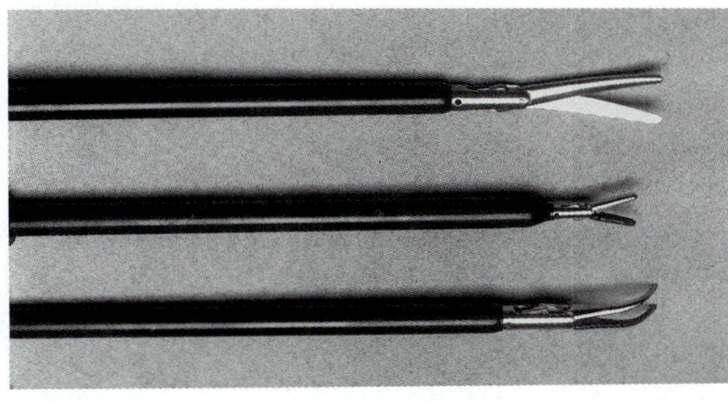

B

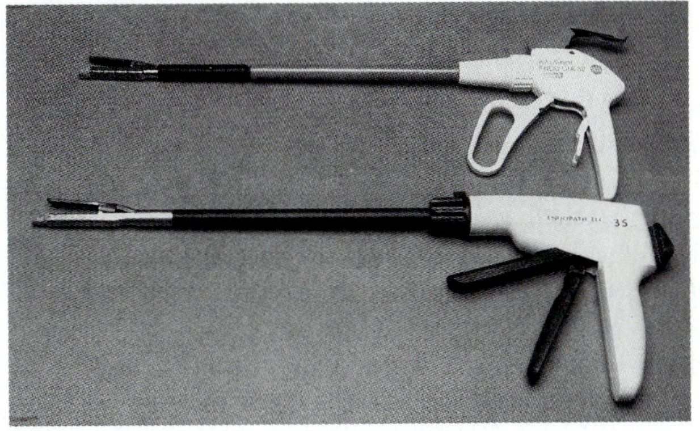

C

**Figure 12A–5.** Thoracoscope equipment: **A.** Grasping forceps designed for lung manipulation. **B.** Scissors, straight hemostat, and curved hemostat. **C.** Endoscopic staplers that apply 3.5-mm staples in multiple rows and cut between the rows. The functional length of the staple line is 3 cm.

dard surgical instruments to be used under primary videoscopic guidance. Intercostal retraction is not used.

Two devices have done much to broaden the scope of VATS interventions; the endostapling devices (Fig. 12A–5C) and the Nd:YAG laser. Endoscopic staplers function similarly to standard stapling devices and tissue between parallel staple lines. Their function is limited by lack of adjustable angles, short staple line length, and restriction of the jaw aperture, which limits the amount of lung tissue that may be included within the jaws. In spite of these limitations, their use enables the resection of many limited-size (<3 cm) peripheral nodules, particularly when the nodules are near a fissure or on the edge of the lung.

The Nd:YAG laser is useful for parenchymal resections that involve deep lesions that cannot be circumscribed with the stapling devices, or for lesions on the broad surfaces of the lung where stapler application is difficult.[9] Introduction of the laser fiber can be undertaken directly through an operating thoracoscope or by a laser control device inserted through a lateral intercostal access site. It is essential that the surgeon be somewhat familiar with laser physics and tissue effects prior to attempting thoracoscopic pulmonary resections with this device.

A standard thoracotomy instrument set should be in the operating room for conversion to an open thoracotomy if a significant complication occurs (i.e., bleeding, tracheal, bronchial, or esophageal injury). Selected "standard" surgical instruments can also be used through the intercostal access sites when necessary to facilitate the VATS procedure.

## Patient Positioning

For most video-assisted procedures, the patient is placed in a full lateral position and surgically prepared for an open thoracotomy. The arm is elevated to expose the axilla and the upper anterior chest. It is sometimes helpful to prep the arm and keep it in the sterile field (covered with a sterile stocking) to allow greater mobility and exposure of the anterior chest, but occasions when this is necessary are rare. The area of sterile skin preparation and exposure by draping is generally wider than for standard thoracotomy, extending to the spine posteriorly, over the shoulder superiorly (with draping to expose the axilla), to the sternum medially and inferiorly to the iliac crest. Lumbar flexion is helpful to permit free motion of the thoracoscope and video camera. This is particularly important in female patients with a wide pelvis, where the iliac crest can impair motion of the thoracoscope and camera (Fig. 12A–6) directed in a cephalad direction. Changes in the table orientation with elevating or lowering the head and tilting left to right will allow gravity to assist with lung displacement from the area of VATS dissection.

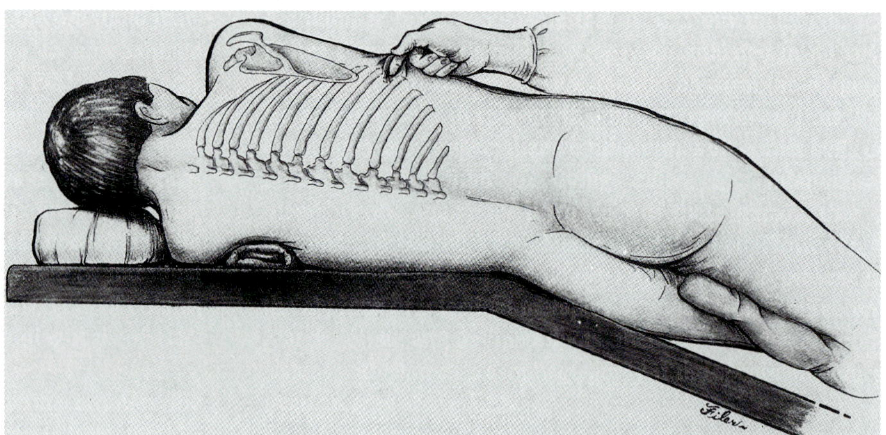

**Figure 12A–6.** Position of a patient in lateral position with hip flexion. This flexion facilitates the insertion of the thoracoscope and instruments. *(From Landreneau RJ, Mack M, Hazelrigg SR, et al: Video-assisted thoracic surgery: Basic technical concepts and intercostai approach strategies. Ann Thorac Surg 54:800–807, 1992, with permission.)*

## Operating Team

The number of individuals needed for a thoracoscopic procedure, and their positioning about the operative field, depends on the complexity of the procedure and equipment necessary. A simple thoracoscopic exploration for an undiagnosed pleural effusion and pleural biopsy can be performed easily by a surgeon and a scrub nurse. Complex procedures may require additional assistants. A first assistant to help with exposure and instrument manipulation and a second assistant to hold the camera and to further assist with exposure may be necessary. The surgeon and first assistant are opposite one another and standing toward the head of the patient. The scrub nurse and second assistant are opposite each other and are located toward the foot of the patient. When the laser is used, the nonsterile laser technician stands by the laser unit, which is most often behind the second assistant, since video monitors will be behind both surgeon and first assistant (Fig. 12A–4).

## Camera and Instrument Orientaticn

The camera position is best at a neutral si·e between the surgeon and assistant.[18] When the direction of view is kept on a line between these two people, in a direct line with the target pathology and the television screen, the anatomic orientation and motion of instruments will seem appropriate. Thus, if all instruments are introduced through sites on the same side of a semicircle that includes the camera site, the orientation of instrument motion will seem appropriate on the monitor (Fig. 12A–7). When instruments are introduced in a direction aiming back toward the viewing lens, the motion on the screen will appear to be backward (or mirrored image), which can cause significant disorientation. Placement of the instrument access sites at an appropriate distance from one another will minimize the interference of the shafts of the instruments with each other and avoid "sword fighting" during the case.

The sixth or seventh intercostal space along the midaxillary line is a good site for initial introduction of the thoracoscope with video camera attachment. Placement of the first trocar is similar to chest tube insertion. Digital palpation ensures a free pleural space and avoids insertion of the trocar into lung parenchyma. The thoracoscope is inserted through this first site. With an adequate pneumothorax and atelectasis of the lung, further intercostal access is achieved under direct thoracoscopic vision (Fig. 12A–8). It is generally wise not to place the thoracoscope access or the sites for instruments too close to the target pathology. This is obviously different from the traditional approach of planning

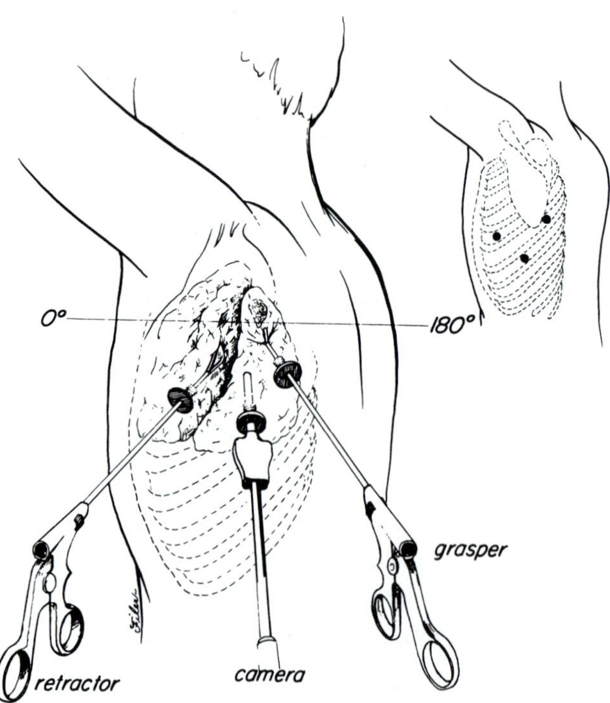


**Figure 12A–7.** The video camera and the instruments should be placed in a semicircular fashion. Adequate spacing between the instruments avoids interference. *(From Landreneau RJ, Mack M, Hazelrigg SR, et al: Video-assisted thoracic surgery: Basic technical concepts and intercostal approach strategies. Ann Thorac Surg 54:800–807, 1992, with permission.)*

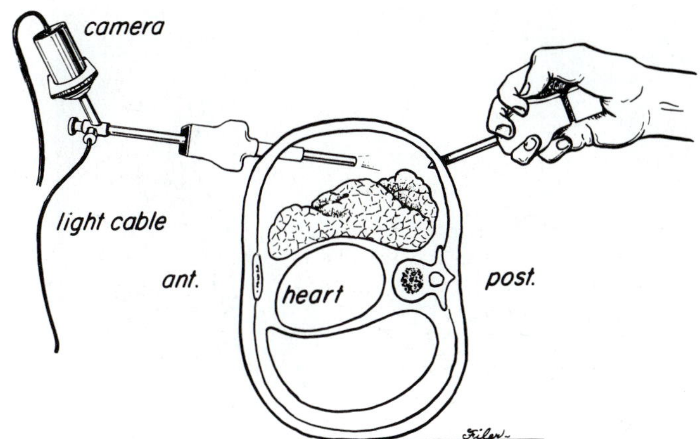


**Figure 12A–8.** After the thoracoscope has been inserted, subsequent stab wounds are made under videoscopic guidance. *(From Landreneau RJ, Mack M, Hazelrigg SR, et al: Video-assisted thoracic surgery: Basic technical concepts and intercostal approach strategies. Ann Thorac Surg 54:800–807, 1992, with permission.)*

the incision as close as possible and directly over the lesion of interest. However, if the camera is too close to the operative site, there is little opportunity to "back away" to enhance orientation and perspective. If the instrument site is close to the target pathology, mobility of the instruments will be impaired limiting dexterity.

The location of the target also dictates optimal location of intercostal access sites. Although placing these sites at a distance from the operative target may enhance visual perspective and instrument mobility, consideration must be given to the angle of instrument "attack" and to visual limitations caused by intervening structures. Structures in the paravertebral area or posterior aspect of the lung, e.g., cannot be seen from anteriorly placed trocar sites, since the lung will be in the way. An anterior site, however, would be ideal for a lung retractor to expose this area. The lung may also compromise the visibility of structures in the superior, posterior mediastinal compartment when a low midaxillary intercostal access site is chosen for the videoscope. This area is further limited by the scapula so that trocar sites may need to be placed either between the scapula and the spine (where the interspaces are narrow) or more anteriorly and in the axilla (usually the better choice). Likewise, it is advantageous to position the videoscope in a more anterior or posterior position to look over the upper lung edge. A 30-degree angled scope may overcome these limitations.

## DIAGNOSTIC THORACOSCOPY (VATS)

### Diagnosis of Pleural Diseases

The origin and development of thoracoscopy centered on evaluation and treatment of pleural disorders. Such problems remain ideally suited for thoracoscopy. When a patient has a pleural effusion, thoracentesis with biochemical, cytologic, and microbiologic analysis of the fluid is the first method of investigation. A transudative effusion suggests an underlying systemic disorder such as congestive heart failure or hepatic or renal insufficiency. Treatment of the underlying organ dysfunction is the primary management. When an exudative fluid is present, further investigation is appropriate.

Causes of exudative effusions are numerous. The most frequent cause is a sterile parapneumonic effusion. With appropriate management of the pulmonary parenchymal infection, these reactive effusions will usually resolve without complication. A minority of these effusions will progress to empyemas. Bacterial infections of the pleural fluid are almost always diagnosed by thoracentesis with Gram's stain and culture. Viral pleuritis with effusion is a diagnosis made by exclusion in the presence of a typical clinical presentation. Tuberculous empyema may elude diagnosis by thoracentesis, but the combination of thoracentesis (for microscopic analysis and culture), plus pleural biopsy with a cutting needle, is 90% accurate in diagnosing pleural tuberculosis.[19] With the exception of the occasional, nonconfirmed case of tuberculous effusion, thoracoscopy has little role in the diagnosis of pleural infection. However, as will be discussed in therapeutic thoracoscopy, there is significant benefit to thoracoscopic pleural debridement when infection is present.

Noninfectious exudative pleural effusions occur from systemic inflammatory diseases such as rheumatoid arthritis, and from primary or metastatic neoplastic pleural involvement. Tissue confirmation is necessary to differentiate between these processes. Direct blind pleural biopsy using specially designed biopsy needles[20,21] will provide the diagnosis in some instances but will be inadequate in up to 40% of cases of malignant pleural effusions.[22,23] When the blind biopsy is inadequate or when potential yield is low, open pleural biopsy is indicated.[19]

In the diagnosis and treatment of malignant pleural effusions, thoracoscopic pleural biopsy provides better visibility than does a limited thoracotomy incision.[24] Pleural involvement with primary or metastatic malignancies tends to be focal rather than uniformly distributed; thus, blind percutaneous pleural biopsy is frequently negative (Fig. 12A–9, 12A–10). Thoracoscopically directed biopsy of

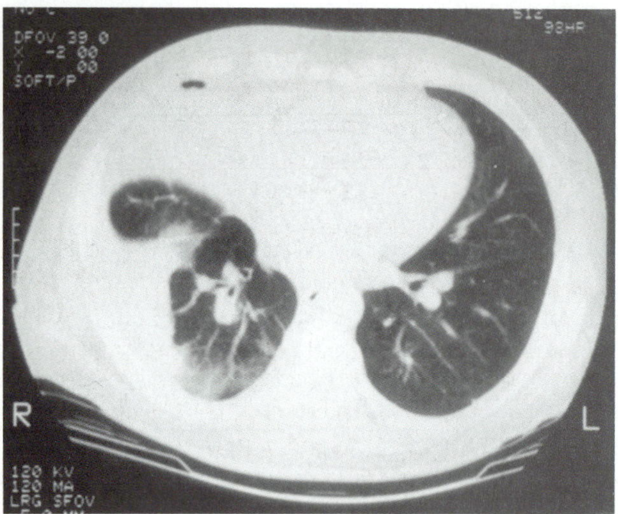


**Figure 12A–9.** CT scan of a patient with an undiagnosed pleural effusion.

pleural seeding enhances the diagnostic yield of such malignancies. The ability of thoracoscopy to diagnose or exclude pleural malignancy in idiopathic pleural effusions exceeds 90%.[23,25]

While less common than effusive pleural processes, pleural based masses can also be diagnosed by thoracoscopically guided biopsy when less invasive diagnostic procedures, such as radiographically guided needle biopsy, have been unsuccessful (Fig. 12A–11). Mesotheliomas involving the pleura are notoriously difficult to diagnose with percutaneous biopsy.[11]

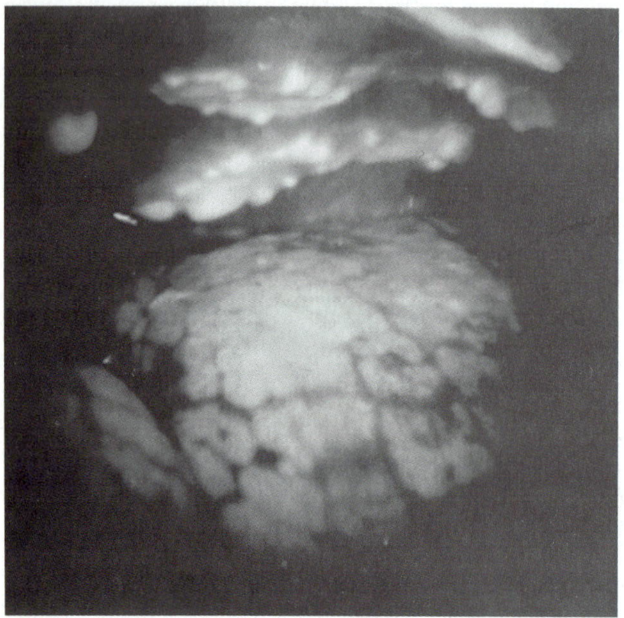

**Figure 12A–10.** Thoracoscopic view of the pleural space of the patient demonstrating pleural mesothelioma. The patchy nature of involvement explains the possibility of negative blind pleural biopsies.

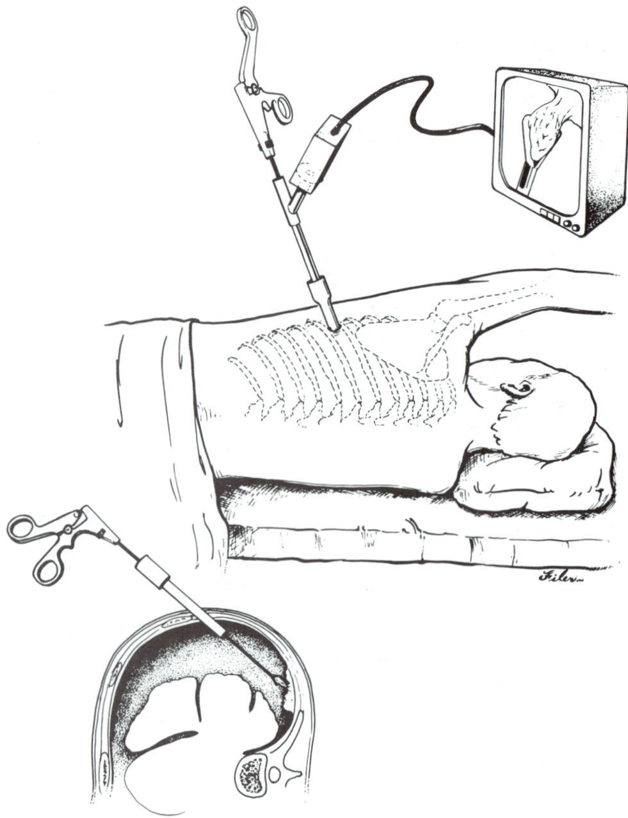

**Figure 12A–11.** Thoracoscopic biopsy of a pleural mass.

## Interstitial Lung Disease and Lung Biopsy

Thoracoscopy is well suited to obtain lung parenchymal biopsies in patients with interstitial lung diseases. Patients with unexplained pulmonary infiltrates will typically have one of two distinct clinical patterns. Less severely ill patients will suffer from chronic progressive dyspnea, while the other group consists of patients who have rapidly progressive radiographic infiltrates, respiratory insufficiency, and suspected sepsis. Patients in this latter group are frequently immunosuppressed following systemic chemotherapy or following transplantation. However, occasional nonimmunosuppressed patients will present with acute pulmonary insufficiency with parenchymal infiltrates, and the severity of the illness will dictate a biopsy (Fig. 12A–12).

Depending on the urgency of obtaining a diagnosis, several procedures may provide a diagnosis without the need for surgical biopsy. Sputum analysis, bronchoscopy with bronchoalveolar lavage and transbronchial biopsy are all useful in the diagnosis of interstitial lung disease. When infection is suspected, sputum analysis with or without bronchoalveolar lavage is the most direct, rewarding proce-

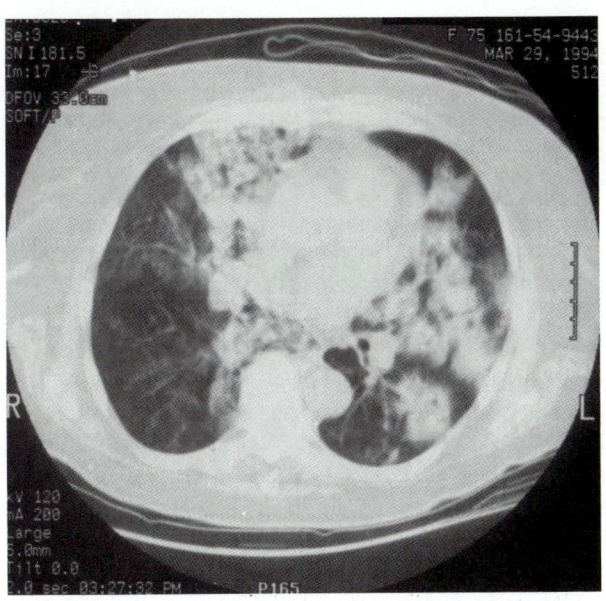


Figure 12A–12. Typical radiographic appearance of a patient with patchy areas of infiltrate that might require surgical biopsy for diagnosis. The enhanced visibility provided by the thoracoscope would permit selection of involved and normal areas for biopsy.

dure. With some noninfectious inflammatory disorders, bronchoscopy can also be useful. The diagnosis of sarcoid, e.g., is often made by transbronchial lung biopsy.[26]

When less invasive methods fail to yield a diagnosis, surgical lung biopsy is indicated. Burt et al[27] compared the results of lung biopsy with synchronously obtained percutaneous aspiration biopsies, cutting needle biopsy, and transbronchial biopsies. A diagnosis was obtained in 94% of the open-lung biopsies as compared with 59% for transbronchial biopsy, 52% for cutting needle biopsy, and 29% for aspiration biopsy. Open-lung biopsy can be performed with low morbidity and mortality. Gaensler et al[28] reported on 502 patients who underwent open-lung biopsy. The diagnostic yield was 92.2%, with a mortality rate of 0.3% and a complication rate of 2.5%. These data strongly support the continued use of surgical lung biopsy for the diagnosis of idiopathic infiltrates among potentially salvageable patients.

The traditional approach to surgical lung biopsy has been to perform a limited thoracotomy incision through which a wedge resection of diseased lung is performed (Fig. 12A–13). The disadvantage of such an incision is that it gives little overall visibility of the lung and pleural cavity, and it limits the accessibility to different areas of the lung parenchyma that may be more involved by the disease. Illustrations in the literature demonstrate generous portions of the lung being delivered through a limited thoracotomy wound for the application of a stapling device, but this is not possible in most circumstances. Lung parenchyma is

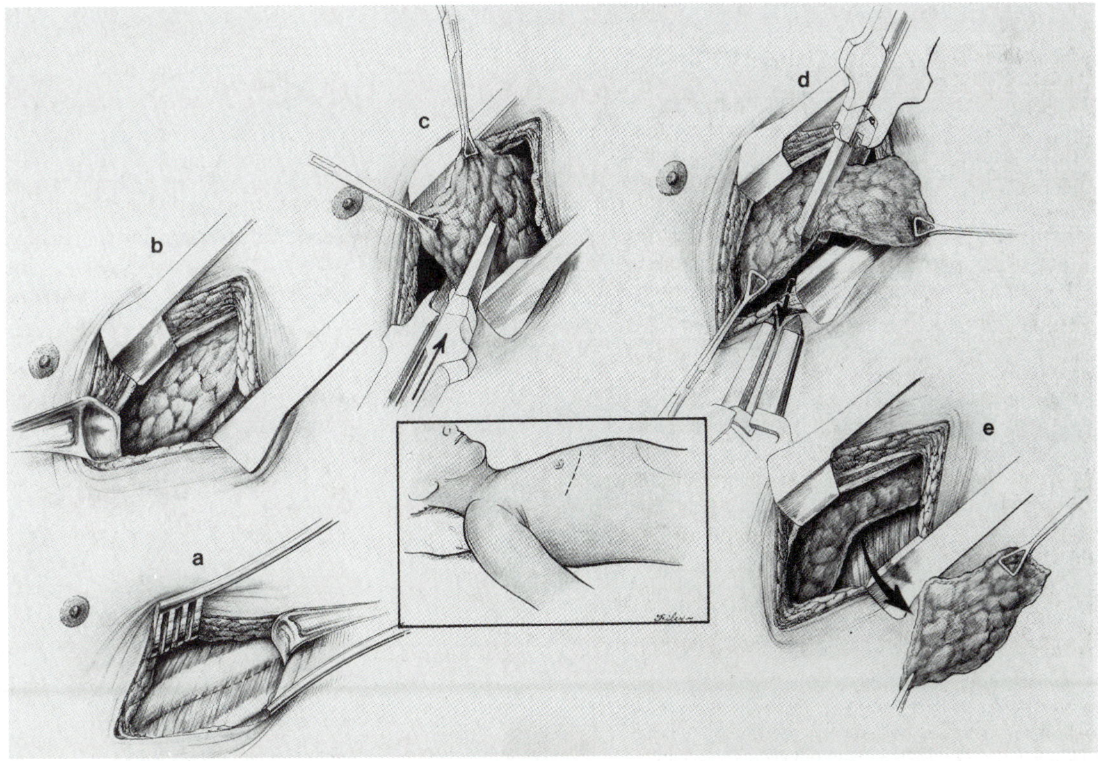


Figure 12A–13. Technique of open-lung biopsy through a small anterior thoracotomy.

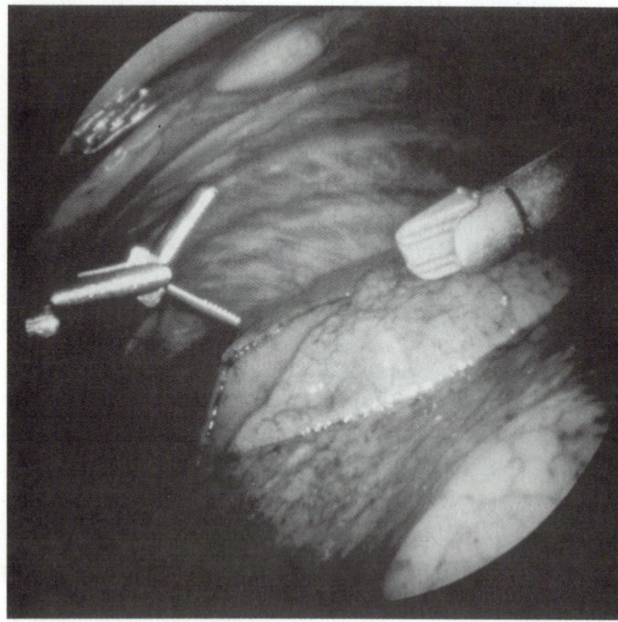

**Figure 12A–14.** Thoracoscopic view of the lung surface as in Figure 12A–16. All three lobes of the right lung are visible and accessible for biopsy sites.

usually noncompliant and unyielding to such manipulation. While the leading edge of the lingula or the middle lobe can be delivered through limited thoracotomy incisions, these areas may not be representative of the disease process, and they have a high risk of showing chronic fibrosis.[26]

As compared with open-lung biopsy, thoracoscopic lung biopsy offers enhanced visibility of nearly the entire surface of the lung (Fig. 12A–14). Biopsies can be taken from areas of lung that are obviously involved with the pathologic process as well as normal areas of the parenchyma. These lung biopsies can be accomplished by using the endoscopic stapling device without causing undue tension on the lung. The tissue biopsy obtained is equivalent to that of wedge resection through an open thoracotomy. The thoracoscopic approach may have less morbidity, at least in the group of patients with chronic progressive infiltrates, as recently reported by our group and others.[29,30]

Two or three sites of intercostal access are sufficient to accomplish VATS wedge resection of the lung. The thoracoscope with video camera is inserted through the seventh or eighth interspace along the midaxillary line. One or two additional intercostal access sites are established in the fifth interspace along the anterior axillary line and/or near the scapula tip. If only one additional access site is used, the grasping forceps can be inserted through the thoracoscope, while the endo-stapler is inserted through the other site. Under these circumstances, it is commonly necessary to exchange the position of the camera with the stapler to place the second intersecting staple line to complete the "V" wedge resection. When a three-intercostal-access approach is used, the grasping forceps is inserted through one site and the stapler through the other. Again, it may be necessary to exchange the location of forceps and the stapler to obtain proper angles to complete the wedge resection (Fig. 12A–15).

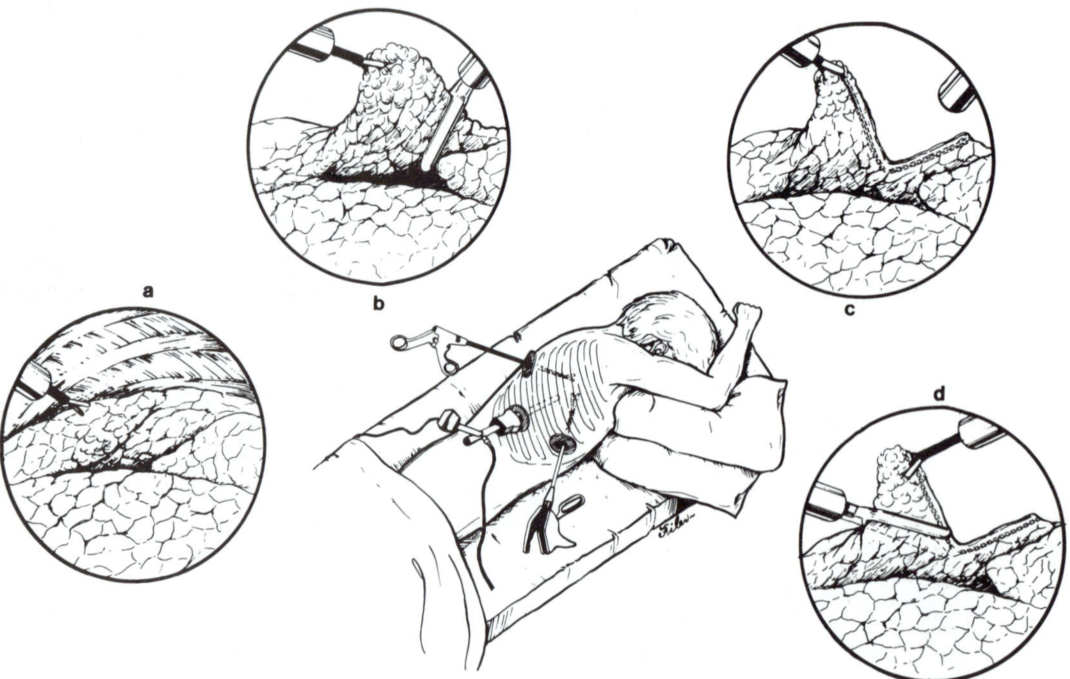


**Figure 12A–15.** Technique of thoracoscopic lung biopsy. *(From Dowling RD, Landreneau RJ, Magee M, et al: Thoracoscopic wedge resection of the lung. Surgical Rounds May: 341–349, 1993, with permission.)*

In our experience, VATS lung biopsy, utilizing general anesthesia with single-lung ventilation, can be performed in nearly all patients with chronic progressive lung disease, even those requiring chronic supplemental oxygen. On the other hand, patients with severe, rapidly progressive respiratory failure, often in the setting of massive sepsis, will typically require high concentrations of inspired oxygen and high levels of PEEP. These patients are not good candidates for thoracoscopic lung biopsy. We find no particular advantage with the use of VATS in these severely ventilator dependent patients since involvement of lung parenchyma is usually widespread and diffuse. The need to exchange the endotracheal tube to a double-lumen variety can be risky. An expeditious wedge resection through a limited thoracotomy, with ventilation through a standard endotracheal tube, is most appropriate.

## Diagnosis of Mediastinal Masses/Adenopathy

Many mediastinal masses should be approached with the intention of performing a resection. There are, however, several clinical settings, such as suspected lymphoma, or for staging of lung cancer, where biopsy of mediastinal masses or lymph nodes is appropriate. Radiographically guided needle biopsy can be helpful with the diagnosis of metastatic carcinoma to the mediastinum.[31] When lymphoma is suspected, the small amount of tissue available from needle biopsy is usually insufficient to obtain an adequate diagnosis and direct subsequent therapy. Surgical biopsy is often indicated to obtain an adequate biopsy.[32]

The anatomic location of the mediastinal lesions influences the approach chosen for biopsy. For masses or lymph nodes in the paratracheal and subcarinal areas, the suprasternal mediastinoscopy as described by Carlens[33] is most appropriate (see Chap. 11). This technique is limited in approaching masses located at the pulmonary hilum, the posterior mediastinum, and the aorto-pulmonary window on the left. For many such lesions, the parasternal-sternal mediastinal exploration has been chosen.[34]

Thoracoscopic evaluation of the mediastinum offers specific advantages as an adjunct to cervical mediastinoscopy and as an alternative to parasternal-sternal exploration for the evaluation of mediastinal adenopathy. Advantages of the VATS approach include the cosmetically superior incisions used compared with the anterior incision for parasternal exploration. Also, the lateral incisions are out of the usual portals used for external beam radiotherapy.[35]

For patients with known or suspected primary lung cancer, thoracoscopy can serve as an adjunct to mediastinoscopy as a prethoracotomy staging procedure. It permits evaluation for regionally advanced disease precluding surgical resection (i.e., pleural implants or direct mediastinal extension (Fig. 12A–16). Additionally, should the exploration and lymph node biopsy dictate further resection, the patient does not need to be repositioned for thoracotomy. For both right- and left-sided resectable lung cancers, preresectional thoracoscopy will permit extended lymph node evaluation beyond that of standard mediastinoscopy (Fig. 12A–17). Lymph nodes in stations 5, 6, 7, and 8 are easily biopsied thoracoscopically with 100% reliability.[36]

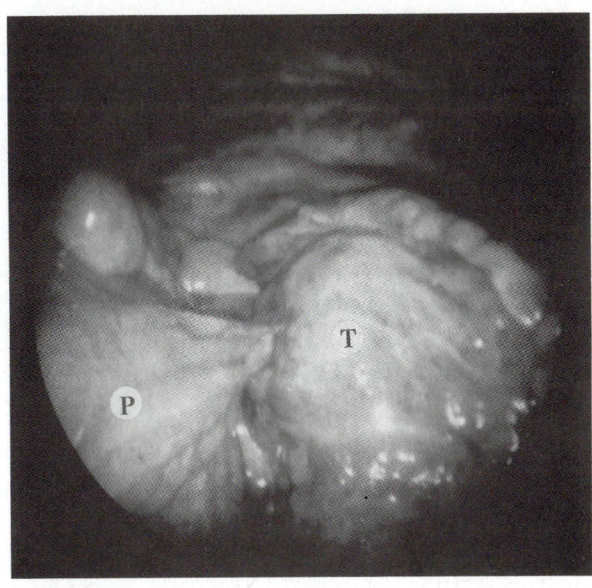


**Figure 12A–16.** Thoracoscopic view showing lung tumor with direct invasion of the pericardium and phrenic nerve (T, tumor in lingula of left upper lobe; P, phrenic nerve along pericardium with invasion of the tumor).

## Indeterminate Pulmonary Nodules

Radiographically visible pulmonary nodules may be solitary or multiple. When a solitary pulmonary nodule is present, the possibility of primary bronchogenic carcinoma is of concern, Higgins et al[37] studied 1134 such patients and found that 32% of such lesions were primary carcinoma. Therefore, there is a compelling reason to obtain a specific diagnosis for such nodules. A similar nodule on old x-rays, or the characteristic but rare appearance of a benign distribution of calcium in the mass, favors a benign nodule. The majority of patients with pulmonary nodules will not have such evidence.

In good-risk patients with a clinically suspicious newly identified pulmonary nodule on x-ray, needle biopsy is of questionable benefit. While the sensitivity of needle biopsy for malignant lesions is high, the diagnosis of malignancy will usually only confirm the clinical impression that resection is required. More importantly, patients with no evidence of malignancy on needle biopsy should also be strongly considered for excisional biopsy, since the false negative rate for "confirming" benignancy is too high. When patients with clinically suspicious lesions, believed to be benign by percutaneous biopsy, are evaluated by thoracotomy or by serial follow-up, malignancy is found in up to 29% of patients.[38,39]

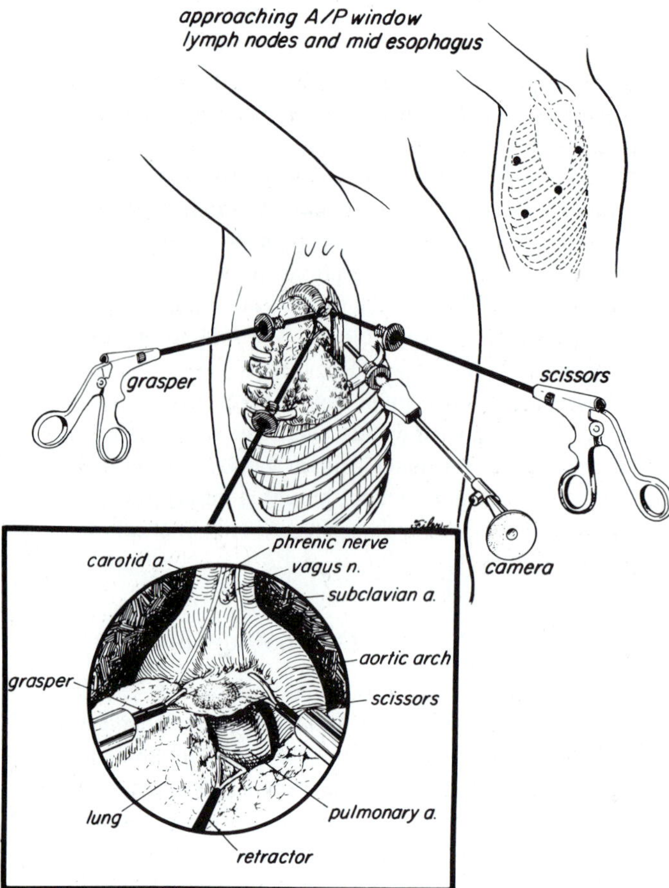


**Figure 12A–17.** Thoracoscopic exposure of the aorto-pulmonary window for lymph node biopsy. A similar approach on the right side will expose the subazygous and the subcarinal lymph nodes. *(From Landreneau RJ, Hazelrigg SR, Mack MJ, et al: Thoracoscopic mediastinal lymph node sampling: Useful for mediastinal lymph node stations inaccessible by cervical mediastinoscopy. J Thorac Cardiovasc Surg 106:554–558, 1993, with permission.)*

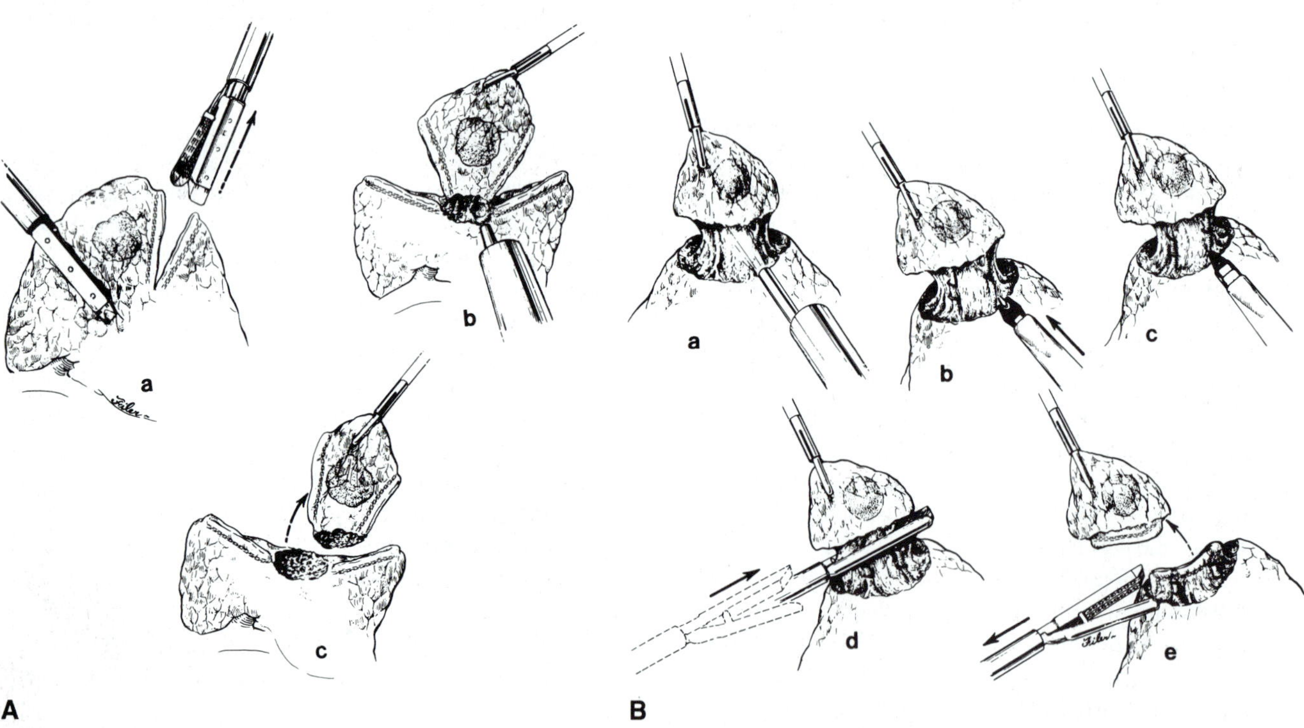


**Figure 12A–18.** Technique of thoracoscopic wedge resection of a solitary pulmonary nodule. After the mass has been palpated with grasping forceps, and suitability for wedge resection has been ascertained, wedge excision is undertaken using either the endoscopic stapling device, the Nd:YAG laser, or a combination of both devices. **A** shows a wedge resection being initiated with the stapler. If the remaining pedicle is too thick to complete with a stapler, the laser can be used to complete the resection. **B** shows the opposite circumstance where the lesion is found on a flat, broad surface of the lung. Initial mobilization with the laser is shown. Individual vessels and bronchi are easily seen and clipped. When a narrow stalk remains, this can be transected with the stapler. *(From Landreneau RJ, Hazelrigg SR, Ferson PF, et al: Thoracoscopic resection of 85 pulmonary lesions. Ann Thorac Surg 54:415–420, 1992, with permission.)*

Even when there is a strong suspicion of primary lung cancer based on risk factors and radiographic appearance, a fine-needle aspiration biopsy is often proposed to attempt to avoid a thoracotomy. Such proposals are motivated by the risk, morbidity, and cost of thoracotomy and lung resection. Thoracoscopic excision of undiagnosed pulmonary masses offers an alternative that precludes sampling error and minimizes morbidity (Fig. 12A–18). Mack et al[40] and Allen et al[41] reported no mortality and minimal morbidity in a large series of patients with indeterminate pulmonary nodules diagnosed by thoracoscopic excisional biopsy. D.agnostic accuracy by such a procedure approached 100%. Those patients with primary lung cancer, who were appropriate candidates for formal resection, had an open thoracotomy at the same operation.

Patients with multiple pulmonary nodules will usually have clinical circumstances suggesting metastatic disease or infection with immunosuppression. When diagnosis cannot be achieved by alternative methods, a similar approach to that of the solitary pulmonary nodule is applicable in these patients.

Selection criteria for thoracoscopic resection of pulmonary nodules include patients with nodules 3 cm in diameter and in the outer third of the lung parenchyma. However, it should be remembered that masses that appear deep to the pleural surface may actually be on a fissure and, thus, be resectable. Figure 12A–19 illustrates a nodule appearing to be deep within the lung parenchyma that actually was in a subpleural location within the major lobar fissure. This nodule was resectable by thoracoscopy resection.

Occasionally, small, subpleural nodules will not be

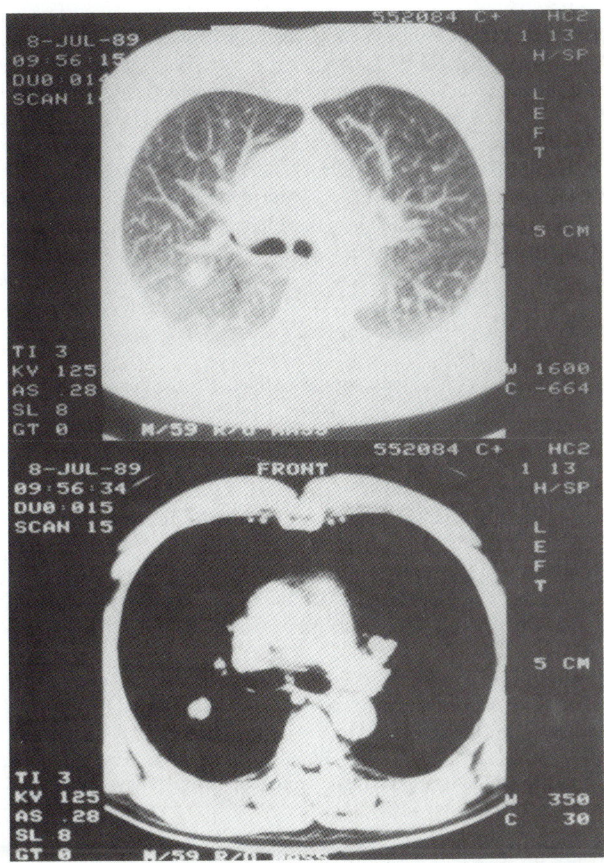


**Figure 12A–19.** CT scan showing a nodule which appears to be deep to the pleural surface. This mass was actually on the pleural surface of the major fissure and was easily resected thoracoscopically.

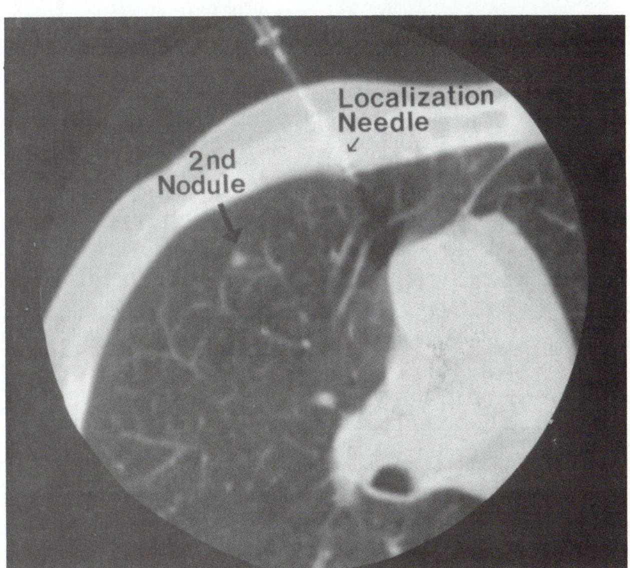


A

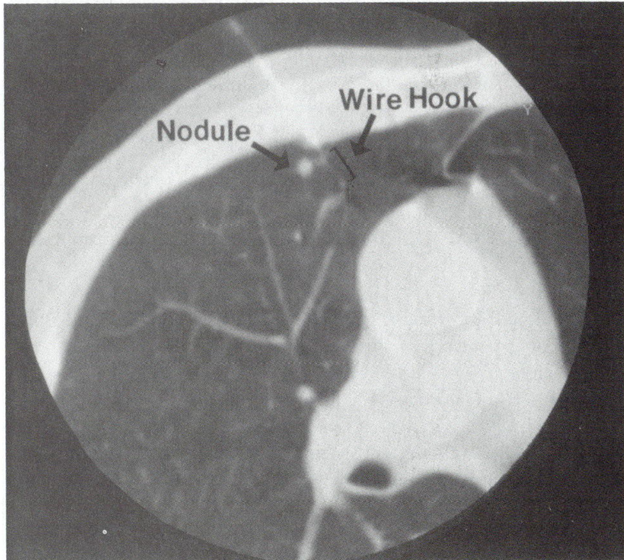


B

**Figure 12A–20.** Technique of wire localization for identification of small pulmonary nodules to be excised thoracoscopically. **A.** Under CT guidance, the nodule is identified, and a localization needle directed into the lung adjacent to the mass. **B.** A hooked wire is inserted through the localization needle and lodged in the lung parenchyma. A small amount (0.1 cc) of methylene blue is also injected. The patient is then taken to the operating room with the wire in place.

visible thoracoscopically. This can lead to a lengthy period of exploration or early conversion to open thoracotomy. When such a dilemma is anticipated, a radiographically placed guide wire with supplemental methylene blue injection can help identify the site for biopsy (Fig. 12A–20). Mack et al[42] and Plunkett et al[43] have demonstrated an accuracy with this technique that approached 100%.

Intraoperative localization of parenchymal pulmonary masses by ultrasound guidance is currently under investigation by us and other investigators.[42,44]

## SUMMARY

Thoracoscopic intervention has provided new techniques for the diagnosis of intrathoracic diseases. There are well-demonstrated advantages for VATS in the investigation of pleural disorders and processes involving the mediastinum and lung parenchyma. After a diagnosis has been made, VATS may be applied when appropriate in the surgical treatment of the disorder.

## REFERENCES

1. Jacobaeus HC: Ueber die Moglichkeit die Zystoskopie bei Untersuchung seroser Hohlungen Anzuwenden. *Munchener Medizinische Wochenschrift* **57**:2090–2092, 1910
2. Jacobaeus HC: The cauterization of adhesions in pneumothorax treatment of tuberculosis. *Surg Gynecol Obstet* 493–500, 1921
3. Smythe WR, Kaiser LR: History of thoracoscopic surgery. In: *Thoracoscopic Surgery.* Little, Brown 1993, pp 1–16
4. Hatch HB, DeCamp PT: Diagnostic thoracoscopy. *Surg Clin* 1405–1410, 1966
5. Miller JI, Hatcher CR Jr: Thoracoscopy: A useful tool in the diagnosis of thoracic disease. *Ann Thorac Surg* 26:68–72, 1978
6. Boutin C, Viallat JR, Cargnino P, Rey F: Thoracoscopic lung biopsy. *Chest* **82**:44–48, 1982
7. Rodgers BM, Talbert JL: Thoracoscopy for diagnosis of intrathoracic lesions in children. *J Pediatr Surg* **11**:703–708, 1976
8. Wakabayashi A: Thoracoscopic ablation of blebs in the treatment of recurrent or persistent spontaneous pneumothorax. *Ann Thorac Surg* **48**:651–653, 1989
9. Landreneau RJ, Hazelrigg SR, Ferson PF, et al: Thoracoscopic resection of 85 pulmonary lesions. *Ann Thorac Surg* **54**:415–420, 1992
10. Landreneau RJ, Herlan DB, Johnson JA, et al: Thoracoscopic NdYAG laser resection of pulmonary nodule. *Ann Thorac Surg* **52**:1–3, 1991
11. Lewis RJ, Caccavale RJ, Sisler GE, Mackenzie JW: One hundred consecutive patients undergoing video-assisted thoracic operations. *Ann Thorac Surg* **54**:421–426, 1992
12. McKenna RJ: Lobectomy by video-assisted thoracic surgery with mediastinal node sampling for lung cancer. *J Thorac Cardiovasc Surg* **107**:879–882, 1994
13. Kirby TJ: Initial experience with video assisted thoracoscopic lobectomy. *Ann Thorac Surg* **56**: 1248–1252, 1993
14. Landreneau RJ, Dowling RD, Castillo W, Ferson PF: Thoracoscopic resection of an anterior mediastinal mass. *Thorac Surg* **54**:142–144, 1992
15. Cuschieri A, Shimi S, Banting S: Endoscopic esophagectomy through a right thoracoscopic approach. *J R Coll Surg* **37**:7–11, 1992
16. Gossot D, Fourquier P, Celerier M: Thoracoscopic esophagectomy: Technique and initial results. *Ann Thorac Surg* **56**:667–670, 1993
17. Ferson PF, Landreneau RJ, Dowling RD, et al: Comparison of open versus thoracoscopic lung biopsy for diffuse infiltrative pulmonary disease. *J Thorac Cardiovasc Surg* **106**:194–199, 1993
18. Landreneau RJ, Mack MJ, Hazelrigg SR, et al: Video-assisted thoracic surgery: Basic technical concepts and intercostal approach strategies. *Ann Thorac Surg* **54**:800–807, 1992
19. Sahn SA: The pleura. *Am Rev Respir Dis* **138**:184–234, 1988
20. Cope C, Orange E: New pleural biopsy needle—preliminary study. *JAMA* **167**:1108, 1958
21. Abrams LD: New inventions: A pleural biopsy punch. *Lancet* **1**:30–31, 1958
22. Poe RH, Israel RH, Utell MJ, et al: Sensitivity, specificity, and predictive values of closed pleural biopsy. *Arch Intern Med* **144**: 325–328, 1984
23. Menzies R, Charbonneau M: Thoracoscopy for the diagnosis of pleural disease. *Ann Int Med* **114**:271–276, 1991
24. Hucker J, Bhatnager NK, Al-Jilaihawi AN, Forrester-Wood CP: Thoracoscopy in the diagnosis and management of recurrent pleural effusions. *Ann Thorac Surg* **52**:1145–1147, 1991
25. Boutin C, Astoul PH, Seitz B: The role of thoracoscopy in the evaluation and management of pleural effusions. *Lung* (suppl):1113–1121, 1990
26. Golden JA: Interstitial (diffuse parenchymal) lung disease: Tissue diagnosis and therapy. In: Gaum GL, Wolinsky E. (eds): *Textbook of Pulmonary Diseases, 5th Ed,* Vol 2. Little, Brown, 1994, pp 1067–1070
27. Burt ME, Flye MW, Webber BL, et al: Prospective evaluation of aspiration needle, cutting needle, transbronchial, and open lung biopsy in patients with pulmonary infiltrates. *Ann Thorac Surg* **32**:146–153, 1981
28. Gaensler EA, Carrington CB: Open biopsy for chronic diffuse infiltrative lung disease: Clinical, roentgenographic, and physiological correlations in 502 patients. *Ann Thorac Surg* **30**:411–426, 1990
29. Ferson PF, Landreneau RJ, Dowling RD, et al: Thoracoscopic vs. open lung biopsy for the diagnosis of diffuse infiltrative lung disease. *J Thorac Cardiovasc Surg* **105**:194–199, 1993
30. Bensard DD, McIntyre RC, Jr, Waring BJ, Simon JS: Comparison of video-assisted lung biopsy to open lung biopsy in the evaluation of interstitial lung disease. *Chest* **103**:765, 1993
31. Weisbrod GL: Transthoracic needle biopsy. *Chest Surg Clin North Am* **2**:631–647, 1992
32. Yellin A: Lymphoproliferative diseases. *Chest Surg Clin North Am* **2**:107–120, 1992
33. Carlens E: Mediastinoscopy: A method for inspection and tissue biopsy in the superior mediastinum. *Dis Chest* **36**:343–352, 1959
34. McNeil TM, Chamberlain JM: Diagnostic anterior mediastinotomy. *Ann Thorac Surg* **2**:532–539, 1966
35. Hazelrigg SR, Mack MJ, Landreneau RJ: Video-assisted thoracic surgery for mediastinal disease. *Chest Surg Clin North Am* **3**:283–297, 1993
36. Landreneau RJ, Hazelrigg SR, Mack MJ, et al: Thoracoscopic mediastinal lymph node sampling: Useful for mediastinal lymph node stations inaccessible by cervical mediastinotomy. *J Thorac Cardiovasc Surg* **106**:554–558, 1993
37. Higgins GA, Shields TW, Keehn RJ: The solitary pulmonary nodule. Ten-year follow-up of Veterans Administration Armed Forces Cooperative Study. *Arch Surg* **110**:570–575, 1975
38. Horrigan TP, Bergin KT, Snow N: Correlation between needle biopsy of lung tumors and histopathologic analysis of resected specimens. *Chest* **90**:638–640, 1986
39. Calhoun P, Feldman P, Armstrong P, et al: The clinical outcome of needle aspirations of the lung when cancer is not diagnosed. *Ann Thorac Surg* **41**:592–596, 1986
40. Mack MJ, Hazelrigg SR, Landreneau RJ, Acuff TE: Thoracoscopy

for the diagnosis of the indeterminate solitary pulmonary nodule. *Ann Thorac Surg* **56:**825–832, 1993

41. Allen MS, Deschamps C, Lee RE, et al: Thoracoscopic wedge excisions for indeterminate pulmonary nodules. *J Thorac Cardiovasc Surg* **106:**1048–1052, 1993
42. Mack MJ, Shennib H, Landreneau RJ, Hazelrigg SR: Techniques for localization of pulmonary nodules for thoracoscopic resection. *J Thorac Cardiovasc Surg* **106:**550–553, 1993
43. Plunkett MB, Peterson MS, Landreneau RJ, et al: CT guided preoperative percutaneous needle localization of peripheral pulmonary nodules. *Radiology* **185:**274–276, 1992
44. Shennib H, Bret P: Intraoperative transthoracic ultrasonographic localization of occult lung lesions. *Ann Thorac Surg* **55:**767–769, 1993

CHAPTER

# 12B

# Thoracoscopy

## *Therapeutic Procedures*

Stephen R. Hazelrigg, Michael J. Mack, and Paul Gordon

### INTRODUCTION

Initially thoracoscopy was a *therapeutic* procedure introduced by Hans Jacobeus[1] to perform pneumolysis as a treatment for tuberculosis. With the introduction of antituberculous therapy and, therefore, a diminished role for thoracoscopy in the treatment of this disease, the procedure was relegated to primarily a diagnostic role.[2] With recent improvements in imaging, lighting, and instrumentation, video-assisted thoracic surgery (VATS) has assumed not only a broader role as a diagnostic procedure but also a significant therapeutic role again.[3] When thoracoscopy is used as a method of access for therapeutic procedures, comparison with standard open approaches is necessary. A surgical procedure should not, of course, be compromised in order to accomplish it by the thoracoscopic approach. The same therapeutic result or end point should be reached by thoracoscopic approach as by open approach.[4] If the procedure has to be compromised solely to accomplish it by a less morbid approach, then conversion to an open procedure should occur. There are multiple therapeutic applications for thoracoscopy, some of which have become accepted in a short period of time as standard therapy, e.g., management of malignant pleural effusions and treatment of recurrent spontaneous pneumothorax. Other applications such as thymectomy for myasthenia gravis have not yet clearly been demonstrated to be effective therapy. This chapter discusses major therapeutic roles for thoracoscopy, as well as the specific operative technique for managing these diseases by the thoracoscopic approach.

### PLEURAL DISEASES

There are several disorders of the pleura that are amenable to treatment utilizing video-assisted thoracic surgical techniques. As a group, pleural disease represents a very common indication for VATS. Diagnosis and treatment of pleural effusions, hemothorax, empyema, and chylothoraces all have been reported using VATS.

#### Pleural Effusions

VATS is frequently used for pleural effusions after failure to achieve a diagnosis with thoracentesis or blind pleural biopsies. VATS has proven to be an excellent diagnostic technique that almost always allows one to determine whether the effusion is malignant in nature.[5–7] In a series of 1000 patients with pleural effusion, over 20% remained undiagnosed after thoracentesis and blind pleural biopsy. Thoracoscopy provided a diagnosis in 96% of these cases.[8] VATS may also play a therapeutic role in the treatment of pleural effusions.

Large malignant effusions may cause significant shortness of breath and disability. Drainage of the fluid alone will result in rapid fluid reaccumulation. Treatment is directed at preventing this reaccumulation, and the method of treatment will vary depending upon when the diagnosis is made (at thoracentesis or at thoracoscopy) and whether or not the lung is "trapped."

For malignant effusions diagnosed by thoracentesis (or blind biopsy) in which the lung will fully re-expand, the treatment has been a chemical pleurodesis after chest tube placement and no operative therapy is required. Various sclerosant agents have been used including tetracycline and its derivatives: quinacrine, bleomycin, nitrogen mustard, and talc. Both bleomycin and talc have had high success rates; however, talc is much cheaper and has had success rates in excess of 90%.[9–12]

When the diagnosis of a malignant effusion is made at thoracoscopy, the method of pleurodesis includes pleurectomy, mechanical abrasion, or any of the chemical sclerosants previously listed. Comparative studies in normal pleura have suggested that both mechanical abrasion and talc create significant adhesions and pleural symphysis.[13,14] Pleurectomy, although effective, is a larger magnitude procedure in a relatively poor risk group of patients. One of the advantages of thoracoscopy in dealing with malignant effusions is the ability to lyse adhesions and break down loculations and, thus, more completely drain the pleural fluid. There presently are no direct comparisons of thoracoscopy to simple chest tube placement and sclerosis.

After draining all of the pleural fluid and freeing the loculations, our preferred method of sclerosis has been the instillation of talc. In an unventilated setting, the talc may be instilled via a bulb syringe, and it will distribute evenly. Another option for talc is to deliver it through an atomizer. Using talc we have achieved success in preventing the recurrence of pleural fluid in 57 of 60 patients with malignant effusions (excluding patients with trapped lung).

Patients with malignant effusions and trapped lung present additional problems. Failure of the lung to expand fully after drainage of pleural fluid may be due to endobronchial obstruction, to tumor encasing the lung, or to the development of a fibrous peel over the lung due to the long-standing fluid. In an effort to prevent the development of trapped lung, we encourage early treatment of malignant effusions. Bronchoscopy should be performed to rule out an endobronchial obstruction.

Trapped lung in a malignant effusion in a debilitated patient may simply be treated by a chest tube with or without sclerosis, if one accepts the fact that fluid will reaccumulate in the remaining space. For better-risk patients, a thoracoscopy may be performed. At times the fibrous peel is loosely adherent to the lung and may be decorticated by video-assisted techniques. We have been successful thoracoscopically at achieving lung expansion in 8 of 17 patients with evidence of trapped lung.

When a thick adherent peel is present, it is generally left in place unless a thoracotomy and decortication seem warranted by the clinical situation. There may be some role for pleural-peritoneal shunts for palliation in patients with trapped lung. Shunts reduce the dyspnea some by limiting the amount of pleural fluid and atelectasis. Shunts work satisfactorily for short periods of time; however, they may become clogged. Shunts also require frequent compression by patients that may be uncomfortable, and patient compliance is very important.

## Empyema

The advent of effective antibiotics to treat pneumonia has decreased the incidence of empyema. However, pneumonia remains the most frequent cause of empyema followed by iatrogenic causes. Empyemas progress from an acute phase where the infected fluid is thin and amenable to tube drainage to a chronic phase where a thick fibrous peel is present around the cavity and the fluid is loculated and viscous. Intermediate between these phases lies a fibropurulent phase where VATS may play a significant therapeutic role.[15] In this phase, where the loculated fluid cannot be adequately treated by tube drainage alone, thoracoscopy allows opening of the loculations and debridement of the thick purulent debris. In some cases a loose fibrinous peel may be removed from the lung to allow re-expansion.

Using thoracoscopic debridement and irrigation along with effective antibiotics, complete resolution of the empyema was achieved by Ridley and Braimbridge in 18 of 30 (60%) patients.[16] Even for some debilitated and septic patients who will require further surgical procedures, this may allow stabilization of the septic state. Chronic empyemas with fibrous encasement will require open decortication or the use of muscle flaps to eradicate the process. Good-risk patients with chronic empyemas may have their overall hospital stays shortened by having decortication performed early.

There is no uniformly accepted correct treatment for empyemas. Thoracoscopic debridement may be successful for fibropurulent empyemas especially if lung re-expansion can be achieved. Failure of VATS does not preclude other surgical procedures, and, in some settings, effective drainage may improve the patient's general condition before further surgical management is attempted.

There has been some success reported with the use of streptokinase (and urokinase) in the treatment of empyemas in the fibropurulent phase.[17] This treatment generally requires daily infusion for at least 1 week. Although treatment must be individualized and enzymatic therapy remains a treatment option, we continue to favor the use of VATS for effective debridement of empyemas in the fibropurulent phase.

## Hemothorax

VATS may play a therapeutic role in the management of hemothorax in several settings. Hemothoraces that are inadequately drained by simple chest tubes carry an increased risk of development of empyema or fibrothorax. Prior to VATS the options for treatment of clotted hemothoraces included enzymatic dissolution or thoracotomy. Early use of VATS has proven successful to evacuate the clot prior to the need for a formal decortication. Thoracoscopy has also proven useful for continued bleeding after chest tube placement in the otherwise stable trauma patient.[18–20] After removal of the clotted blood, the bleeding site may be identified and controlled. Intercostal vessels may be clipped or cauterized, and minor lung lacerations may be sutured or stapled. Occasionally, unsuspected injuries such as diaphragmatic lacerations are identified.

VATS is not a technique to be used in unstable trauma patients; however, much of thoracic trauma can be managed without major operative intervention. A prospective trial included 24 trauma patients (22 penetrating and 2 blunt) and used VATS to treat clotted hemothorax (9 patients), suspected diaphragmatic injury (10), and continued bleeding (5). All but one of the clotted hemothoraces were managed successfully by VATS, and half of the suspected diaphragm injuries were confirmed (four also repaired thoracoscopically). Intercostal artery injury was the source of bleeding in all five cases of continued bleeding, and three were successfully controlled by VATS techniques.[18]

For clotted hemothoraces (that fail nonoperative methods), early intervention has been emphasized. This allows the clotted material to be removed more easily prior to its firm adherence and the need for open decortication.

In most situations the video-assisted technique used includes general anesthesia and a double-lumen endotracheal tube. Instruments such as a ring forceps have worked exceedingly well to extract the clotted material, and two or three trocar sites are required for most procedures. VATS has proven to be a valuable intermediate diagnostic and therapeutic technique for the stable thoracic trauma patient that may help to avert an otherwise necessary thoracotomy.

### Chylothorax

The etiologies for chylothorax include inflammatory or malignant obstruction, trauma, or iatrogenic (postsurgical) causes. Conservative therapy consists of simple drainage and diet modification (modification of dietary fat intake, parenterally administered fluid, and nutritional support). Conservative treatment is successful in the majority of patients, although the success rate is less when the chylothorax is due to surgical injury.[21,22]

If chylothorax does not rapidly resolve with conservative measures, surgical options are considered. Methods of controlling chylothoraces have included direct repair of the injured duct, ligation at the diaphragm, pleurectomy, or pleuroperitoneal shunting. VATS, by being less invasive than a thoracotomy, may encourage earlier surgical intervention and direct repair or ligation of the duct.

Anecdotal reports of repair of chylothorax exist.[23–25] Administration of oral substances (i.e., cream) to stimulate lymph flow aid in identification of the leak. Thoracoscopy allows excellent visualization, and the site of lymph leak is usually readily identified. Suture ligation is the most frequent method of control when direct repair is attempted. Ligation of the duct at the diaphragm through the right chest is often a straightforward method of management. There are presently not enough reports to comment on the expected success rate for VATS treatment of chylothorax.

### Pleural-Based Masses

Biopsy and resection of pleural-based masses are straightforward. The visualization thoracoscopically is excellent and localized masses may be excised (Fig. 12B–1).

## BLEBS AND BULLOUS LUNG DISEASE

Pneumothorax and bullous lung disease are two entities that have the potential for thoracoscopic treatment. Blebs and bullae are disorders that are distinctly different with respect to their pathologic findings and patient population.

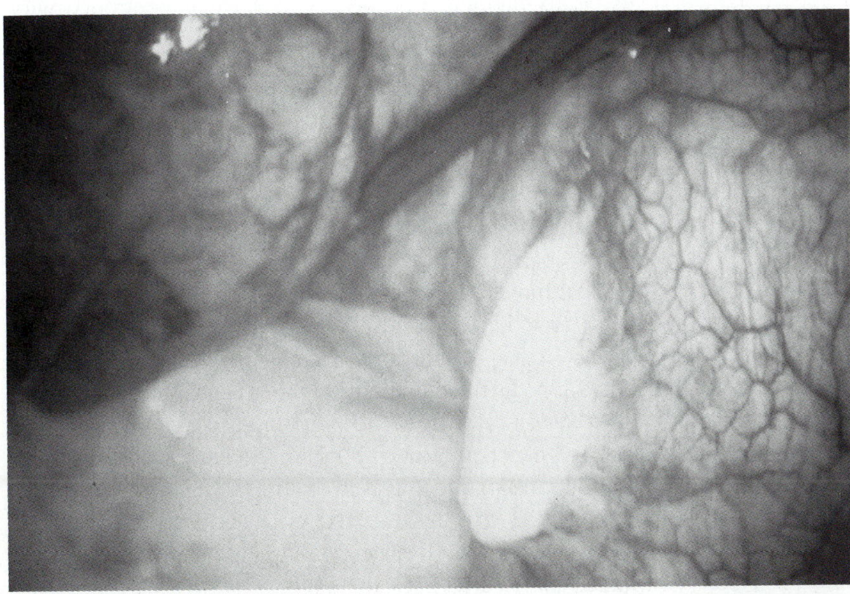

**Figure 12B–1.** Pleural plaque seen at thoracoscopy.

## Spontaneous Pneumothorax

Spontaneous pneumothorax may be primary or secondary. Primary spontaneous pneumothorax (PSP) occurs in patients without underlying lung disease and is usually due to the rupture of an apical bleb. Blebs are small (<1 cm) subpleural air spaces that are the result of alveolar rupture. The relatively young age of these patients and their otherwise normal lung parenchyma allow these patients to tolerate a pneumothorax with relatively minor symptoms in most cases. Dyspnea and pain are the most frequently reported symptoms, and hemothoraces and tension pneumothoraces can occur rarely.

Secondary spontaneous pneumothorax (SSP) occurs in patients with known underlying lung disease. Pneumothorax in these patients is usually due to rupture of an emphysematous bulla. Other etiologies for SSP include infections, interstitial lung disorders, neoplasms, asthma, trauma, congenital cysts, connective tissue disorders (Marfan's disease or Ehlers-Danlos syndrome), lymphangio myomatosis, and endometriosis. Bullae are generally larger than blebs (>1 cm), and the patients are older (mean age 55–65) with poor pulmonary reserve making them more frequently symptomatic even with small pneumothoraces. While surgical treatment of PSP carries little operative risk, the morbidity and mortality in SSP are measurable and are related to the degree of underlying lung disease and the patient's overall health.

Secondary spontaneous pneumothorax (SSP) may also occur in immunocompromised patients. Pneumocystis carinii pneumonia is the most frequent etiology, although tuberculosis and other infectious causes may be responsible. Pneumocystic pneumonia causes alveolar necrosis resulting in pneumothorax. Development of this problem in the acquired immunodeficiency syndrome (AIDS) patient has been shown to be associated with a short remaining life span.[26,27] Mean survival time has been reported to be 147 days after development of a pneumothorax. Bilateral disease is frequent as is recurrence after chest tube therapy alone.

Surgery in immunocompromised patients with SSP is offered in those who fail attempts at treatment with chest tube and pleurodesis or in those where the etiology for the pneumothorax is in question. With pneumonia caused by *Pneumocystis carinii,* the lung is friable and hemorrhagic, which may make thoracoscopic management more difficult. Pleurectomy is advocated when surgery is performed to prevent recurrence.

### Surgical Indications

Surgery is indicated for recurrent pneumothoraces, prolonged air leak, large air cysts, failure to re-expand the lung with a chest tube, hemothorax, and for patients living in remote areas or with specialized vocations or hobbies (i.e., pilots, scuba divers).

The risk of recurrence is estimated to be 20–30% after an initial pneumothorax and rises to over 50% after a second pneumothorax.[28–31] Traditionally, surgical therapy was recommended after the second or third occurrence. The availability of a less morbid surgical approach like VATS may alter this recommendation and move toward intervention with the second occurrence. Since 70–80% of patients can be managed successfully by a chest tube alone with the first pneumothorax, this remains the recommended form of therapy for first-time pneumothoraces. Prolonged air leak has traditionally been defined as 5–7 days. VATS has caused us to recommend intervention earlier in patients with PSP. Our practice has been to offer surgery when an air leak persists for over 72 hours.

### Role of VATS in Spontaneous Pneumothorax

The standard surgical procedure for PSP is resection of the bleb and either apical mechanical abrasion or pleurectomy. Surgery was previously performed most frequently by axillary thoracotomy, although lateral thoracotomy and an approach through the auscultatory triangle have also been used. Although there are reports of success by ablating blebs with cautery, lasers, and endoloop ligatures, the use of the endoscopic stapler has gained the most support, since it mimics the open procedure.[32–43]

Generally three trocars are required, and the entire visceral pleura is inspected carefully for blebs. Often, more than one bleb is identified, and the thoracoscope may need to be placed through more than one trocar site in order to view the entire lung. Blebs are grasped and resected, and the endoscopic stapler is placed across the base of the bleb and resects a small rim of normal tissue (Fig. 12B–2). Mechanical abrasion of the pleural surface may be performed in several ways; our preference has been to introduce an unraveled 4 × 4 sponge and use two grasping instruments to manipulate it over the pleural surface to abrade it[40] (Figs. 12B–3, 12B–4).

Apical pleurectomy may be performed without much difficulty thoracoscopically. Hemostasis is controlled with the electrocautery, and in most instances this can be performed in approximately 30 minutes. Apical pleurectomy is effective; however, it will be accompanied by an occasional case of excessive postoperative bleeding.

Resection of apical blebs may be performed thoracoscopically using local/regional anesthesia. Manipulation of the lung may be more difficult and may produce coughing if the pleura is not completely anesthetized. The induced pneumothorax does not produce as much working space, and it may be difficult to visualize the entire lung surface. Most of our procedures have been performed using general anesthesia and a double-lumen endotracheal tube.

SSP is most frequently due to a ruptured bulla. Bulla that are pedunculated with a discrete "neck" may be handled in a fashion identical to that described for blebs (Figs. 12B–5, 12B–6). For bullae not amenable to simple stapling, other methods have been used including opening of the bulla (and folding back the edges to buttress a staple line)

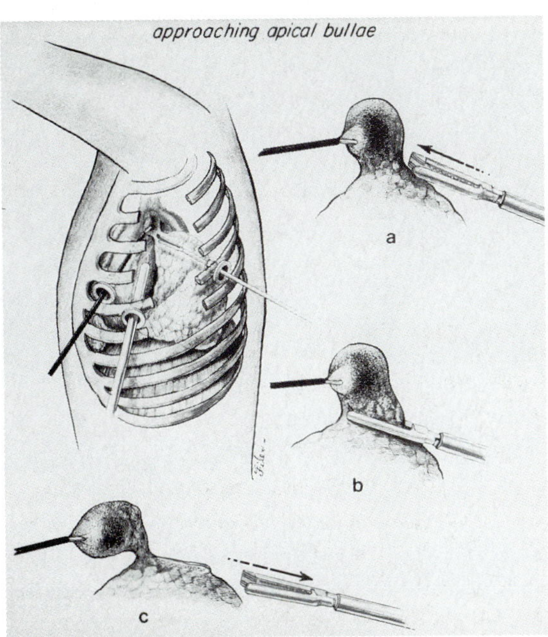


**Figure 12B–2.** Approximate sites of routine trocar placement for spontaneous pneumothorax and demonstration of stapled resection of an apical bleb. The bleb is initially grasped (**A**). The endoscopic stapler is applied with a rim of normal lung tissue (**B**). Each staple application cuts between six rows of staples (**C**). *(From Hazelrigg SR, Landreneau RJ, Mack MJ, et al: Thoracoscopic stapled resection for spontaneous pneumothorax. J Thorac Cardiovasc Surg 105:389–393, 1993, with permission.)*

and utilizing the laser or argon beam coagulator. The laser has been utilized to "shrink" the bulla; however, suturing or stapling may still be required to close the area of rupture. For large bulla an open thoracotomy may be required to manage the problem adequately.

### *Results of VATS Management of Pneumothorax*

There have been reports of the use of lasers ($CO_2$ and Nd:YAG), cautery, sutures and endoloops to treat apical blebs and bullae. Most of these reports have had satisfactory outcomes; however, patient numbers have been small. Wakabayashi and colleagues[33] reported upon the use of the $CO_2$ laser for ablation of blebs and bullae in 12 patients with an initial failure rate of 25%. Torre and Belloni[36] reported results in 14 patients utilizing the Nd:YAG laser to ablate the blebs and perform an apical pleurodesis. Three patients had persistent air leaks for 4 days, and one patient was readmitted for a recurrent pneumothorax.

The endoloop has been described to successfully ligate the bleb, but potential problems include ligating too much lung tissue in the atelectatic lung, thus allowing the endoloop to be extruded when the lung reinflates (or necrosing in the early postoperative period).

Although the use of cautery, laser, and endoloops are often novel, we have preferred the use of the endoscopic stapler, since it allows an operation identical to that usually performed at thoracotomy. We retrospectively reviewed 26 cases performed by VATS and compared them with 20 cases done by an axillary thoracotomy. There were no recurrences with a mean follow-up of 8 months. Mean operative time was less than 1 hour, and the two groups were comparable with respect to chest tube duration. Mean hospital stay was significantly less in the VATS group (2.9 vs. 4.5 days) as was the need for parenteral narcotics after 48 hours. We identified more than two blebs per case thoracoscopically, which we felt was due to superior visualization as compared with an axillary thoracotomy.[40]

Results have been good in treating patients with PSP using VATS techniques. Secondary pneumothoraces have a higher recurrence rate regardless of the surgical route used. For PSP, axillary thoracotomy with stapling of apical blebs

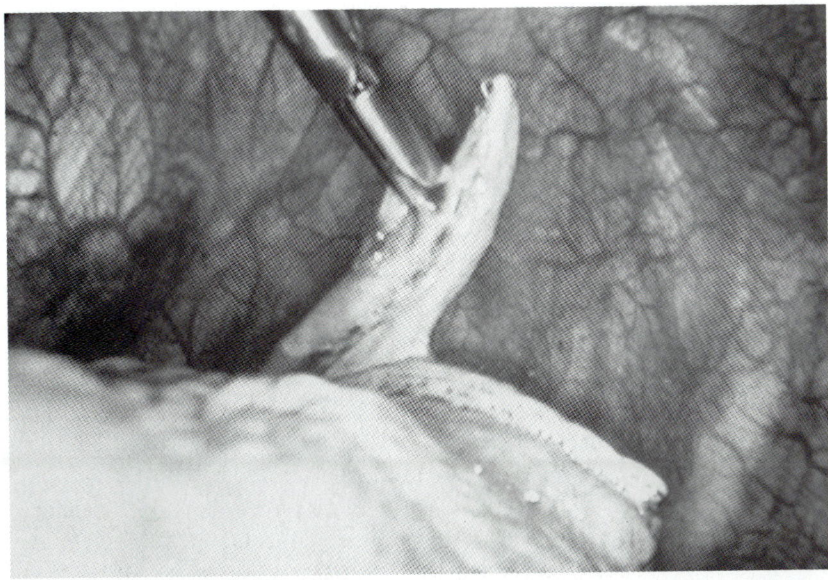

**Figure 12B–3.** Stapled excision of apical bleb in process.

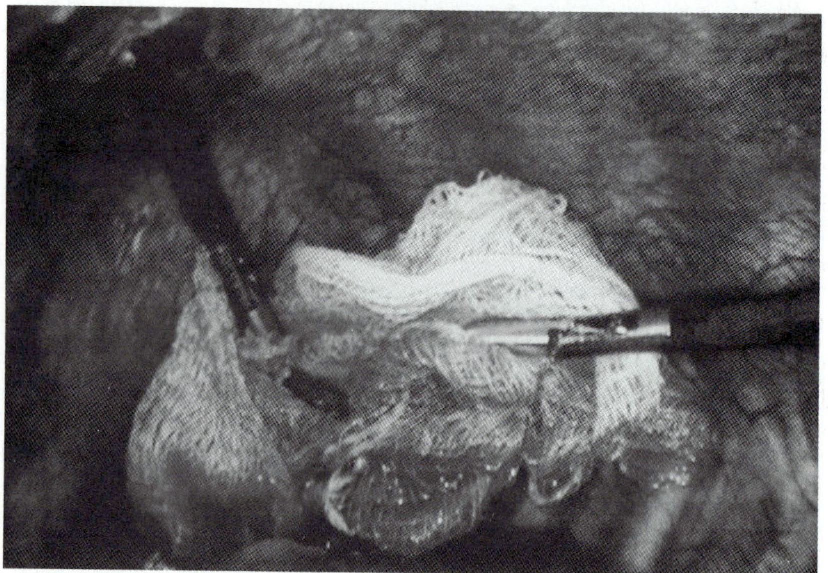

**Figure 12B–4.** Unraveled 4 × 4 gauze sponge manipulated with grasping forceps to create an apical pleural abrasion.

and mechanical abrasion have reported recurrence rates between 1% and 3%.[44–47] For secondary pneumothoraces, rates as high as 12.5% have been noted.[48] One report of VATS treatment for SSP in six patients had two recurrences (33%).[49]

We have reported our results on patients with spontaneous pneumothorax who have been treated by VATS and have a mean of 13 months' follow-up. In 113 patients we have a recurrence rate of 4.3%. Further evaluation of this data reveals that most recurrences occurred in the setting where no apical bleb was identified. For cases where an apical bleb was identified and resected, the recurrence rate was 1.8%.[50]

Our present approach is to use VATS for all patients with PSP. The apical blebs are excised using the endoscopic stapler, and either an apical pleurectomy or abrasion is performed. If no bleb is identified after careful evaluation, we instill saline and attempt to find the air leak with gentle hand ventilation. If no leak is identified (because of our increased recurrence rate in this setting), we recommend either an apical pleurectomy (our preference) or an axillary thoracotomy with further search and apical pleural stripping.

## Diffuse Bullous Emphysema Without Pneumothorax

Surgery for bullous emphysema in patients without pneumothorax has previously been reserved for dyspneic pa-

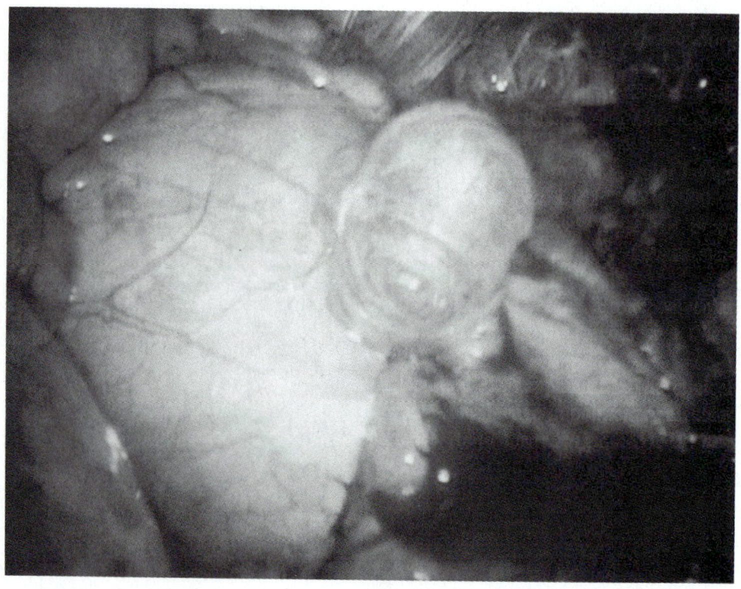

**Figure 12B–5.** Bulla with a discrete "neck" that is amenable to stapled excision.

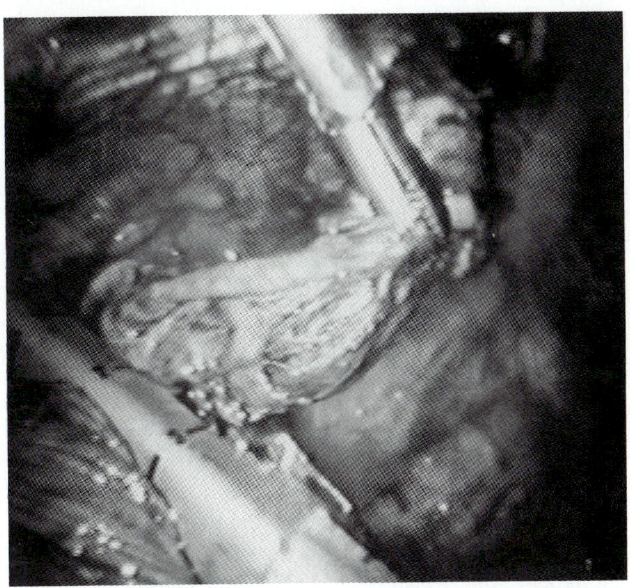

**Figure 12B–6.** Stapled excision of bullous lesion.

tients with local exaggeration of bullous disease and compression of surrounding lung parenchyma. Even in patients with localized disease, it has been difficult to select patients for operative intervention. Ideal characteristics for good results have included large localized bulla encompassing at least one third of the hemithorax with evidence of lung compression in patients otherwise healthy with normal cardiovascular systems. Evidence of a rapid increase in bulla size also correlates with good results. Even in ideally selected patients, the emphysematous process will continue to progress after surgery such that many became dyspneic upon follow-up. Gaensler et al[51] reported that over half of the patients surgically treated were again dyspneic after 5 years.

There has been recent interest in performing reductive surgery on patients with generalized emphysema. Attempts at resecting bullous lung in an effort to decrease the size of the overexpanded lung have been previously reported. Brantigan and Mueller[52] reported in 1957 on performing multiple lung resections along with hilar stripping (denervation to decrease sputum production) via a thoracotomy. He postulated that because of overdistention and increased intrathoracic pressure, the small airways would collapse during expiration. Lung resection would thus restore the outward elastic pull on small airways and reduce expiratory obstruction. Unfortunately, he was unable to quantify his results, and he had a 16% mortality rate.

Present attempts at reducing the overdistention of the lung in this difficult group of patients have included the use of the laser and argon beam coagulator (ABC) through the thoracoscope (along with the endoscopic stapler). The Nd:YAG laser in the contact mode has been the preferred method when the laser is used, and it coagulates the surface of the lung and "shrinks" the bullous tissue. The ABC has a similar effect, although direct comparisons of the two techniques are lacking.

A series of 262 patients was operated upon using VATS Nd:YAG laser bullectomy by Wakabayashi. The mortality rate was 5.3%, and 4.6% required more than one operative procedure. Subjective improvement was noted in the majority of patients, but, only a small percentage of patients had postoperative pulmonary function quantitatively evaluated.[53]

Lewis and colleagues[54] reported on the use of the ABC in eight patients. Six of seven were able to discontinue steroids, and three of six were able to discontinue the need for oxygen. Only three had postoperative pulmonary function testing with a 34% improvement in $FEV_1$. Postoperative complications included pneumonia ($\frac{3}{8}$ = 38%), and the mean hospital stay was >2 weeks.[54]

Cooper et al have recently reported upon the use of median sternotomy and bilateral stapling of the lung to achieve volume reduction.[55] In 20 patients there has been no mortality, and the mean $FEV_1$ has improved by 69%. Problems with postoperative air leaks have been improved by the use of bovine pericardial strips to buttress the staple lines. Mean hospital stay was 15 days, and exercise testing and dyspnea scores have been improved.

The theoretical reasons for improvement in dyspnea with reductive surgery are several. Decreasing the intrathoracic pressure will possibly decrease expiratory obstruction as proposed by Brantigan. Volume reduction may allow the diaphragm to regain its curvature and again participate in respiration. Compressed functional lung may be recruited by removing bullous tissue.

Many questions remain unanswered with respect to this surgery. How do we select patients for this surgery? Which method achieves the best response (laser, ABC, stapling, etc.)? Should this be done unilaterally or bilaterally? How long will any derived benefits last? Until further information is available, surgery for bullous emphysema should be reserved for localized bulla, and any surgery for diffuse bullous disease should remain experimental.

### *Technique of VATS Bullectomy*

The technique for VATS bullectomy using the Nd:YAG laser or ABC is not complicated. At least three trocar sites are required, and the entire lung is carefully evaluated. The ipsilateral lung is disconnected from ventilation, and the bullous areas tend to be the last to have resorptive atelectases and, hence, are readily identified. Areas amenable to stapled resection are so handled. Buttressing the stapling device with bovine pericardium may indeed be a good method of limiting the air leak problems. The Nd:YAG laser in the contact mode has proven a safe method to shrink bullous lung that is not amenable to stapling. Low power settings (5–10 W) are used on contact probes with high surface areas to diffuse the power density. Bullous areas contract causing volume reduction. By manipulating the lung, the entire surface of the lung with bullous disease is "painted." By using the contact Nd:YAG laser, postoperative air leaks have been minimized. A chemical (talc) or mechanical pleurodesis or pleurectomy may be added.

Reductive therapy may be performed using median sternotomy and standard stapling devices. Bullous areas are resected as the lung is sculptured to just fit in each thoracic cavity. Selective ventilation using a double-lumen endotracheal tube is used. The goal of resection has been to reduce the overall volume of each lung by 20–30%.

## LUNG RESECTION

### Indications

Resection of the lung comprises approximately 50% of all VATS procedures performed (Table 12B–1). Thoracoscopic lung resection can be performed as either a nonanatomic wedge resection, a formal lobectomy, or even a pneumonectomy. Current indications for wedge resection include the indeterminate solitary pulmonary nodule,[56] known primary lung cancer in patients with impaired pulmonary function,[57] and as a diagnostic procedure for metastatic disease in the lung.[58] For primary lung cancer, if the clinical situation warrants a lobectomy and the surgeon feels that this is the appropriate surgical procedure, then a VATS lobectomy can be undertaken by the experienced endoscopic surgeon[59–62] (Table 12B–2).

Standard management of the indeterminate solitary pulmonary nodule has traditionally been fine-needle aspiration biopsy (FNAB).[63–66] However, with the advent of minimally invasive pulmonary resective techniques, thoracoscopy has assumed a larger role in the management of the indeterminate nodule.[56] The data of Calhoun et al[67] as well as our own indicate that less than 5% of all patients who undergo FNAB achieve a *specific benign* diagnosis. Since a specific benign diagnosis is the sole result of FNAB that should avoid surgical resection in an otherwise acceptable surgical candidate, we feel that thoracoscopy should assume a larger role in the management of the indeterminate nodule.

**TABLE 12B–1. VATS PROCEDURES: DECEMBER 1990–NOVEMBER 1994**

| | | | |
|---|---|---|---|
| **Lung resection** | 401 | **Mediastinal disease** | 59 |
| Nodule | 279 | Biopsy/staging nodes | 14 |
| Apical blebs/infiltrate | 31 | Mass | 26 |
| Giant bullae | 21 | Cyst | 10 |
| Pneumothorax | 70 | Thymectomy | 9 |
| **Pleural disease** | 165 | Pericardial disease | 38 |
| Effusion | 90 | Sympathectomy | 29 |
| Chylothorax | 3 | Spine procedures | 56 |
| Empyema | 44 | Lobectomy | 24 |
| Hemothorax | 12 | Esophageal procedures | 23 |
| Mass | 16 | Other | 3 |
| Total | 798 | | |

**TABLE 12B–2. ROLE OF VATS IN LUNG CANCER**

| |
|---|
| Diagnosis of indeterminate pulmonary nodule |
| Wedge resection for limited-stage cancer in elderly or compromised patients |
| VATS lobectomy |
| Staging of pleural and mediastinum |
| Treatment of malignant pleural effusions |

In patients with compromised pulmonary function, i.e., an $FEV_1$ of <1.0 L/M, in which a wedge resection would be the standard method of resection by open approach, thoracoscopy offers the ideal method of performing a lung resection.[57]

Although the role of lung resection as therapy in metastatic disease is controversial, thoracoscopy offers the best approach as a diagnostic procedure for the new nodule in a patient with a history of malignant disease.[58] Surgical morbidity is minimal, and the initiation of systemic therapy can be prompt.

Surgical management of stage I carcinoma of the lung is controversial between lobectomy and nonanatomical wedge resection. The results of the Lung Cancer Study Group show that there is no survival benefit to lobectomy compared with wedge resection when performed by the open technique.[68] However, wedge resection was associated with a significantly higher local recurrence rate in this multicenter study.

If the surgeon feels that a lobectomy is the appropriate procedure, it can be performed by VATS technique. Candidate tumors for VATS lobectomy include peripheral stage I tumors 2 cm or less in diameter and preferentially located in the lower lobes. Hilar involvement with either tumor or lymph nodes or an incomplete fissure found at the time of surgical exploration make the lobectomy by the VATS approach technically quite difficult.

### Technique

#### *Wedge Resection*

Standard VATS technique for lung resection involves placement of the ports in a manner similar to the discussion under diagnostic thoracoscopy. The initial port is placed in the seventh intercostal space in the midaxillary line for placement of the endoscope, and two working ports are placed in the fifth and sixth intercostal spaces in the anterior and posterior axillary lines (Fig. 12B–7). Placement of these ports is modified based upon the location of the nodule in the lung. Because digital palpation is sometimes necessary for identifying the location of nodules in the lung, care should be taken to place one port over the area of lung in which the nodule is anticipated to be located so that the probing finger can easily reach the target area (Fig. 12B–8). Standard lung resective techniques involve mainly the endoscopic stapler. Resection is usually best carried out by

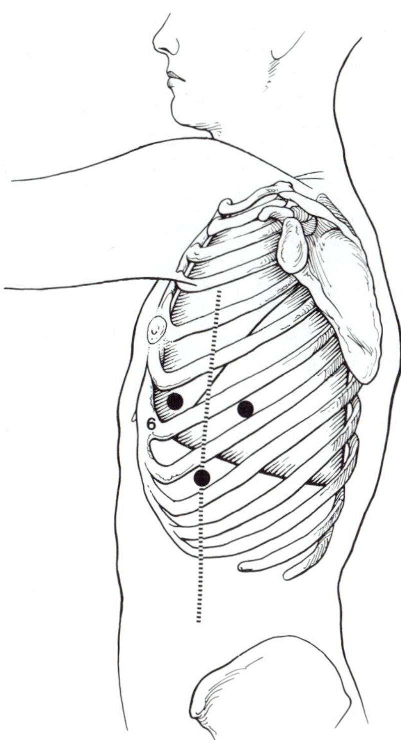


**Figure 12B–7.** Standard port placement for a thoracoscopic wedge resection of the lung.

placing a grasping instrument through one working port and a stapler through the other working port. The stapler fires six rows of staples and cuts the lung between them. After the first firing, it is often helpful to place the stapler through the opposite working portal, and firing again (Fig. 12B–9). Three to four firings of the stapler are sufficient for performing most lung resections. Occasionally the nodule is not adjacent to a margin of the lung but rather against a flat surface, and application of the stapler can be quite difficult. Nodules that are difficult to resect include those on the medial aspect of the upper lobe in the suprahilar area as well as those in the posterior portion of the lower lobes (Fig. 12B–10). In these instances, use of precision electrocautery, the neodymium:YAG laser, or combination of one of these with the stapler is the best method of performing the lung resection. The stapler alone, however, should be sufficient in over 90% of lung resections.

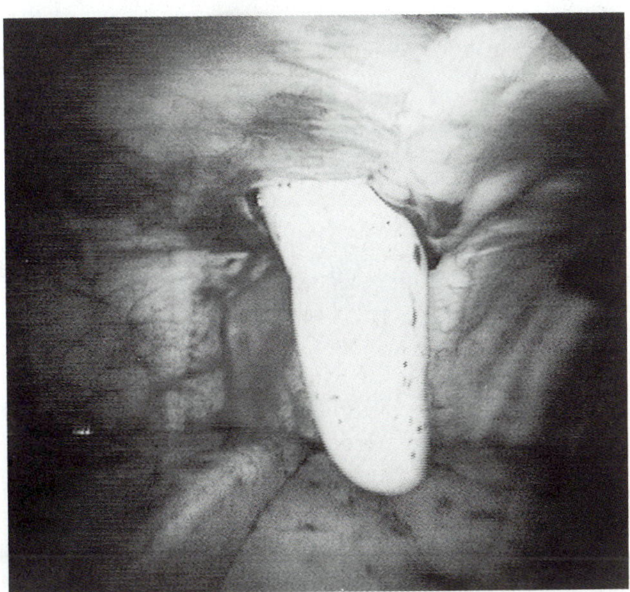

**Figure 12B–8.** Digit placed through trocar site to palpate the adjacent lung to locate an occult nodule.

If there is any potential for malignancy, the specimen should be placed in an endoscopic pouch for extraction so that potential tumor seeding of a trocar site is avoided. The lung is re-expanded, pneumostasis is obtained, and a small size (20 Fr) chest tube is placed.

### *Localization Techniques*

Nodules that are 2 cm or greater and located within 1 cm of the surface of the lung can usually be identified quite simply by visual inspection (Fig. 12B–11A,B) especially if there is any visceral pleural involvement[69] (Table 12B–3). If the visceral pleura is not involved, then effacement of the collapsed lung that occurs around the nodule can give a visual clue to the existence of an underlying nodule. The use of an instrument for palpation or placement of the surgeon's index finger through one of the trocar sites to digitally palpate the lung is also quite helpful (Fig. 12B–8). Careful preoperative examination of the computed tomography (CT) scan, which includes an assessment of whether the nodule is adjacent to a pulmonary fissure, will aid intraoperative identification (Fig. 12B–12A,B). Some nodules that on first glance at the CT scan appear to be deep within the parenchyma of the lung may in fact be located adjacent to one of the fissures and therefore easily identifiable at time of thoracoscopy. If a nodule is <1 cm in diameter and is located >2 cm from the nearest visceral pleural surface, consideration should be given to preoperative needle localization techniques in order to help locate the nodule at the time of surgery[70,71] (Fig. 12B–13). There is limited use of intraoperative ultrasound with the collapsed lung immersed in a fluid filled chest cavity to locate nodules. Although some nodules can be identified by this technique, and ultrasound probes are now adapted for endoscopic procedures, this is not a method that can be routinely recommended. The use of interventional real time magnetic resonance imaging (MRI) offers a *potential* opportunity for identifying the occult pulmonary nodule.

**Air Leaks.** Air leaks can be a significant management problem with thoracoscopic pulmonary resective techniques. Whenever possible, the endoscopic stapler should be used for lung resection. The three rows of staples placed by the endoscopic stapler appear to offer better pneumostasis than the standard open staplers. However, the lung can be torn by traction or by placement of too thick a portion of

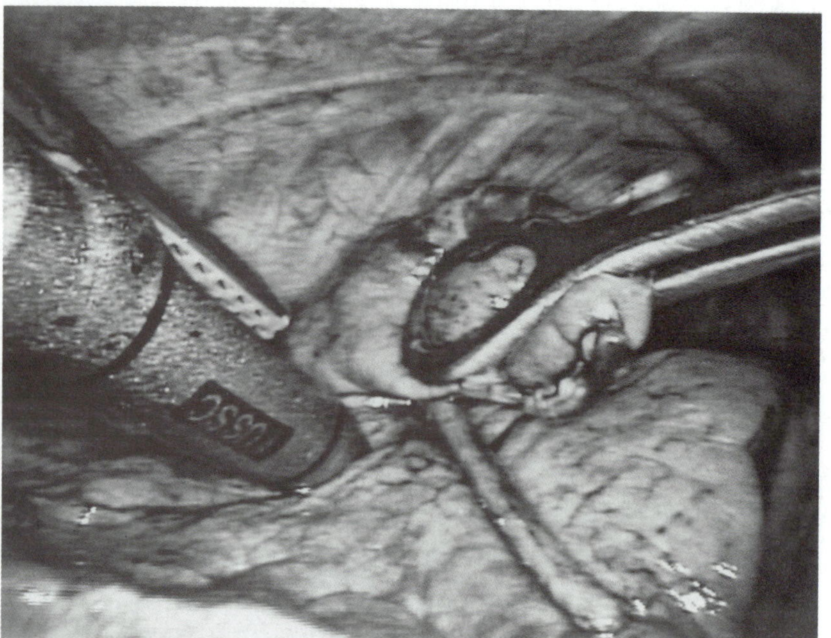

**Figure 12B–9.** Technique of VATS lung resection with grasping instrument and stapler interchanged between ports for the second step of lung resection.

lung within the jaws of the stapler. In addition, significant air leaks can occur due to the presence of underlying bullous emphysema, especially when the lung has been resected by electrocautery or laser techniques. In these instances air leaks should be aggressively managed. The use of endoscopic suturing techniques to oversew leaking lung should be mastered. We have found it quite helpful to use bovine pericardium as reinforcing pledgets to buttress the suture line on leaking lung. In addition, we have used the YAG laser and Argon Beam Coagulator for a coagulative effect on the raw surface of the lung. The addition of fibrin glue placed endoscopically on the raw surface of the lung has also been helpful for managing air leaks in some instances.

### *VATS Lobectomy*

The standard technique for VATS lobectomy involves placement of two trocars as well as a "utility" or "accessory" incision that is used to extract the specimen at the end of the procedure. The placement of this utility incision at the onset can greatly facilitate dissection and resection during the procedure. It is our preference to place this utility incision in the fifth intercostal space (ICS) in the anterior axillary line and the two trocar sites in the seventh and eighth ICSs in the mid- and posterior axillary lines (Fig. 12B–14). If an upper lobectomy is to be performed, placement of one trocar in the fourth intercostal space anteriorly is quite helpful for visualizing the superior aspect of the hilum. Upon initial entry into the chest, exploratory tho-

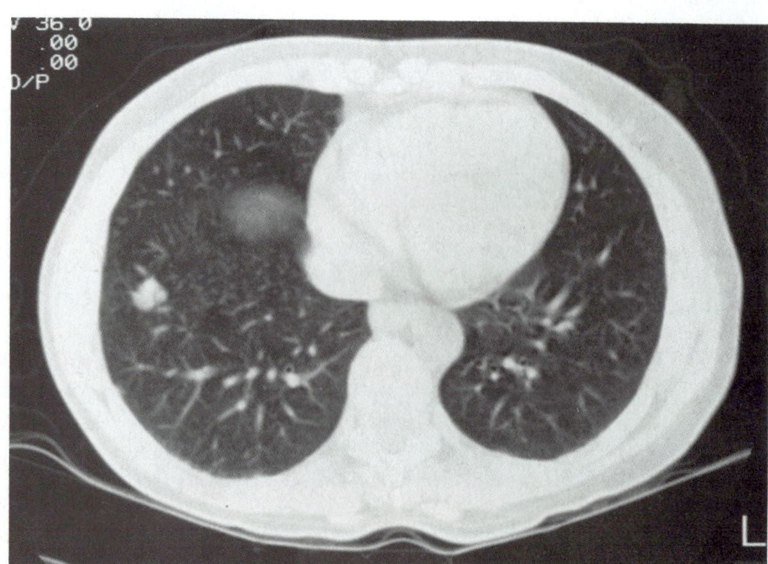

**Figure 12B–10.** Lung nodule that is difficult to resect by VATS because it is fairly deep within the lung parenchyma and is adjacent to a flat surface and not on acute margin of the lung.

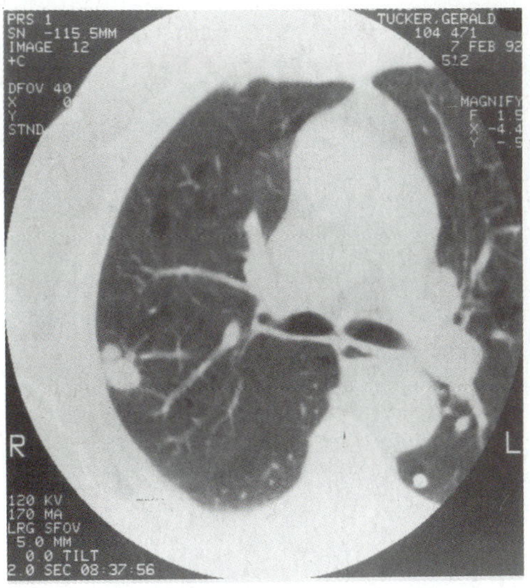


A

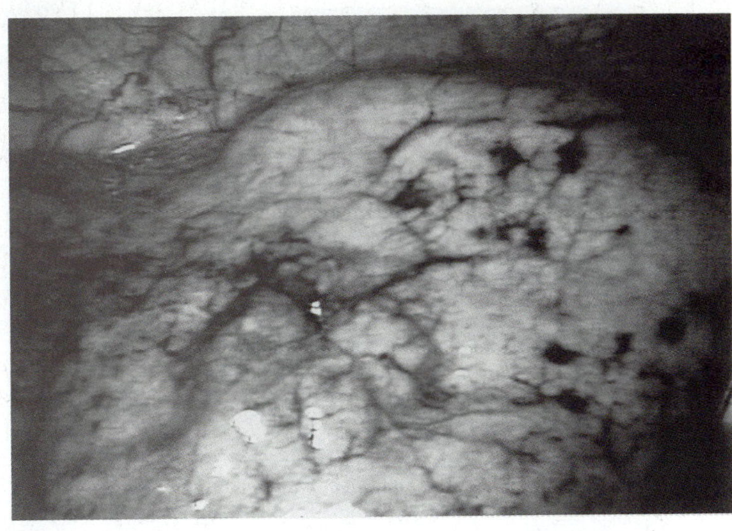

B

**Figure 12B–11. A.** CT scan showing nodule easily identified by thoracoscopy. **B.** Appearance of same nodule at time of VATS resection.

racoscopy is performed to "stage" the cancer and to assure that pleural seeding has not occurred. The mediastinum is examined to be sure that gross N2 disease does not exist. Next the hilum is examined to determine the suitability for resection. Involvement of the hilum with either tumor or lymphadenopathy may make dissection and management of the pulmonary vessels technically difficult, and conversion to an open thoracotomy should occur. In a similar manner, an incomplete fissure makes VATS lobectomy exceedingly difficult, and, again, consideration of conversion to an open procedure should occur.

Lower lobes, especially the left lower lobe, are better suited for resection by VATS techniques than either the middle lobe or either upper lobe (Fig. 12B–15). If, after initial inspection, it is deemed that a VATS lobectomy is possible, the pulmonary vein is managed first. If the lower lobe is to be resected, the inferior pulmonary ligament is divided first, and after careful dissection a traction suture is placed around the inferior pulmonary vein. A vascular endoscopic stapler is then placed across the inferior pulmonary vein and fired (Fig. 12B–16). Care is taken to assure that the proximal end of the vessel can be controlled in case stapler malfunction occurs. Both staple lines are then inspected for hemostasis after the jaws of the stapler are opened and the stapler is removed. Dissection is then carried next into the fissure. In the case of the left lower lobe, the pulmonary arterial branch to the lingula is usually managed separately and divided with an endoscopic vascular stapler. The remaining pulmonary arterial trunk to the lower lobe is divided. The bronchus is divided last with an endoscopic 3.5-mm stapler. The specimen is then removed through the utility incision (Fig. 12B–17). Air leaks are checked for, the lung is re-expanded, and two small diameter (24–28 Fr) chest tubes are placed.

In the case of upper lobe resection, again the pulmonary vein is controlled first and divided with a vascular endoscopic stapler. Division of the segmental pulmonary arteries to the apical and posterior segments followed by the anterior segment are the next easiest vessels to divide. As with a lower lobectomy, the bronchus is divided last. The exception to this is the *left* upper lobe, where it is often easier to divide the upper lobe bronchus before dividing the anterior segmental pulmonary artery.

**TABLE 12B–3. TECHNIQUES FOR LOCATING PULMONARY NODULES FOR VATS RESECTION**

**Preoperative**
- Careful examination of computerized tomogram
- Needle localization
- Methylene blue injection

**Intraoperative**
- Visual inspection for effacement of the collapsed lung around the nodule
- Instrument palpation
- Digital palpation
- Ultrasound

**Future**
- Interventional realtime MR scan

## Results

For the management of the indeterminate solitary pulmonary nodule, thoracoscopy is quite effective. In our own experience in properly selected candidate nodules, thoracoscopy has been uniformly successful in obtaining a diagnostic result.[56] If nodules are deep within the lobe of the

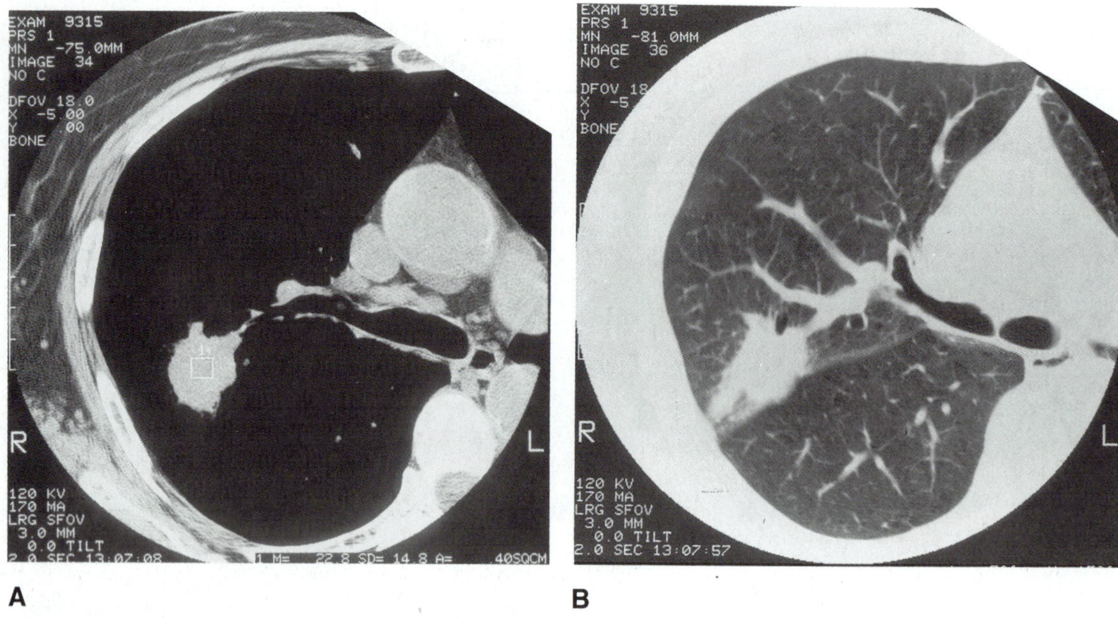


**Figure 12B–12.** **A.** Initial CT exam shows nodule apparently deep within the lung and difficult to identify. **B.** Lung window shows nodule is in fact adjacent to a fissure and, therefore, easy to identify.

lung, then either a fine-needle aspiration biopsy or an open procedure should be undertaken.

If wedge resection is to be used as definitive therapy for stage I lung cancer in patients with compromised pulmonary function, thoracoscopy is the preferred method. In a series by Shennib et al,[57] 50 patients managed by this technique show excellent results.

Four large series of VATS lobectomy now exist (Table 12B–4). A total of 256 patients in these four series has undergone VATS lobectomy with no mortality and no significant morbidity. Four conversions to open thoracotomy were necessary for bleeding, and an additional 10% conversion to open thoracotomy occurred because of technical difficulties primarily due to an incomplete fissure. Although the feasibility of VATS lobectomy and VATS pneumonectomy has been demonstrated, clear benefit over open approaches has not yet been demonstrated.

## Conclusion

Thoracoscopy has become the prime diagnostic modality for the management of the indeterminate nodule in many institutions and has assumed a larger role in those institutions. Pulmonary resective techniques have been well de-

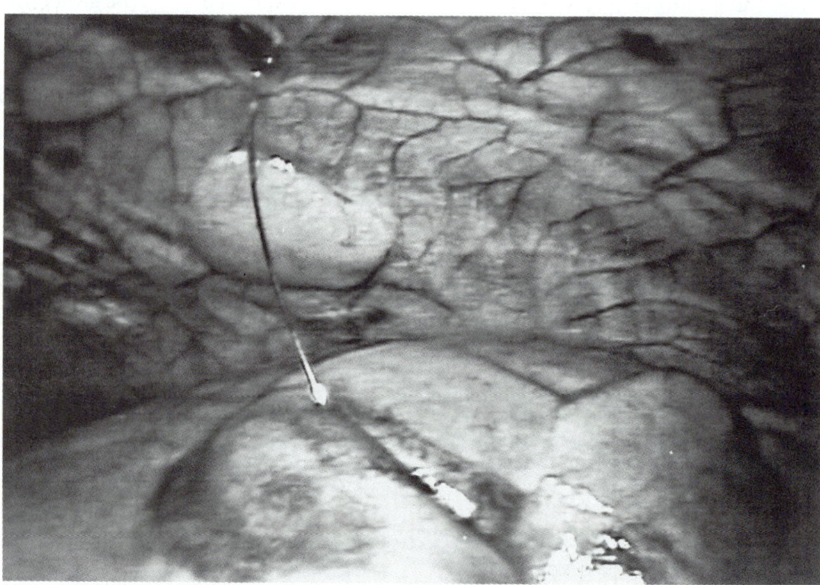

**Figure 12B–13.** Preoperatively placed wire into an occult lung nodule. Note methylene blue lung staining also placed preoperatively.

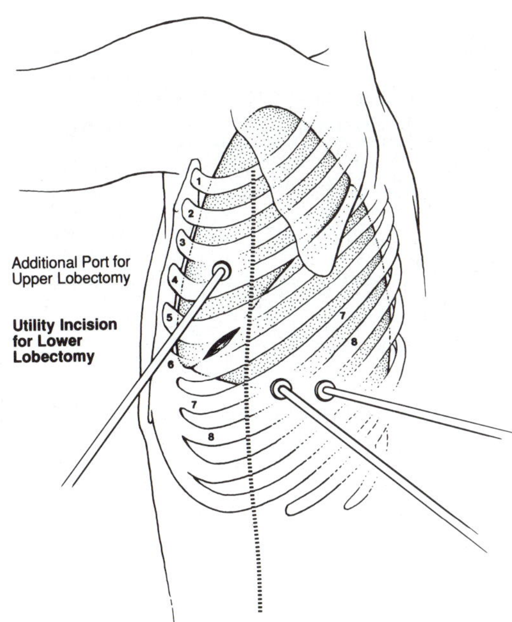


**Figure 12B–14.** Approach strategy for a VATS lobectomy.

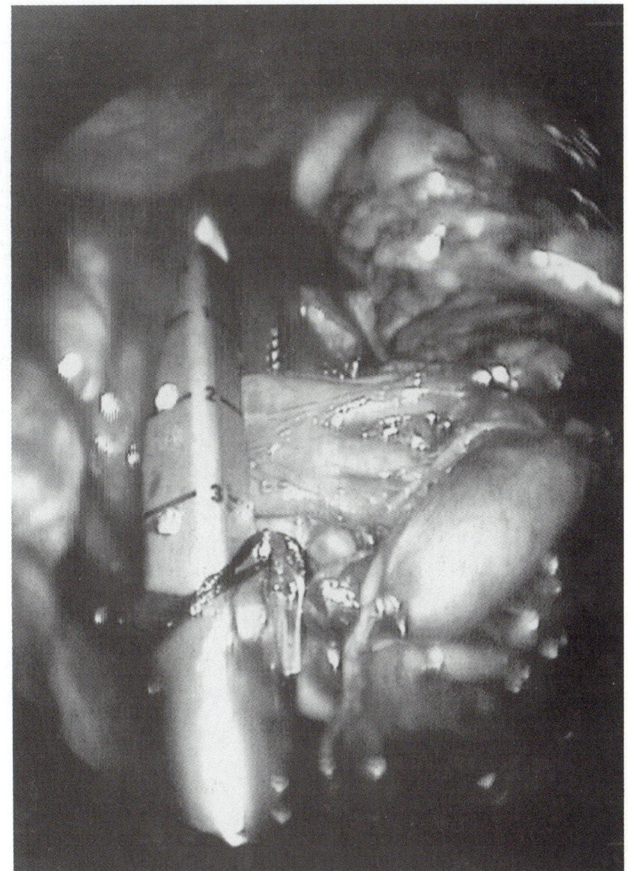

**Figure 12B–16.** Endoscopic vascular stapler placed across the inferior pulmonary vein.

fined and have become standard practice. Wedge resection by VATS has become accepted management for patients with compromised pulmonary function in which the definitive treatment would be a wedge resection if performed by open techniques. The role of wedge resection vs. lobectomy for stage I cancer is still not clearly defined, but if a lobectomy is selected, then VATS can be performed for stage I disease. Feasibility, but not benefit, has been proven.

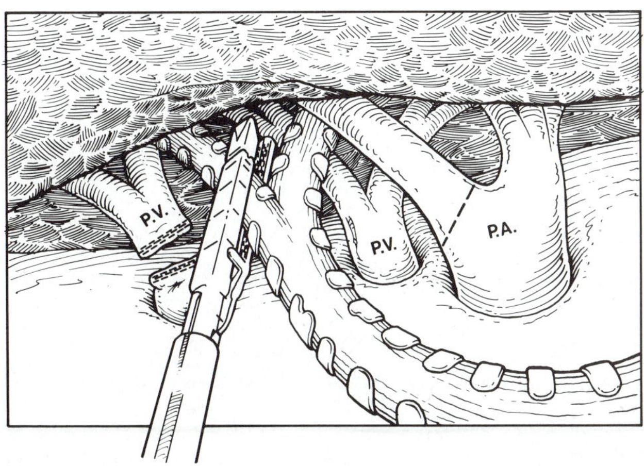


**Figure 12B–15.** Endoscopic view of hilar structures for VATS lobectomy on the left lower lobe.

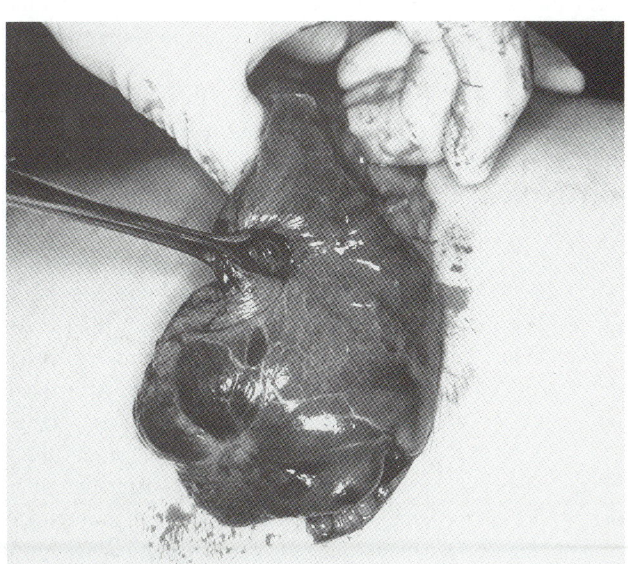

**Figure 12B–17.** Extraction of resected lobe through the "accessory" incision without rib spreading.

**TABLE 12B–4. LOBECTOMY PERFORMED BY VATS**

| Center | | Number | Mortality | Conversion for Bleeding | Conversion for Technical Problems |
|---|---|---|---|---|---|
| Roviaro | (Milan) | 84 | 0 | 2 | 6 |
| McKenna | (Los Angeles) | 45 | 0 | 1 | 2 |
| Walker | (Edinburgh) | 50 | 0 | 0 | 5 |
| Kirby | (Cleveland) | 25 | 0 | 1 | 4 |

## PERICARDIECTOMY

VATS is both diagnostic and therapeutic for pericardial disease. It can be therapeutic for the management of both malignant and benign effusive pericardial disease as well as for purulent pericarditis and radiation-induced pericarditis.[72] The standard techniques for management of effusive pericardial disease include limited anterior or posterolateral thoracotomy,[73] the subxiphoid approach,[74] and now thoracoscopy. Median sternotomy is reserved for constrictive noneffusive pericardial disease.

### Technique

VATS pericardiectomy is performed through either the right or left thoracic cavity. Procedures are performed under general endotracheal anesthesia with the patient in the lateral position. Initial trocar placement when performed on the left side is usually posterior to the midaxillary line to avoid potential injury to the distended pericardial sac (Fig. 12B–18). The left side is usually chosen unless there is an associated pleural effusion or pulmonary nodule on the right side to be managed simultaneously. Advantages to the right side include more room to maneuver the scope and instruments. After initial trocar site is chosen and the scope is placed, two additional working portals are made. The lung is retracted, and the distended pericardium is visualized. Sometimes grasping of the distending pericardium is difficult, especially if a preoperative pericardiocentesis has not been performed. In this case, a pericardiocentesis can be done under direct visualization to decompress the distended pericardial sac or alternatively, and a hook can be used to grasp the pericardium. Once the pericardium has been grasped, a blunt endoscopic scissors is used to incise the pericardium, and the pericardial space is completely drained of fluid. Wide swatches of pericardium are excised both anterior and posterior to the phrenic nerve (Fig. 12B–19). Care is taken to preserve a bridge of pericardium beneath the phrenic nerve to avoid injury. Any bleeding pericardial edge can be managed cautiously with monopolar or biopolar electrocautery once the pericardium has been retracted away from the heart. When adequate pericardium has been excised and the pericardial space completely drained, a chest tube is placed in the pleural cavity.

Because pericardiectomy by the VATS approach can be too invasive for patients with end-stage malignancy, the subxiphoid approach is still a viable alternative. We recently have experience adding video assistance to the subxiphoid approach. A 4-mm videotelescope is placed in the accessory channel of a modified mediastinoscope and placed through the standard subxiphoid incision (Fig. 12B–20). The anterior mediastinal fat is bluntly dissected away from the pericardial surface and the pericardium identified. In a technique similar to that described for the thoracoscopic approach, the pericardium is grasped and incised. The pericardial space is completely drained. A 4 × 4-cm swatch of pericardium can be excised by this approach.

### Results

Our present experience with VATS pericardiectomy comprises over 50 cases. Although we have had no recurrence of the effusive process to date with an average follow-up of

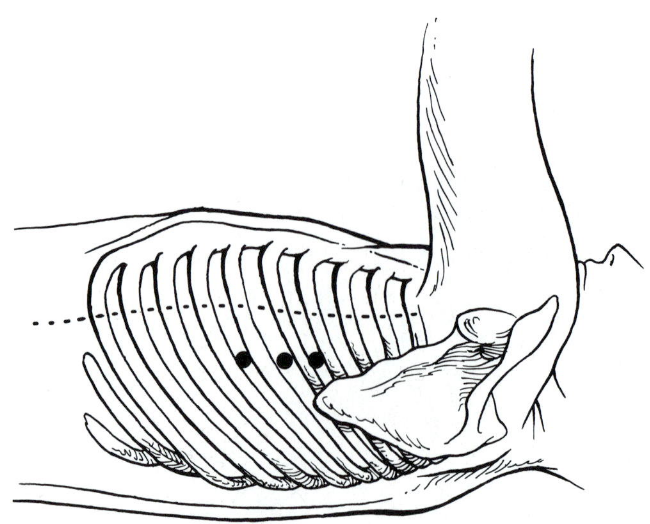

**Figure 12B–18.** Trocar placement for pericardiectomy. Trocars are placed posterior to the midaxillary line to avoid injury and to provide room for maneuverability.

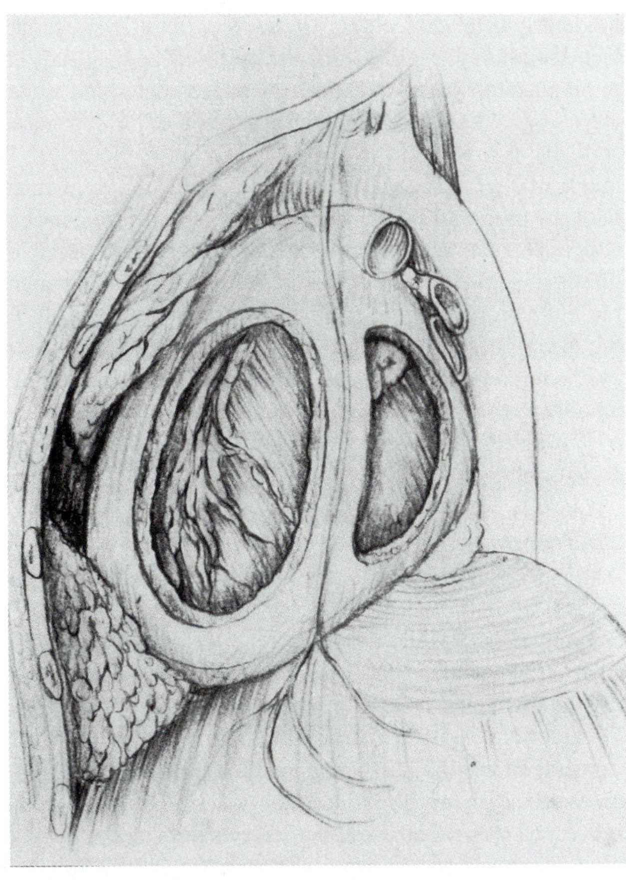

**Figure 12B–19.** Extent of pericardial resection by VATS. *(From Mack MJ, Hazelrigg JR, Landreneau RJ, et al: Video thoracoscopic management of benign and malignant pericardial effusions. Chest 103:390–393S, 1993, with permission.)*

18 months, we have had a number of deaths unrelated to the procedure in the weeks following VATS pericardiectomy in those patients with malignant pericardial involvement.[75] Since the average survival of patients with malignant pericardial involvement from lung cancer is 3–4 months from the time of diagnosis, the least invasive management approach should be entertained in these patients. If catheter pericardiocentesis alone or with sclerosis does not adequately manage the effusive process, then a subxiphoid window rather than a thoracoscopy should be performed for pericardial drainage and resection. Video assistance may allow a wider portion of pericardium to be excised and, therefore, decrease the recurrence rate. For those patients with benign effusive disease or those patients with a good prognosis for malignant disease, e.g., breast cancer or lymphoma, then VATS offers a good approach for pericardiectomy and drainage of the pericardial space.

## MEDIASTINAL DISEASE

### Indications

The indications for thoracoscopy in mediastinal disease include the diagnosis of mediastinal masses,[76–79] staging of lung cancer,[80] and thymectomy.[81] In addition, small, localized, noninvasive masses can be removed from the anterior or posterior mediastinum by the thoracoscopic approach. Mediastinal cysts can also be excised by thoracoscopy.[82] It should be remembered, however, that the presence of a mediastinal cyst does not necessarily mandate removal, since the overwhelming number of mediastinal cysts are benign in nature. However, if symptoms exist due to compression of adjacent structures or if there is concern regarding the benign nature of the cyst, then VATS offers the optimal technique for management of these diseases.

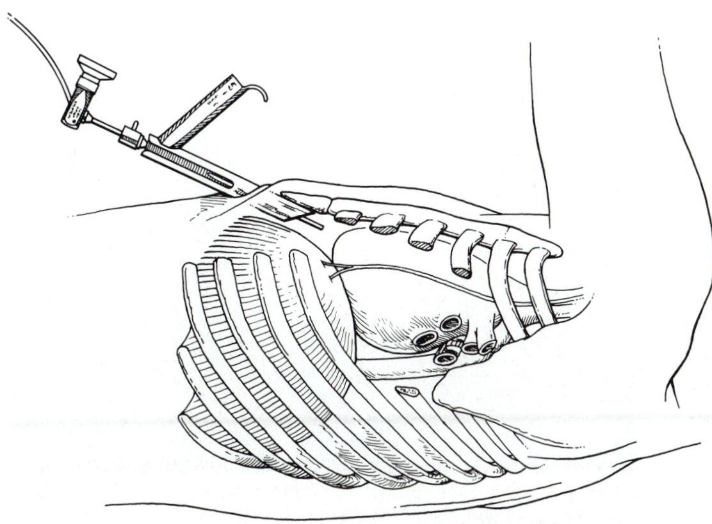

**Figure 12B–20.** Technique of "video" subxiphoid pericardiectomy.

There does appear to be a role for VATS in the role of staging of lung cancer. Cervical mediastinal exploration remains our standard method for staging of right peritracheal lymph nodes. For the staging of left-sided lesions and the aortopulmonary window, levels 4L, 5, 6, and 7, VATS has replaced the Chamberlain procedure as our primary method of staging.

A number of thymectomies for myasthenia gravis either with or without thymoma have been performed. Although total thymic excision can be performed by VATS, the experience and results are limited. For invasive thymoma, an open approach is indicated.

## Technique

### *General*

Port placement is dictated by the area of the mediastinum to be approached. By keeping in mind the general strategy of not placing ports too close to the area to be approached, ports are placed somewhat *anterior* to the midaxillary line for approaching the *posterior* mediastinum.[83] In a similar manner, when one is approaching the *anterior* mediastinum, ports are placed in the *mid-* and *posterior* axillary lines and somewhat lower in the chest, approximately the fifth or sixth interspaces.

### *Posterior Mediastinal Masses*

For posterior mediastinal masses, two ports are typically placed in the anterior axillary line and one in the midaxillary line. The interspace depends upon the level of the mass. Once exploratory thoracoscopy has been performed, the mass is identified, and the parietal pleura adjacent to the mass is scored. Care should be taken to control any segmental vessels that are present immediately adjacent to the mass to be excised, since these can cause bothersome bleeding during the dissection. It should be remembered that the segmental artery and vein traverse the midportion of the vertebral bodies. The segmental vessels can be ligated with endoscopic clips if necessary. Since the overwhelming majority of posterior mediastinal masses are benign, neurogenic tumors, complete excision is usually possible. If concern of malignancy exists, a specimen bag should be used when one is removing the specimen through the chest wall. If the mass is >2 cm in size, slight enlargement of one of the more anterior trocar sites may be necessary to retrieve the specimen from the thoracic cavity. A chest tube is generally not necessary unless inadvertent lung injury has occurred.

### *Cysts*

When there are symptoms due to compression of adjacent structures or there is concern about malignancy, mediastinal cysts should be removed. The thoracoscopic technique for excision is relatively straightforward. Once ports are appropriately placed and the cyst is located within the mediastinum (Fig. 12B–21), dissection planes are usually easiest to identify if the dissection is initiated with the cyst wall intact. Eventually, aspiration of the cyst will be necessary in order to remove the cyst through one of the small trocar sites. Care should be taken upon aspiration of the cyst not to spill the cyst contents in the thoracic cavity. However, as much of the dissection as possible should be performed with the cyst wall intact. Usually, separation from adjacent structures such as pericardium and esophagus is possible; however, if there is an extensive inflammatory component present, complete dissection may be somewhat difficult. In the occasional instance in which complete excision of the cyst is not possible without a significant chance of injury to an adherent vital structure, the remaining small portion of cyst wall can be left and the cyst lining obliterated with electrocautery.

### *Thymectomy*

Although VATS thymectomy is a technically advanced procedure, it can be mastered by the surgeon who has a fair amount of endoscopic surgical experience. Approach can be from either the right or left chest. The side upon which the thymus gland is most prominent is chosen, usually the left side (Fig. 12B–22). Dissection is begun at the left inferior pole of the thymus gland and continued cephalad. The mediastinal pleura is divided just anterior to the phrenic nerve and dissection carried to the origin of the thymic blood supply from the internal mammary artery. We then find that it is easiest to dissect the thymus off of the retrosternal area as far superior and as far to the right as is visible at this stage of the procedure (Fig. 12B–23). Next the thymus gland is dissected off of the pericardium with a combination of sharp and blunt dissection. Any significant vessels are judiciously managed with electrocautery. Resec-

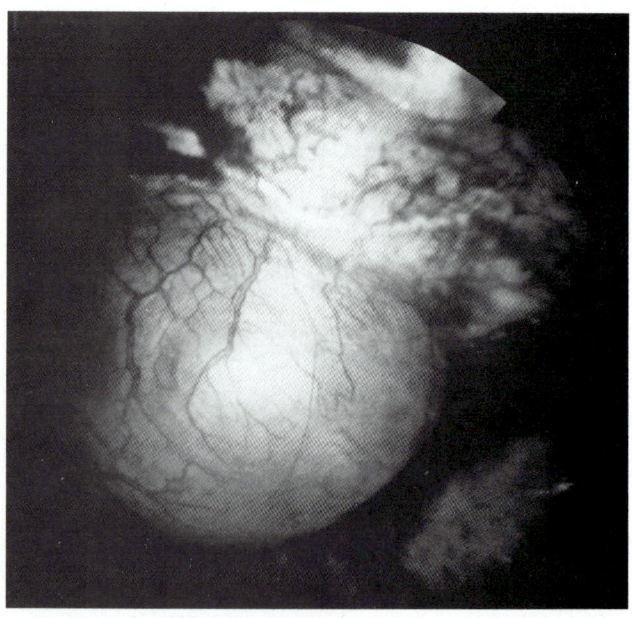

**Figure 12B–21.** VATS appearance of a mediastinal cyst.

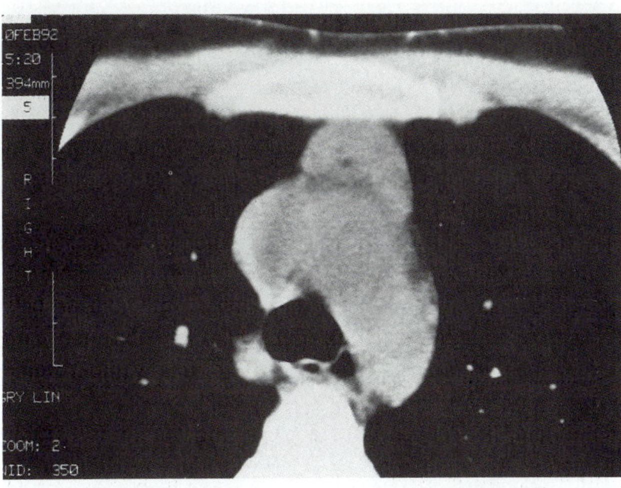


Figure 12B–22. CT scan of patient with myasthenia gravis showing thymic hyperplasia. This is most easily approached from the left side.

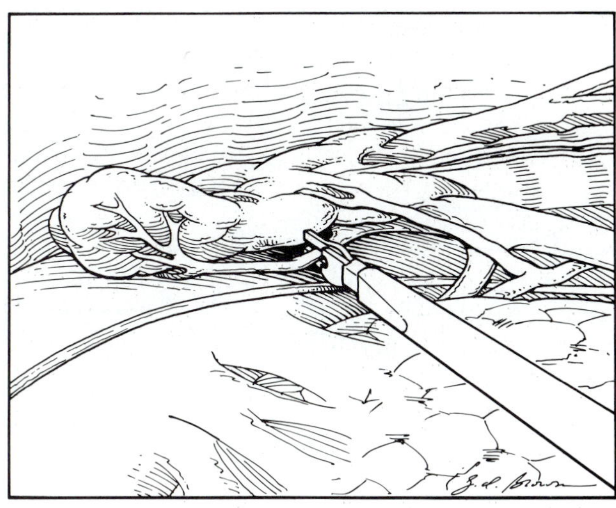

Figure 12B–24. Thymic vein is ligated with an endoscopic clip.

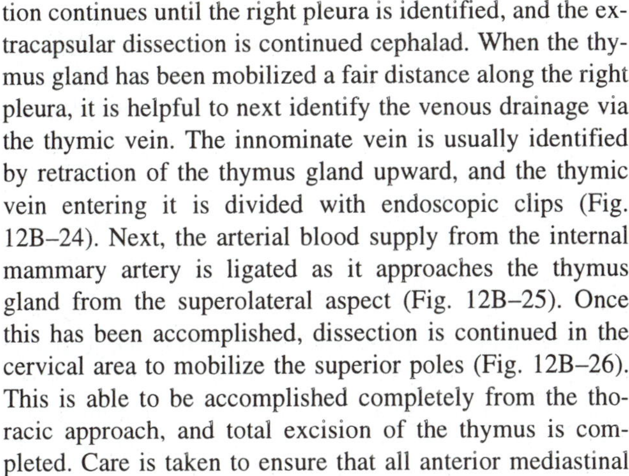

tion continues until the right pleura is identified, and the extracapsular dissection is continued cephalad. When the thymus gland has been mobilized a fair distance along the right pleura, it is helpful to next identify the venous drainage via the thymic vein. The innominate vein is usually identified by retraction of the thymus gland upward, and the thymic vein entering it is divided with endoscopic clips (Fig. 12B–24). Next, the arterial blood supply from the internal mammary artery is ligated as it approaches the thymus gland from the superolateral aspect (Fig. 12B–25). Once this has been accomplished, dissection is continued in the cervical area to mobilize the superior poles (Fig. 12B–26). This is able to be accomplished completely from the thoracic approach, and total excision of the thymus is completed. Care is taken to ensure that all anterior mediastinal tissue is removed because of the potential concern of ectopic thymic gland in the anterior mediastinal tissue. The intact specimen is then removed through one of the anterior trocar sites (Fig. 12B–27). The thymic bed is then checked to assure that hemostasis is obtained, and a chest tube is not usually necessary. Care in an intensive care unit is not necessary, and patients are typically discharged on the day following surgery.

### *Staging*

Mediastinal lymphadenopathy is typically staged prior to lobectomy for lung cancer. For left-sided lesions, three trocars are placed, and careful dissection for lymph nodes is performed in the aortopulmonary window (Fig. 12B–28).

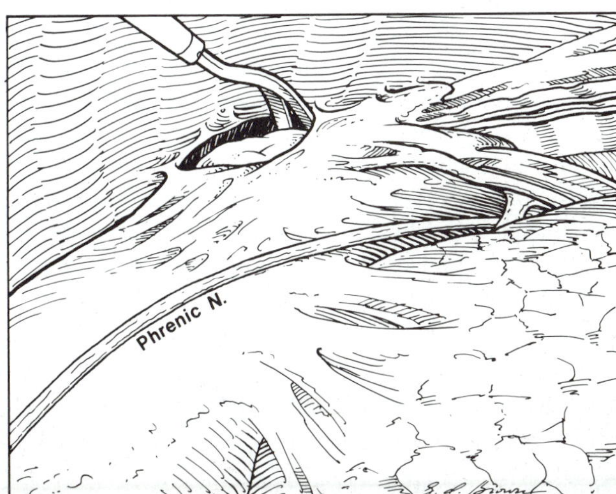


Figure 12B–23. Technique of VATS thymectomy. Thymus is dissected from the retrosternal area.

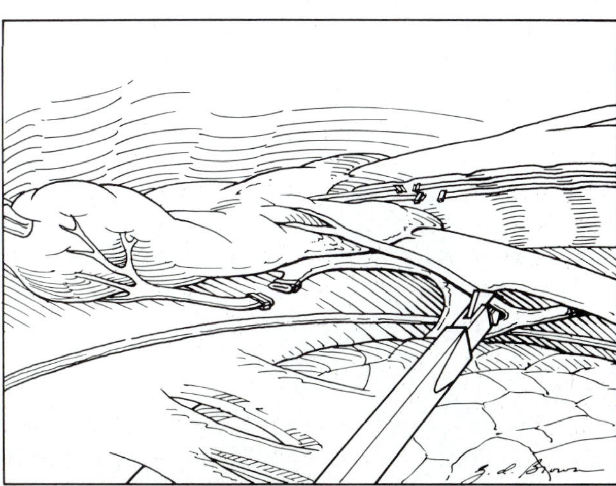

Figure 12B–25. Once the thymic vein has been divided (small arrow), the arterial supply from the internal mammary artery is ligated (large arrow).

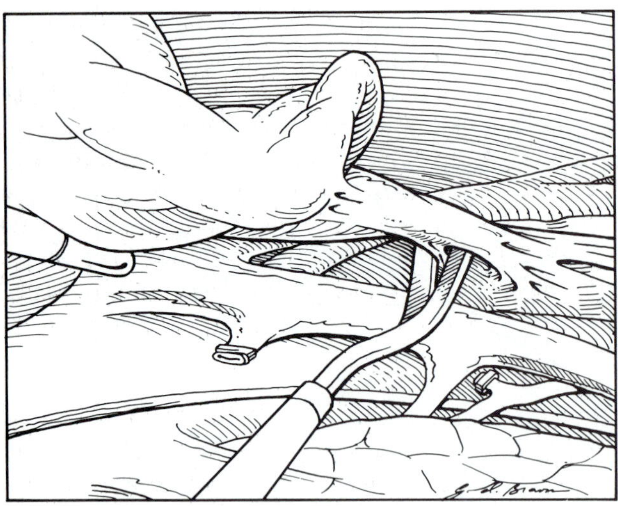

**Figure 12B–26.** Dissection above the innominate vein into the cervical area mobilizes the superior poles of the thymus gland.

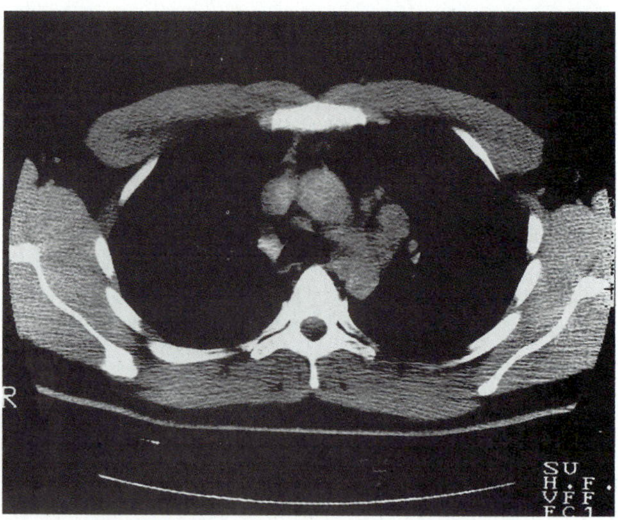

**Figure 12B–28.** CT appearance of aortopulmonary window lymph nodes accessible by VATS.

Better lighting and visualization of the whole aortopulmonary window area allows for an extensive lymph node harvest, and the number of lymph nodes harvested is typically equal or greater to that able to be performed by an open approach. The inferior esophageal nodes (level 8) are also easily dissected by this approach. Subcarinal lymph nodes (level 7) can also be staged, and both levels 4L and 4R can be staged from the appropriate sides.

## Results

Approximately 10% of our VATS procedures are for a mediastinal disease process.[78] The majority of these procedures are diagnostic for mediastinal masses or lymphadenopathy, which usually turns out to be lymphoma. We have been uniformly satisfied with the procedure for the excision of anterior mediastinal cysts. Although the role of VATS for thymectomy is not yet proven, we have performed 10 thymectomies for myasthenia gravis with results equal to the standard transternal approaches.

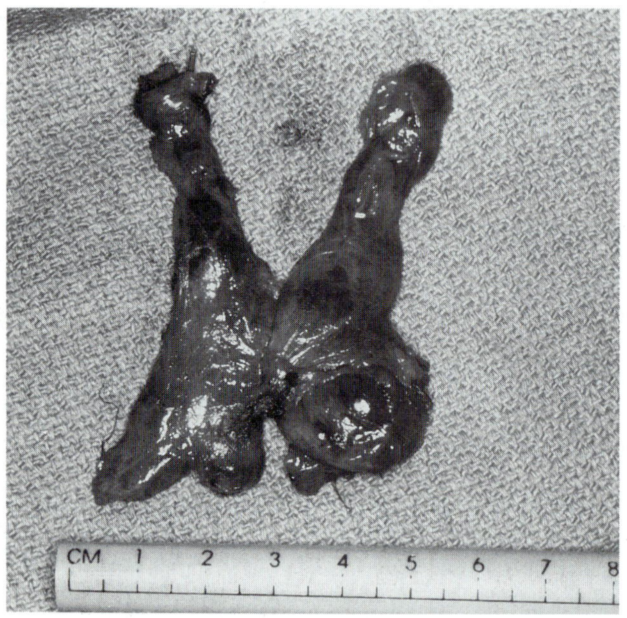


**Figure 12B–27.** Intact thymus gland removed by VATS.

## Conclusions

There is an extensive role for VATS in the management of mediastinal disease. As a diagnostic procedure for anterior mediastinal masses and for mediastinal lymphadenopathy, we still use the cervical mediastinal exploration. However, in instances that we previously would have used the second intercostal space exploration (Chamberlain procedure) for approaching the anterior pulmonary window, we now use VATS. When excision of mediastinal cysts is indicated because of symptoms or concern for malignancy, VATS offers an ideal surgical approach with many procedures able to be performed on an outpatient basis. In addition, the excision of posterior mediastinal masses that most commonly are benign neurogenic tumors are best approached by VATS. Although total thymectomy for myasthenia gravis can be approached by VATS, experience is too small and follow-up is too short to be able to make any legitimate comparison with standard approaches for thymectomy.

# AUTONOMIC NERVOUS SYSTEM

## Thoracic Sympathectomy

Indications for sympathectomy include pain syndromes of the upper extremity (i.e., RSD or causalgia), hyperhidrosis, and occasionally vascular disorders.[84] The ability to perform this procedure endoscopically was reported as early as 1942, but improvements in anesthesia, instruments, and video equipment make it much easier today. Other methods of performing surgical thoracic sympathectomies include cervical, transaxillary, and thoracotomy incisions. Advantages of the cervical approach include good cosmesis and the ability to perform bilateral sympathectomies in one sitting. The potential for injury to many adjacent structures (i.e., phrenic nerve, brachial plexus, subclavian and vertebral arteries) through limited exposure and the inability to excise lower thoracic ganglia (i.e., $T_4$) are disadvantages of the cervical approach. Video-assisted techniques allow excellent visualization of the entire thoracic sympathetic chain while the morbidity of a thoracotomy is avoided (Fig. 12B–29).

Preoperative response to a stellate ganglion block is imperative in order to ensure a good result from sympathectomy.

### Indications

**Hyperhidrosis.** This disorder of unknown etiology results in excessive sweating from eccrine glands and may result in embarrassment and social reclusiveness. Although usually idiopathic, it can be associated with hyperthyroidism, obesity, anxiety disorders, menopause, or pheochromocytoma.

Conservative treatment has included topical creams (i.e., aluminum chloride) and systemic anticholinergic medications. Creams are messy, and medications provide short-term results with frequent side effects. Iontophoresis has had limited success and requires three to six treatments per week. Surgical excision of eccrine glands may be effective if the hyperhidrosis is limited to the axilla. The only effective long-term therapy for most patients is sympathectomy.

The amount of sympathetic chain resected varies depending upon the desired effect. The $T_1$ ganglia supplies innervation to the hand in 10% of cases, but its inclusion in resection requires removal of a portion of the stellate ganglion and the risk of Horner's syndrome.[85,86] If the axilla is to be denervated, then the $T_4$ and $T_5$ ganglia should be included in resection.

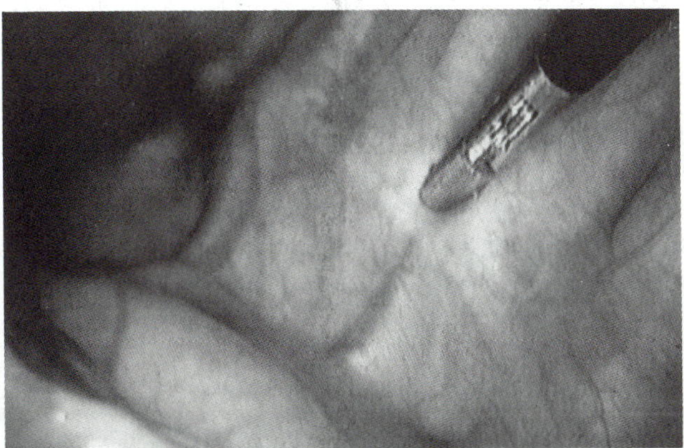

**Figure 12B–29.** Grasping forceps identifies the sympathetic chain in the left chest cavity.

Success rates for sympathectomy in this disorder have been good (85–95%). Potential complications include Horner's syndrome, gustatory sweating, recurrent hyperhidrosis, and compensatory sweating. Compensatory sweating is eventually noted to occur in over 50% of patients, but it is well tolerated and tends to be in the plantar region, which does not produce the embarrassment of palmar sweating.

Kux reported on 59 patients with 54 being satisfied with their results. There were no instances of Horner's syndrome, and two patients developed gustatory sweating.[87] Byrne and colleagues[88] reported on 85 patients with an 85% success rate and an average hospital stay of 3.1 days. Our own experience with VATS sympathectomy parallels these results. We no longer recommend resection of the stellate ganglia but instead recommend resection just below to avoid the risk of Horner's syndrome. The $T_2$ and $T_3$ ganglia are excised for palmar hyperhidrosis and $T_4$ and $T_5$ included if the axilla is involved. Claes et al[89] reported upon 512 patients operated upon for hyperhidrosis with almost 98% having dry palms. They have also abandoned resection of the lower stellate ganglion after Horner's syndrome developed, and it has not affected their success.

**Reflex Sympathetic Dystrophy (RSD).** Posttraumatic pain syndromes (RSD, causalgia, shoulder-hand syndrome, Sudeck's atrophy) have been recognized since prior to World War I. The natural history of RSD is for acute burning pain and muscle spasms in limbs that often have edematous changes that progress to a more chronic disorder with muscular atrophy and even contractures.[90] Although spontaneous resolution may occur in the early phases, most treatments have the best response early and certainly prior to the chronic phase, when it may be irreversible. As many as 50–70% will respond to conservative treatment, which includes physical therapy, medication (i.e., phenoxybenzamine hydrochloride, prazosin, guanethidine) and stellate ganglion blocks.[90] Sympathectomy has demonstrated good results in over 90% of patients, and again results seem better the shorter the time from onset of RSD to sympathectomy.[91–93] Prior to consideration of surgery, patients should demonstrate response to stellate ganglion block.

Sympathectomy is performed to include the $T_4$ ganglion. There is some controversy as to whether the stellate ganglion should be removed. Removal of the stellate ganglion always produces a Horner's syndrome, but failure to excise the stellate ganglion may lead to an infrequent failure of pain relief. We presently excise the sympathetic chain just below the stellate ganglia.

**Vascular Disorders.** Vasospastic vascular disorders have been treated with sympathectomy. Ischemic disorders are better treated with revascularization. Raynaud's phenomenon without collagen vascular disease and drug-resistant Buerger's disease represent rare vascular indications for sympathectomy. Overall, results of sympathectomy have not been as good as for hyperhidrosis and pain syndromes.[94]

### *Technique*

**VATS Sympathectomy.** We have preferred general anesthesia and single-lung ventilation. For unilateral sympathectomies, patients are positioned as for a thoracotomy and tilted slightly forward. Bilateral procedures can be performed in the supine position with the arms extended at 90 degrees.

The procedure is performed with three access sites or ports. Occasionally, a fourth port is required to retract the lung. The camera is inserted in the midaxillary line in the 5th ICS and the other two ports placed in the third ICS in the anterior and posterior axillary line. The sympathetic chain is identified beneath the parietal pleura at the junction of the head of the ribs with the transverse process. The stellate ganglia can usually be recognized overlying the head of the first rib, and it has a snowman or figure eight shape. Resection of the sympathetic chain proceeds from the lowest ganglia up to just below the stellate ganglia. Overlying veins are not infrequent, and they are clipped to prevent bothersome bleeding. Clips generally are not used on the nerves to avoid potential postoperative neuralgias. This dissection generally proceeds quickly, and after its completion the lung is reexpanded. No chest tube is required unless the lung was injured.[83]

We now consider VATS sympathectomy an outpatient procedure. Patients remain in the recovery area for a couple of hours after surgery and receive a chest x-ray to ensure full lung expansion. In our last 14 procedures, all were discharged the same day without complication.

**Thoracic Splanchnicectomy.** The celiac plexus is innervated by the greater splenic nerve ($T_5$–$T_{10}$), lesser splanchnic nerves ($T_{10}$–$T_{11}$) and the least splanchnic nerve ($T_{12}$). A number of reports have suggested that the sympathetic fibers are the primary afferent pathway for pain from the upper abdominal region, and splanchnicectomy has been performed on patients with pancreatic pain from cancer and chronic pancreatitis. Good results have been reported in approximately 70% of cases, although most procedures were done via a thoracotomy.[95] In most situations a left splanchnicectomy is performed and is successful in two thirds of cases. Recurrence of pain tends to be in the right epigastrium and responds to removal of the right sided splanchnic innervation.

In the past the requirement of a thoracotomy was a significant deterrent to splanchnicectomy. Thoracoscopy may rejuvenate enthusiasm for this procedure since it is tolerated so well. The splanchnic nerves can be seen well (especially the greater splanchnic nerve) with the magnified thoracoscopic view. Generally, the procedure is analogous to cervicodorsal sympathectomy except that ports are placed lower in the chest (around the seventh and eighth ICSs) to transect the thoracic ganglia below $T_5$.[96]

Some have advocated the addition of a vagotomy to splanchnicotomy, but this makes development of gastric stasis a potential problem. As with sympathectomy, the procedure may be done as an outpatient surgery, and postoperative complications should be infrequent. Overall, VATS is an excellent technique for sympathectomy or splanchnicotomy.

**Vagotomy.** Thoracoscopic vagotomy would seem to have its greatest potential role in the setting of recurrent ulceration and an incomplete prior vagotomy. The ability to avoid a thoracotomy or recurrent upper abdominal surgery seems to be a great advantage.

There have been multiple case reports of successful VATS vagotomies. Laws and McKernan[97] reported on six patients with recurrent ulceration after prior gastric drainage procedures with incomplete vagotomies. All thoracoscopic vagotomies were successful, and the hospital stay was 3 days or less. Champault and colleagues[98] reported on 21 patients with duodenal ulcers treated primarily by thoracoscopic truncal vagotomy. There was apparently no instances of gastric stasis problems or postvagotomy diarrhea.

Technically, a VATS vagotomy is usually performed from the left chest using general anesthesia and a double-lumen endotracheal tube. Three or four ports are used to approach the distal esophagus. The inferior pulmonary ligament is divided. The video monitors may be placed at the foot of the bed as for esophageal myotomy, which may aid in orientation. Mobilization of the esophagus is required to clearly dissect and transect all vagal fibers. Postoperative chest tubes are not necessary unless lung injury has occurred. The hospital stay will be dependent upon the patient's overall condition more than the operative procedure.[99,100]

## Posterior Mediastinal Neurogenic Lesions

Posterior mediastinal masses account for 25–30% of all mediastinal lesions.[101] In children many posterior masses are malignant, while only 1–4% are in adults. Neurogenic tumors are grouped into three categories: (1) nerve sheath tumors (neurolemma, neurofibroma, neurogenic sarcoma), (2) tumors of the autonomic nervous system (ganglioneuroma, ganglioneuro-blastoma, neuroblastoma), and (3) tumors of the paraganglion system (chemodectoma, pheochromocytoma). Nerve sheath tumors predominate in adults.

Excision is usually recommended for posterior neurogenic tumors, but asymptomatic patients without hypertension or intraspinal extension have been followed. These tu-

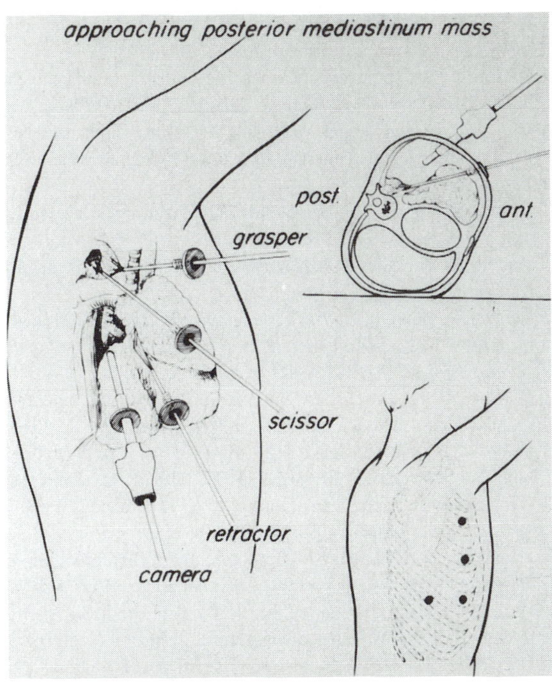


**Figure 12B–30.** Depiction of trocar positions for resection of posterior mediastinal mass. *(From Landreneau RJ, Mack MJ, Hazelrigg JR, et al. Video-assisted thoracic surgery: Basic technical concepts and intercostal approach strategies. Ann Thorac Surg 54:800–807, 1992, with permission.)*

mors tend to be acellular, and, hence, needle biopsies rarely are helpful.

Prior to excision one must rule out intraspinal extension. A CT scan usually allows this determination, but if doubt still exists, magnetic resonance imaging (MRI) has often provided better definition. Thoracoscopy has been used for resection of these lesions on multiple occasions with excellent results.[76–78,82,100] VATS is largely reserved for lesions without intraspinal extensions. Thoracoscopic resection proceeds just as a resection would via a thoracotomy. At least three access sites will be required, and they are generally placed caudad to the tumor (Fig. 12B–30). Technically, control of the neurovascular bundle is the main potential pitfall. Vascular structures are generally controlled with clips and have rarely presented a problem (Fig. 12B–31). If the surgeon is unable to achieve complete excision, then a thoracotomy should be performed. An endoscopic bag should be used for removal of lesions of unknown histology to avoid possible seeding of the trocar site. Chest tube drainage is usually instituted overnight, and overall hospital stay is short. Our mean hospital stay is 1.8 days for resected posterior neurogenic tumors done by VATS, which is certainly shorter than generally achieved after a thoracotomy.

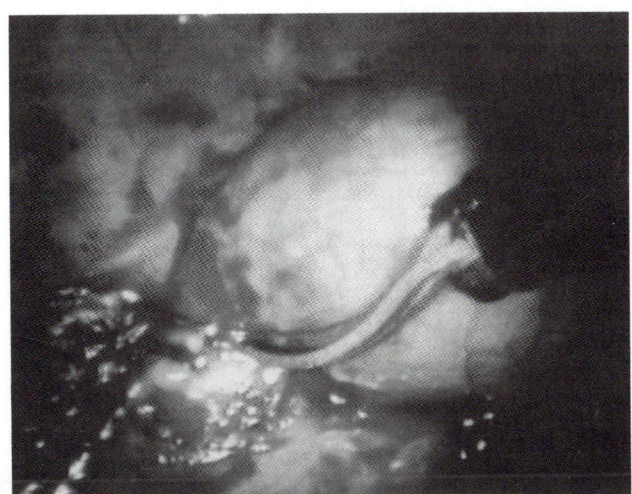

**Figure 12B–31.** Resection of posterior neurogenic tumor with control of intercostal bundle with hemo clips.

## Conclusions

Video-assisted thoracic surgery allows excellent visualization of almost all intrathoracic structures. Many therapeutic procedures can be achieved safely and expeditiously using this technology. Several principles must be adhered to in order for patients to be benefited. No oncologic resection should be compromised in order to complete the procedure thoracoscopically. In general, the only difference in procedures should be in the approach, and the technical details of the remainder of the surgery should mimic those at thoracotomy.

Video-assisted thoracic surgery has thus far been done with remarkably few complications. Training and rapid dispersion of information has been facilitated by the thoracic surgical societies. We must continue to evaluate critically this emerging technology to bring further into focus its precise role in the field of thoracic surgery. Video-assisted thoracic surgery has infused enthusiasm and allowed innovation. Certainly new developments will continue; better instruments, three-dimensional capability, and robotics all seem possible in the near future. We eagerly look for new innovation while maintaining our focus on the goal of improved patient care.

## REFERENCES

1. Jacobaeus HC: The cauterization of adhesions in pneumothorax treatment of tuberculosis. *Surg Gynecol Obstet* **32:**493, 1921
2. Decamp PT, Moseley PW, Scott ML: Diagnostic thoracoscopy. *Ann Thorac Surg* **16:**79, 1973
3. Mack MJ, Aronoff RJ, Acuff TE, et al: Present role of thoracoscopy in the diagnosis and treatment of diseases of the chest. *Ann Thorac Surg* **54:**403–409, 1992
4. Cooper JD: Perspectives on thoracoscopy in general thoracic surgery. *Ann Thorac Surg* **56:**697–700, 1993
5. Daniel TM: Diagnostic thoracoscopy for pleural disease. *Ann Thorac Surg* **56:**639–640, 1993
6. Sharma S, D'Cruz A: Thoracoscopy in the diagnosis of pleural effusion of ambiguous etiology. *J Surg Oncol* **48:**133–135, 1991

7. Daniel TM, Kern JA, Tribble CG, et al: Thoracoscopic surgery for diseases of the lung and pleura. *Ann Surg* **217:**566–575, 1993
8. Boutin C, Astoul PH, Seitz B: The role of thoracoscopy in evaluation and management of pleural effusions. *Lung* (supplement): 1113–1121, 1990
9. Hartman DL, Gaither JM, Kesler KA, et al: Comparison of insufflated talc under thoracoscopic guidance with standard tetracycline and bleomycin pleurodesis for control of malignant pleural effusions. *J Thorac Cardiovasc Surg* **105:**743–747, 1993
10. Daniel TM, Tribble CG, Rodgers BM: Thoracoscopy and talc poudrage for pneumothoraces and effusions. *Ann Thorac Surg* **50:** 186–189, 1990
11. Sanchez-Armengol A, Rodriguez-Panadero F: Survival and talc pleurodesis in metastatic pleural carcinoma, revisited. *Chest* **104:** 1482–1485, 1993
12. Aelony Y, King R, Boutin C: Thoracoscopic talc poudrage pleurodesis for chronic recurrent pleural effusions. *Ann In Med* **115:** 778–782, 1991
13. LoCicero J: Thoracoscopic management of malignant pleural effusion. *Ann Thorac Surg* **56:**641–643, 1993
14. Hucker I, Bhatnagar NK, Al-Jilaihawi AN, Forrester-Wood CP: Thoracoscopy in the diagnosis and management of recurrent pleural effusions. *Ann Thorac Surg* **52:**1145–1147, 1991
15. Ferguson M: Thoracoscopy for empyema, bronchopleural fistula, and chylothorax. *Ann Thorac Surg* **56:**644–645, 1993
16. Ridley PD, Braimbridge MV: Thoracoscopic debridement and pleural irrigation in the management of empyema thoracis. *Ann Thorac Surg* **51:**461–464, 1991
17. Robinson LA, Moulton AL, Fleming WH, et al: Intrapleural fibrinolytic treatment of multiloculated thoracic empyemas. *Ann Thorac Surg* **57:**803–814, 1994
18. Smith RS, Fry WR, Tsoi EK, et al: Preliminary report on videothoracoscopy in the evaluation and treatment of thoracic injury. *Am J Surg* **166:**690–693, 1993
19. Mancini M, Smith LM, Nein A, Buechter KJ: Early evacuation of clotted blood in hemothorax using thoracoscopy: case reports. *J Trauma* **34:**144–147, 1994
20. Graeber GM, Jones DR: The role of thoracoscopy in thoracic trauma. *Ann Thorac Surg* **56:**646–648, 1993
21. Marts BC, Naunheim KS, Fiore AC, Pennington DG: Conservative versus surgical management of chylothorax. *Am J Surg* **164:** 532–535, 1992
22. Ferguson MK, Little AG, Skinner DB: Current concepts in the management of postoperative chylothorax. *Ann Thorac Surg* **40:** 542–545, 1985
23. Inderbitzi RG, Krebs T, Stirnemann P, Althaus U: Treatment of postoperative chylothorax by fibrin glue application under thoracoscopic view with use of local anesthesia. *J Thorac Cardiovasc Surg* **104:**209–210, 1992
24. Hazelrigg SR, Nunchuck SK, LoCicero J, and the Video Assisted Thoracic Surgery Study Group: Video assisted thoracic surgery study group data. *Ann Thorac Surg* **56:**1039–1044, 1993
25. Deslauriers J, Mehran RJ: Role of thoracoscopy in the diagnosis and management of pleural diseases. *Semin Thorac Cardiovasc Surg* **5:**284–293, 1993
26. Gerein AN, Brumwell ML, Lawson LM, et al: Surgical management of pneumothorax in patients with acquired immunodeficiency syndrome. *Arch Surg* **126:**1272–1277, 1991
27. Fleisher AG, McElvaney G, Lawson L, et al: Surgical management of spontaneous pneumothorax in patients with acquired immunodeficiency syndrome. *Ann Thorac Surg* **45:**21–23, 1988
28. Granke K, Fischer CR, Gago O, et al: The efficacy and timing of operative intervention for spontaneous pneumothorax. *Ann Thorac Surg* **43:**540–542, 1986
29. Getz SB Jr, Beasley WE III: Spontaneous pneumothorax. *Am J Surg* **145:**823–827, 1983
30. Saha SP, Arrants JE, Kosa A, et al: Management of spontaneous pneumothorax. *Ann Thorac Surg* **19:**561–564, 1975
31. Gobbel SG Jr, Rhea WG Jr, Nelson IA, et al: Spontaneous pneumothorax. *J Thorac Cardiovasc Surg* **46:**331–345, 1963
32. Hazelrigg SR: Thoracoscopic management of pulmonary blebs and bullae. *Semin Thorac Cardiovasc Surg* **5:**327–331, 1993
33. Wakabayashi A, Brenner M, Wilson AF, et al: Thoracoscopic treatment of spontaneous pneumothorax using carbon dioxide laser. *Ann Thorac Surg* **50:**786–790, 1990
34. Keenan RJ, Ferson PF, Landreneau RJ, Hazelrigg SR: Use of lasers in thoracoscopy. *Semin Thorac Cardiovasc Surg* **5:**294–297, 1993
35. Takeno Y: Thoracoscopic treatment of spontaneous pneumothorax. *Ann Thorac Surg* **56:**688–690, 1993
36. Torre M, Belloni P: Nd:YAG laser pleurodesis through thoracoscopy: New curative therapy in spontaneous pneumothorax. *Ann Thorac Surg* **47:**887–889, 1989
37. Nathanson LK, Shimi SM, Wood RA, Cuschieri A: Videothoracoscopic ligation of bulla and pleurectomy for spontaneous pneumothorax. *Ann Thorac Surg* **52:**316–319, 1991
38. Inderbitzi RG, Furrer M, Striffeler H, Althaus U: Thoracoscopic pleurectomy for treatment of complicated spontaneous pneumothorax. *J Thorac Cardiovasc Surg* **105:**84–88, 1993
39. Yamaguchi A, Shinonaga M, Tatebe S, et al: Thoracoscopic stapled bullectomy supported by suturing. *Ann Thorac Surg* **56:**691–693, 1993
40. Hazelrigg SR, Landreneau RJ, Mack M, et al: Thoracoscopic stapled resection for spontaneous pneumothorax. *J Thorac Cardiovasc Surg* **105:**389–393, 1993
41. Wakabayashi A: Expanded applications of diagnostic and therapeutic thoracoscopy. *J Thorac Cardiovasc Surg* **102:**721–723, 1991
42. Wakabayashi A: Thoracoscopic ablation of blebs in the treatment of recurrent or persistent spontaneous pneumothorax. *Ann Thorac Surg* **48:**651–653, 1989
43. Wakabayashi A, Brenner M, Kayaleh RA, et al: Thoracoscopic carbon dioxide laser treatment of bullous emphysema. *Lancet* **337:** 881–883, 1991
44. Deslauriers J, Beaulier M, Despres JP, et al: Transaxillary pleurectomy for treatment of spontaneous pneumothorax. *Ann Thorac Surg* **30:**569–574, 1980
45. Youmans CR Jr, Williams RD, McMinn MR, Derrick JR: Surgical management of spontaneous pneumothorax by bleb ligation and pleural dry sponge abrasion. *Am J Surg* **120:**644–648, 1970
46. Weeden D, Smith GH: Surgical experience in the management of spontaneous pneumothorax 1972–82. *Thorax* **38:**737–743, 1983
47. Singh SV: The surgical treatment of spontaneous pneumothorax by parietal pleurectomy. *Scand J Thorac Cardiovasc Surg* **16:**75–80, 1982
48. Tanaka F, Itoh M, Esaki H, et al: Secondary spontaneous pneumothorax. *Ann Thorac Surg* **55:**372–376, 1993
49. Cannon WB, Vierra MA, Cannon A: Thoracoscopy for spontaneous pneumothorax. *Ann Thorac Surg* **56:**686–687, 1993
50. Naunheim K, Hazelrigg SR, Landreneau RJ, et al: Safety and efficacy of video-assisted thoracic surgical techniques for the treatment of spontaneous pneumothorax. *J Thorac Cardiovasc Surg*. In press.
51. Gaensler EA, Cugell DW, Knudson RJ, Fitzgerald MX: Surgical management of emphysema. *Clin Chest Med* **4:**443–463, 1983
52. Brantigan OC, Mueller E: Surgical treatment of pulmonary emphysema. *Am Surg* **23:**789–804, 1957
53. Wakabayashi A: Video-assisted laser resection is the best treatment for bullous emphysema. Presented at the 79th Annual Clinical Congress, American College of Surgeons; October 10–15, 1993; San Francisco
54. Lewis RJ, Caccavale RJ, Sisler GE: VATS-argon beam coagulator treatment of diffuse end-stage bilateral bullous disease of the lung. *Ann Thorac Surg* **55:**1394–1399, 1993
55. Cooper JD, Trulock EP, Triantafillou AN, et al: Bilateral pneumectomy for chronic obstructive pulmonary disease. *J Thorac Cardiovasc Surg* **109:**106–119, 1995
56. Mack MJ, Hazelrigg SR, Landreneau RJ, Acuff TE: Thoracoscopy for the diagnosis of the indeterminate solitary pulmonary nodule. *Ann Thorac Surg* **56:**825–832, 1993

57. Shennib H, Landreneau RJ, Mack MJ: Video assisted thoracoscopic wedge resection of T1 lung cancer in high risk patients. *Ann Surg* **218:**555–560, 1993
58. Dowling RD, Keenan RJ, Ferson PF, Landreneau RJ: Video-assisted thoracoscopic resection of pulmonary metastases. *Ann Thorac Surg* **56:**772–775, 1993
59. Kirby TJ, Rice TW: Thoracoscopic lobectomy. *Ann Thorac Surg* **56:**784–786, 1993
60. McKenna RJ Jr: Lobectomy by video-assisted thoracic surgery with mediastinal node sampling for lung cancer. *J Thorac Cardiovasc Surg* **107:**879–882, 1994
61. Roviaro G, Varoli F, Rebuffat C, et al: Major pulmonary resections: Pneumonectomies and lobectomies. *Ann Thorac Surg* **56:**779–783, 1993
62. Kirby TJ, Mack MJ, Landreneau RJ, Rice TR: Lobectomy: VATS vs. thoracotomy. A randomized study. *J Thorac Cardiov Surg* 1995. In press.
63. Westcott JL: Percutaneous transthoracic needle biopsy. *Radiology* **160:**319–327, 1986
64. Khouri NF, Stitik FP, Erozan YS, et al: Transthoracic needle aspiration biopsy of benign and malignant lung lesions. *Am J Roentgenol* **144:**281–288, 1985
65. Berquist TH, Bailey PB, Cortese DA, Miller WE: Transthoracic needle biopsy accuracy and complications in relation to location and type of lesion. *Mayo Clin Proc* **55:**475–481, 1980
66. Khouri FN, Meziane MA, Zerhouni EA, et al: The solitary pulmonary nodule: Assessment, diagnosis and management. *Chest* **91:**128–133, 1987
67. Calhoun P, Feldman PS, Armstrong P, et al: The clinical outcome of needle aspirations of the lung when cancer is not diagnosed. *Ann Thorac Surg* **41:**592–596, 1985
68. Thomas P, Rubinstein L, and the Lung Cancer Study Group. Cancer recurrence after resection: T1N0 non-small cell lung cancer. *Ann Thorac Surg* **59:**242–247, 1990
69. Mack MJ, Shennib H, Landreneau RJ, Hazelrigg SR: Techniques for localization of pulmonary nodules for thoracoscopic resection. *J Thorac Cardiovasc Surg* **106:**550–553, 1993
70. Mack M, Gordon MJ, Postma TW, et al: Percutaneous localization of pulmonary nodules for thoracoscopic lung resection. *Ann Thorac Surg* **53:**1123–1124, 1992
71. Plunkett MB, Peterson MS, Landreneau RJ, et al: CT guided preoperative percutaneous needle localization of peripheral pulmonary nodules. *Radiology* **185:**274–276, 1992
72. Hazelrigg SR, Mack M, Landreneau RJ, et al: Thoracoscopic pericardiectomy for effusive pericardial disease. *Ann Thorac Surg* **56:** 792–795, 1993
73. Piehler JM, Pluth JR, Sehaff HV, et al: Surgical management of effusive pericardial disease. *J Thorac Cardiovasc Surg* **90:**506–516, 1985
74. Naunheim KS, Kesler KA, Fiore AC, et al: Pericardial drainage subxiphoid vs. transthoracic approach. *Eur J Cardio Thorac Surg* **5:**99–104, 1991
75. Hazelrigg SR, Mack M, Landreneau RJ, et al: Thoracoscopic pericardiectomy for effusive pericardial disease. *Ann Thorac Surg* **56:** 792–795, 1993
76. Mack MJ: Thoracoscopy and its role in mediastinal disease and sympathectomy. *Semin Thorac Cardiovasc Surg* **5:**332–336, 1993
77. Hazelrigg SR, Mack MJ, Landreneau RJ: Video-assisted thoracic surgery for mediastinal disease. In: Lewis RJ (ed): *Chest Surgery Clinics of North America.* Philadelphia: Saunders: 1993, pp 283–297
78. Acuff TE, Mack MJ, Hazelrigg SR, et al: Extension of thoracoscopy to management of mediastinal disease. *Chest* **102**(suppl):665, 1992
79. Kern JA, Daniel TM, Tribble CG, Silen ML, Rodgers BM: Thoracoscopic diagnosis and treatment of mediastinal masses. *Ann Thorac Surg* **56:**92–96, 1993
80. Landreneau RJ, Hazelrigg SR, Mack MJ, et al: Thoracoscopic mediastinal lymph node sampling: A useful approach to mediastinal lymph node stations inaccessible to cervical mediastinoscopy. *J Thorac Cardiovasc Surg* **105:**554–558, 1993
81. Sugarbaker DJ: Thoracoscopy in the management of anterior mediastinal masses. *Ann Thorac Surg* **56:**653–656, 1993
82. Hazelrigg SR, Landreneau RJ, Mack M, Acuff TE: Thoracoscopic resection of mediastinal cysts. *Ann Thorac Surg* **56:**659–660, 1993
83. Landreneau RJ, Mack MJ, Hazelrigg SR, et al: Video-assisted thoracic surgery: Basic technical concepts and intercostal approach strategies. *Ann Thorac Surg* **54:**800–807, 1992
84. Hazelrigg SR, Mack MJ: Thoracoscopic surgery. In Kaiser L, Daniel T, eds: *Surgery for Autonomic Disorders.* Little Brown and Co: Boston, 1993, Chap 15; pp 189–202
85. Goetz RH: Sympathectomy for the upper extremities. In: Dale WA (ed): *Management of Arterial Occlusive Disease.* Chicago, Year Book, 1971
86. Haxton HA: The technique and results of upper limb sympathectomy. *J Cardiovasc Surg* 11:27, 1970
87. Kux M: Thoracic endoscopic sympathectomy in palmar and axillary hyperhidrosis. *Arch Surg* **113:**264, 1978
88. Byrne J, Walsh TN, Hederman WP: Endoscopic transthoracic electrocautery of the sympathetic chain for palmar and axillary hyperhidrosis. *Br J Surg* **77:**1046, 1990
89. Claes G, Drott C, Gothberg G: Thoracoscopy for autonomic disorders. *Ann Thorac Surg* **56:**715–716, 1993
90. Drucker WR, et al: Pathogenesis of posttraumatic sympathetic dystrophy. *Am J Surg* **97:**454, 1959
91. Olcott C IV, Etherington LG, Wilcosky BR, et al: Reflex sympathetic dystrophy—The surgeon's role in management. *J Vasc Surg* **14:**488, 1991
92. Mockus MB, et al: Sympathectomy for causalgia. *Arch Surg* **122:** 668, 1987
93. Patman RD, Thompson JE, Persson AV: Management of posttraumatic pain syndromes: Report of 113 cases. *Ann Surg* **177:**780, 1973
94. Roos DB: Sympathectomy for the upper extremities. In: Rutherford R (ed), *Vascular Surgery,* 2nd ed. Philadelphia: Saunders, 1984, pp 725–730
95. Stone HH, Chauvin EJ: Pancreatic denervation for pain relief in chronic alcohol associated pancreatitis. *Br J Surg* **77:**303–305, 1990
96. Worsey J, Ferson PF, Keenan RJ, et al: Thoracoscopic pancreatic denervation for pain control in irresectable pancreatic cancer. *Br J Surg* **80:**1051–1052, 1993
97. Laws HL, McKernan JB: Endoscopic management of peptic ulcer disease. *Ann Surg* **217:**548–556, 1993
98. Champault G, Belhassen A, Rizk N, Boutrlier P: Duodenal ulcer: value of truncal vagotomy through thoracoscopy. *Annales de Chirurgie* **47:**240–243, 1993
99. Chisholm M, Chung SC, Sunderland T, et al: Thoracoscopic vagotomy: A new role for the laparoscope. *Br J Surg* **79:**254, 1992
100. Axford TC, Clair DG, Bertagnolli MM, et al: Staged antrectomy and thoracoscopic truncal vagotomy for perforated peptic ulcer disease. *Ann Thorac Surg* **55:**1571–1573, 1993
101. Naunheim KS: Video thoracoscopy for masses of the posterior mediastinum. *Ann Thorac Surg* **56:**657–658, 1993

CHAPTER

# 13

# Developmental Abnormalities of the Airways and Lungs

## *Thoracic Surgery in Childhood*

Robert J. Touloukian

Developmental abnormalities of the airways and lungs include a wide spectrum of conditions including upper airway obstruction from atresia and stenosis to lesions that affect principally the tertiary bronchi and pulmonary parenchyma. In general, air trapping, resulting in compression of normal adjacent lung with mediastinal shift or secondary infection, are the initial findings. Routine prenatal ultrasound screening has made the diagnosis of congenital cystic lesions possible as early as the 18th to 20th week of gestation, and preparation for eventual surgery actually begins at that time. The future includes the possibility of fetal thoracic surgery with resection of the affected lesion if the prospect of fetal death or severe pulmonary hypoplasia is raised.

The earliest finding of a lung cyst was in a 3-month-old, as reported by Fontanus[1] in 1639. In 1777 Huber[2] described a patient with an apparently normal right lower lobe supplied by a thoracic artery branch—presumably the first known case of an extralobar sequestration.

The first successful operative resection was noted in 1933 by Rienhoff et al[3] for a unilocular right upper lobe lung cyst in a 3-year-old boy. Ten years later Fisher et al[4] reported performing a right upper and middle lobectomy for congenital cystic disease in a 1-month-old infant. In 1946 Gross[5] performed a pneumonectomy in a 3-week-old infant with congenital cystic lung; this marks the advent of the modern era of thoracic surgery in infants and children.

### SURGICAL PRINCIPLES

Surgeons who perform major thoracic operations on a neonate or infant must understand the management of complex respiratory problems unique to this age group. A regional referral center with a neonatal and pediatric intensive care unit provides momentary care, appropriate monitoring, ventilatory support, parenteral nutrition, and support staff trained to recognize and treat acute changes in the patient's condition.

Knowledge of the differences in technique between infant and adult thoracotomy are also essential in achieving a good result. Some general principles are important to emphasize. The incision chosen is modified to achieve appropriate exposure. Mediastinal cysts and tumors can be removed through an anterior thoracotomy, and median sternotomy generally can be avoided. Lobectomy is simplified because of the elasticity of the pulmonary vessels, which are more visible and usually devoid of fat, but an intimate knowledge of developmental anatomy is required to select the appropriate procedure. Tension disturbances from pneumothorax or air block syndromes are common problems in small infants that require emergency management. Most infants with major ventilatory problems on a congenital basis such as lobar emphysema or adenomatoid malformation will rapidly improve following pulmonic resection in the absence of other significant abnormalities. A posterolateral incision is selected to repair esophageal atresia. The extrapleural approach to the esophagus remains popular among pediatric surgeons since the risk of empyema with anastomotic leak is largely avoided. Rib resection in infants is unnecessary, and the chest is easily closed with absorbable pericostal sutures. Since the chest wall is very thin, pleural drainage tubes should be tunneled one interspace to minimize risk of peri-tubal leakage of air and fluid. Major postoperative problems may be unavoidable because of associated life-threatening congenital anomalies and pulmonary immaturity or hypoplasia, but proper pulmonary toilet and monitoring are as important in neonates as in older infants and children to prevent secondary pneumonia. For example, right upper lobe atelectasis is a common complication following thoracotomy for repair of esophageal atresia because of the dependent location of the lobar bronchus and the tendency for mucous secretions to plug the upper airway. To prevent this problem, endotracheal suctioning is routinely performed following chest physiotherapy with the patient prone. Perioperative antibiotic prophylaxis is also appropriate in these small and fragile patients.

Arterial blood gas values are monitored through an umbilical arterial line in the newborn or by radial artery or capillary gas determination in older infants. Transcutaneous oxygen monitoring, a value based on capillary perfusion, is a noninvasive method for trend analysis of the $PO_2$ in critically ill infants. While widely available, caution should be exercised in its use, particularly in the immediate postoperative period, until vasoconstriction or hypovolemia has been corrected. Similarly, the Doppler blood pressure is a useful noninvasive test of systolic blood pressure but is not reliable for diastolic determination. Intra-arterial monitoring is preferred in the unstable patient having rapid fluctuations of blood pressure. Intermittent mandatory ventilation with a "timed" cycle and inspiratory pressure control is used to wean the infant to continuous positive airway pressure prior to extubation. Pulmonary hypoplasia as seen in newborns with a congenital diaphragmatic hernia requires unique ventilatory support with a high-frequency cycle to minimize barotrauma. Extracorporeal membrane oxygenation (ECMO) provides a 5–10-day period of lung rest in these critically ill infants. The success of ECMO is attributed, in large part, to the reversal of pulmonary hypertension and the inherent ability of the neonatal lung for repair and regeneration of alveoli damaged by barotrauma.

## EMBRYOLOGY

The first evidence of the developing respiratory tract appears during the third week of embryonic life as a longitudinal groove on the ventral aspect of the primitive foregut. Separation of the laryngotracheal bud from the esophagus is accomplished by lateral ingrowth of mesenchymal cells beginning at the caudal end of the groove and progressing cephalad to the future laryngeal aperture. The lung bud is, at first, a simple saccule that lengthens caudad and at the fourth week, or 5-mm stage, divides into two branches that are destined to become right and left primary bronchi. The right is the larger; it grows caudad and somewhat dorsally, while the left is more nearly horizontal. The subsequent development of the bronchial tree is asymmetrical. The right bronchus produces a ventral bud and then a more proximal lateral one, which is the eparterial or upper-lobe bronchus (Fig. 13–1). On the left side, this branch appears to be suppressed or perhaps absorbed into the hyparterial bronchus. An acceleration of growth in the fifth and sixth weeks of embryonal life results in the appearance of segmental and subsegmental branches, possibly by a combination of terminal budding and monopodial branching.[6] By the end of the 16th week, about 70% of the subsegmental bronchi that can be recognized in the full-term infant's lung have been formed. Between the 20th and 24th weeks, primitive alveoli appear as canaliculi in the terminal epithelial buds. At about the same time, connective tissue grows between the bronchial branches to form the interlobular septa.[7] Concomitantly, with the formation of the alveoli, there is an active proliferation of capillaries that insinuate themselves among the air passages. As the latter structures enlarge, the original cuboidal lining cells become increasingly attenuated and finally so thin that they are scarcely discernible by light microscopy.

Postnatal growth of new pulmonary tissue increases the volume of neonatal lung by at least 12-fold before puberty.[8] This increase is accomplished by proliferation and enlargement of alveoli and also by elongation and enlargement of the terminal and respiratory bronchioles.

The primitive respiratory tract epithelium is, of course, entodermal in origin, but it is uncertain that this applies to the cells lining the most distal air sacs. Histochemical studies[9] suggest that the alveolar epithelium is derived from coelomic mesenchyme. Changes that occur in these cells during infectious and neoplastic processes of later life tend

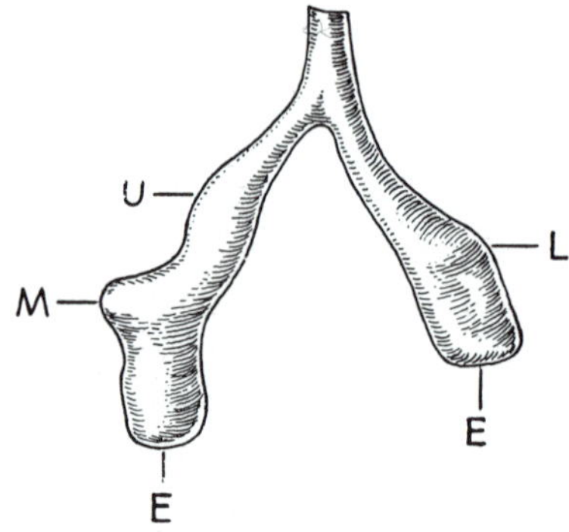


**Figure 13–1.** The human embryonic lungs at the 7-mm stage. Asymmetry is already apparent though the lobar bronchi are mere buds. On the right side are visible upper (U), middle (M), and end or lower (E); on the left side are upper or lateral (L) and lower or end (E) buds.

to support this view. About the 13th week of embryonic development, cilia begin to appear in the pseudostratified columnar epithelium that characterizes the bronchial tree, first in the proximal bronchi and then distally. At about the same time, mucous secretory goblet cells appear. Bronchial cartilages start to develop from precartilage islands around the 10th week, and in the 25th week the condition of cartilaginous plates and rings is approximately that observed at birth. Bronchial mucous glands, which develop as submucosal epithelial buds starting about the 14th week, appear to become functional in the next 6 months.[10] This information helps to understand the following anomalies.

## TRACHEAL AND BRONCHIAL ANOMALIES

### Tracheal Atresia and Stenosis

Tracheal atresia is a uniformly fatal condition that results from a failure of the laryngotracheal bud to develop completely during the critical third to sixth weeks of embryonic life. Associations of tracheal atresia with a fistula of the distal tracheal to the esophagus has also been reported. In a case described by Walcher,[11] the two primary bronchi rose independently from the esophagus. Congenital tracheal stenosis is often associated with other bronchial anomalies including agenesis of the lung. The three types of tracheal stenosis are (1) generalized hypoplasia, (2) funnel-like narrowing, usually tapering to a tight stenosis just above the carina, and (3) segmental stenosis of various lengths that can occur at any level. Harrison et al[12] recently reported a baby undergoing successful resection of a segmental 1.5-cm stenotic lesion just above the carina with end-to-end reconstruction and subsequent normal growth and development when studied 1½ years later. This case illustrates that traditional management by sequential dilatation, local injection of steroids, endotracheal stenting, or electroresection or cryotherapy may not be necessary in carefully selected cases.

### Laryngo-Tracheo-Esophageal Cleft

A failure of the separation of the laryngotracheal bud from the esophagus leads to the rare congenital defect known as a laryngo-tracheo-esophageal cleft (Fig. 13–2). Of the 85 cases reported in the literature, 46 have survived.[13,14] The mortality rate of this condition is high, principally because of continued aspiration from late detection of the anomaly. A cleft should be suspected in an infant with a toneless cry and choking on feeding. On occasion, the anomaly is associated with esophageal atresia and a distal esophageal fistula. Inadvertent passage of a nasogastric tube through the cleft is not uncommon, and its anterior position on lateral chest x-ray should suggest the defect. Confirmation of a laryngeal aperture on barium studies and fiberoptic endoscopy is possible, but diagnostic errors are common because of the massive spillover of contrast and visual difficulty in recognizing the edges of the cleft, which tend to be approximated on expiration. Surgical repair of a partial cleft includes preliminary gastrostomy followed by exposure of the cleft through a cervical incision. Sparing a portion of the esophagus adjacent to the cleft is usually necessary to gain a tension-free closure of the larynx.[15] Interposing autologous tissue, such as a strap muscle between the larynx and esophagus, has been recommended to avoid a recurrent fistula.[16] An indwelling Silastic nasotracheal tube provides a stent for several days until postoperative edema subsides. Tracheostomy can usually be avoided. Repair of a complete laryngotracheoesophageal cleft from larynx to carina was described by Donahoe and Gee.[17] The extent of the anomalie requires exposure of the cleft through both cervical and thoracic approaches, a bifurcated endobronchial tube, and creation of an esophageal flap for closure of the posterior trachea (Fig. 13–3).

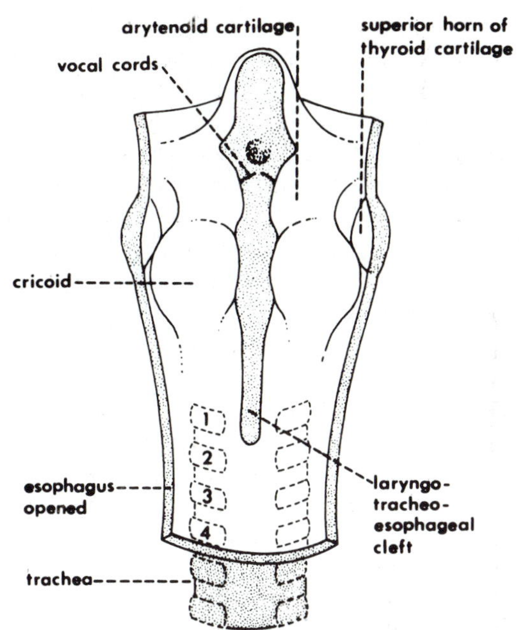


**Figure 13–2.** Anatomy of a laryngotracheoesophageal cleft as seen through the opened esophagus. *(From Burroughs W, Leape LL: Laryngotracheoesophageal cleft: Report of a case successfully treated and review of the literature. Pediatrics 53:516, 1974, with permission.)*

### Tracheomalacia

A failure in formation of the tracheal cartilaginous supporting structure can cause tracheal compression and signs of airway obstruction including severe dyspnea, stridor, and eventually recurrent respiratory infections shortly after birth. The most dramatic and often fatal symptom complex is acute apnea, usually referred to as "dying spells." This condition, known as tracheomalacia, is most often secondary to extrinsic compression of the airway from such le-

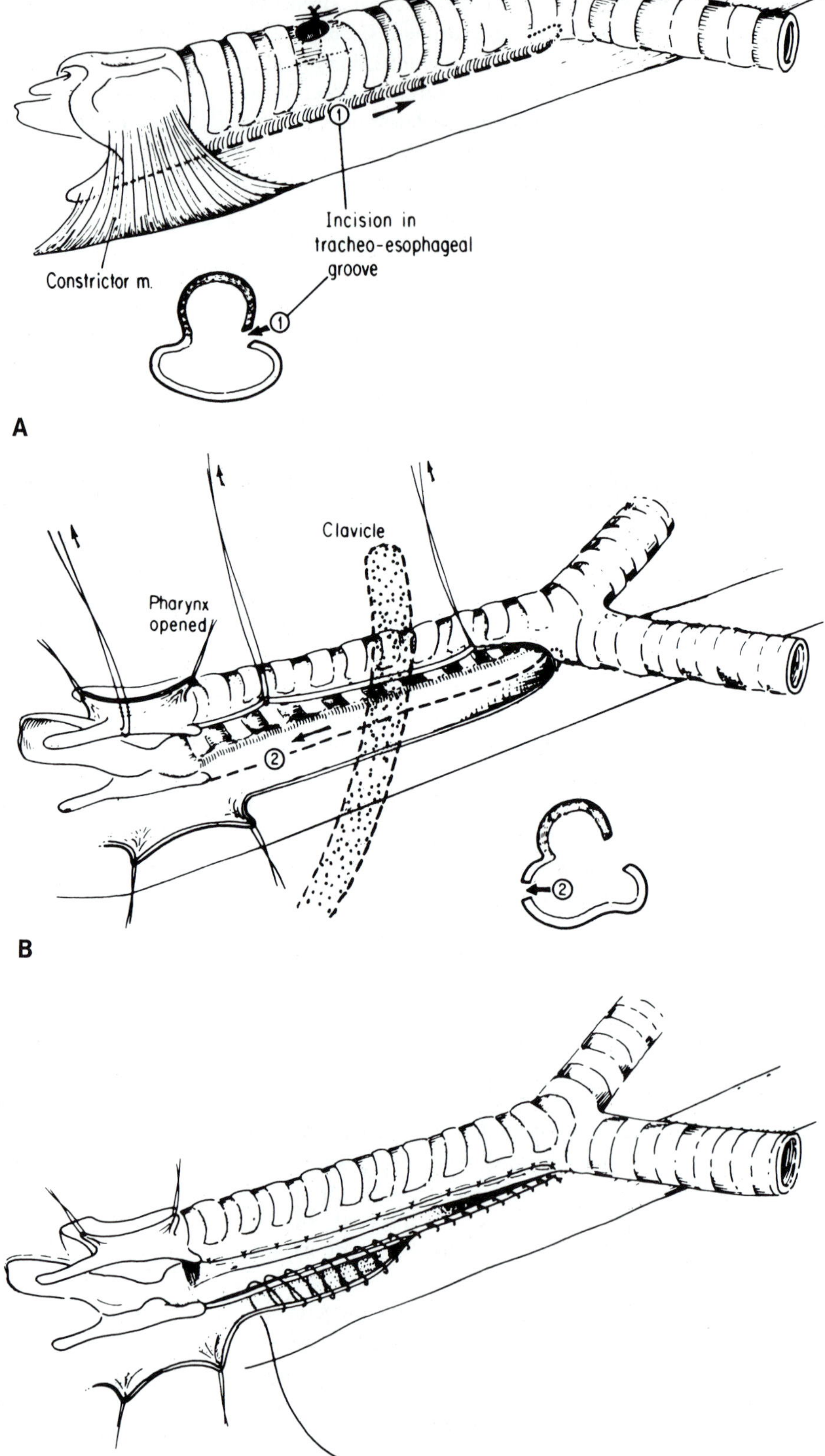


**Figure 13–3.** **A.** Longitudinal incision along right tracheoesophageal groove (dotted line 1) and cross section of laryngotrachea showing the point of division. **B.** Continuation of incision around the distal part of the cleft and through the left wall of the esophagus (dotted line 2) 1 cm down from the left tracheoesophageal groove to create an esophageal flap for closure of the posterior trachea. **C.** Tracheal closure completed with interrupted 6–0 proline sutures. Esophagus repaired with running suture to the level of the inferior cornu of the thyroid. *(From Donahoe PK, Gee PE: Complete laryngotracheoesophageal cleft: Management and repair. J Pediatr Surg 19:143, 1984, with permission.)*

sions as a vascular ring or the dilated and hypertrophied proximal pouch in esophageal atresia.[18] Approximately one quarter of all patients with esophageal atresia have some degree of tracheomalacia that may be suspected in the newborn with visible compression of the trachea by the air or barium-filled upper esophagus (Fig. 13–4). Bronchoscopy reveals a "slitlike" appearance of the distal trachea. Most patients improve with the passage of months as the tracheal cartilages mature and become more stable.[19] Patients who have had major respiratory complications such as "dying spells" may benefit from aortopexy,[20] which aims to provide more space in the upper mediastinum and reduce external compression on the esophagus.

## Pulmonary Agenesis

Bilateral pulmonary agenesis has been reported in a "live" infant with esophageal atresia and first-arch syndrome.[21] The airway ended as a rudimentary lung bud. Unilateral agenesis of the lung is also a great rarity occurring once in every 10,000–15,000 autopsies,[22] but it is compatible with survival and relatively normal growth in the absence of associated major cardiac, gastrointestinal, and other visceral anomalies.[23] The bronchus of the affected lung is a mere dimple or short stump implying an abortive attempt at lung development. A basic developmental defect of genetic or teratogenic origin is likely, but mechanical factors also contribute to the etiology.[24] Compression of the solitary bronchus by anomalous great vessels may give rise to bronchomalacia or bronchial stenosis. Attempts at surgical reconstruction of the obstructed bronchus have been unsuccessful to date.[25] Secondary pulmonary infections, heralded by a high incidence of bronchitis and wheezing followed by pneumonia, are typical in patients who do not survive. In others, the normal lung hypertrophies to fill both hemithoraxes in a manner similar to the outcome after total pneumonectomy. Although respiratory complications are infrequent, growth and development can be delayed because of a mild degree of respiratory insufficiency. X-rays show that the mediastinum is markedly shifted to the contralateral side and the normal lung hyperinflated. There is minimal retraction of the hemithorax as might be seen following pneumonectomy, and the hemidiaphragm is only minimally elevated. When the diagnosis remains in doubt, selective pulmonary angiography is valuable in showing the absence of the pulmonary artery to the affected side. Pulmonary hypertension or emphysema has not been reported in long-term survivors.

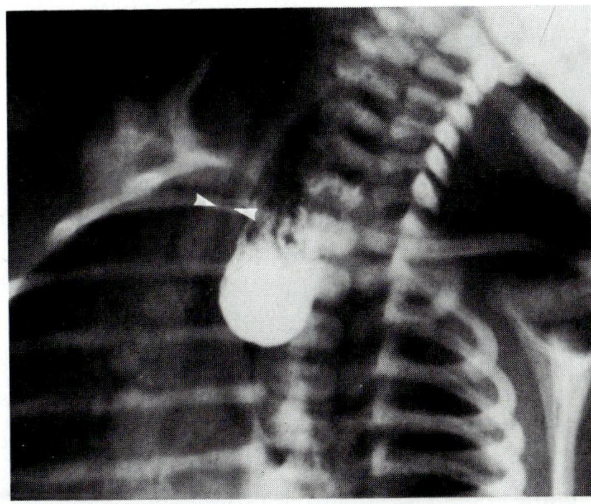

**Figure 13–4.** Tracheomalacia results from chronic in utero compression of the developing tracheal cartilages as seen in this example of a newborn with esophageal atresia.

Approximately 15 cases of pulmonary agenesis with esophageal atresia and tracheoesophageal fistula have been reported. This combination of anomalies carries a particularly high risk of respiratory failure because of tracheomalacia. Tracheostomy has been recommended to provide a tracheal stent following operative repair of the esophageal atresia.[26]

Agenesis of a single lobe is usually well tolerated and discovered during studies performed for other reasons. The only manifestation of the deficient bronchus may be a small diverticulum. Agenesis of the right upper and middle lobes have been observed in association with accessory right hemidiaphragm. No treatment is indicated unless associated vascular malformation or abnormal bronchial communications hamper pulmonary function.

## Bronchial Atresia

Bronchial atresia is a rare condition that may be confused with congenital lobar emphysema.[27] In older infants and children, localized hyperinflation of lung appears in a segmental or lobar distribution, accompanied by a circular or oval parahilar density. Most of these patients have had repeated pulmonary infections or wheezing. Bronchography demonstrates obstruction of the bronchus supplying that part of the lung. Air enters the affected lobe or segment through the patent bronchi and alveoli beyond the atretic segment via the pores of Kohn and the channels of Lambert. This collateral ventilation appears to be more efficient on inspiration giving the confusing picture of the "air block" syndrome, characteristic of lobar emphysema. The circular or parahilar density is in actuality a "mucocele" filling the dilated bronchus just distal to the atresia, an unvarying component of this condition (Fig. 13–5). On occasion, the mucocele may be shaped like a rod or tree but rarely contains an air fluid level. The neonate with bronchial atresia may present with an intrathoracic mass suggesting retained fetal lung fluid in a lobar distribution.[28] The treatment is lobectomy. Congenital bronchial atresia must be distinguished from acquired bronchial stenosis in high-risk neonates who have had endotracheal intubation and mechanical ventilation for many days. The bronchial obstruction is caused by granulation tissue from repeated endotracheal suctioning, and it is likely to produce recurrent

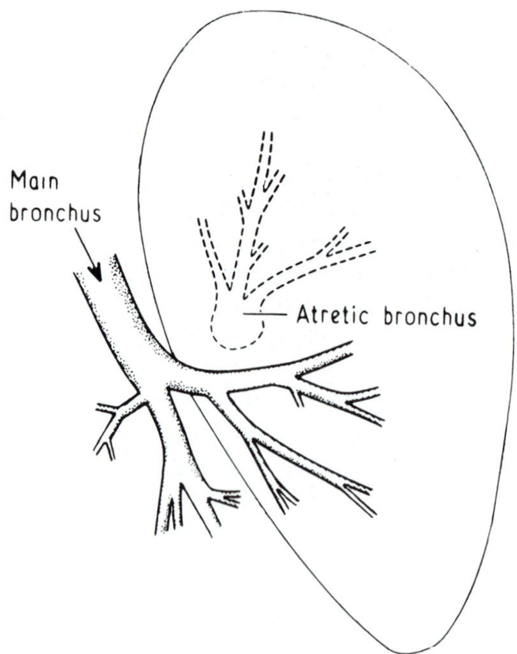


**Figure 13–5.** Diagrammatic representation of the anatomic configuration of the bronchi in a patient with left upper lobe bronchial atresia. The atretic left upper lobe bronchus shows discontinuity in the lumen of the bronchus distal to the site of atresia. The cystic dilatation just beyond the atresia is the site of the "mucocele." *(From Schuster SR, Harris GBC, William A, et al: Bronchial atresia; a recognizable entity in the pediatric age group. J Pediatr Surg 13:682, 1978, with permission.)*

lobal atelectasis. In a recent report, Nagaraj et al[29] described finding nodular and polypoid granulation at the level of the carina and bronchus, and several patients required excision or cauterization of this tissue. This complication can be largely avoided by careful tube placement and fixation to prevent dislodgement. Suctioning should be gentle and the whistle tip or side hole catheters avoided. A program of chest physiotherapy, including vibration of the chest wall and postural drainage, will significantly reduce the need for reintubation and postintubation atelectasis in these infants.

## CONGENITAL LOBAR EMPHYSEMA

Congenital lobar emphysema is a striking pulmonary hyperinflation state that has all the clinical features of an "air block" syndrome similar to obstructive emphysema. The overexpanded lung causes a compression of uninvolved lobes and a marked shift of the labile infantile mediastinum creating a ventilatory crisis characterized by respiratory distress, cyanosis, and sometimes circulatory failure. Approximately 50% of cases present within the first week of life, and another 30% in the subsequent 3 or 4 weeks, while the remainder are distributed in frequency throughout infancy.[30] The left upper lobe is most frequently affected followed by the right middle and upper lobes. Involvement of the lower lobes is rare. In only two of the cases reviewed by Raynor et al[31] was the lesion described as exclusively involving a lower lobe. The differential diagnosis includes pneumothorax, congenital diaphragmatic hernia, tension cysts, and air block syndrome from impacted foreign body, a condition usually found in slightly older patients. The chest x-ray in congenital lobar emphysema shows bronchovascular markings extending to the periphery of the lung, which may be made more obvious by "bright lighting" of the x-ray film. Our experience includes one patient (Fig. 13–6) with an obstructed lobe that slowly became hyperlucent over a few days. "Squame" cells were seen in the alveolar spaces of the surgical specimen. Retention of fetal lung fluid, as illustrated by the example, is a sign of high-grade airway obstruction in the newborn.[32] Further workup, including bronchography or bronchoscopy, is not indicated in the classical cases of hyperlucent lung except in older infants where inhalation of a foreign body is suspected as a cause of bronchial obstruction. Cardiac catheterization may be necessary if there is a suspicion of coexistent congenital heart disease reported as 14% in Murray's[33] review of 166 cases. The primary indication for lobectomy of the hyperinflated lung is progressive signs of tension accompanied by mediastinal displacement. Surgical intervention may be emergent in the neonate with a rapidly enlarging lobe, a situation that has the gravity of a tension pneumothorax. Any attempts at decompression by thoracentesis and intercostal catheter drainage are usually prompted by a misdiagnosis and can be catastrophic by superimposing a pneumothorax.

The operation should be performed under light general anesthesia through a generous anterolateral thoracotomy, rapidly exposing the distended lobe, delivering it from the pleural cavity before one begins the hilar dissection. Excessive positive pressure should be avoided during induction to prevent further distention of the lobe and circulatory embarrassment. Gross and Lewis[34] described the first successful lobectomy in 1945, a procedure that is straightforward in the neonate and carries a low operative morbidity.

Long-term follow-up studies[35] have demonstrated a considerable incidence of chronic bronchitis and asthmatic findings in some patients, but the majority of the infants develop normally without further respiratory tract difficulty. A follow-up[36] of 10–20 years after lobectomy shows that although patients are clinically well, specific pulmonary function abnormalities such as a decrease in airway conductance and forced expiratory volume are detectable.

The pathogenesis remains a subject of considerable interest and controversy, since several etiologic factors have been identified. In the review by Hendren and Mckee[30] of 113 reported cases in 1967, no cause was found in 50% of cases, while 25% had identifiable bronchial cartilaginous dysplasia. In 13% endobronchial obstruction was seen, possibly from a fold of hypertrophic mucous membrane acting as a ball-valve[37] or a tenacious mucous plug.[38] The remain-

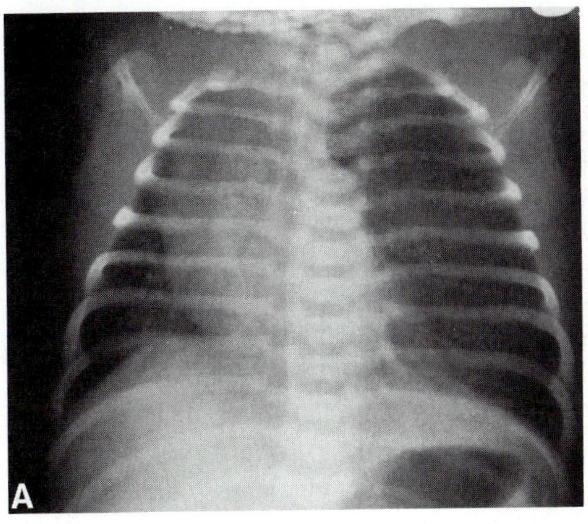


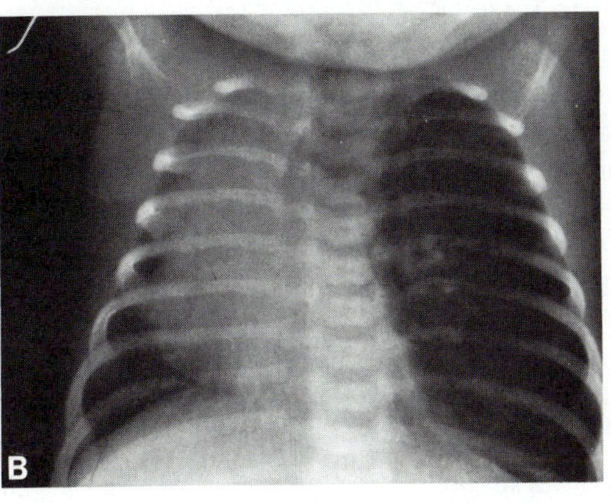


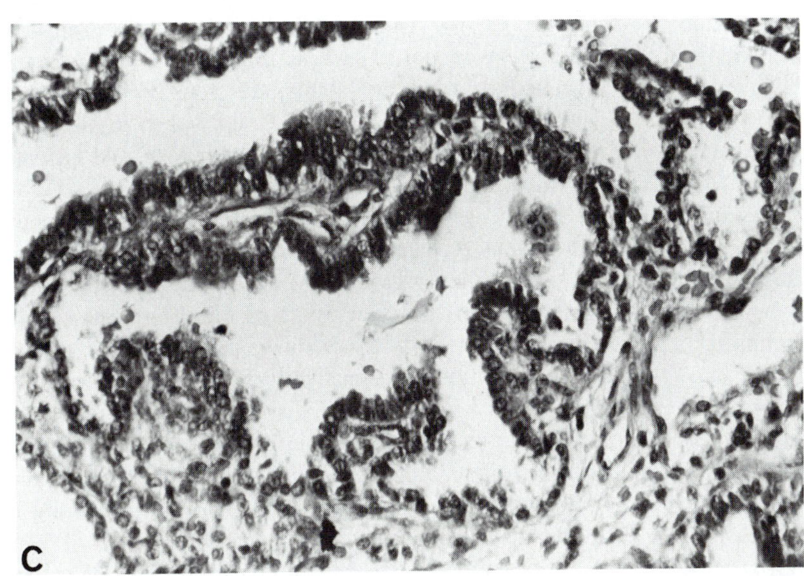


**Figure 13–6.** **A.** Granular density in the obstructed left upper lobe is a sign of retained fetal lung fluid. **B.** Lung becomes hyperlucent 5 days later. X-ray is typical of congenital lobar emphysema. **C.** Retained "squame" cells are seen in the alveolar spaces of the resected lobe.

der had either extrinsic obstruction, possibly from an aberrant artery or fibrous band, or a diffuse bronchial structural deficit. Overstreet[39] in 1939 first described defects in bronchial cartilage with absent or incomplete rings. Lincoln and co-workers[40] found 22 examples of hypoplastic cartilages in 28 cases studied. These investigators conclude that the cartilaginous defect weakens the bronchus, which then collapses on expiration and causes an air-block obstruction with secondary hyperinflation. The cartilaginous abnormalities may be present in the proximal bronchial stump or be destroyed during the preparation of the pathologic material, and, therefore, no etiologic mechanism is found in a significant number of patients. Another particularly interesting cause of congenital lobar emphysema is a poly-alveolar lobe first described by Hislop and Reid[41] in 1970 and subsequently studied by Tapper et al.[36] This entity, which may account for approximately 10% of all cases, is caused by a three- to fivefold increase in the total alveolar number as determined by microscopic point counting of randomly taken lung sections. The number, size, and structure of the airways and arteries are normal for age, suggesting a primary proliferation of alveoli in the affected lobe. The reason why polyalveolar lobes trap air is unknown.

"Acquired" lobar emphysema is a complication of respiratory distress syndrome in premature infants that must be distinguished from congenital causes of lobar emphysema; over 70 cases have been reported.[42] Any lobe may be affected, and the majority of patients have required positive pressure ventilation, oxygen therapy, and endotracheal suctioning, all of which play an important etiologic role. Localization of the disease to one or two lobes following diffuse pulmonary interstitial emphysema is a typical pattern of development.[42] Pathologic changes are characteristic of bronchopulmonary dysplasia and obstructive intra-alveolar emphysema, with air found in the perivascular spaces and a giant cell reaction. In the report by Cooney et al[43] of 10 cases, lobectomy was necessary only in those newborns whose lung scans were characterized by decreased perfusion of the affected lobe, while emphysematous changes resolved in those infants who had normal lung scans. In properly selected patients, pulmonary lobectomy can be successfully performed, but late deaths have been reported because of progressive respiratory insufficiency.[39,44]

## CONGENITAL CYSTIC LESIONS OF THE LUNGS AND BRONCHUS

### Congenital Lung Cyst

Congenital pulmonary cysts are typically located in the lower lobe and are lined by ciliated pseudostratified columnar epithelium in which mucous-secreting cells are present.[45] Smooth muscle and bits of cartilage are frequently seen in the wall of the cyst, which has a distinct fibrous capsule. Many of these cysts are multicompartmented and may represent a simple variant of congenital adenomatoid malformation. Well-documented new cases have not been reported for many years.

Symptoms arise from air trapping, and tension disturbances are not uncommon in neonates and infants. The chest x-ray shows tension with shift of the mediastinum. Lung parenchyma visible about the expanding cyst distinguish it from a tension pneumothorax or congenital lobar emphysema. Treatment is lobectomy, which may be emergent if ventilation of the normal lung is compromised.[46] Aspiration of the cyst prior to lobectomy is indicated, only when cardiovascular disturbances are life-threatening.

In older infants and children, infection of the cyst is more common and may mimic the appearance of a pneumatocele or staphylococcal abscess cavity.[47] Air fluid levels are commonly seen. Even the pathologist may have difficulty in distinguishing an infected congenital cyst from a chronic pulmonary abscess with epithelialization of the wall, cystic bronchiectasis, or a healing tuberculous or mycotic cavity.

## CONGENITAL CYSTIC ADENOMATOID MALFORMATION (CCAM)

Congenital cystic adenomatoid malformation (CCAM) is a relatively rare condition first studied by Ch'in and Tang[48] in 1949, with only 175 cases cited in the English literature prior to 1981.[49] The histology of CCAM was classified by Stocker et al,[50] who correlated findings with lung maturity. Type I CCAM lesions are multicystic with individual cysts often >1 cm in diameter. The walls are lined with ciliated epithelium with some smooth muscle and alveolus-like structure. Cysts in type II are <1 cm and have a thin wall lined by cylindrical to cuboidal epithelium with irregular, smooth muscle bundles. Lungs in type III contain small cysts (<0.5 cm) lined by cuboidal epithelium with little or no smooth muscle or elastic fibers. The latter group is believed to result from arrest in the developing lung bud as early as 35 days' gestation with eventual total lobar involvement. Developmental arrest in later stages of lung development may lead to segmental abnormalities in even more than one lobe.

Several patterns of clinical presentation are found. The first group initially studied by Ch'in and Tang[48] were born prematurely of a pregnancy complicated by hydramnios and were stillborn. Fetal anasarca and major central nervous system anomalies[51] are frequently found in this group. Adzick et al[52] have proposed a new classification (Table 13–1) based on gross anatomy, prenatal ultrasound, and prognosis, since hydramnios exists as a marker for many cases of CCAM. In this classification, microcystic tumors contain cysts <5 mm in diameter and are accompanied by fetal hydrops and a high mortality rate. Prenatal ultrasound findings also include ascites, mediastinal shift, and the non–cystic-type III CCAM (microcystic) lung. Adzick and colleagues[53] have reported success with fetal lobectomy in microcystic lung when hydramnios develops between 24 and 32 weeks' gestation. CCAM resection led to resolution of the hydrops, impressive in utero lung growth, and neonatal survival in four of six recently reported cases.

Macrocystic tumors contain larger cysts, which appear fluid filled by prenatal ultrasound in the absence of hydramnios.[47] In the latter group, severe respiratory distress may begin within the first few hours of life. The cysts expand with air, and the chest x-ray shows a characteristic tension disturbance with mediastinal shift (Fig. 13–7A). The abnormal lung has a multicystic "Swiss chess" configuration that must not be confused with the dilated intestinal loops of congenital diaphragmatic hernia. Abdominal views showing a normal gas pattern will eliminate the possibility of making this diagnostic error.

Approximately one half the reported cases of macrocystic CCAM present with pneumonia and fever in infants and young children.[54,55] The incidence of previously undetected congenital cystic lesions in older children and adults has declined with the advent of prenatal ultrasound screening and greater awareness of this condition in patients with recurrent pneumonia. The initial chest x-ray in macrocystic CCAM often shows an opaque mass consistent with pneumonic consolidation. The clinical course is usually indolent,

**TABLE 13–1. DISTINGUISHING FEATURES OF MICROCYSTIC AND MACROCYSTIC ADENOMATOID MALFORMATION**

| | Microcystic | Macrocystic |
|---|---|---|
| Distribution | Lobar | Lobar or segmental |
| Age at presentation | Fetus | Newborn to infancy |
| Clinical signs | Hydramnios; hydrops | Air trapping; recurrent pneumonia |
| Treatment | ? fetal lobectomy | Lobectomy; segmentectomy |
| Outcome | Usually fatal | Survival |

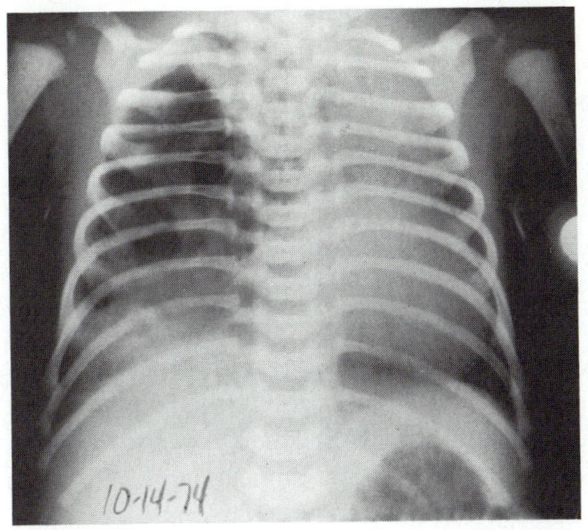


A

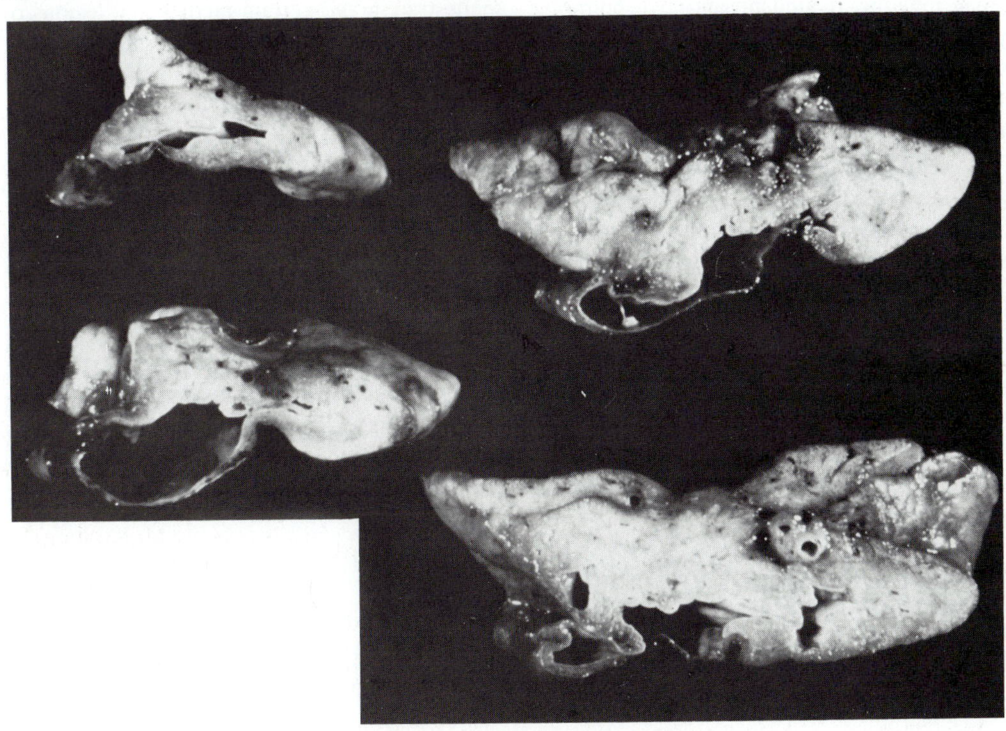

B

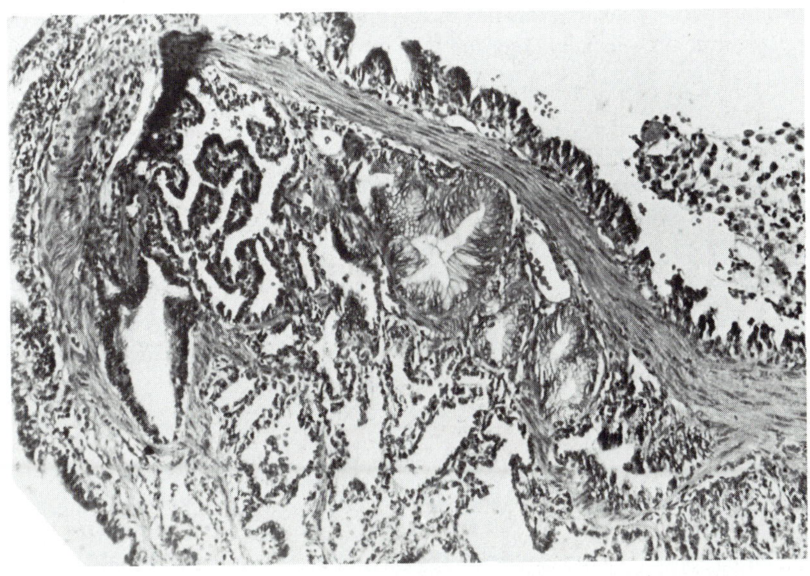

C

**Figure 1[illegible] 7. A.** Multiple air-filled cystic spaces in the right upper lobe of a newborn with congenital adenomatoid malformation cause tension with shift of mediastinum farther to the left. **B.** Serial sections show the typical multicystic spaces found with congenital adenomatoid malformation. **C.** Bronchioles are lined by cuboidal epithelium, and have a polypoid appearance, resembling an adenoma.

and a poor response to systemic antibiotics should raise the suspicion of underlying pathology. Serial x-rays may show either a failure of resolution of the original findings or gradual appearance of multiple cysts. Recurring infection in this group is common and further evidence of a congenital cystic lesion. The characteristic pathologic findings in macrocystic tumors are those of a firm, meaty, multicystic lesion equally affecting the upper and lower lobes of both lungs (Fig. 13–7B) and resemble the pathology described by Stocker (types I and II). The predominant component may be either cystic or solid.[55] Microscopic findings typical for this lesion are a maze of cylindrical or sacular tubules resembling fetal bronchioles lined with cuboidal or columnar respiratory tract epithelium that may be redundant and folded, occasionally having a polypoid appearance resembling an adenoma (Fig. 13–7C). The interstitial tissues may or may not show bits of cartilage, elastic tissue, and smooth muscle. Bronchial-type mucous glands are often present. Some alveoli in aerated portions of the lobe are lined with mucous-secreting cuboidal cells. Pectus excavatum is the most common associated anomaly; cardiac lesions and anomalous pulmonary vessels are very unusual.

Lobectomy is the treatment of choice,[56] but composite resections involving lobectomy plus limited resection of a second lobe is preferred to pneumonectomy in cases of more extensive involvement or chronic inflammation.[57] Occasionally segmentectomy alone will be possible, as in 4 of 32 operated patients reported by Wolf et al.[49] Although anomalous vessels do exist,[58] more recent larger series have shown this finding to be extremely rare, and prevailing opinion is that these were probably unrecognized cases of pulmonary sequestration. The prognosis is excellent, and the patient should survive operation without sequelae.

## PULMONARY SEQUESTRATION

A pulmonary sequestration is an anomalous portion of lung that has no discernible connection with the bronchial tree and receives its blood supply from an ectopic systemic artery instead of the pulmonary artery. Both extralobar and intralobar varieties are believed to have a common embryologic origin, and they should be considered as separate clinical entities. Halasz et al[59] proposed the development of an accessory lung bud caudad to the normal laryngotracheal anlage carrying its blood supply from the original postbranchial segmental vessels and eventually developing in the pleural cavity, diaphragm, or (most often) in the lower pulmonary mesenchyme. This hypothesis is supported by finding occasional patients with pulmonary sequestration who have esophagobronchial communication.[60] Of interest is that heterotopic pancreatic tissue is found in some specimens, lending credence to a common embryogenesis for pulmonary sequestration and certain mediastinal lesions of foregut origin. Gerle et al[61] coined the term *congenital bronchopulmonary foregut malformation* for these various findings and suggested that the time at which the accessory anlage occurs in embryogenesis determines whether the resulting malformation will be an intramural esophageal duplication or an extra- or intrapulmonary sequestration. Utilizing this concept, Tilson and Touloukian[62] reported a case of mediastinal enteric sequestration with aberrant pancreas as a "forme fruste" of the intralobar sequestration. The sequestered tissue is composed of one or more mucous-filled cysts that gradually enlarge and displace the surrounding normal lung. The air seen in the cysts arises from microscopic connections to the lung or via an enteric communication that is the usual source of secondary infection. They described a classification of bronchoenteric cysts (Fig. 13–8).

### Intralobar

An intralobar pulmonary sequestration is invariably located in the posterior basilar region of the lower lobe.[63] The left lung is most frequently involved. The sequestered portion of the lung is supplied by a disproportionately large artery or arteries of systemic elastic type, arising directly from the thoracic aorta in 70% of cases and from the abdominal aorta or its branches in the remainder.[64] The anomalous arteries usually enter the lung through the pulmonary ligament. The

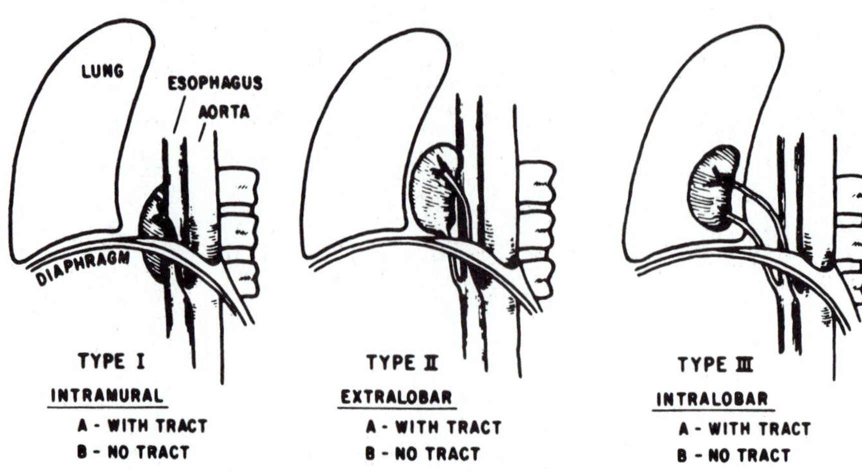


**Figure 13–8.** A proposed classification of broncho-enteric cysts to include pulmonary sequestration. In all cases, there is an anomalous arterial supply from the aorta. Type I represents an intramural lesion, such as an esophageal duplication. Types II and III are characteristic of an extra- or intralobar pulmonary sequestration usually found without a persistent esophago-bronchial communication. *(From Tilson MD, Touloukian RJ, Ann Surg 176:669, 1972, with permission.)*

venous drainage, with extralobar sequestration, is through the azygous or portal vein and by the pulmonary route with intralobar sequestration.

The clinical presentation of an intralobar sequestration is similar to that of congenital adenomatoid malformation in older patients, a condition with which it is often confused. The chest x-ray shows a dense mass that may contain cysts with or without fluid levels, and signs of pulmonary infection are usually present. Preoperative differentiation from other congenital lung cysts requires arteriography. Intralobar sequestration is only rarely associated with other congenital anomalies.

### Extralobar

Extralobar sequestration is likely to be first recognized on routine prenatal ultrasound early in gestation (Fig. 13–9A) or as an unexplained density by chest x-ray during infancy

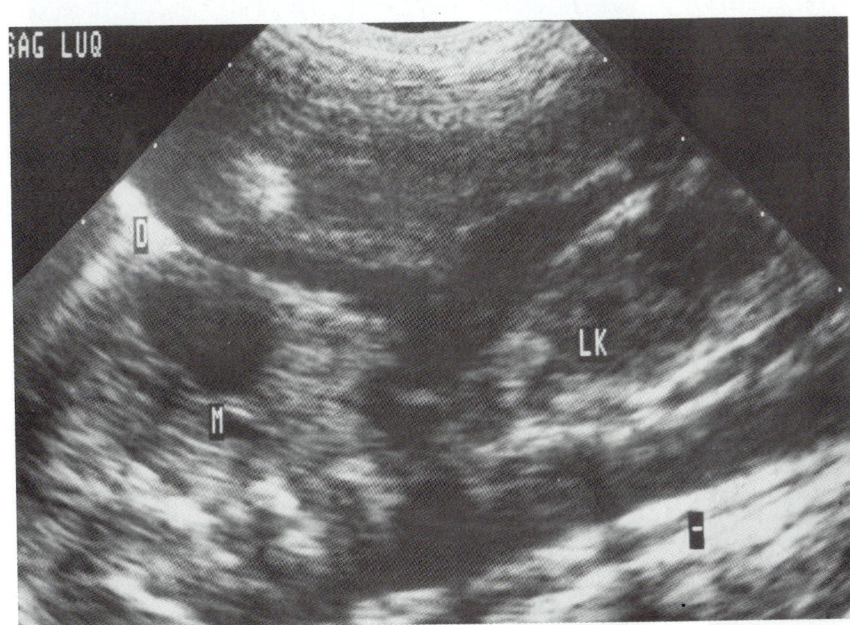


A

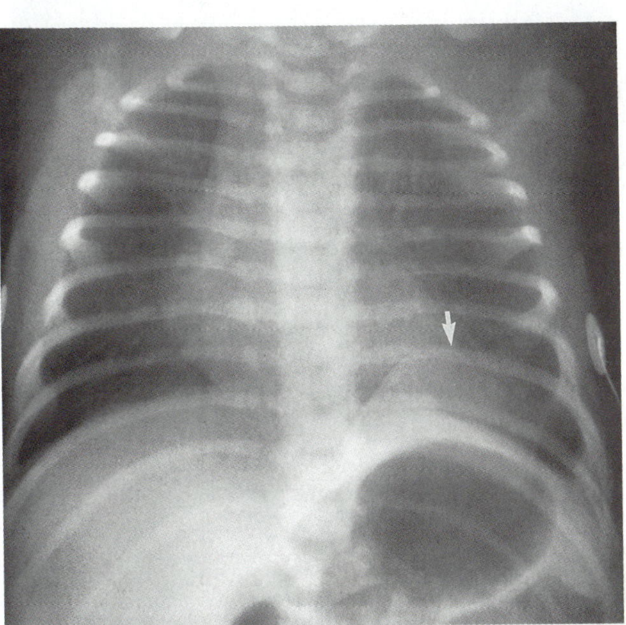

B

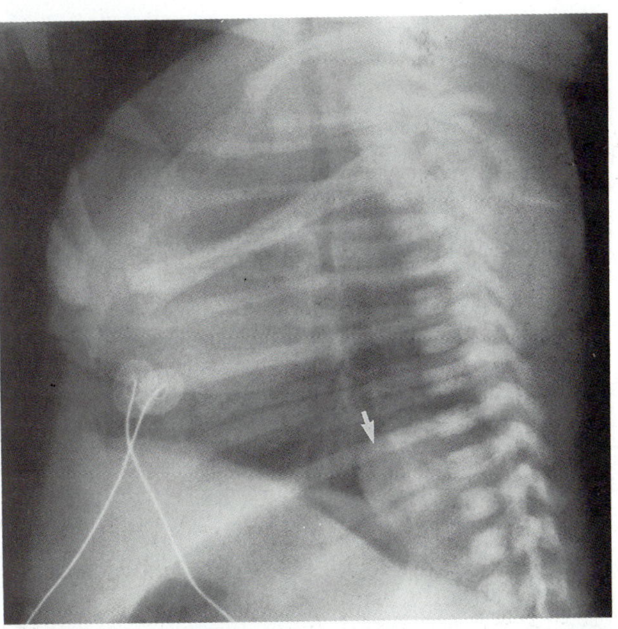

C

**Figure 13–9. A.** Sagittal view of ultrasound in asymptomatic newborn with extralobar pulmonary sequestration, confirming finding of "cystic mass" on prenatal study. Mass lies adjacent to diaphragm. **B, C.** PA and lateral radiographs show the mass located in posterolateral chest (arrows). Sequestration was attached at diaphragm but free of lung, and completely resected.

or childhood (Fig. 13–9B,C). Extralobar sequestration has also been found as an incidental finding in the newborn with a congenital diaphragmatic hernia.[65] Other less commonly associated anomalies include cardiac defects, diaphragmatic eventration, pericardial cysts, and esophageal achalasia. Radiographic examination in the unsuspected case typically demonstrates a triangular-shaped mass close to the pulmonary hilum in the lower lung field (Fig. 13–10A). An arteriogram or computed tomography (CT) scan will delineate the presence of aberrant arterial

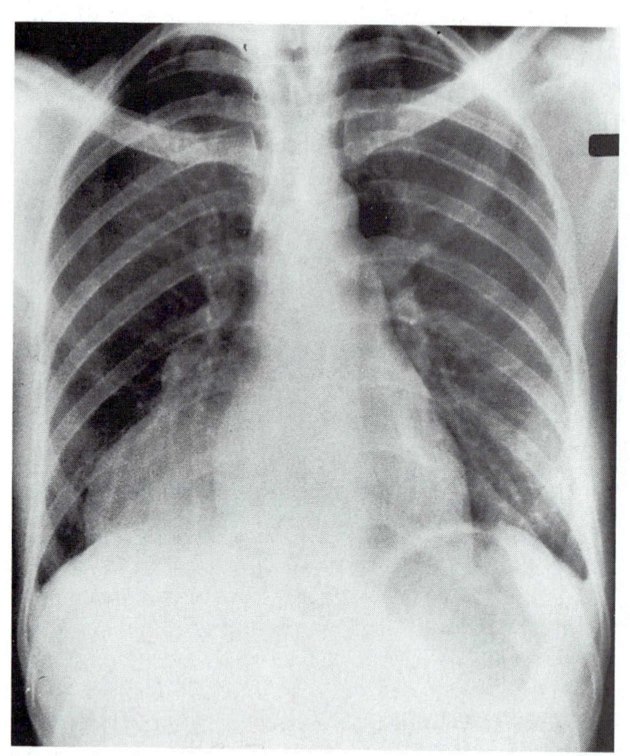

A

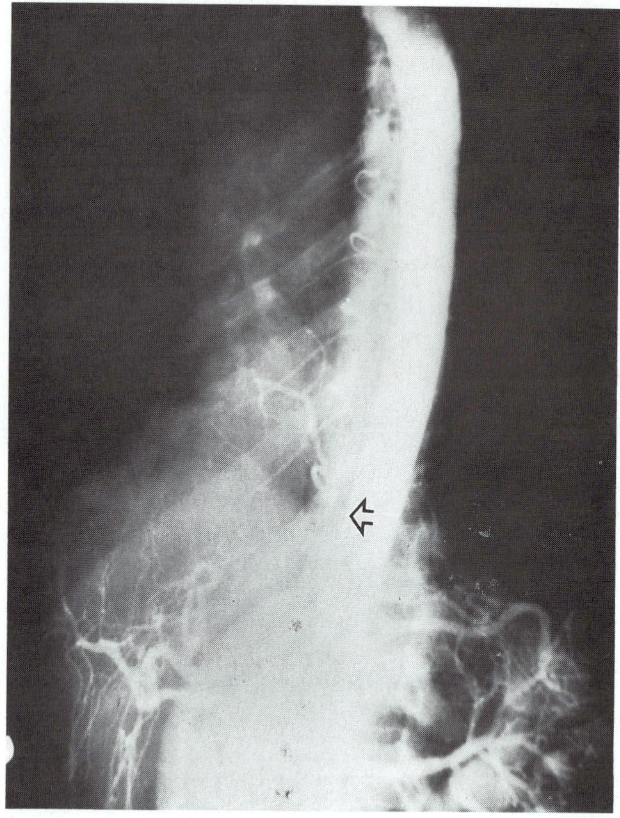

B

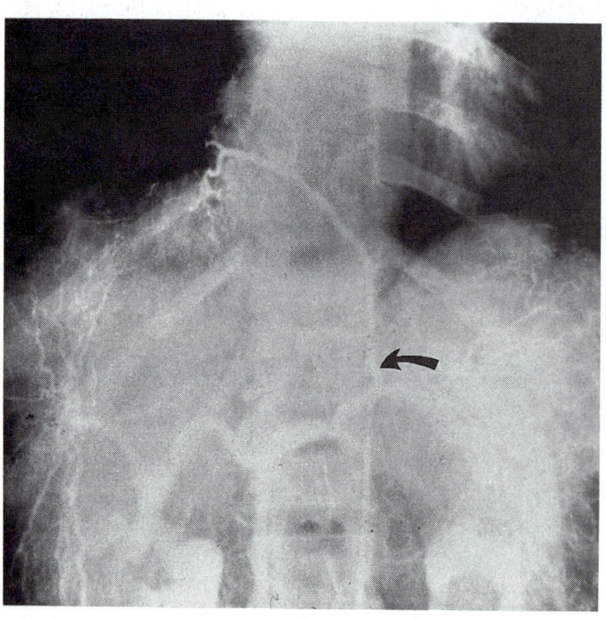

C

**Figure 13–10.** **A.** Ten-year-old girl with an extralobar pulmonary sequestration presented with a multicystic, triangular-shaped mass in the right lower lung field on a chest radiograph obtained during a respiratory tract infection. **B.** Aortogram reveals an aberrant systemic artery arising from the thoracic aorta at the diaphragm. **C.** Venous drainage of the sequestration is to the splenic vein.

branches and the venous drainage (Fig. 13–10B,C). A barium esophagram is useful to identify the unlikely presence of a broncho-enteric communication.

Lobectomy is required treatment for intralobar sequestration while resection of the extralobar sequestration mass without removal of adjacent lung is usually possible. The surgeon must be alert to the existence of the aberrant systemic branches arising from the abdominal or thoracic aorta, which can be inadvertently injured when one is dissecting in the pulmonary ligament, mediastinum, and along the diaphragm. The important distinguishing features of extra and intralobar pulmonary sequestration are summarized in Table 13–2. *Systemic arterialization*[66] of a lower lobe is a rare anomaly, possibly having an embryologic origin similar to sequestration. The systemic artery usually arises from the lower thoracic aorta, but normal lung development and an intact bronchus distinguish this condition from extralobar sequestration. The clinical findings are either high-output congestive heart failure from arteriovenous shunting through the lung, or a murmur, misinterpreted as being cardiac. In carefully studied specimens, the systemic arteries involved have been demonstrated to communicate with pulmonary arteries, not veins. The treatment is division of the shunt with lobectomy reserved for patients having ischemic lung changes or subsequent pulmonary complications.

## STAPHYLOCOCCAL PNEUMONIA AND ITS COMPLICATIONS

*Staphylococcus aureus* is by far the most common organism causing pneumonia in childhood and has been known to occur as a worldwide pandemic in infants, the last outbreak occurring in the mid-1950s.[67] The incidence of pneumococcal, streptococcal, and H-influenza infections causing pneumonia dropped to practically zero in the period immediately following the introduction of systemic antibiotics and may have hastened an overgrowth of the more virulent staphylococcal types that cause pneumonia and its complications. While the overall mortality of staphylococcal pneumonia in infancy and childhood remains below 10% in the so-called poly-antibiotic era, the incidence of major complications remains higher than one encounters in adults. For this reason, a brief summary of the pediatric aspects of staphylococcal pulmonary infection is presented here to supplement information on this subject in another chapter.

**TABLE 13–2. DISTINGUISHING FEATURES OF EXTRA AND INTRALOBAR PULMONARY SEQUESTRATION**

| | Intralobar | Extralobar |
|---|---|---|
| Arterial supply | Thoracic aorta (70%) Abdominal aorta (30%) via pulmonary ligament | Thoracic aorta (70%) Abdominal aorta (30%) via pulmonary ligament |
| Venous drainage | Pulmonary vein | Azygous or portal system |
| Common location | Posterior basal region, usually left lower lobe | Triangular mass lower lung field |
| Presentation | Pulmonic infection with "cystic mass by x-ray" | Dense asymptomatic mass by x-ray |
| Treatment | Lobectomy vs. segmental resection | Lobectomy |

Primary staphylococcal pneumonia usually occurs in infants and presents as a rapidly toxic illness with signs of fever, tachypnea, and cough developing over a few hours' period. The diagnosis is confirmed by the presence of a pulmonary infiltrate by x-ray, which may consolidate over the next day or two. The physical signs are those of any pneumonic infection. The treatment is early aggressive IV methacillin, since the majority of organisms are penicillin resistant.

Serial chest x-rays obtained over the first several days of the acute illness will either show resolution or signs of either *pleural* or *parenchymal* complications.

Empyema is reported in over 50% of patients with staphylococcal pneumonia. In the early stages, the fluid is exudative and not loculated, but it eventually becomes fibropurulent when loculation is common and eventually organizes, forming a thick fibrous peel that may cause lung entrapment. The objective of treatment is early recognition of empyema by decubitus views to distinguish fluid from pulmonic consolidation followed by prompt evacuation of the fluid with closed thoracotomy and negative pressure suction to avoid loculation and cortical scarring.[68] The largest intercostal tube that freely fits the interspace should be inserted in the most dependent position possible along the posterior axillary line. Tube replacement is often necessary; the secretions are very viscous, and insertion of a second or third tube may be required to drain loculated abscesses. With aggressive pleural drainage, only rarely will decortication of a trapped lung be necessary.[69]

The most frequent pulmonary complication is a pneumatocele that is a cluster of air spaces appearing in the previous area of consolidation. In young children without a previous x-ray, the possibility of congenital cystic disease is often raised. The origin of pneumatoceles is primarily from destruction of adjacent alveolar walls by the lytic enzymes produced by the staphylococcus. Ravitch and Fenn suggest that another cause is a breakdown of an intramural end bronchial abscess with direct leakage of air into the parenchyma through a flap valve defect. Most pneumatoceles appear during the resolution phase and gradually disappear over several weeks' or months' convalescent period. The presence of persistent pneumatoceles is not an indication for lobectomy or other surgical procedures. Rarely do a tension pneumatocele or secondary abscess form, but, when recognized, they require prompt tube thoracostomy. A pyopneumothorax, possibly with tension, is a sign of a broncopleural fistula and is an indication to insert both an anterior as well as a more dependent intercostal tube to evacuate air and fluid as quickly as possible and create a seal of the fistula with the parietal pleura. Chronic lung abscess is now rare, but resection of the fibrotic wall is generally indicated to promote full expansion of the lung following long-term thoracostomy drainage. Recurring pneumonia in childhood should raise the question of an immune deficiency such as chronic granulomatous disease or agammaglobulinemia. Mucoviscidosis should also be suspected, and appropriate diagnostic testing is indicated.

## REFERENCES


1. Fontanus N. *N. Responsiorum et curationum medicinalium, book I.* Amsterdam, 1639, p 55
2. Huber JJ. Observations aliquot de arteria singulari pulmoni concessa. *Acta Helvet* **8**:85, 1777
3. Ricinhoff WF Jr, Reichert FL, Heuer GJ: Compensatory changes in the remaining lung following total pneumonectomy. *Bull Johns Hopkins Hosp* **57**:373, 1935
4. Fisher CC, Tropea F Jr, Barley CP: Conbenital pulmonary cysts. *J Pediatr* **23**:219, 1943
5. Gross RE: Congenital cystic lung. *Ann Surg* **123**:229, 1946
6. Arey LA: *Developmental Anatomy. A Textbook and Laboratory Manual of Embryology,* 4th Ed. Philadelphia, Saunders, 1940, p 234
7. Reid L, Rubino M: The connective tissue septa in the foetal human lung. *Thorax* **14**:3, 1959
8. Engel S: *The Child's Lung.* London, Arnold, 1947
9. Waddell WR: Organoid differentiation of the fetal lung. A histologic study of the differentiation of mammalian fetal lung in utero and in transplants. *Arch Pathol* **47**:227, 1949
10. Bucher U, Reid L: Development of the mucus secreting elements in human lung. *Thorax* **16**:219, 1961
11. Walcher K: Angeborener Mangel der Trachea. *Dtsch Z Gericht Med* **12**:292, 1928
12. Harrison MR, Heldt GD, Brosch RC, et al: Resection of distal tracheal stenosis in a baby with agenesis of the lung. *J Pediatr Surg* **15**:938, 1980
13. Burroughs W, Leape LL: Laryngotracheoesophageal cleft; report of a case successfully treated and review of the literature. *Pediatrics* **53**:516, 1974
14. Roth B, Rose KG, Benz-Bolim G, et al: Laryngotracheoesophageal cleft: Clinical features, diagnosis and therapy. *Eur J Pediatr* **140**:41, 1983
15. Donahoe PK, Hendren WH: The surgical management of laryngotracheoesophageal cleft with tracheoesophageal fistula and esophageal atresia. *Surgery* **71**:363, 1972
16. Hendren WH: Repair of laryngotracheoesophageal cleft using interposition of a strap muscle. *J Pediatr Surg* **11**:425, 1976
17. Donahoe P, Gee PE: Complete laryngotracheal cleft; management and repair. *J Pediatr Surg* **19**:143, 1984
18. Fearon B, Shortreed R: Tracheobronchial compression by congenital cardiovascular anomalies in children. Syndrome of apnea. *Ann Otolaryngol* **72**:949, 1963
19. Davies MR, Cywes S: The flaccid trachea and tracheoesophageal congenital anomalies. *J Pediatr Surg* **13**:363, 1978
20. Schwartz MZ, Filler RM: Tracheal compression as a cause of apnea following repair of tracheoesophageal fistula; treatment by aortopexy. *J Pediatr Surg* **15**:842, 1980
21. DeBuse PJ, Movies G: Bilateral pulmonary agenesis, oesophageal atresia, and the first arch syndrome. *Thorax* **28**:526, 1973
22. Olcott CT, Dodey SW: Agenesis of lung in an infant. *Am J Dis Child* **65**:776, 1945
23. Nelson CS, McMillar IKR, Bharucha RK: Tracheal stenosis, pulmonary agenesis and patent ductus arteriosus. *Thorax* **22**:7, 1967
24. Maltz DL, Nadas AS: Agenesis of the lung. Presentation of eight new cases and review of the literature. *Pediatrics* **42**:175, 1968
25. Harrison MR, Hendren WH: Agenesis of the lung complicated by vascular compression and bronchomalacia. *J Pediatr Surg* **10**:813, 1975
26. Black PR, Welch KJ: Pulmonary agenesis (aplasia), esophageal atresia, tracheoesophageal fistula: a different treatment strategy. *J Pediatr Surg* **21**:936, 1986
27. Schuster SR, Harris GBC, Williams A, et al: Bronchial atresia: a recognizable entity in the pediatric age group. *J Pediatr Surg* **13**:682, 1978
28. Waddell JA, Simon G, Reid L: Bronchial atresia of the left upper lobe. *Thorax* **20**:214, 1965
29. Nagaraj HS, Shott R, Fellows R, et al: Recurrent lobar atelectasis due to acquired bronchial stenosis in neonates. *J Pediatr Surg* **15**:411, 1980
30. Hendren WH, McKee DM: Lobar emphysema of infancy. *J Pediatr Surg* **1**:24, 1967
31. Raynor AC, Capp MP, Sealy WC: Lobar emphysema of infancy. Diagnosis, treatment and etiologic aspects. A collective review. *Ann Thorac Surg* **4**:374, 1967
32. Griscom NT, Harris GBC, Wohl MEB, et al: Fluid-filled lung due to airway obstruction in the newborn. *Pediatrics* **43**:383, 1969
33. Murray GF: Collective review. Congenital lobar emphysema. *Surg Gynecol Obstet* **124**:611, 1967
34. Gross RE, Lewis JE Jr: Defect of the anterior mediastinum: successful surgical repair. *Surg Gynecol Obstet* **80**:549, 1945
35. Sloan H: Lobar obstruction emphysema in infancy treated by lobectomy. *J Thorac Surg* **26**:1, 1953
36. Tapper D, Schuster S, McBride J, et al: Polyalveolar lobe: Anatomic and physiologic parameters and their relationship to congenital lobar emphysema. *J Pediatr Surg* **5**:931, 1980
37. Robertson R, James ES: Congenital lobar emphysema. *Pediatrics* **8**:795, 1951
38. Murray GF, Talbert JL, Haller JA Jr: Obstructive lobar emphysema of the newborn infant. Documentation of the "mucus plug syndrome" with successful treatment by bronchotomy. *J Thorac Cardiovasc Surg* **53**:886, 1967
39. Overstreet RM: Emphysema of a portion of the lung in the early months. *Am J Dis Child* **57**:861, 1939
40. Lincoln JCR, Stark J, Subramanian S, et al: Congenital lobar emphysema. *Ann Surg* **173**:55, 1971
41. Hislop A, Reid L: New pathological findings in emphysema of childhood: I. Polyalveolar lobe with emphysema. *Thorax* **25**:682, 1970
42. Martinez-Frontanilla LA, Hernandez J, Haase GM, et al: Surgery of acquired lobar emphysema in the neonate. *J Pediatr Surg* **19**:375, 1984
43. Cooney DR, Minke JA, Allen JE: "Acquired" lobar emphysema: A complication of respiratory distress in premature infants. *J Pediatr Surg* **12**:897, 1977
44. Azizkhan RG, Grimmer DL, Askin FB: Acquired lobar emphysema (overinflation): Clinical and pathological evaluation of infants requiring lobectomy. *J Pediatr Surg* **27**:1145, 1992
45. Fischer CC, Tropea F, Bailey CD: Congenital pulmonary cysts. *J Pediatr* **23**:219, 1943
46. Ravitch MM, Hardy JB: Congenital cystic disease of the lung in infants and children. *Arch Surg* **59**:1, 1949
47. Potts WJ, Riker WL: Differentiation of congenital cysts of the lung and those following staphylococcal pneumonia. *Arch Surg* **61**:684, 1950
48. Ch'in KY, Tang MY: Congenital adenomatoid malformation of one lobe of a lung with general anasarca. *Arch Pathol* **48**:221, 1949

49. Wolf SA, Hertzler HH, Philippart AI: Cystic adenomatoid dysplasia of the lung. *J Pediatr Surg* **15:**925, 1980
50. Stocker JT, Madewell JE, Drake RM: Congenital cystic adenomatoid malformation of the lung: Classification and morphologic spectrum. *Hum Pathol* **8:**155, 1977
51. Taber P, Schwartz DW: Cystic lung lesion in a newborn: Congenital cystic adenomatoid malformation of the lung. *J Pediatr Surg* **7:**366, 1972
52. Adzick NS, Harrison MR, Glick PL: Fetal cystic adenomatoid malformation: Prenatal diagnosis and natural history. *J Pediatr Surg* **20:**483, 1985
53. Adzick NS, Harrison MR, Flake AW: Fetal surgery for cystic adenomatoid malformation of the lung. *J Pediatr Surg* **28:**806, 1993
54. Buntain WL, Isaacs H Jr, Payne VC Jr, et al: Lobar emphysema, cystic adenomatoid malformation, pulmonary sequestration and bronchiogenic cyst in infancy and childhood: a clinical group. *J Pediatr Surg* **9:**85, 1974
55. Bale P: Congenital cystic malformation of the lung. A form of congenital bronchiolar ("adenomatoid") malformation. *Am J Clin Pathol* **71:**411, 1979
56. Holder TM, Christy MG: Cystic adenomatoid malformation of the lung. *J Thorac Cardiovasc Surg* **47:**590, 1964
57. Mentzer SJ, Filler RM, Phillips J: Limited pulmonary resection for congenital cystic adenomatoid malformation of the lung. *J Pediatr Surg* **27:**1410, 1992
58. Hutchin P, Friedman PJ, Saltzstein SL: Congenital cystic adenomatoid with anomalous blood supply. *J Thorac Cardiovasc Surg* **62:**220, 1971
59. Halasz NA, Lindskog GE, Liewbow AA: Esophagobronchial fistula and bronchiopulmonary sequestration. *J Thorac Cardiovasc Surg* **54:**121, 1967
60. Boyden EA, Bill AH, Creighton SA: Presumptive origin of a left lower accessory lung from an esophageal diverticulum. *Surgery* **52:**323, 1962
61. Gerle RD, Jaretzki A III, Ashley CA, et al: Congenital bronchiopulmonary foregut malformation. *N Engl J Med* **278:**1413, 1968
62. Tilson MD, Touloukian RJ: Mediastinal enteric sequestration with aberrant pancreas: A formes frustes of the intralobar sequestration. *Ann Surg* **176:**669, 1972
63. DeParedes CG, Pierce WS, Johnson DG, et al: Pulmonary sequestration in infants and children. *J Pediatr Surg* **5:**136, 1970
64. Buntain WL, Woolley MM, Mahour GH, et al: Pulmonary sequestration in children. A twenty-five year experience. *Surgery* **81:**413, 1977
65. Louw JH, Cywes S: Extralobar pulmonary sequestration communicating with the esophagus and associated with a strangulated congenital diaphragmatic hernia. *Br J Surg* **50:**102, 1962
66. Kirks DR, Kane PE, Free EA, et al: Systemic arterial supply to normal basilar segments of the left lower lobe. *Am J Radiol* **126:**817, 1976
67. Ravitch MM, Fenn R: The changing picture of pneumonia and empyema in infants and children. A review of the experience at the Harriet Lane Home from 1934 through 1958. *JAMA* **175:**1039, 1961
68. Cattaneo SM, Kilman JW: Surgical therapy of empyema in children. *Arch Surg* **106:**564, 1973
69. Sherman MM, Subramanian V, Berger RL: Management of thoracic empyema. *Am J Surg* **133:**474, 1977

CHAPTER

# 14

# Surgical Treatment of Bullous Emphysema

John E. Connolly

Emphysema has been defined as an anatomic alteration of the lung characterized by an abnormal enlargement of the air spaces distal to the terminal nonrespiratory bronchiole, accompanied by destructive changes of the alveolar walls.[1–4] Overdistention of air spaces and alveolar destruction within the secondary lobule is seen. With complete dissolution of one secondary lobule or more, a *bulla* or grossly visible air space (2.5 cm or more in diameter) may be formed. Bullae show no pulmonary vessels with increased radiolucency and are easily recognizable on plain chest films, particularly in full expansion.

Bullous emphysema is usually seen in smokers >40 years of age who exhibit alterations in ventilation, lung volume, intrapulmonary gas distribution, pulmonary gas exchange, and acid-base balance; these smokers often have decreased cardiovascular function. When bullae become large, they can compress relatively normal functioning tissue. Giant bullae are usually multiple and may involve both lungs.

Historically, many surgical approaches have been advocated for large compressive bullae and also for smaller, more diffuse lesions[4] (Table 14–1). The earliest surgical procedures were costochondrectomy and even transverse sternotomy, which were applied because of the mistaken idea that emphysema was the result of a primary skeletal deformity that caused the barrel chest. Costochondrectomy remained in vogue for at least two decades and was performed by such prominent surgeons as Tuffier, Sauerbruch, and Lilienthal.[4] This operation was said to be followed by great relief from dyspnea and an immediate increase in vital capacity.

Recognition that the enlarged thorax and flattened diaphragm were the result and not the cause of the pulmonary disease led to the use of thoracoplasty and pneumonectomy to decrease the volume of the chest. However, the adverse results of these procedures fortunately led to their early abandonment. Another form of therapy touted for the treatment of emphysema was pneumoperitoneum. This modality was discarded after objective measurements showed no correlation with the subjective improvement initially claimed. Later, direct surgical attack on large bullae was advocated, first by thoracentesis with needle aspiration and later by closed Monaldi intracavitary suction. As techniques in operative thoracic surgery improved, local resection of emphysematous bullae by open thoracotomy was developed.

Brantigan et al[5] in 1959 described resection of functionally useless areas of lung so that the emphysematous lung would be reduced in volume to fit or equal the pleural cavity on full expiration, thus restoring the normal physiologic factor of circumferential pull on the bronchioles. They theorized that with the bronchioles held open, air would be permitted an easier flow in and out of the alveoli, thus providing ventilation. Significant morbidity and mortality associated with the procedure along with lack of objective pulmonary function improvement led to its being discarded. This procedure has recently been revived by Cooper et al[6] using a median sternotomy and buttressed stapled excision of portions of both bullous and nonbullous lung to reduce volume. Initial results in a small number of patients are reported to be encouraging; however, further experience with detailed objective pulmonary function improvement and long-term followup is necessary before this procedure can be recommended.

Over the years, evaluation of the various surgical treat-

**TABLE 14–1. HISTORICAL REVIEWS OF SURGICAL PROCEDURES FOR EMPHYSEMA**

| Abnormal Findings | Operation | Rationale for Procedure |
|---|---|---|
| Barrel chest | Costochondrectomy<br>Transverse sternotomy | Restore mobility of thoracic cage<br>Permit further enlargement of lung |
| Hyperinflation | Thoracoplasty<br>Phrenic paralysis | Reduction of lung volumes<br>Diminshed Hering-Breuer reflexes |
| Low, flat, immobile diaphragm | Abdominal belts<br>Pneumoperitoneum | Restore normal motion of diaphragm<br>Reduce lung volume |
| Bullous emphysema | Needle aspiration, injection of irritant<br>Open drainage, Monaldi<br>excision, plication | Reduce tension within bullae<br>Close bronchial communications<br>Permit reexpansion and better function of more normal regions |
| Spontaneous pneumothorax | Closed thoracotomy<br>Open thoracotomy<br>Pleurectomy | Reexpansion of pneumothorax<br>Reinflation of more normal lung |
| Hypovascularity of lung | Parietal pleurectomy or poudrage | New blood supply from chest wall |
| Expiratory collapse of small airways | Resection of peripheral lung tissue | Restore elastic recoil, increase radial tension around airways |
| Expiratory collapse of large airways | Reinforcement of membranous trachea and main bronchi | Prevent expiratory invagination of membranous portion |
| Repeated respiratory infections, $CO_2$ narcosis | Conventional tracheostomy<br>Fenestration | Decrease anatomic dead space |
| Increased respiratory effort due to hypoxemia | Resection of glomus caroticum | Decrease hypoxic respiratory drive |
| Bronchospasm, hypersecretion | Autonomic denervation | Reduce bronchospastic component |
| End-stage emphysema | Lung transplantation | Restoration of function |

ments for emphysema listed above has been difficult because subjective improvement in dyspnea in emphysematous patients often can be attributed to encouragement, moral support, and understanding care. The lack of controlled objective data substantiating improvement eventually led to the demise of these various techniques.

## SELECTION OF PATIENTS FOR SURGERY OF EMPHYSEMA

Some 20% of patients with chest films showing hypertransradiance or absence of "lung markings" have conditions other than bullous emphysema. Hypertransradiance with patent airways is easily separated from bullae by fluoroscopy or inspiration/expiration chest films. In such cases the air trapping and mediastinal shift to the opposite side seen with bullae are not seen. Pneumatoceles from staphylococcal pneumonia usually disappear with time, only occasionally becoming bullae from bronchiole granulation tissue.

Table 14–2 lists the clinical, physiologic, and radiographic findings of both the ideal surgical candidate and the poor candidate. The younger the patient, the presence of a short rapid progression of dyspnea, and cessation of smoking all contribute to a better operative candidate. The best candidates also generally have much reduced, restrictive pattern forced vital capacity (FVC), no response to bronchodilators, and low $PCO_2$, and only slightly reduced $PO_2$. Perhaps the radiographic findings are the most important determinants in the selection of bullous emphysema surgical candidates. Ideal patients show giant bullae of the upper portions of the lungs with basilar crowding of the lower lobes. Angiography and computerized axial tomography can demonstrate intact lower-lobe vasculature with crowding classically into the lower mediastinum. In such cases, removal of bullae will allow good postoperative reexpansion of functioning lung tissue.

Computed tomography (CT) offers advantages over angiography in the preoperative assessment of patients, since it eliminates superimposition of disease and defines individual bullae in three dimensions. CT can also help in the differentiation of pneumothorax from large peripheral bullae.

Because most patients with diffuse emphysema have not tolerated thoracotomy well, it has become widely accepted that such intervention may not be safe and, thus, is indicated only when the function of remaining compressed, relatively normal lung is immediately improved by such operation. Thus, current absolute indications for direct excision of bullae include only those with repeated pneumothorax or giant compressive bullae involving at least 30–50% of a hemithorax.[7,8] Some emphysematous patients with severe impairment and limited life expectancy are also being treated by lung transplantation at a few institutions.

We have reviewed our patients with incapacitating

**TABLE 14–2. INDICATIONS AND CONTRAINDICATIONS FOR BULLECTOMY FOR DYSPNEA**

| | Ideal Case | Relative Contraindications |
|---|---|---|
| **Examination** | | |
| Age | Middle age | Advanced age |
| Smoking | Stopped some time ago | Continues |
| Cough and sputum | Little or none (pink puffer) | Severe (blue bloater) |
| Recurrent infections | None | Common and severe |
| Dyspnea | Rapidly progressive, short history | Slowly progressive, long history |
| Physical examination | No evidence of diffuse emphysema | Severe diffuse emphysema |
| $Alpha_1$-antitrypsin | Normal | Low (rarely) |
| **Physiologic** | | |
| FVC | Much reduced, "restrictive pattern" | Moderately reduced |
| $FEV_1$ and flow rates | Severely reduced | Severely reduced |
| Bronchodilator | No response | Significant increase |
| Helium FRC | High normal, sometimes reduced | Greatly increased |
| Plethysmographic FRC | Much larger than He-test | Slightly larger than He-test |
| Blood gases | Low $Pco_2$, slightly reduced $Po_2$ | Elevated $Pco_2$, much reduced $Po_2$ |
| **Radiographic** | | |
| PA and lateral | Giant bulla or bilateral apical with crowding, no diffuse disease | Poorly defined bullae, diffuse emphysema, no crowding |
| Earlier films | Rapid progression, no infections | Few recent changes, many infections |
| Expiration films | Good chest wall and diaphragmatic motion, marked obscuration of surrounding lung | Little difference from inspiration film |
| Perfusion scan | Well-localized defects | Diffuse multiple defects |
| Angiogram | Well-defined bullae, elsewhere intact vasculature with crowding | Vaguely defined bullae, elsewhere disrupted vasculature, no crowding |
| Computed tomography | Large well-defined bullae with crowded vascularity, signs of praseptal emphysema | Multiple, ill-defined bullae, interspersed much diffuse emphysema, no paraseptal lesions |

dyspnea with unequivocal compression of relatively normal underlung lung tissue that we have treated surgically without mortality, all with documented improvement.[8]

## PATIENTS AND METHODS

All were ambulatory and had unequivocal evidence of compression and displacement by large bullae of relatively uninvolved lung.[7,8] Patients with air spaces or hypertransradiance not due to bullous emphysema, including those with congenital cystic disease, bronchogenic cysts, cystic bronchiectasis, lobar emphysema, or blebs associated with pneumothorax simplex, were excluded from this group. Also excluded were patients with bullae who had tuberculosis, eosinophilic granuloma, and interstitial fibrosis. Seventeen were men, and two were women. All were or had been long-time smokers and were studied with plain chest films, bronchograms, and/or tomograms and angiograms to identify compression of relatively unaffected lung. During the past decade, perfusion lung scans and CT have been added to the diagnostic armamentarium. Before being considered for operation, patients had been intensively treated by medical means with continued incapacitation. Complete pulmonary function studies before and after operation were performed in all patients. Forced vital capacity (FVC) and forced expiratory volume ($FEV_1$) were used to measure ventilatory function, and all patients had preoperative evidence of airway obstruction with $FEV_1$/FVC below 60%.[8] Lung volumes were measured by helium dilution and were one and one half times predicted values or more.

## SURGICAL TECHNIQUE

Cessation of smoking is strongly encouraged. Double-lumen Carlen intubation is now routine. Standard lateral thoracotomy is employed for unilateral disease, while midsternotomy may be used for simultaneous resection of bilateral disease.[9,10] Once bullae are exposed, only the diseased lung is resected, preserving all nonbullous tissue. The bases of the resected bullae are closed with careful stapling, and any gross remaining air leaks are additionally treated with fine absorbable buttressed sutures. If bullae have narrow bases, they can be ligated with a single suture rather than closed with staples. Meticulous closure of the bases of excised bullae is most important, since postoperative air leak is the principle complication of surgery for bullous emphysema. Two large chest tubes are placed, with care taken that at least one reaches the apex of the thorax. Lobectomy is not indicated, in our opinion, since the disease process does not generally totally involve such an anatomic segment, and every attempt to preserve relatively uninvolved lung should be made. Whether laser ablation is superior awaits more experience and supportive data. Two or three chest tubes are often mandatory, and postoperative ventilatory assistance with a respirator may be necessary. Careful attention to tracheal toilet and early postoperative intubation of unresolved air spaces is vigorously pursued. Intermittently changing suction to simple underwater drainage may be helpful in controlling persistent leaks, but suction is always employed initially. Postoperative tracheostomy is rarely necessary and is to be avoided if possible. Bilateral staged operations are ideally spaced at least 4–6 weeks apart and are only performed at the same hospitalization when the remaining disease shifts the mediastum to the operative side, thus necessitating early removal of the opposite upper lobe bullae. Bilateral operation though a midsternotomy may be better tolerated than formerly thought because respiratory function is less deranged and thus may be less invasive than lateral thoracotomy.

## SURGERY FOR PNEUMOTHORAX IN EMPHYSEMA

Approximately one third of patients with bullous emphysema experience pneumothorax that far exceeds its incidence in unselected patients with chronic obstructive pulmonary disease. Pneumothorax in such patients is often a serious complication requiring emergency surgery. In bullous emphysema there is no viable lung tissue to allow healing, resulting in prolonged air leaks unresponsive to closed-tube suction. If bullae are mistaken for pneumothorax and treated by tube suction, severe consequences may result. Stapling of apical bullous leaks can most conservatively be approached by transaxillary incision or even by thoracoscopy.

## MONALDI TUBE DRAINAGE

The initial patient who first sparked our interest in the treatment of bullous emphysema was a bedridden, oxygen-dependent smoker whose chest film showed no lung markings over the right lung field. He was considered to have one large bulla occupying the right hemithorax (Fig. 14–1). Because of skepticism about the safety of thoracotomy in such a poor-risk patient, it was elected to treat the bulla or bullae with Monaldi tube drainage.[11–13] Under local anesthesia a 1-in. piece of midaxillary rib was excised and the wound packed with iodoform gauze. Two weeks later the gauze was removed, and a suction catheter was placed through the adhesed area into the bullae. Over the next week a reaction was noted in the right hemithorax with expansion of the underlying lung. The tube was removed at this time, after which the lower and middle lobes of the right lung were noted to be expanded, filling the hemithorax with normal-appearing lung markings (Fig. 14–2). The patient's improvement was dramatic, and he achieved an exercise tolerance to walking two blocks without oxygen compared with a previous totally bedridden, oxygen-dependent existence. This improvement was sustained for 2 years, at which time the patient was lost to follow-up.

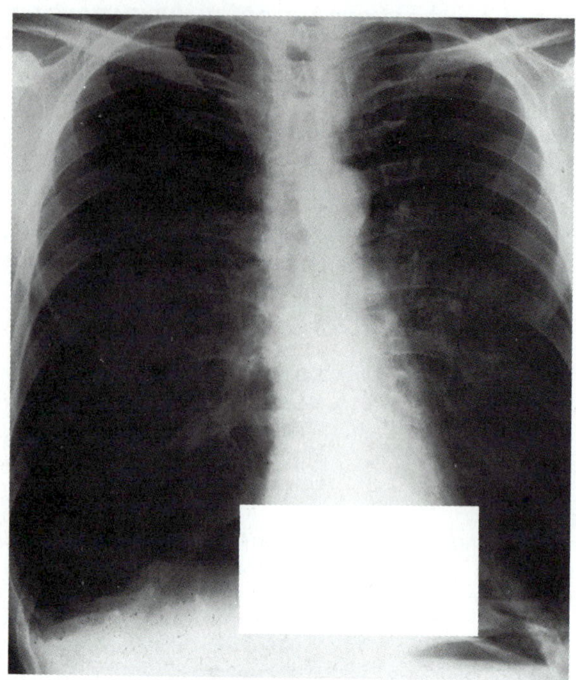

**Figure 14–1.** Chest film showing bullae occupying entire right lung field.

## RESULTS

All 19 patients survived 32 staged operations and were clinically improved, in most cases dramatically so. The clinical improvement was documented by both preoperative and

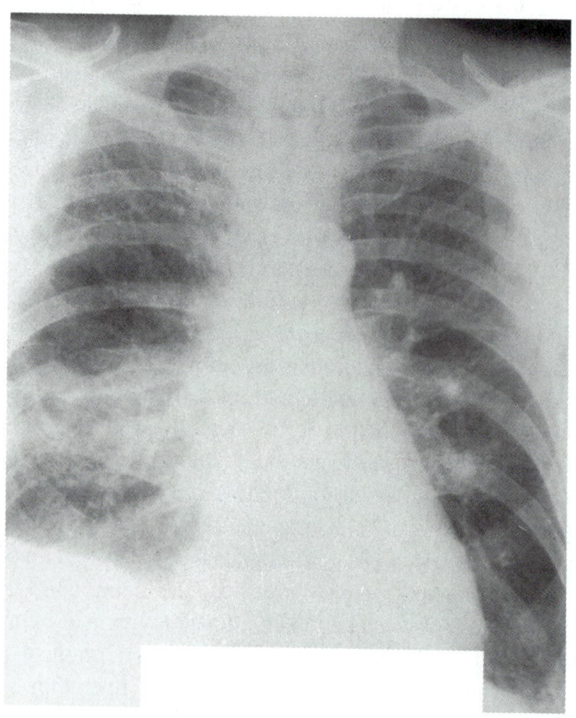

**Figure 14–2.** Full expansion of relatively normal appearing right lung of patient in Figure 14–1, 2 months after Monaldi tube suction.

postoperative pulmonary function testing. Patient follow-up varied from 3 to 22 years, during which time the initial symptomatic improvement in these patients was surprisingly maintained. Three patients have been selected to demonstrate particular features of bullectomy for emphysema.

## ILLUSTRATIVE CASES

### Case 1

This was a 55-year-old male smoker with an 8-year history of dyspnea, especially progressive the last few months. Respirations were labored at 32/min with an enlarged, tender liver. Chest film showed absent markings in both upper lung fields (Fig. 14–3). Pulmonary function studies revealed severe obstructive disease with hyperinflation and volume response to bronchodilation, low diffusing capacity, poor intrapulmonary gas mixing, and mild hypoxemia. Tomograms (Fig. 14–4A) and angiography (Fig. 14–4B) show loss of vascularity of most of the left and right upper lung fields with bilateral compression of normal lower lung tissue. The left lung appeared to be most involved and was selected for operation. At posterolateral thoracotomy, 90% of the left upper lobe and lingula were involved with large bullae (Fig. 14–5). There were also a small number of bullae along the upper margin of the superior segment of the lower lobe. All bullae were excised and their bases closed with staples and oversewn with fine absorbable suture. Air leaks sealed in 7 days. Diagnosis of excised tissue was bullous emphysema and bronchitis. Clinical improvement at 3 months was significant as were postsurgical function tests (Table 14–3).

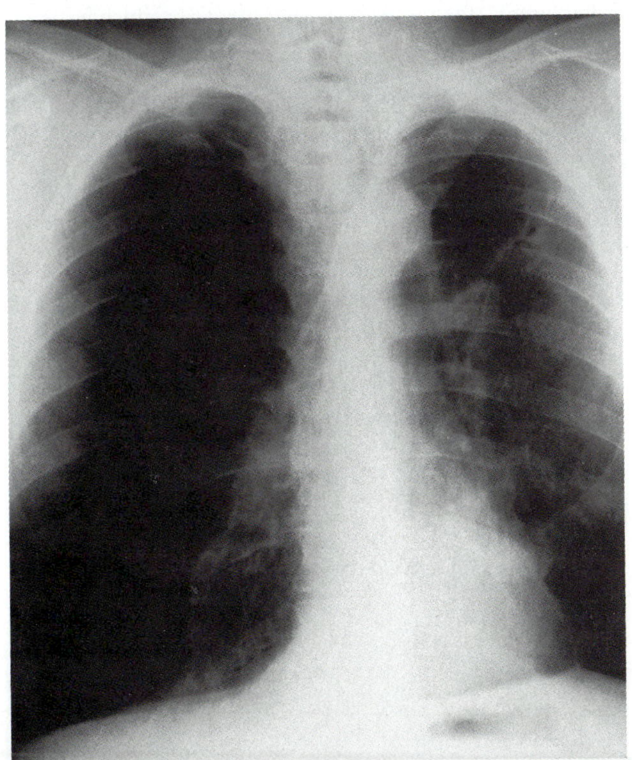

**Figure 14–3.** Preoperative chest film in case 1 showing absence of lung markings in upper halves of chest and suggestion of compression of both lower lobes.

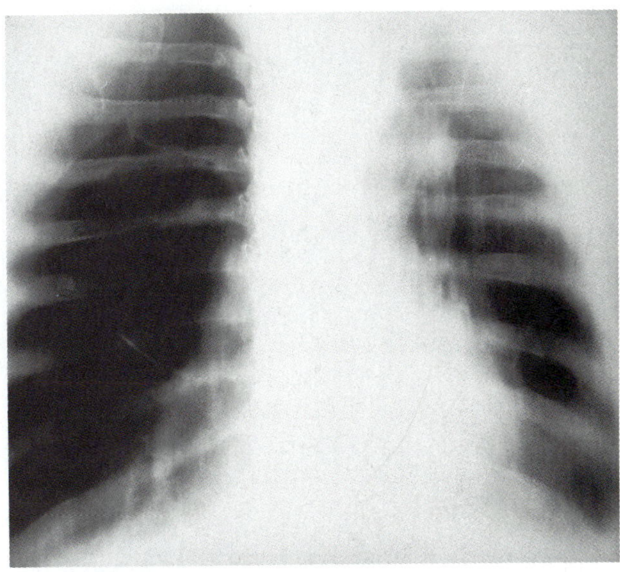

**A**

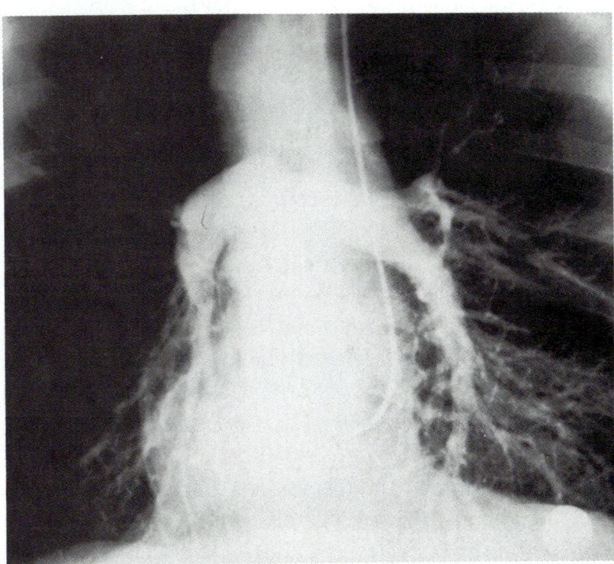

**B**

**Figure 14–4.** Whole lung tomogram (**A**) and pulmonary angiogram (**B**) showing absence of vessels in upper lung fields and compression of vessels of lower lobes.

Twelve years later the patient experienced right pneumothorax that resolved. Angiography showed absent vascularity of the right upper lobe and good but displaced vascularity of the lower lobe. At right thoracotomy, large bullae of the upper lobe and small bullae of the upper margins of the middle and lower lobes were excised. Ventilator assis-

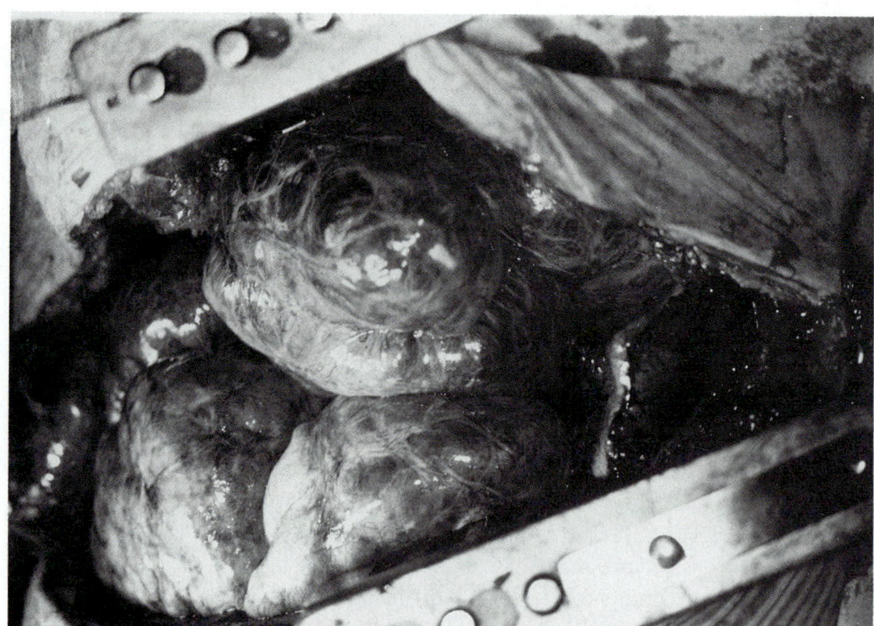

**Figure 14–5.** Large bullae of left upper lobe and lingula. Note tip of normal lower lobe on the right.

tance was required for 4 days and tube suction for 19 days. The patient was doing well 5 years later, 17 years after the first bullectomy. Figure 14–6 is a followup chest film, and Figure 14–7 is the CT scan showing some residual bullae but with relatively normal encompassed lower lobes.

## Case 2

This was a 44-year-old male smoker with a 10-year history of severe dyspnea. The patient could breathe free of pain only when leaning forward (Fig. 14–8). A chest film showed absence of markings in the upper half of both lung fields (Fig. 14–9). Pulmonary function testing and angiograms confirmed the diagnosis of bullous emphysema with crowding of apparently bleb-free lower lobes. Pulmonary function studies are shown in Table 14–4. The more diseased right lung was selected for initial bullectomy. At lateral thoracotomy most of the upper lobe and the upper margins of the middle and lower lobes were involved with "cotton candy" bullous disease. After excision, their bases were closed with staples and simple ligature. Ventilatory assistance was required for 5 days, and air leaks persisted for 10 days. Following the second operation the patient was able to walk 1 mile without stopping but still had shortness of breath with much exertion. Therefore, a left thoracotomy was performed, and, like the right lung, most

**TABLE 14–3. CASE 1: RESULTS OF PULMONARY FUNCTION TESTS**

| | Predicted | Preop | Postop |
|---|---|---|---|
| Date | 9/71 | 9/71 | 12/71 |
| VC (L) | 3.92 | 2.61 | 2.96 |
| $FEV_1$ (L) | 2.98 | 1.18 | 1.79 |
| MVV (L/min) | 137 | 45 | 66 |
| TLC (He) (L) | 5.77 | 6.18 | 5.82 |
| TLC (BB) (L) | 5.77 | — | — |
| $D_LCO$ (mL/mm Hg/min) | 26.1 | 11.1 | 14.8 |
| $Pa{O_2}$ (mm Hg) | 80 | 74 | 88 |

VC = vital capacity; FEV, forced expiratory volume; MVV = maximal voluntary ventilations; TLC = total lung capacity; HE = helium; BB = body box; $D_LCO$ = carbon monoxide diffusion in the lungs; $Pa{O_2}$ = arterial oxygen tension.

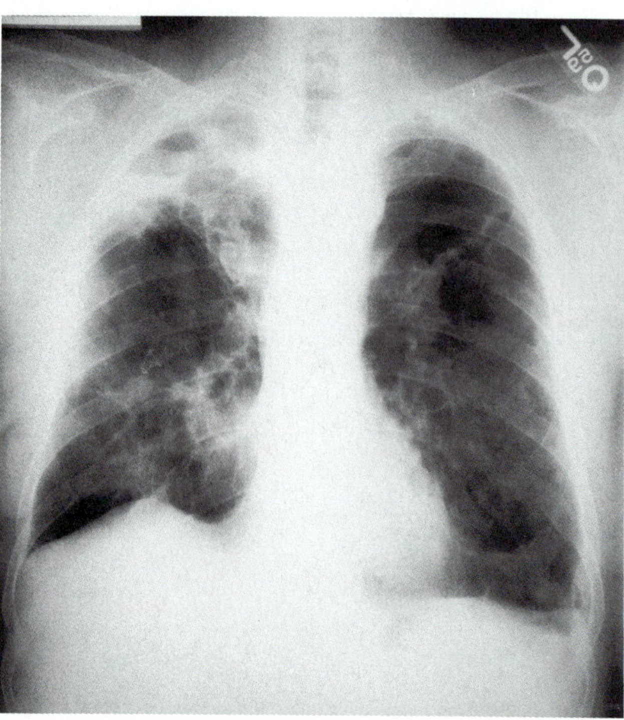

**Figure 14–6.** Chest film in case 1, 17 years after original bilateral bullectomies.

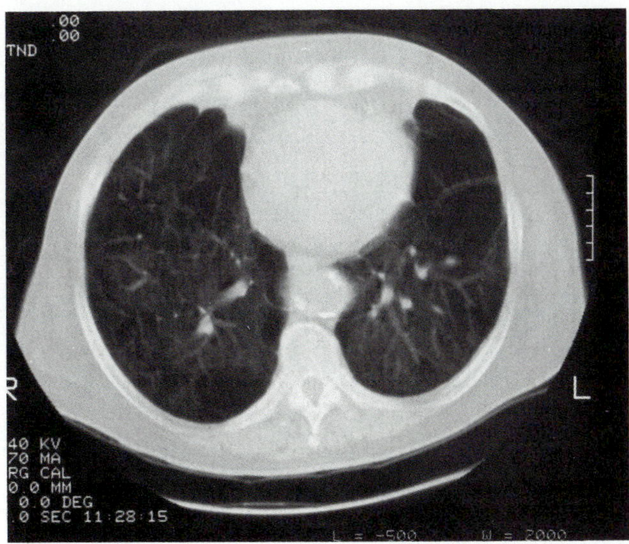


**Figure 14–7.** CT scan 17 years after bilateral bullectomies. Note residual small bullae and relatively normal lower lobes.

of the upper lobe and upper margin of the lower lobe was noted to be involved with bullous disease. Excision and repair were performed as on the right lung. Ventilatory assistance was required for 48 hours and chest tubes for 9 days. Exercise tolerance increased significantly, and he could now climb two flights of stairs without shortness of breath. Pulmonary function studies after both operations are shown in Table 14–4. Five years after operation the patient was still doing well.

## Case 3

A 40-year-old male smoker presented with severe dyspnea. A chest film showed translucency of the upper half of the right-lung field interpreted as pneumothorax (Fig. 14–10). A chest tube was inserted by the medical service without improvement. More careful review of the film suggested bullous emphysema. Figure 14–11 is a computed tomogram showing large bullae in the left upper lobe and smaller bullae in the right upper lobe with lower lobe crowding. Pulmonary function studies showed large residual volume and total lung capacity consistent with bullae (Table 14–5). At right posterolateral thoracotomy, "cotton candy" bullous disease found replacing most of the upper lobe and superior margin of the middle lobe was excised and stapled (Fig. 14–12). Subsequently the patient was completely free of symptoms for a 9-year follow-up period (Fig. 14–13).

## DISCUSSION

Though there is no way in vivo to recognize with certainty the type of emphysema producing bullae of the lung, the term *bullous emphysema* is firmly established in clinical nomenclature. The key to good results in the surgical treatment of bullous emphysema is proper selection of patients.[7,8,14] In all of our operated patients there was unequivocal preoperative evidence of compression and displacement of relatively normal lower-lobe lung tissue. By removal of the nonfunctioning bullous disease, the compressed lower lobes were allowed to expand to increase the patient's ventilatory reserve and thereby result in successful operation. Though there are a number of diagnostic tests to ascertain lower-lobe compression, including bronchograms, lung perfusion studies and CT, angiography,[15] and whole-lung CT,[16] most clearly identify compression or displacement of disease-free lower lobes. Because most patients with bullous emphysema who have symptoms are poor-risk patients, often with cor pulmonale, the small but real risk of angiography[17] favors the use of CT to identify lower-lobe compression.

If the patient's condition is improved by the expansion of compressed functional tissue, even the most ill patients with the poorest reserve can undergo bullectomy with low risk, as shown by case 2. However, if the patient is bedrid-

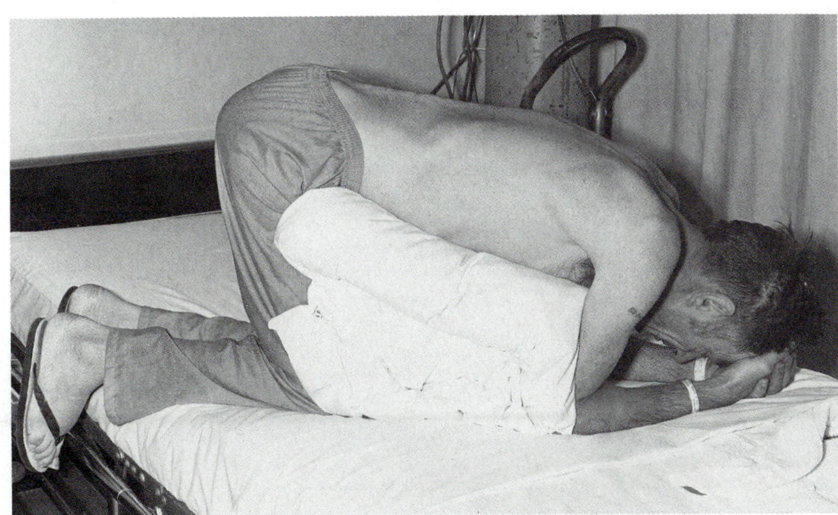

**Figure 14–8.** Preoperative photo of patient 2 showing the only postural position in which breathing was comfortable.

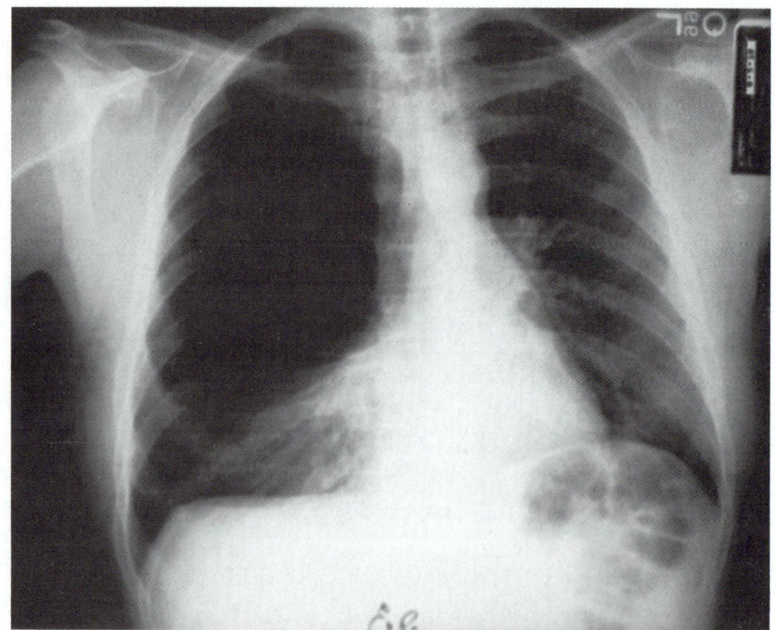

**Figure 14–9.** Chest film of case 2 showing absence of lung markings in upper half of both lung fields consistent with bullous emphysema of upper lobes.

den and receiving continuous oxygen therapy, Monaldi intracavitary suction drainage is a considerably lesser procedure than thoracotomy and may be successful, as seen in patient 1. Monaldi pioneered this procedure to relieve tension in tuberculous cavities.[11] It was first used for emphysematous blebs by Alexander in 1946 and reported by Avery and Head[12] in 1949. Although Monaldi tube suction was initially performed in two to three stages with rib resection and iodoform gauze packing as preliminary steps (as used in our first patient), it can now be performed in one stage. A small piece of rib is resected, and a pursestring absorbable suture is placed that encompasses both the pleura and cyst wall. Within the purse string sutures, a large Foley catheter is inserted and 5–20 Hg suction applied for 36–48 hours, followed by underwater seal for 21 days.[13] Multiple small bronchiolar leaks may close during this period as a result of the inevitable secondary infection with resultant collapse of bullae. The main complication of the technique is a bronchopleural cutaneous fistula, so we prefer to remove the tube as soon as intracavitary inflammation is noted.

In all of our patients, clinical and physiologic early pulmonary improvement was seen and persisted for some years even though most patients continued to smoke. Some eventual deterioration often occurred and was the reason for subsequently removing contralateral bullae.

Wesley et al[18] stated that in their experience, the type of bullae is not as important as whether the bullae significantly embarrassed the function of adjacent lung tissue. They determined this by posteroanterior and lateral chest films on inspiration and expiration, bilateral tomograms, measurements of vital capacity, and forced expiratory volume, as well as transfer factor of carbon dioxide and perfusion lung scans with indium. They had their best surgical results in patients with minimal cough and sputa, localized

**TABLE 14–4. CASE 2: RESULTS OF PULMONARY FUNCTION TESTS**

| | Predicted | Preop | Postop: First Operation (Test 1) | Postop: Second Operation (Test 2) |
|---|---|---|---|---|
| Date | 4/83 | 4/83 | 7/83 | 4/88 |
| VC (L) | 3.31 | 2.18 | 2.84 | 2.97 |
| $FEV_1$ (L) | 2.00 | 0.45 | 1.21 | 0.8 |
| MVV (L/min) | 108 | 26 | 45 | 33 |
| TLC (He) (L) | 5.64 | 4.48 | 4.69 | 4.34 |
| TLC (BB) (L) | 5.64 | 7.62 | 5.47 | 5.91 |
| $D_LCO$ (mL/mmHg/min) | 21.2 | 6.5 | 9.9 | 13.1 |
| $PaO_2$ (mm Hg) | 75 | 67 | 73 | 68 |

For abbreviations see Table 14–3.

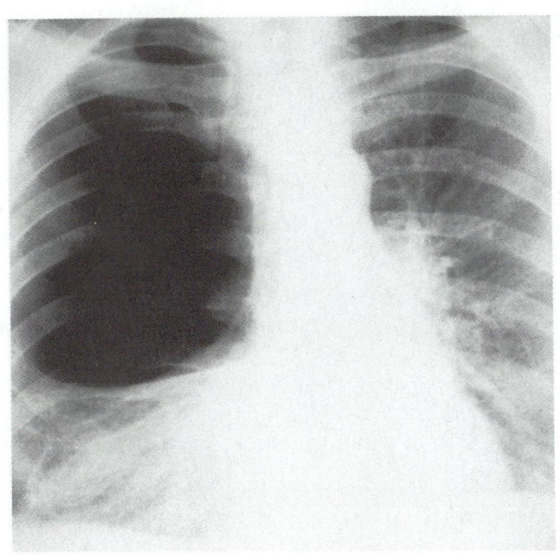

**Figure 14–10.** Chest film of case 3 showing translucency of upper half of right lung field interpreted initially as pneumothorax.

**TABLE 14–5. CASE 3: RESULTS OF PULMONARY FUNCTION**

| | Predicted | Preop | Postop |
|---|---|---|---|
| Date | 12/71 | 12/71 | 10/72 |
| VC (L) | 4.17 | 1.39 | 2.58 |
| $FEV_1$ (L) | 3.32 | 0.56 | 1.19 |
| MVV (L/min) | 151 | 21 | 53 |
| TLC (BB) (L) | 5.77 | — | 5.60 |
| $D_LCO$ (mL/mm Hg/min) | 28.3 | 7.6 | 15.1 |
| $Pao_2$ (mm Hg) | 80 | 51 | 88 |

For abbreviations see Table 14–3.

bullous disease, and evidence of compression of adjacent lung tissue. In such patients, the long-term stability of improved results was impressive.

Fitzgerald and associates[19] reported long-term results in 84 patients who underwent 95 surgical procedures over a period of 23 years. Their best results were with giant bullae simply excised in patients with lesser degrees of obstructive lung disease. Their poorest results were in patients with smaller bullae, diffuse emphysema, and severe bronchitis undergoing lobectomy. They also found that improved function was maintained in some cases for up to 20 years after bullectomy.

Rojas-Miranda and associates[20] reported 108 operations for bullous emphysema, including 14 with bilateral simultaneous lung excisions with no operative deaths. They state that poor-risk patients are acceptable if there is demonstrable compression of normal lung, and six of their patients underwent emergency operation.

Potgieter and colleagues[21] stated that in their 20 surgical patients, improvement was due to allowing compressed lung tissue to reexpand and less commonly by reducing functional residual capacity or by removing dead space. Their conclusion was that operation was justified if patients have symptoms and there is good evidence of compression.

Pearson and Ogilvie[22] reported on 12 patients undergoing bullectomy with a 5–10-year follow-up. Half of their patients had a preoperative $FEV_1$ of less than 1 L. They found that in most patients the benefit lasted more than 5 years and that removal of bullae did not hasten the progress of the underlying emphysema.

With the advent of video-directed thoracoscopic surgical techniques, some investigators[23–25] have recently revisited the surgical approach to patients with more diffuse emphysema. Bullae of various sizes have been excised,

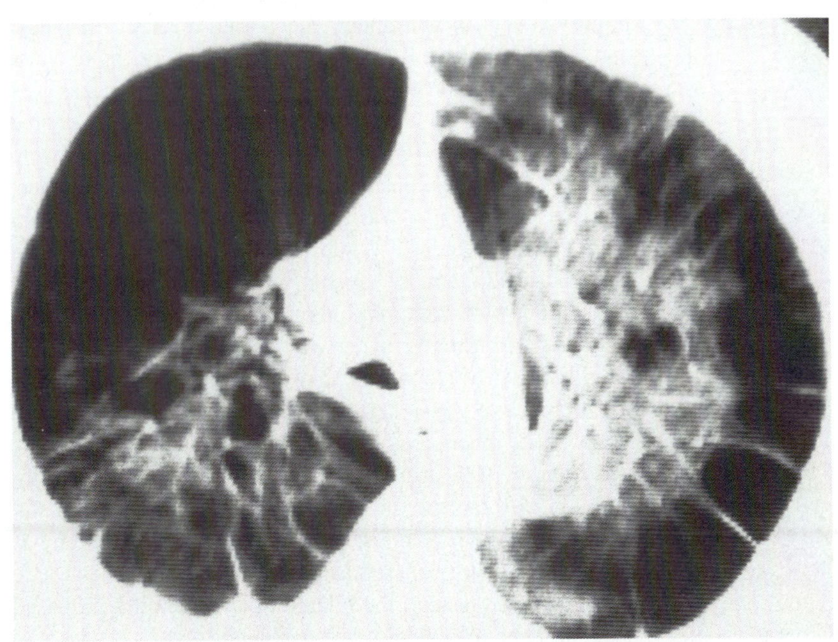

**Figure 14–11.** Computed tomogram of case 2 showing large bullae of left upper lobe and smaller bullae of right upper lobe, both with lower-lobe compression.

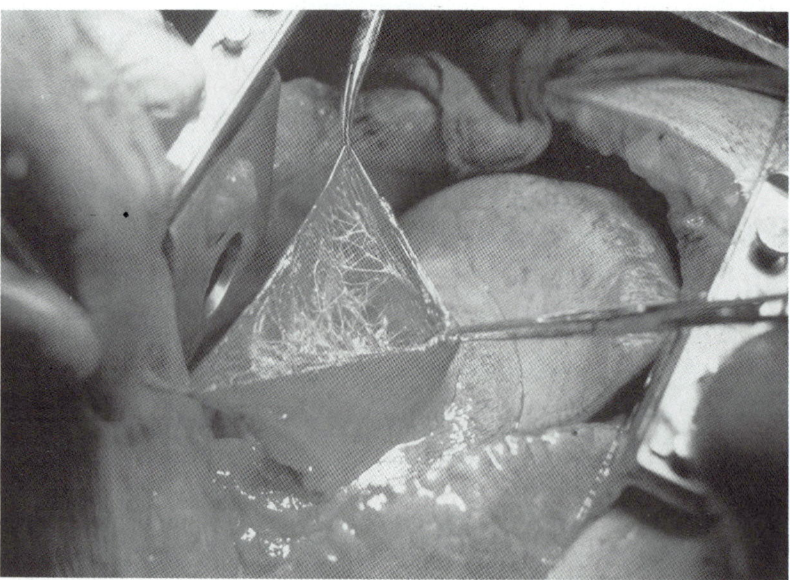

**Figure 14–12.** Cotton-candy-like bullae of right upper lobe in case 3.

destroyed, or plicated with various types of lasers and also by conventional direct ligation or stapling through a thoracoscope. While this technique obviously can be supported as an alternative method for excision of giant bullae that compress relatively normal lung, expanded application to patients with multiple bullae and underlying general emphysema is not yet clear. Early experience has indicated subjective improvement, but adequate data regarding objective improvement is still scant. Brenner and associates[26] have attempted to define criteria for selection of patients who may benefit from resection of less defined bullous disease. To do so, they extensively studied 19 survivors of 24 patients who underwent thorascopic carbon dioxide laser ablation of bullous emphysema. As might have been predicted, patients with large bullae accompanied by crowding of adjacent lung structures, upper-lobe predominance, and minimal emphysema had the greatest improvement from laser bullectomy. However, some patients with multiple smaller bullae and diffuse emphysema also demonstrated objective improvement after operation.

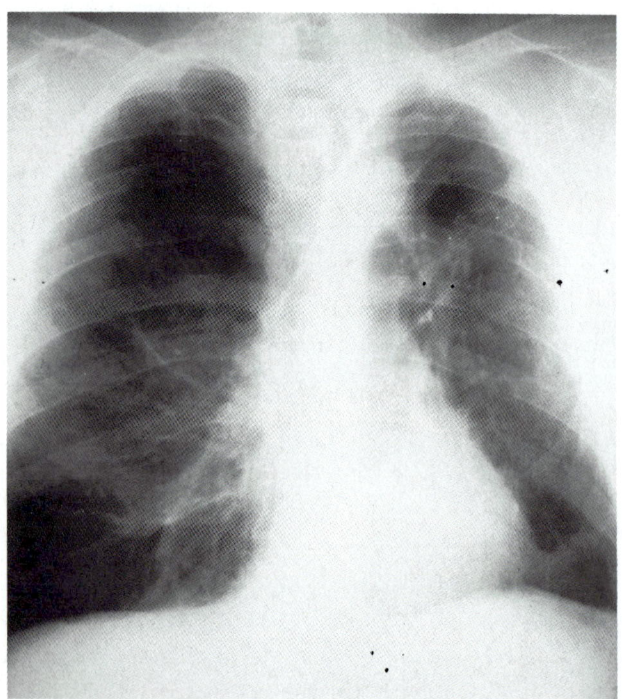

**Figure 14–13.** Nine-year follow-up chest film in case 3.

Pulmonary function testing in these patients showed improvements in spirometry, decreased airway resistance, and decreased specific conductance; however, there were no significant changes in resting gas exchange. Air leak was the major cause of morbidity. All patients had some degree of air leak lasting from 1 to 37 days. Three patients were discharged from the hospital with Heimlich valves in place. Median hospital stay was 26 days with an average of 6.5 days in intensive care. While aggressive extension of thorascopic techniques to patients who do not have classical large bullae with compression of relatively nonemphysematous lung is currently underway by several groups,[23–25] it would appear prudent to reserve such operations until thorough objective physiologic data is available to substantiate the benefits of procedures that currently may carry a mortality rate of 10% or higher. Also, it is not clear if laser ablation is preferable to simple bleb ligation or buttressed stapling, and whether thoracoscopic or open thoracotomy is the preferred surgical approach to the bullae.

As stated earlier, the bilateral pneumectomy proposed by Cooper et al[6] may also be worthwhile.

## REFERENCES


1. American Thoracic Society: Chronic bronchitis, asthma, and pulmonary emphysema: A statement by the Committee on Diagnostic Standards for Non-Tuberculosis Respiratory Disease. *Am Rev Respir Dis* **85**:762–768, 1962
2. Thurlbeck WM: Morphology of emphysema and emphysema-like conditions in chronic airflow obstructions in lung disease. In: *Chronic Airflow Obstruction in Lung Disease.* Philadelphia, Saunders, 1976, pp 96–234
3. Gaensler EA, Jederlinic PJ, Fitzgerald MX: Patient work-up for bullectomy. *J Thorac Imaging* **1**:75–93, 1986
4. Knudson RJ, Gaensler EA: Surgery for emphysema. *Ann Thorac Surg* **1**:332–362, 1965
5. Brantigan OE, Muller E, Dress MO: A surgical approach to bullous emphysema. *Am Rev Resp Dis* **80**:194–204, 1959
6. Cooper JD, Trulock EP, Triantafillou AN, Patterson GA, Pohl MS, Deloney RN, Sundaresan RS, Roper CL: Bilateral pneumectomy (volume reduction) for chronic obstructive pulmonary disease. *J Thorac Cardiovasc Surg* **109**:106–119, 1995
7. Laros CD, Gelissen HJ, Bergstein PGM, et al: Bullectomy for giant bullae in emphysema. *J Thorac Cardiovasc Surg* **91**:63–70, 1986
8. Connolly JE, Wilson A: The current status of surgery for bullous emphysema. *J Thorac Cardiovasc Surg* **97**:351–361, 1989
9. Iwa T, Watanabe Y, Fukatain G: Simultaneous bilateral operations for bullous emphysema by median sternotomy. *J Thorac Cardiovasc Surg* **81**:732–737, 1981
10. Lima O, Ramos L, DiBiasi P, Judice L, Cooper JD: Median sternotomy for bilateral resection of emphysematous bullae. *J Thorac Cardiovasc Surg* **8**:892–897, 1981
11. Monaldi V: Endocavitary aspiration: Its practical applications. *Tubercule* 28:223–228, 1947
12. Head JR, Avery EF: Intracavitary suction (Monaldi) in the treatment of emphysematous bullae and blebs. *J Thorac Surg* **18**:761–776, 1949
13. MacArthur AM, Fountain SW: Intracavitary suction and drainage in the treatment of emphysematous bullae. *Thorax* **32**:668–672, 1977
14. Hugh-Jones P, Whimster W: The etiology and management of disabling emphysema. *Am Rev Respir Dis* **117**:343–378, 1978
15. Jensen KM, Miscall L, Steinberg I: Angiocardiography in bullous emphysema: its role in selection of the case suitable for surgery. *Am J Roentgenol* **85**:229–245, 1961
16. Bergin CJ, Muller NL, Miller RR: CT in the qualitative assessment of emphysema. *J Thorac Imaging* **1**:94–103, 1986
17. Stein MA, Winter J, Grollman JR Jr: The value of the pulmonary-artery seeking catheter in percutaneous selective pulmonary arteriography. *Radiology* **114**:299–304, 1975
18. Wesley JR, Macleod WM, Mullard KS: Evaluation and surgery of bullous emphysema. *J Thorac Cardiovasc Surg* **63**:945–955, 1972
19. Fitzgerald MX, Keelan PJ, Cugell DW, Gaensler EA: Long-term results of surgery for bullous emphysema. *J Thorac Cardiovasc Surg* **68**:566–587, 1974
20. Rojas-Miranda A, Ranson-Bilker B, Levasseur P, et al: Chirurgie de l'emphyseme bulleux de l' adulte: A propos de 95 cas. *Ann Chir Thorac Cardiovasc* **13**:143–153, 1974
21. Potgieter PD, Benatar SR, Hewiston R, Ferguson AD: Surgical treatment of bullous lung disease. *Thorax* **36**:885–890, 1981
22. Pearson MG, Ogilvie C: Surgical treatment of emphysematous bullae: Late outcome. *Thorax* **38**:134–137, 1983
23. Wakabayashi A, Brenner M, Kayaleh RA, et al: Thoracoscopic carbon dioxide laser treatment of bullous emphysema. *Lancet* **337**: 881–883, 1991
24. Wakabayashi A: Surgical technique for management of giant bullous lung disease. *Ann Thorac Surg* **56**:708–712, 1993
25. Lewis RJ, Caccavale RJ, Sisler GE: VATS-Argon beam coagulator treatment of diffuse end-stage bilateral bullous disease of the lung. *Ann Thorac Surg* **55**:1394–1399, 1993
26. Brenner M, Kayaleh RA, Milne E, et al: Thoracoscopic laser ablation of pulmonary bullae. *J Thorac Cardiovasc Surg* **107**:883–890, 1994

CHAPTER

15

# Diagnosis of Benign, Diffuse Pulmonary Disease

Thomas M. Hyers and Carlos W.M. Bedrossian

## INTRODUCTION AND HISTORICAL ASPECTS

The cardiothoracic surgeon usually encounters benign diffuse pulmonary disease in two settings. The first involves the surgeon's hospitalized patient who unfortunately develops an acute process such as diffuse pneumonia, cardiogenic pulmonary edema, or acute respiratory distress syndrome (ARDS). In this setting the surgeon's diagnostic and treating skills are necessary to ensure proper care of the patient, although a surgical procedure will likely not be necessary. In the second setting, the cardiothoracic surgeon is called to consult on a patient with an acute undiagnosed diffuse pulmonary infiltrate or on an outpatient with a baffling, chronic diffuse infiltrate. Often in this setting, less invasive diagnostic procedures will have already been performed and been unrevealing. The cardiothoracic surgeon will be asked to perform a bronchoscopy or an open-lung biopsy. In considering open-lung biopsy, the cardiothoracic surgeon must be familiar with the differential diagnosis of acute and chronic diffuse pulmonary diseases. Furthermore, the surgeon must understand the variety of biochemical, microbiologic, histologic, cytologic, and ultrastructural techniques available to aid in the diagnosis and be prepared to work closely with the pathologist and others to ensure proper procurement and handling of the specimens.

The historical aspects of the diagnosis of diffuse pulmonary disease are instructive. Until the introduction of fiberoptic bronchoscopy and transbronchial lung biopsy some 30 years ago, thoracotomy was the only reliable way to obtain lung tissue for diagnosis. The procedure was associated with enough morbidity and mortality that it was infrequently performed and then only in relatively stable patients. The advent of transbronchial lung biopsy greatly enlarged the indications for lung biopsy, but the procedure is limited by the small amount of tissue obtained and by the operator's inability to see the area being biopsied. In the last 15 years fine-needle aspiration (FNA) with computerized tomographic guidance has further revolutionized our capability for pulmonary diagnosis, but this technique is mainly limited to cytologic and microbiologic specimens. As these newer diagnostic procedures were being developed, the wider application of organ transplantation resulted in a large increase in immunosuppressed patients, some of whom develop opportunistic infections and other types of pulmonary infiltrative diseases. The need for larger histologic as well as cytologic and microbiologic specimens in these and other patients was not adequately met until the widespread use of thoracoscopic lung biopsy in the past few years. These procedures together offer unprecedented access to lung tissue for diagnosis and to guide therapy. With the advent of molecular and genetic diagnostic techniques, these procedures will find even greater application. This chapter is intended to give the reader an approach to the differential diagnosis of these diseases and to procedures and techniques used in their diagnosis.

## THE COMPREHENSIVE APPROACH TO DIAGNOSIS

In order to arrive at an accurate diagnosis, the surgeon has to interpret correctly physical signs and symptoms, laboratory data, and the results of a myriad of special studies. These range from noninvasive imaging techniques to invasive and semi-invasive procedures to obtain fluids, cells, and tissues from the lung. In this endeavor the surgeon works closely with the radiologist, who should be familiar with the intricate anatomy of the thorax, and the pathologist, who should be versed in pulmonary microbiology, cytopathology, and histopathology.[1] In a select number of diseases, specialized diagnostic techniques are required such as electron microscopy, immunocytochemistry, image analysis, and flow cytometry. Both old and new techniques have their advantages and disadvantages, and it is our purpose to explore the usefulness of the various methods in the diagnosis of lung diseases. Major areas to be addressed include (1) role of history and physical examination in diagnosis, (2) routine laboratory testing and interpretation, (3) the classification of diffuse benign pulmonary diseases, and (4) specialized diagnostic techniques and their applications. As noted throughout the chapter, correlation between clinical data and pathologic findings is crucial for the understanding of disease processes and the institution of effective therapy. Cooperation between surgeon and pathologist starts with a preprocedural discussion of the most adequate strategy to follow in a given clinical situation. It extends to assisted collection of specimens such as thoracoscopic, bronchoscopic, and transcutaneous fine-needle aspiration (FNA) biopsies, which should be handled expeditiously in order to be of significance in patient management. And it culminates with discussion of the findings, often over the double-headed microscope, so that the histologic and cytologic features can be correlated lucidly to the patient's symptoms. This clinicopathologic approach is enriched by frequent meetings, which include the participation of surgeons, radiologists, and other specialists interested in lung disease.

## THE HISTORY AND PHYSICAL EXAMINATION

A careful log of occupational exposures, drug use, and family history is essential in patients with diffuse pulmonary disease. The history is often the only way the duration of the process can be gauged, and it is also the best way to judge its severity. The history frequently gives clues to etiology as well. This occupational history should include work extending back 20 or 30 years because of the long latency period of the pneumoconioses. Inhalation of chemicals or organic dust can cause wheezing and asthma-like symptoms. The breathing of respirable particles from the grinding or cutting of heavy metal or inhaling of silica or asbestos fibers can initiate a diffuse interstitial pulmonary process over years. The drug history should focus particularly on the use of any antineoplastic drugs, antiarrhythmics, antibiotics, and thiazide diuretics. However, a drug as seemingly innocuous as aspirin can also cause interstitial lung disease and pulmonary edema, and a careful history of the use of over-the-counter preparations is therefore essential. Asthma and chronic obstructive pulmonary disease (COPD), particularly when associated with $\alpha_1$-antitrypsin deficiency, tend to cluster in families. There are congenital and familial clusters of interstitial lung disease as well. A family history of recurrent infections, fetal wastage, or neonatal death can help in the diagnosis of such diseases as cystic fibrosis or Kartagener's syndrome, which can lead to bronchiectasis and chronic lung disease. The smoking history should be quantified as to number of packs smoked daily over years. It is essential to document the use of other tobacco products, because snuff has been associated with cancer of the upper aero-digestive tract. Marijuana, too, has been associated with chronic bronchitis, and other illicit drugs, particularly when injected intravenously, can cause pulmonary vasculitis and interstitial disease.

### Respiratory Symptoms

Dyspnea and cough are the most common respiratory symptoms. Chest pain, wheezing, and hemoptysis also are frequent complaints. Dyspnea should be assessed semiquantitatively as to the extent of exercise necessary to provoke it. Changes in dyspnea patterns are important to judge progression of disease. Many more people with asthma cough than wheeze, and, for the most part, chronic cough should not be dismissed as psychogenic until the common physical causes have been investigated. Chest pain is less likely to be ignored by the patient than are dyspnea and cough. Pleuritic pain can be caused by processes that involve the pleural space and by those that involve the visceral pleura with adjacent irritation of the parietal pleura, where most of the pain receptors reside. Pain associated with pulmonary embolism can be pleuritic in nature or can mimic angina and must be distinguished from acute myocardial ischemia. Pain emanating from soft tissue, bone, or cartilage inflammation or from reflux of stomach acid into the esophagus can also mimic angina.

Hemoptysis is a frightening symptom and should always be investigated. Although it is most frequently associated with bronchitis in smokers, the finding of hemoptysis necessitates upper airway examination, indirect laryngoscopy, and bronchoscopy, unless it is clearly associated with a process such as acute pneumonia. The quantity and quality of the hemoptysis can vary from the rusty colored sputum of acute pneumonia to frank bleeding associated with bronchiectasis or with a fungus ball in a residual lung cavity. Vomited blood from the gastrointestinal tract can also be aspirated and expectorated. Consequently, when the usual diagnostic tests for unexplained hemoptysis have been negative, the upper gastrointestinal tract should also be investigated. Finally, focal bleeding, such as hemoptysis, that develops in a patient being anticoagulated for another reason should be investigated. Anticoagulants can cause bleeding from occult tumors, and the onset of hemoptysis may be the first sign of bronchogenic carcinoma in a patient receiving anticoagulants for deep venous thrombosis or another indication.

### Physical Examination

Many times more information can be gained from simply watching the patient's breathing pattern than from any other aspect of the physical examination. A rapid, shallow respiratory rate associated with flairing of the nasal alae, intercostal retractions, and strenuous use of the accessory respiratory muscles can indicate impending respiratory failure. A dyspneic patient leaning forward with hands fixed on thighs or with elbows braced against his or her bedside table and breathing shallowly with pursed lips often makes the diagnosis of emphysema for the examiner. Is the trachea midline? Do the chest walls expand and contract symmetrically? All this information can be obtained by inspection and will guide the examiner to a more precise completion of the chest physical examination. Palpation is useful for detecting areas of tenderness, uncovering adenopathy and assessing fremitus. Fremitus is simply the palpation of sound waves. In instances in which the auscultator hears increased transmission of sound, fremitus should also be increased; consequently, fremitus can be used to confirm the auscultated sounds in the physical examination. Percussion and auscultation should be performed horizontally across the chest and back rather than vertically, so that the examiner can test comparable areas of each lung. As can be seen from Table 15–1, careful utilization of the four components of the physical examination of the chest can usually distinguish most common pathologic abnormalities with the exception that a pleural effusion cannot be distinguished from an atelectatic or edematous portion of the lung that does not exchange air because of an occluded bronchus. The chest x-ray is an extension of the pulmonary physical examination. It is used to help confirm the examiner's suspicions derived from the physical examination and history. In the example cited above, it is particularly useful for distinguishing pleural effusion from atelectatic lung. Consequently, the physical examiner is truly accomplished when he or she has obtained some experience in interpreting the chest x-ray as well. This expertise is particularly important in the evaluation of the interstitial lung diseases, since the physical exam typically reveals little in these patients.

The physical examination of the lungs must be correlated to the remainder of the exam. The heart must be examined to assess for heart failure. Left heart failure typically presents with evidence of pulmonary congestion, whereas right heart failure presents with hepatomegaly, hepatojugular reflux, and peripheral edema. In a bedridden patient, peripheral edema may accumulate presacrally rather than in the legs. Cyanosis usually indicates 4–5 g of unsaturated hemoglobin per 100 mL of blood. Consequently, it is not well seen in anemic people who are hypoxemic, and it is not well seen in darkly pigmented people. In the latter it can be appreciated by examining the mucus membranes of the mouth. Clubbing of the fingertips is seen with non–small-cell carcinoma of the lung; with chronic suppurative lung processes such as bronchiectasis or lung abscess; and with certain of the interstitial pneumonias, particularly idiopathic fibrosis and asbestosis. It is also seen in any individual with a longstanding right to left shunt, either at the cardiac level or in an arteriovenous malformation in the lung. Clubbing is not seen with COPD or asthma and when present in these patients, another diagnosis must be entertained.

## ROUTINE AND SPECIALIZED LABORATORY TESTING

The triad of sputum, complete blood count, and urinalysis may reveal useful information in the diagnosis of lung disease. Overtly purulent, foul-smelling sputum is helpful to diagnose pneumonia or its complications, depending on the radiographic appearance of the chest. An increase in polymorphonuclear leukocytes in the peripheral blood is further corroboration of infection with pus-forming bacteria, while lymphocytosis favors viral infection or immunologic abnormalities. Tuberculosis and fungal infections commonly involve the lungs and are characterized by a mixed acute and chronic inflammatory response depending on whether the process is quiescent or reactivated. For the most part microbiologic procedures such as culture and direct smears are

**TABLE 15–1. PHYSICAL EXAMINATION OF THE THORAX**

| Abnormal Process | Inspection | Palpation | Percussion | Auscultation |
|---|---|---|---|---|
| Chronic interstitial lung disease | Hyperpnea | Normal function | Normal resonance | Normal or crackles |
| Acute pneumonia or pulmonary edema | Hyperpnea, splinting | ↑ Fremitus | Dullness | Bronchial sounds |
| Pleural effusion | Ipsilateral excursion | ↓ Fremitus | Dullness | ↓ Sounds |
| Atelectasis | Ipsilateral excursion | ↓ Fremitus | Dullness | ↓ Sounds |
| Asthma | Hyperpnea, nasal flaring | ↓ Fremitus | ↑ Resonance | Wheezing |
| Coronary obstructive pulmonary disease | ↑ AP diameter | ↓ Fremitus | ↑ Resonance | Wheezing |
| Pneumothorax | Ipsilateral ↓ excursion | ↓ Fremitus | Tympanic | ↓ Sounds |

needed to identify the mycobacterial and fungal species responsible for the infection. In certain circumstances the clinician may have to be able to perform and interpret the Gram's stain of sputum specimens. The finding of bacteria by Gram's stain of sputum is only significant if collection minimizes contamination from the upper airway.

Urinalysis is useful in the diagnosis of diseases with associated pulmonary and renal involvement such as the vasculitides, Wegener's granulomatosis, and Goodpasture's syndrome.[2] Patients in severe renal failure may develop uremic pneumonitis. In renal transplant patients pulmonary involvement is due mainly to opportunistic infections, but it may also result from immunosuppressive drugs the patient is receiving.[3] With the advent of cyclosporin this latter complication is much less frequent, even though the lung may be the site of graft versus host disease in kidney, heart, and bone marrow transplants.[4]

The laboratory examination in patients with diffuse interstitial pulmonary disease should include a complete blood count, a platelet count, and a urinalysis. Many times liver function tests and assessment of nutritional status are essential as well, so that an SMA-12 is often performed. In individuals with interstitial lung disease an anti-nuclear antibody, a rheumatoid factor, and an erythrocyte sedimentation rate can help to rule out connective tissue disease.[5] A white blood cell count differential is essential in these patients even if the white cell count is within normal limits because of the possibility of an eosinophilia-related syndrome. In this regard, a total eosinophil count is more sensitive in finding eosinophilia than is a routine differential count. Serum $\alpha_1$-antitrypsin and angiotensin converting enzyme (ACE) levels are useful in the diagnosis of emphysema and sarcoidosis, respectively.[6] In every case laboratory information must be correlated with the history and physical examination. After performance of a correlative analysis of this data, specialized tests may be necessary to complete the diagnostic workup.

Special tests include computerized tomography (CT) or magnetic resonance imaging (MRI), ultrasound examination of the thoracic content, fiberoptic bronchoscopy, thorascopic lung biopsy, fine-needle aspiration for diagnosis of infection, or cytology with a variety of attendant techniques. Computed tomography and magnetic resonance imaging (MRI) have revolutionized the noninvasive examination of the chest contents. Fiberoptic bronchoscopy has become even more specialized with the application of bronchoalveolar lavage[7] to corroborate the diagnosis of several interstitial diseases and the use of transbronchial fine-needle aspirates for the cytologic diagnosis of neoplasms.[8] Percutaneous fine-needle aspiration of the lung for cytologic and bacteriologic specimens utilizing CT or fluoroscopic guidance is now routine. Careful collaboration with professionals from pathology, cytology, and microbiology departments is essential to obtain maximal information from these studies. Lung cancer continues to be the most common neoplasm in males and has now surpassed breast cancer as a cause of death in females. These tumors may present as a mass, in a bronchioloalveolar neoplasm or in a lymphangitic pattern, and the latter two patterns should enter the differential diagnosis of diffuse pulmonary processes. The acquired immunodeficiency syndrome (AIDS) has become the most common cause of immunosuppression.[9] In addition, the increased use of immunosuppressive drugs, as organ transplantation becomes commonplace, has led to a constantly increasing incidence of opportunistic infection in the immunosuppressed host.[10] Open-lung biopsy remains the most definitive diagnostic procedure in many cases, and the cardiothoracic surgeon is often called on to obtain tissue for diagnosis in the immunosuppressed and in individuals with idiopathic interstitial pneumonia. In this regard, the advent of thoracoscopic lung biopsy has greatly reduced the morbidity associated with open-lung biopsy and given much greater access to lung tissue for diagnostic purposes.[11–14] In contrast, the diagnosis of lung cancer can be arrived at with more conservative approaches such as sputum cytology, bronchoscopic washing, brushings, aspirates, or biopsy, none of which require thoracotomy. Mediastinoscopy is necessary to ascertain the extent of neoplasia, but a combination of CT scan with FNA biopsy may obviate this invasive approach.[15] Transbronchial FNA, the so-called Wang needle biopsy, is also useful in the assessment of mediastinal disease but requires special skill in its performance.[16] This technique is also being investigated in the assessment of diffuse interstitial lung disease, but the catheter is difficult to position accurately in the lung periphery, and it only yields a cytology specimen. With transbronchial forceps biopsy, peribronchial tissues can be adequately sampled, but these areas may not accurately reflect the nature of the disease process affecting the alveolar portion of the lung. Diffuse interstitial pulmonary disease has a tendency for patchy pulmonary involvement and marked variation of the severity in different portions of the lung. For these reasons transbronchial biopsies may not accurately reflect disease activity and may even be misleading, as in the case of desquamative interstitial pneumonia-like reactions accompanying localized lung lesions.[17]

Fine-needle aspiration biopsy (FNAB) of isolated lung lesions has dramatically changed cytopathology practice by providing a quick, reliable, and cost-effective diagnostic modality. The method renders itself well for the identification and classification of tumor cells but is also of value in the diagnosis of diffuse pulmonary infections.[18] This is particularly true when the infection presents in a localized fashion such as a granuloma or a fluid-filled cavity. For diffuse processes we prefer an open-lung biopsy utilizing the thoracoscope because of the need to estimate the extent of involvement in interstitial pulmonary disease. For maximum success of FNAs, rapid microscopic assessment of adequacy of the specimen should follow each pass of the needle. This service is becoming more widely available not only for transthoracic FNABs, but for transbronchial needle biopsies as well. Material is collected for a number of specialized examinations such as cytologic evaluation of filters and smears; histopathologic assessment of cell blocks; ultrastructural evaluation of cell suspensions by electron microscopy[19]; immunocytochemistry; and, in selected cases, flow cytometry. Flow cytometry is very useful in the identification of malignancy, as, e.g., in the differential diagnosis of mesothelial hyperplasia and malignant mesothelioma associated with a pleural effusion.[20] Immunocytochemistry can also be used in such cases and has the added advantage of identifying the site of origin of the primary neoplasm in these sites for which specific cell markers are available.[21] The diagnosis of specific viral infections in cytologic specimens is possible by both immunocytochemistry and electron microscopy.[22]

Bronchoalveolar lavage involves wedging the tip of the fiberoptic bronchoscope into a segment or subsegment of the lung and repetitively lavaging the isolated distal portion of the lung. The return of fluid is pooled, and cells are separated by centrifugation.[23] The supernatant is utilized for biochemical evaluation of protein and lipid fractions, particularly surface-active phospholipids. The cell-rich sediment is fixed in an alcohol-based solution, and a number of examinations can be performed on separate aliquots. For cell differential counts, 100 μL of fluid are cytocentrifuged and stained with Wright-Giemsa. Cell counts are performed in a hemocytometer chamber and results expressed in number of cells per milliliter. The differential count should include identification of macrophages, neutrophils, lymphocytes, and eosinophils. Epithelial cells are also present in small numbers in bronchoalveolar lavage (BAL) fluid but are not included in the differential count. For certain conditions, one aliquot of the BAL fluid is processed for electron microscopy. In this fashion, the diagnosis of amiodarone-induced pulmonary toxicity can be strongly suggested by the detection of characteristic, lipid-filled alveolar macrophages that display prominent osmiophilic inclusions in the cytoplasm. Opportunistic infections by agents such as protozoal *(Pneumocystis, Toxoplasma)*, fungal *(Cryptococcus, Aspergillus)*, helminthic *(Strongyloids, Ascaris)*, and bacterial *(Mycobacterium aviae intracellulare, Legionella)* pathogens are easily diagnosed by BAL fluid examination. The greatest application of BAL fluid analysis, however, is in the estimation of disease activity in interstitial processes such as idiopathic pulmonary fibrosis, sarcoidosis, and other immunologic pneumopathies.[24] In these cases not only the differential counts, but also the subsets of T and B lymphocytes are important to elucidate pathogenesis, disease activity, and to guide effective therapy.

## Classification of Benign, Diffuse Pulmonary Diseases

While a number of arbitrary classifications exist, a scheme the authors have found clinically useful involves both a judgment about acuteness and some knowledge of radiographic interpretation (Table 15–2). The acuteness or chronicity of a process is judged almost exclusively by the history. If the onset of symptoms is within 7 days, the process is considered acute. If it is between 7 days and 1 month, it is arbitrarily called subacute, and symptoms of longer than 1 month's duration indicate a chronic process.

**TABLE 15–2. PATHOLOGIC PROCESSES AND TYPICAL RADIOGRAPHIC APPEARANCES**

| Acute | Chronic |
|---|---|
| **Acinar** | |
| Infectious pneumonias | Eosinophilic pneumonia |
| Acute respiratory distress syndrome | Pulmonary alveolar proteinosis |
| Cardiogenic pulmonary edema | Idiopathic pulmonary hemosiderosis |
| Vasculitic and connective tissue disease | Infections (tuberculosis, viral) |
| Goodpasture's syndrome | Bronchioloalveolar carcinoma |
| Drug reactions (aspirin) | |
| **Interstitial** | |
| Atypical pneumonias (viral, etc.) | Idiopathic pulmonary fibrosis |
| Cardiogenic pulmonary edema (early) | Sarcoidosis |
| Acute respiratory distress syndrome (early) | Connective tissue disease |
| | Hypersensitivity pneumonias |
| | Pneumoconiosis |
| | Drug reactions |
| | Eosinophilic granuloma |
| | Irradiation lung injury |
| | Congenital (neurofibromatosis, tuberous sclerosis) |
| | Neoplastic (lymphoma, leukemia, Waldenstrom's macroglobulinemia) |
| | Cystic fibrosis |
| | Chronic cardiogenic pulmonary edema (rare) |

The radiographic classification of diffuse pulmonary disease depends on the interpretation of the chest x-ray as showing either an acinar (alveolar) pattern, or an interstitial (reticulo-nodular) pattern. The acinar pattern is characterized by confluent densities that obliterate adjacent blood-filled structures such as the mediastinum, heart borders, and diaphragm or by the presence of air bronchograms that signify fluid in air-filled structures adjacent to patent bronchi in the lung fields. In contrast, interstitial infiltrates do not obliterate adjacent fluid-filled structures or show air bronchograms. There is some overlap between the two patterns, but an understanding of the difference in the patterns can be useful in the differential diagnosis of benign, diffuse pulmonary diseases.

### *Acute, Diffuse, Benign Pulmonary Diseases*

These diseases are almost always acinar in their appearance on chest roentgenogram. The few exceptions to this rule include interstitial infections or immunologic processes that start with an increase of the interstitial markings but eventually become confluent and acinar in appearance. The acute processes can be divided conveniently into four major groups: (1) acute infectious pneumonias; (2) the acute respiratory distress syndrome (ARDS), including its infectious causes; (3) acute cardiogenic pulmonary edema; and (4) a number of vasculitic-immunologic syndromes.

The acute respiratory distress syndrome is an enhanced permeability pulmonary edema that follows a variety of direct lung insults or severe systemic processes.[25] It develops explosively and is usually heralded by the rapid onset of dyspnea and hypoxemia followed by the appearance of widespread confluent pulmonary infiltrates. Although scores of causes of ARDS have been described, fully three fourths of cases can be accounted for by aspiration of gastric contents, acute bacterial infections either of the lung or a distant site associated with the clinical picture of sepsis, and extensive trauma often associated with shock and massive blood transfusions (Table 15–3). Shock is often a harbinger of the onset of ARDS. The syndrome typically occurs within 72 hours of the predisposing risk factor. Despite current standards of critical care, the syndrome continues to carry a mortality rate between 40% and 60%. The onset of the syndrome signifies respiratory failure, and, when caused by infection, it is often associated with the failure of other target organs, notably the kidneys, cardiovascular system, gut, hematologic, and hepatic systems. Histologically the acute phase of the syndrome is characterized by diffuse alveolar damage, proteinaceous pulmonary edema and an acute inflammatory response.[26] As the syndrome progresses, type II pneumonocyte hyperplasia occurs, and monocytes and lymphocytes infiltrate the lungs. The long-term outlook is generally good if the patient survives 2–3 weeks. In those who survive, only a minority will have significant long-term sequela either of a fibrotic or an obstructive nature.

**TABLE 15–3. IMPORTANT CAUSES OF DIFFUSE ALVEOLAR DAMAGE IN ARDS**

| Direct Lung Insults | Nonthoracic (Systemic) Process |
|---|---|
| **Aspiration** | **Shock** |
| Gastric contents | Traumatic |
| Near drowning | Hemorrhagic |
| Lighter hydrocarbons | Septic |
| Paraquat | Neurogenic |
| **Inhalation** | **Other** |
| Oxygen | Acute pancreatitis |
| Nitrogen dioxide | Air embolism |
| Sulfur dioxide | Uremia |
| Smoke | Heat |
| Other noxious gases, vapors, or fumes | High altitude |
| | Molar pregnancy |
| **Infection** | Disseminated intravascular coagulation |
| Gram-negative bacteria | Amniotic fluid embolism |
| Staphylococcus | Drug overdose |
| Viruses | |
| Mycoplasma | |
| Pneumocystis (especially in the immunosuppressed host) | |
| Other | |
| **Iatrogenic** | |
| Blood transfusion | |
| Cardiopulmonary bypass | |
| Radiation | |
| Chemotherapeutic agents | |
| Other agents | |

The pathophysiology of ARDS is not well understood, but the syndrome can be initiated from either the airway or the vascular sides of the terminal air units of the lung. The respiratory initiation of the process generally occurs after aspiration of acidic gastric contents, inhalation of noxious gases, vapors or fumes,[27] or infection. Systemic processes that affect the lung, presumably from the vascular side, include sepsis, trauma, hypotension and shock, pancreatitis, drug overdose, disseminated intravascular coagulation, and acute central nervous system catastrophes (Table 15–3). The cause of the enhanced capillary permeability is multifactorial. Contributing factors appear to include polymorphonuclear leukocyte-borne proteases and a number of oxygen radical species. In addition, monocytes and macrophages likely add to the endothelial injury by the production of leukotrienes, oxygen radicals, platelet activating factor, and other permeability enhancing substances. The coagulation and complement systems have also been secondarily implicated.

Infection, particularly with gram-negative aerobic rods or *Staphylococcus aureus,* is the most common cause of ARDS. Even those patients with ARDS from noninfectious causes, such as pancreatitis or trauma and hypotension, are prone to get nosocomial infection. This secondary infection occurs most often in the lung or at the site of trauma. It is extremely difficult to diagnose and treat nosocomial pneumonia in these patients, but the treatment of infection with antibiotics and drainage of pus in closed spaces is essential for the recovery of the lung, since there is as yet no specific treatment for ARDS.

A number of vasculitic-immunologic processes can cause acute lung injury. Examples are acute lupus pneumonia[28] and Goodpasture's syndrome,[29] which may present as a bilateral, diffuse acinar infiltrate on the chest x-ray. While the clinical and pathophysiologic presentation is often identical to that of ARDS, the pathogenesis is different, and these syndromes should be considered separately from ARDS. In many instances, the open lung biopsy incorporating careful pathologic, cytologic, and microbiologic analysis of the tissue is needed to differentiate these syndromes from ARDS. In acute lupus pneumonia, the salient feature is capillaritis characterized by the accumulation of neutrophils in alveolar capillaries and the surrounding alveolar walls without extravasation into alveolar spaces. The intra-alveolar material in Goodpasture's syndrome consists mostly of fresh and old blood represented by red blood cells and hemosiderin-laden macrophages.[29] In idiopathic pulmonary hemosiderosis, the pathologic features in the lung are similar to Goodpasture's syndrome, but the kidneys are unaffected.[30]

The acute onset of congestive heart failure can mimic ARDS or the vasculitic-immunologic syndromes. Congestive heart failure with cardiogenic pulmonary edema is more common than the other two syndromes, but it is usually differentiated on the basis of the clinical presentation, physical exam, and routine laboratory tests. The major physiologic differentiator of cardiogenic pulmonary edema from the other two syndromes is the pulmonary arterial occlusion pressure (capillary wedge pressure). This pressure, when properly measured, is generally 18 mm Hg or greater in cardiogenic pulmonary edema, whereas it is <18 mm Hg in ARDS and in the vasculitic-immunologic syndromes.

### *Chronic Diffuse Benign Pulmonary Diseases*

These processes can present as a reticulo-nodular (interstitial) pattern, as acinar (alveolar) pattern, or as a combination of these two roentgenographic patterns. The causes of the interstitial pattern may be grouped into 10 major categories. Although more than 50 disease processes have been reported to cause chronic interstitial pneumonitis, the 10 processes listed in Table 15–4 will account for greater than 80% of the known causes of interstitial pneumonitis. It is extremely important to work through the known causes before one labels the process idiopathic interstitial fibrosis[31] (North American terminology) or cryptogenic fibrosing alveolitis[32] (British terminology).

### *Interstitial Pneumonias*

This process affects the supportive structure of the alveolar walls and the terminal airways. The most common presenting symptoms are chronic dyspnea and nonproductive cough. There is a great overlap of appearance among the various subtypes on the chest roentgenogram, and there are consistent derangements in pulmonary physiology characterized by a restrictive defect on lung volumes; a decreased diffusing capacity of carbon monoxide (DLCO); and a stiff, noncompliant lung. The most common cause of interstitial pneumonia is sarcoidosis.[33] The title is a misnomer, because Boeck, the individual who originally described the process, thought it resembled a sarcoma. Sarcoid is an idiopathic multisystem disease characterized by noncaseating, granulomatous inflammation of parenchymal organs and lymph nodes. The respiratory tract is most often the target organ, suggesting that some inhaled substance is the inciting antigen. The process affects mainly the peribronchial and peribronchiolar tissues but eventually extends to the perivascular sheaths and the alveoli.[34] However, the liver, skin, bone, heart, eyes, and central nervous system can also be affected. The chest roentgenogram is often distinctive with symmetrical hilar adenopathy and apparently clear lung fields. As the disease progresses, the adenopathy may remain or regress and interstitial reticulo-nodular changes appear. Lymphocytes are the characteristic inflammatory cell, and specifically the CD-4 helper lymphocyte seems to be the predominant cell around the granulomatous lesions. The granulomas lack an overtly necrotic center, and the giant cells contain asteroid inclusion bodies. The diagnosis is often made clinically, supported by the characteristic chest roentgenographic appearance and the confirmatory findings of noncaseating, granulomatous inflammation on transbronchial lung biopsy.[35] Lymphocytosis and an increased number of CD-4 helper lymphocytes are noted in bronchoalveolar lavage specimens.[36] The disease runs a variable course with numerous episodes of spontaneous remission. In a minority of patients, it can be progressive and culminate in pulmonary fibrosis and chronic respiratory failure. Sudden death may also rarely result from strategically located granulomas that interfere with the conductive system of the heart.[37]

**TABLE 15–4. THE TEN MAJOR CAUSES OF CHRONIC INTERSTITIAL LUNG DISEASE**

| |
|---|
| Sarcoidosis |
| Hypersensitivity pneumonitis (organic dusts) |
| Pneumoconiosis (inorganic dusts) |
| Connective tissue diseases |
| Lung irradiation |
| Drug-induced toxicity |
| Eosinophilic granuloma |
| Congenital (neurofibromatosis, tuberous sclerosis) |
| Cancer with lymphangitic spread |
| Congestive heart failure (chronic and mild) |

The pathologist recognizes certain types of interstitial pneumonia that have some prognostic significance.[38] The prototype of these processes is known as usual interstitial pneumonia (UIP) and is characterized by thickening of the alveolar walls by fibrosis and an inflammatory exudate composed mainly of mononuclear cells (Fig. 15–1). Ultrastructurally, there is a combination of edema and collagen deposition of the alveolar walls and varying degrees of epithelial and endothelial cell damage (Fig. 15–2). Desquamative interstitial pneumonia (DIP) refers to a histologic pattern represented by a large number of alveolar macrophages that gain access to the alveoli by diapedesis from the alveolar capillaries (Fig. 15–3). DIP, however, may represent only a stage in the development of more mundane forms of interstitial pneumonias such as those that precede fibrosing alveolitis.[39] The term *desquamative* was originated because Liebow, who first described this entity, believed these cells were type II alveolar pneumonocytes. Ultrastructural studies, however, clearly identify the intra-alveolar cells as macrophages[40] (Fig. 15–4). Glucocorticoid therapy is followed by dramatic recovery, because in DIP the underlying lung architecture is preserved, and the macrophage migration is responsive to the anti-inflammatory actions of the drug. A histopathologic picture indistinguishable from DIP has also been recognized in association with eosinophilic granuloma and other space-occupying localized lesions of the lung[17] (Table 15–5).

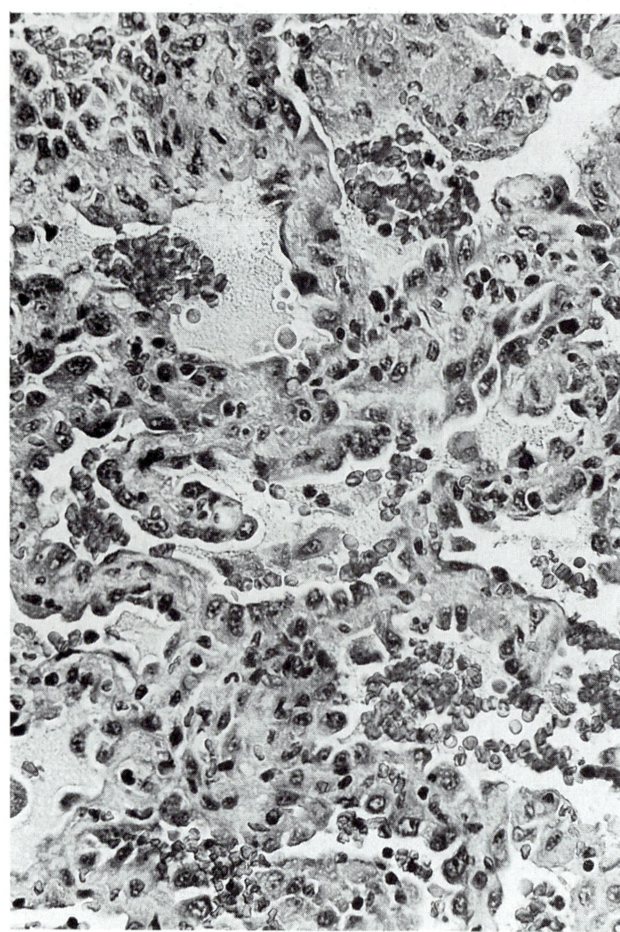

**Figure 15–1.** Subacute phase of diffuse alveolar damage showing usual interstitial pneumonia. Note inflammatory cells, fresh hemorrhage, early fibrosis, and hyperplastic cells lining the distal air spaces.

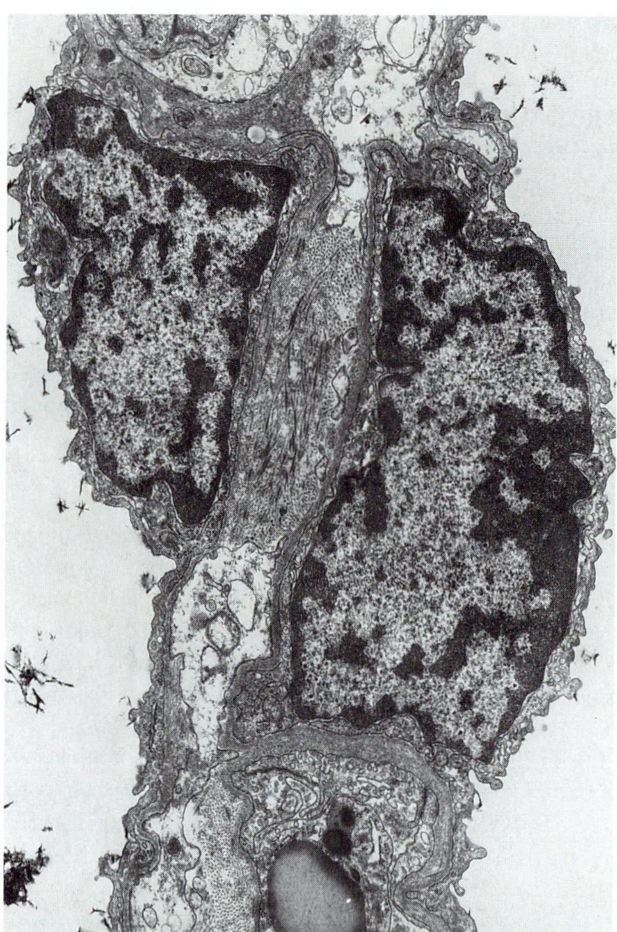

**Figure 15–2.** Early stage of usual interstitial pneumonia. Note alveolar wall lined on both sides by flattened, Type I pneumonocytes. Basement membranes are intact but slight edema and collagen deposition is evident in the interstitium.

Since the description of DIP by Leibow et al[41] and the description of DIP-like reactions by Bedrossiak et al,[17] a number of causes have been associated with both of these conditions (Table 15–6). In addition to obtaining a careful history to elicit an etiology for the process, the pathologist should examine the tissue to determine whether the desquamative process, the pathologist should examine the tissue to determine whether the desquamative process is superimposed on UIP (Fig. 15–5). In lymphocytic interstitial pneumonia (LIP), lymphocytes accumulate around bronchioles and blood vessels and within the substance of the alveolar walls.[42] Some of these patients have a high number of plasma cells in the infiltrate and develop a monoclonal gammopathy that can be detected by serum electrophoresis.[43] The response to steroids is only partial and unpredictable, and many patients go on to a picture of florid lymphoid hyperplasia (pseudolymphoma) or full-blown lymphoma affecting the lungs. Other causes of heavy lymphoplasmocytic infiltration of the lung include AIDS,[44] Sjogren's syndrome,[45] the early phase of sarcoidosis, and rheumatoid lung. If the diagnosis of giant cell interstitial pneumonia (GIP)[46] is rendered one should search carefully for undetected exposure to some obscure dust—most notably wood powder, cobalt, tungsten, or other hard metals—responsible for mixed dust pneumoconioses.[47] Viral pneumonia should be ruled out when this pattern is found in a lung biopsy.[48] The last of Liebow's interstitial pneumonias is characterized by progressive small airway disease secondary to bronchiolitis obliterans. Termed bronchiolitis obliterans interstitial pneumonia (BIP), this diagnosis did not gain popularity and has been supplanted by the term bronchiolitis obliterans (BO). BO is a nonspecific response of the distal air spaces to a variety of inhalational, infectious, immunologic, iatrogenic, and miscellaneous causes (Table 15–7). In its final stage, the diagnosis of BO is difficult to establish because the component of interstitial fibrosis may override the involvement of small airways. The process is nonresponsive to steroids. BO has been associated with rheumatoid arthritis and other collagen diseases so that a biopsy with this finding warrants further evalua-

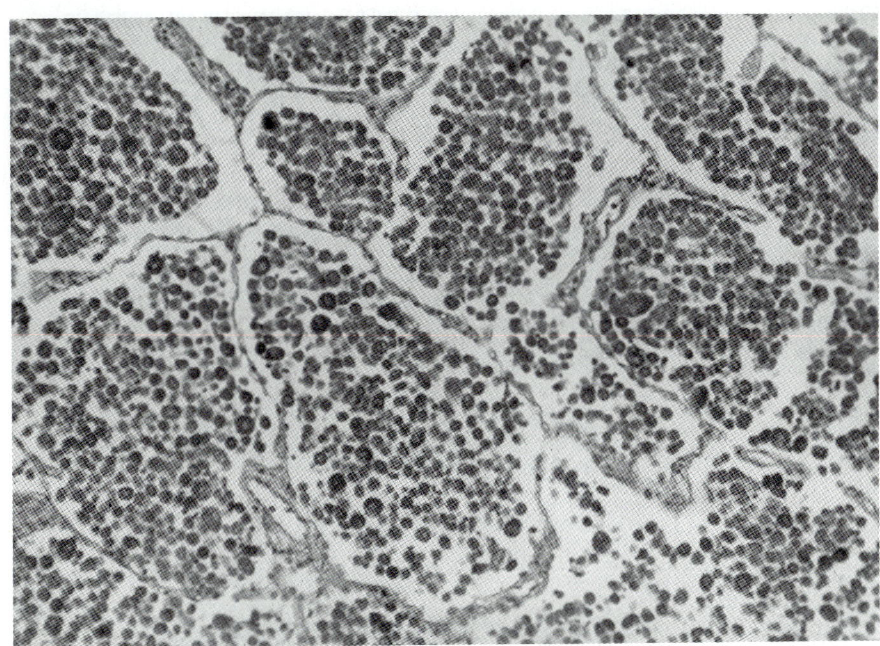

**Figure 15–3.** Desquamative interstitial pneumonia. (Top) DIP— The airspaces are filled by large, almost coalesced macrophages. The alveolar walls are delicate, unaffected by fibrosis or epithelial hyperplasia. (Bottom) UIP—In contrast to DIP, the alveolar lumens are clear, but the alveolar walls are thickened by fibrosis.

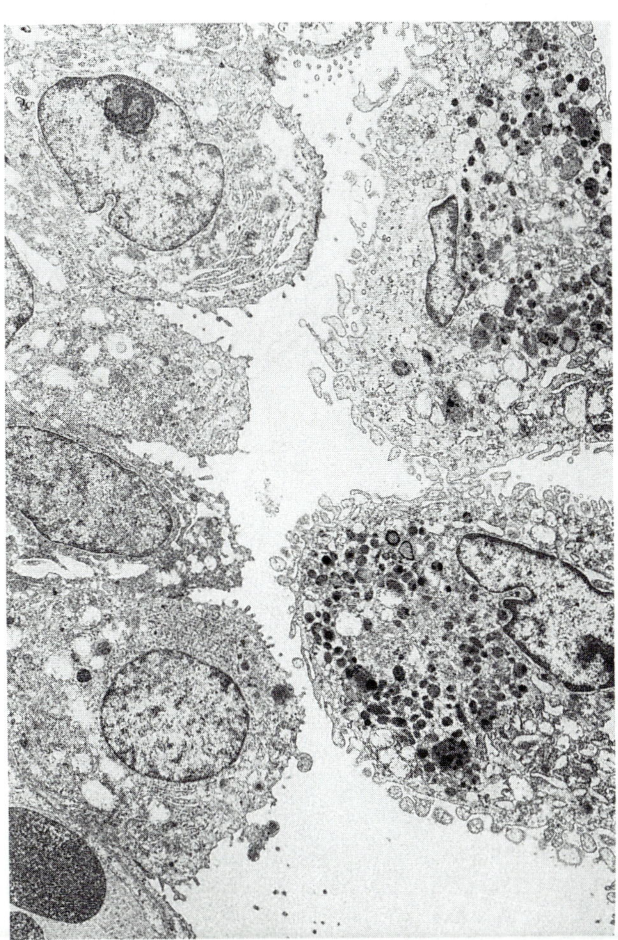

**Figure 15–4.** Ultrastructure of DIP. The cells lining the alveoli are Type II pneumonocytes with characteristic myelinoid bodies. Within the alveoli, macrophages show numerous lysosomes.

tion of rheumatoid factor, antinuclear antibody (ANA), and other serologic tests.[50] BIP has also been associated with graft-vs.-host reaction,[51] rejection of heart-lung transplants,[52] and infection by adenoviruses and *Hemophilus influenza.*[53] The process may also be related to smoking or result from the effect of penicillamine in the lung.[54] A new arrival to the constellation of interstitial pulmonary processes is represented by bronchiolitis obliterans organizing pneumonia (BOOP), first described by Epler et al[55] in 1985. The concept received such a wide popularity that it mushroomed into an international congress to discuss the clinicopathologic features of BOOP in Kyoto, Japan, in 1990.[56] The disease shows some clinical overlap with UIP and small airway disease due to its underlying pathologic

**TABLE 15–5. HISTOPATHOLOGIC FEATURES OF USUAL AND DESQUAMATIVE FORMS OF INTERSTITIAL PNEUMONIAS**

| | UIP | DIP | DIP-like Reaction |
|---|---|---|---|
| Distribution | Patchy | Uniform | Around solid lesions |
| Location | Interstitial | Intra-alveolar | Intra-alveolar |
| Interstitial fibrosis | Common, honeycomb is frequent | Less common, honeycomb infrequent | Depends on the primary process |
| Time element | Lesions of various ages | Uniform age | Variable age |
| Response to steroids | Minimal | Excellent | Variable |

UIP, usual interstitial pneumonia; DIP, desquamative interstitial pneumonia.

**TABLE 15–6. CAUSES OF DIP AND CONDITIONS ASSOCIATED WITH DIP-LIKE REACTIONS OF THE LUNG**

| DIP | DIP-like Reactions |
|---|---|
| Nitrofurantoin | Eosinophilic granuloma |
| Aluminum shavings | Rheumatoid nodule |
| Asbestosis | Tuberculous granuloma |
| Talc | Mycetoma |
| Hard metals | Solitary pulmonary nodule |
| Wood dust | Hamartoma |
| Silica | Intraparenchymal lymph node |
| Silicates | Respiratory bronchiolitis |

features.[57] BOOP, in contrast to BO, is responsive to steroids and is not accompanied by severe interstitial fibrosis. In open-lung biopsies, the process is characterized by plugs of recently found fibrous tissue ("Masson bodies") in the distal airways, extending peripherally into alveolar ducts and alveoli[58] (Fig. 15–6). As with other pathologically defined entities, BOOP has been associated with an increasing array of conditions leading to interstitial lung

**TABLE 15–7. CAUSES OF BRONCHIOLITIS OBLITERANS**

| Inhalation | Collagen-Vascular Disease |
|---|---|
| Thermal injury | Rheumatoid arthritis |
| Chlorine | Sjögren syndrome |
| Ammonia | Systemic lupus erythematosus |
| Hydrochloric acid | Eosinophilic fasciitis |
| Mustard gas | Scleroderma |
| Nitrogen dioxide | Ankylosing spondylitis |
| Sulfuric acid | **Transplantation** |
| Hypersensitivity | Heart-lung transplant |
| **Infection** | Bone marrow transplant |
| Respiratory syncytial virus | **Drugs** |
| Adenovirus types, 1,3,7,21 | Penicillamine |
| Influenza | Sulfa drugs |
| *Bordetella pertussis* | Methotrexate |
| *Mycoplasma pneumoniae* | **Miscellaneous** |
| *Chlamydia* spp. | Aspiration |
| Measles | Lymphoma-leukemia |
| *Haemophilus influenzae* | Cystic fibrosis |
| | Diffuse alveolar damage |
| | Idiopathic |

*(From Yousem SA: Small air disease. In Saldaña MJ (ed): Pathology of Pulmonary Disease. Philadelphia, Lippincott, 1994, p 318, with permission.)*

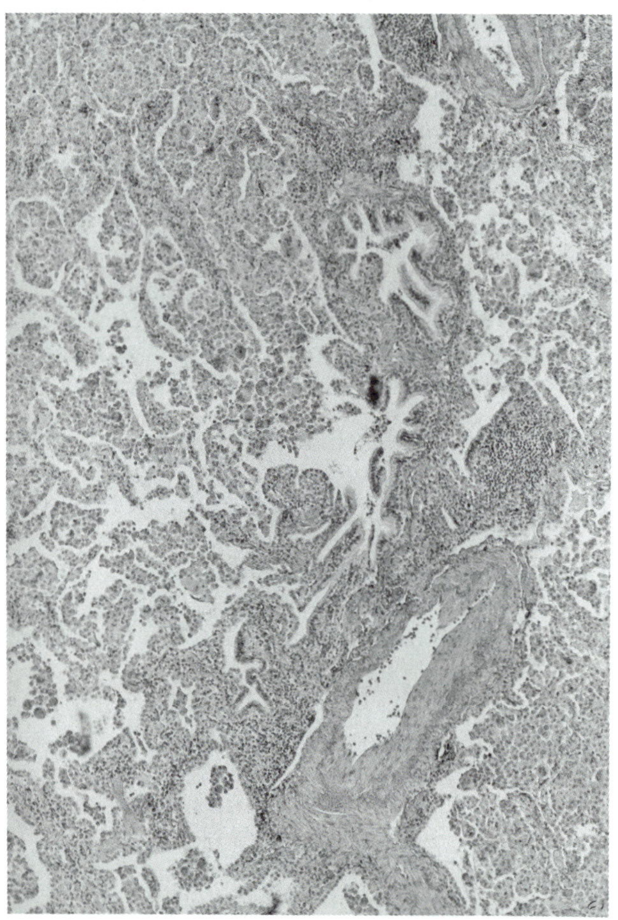

**Figure 15–5.** DIP superimposed on UIP. In addition to the many macrophages filling the air spaces, notice fibrous thickening of the alveolar walls.

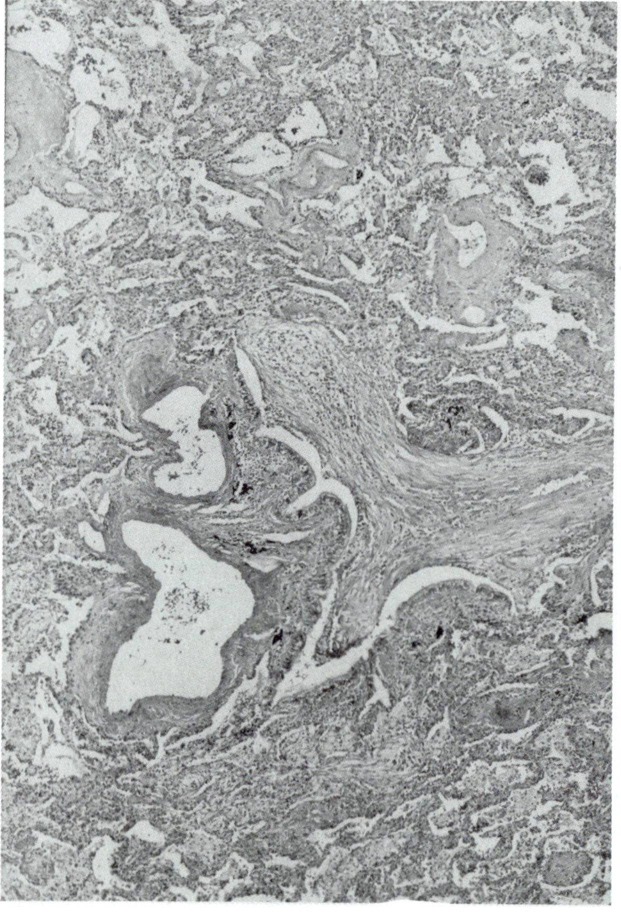

**Figure 15–6.** BOOP—A branching fibrous plug fills the lumen of a small airway near a bifurcation. The adjacent air spaces contain a fibrinous exudate.

disease (Table 15–8). In many cases, however, the condition is idiopathic.[59]

### Hypersensitivity Pneumonitides

Hypersensitivity pneumonitis, also known as extrinsic allergic alveolitis by the British,[60] involves an immunologic aberration characterized by the increase in the lung of a class T lymphocyte, the CD-8 suppressor cell. The process generally evolves in response to the inhalation of exogenous organic antigens. Common sources include avian proteins in bird fanciers, fungal elements of thermophilic actinomyces, and a number of peculiar organic substances from many sources in various hobbies and occupations (Table 15–9). The disease is manifested by the onset of dyspnea and nonproductive cough. Fever and wheezing can be variably present. The biopsy shows noncaseating granulomata typically around terminal bronchioles and a mixed inflammatory infiltrate of the alveolar walls.[61] In late stages there is progression to fibrosis. The disease can be confused with sarcoid, and the history and the classification of the T-cell subclass population on bronchoalveolar lavage are both independently important to differentiate the two processes.[62] Polarization of the biopsy material will reveal birefringent fibrous or particulate matter, but the exact significance of this finding is not known.[63] In cytologic specimens, pullularia, alternaria, and other airborne fungi can be identified, but, again, no direct relationship with the disease process can be ascertained due to possible contamination of the specimen. In bronchoscopic washings or BAL fluid as well as in the serum, the presence of a precipitating antibody that reacts with a suspected offending antigen indicates exposure but not necessarily disease.[64] Skin tests and bronchial inhalation challenge have also been performed in hypersensitivity pneumonitides with various degrees of diagnostic success. In allergic bronchopulmonary aspergillosis, the infiltrate is more interstitial and parallels markings of the bronchovasculature, but acute exacerbations may also result in acinar patterns on the chest x-ray.

### Inorganic Pneumonoconiosis

The inhalation of nonorganic dusts and fibers can result in chronic interstitial lung disease.[65] These dusts and fibers are most often inhaled in the course of various occupational and environmental exposures. The three most common occupational lung diseases are silicosis, coal worker's pneumoconiosis, and asbestosis (Tables 15–6, 15–10). Silicosis results from the immunologic and cellular response to the inhalation of respirable crystalline silica particles.[66] Occupations at high risk for silicosis include sandblasters, foundry workers, quarry workers, glass workers, and underground miners in general. Coal worker's pneumoconiosis has many features similar to silicosis, but it has been given a separate pathologic status. The main difference is noted in early stages of the two conditions. In coal worker's pneumoconiosis, there may be only a mild bronchiolitis, whereas silicosis starts as an interstitial pneumonitis. Subsequently, silicosis may evolve to either silicotic nodules or progressive massive fibrosis with ominous consequences.[67] Both processes seem to predispose to tuberculosis and an unusual rheumatologic disorder known as Caplan's syndrome.[67] Exposure to respirable particles over decades is usually necessary for the rheumatologic syndrome to develop; however, in silicosis an acute pneumonic syndrome that mimics pulmonary alveolar proteinosis has also been described.[68]

The environmental agent that is currently receiving the most attention with regard to the lung is asbestos.[69] Despite its large size (50–100 μm), this fiber is inhaled as respirable particles because of its small cross-sectional diameter. Once in the lung, the long fibers are only partially engulfed by pulmonary alveolar macrophages. However, asbestos is not metabolized, and it is not cleared by the lung in any appreciable manner. Workers in production of asbestos insulation materials have received the most exposure followed by insulators, boilermakers, pipe fitters, and sheet metal workers. However, anyone who has worked in the construction or ship building industry in the last 20–30 years has likely had appreciable exposure to asbestos fibers. In addition, instances of asbestos-related diseases have been described in spouses and other close relatives of workers who are exposed to asbestos.[70] There is a long latent period between the onset of asbestos exposure and the development of clinical markers of asbestos exposure. The latter may or may not lead to more severe asbestos-related diseases, and, again, the process may take many years. Circumscribed, flat, pleural plaques along the chest wall and the diaphragm that occasionally calcify in a linear fashion are taken as evidence of asbestos exposure when the history is appropriate.[71] Malignant mesothelioma of the pleura and peritoneum is clearly related to asbestos exposure.[72] Development of this rare neoplasm is not caused by cigarette smoking to the same extent as is lung carcinoma. In contrast to mesothelioma, the pathogenesis of lung carcinoma is synergistically influenced by cigarette smoking and asbestos exposure.[73] Asbestosis, the debilitating interstitial pneumonitis related to asbestos exposure, typically affects the lower lung fields and can be associated with circumscribed visceral pleural thickening. The process, when ad-

**TABLE 15–8. CONDITIONS ASSOCIATED WITH BRONCHIOLITIS OBLITERANS ORGANIZING PNEUMONIA (BOOP)**

| Infections | Noninfectious |
|---|---|
| Mycoplasma | Wegener's granulomatosis |
| Pneumocystis | Drug reactions |
| Adenovirus | Toxic fumes |
| Bacteria | Aspiration pneumonia |
| Fungi | Hypersensitivity pneumonitis |
| | Chronic eosinophilic pneumonia |
| | Heart–lung transplantation |
| | Bone marrow graft |

**TABLE 15–9. CAUSES OF HYPERSENSITIVITY PNEUMONITIS**

| Disease | Antigen | Sources of Antigen |
|---|---|---|
| **Bacteria** | | |
| Farmer's lung | *Micropolyspora faeni* | Moldy hay, grain, silage |
| Ventilation pneumonitis | *Thermoactinomyces candidus* | Contaminated forced-air systems |
| Bagassosis | *T. vulgaris* | Moldy sugarcane (bagasse) |
| Mushroom worker's lung | *T. sacchari* | Moldy mushroom compost |
| Suberosis | *T. viridis* | Cork dust mold |
| **Fungi** | | |
| Malt worker's lung | *Aspergillus fumigatus*<br>*Aspergillus clavus* | Moldy barley |
| Sequoiosis | *Graphium, Pullularia* | Moldy wood dust |
| Maple bark disease | *Cryptostroma corticale* | Moldy maple bark |
| Cheese washer's lung | *Aspergillus clavatus* | Moldy cheese |
| Woodworker's lung | *Alternaria* | Oak, cedar and mahogany dust; pine and spruce pulp |
| Cheese worker's lung | *Penicillum casei* | Cheese mold |
| Paprika slicer's lung | *Mucor stolonifer* | Moldy paprika pods |
| Summer pneumonitis | *Trichosporon cutaneum* | "Contaminated old houses" |
| **Animal protein** | | |
| Bird fancier's, breeder's, or handler's lung | Avian droppings, feathers, serum, etc. | Parakeets, burdgerigars, pigeons, chickens, turkeys |
| Pituitary snuff taker's lung | Pituitary snuff | Bovine and porcine pituitary proteins |
| Fish meal worker's lung | Fish meal | Fish meal dust |
| Furrier's lung | Animal fur dust | Animal pelts |
| Bat lung | Bat serum protein | Bat droppings |
| **Insect proteins** | | |
| Miller's lung | Sitophilus granarius (wheat weevil) | Dust-contaminated grain |
| Lycoperdonosis | Puffball spores | Lycoperdon puffballs |
| **Unknown** | | |
| Sauna taker's lung | | Contaminated sauna water |
| Coptic lung | | Cloth wrappings of mummies |
| Grain measurer's lung | | Cereal grain |
| Coffee worker's lung | | Coffee bean dust |
| Thatched roof lung | | Dead grasses and leaves |
| Tea grower's lung | | Tea plants |
| Tobacco grower's lung | | Tobacco plants |

*(From Hammar SP: Extrinsic allergic alveolitis. In: Dail DA, Hammar SP (eds); Pulmonary Pathology, New York, Springer Verlag, 1988, chap 14, p 381, with permission.)*

**TABLE 15–10. PULMONARY REACTIONS TO CHRONIC INORGANIC DUST EXPOSURE**

| Reaction | Examples |
|---|---|
| **Fibrogenic dusts** | |
| Concentric hyaline nodules | Silica (nodular silicosis) |
| Stellate interstitial nodules | Silica and inert dust (mixed dust pneumoconiosis) |
| Alveolar proteinosis-like lesion | Silica (acute silicosis) |
| Diffuse interstitial fibrosis | Asbestos (asbestosis) |
| Granulomatous inflammation | Beryllium (beryllium disease) |
| Progressive massive fibrosis | Talc (talc pneumoconiosis) |
| | Silica (complicated silicosis, complicated coal worker's pneumoconiosis, silicotuberculosis) |
| **Inert dusts** | |
| Dust macule (peribronchiolar or perivascular collections of dust and dust-laden macrophages, minimal fibrosis) | Coal dust (uncomplicated coal worker's pneumoconiosis)<br>Iron (siderosis) |

*(From Katzenstein AL, Askin F: Surgical Pathology of Non-neoplastic Lung Disease, Philadelphia, Saunders, 1982, p 74, with permission.)*

vanced, is also characterized by a restrictive pattern on pulmonary function tests, crackles on auscultation of the chest and dyspnea with exertion. Ferruginous (asbestos) bodies found in cytologic specimens or tissue biopsies may be helpful in the diagnosis of asbestosis, but the absence of these bodies does not exclude the diagnosis.[74] Currently, exposure to asbestos insulation has been greatly reduced, and even when exposure is unavoidable, extreme caution is exercised to avoid respirable particles. However, because of the long latent period of the disease, patients with newly diagnosed asbestos-related pulmonary problems continue to be seen, and their cases are often involved in litigation. Quantitative assessment of fibers in the lung digests[75] and specialized x-ray diffraction analysis of lung tissue[76] are sometimes useful to settle such disputes.

### *Connective Tissue Diseases*

Connective tissue diseases are all associated with interstitial lung disease.[77] In rheumatoid arthritis[78] and systemic lupus erythematosus (SLE),[79] the interstitial lung disease is typically associated with pleural thickening or effusions. Inter-

**TABLE 15–11. PLEUROPULMONARY LESIONS IN CONNECTIVE TISSUE DISEASES**

| |
|---|
| Pleuritis and/or pleural effusion |
| Interstitial pneumonitis or fibrosis |
| Pulmonary hemorrhage and/or hemosiderosis |
| Pulmonary hypertension with or without vasculitis |
| Obliterative bronchiolitis |
| Inflammation and degeneration of cartilage |
| Apical fibrobullous disease |
| Necrobiotic nodules or cavities |
| Bronchiectasis |
| Amyloidosis |
| Various drug therapy effects |
| Infection (pneumonia, abscess, or empyema) |
| Malignant neoplasms, especially carcinoma and lymphoma |

*(From Stanford RE: Connective tissue disease. In: Dail DH, Hammar SP (eds); Pulmonary Pathology, New York, Springer Verlag, 1988, Chap 17, p 472, with permission.)*

stitial lung disease can also be seen with scleroderma,[80] polymyositis,[81] and mixed connective tissue disease[82] albeit less frequently. In rare instances the pulmonary problem may precede the rheumatologic manifestations of these diseases. Except for the rheumatoid nodule, which has a characteristic histologic appearance, the other manifestations do not allow differentiation of one collagen disease from another based on a biopsy specimen. A severe vasculitis may be noted in SLE but is indistinguishable from that noted in polyarteritis nodosa and also may be clinically confused with chronic thromboembolism.[83] Patients with connective tissue diseases often suffer from immunologic abnormalities or may become immunosuppressed due to prolonged steroid therapy. As a result they may develop infections, neoplasms, or drug reactions associated with their complex disease state (Tables 15–10, 15–11). Immune complexes play a role in the pathogenesis of connective tissue disease and have been recovered in the serum and BAL fluid of patients with pulmonary manifestations.[84] Others have expressed skepticism as to the role of these complexes, and consequently the pathogenesis remains obscure. A connective tissue disorder should be suspected in any patient with a diffuse, bilateral infiltrate on chest x-ray and unexplained multisystem symptoms.

### *Pulmonary Drug Toxicity*

Drugs are common causes of iatrogenic interstitial lung disease.[85] A large number of drugs used in cancer chemotherapy have been implicated in the pathogenesis of interstitial lung disease.[86] In addition, commonly used agents such as nitrofurantoin, penicillamine, gold salts, antiarrhythmics, thiazide diuretics, and an increasing number of other drugs

**TABLE 15–12. DRUGS PRODUCING DIFFUSE ALVEOLAR DAMAGE THAT MAY PROGRESS TO USUAL INTERSTITIAL PNEUMONIA**

| Cytotoxic Drugs | Noncytotoxic Drugs | |
|---|---|---|
| **Antibiotics** | **Antibacterial agents** | **Antihypertensive agents** |
| Bleomycin | Nitrofurantoin | Hexamethonium |
| Mitomycin | Amphotericin | Pentolinium |
| Necarzinostatin | Sulfadimethoxine | Mecamylamine |
| | PAS | Hydralazine |
| | Sulfachryseindine | |
| | Sulfasalazine | |
| **Alkylating agents** | **Analgesics** | **Diuretics** |
| Busulfan | Acetylsalicylic acid | Hydrochlorothiazide |
| Cyclophosphamide | | |
| Chlorambucil | | |
| Melphalan | | |
| **Nitrosoureas** | **Opiates** | **Antiarrythmics** |
| Carmustine (BCNU) | Heroin | Amiodarone |
| Semustine (methyl CCNU) | Propoxyphene | Lidocaine |
| Lomustine (CCNU) | Methadone | Tocanide |
| Chlorozotocin | | Procainamide |
| **Antimetabolites** | **Sedatives** | **Anticonvulsants** |
| Methotrexate | Ethchlorvynol | Diphenylhydantoin |
| Azathioprine | Chlorpromazine | Carbamazepine |
| Mercaptopurine | | |
| Cytosine arabinoside | | |
| **Miscellaneous** | **Major tranquilizers** | **Miscellaneous** |
| Procarbazine | Haloperidol | Gold salts |
| VM-26 | Fluphenazine | Penicillamine |
| Vinblastine | Chlordiazepoxide | Colchicine |
| Vindesine | | Cromolyn sodium |
| | | Methysergide |

*PAS = paramino salicylic acid.*
*(From Cooper JAD Jr, White DA, Matthay RA: Drug-induced pulmonary disease. Am Rev Respir Dis 133:321–340, 1986, with permission.)*

have been implicated in this process (Table 15–12). A careful history of all prescription and over-the-counter drugs used in the previous 5–10 years must be elicited in every patient with unexplained interstitial lung disease. Likewise, diffuse alveolar damage, interstitial pneumonias, and interstitial fibrosis when encountered in a biopsy specimen should trigger a search for a possible drug administration that escaped the interviewer during the initial history obtained from the patient.[87] Certain cytologic abnormalities are highly characteristic of pulmonary drug toxicity but do not allow the recognition of the specific offending agent.[88] The presence of large foamy cells in distal air spaces is a common effect of amiodarone (Fig. 15–7). The osmiophilic inclusions found in pulmonary alveolar macrophages of patients who receive amiodarone are a reliable indicator of the effect of this drug (Fig. 15–8). But the extent of the disease has to be evaluated by history, chest x-ray, and pulmonary function tests prior to one's making a diagnosis of drug toxicity.[88] Direct toxic effects due to oxidant lung injury, hypersensitivity phenomena, and idiosyncrasy play a role in

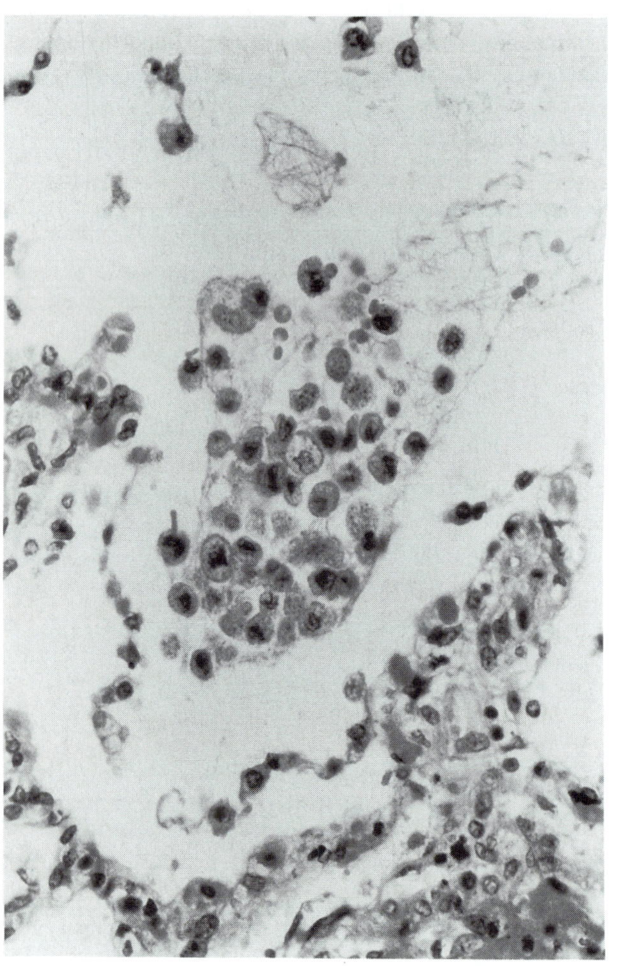

**Figure 15–7.** Distal air spaces in amiodarone toxicity. The lumen is filled with foamy macrophages and the alveolar walls are edematous.

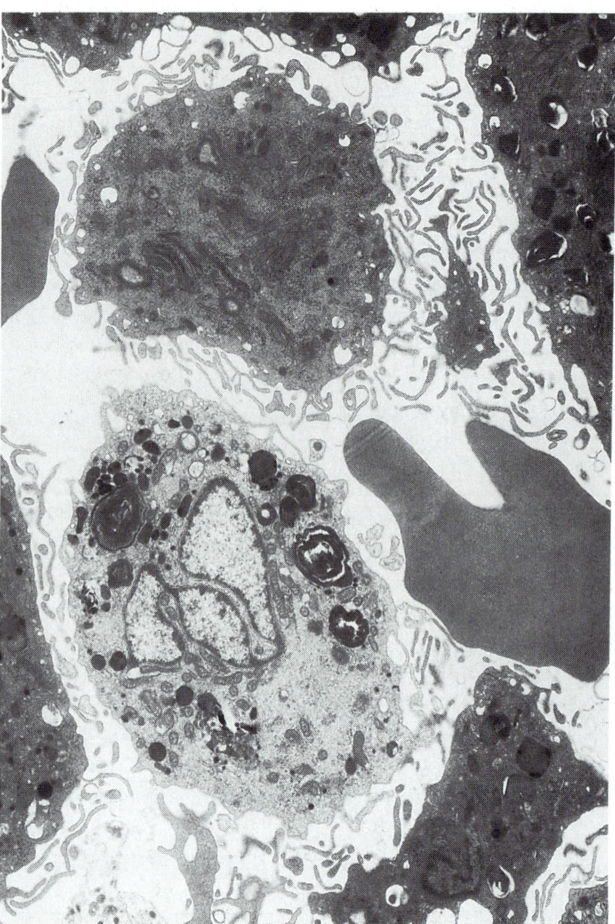

**Figure 15–8.** Ultrastructure of the lung in amiodarone toxicity. Note eosinophilic inclusions within lysosomes of macrophages, which display long pseudopods.

the development of pulmonary reactions to drugs (Table 15–13). These processes benefit from removal of the offending drug with or without the administration of glucocorticoids. Other patients develop pulmonary symptoms due to a SLE-like syndrome that need not be restricted to the lungs but may affect the kidneys, the skin, and the lymph nodes.[89]

### *Chronic Eosinophilic Pneumonia*

This process can have elements of both interstitial and acinar infiltrates on chest x-ray. It can appear in all age groups and is sometimes associated with a peripheral eosinophilia. The hallmark of the diagnosis is a chronic organizing pneumonia with eosinophils on histology and no obvious evidence of infection.[90] The chest x-ray classically shows a "reverse negative" pattern in which the infiltrate, rather than predominating centrally around the hilar structures, is seen peripherally along both chest walls[91] (Fig. 15–9). However, there is no specific roentgenographic or clinical presentation for this syndrome. Clinical presentation can range from a completely asymptomatic chronic condition to

**TABLE 15–13. MECHANISMS OF DRUG-INDUCED LUNG DISEASE**

| Mechanism | Clinical Features | Pulmonary Pathology |
|---|---|---|
| Direct toxicity (oxidant lung injury) | Dose-dependent<br>Cumulative effect<br>Poor response to steroids<br>May become chronic | Diffuse alveolar damage; may progress to usual interstitial pneumonia |
| Allergic reaction (hypersensitivity phenomenon) | Non-dose related<br>Requires induction period<br>Usually acute<br>Responds to steroids<br>Good prognosis | Extrinsic allergic alveolitis; poorly formed granulomas; eosinophilic infiltrates |
| Drug idiosyncrasy (individual susceptibility) | Non-dose related<br>No induction period<br>Usually acute<br>May respond to steroids<br>May be fatal | Variable; may start as noncardiogenic pulmonary edema |

*(From Bedrossian CWM: Iatrogenic and toxic injury. In: Dail DH, Hammar SP (eds); Pulmonary Pathology. New York, Springer Verlag, 1988, chap 19, p 512, with permission.)*

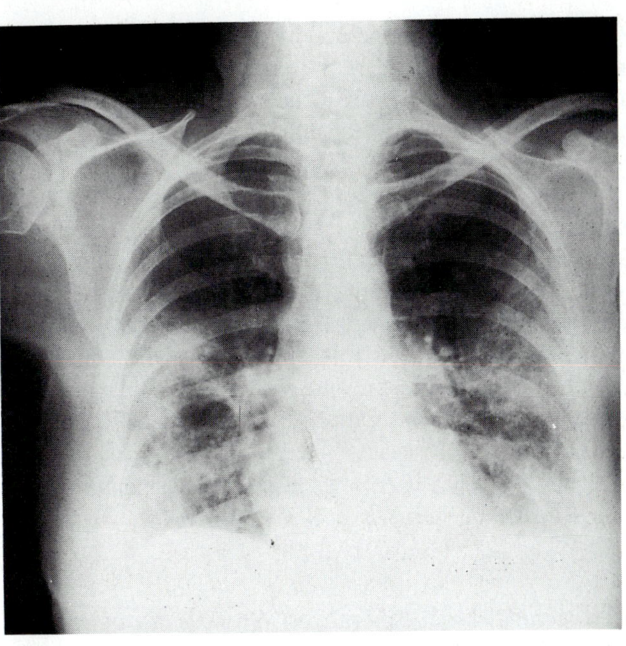

**Figure 15–9.** Chest x-ray of eosinophilic pneumonia. Note the butterfly wing distribution, which is the reverse of pulmonary edema.

**TABLE 15–14. SOME IDENTIFIABLE CAUSES OF EOSINOPHILIC PNEUMONIA**

| Parasites | Drugs | | Other |
|---|---|---|---|
| **Nematodes (roundworms)**<br>*Ascaris*<br>*Strongyloides*<br>*Ancylostoma*<br>*Necator*<br>*Toxocara*<br>*Trichinella* | **Antibiotics**<br>Penicillin<br>Sulfa<br>Nitrofurantoin<br>Streptomycin<br>Tetracycline<br>Isoniazid<br>Aminosalicylic acid<br>Para-aminosalicylic acid | **Antihyperglycemic**<br>Chlorpropamide<br>Tolbutamide | **Bacteria**<br>*Brucella*<br>*Staphylococcus*<br>*Pneumococci*<br>*Proteus*<br>*Escherichia coli*<br>*?Tuberculosis* |
| **Filarial nematodes**<br>*Wuchereria*<br>*Brugia*<br>*Dirofilaria* | **Antineoplastic**<br>Azathioprine<br>Methotrexate<br>Bleomycin<br>Procarbazine | **Antihypertensive**<br>Hydralazine<br>Mecamylamine | **Fungi**<br>*Aspergillus*<br>*Coccidioidomycen*<br>*Candida*<br>*Sporothrix* |
| **Trematodes (flatworms or flukes)**<br>*Schistosoma*<br>*Fasciola* | **Anti-inflammatory**<br>Aspirin<br>Beclomethasone<br>Naproxen<br>Gold salts<br>Cromoglycate | **CNS-effective**<br>Chlorpromazine<br>Imipramine<br>Methylphenidate<br>Carbamazepine<br>Mephenesin | **Viruses**<br>?In children |
| **Cestodes (tapeworms)**<br>*Echinococcus*<br>*Taenia* | | **Other Drugs**<br>Adrenalin<br>Dantrolene | **Other Allergens**<br>Pollen<br>Beeswax<br>Desaturated croton oils<br>**Metals**<br>Nickel<br>Beryllium<br>Zinc<br>Fumes (probably nickel and chromium) |

*(From Dail DH: Eosinophilic infiltrates. In: Dail DH, Hammar SP (eds): Pulmonary Pathology. New York, Springer Verlag, 1988, chap 13, p 363, with permission.)*

the acute onset of a febrile illness with dry cough and wheezing. The syndrome has been associated with various fungi, parasites, and drugs (Tables 15–8, 15–14). Many times the etiology is unclear. In its early stages it is exquisitely sensitive to glucocorticoid therapy.

The diagnosis is made when peripheral blood eosinophilia is matched by a cytologic or a biopsy specimen showing eosinophils and Charcot-Leyden crystals in the absence of epithelial hyperplasia. These patients are rarely ill enough to warrant an open-lung biopsy so that the complete histopathologic picture is not commonly appreciated. In one of these rare instances, the lung tissue showed a large number of eosinophils, in capillaries, in the alveolar walls and even free in alveolar spaces[92] (Fig. 15–10). By electron microscopy, the characteristic inclusions of eosinophils were noted in the interstitial spaces or even phagocytosed by macrophages.

### *Pulmonary Vasculitides and Granulomatoses*

Several relatively rare granulomatous or immunologic processes can result in diffuse acinar patterns in the lung.

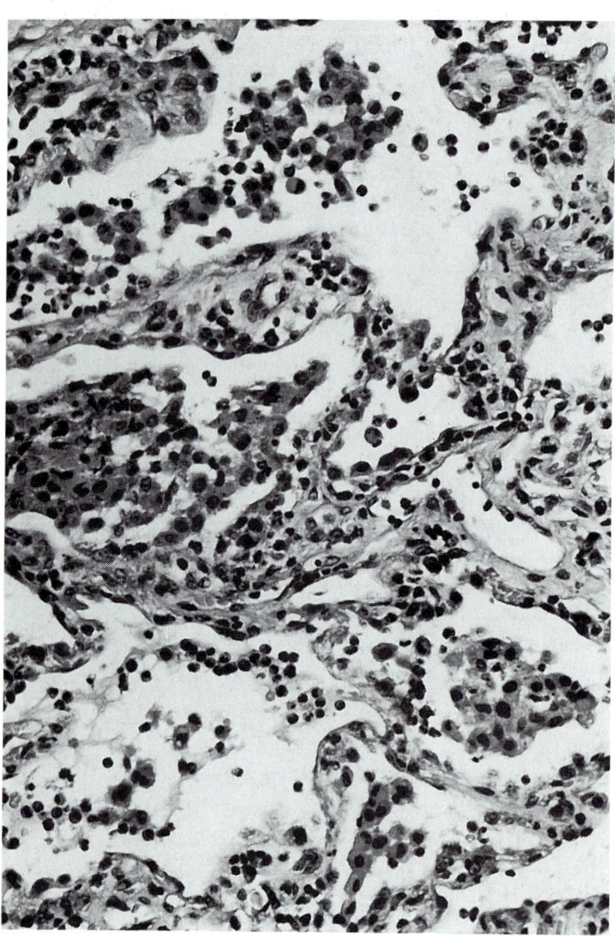

**Figure 15–10.** Distal air spaces in eosinophilic pneumonia. The alveolar walls and the air spaces contain numerous eosinophils but their structure is the most intact.

These include pulmonary alveolar proteinosis,[93] chronic pulmonary hemosiderosis,[94] Wegener's granulomatosis,[95] Churg-Strauss syndrome,[96] and a number of other vasculitic processes[97] that can affect the lung. These diseases are seen infrequently, and the physical signs, history, chest x-ray, and routine laboratory data are usually nonspecific. Open-lung biopsy by thorascopic thoracotomy is often necessary for the diagnosis. Despite an adequate specimen, the diagnosis depends on close clinical and pathologic correlation and is often fraught with subjectivity (Table 15–15). Distinction between angiocentric and bronchocentric processes requires an open-lung biopsy, which should be properly examined by special stains that outline bronchi and blood vessels as well as the remnants of alveoli in areas of extensive necrosis. These studies include Wilder's reticulum stain and Verhoeff-van-Gieson for elastic fibers. It is important to separate the necrotizing vasculitides from the lymphoproliferative processes.[98] While the necrotizing processes may be rather severe and extend even beyond the lungs, they respond relatively well to immunosuppressive and cytotoxic therapy. In contrast, the lymphoproliferative disorders are refractory to treatment and tend to progress to overt lymphoma except for the benign lymphocytic angiitis described by Saldana et al[99] in 1977. Mucoid impaction is a complication of asthma that can be easily treated with bronchodilators and chest physical therapy.[100] Allergic bronchopulmonary aspergillosis (ABPA) requires more vigor-

**TABLE 15–15. PULMONARY VASCULOPATHIES AND GRANULOMATOSES**

| |
|---|
| **Group I** |
| Necrotizing granulomatous vasculitides |
| Wegener's granulomatosis ("classic" and "limited" variants) |
| Allergic granulomatosis and angiitis (Churg-Strauss syndrome) |
| Necrotizing sarcoid granulomatosis |
| **Group II** |
| Angiocentric lymphoproliferative processes |
| Benign lymphocytic angiitis and granulomatosis |
| Lymphomatoid granulomatosis |
| Angiocentric large cell lymphomas |
| **Group III** |
| Miscellaneous vasculitides |
| Classic polyarteritis nodosa |
| Hypersensitivity vasculitis |
| Pulmonary infections |
| Intravenous drug addiction |
| Behçet's disease |
| Hughes-Stovin syndrome |
| Pulmonary hypertension |
| **Group IV** |
| Bronchocentric processes |
| Bronchocentric granulomatosis |
| Bronchiolitis obliterans |
| Mucoid impaction of the lung |
| Allergic bronchopulmonary aspergillosis |

*(From Saldaña M: Pulmonary vasculitides and angiocentric lymphoproliferative processes. In: Dail DH, Hammar SP (eds): Pulmonary Pathology. New York, Springer Verlag, 1988, p 448, with permission.)*

ous treatment with bronchodilators and glucocorticoids.[101] It is imperative to rule out infective granulomas in all vasculitides and granulomatoses prior to the initiation of glucocorticoid therapy, since a number of cases initially treated as vasculitides were subsequently found to result from infections by fungi and mycobacteria.[102,103]

### *Other Causes of Interstitial Lung Disease*

Lymphangitic spread of adenocarcinoma, certain chronic infections, and a number of relatively rare processes of unknown etiology must be considered in the differential diagnosis of chronic acinar patterns of diffuse pulmonary disease. There is clearly some overlap between these syndromes and those that result in the purely interstitial or reticular nodular patterns, and sometimes a clear distinction between the two patterns cannot be discerned on the chest x-ray. In such cases, involvement of the lymphatics should be suspected.

Lymphangitic spread of adenocarcinoma from a number of sites can result in a widespread acinar and interstitial pattern on the chest x-ray.[104] Common sites of origin for the neoplasm include the lung, breast, stomach, colon, and kidney. Patients are usually quite dyspneic and hypoxemic, and the disease is rapidly progressive. The diagnosis is best made by fiberoptic bronchoscopy and transbronchial lung biopsy, which shows peribronchial lymphatics studded with tumor cells. Bronchiolar alveolar cell carcinoma of the lung can also present as a diffuse acinar pattern.[105] Typically, it is more likely to be focal in its onset, but then it spreads into a more diffuse pattern. Diagnosis of this process is best made with expectorated sputum cytology or by fiberoptic bronchoscopy.[106] Fine-needle aspiration may also yield diagnostic material. Electron microscopy allows the demonstration of histogenesis from mucinous and nonmucinous cells such as Clara cells and alveolar type II pneumonocytes.[107] A number of infections can present as confluent fibronodular or acinar infiltrates. These include tuberculosis in both the immunocompetent and the immunocompromised host; actinomycosis in the immunocompetent patient; and fungal infections, nocardiosis, *Pneumocystis carinii* pneumonia, and certain viral pneumonias in immunosuppressed patients.[108]

Pulmonary alveolar proteinosis is characterized by the presence of lipoproteins in the distal air spaces. There is no significant inflammation, and the alveolar walls are nearly intact (Fig. 15–11). Pulmonary alveolar proteinosis may occur in a primary idiopathic form, initially described by Rosen et al[109] in 1967, or a secondary variety as a result of immunosuppression induced by drugs and/or lymphoreticular malignancies.[110] Because the secondary process is often accompanied by opportunistic infections, special stains should be used in order to rule out the presence of fungi, *Nocardia,* mycobacteria, and *P. carinii* in the thick proteinaceous fluid accumulated in distal air spaces. Most of this material is surfactant related and can be demonstrated

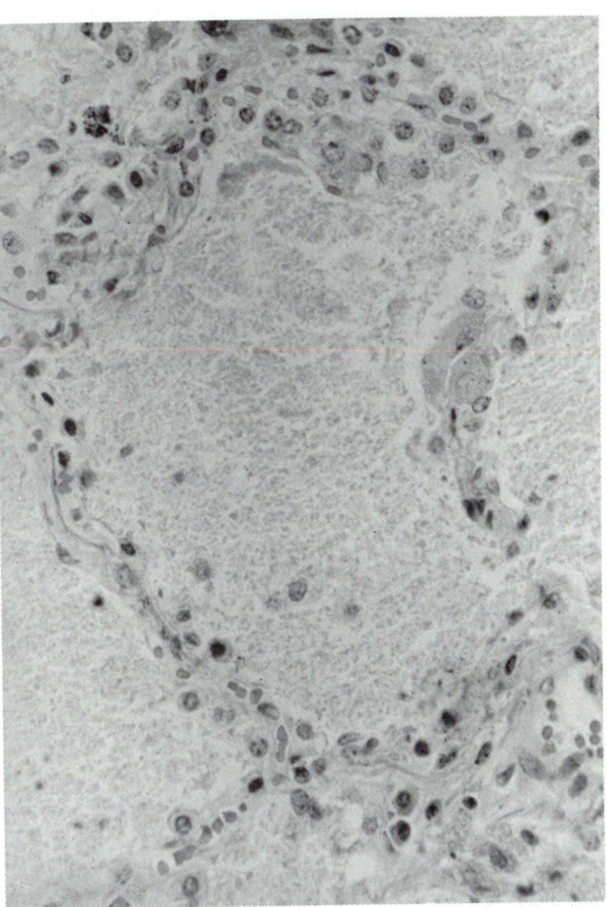

**Figure 15–11.** Pulmonary alveolar proteinosis. A granular material fills the distal air spaces. The alveolar walls show only minimal involvement.

by means of anti-apoprotein antibodies, which are helpful in distinguishing the primary form from the secondary form of alveolar proteinosis.[111] Lymphangioleiomyomatosis is a rare condition characterized by the florid proliferation of smooth muscle in the walls of lymphatics, blood vessels, bronchioles, and alveoli, resulting in multiple cystic spaces in the lung parenchyma.[112] There is usually an associated chylous pleural effusion or ascites, which attests to the extrapulmonary involvement of the condition. The etiology is unknown, but lymphangioleiomyomatosis occurs almost exclusively in women of childbearing age and is benefited by oophorectomy[113] and the administration of progesterone.[114] Other cases with similar lesions in the lung have been associated with tuberous sclerosis.[115]

In addition to these causes of interstitial lung disease, ionizing radiation,[116] eosinophilic granuloma,[117] lipid inhalation,[118] ankylosing spondylitis,[119] and certain congenital and metabolic causes including neurofibromatosis,[120] Gaucher's disease,[121] myxedema,[122] and amyloidosis[123] can cause interstitial lung disease. The clinician who is careful about ruling out the known causes of interstitial lung disease can account for the etiology of approximately

70% of interstitial lung disease. When all of these more common causes of interstitial lung disease are ruled out, the clinician is then left with a much stronger likelihood that the disease is truly idiopathic.

### *Idiopathic Pulmonary Fibrosis*

Idiopathic pulmonary fibrosis or cryptogenic fibrosing alveolitis, as it is known in the United Kingdom, accounts for between 20% and 30% of all interstitial lung disease.[124] The idiopathic syndrome occurs slightly more frequently in men and is generally a diagnosis of the middle-aged man without a history of exposure to known pulmonary toxins. It presents with dyspnea and chronic nonproductive cough. Clubbing of the fingers may be present, and hypoxemia and cyanosis are prominent in more advanced disease. The complaint of arthralgias is prominent, but frank arthritis is rare and, when it is present, should suggest either sarcoidosis or connective tissue disease. The examination of the chest is remarkable for the presence of coarse crackles on auscultation throughout the lung fields. Laboratory workup is generally unremarkable, but routine laboratory screening should be performed. The erythrocyte sedimentation rate (ESR) is typically elevated up to 50 mm/h. Mild abnormalities of the antinuclear antibody titer and the rheumatoid factor titer up to 1:160 are often seen. Higher elevations of these titers should suggest a connective tissue disease. Early in the progression of the disease, lung biopsy will show little collagen deposition, but inflammatory cells such as polymorphonuclear leukocytes and alveolar macrophages will often be present in excess. Later the intra-alveolar exudate is invaded by fibroblasts, and the combination of interstitial and intra-alveolar fibrosis leads to a subcrepitant lung (Fig. 15–12). As the disease progresses, more collagen deposition is seen, and there is gross distortion of the lung architecture resulting in areas of atelectasis alternating with overexpansion (Fig. 15–13). Concomitantly, the intensity of the inflammatory cellular infiltrate begins to wane. Survival is quite variable, but the average duration of the disease is around 4–5 years following diagnosis. In many patients the disease is slowly progressive, and some patients live in ex-

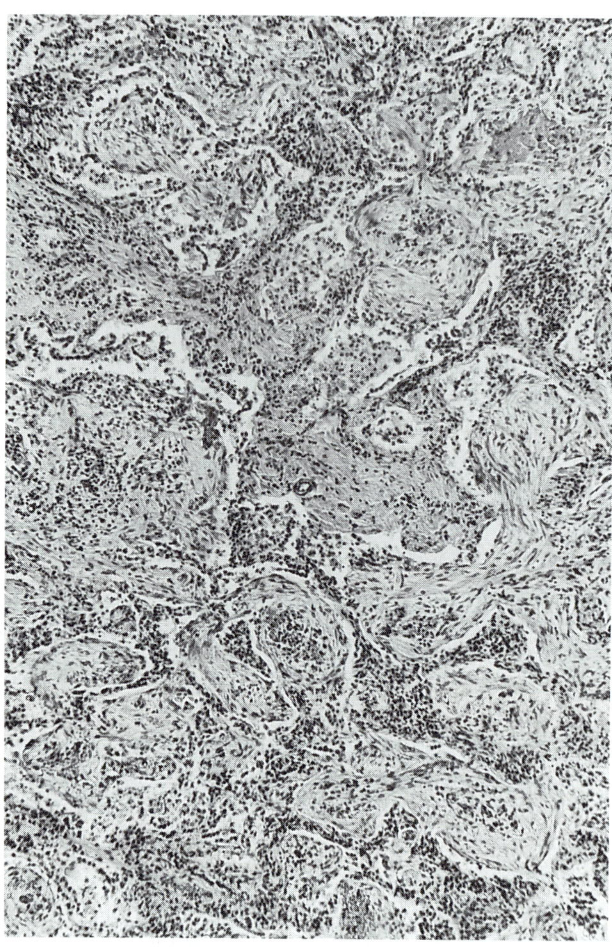

**Figure 15–12.** Distal portion of lung in pulmonary fibrosis. Note pronounced inflammation and combination of intraalveolar and interstitial fibrosis.

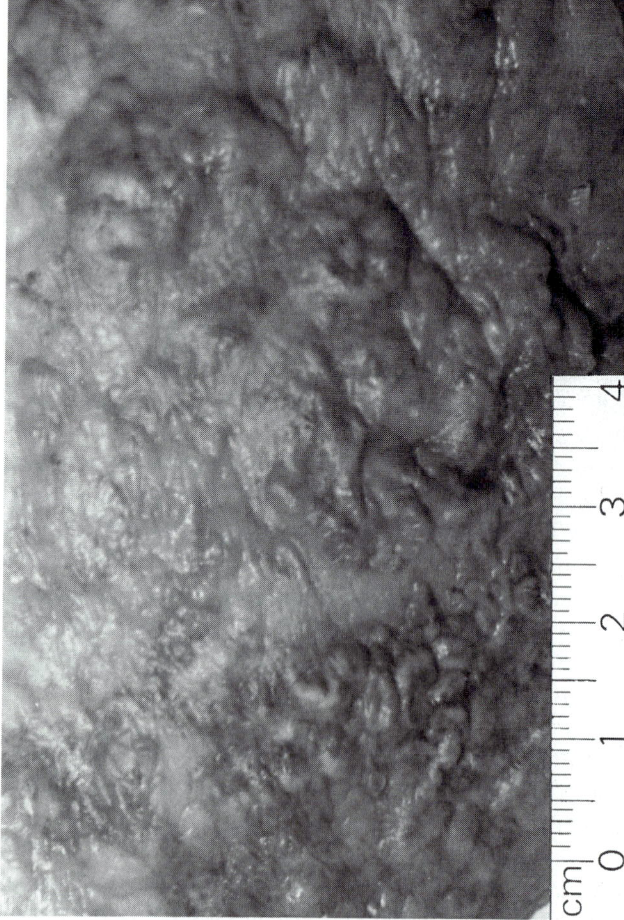


**Figure 15–13.** Pleural aspect of lung with diffuse interstitial pulmonary fibrosis. Areas of retraction alternate with raised areas overlying cystic spaces. The overall configuration resembles the surface of cirrhotic liver.

cess of 20 years with the diagnosis. A rapidly progressive form of idiopathic pulmonary fibrosis is referred to as the Hamman-Rich syndrome after the individuals who first described it in 1935.[125] No matter how rapid the process, in its final stages the lung assumes the appearance of a honeycomb on the chest x-ray as well as at gross examination at the pathologist's bench (Fig. 15–14). This pattern is nonspecific and is seen in all end-stage interstitial pneumonitis, regardless of cause. Fibrosis may be accompanied by a florid epithelial hyperplasia that may even evolve into carcinoma (Fig. 15–15). Because fibrosis is irreversible, the prognosis is generally poor.

The pathophysiology of the syndrome is under intense study. Clearly, immunologic abnormalities contribute to the pathogenesis of idiopathic pulmonary fibrosis. The polymorphonuclear leukocyte and the alveolar macrophage appear to play a prominent role in triggering the disease. Immune complexes have been implicated in the pathogenesis as stimulators of neutrophil and macrophage function.[126] The activated neutrophils and macrophages then release various pro-inflammatory substances, which can result over time in a fibrotic reaction. Proteases, oxygen radicals, leukotrienes, and cytokines are all thought to be involved. A familial type of idiopathic pulmonary fibrosis has been described and offers the opportunity for concentrated study of this syndrome, particularly by the serial exam of BAL fluid. In contrast to sarcoidosis and other types of lymphocyte-mediated interstitial lung disease, idiopathic pulmonary fibrosis is characterized by an increase of neutrophils and macrophages in the differential count.[127] Paradoxically, these cells are not conspicuous in the biopsied lung tissue, which contains more of a chronic inflammatory infiltrate than a purulent exudate. Macrophages may be accumulated in the air spaces in the form of DIP-like reaction, while lymphocytes, plasma cells, and a small number of eosinophils are found in the lung interstitium. If such a cellular response is noted in the biopsy, the prognosis is more favorable because the process tends to respond at least partially to glucocorticoid administration. If fibrosis predominates, the response to glucocorticoid is poor. However,

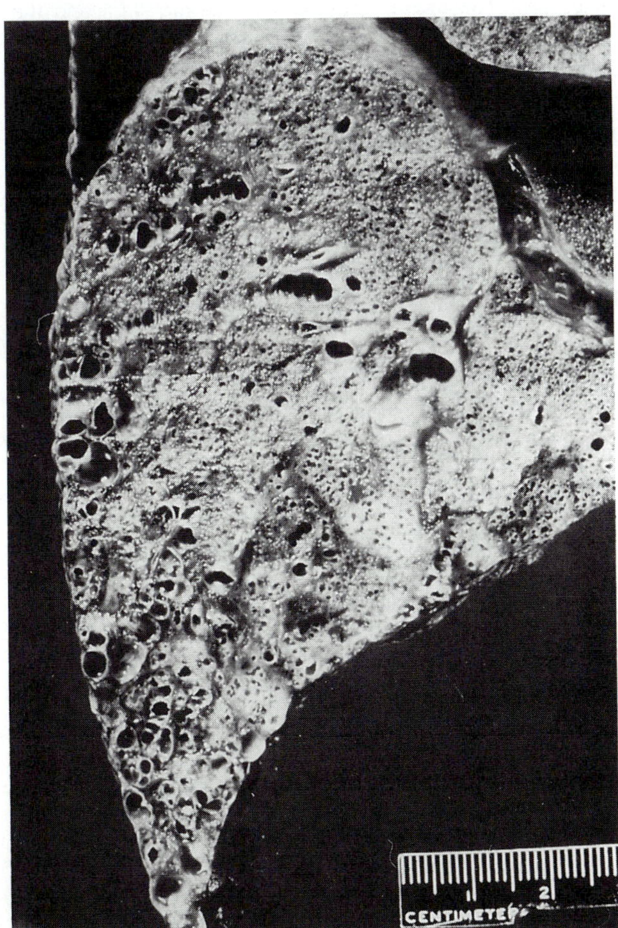


**Figure 15–14.** Diffuse interstitial pulmonary fibrosis. The lung shows cystic spaces at the base and along the posterior subpleural border. Note whitish areas of fibrosis among the cysts.

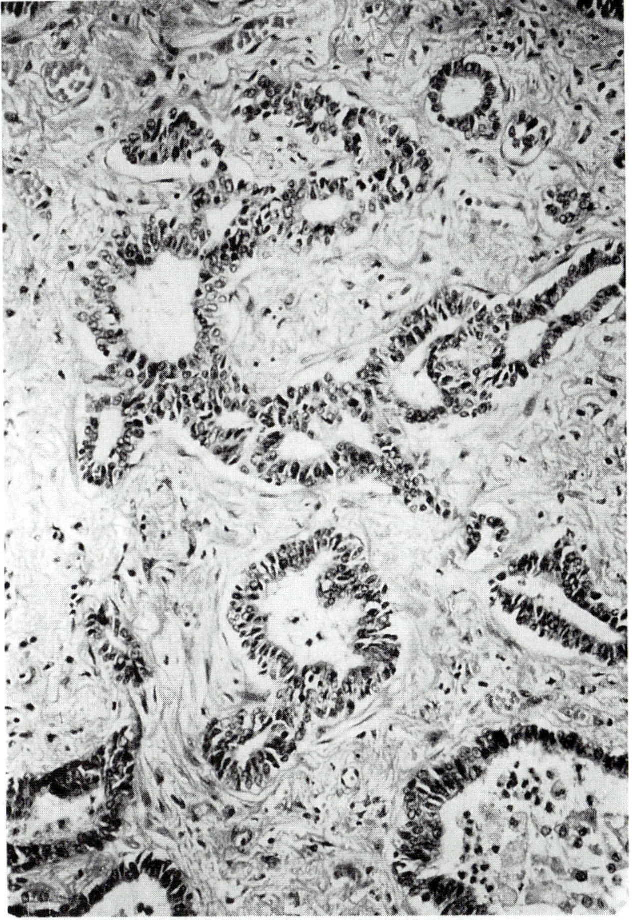

**Figure 15–15.** Histologic section from cystic areas in the Hamman-Rich syndrome. The cysts are lined by hyperplastic epithelium and contain cellular debris.

the drug still should be tried in a 4–6-week test with follow-up because of the patchy nature of the process and the fact that even open-lung biopsies may not be representative of the extent and severity of the process as a whole.

## SUMMARY

The surgeon makes many choices to select the correct diagnostic procedure for a variety of benign, diffuse pulmonary diseases. Following a careful history and a thorough physical exam, the chest x-ray is the most useful diagnostic tool to determine the extent of the process and to classify it in a general category such as localized or diffuse. For diffuse processes, further classification into acinar and interstitial is very useful even though not possible at all times. Bronchoscopy to obtain BAL fluid or a biopsy specimen constitutes the next useful step. For intra-alveolar processes where the suspicion is an infection or an immunologic phenomenon, BAL may suffice. Where one suspects a peribronchial lymphatic malignancy, or in cases of more localized peribronchial involvement, Wang needle aspirate is preferred. When the presumptive diagnosis is sarcoidosis or another benign interstitial process, one should first attempt a transbronchial biopsy. Whenever there is life-threatening respiratory failure, as, e.g., in the immunosuppressed host, or when the transbronchial biopsy is unrevealing, an open-lung biopsy is usually performed. Open-lung biopsies are increasingly being performed with the thoracoscope.[11–14]

A close communication between surgeon and pathologist is essential for the correct handling of the specimen. The choice of techniques to examine the specimen should be tailored to the clinical impression. Routine stains and light microscopy alone are insufficient for a comprehensive assessment of the tissue. Polarization microscopy is needed to rule out environmental exposure. Special stains for microorganisms are essential to rule out infection. For bacteria, the staining methods of Kenyoun (acid-fast bacilli) and Brown and Bren (Gram-stainable bacilli and cocci) work well in tissue biopsies. Viruses need immunologic techniques for a more precise identification of the offending agent, while the Gomori methenamine silver (GMS) method is very useful in the detection of fungi and *P. carinii.*[128] For the latter, examination of Papanicolaou-stained smears with fluorescent light provides a quick method of identification of the cyst walls.[129] In BAL fluid, a Wright-Giemsa stain reveals the internal structures of trophozoites.[130] All of these stains can be applied to imprint smears, which should be part of the examination of open-lung biopsies. If a more definitive identification of acid-fast bacteria is needed, the auramine-rhodamine fluorescent technique should be utilized. Electron microscopic examination of specimens is commonly used whenever the possibilities of drug toxicity,[131] bronchioloalveolar carcinoma, and small-cell carcinoma exist. For the differentiation between mesothelioma and adenocarcinoma, it is preferable to employ the combination of special stains, immunocytochemistry, and electron microscopy. Often the pathologist is faced with a biopsy specimen that shows neither an obvious tumor nor an easily diagnosable infection, and yet the patient is very ill, and the clinicians anxiously await some guidance in management. In these cases the pathologist should carefully evaluate the character and distribution of the inflammatory infiltrate and provide an account of the presence and extent of fibrosis. The epithelial response is important as well, because it may reflect viral infections in the shape of intracellular inclusions or drug toxicity in the form of metaplastic and atypical changes.[22,79] In the broad category of allergic-immunologic phenomena, it is important to search for eosinophils, which, even in small numbers, serve as an indicator for employing glucocorticoid therapy. If alerted to this possibility, the pathologist should collect frozen tissue for fluorescence microscopy. In diffuse interstitial processes, both the presence of an intra-alveolar "desquamative" component and the persistence of a cellular inflammatory reaction imply a better prognosis and possible success in the administration of glucocorticoids. In contrast, diffuse fibrosis with marked collagenization is a poor prognostic sign. The use of Masson's trichrome stain and the observation of plump, young fibroblasts are useful in the separation of early and late fibrosis. In any process with necrosis of the lung tissue, infection should be ruled out by special stains and appropriate bacteriologic methods prior to the institution of glucocorticoids.

## REFERENCES

1. Churg A: Pulmonologist and pathologist: Ever the two shall meet. *Hum Pathol* **17:**763–764, 1986
2. Rackow E, Fein I, Sprung C, Grodman R: Uremic pulmonary edema. *Am J Med* **64:**1084–1088, 1978
3. Bedrossian CWM, Sussmann J, Conklin RH, Kahan B: Azathioprine-associated interstitial pneumonitis. *Am J Clin Pathol* **82:**148–154, 1983
4. Beschorner WE, Saral R, Hutchins GM, et al: Lymphocytic bronchitis associated with graft-versus-host disease in recipients of bone marrow transplants. *N Engl J Med* **299:**1030–1036, 1978
5. Hunninghake GW, Fanci AS: Pulmonary involvement in the collagen vascular diseases. *Am Rev Res Dis* **119:**471–503, 1979
6. Schultz T, Miller WC, Bedrossian CWM: Clinical application of the measurement of A.C.E. level. *JAMA* **242:**439–441, 1979
7. Daniele RP, Elias JA, Epstein PE, Rossman MD: Bronchoalveolar lavage: Role in the pathogenesis, diagnosis and management of interstitial lung disease. *Ann Int Med* **102:**93–108, 1985
8. Shure D, Fedullo PF: Transbronchial needle aspiration of peripheral lung masses. *Am Rev Res Dis* **128:**1090–1092, 1983
9. Curran JW, Morgan WM, Hardy AM, et al: The epidemiology of AIDS: current status and future prospects. *Science* **229:**1352–1357, 1985
10. Bedrossian CWM, Conklin RH, Kahan B: Pulmonary cytopathology of the renal transplant patient: comparison with histopathology and ultrastructure. *Acta Cytol* **25:**58–59, 1981
11. Hazelrigg SR, Nunchuck SK, LoCicero III J, and The Video As-

sisted Thoracic Surgery Study Group: Video assisted thoracic surgery study group data. *Ann Thorac Surg* **56:**1039–1044, 1993
12. Ferguson MK: Thoracoscopy for diagnosis of diffuse lung disease. *Ann Thorac Surg* **56:**694–696, 1993
13. Dowling RD, Ferson PF, Landreneau RJ: Thoracoscopic resection of pulmonary metastases. *Chest* **102:**1450–1454, 1992
14. Mack MJ, Hazelrigg SR, Landreneau RJ, Acuff TE: Thoracoscopy for the diagnosis of the indeterminate solitary pulmonary nodule. *Ann Thorac Surg* **56:**825–832, 1993
15. Tao LC, Sanders DE, Weisbrod GL, et al: Value and limitations of transthoracic and transabdominal FNA cytology in the clinical practice. *Diagn Cytopathol* **2:**271–276, 1986
16. Wang KP, Marsh BR, Summer WR, et al: Transbronchial needle aspiration for diagnosis of lung cancer. *Chest* **80:**48–50, 1981
17. Bedrossian CWM, Kuhn C III, Luna MA, et al: Desquamative interstitial pneumonia-like reaction accompanying pulmonary lesions. *Chest* **72:**166–169, 1977
18. Bedrossian CWM, Accetta P, Kelly L: Cytopathology on nonneoplastic pulmonary diseases. *Lab Med* **14:**86–95, 1983
19. Bedrossian CWM, Glick AD, Graham S, Mitchell L: Cytopathology and electron microscopy in the diagnosis of lung cancer by FNA biopsies. *Patologia (Mex City)* **22:**367–386, 1984
20. Unger H, Stein DA, Barlogie B, Bedrossian CWM: Analysis of pleural effusion by pulse cytophotometry. *Cancer* **52:**873–877, 1983
21. Mason M, Bedrossian CWM, Fahey C: Value of immunocytochemistry in the study of malignant effusion. *Diagn Cytopathol* **3:**215–221, 1987
22. Bedrossian CWM, DeArce EL, Bedrossian UK, Kelly LV-H: Herpetic tracheobronchitis detected at bronchoscopy: cytologic diagnosis by the immunoperoxidase method. *Diagn Cytopathol* **1:**292–299, 1985
23. Reynolds HY, Newball HH: Analysis of proteins and respiratory cells obtained from human lungs by bronchoalveolar lavage. *J Lab Clin Med* **84:**559–573, 1974
24. Rudd RM, Haslann PL, Turner-Warwick M: Cryptogenic fibrosing alveolitis: relationships of pulmonary physiology and BAL for response to treatment and prognosis. *Am Rev Res Dis* **124:**1–8, 1981
25. Katzenstein ALA, Bloor CM, Liebow AA: Diffuse alveolar damage—the role of oxygen, shock, and related factors. A review. *Am J Pathol* **85:**210–228, 1976
26. Nash G, Foley FD, Langlinais PC: Pulmonary interstitial edema and hyaline membranes in adult burn patients. Electron microscopic observations. *Hum Pathol* **5:**149–160, 1974
27. Eade NR, Taussig IM, Marks MI: Hydrocarbon pneumonitis. *Pediatrics* **54:**351–357, 1974
28. Myers JL, Katzenstein AA: Microangiitis in lupus-induced pulmonary hemorrhage. *Am J Clin Pathol* **85:**552–556, 1986
29. Botting AJ, Brown AL, Divertie MD: The pulmonary lesion in Goodpasture's Syndrome as studied with the electron microscope. *Am J Clin Pathol* **42:**387–394, 1964
30. Morgan PGM, Turner-Warwick M: Pulmonary haemosiderosis and pulmonary hemorrhage. *Br J Dis Chest* **75:**225–242, 1981
31. Hammar SP: Idiopathic interstitial fibrosis. In Dail DH, Hammar SP (eds): *Pulmonary Pathology.* New York, Springer Verlag, 1988, Chap 18, pp 483–510
32. Scadding JG, Hinson KFW: Diffuse fibrosing alveolitis: correlation of histology at biopsy with prognosis. *Thorax* **22:**291–304, 1967
33. Carrington CB, Gaensler EA: Clinical-pathologic approach to diffuse infiltration lung disease. In Thurlbeck WM (ed): *The Lung: Structure, Function and Disease.* Baltimore, Williams & Wilkins, 1979, Chap 4, pp 58–87
34. Woodard BH, Rosenberg SL, Farnham R, Hams DO: Incidence and nature of primary granulomatous inflammation in surgically removed material. *Am J Surg Pathol* **6:**119–129, 1982
35. James DG, Williams WJ: Intrathoracic and upper respiratory tract. In Smith Jr LH (ed): *Sarcoidosis and Other Granulomatous Disorders,* Vol 24. Saunders, Philadelphia, 1985, Chap 5, pp 49–76
36. Baughman R, Strohofer S, Kim CK: Variation of differential cell counts of bronchoalveolar lavage fluid. *Arch Pathol Lab Med* **110:**341–343, 1986
37. Stork WJ, Greenberg SD, Bedrossian CWM: Fatal sarcoidosis. In Iwai H, Hosoda Y (eds): *Proceedings of the VI International Conference on Sarcoidosis.* Tokyo, University Park Press, 1987, pp 462–474
38. Liebow AA: Definition and classification of interstitial pneumonias in human pathology. *Prog Resp Res* **8:**1–33, 1975
39. Bedrossian CWM: Desquamative interstitial pneumonia versus usual interstitial pneumonia. *Chest* **73:**559–560, 1978
40. Valdivia E, Hensely G, Wu J, et al: Morphology and pathogenesis of desquamative interstitial pneumonitis. *Thorax* **32:**7–18, 1977
41. Liebow AA, Steer A, Billingsley JG. Desquamative interstitial pneumonia. *Am J Med* **39:**369–404, 1965
42. Kradin RL, Mark EJ: Benign lymphoid disorders of the lung with a theory regarding their development. *Hum Pathol* **14:**857–867, 1983
43. Liebow AA, Carrington CB: Diffuse pulmonary lymphoreticular infiltrations associated with dysproteinemia. *Med Clin North Am* **57:**809–843, 1973
44. Grieco MH, Chinog-Acharya P: Lymphoid interstitial pneumonia associated with the acquired immune deficiency syndrome. *Am Rev Res Dis* **131:**952–955, 1985
45. Fairfax AJ, Haslam PL, Pavia D, et al: Pulmonary disorders associated with Sjogren's syndrome. *Q J Med* **50:**279–295, 1981
46. Reddy PA, Gorelich DF, Christianson CS: Giant cell interstitial pneumonia (GIP). *Chest* **58:**319–325, 1970
47. Sprince NL, Chamberlin RI, Hales CA, et al: Respiratory disease in tungsten carbide production workers. *Chest* **84:**549–557, 1984
48. Haran K, Jacobsen K: Measles and its relationship to giant cell pneumonia (Hecht pneumonia). *Acta Pathol Microbiol Immunol Scand Sect A Pathol* **81:**761–769, 1973
49. Yousem SA, Colby TV, Gaensler EA. Respiration bronchiolitis-associated interstitial lung disease: A clinico-pathologic study of six cases. *Mayo Clin Proc* **64:**1373–1377, 1989
50. McCann BG, Hart GJ, Stokes TC, Harrison BDW: Obliterative bronchitis and upper zone pulmonary consolidation in rheumatoid arthritis. *Thorax* **38:**73–74, 1983
51. Wyatt SE, Nunn P, Hows JM, et al: Airways and obstruction associated with graft-versus-host disease after bone marrow transplantation. *Thorax* **39:**887–894, 1984
52. Burke CM, Theodore J, Dawkins KD: Post-transplant obliterative bronchiolitis and other late lung sequelae in human heart-lung transplantation. *Chest* **86:**824–829, 1984
53. Johnson WD, Kaye D, Hook EW: Hemophilus influenza pneumonia in adults. Report of nine cases and review of the literature. *Am Rev Res Dis* **97:**1112–1117, 1968
54. Lyle WH. D-Penicillamine and fatal obliterative bronchiolitis. *Br Med J* **1:**105–109, 1977
55. Epler GR, Colby TV, McLoud TC, et al: Bronchiolitis obliterans organizing pneumonia. *N Engl J Med* **312:**152, 1985
56. Izumi T, ed. Proceedings of the International Congress on Bronchiolitis obliterans organizing pneumonia. *Chest* **102**(suppl):1, 1992
57. Guerry-Force ML, Müller NL, Wright JL, et al. A comparison of bronchiolitis obliterans with organizing pneumonia, usual interstitial pneumonia and small airways disease. *Am Rev Respir Dis* **135:**705, 1987
58. Wright JL, Cagle P, Churg A, et al: Diseases of the small airways. *Am Rev Respir Dis* **146:**240, 1992
59. Wohl MEB, Cherniack V: Bronchiolitis. *Am Rev Res Dis* **118:**759–781, 1978
60. Salvaggio J, Harr R: Hypersensitivity pneumonitis: state-of-the-art. *Chest* **75:**270–276, 1979
61. Costabel V, Bross KJ, Marxen MA, Matthys H: T-lymphocytosis in BAL fluid of hypersensitivity pneumonitis: Changes in profile of T-cell subsets during the course of disease. *Chest* **85:**514–518, 1985
62. Hammar S: Hypersensitivity pneumonitis. *Pathol Annu* **23:**195–216, 1988

63. Pennington J: Aspergillus lung disease. *Med Clin North Am* **64:**475–490, 1980
64. Fitzgerald MX, Carrington CB, Gaeryler EA: Environmental lung disease. *Med Clin North Am* **57:**593–616, 1973
65. Graighead JE, Vallyathan NV: Lyptic pulmonary lesions in workers occupationally exposed to dusts containing silica. *JAMA* **233:**1939–1946, 1980
66. Kleinerman J, Green F, Laquer W, et al: Pathology standards for coal worker's pneumonoconiosis. *Am Pathol Lab Med* **103:** 375–432, 1979
67. Gaensler EA: Pathological, physiological and radiological correlations in the pneumoconiosis. *Ann N Y Acad Sci* **200:**574–607, 1972
68. Buednner HA, Ansari A: Acute silicoproteinosis: A new pathologic variant of acute silicosis in sand blasters characterized by histologic features resembling alveolar proteinosis. *Dis Chest* **55:**274–284, 1969
69. Bedrossian CWM. Asbestos-related diseases: A historical and mineralogic perspective. *Semin Diag Pathol* **9:**91–96, 1992
70. Anderson HA, Lillis R, Daum SM, et al: Household contact asbestos neoplastic risk. *Ann N Y Acad Sci* **271:**311–323, 1976
71. Varkey B, Kumar VU: Asbestos-related diseases of lung and pleura. *Postgrad Med* **63:**48–59, 1978
72. Kannerstein M, Churg J, McCauphey WTE: Asbestos and mesothelioma: A review. *Pathol Ann* **13:**81–103, 1978
73. Selikoff IJ, Hammond EC: Asbestos and smoking. *JAMA* **242:**458–459, 1979
74. Roggli VL, Greenberg S, McLarty JL, et al: Comparison of sputum and lung asbestos body counts in former asbestos workers. *Am Rev Resp Dis* **122:**941–945, 1981
75. Roggli VL, Pratt PC, Brody AR: Asbestos content of lung tissue in asbestos-associated diseases: a study of 110 cases. *Br J Indust Med* **43:**18–26, 1986
76. Abraham JL: Recent advances in pneumoconiosis—the pathologist's role in etiologic diagnosis. In Thurlbeck WM, Abell MR (eds): *The Lung: Structure, Function and Disease.* Baltimore, Williams & Wilkins, 1978, pp 96–137
77. Stanford RE: Rheumatoid and other collagen lung diseases. *Semin Resp Med* **4:**107–112, 1981
78. Yousem SA, Colby TV, Carrington CB: Lung biopsy in rheumatoid arthritis. *Am Rev Respir Dis* **131:**770–777, 1985
79. Segal AM, Calabrese LH, Ahinad M, et al: The pulmonary manifestation of systemic lupus erythematosus. *Semin Arthritis Rheum* **14:**202–224, 1985
80. Edelson JD, Hyland RH, Ramsden M, et al: Lung inflammation in scleroderma: Clinical, radiographic, physiologic and cytopathologic features. *J Rheumatol* **12:**957–963, 1985
81. Salmeron G, Greenberg SK, Lidsky MD: Polymyositis and diffuse interstitial lung disease: a review of the pulmonary histopathologic findings. *Arch Int Med* **14:**1005–1010, 1981
82. Prakash UB, Luthra HS, Divertie MD: Intrathoracic manifestations in mixed connective tissue disease. *Mayo Clin Proc* **60:**813–821, 1985
83. Sack KE, Kekheit S, Fadem SZ, Bedrossian CWM: Severe pulmonary vascular disease in S.L.E. *South Med J* **72:**1016–1018, 1979
84. Martinet Y, Haslam PL, Turner-Warwick M: Clinical significance of circulating immune complexes in "lone" cryptogenic fibrosis alveolitis and those with associated connective tissue disorders. *Clin Allergy* **14:**491–497, 1984
85. Bedrossian CWM: Iatrogenic and toxic injury. In Dail DH, Hammar SP (eds): *Pulmonary Pathology.* New York, Springer Verlag 1988, pp 511–534
86. Bedrossian CWM: Pathology of drug-induced lung diseases. *Semin Respir Med* **4:**98–102, 1982
87. Bedrossian CWM, Corey BVJ: Abnormal sputum cytology during chemotherapy with bleomycin. *Acta Cytol* **22:**202–207, 1978
88. Liu FL-W, Cohen RD, Downar E, et al: Amiodarone toxicity: functional and ultrastructural evaluation. *Thorax* **41:**100–105, 1986
89. Alarcon-Segovia D: Drug-induced lupus syndromes. *Mayo Clin Proc* **44:**664–681, 1969
90. Schatz M, Wasserman S, Patterson K: Eosinophils and immunologic lung disease. *Med Clin North Am* **65:**1055–1071, 1981
91. Gaensler EA, Carrington CB: Peripheral opacities in chronic eosinophilic pneumonia: the photographic negative of pulmonary edema. *Am J Roentgenol* **128:**1–13, 1977
92. Bedrossian CWM, Greenberg SD, Williams LJ: Ultrastructure of the lung in Loeffler's pneumonitis. *Am J Med* **58:**438–443, 1975
93. McClenahan JB, Mussenden R: Pulmonary alveolar proteinosis. *Arch Intern Med* **133:**284–287, 1974
94. Morgan PGH, Turner-Warwick M: Pulmonary hemosiderosis and pulmonary hemorrhage. *Br J Dis Chest* **75:**225–242, 1981
95. Haworth SJ, Savage CO, Carr D, et al: Pulmonary hemorrhage complicating Wegener's granulomatosis and microscopic polyarteritis. *Br Med J* **290:**1775–1778, 1985
96. Koss MN, Antonovych T, Hochholzer L: Allergic granulomatosis (Churg Strauss syndrome): Report and analysis of 30 cases. *Mayo Clinic Proc* **52:**477–484, 1977
97. Leatherman JW, Davies SF, Hoidal JR: Alveolar hemorrhage syndromes: Diffuse microvascular lung hemorrhage in immune and idiopathic disorders. *Medicine* **63:**343–361, 1984
98. Katzenstein A: The histologic spectrum and differential diagnosis of necrotizing granulomatous inflammation in the lung. In Fenoglio M, Wolff M (eds): *Progress in Surgical Pathology,* Vol. II. New York, Masson, 1980, pp 42–70
99. Saldana MJ, Patchefsky AS, Israel HL, et al: Pulmonary angiitis and granulomatosis. The relationship between histologic features, organ involvement and response to treatment. *Hum Pathol* **8:**391–409, 1977
100. Jelikovsky T: The structure of bronchial plugs in mucoid impaction, bronchocentric granulomatosis and asthma. *Histopathology* **7:**153–168, 1983
101. Rosenberg M, Patteron R, Mintzer R, et al: Clinical and immunologic criteria for the diagnosis of allergic bronchopulmonary aspergillosis. *Ann Intern Med* **86:**405–410, 1977
102. Ulbright T, Katzenstein A: Solitary necrotizing granulomas of the lung: differentiating features and etiology. *Am J Surg Pathol* **4:**13–28, 1980
103. Myers JL, Katzenstein A-LA: Granulomatous infection mimicking bronchocentric granulomatosis. *Am J Surg Pathol* **10:**317–322, 1986
104. Yang SP, Lin CC: Lymphangitic carcinomatosis of the lungs: The clinical significance of its roentgenologic classification. *Chest* **62:**179–187, 1972
105. Clayton F: Bronchioloalveolar carcinomas: Cell patterns of growth and prognostic types correlates. *Cancer* **57:**1555–1564, 1986
106. Silverman J, Finely JL, Park K, et al: Psammoma bodies and optically clear nuclei in bronchiolo-alveolar cell carcinoma. *Diagn Cytopathol* **1:**205–215, 1985
107. Bedrossian CWM, Weilbaecher DG, et al: Ultrastructure of human bronchioloalveolar cell carcinoma. *Cancer* **36:**1399–1413, 1975
108. McLoud TC, Carrington CB, Gaensler EA: Diffuse infiltrative lung disease: A new scheme for description. *Radiology* **149:**353–363, 1983
109. Rosen SH, Castleman B, Liebow AA: Pulmonary alveolar proteinosis. *N Engl J Med* **258:**1123–1142, 1958
110. Bedrossian CWM, Luna MA, Conklin RH, et al: Alveolar proteinosis as a consequence of immunosuppression: A hypothesis based on clinical and pathologic observations. *Human Pathol* **11:**527–535, 1980
111. Singh G, Katyal SL, Bedrossian CWM, et al: Pulmonary alveolar proteinosis: Staining for surfactant apoprotein in alveolar proteinosis and conditions simulating it. *Chest* **83:**82–86, 1983
112. Corrin B, Liebow AA, Friedman PJ: Pulmonary lymphangioleiomyomatous: A review. *Am J Pathol* **79:**348–382, 1975
113. Kitzsteiner KA, Mallan RG: Pulmonary lymphangioleiomyomatosis: Treatment with castration. *Cancer* **46:**2248–2251, 1980

114. McCarty KS, Jr, Mossler JA, McLelland R, et al: Pulmonary lymphangioleiomyomatosis responsive to progesterone. *N Engl J Med* **303:**1461–1463, 1980

115. Lie JT, Miller RD, Williams DE: Cystic disease of the lung in tuberous sclerosis: Clinicopathologic correlation including body plethysmographic lung function tests. *Mayo Clin Proc* **55:**547–553, 1980

116. Fajardo LF, Bewrthrong M: Radiation injury in surgical pathology—part I. *Am J Surg Pathol* **2:**159–199, 1978

117. Colby TV, Lomard C: Histiocytosis of the lung. *Human Pathol* **14:**847–856, 1983

118. Lipinski J, Weisbrod G, Sanders D: Exogenous lipoid pneumonitis. *Am J Roentgenol* **136:**931–938, 1981

119. Rosenow EC III, Strimlan CV, Muhm JR, et al: Pleuropulmonary manifestations of ankylosing spondylitis. *Mayo Clin Proc* **52:** 641–649, 1977

120. Davis SA, Kaplan RL: Neurofibromatosis and interstitial lung disease. *Arch Dermatol* **114:**1368–1369, 1978

121. Schneider EL, Epstein CJ, Kaback MJ, et al: Severe pulmonary involvement in adult Gaucher's disease: report of three cases and review of the literature. *Am J Med* **63:**475–480, 1977

122. Naeiye RL: Capillary and various lesions in myxederma. *Lab Invest* **12:**465–470, 1963

123. Celli BR, Rubinow A, Cohen AS, Brody JS: Patterns of pulmonary involvement in systemic amyloidosis. *Chest* **74:**593–597, 1978

124. Crystal RG, Gadek JE, Ferrous VJ, et al: Interstitial lung disease: current concepts of pathogenesis, staging and therapy. *Am J Med* **70:**542–568, 1981

125. Hamman L, Rich AR: Acute diffuse interstitial fibrosis of the lungs. *Bull Johns Hopkins Hosp* **74:**177–212, 1944

126. Dreisen RB, Schwarz MI, Theophilopoulos AN, et al: Circulating immune complexes in the idiopathic interstitial pneumonias. *N Engl J Med* **298:**353–357, 1978

127. Haslam PL, Turton CWG, Heard B, et al: Bronchoalveolar lavage in pulmonary fibrosis: comparison of cells obtained with lung biopsy and clinical features. *Thorax* **35:**9–18, 1980

128. Sunt T, Chess Q, Tannembaum B: Morphologic criteria for the identification of *Pneumocystis carinii* in Papanicolaou stained preparations. *Acta Cytol* **30:**80–82, 1986

129. Bedrossian CWM, Mason MR, Gupta P. Rapid cytologic diagnosis of pneumoncystis: A comparison of effective techniques. *Semin Diagn Pathol* **6:**245–261, 1989

130. Golden J, Hollander H, Stulbarg M, et al: BAL as the exclusive diagnostic modality for pneumocystis Carinii pneumonia: a prospective study among patients with AIDS. *Chest* **90:**18–22, 1986

131. Bedrossian CWM, Warren C, Ohar J, et al: Amiodarone pulmonary toxicity: BAL, cytopathology, ultrastructure and immunocytochemistry. *Hum Pathol* In press.

CHAPTER

# 16

# Pneumonia, Bronchiectasis, and Lung Abscess

James B.D. Mark and Norman W. Rizk

## HISTORY

The existence and clinical presentations of suppurative diseases of the lungs have been known for many centuries. Detailed accounts abound of patients and their illnesses with outcomes both successful and fatal. External drainage of lung abscess was practiced as early as the time of Hippocrates and was undoubtedly lifesaving in some instances. However, the accurate diagnosis of pyogenic lung abscess and bronchiectasis, and the differentiation of these problems from the ever-present pulmonary tuberculosis, awaited the introduction of the stethoscope by Laennec in 1819, the x-ray by Roentgen in 1895, iodized oil bronchography by Sicard and Forestier in 1922, and accurate bronchoscopy by Koch and others.[1,2] Improvements in the treatment of these entities followed their accurate anatomic and pathologic delineation by Brock, Churchill, and others.[3,4]

## PNEUMONIA

In the United States currently, pneumonia is the sixth leading cause of death and the most common infectious cause.[5] It occurs when either a virulent infectious inoculum or a defect in immunologic host mechanisms breaches the normal anatomic and cellular defenses that maintain sterility of the lower tracheobronchial tree. A specific microbiologic etiology of pneumonia may be identified by culture or serologic assays, but in as many as 50% of patients the responsible pathogen is not discovered despite extensive testing.[6] Formulating a diagnostic strategy and selecting empiric therapy for the remainder of the patients is dependent upon whether the pneumonia is community or hospital acquired, on the immunocompetency of the host, and on whether it was due to gross aspiration.

### Community-Acquired Pneumonia

Approximately 4 million cases of community-acquired pneumonia (CAP) occur annually in the United States. Of these about one fifth require hospitalization,[5] and as many as 25% of the hospitalized patients die of it. CAP is increasingly encountered in patients with advanced age and comorbidity, particularly congestive heart failure, chronic renal failure, diabetes mellitus, and chronic obstructive lung disease. In large surveys, the most common etiologies are *Streptococcus pneumoniae, Mycoplasma pneumoniae* (in patients under age 60), *Chlamydia pneumoniae,* respiratory viruses, and gram negative bacilli, especially *Legionella* species and *Hemophilus influenzae.*[6]

Appropriate diagnostic studies include cultures of blood, sputum, and, when possible, of pleural fluid. Unfortunately the sensitivity and specificity of sputum cultures are poor, and only the most severely ill patients have positive blood or pleural fluid cultures. Gram staining of expectorated sputum is problematic as well, since it does not correlate well with cultures of alveolar material, even when controls like fewer than five squamous epithelial cells per low-power microscopy field are imposed. Serologic testing and cold agglutinin assays are occasionally useful but should not be routinely performed; their main value resides in confirming a specific etiology suspected clinically.[6] Use of complement fixation testing for *M. pneumoniae* or immunodiffusion assays for coccidiomycosis are examples of this.

Invasive diagnostic measures, including transtracheal

aspiration, bronchoscopy with protected brush or bronchoalveolar lavage sampling, and fine-needle aspiration, should be reserved for gravely ill patients or patients with unresolving pneumonia. In the absence of a specific positive culture, younger, less severely ill patients can be treated with macrolides, i.e., erythromycin.[6] Clarithromycin and azithromycin are useful for those intolerant of erythromycin. Older and sicker patients should receive a second-generation cephalosporin, trimethoprim-sulfamethoxazole, or a beta-lactam/beta-lactam inhibitor, possibly with a macrolide.[6] Gravely ill hospitalized patients may be treated with a macrolide plus a third-generation cephalosporin with anti-pseudomonal activity, ciprofloxacin, or imipenem/cilastin.[6]

## Hospital-Acquired Pneumonia

Nationwide surveys of the etiology of nosocomial pneumonias have revealed that *Pseudomonas aeruginosa* and *Staphylococcus aureus* remain the most frequent isolates from patients with pneumonia. Also commonly encountered are *Enterobacter* species, *Klebsiella pneumoniae,* and *Escherichia coli.*[7] In patients with in-dwelling central lines, particularly parenteral nutrition lines, Candidal species are a frequent pathogen. Ventilator-associated pneumonia carries a particularly poor prognosis, with a fatality rate as high as 23%[8]; ventilator-associated pneumonia is also difficult to diagnose, since many ventilated patients have other explanations for pulmonary infiltrates, like pulmonary edema, atelectasis, or hemorrhage. In fact, some studies have indicated that even the constellation of purulent sputum, fever, leukocytosis, and radiographic infiltrates has a poor specificity for pneumonia in this setting.[9,10] In one report, only 22 of 75 mechanically ventilated patients with all of these findings actually had pneumonia, as judged by quantitative cultures from protected brush specimens.[9] The low specificity of the clinical findings was further confirmed in this study by withholding antibiotics from the patients with negative quantitative protected brush cultures, with no adverse clinical outcomes. Because of this, some investigators advocate quantitative bronchoalveolar lavage or protected brush cultures in all ventilated patients being evaluated for pneumonia.[11,12] However, in most centers a wary clinical approach, rather than an invasive diagnostic one, is still the most common method. Empiric therapy, based on the likely nosocomial pathogens, might include third generation cephalosporins and extended range penicillins, perhaps with an aminoglycoside or imipenen/cilastin.[13]

## Pneumonia Associated with Aspiration

Aspiration may occur perioperatively or at any time when the state of consciousness and gag reflex are impaired. Chemical injury and obstruction usually cause acute symptoms, but the establishment of true aspiration pneumonia ordinarily occurs several days later.

Anaerobes should be actively sought in the bacteriologic workup, since they are more common than and frequently coexist with aerobes in these pneumonias. *Bacteroides melanogenicus, Fusobacteria,* and anaerobic streptococci are the most common anaerobes in this setting. When the aspiration occurs outside the hospital, streptococci are the most common aerobes; in hospital, *Staphylococcus aureus* and gram-negative bacilli predominate. Out of hospital aspiration can be treated by clindamycin or penicillin alone. In hospital aspiration requires a broader-spectrum penicillin like piperacillin or ticarcillin, and an aminoglycoside.

## Pneumonia in Immunocompromised Hosts

The spectrum of potential pathogens increases greatly with immunosuppression. In particular, neutropenic hosts have a high frequency of fungal—particularly *Aspergillus*—infections in addition to gram-negative bacilli and staphylococcal isolates. Patients with lymphoid line defects are at particular risk for *Pneumocystis carinii* and viral infections. Corticosteroids predispose to *P. carinii,* fungal disorders, nocardial disease, and *Legionella* species. Bone marrow transplant recipients are at major risk for cytomegalovirus pneumonitis at 5–10 weeks' posttransplant, and for diffuse alveolar hemorrhage while thrombocytopenic. Because of the wide differential diagnosis in immunocompromised hosts, an algorithmic approach that encompasses radiographic findings, risks of procedures, and tempo of progression of infection is useful. In the last few years, thoracoscopic video-assisted biopsy has largely replaced open biopsy, except in patients with uncorrectable coagulopathies or sealed pleural spaces.

## Characteristics of Unresolved Pneumonia

Unresolved pneumonia may be defined as a segmental or lobar infiltrative process that persists more than 2 weeks with proper treatment. When accurately diagnosed and adequately treated, acute inflammatory processes in the lung should show discernable clinical and radiographic improvement. Should a pneumonia fail to improve within 2 weeks, certain questions should be asked and answered[14]:

1. Has the proper diagnostic information been obtained, as described earlier, for cultures?
2. Are the proper antibiotics being used?
3. Has there been a change in organism or superinfection?
4. Is this a nonbacterial infection (such as fungal, viral, or protozoal infection), tuberculosis, mycoplasma, or *Legionella*?

A particularly common, important, and easily diagnosed reason for unresolved pneumonia is lobar or segmental bronchial obstruction. Obstruction, particularly by a tumor or foreign body, may precede pneumonia and be related to its occurrence, as well as to its failure to clear. Extrinsic obstruction by enlarged lymph nodes or intrinsic obstruction by granulation tissue or scarring is less common, though well described.

In children, especially those under 5 years of age, unresolved pneumonia should lead to the suspicion of foreign body aspiration. Nonradiopaque foreign bodies, such as peanuts or other food, small pieces of plastic, vegetable matter such as Timothy grass,[15] or crayons, may easily escape detection. A careful history taken from the parents concerning choking or coughing episodes is generally helpful. Bronchoscopy should be done in every child with unresolved pneumonia by an endoscopist skilled in the use of rigid instruments and in the techniques of foreign-body removal.

In middle-aged patients with localized unresolved pneumonitis, there must be a high index of suspicion for carcinoma. Careful bronchoscopy is the definitive diagnostic procedure in such circumstances. Bronchograpy is rarely positive when bronchoscopy is negative for tumor, and it is not of additional benefit when bronchoscopy is positive. Computed tomography (CT) scanning, because of its volume averaging, is not a sensitive tool for endobronchial disease and therefore not a substitute for endoscopy.

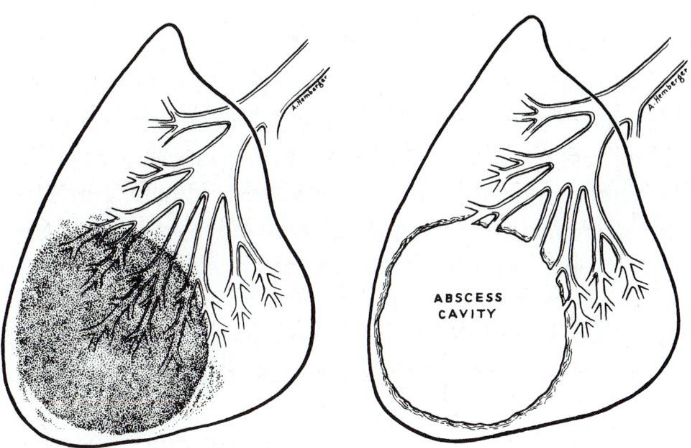


**Figure 16–1.** Diagram to illustrate the pathogenesis of pulmonary abscess. The lobe at the left shows a large zone of necrotizing pneumonitis involving numerous bronchi in "cross-country" fashion. At the right, the contents of the abscess have been evacuated, and healing is indicated in the margins of the residual cavity. The latter remains in communication with several bronchi from which an ingrowth of epithelium may proceed. Ultimately, epithelization can become complete. The outer wall is a condensate of scarred lung tissue in which proliferated smooth muscle is often so prominent that confusion with congenital cysts can occur.

## LUNG ABSCESS

In 1936, when Neuhoff and Touroff[16] reported their extensive personal experience with surgical treatment of lung abscess in the preantibiotic era, they concluded that "the great majority of the graver lesions should be subjected to operation" and that "the seriousness of acute pulmonary abscess can be appreciated only if the sequelae of the policy of delay and the complication with their mortality are borne in mind." Supportive measures, including nutrition and postural drainage, were important elements of therapy then, and the great strides made in nutritional support and chest physiotherapy make them even more valuable in the present day; but it was the introduction of antibiotics that transformed our approach to the treatment of lung abscess.

### General Characteristics of Lung Abscess

Lung abscess may be defined as a suppurative and destructive process occurring within the pulmonary parenchyma caused by pyogenic organisms. The frequency and occurrence of lung abscess, particularly following pneumonia, has diminished sharply since the advent of antibiotics. Abscess still occurs with some frequency in alcoholics and other patients who aspirate gastric contents and other material into the tracheobronchial tree. Pyogenic abscess must be carefully differentiated from cavitary tuberculosis and cavitary carcinoma.

### Pathology

The pathologic process of abscess formation results in the destruction of pulmonary parenchyma (Fig. 16–1). The inner wall of an acute abscess is lined by fibrinopurulent material that merges with surrounding consolidated pulmonary tissue. Pulmonary vessels in the abscess are generally destroyed or thrombosed and may rupture, causing bleeding of varying degree.

Mild to moderate hemoptysis is not unusual in lung abscess, and massive hemoptysis may occur. Although usually confined to a single lobe, the pathologic process is not confined by segmental boundaries. Abscesses, especially those caused by staphylococci, may be multiple and may occur in more than one lobe simultaneously. This is particularly true when the abscess follows a major aspiration resulting in soilage of multiple areas of the lung. It should be remembered that bronchial communication is the rule, and this is the reason for the frequent finding of an air–fluid level on the upright chest radiograph.

As an abscess becomes chronic, the acute inflammatory process lining the cavity gives way to granulation tissue, and this inflammation evolves into the "golden pneumonia" that is characterized microscopically by the presence of lipid-laden macrophages. Later in the pathologic process, the wall of the abscess may become lined with low cuboidal or even pseudostratified columnar epithelium. By such time, the surrounding inflammatory process has yielded to scar tissue, which contracts and obliterates the abscess cavity.

In the acute phase, an abscess may extend to the pleural surface, causing pleuritis, pleural effusion, or empyema. If an abscess perforates into the pleural cavity, pyopneumothorax with or without tension may result. A far advanced or neglected abscess may rupture into the mediastinum, the pericardium, or transdiaphragmatically into the abdomen.

## Abscess of Aspirative Origin

Aspiration is the most common causative mechanism for lung abscess.[17] The combination of vomiting and unconsciousness produced by alcohol or drug ingestion is particularly incriminated in this etiology; head trauma, convulsive disorders, and general anesthesia are other precipitating factors. Esophageal disorders causing obstruction, such as incoordination of swallowing, achalasia, stricture, carcinoma, or reflux, are less common causes of lung abscess. However, these may lead to recurrent episodes of pneumonitis, particularly in the lower lobes.

Lung abscess has been associated with "metastatic" infection from the head and neck, and patients with lung abscess do frequently have poor orodental hygiene.[18] Bronchial obstruction by a foreign body should be considered as another etiology of lung abscess, especially in children.

More than 40 years ago, Brock[19] clearly defined the mode of aspiration in the lungs and related this to the position of the patient at the time of aspiration. One generally thinks of the basilar segments of the lower lobes as being the most dependent portions of the lungs, but this is only true when the patient is erect. When the patient is supine, the superior segmental orifices of the lower lobes are the ones that are most dependent (Fig. 16–2). The upper lobe orifices are dependent when the patient is in the lateral decubitus position.

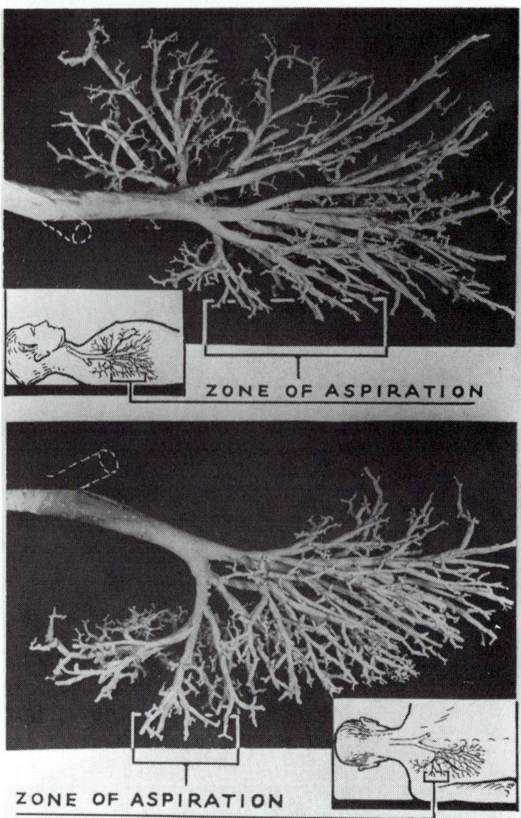


**Figure 16–2.** Mechanism of bronchial aspiration in the pathogenesis of lung abscess illustrated by a bronchial cast of a left lung. Upper frame: In the supine position, aspirated material gravitating down the trachea and main bronchus will enter the first dorsally directed (dependent) bronchus, that supplying the superior segment of the lower lobe. Lower frame: In the lateral decubitus position, the most dependent regions and the first to receive foreign material are the axillary subsegments of the posterior ($B_3$) and anterior ($B_2$) segments of the upper lobe.

## Abscess Associated with Infarction

In the past, infarction was thought to be the most common etiology for lung abscess, but this was probably never the case. The theory of aspiration described above is much more plausible, and it correlates with the anatomic and pathologic observations. There is no question, however, that septic emboli can cause lung abscess.[20] These emboli can arise from pelvic veins following a septic abortion or prostatitis; from septic peripheral thrombophlebitis; from osteomyelitis; or from truncal veins containing infected thrombi following liver abscess, suppurative pancreatitis, or peritonitis. Antibiotics have rendered most of the aforementioned entities quite rare, and septic emboli thus occur much less frequently than in the past.

## Abscess Following Trauma

Lung abscess may occasionally follow penetrating or blunt trauma. A hematoma of the lung following trauma may become infected by blood-borne or aspirated organisms, or through the presence of a foreign body. Victims of nonthoracic trauma, which has resulted in prolonged hospitalization with unconsciousness, immobilization, or sepsis, not infrequently develop pulmonary complications, usually atelectasis or pneumonia, and sometimes they develop lung abscess. Such an abscess is often due to hospital-acquired organisms and may be very difficult to treat successfully. In such cases, awareness of the possibility of such infection and its successful prevention are extremely important.

## Extension from the Abdomen or Mediastinum

The pleuropulmonary complication that most often follows subdiaphragmatic or mediastinal infection is empyema. However, if pleural adhesions are dense, and if the lung is tightly adherent to adjacent parietal structures, a mediastinal or subdiaphragmatic infection may penetrate into the lung and cause an abscess. Such abscesses may follow amoebic or pyogenic liver abscess, subdiaphragmatic abscess from any cause, or mediastinitis, most often due to esophageal perforation. The successful treatment of lung abscesses related to other such diseases in the mediastinum or abdomen depends largely upon the successful treatment of the underlying problem.

### Abscess Associated with Bronchial Obstruction

Bronchial obstruction, most often due to tumor or foreign body, and less often to such unusual entities as broncholithiasis or inflammatory bronchostenosis, may lead to distal infection through poor lobar or segmental drainage (Fig. 16–3). This type of infection is usually pneumonia, superimposed on atelectasis, and it may progress to lung abscess. Because bronchial obstruction may lead to abscess, bronchoscopy should be done in any patient whose abscess fails to clear promptly with appropriate antibiotic and supportive treatment.

### Abscess Following Necrotizing Pneumonia

Pneumonias caused by *S. aureus,* type III pneumonococcus, *P. aeruginosa,* and *K. pneumoniae* are apt to result in the early necrosis of pulmonary parenchyma and abscess formation. Staphylococcal infection may occur as a primary process, especially in children. Pneumococcal pneumonia tends to occur primarily in the elderly. However, hospital-acquired infections, particularly those with gram-negative organisms, frequently occur in patients sustaining trauma or undergoing major surgery. As outlined earlier, nosocomial infections are especially frequent in immunocompromised hosts. It should be remembered that pneumonia and abscess may lead very quickly to sepsis and death in these patients whose immune and/or nutritional status is significantly impaired.[21]

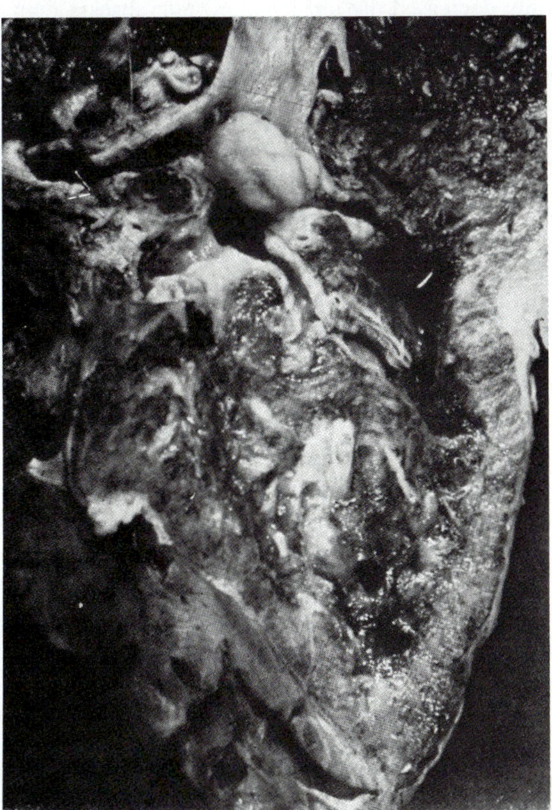

**Figure 16–3.** Surgical specimen showing an abscess distal to an obstructing bronchial chondroma. Two bronchi are seen to enter the large cavity, which has additional ramifications in the basilar segments of the lobe, here largely obscured by the organizing pneumonitis.

### Abscess in Preexisting Pulmonary Lesions

Secondary infection of intrapulmonary bronchogenic cysts or acquired bullae may produce a febrile illness in a patient with an "abscess" by chest radiograph. If the cyst or bulla has been known to exist prior to the infection, and/or the air–fluid level is contained in a sharply delineated perimeter surrounded by little evidence for pulmonary infiltration, a pyocyst or infected bulla should be strongly suspected. Such lesions may be aspirated under fluoroscopic guidance via the transbronchial route, using a plastic catheter with a guidewire passed through the flexible bronchoscope.[22,23] Less commonly, abscess formation may result from the secondary infection of bronchopulmonary sequestrations. These lesions do not respond completely to nonoperative treatment alone. If such a lesion is suspected, a chest CT scan with contrast or a magnetic resonance imaging (MRI) scan may demonstrate the anomalous blood supply. If any question remains, a thoracic aortogram should be carried out. This is the definitive procedure. Identification of anomalous blood supply will help in the prevention of serious hemorrhage at the time of operation.

### Carcinomatous Abscess

Cavitating carcinoma of the lung is the most common reason for lung abscess in middle-aged smokers.[24] While it is impossible to differentiate the pyogenic from the carinomatous abscess by radiographic means alone, carcinomatous abscesses tend to have thick and irregular walls and may demonstrate umbilication. The patient may not have a history to suggest infection or aspiration. Knowledge of these facts will lead to earlier additional studies such as bronchoscopy and fine-needle aspiration. If a carcinoma is identified early, a better chance of long-term survival may accompany earlier appropriate treatment.

## CLINICAL MANIFESTATIONS

### Symptoms

Since there are several different causes of lung abscess, the clinical symptoms vary in severity and acuity. Fever and sputum production may worsen immediately following an episode of pneumonia, or there may be a latent period of several days or weeks following an aspirative episode before fever and sputum production begin. The sputum is generally purulent and is frequently tinged with blood. It may be voluminous and fetid. A frequent clinical observation is the layering of sputum in a container, with gray-green portion at the bottom, a mucoid midzone, and a frothy superficial layer. Chest pain, pleuritic or steady in nature, is often seen in patients with lung abscess. However, there is nothing in the symptom complex that clearly differentiates lung abscess from other pyogenic or cavitating pulmonary problems.

### Physical Signs

Patients with acute, untreated lung abscess usually appear ill, with fever, tachycardia, and tachypnea. The patient's breath may be malodorous, and gingivodental hygiene is often poor. There may be tenderness on palpation of the chest wall over the affected area of the lung. The examiner frequently notes dullness to percussion and diminished breath sounds, but rales are not always present. If there is free connection of the abscess to the bronchus, the breath sounds are apt to be tubular; moist rales and rhonchi are generally heard. Because physical signs in the chest may change from day to day, depending upon the state of bronchial communication, frequent, careful examination of the chest is necessary. Clubbing of the fingers, a finding in many patients with chronic hypoxic pulmonary disease, may become evident as early as 2 weeks after the onset of a lung abscess. Clubbing generally regresses as the abscess resolves.

### Radiographic Findings

In his well-known monograph, Lord Brock noted that "the abscess cavity usually lies within less than a centimetre of the surface of presentation; even though an incorrect surgical approach may not uncover the most superficial area of presentation."[19] To be sure, this fact critically affects surgical decision making in the drainage of lung abscess.[25]

Prior to communication between the lung abscess and the tracheobronchial tree, the chest radiograph will not show the characteristic and expected air–fluid level. Instead, there is an area of infiltrate, with or without atelectasis, involving one or more pulmonary segments or an entire lobe. Once bronchial communication is established, an air–fluid level will be seen on upright and lateral decubitus chest radiographs or on CT scan (Fig. 16–4). Any supine or prone x-ray (except for CT scan) will fail to show an air–fluid level and, therefore, may be misleading to the unwary. Abscesses characteristically have a surrounding zone of parenchymal infiltration. Thin-walled and expanding abscesses suggest a diagnosis of pyocyst or pneumatocele. Thickening and nodularity of the cavity wall suggest the possibility of cavitating carcinoma. Significant enlargement of hilar or mediastinal lymph nodes may be associated with pyogenic abscess or with carcinoma. It may occasionally be difficult to differentiate an abscess from an empyema with bronchopleural fistula. Ultrasound and especially CT frequently help in this differentiation.[26,27]

An underutilized, relatively inexpensive, and frequently helpful radiographic study in patients with lung abscess or recurrent pneumonia is the barium esophagogram. Gastric reflux or esophageal obstruction due to tumor, stricture, or achalasia may lead to aspiration into the tracheobronchial tree, resulting in pneumonia or abscess. This association is particularly well known in children.

### Differential Diagnosis

Cavitating bronchogenic carcinoma, tuberculosis, empyema with bronchopleural fistula, pyocyst, and cavitating mycotic lesions must be differentiated from pyogenic lung abscess. As the incidence of carcinoma continues to rise, especially in women, cancer assumes a primary place in the differential diagnosis of lung abscess, particularly in smokers in their middle years without a history of factors predisposing to pyogenic lung abscess.

### Treatment

It is true today as it was 50 years ago that general supportive care, including nutritional support and chest physiotherapy with vigorous postural drainage, are important and effective aspects of the treatment of patients with lung abscess.[28] However, the appropriate use of antibiotics has not only decreased the incidence of lung abscess dramatically but also has changed the mode of treatment and outcome expectations. Before antibiotics, the conservative measures in the treatment of lung abscess consisted of the supportive care mentioned above and bronchoscopy. Patients who failed to improve on this regimen required surgical drainage (Monaldi drainage) in two stages or, later, one stage. Morbidity and mortality were high, and long-term successful outcome was the exception rather than the rule. Today, although aggressive pulmonary toilet, appropriate nutritional support, transfusions of blood when indicated, and attention to any etiologic factors that may be present—such as poor oral hygiene, causes of aspiration, and alcoholism—continue to be important, antibiotics have made the clinical cure of lung abscess, without the need for external drainage or surgical resection, clearly the rule. As succinctly stated by LeRoux and coworkers,[29] proper management consists of "administration of an appropriate antibiotic, drainage of the pus by some means, and pulmonary resection in cases where there is permanent lung damage with symptoms, or a threat to life, such as massive hemoptysis."

When the diagnosis of lung abscess is made, appropriate sputum cultures and smears should be obtained in order to accurately identify the offending organism(s). Most often, a mixed, oral flora will be found, lending further support to the aspirative theory for the etiology of lung abscess. For complete identification of bacteria, both aerobic and anaerobic cultures should be obtained. The latter requires direct access to the tracheobronchial tree by transtracheal aspiration, proper bronchoscopy using techniques to avoid oral contamination, or direct percutaneous aspiration of the

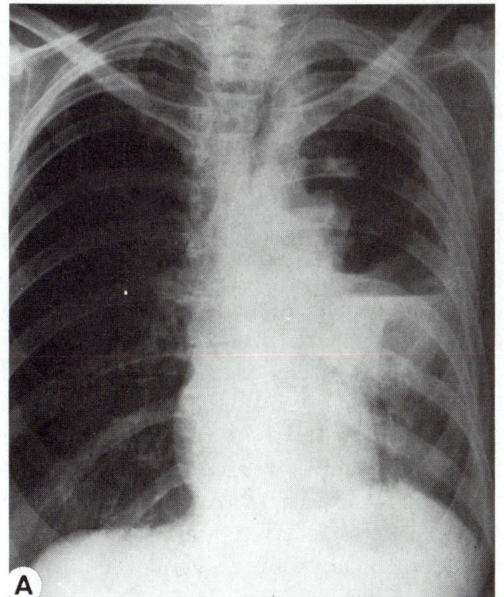

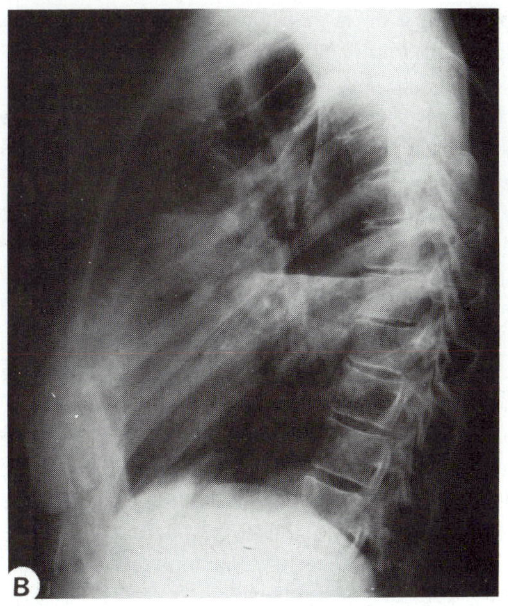

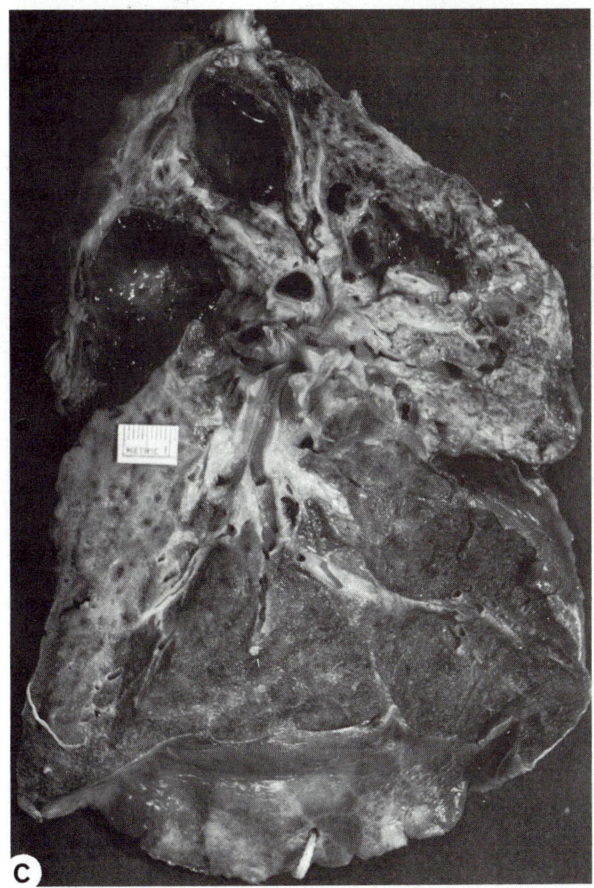

**Figure 16–4.** Multiple chronic abscesses involving both lobes of the left lung. The patient was an alcoholic divorcee with poor orodental hygiene. Three years before admission, she had pneumonia that was followed by a persistent cough and purulent sputum. Four months prior to hospitalization, she experienced a series of brisk hemoptyses with fever and night sweats. **A.** PA roentgenogram at admission, demonstrating a contracted left chest and lung, an elevated left hemidiaphragm, and multiple cavities with air–fluid levels in the upper and midlung fields. **B.** The lateral projection localizes a large cavity in the superior segment ($B_6$) of the lower lobe and a larger multilocular abscess involving much of the upper lobe. After 3 weeks of treatment with antibiotics, bronchoscopy, and transfusions, a left total pneumonectomy was performed. **C.** Sagittal section of the resected lung shows the cavities described above. Below the cavity in the lower lobe is an area of pulmonary consolidation chiefly by fat-filled phagocytes, the so-called golden pneumonia.

abscess under CT or fluoroscopic guidance. Examination of the material for fungi, acid-fast bacilli, and cancer cells is essential. The immediate use of high-dose IV penicillin or clindamycin is indicated in the treatment of lung abscess, unless or until bacteriologic evidence mandates the use of different antibiotics (such as vancomycin for *S. aureus*).[30,31] Precise and proper antibiotic use, along with supportive measures, should result in significant clinical improvement within several days to 1 week. Prolonged antibiotic use for weeks or even months is required in some cases until radiographic evidence shows healing to be well on its way to completion. It should be noted that clinical improvement usually precedes radiographic improvement by days or even weeks. If the patient is improving clinically, the persistence of an air–fluid level, with or without surrounding infiltration, is not an indication for surgical resection.

Bronchoscopy is no longer carried out in all patients with lung abscess. It should be done, however, in abscesses that resolve slowly or when tumor or foreign body are suspected. The endoscopist should be skilled in both flexible and rigid bronchoscopy since flooding of the tracheobronchial tree may occur. Repeated bronchoscopy may be necessary during the course of treatment if improvement and/or radiographic resolution do not occur.

With antibiotic and supportive treatment as described, the mortality rate from acute lung abscess in the nonimmunocompromised host has declined dramatically, and clinical cure is now the rule than the exception. Overall, 80–90% of patients with lung abscess should be cured without surgical intervention.[32–37] However, this remains a serious illness, where mortality is still seen and where hospitalization for 1–3 weeks is the norm.[38–40]

## Decision for Surgery

Surgical drainage may be internal (bronchoscopic) or external. More definitive drainage should be undertaken when a patient remains febrile more than 10 days–2 weeks, when there has been no radiographic progress in 3–4 weeks, or when surgical complications such as hemoptysis, empyema, or bronchopleural fistula occur.[41,42] The dramatic advances in interventional radiology have shown the effectiveness of percutaneous drainage of lung abscess using catheters (approximate 8–10 French) placed under fluoroscopic, CT, or ultrasound guidance.[28,29,43,44] It has been shown that empyema is not more common after percutaneous drainage.[40] Percutaneous drainage has even been accomplished successfully in the setting of positive pressure ventilation.[45]

In certain cases, one should consider percutaneous drainage even earlier in the course of treatment. It has been shown that young children (less than 7 years) rarely respond to conservative treatment and should undergo early percutaneous drainage.[25] Furthermore, patients with so-called giant lung abscess should undergo percutaneous drainage early on.[46] Brock's observation that nearly all lung abscesses will be seen to abut the chest wall when adequate radiographic views are obtained further corroborates the validity of this mode of drainage.[19]

## Surgical Treatment

### *Direct Tube Drainage (Pneumonotomy or Monaldi drainage)*

If direct tube drainage of an acute abscess is necessary, one must keep in mind two important principles. First, accurate topical localization of the abscess is imperative. Usually, this is readily accomplished by posteroanterior and lateral, and, if necessary, oblique chest radiographs, and the careful counting of overlying ribs by the surgeon. If there is any doubt, fluoroscopy, ultrasound, or CT localization can be done with a radiopaque marker on the skin at the proposed drainage site. Appropriate adjustments can then be made in the operating room.

Second, one must be as certain as possible that the lung in the area of the abscess is adherent to the overlying parietal pleura. With proper localization, this is usually the case, and this circumstance will prevent spillage of abscess contents into the free pleural cavity.

Local or general anesthesia may be used. We prefer the latter, administered through a properly placed double-lumen endotracheal tube in order to prevent bronchial flooding should the abscess drain into the tracheobronchial tree during manipulation. A 5- or 6-cm segment of the appropriate rib is removed subperiosteally, with care being taken by the surgeon not to enter the pleural space. If the proper location has been chosen, the pleura will be thickened and opaque. The abscess should then be aspirated by needle to confirm its location and depth and to obtain a specimen for smear and cultures, both aerobic and anaerobic. Fungal and tuberculosis studies should be done if such an etiology is suspected.

For entry into the abscess, lung tissue over the abscess may be incised with electrocautery. Suction and gentle mechanical debridement should be carried out. A large (36–40 French) Malecot or mushroom catheter should then be inserted, affixed to the skin with one or two sutures of heavy silk, and attached, through an underwater seal, to a suction of –20 cm $H_2O$. The suction should be continued until marked radiographic clearing and clinical improvement are apparent.

Such drainage of a lung abscess may result in prompt and dramatic clinical improvement, with a decrease in sputum production and defervescence. The drainage, which may initially be voluminous, will gradually diminish. An air leak is to be expected at the outset, but this usually disappears within several days to 2 weeks, as healing progresses. If the patient is doing well and the air leak has ceased, suction may be discontinued and the tube cut short so that a dressing may be worn over it, and the patient may be freely ambulatory. The tube should be further secured to the skin at this time, usually with a safety pin and tape. The tube is usually left in place for several weeks, although the patient may be discharged from the hospital much sooner than that.

Careful outpatient follow-up is important. Irrigation of the drainage tube in lung abscess, unlike empyema, is usually inadvisable because of the bronchial connections. Once the patient is better and the x-ray appearance has improved, the tube may be removed. The remaining tract generally heals without much difficulty over a period of 1 or more weeks.

Tube drainage is not free of potential problems. Secondary hemorrhage, pyopneumothorax, and cerebral abscess may all result from the abscess itself or from the operative procedure. Nevertheless, tube drainage may be lifesaving for the desperately ill patient with a large abscess. Late bronchiectasis and bronchopleural fistula are surprisingly rare following tube drainage of an abscess.[46]

### Pulmonary Resection

While most lung abscesses heal satisfactorily with antibiotic treatment, with or without drainage, the occasional acute lung abscess will progress to a chronic stage, with a thick-walled cavity; irreversible changes in the surrounding lung tissues; and continuing symptoms of fever, cough, and sputum production (Fig. 16–5). Factors favoring chronicity are poorly drained loculations, bronchostenosis, and empyema associated with perforation into the pleura. Such occurrences usually necessitate pulmonary resection by lobectomy, in order to affect a cure. Other indications for resection of a chronic abscess are massive hemorrhage or recurrent significant hemoptysis[47,48] (Fig. 16–6).

A wedge or segmental resection of a chronic lung abscess will rarely result in an uncomplicated cure. Not only is there generally enough destruction of adjacent pulmonary parenchyma to render attempts to save portions of a lobe fruitless, but such efforts are also associated with a higher incidence of persistent air leak and empyema than is lobectomy. In most instances, quantitative ventilation-perfusion scans (or perfusion scans alone) will be reassuring; these most often demonstrate the lack of function of an entire lobe in cases in which there is a clinical indication for pulmonary resection.

The presence of a lung abscess, even a chronic one necessitating resection, is an indication for the use of a double-lumen endotracheal tube in order to prevent spillage of pus into the contralateral lung or into another lobe or lobes on the ipsilateral side. The surgeon should be prepared for rigid bronchoscopy before and/or after the operation, if this is indicated by the presence of pus or blood in the tracheobronchial tree.

Dense and vascular pleural and hilar adhesions may be present. If an empyema cavity or tense lung abscess is present, suction decompression will generally make the operation technically safer. Bronchial vessels are sometimes enlarged and tortuous. Lymph nodes may be densely adherent, not only to the bronchi but also to the pulmonary artery and its branches. Particular care in hilar dissection is important in order to prevent major hemorrhage. Meticulous hemostasis is especially important, since what appears to be oozing or minor bleeding from lymph nodes or adhesions is usually from small systemic arteries rather than from a pulmonary vessel. Because of higher pressure in the systemic circuit, bleeding may not stop spontaneously. The pleural cavity should be generously drained with at least two large-caliber tubes in order to encourage prompt expansion of the remaining lobe or lobes, to help stop air leaks, and to give the best assurance against postoperative empyema. The successful resection of a chronic lung abscess should not only improve the patient's chronic symp-

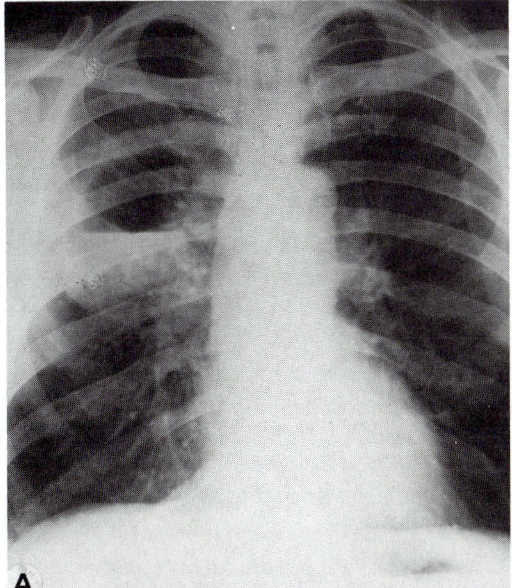


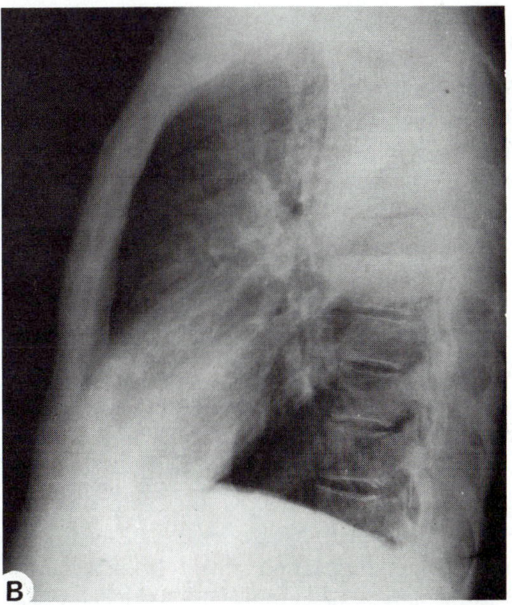


**Figure 16–5.** Transfissural extension of an acute lung abscess. **A.** Admission roentgenogram shows a huge, unilocular and thin-walled abscess in the right midlung field, with an air–fluid interface clearly demarcated. **B.** In the lateral projection the abscess centers on the posterior aspect of the oblique fissure. At operation it involved both upper and lower lobes. An upper lobectomy and resection of the superior segment of the lower lobe were performed, since the therapeutic response to antibiotics and bronchoscopy was poor; furthermore, the bilobar extension suggested that simple pneumonotomy and drainage might not be adequate.

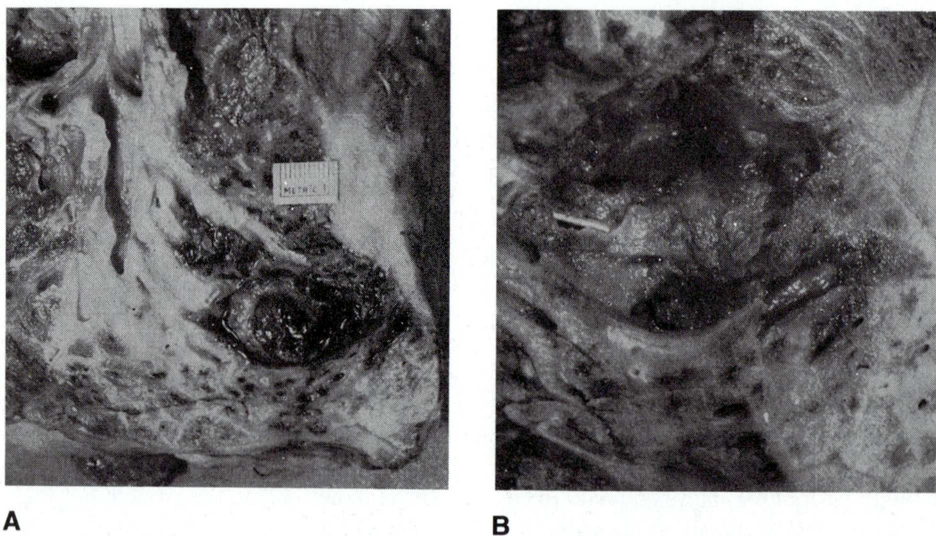

**Figure 16–6.** Specimen from a case with massive hemoptysis caused by a lung abscess. **A.** The abscess, situated in the posterior basilar segment ($B_{10}$) of the right lower lobe, is filled with clotted blood. **B.** A closer view of the cavity after the clot had been removed and a probe inserted into a ruptured thin-walled aneurysm of the subsegmental pulmonary arterial branch. Abscess may be a cause of lethal hemorrhage.

toms but also help to prevent recurrent abscess by removing a diseased focus of lung.

## BRONCHIECTASIS

### History

Laennec first described bronchiectasis in 1819, but it remained for Sicard and Forestier in 1922 to establish a method for accurately diagnosing the disease.[4] They took Lipiodol, an organically bound iodine preparation described by Lafay in 1901, and instilled it into the tracheobronchial tree by direct transcricoid needle puncture. Chest x-rays then demonstrated the radiopaque oil coating the tracheobronchial tree. Modifications in contrast media and technique have occurred, but the basic concept of this method remains.

### Pathology

Bronchiectasis is a chronic disease of the lungs characterized by bronchial dilatation with associated infection of bronchial walls and of surrounding pulmonary parenchyma. The causative infection may be active or inactive at any given time, but once the disease is established, the bronchial dilatation and destruction remain. Bronchiectasis is described as cylindrical or saccular, the latter being the more advanced stage.

The incidence of bronchiectasis at autopsy is considerably greater than the number of cases observed during life, suggesting that many cases remain asymptomatic. While bronchiectasis may be associated with bronchial obstruction due to tumor, foreign body, external compression, or bronchostenosis, and may then occur in any lobe, the vast majority of cases are unassociated with obstruction and occur in dependent portions of the lung—basilar segments of the lower lobes, middle lobe, and lingula. Upper-lobe bronchiectasis is seen in association with universal bronchiectasis, which is usually congenital in nature; isolated upper-lobe bronchiectasis—which is rare—is commonly associated with tuberculosis, generally inactive, or obstruction. About one third of bronchiectasis is unilobar, but about one third is unilateral but bilobar, and one third is bilateral. Severe universal bronchiectasis is ordinarily incompatible with long life.

Bronchiectasis usually involves the second- to fourth-order segmental bronchi rather than lobar or even primary segmental bronchi. This fact is most apparent at the time of bronchography or pathologic examination of a resected lobe, and it explains the fact that the major findings of bronchiectasis are not visible at bronchoscopy, even with the flexible instrument. Pitting and trabeculation of the bronchial mucosa—characteristic of chronic bronchitis—may be seen endoscopically, and pus may be seen extruding from involved bronchial orifices. Gross examination of properly bisected resected lobes reveals tubular or saccular dilatation of bronchi (Fig. 16–7). These bronchi may be filled with mucus, pus, or, on occasion, broncholiths, representing mucoid concretions or calcified peribronchial lymph nodes that have eroded into the bronchial lumen (Fig. 16–8). The affected lobe is shrunken, scarred, and relatively airless. Shiny, thinned-out bronchial mucosa may protrude between the more rigid cartilages of small bronchi.

Microscopic examination reveals the dilated bronchi to be lined by an intact mucous membrane of pseudostratified

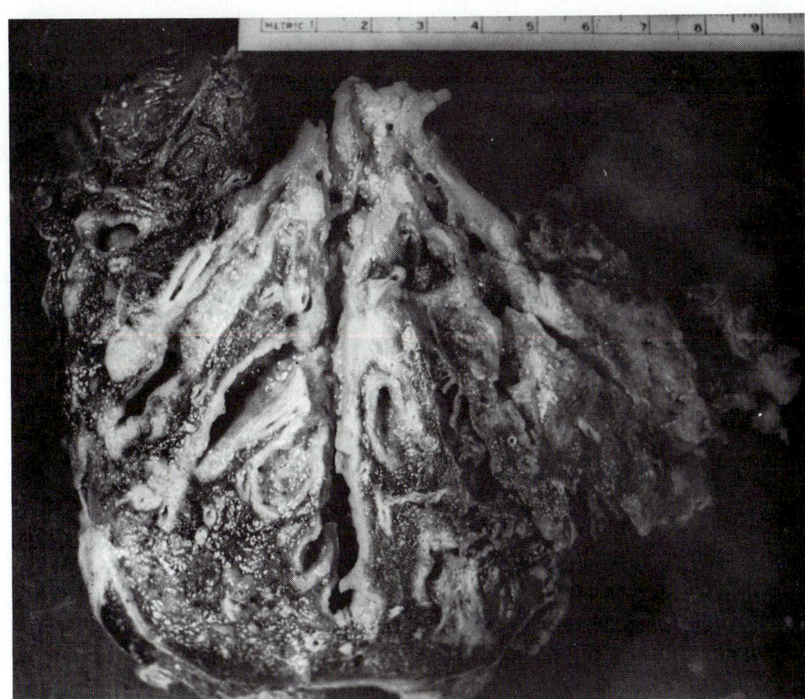

**Figure 16–7.** Bronchiectasis of the right lower and middle lobes, treated by bilobectomy. There is bronchiectasis in all segments of both lobes except the upper part of the lower lobe superior segment, $B_6$ (at upper left of photograph). The ectasia involves the second- to fourth-order branches of the segmental bronchi. Aerated parenchyma still surrounds the ectatic basal bronchi, being supplied by collateral ventilation from normal parts of the superior segment. Atelectasis of the middle lobe is complete in the absence of collateral ventilation. Note that the middle-lobe bronchus and that to the superior segment of the lower lobe originate at approximately the same level.

columnar epithelium and mucus-producing cells. Alteration of the mucosa, if present at all, is scattered and superficial. In surgical specimens, there is evidence of chronic infection, with scarring, round-cell infiltration, and bronchiolar obliteration. Bronchial arteries are hypertrophied and dilated as a consequence of the inflammatory process. The rich bronchial circulation and bronchopulmonary shunting may lead to hemoptysis.

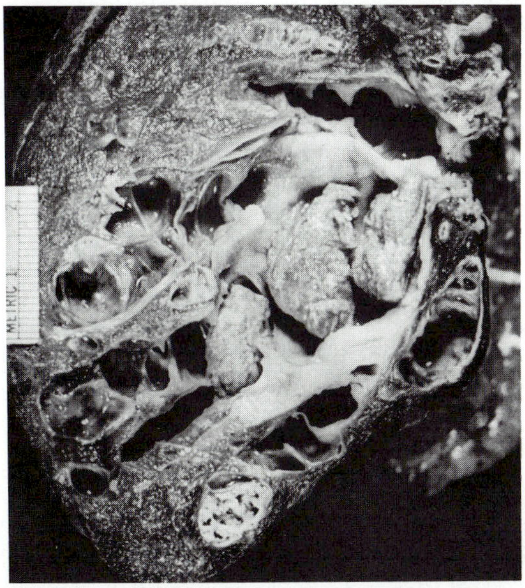

**Figure 16–8.** Broncholithiasis. The multiple, soft intrabronchial concretions have the characteristics of inspissated mucus. Their surfaces are marked with ridges corresponding to the adjacent bronchial laminae.

## Pathogenesis

There are numerous theories of the pathogenesis of bronchiectasis; at least two etiologies are operative. Acquired infection of the lung plays a part in both instances.

## Congenital

Truly congenital bronchiectasis is rare. Even when bronchiectasis occurs in early childhood, it is usually the result of a severe but localized infection and its sequelae. Congenital bronchiectasis is probably due to developmental arrest in the tracheobronchial tree and may be unilateral or universal. More recently, various states of immune deficiency[49,50] and congenital defects in the action of respiratory cilia[51,52] have been associated with the development of bronchiectasis. The ciliary defects have been particularly implicated in the development of Kartagener's syndrome, which consists of situs inversus, pansinusitis, and bronchiectasis. Patients with congenital IgA deficiency or with congenital or acquired hypogammaglobulinemia are susceptible to bronchiectasis because of their lack of resistance to infections of various sorts. Bronchiectasis is a rare complication of acquired immunodeficiency (AIDS)[53] and $\alpha_1$-antitrypsin deficiency is occasionally implicated in the development of extensive bronchiectasis, although it is more often associated with panacinar emphysema.[54–56] Congenital defects in bronchial cartilage and chronic inflammation and infection are associated with the development of bronchiectasis in cystic fibrosis, and bronchiectasis, often extensive and bilateral, is a salient feature of cystic fibrosis lung disease.

### Traction

The traction theory best explains the pathogenesis in the vast majority of cases of bronchiectasis (Fig. 16–9). Destructive pneumonitis may follow bacterial or viral infection of the lung or, in some instances, foreign body aspiration. The pneumonitis that leads to bronchiectasis may sometimes be undiagnosed or inadequately treated, but it tends to be severe. As the destructive process, which actually occurs distal to the bronchiectasis, heals, there is scarring and contraction of the pulmonary parenchyma, leading to volume loss in the lobe and to circumferential traction on bronchi from scar contraction. The affected second- to fourth-order bronchi, already damaged by the inflammatory process, become dilated in a tubular or saccular fashion (Fig. 16–10). While the acute inflammatory process generally heals with time, the secretions, which pool in the dilated, dependent, poorly functioning bronchi, lead to obstruction and infection. Coughing is less than completely effective in clearing these secretions, since there is no propulsive force of air behind the secretions in these contracted lobes and segments.

Cylindrical bronchial dilatation occurs as part of the healing process in many types of pneumonias and may mimic bronchiectasis on bronchograms performed within several weeks following the pneumonic episode.[57] This dilatation is reversible and should not lead to the need for surgical treatment. One should, therefore, wait 3 months after an acute episode of pneumonia before performing a bronchogram or diagnostic CT scan in order to avoid this confusion.

### Middle-Lobe Syndrome

Middle-lobe syndrome, which may be confused with bronchiectasis, is a condition of chronic atelectasis of the middle lobe due to intrinsic or extrinsic obstruction of the middle-lobe bronchus.[58] This bronchus is relatively long, subtends an acute angle with the intermediate bronchus, and is surrounded by a collar of lymph nodes distal to its takeoff, but proximal to its first division into lateral and medial segments. When these lymph nodes become enlarged due to infection of the middle or lower lobe, or when they become scarred or even calcified secondary to chronic granulomatous disease, they may cause obstruction of the middle-lobe bronchus, leading to atelectasis with or without infection. If there is little or no infection, this chronic atelectasis and middle-lobe syndrome may persist for years in an asymptomatic patient. In other patients, middle-lobe syndrome may lead to chronic cough even in the absence of infection. Should the lobe become infected, bronchiectasis may ensue. The integrity of the horizontal fissure is said to play a major part in middle-lobe syndrome.[59] When this fissure is incomplete, collateral ventilation occurs across the fissure, and atelectasis is less likely to occur.

### Association with Paranasal Sinusitis

The association of bronchiectasis with paranasal sinusitis is well known, but it is unclear which condition is primary. Conventional wisdom holds that the sinusitis occurs first, with bronchiectasis occurring later, due to the aspiration of infected material from the sinuses into the tracheobronchial tree. However, in one series of patients with bronchiectasis, only 15% of patients who had the disease for 5 years or less had sinusitis, as compared with 44% of the group as a whole, suggesting that the bronchiectasis might have been the primary disease.[60]

### Kartagener's Syndrome

Kartagener's syndrome is a rare but well-described association of sinusitis, situs inversus, and bronchiectasis (Fig. 16–11). It is surprising how confusing physical examination and x-rays can be in this disease, even when its presence is

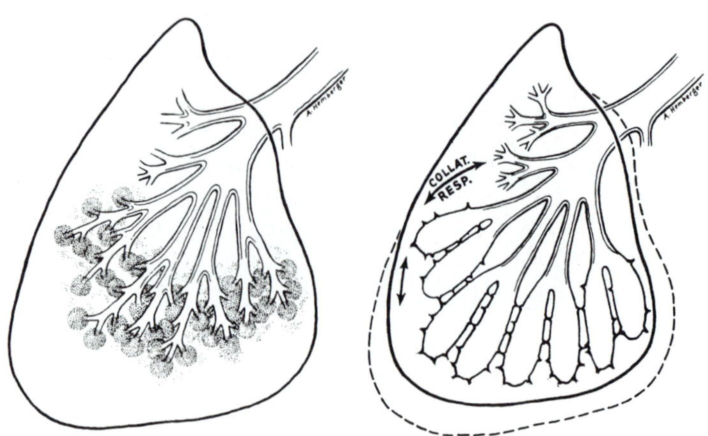


**Figure 16–9.** Diagram to illustrate the traction mechanism of bronchiectasis. In the left-hand drawing, finely dotted zones indicate focally distributed areas of necrotizing bronchitis and pneumonitis around branches of segmental bronchi; some are already confluent. As organization proceeds, the smaller bronchi are largely obliterated. As the resultant scars contract, they exert a pull on the more proximal bronchi, with consequent ectasia, as shown in the right-hand diagram. The involved lobe shrinks; the broken line indicates the original volume. The bronchiectatic sacs end blindly, having been isolated from the aerated parenchyma of the basal segments. Ventilation of the latter is partially maintained through collateral pathways from uninvolved bronchi in the superior segment, as suggested by the arrows.

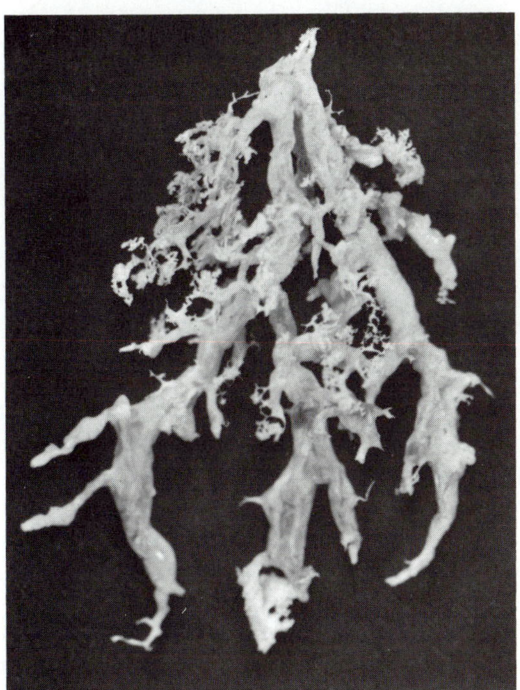

**Figure 16–10.** Vinylite bronchial cast of a bronchiectatic lobe provides evidence in support of the traction theory of pathogenesis. Clearly demonstrable are numerous minute funnel-shaped projections from the ectatic sacs. The former represent persistent channels within branch bronchi that have been narrowed by constricting bronchiolitis and by the contraction of surrounding pneumonic tissue as it organizes.

known. Diagnostic and therapeutic measures in Kartagener's syndrome are the same as those in patients without situs inversus.

## Complications of Bronchiectasis

Recurrent pulmonary infection, metastatic infection (especially to the central nervous system), and hemoptysis are the major complications of bronchiectasis. Areas of lung involved with bronchiectasis are readily reinfected, even when nonoperative treatment has been appropriately aggressive. Secondary infection of other lung areas, due to the direct or hematogenous spread of infection, is a real danger. Even with antibiotic treatment, infection may spread. Hemoptysis, while usually not of dangerous magnitude, may be massive. It is well to remember that systemic vessels—the bronchial arteries—are the sources of bleeding in these patients, and that control of hemorrhage can on occasion be a major problem.[61] If the source of even minor bleeding can be identified, surgical resection of the involved area should be strongly considered. In the patient who is not a candidate for operation, bronchial arterial embolization may be carried out in an attempt to control bleeding.

## Clinical Aspects

The incidence of bronchiectasis has decreased dramatically since the advent of antibiotics leading to the more effective treatment of pulmonary infections. Similarly, certain diseases of childhood such as pertussis, which in some cases led to bronchiectasis, have almost disappeared in the United States due to effective immunization.

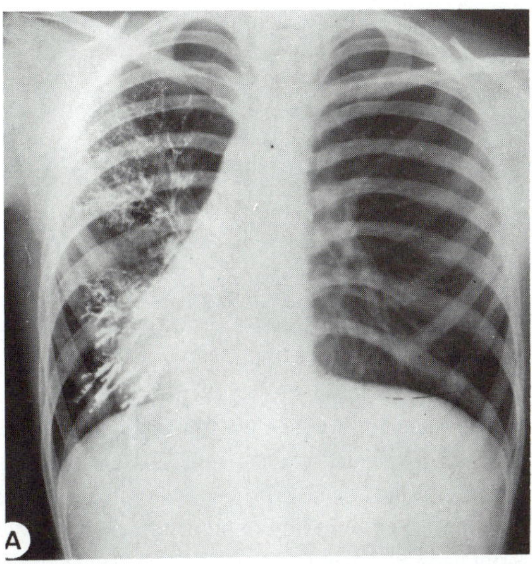



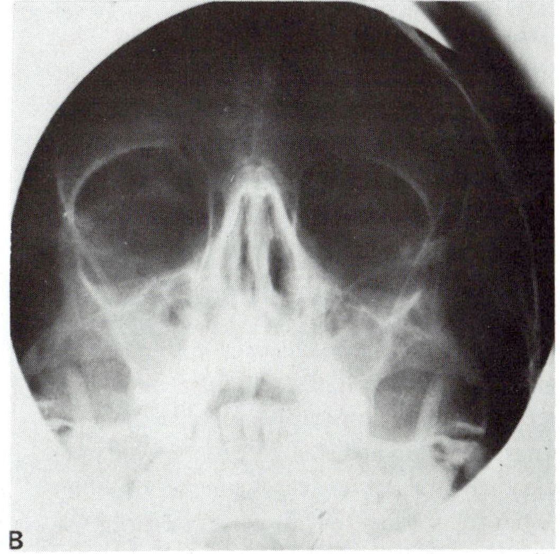



**Figure 16–11.** Roentgenograms from a case of Kartagener's syndrome. **A.** An iodized oil bronchogram demonstrates bronchiectasis in the right (transposed left) lower lobe and lingula. The transposed heart is shifted further to the right because of atelectasis in the lower lobe. **B.** Roentgenogram of the skull reveals agenesis of the frontal sinuses and clouding of the maxillary antra. The bronchiectasis was treated by lower lobectomy and lingulectomy.

The usual case history of bronchiectasis is characterized by recurring cough, mucopurulent sputum, fever, and often hemoptysis. Other manifestations include fatigability, anorexia, gastrointestinal disturbances, joint pains, and retarded physical development. The onset of the disease may be dated in many cases to infancy or early childhood, when recurring episodes of bronchitis or bronchopneumonia, particularly in the winter months, follow a severe, acute respiratory infection. Each severe episode, even if adequately treated with antibiotics, takes its toll, leaving the patient weakened and susceptible to further infection.

Cough varies in frequency and intensity; it is typically most severe in the early morning hours and subsides later in the day, after the bronchi are cleared of accumulated secretions. The sputum volume varies, even in the same individual, from a few milliliters a day to as much as 500 or 1000 mL daily. Usually, the sputum is mucopurulent, gray-green, or yellow in color. It is often musty or fetid, so that some patients complain of a bad taste and others of a bad odor. The amount may be difficult or impossible to estimate in children. Blood streaking or frank hemoptysis occurs in about 50% of cases; it is of major proportions in perhaps 10% but is rarely lethal. Hemoptysis usually appears late in the course of bronchiectasis, since it depends on the development of enlarged bronchial-pulmonary vascular communications. Bleeding from the lungs may be associated with the onset of the menses. Massive bleeding is not relatively as frequent as in pulmonary abscess.

Fever is usually low-grade but may be alarmingly high and associated with chills. Chest pain is usually not prominent but may occasionally be pleuritic. Prolonged fever and episodes of coughing may cause anorexia and vomiting, with a resulting weight loss. Diarrhea is a sign of amyloidosis in rare cases. Retarded physical development and delayed sexual maturity are common in children. Painful swelling of joints and tenderness of the shins are manifestations of pulmonary hypertrophic osteoarthropathy.

Dyspnea is not a common complaint in bronchiectasis; its presence suggests the possibility of diffuse disease, with emphysema or cor pulmonale. Bronchiectatic patients may have difficulties in personal adjustment because of frequent cough, fetor oris, and an appearance of chronic illness.

## Physical Signs

Most patients with bronchiectasis show stigmata of their chronic illness. Children may be small for their age or poorly developed. Adults who have had the disease since childhood are apt to be thin and small. Tenderness may be elicited by palpation over the paranasal sinuses. Clubbing of fingers and toes (pulmonary hypertrophic osteoarthropathy) is not unusual, but cyanosis is rare.

Examination of the chest may show asymmetry, with flattening and decreased respiratory excursions on the affected side. Auscultatory findings vary according to the effectiveness of bronchial drainage and the presence or absence of active pneumonitis. Even when the disease is relatively quiescent, midinspiratory crackling rales may be heard over the affected areas. The breath sounds in the same region may be coarse or diminished.

Auscultatory and even standard radiographic findings correlate poorly with the extent of disease. CT scans or even bronchography may be necessary to make this determination.

## Laboratory Studies

Mild anemia is common in patients with bronchiectasis, and the erythrocyte sedimentation rate is increased. The white cell count is elevated during episodes of acute pneumonia.

Sputum smears and cultures may show a normal flora, even in the presence of acute pneumonia. Careful culture and sensitivity data should be obtained in every case, so that antibiotic treatment can be specific.

In selected cases, particularly children, causes for diminished resistance to infection should be sought. Plasma protein immunoelectrophoresis, sweat chloride studies, and determination of serum $\alpha_1$-antitrypsin levels may give a clue to an important underlying cause of bronchiectasis in some patients.

## Radiographic Findings

Abnormalities seen on standard posteroanterior and lateral roentgenographs of the chest are never sufficient to establish the diagnosis or extent of bronchiectasis with certainty. Saccular lesions, honeycombing, blurring of the diaphragmatic silhouette or heart border, linear streaking or stranding, and even small air–fluid levels may be seen on plain films, and, with the history and physical findings, suggest the presence of bronchiectasis. However, these findings are not diagnostic. Segmental or lobar atelectasis associated with mediastinal shift, as well as other radiographic signs of volume loss and compensation, are present in some instances. All of these radiographic changes are more frequent in the lower lung zones, which are the dominant sites of the disease.

## Bronchoscopy

Diagnostic bronchoscopy should be done in most, if not all, patients with bronchiectasis.[62]

While the bronchoscopic findings of a reddened, edematous mucosa, pitting of the mucosa due to dilatation of the ostia of bronchial glands, and pus coming from specific segmental bronchial orifices, are typical in bronchiectasis, they are, like the radiographic findings, not diagnostic. Material aspirated from the bronchi should be carefully stained and cultured both aerobically and anaerobically. A careful examination for bronchial obstruction should be done and any obstruction alleviated, if possible. Thorough suctioning of the tracheobronchial tree and irrigation with normal saline are usually of symptomatic benefit, sometimes for quite a long time.

In some instances, bronchoscopy should be repeated in order to clean out the tracheobronchial tree as thoroughly as possible. This will permit the best possible aeration of atelectatic lung areas and, possibly, decrease the bacterial population, thereby allowing antibiotics to do their work more effectively.

### Computed Tomographic Scanning

In recent years, CT scanning has almost replaced bronchography as a radiographic method for localization of areas of bronchiectasis. In both children and adults, CT scanning effectively localizes bronchiectasis in almost all instances[63–65] (Fig. 16–12). It is probably still too early to say that bronchography is never necessary in the diagnostic evaluation of patients with bronchiectasis, but this may soon be the case. Even in patients with bilateral disease, CT scanning may be sufficient for the delineation of the extent of disease.

### Bronchography

When bronchography is used, Propylodone in oil (Dionosil) is the most popular currently used material. It is reasonably well tolerated by the lungs, coats the tracheobronchial tree well, produces good quality roentgenographs, and is readily available.

Sicard and Forestier originally used transcricoid needle puncture and direct instillation of dye into the tracheobronchial tree. This method may still be used, particularly in children, but it is not widely practiced. Transcricoid placement of a small catheter allows for a more selective study, but Dionosil is quite viscous and does not flow well through a small catheter.

In adults, we prefer to inject the contrast material through an endotracheal catheter (14–16 French) inserted under topical anesthesia in adults and general anesthesia in children. The procedure may be combined with bronchoscopy in either age group. The lower, as well as the upper, airway must be well anesthetized in order to prevent coughing during the procedure, which is always done in close consultation with a radiologist. Under fluoroscopic control with image intensifier monitoring, Dionosil is gradually instilled first into the major area in question and then sequentially into all lobes and segments on the side of dominant disease. Multiple-spot films in different projections should be obtained during the injection, with final overhead films in the anteroposterior and lateral projections. If the procedure has been skillfully done, and especially if the anesthetic has been effective, a complete unilateral bronchogram, without the alveolarization of contrast material, should be available for study (Figs. 16–13, 16–14).

The question sometimes arises of performing bilateral bronchograms at one sitting. We usually advise against it. Lateral films of the second side are unsatisfactory because the opacified bronchial trees overlap; however, without films in all projections, the study may well be incomplete. Furthermore, bilateral bronchography is frequently a prolonged procedure, trying the tolerance of even a cooperative patient. Perhaps most important, the amount of Dionosil necessary for a bilateral bronchogram (sometimes up to 50 mL) may cause significant interference with respiratory gas exchange, leading to respiratory distress and hypoxia.[66]

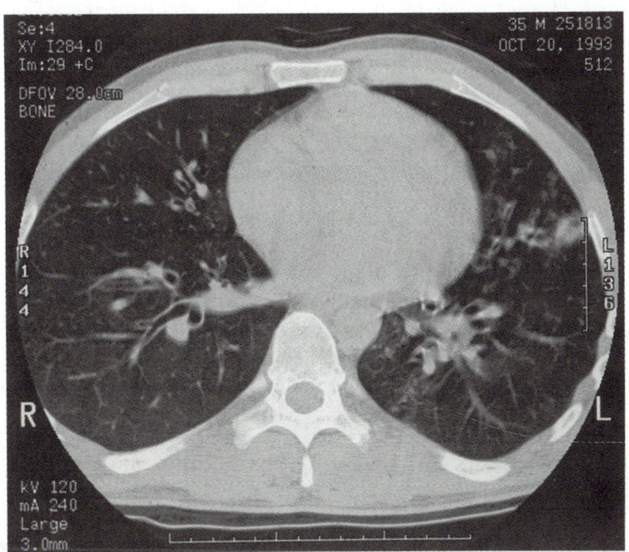


A

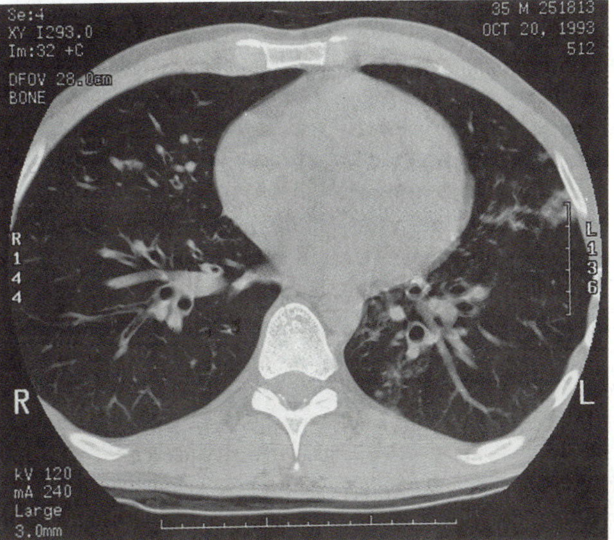


B

**Figure 16–12. A,B.** CT scan showing peripheral cylindrical bronchiectasis in the lingular segments of the left upper lobe, basal segments of the left lower lobe and less extensively in middle lobe on the right.

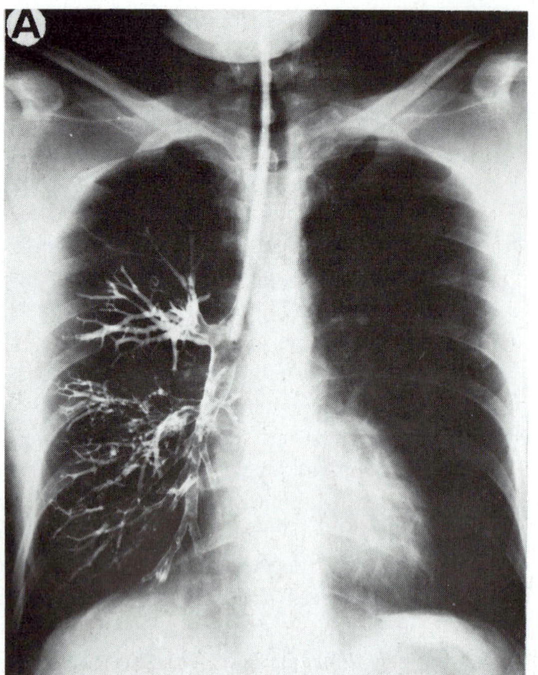

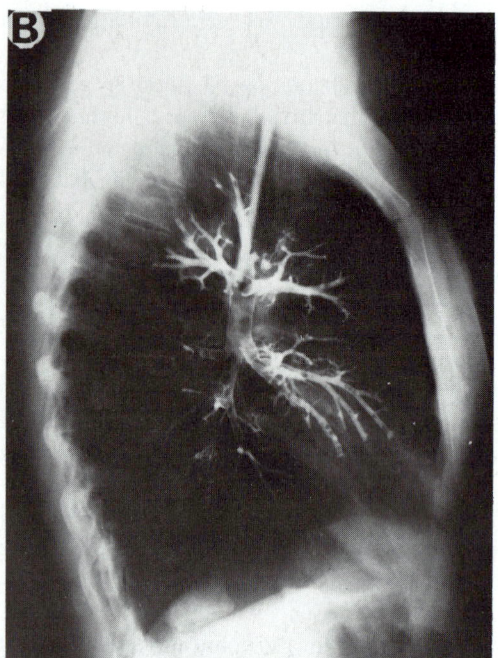

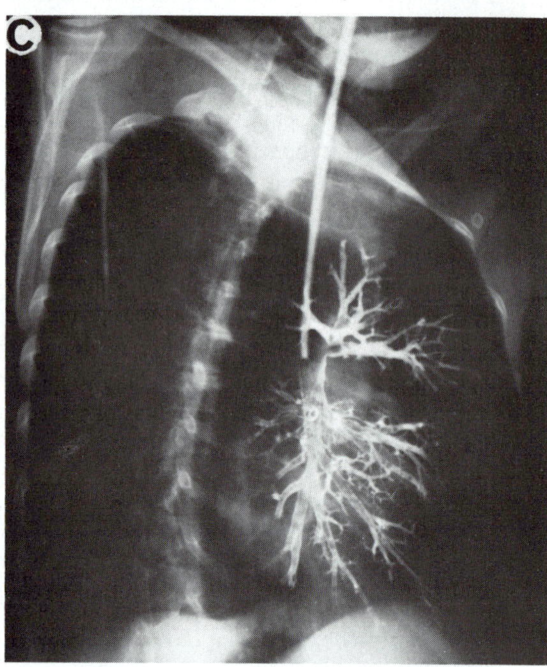

**Figure 16–13.** A selective iodized oil bronchogram of the right lung. **A.** Posteroanterior roentgenogram. **B.** Lateral projection. **C.** Oblique projection. This is particularly useful when there is contrast medium in the contralateral lung.

Additionally, there may be a febrile response following bronchography. This is probably due to chemical or bacterial pneumonitis or to a combination of the two.

Following bronchography, postural drainage and percussion should be instituted in order to empty the lungs of contrast material. Patients should be cautioned not to eat or drink anything for 2–3 hours following procedures done under topical anesthesia in order to prevent aspiration.

Two points deserve reemphasis. First, bronchography should not be done within 3 months of an acute episode of pneumonia, in order to avoid interpreting an area of bronchial dilatation as permanent when it may be reversible, and to decrease the possibility of postbronchographic pneumonia. Second, if CT scanning is not sufficiently specific, complete bilateral bronchography, usually done at two sittings several weeks apart, is essential before a proper decision can be made concerning the advisability and extent of surgical resection.

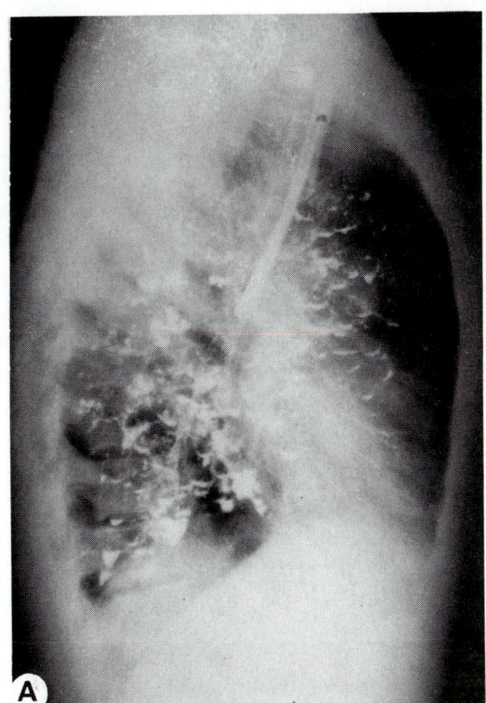

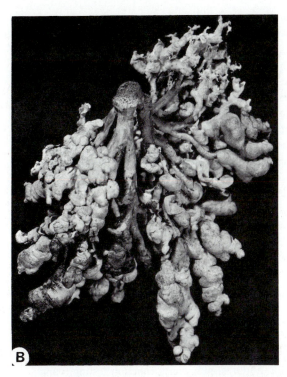


**Figure 16–14. A.** Bronchogram from a case of total left lung bronchiectasis. There is a marked "puddling" of contrast medium in the numerous sacs. (Print reversed to correspond with cast). **B.** Vinylite cast prepared from the resected lung. Despite extensive disease distally, the proximal bronchi are of normal caliber and show a usual pattern of branching. Bronchiectatic changes are most severe in the lingular and basilar segments and less pronounced in the apical and superior segments. The sacculation involves chiefly third- and fourth-order branches of the segmental bronchi. These seem to end blindly, producing the "leafless tree" appearance. The surrounding pulmonary parenchyma showed dense fibrosis. *(From Liebow AA, Hales MR, Lindskog MR, et al: Bull Int Assoc Med Museums 27:116, 1947, with permission.)*

## Treatment

The initial management of patients with bronchiectasis should be nonoperative.[67,68] This does not mean that aggressive management is not required but only that the surgical resection of diseased lung is not usually necessary. Nonoperative treatment is generally begun after initial diagnostic studies, including a careful search for specific etiologic factors, sputum cultures, and usually bronchoscopy. In many instances, symptoms will be controlled adequately, and no operation will be necessary. If, however, the patient has recurrent pneumonia, complications of pulmonary infections, continuing copious sputum, hemoptysis, or, in children, significant failure of growth or development, operative treatment should be considered. It is at this time that bronchography should be done if it has not been done previously.

Surgery for bronchiectasis should not be done prematurely. Equally certainly, it should not be delayed so long that irreversible physical, psychologic, or social changes have occurred.

## Conservative Treatment

The conservative treatment of bronchiectasis consists of general and nutritional support, postural drainage with percussion, and sometimes therapeutic bronchoscopy. Systemic antibiotics, chosen on the basis of recent culture and sensitivity data, should be used for the treatment of any episode of pneumonia, or even severe symptomatic bronchitis. Febrile episodes, even without a change in symptoms or x-rays, require antibiotic treatment. The length of conservative treatment for bronchiectasis depends on a number of factors. Poor control of symptoms, especially in a child or young adult with relatively localized disease, and hemoptysis from a localized source are indications for resection of the disease lobe or segment. Patients with generalized disease and those with cystic fibrosis are generally poor candidates for operation.

## Surgical Treatment

### *Historical Aspects*

Many of the early multistage resections and drainages of pulmonary tissue were for bronchiectasis. It remained for Brunn[69] in 1929 to show that one-stage lobectomy could be performed with relative safety. He had five patients with bronchiectasis and one with cancer treated by lobectomy, with one hospital death. Perhaps the secret of his success was adequate tube drainage of the pleural cavity in the postoperative period, a practice not widely done at that time.

Major advances in surgical technique for pulmonary resection were made by Churchill and Belsey[70] in 1939, and by Blades and Kent[71] in 1940, when they demonstrated the feasibility and advantages of precise anatomic dissection of the bronchovascular structures in the pulmonary hilum, with individual suture of each structure rather than mass ligation, as had been the practice until that time. The newer techniques led to fewer operative complications and certainly resulted in a significant decrease in postoperative hemorrhage, empyema, bronchopleural fistula, and mortality. Improvements in anesthetic management, the use of double-lumen endotracheal tubes, improved prevention and treatment of abnormalities in fluids and electrolytes, intensive care units, the use of stapling devices, and other modifications of management have continued to help in reducing morbidity and mortality following all types of surgical resection.

### *Operative Treatment*

The extent of surgical resection for bronchiectasis should be planned well in advance on the basis of CT scanning, bronchoscopic findings, pulmonary function testing, ventilation perfusion scans, and, if necessary, bronchography.[72] In most cases, unilateral resection will suffice, but in about 10% of patients, bilateral resection will be necessary.[73] A detailed evaluation of pulmonary function is especially important in this group. In many instances bilateral resection can be carried out in one operation by using a median sternotomy incision. If a bilateral procedure is planned, the most seriously involved side should be resected first. The patient should be prepared for operation with careful tracheobronchial toilet, including bronchoscopy, if necessary, and specific antibiotics.

The techniques of surgical resection for bronchiectasis are similar to those used for other lung diseases. A thorough knowledge of segmental anatomy and the technique of segmental resection is necessary if all disease is to be removed while preserving all normal pulmonary parenchyma—the goal of this kind of surgery. Peripheral adhesions are frequently present in areas of disease but are not usually troublesome. Adhesions across fissures must be divided early in the dissection in order to gain wide exposure of the hilar vessels. Dense adhesions are frequently present in the lobar hilum, and dissection must proceed carefully. Meticulous hemostasis is mandatory; troublesome operative and postoperative bleeding may occur from bronchial vessels. After careful ligation and division of the pulmonary vessels, the appropriate bronchus or bronchi are divided. It is especially important not to leave long bronchial stumps in patients with bronchiectasis. We use the stapling device for bronchial closure and have been pleased with it. We cover the bronchial stump with a pedicled flap of parietal pleura whenever possible. Intercostal tube drainage is mandatory until expansion of the remaining lung is complete, air leaks have stopped, and fluid drainage is minimal. Most patients are ready for discharge from the hospital within 5–7 days following operation.

Bronchiectasis is a disease of anatomic bronchial segments and may involve one or all bronchopulmonary segments. Anatomic resection of the involved segment or combination of segments is the usual planned surgical treatment for bronchiectasis. Single segmental resection is rarely indicated. Resection of two segments, specifically right middle lobectomy or lingulectomy, is not uncommon. Since bronchiectasis frequently involves one or more basilar segments of the lower lobes, the question of resection of one or more basilar segments without resection of the remainder of the lower lobe sometimes arises. We would advise against subtotal basilar segmentectomy. The anatomy of the basilar segments is variable enough that resection of one or two segments while one is trying to preserve one or two others may turn into a triumph of technique over judgment. Subtotal involvement of basilar segments is unusual. The advantage of preserving one or two basilar segments is questionable. Resection of all of the basilar segments while one is preserving the superior segment of the lower lobe is, on the other hand, not a rare circumstance. Since the superior segment tends to have a better drainage pattern than do the basilar segments, it may be free of bronchiectasis even when all other lower lobe segments are involved. In this circumstance, preservation of the superior segment is desirable, particularly if it is a fairly large segment. Technically, this is not particularly difficult from the anatomic standpoint, but the dissection may be tedious and must proceed carefully because of surrounding inflammation, adhesions, and the danger of bleeding. After the successful basilar segmentectomy, one must be certain that there is no torsion of the remaining superior segment around its bronchovascular pedicle. If the long fissure between the superior segment of the lower lobe and the posterior segment of the upper lobe is incomplete, it should not be divided if only basilar segmental resection is planned. Attachment of these segments in this manner will not only prevent torsion of the superior segment but may prevent its sagging or late rotation, which could lead to the subsequent development of bronchiectasis in a now dependent segment.

### *Results of Treatment*

In properly selected and managed patients, the mortality following resection for bronchiectasis should be 1% or less, as has been the case in several recent series.[74,75] Major postoperative morbidity, due chiefly to empyema, can be minimized by careful attention to preoperative, operative, and postoperative details in management. Careful selection of cases, optimum preoperative preparation, meticulous surgical techniques—including the removal of all diseased tissue and care to avoid injury to remaining, normal lung—and attentive postoperative management—including careful pulmonary toilet, full re-expansions of remaining lobes and segments, and proper antibiotic administration—will all help to minimize postoperative morbidity and mortality.

One would expect about 80% of patients to become asymptomatic postoperatively. About 15% will be improved but still have residual symptoms. Five percent will be unimproved or worse. Even in patients with bilateral disease, the expectation for improvement should be in a similar range. Most patients are extremely grateful following pulmonary resection for bronchiectasis, and they often express the wish that they had undergone operation earlier in the course of their disease.

## REFERENCES


1. Hochberg LA: *Thoracic Surgery Before the 20th Century.* New York, Vantage, 1960
2. Mead RH: *A History of Thoracic Surgery.* Springfield, Illinois, Thomas, 1961
3. Alexander JC Jr, Wolfe WG: Lung abscess and empyema of the thorax. *Surg Clin North Am* **60:**835, 1980
4. Takara, T, Scott SM, Bridgman AH, et al: Suppurative diseases of the lungs, pleurae, and pericardium. *Curr Probl Surg* **14:**6, 1977
5. Garibaldi RA. Epidemiology of community-acquired respiratory trait infections in adults: Incidence, etiology, and impact. *Am J Med* **78**(suppl 6B):32–37S, 1985
6. Niederman MS, Bass JB, Campbell GD, et al: Guidelines for the initial management of adults with community acquired pneumonia: diagnosis, assessment of severity, and initial antimicrobial therapy (Official American Thoracic Society Statement). *Am Rev Resp Dis* **148:**1418–1426, 1993
7. Schaberg DR, Culver DH, Gaynes RP: Major trends in the microbial etiology of nosocomial infection. *Am J Med* **91**(suppl 3B):7S–11S, 1991
8. Torres A, Aznar R, Gatell JM, et al: Incidence, risk, and prognosis factors of nosocomial pneumonia in mechanically ventilated patients. *Am Rev Respir Dis* **142:**523–528, 1990
9. Fagon JY, Chastre J, Hance AJ, et al: Detection of nosocomial lung infection in ventilated patients. *Am Rev Resp Dis* **138:**110–116, 1988
10. Meduri GU, Wanderink RG, Leeper KV, Beals DH: Management of bacterial pneumonia in ventilated patients. *Chest* **101:**500–508, 1992
11. Meduri GU: Ventilator-associated pneumonia in patients with respiratory failure. *Chest* **97:**1208–1219, 1990
12. Johanson WG: Ventilator-associated pneumonia: Light at the end of the tunnel? *Chest* **97:**1026, 1990
13. Lynch JP: Nosocomial pneumonia: which agent(s) to use? *J Respir Dis* **13:**1123–1138, 1992
14. Bulmer SR, Lamb D, McCormack RJ, et al: Aetiology of unresolved pneumonia. *Thorax* **33:**307, 1978
15. Hilman BC, Kurzweg FT, McCook WW Jr, et al: Foreign body aspirate of grass inflorescences as a cause of hemoptysis, *Chest* **78:**306, 1980
16. Neuhof H, Touroff AS: Acute putrid abscess of the lung: principles of operative treatment. *Surg Gynecol Obstet* **63:**353, 1936
17. Wilkins EW Jr: Acute putrid abscess of the lung. *Ann Thorac Surg* **44:**560–561, 1987
18. Shanks GD, Berman JD: Anaerobic pulmonary abscesses. *Clin Pediatr* **25:**520–522, 1986
19. Brock RC: *Lung Abscess.* Springfield, Illinois, Thomas, 1952
20. Vidal E. LeVeen HH, Yarnoz M, et al: Lung abscess secondary to pulmonary infarction. *Ann Thorac Surg* **11:**557, 1971
21. Baldwin JC, Mark JBD: Pulmonary diseases associated with immunosuppression. In Pickard LR (ed): *Decision Making in Cardiothoracic Surgery.* Philadelphia, Saunders, 1988
22. Connors JP, Roper CL, Ferguson TB: Transbronchial catheterization of pulmonary abscesses. *Ann Thorac Surg* **19:**254,1975
23. Rowe LD, Keane WM, Jafek BW, et al: Trnsbronchial drainage of pulmonary abscesses with the flexible fiberoptic bronchoscope. *Laryngoscope* **89:**122, 1979
24. Wallace RJ Jr, Cohen A, Awe RJ, et al: Carcinomatous lung abscess—Diagnosis by bronchoscopy and cytopathology. *JAMA* **242:**521, 1979
25. Kosloske AM, Ball WS Jr., Butler C, Musemeche CA: Drainage of pediatric lung abscess by cough catheter, or complete resection. *J Pediatr Surg* **21:**596–600, 1986
26. Adams FV, Kolodny E: M-mode ultrasonic localization and identification and fluid-containing pulmonary cysts. *Chest* **75:**330, 1979
27. Baber CE, Hedlund LW, Oddson TE, et al: Differentiating empyemas and peripheral pulmonary abscesses—The value of computed tomography. *Radiology* **135:**755, 1980
28. Parker LA, Nelton JW, Delany DJ, Yankaskas BC: Percutaneous small bore catheter drainage in the management of lung abscesses. *Chest* **92:**213–218, 1987
29. LeRoux BT, Mohlala ML, Odell JA, Whitton ID: Suppurative diseases of the lung and pleural space. *Part I: Empyema Thoracic and Lung Abscess.* Chicago, Year Book, 1986
30. Bartlett JG, Gorbach SL, Tally FP, et al: Bacteriology and treatment of primary lung abscess. *Am Rev Respir Dis* **109:**510, 1974
31. Brook I, Finegold SM: Bacteriology and therapy of lung abscess in children. *J Pediatr* **94:**10, 1979
32. Weiss, W, Cherniak NS: Acute nonspecific lung abscess: A controlled study comparing orally and parenterally administered penicillin G. *Chest* **66:**348, 1974
33. Mark JBD: Lung abscess. In Fries JF, Ehrlich GE (eds): *Prognosis: Contemporary Outcomes of Disease.* Bowie, Maryland: Charles Press, 1981, pp 232–234
34. Chidi CC, Mendelsohn HJ: Lung abscess. A study of the results of treatment based on 90 consecutive cases. *J. Thorac Cardiovasc Surg* **68:**168, 1974
35. Estrera AS, Platt MR, Mills LJ, et al: Primary lung abscess. *J Thorac Cardiovasc Surg* **79:**275, 1980
36. Gopalakrishna KV, Lerner PI: Primary lung abscess: Analysis of 66 cases. *Cleve Clin Q* **42:**3, 1975
37. Hagan JL, Hardy JD: Lung abscess revisited. *Ann Surg* **197:**755–762, 1983
38. Delarue NC, Pearson FG, Nelems JM, Cooper JD: Lung abscess: Surgical implications. *Can J Surg* **23:**297–302, 1980
39. Mori T, Ebe T, Takahaski M, et al: Lung abscess: Analysis of 66 cases from 1979 to 1991. *Int Med* **32:**278–284, 1993
40. Brook I: Lung abscesses and pleural empyema in children. *Adv Pediatr Infect Dis* **8:**159–176, 1993
41. Weissberg D: Percutaneous drainage of lung abscess. *J Thorac Cardiovasc Surg* **87:**308–312, 1984
42. Mengoli L: Giant lung abscess treated by tube thoracostomy. *J Thorac Cardiovasc Surg* **90:**186–194, 1985
43. Ha HK, Kang MW, Park JM et al: Lung abscess. Percutaneous catheter therapy. *Acta Radiologica* **34:**362–365, 1993
44. Lambiase RE, Deyoe L, Cronan JJ, Dorman GS: Percutaneous drainage of 335 consecutive abscesses: Results of primary drainage with 1-year follow-up. *Radiology* **184:**167–179, 1992
45. Dean NC, Stein MG, Stalbarg MS: Percutaneous drainage of an infected lung bulla in a patient receiving positive pressure ventilation. *Chest* **91:**928–930, 1987
46. Lawrence GH, Rubin SL: Management of giant lung abscess. *Am J Surg* **136:**134, 1978
47. Thoms NW, Wilson RF, Puro HE, et al: Life-threatening hemoptysis in primary lung abscess. *Ann Thorac Surg* **14:**347, 1972
48. Philpott NJ, Woodhead MA, Wilson AG, Millard FJ: Lung abscess: A neglected cause of left threatening haemoptysis. *Thorax* **48:** 674–675, 1993
49 Chipps BE, Talamo RC, Winkelstein JA: IgA deficiency, recurrent pneumonitis and bronchiectasis. *Chest* **73:**419, 1978
50. Hilton AM, Doyle L: Immunological abnormalities in bronchiectasis with chronic bronchial suppuration. *Br J Dis Chest* **72:**207, 1978

51. Eliasson R, Mossberg B, Camner P, et al: The immotile-cilia syndrome. A congenital ciliary abnormality as an etiologic factor in chronic airway infections and male sterility. *N Engl J Med* **297**:1, 1977
52. Rossman CM, Forrest JB, Ruffin RE, et al: Immotile cilia syndrome in persons with and without Kartagener's syndrome. *Am Rev Respir Dis* **121**:1011, 1980
53. McGuinness G, Naidich DP, Garay S, et al: AIDS associated bronchiectasis: CT features. *J Comput Assist Tomog* **17**:260–266, 1993
54. Longstreth GF, Weitzman SA, Browing RJ, et al: Bronchiectasis and homozygous alpha1 antitrypsin deficiency. *Chest* **67**:233, 1975
55. Varpela E, Koistinen J, Korhola O, et al: Deficiency of alpha1-antitrypsin and bronchiectasis. *Ann Clin Res* **10**:79, 1978
56. Shin MS, Ho KJ: Bronchiectasis in patients with alpha1-antitrypsin deficiency. A rare occurrence? *Chest* **104**:1384–1386, 1993
57. Blades B, Dugan D: Pseudobronchiectasis. *J Thorac Surg* **13**:40, 1944
58. Linkskog GE, Spear HC: Middle-lobe syndrome. *N Engl J Med* **253**:489, 1955
59. Bradham RR, Sealy WC, Young WG Jr: Chronic middle lobe infection: Factors responsible for its development. *Ann Thorac Surg* **2**:612, 1966
60. Linkskog GE, Hubbell DS: An analysis of 215 cases of bronchiectasis. *Surg Gynecol Obstet* **100**:643, 1955
61. Liebow AA, Hales MR, Linkskog GE: Enlargement of the bronchial arteries and their anastomoses with the pulmonary arteries in bronchiectasis. *Am J Pathol* **25**:211, 1949
62. Schoenbaum SW, Pinsker KL, Rakoff SJ, et al: Fiberoptic bronchoscopy: Complete evaluation of the tracheobronchial tree in the radiology department. *Radiology* **109**:571, 1973
63. Herman M, Michalkova K, Kopriva E: High-resolution CT in the assessment of bronchiectasis in children. *Pediatr Radiol* **23**:376–379, 1993
64. Kornriech L, Horev G, Ziv N, Grunebaum M: Bronchiectasis in children: Assessment by CT. *Pediatr Radiol* **23**:120–123, 1993
65. McGuiness G, Naidich DP, Leitman BS, McCauley DI: Bronchiectasis: CT evaluation. *Am J Roentgenol* **160**:253–259, 1993
66. Christoforidis AJ, Nelson SW, Tomashefski FJ: Effects of bronchography on pulmonary function. *Am Rev Respir Dis* **85**:127, 1962
67. Bolman RM III, Wolfe WG: Bronchiectasis and bronchopulmonary sequestration. *Surg Clin North Am* **60**:867, 1980
68. Sanderson JM, Kennedy MCS, Johnson JF, et al: Bronchiectasis: Results of surgical and conservative management—A review of 393 cases. *Thorax* **29**:407, 1974
69. Brunn H: Surgical principles underlying one-stage lobectomy. *Arch Surg* **18**:490, 1929 (Part II)
70. Churchill ED, Belsey R: Segmental pneumonectomy in bronchiectasis; the lingula segment of the left upper lobe. *Ann Surg* **109**:481, 1939
71. Blades B, Kent EM: Individual ligation technique for lower lobe lobectomy. *J Thorac Surg* **10**:84, 1940
72. Wernly JA, DeMeester TR, Kirchner PT, et al: Clinical value of quantitative ventilation-perfusion scans in the surgical management of bronchogenic carcinoma. *J Thorac Cardiovasc Surg* **80**:535, 1980
73. George SA, Leonardi HK, Overholt RH: Bilateral pulmonary resection of bronchiectasis. A 40-year experience. *Ann Thorac Surg* **28**:48, 1979
74. Ripe E: Bronchiectasis: I. A follow-up study after surgical treatment. *Scand J Respir Dis* **52**:96, 1971
75. Sealy WB, Bradham RR, Young WG Jr: The surgical treatment of multisegmental and localized bronchiectasis. *Surg Gynecol Obstet* **123**:80, 1966

CHAPTER

17

# Thoracic Infections Caused by Actinomycetes, Fungi, Opportunistic Organisms, and Echinococcus

Stewart M. Scott, Timothy Takaro, and Robert Duane Davis

## ACTINOMYCETES INFECTIONS

Actinomycosis and nocardiosis are bacterial infections caused by organisms with branching hyphae that resemble and were once mistaken for fungi. The distinction is clinically important because these organisms respond to antibiotics but not to antifungal drugs.

### Actinomycosis

Actinomycosis is a chronic infection characterized by suppuration, abscess formation, sinuses, and dense scarring. In 1877, Bollinger identified the organism as the cause of lumpy jaw in cattle. Harz in 1879 named the organism *Actinomyces bovis* because he thought the organism with its raylike appearance was a fungus. Israel in 1878 isolated actinomycetes from a human. Actinomycosis in humans is usually caused by *Actinomyces israelii,* a gram-positive, microaerophilic organism that must be cultured under anaerobic conditions.[1]

The sites of clinical manifestations of actinomycosis are cervicofacial, thoracic, and abdominal. Cervicofacial infections are the most common. Actinomycetes are part of the normal human oropharyngeal flora. Infection begins in the soft tissues of the mouth and throat and manifests itself as a submandibular mass with chronic draining sinuses. Infection spreads by direct extension across fascial planes and can extend into the mediastinum directly from the neck. Thoracic actinomycosis, however, most commonly occurs when organisms are aspirated from a colonized oropharynx. Symptoms may be few at first until there is pleural or chest-wall involvement. Empyema and chronically draining chest-wall sinuses are characteristic, but they are usually late stages of the pulmonary process. The latter may take the form of a non-specific–appearing pulmonary infiltration, consolidation, or hilar mass. The resemblance to bronchogenic carcinoma is sometimes striking (Fig. 17–1).[2] Helpful radiographic clues are findings of pleural fluid, chest-wall involvement (including the ribs and/or periosteum), penetration of interlobar fissures, and vertebral destruction. The infection may even extend into the pericardium.[3]

In about 20% of patients, actinomycosis occurs in the abdomen or pelvis.[4] It has been found in association with intrauterine devices. It also occurs in the brain, liver, kidney, and skeletal system, and it has been identified in association with the acquired immunodeficiency syndrome (AIDS).[5]

The diagnosis must be made by histopathologic examination and culture of material from draining sinuses and abscesses. Characteristic yellow-brown mycelial granules called "sulfur granules" are found in the tissues (Fig. 17–2)

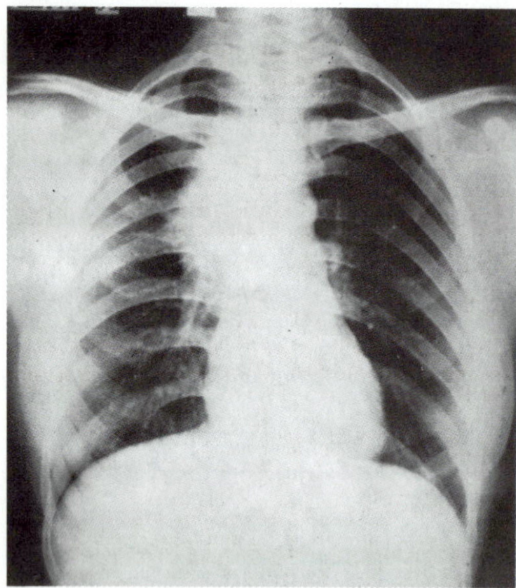

**Figure 17–1.** Chest x-ray of a patient with actinomycosis. The picture is suggestive of bronchogenic carcinoma; however, this was from a young woman who developed pleural empyema and a draining chest-wall sinus that was biopsied. This showed *A. israelii.* Recovery followed treatment with sulfamerazine.

and are composed of branching filamentous rods that stain positive with Gram stain. Anaerobic cultural characteristics are used to identify the organism.

Penicillin is the drug of choice for treating actinomycosis, although other antibiotics have been used successfully.[6] Very high doses of antibiotics must be used for long periods of time: 20 million U penicillin daily for 1–3 months because of the dense fibrous tissue surrounding the colonies of organisms. The prognosis after effective treatment is good. The most common indication for surgery for actinomycosis is thoracotomy for possible carcinoma. Adequate and prolonged drug therapy is important after surgery

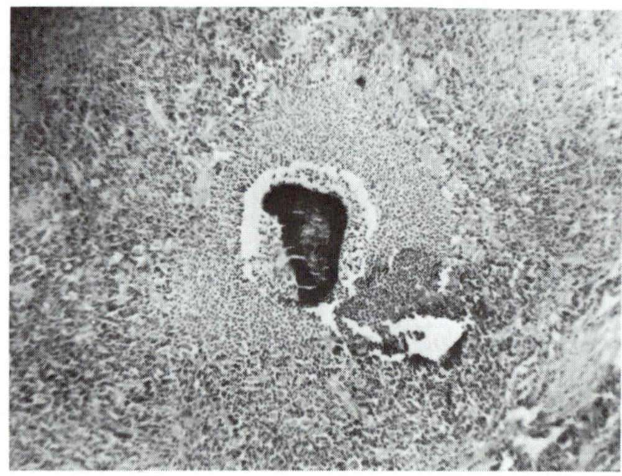

**Figure 17–2.** Characteristic actinomycetic granule in a microabscess from a patient with actinomycosis (PAS, ×85). *(From Takaro T: In Goldsmith HS (ed): Practice of Surgery, 1978, courtesy of Harper and Row, with permission.)*

to prevent reactivation of disease or the development of empyema.

## Nocardiosis

Nocardiosis is a chronic infection most often caused by *Nocardia asteroides* and is characterized by pulmonary involvement with or without secondary hematogenous dissemination to other organs, especially the central nervous system.[7] It may occasionally present as a cutaneous lesion. Nocardiosis is sometimes difficult to recognize, and the infection can be fatal without adequate, specific treatment. Nocardiosis is an opportunistic infection occurring in patients with disordered immune systems associated with malignancy, organ transplantation, and immunosuppressive therapy.[8] It has been observed in patients with AIDS.[9] In these patients, the diagnosis can be obscured by the presence of *Pneumocystis carinii. N. asteroides,* like *A. israelii,* occurs in pathologic material in clumps or granules. The short but sometimes long-branching filaments are gram-positive, aerobic, and mildly acid-fast and may be confused with *Mycobacterium tuberculosis.*

Subcutaneous abscesses and draining sinuses on or near the chest wall that exude sulfur granules similar to those observed in actinomycosis are characteristic. Nonspecific flulike symptoms (cough, malaise, fever), weight loss, and occasionally hemoptysis and pleuritic chest pain are noted in an immunosuppressed patient. Chest x-rays may reveal solitary nodules, nonspecific infiltrates (Fig. 17–3A), or cavitary disease resembling pulmonary tuberculosis. Since both the symptoms and the x-rays in nocardiosis can suggest pulmonary tuberculosis, these two diseases have been and still are occasionally confused. Localized pneumonic or infiltrative lesions may also suggest bronchogenic carcinoma. In the opportunistic form of the disease, pulmonary cavitation or dissemination may occur, and empyema develops in up to 25% of cases with formation of fistulous tracts.

Nocardiosis was originally described in cattle by Nocard in 1888. The organism is widely distributed in nature, but its morphology is typical enough that it can be distinguished from other bacteria and fungi. If *Nocardia* is recovered from the sputum of a patient with an abnormal chest x-ray, or from an abscess or a closed space (such as the pleura), or from surgically excised material, one can be secure in the diagnosis. In doubtful circumstances, culture is reliable and will serve to identify the *Nocardia* species (Fig. 17–3B). This is important since all are penicillin resistant.

Sulfadiazine, 4.0–8.0 g daily, or sulfisoxazole (Gantrisin), in divided doses totaling 12.0 g daily, are the drugs of choice in treating nocardiosis. A minimum of 2–3 months is usually necessary, but treatment may have to be prolonged (up to 6–8 months). Minocycline hydrochloride also is effective. The combination of trimethoprim and sulfamethoxazole is effective in high doses.[10]

Adjunctive surgical treatment may be required to ef-

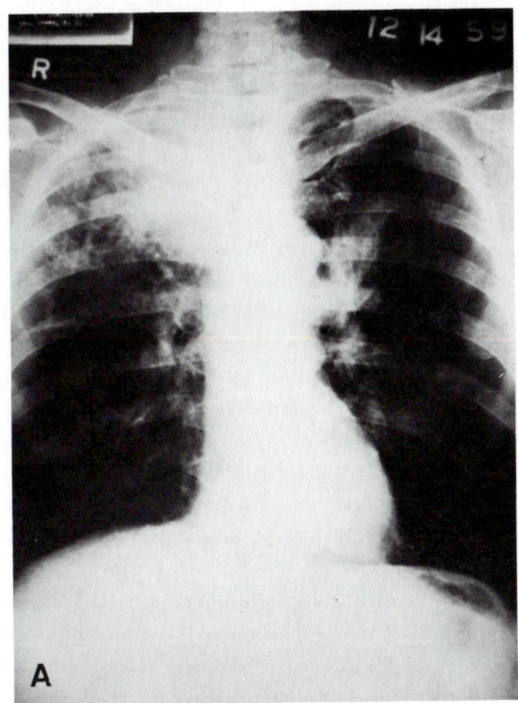


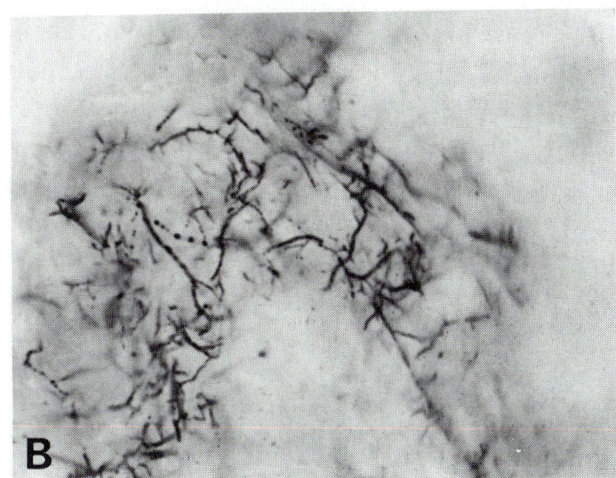


**Figure 17–3. A.** Chest x-ray showing pneumonic infiltrate, right and left upper lung fields. **B.** *Nocardia asteroides* was cultured from the sputum. The patient received a course of sulfadiazine and recovered (Gram stain, ×680). *(From Takaro T: In Goldsmith HS (ed), Practice of Surgery, 1978, courtesy of Harper and Row, with permission.)*

fect a cure or to provide biopsy material. In immunosuppressed patients, bronchial brushings or percutaneous transthoracic needle aspiration biopsy of the lung may help establish the diagnosis and avoid the need for thoracotomy. Drainage of empyemas or abscesses that may be present is indicated and should be carried out with specific drug coverage. Pulmonary resection for previously diagnosed *Nocardia* infection is rarely indicated; for unrecognized nocardiosis, it can be done safely without drug coverage, provided the diagnosis is made on the resected material, and an adequate course of a sulfonamide is given following operation.

## THORACIC MYCOTIC INFECTIONS

There are over 100,000 species of fungi. Only a few are known to cause disease in humans (Table 17–1). The thoracic surgeon should be familiar with these diseases, because they often mimic bronchogenic carcinoma and pulmonary tuberculosis. Almost all organisms causing fungal infections were isolated and named in the latter part of the 19th century, when such diseases were considered fatal. Today, subclinical forms of histoplasmosis, blastomycosis, and coccidioidomycosis are known to be common. These and other fungi also have been identified with increasing frequency as organisms causing opportunistic infections in immunocompromised patients, a subject discussed later in this chapter.

The diagnosis of a mycotic infection requires identification of the organism in either tissue, sputum, or other body fluid. Special stains and special culture methods are required. Some fungi occur as yeasts, having single, budding cells. Others occur as molds with branching hyphae. *Histoplasma, Blastomyces, Sporotrichum, Coccidioides,* and *Paracoccidioides* are dimorphic. In tissue they appear as yeast cells, but when cultured at room temperature they become filamentous molds. With rare exception, mycoses are not transmissible from patient to patient. However, *Coccidioides* and *Histoplasma* are infectious in the mold form, so these organisms must be handled with care.

**TABLE 17–1. FUNGI NORMALLY PATHOGENIC IN HUMANS THAT CAUSE PULMONARY INFECTIONS**

| Organism | Morphology | Appearance in Tissue | Endemicity |
|---|---|---|---|
| *Blastomyces dermatitidis* | Dimorphic | Large budding yeast, 8–20 μm | Central and Southeastern United States |
| *Coccidioides immitis* | Dimorphic | Spherules with endospores, 30–60 μm | Southwestern United States and Mexico |
| *Histoplasma capsulatum* | Dimorphic | Small intracellular yeasts, 1.5–3.5 μm | Central United States |
| *Cryptococcus neoformans* | Yeast | Budding yeast with thick capsule, 5–20 μm | Pandemic |
| *Paracoccidioides brasiliensis* | Dimorphic | Large budding yeasts—"pilot wheel," 10–40 μm | South and Central America and Mexico |
| *Sporothrix schenckii* | Dimorphic | Small ovoid budding yeast, 3–6 μm | Pandemic |

The most commonly encountered fungus infections—histoplasmosis, blastomycosis, and coccidioidomycosis—are also endemic to certain parts of the United States. Fungi live in soil and water and on plants. *Candida* is the only fungus causing systemic mycosis that lives normally in man.

## Histoplasmosis

Histoplasmosis is a systemic disease caused by *Histoplasma capsulatum.* This organism was first identified in Panama in 1905 by Darling, who named it inappropriately, thinking the organism he saw was a plasmodium encapsulated in a histiocyte. Thirty years later, de Monbreun demonstrated its true identity as a biphasic fungus by isolating it in culture. Histoplasmosis was thought to be a rare and fatal disease before Christie and Peterson[11] showed in 1945 that it was a very common and usually benign disease. (There are excellent reviews of *Histoplasmosis* by Goodwin et al.[12]) It is estimated that some 50 million people in the United States have been infected with *H. capsulatum,* most of whom live along the Mississippi, Missouri, and Ohio rivers. Active disease is uncommon, and only 1 person in 2000 develops manifestations of chronic pulmonary disease. Epidemics of acute histoplasmosis occur in association with exposure to dusty soil contaminated with the excreta of birds, pigeons, chickens, and bats. Bats become infected with the organism, but birds, because of their high body temperature, do not. The organism derives nutrients from the contaminated soil and thrives especially well in a warm, moist environment. Although the disease is endemic in central and eastern United States, it occurs throughout the world.

An acute infection occurs when spores from the mycelial form of *H. capsulatum* are inhaled into the lung, where they germinate and release yeast cells. The yeast cells are phagocytosed by macrophages and transported to mediastinal lymph nodes, liver, and spleen. An inflammatory response in the lung and adjacent lymph nodes results similar to the once familiar Ghon complex of primary pulmonary tuberculosis. Most patients are asymptomatic and are identified only later from positive skin tests and pulmonary calcifications on chest x-rays. In the normal host, symptoms are mild fatigue, myalgia, and fever. In patients with AIDS, the disease is severe and often fatal unless aggressively treated.[13] Physical findings are few. The chest x-ray is either normal in appearance or may show scattered infiltrates and hilar adenopathy.

Chronic histoplasmosis occurs in patients with previously abnormal lung tissue. Chronic progressive disseminated histoplasmosis is rare but does occur in elderly patients with impaired immune defenses. A diagnosis can be made from biopsy of the oropharyngeal ulcer, which is commonly present.[14]

Inactive or healed forms of histoplasmosis include multiple pulmonary calcifications, fibronodular scarring, solitary (sometimes multiple) nodules or histoplasmomas, and mediastinal fibrosis. Histoplasmomas are characteristically dense with central calcification, but if calcification is absent, they may be difficult to distinguish from neoplasms (Fig. 17–4).

Mediastinal fibrosis results when acute histoplasmosis involves the hilar lymph nodes. The fibrosis may be intense, resulting in obstruction of the superior vena cava, main bronchi, and the pulmonary vessels.[15]

Diagnosis depends upon the demonstration of *H. capsulatum* in cultures of sputum or bronchial secretions, or upon the identification of organisms in tissue specimens or gastric secretions or in the urine[16–18] (Fig. 17–5). A positive histoplasmin skin test does not indicate active disease. Moreover, even in patients with bacteriologically proven disease, there is a 20% incidence of false-negative reactions. Histoplasmin skin testing will boost *Histoplasma* antibodies and should not be done if serologic tests are contemplated. Radioimmunoassay (RIA) and enzyme immunoassay (EIA) are highly sensitive and useful as screening tests but must be confirmed with the more specific complement fixation.

Acute pulmonary histoplasmosis is self-limited and rarely requires antifungal therapy. For severe or prolonged illness, amphotericin B, 40–50 mg daily for 2–3 weeks, or ketoconazole, 400 mg by mouth daily, may be necessary.[19] Itraconazole is also effective. Amphotericin B is the drug of

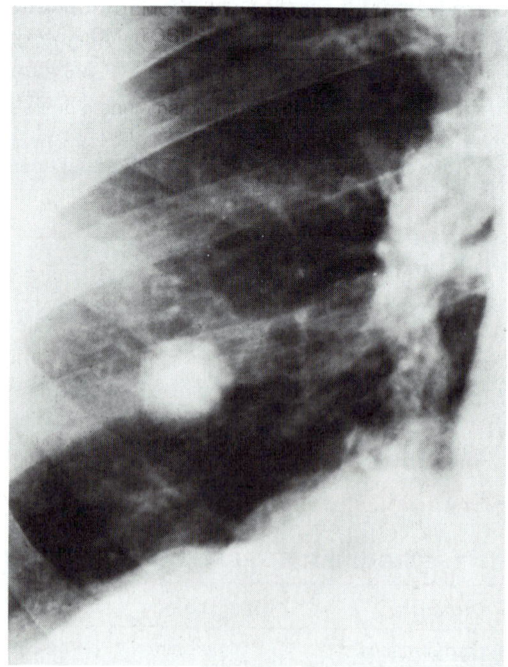

**Figure 17–4.** Solitary pulmonary nodule, probably a *Histoplasma* granuloma, from a patient in the endemic area. This was first noted in 1968 in a 45-year-old male with chronic obstructive lung disease. The lesion has a dense, laminated, calcific center. There was no change over a 10-year period.

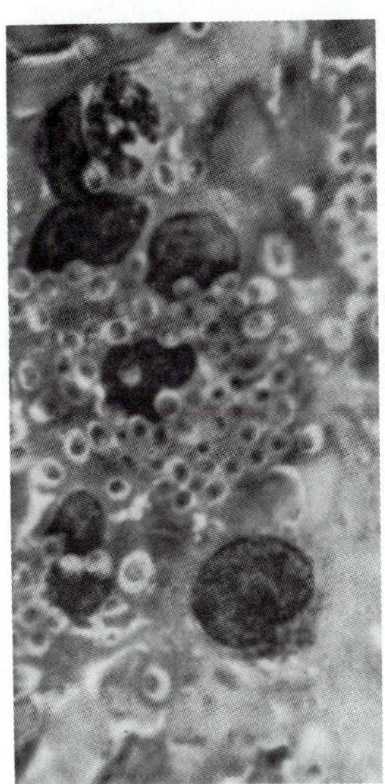


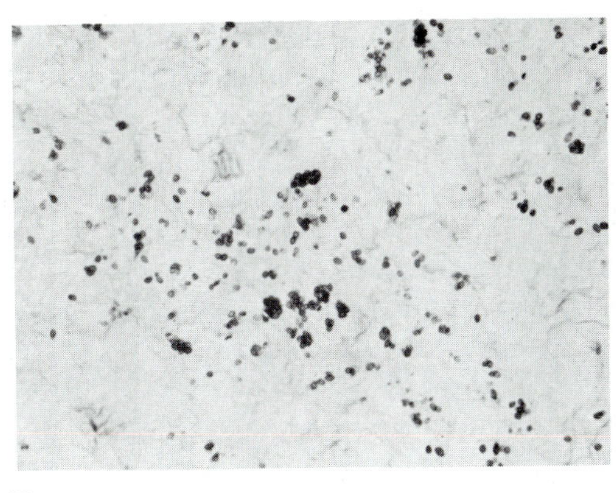


**Figure 17–5.** Forms of *Histoplasma capsulatum* found in the tissues: **A.** Intracellular organisms (Giemsa, ×1000). **B.** Nonviable capsules of *H. capsulatum* in necrotic center of a histoplasmoma (Gomori, ×630).

choice for chronic histoplasmosis. For disseminated disease, amphotericin B is urgently needed, and the dose should be at least 25 mg/kg body weight daily for a total dose of 2.5–3.5 g. The azole drugs can provide effective alternative or suppressive treatment in patients with AIDS.[20,21] The pharmacologic effects of antimycotic agents, their toxicity, and the methods of their administration are well described.[22]

Management of the solitary pulmonary nodule requires exploratory thoracotomy, unless the diagnosis can be made by transbronchial brushing, needle biopsy, or from the characteristic calcification or if the lesion has been present and unchanged for several years, in which case neither thoracotomy nor drug therapy is necessary.[23]

Cavitary histoplasmosis, proven by culture, should be treated primarily with amphotericin B. Surgery does not improve survival or prevent relapse even in conjunction with amphotericin B.[24] Resectional surgery, if undertaken, should be accompanied by amphotericin B or ketoconazole.[25]

Surgery may be necessary for life-threatening tracheobronchial and esophageal obstruction and bronchoesophageal fistulae.[15] Enlarged lymph nodes can cause compression of the trachea, bronchi, or esophagus, and caseous nodes can result in traction diverticuli of the esophagus or bronchoesophageal fistulae. Coalescence of mediastinal nodes may produce large granulomas with thick fibrotic capsules formed in response to the *Histoplasma* antigen. This reaction can extend into adjacent normal tissue with devastating effect. Stenosis of pulmonary arteries, pulmonary veins, or superior vena cava can occur.

Excision of mediastinal granulomas may avert development of a fibrocalcific mediastinum. Vena caval obstruction has been successfully treated with a bypass graft constructed from a spiral of autogenous saphenous vein.[26] Pleural effusion, pericarditis, and endocarditis are rare complications that may require surgical management. Endocarditis has been observed on both native and prosthetic heart valves.[27] Infection of the native heart valve should be treated with amphotericin B and long-term ketoconazole, although valve replacement may be required for valvular insufficiency. Infected prostheses should be replaced promptly.

Broncholithiasis results when a calcified node erodes into a bronchus. In a report describing 40 patients with broncholithiasis and living in an endemic area for histoplasmosis, 21% of the patients required no treatment, 19% were treated successfully with endoscopic extraction, and the remaining patients required thoracotomies for successful management.[28]

## Coccidioidomycosis

The responsible organism, *Coccidioides immitis,* was first correctly identified as a fungus by Ophuls and Moffit in 1900. Initially, only severe and usually fatal forms of the disease were recognized. In 1937, Dickson described San Joaquin "valley fever," an acute, mild, self-limited form of the disease. San Joaquin Valley is in the arid southwestern United States, where coccidioidomycosis is endemic. Infection takes place by inhalation of spore-laden dust and is estimated to occur in about 100,000 people in the United States annually, especially among agricultural and other outside workers. A 10-fold increase in the number of reported cases in California was reported in 1992.[29] Excellent reviews of this disease are provided by Catanzaro[30] and Stevens.[31]

The gross pathologic lesions resemble those of pulmonary tuberculosis, with a primary complex of pneumonitis and regional lymph node involvement. With reactivation, granuloma formation, caseation, and cavitation may occur (Fig. 17–6). Extrapulmonary dissemination is more likely to result during the primary rather than in the reinfection phase.

Most cases of primary infection are asymptomatic. The x-ray findings are nonspecific. In the acute stage, miliary lesions, pneumonic infiltrates, hilar adenopathy, or pleural and pericardial effusions may be observed. With chronic coccidioidomycosis, manifestations may include solitary nodules; thin-walled cavities, sometimes with a fluid level; pneumothorax; fibrosis; or empyema. Pericarditis has also been reported.[32] Immunocompromised patients are four times more likely to develop a primary infection when exposed to *C. immitis* than immunocompetent patients. The risk to renal and cardiac transplant patients in endemic areas is 3–6% per year.[33] The risk to AIDS patients is 2.7% per year, whereas in a normal population, the risk should not exceed 0.4% per year.[34] Also, risk of dissemination is greater in the immunocompromised patient (50–80%) than in the immunocompetent patient (15%).[35]

A positive culture of sputum (or other body fluid or tissue) is necessary for a diagnosis. In cases with pleural effusion, cultures of pleural biopsy specimens can be more rewarding than culture of the fluid exudate. *C. immitis* is a dimorphic fungus without a yeast phase. The saprophytic cycle produces spherules with endospores that can be iden-

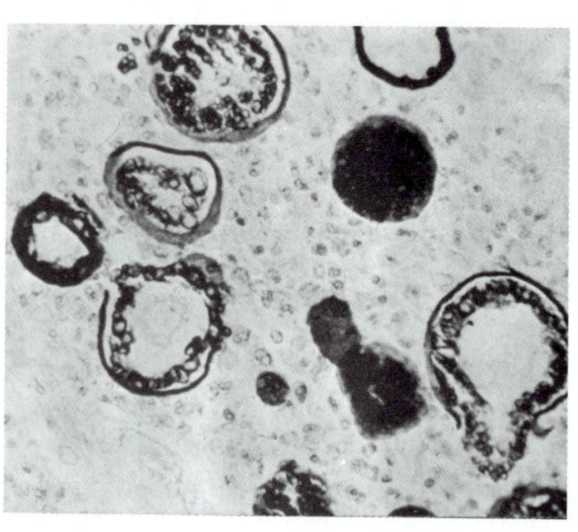

**Figure 17–6.** Histologic section of lung. Stages in formation and maturation of spherules of *C. immitis* (most of them containing endospores) (Grocott stain). Chest x-rays showing thin-walled cavity with varying fluid levels over a period of several months (**A**—May 26, **B**—June 1, **C**—October 13) in a young man with recurrent episodes of hemoptysis. Sputum was positive for *C. immitis*. The cavity was surgically resected. *(From Sagel SS: Common fungal diseases of the lungs. I: Coccidioidomycosis. Radiol Clin North Am 11:153, 1973, with permission.)*

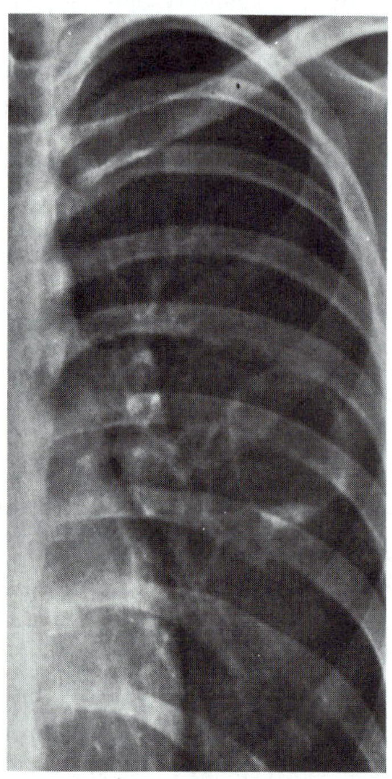

**A**

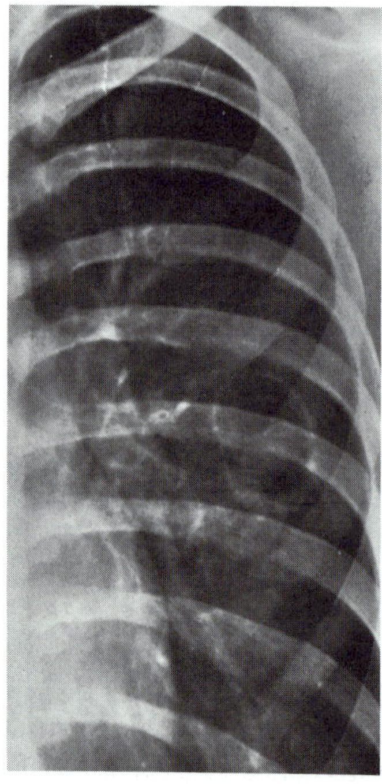

**B**

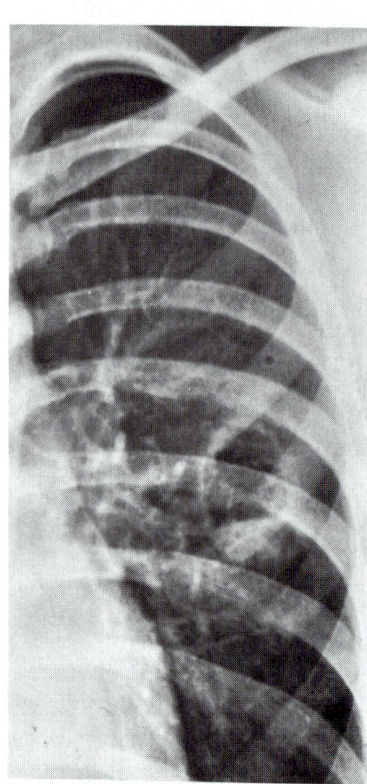

**C**

tified in sputum (10% potassium hydroxide) and tissue (H and E, periodic acid-Schiff [PAS], or methenamine silver stains). Hyphae may be seen at times in the tissue from cavitary lesions, and there are rare reports of cavitary lesions with coccidioidal mycetomas.[36]

A skin test should be done if coccidioidomycosis is suspected. A recent conversion to positive is strongly suggestive of the diagnosis. Serologic testing is useful. Early infections may be detected using an immunodiffusion test, which detects IgM antibodies. The complement fixation test, which identifies IgG antibodies, is especially useful for monitoring the severity of the disease. A rising titer means severe disease or possible dissemination; a falling titer suggests regression or improvement.

Many cases of coccidioidomycosis require no treatment. The most effective agent is amphotericin B, but because of the drug's toxicity, specific indications for its use are needed.[37] These are control of severe acute disease; prevention of dissemination, as indicated from a continuous elevation of the titer of the complement fixation test (1:64 or higher); control of cavitary disease in cases with a sputum culture positive for *C. immitis;* arrest of disseminated disease; control of progressive chronic pulmonary lesions; surgical coverage during pulmonary resection, excision, or drainage of diseased foci; and preventive medical coverage in the diabetic or pregnant patient with active coccidioidomycosis, or during corticosteroid therapy for whatever reason.[38] Itraconazole, ketoconazole, and fluconazole are for some patients effective alternatives to amphotericin B.

Surgical resection of the undiagnosed pulmonary nodule is indicated to exclude carcinoma, especially in patients over 40 years of age with a smoking history. A granuloma that is known to be coccidioidal does not require resection. A complication rate of 10% has been reported after resection of localized lesions. Fine-needle aspiration biopsy will sometimes prevent the need for thoracotomy.[39]

The indications for surgery for cavitary lesions include persisting cavities 2 cm or greater in diameter; cavities that are enlarging, thick-walled, or ruptured; cavities associated with severe or recurring hemoptysis; those occurring in diabetic or pregnant patients; and those coexisting with pulmonary tuberculosis.[36,40,41] Drug coverage with amphotericin B is recommended, but it is not clear that use of amphotericin B has resulted in significantly fewer complications of bronchopleural fistula, empyema, or recurrent cavitation. Ketoconazole, itraconazole, or fluconazole may be used in reactivated cases, and in patients with human immune deficiency virus (HIV) infection.[42]

## Blastomycosis

Blastomycosis is a pyogranulomatous infectious disease caused by *Blastomyces dermatitidis.* It was first described by Gilchrist in 1894 and initially was thought to be a disease limited to the skin. Subsequently, it has been shown that the lung is the primary site of infection and that skin lesions, as well as lesions in the bone, prostate, and meninges, are due to secondary dissemination.

Blastomycosis is endemic in central and southeastern United States and Canada, in areas bordering the Mississippi and Ohio Rivers and the Great Lakes. It is endemic also in parts of Central and South America, Africa, and Asia. The organism grows as a mold in soil contaminated with animal feces and bird droppings.[43]

The mycelial form of the fungus produces arthrospores, which become airborne when the soil in which they are growing is disturbed. They are inhaled and lodge in the alveoli of the lung, where they convert to yeast forms and produce a pneumonitis. As the pneumonitis heals, fibrosis usually occurs. The pulmonary events are highly variable, however, and microabscesses, cavitation, giant cells, or caseation may be seen. Pleural involvement is common; if it is very extensive, the prognosis is poor.[44]

The patient may be asymptomatic or may complain of chest pain, cough, malaise, weight loss, weakness, or hemoptysis. Physical signs are not helpful. Pulmonary consolidation is characteristic; however, fibronodular lesions, with or without cavitation and resembling pulmonary tuberculosis, are also common, and lesions resembling bronchogenic carcinoma may occur.

Extrapulmonary blastomycosis may be present when a pulmonary infection occurs, or it may appear after pulmonary disease has resolved.[45] The most common extrapulmonary manifestations are cutaneous ulcers (Fig. 17–7). Cases of pulmonary blastomycosis are being reported with increasing frequency in immunocompromised patients, including cardiac transplant patients.[46]

The diagnosis is made by cytologic or cultural demonstration of the organism in sputum, or by culturing the organism from biopsy material, pus, or urine (Fig. 17–7). Although the large (8–20 μm), thick-walled yeast cells can be recognized on routine hematoxylin- and eosin-stained sections, silver-methenamine is most often used to identify the fungus, staining its cell wall black.[47] Skin and serologic tests are not helpful.

In some patients pulmonary blastomycosis is a self-limited disease that may not require chemotherapy. These patients may be followed clinically and radiographically.[48] Patients with severe symptoms, or who show no signs of resolution, or who have extrapulmonary lesions should be treated. A presumptive diagnosis is not an adequate basis for beginning chemotherapy. Transbronchial, transthoracic, or open-lung biopsy may be necessary that unfortunately is occasionally followed by dissemination of the disease.

Amphotericin B is effective treatment for all forms of blastomycosis. Ketoconazole and itraconazole are both excellent alternative drugs that may be given orally.[49]

Surgery is indicated if bronchogenic carcinoma is suspected after efforts have been made to rule out blastomycosis, especially in endemic areas. Amphotericin B should be given after surgery if the diagnosis is made at thoracotomy. Resection of known blastomycotic cavitary lesions is indi-

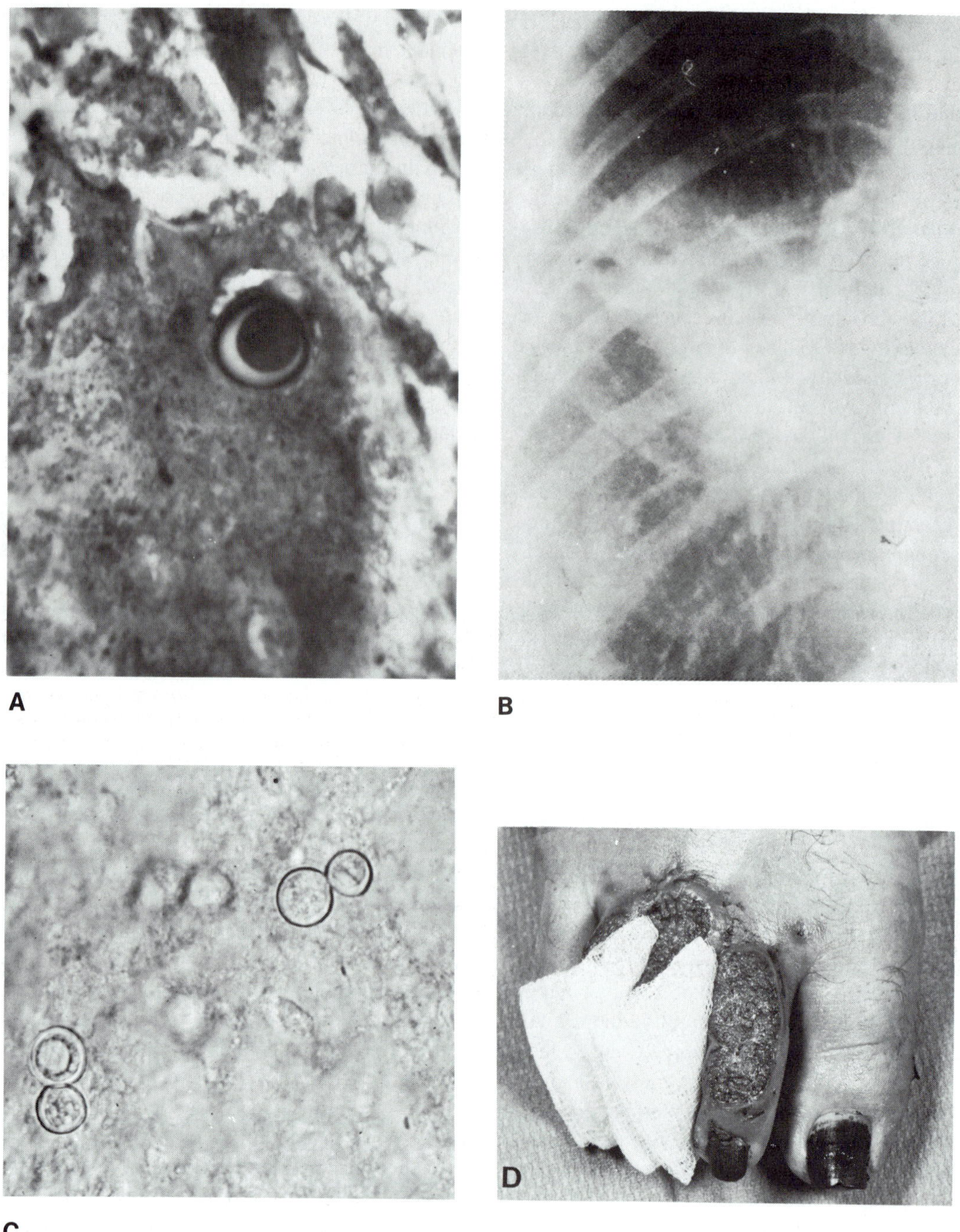

**Figure 17–7.** Examples of *B. dermatitidis* organisms. **A.** From resected lung tissue, showing thick-walled yeast cell (PAS, ×1133). *(From Takaro T: In Goldsmith HS (ed), Practice of Surgery, 1978, courtesy of Harper and Row, with permission.)* **B.** Chest x-ray of a 44-year-old female showing perihilar lesion subsequently proven to be due to North American blastomycosis. **C.** From sputum: fresh specimen unstained, mixed with 10% potassium hydroxide, showing characteristic figure-eight appearance of budding organisms (×354). *(Courtesy of Basil Varkey, MD, VA Medical Center, Wood, Wisconsin, In: Chest 77:789, 1980, with permission.)* **D.** Skin lesions of blastomycosis on the foot of a male patient. The toes have been separated by gauze pads. Note characteristic elevated edges of lesions. Biopsy of these areas showed microabscesses with giant cells containing *B. dermatitidis*. *(From Takaro T: In Goldsmith HS (ed), Practice of Surgery, 1978, courtesy of Harper and Row, with permission.)*

cated if they persist after adequate drug treatment (a total of at least 2 g of amphotericin B), because the likelihood of viable organisms persisting in such lesions is great, even if they cannot be recovered from the sputum.

Pulmonary blastomycosis is a serious disease with, in the past, a 5-year mortality rate of approximately 20%, but now with the availability of ketoconazole and itraconazole, the prognosis after treatment of blastomycosis should improve.

## Cryptococcosis

Cryptococcosis is a subacute or chronic infection caused by *Cryptococcus neoformans* (formerly known as *Torula histolytica*), which has a predilection for the bronchopulmonary and the central nervous systems. In the United States and Europe, it is more likely to occur as an opportunistic infection in debilitated or immunocompromised patients. Although the organism is neurotrophic, dissemination occurs to all parts of the body, especially in immunocompromised patients. In addition to the bronchopulmonary and central nervous systems, the most common sites of dissemination are skin, skeletal tissue, and the urinary tract. Cryptococci occur throughout the world and are present in soil and dust contaminated by pigeon and bird droppings. Serotype A and D organisms are most commonly associated with human infection and are identifiable in soil. Serotype B and C cryptococci, which appear to be endemic to southern California, Mexico, and Oklahoma, are difficult to find in their natural environment.[50]

*C. neoformans* is a round, budding yeast, 5–20 μm in diameter, the most distinctive feature of which is the wide, unstained, gelatinous, polysaccharide capsule that surrounds the organism (Fig. 17–8). Four serotypes (A, B, C, and D) of this capsule have been identified. The capsule surrounds the cell and inhibits phagocytosis by white blood cells by covering its binding sites for complement. Complement is necessary for phagocytosis of the organism, and the absence of complement from cerebrospinal fluid helps explain the predilection of this encapsulated organism for the central nervous system.[51]

The respiratory tract is the organism's portal of entry. A primary granulomatous complex with hilar node involvement, as in pulmonary tuberculosis, but with little acute inflammatory response, is characteristic of cryptococcosis. The lesions are often solid, with a bright or shiny cut surface, as seen in mucoid carcinoma. Central necrosis, cavitation, and calcification are uncommon. Pleural effusions and empyemas are seen. The pulmonary symptoms of the disease are nonspecific, insidious, or absent. Spontaneous remission probably occurs. In the majority of patients, cryptococcosis is seen as an opportunistic infection. The manifestations of the primary disease may overshadow the effects specifically known to be caused by *Cryptococcus*, and the diagnosis may become apparent only after abnormalities on the thoracic x-rays call attention to the lungs or symptoms referable to the central nervous system suggest meningitis.

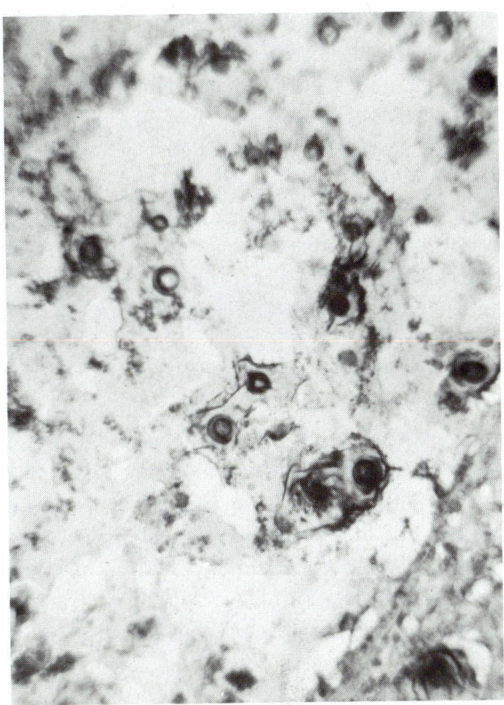

**Figure 17–8.** Cryptococcosis. Organisms of *C. neoformans* in resected lung tissue, showing thick unstained capsule surrounding the organisms (Mucicarmine, ×845). *(From Takaro T: In Goldsmith HS (ed), Practice of Surgery, 1978, courtesy of Harper and Row, with permission.)*

The roentgenographic features of pulmonary cryptococcosis are not sufficiently characteristic to be of diagnostic help. Autopsy studies have revealed four distinct histologic types of infection: peripheral pulmonary granuloma, granulomatous pneumonia, intracapillary-interstitial infection, and massive pulmonary involvement. Pleural effusion may be present.[52]

The causative organism may be isolated from sputum, bronchial washings, bronchial brushing, or fine-needle aspiration specimens, as well as from cerebrospinal fluid, where it should be specifically sought. Often the diagnosis is made from a resected lung specimen or at autopsy. Gomori's methenamine silver, PAS, and Mayer's mucicarmine are stains useful in distinguishing cryptococcus from other yeasts and from *P. carinii.* Culture requires 2–7 days. Cryptococci in the cerebrospinal fluid are usually identified on India ink preparations. Cryptococcosis skin tests are not reliable. The latex cryptococcal agglutination test is rapid and the most reliable serologic test, but some false positives do occur.[53]

The antifungal agents effective against *C. neoformans* are amphotericin B and 5-fluorocytosine. Like histoplasmosis, cryptococcosis was formerly thought to be a rare and invariably fatal infection, with meningitis the most prominent feature. However, it is now apparent that benign forms of bronchopulmonary disease are much more common than the dreaded meningeal form. Since the introduction of amphotericin B and 5-fluorocytosine, even the meningeal form of the disease can be brought under control and is no longer fatal.[54] Recovery with drug therapy is the rule rather than the exception. Also, the number of patients with opportunistic infection continues to increase. These patients are particularly susceptible to recurrence and dissemination. Any patient with immune deficiency, pulmonary lesions, and *C. neoformans* isolated from the respiratory tract should receive drug treatment. In fact, all patients with proven cryptococcosis should receive antifungal therapy, since experience indicates that patients receiving therapy do not develop meningitis. A less toxic regimen is made possible by using orally administered 5-fluorocytosine together with low doses of amphotericin B (0.3 mg/kg).

In the unusual event that the diagnosis of pulmonary cryptococcosis has been firmly established prior to surgery, and pulmonary resection is being considered, the combination of drug treatment noted earlier should be undertaken first (4 weeks is probably sufficient).[55]

## Sporotrichosis

Sporotrichosis is caused by a dimorphic fungus, *Sporothrix schenckii.* This organism, first described by Link in 1809, is a protean saprophyte of plants, insects, animals, and man. Its pathogenicity for man was demonstrated by Schenck in 1898. Ordinarily it is characterized by cutaneous and lymphatic involvement and only rarely as a pulmonary disease. In ambient temperatures the organism grows as a mold, but at 37°C it is a yeast appearing as basophilic short rods or as ovoid bodies with pale capsules, which occur singly or in clusters, free or phagocytized, and stain bright red with PAS stain (Fig. 17–9).

The symptoms of pulmonary sporotrichosis resemble those of pulmonary tuberculosis. Localized cavitary disease with surrounding parenchymal involvement is the most common x-ray finding, but other types of pathology including hilar lymphadenopathy, pleural effusion, lobular consolidation, fibrosis, and multiple nodules have also been reported.[56]

A definitive diagnosis can be made by fluorescent antibody staining or by culture of the organism. Serum agglutination with coated latex antigens is highly specific. Skin tests are of little value.

Chemotherapy for pulmonary and other visceral or disseminated forms of sporotrichosis has been disappointing.[57] Surgical resection is the most effective therapy for pulmonary sporotrichosis; cures are obtained twice as often with surgery as with drug therapy alone.[58] Perioperative chemotherapy with potassium iodide (SSKI) may be helpful. Amphotericin B is reserved for treatment failures, ex-

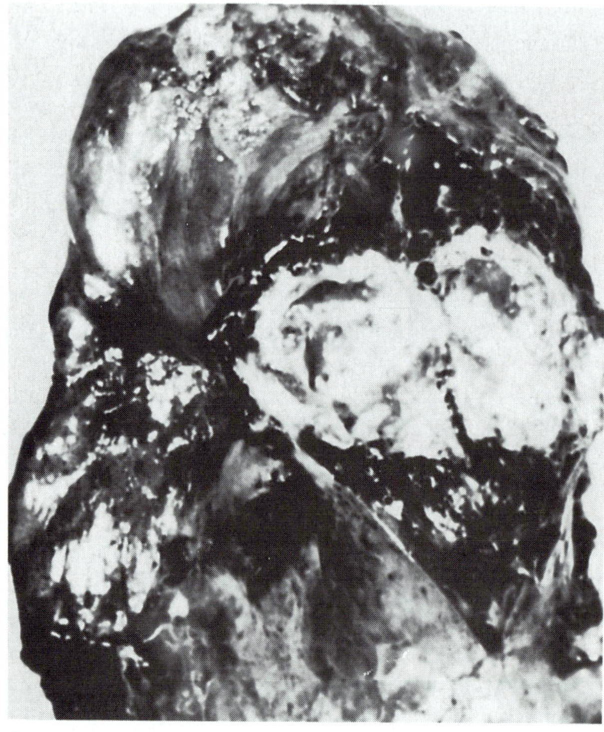

A

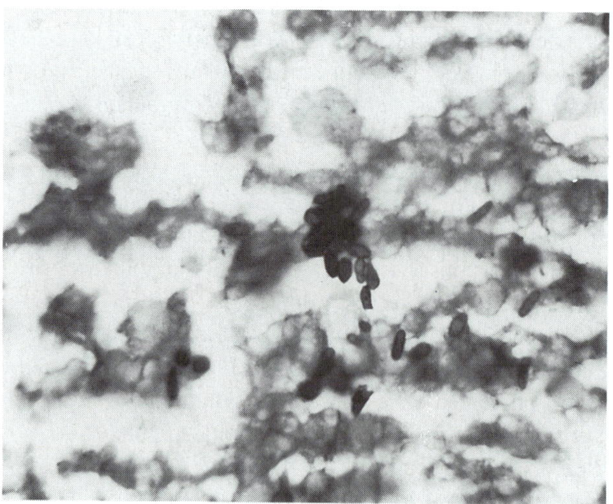

B

**Figure 17–9.** Sporotrichosis. **A.** Gross specimen of surgically resected upper lobe incised to show cavitary lesion of pulmonary sporotrichosis. **B.** Cigar-shaped organisms of *S. schenckii* seen in resected lung lesion (PAS stain, ×814). *(From Scott SM, Peasley ED, Crymes TP: Pulmonary sporotrichosis: A report of two cases with cavitation, N Engl J M 265:453, 1961, with permission.)*

tensive disease, and severely immunocompromised patients. While results using ketoconazole have not been uniformly good, itraconazole administered to some patients has been effective.[59] Spontaneous remission has been reported.[60]

### Paracoccidioidomycosis (South American Blastomycosis)

Paracoccidioidomycosis is the most common systemic deep mycosis occurring in Latin America.[61] It is a chronic granulomatous infection of the lung, oropharynx, skin, mucous membranes, lymph nodes, and other visceral organs. The disease is caused by *Paracoccidioides brasiliensis,* a soil saprophyte that is endemic to South and Central America and Mexico and that has only rarely been found in other areas.

Infection results almost always from inhalation of the organism's conidia. In approximately one third of patients, the disease is limited to the lungs and often resolves spontaneously. In some patients residual pulmonary nodules or calcifications remain. In sputum and in tissue specimens large (6–39 μm) budding yeast forms with a characteristic pilot-wheel appearance may be seen (Fig. 17–10). Cultures require 3–4 weeks and are usually positive. Both skin and serologic tests are helpful in making a diagnosis.

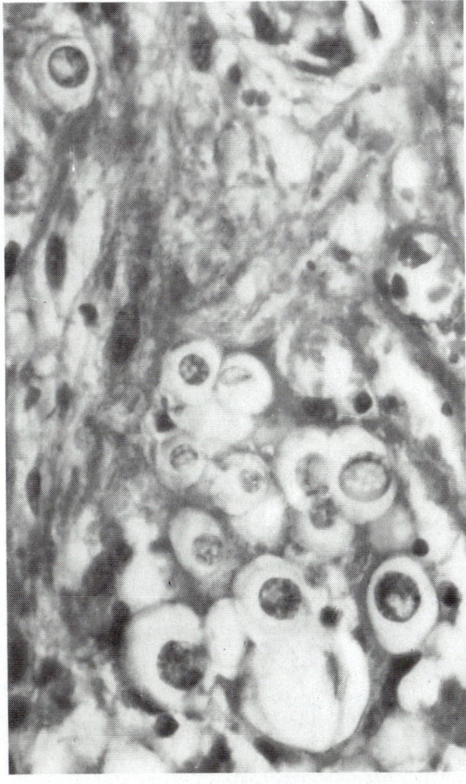

**Figure 17–10.** Paracoccidioidomycosis (South American blastomycosis). Organisms of *P. brasiliensis,* in tissue. Note resemblance to *B. dermatitidis. (From Takaro T: In Goldsmith HS (ed), Practice of Surgery, 1978, courtesy of Harper and Row, with permission.)*

The present treatment of choice is itraconazole.[62] The role of surgery is limited to the occasional lung biopsy.

## OPPORTUNISTIC FUNGAL INFECTIONS

The opportunistic fungi, *Aspergillus, Candida,* the *Zygomycetes, Pseudallescheria,* and other less common organisms, are of low virulence and exist as saprophytes in immunocompetent individuals without causing disease. They differ from the normally pathogenic species, *Histoplasma, Blastomyces, Coccidioides, Paracoccidioides,* and *Sporothrix,* which are dimorphic and exist in nature as molds but in hosts as yeasts (or spherules in the case of *Coccidioides*) that are resistant to phagocytosis by polymorphonuclear leukocytes (PMN).[63] The opportunistic fungi do not cause disease in normal hosts, possibly because they are susceptible to PMN phagocytosis; they do cause disease in neutropenic patients. Both pathogenic and opportunistic fungi cause infection in patients with severely depressed cell-mediated immunity.

### Aspergillosis

Aspergillosis is caused by an ubiquitous, saprophytic mold, *Aspergillus,* of which there are over 200 species that grow on organic debris, especially around barns and stables. The most pathogenic species, *A. fumigatus,* grows well at higher temperatures, which explain why it is found in abundance in stored hay and grains. The isolated organisms are filamentous fungi that produce airborne spores. In pathologic materials, usually only coarse, fragmented, septate, branching hyphae are found, either as short strands or ball-like clusters.[64]

There are three distinctly different clinical syndromes: aspergillus bronchitis, chronic mycetoma (aspergilloma), and invasive aspergillosis. The first is an allergic or hypersensitivity manifestation.[64] The last occurs as an opportunistic infection. Because of its increasing incidence, aspergillosis is now the third most common systemic fungus infection requiring hospital care. The mycetoma, or "fungus ball," is of special interest to the surgeon (Fig. 17–11).

An aspergilloma may exist for years without symptoms. The most common symptom, however, is hemoptysis, which may be mild or severe, even exsanguinating. Physical findings are few and are more likely related to an underlying chronic lung disease due to tuberculosis, sarcoidosis, histoplasmosis, bronchiectasis, bronchogenic cyst, chronic lung abscess, or cavitating bronchogenic carcinoma. Aspergillomas may be simple (occurring in a thin-walled, epithelium-lined cyst without surrounding parenchymal disease), or complex (occurring in a thick-walled cavity with surrounding parenchymal disease) (Fig. 17–12). The fungus ball is a round, friable, necrotic-looking mass of hyphae,

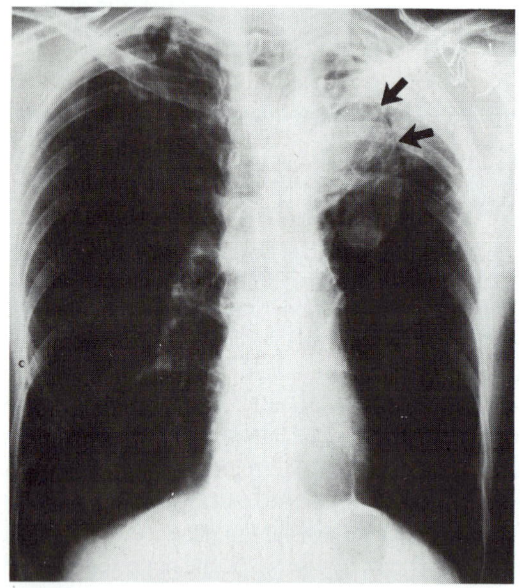

**Figure 17–11.** Aspergillosis. Chest x-ray of a 50-year-old male with a history of pulmonary tuberculosis 20 years earlier. Thoracic aortic aneurysm was first suspected, but the thin rim of air between the mass and the wall of the cavity in which it resides (arrows) is characteristic of a fungus ball.

fibrin, and inflammatory cells. It will shift position within the cavity when the patient changes position. A chest x-ray with the patient in the upright position is often characteristic, having a crescentic radiolucency above a rounded radiopaque lesion (Fig. 17–11).

The finding of a species of *Aspergillus* in the sputum does not of itself justify the diagnosis of aspergillosis. However, sputum cultures positive for *Aspergillus* render the diagnosis probable. Transtracheal or direct lung aspirates taken with thin-walled, 19-gauge needles may provide a definitive diagnosis and are especially useful in immunosuppressed patients with pulmonary aspergillosis. Precipitating antibodies against *A. fumigatus* in the serum, skin sensitivity to *Aspergillus* antigen, or a characteristic chest x-ray are confirmatory evidence.

The medical treatment of aspergillosis has been unsatisfactory, but isolated cures of aspergillomas have been reported with amphotericin B, which is the drug of choice. Itraconazole is being evaluated. Amphotericin B is the drug of choice for invasive aspergillosis, which has a mortality in excess of 80%.[65]

Resection is the only sure method of curing aspergilloma,[66] although many patients spontaneously resolve their symptoms. In a review of the Mayo clinic experience with 53 patients, operative mortality was 34% for

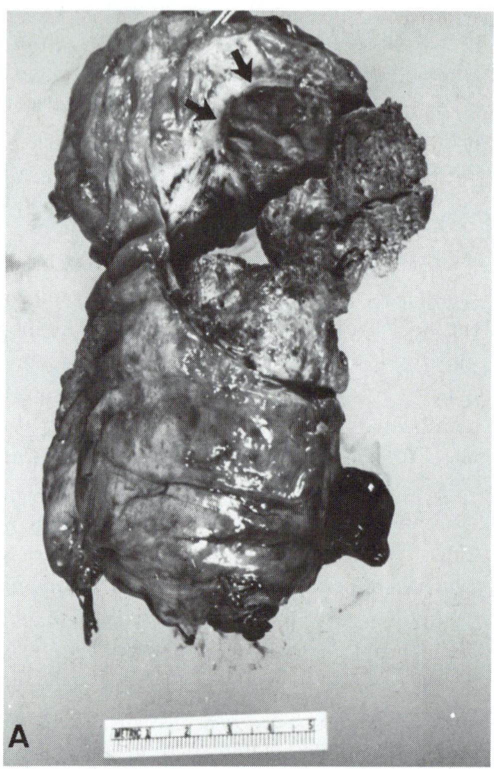



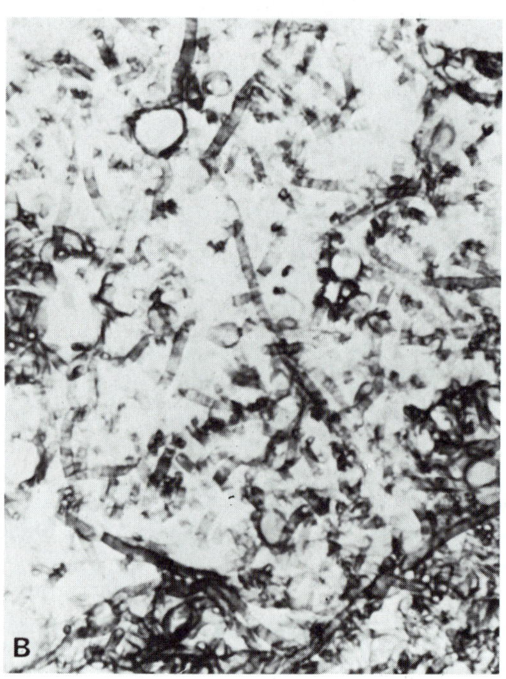



**Figure 17–12.** **A.** Gross appearance of the resected specimen illustrated in Figure 17–11. Note thick-walled cavity (arrows) that the necrotic material comprising the "fungus ball," on the right, almost completely filled. **B.** Coarse, fragmented septate mycelia of *A. fumigatus*. Round bodies are mycelia seen end-on (Gomori, ×741). *(Courtesy of Dr. William Wyatt, with permission.)*

complex aspergilloma and 5% for simple aspergillomas. Complications occurred in 78% of patients with complex aspergillomas and in 33% of patients with simple aspergillomas.[67] This experience suggests that surgery is indicated for patients with complex aspergillomas only if they continue to have symptoms after medical therapy or if they have undiagnosed pulmonary masses. Since patients with simple aspergillomas have the potential for massive hemorrhage and death and their surgical risk is low, resection is indicated for these patients if they are otherwise in good health.

Serious hemoptysis may be life-threatening due to asphyxiation from airway obstruction. Management includes positioning the patient with the normal side uppermost or in the semisetting position, blood replacement, radiotherapy, and transbronchoscopic tamponade.[68,69] Localization of the bleeding site by flexible fiberoptic bronchoscopy, for lesser degrees of bleeding, or by rigid bronchoscopy, for massive hemoptysis (600 mL in 24 hours), is essential if the chest x-ray does not permit identification of the site of bleeding. Endotracheal intubation with a double-lumen tube allows ventilation of the unaffected lung and the aspiration of blood clots. An emergency thoracotomy and resection are sometimes necessary to control pulmonary bleeding in aspergillosis; however, percutaneous intracavitary instillation of amphotericin B will often (76%) control hemorrhage and induce resolution (57%) of disease.[70]

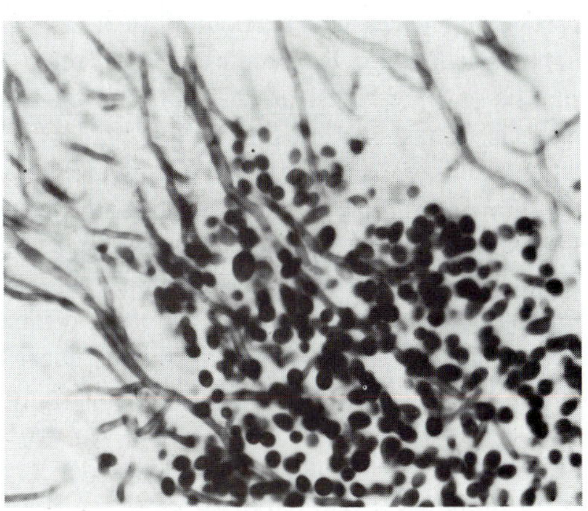

**Figure 17–13.** *C. albicans* organisms invading esophageal wall. Note presence of both yeast and mycelial forms (Gomori, ×690). *(From Takaro T: In Goldsmith HS (ed), Practice of Surgery, 1978, courtesy of Harper and Row, with permission.)*

## Candidiasis (Moniliasis)

Candidiasis is an acute, subacute, or chronic superficial infection of the skin or the oral, bronchial, or vaginal mucosa caused by *Candida,* usually *C. albicans.* Rarely, the infection is deep or systemic, involving the lungs, bloodstream, endocardium, meninges, or almost any other organ. Other fungi of this species are occasionally human pathogens. These organisms are commensal in humans but become invasive when normal immune defenses are altered. *C. parapsilosis,* which frequently causes infection associated with long-term, in-dwelling IV catheters and in IV drug users, may be an exception in that it can originate as a contaminant.[71] *C. tropicalis* is said to be the most pathogenic of the species.

The organism responsible for thrush was identified as a fungus by Bergin in 1841 and is now known as *C. albicans* or, less commonly, *Monilia albicans. Candida* organisms appear in fresh or fixed tissues as small (2.5–4 μm), oval, thin-walled, budding yeast cells with or without mycelial elements (Fig. 17–13). Infection may precipitate an acute or chronic granulomatous reaction. In systemic infections, both mycelial and yeast forms may be seen in clusters surrounded by polymorphonuclear leukocytes, forming microabscesses. The fungi also may be observed invading tissues and blood vessel walls, with very little evidence of inflammatory reaction in some instances. Osteomyelitis of the sternum and mediastinitis both caused by *Candida* have been reported.[72]

Aside from the fact that it is the most common of fungal infections, the importance of candidiasis as an opportunistic infection lies in the steadily increasing incidence of bloodstream infections and disseminated disease due to *Candida* sp., particularly since the advent of antibiotics in the 1940s and the subsequent use of immunosuppressive drugs. This is essentially an iatrogenic phenomenon resulting in dissemination to internal organs, fungemia, and endocarditis—previously almost unheard of. Intensive or prolonged antibiotic therapy, especially with multiple drugs, or immunosuppressive therapy following organ transplantation may suppress the normal bacterial flora, allowing an overgrowth of *Candida* sp., which normally inhabit the gastrointestinal tract and the female genital tract. Invasion takes place across the mucosal barrier or through any portal, needles, IV cannulae, or urinary bladder catheters. In the presence of altered host immunity or an inhibited inflammatory response for any of a variety of reasons, *Candida* pneumonia, abscess, or septicemia and generalized infection may result, often with a fatal outcome. The overall mortality is 52% and tends to increase with the age of the patient.[73]

Patients with cell-mediated immunity (CMI) defects, as seen in patients with AIDS, are predisposed to chronic mucocutaneous candidiasis but not to hematogenous dissemination. Neutropenic patients are at high risk for hematogenous spread, especially by *C. tropicalis.* Thus, although the presence of *Candida* species in the sputum of many healthy persons ordinarily is of no diagnostic or prognostic importance, the same cannot be said for the finding of these organisms in bronchial or lung biopsies, in the bloodstream, or in deep tissue spaces, especially in immunosuppressed or otherwise compromised patients who have symptoms and signs of pneumonia or septicemia. In such cases, one must assume the possibility of *Candida* septicemia or pneumonia. IV needles or lines and urinary catheters must be removed or changed, and therapy with amphotericin B must be started promptly.[74]

Of special interest to cardiac surgeons is fungal endocarditis following cardiac surgery[75] and pacemaker implantation.[76]

Pregnancy and diabetes are also risk factors. A diagnosis of systemic candidiasis requires culture and identification of the organism from a biopsy specimen, but if biopsy material is not available, a presumptive diagnosis may be based on the presence of endophthalmitis, positive blood cultures 24 hours after removal of intravascular lines, and culture of *Candida* from three or more separate body sites.[77]

The treatment of systemic candidiasis is amphotericin B. For patients morbidly ill or with *Candida* pneumonia, flucytosine should be added. A *Candida* infection involving the wall of a peripheral vessel, a native heart valve, or a heart valve prosthesis or lung abscess may require surgical excision.

### Zygomycosis (Mucormycosis)

Zygomycosis is an opportunistic infection caused by fungi from the orders *Mucorales* and *Entomophthorales* in the class *Zygomycetes.*[78] These fungi are characterized structurally by broad (6–50 μm), nonseptate hyphae. Among disease-causing organisms in this group are *Rhizopus, Mucor, Absidia, Cunninghamella,* and *Conidiobolus.* They are saprophytic and occur as woolly molds on manure and decaying fruit and vegetable matter and produce small spores that may be inhaled. These organisms do not invade a normal host. Characteristically an infection comprises blood vessel invasion, thrombosis, and infarction of invaded organs with marked tissue destruction and cavitation.

Zygomycosis manifests clinically in five different ways. Rhinocerebral infections tend to occur in diabetic and acidotic patients and cause extensive necrosis of the paranasal sinuses and the orbits of the eyes, often extending into the brain, and are rapidly fatal. Zygomycosis of the skin and soft tissues also is found in diabetics and may be rapidly fatal when occurring in association with burn wounds. Gastrointestinal involvement is usually the result of malnutrition or uremia. Pulmonary zygomycosis most often occurs in patients with leukemia, lymphoma, and neutropenia. It has been found also in patients undergoing cancer chemotherapy and renal transplantation and in patients with renal failure. Pulmonary zygomycosis in leukemic or neutropenic patients presents as a pneumonitis with diffuse infiltration similar to and sometimes indistinguishable from aspergillosis.[79] In diabetic patients, mucormycosis may appear as a nodule, pulmonary infarction, abscess, mycetoma, or infiltrate. Hemoptysis is not common, although fatal pulmonary hemorrhage has been reported.[80] Zygomycosis has been reported involving the mediastinum, heart, and even the chest wall following aortocoronary bypass surgery.[81]

Diagnosis depends on histologic identification of characteristic hyphae in and around thrombosed blood vessels (Fig. 17–14). Antemortem diagnosis of pulmonary and disseminated disease is difficult to make because cultures are usually negative.

The incidence of zygomycosis, like most opportunistic infections, is increasing; however, the prognosis with treatment has improved since 1970 from a dismal 6% survival rate to 73%.[82] This has been attributed to improved diagnosis, amphotericin B,[83] and aggressive surgery.[84–87]

### Pseudallescheriasis (Monosporiosis)

Pseudallescheriasis is caused by *P. boydii,* a ubiquitous soil inhabitant that acts as a secondary invader of previously damaged lung tissue such as a tuberculous cavity, a cyst, or a bronchial saccule. It may form a fungus ball in a preexisting pulmonary cavity resulting in life-threatening hemorrhage. It is often mistaken for infection caused by *Aspergillus,* since it occurs throughout the human body. *P. boydii* was first isolated in its imperfect form in 1900 and was named *Monosporium apiospermum.* Consequently, the disease has been known also as monosporiosis. Two other synonyms are petriellidiosis and allescheriasis. *P. boydii* is the most common cause of mycetoma, a chronic necrotizing infection usually occurring on an extremity. Pulmonary and systemic pseudallescheriasis almost never occur in an immunocompetent host.

The thin septate hyphae of *P. boydii* resemble those of *Aspergillus.* Diagnosis requires culture to identify the organism.[88] The organism is resistant to both amphotericin B and 5-fluorocytosine, although some patients have responded to miconazole, ketoconazole, and itraconazole.[89,90] Surgery is indicated for cavitary lung disease and when pulmonary resection is necessary to establish the diagnosis.[91]

## PROTOZOAN INFECTIONS

Protozoa are single-cell organisms responsible for many well-known human diseases such as amebiasis, malaria, leishmaniasis, Chagas' disease, and African sleeping sickness (trypanosomiasis). Other less prominent protozoan species have become notable for being pathogens in immunocompromised patients; these are *P. carinii, Toxoplasma gondii,* and *Cryptosporidium,* opportunistic infections that occur in patients with AIDS.

Pneumocystosis is a diffuse interstitial pneumonitis that occurs in patients who are congenitally immunodeficient, pharmacologically immunosuppressed, or who have acquired immunodeficiency. It was first described by Chagas in 1909 and came to be recognized in epidemic form during World War II among malnourished children in

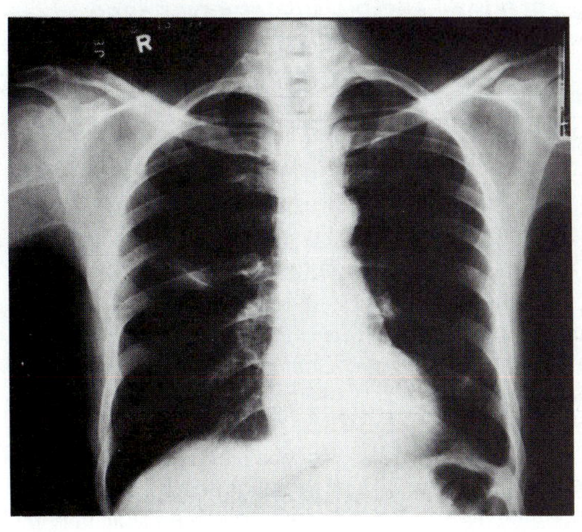


A

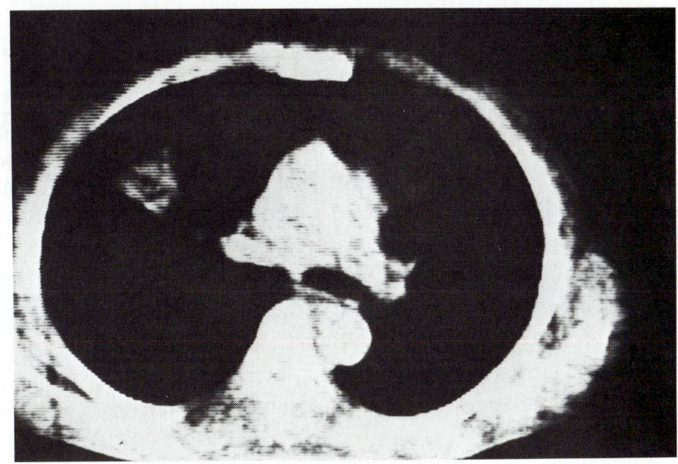

B

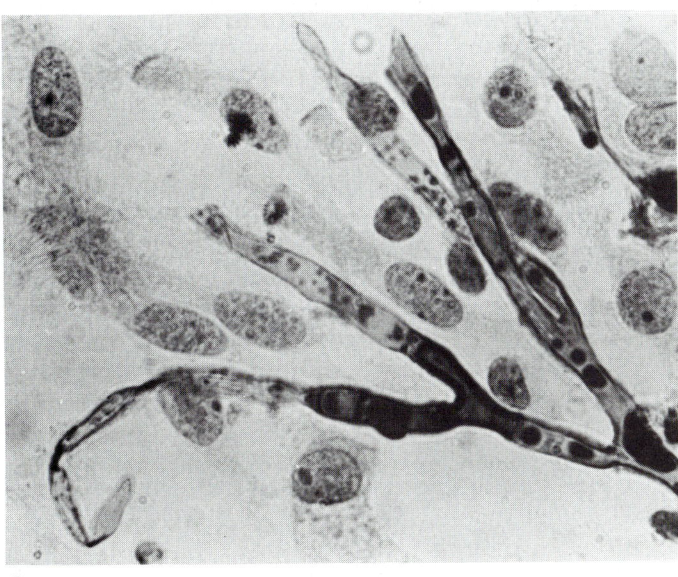

C

**Figure 17–14.** Mucormycosis. **A.** Chest x-ray. **B.** Whole-lung computed tomogram showing mass lesion with central radiolucency, in a patient with localized mucormycosis. **C.** Bronchial brushings from the right upper lobe, showing nonseptate branching hyphae. *(From DeSouza R, MacKinnon S, Spagnolo SV, Fossieck BE Jr: South Med J 72:609, 1979, with permission.)*

central European orphanages. The causative organism, *P. carinii,* exists in the lung as trophozoites or in thin- or thick-walled cystic forms of 5–12 μm diameter. Cysts have a double-walled outer membrane; within this are from three to eight intracystic bodies. The organism stains like a fungus with silver methenamine. However, it responds to antiprotozoan drugs.

*P. carinii* exists as a saprophyte in the lungs of many animals throughout the world, including humans. There is evidence suggesting that infestation occurs in early childhood and that the organism remains latent until the host becomes immunodeficient.

X-ray findings include diffuse infiltrates radiating from the hilum, or localized areas of pneumonitis (Fig. 17–15). Cavitation, large pleural effusion, and hilar adenopathy are not present unless due to associated disease. Marked hypoxemia and hypocapnia characterize the clinical picture. Diagnosis of the disease depends upon the demonstration of the organisms. It is because of the frequent need for open-lung biopsy for diagnosis that the thoracic surgeon is often called upon.

If the diagnosis is made, pentamidine isethionate or trimethoprim-sulfamethoxazole should be initiated. Both drugs are toxic to 50% of patients and are about equally effective against *P. carinii.* The drugs should not be given simultaneously. For patients with a $PO_2$ of <70 mm Hg, administration of prednisone has been shown to be beneficial. Untreated *P. carinii* pneumonia is often fatal, but when treated early and adequately, approximately 65–75% of patients may survive.

## THE IMMUNODEFICIENT PATIENT

It is important to recognize the likely causes of thoracic disease in patients with abnormal immune function. The most common causes of immune dysfunction include the human immunodeficiency virus (HIV), the etiologic agent of AIDS, chemotherapy administration, and antirejection therapy associated with solid organ and bone marrow transplantation. Over 350,000 cases of AIDS have been reported to the Centers for Disease Control (CDC), while over 1 million Americans are thought to be infected with HIV. In the United States, over 18,000 solid organ transplants were performed in 1993. In addition, the use of bone marrow transplantation has continued to increase, as has the application of chemotherapy in the treatment of malignancies. Because the immune defects differ among the various causes of immunodeficient states, a spectrum of pleuropulmonary and esophageal diseases exists.

## Infection with the Human Immune Deficiency Virus

In HIV infections, the virus preferentially binds to the CD-4 molecule that is present on T-helper cells (CD-4 lymphocyte), macrophages, and monocytes. The final phase of illness is manifest by opportunistic infections and malignancies and is associated with CD-4 lymphocyte counts <200/mm.[92] A variety of opportunistic infections is associated with a diverse spectrum of pulmonary parenchymal, pleural, or esophageal disorders. The common causes of pulmonary, pleural, and esophageal lesions are listed in Table 17–2.

The importance of differentiating focal infiltrates from

**TABLE 17–2. PLEURAL AND PULMONARY DISEASES IN IMMUNOCOMPROMISED PATIENTS**

| Infectious Etiologies | Noninfectious Etiologies |
|---|---|
| Focal Infiltrates | |
| Bacterial | Pulmonary emboli |
| Fungal | Pulmonary infarction |
| Mycobacterial | Lymphoma, Kaposi's sarcoma metastatic tumors, lymphoid interstitial pneumonitis |
| Diffuse Infiltrates | |
| Protozoal-Pneumocystosis, toxoplasmosis | Chemotherapeutic agents |
| Viral | Radiation injury |
| Fungal | Graft-vs.-host reaction |
| Mycobacterial | Congestive heart failure, lymphoma, Kaposi's sarcoma, metastatic tumors, lymphoid interstitial pneumonitis |
| Pleural effusions | |
| Bacterial | Lymphoma, Kaposi's sarcoma, metastatic tumors, pulmonary infarction |

Most common bacteria: gram-negative organisms, *Pneumococcus pneumoniae, Staphylococcus, Nocardia, Legionella.*
Most common fungi: *Aspergillus, Coccidioides, Histoplasma, Cryptococcus, Mucor, Pseudallescheria.*
Most common viruses: CMV, cytomegalovirus; HSV, herpes simplex virus; RSV, respiratory syncytial virus; EBV, Epstein-Barr virus.

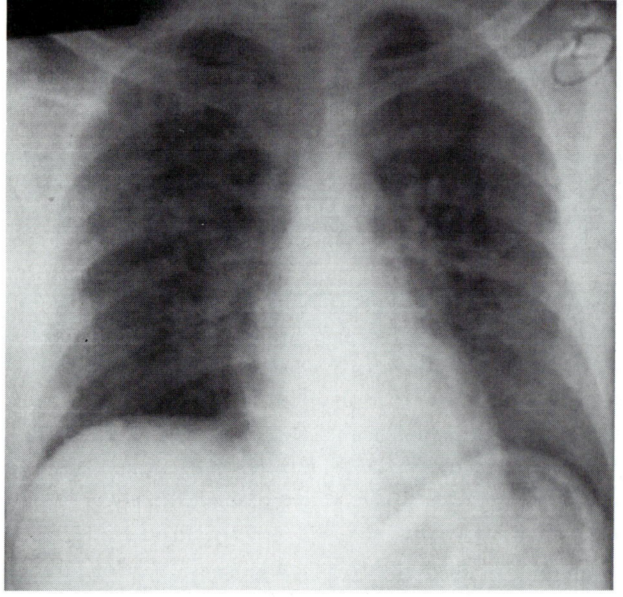
A

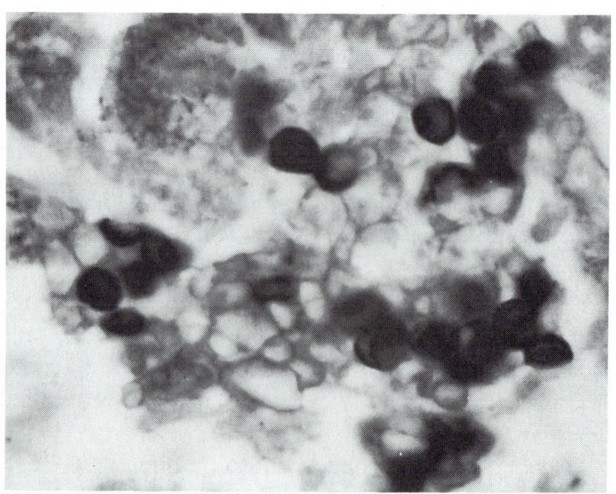
B

**Figure 17–15. A.** Chest x-ray of a 35-year-old male with AIDS and diffuse bilateral pneumonitis caused by *P. carinii.* **B.** Darkly stained cysts of *P. carinii* filling alveolus of lung specimen that has been stained with Gomori's methenamine silver nitrate. Trophozoites within the cysts cannot be seen in this preparation, which preferentially stains the cyst's capsule.

diffuse infiltrates is related to the prevalence of *P. carinii,* which has already been described and is the most common cause of diffuse involvement. However, fungi, mycobacteria, and Kaposi's sarcoma may cause either focal or diffuse infiltrates. Early in the symptomatic phase of HIV infection, *Pneumococcus pneumoniae* or *Hemophilus influenza* may be the etiology of focal infiltrates. Lymphoma may present as a focal infiltrate but more often causes hilar adenopathy. Common fungal infections in these patients include cryptococcosis, histoplasmosis, coccidiodomycosis, and aspergillosis. In children with HIV infections, the most common cause of diffuse pulmonary involvement is lymphoid interstitial pneumonitis, which is probably related to Epstein-Barr virus (EBV) infection.

Generalized lymphadenopathy is common during the asymptomatic phase of HIV infection. Mycobacteria, fungi, lymphomas, and Kaposi's sarcoma should be included in the differential diagnosis.

Because of the numerous etiologies and the vastly different therapies required for proper treatment, accurate diagnosis is important. For patients in whom a diagnosis is in question, thoracoscopic or open-lung biopsy may be necessary.

Pleural involvement in patients with HIV infections may present with effusions or pneumothoraces. Bacterial, fungal, tubercular, and malignant effusions occur commonly. Fungal infections are usually due to *Cryptococcus* or *Aspergillus.*

Pneumothorax in patients with HIV infection is not uncommon. This is often related to pneumocystic infection, which may cause severe alveolar damage leading to subpleural emphysematous blebs or pneumatoceles as well as parenchymal necrosis. In patients with a unilateral pneumothorax tube, thoracostomy and appropriate antimicrobial therapy are frequently successful. Patients with bilateral disease, which is not uncommon, frequently fail therapy using tube drainage and antibiotics, and may require bilateral stapling or pleurodesis.[93] In approximately 20% of the patients, progressive clinical deterioration occurs with early mortality despite appropriate therapy.

## Organ Transplantation

Bacterial, fungal, and viral infections are the most common causes of complications and deaths in transplant patients. Immunosuppressives used include cyclosporine, Imuran, and corticosteroids. A combined suppression of cellular, humoral, and leukocyte immunity results. Induction or rejection therapy using T-cell cytolytics, which include polyclonal, antithymocyte globulin and monoclonal agents such as OKT-3, profoundly affect cellular immunity. OKT-3 causes a greater impairment in immune function. Treatment of rejection episodes using bolus corticosteroids impairs leukocyte function, humoral immunity, and reticuloendothelial function.

The etiology, site, and severity of thoracic infections are dependent on the organ transplanted and the temporal relationship to the transplant. Lung transplant patients are particularly at risk for infections of the lung allograft. The lung allograft is denervated and lacks a systemic blood supply. Mucociliary function is markedly impaired. Because of denervation, stimulation of the distal airways by foreign matter or secretions does not elicit the protective cough mechanism.

The time course of infections involving thoracic organisms following transplantation is depicted in Figure 17–16. Bacterial organisms are the most common cause of infection any time following transplant. During the first weeks following transplant, pneumonia is rarely due to nonbacterial causes. Nosocomial gram-negative organisms predominate. In lung transplant patients, an infiltrate demonstrated by chest x-ray may be due to parenchymal injury caused by brain death; ischemia and reperfusion; atelectasis, often due to mucus plugging; or rejection. In lung transplant patients, bacterial pneumonia early after transplant is usually due to organisms that colonized the airway of the donor or the recipient.[92,94] Late bacterial infections are often associated with augmented immunosuppression during treatment of rejection episodes, or in lung transplant patients, following the development of the obliterative bronchiolitis syndrome.

Cytomegalovirus (CMV) is the most common and consequential viral pathogen. CMV infections vary in severity from asymptomatic shedding of virus, to CMV syndrome, to CMV pneumonitis. The incidence and severity of the infection is dependent on a number of variables. Recipients who are seronegative for CMV who receive an allograft from a CMV seropositive donor are at the greatest risk for development of CMV infection (approximately 90% in one series).[95] Cytolytic therapy, particularly utilizing OKT-3 as compared with the polyclonal antithymocyte globulin, is associated with significant increases in CMV incidence and severity. Prophylaxis for CMV infections includes the use of a variety of antiviral agents. A suggested regimen is shown in Table 17–3.

Herpes simplex pneumonia presents in a similar fashion to CMV infections. Differentiation is based on the viral culture, as well as immunostaining. Acyclovir is used for treatment and prophylaxis. Infection with EBV may cause a mononucleosis syndrome with fever, malaise, adenopathy, and pharyngitis. More ominous is the association between EBV and lymphoproliferative disease in which B-cell lymphomatous infiltrates may develop in any organ. Lung allografts are particularly likely to be involved. Treatment is not standardized. However, reduction in immunosuppression and administration of acyclovir is usually initiated. Histologically aggressive lymphoma has been treated with a variety of chemotherapeutic regimens and lymphoid irradiation with good initial response. Unfortunately relapses are common.

Fungal infections occur infrequently but are associated with a high mortality. The peak incidence of infection is be-

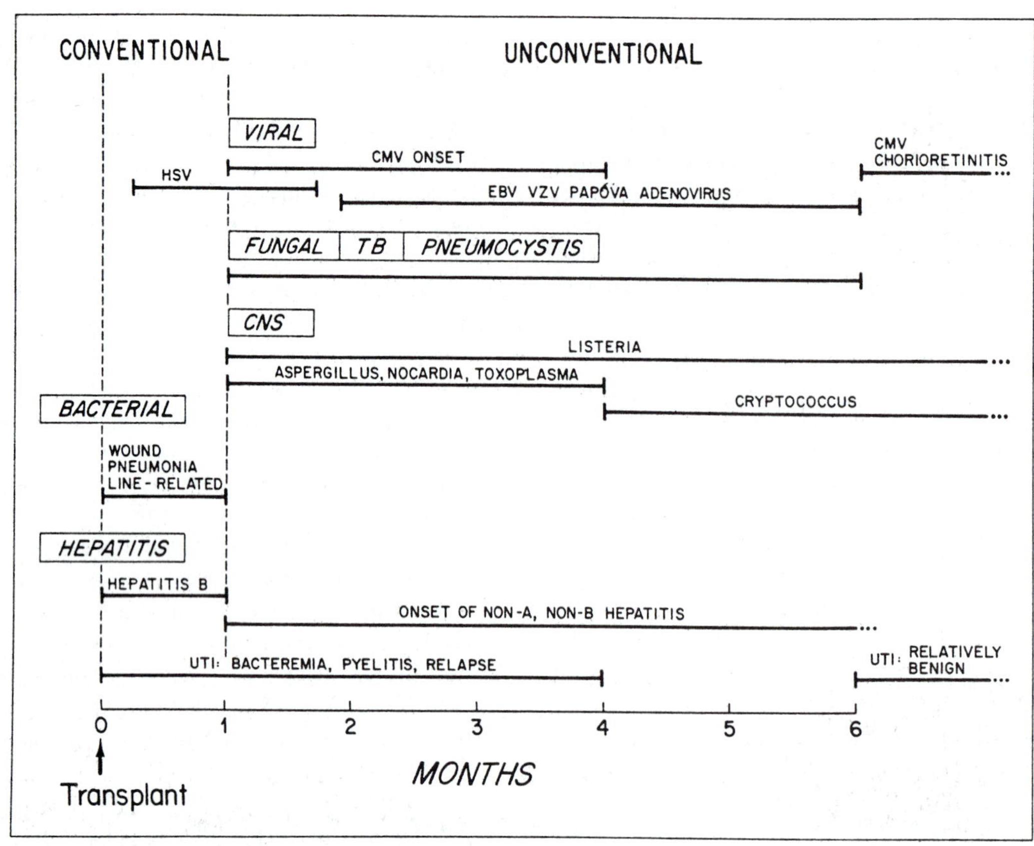


**Figure 17–16.** Timetable for the occurrence of infection in recipients. CMV = cytomegalovirus; HSV = herpes simplex virus; EBV = Epstein-Barr virus; VZV = varicella-zoster virus; CNS = central nervous system; UTI = urinary tract infection. *(From Rubin RH, Wolfon JS, Cosimi AB, Tolkoff-Rubin NE: Infection in the renal transplant patient. Am J Med 70:405, 1981, with permission.)*

tween 10 days and 2 months following transplant. Colonization of the airways with *Candida* species occurs frequently, but invasive pneumonitis due to *Candida* is uncommon. Systemic candidiasis develops most often in patients treated with prolonged courses of broad-spectrum antibiotics. Although infection of a vascular anastomosis is infrequent, it is highly lethal. Treatment of *Candida albicans* with fluconazole is usually successful. However, non-*C. albicans* species and resistant species require treatment with IV amphotericin-B.

**TABLE 17–3. VIRAL PROPHYLAXIS—DUKE LUNG TRANSPLANT PROGRAM**

| CMV Status[a] | Regimen |
|---|---|
| Donor positive/recipient negative | Ganciclovir 5 mg/kg q 12 h × 2 wk then 5 mg/kg q 24 h × 2 wk<br>IVIG 10% 0.5 g/kg on days 1, 14, 28, then 0.25 g/kg on days 42, 56<br>Acyclovir 800 mg qid from days 30–90 |
| Donor positive or negative/recipient positive | Ganciclovir 5 mg/kg q 12 h × 14 day, then acyclovir 800 mg qid days 15–90 |
| Donor negative/recipient negative | |
| HSV donor or recipient positive | Acyclovir 200 g po × 12 weeks |
| HSV donor and recipient negative | None |

CMV, cytomegalovirus; HSV, *Herpes simplex* virus.
[a]Seropositive or seronegative for CMV.

*Aspergillus* species may colonize an airway, cause an erosive tracheobronchitis, or lead to a disseminated infection. In patients with *Aspergillus* growing from bronchial washings without evidence of ulcerative lesions in the airway or invasive disease on biopsy, observation is adequate; otherwise, therapy with itraconazole is initiated. Amphotericin-B is often used in conjunction, particularly with invasive or progressive disease. Although disseminated disease is usually fatal, early disease is frequently treatable. The use of liposomal encapsulated amphotericin-B has been shown to minimize nephrotoxic complications.[96]

Infections due to *Pseudallescheria* may be difficult to differentiate from *Aspergillus* species due to the similar clinical manifestations and histologic appearance with branched septate hyphae. However, the differentiation by culture is imperative, because most *Pseudallescheria* species are resistant to amphotericin. Miconazole and itraconazole have the most activity against this organism. Infections with *C. neoformans* have been rare.

*P. carinii* pneumonia occurred in >85% of lung transplant patients and in 10–40% of heart transplant patients prior to the routine institution of antibiotic prophylaxis.[97,98] Infections occur after the seventh week following transplant. Prophylaxis using Trimethoprim-sulfa three times a week, or monthly inhalation treatment of pentamidine, essentially has eliminated this complication. Although the period of highest risk is the first year after transplant, infections occur late after transplant, and most programs continue prophylaxis indefinitely.

### Immunosuppression from Chemotherapy

Immunosuppression from chemotherapy is primarily due to decreases in leukocyte function that directly correlate with the absolute granulocyte count. Pulmonary parenchymal, pleural, and esophageal infections are usually secondary to bacterial and fungal organisms. Numerous noninfectious etiologies also may cause focal or diffuse parenchymal processes (Table 17–2). The most common chemotherapeutic agents causing direct parenchymal injury are bleomycin, methotrexate, cyclophosphamide, busulfan, nitrosureas (carmustine, lomustine, semustine), methotrexate, and mitomycin. Differentiation among these various etiologies is imperative to enable the selection of appropriate therapy.

### Esophagitis in Immunosuppressed Patients

Esophageal involvement in immunocompromised patients is common. The most frequent infectious etiologies include *C. albicans,* Herpes simplex virus (HSV), and CMV. Noninfectious causes include malignancy and reflux. The physical examination may suggest the cause of the esophageal pathology. Patients with *Candida* esophagitis frequently have oral thrush. In patients with HSV esophagitis, oral lesions demonstrate shallow ulcerations. Unfortunately, patients with CMV esophagitis rarely have stigmata apparent by physical examination. However, CMV retinitis may be present. Based on clinical suspicion, empiric therapy is usually initiated. In patients with *Candida* esophagitis, fluconazole 100–200 mg/day or ketoconazole 400 mg/day is administered for 1 week. If clinical improvement occurs, therapy is continued for an additional 2 weeks. If herpetic esophagitis is presumed, acyclovir 400 mg five times daily is administered. If clinical symptoms improve, then 200 mg five times daily is administered for an additional 2 weeks. If empiric therapy is not associated with improvement or if CMV esophagitis is presumed, endoscopy with biopsy of ulcers is indicated. The biopsy specimen should be sent for fungal and viral cultures as well as immuno-stained for viral and fungal organisms. CMV esophagitis requires parenteral therapy with either ganciclovir or foscarnet. An oral agent effective against CMV is not currently available. Prophylaxis using oral Nystatin solution or Mycostatin troche decreases the incidence of Candida esophagitis.

## PULMONARY ECHINOCOCCOSIS (CYSTIC HYDATID DISEASE OF THE LUNG)

Pulmonary *echinococcosis,* cystic hydatid disease (CHD), is caused by the small tapeworm, *Taenia echinococcus,* or *Echinococcus granulosus,* which spends part of its parasitic life cycle in dogs and sheep.

Echinococcosis is rather rare in North America, but common in many other parts of the world where large numbers of sheep, cattle, and dogs are encountered and where the custom of feeding offal to dogs prevails. In Australia, New Zealand, South America, Iceland, and the countries bordering the Mediterranean Sea, echinococcosis remains a serious problem.[99] In the United States, most cases are found in immigrants from endemic areas, but sporadic indigenous cases have been identified.[100–103] A more benign, sylvatic form of *E. granulosus,* occurring in Alaska and Canada, has been recognized by Wilson et al.[104]

A less common but more lethal form of echinococcosis is alveolar hydatid disease (AHD), which is caused by *E. multilocularis.* This organism is found in the foxes and rodents of Siberia, Alaska, and central Europe, where it is endemic. When untreated, mortality from this infection approaches 90%.[105]

The echinococcal cyst itself consists of a germinal layer and of cyst fluid containing brood capsules and scolices of the worm (Fig. 17–17). A succession of acellular, white hyaline layers is laid down outside the cyst, which is thus enclosed by a laminated cyst membrane. As the cyst enlarges, it usually reaches the pleural surface. Compression of the surrounding lung produces a thin, fibrous layer of atelectatic lung around the hydatid; this layer is variously called a "capsule," "adventitia," or "pericyst."

The cyst may remain dormant for many years. However, it poses a hazard to the patient because it may rupture at any time, resulting either in the formation of daughter cysts or, uncommonly, in death due to asphyxiation or to a hypersensitivity reaction to the cyst contents. In any event, a ruptured cyst may become infected, forming a chronic lung abscess or a localized bronchiectatic area. The diagnosis is made most commonly by the characteristic roentgenographic appearance of round or oval, radiopaque shadows of a very homogeneous, waterlike density, with clear-cut borders and little or no evidence of reaction around them (Fig. 17–18). These shadows are usually located in the mid- or lower-lung fields. When air enters the perivesicular space, a characteristic, thin crescentic shadow is seen that is quite unlike the semilunar shadow seen with aspergillomas. The most unusual and unique roentgenographic sign of pulmonary echinococcosis—the "water lily" sign—consists of a lenticular shadow rising from a fluid level in a cyst. This is seen after rupture of the cyst and partial evacuation of its contents, with the torn vesicular or germinal layer floating on the surface of the retained fluid. The Casoni skin test for echinococcosis is not completely reliable.

Symptoms are minimal until significant compression

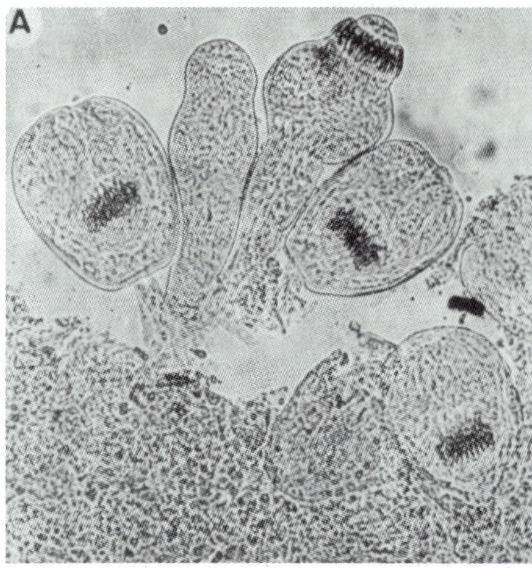


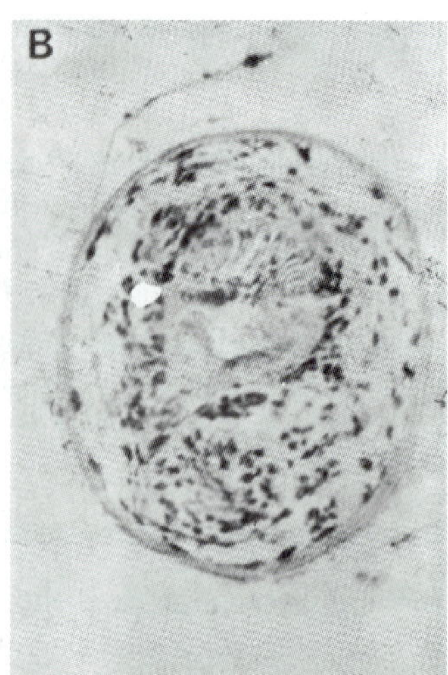


**Figure 17–17.** Pulmonary echinococcosis. **A.** Larval scolices of *E. granulosus,* from lung cyst, unstained. **B.** Scolex in histologic section. (Hematoxylin and eosin, H & E, stain.)

of an airway or a mediastinal structure such as the esophagus or the great veins occurs, or unless the cyst ruptures. At such a time, there may be dramatic expectoration of cyst fluid, followed by an allergic rash, and sometimes by fever. If secondary infection occurs, the symptoms of lung abscess or bronchiectasis predominate.

The diagnosis of such a lesion in a patient from a geographic area where "pastoral" (as opposed to "sylvatic") echinococcosis is found—i.e., where sheep and cattle are raised—is an indication for surgery. Conservative operations are advocated wherever possible. There are differences of opinion about the appropriate procedure for removal of the cysts.[106] Peschiera[106] is certain that the best method is partial aspiration of the cyst at open thoracotomy, with instillation of formalin into the cyst. After that, the cyst is opened and removed, together with the adventitial pericyst formed by the patient's own lung. Others favor enucleation of the intact cyst, especially if it is not under tension.[99,107,108] In this procedure, the nonadherent cleavage plane between the cyst and pericyst is first widely opened. Then the lung is inflated by the anesthetists, allowing the fragile, intact cyst to be extruded into a waiting spoon, hand, or basin. There is no need to grasp or touch the cyst. Occasionally, 10 mL of 10% NaCl solution is instilled into the cyst as a preliminary maneuver. In both surgical methods, the remaining space in the lung parenchyma is obliterated, after careful control of small and large bronchial fistulae, with or without removal of the fibrous pericyst. Segmental resection or lobectomy may prove necessary, after removal of the cyst, if lung tissue has been destroyed by prolonged compression or infection.[109] Nonoperative treatment is recommended for the asymptomatic patient with the less common sylvatic or forest type of echinococcosis. Mebendazole has been used with success in the treatment of nonresectable lesions.[110,111]

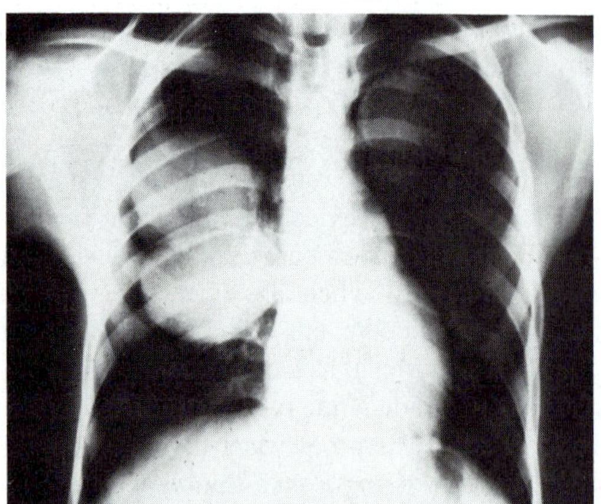

**Figure 17–18.** Chest x-ray showing echinococcus cysts, multiple and bilateral. Characteristic are large, rounded shadows of homogeneous density with clear-cut borders. *(From Wolcott MW, et al: J Thorac Cardiovasc Surg 62:465, 1971, with permission.)*

Historically, echinococcosis has been a surgical disease, the only effective treatment being surgical excision and sometimes radical excision. However, experience with several benzimidazole derivatives, especially mebendazole and albendazole in the past decade, indicates that in certain circumstances, chemotherapy may replace surgery.[112]

## REFERENCES


1. Rippon JW (ed): *Medical Mycology,* Philadelphia, Saunders, 1988, pp 30–52
2. Jensen BM, Kruse-Anderson S, Andersen K: Thoracic actinomycosis. *Scan J Thorac Cardiovasc Surg* **23:**181, 1989
3. Fife TD, Finegold SM, Grennan T: Pericardial actinomycosis. Case report and review. *Rev Infect Dis* **13:**120, 1991
4. Wohlgemuth SD, Gaddy MC: Surgical implications of actinomycosis. *South Med J* **79:**1574, 1986
5. Yeager BA, Hoxie J, Weisman RA, et al: Actinomycosis in the acquired immunodeficiency syndrome-related complex. *Arch Otolaryngol Head Neck Surg* **112:**1293, 1986

6. Filice GA: Actinomycosis. In Sarosi GA, Davis SF (eds): *Fungal Diseases of the Lung*. New York, Raven Press, 1993, pp 181–190
7. Conant EF, Wechsler RJ: Actinomycosis and nocardiosis of the lung. *J Thorac Imaging* **7**:75, 1992
8. Arduino RC, Johnson PC, Miranda AG: Nocardiosis in renal transplant recipients undergoing immunosuppression with cyclosporine. *Clin Infect Dis* **16**:505, 1993
9. Coker RJ, Gignardi G, Horner P, et al: Nocardia infection in AIDS: A clinical and microbiological challenge. *J Clin Pathol* **45**:821, 1992
10. Filice GA: Nocardiosis. In Sarosi GA, Davies SF (eds): *Fungal Diseases of the Lung*. New York, Raven Press, 1993, pp 191–204
11. Christie A, Peterson JC: Pulmonary calcification in negative reactors to tuberculin. *Am J Public Health* **35**:1131, 1945
12. Goodwin RA Jr, Loyd JE, Des Prez RM: Histoplasmosis in normal hosts. *Medicine* **60**:231, 1981
13. Mandell W, Goldberg DM, Neu HC: Histoplasmosis in patients with the acquired immune deficiency syndrome. *Am J Med* **81**:974, 1986
14. Samuel J, Wolff L: Otolaryngeal histoplasmosis. *J Laryngol Otol* **100**:587, 1986
15. Garrett HE, Roper CL: Surgical intervention in histoplasmosis. *Ann Thorac Surg* **42**:711, 1986
16. Klatt EC, Cosgrove M, Meyer PR: Rapid diagnosis of disseminated histoplasmosis in tissues. *Arch Pathol Lab Med* **110**:1173, 1986
17. Wheat LJ, Kohler RB, Tewari RP: Diagnosis of disseminated histoplasmosis by detection of *Histoplasma capsulatum* antigen in serum and urine specimens. *N Engl J Med* **314**:83, 1986
18. Prechter GC, Prakash UBS: Bronchoscopy in the diagnosis of pulmonary histoplasmosis. *Chest* **95**:1033, 1989.
19. Stamm AM, Dismukes WE: Current therapy of pulmonary and disseminated fungal diseases. *Chest* **83**:911, 1983
20. Sharkey-Mathis PK, Velez J, Fetchick R, Graybill JR: Histoplasmosis in the acquired immunodeficiency syndrome (AIDS): Treatment with itraconazole and fluconazole. *J Acquired Immune Def* **6**:809, 1993
21. Wheat J, Hafner R, Wulfsohn M, et al: Prevention of relapse of histoplasmosis with itraconazole in patients with the acquired immunodeficiency syndrome. *Ann Intern Med* **118**:610, 1993
22. Borgers M, Bossche HV, Cauwenbergh G: The pharmacology of agents used in the treatment of pulmonary mycoses. *Clin Chest Med* **7**:439, 1986
23. Godwin JD: The solitary pulmonary nodule. *Radiol Clin North Am* **21**:709, 1983
24. Parker JD, Sarosi GA, Dota IL, et al: Treatment of chronic pulmonary histoplasmosis. A National Communicable Disease Center Cooperative Mycoses Study. *N Engl J Med* **283**:225, 1979
25. Terrell CL, Hughes CE: Antifungal agents used for deep-seated mycotic infections. *Mayo Clin Proc* **67**:69–91, 1992
26. Levitt RG, Glazer HS, Gutierrez F, Moran J: Magnetic resonance imaging of spiral vein graft bypass of superior vena cava in fibrosing mediastinitis. *Chest* **90**:676, 1986
27. Svirbely JR, Ayers LW, Bueshing WJ: Filamentous *Histoplasma capsulatum* endocarditis involving mitral and aortic valve porcine bioprostheses. *Arch Pathol Lab Med* **109**:273, 1985
28. Cole FH, Cole FH Jr, Khandekar A, Watson DC: Management of broncholithiasis: Is thoracotomy necessary? *Ann Thorac Surg* **42**:255, 1986
29. Pappagianis D, Sun RK, Werner SB, et al: Coccidioidomycosis—United States, 1991–1992. *MMWR* **42**:21–24, 1993
30. Catanzaro A: Coccidioidomycosis. In Sarosi GA, Davies SF (eds): *Fungal Diseases of the Lung*. New York, Raven Press, 1993, pp 65–83
31. Stevens DA: Coccidioides immitis. In Mandell GL, Douglas RG, Bennett JE (eds): *Principles and Practice of Infectious Diseases*, 2nd Ed. New York, Wiley, 1985, pp 1485–1492
32. Amundson DE: Perplexing pericarditis caused by coccidioidomycosis. *South Med J* **86**:694, 1993
33. Hall KA, Sethi GK, Rosado LJ, Martinez, et al: Coccidioidomycosis and heart transplantation. *J Heart Lung Transplant* **12**:525, 1993
34. Bronnimann DA, Adam RD, Galgiani JN, et al: Coccidioidomycosis in the acquired immunodeficiency syndrome. *Ann Intern Med* **106**:372, 1987
35. Seltzer J, Broaddus VC, Jacobs R, Golder JA: Reactivation of *Coccidioides* infection. *West J Med* **145**:96, 1986
36. Rohatgi PK, Schmitt RG: Pulmonary coccidioidal mycetoma. *Am J Med Sci* **287**:27, 1984
37. Graybill JR: Azole antifungal drugs in treatment of coccidioidomycosis. *Semin Respir Infect* **1**:53, 1986
38. Baker EJ, Hawkins JA, Waskow EA: Surgery for coccidioidomycosis in 52 diabetic patients with special reference to related immunologic factors. *J Thorac Cardiovasc Surg* **75**:680, 1978
39. Raab SS, Silverman JF, Zimmerman KG: Fine-needle aspiration biopsy of pulmonary coccidioidomycosis. *Am J Clin Pathol* **99**:582, 1993
40. Cunningham RT, Einstein H: Coccidioidal pulmonary cavities with rupture. *J Thorac Cardiovasc Surg* **84**:172, 1982
41. Nelson AR: The surgical treatment of pulmonary coccidioidomycosis. *Curr Probl Surg*, 1–48, 1974
42. Fish DG, Ampel NM, Galgiani JN, et al: Coccidioidomycosis during human immunodeficiency virus infection. *Medicine* **69**:384, 1990
43. Klein BS, Vergeront JM, Weeks RJ, et al: Isolation of *Blastomyces dermatitidis* in soil associated with a large outbreak of blastomycosis in Wisconsin. *N Engl J Med* **314**:529, 1986
44. Kinasewitz GT, Penn RL, George RB: The spectrum and significance of pleural disease in blastomycosis. *Chest* **86**:580, 1984
45. Davies SF, Sarosi GA: Blastomycosis. In Sarosi GA, Davies SF (eds): *Fungal Diseases of the Lung*, New York, Raven Press, 1993, pp 51–63
46. Pappas PG, Ghrelkeld MG, Bedsole GD, et al: Blastomycosis in immunocompromised patients. *Medicine* **72**:311–325, 1993
47. O'Hara M: Histopathologic diagnosis of fungal diseases. *Infect Control* **7**:78, 1986
48. Sarosi GA, Davies SF, Phillips JR: Self-limited blastomycosis: A report of 39 cases. *Semin Respir Infect* **1**:40, 1986
49. Bradsher RW: Blastomycosis. *CID* **14**:582, 1992
50. Bottone EG, Kirschner PA, Salkin IF: Isolation of highly encapsulated *Cryptococcus neoformans* serotype B from a patient in New York City. *J Clin Microbiol* **23**:186, 1986
51. Levitz SM: The ecology of *Cryptococcus neoformans* and the epidemiology of cryptococcosis. *Rev Infect Dis* **13**:1163, 1991
52. McDonnell JM, Hutchins GM: Pulmonary cryptococcosis. *Hum Pathol* **16**:121, 1985
53. Kerkering TM, Turik MA: Pulmonary cryptococcosis. In Sarosi GA, Davies SF (eds): *Fungal Diseases of the Lung*. New York, Raven Press, 1993, p 95
54. Sabetta JR, Andriole VT: Cryptococcal infection of the central nervous system. *Med Clin North Am* **69**:333, 1985
55. Smith FS, Gibson P, Nicholls TT, Simpson JA: Pulmonary resection for localized lesions of cryptococcosis (torulosis): A review of eight cases. *Thorax* **31**:121, 1976
56. England DM, Hochholzer L: Primary pulmonary sporotrichosis. Report of eight cases with clinicopathologic review. *Am J Surg Pathol* **9**:193, 1985
57. Pluss JL, Opal SM: Pulmonary sporotrichosis: Review of treatment and outcome. *Medicine* **65**:143, 1986
58. Scott SM, Peasley ED, Crymes TP: Pulmonary sporotrichosis. Report of two cases with cavitation. *N Engl J Med* **265**:453, 1961
59. Breeling JL, Weinstein L: Pulmonary sporotrichosis treated with itraconazole. *Chest* **103**:313, 1993
60. Pueringer RJ, Iber C, Deike MA, Davies SF: Spontaneous remission of extensive pulmonary sporotrichosis. *Ann Intern Med* **104**:366, 1986
61. Tuder RM, El Ibrahim R, Godoy CE, De Brito T: Pathology of the human pulmonary paracoccidioidomycosis. *Mycopathologia* **92**:179, 1985

62. Brummer E, Castaneda E, Restrepo A: Paracoccidioidomycosis: An update. *Clin Microbiol Rev* **6**:89, 1993
63. Murphy JW: Mechanisms of natural resistance to human pathogenic fungi. *Ann Rev Microbiol* **45**:509, 1991
64. Iber C: Allergic bronchopulmonary aspergillosis. In Sarosi GA, Davies SF (eds): *Fungal Diseases of the Lung.* New York, Raven Press, 1993, pp 205–214
65. Pennington JE: Aspergillus. In Sarosi GA, Davis SF (eds): *Fungal Diseases of the Lung.* New York, Raven Press, 1993, pp 133–148
66. Battaglini JW, Murray GF, Keagy BA, et al: Surgical management of symptomatic pulmonary aspergilloma. *Ann Thorac Surg* **39**:512, 1985
67. Daly RC, Pairolero PC, Piehler JM, et al: Pulmonary aspergilloma. Results of surgical treatment. *J Thorac Cardiovasc Surg* **92**:981, 1986
68. Conlan AA, Hurwitz SS: Management of massive hemoptysis with the rigid bronchoscope and cold saline lavage. *Thorax* **35**:901, 1980
69. Shneerson JM, Emerson PA, Phillips RH: Radiotherapy for massive hemoptysis from an aspergilloma. *Thorax* **35**:953, 1980
70. Lee KS, Kim HT, Kim YH, Choe KO: Treatment of hemoptysis in patients with cavitary aspergilloma of the lung: value of percutaneous instillation of amphotericin B. *AJR* **161**:727, 1993
71. Chu FE, Armstrong D: *Candida* species pneumonia. In Sarosi GA, Davies SF (eds): *Fungal Disease of the Lung.* New York, Raven Press, 1993, pp 125–131
72. Williams CD, Cunningham JN, Falk EA, et al: Chronic infection of the costal cartilages after thoracic surgical procedures. *J Thorac Cardiovasc Surg* **66**:592, 1973
73. Duess DL, Garrison NR, Fry DE: Candida sepsis. *Arch Surg* **120**:345, 1985
74. Strinden WD, Helgerson RB, Maki DG: Candida septic thrombosis of the great central veins associated with central catheters. *Ann Surg* **202**:653, 1985
75. Norenberg RG, Sethi GK, Scott SM, Takaro T: Opportunistic endocarditis following open-heart surgery. *Ann Thorac Surg* **19**:592, 1975
76. Wilson HA, Downes TR, Julian JS, White WL, et al: Candida endocarditis. A treatable form of pacemaker infection. *Chest* **103**:283, 1993
77. Soutter DI, Todd TRJ: Systemic candidiasis in a surgical intensive care unit. *Can J Surg* **29**:197, 1986
78. Walsh TJ, Rinaldi MR, Pizzo PA: Zygomycosis of the respiratory tract. In: Sarosi GA, Davies SF (eds): *Fungal Diseases of the Lung.* New York, Raven Press, 1993, pp 149–170
79. Bigby TD, Serota ML, Tierney LM Jr, et al: Clinical spectrum of pulmonary mucormycosis. *Chest* **89**:435, 1986
80. Murray HW: Pulmonary mucormycosis with massive fatal hemoptysis. *Chest* **68**:65, 1975
81. Gartenberg G, Bottone EJ, Keusch GT, Weitzman I: Hospital-acquired mucormycosis (*Rhizopus rhizopodiformis*) of skin and subcutaneous tissue. *N Engl J Med* **299**:1115, 1978
82. Parfrey NA: Improved diagnosis and prognosis of mucormycosis. *Medicine* **65**:113, 1986
83. Berns JS, Lederman MM, Greene BM: Nonsurgical cure of pulmonary mucormycosis. *Am J Med Sci* **287**:42, 1984
84. Coffey MJ, Fantone J, Stirling MC, Lynch JP: Pseudoaneurysm of pulmonary artery in mucormycosis. *Am Rev Respir Dis* **145**:1487, 1992
85. Brown RB, Johnson JH, Kessinger JM, Sealy WC: Bronchovascular mucormycosis in the diabetic: An urgent surgical problem. *Ann Thorac Surg* **53**:854, 1992
86. Majid AA, Yii NW: Granulomatous pulmonary zygomycosis in a patient without underlying illness. *Chest* **100**:560, 1991
87. Tedder M, Spratt JA, Anstadt MP, Hegde SS, et al: Pulmonary mucormycosis: Results of medical and surgical therapy. *Ann Thorac Surg* **57**:1044, 1994.
88. Travis LB, Roberts GD, Wilson WR: Clinical significance of *Pseudallescheria boydii:* A review of 10 years' experience. *Mayo Clin Proc* **60**:531, 1985
89. Mesnard R, Lamy T, Dauriac C, LePrise PY: Lung abscess due to *Pseudallescheria boydii* in the course of acute leukaemia. *Acta Haematol* **87**:78, 1992
90. Stolk-Engelaar MVM, Cox NJM: Successful treatment of pulmonary pseudallescheriasis with itraconazole. *Eur J Clin Microbiol Infect Dis* **12**:142, 1993
91. Jung JY, Salas R, Almond CH, et al: The role of surgery in the management of pulmonary monosporiosis. A collective review. *J Thorac Cardiovasc Surg* **73**:139, 1977
92. Low DE, Kaiser LR, Haydock DA, Trulock E: The donor lung: Infectious and pathologic factors affecting outcome in lung transplantation. *J Thorac Cardiovasc Surg* **106**:614, 1993
93. Gerein AN, Brumwell ML, Lawson LM, Chan NH, et al: Surgical management of patients with acquired immunodeficiency syndrome. *Arch Surg* **126**:1272, 1991
94. Doweling A, Yousem S, et al: Donor-transmitted pneumonia in experimental lung allografts. *J Thorac Cardiovasc Surg* **103**:767, 1992
95. Griffith B, Bando K, Armitage J, Hattler B, et al: Lung transplantation at the University of Pittsburgh. *Clinical-Transplant* 149–159, 1992
96. Katz NM, Pierce PF, Anzeck PA, Visner MS, et al: Liposomal amphotericin B for treatment of pulmonary aspergillosis in a heart transplant patient. *J Heart Transplant* **9**:14, 1990
97. Kramer MR, Stoehr C, Lewiston NJ, et al: Trimethoprim-sulfamethoxazole prophylaxis for *Pneumocystis carinii* infection in heart-lung and lung transplantation. How effective and for how long? *Transplantation* **53**:586, 1992
98. Olsen SL, Renlund DG, O'Connell JB, et al: Prevention of *Pneumocystis carinii* pneumonia in cardiac transplant recipients by Trimethoprim-sulfamethoxazole. *Transplantation* **56**:359, 1993
99. Burgos L, Baquerizo A, Munoz W, et al: Experience in the surgical treatment of 331 patients with pulmonary hydatidosis. *J Thorac Cardiovasc Surg* **102**:427, 1991
100. Spruance SL, Klock LE, Chang F, et al: Endemic hydatid disease in Utah. *Rocky Mt Med J* **71**:17, 1974
101. Katz R, Murphy S, Kosloske A: Pulmonary echinococcosis: A pediatric disease in the Southwestern United States. *Pediatrics* **65**:1003, 1980
102. Kennedy D, Sharma OP: An unusual presentation of hydatid disease of the lungs. *Chest* **97**:997, 1990
103. Burlew BP, Cook EW, Thiele JS: Asymptomatic pulmonary cyst in a college student. *Chest* **98**:455, 1990
104. Wilson JF, Diddams AC, Rausch RL: Cystic hydatid disease in Alaska. A review of 101 autochthonous cases of *Echinococcus granulosus* infection. *Am Rev Respir Dis* **98**:1, 1968
105. Schantz PM: Effective medical treatment for hydatid disease? *JAMA* **253**:2095, 1985
106. Peschiera C: Hydatid cysts of the lung. In Steele J (ed): *Treatment of Mycotic and Parasitic Diseases of the Chest.* Springfield, Illinois, Charles C Thomas, 1964
107. Lichter I: Surgery of pulmonary hydatid cyst—The Barrett technique. *Thorax* **27**:529, 1972
108. Xanthakis D, Efthimiadis M, Papadakis G, et al: Hydatid disease of the chest. Report of 91 patients surgically treated. *Thorax* **27**:517, 1972
109. Perianayagam WJ, Freitas E, Sharma SS, et al: Pulmonary hydatid cyst: A 25-year experience. *Aust N Z J Surg* **49**:450, 1979
110. Wilson JB, Davidson M, Rausch RL: A clinical trial of mebendazole in the treatment of alveolar hydatid disease. *Am Rev Respir Dis* **118**:747, 1978
111. Morris DL, Dykes PW, Marriner S, et al: Albendazole—Objective evidence of response in human hydatid disease. *JAMA* **253**:2053, 1985
112. Messaritakis J, Psychou P, Nicolaidou P, Karpathios T, et al: High mebendazole doses in pulmonary and hepatic hydatid disease. *Arch Dis Child* **66**:532, 1991

CHAPTER

# 18

# Surgical Treatment of Tuberculosis and Other Pulmonary Mycobacterial Infections

Marvin Pomerantz

## INTRODUCTION

Tuberculosis is one of the oldest recorded diseases. *Mycobacterium tuberculosis* pulmonary infections are virulent, easily transmitted by airborne droplets, and when untreated are rapidly destructive to previously normal lung tissue. Tuberculosis is a disease of poverty, overcrowding, and inadequate nutrition associated with substandard public health conditions.

There are 3,000,000 deaths yearly worldwide from tuberculosis, and approximately one-third of the world's population (1.7 billion) are infected with tuberculosis, although only 10% may manifest the disease.[1]

After a steady decline in the incidence of tuberculosis in the United States beginning in 1985, the occurrence of new cases has begun to rise. Currently, there are over 26,000 new cases in the United States each year.[1] Nationally in the first quarter of 1991, 3% of new tuberculosis cases and 6.9% of recurrent cases were found to be multidrug resistant.[1] In some parts of the United States, multidrug resistance is considerably greater, reaching as high as 56%.[2,3] The incidence of multidrug resistance in other parts of the world is variable but may be considerably higher than in the United States. The reasons for the increase in tuberculosis are multifactored. The appearance of acquired immune deficiency syndrome with its immunocompromised host is a major factor. Other factors include immigration patterns, some complacency in the medical community, and an increase in poverty areas with associated overcrowding and poor sanitation. Furthermore, there have been no new drugs introduced that are highly effective in the treatment of tuberculosis during the past 20 years, rifampin being introduced in 1971.

Associated with the increase in tuberculosis has been a rise in pulmonary infection due to mycobacteria other than tuberculosis (MOTT). Some of this increase may be due to better recognition and diagnosis, but there appears to also be an absolute increase in the number of these infections.[4] These MOTT infections are usually more indolent and more often attack previously diseased lung tissue, while tuberculosis is more virulent and can attack healthy tissue. The most significant MOTT infection is by the *Mycobacterium avium* complex (MAC) organisms. Other MOTT organisms include kansasii, chelonae, fortuitum, xenopi, and a number of less common MOTT infections.

## HISTORY OF TREATMENT

The tuberculosis bacillus was isolated by Koch[5] in 1882. Prior to that time in 1850, the sanitorium system was begun in Europe and later in the United States. Treatment consisted of bed rest, improved diet, and fresh mountain air. Results were variable and often took years.

Collapse therapy was started by Folanini[6] in 1895 using artificial pneumothorax. The principle behind collapse therapy was to compress the cavities and prevent oxygen from entering, thus killing the tuberculosis organism, an obligate aerobe. The most common form of collapse therapy utilized was thoracoplasty popularized beginning in the 1930s (Fig. 18–1). Other forms of collapse therapy included plombage with either paraffin or plastic balls, phrenic nerve paralysis, or pneumoperitoneum (Figs. 18–2, 18–3, 18–4).

With the advent of resectional surgery, collapse therapy was abandoned, and, with the introduction of chemotherapy, resectional surgery was gradually replaced. Currently, with the appearance of drug resistance and in certain MOTT infections, resectional surgery is once again being utilized as an adjunct to medical therapy.

## DIAGNOSIS

Classic symptoms of tuberculosis include fever; night sweats; a persistent cold; weight loss; cough; and, in some cases, hemoptysis. A positive skin test may be helpful, but it is only a sign of exposure to the tuberculosis organism at some time and is not synonymous with the active disease. The most commonly used skin test is the purified protein derivative (PPD) injected intradermally. A positive test will produce an indurated erythematous swelling at 48–72 hours. A 5-mm area of induration is considered positive if the individual has been in close contact to patients with infectious tuberculosis or is HIV positive.

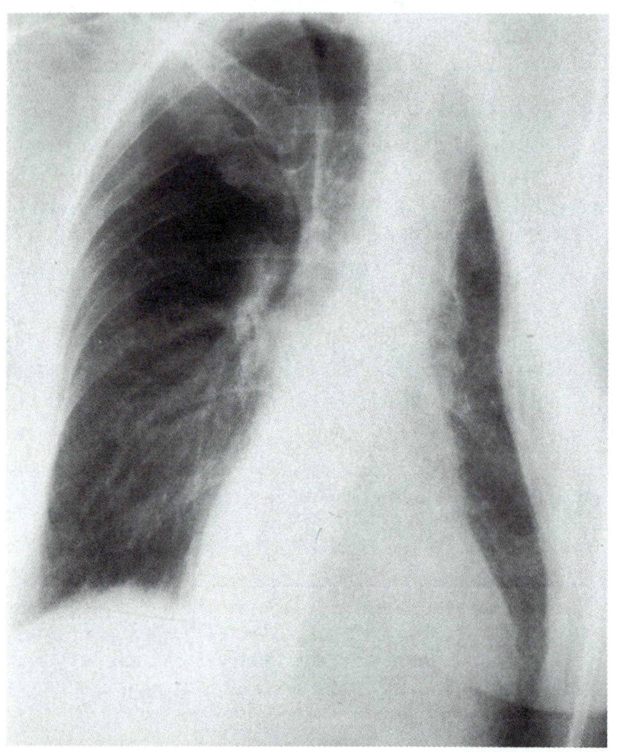

**Figure 18–1.** Total left thoracoplasty for tuberculosis.

A 10-mm indurated area is positive in individuals if they come from high-prevalence countries or poverty areas, are IV drug users, have other medical factors that increase the risk, are in long-term care facilities, or in some cases are health care workers. If there are no risk factors, 15 mm induration is needed to be considered positive.

In patients who are immunocompromised, any new pulmonary infiltrate should be considered to be tuberculosis until this is ruled out.

The definitive diagnosis for tuberculosis is made by smear and culture of the sputum. The finding of acid-fast bacilli on sputum smears could dictate immediate therapy while one awaits specific culture reports regarding sensitivities and typing. Usually, coverage with isoniazid, rifampin, and pyrazinamide is adequate until culture reports are returned.

## TUBERCULOSIS PRESENTATION

Primary tuberculosis is the initial infection with the tuberculosis organism. It is caused by the inhalation of airborne droplets from an infected source. Infection may be totally asymptomatic or present as a febrile illness. The body's defenses usually contain the infection, and the end result will be a Ghon complex consisting of a peripheral lesion and hilar adenopathy.

Miliary tuberculosis is produced by the dissemination of mycobacterium into the bloodstream. Miliary tuberculosis is more commonly found in the older, debilitated patient or in one who is immunocompromised.

Treatment of primary tuberculosis and miliary tuberculosis is with chemotherapy. Surgery is used only when complications develop that require intervention.

Pulmonary tuberculosis that is not contained by the host's defenses may progress rapidly with the destruction of considerable lung tissue. In addition, previously dormant lesions may break down and reactivate as the host loses its cellular mediated immunity either through disease or advancing age. The initial treatment of these patients, as with primary and miliary tuberculosis, is chemotherapy.

## MYCOBACTERIUM OTHER THAN TUBERCULOSIS (MOTT)

The epidemiology of MOTT infections is not as straightforward as with tuberculosis. It is not felt to be transmitted from one person to another. While tuberculosis can infect and destroy normal lung tissue, MOTT infections usually occur in lungs that have sustained prior damage. Often this has been due to tuberculosis but may be secondary to other destructive lung conditions. A specific group of patients have MOTT infections of the middle lobe and/or lingula. In

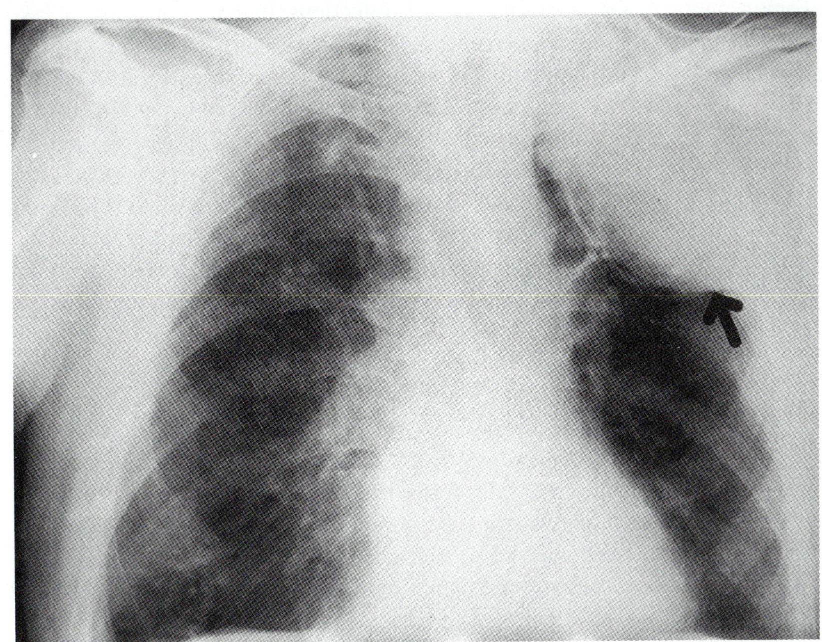

**Figure 18–2.** Collapse therapy using paraffin plombage.

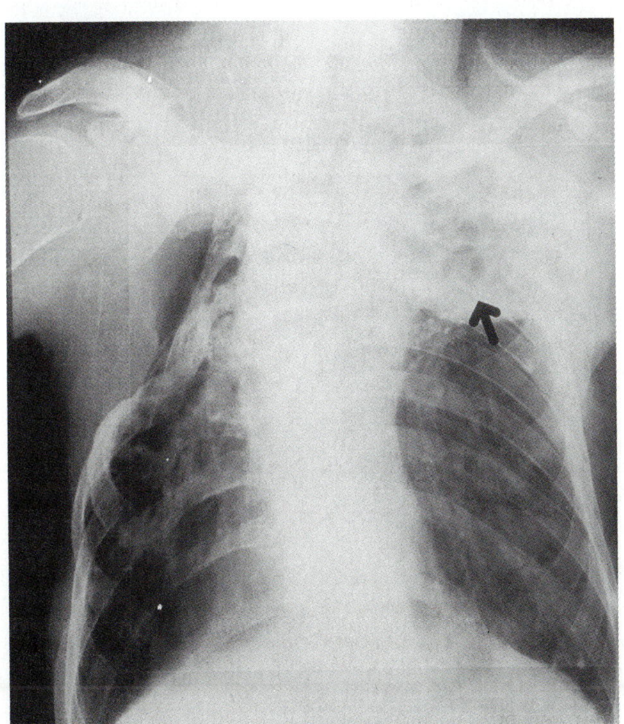

**Figure 18–3.** Collapse therapy using a thoracoplasty on the right and Lucite ball plombage on the left.

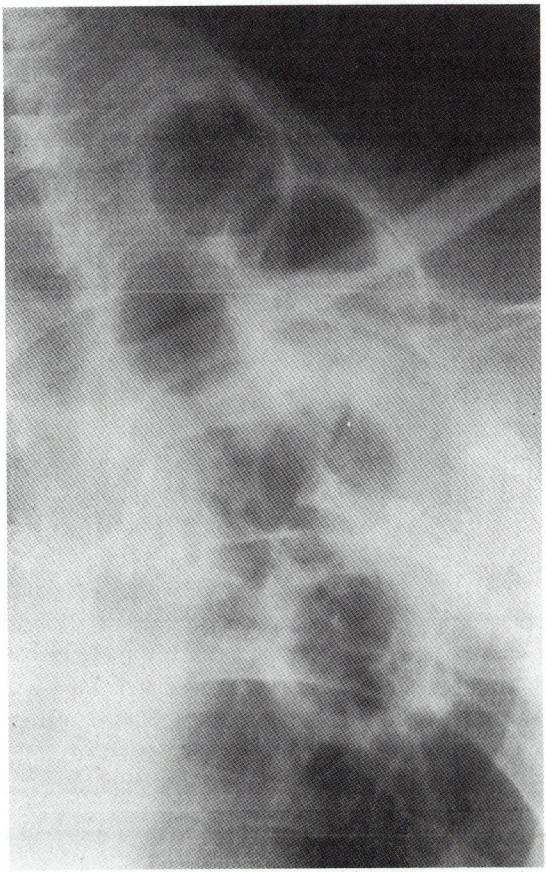

**Figure 18–4.** Close up of Lucite balls with air fluid level from which tuberculosis was cultured.

our experience, these patients have all been women and usually are of slender body habitus. Bronchiectasis is invariably present, and often there are skeletal abnormalities.

## MEDICAL TREATMENT

The initial management of tuberculosis is medical. There are five first-line drugs: isoniazid, rifampin, ethambutol, pyrazinamide, and streptomycin. All have side effects and toxicity that must be monitored. Isoniazid can produce a peripheral neuritis as well as cause hepatitis. Rifampin and pyrazinamide are both hepatotoxic, while ethambutol can cause an optic neuritis. Streptomycin is both ototoxic and toxic to the vestibular apparatus. Second and third line drugs are usually more expensive, less effective, and more toxic. Some of these are kanamycin, capreomycin, ethionamide, cycloserine, para-aminosalycitic acid, ofloxicin, ciprofloxicin, amikacin, and rifabutin.

Treatment should be begun with a minimum of three drugs as soon as the diagnosis is made. The preferred regimen is isoniazid and rifampin for 6 months and pyrazinamide for 2 months. Ethambutol can be added in patients from areas where there is a high incidence of multidrug resistance until specific drug sensitivities can be obtained.

If after 3 months of therapy, the patient still has positive sputum, one should consider that the patient is noncompliant, has multidrug resistant organisms, or that the organism has been misidentified, is a MOTT organism, and the patient has been on inappropriate therapy. Cultures should be repeated and appropriate antibiotic treatment instituted.

## SURGICAL THERAPY

The most common indication for surgery is the development of multidrug resistant tuberculosis in patients with localized disease and adequate pulmonary reserve.[7] These patients often have such poor drug sensitivities that even if the sputum initially becomes negative, the chances of relapse are quite high. With surgical resection in these patients along with continued chemotherapy, the cure rate is over 90%.

Other indications for surgery include bronchopleural fistula, massive hemoptysis (>600 cc/24 h), bronchial stenosis, empyema, and to rule out cancer.

The preoperative workup should include the standard tests done for most pulmonary surgical patients. Particular emphasis is placed on the findings from computed tomography (CT) ventilation perfusion scans and pulmonary function tests. Accurate calculation of the remaining functioning lung following proposed resection is mandatory. When possible, it is advisable to leave an $FEV_1$ of 800–1000 cc. It is also important to resect all the grossly diseased nonfunctioning lung in patients with multidrug resistant tuberculosis or severe MOTT infections if antibiotics are to cure residual microscopic disease invariably left behind.

Attention should be paid preoperatively to nutrition. Many of these patients are catabolic, and hyperalimentation is useful in achieving an anabolic condition at the time of surgery. In patients who are to undergo surgery, decreasing the mycobacterial count is important. This often requires an intensive course of drug specific therapy for 3 months.

In all surgical procedures, double-lumen endobronchial tubes are used. An additional technical point is the use of bronchoscopy. The bronchial anatomy should be visualized prior to thoracotomy. If significant purulent secretions are noted, bronchoscopy should be repeated after completion of the resection to clean out any spilled secretions. Characteristically in MOTT infections of the middle lobe, there is usually a significant amount of purulent white secretions coming from the middle-lobe orifice. These secretions may be spread into the bronchus intermedius during lobectomy and if not removed at the end of the procedure could contaminate the remaining right lung.

Surgery for patients with multidrug resistant tuberculosis includes resection of the maximally diseased portion of the lung. When an entire lung has been destroyed, a pattern of selective left lung destruction has been noted[8] (Fig. 18–5). Operation upon these patients usually requires extrapleural pneumonectomy. Cavitary disease as in the past is another indication for resection in patients with multidrug resistant tuberculosis and localized disease.

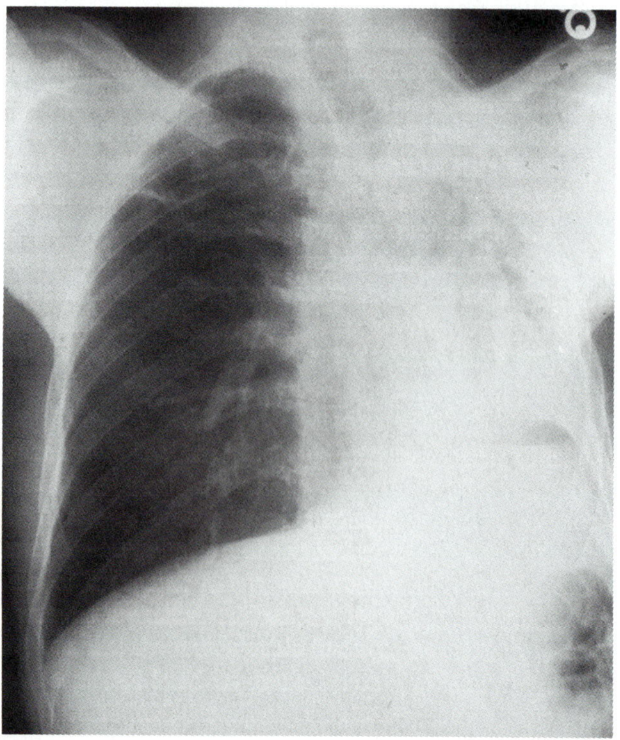

**Figure 18–5.** Destroyed left lung due to multidrug resistant tuberculosis.

Massive hemoptysis may necessitate resectional surgery. The source of hemoptysis may be obvious, but in some cases endoscopy or angiography will be required to localize the site of bleeding.

Local bronchial stenosis occasionally can be treated by resection and end-to-end repair. However, resection of the distal lung is more often necessary.

In patients with tuberculous empyemas, frequent aspiration is preferable to tube drainage, since the latter may convert a pure tuberculous empyema to an infection with mixed flora, which is more difficult to treat. Malignancies can develop in old tuberculous scars, and, when cancer cannot be ruled out, resection is also justified.

Patients with MOTT infections have similar indications for surgery as those who have tuberculosis. MOTT infections are usually more indolent and often are referred later for surgery when extensive parenchymal damage has occurred. The pattern of MOTT infections in the middle lobe and/or lingula (Fig. 18–6) is not seen in patients with tuberculosis. If associated with significant bronchiectasis and/or atelectasis, lobectomy in addition to continued medical therapy is necessary.

To supplement resectional surgery for mycobacterial disease, muscle flaps have been used to buttress prophylactically the bronchial stump and as a space filler rather than to perform a thoracoplasty.[8] Specific indications for the use of a muscle flap include positive sputum at the time of surgery, preexisting bronchopleural fistula, and extensive polymicrobial contamination as well as to fill the space anticipated after some lobectomies. The latissimus dorsi muscle is the muscle most frequently used. The serratus anterior and pectoralis major muscles can also be used. Intercostal muscle in these patients is usually too small to be of much use.

In properly prepared patients, operative mortality should be less than 5%. Complications may be high particularly in the malnourished patient. Bronchopleural fistulas are more common following right pneumonectomy than left pneumonectomy. The combination of a MOTT patient, malnourished with polymicrobial contamination and a destroyed right lung, is particularly susceptible to stump breakdown even if muscle flaps are used. Other complications include wound breakdown particularly in catabolic patients and recurrent nerve injury following extrapleural left pneumonectomy. When one is using muscle flaps for expected space problems after lobectomy, prolonged air leaks are uncommon.

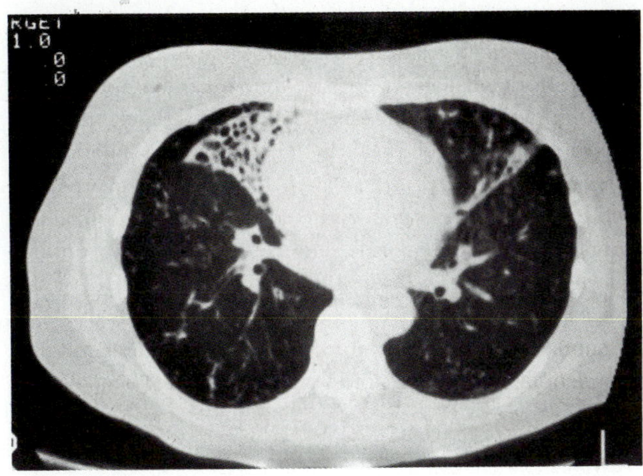

**Figure 18–6.** Bronchiectasis of middle lobe and lingula in a patient infected with myobacterium avium complex (MAC).

In summary, tuberculosis is still a major health hazard causing considerable morbidity and mortality in the world. It has been on the rise in the United States since 1985. Resistant organisms present a particularly difficult treatment situation. MOTT infections are also increasing. While not a contagious problem, they represent a considerable health problem to those infected. Surgery has played an important role in the evolution of treatment for mycobacterial pulmonary disease. Once again, surgery in specific cases should be used along with continued medical therapy.

## REFERENCES


1. Turett GS, Telzak EE, Gold JWM: Strategies to manage resurgent TB. *Int Med* **15:**50, 1994
2. Goble M, Iseman M, Madsen LA, et al: Treatment of 171 patients with pulmonary tuberculosis resistant to Isoniazid and Rifampin. *New Engl J Med* **328:**527, 1993
3. Neville K, Bromberg A, Bromberg R, et al: The third epidemic—multidrug resistant tuberculosis. *Chest* **105:**45, 1994
4. Iseman M: *Nontuberculosis Mycobacterial Infections: Infectious Diseases.* Philadelphia, Saunders, 1992, pp 1246–1256
5. Koch R: Die Aetiologie der Tuberkulose. *Berl Klin Wschr* **19:**221, 1882 (trans: *Med Classics* **821,** 1938)
6. Folanini C: As cited by Alexander J: *The Collapse Therapy of Pulmonary Tuberculosis.* Springfield, Illinois, Charles C. Thomas, 1937
7. Pomerantz M: Surgery for tuberculosis. In Pomerantz M (ed): *Chest Surgery Clinics of North America.* Philadelphia, WB Saunders, 1993, pp 723–727
8. Pomerantz M, Madsen L, Goble M, Iseman M: Surgical management of resistant mycobacterial tuberculosis and other mycobacterial pulmonary infections. *Ann Thorac Surg* **52:**1108, 1991

CHAPTER

# 19

# Molecular Biology and Immunology of Lung and Esophageal Cancer

David S. Schrump and Jack A. Roth

## INTRODUCTION

Tobacco consumption is believed to be responsible for >90% of lung cancers in men and approximately 80% of such neoplasms in women.[1] Presently the relative risk of lung cancer in smokers exceeds 20 for men and 10 for women compared with nonsmokers, and is proportional to the cumulative amount of tobacco exposure.[2] Tobacco consumption has also been implicated in the pathogenesis of esophageal squamous cell carcinomas, interacting in a synergistic or additive manner with ethanol consumption and cultural dietary practices, respectively, in high-incidence areas throughout Asia, South Africa, South America, and western Europe.[3] However, the fact that only a minority of smokers develop lung or esophageal cancer implies that additional genetic or environmental factors contribute to the pathogenesis of these neoplasms.

Epidemiologic studies have demonstrated a familial risk of lung cancer and suggest that the development of this disease at an early age (<50 years) is related to mendelian inheritance of a rare autosomal codominant allele, although this phenomenon has been observed less frequently in more typical elderly patients.[4,5] Mendelian inheritance of an autosomal recessive allele may predispose some individuals to the development of squamous cell esophageal cancer in high-risk areas in Asia.[6] Currently, a major focus of molecular epidemiology research involves the elucidation of genetic markers associated with lung and esophageal cancers that might be utilized to identify individuals who are at high risk of developing these neoplasms.[7]

In the United States, the incidence of esophageal adenocarcinoma has risen faster than any other malignancy in recent years[3,8] and presently represents the major histologic type of esophageal cancer observed in several institutions. In contrast to squamous cell cancers, esophageal adenocarcinomas tend to occur in relatively young male patients with no significant history of cigarette or ethanol abuse. Chronic gastroesophageal reflux, hiatal hernia, and Barrett's esophagus have been cited as predisposing to esophageal adenocarcinoma[3,9]; however, the precise etiology of this malignancy and the epidemiologic variables responsible for its dramatically increasing incidence remain obscure.

Barrett's esophagus, particularly the specialized subtype, increases the risk of developing esophageal cancer 40-fold, although the rate of malignant transformation still may be quite low (estimated to be approximately 1:100–1:440 patient years).[10,11] Flow cytometric analysis has documented increasingly severe genomic instability and aneuploidy correlating with progression to invasive carcinoma in Barrett's epithelia.[12] In some cases genomic instability antecedes histologic alterations observed in standard biopsy specimens.

Appreciation of the molecular events associated with carcinogenesis in the aerodigestive tract may improve the diagnosis and clinical management of patients with advanced disease and may provide an experimental foundation upon which to base preventative interventions in high-risk individuals. This chapter will emphasize aspects of the molecular biology of lung and esophageal cancers that may be of clinical significance in the near future.

## CELL CYCLE

Cell proliferation normally proceeds through finely orchestrated phases, thus ensuring fidelity of deoxyribonucleic acid (DNA) replication[13,14] (Fig. 19–1). Growth factor stimulation induces the movement of quiescent (GO phase) cells into G1, thereby activating genes encoding regulatory proteins involved in DNA synthesis. Following DNA replication in S phase, cells proceed into G2, during which the mitotic spindle apparatus is constructed, and ultimately progress into M phase, whereby cell division occurs. Check points at the G1/S and G2/M transitions normally prevent replication of damaged DNA and improper chromosomal segregation, respectively.

The individual phases of the cell cycle are characterized by the appearance of discrete types of enzymes referred to as cyclins,[15] which associate with their respective cyclin-dependent kinases[16] to activate multiple regulatory proteins involved in cell proliferation. Cyclins A and B are involved in regulating progression through the S and G2 phases of the cell cycle. During G1, D type cyclins appear to function as growth factor sensors for the cell cycle machinery, whereas cyclin E accumulation coincides with G1/S transition; thus, D- and E-type cyclins appear to be critical regulators of G1 to S phase progression in normal cells.[13] Perturbation of cell cycle integrity via alterations in cyclin levels or disruption of physiologic check points (due to mutations involving oncogenes or tumor suppressor genes) induces genomic instability, DNA amplification, and malignant transformation.[17,18]

## DOMINANT AND RECESSIVE ONCOGENES

Mutations associated with carcinogenesis may occur in dominant or recessive (tumor suppressor) genes. Dominant oncogenes are genes in which mutation in one allele results in constitutive growth stimulation. Myc, ras, and a variety of growth factor receptor genes are dominant oncogenes, some of which can directly transform cells in tissue culture. In contrast, tumor suppressor genes tend to control cell proliferation; loss of both alleles by mutation or chromosomal deletion is necessary to abrogate the growth inhibitory effects of these genes. In general mutant tumor suppressor genes are incapable of inducing cell transformation, although they may facilitate transformation by dominant oncogenes.

## GROWTH FACTORS AND GROWTH FACTOR RECEPTORS

Lung and esophageal cancers have been associated with abnormal expression of a variety of growth factors and growth factor receptors that may be relevant to the biology and treatment of these neoplasms (Table 19–1). Constitutive stimulation of a growth factor receptor by abnormal expression of the receptor ligand or by mutation of the receptor molecule may cause it to function as a dominant oncogene. Growth factors secreted by tumor cells may influence distant cells (endocrine stimulation) or adjacent cells (paracrine stimulation), or they may stimulate proliferation of the cell from which they have been secreted by autocrine mechanisms. Cells that replicate independent of growth factor support are termed *acrine*.

### Gastrin-Releasing Peptide

Gastrin-releasing peptide (GRP) is a 27-amino acid homolog of an amphibian hormone referred to as bombesin, which has been found in neural, bronchial endocrine, and fetal lung tissues.[19,20] High-affinity GRP receptors are present on small-cell but are absent on non–small cell lung cancer cells.[21,22] Classic, but not variant small cell lung cancer lines, secrete GRP, which is mitogenic for small cell lung cancers as well as normal human bronchial epithelial cells.[23] In vitro proliferation and tumorigenicity of small-cell lung cancer can be inhibited by antibombesin monoclonal antibodies or by pharmacologic antagonists of bombesin, thereby implicating GRP in autocrine mediated growth of small cell lung cancer.[24]

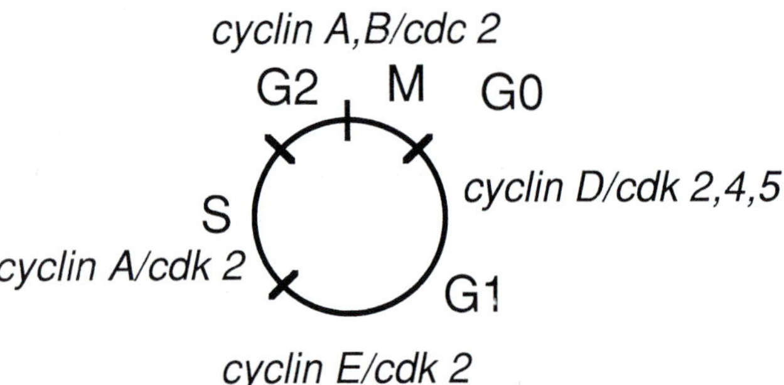


**Figure 19–1.** Eukaryotic cell cycle.

**TABLE 19–1. GROWTH FACTORS, ONCOGENES, AND TUMOR SUPPRESSOR GENES ASSOCIATED WITH LUNG AND ESOPHAGEAL CANCERS**

| Growth Factors | Oncogenes | Tumor Suppressor Genes |
|---|---|---|
| GRP | myc | 3p |
| TGF-α | ras | Rb |
| PDGF | EGFr | p53 |
| IGF | ErbB2 | APC/MCC |
| | Cyclin D | DCC |
| | | p16 |

## Epidermal Growth Factor Receptor

The epidermal growth factor receptor (EGFr) is a 170-kd tyrosine kinase glycoprotein consisting of extracellular, transmembrane, and intracellular domains.[25] Activation of the EGFr by ligand binding results in receptor dimerization, auto-phosphorylation, and subsequent activation of early response genes leading to cell proliferation.[26] Overexpression of normal EGFr is sufficient to transform NIH 3T3 cells.[27]

Aberrant EGFr expression resulting from gene amplification or overexpression of a normal or mutant epidermal growth factor receptor gene product has been observed in cell lines or specimens derived from primary lung and esophageal cancers.[28–30] Approximately 45% of lung cancers overexpress EGFr, and whereas no EGF has been detected in normal or cancerous lung tissues, approximately 60% of tumors express TGF alpha.[31] This substance is structurally similar to EGF and functions as a ligand for cell surface as well as intracellular autocrine stimulation of the EGFr.[32] EGFr overexpression has been observed in adenocarcinomas as well as squamous cell cancers, and recent studies have revealed a statistically significant association between EGFr overexpression and diminished survival in non–small cell lung cancer patients.[33,34]

Although less extensively analyzed, EGFr overexpression has been identified in approximately 80% of esophageal squamous cell cancers and a minority of esophageal adenocarcinomas.[30,35] Expression of TGF alpha has been observed in the majority of squamous cell esophageal cancer lines that have been studied thus far.[36] EGF receptor overexpression independent of pathologic staging criteria adversely affects survival in a statistically significant fashion in patients with squamous cell esophageal cancers.[37,38]

## ErbB2/Neu

The erbB2/neu gene encodes a 185-kd transmembrane tyrosine kinase receptor molecule structurally related to the epidermal growth factor receptor that is present on normal ciliated epithelium, mucous cells, and type II pneumocytes of the adult lung.[39] It does not appear to be expressed in adult esophageal mucosa. Small polypeptides designated heregulins are the naturally occurring ligands for p185, stimulating proliferation of some but not all cells containing this receptor molecule[40]; overexpression of erbB2 can induce transformation of NIH 3T3 cells.[41]

Overexpression of erbB2 has been reported in squamous cell cancers and adenocarcinomas of the lung as well as esophageal adenocarcinomas, although the precise mechanisms responsible for this overexpression are unclear; gene amplification appears to be involved in only a small percentage of cancers.[42] Increased immunoreactivity indicative of p185 overexpression has been detected in approximately 40% of pulmonary adenocarcinomas and squamous cell cancers, as well as 60% of esophageal adenocarcinomas.[35,43] Interestingly, p185 expression has been observed in Barrett's epithelia, thereby suggesting that p185 may contribute to malignant transformation is esophageal tissues.[35] Multivariate analysis has revealed that p185 expression is associated with reduced survival independent of tumor stage for pulmonary adenocarcinomas but not squamous cell cancers[43]; the prognostic significance of p185 expression in esophageal cancers has not been ascertained. Recent observations that erbB2 expression correlates with in vitro drug resistance[44] substantiate the biologic and clinical relevance of erbB2 in non–small-cell lung and esophageal cancers.

## Platelet-derived and Insulin-like Growth Factors and Their Respective Receptors

The interactions of platelet-derived growth factor receptor (PDGFr) and insulin-like growth factor receptor (IGFr) with their respective ligands are critical determinants of cell cycle progression in mammalian cells.[14] PDGFr occurs either as a homodimer or a heterodimer of two structurally related proteins (alpha and beta), whereas the platelet-derived growth factor ligand may exist as a homo- or heterodimer of A and B chains that determine the specificity and affinity of receptor–ligand binding. Platelet-derived growth factor induces receptor dimerization and mitogenic stimulation of a variety of cell types.[45]

Several studies have documented expression PDGF, PDGFr, or both in lung and esophageal cancer lines,[46,47] and significantly elevated levels of PDGF have been detected in metastatic pleural effusions associated with adeno but not squamous cell lung cancers.[48] Normal pulmonary epithelial cells do not express PDGF ligand or receptor transcripts, whereas lung cancer cells express PDGF as well as PDGF receptors.[49] PDGF and PDGF receptor expression can be induced in epithelial tissues by trauma[50]; conceivably, expression of these molecules could be induced in bronchial epithelia by noxious stimuli, thereby resulting in autocrine stimulation of preneoplastic and cancerous lung tissues. A similar autocrine growth mechanism may also be relevant with respect to esophageal carcinogenesis, although this has not been evaluated.

Insulin growth factors I and II are structurally similar to proinsulin, and function in growth and metabolism of a variety of tissues.[51] The IGF-I receptor is similar to the insulin receptor, and mitogenic activities of IGF-I, IGF-II, and insulin in cancers occur via these receptors.[52] Activation of the IGF-I receptor by its ligand appears to be a crucial initiator of cell cycle progression in quiescent cells, and constitutive expression of IGF-I receptor and IGF-I ligand negates requirements for exogenous growth factor support in tissue culture.[53] Insulin growth factor ligands and receptors have been identified in lung and esophageal cancer lines,[54,55] and enhanced expression of these molecules in lung cancers relative to normal lung tissues has been observed.[56] Furthermore, IGF-I, IGF-II, or insulin-stimulated mitogenesis in lung or esophageal cancer lines can be competitively inhibited by monoclonal antibodies directed against IGF-I receptors or ligands, thereby establishing the role of these molecules in autocrine mediated growth of these cancer cells.[54,55]

## CYCLIN D

Several genes mapping to 11q13 are known to be amplified or overexpressed in lung and esophageal cancers. The HST-1 and INT-2 genes, encoding acidic fibroblast growth factors and heparin binding growth factors, respectively, are co-amplified in a small percentage of lung cancers and approximately 50% of esophageal squamous cancers[57]; however, expression of these genes has not been observed, therefore suggesting that additional genes present within the 11q13 region are involved in lung and esophageal carcinogenesis.

The cyclin D (prad-1) gene appears to be amplified but not expressed in approximately 10% of large cell and squamous cell lung cancers.[58] In contrast, amplification and overexpression of the cyclin D gene has been observed in approximately 32% of squamous cell esophageal cancers.[59] Cyclin D and its associated cyclin-dependent kinase (cdk-4) phosphorylate thus inactivate the Rb protein,[60,61] thereby releasing G1 constraints enabling progression through the G1/S cell cycle check point (Fig. 19–2). Overexpression of cyclin D disrupts G1 cell cycle kinetics, resulting in premature G1/S transition, replication of damaged DNA, and malignant transformation in preneoplastic tissues.[62]

## RAS

The H, K and N-ras genes are members of an evolutionarily conserved super-gene family encoding 21-kd proteins that are localized to the inner plasma membrane and play a pivotal role in signal transduction from cell surface receptors to early-response genes involved in mitogen-induced proliferation.[63] Ras proteins exhibit GTP-binding and intrinsic GTPase activities. Inactive ras binds GDP; activation of ras involves GTP-GDP exchange, and conformational alterations with subsequent activation of downstream effector molecules.[64,65] Intrinsic GTPase activity then hydrolyzes GTP to GDP, thereby restoring ras to its inactive conformation. Ras activation is normally tightly regulated by positive and negative control mechanisms. Mutations involving ras stabilize the activated conformation, resulting in unabated growth stimulation.[66]

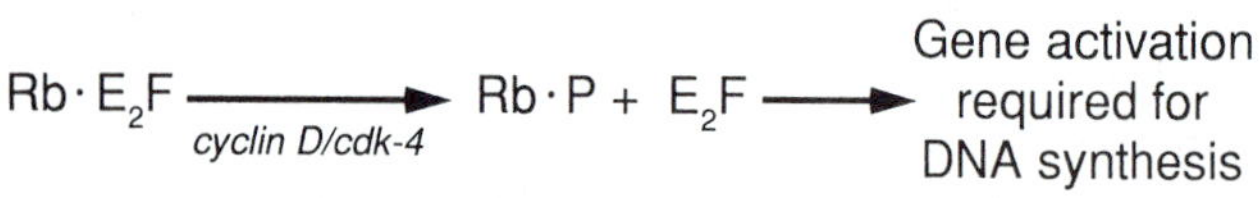

Ras mutations are among the most common oncogene defects recorded in human cancers, and individual ras genes appear to be preferentially activated in tumors of different histologic types.[67] Essentially all relevant mutations occur in codons 12, 13, and 61 of these genes. As a dominant oncogene, mutation in one ras allele is sufficient to induce transformation of mammalian cells either alone or in concert with additional activated oncogenes; vH-ras can transform normal human bronchial epithelial cells in culture.[68]

Ras mutations do not occur in esophageal or small-cell lung cancers and have been observed only sporadically in squamous, adeno-squamous, or large-cell lung cancers. However, K-ras mutations are relatively common in pulmonary adenocarcinomas, particularly in those patients with tobacco exposure. A recent comprehensive analysis[69] revealed that 30% of adenocarcinomas from patients who smoked had K-ras mutations, the majority of which were G → T transversions involving codon 12; benzo-a-pyrene contained in cigarette smoke is known to induce such mutations. In contrast only 5% of adenocarcinomas from nonsmokers had K-ras mutations. Additional investigations have confirmed these observations, demonstrating statistically significant associations between pulmonary adenocarcinomas and K-ras mutations, and smoking and K-ras mutations.[70] Although no correlation between K-ras mutations and clinical stage has been observed, patients with tumors containing these mutations have significantly reduced overall survival relative to similarly staged patients with adenocarcinomas containing wild-type K-ras alleles.[69]

Ras proteins are synthesized as cytosolic precursors that become localized to the inner-plasma membrane following farnesylation of the carboxy terminus in a reaction that is catalyzed by farnesyl protein transferase (FPTase). Farnesylation is critical for membrane localization, which is essential for normal as well as mutant ras function. Pharmacologic reagents that inhibit farnesylation can selectively suppress the growth and malignant phenotype of ras-transformed cells,[71,72] and in all likelihood further investigation will identify agents that will be applicable to the clinical management of lung as well as other cancers containing ras mutations.

Rb · $E_2F$ —(cyclin D/cdk-4)→ Rb · P + $E_2F$ → Gene activation required for DNA synthesis

**Figure 19–2.** Cell cycle regulation by Rb, cyclin D, and CDK-4.

## Myc

The myc gene family consists of three closely related genes (C, L, N) that are differentially expressed during mammalian development and human carcinogenesis.[73] These genes encode DNA transcription factors that are critical for initiating movement of quiescent (G0) cells into and through the G1 phase of the cell cycle; activation of myc appears to be sufficient to initiate DNA synthesis.[74] Reduction of C myc correlates with terminal differentiation in a variety of cells lines, and enforced expression of myc can prevent differentiation in these cells.[75]

Myc expression is predominately deregulated by gene amplification; however, more subtle disturbances in transcriptional control may also be relevant; as such, messenger RNA levels may not necessarily correlate with gene amplification.[76] Whereas no interchromosomal recombinations involving myc genes have been observed in lung cancers, complex intrachromosomal rearrangements have been shown to deregulate L-myc, preceding DNA amplification in those tumors overexpressing this gene.[77]

Although occasionally observed in non–small-cell lung and esophageal cancers, aberrant myc expression has been documented primarily in specimens or cell lines derived from small-cell lung cancers. Initial studies detected amplification of C-myc in 7 of 13 small-cell lung cancer lines, 5 of which were small-cell lung cancer variant cell lines,[78] whereas L- or N-myc overexpression was detected in approximately 20% of classic small-cell lung cancer lines.[79,80] Subsequent studies have determined that different myc genes are not co-expressed within a given tumor, and rather than correlating with histologic subtype per se, myc gene overexpression appears associated with exposure to chemotherapy. Comprehensive analysis revealed myc amplification in approximately 10% of cell lines or specimens obtained from patients prior to chemotherapy compared with 33% of cell lines or tumors obtained from patients subsequent of treatment[81]; myc amplification tended to occur more frequently in those patients receiving cyclophosphamide based regimens as opposed to etoposide-cisplatin therapy. Whereas those patients with c-myc amplification have statistically significant reduction in overall survival relative to those patients without such amplification, no prognostic value has been ascribed to L- or N-myc abnormalities in small-cell lung cancer.[80,81]

Although the precise mechanisms remain obscure, available data suggest that myc amplification occurs relatively late in the course of carcinogenesis, enhancing tumor progression and metastasis.[82] Because myc expression is regulated by a variety of growth factors and tumor suppressor genes,[83] multiple mechanisms exist by which mutations involving oncogenes or tumor suppressor genes may deregulate myc expression, thereby conferring upon the malignant cell a more aggressive, metastatic phenotype.

## TUMOR SUPPRESSOR GENES

### 3p

Cytogenetic analysis has confirmed that lung and esophageal cancers are associated with multiple genetic alterations. The majority of these neoplasms are aneuploid with complex karyotypes; however, nonrandom chromosomal abnormalities have been observed in primary lung cancer specimens, irradiated bronchial epithelial cells, and esophageal cancer cells, suggesting that these events are causally related to carcinogenesis. In addition to trisomy seven, commonly detected abnormalities in these neoplasms include 1p, 3p, 5q, 7q, 9p, 11q, 11p, 13q, and 17p.[84–86]

Deletions involving 3p have been detected in nearly 100% of small-cell lung cancers, greater than 50% of non–small-cell lung carcinomas, and approximately 70% of esophageal cancers. Whereas the region of deletion in non–small-cell lung cancers appears to be 3p21, deletions in small-cell lung cancers have been observed in 3p14-cen, 3p21.3, and 3p25[85,87]; 3p deletions in esophageal cancers involve long chromosomal segments commencing at or proximal to p14.[86] Intensive effects are underway to isolate putative tumor suppressor genes on 3p that are believed to be mutated or deleted early in the course of malignant transformation in a variety of epithelial tissues.

### Rb

The Rb gene is located on 13q14 and encodes a 105-kd nuclear phosphoprotein that is intimately involved in regulation of the G1/S cell cycle check point.[88,89] The Rb protein has complex interactions with a variety of regulatory proteins including cyclin-dependent kinases, transcription factors, and cellular as well as viral oncoproteins.[90–92] The association of Rb with the transcription factor E2F inhibits transcription of genes required for S phase; phosphorylation of Rb by cyclin D/cdk4 or binding of Rb to viral oncoproteins dissociates the Rb/E2F complex, thus permitting E2F-mediated gene transcription and cell cycle progression in normal as well as virally infected cells (Fig. 19–2). Loss of Rb protein expression disrupts the normal regulatory mechanisms governing the G1/S cell cycle checkpoint, thus facilitating premature DNA replication and malignant transformation; restoration of Rb expression via gene transfer techniques diminishes the proliferation and tumorigenicity of cancer cells bearing these mutations.[93]

The mechanisms of acquired Rb gene inactivation in lung and esophageal cancers are complex, often involving subtle point mutations or deletions that are manifested by an inability of the cell to synthesize an intact Rb protein. Approximately 90% of small-cell lung carcinomas lack Rb protein expression, and a similar phenomenon has been observed in approximately 20%, 40%, and 60% of adeno, squamous, and large-cell lung cancers, respectively.[94,95]

Although insufficient data exist regarding Rb inactivation in Barrett's epithelia, Rb mutations have been observed in 30–40% of adeno and squamous cell esophageal cancers.[59,96] Interestingly, although investigation has been limited, esophageal cancers with Rb mutations appear to have normal cyclin D levels, whereas those tumors with cyclin D amplification have normal Rb gene function,[59] therefore suggesting that abrogation of Rb-mediated G1/S checkpoint control may occur via several mechanisms with similar consequences with regard to esophageal carcinogenesis. Presently no significant correlation between Rb inactivation and clinical outcome in patients with lung and esophageal cancers has been reported; thus, the clinical implications of Rb mutations in these neoplasms await further investigation.

## p53

The p53 gene encodes a 53-Kd nuclear phosphoprotein that regulates G1/S cell cycle progression in normal and malignant cells via multiple complex mechanisms involving sequence specific DNA binding, transcriptional activation and repression activities, and protein interactions, some of which affect expression of other oncoproteins.[97–99] DNA damage from a variety of physical or chemical agents induces p53 expression (Fig. 19–3). A nonspecific DNA binding domain in the carboxyterminal region of p53 interacts with single-strand DNA; depending upon the extent of DNA damage, a sequence-specific DNA binding site in the central region of p53 mediates either G1 arrest and activation of DNA repair mechanisms, or commits the cell to an apoptotic (programmed cell death) pathway.[100,101] Although a detailed discussion of this issue is beyond the scope of this text, determination of the molecular mechanisms by which p53 regulates G1 arrest and apoptosis in normal and transformed cells may have profound implications with regard to future pharmacologic interventions in a variety of malignant and preneoplastic conditions.

The majority of p53 mutations identified to date are base substitutions occurring at evolutionarily conserved residues that disrupt the sequence-specific DNA binding region; however, mutations outside these areas have been noted with relative frequency in lung cancer specimens.[102,103] A significant number of p53 mutations in non–small-cell lung cancers involve G:C → T:A transversions; benzo (a) pyrene contained in cigarette smoke can induce such mutations. In comparison, G:C → A:T transitions are relatively common in small-cell lung cancers. In contrast to lung cancers, transversions occurring at G:C and A:T pairs occur with equal frequencies in esophageal cancers, and many of these mutations are chain-terminating events.[102] Transitions at CpC dinucleotides, believed to be indicative of spontaneous mutations, have been observed in 10% and 31% of non–small-cell and small-cell lung cancers, respectively, and in 20% of esophageal cancers. In all likelihood, the specific nature of p53 mutations in lung and esophageal cancers reflects carcinogen exposure and may be relevant concerning the pathogenesis of these diseases.

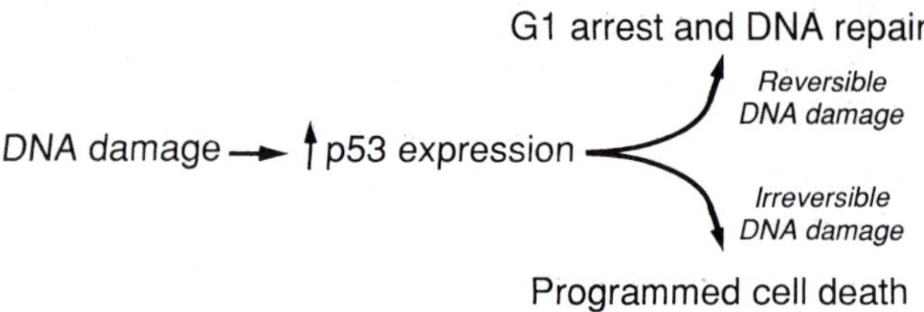


**Figure 19–3.** Cell cycle regulation by p53.

Nucleic acid sequence analyses, as well as immunohistochemical studies of protein expression* have revealed that approximately 70% of small-cell and 50% of non–small-cell lung cancers contain p53 mutations.[103,104] Similar analyses have revealed p53 mutations in 50% of esophageal squamous cell cancers and 40% of esophageal adenocarcinomas.[96,105] Although not associated with disease extent or survival in patients with small-cell lung cancer,[106] and its prognostic significance in esophageal cancers is not known, aberrant p53 expression appears to correlate with nodal metastases and reduced survival in patients with non–small-cell lung cancer.[107,108] Analysis of non–small-cell lung cancers using nucleic acid and immunohistochemical techniques revealed that 0 of 13 tumors negative for p53 mutations by both methods were metastatic, whereas 17 of 17 metastatic tumors had p53 mutations.[107] A large retrospective study of stage I and stage II non–small-cell lung cancer cases utilizing immunohistochemistry techniques identified abnormal p53 expression in 40% of adeno and squamous cell cancers. p53 expression correlated significantly with reduced patient survival irrespective of pathologic stage. Furthermore, seven stage II patients had negligible p53 immunoreactivity in their primary tumors but had abnormal p53 expression in metastatic lymph nodes; these patients had a mean survival time of 11 months compared with 34 months for stage II patients whose tumors and lymph nodes had normal p53 expression.[108] These data have been confirmed by other investigators who have observed that p53 mutations in primary non–small-cell lung cancer as determined by biochemical analysis correlated significantly with reduced patient survival independent of pathologic stage.[109]

Several studies have demonstrated the presence of p53 mutations in preneoplastic lung tissues, thereby suggesting that these mutations occur relatively early in the course of bronchial neoplasia.[110,111] In addition, aberrant p53 expression has been observed in histologically normal epithelium adjacent to squamous cell esophageal cancers,[112] and 5% of Barrett's epithelia without dysplasia, 15% of Barrett's epithelia with low-grade dysplasia, 45% of Barrett's epithelia with high-grade dysplasia, and 53% of Barrett's adenocarcinomas,[113] therefore indicating that p53 mutations are early events with respect to malignant transformation in esophageal tissues. However, additional investigations involving lung cancer specimens have suggested that p53 mutations may also occur late in the clinical course of this disease.[108] In all likelihood, mutations involving p53 facilitate

*Mutations tend to stabilize and prolong the half-life of the p53 protein. As such, p53 mutations can be evidenced in tissue sections by quantitatively enhanced reactivity with monoclonal antibodies recognizing both wild-type and mutant proteins, or they may be detected by monoclonal antibodies recognizing epitopes contained only on mutant proteins.

additional destabilizing genetic events that culminate in malignant transformation of preneoplastic cells,[18] whereas p53 mutations occurring in the context of an established malignancy may act as progression factors, thereby enhancing metastatic potential. In this regard p53 mutations may profoundly influence the clinical course of lung and esophageal cancers regardless of the timing of such events in these conditions.

## APC/MCC and DCC

APC and MCC are two closely linked genes on 5q21 encoding proteins involved in signal transduction that are deleted or mutated in familial as well as sporadic colon cancers.[114,115] An additional locus-designated DCC encoding a cell surface adhesion molecule is present on 18q21 and is also frequently mutated in colon cancers.[116] Although not extensively analyzed, mutations involving APC/MCC loci have been observed in approximately 80% of small-cell lung carcinomas, 40% of non–small-cell lung carcinomas, and 65% of esophageal cancers[117–119]; abnormal DCC gene sequences have been detected in 25% of esophageal cancer specimens.[119] Clonal analysis of Barrett's epithelia and Barrett's carcinomas suggests that p53 mutations precede those involving loci at 5q.[120] The precise roles of these tumor suppressor genes in the pathogenesis of lung and esophageal cancers are unclear at present.

## p16

p16 is a 16-kd protein encoded on 9p21 that acts to sequester cdk4, inhibiting formation of the cyclin D/cdk4 complex, thus preventing Rb phosphorylation and cell cycle progression. Recently, mutations involving p16 loci have been detected in nearly 50% of cancer cell lines derived from a variety of tissues, including 25% of lung cancers.[121,122] Although analysis has been limited, initial data suggest that the incidence of p16 mutations may exceed that of p53 abnormalities in human cancers, and they demonstrate the critical relationship between cell cycle integrity, tumor suppressor genes, and malignant transformation.

## Conclusion

Whereas our appreciation of the complexities of the molecular events in lung and esophageal cancer is fragmentary, current approaches to the clinical management of these neoplasms can be refined based on available information. For instance, the identification of particular molecular genetic defects such as C-myc amplification in primary small-cell lung cancer, or abnormal expression of ras, EGFr, p185, or p53 in non–small-cell lung or esophageal cancers may identify patients at high risk of failing conventional treatments who should be considered for aggressive investigational protocols. Furthermore, the specific targeting of growth factor receptors such as GRP in small-cell lung cancer, or EGFr and p185 in non–small-cell lung and esophageal cancers may enhance the specificity of cytostatic or cytocidal agents in the management with these neoplasms.[123] Without question, much work is still needed to define the relevance of individual genetic aberrations in premalignant lesions so as to identify individuals at high risk of developing invasive cancers who might benefit from preventative interventions.

Although cancer is a multistep process involving separate genetic events, correction of one or perhaps two critical defects may be sufficient to inhibit the relentless proliferation of malignant cells. Targeting of activated oncogenes necessitates inhibition of expression of the mutant genes, whereas correction of tumor suppressor gene defects requires the delivery of wild-type gene sequences to tumor cells.

Dominant oncogene expression can be inhibited using antisense technology. In brief, gene transcription involves messenger ribonucleic acid (RNA) synthesis from a single DNA strand (sense strand); the complementary (antisense) strand is not normally transcribed. Delivery to tumor cells of gene sequences in which this previously inactive strand is transcribed results in the production of complementary messenger RNAs that anneal and are rapidly degraded by ribonuclease enzymes, thus preventing translation of the messenger RNA corresponding to the mutated (activated) oncogene allele.[124]

This strategy has been used to target K-ras mutations in lung cancer. Recent experiments have utilized a replication defective retrovirus (LNSX) to deliver an antisense K-ras gene construct to lung cancer cells bearing K-ras mutations. These experiments revealed that K-ras expression could be specifically inhibited, resulting in an 80–90% inhibition of in vitro proliferation of the transduced cells. Tumorigenicity of transduced lung cancer cells in nude mice was similarly reduced in a statistically significant manner.[125] Additional studies demonstrated that this antisense K-ras construct prevented the outgrowth of lung cancer cells in an orthotopic lung cancer model in nude mice, thereby demonstrating the potential applicability of antisense K-ras constructs in the clinical management of human lung cancers.[126]

Additional studies have focused on the targeting of p53 mutations in lung cancer. Wild-type p53 gene sequences have been delivered to lung cancer cells containing point-mutated, null, or wild-type p53 alleles, via retroviral or adenoviral vectors. Virally delivered p53 significantly inhibited the proliferation and tumorigenicity of cancer cells bearing p53 mutations while having minimal effect on cells with normal p53 gene expression.[127,128]

Recent data also demonstrate that p53 markedly enhances the response of cancer cells to cytotoxic agents presumably via induction of apoptosis in response to DNA damage.[129] Thus, p53 gene therapy may enhance the efficacy of chemotherapeutic regimens currently used in the management of lung and esophageal cancer patients. Conceivably, precise targeting of molecular defects in lung and esophageal cancers via gene therapy may significantly alter the clinical course of patients with advanced thoracic malignancies, as well as those individuals with premalignant lesions who are at high risk of developing these neoplasms.

## IMMUNOLOGY OF LUNG CANCER

Although esophageal cancer frequently presents in debilitated patients, and esophageal cancer cells secrete an immunosuppressive factor,[130] immune function of esophageal cancer patients and immunotherapeutic intervention in these individuals have not been extensively analyzed and, thus, will not be addressed in this chapter. In contrast, a variety of defects involving cellular and humoral immune mechanisms have been observed in lung cancer patients including alterations in lymphocyte counts and populations, disproportionate infiltration of tumors by suppressor T cells, and impaired T- and B-cell responses to recall antigens, suggesting that immune dysfunction contributes to the pathogenesis of this disease.[131,132]

Observations linking bacterial infections (particularly erysipelas) and inflammatory response to tumors dating back to the 1800s suggested that microbial products could induce the resolution of cancer.[133] In 1882, Fehleisen deliberately inoculated cancer patients with viable strep, the causative agent of erysipelas. Subsequently, William Coley developed a vaccine containing heat-killed *Streptococcus pyogenes* and *Serratia marcescens* that produced symptoms of active bacterial infection. This vaccine, known as Coley's toxin, was used in hundreds of cancer patients prior to the modern era of chemo- and radiation therapy.[133,134]

Coley's daughter, Helen Coley Nauts, summarized the reported experience of spontaneous or experimentally induced bacterial infections in cancer patients.[133] Although most recorded cases involved sarcomas, melanomas, or renal cell cancers, several lung cancer patients were described including a 37-year-old male with advanced squamous cell lung cancer who developed a postthoracotomy empyema resulting in complete regression of his cancer.[135]

Anecdotal reports of tumor regression in lung cancer patients following bacterial infections were validated by laboratory evidence of systemic immunopotentiation by microbial cell wall products. Old et al[136] observed that bacillus Calmette-Guérin (BCG) administration enhanced resistance of laboratory animals to challenge with tumor cells. Subsequently, multiple clinical trials were initiated to evaluate the efficacy of nonspecific immunopotentiating agents in lung cancer patients. BCG administered via intrapleural, intradermal, intralesional, or aerosolized routes produced inconsistent results regarding patient survival. Similarly, other nonspecific immunostimulants including levamisole, transfer factor, and interferon did not improve the clinical outcome of lung cancer patients.[137,138] More recently, clinical trials utilizing IL-2–based therapies designed specifically to bolster cellular immune reactivity to established lung cancers have been unsuccessful,[139,140] thus questioning the clinical relevance of immune response to lung cancer.

Initial investigation of immune recognition in lung cancer patients revealed that in vitro reactivity of lymphocytes with autologous tumor cells correlated significantly with overall survival in those patients without metastatic disease at the time of treatment; furthermore, these studies suggested that lung cancers are nearly as immunogenic as melanomas and renal cell carcinomas.[141] More recently Uchida et al[142] evaluated the prognostic significance of in vitro autologous tumor response in 32 stage I and 18 stage II non–small-cell lung cancer patients undergoing curative resection. Peripheral blood lymphocytes were analyzed for autologous tumor-killing (ATK) activity and T-cell recognition of tumor cells, using standard chromium release and proliferation assays, respectively. ATK was observed in 59% of stage I and 44% of stage II patients, which was independent of the histology of the primary cancer. Twenty-three of 27 patients with ATK were alive at 5 years; in contrast, 23 patients without ATK recurred within 18 months and were dead by 42 months. The differences with regard to disease-free interval and overall survival for those patients with and without ATK were statistically significant. A similar phenomenon was observed with respect to those patients with and without response to tumor in the T-cell proliferation assays.

Hollingshead et al[143,144] used tumor cell extracts as adjuvant therapy in surgically resected stage 1 and stage 2 lung cancer patients. Standard delayed-type hypersensitivity (DTH) assays (analogous to TB skin testing) were utilized to isolate several immunogenic proteins preferentially associated with either adeno or squamous cell lung cancers. Subsequent clinical trials revealed that DTH and serologic reactivity to these proteins could be induced in lung cancer patients. Seventy-five percent of patients receiving adjuvant specific immunotherapy survived 5 years compared with only 30% of control patients, with the major survival benefit being observed in stage I patients. A more recent study by Takita et al[145] confirmed a significantly improved survival in lung cancer patients receiving specific immunotherapy. Although somewhat imperfect with regard to experimental design and data analysis, these studies suggest a possible role for adjuvant specific immunotherapy in lung cancer patients, and mandate additional stringently controlled investigation.

Extensive animal data substantiate a role for T cells in tumor immunity,[146] and recently the molecular basis of antigen recognition by T cells has been elucidated.[147] Peptide antigens are normally processed and presented in the context of class 1 or class 2 major histocompatibility complex (MHC) antigens to naive or activated T cells (Fig. 19–4). Optimal antigen presentation necessitates co-stimulation of the CD28 molecule on T cells by the B7 ligand of

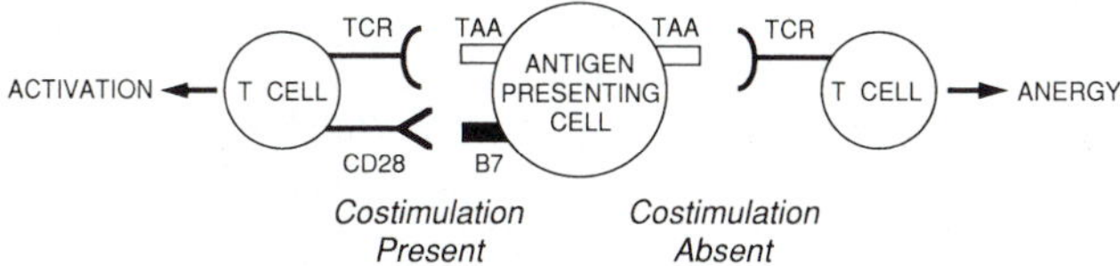


**Figure 19–4.** Mechanisms of T-cell immune response to tumor.

the antigen presenting cells (dendritic cells, macrophages, or activated B cells).[148] In the absence of B7 co-stimulation such as may occur in the context of tumor-associated antigen presented by an epithelial cell that does not normally express B7, T cells fail to proliferate and achieve effector function in response to antigen recognition, resulting in T-cell inactivation or anergy.[149] Immunologic response to tumor-associated antigens is dependent on the dose of these antigens, MHC genotype, and the milieu of cytokines in the tumor microenvironment; and tumor-induced proliferation of suppressor T cells may polarize the immune response, thus specifically inhibiting tumor rejection despite active recognition by the host.[146,147]

It is now evident that multiple mechanisms exist whereby tumors may escape immunologically mediated destruction (Table 19–2). In contrast to virally or chemically induced animal tumors, human epithelial cancers in general are poorly immunogenic, possibly due to the level of carcinogen exposure and the duration of the preclinical phases of these malignancies. Selective loss of MHC expression or modulation of tumor-associated antigens may allow the tumor to "sneak through" immunosurveillance networks. Furthermore, failure of immunogenic tumor-associated antigens to be presented in the proper context with requisite co-stimulatory signals may result in tumor specific anergy or tumor-induced immunosuppression. Eventually, excessive tumor burden may simply overwhelm the capacity of the immune system to contain the cancer.[134,146,150]

The elucidation of the molecular basis of immune recognition including the identification of cytokines involved in tumor immunity, and the availability of reliable gene transfer techniques have ushered in a new era of sophisticated immune intervention in malignant diseases.[147,151] Recent experiments demonstrated that murine lung cancer cells engineered to express IL-2, IL-4, or IL-6 cytokine genes induced potent immunity against nontransfected, normally nonimmunogenic lung cancer cells.[152,153] Vaccination of mice with CMS-5 cells transduced with interferon-gamma, which upregulates MHC expression, resulted in prolonged T-cell immunity against poorly immunogenic parental CMS-5 cells, evidenced by resistance to tumor challenge and specific anti-CMS-5 reactivity in the immunized mice.[154] More recently, Townsend and Allison[155] observed that immunization of mice with B7-transfected melanoma cells protected against challenge with parental cells, therefore demonstrating that B7 was able to provide sufficient co-stimulation to activate cytolytic T cells against melanoma cells that are normally poorly immunogenic.

**TABLE 19–2. POSSIBLE MECHANISMS BY WHICH TUMORS ESCAPE IMMUNOLOGICALLY MEDIATED DESTRUCTION**

1. Poorly immunogenic tumor associated antigens (TAA)
2. Modulation of TAA
3. Loss of MHC expression
4. Lack of costimulation
5. Nonspecific immunosuppression by tumor-related cytokines
6. Excessive tumor burden

T-cell cloning techniques now enable precise biochemical dissection of immune recognition in cancer patients that previously was achieved only via serologic methods.[156,157] Recently, cytolytic T-cell (CTL) clones from melanoma patients identified a protein antigen designated MZ2-E, which is presented in the context of HLA-A1 (class I MHC) molecules.[158,159] MZ2-E is encoded by the human gene MAGE-1 belonging to a family of 12 closely related genes. A second antigen that is encoded by the MAGE-3 gene is also presented on HLA-A1 molecules. Whereas MAGE 1, 2, and 3 genes are not actively transcribed in any normal tissues except testes, 48% of lung cancers express one or more of these three genes (35% of lung cancers express MAGE-1).[160] Since the HLA-A1 allele is expressed in 26% of caucasians, approximately 9% of lung cancers could be expected to express the MZ2-E antigen. Furthermore, additional peptides derived from MAGE-1 can be presented by HLA-C molecules. These exciting data suggest that tumor-associated peptides encoded by MAGE genes exist on the surface of cancer cells that might be exploited for immunotherapy of lung cancer patients.

Intracellular peptides such as ras and p53 are processed and presented at the cell surface, and as such, mutant oncoproteins can be targets for specific immune intervention in lung cancer patients. Jung and Schluesener[161] generated T-cell clones from normal individuals that specifically recognized a synthetic ras peptide corresponding to a codon 12 gly → val mutation, demonstrating the capacity of normal individuals to recognize mutant ras proteins. More recently, Fossum et al[162] isolated a T-cell clone from a patient with colorectal cancer that reacted with a synthetic ras peptide corresponding to a codon 13 gly → asp mutation. This clone did not cross-react with a panel of synthetic peptides corresponding to other mutant or normal ras sequences. Analysis of the primary cancer revealed no ras mutations, suggesting that immunoselection eliminated tumor clones bearing these defects. The fact that no anti-ras reactivity has been observed in 17 patients with pancreatic cancer,[162] the vast majority of which contain ras mutations, implies that the capacity of the tumor-bearing host to recognize mutant ras proteins may influence the cancer phenotype.

Preliminary evaluation of polyclonal sera has revealed that 13% of lung cancer patients have antibodies recognizing both wild-type and mutant p53.[163] Interestingly, many of the p53 mutations in lung cancer specimens cannot be presented by HLA class I molecules, due either to mutations external to HLA binding domains in the p53 molecule, or loss of HLA class one expression by the cancer cells, suggesting selective outgrowth of p53 mutant tumors that escape immunologic surveillance.[164] Much work is needed to evaluate the significance of ras and p53 reactivity in animal models and human cancer patients, and the targeting of mutant oncoproteins in established human cancers and premalignant conditions should be rigorously addressed.

The failure of previous immunotherapy trials in lung cancer patients is related most likely to tumor burden of patients entered into protocols, and an inadequate appreciation of the complexities of immune dysfunction in these individuals. Continued refinement of our understanding of immune response in cancer patients may eventually enable successful immune intervention utilizing gene therapy techniques to deliver physiologically appropriate cytokines or co-stimulatory molecules to tumor sites to facilitate rejection of established tumors.[165,166] Ultimately, immunotherapy in lung cancer patients may prove to be most efficacious in situations involving vaccine prophylaxis for premalignant conditions, or adjuvant therapy for surgically resected patients to promote immune destruction of micrometastases.

## REFERENCES


1. Shopland DR, Eyre HJ, Pechacek TF: Smoking attributable cancer mortality in 1991: Is lung cancer now the leading cause of death among smokers in the United States? *J Natl Cancer Inst* **83:**1142–1148, 1991
2. Osann KE, Anton-Culver LT, Kurosak T, Taylor T: Sex differences in lung cancer risk associated with cigarette smoking. *Int J Cancer* **54:**44–48, 1993
3. Kelsen D, Laufer I, Leichman L, et al: Alarming trends in esophageal cancer. *Patient Care* 72–122, 1992
4. Ooi WL, Elston RC, Chen VW, et al: Increased familial risk for lung cancer. *J Natl Cancer Inst* **76:**217–222, 1986
5. Sellers TA, Bailey-Wilson JE, Elston RC, et al: Evidence for mendelian inheritance in the pathogenesis of lung cancer. *J Natl Cancer Inst* **82:**1272–1279, 1990
6. Carter CL, Hu N, Wu M, et al: Segregation analysis of esophageal cancer in 221 high-risk Chinese families. *J Natl Cancer Inst* **84:**771–776, 1992
7. Amos CI, Caporaso NF, Weston A: Host factors in lung cancer risk: A review of interdisciplinary studies. *CEBP* **1:**505–513, 1992
8. Blot WJ, Devesa SS, Kneller RW, Fraumeni JF Jr: Rising incidence of adenocarcinoma of the esophagus and gastric cardia. *JAMA* **265:**1287–1289, 1991
9. Roth JA, Putnam JB, Lichter AS, Forastiere AA: Cancer of the esophagus. In: Devita V, Hellman JS, Rosenberg S (eds): *Cancer—Principles and Practice of Oncology*, Philadelphia, Lippincott, 1993, pp 776–817
10. Spechler SJ, Goyal RK: Barrett's esophagus. *N Engl J Med* **315:**362–371, 1987
11. Polepalle SC, McCallum RW: Barrett's esophagus. *Gastro Clin North Am*, **19:**733–744, 1990
12. Rabinovitch PS, Reid BJ, Haggitt RC, et al: Progression to cancer in Barrett's esophagus is associated wtih genomic instability. *Lab Invest* **60:**65–71, 1988
13. Marx J: How cells cycle toward center. *Science* **263:**319–321, 1994
14. Baserga R, Rubin R: Cell cycle and growth control. *Crit Rev Eukaryot Gene Exp* **3:**47–61, 1993
15. Sherr CJ: Mammalian G1 cyclins. *Cell* **73:**1059–1065, 1993
16. Nigg EA: Targets of cyclin-dependent protein kinases. *Curr Biol* **5:**187–193, 1993
17. Hartwell L: Defects in a cell cycle checkpoint may be responsible for the genomic instability of cancer cells. *Cell* **71:**543–546, 1992
18. Weinert T, Lydall D: Cell cycle checkpoints, genetic instability and cancer. *Semin Cancer Biol* **4:**129–140, 1993
19. Wharton J, Polak JM, Bloom SR, et al: Bombesin-like immunoreactivity in the lung. *Nature* **273:**769–770, 1978
20. Yamaguchi K, Abe K, Kameya T, et al: Production and molecular size heterogeneity of immunoreactive gastrin-releasing peptide in fetal and adult lungs and primary lung tumors. *Cancer Res* **43:**3932–3939, 1983
21. Moody TW, Bertness V, Carney DN: Bombesin-like peptides and receptors in human tumor cell lines. *Peptides* **4:**683–686, 1983
22. Moody TW, Carney DN, Cuttitta F, et al: High affinity receptors for bombesin/GRP-like peptides on human small-cell lung cancer. *Life Sci* **37:**105–113, 1985
23. Carney DN, Cuttitta F, Moody TW, Minna JD: Selective stimulation of small-cell lung cancer clonal growth by bombesin and gastrin-releasing peptide. *Cancer Res* **47:**821–825, 1987
24. Layton JE, Scanlon DB, Soveny C, Morstyn G: Effects of bombesin antagonists on the growth of small cell lung cancer cells in vitro. *Cancer Res* **48:**4783–4789, 1988
25. Hunter T. The epidermal growth factor gene and its product. *Nature* **311:**414–416, 1984
26. Buday L, Downward J: Epidermal growth factor regulates p21 ras through the formation of a complex of receptor, Grb2 adapter protein, and Sos nucleotide exchange factor. *Cell* **73:**611–620, 1993
27. Reidel H, Massoglia S, Schlessinger J, Ullrich A: Ligand activation of overexpressed epidermal growth factor receptors transforms NIH3T3 mouse fibroblasts. *Proc Natl Acad Sci U S A* **85:**1477–1481, 1988
28. Veale D, Kerr N, Gibson GJ, Harris AL: Characterization of epidermal growth factor receptor in primary human non-small cell lung cancer. *Cancer Res* **49:**1313–1317, 1989
29. Garcia de Palazzo IE, Adams GP, Sundareshan P, et al: Expression of mutated epidermal growth factor receptor by non-small cell lung carcinomas. *Cancer Res* **53:**3217–3220, 1993
30. Lu S-H, Hsieh L-L, Luo F-C, Weinstein IB: Amplification of the EGF receptor and c-myc genes in human esophageal cancers. *Int J Cancer* **52:**502–505, 1988
31. Rusch V, Baselga J, Cordon-Cardo C, et al: Differential expression of the epidermal growth factor receptor and its ligands in primary non-small cell lung cancers and adjacent benign lung. *Cancer Res* **53:**2379–2385, 1993
32. Putnam EA, Yen N, Gallick GE, et al: Heterogeneity of autocrine growth stimulation mechanisms by transforming growth factor-α in human non-small cell lung cancer. *Surg Oncol* **1:**49–60, 1992
33. Veale D, Kerr N, Gibson GJ, et al: The relationship of quantitative epidermal growth factor receptor expression in non-small cell lung cancer to long term survival. *Br J Cancer* **68:**162–165, 1993
34. Volm M, Drings P, Wodrich W: Prognostic significance of the expression of c-fos, c-jun and c-erbB-1 oncogene products in human squamous cell lung carcinomas. *J Cancer Res Clin Oncol* **119:**507–510, 1993
35. Al-Kasspooles M, Moore JH, Orringer MB, Beer DG: Amplification and over-expression of the EGFR and erbB-2 genes in human esophageal adenocarcinomas. *Int J Cancer* **54:**213–219, 1993
36. Yoshida K, Kyo E, Tsuda T, et al: EGF and TGF-α, the ligands of hyperproduced EGFR in human esophageal carcinoma cells, act as autocrine growth factors. *Int J Cancer* **45:**131–135, 1990
37. Ozawa S, Ueda M, Ando N, et al: Prognostic significance of epidermal growth factor receptor in esophageal squamous cell carcinomas. *Cancer* **63:**2169–2173, 1989

38. Mukaida H, Masakazu T, Toshihiro H, et al: Clinical significance of the expression of epidermal growth factor and its receptor in esophageal cancer. *Cancer* **68:**142–148, 1991
39. Bargmann CI, Hung M-C, Weinberg RA: The neu oncogene encodes on epidermal growth factor receptor-related protein. *Nature* **319:**226–230, 1986
40. Holmes WE, Sliwkowski MX, Akita RW, et al: Identification of heregulin, a specific activator of p185erbB-2. *Science* **256:** 1205–1210, 1992
41. DiFiore PP, Pierce JH, Kraus MH, et al: ErbB-2 is a potent oncogene when overexpressed in NIH-3T3 cells. *Science* **237:**178–182, 1987
42. Schneider PM, Hung M-C, Chiocca SM, et al: Differential expression of the c-erbB-2 gene in human small cell and non-small cell lung cancer. *Cancer Res* **49:**4968–4971, 1989
43. Kern JA, Schwartz DA, Nordberg JE, et al: p185neu expression in human lung adenocarcinomas predicts shortened survival. *Cancer Res* **50:**5184–5191, 1990
44. Tsai C-M, Chang K-T, Perng, R-P, et al: Correlation of intrinsic chemoresistance of non-small cell lung cancer cell lines with HER-2/neu gene expression but not with ras gene mutations. *J Natl Cancer Inst* **85:**897–901, 1993
45. Heldin C-H, Westermark B: Platelet-derived growth factor: Mechanism of action and possible in vivo function. *Cell Regulation* **1:**555–566, 1990
46. Betsholtz C, Bergh J, Bywater M, et al: Expression of multiple growth factors in a human lung-cancer cell line. *Int J Cancer* **39:**502–507, 1987
47. Altorki N, Schwartz GK, Blundell M, et al: Characterization of cell lines established from human gastric—esophageal adenocarcinomas. *Cancer* **72:**649–657, 1993
48. Safi A, Sadmi M, Martinet N, et al: Presence of elevated levels of platelet-derived growth factor (PDGF) in lung adenocarcinoma pleural effusions. *Chest* **102:**204–207, 1992
49. Antoniades HN, Galanopoulos T, Neville-Golden J, O'Hara CJ: Malignant epithelial cells in primary human lung carcinomas coexpress in vivo platelet-derived growth factor (PDGF) and PDGF receptor mRNAs and their protein products. *Proc Natl Acad Sci U S A* **89:**3942–3946, 1992
50. Antoniades HR, Galanopoulos T, Neville-Golden J, et al: Injury induces in vivo expression of platelet derived growth factor (PDGF) and PDGF receptor mRNAs in skin epithelial cells and PDGF and mRNA in connective tissue fibroblasts. *Proc Natl Acad Sci U S A* **84:**565–569, 1991
51. Froesch ER, Schmid C, Schwander J, Zapf J: Actions of insulin-like growth factors. *Annu Rev Physiol* **47:**443–467, 1985
52. Nakanishi Y, Mulshine JL, Kasprzyk PG, et al: Insulin-like growth factor-1 can mediate autocrine proliferation of human small cell lung cancer cell lines in vitro. *J Clin Invest* **82:**354–359, 1988
53. Piertrzkowski Z, Lammers R, Carpenter G, et al: Constitutive expression of insulin-like growth factor 1 and insulin-like growth factor 1 receptor abrogates all requirements for exogenous growth factors. *Cell Growth Differ* **3:**199, 1992
54. Macaulay VM, Everard MJ, Teale JD, et al: Autocrine function for insulin-like growth factor I in human small cell lung cancer cell lines and fresh tumor cells. *Cancer Res* **50:**2511–2517, 1990
55. Oku K, Tanaka A, Yamanishi H, et al: Effects of various growth factors on growth of a cloned human esophageal squamous cancer cell line in a protein-free medium. *Anticancer Res* **11:**1591–1596, 1991
56. Kaiser U, Schardt C, Brandscheidt D, et al: Expression of insulin-like growth factor receptors I and II in normal human lung and in lung cancer. *J Cancer Res Clin Oncol* **119:**665–668, 1993
57. Tsuda T, Tahara E, Kajiyama G, et al: High incidence of coamplification of hst-1 and int-2 genes in human esophageal carcinomas. *Cancer Res* **49:**5505–5508, 1989
58. Berenson JR, Koga H, Yang J, et al, and the Lung Cancer Study Group: Frequent amplification of the bcl-1 locus in poorly differentiated squamous cell carcinoma of the lung. *Oncogene* **5:**1343–1348, 1990
59. Jiang W, Zhang Y, Kahn SM, et al: Altered expression of the cyclin D1 and retinoblastoma genes in human esophageal cancer. *Proc Natl Acad Sci U S A* **90:**9026–9030, 1993
60. Ewen ME, Sluss HK, Sherr CJ, et al: Functional interactions of the retinoblastoma protein with mammalian D-type cyclins. *Cell* **73:**487–497, 1993
61. Dowdy SF, Hinds PW, Louie K, et al: Physical interaction of the retinoblastoma protein with human D cyclins. *Cell* **73:**499–511, 1993
62. Hinds PW, Dowdy SF, Eaton EN, et al: Function of a human cyclin gene as an oncogene. *Proc Natl Acad Sci U S A* **91:**709–713, 1993
63. Barbacid M: Ras genes. *Annu Rev Biochem* **56:**799–827, 1987
64. McCormick F: How receptors turn ras on. *Nature* **363:**15–16, 1993
65. Blenis J: Signal transduction via the map kinases: Proceed at your own rsk. *Proc Natl Acad Sci U S A* **90:**5889–5892, 1993
66. Feig LA: The many roads that lead to ras. *Science* **260:**767–768, 1993
67. Rodenhuis S: Ras and human tumors. *Cancer Biol* **3:**241–247, 1992
68. Yoakum GH, Lechner JF, Gabrielson EW, et al: Transformation of human bronchial epithelial cells transfected by Harvey ras oncogene. *Science* **227:**1174–1179, 1985
69. Rodenhuis S, Slebos RJ: Clinical significance of ras oncogene activation in human lung cancer. *Cancer Res* **52:**2665–2669, 1992
70. Slebos RJC, Hruban RH, Dalesio O, et al: Relationship between K-ras oncogene activation and smoking in adenocarcinoma of the human being. *J Natl Cancer Inst* **83:**1024–1027, 1991
71. Kohl NE, Masser SD, deSolms SJ, et al: Selective inhibition of ras-dependent transformation by a farnesyl transferase inhibitor. *Science* **260:**1934–1937, 1993
72. James GL, Goldstein JL, Brown MS, et al: Benzodiazepene peptidomimetics: Potent inhibitors of ras farnesylation in animals cells. *Science* **260:**1937–1942, 1993
73. Marcu KB, Bossone SA, Patel AJ: Myc function and regulation. *Annu Rev Biochem* **61:**809–860, 1992
74. Koskinen PJ, Alitalo K: Role of myc amplification and overexpression in cell growth, differentiation and death. *Cancer Biol* **4:**3–12, 1993
75. Birrer MJ, Raveh L, Dosaka H, Segal S: A transfected 1-myc gene can substitute for c-myc in blocking murine erythroleukemia differentiation. *Mol Cell Biol* **9:**2734–2737, 1989
76. Krystal G, Birrer M, Way J, et al: Multiple mechanisms for transcriptional regulation of the myc gene family in small-cell lung cancer. *Mol Cell Biol* **8:**3373–3381, 1988
77. Sekido Y, Takahaski T, Makela TP, et al: Complex intrachromosomal rearrangements in the process of amplification of the 1-myc gene in small-cell lung cancer. *Mol Cell Biol* **12:**1747–1754, 1992
78. Little CD, Nau MM, Carney DN, et al: Amplification and expression of the C-myc oncogene in human lung cancer cell lines. *Nature* **306:**194–196, 1983
79. Nau MM, Brooks BJ, Battey J, et al: L-myc, a new myc-related gene amplified and expressed in human small cell lung cancer. *Nature* **318:**69–73, 1985
80. Nau MM, Brooks BJ, Carney DN, et al: Human small-cell lung cancers show amplification and expression of the N-myc gene. *Proc Natl Acad Sci U S A* **83:**1092–1096, 1986
81. Brennan J, O'Connor T, Makuch RW, et al: Myc family dna amplification in 107 tumor and tumor cell lines from patients with small cell lung cancer treated with different combination chemotherapy regimens. *Cancer Res* **51:**1708–1712, 1991
82. Garte SJ: The c-myc oncogene in tumor progression. *Crit Rev Oncogenesis* **4:**435–449, 1993
83. Postel EH, Berberich SJ, Flint SJ, Ferrone CA: Human c-myc transcription factor PuF identified as nm23-H2 nucleoside diphosphate kinase, a candidate suppressor of tumor metastasis. *Science* **261:**478–480, 1993

84. Willey JC, Hei TK, Piao CQ, et al: Radiation-induced deletion of chromosomal regions containing tumor suppressor genes in human bronchial epithelial cells. *Carcinogenesis* **14:**1181–1188, 1993
85. Whang-Peng J, Knutsen T, Gazdar A, et al: Nonrandom structural and numerical chromosome changes in non-small-cell lung cancer. *Genes Chromosom Cancer* **3:**168–188, 1991
86. Whang-Peng J, Banks-Schlegal SP, Lee EC: Cytogenetic studies of esophageal carcinoma cell lines. *Cancer Genet Cytogenet* **45:** 101–120, 1990
87. Hibi K, Takahashi T, Yamakawa K, et al: Three distinct regions involved in 3p deletion in human lung cancer. *Oncogene* **7:**445–449, 1992
88. Weinberg RA: The retinoblastoma gene and gene product. *Cancer Surv* **12:**43–57, 1992
89. Hollinsworth RE Jr, Chen P-L, Lee W-H: Integration of cell cycle control with transcriptional regulation by the retinoblastoma protein. *Curr Opin Cell Biol* **5:**194–200, 1993
90. Hu QJ, Lees JA, Buchkovich KJ, Harlow E: The retinoblastoma protein physically associates with the human cdc2 kinase. *Mol Cell Biol* **12:**971–980, 1992
91. Nevins JR. E2F: A link between the rb tumor suppressor protein and viral oncoproteins. *Science* **258:**424–429, 1992
92. Chellappan S, Kraus VB, Kroger B, et al: Adenovirus E1a, simian virus 40 tumor antigen, and human papilloma virus E7 protein share the capacity to disrupt the interaction between transcription factor E2F and the retinoblastoma gene product. *Proc Natl Acad Sci U S A* **89:**4589–4553, 1992
93. Ookawa K, Shiseki M, Takahashi R, et al: Reconstitution of the rb gene suppresses the growth of small-cell lung carcinoma cells carrying multiple genetic alterations. *Oncogene* **8:**2175–2181, 1993
94. Harbour JW, Lai S-L, Whang-Peng J, et al: Abnormalities in structure and expression of the human retinoblastoma gene in sclc. *Science* **241:**353–357, 1988
95. Reissmann PT, Koga H, Takahashi R, et al, and Lung Cancer Study Group: Inactivation of the retinoblastoma susceptibility gene in non-small-cell lung cancer. *Oncogene* **8:**1913–1919, 1993
96. Huang Y, Roynton RF, Blount PL, et al: Loss of heterozygosity involves multiple tumor suppressor genes in human esophageal cancers. *Cancer Res* **52:**6525–6530, 1992
97. Levine AJ: The p53 tumour suppressor gene and product. *Cancer Surv* **12:**59–78, 1992
98. Shiio Y, Yamamoto T, Yamaguchi N: Negative regulation of Rb expression by the p53 gene product. *Proc Natl Acad Sci U S A* **89:**5206–5210, 1992
99. Donehower LA, Bradley A: The tumor suppressor p53. *Biochim Biophys Acta* **1155:**181–205, 1993
100. Kuerbitz SJ, Plunkett BS, Walsh WV, Kastan MB: Wild-type p53 is a cell cycle checkpoint determinant following irradiation. *Proc Natl Acad Sci U S A* **89:**7491–7495, 1992
101. Yonish-Rouach E, Grunwald D, Wilder S, et al: p53-mediated cell death: relationship to cell cycle control. *Mol Cell Biol* **13:**1415–1423, 1993
102. Hollstein M, Sidransky D, Vogelstein B, Haris CC: p53 mutations in human cancers. *Science* **253:**49–53, 1991
103. D'Amico D, Carbone D, Mitsudomi T, et al: High frequency of somatically acquired p53 mutations in small-cell lung cancer cell lines and tumors. *Oncogene* **7:**339–346, 1992
104. Chiba I, Takahashi T, Nau MM, et al: Mutations in the p53 gene are frequent in primary, resected non-small cell lung cancer. *Oncogene* **5:**1603–1610, 1990
105. Huang Y, Meltzer SJ, Yin J, et al: Altered messenger RNA and unique mutational profiles p53 and Rb in human esophageal carcinomas. *Cancer Res* **53:**1889–1894, 1993
106. Lohmann D, Putz B, Reich U, et al: Mutational spectrum of the p53 gene in human small-cell lung cancer and relationship to clinicopathological data. *Am J Pathol* **142:**907–915, 1993
107. Marchetti A, Buttitta F, Merlo G, et al: p53 alterations in non-small cell lung cancers correlate with metastatic involvement of hilar and mediastinal lymph nodes. *Cancer Res* **53:**2846–2851, 1993
108. Quinlan D, Davidson AG, Summers CL, et al: Accumulation of p53 protein correlates with a poor prognosis in human lung cancer. *Cancer Res* **52:**4828–4831, 1992
109. Horio Y, Takahashi T, Kuroishi T, et al: Prognostic significance of p53 mutations and 3p deletions in primary resected non-small cell lung cancer. *Cancer Res* **53:**1–4, 1993
110. Bennett WP, Colby TV, Travis WD, et al: p53 protein accumulates frequently in early bronchial neoplasia. *Cancer Res* **53:**4817–4822, 1993
111. Sundaresan V, Ganly P, Hasleton P, et al: p53 and chromosome 3 abnormalities, characteristic of malignant lung tumours, are detectable in preinvasive lesions of the bronchus. *Oncogene* **7:**1989–1997, 1992
112. Wang L-D, Hong J-Y, Qiu S-L, et al: Accumulation of p53 protein in human esophageal precancerous lesions: A possible early biomarker for carcinogenesis. *Cancer Res* **53:**1783–1787, 1991
113. Ramel S, Reid BJ, Sanchez CA, et al: Evaluation of p53 protein expression in Barrett's esophagus by two-parameter flow cytometry. *Gastroenterology* **102:**1220–1228, 1992
114. Nishisho I, Nakamura Y, Miyoshi Y, et al: Mutations of chromosome 5q21 genes in FAP and colorectal cancer patients. *Science* **253:**665–669, 1991
115. Kinzler KW, Nilbert MC, Vogelstein B, et al: Identification of a gene located at chromosome 5q21 that is mutated in colorectal cancers. *Science* **251:**1366–1370, 1991
116. Fearon ER, Cho KR, Nigro JM, et al: Identification of a chromosome 18q gene that is altered in colorectal cancers. *Science* **247:**49–56, 1990
117. Ashton-Rickard PG, Wyllie AG, Bird CC, et al: MCC, a candidate familial polyposis gene in 5q21, shows frequent allele loss in colorectal and lung cancer. *Oncogene* **6:**1881–1886, 1991
118. D'Amico D, Carbone DP, Johnson BE, et al: Polymorphic sites within the MCC and APC loci reveal very frequent loss of heterozygosity in human small cell lung cancer. *Cancer Res* **52:**1996–1999, 1992
119. Boynton RF, Blunt PL, Yin J, et al: Loss of heterozygosity involving the APC and MCC genetic loci occurs in the majority of human esophageal cancers. *Proc Natl Acad Sci U S A* **89:**3385–3388, 1992
120. Blount PL, Meltzer SJ, Yin J, et al: Clonal ordering of 17p and 5q allelic losses in Barrett dysplasia and adenocarcinoma. *Proc Natl Acad Sci U S A* **90:**3221–3225, 1993
121. Kamb A, Gruis NA, Weaver-Feldhaus J, et al: A cell cycle regulator potentially involved in genesis of many tumor types. *Science* **264:**436–440, 1994
122. Marx J: New tumor suppressor may rival p53. *Science* **264:**344–345, 1994
123. Baselga J, Norton L, Masui H, et al: Antitumor effects of doxorubicin in combination with anti-epidermal growth factor receptor monoclonal antibodies. *J Natl Cancer Inst* **85:**1327–1333, 1993
124. Eguchi Y, Itoh T, Tomizawa J: Antisense rna. *Annu Rev Biochem* **60:**631–652, 1991
125. Zhang Y, Mukhopadhyay T, Donehower LA, et al: Retroviral vector-mediated transduction of K-ras antisense rna into human lung cancer cells inhibits expression of the malignant phenotype. *Hum Gene Ther* **4:**451–460, 1993
126. Georges RN, Mukhopadhyay T, Zhang Y, et al: Prevention of orthotopic human lung cancer growth by intratracheal instillation of a retroviral antisense K-ras construct. *Cancer Res* **53:**1743–1746, 1993
127. Cai DW, Mukhopadhyay T, Liu Y, et al: Stable expression of the wild-type p53 gene in human lung cancer cells after retrovirus-mediated gene transfer. *Hum Gene Ther* **4:**617–724, 1993
128. Zhang W-W, Fang X, Mazur W, et al: High-efficiency gene transfer

and high-level expression of wild-type p53 in human lung cancer cells mediated by recombinant adenovirus. *Cancer Gene Ther* **1**:1–10, 1994

129. Lowe SW, Ruley HE, Jacks T, et al: p53-dependent apoptosis modulates the cytotoxicity of anticancer agents. *Cell* **74**:957–967, 1993
130. O'Mahoney AM, O'Sullivan GC, O'Connel J, et al: An immune suppressive factor derived from esophageal squamous carcinoma induces apoptosis in normal and transformed cells of lymphoid lineage. *J Immunol* **151**:4847–4856, 1993
131. Holmes EC, Golub SH. Immunologic defects in lung cancer patients. *J Thorac Cardiovasc Surg* **71**:161–168, 1976
132. Han T, Takita H: Immunologic impairment in bronchogenic carcinoma: A study of lymphocyte response to phytohemagglutinin. *Cancer* **30**:616–620, 1972
133. Nauts HC: *The Beneficial Effects of Bacterial Infections on Host Resistance to Cancer End Results in 449 Cases.* New York, Cancer Research Institute, Inc, 1980
134. Old LJ, Tumor immunology: The first century. *Curr Opin Immunol* **4**:603–607, 1992
135. Bell JW, Jesseph JF, Leighton RS: Spontaneous regression of bronchogenic carcinoma with five year survival. *J Thorac Cardiovasc Surg* **48**:984–990, 1964
136. Old LJ, Clarke DA, Banaceraff B: Effects of bacillus calmette-guerin on transplanted tumors in the mouse. *Nature* **184**:291–292, 1959
137. Fishbein GE: Immunotherapy of lung cancer. *Semin Oncol* **20**:351–358, 1993
138. Sarna G, Figlin R, Callaghan M: (human leukocyte)-interferon as treatment for non-small cell carcinoma of the lung: a phase II trial. *J Biol Response Mod* **2**:343–347, 1983
139. Bernstein ZP, Goldrosen MH, Vaickus L, et al: Interleukin-2 with ex vivo activated killer cells: Therapy of advanced non-small cell lung cancer. *J Immunother* **10**:383–387, 1991
140. Kradin RL, Boyle LA, Preffer FI, et al: Tumor-derived interleukin-2-dependent lymphocytes in adoptive immunotherapy of lung cancer. *Cancer Immunol Immunother* **24**:76–85, 1987
141. Vanky JF, Peterffy A, Book K, et al: Correlation between lymphocyte-mediated auto-tumor reactivities and the clinical course. *Cancer Immunol Immunother* **16**:17–22, 1983
142. Uchida A, Kariya Y, Okamoto N, et al: Prediction of postoperative clinical course by autologous tumor-killing activity in lung cancer patients. *J Natl Cancer Inst* **82**:1697–1701, 1990
143. Hollinshead A, Steward THM, Takita H, et al: Adjuvant specific active lung cancer immunotherapy trials. *Cancer* **60**:1249–1262, 1987
144. Hollinshead A, Takita H, Stewart T, Raman S: Specific active lung cancer immunotherapy. *Cancer* **62**:1662–1671, 1988
145. Takita H, Hollinshead AC, Adler RH, et al: Adjuvant specific active immunotherapy for resectable squamous cell lung carcinoma: A 5-year survival analysis. *J Surg Oncol* **46**:9–14, 1991
146. Schrieber H: Tumor immunology. In Paul WE (ed): *Fundamental Immunology*, 3rd Ed. New York, Raven Press, 1993, pp 1143–1178
147. Lanzavecchia A: Identifying strategies for immune intervention. *Science* **260**:937–94, 1993
148. Liu Y, Linsley PS: Costimulation of T-cell growth. *Curr Opin Immunol* **4**:265–270, 1992
149. Schwartz RH: A cell culture model for T lymphocyte clonal anergy. *Science* **248**:1349–1356, 1990
150. Browning MJ, Bodmer WF: MHC antigens and cancer: Implications for T-cell surveillance. *Current Biology* **4**:613–618, 1992
151. Zhang W-W, Fujiwara T, Grimm EA, Roth JA: *Advances in Cancer Gene Therapy.* Academic Press, Inc. In press.
152. Ohe Y, Podack ER, Olsen KJ, et al: Combination effect on vaccination with IL2 and IL4 cDNA transfected cells on the induction of a therapeutic immune response against Lewis lung carcinoma cells. *Int J Cancer* **53**:432–437, 1993
153. Porgador A, Tzehoval E, Katz A, et al: Interleukin 6 gene transfection into Lewis lung carcinoma tumor cells suppresses the malignant phenotype and confers immunotherapeutic competence against parental metastatic cells. *Cancer Res* **52**:3679–3686, 1992
154. Gansbacher B, Bannerji R, Daniels B, et al: Retroviral vector-mediated γ-interferon gene transfer into tumor cells generates potent and long lasting antitumor immunity. *Cancer Res* **50**:7820–7825, 1990
155. Townsend SE, Allison JP: Tumor rejection after direct costimulation of CD3+ T cells by B7-transfected melanoma cells. *Science* **259**:368–370, 1993
156. Boon T: Tumor antigens recognized by cytoloytic T lymphocytes: Present perspectives for specific immunotherapy. *Int J Cancer* **54**:177–180, 1993
157. van der Bruggen P, Van den Eynde B: Molecular definition of tumor antigens recognized by T lumphocytes. *Curr Biol* **4**:608–612, 1992
158. van der Bruggen P, Traversari C, Chomez P, et al: A Gene encoding an antigen recognized by cytolytic T lymphocytes on a human melanoma. *Science* **254**:1643–1647, 1991
159. Traversari C, van der Bruggen P, Luescher IF, et al: A nonapeptide encoded by human gene MAGE-1 is recognized on HLA-A1 by cytolytic T lymphocytes directed against tumor antigen MZ2-E. *J Exper Med* **176**:1453–1457, 1992
160. Weynants P, Lethe B, Brasseur F, et al: Expression of MAGE genes by non-small-cell lung carcinomas. *Int J Cancer* **56**:826–829, 1994
161. Jung S, Schluesener HJ: Single point-mutated, oncogenic ras proteins. *J Exper Med* **173**:273–276, 1991
162. Fossum B, Gedde-Dahl T III, Breivik J, et al: p21-ras-peptide-specific T-cell responses in a patient with colorectal cancer. CD4+ and CD8+ T cells recognize a peptide corresponding to a common mutation. *Int J Cancer* **56**:40–45, 1994
163. Winter SF, Minna JD, Johnson BE, et al: Development of antibodies against p53 in lung cancer patients appears to be dependent on the type of p53 mutation. *Cancer Res* **52**:4168–4174, 1992
164. Wiedenfeld EA, Fernandez-Vina M, Berzofsky JA, Carbone P. Evidence for selection against human lung cancers bearing p53 missense mutations which occur within the HLA A *0201 peptide consensus motif. *Cancer Res* **54**:1175–1177, 1994
165. Pardoll D: New strategies for active immunotherapy with genetically engineered tumor cells. *Curr Opin Immunol* **4**:619–623, 1992
166. Fujiwara T, Grimm EA, Roth JA: Gene therapeutics and gene therapy for cancer. *Curr Opin Oncol* **6**:96–105, 1994

CHAPTER

20

# Benign Tumors of the Lower Respiratory Tract

Joseph I. Miller, Jr.

## INTRODUCTION

The practicing cardiothoracic surgeon must have a clear basic knowledge of both benign and malignant disease of the cardiorespiratory system. Specific knowledge of the natural history of the disease as well as a firm foundation in gross pulmonary pathology and microscopic diagnoses will aid the thoracic surgeon in pursuing the best course of therapy for his patient.

## HISTORY OF PULMONARY PATHOLOGY

### Historical Aspects

The development of a subspecialty of pulmonary pathology was firmly established in the late 1950s, when Dr. Averill A. Liebow[1] at Yale University and Dr. Herbert Spencer[2] in England first described in articles and later pathology texts the many and varied benign diseases of the lung. Liebow at Yale and later at the University of California at San Diego is most noted for his description of the benign idiopathic disorders of the lung, particularly the interstitial disease processes. He and his associates helped to describe chronic eosinophilic pneumonia, bronchoconcentric granulomatosis, pulmonary alveolar proteinosis, desquamative interstitial pneumonitis, giant interstitial pneumonia, interstitial pneumonia with bronchiolitis obliterans, and lymphocytic interstitial pneumonia. In addition, they described such entities as small chemodectomas of the lung, sclerosing hemangiomas, plasma cell granuloma, and pulmonary hyalinizing granuloma. They also provided descriptions of the basic aspects of Wegener's granulomatosis, diffuse alveolar proteinosis, and pulmonary histiocytosis. Many world-renowned pathologists have studied under Liebow and have further contributed to our knowledge of these disease processes. Dr. Herbert Spencer was born and worked in England, where he published an exquisite two-volume treatise on surgical pathology of the lung in 1962 with the latest edition in 1985.[2] He described pulmonary blastoma as well as many other conditions. To date there are five or six outstanding pathologists who deal with benign diseases of the lung. They have each published or edited acknowledged texts in this field. Noted are texts in pulmonary pathology by Dail and Hammar,[3] Thurlbeck,[4] Colby et al,[5] and Katzenstein and Askin.[6] Through efforts of these authors, the development of the specialty of pulmonary pathology has become well recognized.

## BENIGN TUMORS OF THE LUNG

Benign tumors of the lung and tracheobronchial tree comprise approximately 5% of all bronchopulmonary neoplasms.[7] Steele[8] pointed out that solitary benign tumors of the tracheobronchial tree comprised 8–15% of all solitary pulmonary lesions. Most of these lesions are found within the lung parenchyma, with only 6% occurring endobronchially. These lesions seldom cause symptoms unless endobronchial extension produces signs and symptoms of bronchial obstruction. The diagnosis of a benign tumor of the tracheobronchial tree implies cure following resection with an excellent long-term prognosis. The hallmark of surgical treatment of benign lesions remains conservative resection, whenever possible.

## CLASSIFICATION OF BENIGN TUMORS OF THE LUNG AND TRACHEOBRONCHIAL TREE[9] (TABLE 20–1)

Classification of benign tumors of the lung and tracheobronchial tree has been controversial because of the difficulty in determining the cell of origin and natural history of many of these lesions. Recent developments in electron microscopy have further elucidated the cell origin of many of these lesions, and the classification presented by the World Health Organization modified from Liebow[1] is the one most commonly employed today. There are only two series in the literature that include a significant number of benign lesions seen at one institution.[10,11] Most are isolated case reports with a review of the literature. The classification by Liebow[1] has been modified to include new terminology on the basis of new information and to exclude some favored terms of the past. Greenfield[9] has revised this in a detailed classification of benign tumors of the tracheobronchial tree based on their cell of origin, whenever possible. Tumors previously thought to be benign, such as bronchial adenomas, including carcinoid, cylindromas, and mucoepidermoid carcinomas, have been excluded from this classification, since they are now known to be malignant. Pulmonary blastoma, tumorlets, and hemangiopericytomas were formerly considered benign, but they are now considered malignant and are excluded from this classification.

**TABLE 20–1. BENIGN TUMORS OF THE LUNG AND TRACHEOBRONCHIAL TREE**

1. Epithelial tumors
   - Papilloma
   - Polyps
2. Mesodermal
   - A. Vascular
     1. Angioma
        - Hemangioma
        - Lymphangioma
        - Hemangioendothelioma
        - Hemangiopericytoma
     2. Lymphangiomyomatosis
     3. Pulmonary arteriovenous fistula
   - B. Bronchial tumors
     - Fibroma
     - Chondroma, osteochondroma
     - Lipoma
     - Granular cell myoblastoma
     - Leiomyoma
     - Neurogenic tumor
3. Developmental *or* unknown origin tumors
   - Hamartoma
   - Teratoma
   - Chemodectoma
   - Clear cell tumor
   - Thymoma
4. Inflammatory and other pseudotumors
   - Plasma cell granuloma (histiocytoma)
   - Pseudolymphoma
   - Xanthoma
   - Amyloid
   - Tracheobronchopathia osteoplastica

## CLINICAL FEATURES

The mode of presentation of a benign tumor of the lung or tracheobronchial tree depends on the location and size. The majority of peripheral tumors are asymptomatic and are detected most often by plain chest roentgenography. Arrigoni et al[10] reported this method of presentation in 60% of their patients who were free of chest symptoms. They also pointed out, in the cases of peripheral lesions, the problem of differential diagnosis of a solitary coin lesion of the lung. Peripheral lesions must be diagnosed histologically to provide appropriate treatment and to exclude the possibility of an early carcinoma. In the remaining 40% of their patients who had thoracic complaints, chronic cough or vague chest pain was the most common pulmonary symptom.

Respiratory symptoms can usually be attributed to bronchial obstruction and secondary pneumonitis. Symptomatic lesions are more centrally located and may behave as a ball valve, depending on their size and mobility. This may produce audible wheezing on physical examination. Partial bronchial obstruction impairs clearance of secretions, contributing to recurrent bouts of pneumonia, bronchitis, bronchiectasis, or abscess formation. Progression to complete bronchial obstruction usually results in atelectasis and necrosis of the distal lung.[9] Hemoptysis occurs in less than 3% of all benign lung cases. In contrast to peripheral lung lesions, 87% of those lesions presenting endobronchially will produce symptoms.[6] The presenting symptoms in these patients have been cough, 46%, and hoarseness, 36%. Twenty-eight percent presented with symptoms of pulmonary infection, including pneumonitis, bronchitis, bronchiectasis, and empyema.[11]

The diagnosis of a benign tumor of the tracheobronchial tree may be suggested by radiographic findings on chest x-ray, chest tomography, or computerized axial tomography of the chest. Certain lesions have a characteristic roentgenographic appearance, such as the "popcorn" calcification, as classically described in hamartomas of the lung. However, more frequently, these lesions merely present as an asymptomatic lesion. Whether it is a peripheral lung lesion or an endobronchial lesion, definitive diagnosis must be made on pathologic examination of tissue. When the lesion presents endobronchially, the diagnosis can be made by fiberoptic bronchoscopy. Many endobronchial lesions look the same, and definitive diagnosis requires pathologic examination. If a bronchial adenoma is suspected, care should be taken in performing biopsies, since these lesions tend to be quite vascular, and fatal bleeding has ensued in a small number of reported cases. If the lesion is a peripheral lung lesion, either needle biopsy or open thoracotomy is generally required for definitive diagnosis.

Conservative resection with preservation of pulmonary parenchyma is the surgical treatment of choice of all benign tumors of the lung. When the lesion occurs endobronchially, it can frequently be excised utilizing the Jackson-type forceps or with Neodymium:YAG laser therapy. In those areas in which there is destruction of lung tissue or obstruction of a lobe with bronchiectasis or abscess, a more radical resection, such as lobectomy or, rarely, pneumonectomy may be required even though the lesion is benign. For peripheral lesions on the surface of the lung or just under the surface, complete wedge excision can often be accomplished by thoracoscopy or by a minithoracotomy (see Chap. 12).

We will review each of the common benign lung tumors for pertinent aspects of diagnosis, pathology, and surgical therapy.

## TUMORS OF EPITHELIAL ORIGIN

### Papillomas of the Tracheobronchial Tree

Papillomas are the most common laryngeal tumor seen in children but are rarely seen in adults. Lesions may be single, multiple, or present as a diffuse papillomatosis extending down the tracheobronchial tree into the lungs obstructing the airways. The lesion is generally confined to the larynx or upper trachea. Recent review of the literature revealed only 10 well-documented cases in which the lesions extended into the mainstem bronchi and beyond.[12]

Spencer[2] subclassified papillomas as follows: (1) solitary benign papillomas, (2) multiple benign papillomas, (3) benign combined bronchial mucous gland and surface papillary tumors, (4) papillary bronchial carcinoma in situ, and (5) bronchial papillomas. The more proximal lesions consist of squamous cell epithelium on a tissue stalk (Fig. 20–1) originating in the larynx or trachea. More distal papillomas may have lining cells resembling clear cells or may be covered by a mixture of epithelial type cells. While the exact etiology is unknown, the theory is that the majority of benign papillomatosis in the larynx and upper trachea is related to a viral type of infection, and the more distant multiple and recurrent papillomas can be attributed to a multifocal neoplastic process affecting an extensive epithelial surface. Bronchial papillomas very rarely precede laryngeal or tracheal lesions or develop in their absence.

Bronchial papillomas in adults are often solitary growths but may be associated with papillomas elsewhere in the bronchial tree, and also carcinoma in situ changes in adjacent portions of bronchial epithelium. Approximately 50% of solitary bronchial papillomas are ultimately associated with a lung cancer.

Pathologically, papillomas contain a core of vascular connected tissue covered by stratified squamous epithelium and occasionally by a surface layer of ciliated respiratory columnar epithelium. Microscopically, the tumor is a wart-like growth into the bronchial lumen, though tumors arising from terminal air passage may present as cystic masses. The bronchial papilloma consists of connective tissue stroma infiltrated with lymphocytes covered entirely with either cuboidal or squamous epithelium and by a mixture of cili-

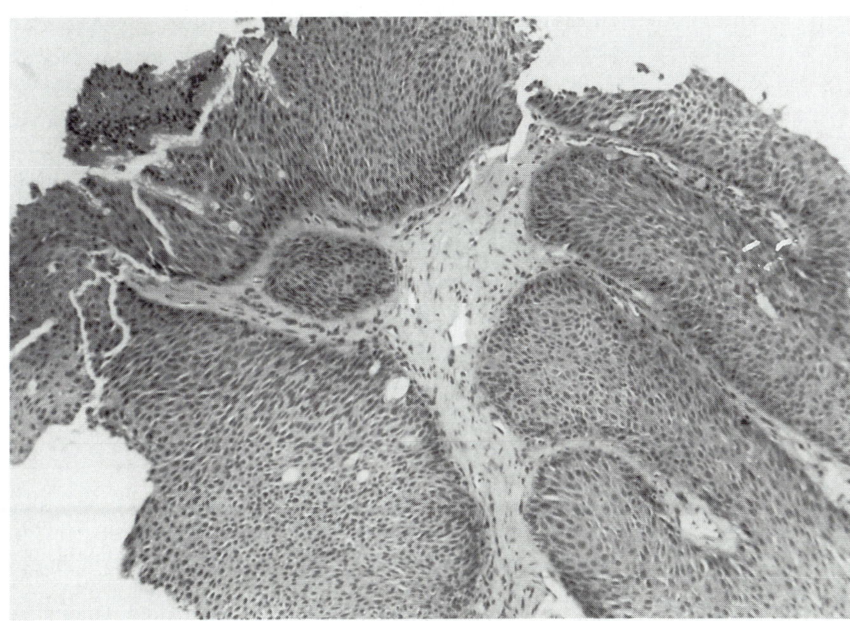

**Figure 20–1.** Bronchial squamous papilloma. This low-power view shows well-differentiated, nonkeratinizing squamous epithelium supported by an arborizing fibrovascular connective tissue stalk (40×).

ated and nonciliated cuboidal nonsquamous epithelium (Fig. 20–1). The predominant etiologic theory is that they are of viral origin, and malignant change may occur in 2–3%.

Roentgenographically, the manifestations are variable and range from airway obstruction detected by peripheral atelectasis and obstructive pneumonitis to a completely normal chest x-ray.

Clinically, the lesion generally presents with a history of chronic cough, hemoptysis, wheeze, asthmalike symptoms, recurrent pneumonia, or symptoms of distal obstruction. The diagnosis can generally be made easily on endoscopic examination by fiber-optic bronchoscopy and biopsy.

Treatment generally consists of bronchoscopic resection, although the recurrence rate is very high. These patients must be followed very carefully by frequent endoscopy because malignant transformation may occur rarely. With more severe forms of papillomatosis, tracheostomy may occasionally be required. In those cases of distal papillomatosis involving a segmental area with distal obstruction and atelectasis, resectional surgery of the involved area of the lung may be required if the patient is in appropriate physiologic condition.

In recent years, the treatment of benign laryngeal and tracheal papillomatosis has also utilized the carbon dioxide and neodymium:YAG lasers in selected cases.

#### *Polyps*

Benign inflammatory polyps of the tracheobronchial tree are relatively uncommon, with only a few case reports. These generally involve the upper respiratory tract, being found in the trachea or mainstem bronchi. These are covered by squamous ciliated columnar epithelium and granulation tissue. Bronchoscopic removal is generally successful, and recurrence is rare.[3]

## TUMORS OF MESODERMAL ORIGIN

### Hemangioma

A hemangioma is a benign tumor consisting of a mass of thin-walled vessels with a little supporting stroma. It infrequently occurs in the lung and is more frequently seen in the trachea and mainstem bronchi. The lesion may sclerose, forming hyalinized connective tissue—thus, the designation "sclerosing hemangioma" applied by Liebow and Hubble.[13] Some authors do not accept "sclerosing hemangiomas" as vascular in origin and refer to such lesions as fibrous histiocytomas.

The hemangiomas may develop in peripheral lung parenchyma, commonly subpleural. Occasionally, the lesion may involve the wall of the bronchus but rarely invades the mucosa or protrudes into the lumen. The individual mass lesions tend to be sharply circumscribed with a round margin averaging 3 cm in diameter.

Pulmonary hemangiomas are multiple lesions in about one third of all cases.[2] In 8% of cases, the lesions are bilateral, and in approximately 4% there is a systemic arterial supply. In about one half of the cases with multiple angiomas, the lesions are unilateral. In 60% of cases, pulmonary angiomas form part of the generalized disorder of hereditary telangiectasia (the Osler-Rendu-Weber disease) and may be the first manifestation of this disease.

The surgical treatment of choice for parenchymal hemangioma is conservative surgical resection with preservation of lung tissue. For those lesions in the endobronchial tree, the treatment of choice is YAG laser therapy followed by radiation therapy for any residual disease. Endoscopic removal of hemangiomas should not be attempted because of the risk of severe bleeding. These can be easily obliterated with Nd:YAG laser therapy with radiation therapy given for any remaining portion of the hemangioma not amenable to laser therapy.

### Lymphangioma

A lymphangioma is an extremely rare tumor occurring in the trachea and is generally found in infancy. The lesion may be seen in association with cystic hygroma and hemangioendothelioma in the neck. It may require surgical excision.[2]

### Hemangioendothelioma

Hemangioendothelioma is an extremely rare, benign tumor known also as angiosarcoma. It predominantly occurs in patients with congenital cardiac defects. It generally presents as a solitary pulmonary nodule and may be associated with hemothorax or hypertrophic pulmonary osteoarthropathy.[14]

### Hemangiopericytoma

This tumor may arise anywhere in the body. In one study of 247 cases, 28 involved the lung.[15] The lesions are generally large, and about 50% may be malignant. The tumors originate from the capillary endothelium and possess phagocytic properties. In the lung, these neoplasms are usually centrally located and well encapsulated but may grow so large as to reach the visceral pleura. Microscopically, the tumor is highly vascular with peritheliomatous arrangement of tumor cells mixed with fine reticulum fiber and fibrels (Fig. 20–2). Approximately one half of the patients are asymptomatic when the tumor is discovered. When present, symptoms include endobronchial obstruction with cough and hemoptysis and chest pain if the tumor involves a visceral pleura. Treatment is conservative surgical therapy, except when malignancy is present.

### Pulmonary Lymphangiomyomatosis

Pulmonary lymphangiomyomatosis (also called lymphangioleiomyomatosis) is a rare disorder that occurs in all races

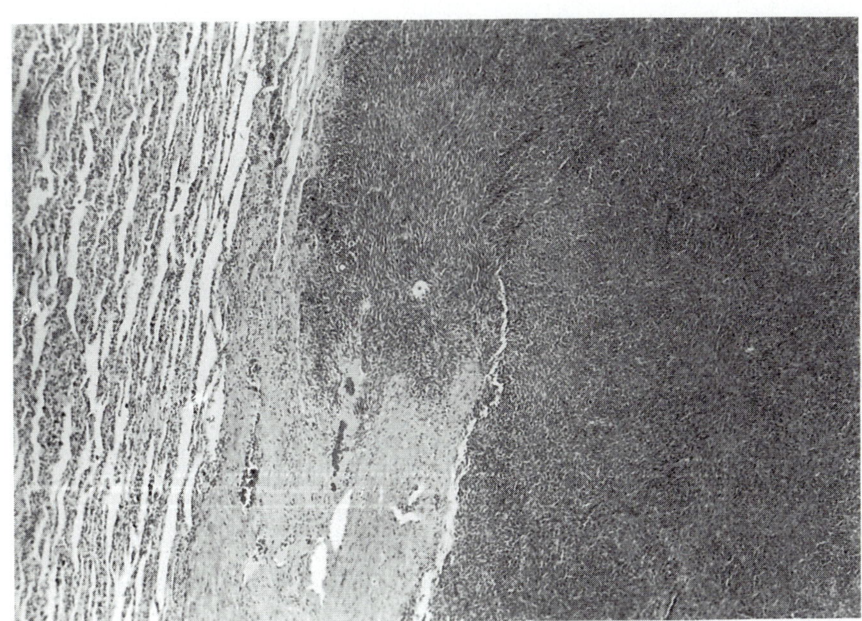

**Figure 20–2.** Hemangiopericytoma. Sheets of polygonal and spindle cells with little cytoplasm assume a perivascular localization (best seen in a reticulum stain). These tumors are well demarcated from surrounding lung (20×).

and forms a part of a much more extensive hamartomatous development of smooth muscle involving the lungs, lymphatics, hilar, abdominal and lower cervical lymph nodes. It is defined as a progressive disorder of women of childbearing age, marked by nodular and diffuse interstitial proliferation of smooth muscle in the lungs, lymph nodes, and thoracic duct. Corrin et al[16] in 1975, in the most extensive report to date, reviewed 34 previously published cases and added 23 new cases that they had collected. All the patients were women, generally between 30 and 50 years old. Roentgenographically, it is characterized by fine multinodular lesions in the lung bases with subsequent loss of parenchyma and honeycombing. Microscopically, in well-established cases, the lungs present a honeycombed appearance with thickened pleura and septa surrounding air-distended spaces. Pulmonary lymphangiomyomatosis is characterized by the presence of nodular, interstitial proliferation of plain muscle tissue in the lobar septa, pleura, the walls of the alveoli, and in the walls of the smaller bronchi and bronchioles (Fig. 20–3). The lesions are similar to those in patients with tubular sclerosis, and there may be a causal relationship between the two.[16] The lesions can produce shortness of breath, emphysema, pneumothoraces, pulmonary hemorrhage with hemoptysis, and chylothorax. Tissue should be obtained for steroid receptor assay.[17] Because of the association of lymphangiomyomatosis in women, it has been suggested that estrogens may play some role in the genesis of this lesion. Treatment with pleurodesis, tamoxifen, and tetracycline has been helpful.[18] However, a definite causal relationship has not been found. Conservative surgical resection is recommended whenever possible, although the lesions are generally larger sized and may require a more radical resection than simple wedge resection. Often the lesions are bilateral and not resectable. Adamson et al[19] and Banner et al[20] suggest that hormonal manipulation or oophorectomy may be helpful. The disease may be slowly progressive and result in respiratory insufficiency and death within 10 years.

### Pulmonary Arteriovenous Malformations

Pulmonary arteriovenous (AV) fistula (malformation) is mentioned for completeness. Although not a true tumor, it is considered a vascular malformation with anomalous AV connections. Some individuals have considered it to be a vascular type of hamartoma resulting from incomplete fusion of venous and arterial septa.[21] In general, it occurs as an asymptomatic solitary pulmonary nodule, usually with two large vascular markings seen on chest roentgenograpy. A contrast thoracoabdominal computed tomography (CT) scan will show the entrance of the arterial and venous sides of the AV malformation. In occasional cases, it may be associated with large right-to-left shunts from pulmonary artery to vein, producing cyanosis, clubbing, polycythemia, and a pulmonary murmur.[2] Occasional cases are associated with brain abscess and systemic embolization. AV malformations are most frequently seen in the lower lobes and are frequently associated with hereditary hemorrhagic telangiectasia (the Osler-Rendu-Weber syndrome). Surgical resection of the lesion is by conservative resection, since occasional lesions may be multiple.

## BRONCHIAL TUMORS

### Fibroma

Benign fibromas may arise from the peripheral parenchyma of the lung or from the walls of the trachea and bronchi. They are an extremely rare neoplasm but are more common than other benign tumors of mesenchymal origin in the pediatric and adult age group. As with other mesenchymal

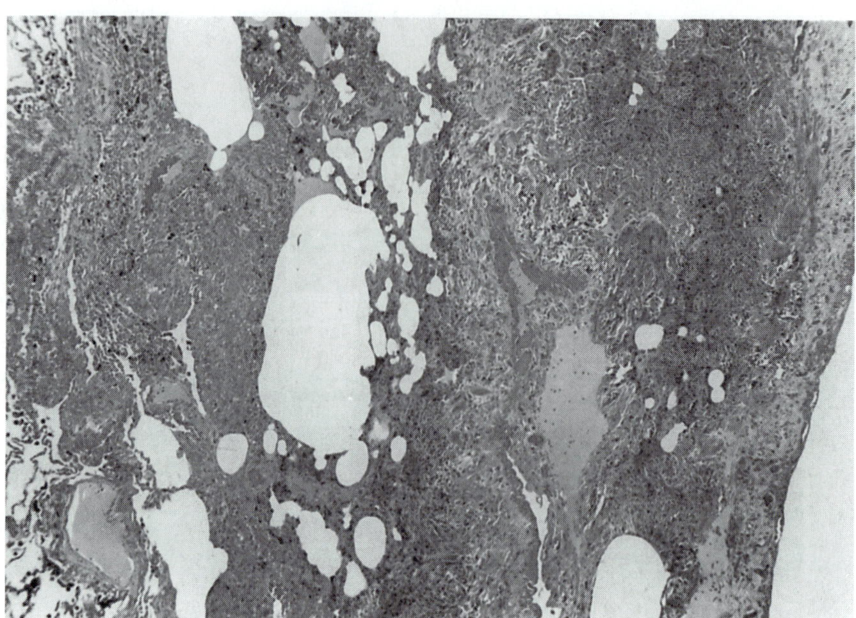

**Figure 20–3.** Pulmonary lymphangiomyomatosis. There is a disorganized proliferation of benign appearing smooth muscle involving the interstitium of the lung, blood vessels, and bronchioles. Partially obstructed small airways produce cystic air trapping. Fibrosis may result in part from vascular occlusion (20×).

lung neoplasms, various combinations of tissues may be present, and it is difficult to establish a precise descriptive histologic terminology.[22] In 1963, only 16 cases of intrapulmonary fibroma had been reported.[22]

The x-ray findings are not characteristic. Peripheral fibromas may present as a solitary nodule, and endobronchial lesions may or may not cause endobronchial obstruction. Peripheral fibromas are generally asymptomatic, and those occurring endobronchially generally present with symptoms of respiratory tract obstruction. The therapy of choice is bronchoscopic removal or YAG laser therapy for endobronchial lesions, and conservative parenchymal resection of the tumor for those peripheral benign fibromas.

### Chondroma and Osteochondroma

Chondroma and osteochondroma are the second most common types of mesodermal tumor. They may occur in the lung parenchyma or in the bronchial wall. They are most commonly seen as an endobronchial lesion embedded in the cartilaginous bronchial wall. Histologically, the lesion consists of cartilage covered with epithelium without glands or other elements. The majority of endobronchial lesions are in the middle third of the tracheobronchial tree adjacent to a large bronchus. The presence of symptoms depends upon the presence or absence of endobronchial obstruction. The endobronchial chondroma may be difficult to distinguish from a cartilaginous hamartoma, but pathologically it lacks the other germ cell elements characteristic of a hamartoma.

Treatment is endobronchial resection or conservative wedge resection of the peripheral chondromas.

### Lipoma

Benign lipomas are among the least common benign lung tumors. They may occur endobronchially or in the pulmonary parenchyma. As recently as 1979, there were only 50 endobronchial lipomas reported in the English literature.[23] Other investigators have estimated that fibrolipomas account for 4.6% of all benign tumors of the lung.[24]

This lesion was first reported in a submucous endobronchial location by Rokitansky in 1854.[25] Eighty percent of the lesions occur endobronchially and 20% in the pulmonary parenchyma. The lesions are generally slow-growing and are histologically benign. Many endobronchial lipomas are of a dumbbell shape with the narrow neck lying between the submucosa and luminal portions. They may contain fibrous tissue as well as fat. The majority lies in the right cardiophrenic angle. Ninety percent of the lesions occur in middle-aged males, although the tumors have occasionally been noted in females. They are usually yellow or gray in appearance and can be confused endoscopically with bronchial adenoma.

Radiographically, the parenchymal, subpleural, and small endobronchial lipomas typically present as solitary nodules. Major obstruction of a bronchus presents with the typical characteristics of endobronchial obstructive lesions. The peripheral lipoma is asymptomatic, and those endobronchially may or may not present with symptoms of endobronchial obstruction. Therapy consists of removal of the tumor. In about 50% of cases, this can be performed by endoscopic resection.[26] Treatment of peripheral lipomas is by surgical resection. The long-term outlook is excellent, and the majority of patients do extremely well.

### Granular Cell Myoblastoma

These tumors most frequently arise in the tongue, skin, subcutaneous breast tissue, and occasionally in the lungs. Abrikossoff[27] was the first to recognize this tumor and reported it arising in the tongue in 1926. When occurring in the lung, the lesion generally appears in the larger bronchi producing obstructive symptoms, and diagnosis is made by endobronchial biopsy. Abrikossoff hypothesized that these lesions resulted from regenerative processes in striated muscle following trauma or inflammation. Kramer[28] described the first case of granular cell myoblastoma of the bronchus in 1939. Only 6% of these tumors occurred endobronchially, and the reported world experience by Valenstein and Thurer[29] in 1978 was confined to 46 solitary endobronchial lesions and 2 multiple lesions.

Granular cell myoblastomas are not encapsulated. They are composed of large ovoid or polygonal cells that contain abundant fine granular eosinophilic cytoplasm that stains with periodic acid-Schiff (PAS). They may occur in either lung but, in general, arise in the walls of a larger bronchus. Symptoms depend upon the degree of endobronchial obstruction.

Treatment is dictated by the size of the endobronchial lesion and the degree of invasion of the bronchial wall. When the lesion is <8 mm in diameter, it may be removed by endoscopic resection with the bronchoscope or neodymium:YAG laser. When the depth of invasion of the bronchial wall is significant, as shown on axial computed tomography (CT), then conservative pulmonary resection is the treatment of choice, and the recurrence rate is low. The majority of these lesions will require pulmonary resection in order to prevent recurrence of the lesion, since the recurrence rate is quite high if not completely excised.

### Leiomyoma

Leiomyoma of the lung is a rare benign tumor of mesodermal origin, often discovered on routine chest x-ray. Only 52 cases have been recorded.[30] Leiomyoma was first reported by Farkel[31] in 1910. Leiomyomas in the respiratory system rank fourth in frequency among benign mesodermal tumors of the lung,[32] preceded by fibromas, chondromas, and lipomas. Leiomyomas are less than 17% of reported benign primary lung tumors.[33] Females are involved more often than males by a ratio of 3:2. Age range varied from 6 to 67 years (average 35 years).

There are no characteristic signs or symptoms associated with this lesion. Presenting complaints may include cough, hemoptysis, chest pain, chills, fever, dyspnea, or weight loss. The symptoms are most pronounced with bronchial obstruction or pneumonitis. Physical findings are related to the size and location of the tumor. Chest x-ray usually portrays an ovoid, well-defined mass, which may be associated with a contiguous area of atelectasis. The lesions have not been noted to exhibit any predilection for either side of the chest. Pathologically, leiomyoma is a primary neoplasm of muscular origin that may include involvement of the lung. Grossly, the tumor has a yellow-gray white surface with normal intact mucosa. It is firm, spherical and often encapsulated. On cut section, a grayish white color in the interlacing whorls of tissue is characteristic. Microscopically, sheets of smooth muscle predominate with white interlacing whorls of tissue, spindle-shaped in nature, and occasionally mixed with flecks of calcium. To date, there are no reports of malignant transformation of a leiomyoma.[34]

Resection of the tumor is the treatment of choice. A conservative approach is generally advocated, but the site of origin and the presence of secondary complications may necessitate a lobar or segmental resection. If the tumor is small and confined to the periphery, a local wide resection is adequate. However, in the presence of extended pulmonary disease or proximal bronchial obstruction, a lobectomy or more extensive pulmonary resection may be required.

## NEUROGENIC TUMORS

Neurogenic tumors are extremely rare in the lungs although found with great frequency in the posterior mediastinum. They arise from neurogenic tissue and include neuroma, neurofibroma, and neurilemmoma. They may occur in either the benign state as neurilemmoma or neurofibroma or in the malignant form as a neurogenic sarcoma. Strauss and Guckien[35] reported a polypoid schwannoma removed endoscopically in 1951. Tolin and Good[36] reported a neuroma of the bronchus treated by bronchoscopic fulguration and subsequently by lobectomy in 1954. These neoplasma may arise in the peripheral lung parenchyma and appear as a solitary nodule. Treatment is by conservative resection when in the lung parenchyma, or endoscopic removal in the bronchial tree.

## TUMORS OF DEVELOPMENTAL OR UNKNOWN ORIGIN

### Hamartoma

Hamartomas are the most common benign lung tumor, comprising 75% of all benign tumors of the lung.[10] Hamartomas constitute approximately 80% of all pulmonary coin lesions.[8] They appear in approximately 0.25% of the general population.[37] The term *hamartoma* is credited to Albrecht,[38] who in 1904 described a disorganized arrangement of tissues normally present in an organ. Hamartomas are thought to be derived from embryologic remnants, representing an abnormal mixture of normal components of the organ in which they are found (Fig. 20–4). They are slightly more frequent in males than females with a ratio of 2.5:1. The tumors consist of a disorganized collection of smooth muscle and collagen and, thus, appear to fulfill the definition of hamartomas. However, this is extremely rare. The tumor generally appears on routine chest x-ray as an asymptomatic coin lesion in patients around 50 years old. Ninety percent of these appear in the lung periphery, with less than 10% occurring endobronchially.[39] The tumors are thought to arise in the connective tissue of the small bronchi. They tend to be well circumscribed and slightly

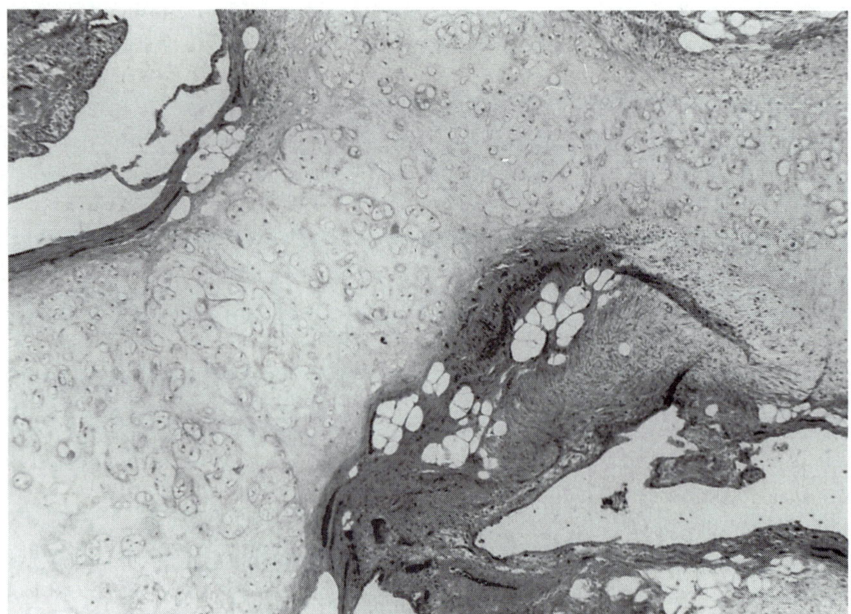

**Figure 20–4.** Chondromatous hamartoma. Benign cartilage, adipose, fibrous, and epithelial elements are arranged in a disorganized architectural pattern. Cartilage and adipose tissue are well represented. Epithelium is present in peripheral somewhat cystic spaces (40×).

lobulated; contiguous lung parenchyma is compressed. Cartilage is almost always present and often predominates, although it bears no relationship to the cartilaginous lining of the conducting airways. In certain cases, leiomyomatous tissue may predominate (Fig. 20–5). In the periphery, the tumors are round or lobulated with or without calcification. When in the lung parenchyma, the lesions are usually asymptomatic and only in cases with endobronchial extension do the lesions cause symptoms. Hamartomas may be multiple and occurring in different sites in the same lung or contralateral lung. Hamartomas are most frequently found in a subpleural location, and at the time of surgery can generally be shelled out quite easily. When a tumor in the deeper lung parenchyma, treatment is by conservative wedge resection.

A second type of hamartoma occasionally encountered in the newborn is a massive tumor involving a lobe or an entire lung.[9] This type of hamartoma is extremely rare and has been referred to as a cystic or congenital adenomatoid malformation. These may be associated with other congenital abnormalities.

The majority are discovered on routine chest roentgenography as an asymptomatic coin lesion. Radiographically, they are characterized as being round or lobu-

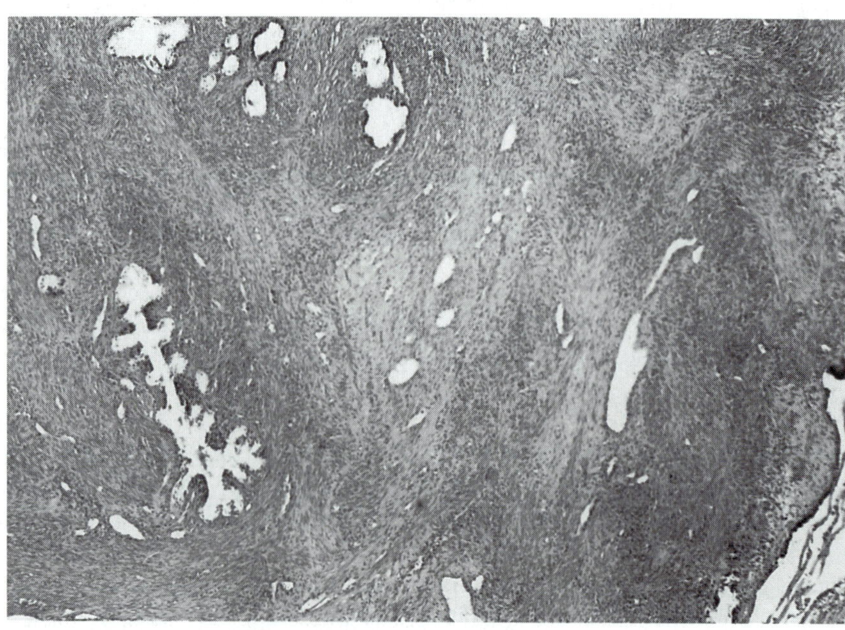

**Figure 20–5.** Leiomyomatous hamartoma. This interstitial and somewhat nodular proliferation of smooth muscle is well differentiated and in no area suggests sarcoma. The lesion is well demarcated and has incorporated several bronchioles (40×).

lated with a smooth and sharply demarcated border. Some may contain calcium or bone in sufficient quantities to be demonstrated on an ordinary chest x-ray. More frequently, chest tomography or CT helps in distinguishing a differential diagnosis. Specific popcorn-type calcifications are almost pathognomonic for a pulmonary hamartoma. The major difficulty with hamartomas is distinguishing them from inflammatory and metastatic lesions. They must also be differentiated from small primary bronchogenic carcinomas. Unless an absolute diagnosis of hamartoma can be made, conservative resection is the treatment of choice. Recurrence is rare.

### Pulmonary Teratoma

Intrapulmonary or tracheobronchial teratomas are extremely rare, with only 18 cases of primary intrapulmonary teratomas being documented by 1969.[40] The majority of these were in the left upper lobe, and all were benign. Most commonly, these contained nonmalignant tissue from one or more of the three germ layers, including skin, hair, or other dermal appendages and pancreatic or osteoid tissue. The roentgenographic appearance of calcification and of peripheral cavity in a tumor may be a clue to the diagnosis. These tumors show differentiated tissue from all germ layers and must be distinguished from metastatic lesions from a testicular tumor or extension from the mediastinum where they are more commonly found.

### Chemodectoma

Primary chemodectoma arising in the lung is an extremely rare neoplasm. A chemodectoma is a nonchromaffin paraganglioma. This lesion occurs with much more frequency in the mediastinum than in the lungs per se. Most lung chemodectomas are solitary and may be very large, the diameter ranging from 1 to 17 cm.[41] They are composed of ovoid or round cells with abundant cytoplasm arranged in sheets and nests. These nests are divided by thin strands of connective tissue and dilated, congested, vascular channels.[2] These tumors cause symptoms only when they compress adjacent structures or cause endobronchial compression.

## CLEAR CELL TUMOR AND THYMOMA

This tumor was originally described by Liebow and Castleman[42] in 1971. Histologically, it resembles a hypernephroma but shows abundant glycogen content on PF staining. The presence of a dense core of neurosecretory type granules suggests that this rare tumor may originate in Kulchitsky cells and be related to carcinoid tumors.

Rarely, ectopic thymic tissue has been reported to occur both in hilar and peripheral lung locations.[9]

## INFLAMMATORY AND OTHER PSEUDOTUMORS OF THE LUNG

### Plasma Cell Granuloma (Histiocytoma)

Plasma cell granuloma or histiocytoma of the lung is a rare benign tumor occurring mostly in younger patients. It is typically composed of plasma cells, lymphocytes, and various amounts of fibrous tissue with a variable vascular component. These tumors have been referred to as plasma cell tumors or plasmacytomas, histiocytomas, plasma cell granulomas, xanthomas, and pseudoinflammatory tumors.[2]

Bahadori and Liebow[43] reported 40 cases of plasma cell granuloma of the lung in 1973. They found that the lesion generally occurred as an isolated primary tumor in children under 16 years of age. Twenty-five of the 40 patients were females, ranging from 13 to 68 years. In 24 patients, the lesion was discovered on a routine chest x-ray with no previous history of related illness.

Laboratory findings are nonspecific, with a normal white cell count and absence of a typical myeloma electrophoretic pattern. In 23 of the 40 patients, the lesion presented as a solitary circumscribed tumorlike mass with 10 being described with the term *coin lesion.* The lesion was peripheral in the majority of cases with a parenchymal mass measuring up to 12 cm in diameter. On gross examination, the tumor is usually firm, with a characteristic yellow-white color. Histologically, mature plasma cells are the major and constant component of the cellular population, being predominant in 25 of the 40 cases.[43] Most were mature and occasionally multinucleated, and scattered Russell bodies were present. These tumors represent localized proliferations of mature plasma cells mixed with Russell bodies and reticuloendothelial cells in intermediate forms, supported by stroma. Other cellular elements, including lymphocytes and large mononuclear cells, may be present. The lesions are usually asymptomatic and are most commonly detected in chest x-rays as a circumscribed coin lesion or a large mass. They may be static or slowly increase in size. More than two thirds of the patients are <30 years of age.

Treatment is by surgical resection, generally either lobectomy, conservative wedge, or segmental resection being appropriate. If the lesions are unresponsive to antibiotics or steroids, patients may receive chemotherapy.

The etiology of plasmacytoma is unknown. A virus etiology, an inflammatory response, or neoplastic degeneration of normal cellular elements have been postulated. An immunologic cause must be considered in any lesion containing a large number of plasma cells.[39] Prognosis is extremely good following resection, and long-term survival can be anticipated.

### Pseudolymphoma of the Lung

Pulmonary pseudolymphoma is rare with only 30 cases being reported.[44] It presents as a solitary nodule that clinically and roentgenographically can resemble a primary bronchogenic carcinoma. The lesion is distinguishable histologically from lymphocytic lymphoma by criteria established by Salzstein.[45] Initially regarded as an inflammatory pseudotumor, it was thought to be completely benign. However, of the 30 cases originally reported by Fisher et al,[44] 4 have developed malignant lymphoma at various sites up to 4 years after the initial diagnosis.

The lesion resembles lymphoid interstitial pneumonitis histologically but is a discrete localized mass and does not involve both lungs. Pseudolymphomas are composed of a mixture of lymphoid cells including mature lymphocytes and plasma cells (Fig. 20–6). A diagnostic feature is the presence of well defined germinal centers, (Fig. 20–7), and the regional lymph nodes show reactive changes only. The infiltrates tend to be peribronchial, but in contrast to malignant lymphoma, bronchial cartilage is spared, and the mucosa is usually intact. Grossly, there is no distinguishing feature from a malignant lymphoma. Histologically, this condition is identical to lymphoid interstitial pneumonitis, which is a diffuse pulmonary disease usually, but not always, affecting both lungs. The term *pseudolymphoma* implies a discrete localized mass with the aforementioned histologic characteristics, but in published cases a clear distinction has not always been made between lymphocytic interstitial pneumonitis and pseudolymphoma. In Fisher's review,[44] 27 patients had a solitary nodule, and 3 had more than one lesion.

Treatment is by lobectomy or segmental resection of the lesion, since the prognosis of unresected pseudolymphoma is not known. Hilar lymph nodes should also be removed, since their noninvolvement of lymphoma is probably the single most important diagnostic and pathologic feature. Most of the original cases had no recurrence up to 13 years later, but four had progression to malignant lymphoma. This raises the possibility that pseudolymphoma is not always a benign condition and may lead to malignant lymphoma. Prolonged follow-up is recommended. Recurrent lesions have been treated with chemotherapy and radiation therapy with good responses.[40]

## Xanthoma

Carter et al[46] in 1968 reported 38 cases of primary xanthoma of the lung. These lesions characteristically show an encapsulated yellow mass with foam cells, spindle cells, and lymphocytes microscopically. Almost all these are in the lung parenchyma, and conservative surgical resection is the treatment of choice.

## Amyloid Tumors

Primary amyloidosis of the lung may be divided into the following forms[8]: (1) a localized deposit in the bronchus, (2) multiple or diffuse bronchial deposits, (3) localized or multiple parenchymal deposits, or (4) diffuse parenchymal amyloid infiltration of the alveolar walls and blood vessels in the lungs. Pulmonary amyloidosis occurs mainly in individuals >60 years of age and affects both sexes equally. It may occur in patients with a neoplasm located elsewhere in the body. Endobronchial amyloidosis may be found most frequently in the orifices of segmental branches and appear as round, smooth, grayish white sessile tumors in the lumen. Most cases of diffuse amyloidosis are associated with deposits in the larynx and trachea causing hoarseness. Single amyloid tumors in the bronchi may be treated by endoscopic resection or laser therapy, but diffuse involvement

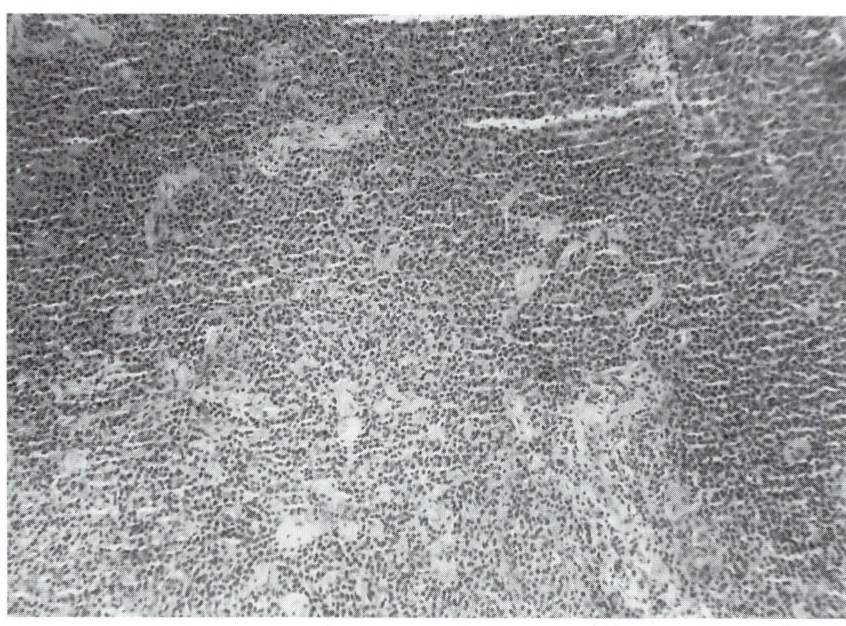

**Figure 20–6.** Pseudolymphoma. The lymphocytes are well differentiated. A few plasma cells are present. In the right upper aspect of this photograph is a germinal center (100×).

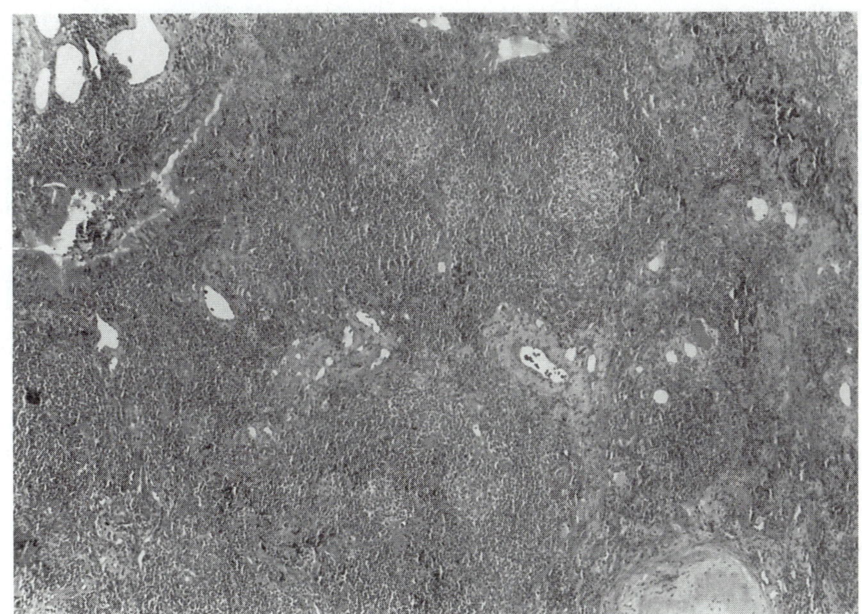

**Figure 20–7.** Pseudolymphoma. Prominent germinal centers in a background of mature lymphocytes is a diagnostic feature of pseudolymphoma (40×).

often leads to obstruction and consequent obstructing pneumonitis, which may require fairly extensive resective surgery.

Nodular pulmonary amyloidosis in the lung may be single or multiple and is often discovered on postmortem examination. Bronchial deposits are not necessarily present.

These amyloid deposits may be single or multiple, appearing usually as a transient, gray tumor mass varying in size up to about 8 cm in diameter. Diagnosis is generally made at the time of thoracotomy for a suspected pulmonary neoplasm, and treatment is by conservative surgical resection. The tumor mass is usually shelled out readily from the surrounding compressed lung. Although the clinical progress of these cases may be slow, the disease may eventually prove fatal.

### Tracheobroncheopathia Osteoplastica

This lesion is a more common submucosal growth, apparently arising from tracheal cartilages as well as endochondrosis that can ossify. There are multiple tumors underlying the mucosa between cartilaginous rings extending the entire length of the trachea. The cartilages of the trachea often appear to be formed and covered by an intact mucous membrane. After closer examination, however, multiple small sessile to plaquelike nodules can be seen projecting into the bronchial lumen. The wall of the trachea is extremely hard and thickened, but the predominant part of the ossification process is confined to the cartilaginous walls with the membranous portion being relatively normal. The process usually begins several centimeters below the vocal chords and extends down to and involves the tracheal bifurcation. In occasional patients, the bronchi may likewise be affected. In general, the diameter of the lumen of the trachea or the bronchus is decreased significantly but does not interfere with normal breathing. There is no known treatment other than bronchoscopic removal, but the lesions are fairly extensive, and major surgical resection of the tracheobronchial tree is not indicated.

## SUMMARY

Benign tumors of the tracheobronchial tree are rare compared with their malignant counterparts. Hamartoma is by far the most common benign tumor. The lesions are gener-

**TABLE 20–2. EXPERIENCE WITH BENIGN LESIONS**

| | Arrigoni et al[10] | Caldarola et al[11] | Miller[a] |
|---|---|---|---|
| Hamartoma | 100 | 7 | 41 |
| Papilloma | | 26 | 2 |
| Benign mesothelioma | 16 | | |
| Tracheopathia osteoplastica | | 11 | 1 |
| Inflammatory pseudotumor | 7 | | 3 |
| Fibrous polyp | | 7 | 2 |
| Lipoma | 2 | 6 | 1 |
| Myoblastoma | | 2 | |
| Leiomyoma | 2 | 1 | 1 |
| Amyloid | | 2 | 2 |
| Hemangioma | 1 | | 1 |
| Xanthoma | | 1 | 1 |
| Adenoma of mucous glands | 1 | | |
| Pseudolymphoma | | | 2 |
| Mixed tumor | 1 | | |
| Plasmacytoma | | | 1 |
| Hemangiopericytoma | | | 1 |
| Total | 130 | 63 | 59 |

[a]Unpublished.

ally asymptomatic when occurring peripherally, and they cause symptoms of bronchial obstruction when occurring centrally. Radiographic techniques of tomography and axial CT are helpful in establishing the diagnosis. Pathologic confirmation of tissue is required to establish a definitive diagnosis. Treatment is with endoscopic resection, laser therapy, or conservative surgical resection in the majority of cases. Table 20–2 lists the author's experience with benign lesions compared with two other series.[10,11]

## ACKNOWLEDGMENT

I wish to thank Dr. John Nickerson, chief of the Department of Pathology, Crawford W. Long Hospital of Emory University for his valuable assistance in pathology interpretation.

## REFERENCES

1. Liebow AA: Tumors of the lower respiratory tract. In: *Atlas of Tumor Pathology,* Sec. V, Fasc. 17. Washington, DC, Armed Forces Institute of Pathology, 1952
2. Spencer H: *Pathology of the Lung,* 4th Ed., Philadelphia, Saunders, 1985
3. Dail DH, Hammar SP: *Pulmonary Pathology.* New York, Springer-Verlag, 1988
4. Thurlbeck W: *Pathology of the Lung.* Stuttgart, Thieme Medical, 1988
5. Colby TV, Lombard C, Yousem SA, Kitaich M: *Atlas of Pulmonary Surgical Pathology.* Philadelphia, Saunders, 1991
6. Katzenstein ALA, Askin FB: *Surgical Pathology of Nonneoplastic Lung Disease,* 2nd Ed. Philadelphia, Saunders, 1990
7. Claggett OT, Ellen TH, Payne WS, et al: The surgical treatment of pulmonary neoplasms—A ten year experience. *J Thorac Cardiovasc Surg* **48:**391, 1964
8. Steele JD: The solitary pulmonary nodule: Report of a cooperative study of resected asymptomatic solitary pulmonary nodules in males. *J Thorac Cardiovasc Surg* **46:**21, 1963
9. Greenfield LJ: Benign tumors of the lung and bronchi. In: Sabiston D (ed): *Surgery of the Chest,* 5th Ed. Philadelphia, Saunders, 1980
10. Arrigoni MG, Woolner LB, Bernatz PE, et al: Benign tumors of the lung: A ten-year surgical experience. *J Thorac Cardiovasc Surg* **60:**589, 1970
11. Caldarola VT, Harrison EG, Clagett OT: Benign tumors and tumor like conditions of the trachea and bronchi. *Ann Otol* **73:**1042, 1964
12. Singer DB, Greenberg SD, Harrison GM: Papillomatosis of the lung. *Am Rev Resp Dis* **94:**777, 1966
13. Liebow A, Hubbell DF: Sclerosing hemangioma of the lung. *Cancer* **9:**53, 1956
14. Tralka GA, Katz S: Hemangioendothelioma of the lung. *Am Rev Resp Dis* **87:**107, 1963
15. Meade JB, Whitwell F, Bickford BJ, et al: Primary hemangiopericytoma of the lung. *Thorax* **29:**1, 1974
16. Corrin B, Liebow AA, Friedman PJ: Pulmonary lymphangiomyomatosis. *Am J Pathol* **78:**348, 1975
17. Graham ML, Spelsberg TC, Dines DE, et al. Pulmonary lymphangiomyomatosis: with particular reference to steroid-receptor assay studies and pathologic correlation. *Mayo Clin Proc* **59:**3, 1984
18. Luna CM, Jolly EC, Defranchi HA, et al: Pulmonary LAM associated with tuberous sclerosis: treatment with tamoxifen and tetracycline pleurodesis. *Chest* **88:**473, 1985
19. Adamson D, Heinricks WL, Raybin DM, et al: Successful treatment of pulmonary LAM with oophorectomy and progesterone. *Am Rev Respir Dis* **132:**916, 1985
20. Banner AS, Carrington CB, Emory WB, et al: Efficacy of oophorectomy in lymphangioleiomyomatosis and benign metastasizing leiomyoma. *N Engl J Med* **305:**204, 1981
21. LeRoux BT: Pulmonary hamartoma. *Thorax* **19:**236, 1964
22. Kovarik JL, Prather, Ashe SM: Intrapulmonary fibroma. *Am Rev Resp Dis* **88:**539, 1963
23. Politis J, Funahashi A, Gehlsen JA, et al: Intrathoracic lipomas: Report of 3 cases and review of the literature with emphasis on endobronchial lipoma. *J Thorac Cardiovasc Surg* **77:**550, 1979
24. Jensen MS, Pattersen AH: Bronchial lipoma: *J Thorac Cardiovasc Surg* **4:**131, 1970
25. Watts CF, Clagett OT, McDonald JR: Lipoma of the bronchus: Discussion of benign neoplasms and report of a case of endobronchial lipoma. *J Thorac Surg* **15:**32, 1946
26. Spinelli P, Pizzetti P, LoGollo C, et al: Resection of obstructive bronchial fibrolipoma through the flexible fiberoptic bronchoscope. *Endoscopy* **14:**61, 1982
27. Abrikossoff A: Uber myome, ausgehenol von der quergestreiften willkorlichen muskolatur. *Virchous Arch* **260:**215, 1926
28. Kramer R: Myoblastoma of the bronchus. *Ann Otol Rhinol Laryngol* **48:**1083, 1939
29. Valenstein SL, Thurer RJ: Granular cell myoblastoma of the bronchus. *J Thorac Cardiovasc Surg* **76:**465, 1978
30. Orlowski TM, Stasiak K, Kilodzie J: Leiomyoma of the lung. *J Thorac Cardiovasc Surg* **76:**257, 1978
31. Farkel W: Ein fall von fibroleiomycm der lunge. *Ztschr J Krebsfersch* **8:**390, 1910
32. Baum GL: *Textbook of Pulmonary Disease,* 2nd ed. Boston, Little, Brown, 1974, p 794
33. Peleq H, Pauzher Y: Benign tumors of the lung. *Dis Chest* **47:**179, 1965
34. Defore WW, Miller JI: Leiomyoma of the lung: Case report and review of the literature. *J Miss State Med Assoc* **22:**49, 1981
35. Straus GD, Guckien JL: Schwannoma of the tracheobronchial tree: case report. *Ann Otol Rhinol Laryngol* **60:**242, 1951
36. Tolin DJ, Good RE: Nonmalignant tumors of bronchus. *N Y J Med* **54:**1771, 1954
37. McDonald JR, Harrington SW, Claggett OT: Hamartoma of the lung. *J Thorac Surg* **14:**128, 1945
38. Albrecht E: Veber hamartoma. *Verh Dtsch Ges Pathol* **7:**153, 1904
39. Carter D: The pathology of tumors of the lower respiratory tract. In: Glenn WH, et al (eds). *Thoracic and Cardiovascular Surgery,* 4th Ed. Norwalk, Connecticut, Appleton-Century-Crofts, 1983, p 387
40. Gawtam HP: Intrapulmonary malignant teratoma. *Am Rev Resp Dis* **100:**863, 1969
41. Mostecky H, Lichtenberg J, Kalus M: A non-chromaffin paraganglioma of the lung. *Thorax* **21:**205, 1966
42. Liebow AA, Castleman B: Benign clear cell (sugar) tumors of the lung. *Yale J Biol Med* **43:**213, 1971
43. Bahadori M, Liebow AA: Plasma cell granulomas of the lung. *Cancer* **31:**191, 1973
44. Fisher C, Grubb C, Kenning B, et al: Pseudolymphoma of the lung: a rare case of a solitary nodule. *J Thorac Cardiovasc Surg* **80:**11, 1980
45. Saltzstein SL: Pulmonary malignant lymphoma and pseudolymphoma: Classification, therapy and prognosis. *Cancer* **16:**928, 1963
46. Carter R, Wareham EE, Bullock WK, et al: Intrathoracic fibroxanthomatous pseudo-tumors: Report of 10 cases and review of the literature. *Ann Thorac Surg* **5:**97, 1968

CHAPTER

# 21

# Lung Carcinomas

John R. Benfield and Liisa A. Russell

Two basic observations about neoplasms of the lung are important: Most tumors are malignant, and most neoplasms are metastatic from extrapulmonary primary sites. Cancers of the gastrointestinal tract and breast are the most common tumors to metastasize to the lung, but virtually any of the carcinomas or sarcomas can be the primary source. This chapter focuses on primary lung neoplasms.

## EPIDEMIOLOGY

Primary lung cancer strikes about 900,000 people yearly, and it is the most common cause of death for men in the entire world;[1] in the United States it kills more men and women than any other cancer.[1] However, the incidence of lung cancer is even higher elsewhere in the world; the lung cancer death rate of men in the United States ranked in the 10th place in the world in 1990. Hungary and the former Czechoslovakia had the two highest overall lung cancer death rates.[2]

Since 1930 more people have succumbed to lung cancer than to all other types of cancer combined. In 1991, more than 143,000 people died of lung cancer in the United States. In 1994, the estimate for *new* cases is more than 170,000 (101,000 men, 60,000 women); of these, 153,000 are expected to die of the disease.[3] In the year 2000, it is expected that 295,000 new lung cancer cases will occur in the United States and that 33% of all deaths from cancer in men and 23% of deaths in women will be caused by cancers of the lung.

### Lung Cancer in Men

In men, the lung cancer rate has increased from 5 per 100,000 in the early 1930s to 57 per 100,000 in 1990. Presumably as the result of earlier diagnosis and better treatment, lung cancer mortality rates started to decline in younger men in the early 1970s. Death rates from 1983 to 1989 decreased an additional 4% in men aged 35–54 years; however, deaths from lung cancer increased 7% in men aged 55–74 years and 28% in men 75 years and older.

### Lung Cancer in Women

The death rate of women from lung cancer in the United States has been steadily increasing; it now ranks in second place after Scotland. Worldwide, the lung cancer incidence in women has risen dramatically. Between 1965 and 1990 the lung cancer rate in women increased eightfold during the same period as the incidence of stomach and colorectal cancer decreased and the occurrence of breast cancer increased only slightly. Lung cancer is now the leading cause of deaths from cancer in women between the ages of 55 and 74 and is second only to breast cancer as the cause of cancer deaths in women between the ages of 35 and 54.[3] In a Canadian study based on data from the Saskatchewan Cancer Foundation Tumor Registry,[4] 42% of the women and 25.6% of the men ($P$ = .001) were diagnosed before the age of 60. Women were more likely to be nonsmokers than men (23% vs .3.7%; $P$ = .05), and women developed lung cancers after shorter duration of smoking than men.

### Lung Cancer in Young Adults

Less than 5% of lung cancer patients have been younger than 40 years of age.[5] Lung cancer patients in various geographic locations exhibit differences in clinical and pathologic features when older and younger patients are compared. Our experience indicates that cancers in young men are inordinately aggressive.[6] In general, the male to female ratio is reported to be lower in younger patients, and adenocarcinomas and small cell undifferentiated lung carcinomas

(SCLC) have been more common among young patients. In Canada, of 2800 lung cancer cases, 187 patients (101 men and 86 women) were <50 years old.[7] The male to female ratio in the younger group was 1.7:1 vs. 3.47:1 in the older group. The most frequent tumor type in the younger patient group was adenocarcinoma. In China between 1958 and 1987, 1.73% of lung cancers were diagnosed in patients <30 years of age; between 1983 and 1987, 29.5% of cancers in patients <30 years of age were lung carcinomas, and 45.6% of these were SCLC.[8]

## ETIOLOGY

### Tobacco Smoking

The carcinogenic effects of tobacco were first recognized 200 years ago, and now it is well known that about 90% of all lung cancers occur in cigarette smokers. There is compelling evidence to indicate that tobacco smoking is the most important etiologic contributor to the development of lung cancer. In 1941, Ochsner and DeBakey[9] pointed out the connection between rising lung cancer rates and increased cigarette consumption, but it was the classic 1950 paper of Wynder and Graham[10] that correlated tobacco smoking and lung cancer. The study of Kabat and Wynder[11] et al of 2668 lung cancer patients reported that only 1.9% of men and 13.0% of women were nonsmokers. It is thought that there is a latent period of 20–25 years between the initiation of smoking and clinically apparent lung cancer. This time span would explain the high incidence of lung cancer among cigarette smokers who are 45–70 years old.

There are data to show convincingly that the incidence of lung cancer in cigarette smokers is dose-related.[12] Heavy smokers have 25 times as many lung cancers as nonsmokers. The risk of lung cancer is directly related to the number of cigarettes smoked, the duration of smoking, the depth of inhalation, and the amount of tar and nicotine in the cigarettes smoked. The reversibility of precancerous changes in the bronchial epithelium is suggested by the observation that the rate of lung cancer is reduced in ex-smokers[13] and by our experimental studies in animals wherein precancerous lesions caused by chemical carcinogens were reversible.[14,15]

The incidence of lung cancer is expected to continue to rise through the 1990s. Even though lung cancer deaths among men are expected to decline, deaths among women are expected to continue to increase at least into the 21st century. It has been suggested that cigarette smoking is the most serious and widespread drug addiction in the world.[16]

### Components of Cigarette Smoke

Cigarette tar contains more than 4000 components, many of which have been identified as *tumor initiators; tumor promoters* or cocarcinogens; and *complete carcinogens.* The particulate phase of tobacco smoke is central to tobacco smoke's carcinogenic activity. In experimental animals, the carcinogenic activity of the particulate matter in tobacco smoke is greater than the sum of the effects of component carcinogens.

There are at least two dozen polycyclic aromatic hydrocarbons including benzo(a)pyrene that serve as tumor initiators at the dose levels found in tobacco tar. Azarenes and methylated three-ring aromatic hydrocarbons (e.g., 1.4-dimethylphenanthrene) are procarcinogens that require metabolic activation.

*Tumor promoters* in tobacco smoke include fatty acids, phenols, N-methylated indoles, carbazoles, and agricultural chemicals such as residual insecticides and pesticides. Low-dose nicotine also acts as a tumor promoter.

Tobacco smoke contains three broad types of N-nitrosamines: volatile N-nitrosamines, nitrosamines derived from agricultural chemicals used in tobacco growing, and tobacco-specific nitrosamines. Practically all volatile nitrosamines in tobacco smoke appear to be retained by the respiratory system upon inhalation. All the volatile N-nitrosamines in tobacco and tobacco smoke have been shown to be moderately organ specific.

Other agents such as radioactive plutonium, nickel, and arsenic are present in tobacco smoke and are carcinogenic in experimental animals. Smoking two packs of cigarettes per day for 40 years gives an estimated dose of 1300 rem from polonium,[210] enough to cause lung cancer. The total dose may be much greater (up to 2000 rem) when indoor radon decay products are included.[17] There are now also well-characterized experimental models of focally originating bronchial non-small cell cancers of all histologic types induced by chemical carcinogens of the type that are found in cigarette smoke.[18]

Although the relationship between smoking and lung cancer has been recognized by health care professionals for decades, and education aimed at the public at large has resulted in cessation of smoking by an estimated 40 million people in the United States, there are still about 50 million people who are smoking. Globally, the tobacco abuse problem is far from being solved; it is merely being transferred from rich to poor countries.[19]

### Secondhand Tobacco Smoke

Most of the chemical constituents of mainstream smoke are also present in side-stream smoke. Some compounds such as volatile nitrosamines and nitrogen oxides are present in markedly higher concentrations in side-stream smoke. In mouse skin turmorigenesis assays, side-stream smoke condensate has been found more tumorigenic per unit weight than mainstream smoke. Secondhand smoke includes particles with attached charged radon progeny that increase the carcinogenicity as compared with mainstream smoke.[20] Claxton et al[21] estimated that 40% of the mutagenity from cigarette smoke was in side-stream particulates, 30% in mainstream particulates, 20% in side-stream semivolatile components, and 10% in the mainstream semivolatile fraction.

Approximately 15% of lung cancers occur in nonsmokers, and the cancer incidence in this population is increasing. Janerich et al,[22] with a population-based study of 191 lung cancer patients who had never smoked, found that household exposure to 25 or more years of secondhand smoke during childhood and adolescence doubled the risk of lung cancer. They concluded that about 17% of the lung cancers among nonsmokers can be attributed to high levels of exposure to tobacco smoke during childhood and adolescence. The Surgeon General's Report[23] in 1989 concluded that passive smoke exposure was related to respiratory symptoms and illnesses in children, and the National Research Council[24] estimated in 1986 that the adjusted lung cancer risk among nonsmokers was enhanced 25% by passive smoke exposure. Despite evidence linking carcinogenesis with secondhand smoke, proposed antismoking ordinances for workplaces and public buildings have met with stiff resistance from smokers and tobacco producers.

### Occupational and Industrial Exposure

There is ample epidemiologic evidence that lung cancer is increased among workers that are exposed to industrial agents. Examples of these toxins include arsenic, chromates, nickel, asbestos, silica and other fibrogenic dusts, beryllium, iron, coal, and mustard gas. Organic chemicals such as benzopyrene, vinyl chloride, and chloromethyl ether as well as radioactive emissions are known to be carcinogenic. For example, nonsmoking uranium miners have four times as high and smoking uranium miners have 10 times as high rates of cancer as the general population.[25] Newspaper workers, halothane workers, and miners are occupational groups with a known increased lung cancer risk.

Reports linking asbestos and lung cancer have been published since 1934.[26] This relationship has been scrutinized extensively because of the litigation in possible asbestos-related lung cancer cases and the difficult question of assessing asbestos-related lung cancer risk among patients who are also heavy smokers.[27] A carcinogenic synergism between cigarette smoking and asbestos exposure has been shown[28,29]; asbestos workers who smoked had a 50–90 times greater risk of developing lung cancer than did non-smoking control populations. Approximately one fifth of the deaths among asbestos workers were from bronchogenic carcinoma, one tenth from pleural or peritoneal mesotheliomas, and one tenth from gastrointestinal cancers.[30]

### Atmospheric Pollution

Urban air contains an increasingly complex mixture of carcinogenic pollutants such as polycyclic aromatic hydrocarbons, noncombustible aliphatic hydrocarbons, radioactive substances and arsenic, chromium, and nickel compounds. When different smoking habits are taken into consideration, mortality from lung cancer is higher in urban areas than in rural communities. The combined effect of air pollutants and passive smoking is perhaps the reason for the increasing incidence of lung cancer in nonsmokers.

Long-term lung cancer risk from atom bomb fallout, nuclear testing, and reactor accidents is only partially known. The effects of the recent tragic accident in Chernobyl will not become fully known for years because of the long latent period before lung cancer develops.[31] An increased lung cancer rate in Hungary has been attributed to the Chernobyl accident,[32] and an increased lung cancer incidence has been reported among the survivors of Hiroshima and Nagasaki.

Attention has also been focused on the problem of "indoor air pollution," particularly from radon leaking into buildings.[33] The carcinogenic mechanism is thought to be inhalation of radioactive decay products that become attached to respirable particulate matter and aerosols that are deposited on the airway epithelium. Some investigators have attributed the increase in lung cancer rates in nonsmokers to low-level indoor exposure to radon in areas that have a high radon concentration in the soil.

### Genetic Factors and Lung Cancer

The role of genetics in the development of cancer is currently among the most active areas of research. Even though the genetic basis for familiar cancer of some organs such as colon, ovary, and breast has been established and chromosome patterns among lung cancer patients have been found,[34] lung cancer is not considered to be an inherited disease and specific lung cancer genes have yet to be discovered. There is increasing information about the genetic regulation of deoxyribonucleic acid (DNA) repair, cellular growth, and enzyme metabolism pertaining to handling of environmental chemicals. The family of *ras*- and *myc*-oncogenes is associated with growth regulation. One example of genetic regulation of enzyme activity is the single gene that controls the ability to induce aryl hydrocarbon hydroxylase (AHH) that converts polycyclic hydrocarbons into highly carcinogenic epoxides. Individuals with high levels of AHH have a greater risk of developing lung cancer.[35,36] Genes that encode the cytochrome P-450 enzymes are also interesting, and it has been suggested that polymorphism at one of the P-450 loci is associated with increased susceptibility to lung cancer in cigarette smokers.[37]

The role and interaction of carcinogens, tumor viruses, genetic factors, dominant and recessive oncogenes, growth promoters, and suppressors in the development of cancer is increasing too rapidly to provide a timely and complete summary within the scope of this chapter, but molecular biology and genetics promise to hold the keys to understanding the development of cancer. Chapter 19 in this volume is devoted to the impact of these sciences upon thoracic surgery.

## HISTOGENESIS AND PATHOGENESIS OF LUNG CANCER

All cells in the bronchial epithelium have their origin in the endoderm. Histogenetically, it seems most likely that the cell of origin for all lung cancers is derived from endoderm, and accordingly a stem cell theory has been proposed.[38] This theory explains the common finding of tumors with mixed histologic patterns. Yesner and Carter[39] proposed that lung cancer may differentiate and lose differentiation in ongoing fashion and that this process can be depicted with "Y diagram." In this diagram, SCLC is at the bottom, large cell cancer is at the fork, epidermoid (squamous) carcinoma is at the top of one arm of the Y, and adenocarcinoma is at the top of the other. This concept was designed to be consistent with the high incidence of lung cancers of mixed cell type and with the knowledge that large cell cancers are often highly malignant to a degree that may approach the behavior of SCLC. We recently advanced evidence from human lung cancers and from animal models in favor of a potentially unifying oncofetal concept of carcinogenesis.[40]

It is clear that cell type is not a fully reliable indicator of biologic behavior. There is experimental evidence obtained from transgenic mouse mammary carcinoma model linking a mutation in a particular oncogene (*ras, myc,* or *neu*) with a particular type of tumor pattern.[41] This evidence suggests the possibility that the histologic type of lung cancer may be determined by the action of a certain type of carcinogen and by the type of mutation that takes place in the stem cell. The type of differentiation that occurs during carcinogenesis may be further influenced by growth factors or by genetic disposition.

The pulmonary epithelial cells have a limited range of initial responses to a variety of noxious agents: (1) basal cell hyperplasia with metaplasia and differentiation toward squamous or goblet cells, (2) proliferation of Kulchitsky cells, and (3) proliferation of type II pneumocytes. The same reactions occur in response to many kinds of injuries and may be followed by increasing nuclear atypia. However, in the absence of carcinogenesis, the nuclear atypia is reversible in animal models and thought to be reversible also in humans.[15,18,42]

### The Stages of Carcinogenesis

Carcinogenesis is a stepwise process that includes initiation, promotion, invasion, and metastasis. Initiation is an irreversible event that is thought to be rapid and caused by a genotoxic agent. Promotion is a reversible process that is a long-lasting event that includes clonal expansion of the abnormally affected cells that have undergone initiation.

Progression, invasion, and metastasis are processes that are clinically evident without full understanding of the factors that control their rate of progress. The stages of bronchial carcinogenesis have been observed in humans and described in detail in experimental animals.[18,43,44] The following changes are common in the development of epidermoid cancers and analogous, but less well-defined changes are seen during the development of adenocarcinomas. During squamous cell carcinogenesis there is a gradual change from normal to malignant cell populations that pass through the following stages of increasingly severe morphologic atypia: hyperplasia, metaplasia, dysplasia, carcinoma in situ (Fig. 21–1), and invasive carcinoma.

*Hyperplasia* is the first response of the respiratory epithelium to injury. The number of basal (reserve) cells increases as a result of effects of growth factors on bronchial epithelial cells. The cells appear benign and respond to normal cellular control mechanisms, but hyperplasia provides the setting for neoplastic development. Hyperplasia is common in patients who have been chronically exposed to carcinogens, i.e., long-term smokers who also often have chronic bronchitis.

*Metaplasia* is a reversible change in which normal ciliated bronchial epithelial cells are replaced by goblet cells or squamous cells. The cells are morphologically benign, but reactive nuclear changes are often present. Metaplasia represents an adaptive substitution that is undesirable, because it often predisposes to cancer. Like hyperplasia, squamous metaplasia is common in chronic bronchitis and in the bronchi of long-term smokers. Goblet cell metaplasia occurs in asthma and chronic bronchitis.

*Dysplasia* is characterized by a thickened epithelium where the cellular orientation and maturation are disordered, but some maturation toward the surface is present. In contrast to simple hyperplasia and metaplasia, cytologic features are abnormal in dysplasia, and the nuclear to cytoplasmic ratio is increased. The nuclei are hyperchromatic and pleomorphic, the nuclear membranes may be thickened, and they may have folds and indentations. Their proliferation rate is increased. This is demonstrated by increased nuclear basophilia and increased mitoses. Dysplasia can be graded as mild, moderate, or severe and is considered a potential precursor of cancer. Dysplasia may be reversed when the cause is removed.

There has been considerable effort spent in trying to identify those dysplasias that are premalignant. Quantitative deoxyribonuleic acid (DNA) analysis by image analysis and flow cytometry have been used to assess total DNA or ploidy.[44–47] As shown in Figure 21–2, a progressive increase in mean DNA values during bronchial carcinogenesis in humans, dogs, and hamsters has correlated with the progression of the morphologic changes toward cancer; the identification of mutations in oncogenes and regulatory genes is reported to be a useful additional tool in identifying those cases of dysplasia with a high risk for developing an invasive cancer (see Chap. 19).

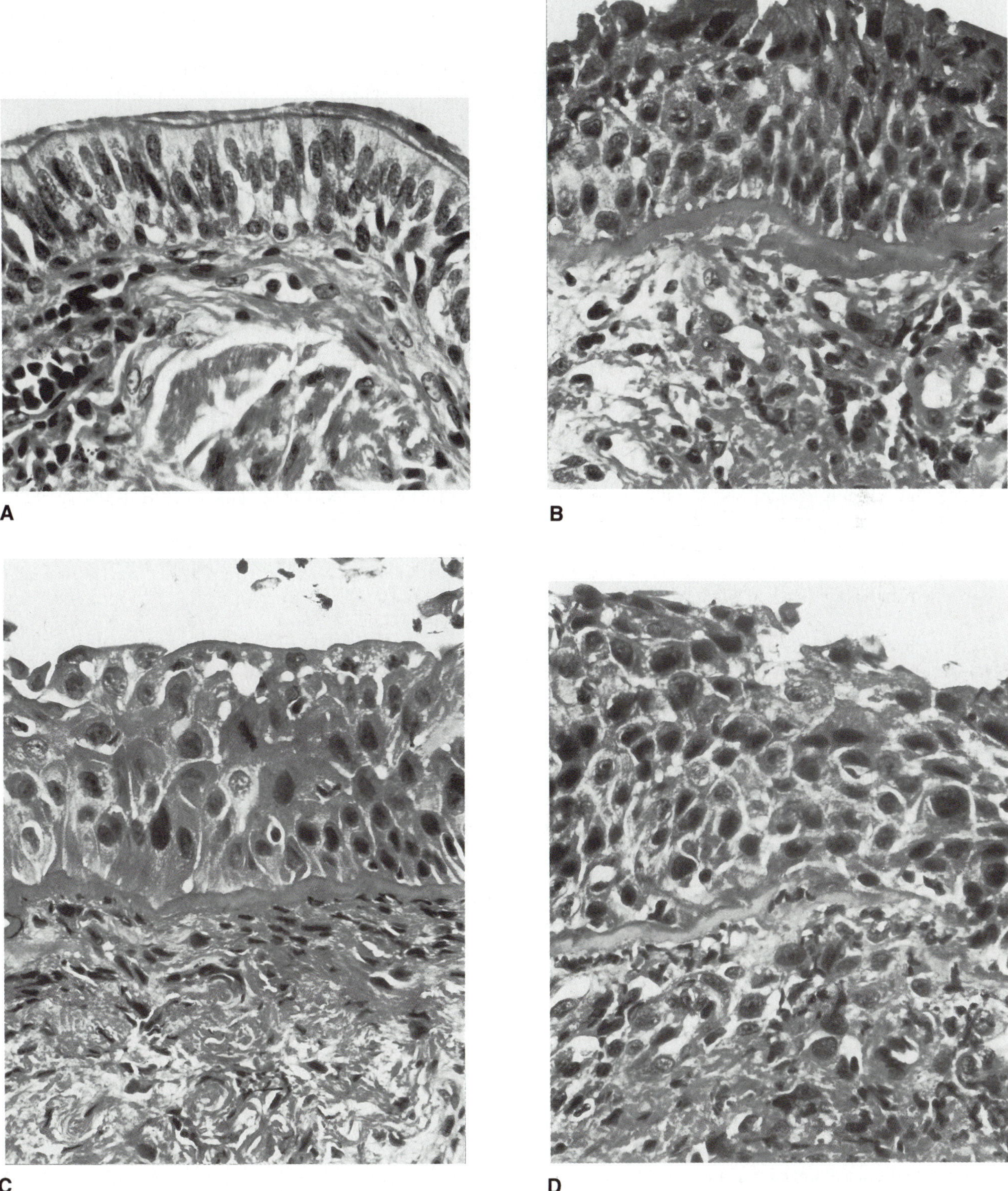


**Figure 21–1.** *Stages of carcinogenesis.* **A.** Normal pseudostratified columnar bronchial epithelium. Note a thin layer of mucus on top of the cilia. Bronchial biopsy. H&E, 360×; **B.** Basal cell hyperplasia. There is no nuclear enlargement or atypia, and the surface is covered by columnar cells. Note the thickened basement membrane and subepithelial mixed inflammatory infiltrate. Bronchial biopsy. H&E, 360×; **C.** Squamous metaplasia with moderate to severe atypia. The epithelium is thickened. There is nuclear enlargement and pleomorphism, and mitotic figures are present in the upper half of the epithelium. The cellular polarity is disturbed. The basement membrane is thickened, and the underlying stroma is chronically inflamed and fibrotic. Bronchial biopsy. H&E, 360×; **D.** Squamous carcinoma in situ. The epithelium is thickened. The cellular polarity is disturbed and the nuclei are enlarged, hyperchromatic, and pleomorphic. There is no maturation toward the surface. Bronchial biopsy. H&E, 360×.

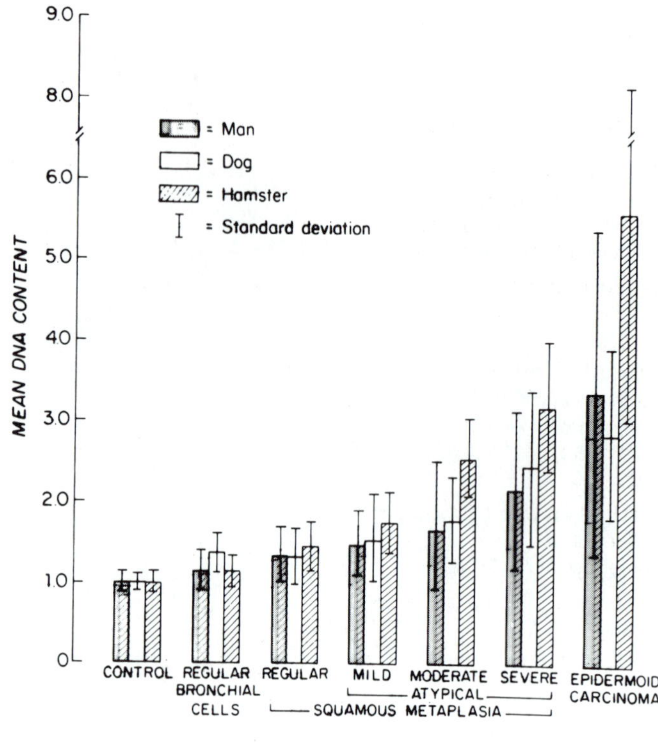


**Figure 21–2.** *Quantitative DNA* (ploidy) during carcinogenesis in humans, dogs, and hamsters.[47] Note the progressive increase in ploidy in all three species as the sequential process of carcinogenesis proceeds. *(Reprinted with permission of Mosby-Yearbook, Inc.)*

### *Carcinoma In Situ*

The characteristic feature of carcinoma in situ (CIS) is a thickened, severely atypical epithelium in which the abnormality extends throughout the thickness of the epithelium. The orientation of the epithelial cells is disordered, and there is no maturation toward the surface. The cytologic features in CIS are more atypical than in dysplasia, and they include increased nuclear to cytoplasmic ratio, nuclear hyperchromasia and pleomorphism, and increasingly severe nuclear membrane abnormalities. The proliferation rate is also increased. The nuclear basophilia and the mitotic rate are increased, and mitoses are found in all layers of epithelium. The cellular features of CIS are similar to those of carcinoma, but the important difference is that there is no invasion through the basement membrane. Long-term smokers may have multiple CIS lesions in their airways. It is also common to find several foci of dysplasia outside the tumor in lungs resected for lung cancer. The lag time between the development of CIS and invasive cancer is not known.

Recent studies have linked mutations in the genes regulating the growth and differentiation process with the onset of invasion and one such gene, nm23, has attracted attention.[48] In murine cancer models, high expression of nm23 was associated with low metastatic potential, whereas low expressions of nm23 was associated with high metastatic potential. In human breast cancer, the nm23 levels were highest in tumors that had three or fewer metastases and uniformly low in tumors with extensive nodal involvement.[49] It is not clear, however, if these findings apply to other tumors.

## CLASSIFICATION OF LUNG TUMORS

Histologic and cytologic features of lung carcinomas depend on the degree of differentiation. In other words, the more the cancer cell resembles its benign counterpart, the higher the degree of differentiation. The degree of differentiation may vary considerably within any given tumor. Roggli et al[50] reported that 45% of 100 consecutive lung cancers had mixed histologic pattern by light microscopic examination when the tumor was carefully sampled. Immunopathologic studies similarly reveal mixed differentiation patterns in more than half of the cases if the tumors are thoroughly studied.

The World Health Organization Histologic Classification of Lung Tumors separates primary lung tumors into usual and rare tumors.[51] Usual tumors account for 95% of all primary neoplasms, and this group consists of seven histologic types (Table 21–1).

## STAGING OF LUNG CANCER

The tumor, nodes, and metastases (TNM) staging system is widely used to assess the extent of disease and to evaluate

**TABLE 21–1. CLASSIFICATION OF LUNG TUMORS**

| Bronchogenic Carcinoma | Proportion of Bronchogenic Carcinomas (%) |
|---|---|
| Squamous cell carcinoma | 30–50 |
| Well differentiated | |
| Moderately differentiated | |
| Poorly differentiated | |
| Adenocarcinoma | 15–35 |
| Well differentiated | |
| Poorly differentiated | |
| Bronchioloalveolar | |
| Large cell undifferentiated carcinoma | 10–15 |
| Undifferentiated | |
| Giant cell | |
| Clear cell | |
| Small cell undifferentiated carcinoma | 20–25 |
| Oat cell type | |
| Intermediate cell type | |
| Combined squamous and adenocarcinoma | 1.5 |

resectability, assess prognosis, plan treatment, and evaluate therapeutic outcomes.

The American Joint Committee for Cancer Staging and End Results Reporting (AJC) and the Union Internationale Contre Cancer (UICC) have accepted a staging nomenclature that is currently used almost universally.[52] Details are given elsewhere in this volume, but the following summary is provided to facilitate description of pulmonary pathology:

### Primary Tumor (T)

- TX: Tumor proven by the presence of malignant cells in secretions, but not localized
- T0: No evidence of primary tumor
- TIS: Carcinoma in situ
- T1: Tumor <3.0 cm in greatest diameter without evidence of invasion proximal to a lobar bronchus
- T2: Tumor >3.0 cm in greatest diameter that is >2 cm from the carina, tumor of any size that has invaded the visceral pleura, or tumor of any size associated with atelectasis or obstructive pneumonia that extends to the hilar region but involves less than the entire lung *and* that is not associated with a malignant pleural effusion
- T3: Tumor of any size with direct extension into contiguous structures, e.g., chest wall without invasion of the heart, great vessels, trachea, esophagus, or vertebral body *or* tumor involving a main bronchus <2.0 cm distal to the tracheal carina but not involving the carina
- T4: Tumor that involves the mediastinum, heart, great vessels, trachea, esophagus, or vertebral body *or* tumor associated with a malignant pleural effusion

### Nodal Involvement (N)

- N0: No demonstrable metastasis to regional lymph nodes
- N1: Metastasis or extension to ipsilateral hilar lymph nodes
- N2: Metastasis to ipsilateral mediastinal or subcarinal lymph nodes
- N3: Metastasis to contralateral, scalene, or supraclavicular lymph nodes

### Distant Metastasis (M)

- MX: Not assessed
- M0: No known distant metastasis
- M1: Distant metastasis present

### Lung Cancer Stages Based on These TNM Characteristics

- Occult carcinoma: TX N0 M0
- Stage 0: TIS N0 M0
- Stage I: T1 N0 M0; T2 N0 M0
- Stage II: T1 N1 M0: T2 N1 M0
- Stage IIIA: T3 N0–1, M0; T1–3 N2 M0
- Stage IIIB: Any T N3 M0; T4 any N M0
- Stage IV: Any T any N M1

## SQUAMOUS CELL CARCINOMA

About 90% of squamous cell carcinomas arise in segmental or larger bronchi, and 10% are peripheral in the lung in small bronchi. These tumors characteristically appear as fungating gray, white, or yellow, slow-growing masses. They grow endobronchially and invade the peribronchial soft tissue, lung parenchyma, and adjacent lymph nodes (Fig. 21–3A). The pulmonary artery and vein are often compressed. Endobronchial tumor growth results in secondary changes in the distal lung such as atelectasis, bronchopneumonia, obstructive pneumonia, lipoid pneumonia, and organizing pneumonia.

Central squamous cell carcinomas can often be diagnosed by sputum cytology, and a definitive diagnosis by bronchoscopy is usually possible using bronchial brushing and washing as well as bronchoscopic biopsy as part of this technique. Squamous cell carcinoma was the most common neoplasm detected under the National Cancer Institute-sponsored early detection program.[53] TX lesions that were eventually found or lesions that recurred were frequently multicentric, and multicentricity was a common reason for ultimate treatment failure despite early detection.

Squamous cell carcinomas of the lung typically spread and metastasize within the thorax with involvement of hilar and mediastinal lymph nodes, pleura, diaphragm, and contralateral lung. Metastasis to extrathoracic sites, including liver, adrenals, kidneys, and central nervous system, occur

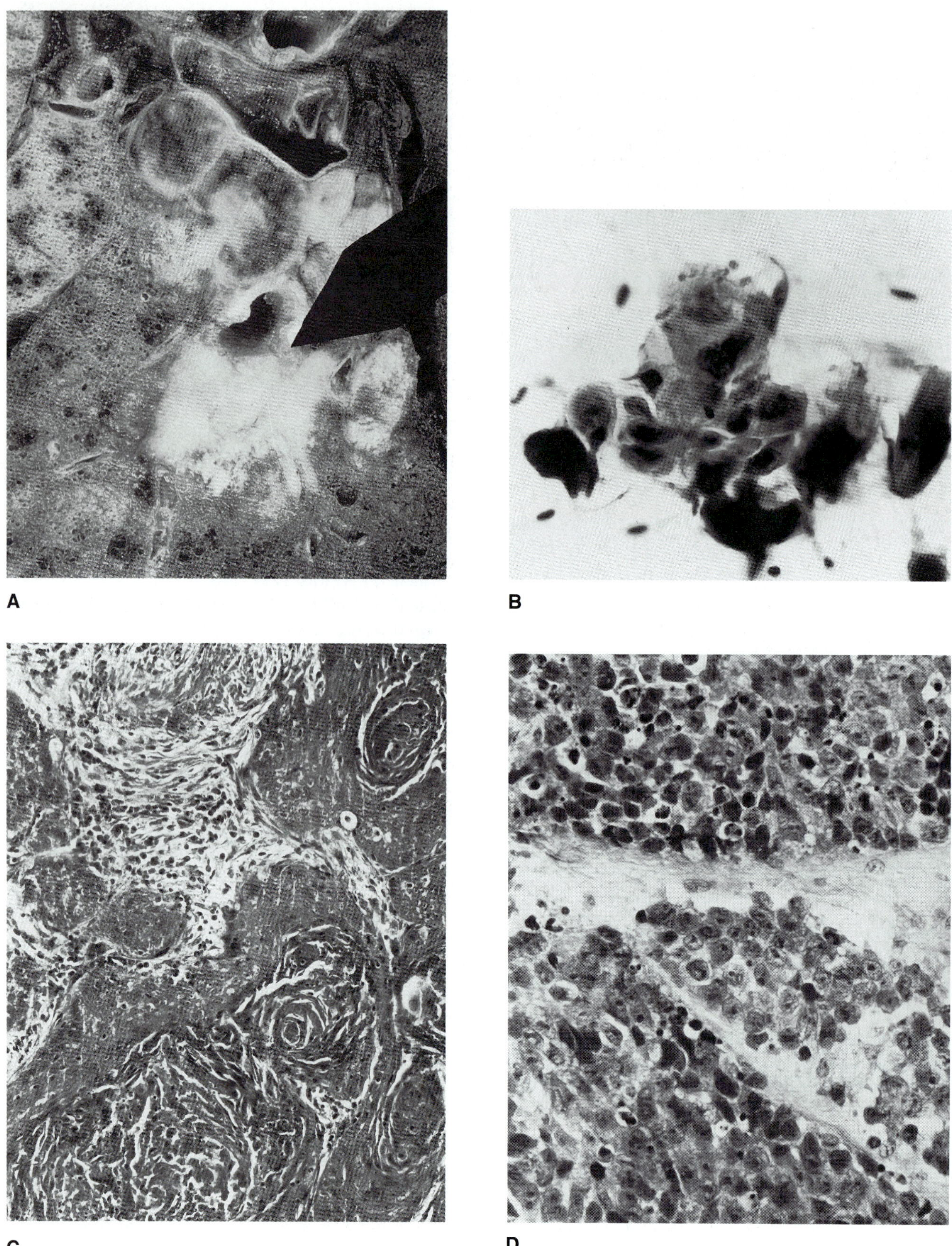

**Figure 21–3.** *Squamous cell carcinoma.* **A.** Infiltrating squamous cell carcinoma arising in a mainstem bronchus. Note tumor invasion into hilar lymph nodes. **B.** Well-differentiated keratinizing squamous cell carcinoma. Fine-needle aspiration biopsy of a peripheral lung mass. Papanicolaou-stained smear, 238×. **C.** Well-differentiated infiltrating squamous cell carcinoma. Note intracytoplasmic keratinization and keratin "pearls." H&E, 136×. **D.** Poorly differentiated infiltrating squamous cell carcinoma. The N:C ratio is increased, and there are many mitoses and foci of necrosis. H&E, 360×. *(Continued.)*

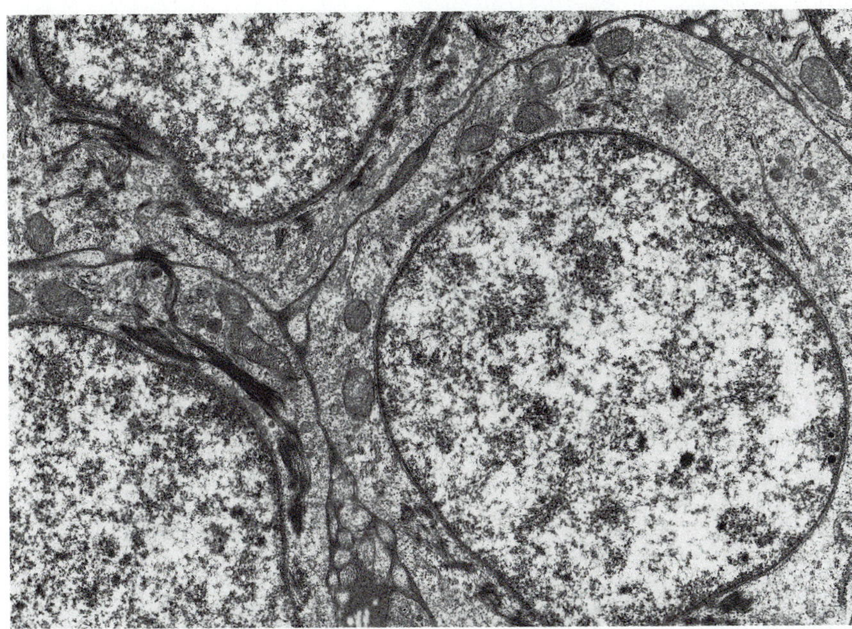

E

**Figure 21–3.** *(Continued.)* **E.** Transmission electron micrograph of squamous cell carcinoma. Note desmosomes and tonofilaments. TEM, 3960×.

only in 20–25% of well- and moderately differentiated tumors.[54] In spite of pleural involvement in approximately one third of the cases, it is not common to see squamous cancer cells in pleural effusions.

We nearly always perform bronchoscopy before mediastinoscopy or thoracotomy, in part to ascertain that there has been no change since previous examination by another observer and in part to evaluate the potential site of bronchial transection.

Peripheral squamous cell carcinomas are often well differentiated, and they have a tendency to form large pools of keratin and may cavitate. They are often synchronous with cancers of the head and neck.[55] In our experience it may be impossible to distinguish a peripherally located, well-differentiated primary squamous cell carcinoma from a solitary metastasis from the head and neck area by available techniques. The prognosis is very poor for patients who have upper airway cancer and lung cancer when the lung cancer is symptomatic, but cure can be achieved if the lung cancer is asymptomatic and in stages I or II. We use segmentectomy as the resection method, because patients with upper and lower airway cancers often have impaired respiratory function and are at high risk for additional metastatic or primary lung cancer.

Superior sulcus carcinomas, with or without Horner's syndrome, are curable in about 35% of the cases if they are in stage IIIA (T3N0M0).[56] The pervious belief that superior sulcus neoplasms were always squamous cell carcinomas has proved incorrect. Adenocarcinomas are almost as common as squamous cell cancers in this location. Because cures are rarely if ever achieved when there are any lymphatic metastases indicating systemic disease, we believe that superior sulcus cancers that are stage IIIB should be entered into induction therapy protocols or treated primarily to achieve palliation.

### Histologic Features

Well-differentiated squamous cell carcinoma (Fig. 21–3B,C) is composed of cells that have keratinized; "glassy" cytoplasm, and oval, elongated, often angular nuclei that show "margination" of chromatin in histologic sections. The nuclei often contain multiple nucleoli. Intercellular bridges are evident, and there are multiple keratin pearls. Moderately differentiated squamous cell carcinomas show less evidence of keratinization, but intercellular bridges can usually be found.

Poorly differentiated squamous cell carcinomas (Fig. 21–3D) have large, poorly differentiated cells. Intercellular bridges may be present but are not obvious, and cells with cytoplasmic keratinization may be difficult to find. Mitoses are common, and the tumor frequently contains necrotic areas. Immunocytochemical studies are helpful in establishing a correct diagnosis and characteristically reveal high molecular weight cytokeratin in the tumor cell cytoplasm in a typical granular perinuclear pattern. Electron-microscopic studies reveal tonofilaments and desmosomes (Fig. 21–3E).

## ADENOCARCINOMA

The incidence of adenocarcinoma is increasing in both women and men. It is the most common type of lung cancer in women in the United States and the most common lung tumor in Japan in both sexes.[57] Approximately 30% of adenocarcinomas arise in the surface epithelium and submu-

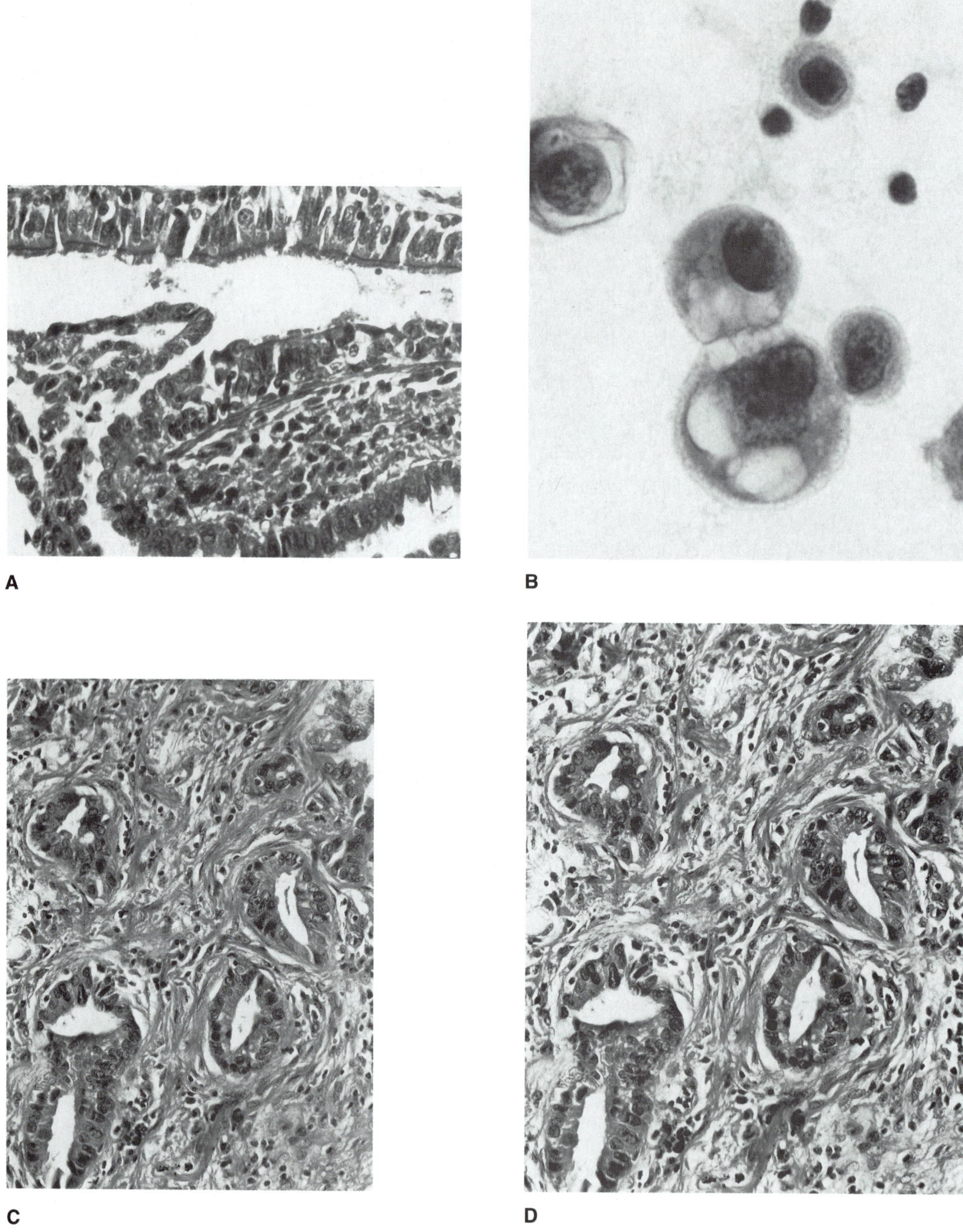


**Figure 21–4.** *Adenocarcinoma.* **A.** Columnar cell atypia in bronchial epithelium adjacent to a papillary adenocarcinoma arising in a bronchial wall. H&E, 297×. (see color slides.) **B.** Mucin secreting adenocarcinoma cells in pleural fluid. Papanicolaou stain, 429×. **C.** FNA biopsy of a peripheral lung mass shows preservation of the acinar configuration. Papanicolaou-stained smear, 520×. **D.** Typical adenocarcinoma. Note irregular glandular spaces and the fibrotic stroma with lymphocytic infiltration. H&E, 320×. *(Continued.)*

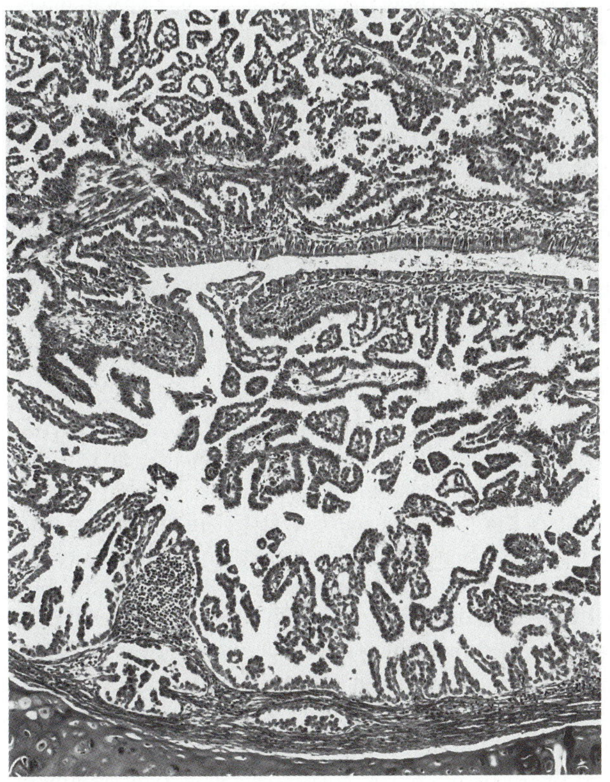

E

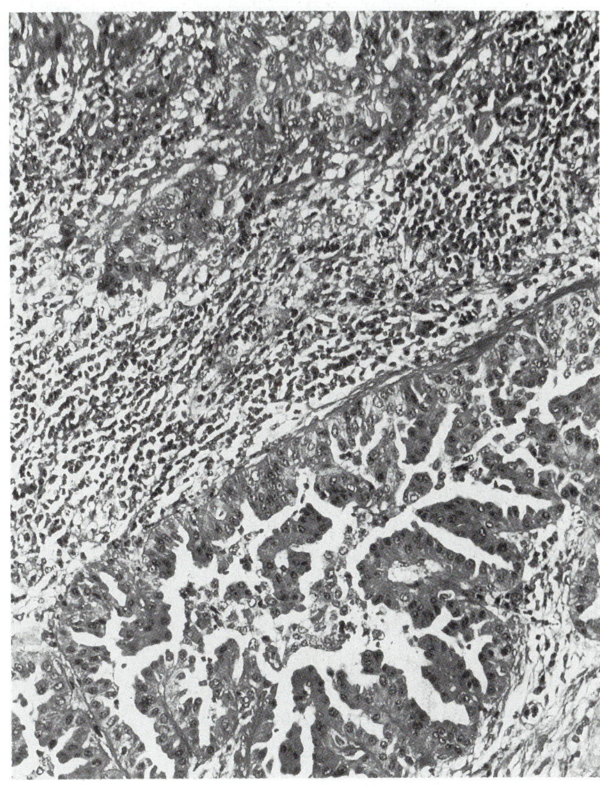

F

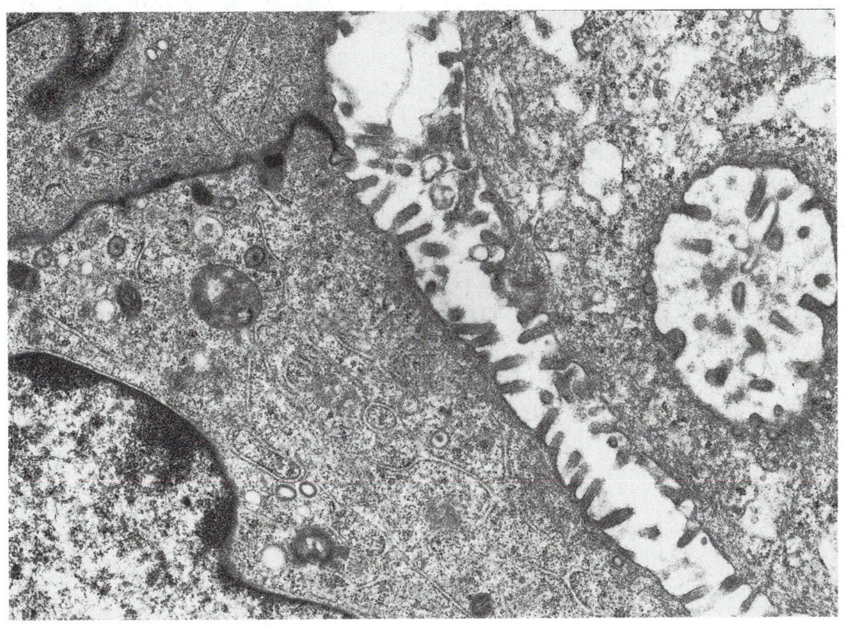

G

**Figure 21–4.** *(Continued.)* **E.** Papillary adenocarcinoma arising in a bronchial wall. H&E, 80×. **F.** Adenocarcinoma with a well-differentiated papillary and a poorly differentiated solid pattern. Note the stroma with dense lymphoid infiltrates. H&E, 136×. **G.** Transmission electron micrograph of an adenocarcinoma. Note short, stubby microvilli, intracytoplasmic lumen, and a junctional complex (J). TEM, 5082×.

cosal glands of bronchi, which are smaller than those in which squamous cell carcinoma arise. Atypia and dysplasia are commonly present in the adjacent epithelium (Fig. 21–4A). Some electron-microscopic surveys of adenocarcinomas suggest that a cell resembling the nonciliated bronchiolar epithelial cell (Clara cell) may be the common cell of origin for any type of adenocarcinoma. The tumor appears characteristically as a hard gray or white mass in the periphery of the lung covered by fibrotic, puckered pleura. Extensive necrosis can occur, but cavitation is rare. Adenocarcinomas typically elicit a desmoplastic (fibrotic) response. These tumors grow more rapidly than squamous cell carcinomas, and they metastasize readily. Extrapulmonary metastases to mediastinal, periaortic, axillary, supraclavicular, and neck lymph nodes are more common in adenocarcinoma than in squamous cell carcinoma. Pleural involvement is common and leads usually to pleural effusion (Fig. 21–4B). More than 80% of the tumors present with extra thoracic mestastases, and adrenals, liver, bone, and brain are the most often involved organs.[54]

*Clinically,* the common type of bronchogenic adenocarcinoma is an asymptomatic masses in the lung periphery are more likely to be adenocarcinoma than another cancer. Such a lesion may be difficult to differentiate from metastatic cancer of extrathoracic origin. Chronic bronchitis with cough and postobstructive pneumonia usually without hemoptysis may be manifestations of adenocarcinomas, even if they are in the lung periphery. Fine-needle aspiration (FNA) (Fig. 21–4C) is probably the most common method of diagnosis. Occult metastases in the mediastinal lymph nodes, liver, and brain account for many of the treatment failures. However, routine preoperative brain scanning in asymptomatic lung cancer patients without neurologic findings is not recommended because of the low cost:benefit ratio.

Differential diagnosis between primary and metastatic pulmonary adenocarcinoma may be difficult, even with special staining methods and electron microscopy. Any symptoms or findings that may lead to the discovery of an extrathoracic primary cancer should be vigorously pursued. However, search for an extrapulmonary primary in asymptomatic patients without abnormal findings is generally not useful and therefore not recommended. Molecular biologic methods promise to assist in this aspect of diagnosis, as illustrated by our finding of different methylation patterns when histologically similar primary and metastatic adenocarcinomas were compared using restriction enzymatic methods.[58]

### Histologic Features

The acinar subtype is the most common, but papillary and solid mucin-producing adenocarcinomas also occur, and most adenocarcinomas show more than one histologic pattern. Figure 21–4 shows some of the characteristic microscopic features of adenocarcinoma. Well-differentiated adenocarcinomas are composed of well-formed glands surrounded by a variable amount of fibrotic stroma. Columnar or cuboidal tumor cells have round or oval, sometimes vesicular, nuclei and prominent acidophilic nucleoli. The tumor cell cytoplasm may be vacuolated indicating mucin production.

In moderately differentiated adenocarcinomas, the gland formation is less obvious but still recognizable. The cytoplasmic and nuclear features are similar to those seen in the well-differentiated adenocarcinomas, except that there is more nuclear atypia.

Poorly differentiated adenocarcinomas have no well-formed glands. The nuclei are vesicular with well-defined nuclear membranes and prominent acidophilic nucleoli. Mucin stains may show the presence of cytoplasmic mucin droplets or highlight the glycocalyx. Immunocytochemical studies reveal low molecular weight cytokeratin, mucin, or special secretory products. Electron microscopy reveals junctional complexes and tight junctions. Microvilli, intracellular lumens, and secretory vesicles are also helpful features in identification of adenocarcinomas (Fig. 21–4G).

## BRONCHOALVEOLAR (BRONCHIOLAR) CARCINOMA

The incidence of bronchoalveolar (bronchiolar) carcinoma (BAC) has increased worldwide during the past few years.[57] Between 1978 and 1989, the incidence of bronchoalveolar carcinoma more than doubled from 9.3% to 20.3%. A study of lung cancer cases among nonsmokers and former smokers showed a decrease of large airway and an increase of peripheral carcinomas. BAC is equally common in men and women, although in some series, 75% of BACs are diagnosed in women.[59] It almost always arises in the periphery of the lung in the terminal bronchoalveolar region and tends to be multicentric at the time of diagnosis. It may present radiographically with pneumonia-like infiltrates rather than a mass. BAC starts as a local nodule or infiltrate and frequently appears unchanged for years. Because of this, BAC may be misdiagnosed as scar, tuberculosis, lung impact, or chronic pneumonia. BAC frequently arises in a field of alveolar hyperplasia or adjacent to alveolar hyperplasia atypia. Care must be taken to not diagnose the latter two entities as BAC. The relationship between BAC and smoking is debated, and the increased incidence has been attributed by some to the increasing atmospheric pollution.

It is a misconception that this kind of cancer is less aggressive and less likely to metastasize than other forms of non-small cell lung cancer (NSCLC). In our experience, bronchorrhea has been rare. Because bronchiolar cancer cells line the alveoli (Fig. 21–5), progressive respiratory failure may be the end stage of this disease. Accordingly, we favor segmentectomy as the treatment of choice for bronchiolar carcinoma whenever this operation will result in complete removal and cancer-free margins of resection.

### Histologic Features

BAC is a subtype of adenocarcinoma and nonciliated Clara cells, and type II pneumocytes are the cells of origin. The tumor cells grow along intact alveolar septa in lepidic (from lepidoptera), a so-called growth pattern, and may form papillary projections into the alveolar spaces. Three morphologically different cell types are recognized: (1) well-differentiated, tall columnar cells with basally located nuclei and abundant clear cytoplasm; (2) tall columnar cells with cytoplasmic caps in a "hobnail" pattern; and (3) cuboidal cells with granular cytoplasm. Intranuclear inclusions are often

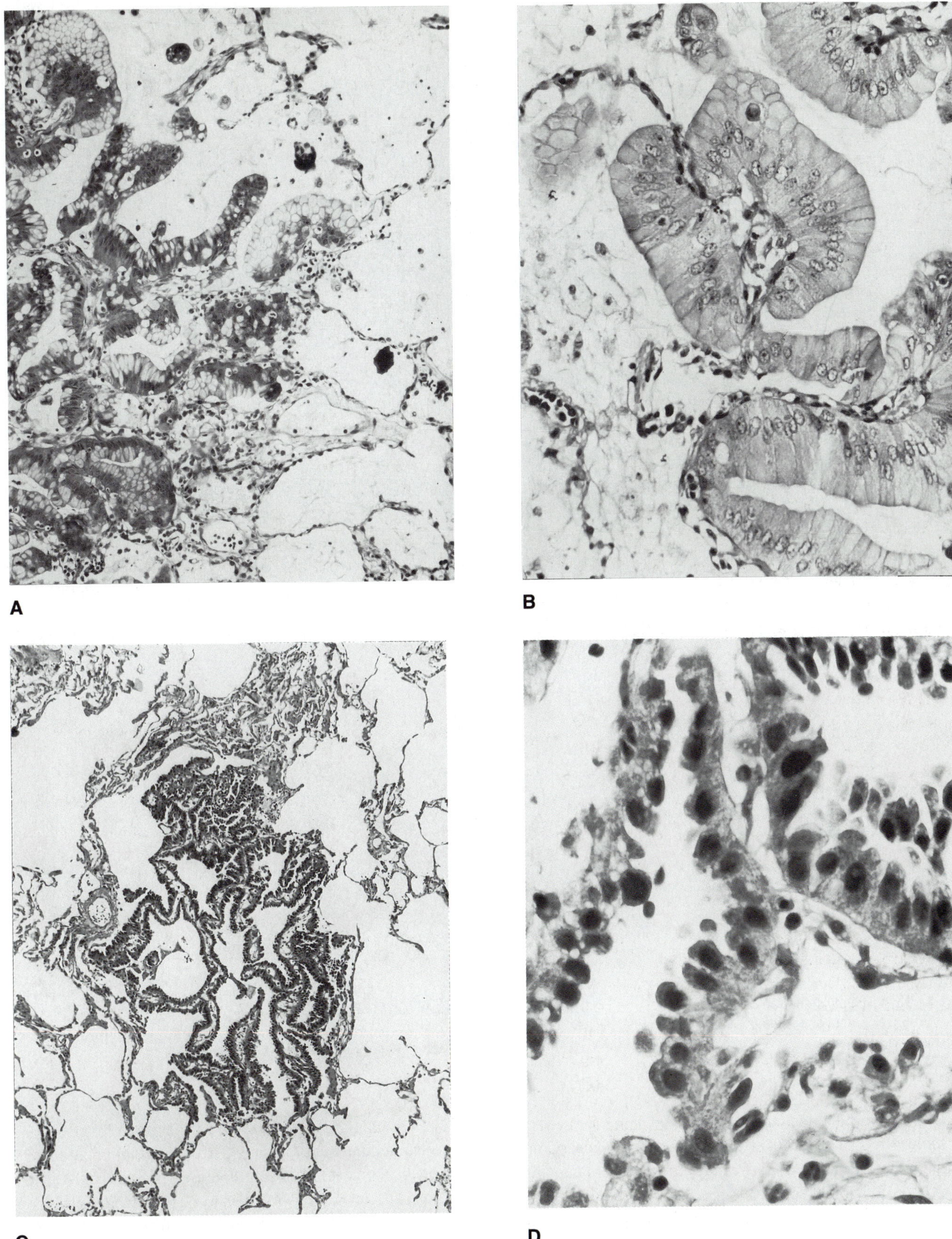

**Figure 21–5.** *Bronchioloalveolar (bronchiolar) carcinoma,* a subtype of adenocarcinoma. **A.** The tumor cells grow along intact, slightly thickened alveolar septa. Note small groups of tumor cells floating in the alveoli outside the tumor margin. H&E, 136×. **B.** Note well-differentiated, tall columnar tumor cells with large amount of cytoplasm. H&E, 320×. **C.** This cancer, found outside of the main tumor seen in Figure 21–4A, B, has different cellular morphology and represents a separate primary neoplastic focus. The severe nuclear atypia and mitosis warrant the diagnosis of carcinoma rather than dysplasia. H&E, 80×. **D.** Note the secretory "caps" in the apex of the tumor cells. H&E, 320×. *(Continued.)*

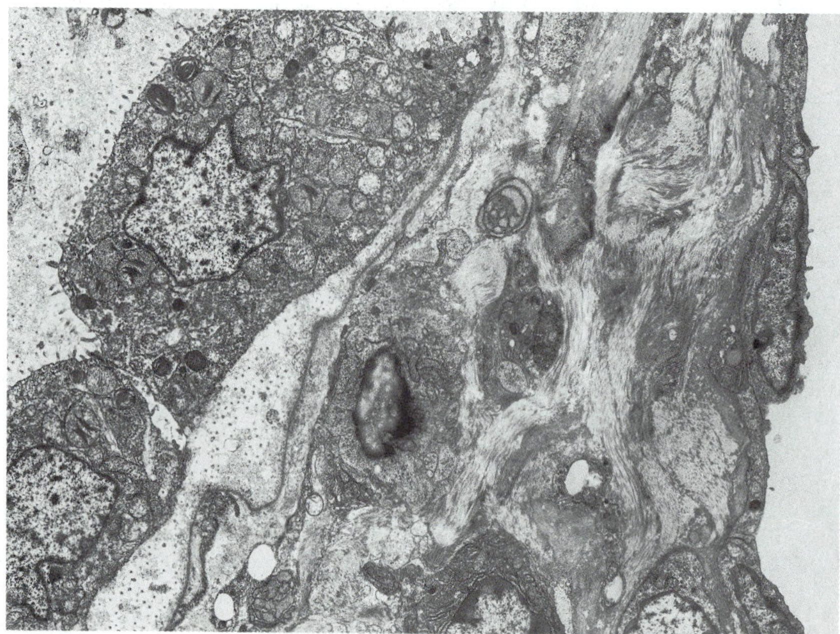

E

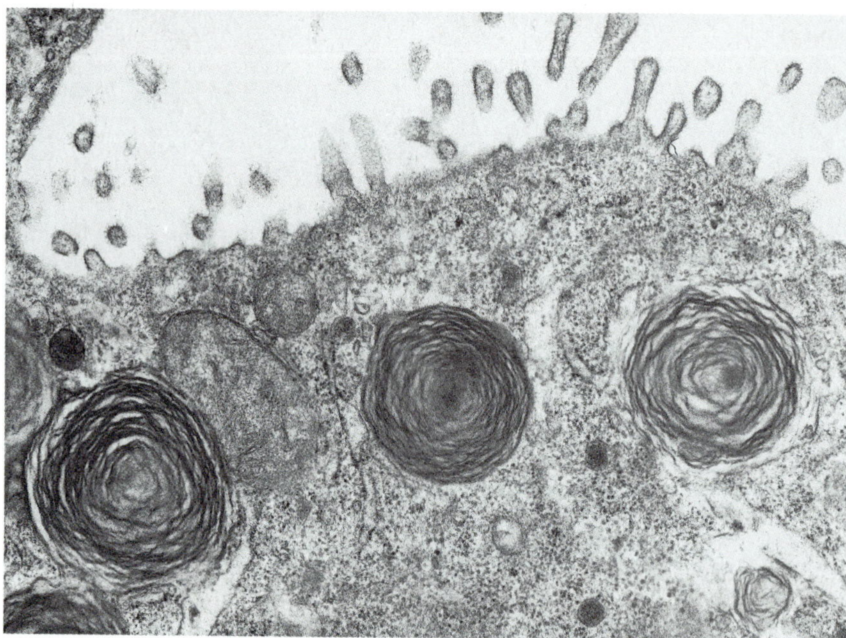

F

**Figure 21–5.** *(Continued.)* **E.** Transmission electron micrograph. The fibrotic alveolar wall contains inflammatory cells, fibrinoblasts, and collagen. It is lined on the left side by cancer cells and on the right side by benign type I cells. Note lamellar bodies and short, stubby microvilli in the tumor cells. TEM, 1089×. **F.** Lamellar bodies, a source of surfactant. TEM, 8250×.

found. Mucin production can sometimes be demonstrated in the tumor cells, and electron micrographs reveal lamellar bodies in the cytoplasm of particularly those tumors that are composed of cuboidal cells.

## LARGE CELL UNDIFFERENTIATED CARCINOMA

Large cell undifferentiated tumors are bulky, soft gray, tan, or pink masses, usually with extensive necrosis. Approximately 50% of large cell cancers arise in subsegmental or larger bronchi, i.e., this location of large cell cancers is less frequent than that of squamous cell carcinoma but more frequent than that of adenocarcinomas. Approximately 50% of these cancers are peripheral and subpleural in location and macroscopically indistinguishable from adencarcinomas.

*Clinically,* these cancers are aggressive and grow rapidly. Patients often have stage III or stage IV lesions at time of presentation, and lesions in stage II tend to be <3 cm (T2). Large cell undifferentiated cancers have a very poor prognosis.

### Histologic Features

Undifferentiated large cell carcinomas (Fig. 21–6) are composed of round to ovoid, polygonal, or spindle-shaped cells with irregular, pleomorphic nuclei and big nucleoli. The tumor cells grow in sheets without organization or pattern. There is no evidence of maturation toward squamous cell or adenocarcinoma by light microscopy. Necroses and hemorrhage may be prominent features of the tumor.

The giant cell variant is composed of very large, polygonal, or spindle-shaped cells with bizarre, sometimes multiple nuclei that contain prominent nucleoli. Nuclear inclusions are sometimes noted.

The clear cell variant has the same anaplastic features described earlier and in addition has abundant clear cytoplasm. With immunohistochemistry and electron microscopy, most undifferentiated large cell carcinomas can be shown to have features of squamous carcinoma or adenocarcinoma or both. There is a small subset of tumors that truly shows no differentiating characteristics.

## COMBINATION CARCINOMAS

A thorough examination of multiple samples from any given cancer reveals evidence of a variation of histologic pattern and cell type at least 45–50% of the time. When immunohistochemical and electron microscopic studies are performed, the proportion of combination tumors is even greater. Adenocarcinoma with squamous carcinoma is the most common combination (Fig. 21–7), but virtually any combination can occur.

From the clinical viewpoint, it is appropriate to expect a given cancer to behave like the most malignant portion of the neoplasm. For example, if an adenocarcinoma contains elements of large cell undifferentiated carcinoma, the cancer will likely be as highly malignant as a relatively pure large cell neoplasm. An important variety of combination cancer consists of elements of large cell undifferentiated and SCLC; the latter variety should generally be treated as if it were SCLC in a more pure form.

## SCAR CARCINOMA

About one third of adenocarcinomas and one fifth of squamous cell carcinomas have sufficient scar tissue to raise the question of whether the cancer arose in preexisting scar or whether the scar formation was part of a desmoplastic response to the cancer cells. Approximately 50% of scar carcinomas are associated with healed infarcts or arrested granulomatous lesions, and about 25% are seen with miscellaneous scars, e.g., pneumoconiosis, posttraumatic scar, fibrosis secondary to foreign bodies, or idiopathic scarring.

*Clinically,* scar carcinoma is found most often in the upper lobes. It is a diagnostic challenge in at least two ways: (1) the radiographic appearance of a scar from a known and arrested inflammatory lesion such as treated tuberculosis may change slightly; the question is whether or not excision of a long-standing scar is indicated; or (2) a fine-needle aspirate of a new pulmonary mass reveals scar tissue and no malignant cells and creates the classic dilemma of representative vs. nonrepresentative sample. The concern is that they may be an adjacent focus of carcinoma.

## NEUROENDOCRINE (KULCHITSKY CELL) CARCINOMAS

The evolution of terminology that has been applied within the past five decades to this group of neoplasms reflects increasing understanding of their clinical behavior and accumulated knowledge about their morphologic, immunohistochemical, and cytogenetic characteristics. An important first step was recognition of *atypical carcinoid* as an aggressive variant of *typical carcinoid.*[60] Next came the recognition that there were biochemical indicators of these tumors when they were included with other neoplasms that were included within the amine precursor uptake derivative (APUD) spectrum.[47] This included the first evidence that total DNA content (ploidy) correlates at least to some degree with the relative aggressiveness of variants within this group of cancers. The label *neuroendocrine tumors* was applied as a result of detailed studies of the ultrastructure and immunohistochemical properties of this group of cancers.[61] Shortly thereafter, the term *Kulchitsky cell carcinoma* (KCC) was initiated.[62] The *KCC nomenclature* was intended to highlight a common cell of origin among cancers in this group and to recognize evidence from long-term follow-up studies that showed that nearly 10% of patients thought to have had carcinoid eventually proved to have had *small cell undifferentiated carcinoma* (SCLC) of the lung. Consistent with this concept is the notion that SCLC is a genetic variant of carcinoid. An excellent, relatively recent summary of the various terminologies that have been applied to this group of neoplasms was provided by Travis et al.[63]

### Carcinoid, Typical (KCC I), and Atypical (KCC II)

Three to five percent of all lung tumors are carcinoids (KCC I and II). They are not associated with smoking, and there is no sex difference in incidence. The cell of origin is the neuroendocrine (Kulchitsky) cell of the bronchial mucosa. Electron microscopic examination reveals dense core granules in the cytoplasm of the tumor cells (Fig. 21–8F). Carcinoids secrete hormonally active polypeptides that can be identified by immunohistochemical methods and may occur alone or as a component of multiple endocrine neoplasia syndrome. Ninety percent of carcinoids are *central* and arise in main, lobar, or segmental bronchi and grow in a

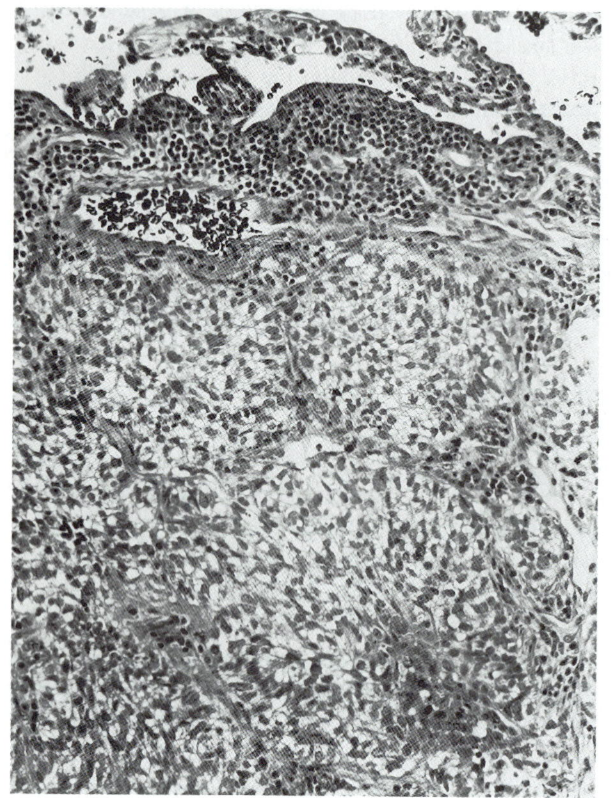

A

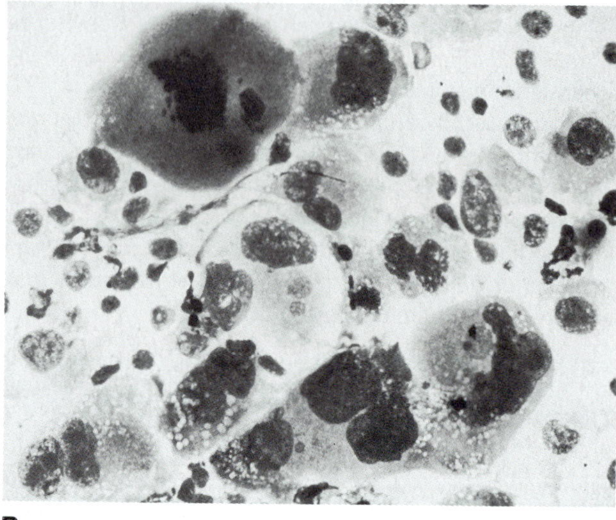

B

C

**Figure 21–6.** *Large cell undifferentiated carcinoma.* **A.** The clear cell variant. Note that gland formation or cytoplasmic keratinization is not evident by light microscopy. There are dense lymphocytic infiltrates surrounding the tumor and in the adjacent alveolar walls. H&E, 136×. **B.** The giant cell variant has large, bizarre, multinucleated cells and abundant cytoplasm. H&E, 136×. **C.** Transmission electron-microscopic features of junctional complexes (J), microvilli (M), and intracytoplasmic lumina (L) are consistent with adenocarcinoma. TEM, 5082×.

polypoid, exophytic manner, projecting into the bronchial lumen (Fig. 21–8A—see Color Plates following page XXX). Ten percent of carcinoids are *peripheral* with no apparent connection to bronchi.

Carcinoid appears macroscopically as a smooth, bosselated, well-vascularized, fleshy unencapsulated endobronchial mass (Fig. 21–8B). Central carcinoids are covered by an intact bronchial mucosa and usually grow slowly (Fig. 21–8C). Most tumors measure 2–4 cm in diameter at the time of diagnosis. Approximately 5% of carcinoids metastasize, usually to regional lymph nodes, but distant metastases to liver and bone and elsewhere may occur.

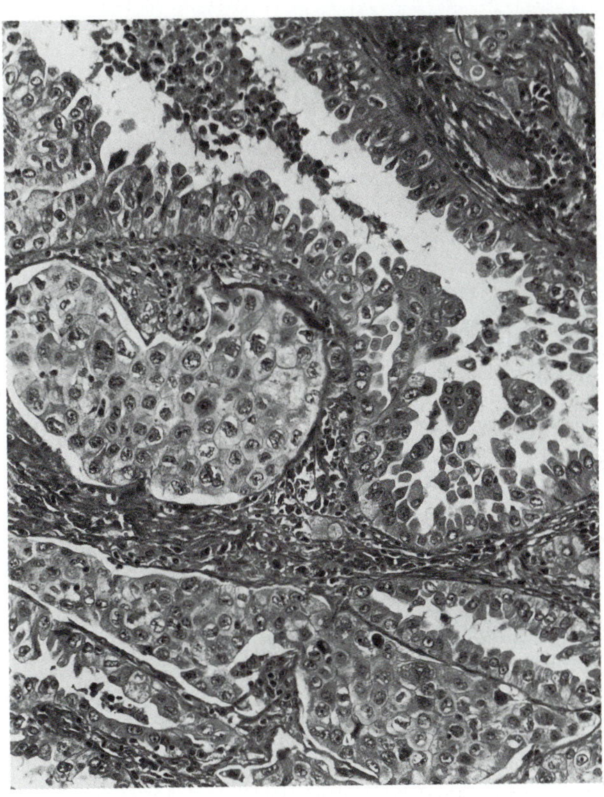

A

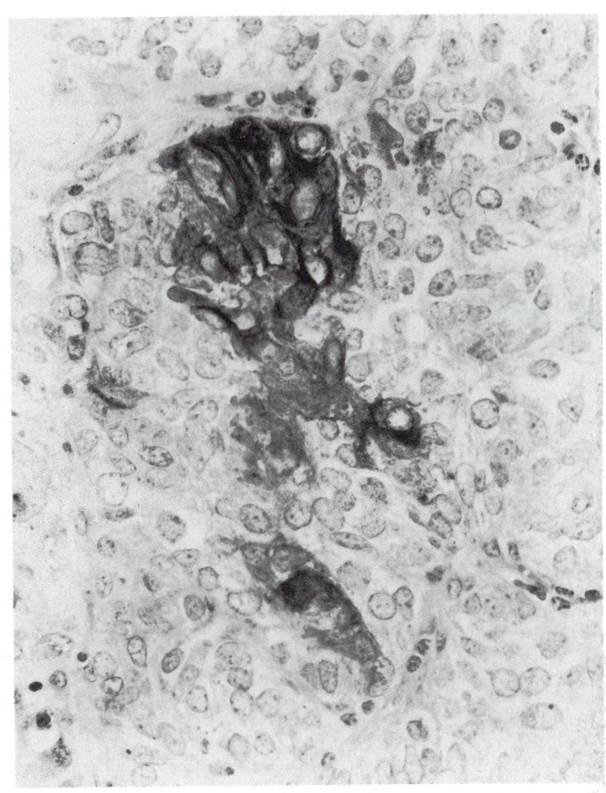

B

**Figure 21–7.** *Combination carcinoma.* **A.** Both squamous and glandular differentiation are present. H&E, 136×. **B.** A group of cells on a field of poorly differentiated adenocarcinoma stains positively for high molecular weight cytokeratin indicating squamous differentiation. Dilute hematoxylin counterstain, 320×.

Large carcinoids (>4 cm) often have atypical histology, and 70% of T2–3 carcinoids develop metastases. It is noteworthy that perfectly benign histologic features may be associated with metastases.

*Clinically,* typical carcinoid (KCC I) has the least malignant behavior among neuroendocrine neoplasms and may manifest itself only with hemoptysis without an abnormal chest radiograph or obstructive pneumonia. A typical endobronchial neoplasm is seen at bronchoscopy (Fig. 21–8). Biopsy can almost always be safely done, and complete excision with a conservative resection is recommended. Sleeve resection is often useful for the purpose of preserving parenchyma, particularly when the neoplasm occurs in a mainstem bronchus. Endoscopic laser ablation is not recommended, because these neoplasms extend deep to the mucosa.

Typical carcinoid is a true cancer that will eventually metastasize and cause death; long-term follow-up has shown it rarely to be precursor of SCLC.[64] This low-grade cancer has an excellent prognosis (a 94–100% 5-year survival rate) with complete removal, often utilizing bronchoplastic reconstruction, and sleeve resections. *Carcinoid syndrome* occurs in less than 3% of patients.[62] Carcinoid crisis prompted by biopsy has been reported,[65] but generally neither this syndrome nor serious bleeding is a problem as the result of taking biopsies.

Atypical carcinoma is the most malignant form of carcinoid tumors. Stage 1 lesions are usually curable with complete but conservative resections. However, 46% of such lesions present with lymph node metastases in stages II or III, and nearly 20% of patients had M1 disease. We have treated and apparently cured bilateral atypical carcinoid; we and others have repeatedly experienced referral of patients with erroneous original diagnosis of SCLC who eventually proved to have atypical carcinoid.[64,66,67] The outcome of treatment for atypical carcinoma is stage related and similar to the outcome for NSCLC. In our experience, the mean survival time was 25 (0–47) months, with 27% of patients dying of their cancers. Chemotherapy for advanced disease is similar to that given for SCLC.

## Histologic Features

*Typical carcinoid (KCC I)* tumor (Fig. 21–8B–D) is composed of uniform cells with abundant eosinophilic cytoplasm. The tumor cells have round or oval, centrally placed nuclei with well-defined membranes and finely dispersed chromatin. Mitoses are absent or very rare. The tumor grows in

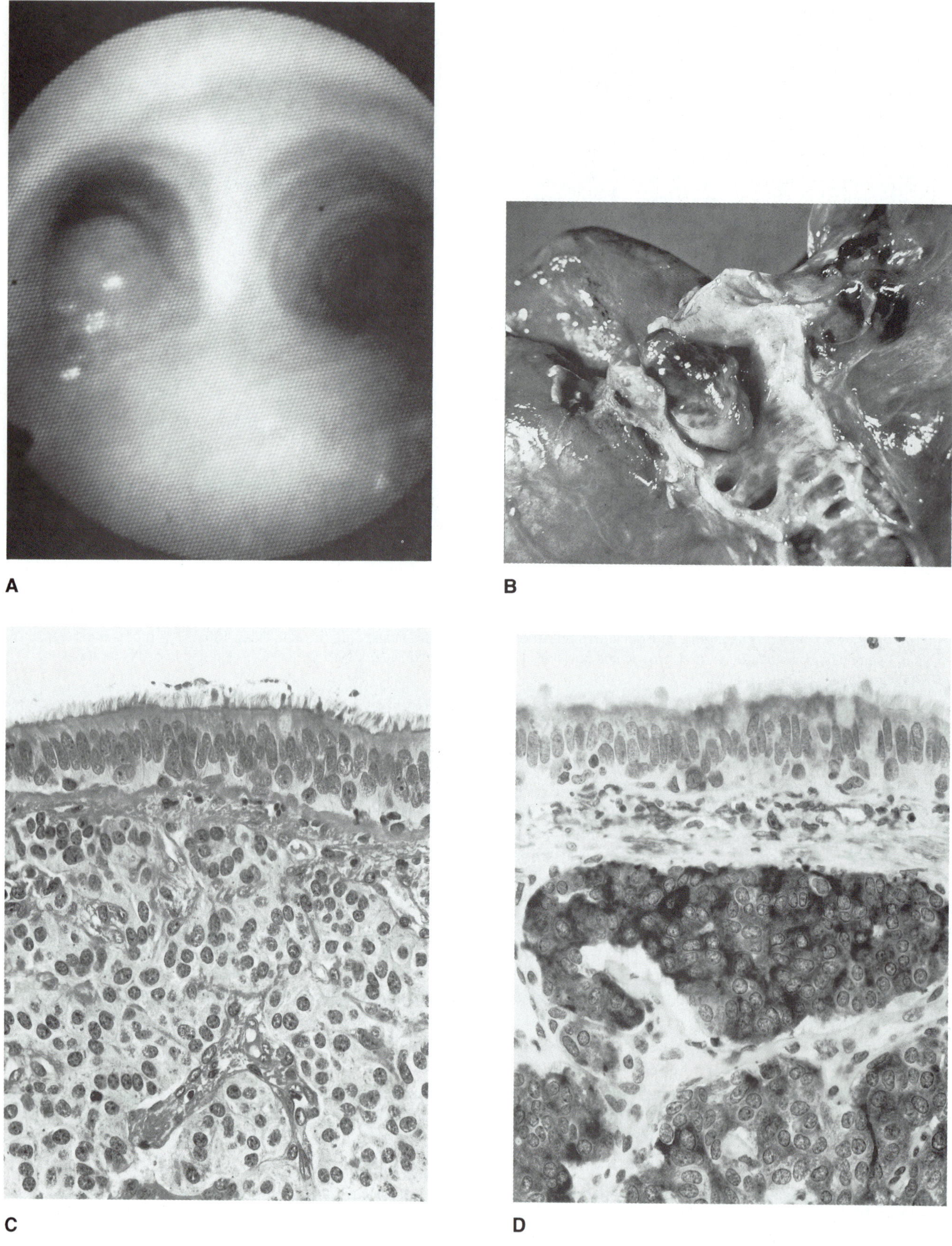


**Figure 21–8.** *Bronchial carcinoid* (KCC I). **A.** Typical tumor in left mainstem bronchus seen by bronchoscopy. (See also Color Plates, following page 608.)**B.** Macroscopic appearance of typical carcinoid. **C.** This exophytic tumor is covered by intact bronchial epithelium. The tumor cells have round uniform "endocrine" nuclei and abundant cytoplasm. H&E, 200×. **D.** The neoplastic cells are strongly positive for chromogranin-A. Dilute hematoxylin counterstain, 200×. *(Continued.)*

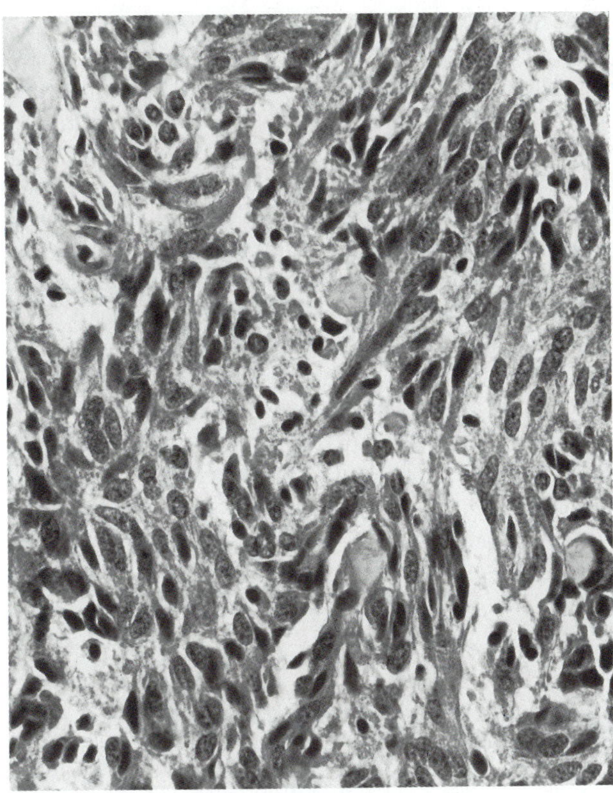

E

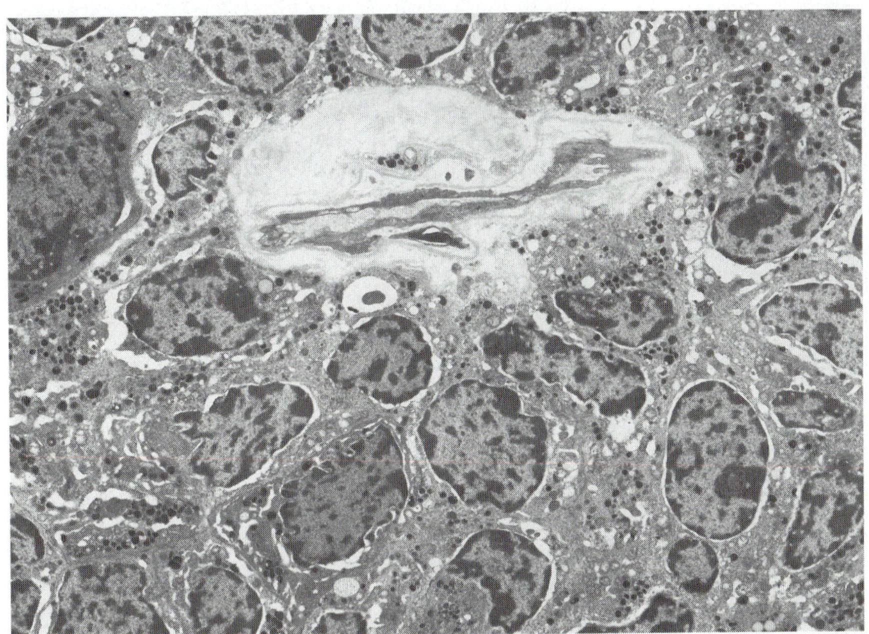

F

**Figure 21–8.** *(Continued.)* **E.** Atypical spindle cell carcinoid (KCC II). Note nuclear pleomorphism and small foci of necrosis. H&E, 160×. **F.** Transmission electron micrograph of typical carcinoid (KCC I). The tumor cells form a rosette-like structure and contain many dense core neurosecretory granules. TEM, 1089×.

a mosaic pattern composed of nests, cords, ribbons, and trabeculae separated by delicate fibrovascular stroma. Acinar arrangement is less common. Tumor stroma may undergo hyalinization and occasionally bony metaplasia. Mucus production may be present in areas with acinar configuration. Typical carcinoids are most often centrally located.

*Atypical carcinoids (KCC II)* comprise approximately 10% of carcinoids. The tumor cells have pleomorphic, large, hyperchromatic nuclei; frequent mitoses; and foci of necrosis. These tumors behave aggressively and metastasize to regional lymph nodes and systemically. Differential diagnosis between an atypical carcinoid and SCLC (KCC III) may be difficult sometimes, particularly if there is only cytologic material obtained by percutaneous fine-needle aspiration.

*Spindle cell carcinoid* (Fig. 21–8E) cells resemble neural or smooth muscle cells. The tumor cell nuclei are more pleomorphic, and mitoses are more frequent than in a typical carcinoid. Spindle cell carcinoids are more often peripherally located than typical carcinoids.

## Small Cell Undifferentiated Carcinoma

SCLC tumors arise from small basal cells of the bronchial epithelium and show neuroendocrine differentiation. Small cell carcinomas metastasize early and widely, so that clinical manifestations are frequently due to metastases rather than to the primary lesion. Even in the presence of extensive invasion, endobronchial changes may be minimal or absent. The tumor starts in the bronchial mucosa and extends centrifugally to involve the walls of bronchi, peribronchial spaces, and lung parenchyma. Hilar and mediastinal lymph nodes are enlarged and appear totally replaced by soft white or gray friable tissue. Invasion and obstruction of the superior vena cava is frequent. Bone marrow metastases are common. Treatment may cause SCLC to "mature" into squamous cell carcinoma. Instead of maturation, it seems likely to us that this transformation may come from therapy-induced complete remission of SCLC, leaving a residual of chemotherapy-resistant squamous cell carcinoma in cancers that were originally combination carcinomas.

*Clinically,* it may be treacherous to establish a definitive diagnosis of SCLC because of small tissue samples that characteristically have crush artefact (Fig. 21–9). Histologic and cytologic specimens may be difficult to interpret differentially from atypical carcinoid (neuroendocrine carcinoma, Kulchitsky cell carcinoma, grade 2, or from lymphoproliferative lesions). We and others have repeatedly cared for patients thought initially to have SCLC whose ultimate diagnosis proved to be KCC II (atypical carcinoid).[64,66,67]

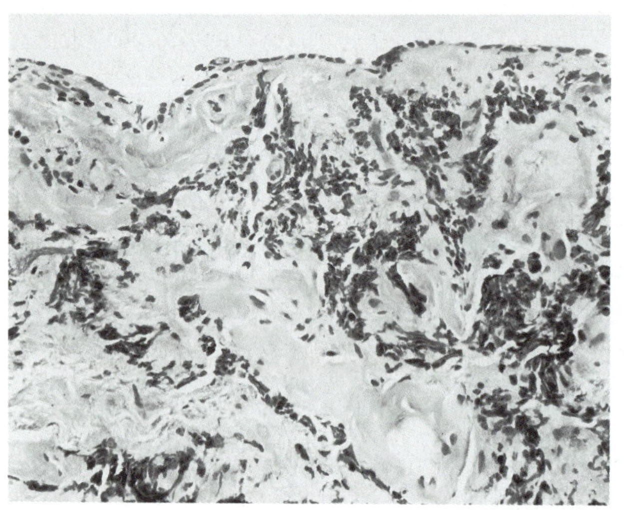

A

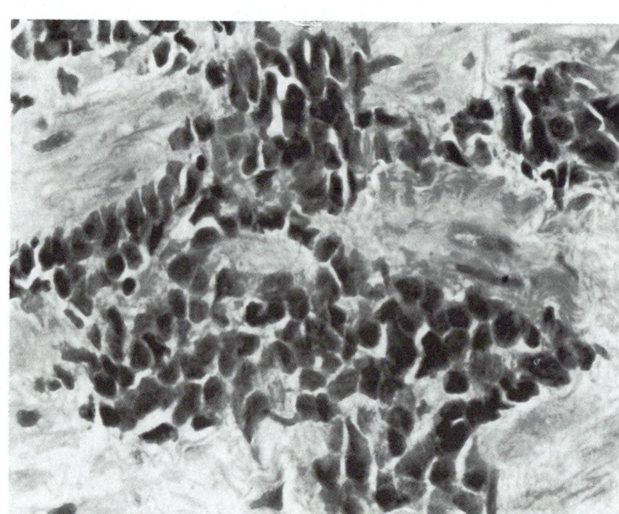

B

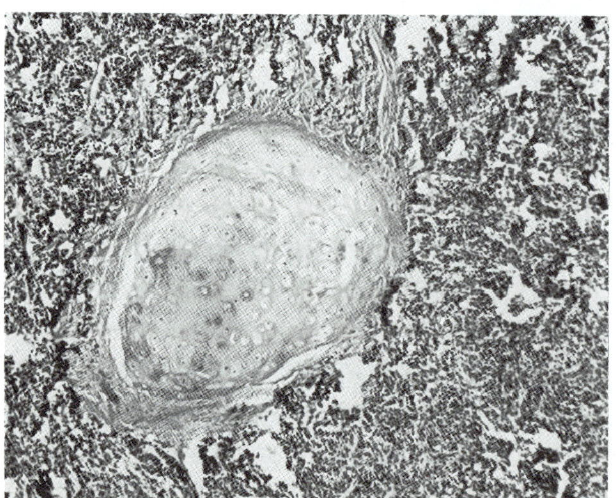

C

**Figure 21–9.** *Small cell undifferentiated carcinoma* (KCC III). **A.** The surface is covered by an intact, attenuated epithelium. Note the "diagnostic" crush artefact and "streaming" nuclei that are commonly noted in small bronchial biopsy samples. H&E, 109×. **B.** The cancer cells have small, hyperchromatic, "salt and pepper" nuclei that exhibit molding. The cytoplasm is scanty and poorly defined. H&E, 292×. **C.** Oat cell type completely destroying bronchial wall. H&E, 65×.

We have also had patients with neoplasms originally thought to be SCLC who ultimately were proved to have lymphoproliferative lesions. Never in the practice of oncology is it more important than with SCLC to *obtain adequate biopsy material to establish a secure diagnosis.*

Staging evaluation regularly includes imaging of the brain and bone marrow biopsy because SCLC is usually systemic. Despite controversy about the role of resection,[68,69] there is evidence that patients with SCLC, stage I, may be cured with resection plus adjuvant chemotherapy.[70] It seems likely that SCLC in stage II can only be cured when systemic therapy is added to a method of local control. There is currently insufficient evidence to recommend resection of SCLC in stage III.

### Histologic Features

The term *oat cell cancer* has been inappropriately used as a synonym for all SCLCs. The classic SCLC of the oat cell type has small lymphocyte-like fragile tumor cells with oval- to spindle-shaped nuclei that measure 1.5–2 times the diameter of a lymphocyte nucleus. Nucleoli are indistinct, and coarsely granular "salt and pepper" chromatin is a characteristic feature. Necrosis is common in this variety of SCLC. Immunohistochemical stains for one or more neuroendocrine markers (L-dopa decarboxylase, neuron-specific enolase, synaptophysin, chromogranin A, serotonin, creatine kinase, bombesin, calcitonin, and various pituitary and brain-gut peptide hormones) are characteristically positive. Some SCLCs are also positive for Leu-7, which stains natural killer cells. Electron microscopy reveals membrane-bound, dense-core secretory granules, 100–200 nm in diameter, poorly formed tonofilaments, and occasional desmosomes.

The intermediate cell type of SCLC is characterized by polygonal or spindle-shaped cells that are larger than oat cells. The nuclei measure less than three times the diameter of a lymphocyte nucleus, and nucleoli are indistinct. Usually a small amount of eosinophilic cytoplasm is present. Mitoses are more readily identified in this variety of SCLC than in the classic oat cell tumors.

The new histologic classification proposed by the Pathology Panel of the International Association for the Study of Lung Cancer[71] divides SCLC into three groups based partly on functional parameters such as enzyme and peptide hormone content and expression of oncogenes, and in part upon the degree of radiosensitivity of the neoplasms. The subdivisions are as follows: small cell carcinoma, pure; small cell carcinoma with large cell component; and combined small cell carcinoma.

### Large Cell Neuroendocrine Carcinoma (Intermediately Differentiated Neuroendocrine Carcinoma)

*Clinically,* we have most often encountered the diagnosis of large cell neuroendocrine carcinoma (LCNEC) after excision of the lesion, although it can also be made from biopsies taken during the process of staging. In our experience, such tumors have often been at least T2 in size, usually in at least stage II, and often in stage III or IV at the time of presentation. The prognosis of LCNEC is somewhere between that of atypical carcinoid (KCC II) and SCLC (KCC III).

### Histologic Features

Detailed study of this neoplasm has been made by Travis et al,[63] who used immunohistochemistry, electron microscopy, and flow cytometry extensively. In the final analysis they found no advantage over light microscopy from these modalities, except for the purpose of characterizing the neoplasms and demonstrating their neuroendocrine properties.

Light microscopy reveals a high-grade carcinoma with neuroendocrine appearance. The tumor cells are large and polygonal in shape and arranged in a trabecular or insular pattern (Fig. 21–10B). The cells have abundant cytoplasm, and the nuclei contain coarse chromatin and prominent nucleoli. The mitotic rate is high, and immunohistochemistry (Fig. 21–10C) and electron microscopy demonstrate neuroendocrine features. If all the above criteria are met, the label of LCNEC is appropriate.

### Non-small Cell Carcinomas with Neuroendocrine Features

Neuroendocrine markers can be demonstrated by immunohistochemistry or electron microscopy in some lung tumors that otherwise have the light microscopic features of squamous-, adeno-, or large cell undifferentiated carcinoma. It has been speculated that these tumors may be more aggressive and have a poorer prognosis than other NSCLCs and that they also respond differently to chemotherapy. However, the clinical and therapeutic significance of neuroendocrine features in this group of lung carcinomas is yet to be determined.[66]

## OTHER NEOPLASMS OF THE RESPIRATORY TRACT

### Mucus Gland Carcinomas

This group of neoplasms (Fig. 21–11) includes adenoid cystic carcinoma and mucoepidermoid carcinoma.

*Adenoid cystic carcinoma* (previously called "cylindroma") typically occurs in a mainstem bronchus or at least in a major bronchus. It is characterized by submucosal creeping and perineural and perivascular invasion, and, therefore, a careful frozen section evaluation of margins of resection is an important part of management. Complete excision, often with a sleeve resection, can result in cure. However, some tumors have a slow but relentless course,

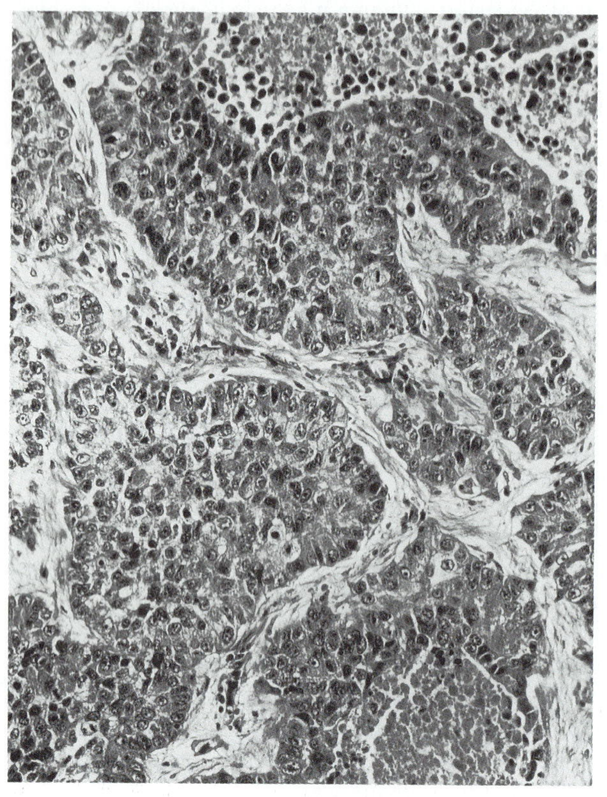

A

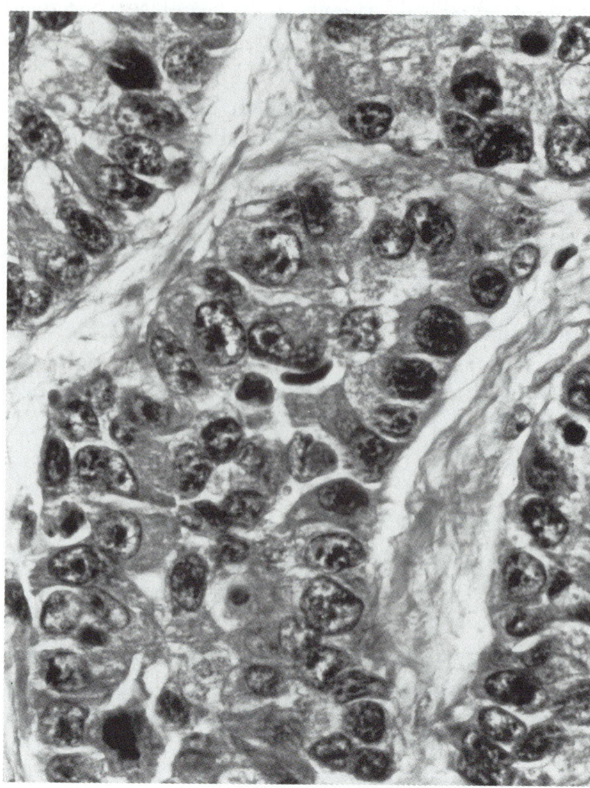

B

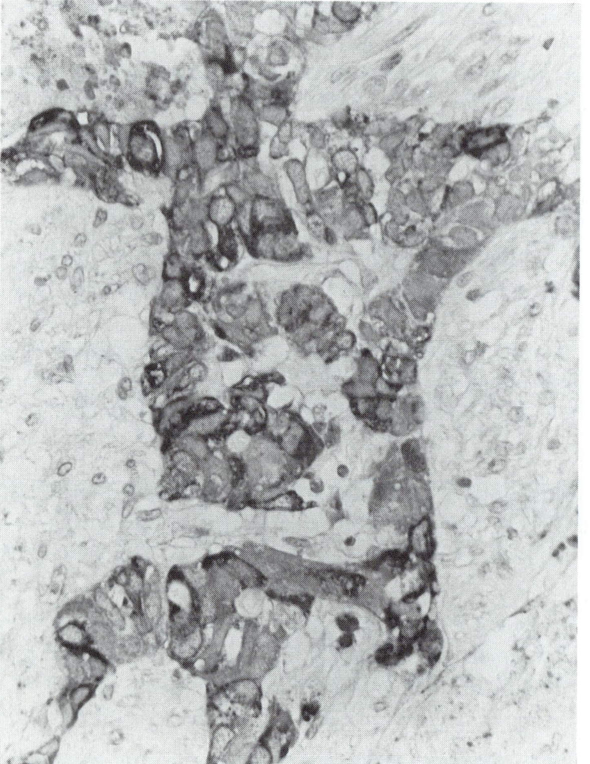

C

**Figure 21–10.** *Large cell neuroendocrine carcinoma.* The neuroendocrine features may be overlooked, and without special studies this tumor may be diagnosed as poorly differentiated adenocarcinoma or large cell undifferentiated carcinoma. **A.** The tumor cells show palisading in the periphery of the nests and islands. Mitotic rate is high, and necrosis is common. H&E, 136×. **B.** The tumor grows in a trabecular pattern and is composed of large malignant cells with pleomorphic, large nuclei, and macronucleoli. Mitoses are common and often abnormal. H&E, 520×. **C.** The tumor cells stain positively for chromogranin-A. Weak hematoxylin counterstain, 136×.

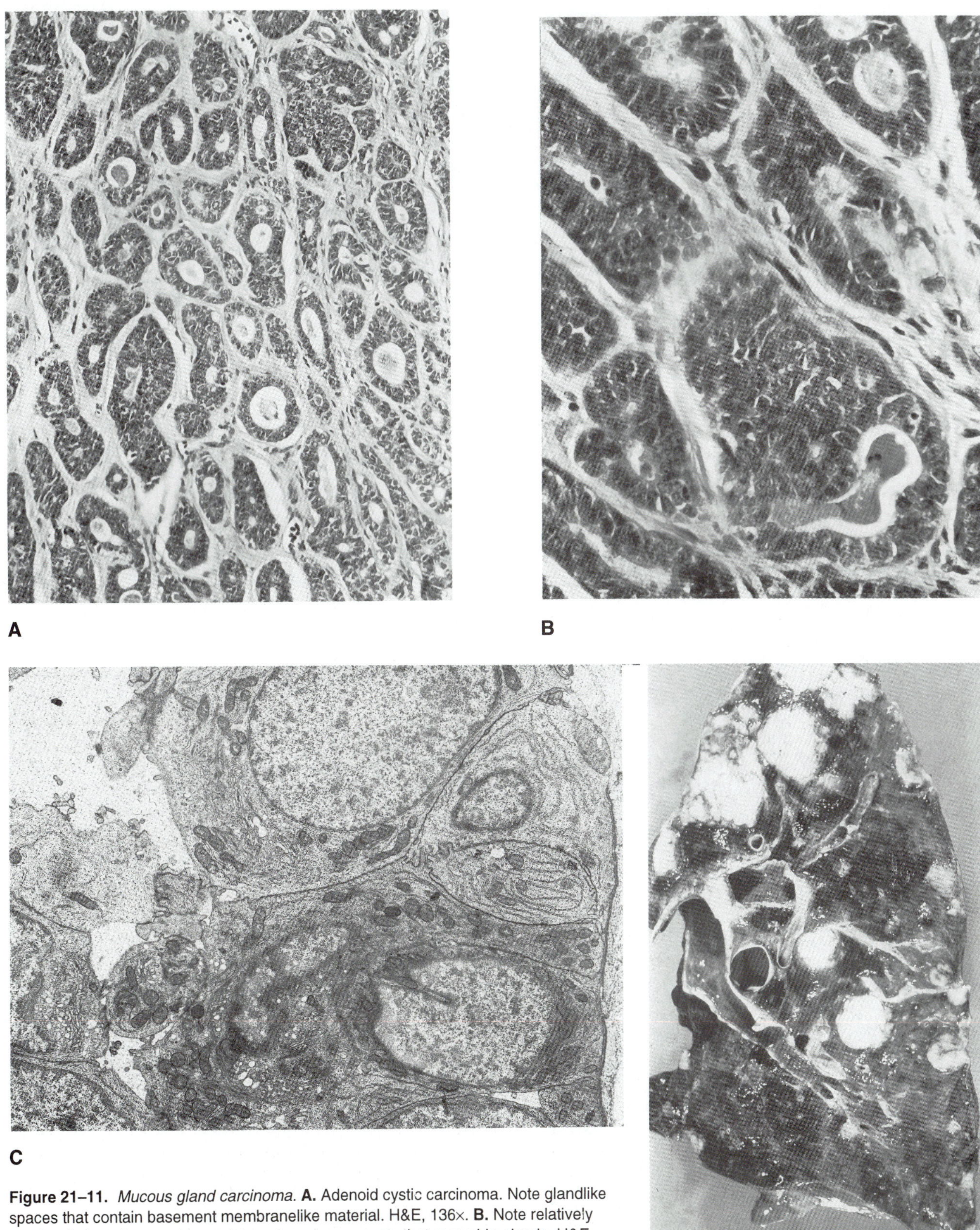



**Figure 21–11.** *Mucous gland carcinoma.* **A.** Adenoid cystic carcinoma. Note glandlike spaces that contain basement membranelike material. H&E, 136×. **B.** Note relatively small cell size, pleomorphic nuclei, and carcinoma nests that resemble glands. H&E, 200×. **C.** Transmission electron micrograph of adenoid cystic carcinoma. Note tight junctions between tumor cells. TEM, 2310×. **D.** Metastatic adenoid cystic carcinoma. Note multiple masses that were in the contralateral lung.

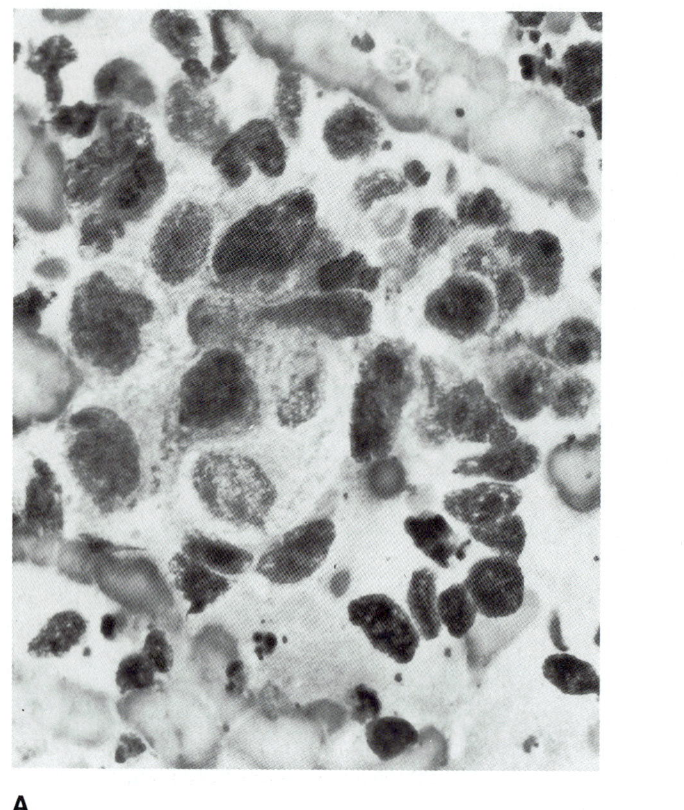

A

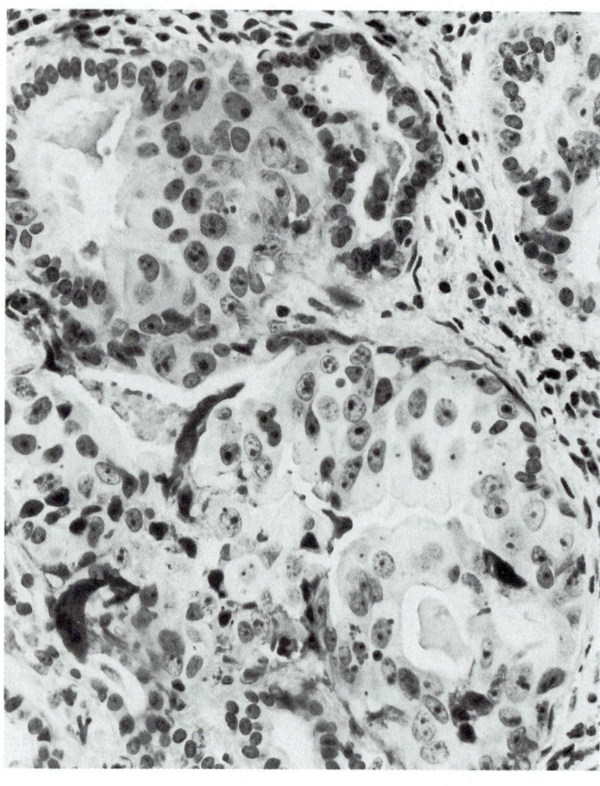

B

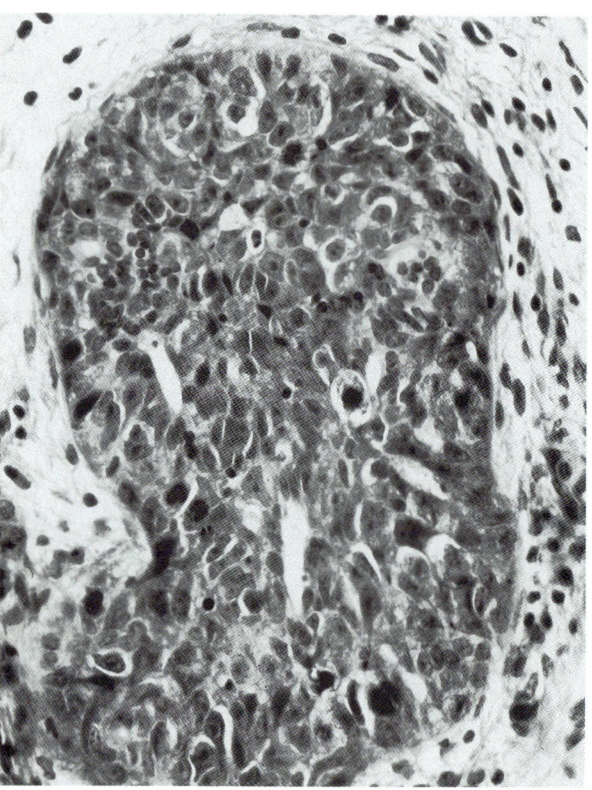

C

**Figure 21–12.** *Mucous gland carcinoma* **A.** Mucoepidermoid carcinoma. Fine-needle aspiration biopsy. Note two types of cells: larger squamous cells and intercellular pipioles and smaller granular cells in acinar configuration. Wright-Giemsa, 520×. **B.** Well-differentiated tumor with glandular and squamoid differentiation. H&E, 360×. **C.** Poorly differentiated area that, by itself, is indistinguishable from squamous cell carcinoma, H&E, 200×. *(Continued.)*

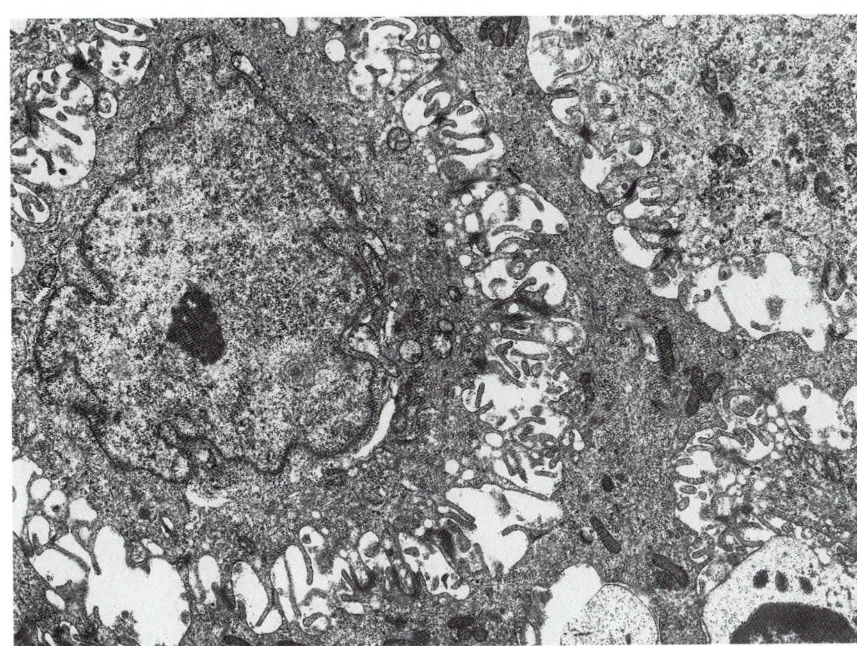

D

**Figure 21–12.** *(Continued.)* **D.** Transmission electron micrograph of mucoepidermoid carcinoma. Note desmosomes and microvilli. TEM, 3036×.

and multiple local recurrences may occur many years after the original resection. We have seen an adenoid cystic carcinoma recur 20 years after an apparent cure. This cancer metastasized to the contralateral lung parenchyma (Fig. 21–11D) and to the lymphatics. When local control by resection is no longer possible, radiotherapy has temporarily controlled this neoplasm.

The histologic features of adenoid cystic carcinoma of the lung and salivary gland are similar (Fig. 21–11A,B). The tumor is composed of islands, nests, and cords of polygonal cells with a moderate amount of cytoplasm. Glandlike cystic spaces in the tumor nests create a cribriform pattern and contain eosinophilic material that does not stain with mucin stains and resembles basement membrane by electron microscopy (Fig. 21–11C).

*Mucoepidermoid carcinoma* was previously referred to as mucoepidermoid tumor because of the mistaken impression that it was a benign lesion. The majority of these carcinomas are low-grade, slowly growing tumors that are composed of mixed populations of cells showing glandular or squamous differentiation or both[72] (Fig. 21–12A–C). A variety of histologic patterns are typically present ranging from mucin-filled cysts lined by mucinous cells to solid sheets of squamoid (intermediate) cells that are interspersed by goblet cells. Cytoplasmic keratinization and keratin pearls are not a feature. The tumor cell nuclei are relatively bland, and mitotic figures are not frequent in the low-grade tumors (Fig. 21–12B). In high-grade tumors (Fig. 21–12C) a transition from low to high grade should be evident, otherwise the tumor should be classified as adenosquamous carcinoma. High-grade neuroepidermoid carcinomas may be difficult to differentiate from nonmetastasizing squamous cell carcinomas in small biopsy samples (Fig. 21–12C). Electron micrographs reveal features intermediate between adeno- and squamous-cell carcinomas with microvilli, prominent desmosomes, and intracytoplasmic lumens (Fig. 21–12D).

## Carcinosarcoma

Carcinosarcoma is a malignant tumor with carcinomatous and sarcomatous differentiation. The tumor may be endobronchial or parenchymal and typically shows both "mature" carcinoma and "mature" sarcoma. Any combination of squamous cell-, adeno-, large cell undifferentiated-, or SCLC may occur with any type of sarcoma, including malignant fibrous histiocytoma. The most frequent combination is squamous cell or adenocarcinoma with fibrosarcoma or malignant fibrous histiocytoma. The theories for the pathogenesis of these tumors include metaplastic sarcomatous development, collision tumors, and biphasic differentiation of primitive totipotential cells.

## Miscellaneous Malignant Tumors

This complex group of neoplasms includes pulmonary blastoma and malignant mesenchymal tumors such as fibrosarcoma, leiomyosarcoma (Fig. 21–12), hemangiopericytoma, and pulmonary lymphomas.

Primary lung lymphomas cannot, by current methods, be definitively diagnosed by fine-needle aspiration. The previous term *pseudolymphoma* is no longer meaningful. Resection is the first treatment of choice.[73,74] Careful light microscopic evaluation of adequate tissue samples and immunohistochemical study is required to differentiate among three major types of pulmonary lymphoma, each of which

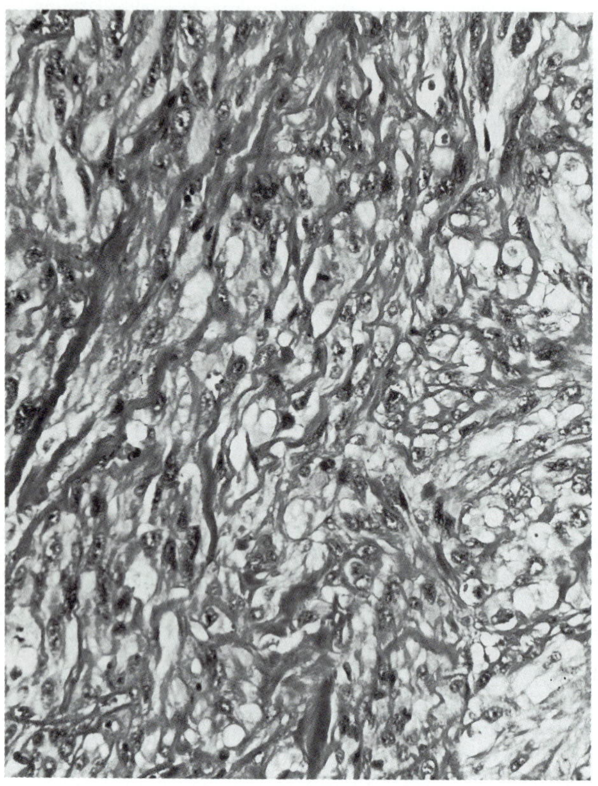

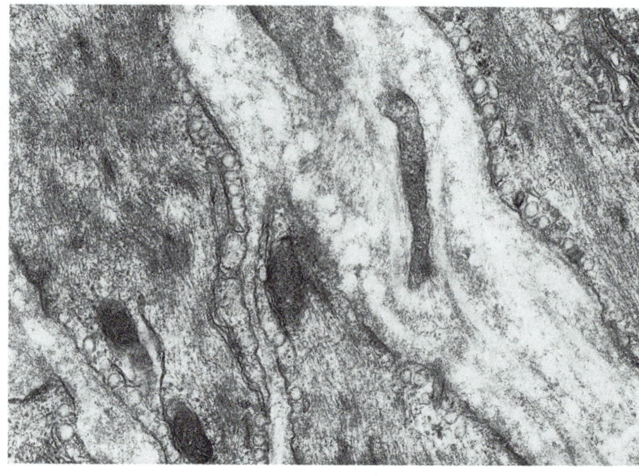

A B

**Figure 21–13.** *Pulmonary leiomyosarcoma.* **A.** The tumor is composed of bundles of spindle-shaped cells that have fairly bland-appearing nuclei. The perceived difference in the cell shape is mostly due to the angle of sectioning relative to the orientation of the tumor cells. Note mitotic figures. H&E, 136. **B.** Note cytoplasmic dense bodies (D) and caveoli (pinocytic vesicles) at the edges of the tumor cells. TEM 7755×.

has a different prognosis. Overall mean survival of patients with pulmonary lymphoma after complete conservative resection of mass lesions is about 117 months. "Lymphomatoid granulomatosis" is a lymphoma that is characterized by pulmonary infiltrates in an angiocentric pattern composed of a mixed population of atypical lymphoid cells.

## PARANEOPLASTIC SYNDROMES

Lung neoplasms are sometimes associated with extrapulmonary manifestations, which are referred to as paraneoplastic syndromes.[75] The syndromes that are known to be associated with hormone production are summarized in Table 21–2. The endocrine properties of SCLC are carcinoids (Kulchitsky cell or neuroendocrine carcinomas) have been emphasized because they have been studied extensively and have been found to secrete more than one hormone. However, based on evidence that is beyond the scope of this chapter, there is reason to believe that virtually all primary lung cancers may have endocrine properties.

Other occasional paraneoplastic manifestations of primary lung cancers include myasthenia gravis, Eaton-Lambert syndrome, and Trousseau's syndrome (hypercoagulability and migratory thrombophlebitis). Peripheral neuropathy, leukemoid reactions, acanthosis nigricans, and hypertrophic pulmonary osteoarthropathy may all occur as manifestations of primary lung cancers.

**TABLE 21–2. PARANEOPLASTIC SYNDROMES**

| Hormones or Hormonelike Substances | Symptoms | Signs |
|---|---|---|
| ADH | Hyponatremia | Small cell carcinoma |
| Adrenocorticotrophic hormone (ACTH) | Cushing's syndrome | Small cell carcinoma |
| Parathyroid hormone, (PTH)-like substances, and PGE | Hypercalcemia | Squamous carcinoma |
| Calcitonin | Hypocalcemia | Squamous carcinoma |
| Gonadotropins | Gynecomastia | Any tumor |
| Serotonin | Carcinoid syndrome | Carcinoid, small cell carcinoma |

ADH, antidiuretic hormone; PGE, prostaglandin E.

## SELECTED DIAGNOSTIC PITFALLS

The common diagnostic problems fall into four basic categories: detection, localization, sampling, and interpretation. These problems are illustrated in Figure 21–14.

Once a pulmonary mass or otherwise suspicious lesion is detected, a specific tissue diagnosis can usually be made if the cytologic or biopsy material obtained by bronchoscopy, fine-needle aspiration biopsy, or incisional biopsy is representative and adequate. Sampling problems, i.e., failure to provide the pathologist with material that is adequate for definitive diagnosis, can result from such things as inability to advance a bronchoscope to the level of tumor because of mucosal edema and/or inflammation, failure to "hit" a small cancer that is surrounded by massive inflammation with an aspiration needle or failure to obtain recognizable tissue from a necrotic tumor. It may be impossible to select the "correct" biopsy site in patients with mul-

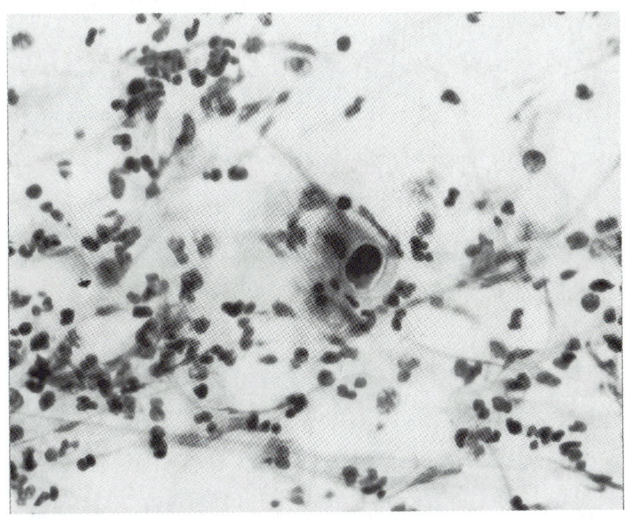

A

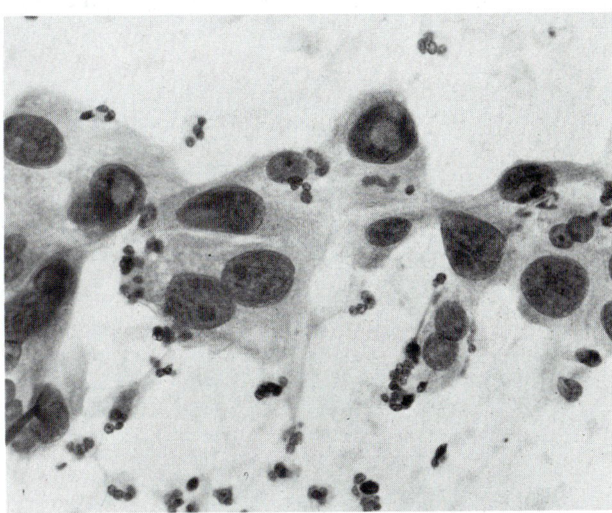

B

C

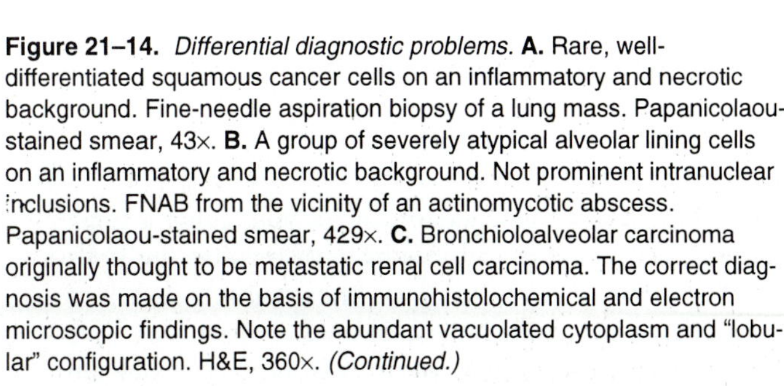

**Figure 21–14.** *Differential diagnostic problems.* **A.** Rare, well-differentiated squamous cancer cells on an inflammatory and necrotic background. Fine-needle aspiration biopsy of a lung mass. Papanicolaou-stained smear, 43×. **B.** A group of severely atypical alveolar lining cells on an inflammatory and necrotic background. Not prominent intranuclear inclusions. FNAB from the vicinity of an actinomycotic abscess. Papanicolaou-stained smear, 429×. **C.** Bronchioloalveolar carcinoma originally thought to be metastatic renal cell carcinoma. The correct diagnosis was made on the basis of immunohistolochemical and electron microscopic findings. Note the abundant vacuolated cytoplasm and "lobular" configuration. H&E, 360×. *(Continued.)*

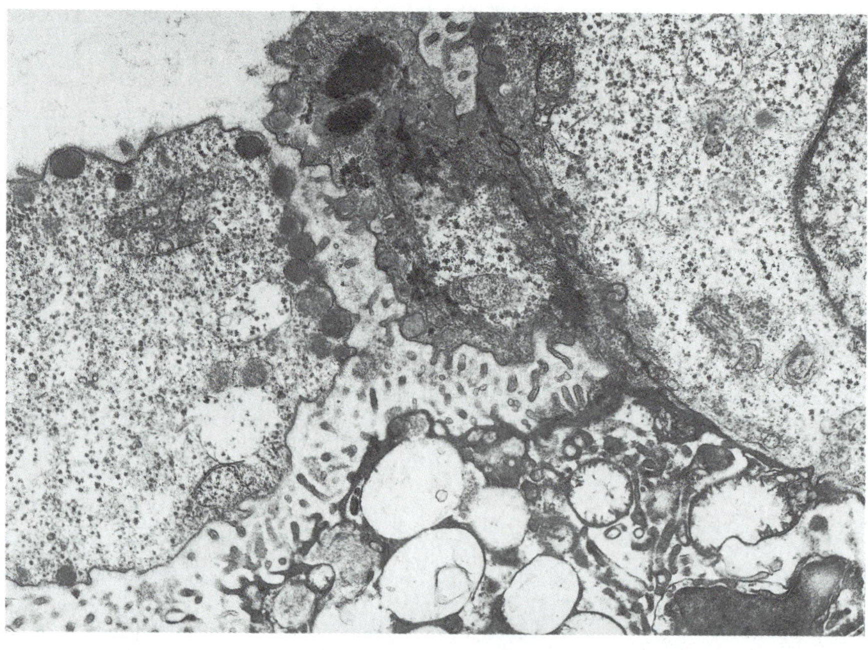

D

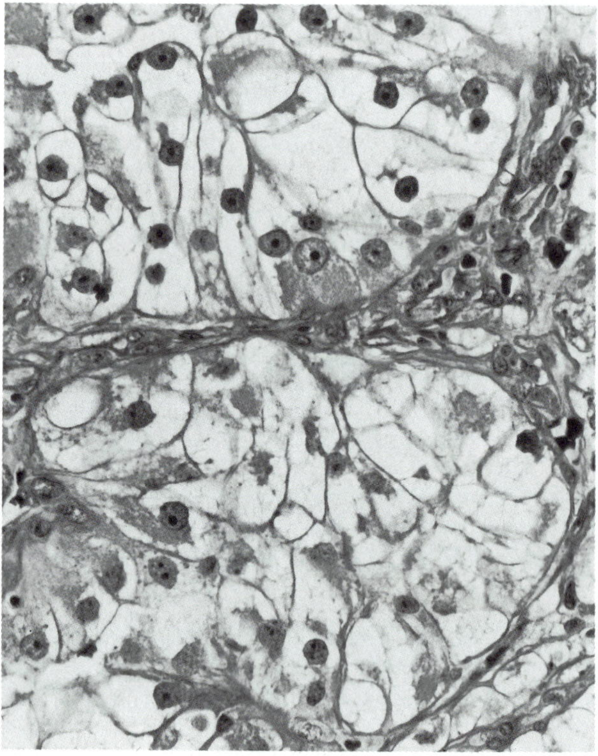

E

**Figure 21–14.** *(Continued.)* **D.** Transmission electron micrograph of a bronchioloalveolar carcinoma. Note junctional complexes, microvilli, lamellar bodies, and mucin droplets. TEM, 3036. **E.** Renal cell carcinoma originally thought to represent an adenocarcinoma. The correct diagnosis was made on the basis of immunohistolochemical and electron microscopic findings. Note large, pleomorphic nuclei of variable size, macronucleoli, and abundant clear or vacuolated cytoplasm. H&E, 360×. *(Continued.)*

tiple apparent scars, any one of which could harbor a small cancer. Crush or cautery artefact may make tissues and cells difficult or impossible to interpret, thus resulting in risk of delayed or even incorrect diagnosis. After specimens have been obtained, they are subject to deterioration if they are not treated promptly and well with an appropriate fixative. It cannot be stressed enough that the diagnosis can be only as good as the sample, and multiple, properly handled samples from several areas of the lesion minimize the problem of inadequate diagnostic material.

*Clinically,* there are practical guidelines that have evolved. During bronchoscopy, neoplasms may be coated

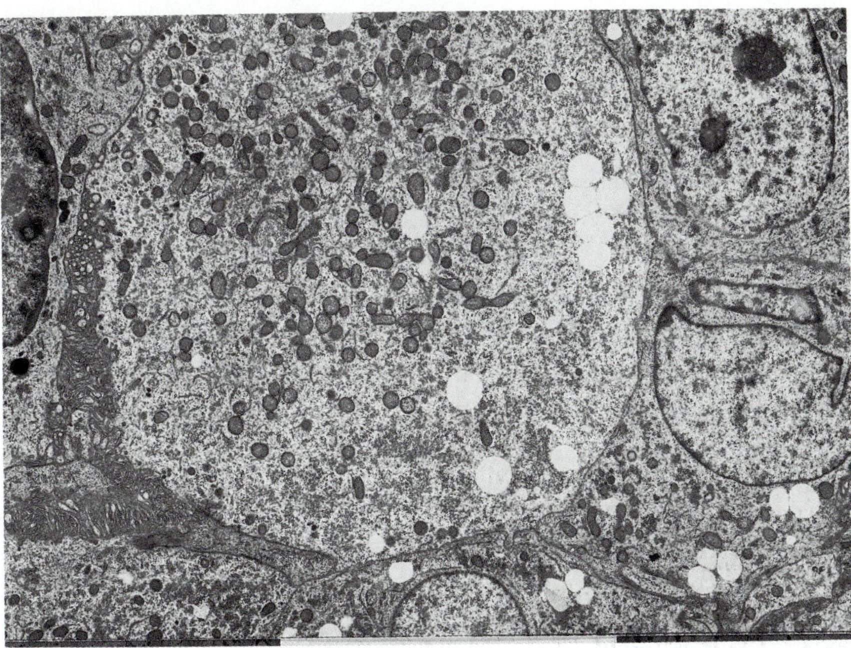

F

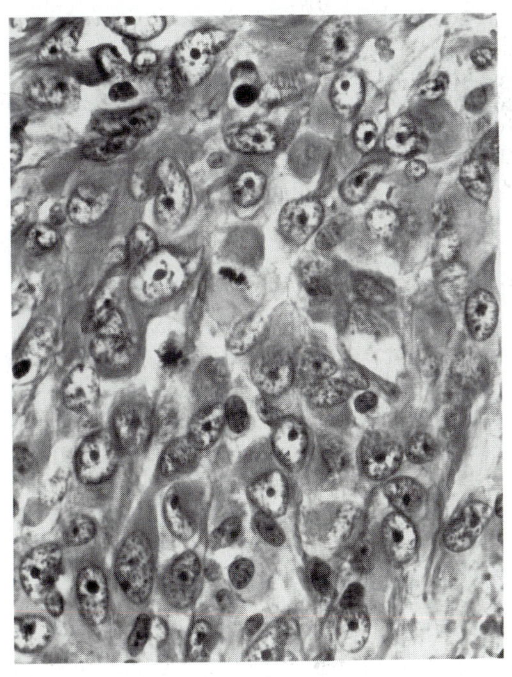

G

**Figure 21–14.** *(Continued.)* **F.** Transmission electron micrograph of renal cell carcinoma. Note fat droplets, abundant mitochondria, and complex interdigitation of the plasma membrane. TEM, 3036×. **G.** Malignant mesothelioma originally thought to represent a poorly differentiated adenocarcinoma. The correct diagnosis was based on immunohistologic and electron microscopic findings. Note large, pleomorphic nuclei, centrally placed macronucleoli, and abundant cytoplasm. H&E, 520×.

with an exudate. On histologic section cancers may be deep-to-normal or near normal mucosa. A classic example of this is small cell undifferentiated carcinoma. Accordingly, several biopsy specimens are recommended when possible. Bronchoscopic biopsy specimens are usually small, and, therefore, we may defer therapeutic decisions until permanent sections are available. Only occasionally will we ask the pathologist for a diagnosis based on frozen sections. The same general principle holds true for specimens obtained by mediastinoscopy. However, frozen section is requested when there is a need to know whether or not the biopsy material is adequate for diagnosis during the course of an operation. Fine-needle aspiration specimens should be interpreted preferably by a cytopathologist. This evaluation will determine whether or not additional needle aspirations need to be done. Despite best efforts, sampling inadequacies will never be eliminated, but they can be reduced to a minimum. To accomplish this, our usual intraop-

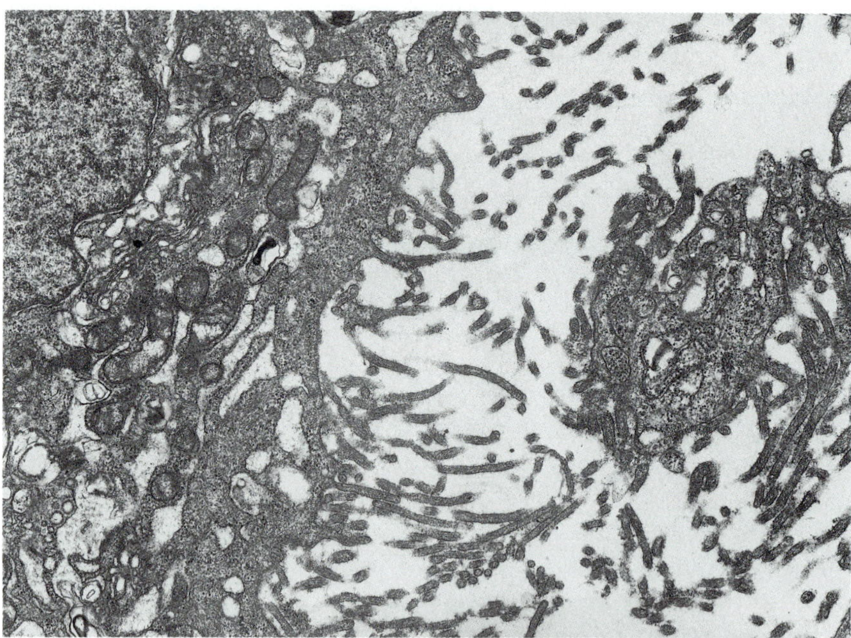

H

**Figure 21–14.** *(Continued.)* **H.** Transmission electron micrograph of malignant mesothelioma. Note long, slender microvilli. TEM 5082×.

erative question to the pathologist is, "Do you have enough material for eventual definitive diagnosis?"

Infectious or inflammatory processes sometimes present a sampling and differential diagnostic problem. Pneumonia may sometimes mask a carcinoma that is narrowing or obstructing the airway. Figure 21–14A illustrates this with an FNA biopsy from a middle-aged smoker who had recurrent pneumonia and an unresolving lung infiltrate. Repeated biopsies, bronchial brushings, and washings contained only necrotic material and numerous acute inflammatory cells, and only very rare, atypical but well-differentiated keratinized squamous cells were found after a diligent search in the second fine-needle aspiration biopsy. The cytologic interpretation was ". . . suspicious but not diagnostic for cancer." At thoracotomy, a moderately differentiated keratinizing and largely necrotic squamous cell carcinoma surrounded by acute and chronic pneumonia was found. It could be argued that the significance of the cells with nuclear atypia had not been fully appreciated.

The converse of the earlier situation may arise from cellular atypia and dysplasia associated with inflammation. Squamous metaplasia is not an uncommon finding in airways, and, even in lung parenchyma a chronic or organizing pneumonia, the squamous cells may often exhibit reactive nuclear atypia. Fungal infection is notorious for associated cellular atypia. Figure 21–14B shows a group of severely atypical alveolar cells from a fine-needle aspiration biopsy of a lung mass in a middle-aged patient with a history of smoking. The classical and radiographic findings were suspicious for cancer. The fine-needle aspiration sample contained groups and individual atypical cells on an inflammatory and necrotic background. Two pathologists called the atypical cells cancer, and a third pathologist called them highly suspicious for malignancy. A lobectomy specimen revealed a poorly demarcated 3- × 6-cm mass composed of multiple conjoining actinomycotic abscesses surrounded by extensive organizing pneumonia. The specimen contained bronchiolar and alveolar cells with atypia, but no carcinoma was found.

The distinction between a primary and a metastatic neoplasm in the lung may be difficult. If no bronchial origin for a carcinoma can be demonstrated and the histologic features are not typical enough to allow a specific diagnosis, the possibility of an extrathoracic primary cancer must be considered. Prime candidates for metastatic pulmonary carcinomas include adenocarcinomas of any organ, head and neck cancers, and amelanotic melanomas. Conversely, patients with previous extrathoracic carcinomas may have unrelated, new primary, potentially curable lung cancers. Figure 21–14C,D shows a primary pulmonary bronchiolar carcinoma that mimicked a metastatic renal cell carcinoma. The patient had unrelated kidney and adrenal lesions. Figure 21–14E,F shows a renal cell carcinoma originally thought to be primary in the lung. Melanoma is considered the great histologic mimicker, and this neoplasm may also be mistaken for primary lung cancer; this conundrum is particularly likely to occur if no cytoplasmic pigment is noted. In short, there are numerous histologic "look-alikes" that need to be separated from one another.

To distinguish a well-differentiated adenocarcinoma metastatic to the pleura from mesothelioma and from reactive hyperplasia of mesothelial cells is sometimes problematic (Fig. 21–14G,H). This is true particularly if the patient has had a prior diagnosis of carcinoma. Chronic pleural effusions can result in an exuberant mesothelial proliferation, and a correct diagnosis may require further studies. An epithelioid mesothelioma can sometimes present as a pleural-based peripheral pulmonary mass and be mistaken for a poorly differentiated adenocarcinoma. There are no mesothelioma-specific immunohistochemical markers, and, therefore, a correct diagnosis often requires a panel of immunohistochemical studies (Table 21–3). Electron micrographs characteristically reveal long, slender microvilli with a length-to-width ratio of 10:15 (Fig. 21–14H), which is considerably greater than the length-to-width ratio of the microvilli of adenocarcinomas. In contrast to adenocarcinomas, mesotheliomas also lack the fuzzy glycocalyx of adenocarcinomas. Instead of junctional complexes, mesothelial cells are connected to each other by large desmosomes, into which intermediate filaments are inserted. In our experience, mucin and alcian blue stains with and without hyaluronidase are next to useless.

*Clinically,* we have evolved the following guidelines. When the distinction of infectious or inflammatory processes presents a diagnostic problem, we usually pursue a definitive diagnosis until it is achieved. Often this requires pulmonary resection, which we consider to be the conservative approach to an indeterminate lung lesion. Occasionally the clinical circumstances may dictate expectant management or a trial of nonoperative therapy, but generally we do not favor deferring definitive diagnosis. With regard to the distinction between primary and a metastatic neoplasm in the lung, in doubtful situations we favor considering the neoplasms as potentially curable new lung cancers that are worthy of resection. This view is based on the fact that excision is clearly the best treatment for primary T1–2 lung cancers, and it is also the best currently available treatment for solitary pulmonary metastasis from a number of extrathoracic cancers, providing that the original neoplasm remains under local control. When a lung cancer that could be metastatic from outside the chest has been biopsied or excised, we resist an exhaustive and expensive search for a primary carcinoma. If there are truly no symptoms of bowel abnormalities, and examination of the stool for occult blood is negative, and sigmoidoscopy as well as urinalysis are negative, we feel comfortable in accepting the lung cancer as a primary bronchogenic neoplasm. Conversely, even subtle symptoms or findings suggestive of an occult extrathoracic primary are pursued in a focused fashion. To distinguish a well-differentiated adenocarcinoma metastatic to the pleura from mesothelioma and from reactive hyperplasia of mesothelial cells, we rely on the pathologists' best efforts. We use video-assisted thoracotomy liberally for the purpose of obtaining adequate tissue samples.

**TABLE 21–3. STAINING METHODS TO DIFFERENTIATE MESOTHELIOMA AND ADENOCARCINOMA[a]**

| Stain | Mesothelioma | Adenocarcinoma |
|---|---|---|
| Mucicarmine | Negative | Positive |
| PAS/diastase | Negative | Positive (66%) |
| Cytokeratin | Positive | Positive |
| CEA | Negative | Positive (84%) |
| LeuM1 | Negative | Positive (80%) |
| BER-EP4 | Negative | Positive (86%) |
| B72.3 | Negative | Positive (88%) |

[a]The presence of mucin is incompatible with a diagnosis of mesothelioma. Sarcomatoid mesotheliomas express cytokeratin as opposed to pleural or pulmonary sarcomas which lack keratin. Epithelial malignant mesotheliomas express cytokeratin but stain negatively with antibodies to CEA, LeuM1, BER-EP4, and B72.3.

## REFERENCES


1. Boffetta P, Parkin M: Cancer statistics. *CA Cancer J Clin* **44:**81, 1994
2. Levi F, Lucchini F, La Vecchia C: Worldwide patterns of cancer mortality, 1985–89. *Eur J Cancer Prev* **3:**109, 1994
3. Boring CC, Squires TS, Tong T, Mongomery S: Cancer statistics. *CA Cancer J Clin* **44:**9, 1994
4. McDuffie HH, Klaassen DJ, Dosman JA: Female-male differences in patients with primary lung cancer. *Cancer* **59:**1825, 1987
5. Feliu J, Gonzalez Baron M, Berrocal A, et al: Lung cancer in patients under 40 years of age: A different problem? *Med Clin* **97:**373, 1991
6. DeCaro L, Benfield JR: Lung cancer in young persons. *J Thorac Cardiovasc Surg* **83:**372, 1982
7. McDuffie HH, Klassen DJ, Dosman JA: Characteristics of patients with primary lung cancer diagnosed at age of 50 years or younger. *Chest* **96:**1298, 1989
8. Lu GM: Lung cancer in the young—x-ray manifestations in 135 cases. *Chung-Hua Chung Liu Tsa Chih [Chinese J Oncol]* **12:**148, 1990
9. Ochsner A, DeBakey M: Carcinoma of the lung. *Arch Surg* **42:**209, 1941
10. Wynder EL, Graham EA: Tobacco smoking as a possible etiologic factor in bronchiogenic carcinoma; study of 684 proved cases. *JAMA* **143:**329, 1950
11. Kabat GC, Wynder EL: Lung cancer in nonsmokers. *Cancer* **53:**1214, 1984
12. Zang EA, Wynder EL: Cumulative tar exposure. A new index for estimating lung cancer risk among cigarette smokers. *Cancer* **70:**69, 1992
13. Sobue T, Suzuki T, Fujimoto I, et al: Lung cancer risk among exsmokers. *Jpn J Cancer Res* **82:**273, 1991
14. Hammond WG, Teplitz RL, Benfield JR: Variable regression of experimental bronchial preneoplasia during carcinogenesis. *J Thorac Cardiovasc Surg* **101:**800, 1991
15. Sawyer RW, Hammond WG, Teplitz RL, Benfield JR, et al: Regression of bronchial epithelial cancer in hamsters. *Ann Thorac Surg* **56:**74, 1993
16. Pollin W, Ravenholt RT: Tobacco addiction and tobacco mortality. Implications for death certification. *JAMA* **252:**2849, 1984
17. Samet JM, Hornung RW: Review of radon and lung cancer risk. *Risk Anal* **10:**65, 1990
18. Benfield JR, Hammond WG: Bronchial and pulmonary carcinogenesis at focal sites in dogs and hamsters. *Cancer Res* **52:**2687s, 1992
19. Mackay JL: The fight against tobacco in developing countries. *Tuber Lung Dis* **75:**8, 1994

20. Repace J, Lowrey AH: An enforceable indoor air quality standard for environmental tobacco smoke in the workplace. *Risk Anal* **13:**463, 1993
21. Claxton LD, Morin RS, Highes TJ, Lewtas J: A genotoxic assessment of environmental tobacco smoke using bacterial bioassays. *Mutat Res* **222:** 81, 1989
22. Janerich DT, Thompson WD, Varela LR, et al: Lung cancer and exposure to tobacco smoke in the household. *N Engl J Med* **323:**632, 1990
23. *Reducing the Health Consequences of Smoking: 25 Years of Progress: A Report of the Surgeon General: 1989 Executive Summary.* Rockville, Maryland, DHSS, 1989
24. National Research Council Committee on Passive Smoking: *Environmental Tobacco Smoke: Measuring Exposures and Assessing Health Effects.* Washington, DC: National Academy Press, 1986
25. Saccomano G, Archer VE, Auerbach O, et al: Histologic types of lung cancers among uranium miners. *Cancer* **27:**515, 1971
26. Allen ML: Associated bronchogenic carcinoma: 2 cases. *J Industr Hygiene* **16:**346, 1934
27. Siskind FB: The cost of compensating asbestos victims under the Occupational Disease Compensation Act of 1983. *Risk Anal* **7:**59, 1987
28. Frank AL: Asbestos as an air pollutant and synergism with smoking. *Cancer Detect Prev* **9:**337, 1986
29. Reif AE: Synergism in carcinogenesis. *J Natl Cancer Inst* **73:**25, 1984
30. Churg A: Neoplastic asbestos-induced diseases. In Churg A, Green F (eds): *Pathology of Occupational Lung Disease.* New York, Igaku-Shoin, 1988, p. 279
31. Guda V, Kozak R: [The medical problems of the aftermath of the accident at the Chernobyl Atomic Electric Power Station.] *Vrachebnoe Delo* **10–12:**21, 1993
32. Abraham E, Karacsonyi L, Dinya E: [Possible cause of the increased incidence of lung cancer in 1987 in the 10th District of Budapest.] *Orv Hetil* **131:**2877, 1990
33. Hei TK, Piao CQ, Willey JC, et al: Malignant transformation of human bronchial epithelial cells by radon-stimulated alpha-particles. *Carcinogenesis* **15:**431, 1994
34. Sandberg AA, Weinberg RA, Mittleman F: Chromosomes, genes and cancer, *CA Cancer J Clin* **44:**136, 1994
35. Kellerman G, et al: Arylhydrocarbon hydroxylase inducibility in bronchogenic carcinoma. *N Engl J Med* **289:**934, 1973
36. Karki NT, Pokela R, Nuutinen L, Pelkonen O: Arylhydrocarbon hydroxylase in lymphocytes and lung tissue from lung cancer patients and controls. *Int J Cancer* **39:**565, 1987
37. Gough AC, Miles JS, Spurr NK, et al: Identification of the primary gene defect at the cytochrome P450 CYP2D locus. *Nature* **347:**773, 1990
38. Sell S, Pierce GB: Mutation arrest of stem cell differentiation is a common pathway for the cellular origin of teratocarcinomas and epithelial cancers. *Lab Invest* **70:**6, 1994
39. Yesner R, Carter D: Pathology of carcinoma of the lung. Changing patterns. *Clin Chest Med* **3:**257, 1982
40. Ten Have-Opbroek AAW, Benfield JR, Hammond WG, et al: In favour of an oncofoetal concept of bronchogenic carcinoma and development. *Histol Histopathol* **9:**375, 1994
41. Cardiff RD, Sinn E, Muller W, Leder: Transgenic oncogene mice. Tumor phenotype predicts genotype. *Am J Pathol* **139:**495, 1991
42. Roby TJ, Swan GE, Sorensen KW, et al: Discriminant analysis of lower respiratory tract components associated with cigarette smoking, based on quantitative sputum cytology. *Acta Cytol* **34:**147, 1990
43. Marchevsky AM: Pathogenesis and experimental models of lung cancer. In Marchevsky AM (ed.): *Surgical Pathology of Lung Neoplasms.* New York, Marcel Dekker, 1990, p. 7
44. Teplitz RL, Pak HY, Benfield JR, et al: Quantitative DNA. Comparative studies of cellular marker for bronchogenic carcinoma. *JAMA* **249:**1046, 1983
45. Carey FA, Prasad US, Walker WS, et al: Prognostic significance of tumor deoxyribonucleic acid content in surgically resected small cell carcinoma of lung. *J Thorac Cardiovasc Surg* **103:**1214, 1992
46. Rice TW, Bauer TW, Gephardt GW, et al: Prognostic significance of flow cytometry in non-small lung cancer. *J Thorac Cardiovasc Surg* **106:**210, 1993
47. DeCaro LR, Paladugu RR, Benfield JR, et al: Typical and atypical carcinoids within the pulmonary APUD spectrum. *J Thorac Cardiovasc Surg* **86:**528, 1983
48. Myeroff LL, Markowitz SD: Increased nm23-H1 and nm23-H2 mRNA expression and absence of mutations in colon carcinomas of low and high metastatic potential. *J Natl Cancer Inst* **85:**147, 1993
49. Hart IR, Easty D: Identification of genes controlling metastatic behavior. *Br J Cancer* **63:**9, 1991
50. Roggli VL, Vollmer RT, Greenberg SD: Lung cancer heterogeneity: A blinded and randomized study of 100 consecutive cases. *Hum Pathol* **16:**569, 1985
51. World Health Organization. *Histological Typing of Lung Tumours,* 2nd Ed. Geneva, WHO, 1981
52. Mountain CF: A new international staging system for lung cancer. *Chest* **89:**225s, 1986
53. National Cancer Institute Cooperative: Early Lung Cancer Detection Program—summary and conclusion. *Am Rev Respir Dis* **130:**565, 1984
54. Matthews MJ: Problems in morphology and behavior of bronchopulmonary malignant disease. In Israel and Chabinian (eds): *Lung Cancer. Natural History, Prognosis, and Therapy.* New York, Academic Press, 1976, p. 23
55. Yellin A, Hill LR, Benfield JR: Bronchogenic carcinoma associated with upper aerodigestive cancers. *J Thorac Cardiovasc Surg* **91:**674, 1986
56. Paulson DL: the "superior sulcus" lesion. In Delarue NC, Eschapasse H (eds): *Lung Cancer. International Trends in General Surgery.* Philadelphia, Saunders, 1985, pp. 121–131
57. Auerbach O, Garfinkel L: The changing pattern of lung carcinoma. *Cancer* **68:**1973, 1991
58. Wain JC, Wilkins SJ, Benfield JR, Smith SS: Altered DNA methylation patterns in human lung carcinomas. *Curr Surg* **43:**489, 1986
59. Greco RJ, Steiner RM, Goldman S, et al: Bronchoalveolar cell carcinoma of the lung. *Ann Thorac Surg* **41:**652, 1986
60. Arrigoni MG, Woolner LB, Bernatz PE: Atypical carcinoid tumor of the lung. *J Thorac Cardiovasc Surg* **64:**413, 1972
61. Gould VE, Linnoila RI, Memoli VA, Warren WH: Neuroendocrine components of the bronchopulmonary tract: hyperplasias, dysplasias and neoplasms. *Lab Invest* **49:**519, 1983
62. Paladugu RR, Benfield JR, Pak HY, et al: Kultchisky cell carcinomas. A new classification scheme for typical and atypical carcinoids. *Cancer* **55:**1303, 1985
63. Travis WD, Linnoila RL, Tsokos MG, et al: Neuroendocrine tumors of the lung with proposed criteria for large cell neuroendocrine carcinoma. An ultrastructural immunohistochemical and flow cytometric study of 35 cases. *Am J Surg Pathol* **15:**529, 1991
64. Yellin A, Benfield JR: The pulmonary Kultchisky cell (neuroendocrine) cancers: from carcinoid to small cell carcinoma. *Curr Probl Cancer* **9:**1, 1985
65. Karmy-Jones R, Vallieres E: Carcinoid crisis after biopsy of a bronchial carcinoid. *Ann Thorac Surg* **56:**1403, 1993
66. Warren WH, Faber LP, Gould VE: Neuroendocrine neoplasms of the lung. *J Thorac Cardiovasc Surg* **98:**321, 1989
67. Warren WH, Memoli VA, Jordan AG, et al: Reevaluation of pulmonary neoplasms resected as small cell carcinomas. Significance of distinguishing between well differentiated and small cell neuroendocrine carcinoma. *Cancer* **65:**1003, 1990
68. Bunn PA Jr: Operation for stage III, a small cell lung cancer. *Ann Thorac Surg* **49:**691, 1990
69. Ginsberg RJ: Operation for small cell lung cancer—where are we? *Ann Thorac Surg* **49:**692, 1990

70. Salzer GM, Mueller LC, Huber H, et al: Operations for N2 small cell lung carcinoma. *Ann Thorac Surg* **49:**759, 1990
71. Hirsch FR, Matthews MJ, Aisner S, et al: Histopathologic classification of small cell lung cancer. Changing concepts and terminology. *Cancer* **62:**973, 1988
72. Dowling EA, et al: Mucoepidermoid tumors of the bronchi. *Surgery* **52:**600, 1962
73. Kennedy JL, Nathwani BN, Burke JS, et al. Pulmonary lymphomas and other pulmonary lymphoid lesions. A clinicopathologic and immunologic study of 645 patients. *Cancer* **56**:539, 1985
74. Yellin A, Pak HY, Benfield JR, et al: Surgical management of lymphomas involving the chest. *Ann Thorac Surg* **44:**363, 1987
75. Abeloff MD: Paraneoplastic syndromes. *N Engl J Med* **317:**1598, 1987

CHAPTER

# 22

# Diagnosis and Staging of Lung Cancer

Thomas W. Shields

The goals of the evaluation of the patient suspected of having lung cancer are to establish the cell type of the tumor, to determine the extent of the disease process, and to determine the functional status of the patient so that the appropriate therapeutic decisions may be made. Prior to the 1970s, tissue for diagnosis and for rudimentary staging was obtained by rigid bronchoscopy and infrequently mediastinoscopy.[1] Most patients, however, with the exception of those with obvious distant metastasis, underwent exploratory thoracotomy in hopes that a resection could be performed. Unfortunately, in approximately 50% of the patients, the disease could not be removed. During the past 30 years, however, newer techniques for diagnosis and the development of appropriate anatomic staging systems for both non-small cell and small cell lung cancers have been developed so that unrewarding exploratory thoracotomies have been reduced to less than 5% in most surgical centers, although rates as high as 10% are still reported.

The initial staging system was developed by the Union International Contra le Cancerium (UICC) based on the suggestion of Denoix[2] that the extent of the tumor be codified by the descriptor T, the presence of lymph node metastases by the descriptor N, and the presence of distant metastasis by the descriptor M. The patients with varying combinations of the TNM designations were then placed into stage categories to denote the extent of the disease process. In North America the first system adopted by the surgical community was that advocated by the American Joint Committee for Cancer Staging and End Results Reporting in 1973.[3] Numerous flaws unfortunately were present, and, in addition, the system was not completely compatible with the systems used by radiation oncologists and by surgeons in Europe and Japan. Through consultation and international cooperation, a new international staging system was agreed upon and published in 1986.[4] This system is now accepted for the staging of non-small cell lung cancer by almost all workers in the field. In patients with small cell lung cancer, this system has very limited applicability, and a less sophisticated system of limited and extensive disease categories, as initially suggested by the Veterans Administration Lung Cancer Study Group, is used.[5] Both systems will be discussed in detail after the consideration of the various methods of obtaining a histologic diagnosis in those patients suspected of having a lung cancer.

## THE STAGING PROCESS

Once a patient is identified as possibly having a carcinoma of the lung, a tissue diagnosis is required, the extent of the disease must be determined, and the functional status of the patient must be evaluated. The determination of these parameters may be regarded as the "staging process." Each of these three areas requires the use of various noninvasive and invasive techniques. The studies required must be used in a selective manner to best establish the overall status of the patient and to determine the appropriate therapeutic approach.

## HISTOLOGIC STAGING

Pathologically, the tumor may be classified as either a non-small cell carcinoma or a small cell carcinoma (Table 22–1). This determination has therapeutic importance, since almost all surgical candidates have one of the three major

**TABLE 22–1. HISTOLOGIC CLASSIFICATION OF BRONCHIAL CARCINOMA**

| |
|---|
| **Non-small Cell Carcinoma** |
| Squamous cell (epidermoid) carcinoma |
| Spindle cell (squamous) variant |
| Adenocarcinoma |
| Acinar adenocarcinoma |
| Papillary adenocarcinoma |
| Bronchioloalveolar carcinoma |
| Solid carcinoma with mucus formation |
| Large cell undifferentiated carcinoma |
| Giant cell variant |
| Clear cell variant |
| Adenosquamous carcinoma |
| **Undifferentiated Small Cell Carcinoma** |
| Oat cell (typical small cell) carcinoma |
| Intermediate (polygonal, fusiform) cell type |
| Combined (mixed) cell type |

non-small cell tumors, whereas almost all patients with small cell lesions are not surgical candidates and require chemotherapy as the major therapeutic modality.

A histologic or cytologic diagnosis may be obtained by sputum cytology, bronchoscopic biopsy of the tumor, or by needle aspiration or biopsy of the primary tumor or of a metastatic site. Open-surgical biopsy may be required occasionally in a few patients, and histologic diagnosis may not be established until thoracotomy.

## SPUTUM CYTOLOGIC EXAMINATION

With appropriate cytologic study of several sputum specimens, tumor cells may be found in 20% to as many as 74% of the lung cancer patients. In one study of patients with primary lung cancer, one or two sputum samples resulted in a 59% positive yield, three sputa a 69% positive yield, and four samples an 85% positive yield.[6] A false-positive incidence of less than 1% was observed. The location of the tumor is important relative to the incidence of a positive yield. Central lesions are more apt to have positive sputum cytology than peripheral ones (75% vs 45%).[7] Larger peripheral tumors may have positive sputum cytology in as high as 50% of instances, whereas smaller peripheral tumors have been noted to have less than a 5% positive yield.[8] Cell type also influences the incidence of positive findings. Cytology is most apt to be positive in patients with squamous cell carcinoma, least in those with small cell carcinoma, and intermediate in those with adenocarcinoma or large cell tumors.

Cell type as determined by cytologic study agrees with that of the final histologic diagnosis in approximately 85% of patients. A comparison of cytologic and histologic diagnosis in a group of lung carcinomas showed that well-differentiated epidermoid carcinomas, undifferentiated small cell carcinomas, and adenocarcinomas could be effectively typed by cytology. The accuracy of cytologic diagnosis—reactive to definitive histologic diagnosis—is 90–100% in small cell carcinoma, 92–96% in squamous cell carcinoma, and 87–97% in adenocarcinoma.[7] The undifferentiated carcinomas, the poorly differentiated epidermoid carcinomas, and the combined carcinomas are more difficult to type correctly.

In an attempt to improve the yield in patients with more peripherally placed lesions, bronchial brushing has been carried out via the use of a bronchial catheter under fluoroscopic, image intensifier guidance systems and during fiber-optic bronchoscopic examination. Many investigators have reported excellent results with these techniques.[9–11] The rate of diagnostic accuracy has been reported to be as high as 75% in patients with peripheral lesions <2 cm in size and approximately 83% in those lesions 2 cm or more in greatest dimension.[12] Minor bleeding may occur in a small percentage of patients after this examination.

In those patients with occult tumors (positive cytology and negative chest roentgenographs), approximately 90% are squamous cell tumors.[13] Three fourths of these occult tumors can be readily identified on initial bronchoscopy; the others require more extensive investigation.[14] The use of a lung imaging fluoresence endoscope (LIFE) device may be useful in this regard.[15]

An extension of cytologic studies may be the use of immunochemical analyses of sputum specimens.[16,17] Lung cancer-associated monoclonal antibodies and molecular alterations in cells are being investigated as markers for cancer cell types. These markers in the future may be developed as screening modalities for the detection of early lung cancer.[18]

## BRONCHOSCOPIC BIOPSY

Examination of the tracheobronchial tree with the flexible fiberoptic bronchoscope, only occasionally with the rigid bronchoscope, is done in all patients suspected of having a tumor of the lung. An exception may be made in those patients with a small, peripheral lesion with no evidence of hilar or mediastinal lymphadenopathy on roentgenographic examination of the chest. Bronchoscopy, however, should be done in this group of patients at the time of thoracotomy or video-assisted thoracoscopic removal.

Direct visualization of the tumor, or positive biopsy findings, or both are obtained in 25–50% of the patients with lung cancer. A higher positive diagnostic yield may be secured if a large number of patients with central tumors or far advanced disease are included in any given series. When the lesion can be visualized endobronchially, the yield is as high as 95%. Also, cell type influences the rate of positive findings. Small cell tumors are identified proportionately more often than are squamous cell or large cell undifferentiated tumors. Adenocarcinomas are identified least frequently of all.

At endoscopy, changes in the bronchial wall may be due directly to presence of the tumor or as a result of its infiltration in the layers of the bronchial wall. Changes in the size of the bronchial lumen as the result of stenosis or obstruction due to the tumor, its infiltration, or external compression by the tumor may be observed. In centrally located squamous cell carcinomas, the tumor is either completely or partially exposed in the bronchial mucosa in most instances, whereas most small cell tumors (three quarters) tend to be submucosal in location.[19] Adenocarcinomas also tend to be submucosal in location, although some may be exposed in the bronchial mucosa as well (see Chapter 10).

## NEEDLE ASPIRATION BIOPSY

Fine-needle aspiration for cytologic evaluation may be accomplished via the fiber-optic bronchoscope (transbronchial aspiration cytology) or percutaneously. Both methods may be used to biopsy the primary tumor or to biopsy a suspected metastatic site.

Transbronchoscopic fine-needle aspiration is indicated in patients with extrabronchial lesions with no pathologic changes in the bronchial wall as well as in those in whom only compression or stenosis of the bronchial wall is noted. The technique also has been used to obtain a diagnosis in peripheral lesions; however, percutaneous biopsy is more often done in this situation. Many authors have found this latter procedure to be more accurate than the use of the flexible fiberoptic bronchoscope in patients with peripherally placed lesions.[20,21] The ability to biopsy the lesion has been greatly enhanced with the use of computed tomography (CT)-guided fine-needle aspiration of the peripheral lesion. However, lesions <1 cm in size are believed by most to be a contraindication for the use of any fine-needle aspiration technique.

The accuracy of diagnosis of peripheral tumors with percutaneous fine-needle aspiration is in the range of 84–95%. False-positive results are rare. In indeterminate peripheral lesions that are initially considered to be benign or nondiagnostic on fine-needle aspiration, the incidence of tumor has been reported to be subsequently as high as 29%.[22] Thus, the report of malignancy not being present on fine-needle aspiration cannot be considered as absolute unless a specific nonmalignant diagnosis has been established; tuberculoma and hamartoma are two examples. It has been estimated that a specific nonmalignant diagnosis is established by fine-needle aspiration in only 14–16% of patients with indeterminate peripheral nodules.

Despite these latter observations, the practice of needle aspiration of a peripheral lung mass has almost become routine. This practice is often unnecessary unless one is attempting to obtain a diagnosis in a patient who declines the recommendation for surgery or who is medically unfit for an operative procedure. In a medically fit patient with an indeterminate peripheral mass that is more likely to be benign than malignant, a video-assisted thorascopic removal for histologic evaluation is often the more appropriate procedure.[23] In those patients in whom the lesion is most likely to be a malignant tumor (size >3 cm, spiculated margins, and the patient has a long history of smoking), it is not unreasonable to proceed directly to a thoracotomy. It should be emphasized that whether or not a fine-needle biopsy is positive for tumor, most patients with an indeterminate peripheral lesion will eventually be explored.

Fine-needle aspiration also may be used for the biopsy of suspected metastatic sites. These include enlarged mediastinal nodes (particularly those that are paratracheal or subcarinal in location), enlarged supraclavicular nodes, and suspected liver or adrenal metastases. Since the presence of tumor in the mediastinal lymph nodes greatly affects the therapeutic approach, CT should be done prior to bronchoscopy in patients with suspected lung cancer so that enlarged nodes can be identified when present to facilitate the fine-needle aspiration of such nodes at the time of bronchoscopy.[24,25] The diagnostic sensitivity of fine-needle aspiration of enlarged nodes in patients with non-small cell cancer has been reported to be as high as 82%[24] (see Chapter 8).

Cutting-needle biopsy is used infrequently at present. A major indication for its use is a mass fixed to or involving the chest wall. In the presence of a pleural effusion, a cutting needle may be used to obtain an adequate pleural biopsy to determine the presence or absence of metastatic involvement of the pleura. Multiple specimens should be obtained in this situation.

## VIDEO-ASSISTED THORACOSCOPY

With the development of video-assisted thorascopic surgical (VATS) techniques (see Chapter 12), excision of a peripheral nodule, biopsy of specific nodal stations, as will be subsequently noted, and evaluation of suspected malignant pleural effusions by these techniques is practiced by most thoracic surgeons in lieu of many older techniques that formerly have been used.[26]

## THORACOTOMY

Infrequently, open-surgical biopsy is necessary to obtain tissue for a histologic diagnosis. Most often, however, one of the less invasive biopsy techniques such as mediastinoscopy, mediastinotomy, or video-assisted thoracoscopy is used primarily to obtain the necessary tissue diagnosis.

Infrequently, a histologic diagnosis will not be obtained in a variable number of patients prior to thoracotomy for definitive treatment. A few of these patients will be those with peripheral nodules in whom a video-assisted thoracoscopic removal or a fine-needle aspiration biopsy was either not done or in whom the latter diagnostic procedure did not yield a definitive diagnosis. A small number of patients in whom a prethoracotomy diagnosis has not been obtained will have central lesions from which diagnostic tissue was not recovered by bronchoscopy, needle aspiration, or mediastinal exploration.

When the diagnosis is unknown prior to thoracotomy, a definitive therapeutic resection may be done without a final tissue diagnosis when the procedure is no greater than a lobectomy or is of lesser extent (a segmentectomy or wedge resection). However, when the planned procedure is a pneumonectomy or entails an en bloc resection of an adjacent structure such as the chest wall, a tissue diagnosis is mandatory prior to the procedure. Tissue may be obtained by an intraoperative fine-needle aspiration of the lesion,[27] a wedge resection of the mass, or even at times an incisional biopsy of the suspected tumor. A thoracotomy for the purpose of obtaining only a tissue diagnosis in a patient who has nonresectable disease or known distant metastases should be avoided, since such a procedure confers no benefit to the patient (Fig. 22–1).

## STAGING THE EXTENT OF DISEASE

The extent of the disease process at the time of initial diagnosis is of great importance in determining the therapeutic plan and the prognostic outlook of the patient in both the non-small cell and small cell histologic subgroups. As noted, rather precise classification has been developed for the staging of patients with non-small cell tumors, whereas a relatively broad classification generally has been utilized for those patients with small cell tumors.

## THE STAGE CLASSIFICATION

The presently used classification to categorize and stage-group patients with non-small cell tumors is the new International Staging System.[4] In this classification (Table 22–2), as in the initial AJC classification, the T descriptor relates to the site, size, and local extent of the primary tumor; N denotes the presence and location of regional lymph node involvement, and M indicates the documented presence or absence of distant metastases beyond the ipsilateral hemithorax.

In the new international classification, the descriptors T1 and T2 remain the same as in the original AJC classification. The new T3 descriptor now includes only those tumors that have invaded locally beyond the visceral pleura into structures that are surgically resectable by conventional criteria (Fig. 22–2A,B). A T4 descriptor has been added to designate those locally invasive tumors that involve structures that preclude complete surgical resection (Fig. 22–3A,B) or those that are associated with a malignant pleural effusion. Several special circumstances occur in which questions arise as to the appropriate T designation. It has been suggested that discontinuous tumor deposits on the visceral or parietal pleura, recurrent nerve involvement, and the presence of multiple intraparenchymal nodules in addition to the primary tumor in a different but ipsilateral lobe be designated as T4 disease; multiple nodules in the same lobe are designated as T3 disease.[28]

The descriptors N0 and N1 remain unchanged and describe the absence of lymph node metastases (N0) or the presence of ipsilateral lobar or hilar lymph node involvement (N1). However, the descriptor N2 is now used only to signify the presence of metastatic or direct involvement of ipsilateral or subcarinal mediastinal lymph nodes. The new N3 descriptor is used to denote metastatic involvement of the contralateral mediastinal or hilar lymph nodes, and it also is used to describe metastasis to either ipsilateral or contralateral supraclavicular lymph nodes. Supraclavicular lymph node involvement was previously considered to be distant metastasis (M1), but, in fact, this metastatic involvement represents local-regional disease extension. With this later exception, the descriptors M0 (no distant metastases) and M1 (known distant metastases present) remain unchanged.

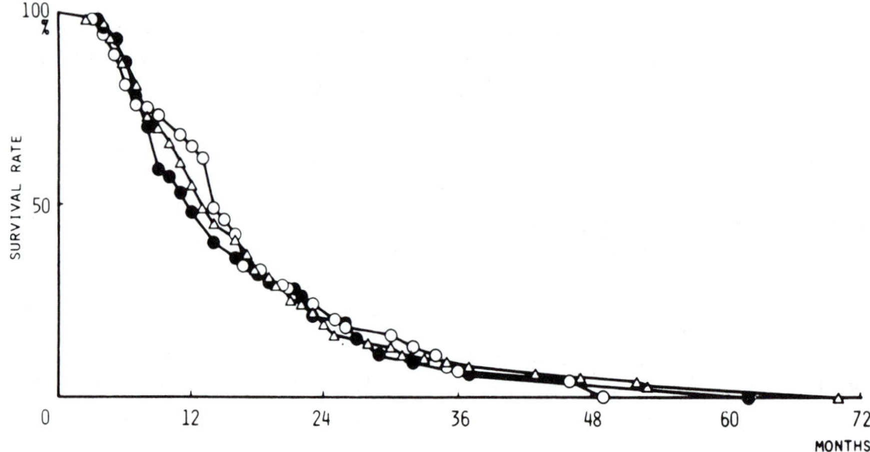


**Figure 22–1.** Survival curves of patients with stage III carcinoma of the lung who underwent a palliative resection (○; 54 patients) thoracotomy only (●; 54 patients), or no surgical intervention (△; 113 patients). Survival of each group is essentially the same. *(From Hara N et al: Assessment of the role of surgery for Stage III bronchogenic carcinoma. J Surg Oncol 25:153, 1984, with permission.)*

**TABLE 22–2. DEFINITIONS OF T, N, AND M CATEGORIES FOR CARCINOMA OF THE LUNG**

| Category | Definition |
|---|---|
| **T Primary Tumors** | |
| TX | Tumor proven by the presence of malignant cells in bronchopulmonary secretions but not visualized roentgenographically or bronchoscopically, or any tumor that cannot be assessed as in a retreatment staging. |
| TO | No evidence of primary tumor. |
| TIS | Carcinoma in situ. |
| T1 | A tumor that is 3.0 cm or less in greatest dimension, surrounded by lung or visceral pleura, and without evidence of invasion proximal to a lobar bronchus at bronchoscopy. |
| T2 | A tumor more than 3.0 cm in greatest dimension, or a tumor of any size that either invades the visceral pleura or has associated atelectasis or obstructive pneumonitis extending to the hilar region. At bronchoscopy, the proximal extent of demonstrable tumor must be within a lobar bronchus or at least 2.0 cm distal to the carina. Any associated atelectasis or obstructive pneumonitis must involve less than an entire lung. |
| T3 | A tumor of any size with direct extension into the chest wall (including superior sulcus tumors), diaphragm, or the mediastinal pleura or pericardium without involving the heart, great vessels, trachea, esophagus, or vertebral body, or a tumor in the main bronchus within 2 cm of the carina without involving the carina. |
| T4 | A tumor of any size with invasion of the mediastinum or involving heart, great vessels, trachea, esophagus or vertebral body or carina or presence of malignant pleural effusion. |
| **N Nodal Involvement** | |
| NO | No demonstrable metastasis to regional lymph nodes. |
| N1 | Metastasis to lymph nodes in the peribronchial or the ipsilateral hilar region, or both, including direct extension. |
| N2 | Metastasis to ipsilateral mediastinal lymph nodes or subcarinal lymph nodes. |
| N3 | Metastasis to contralateral mediastinal lymph nodes, contralateral hilar lymph nodes, ipsilateral or contralateral scalene or supraclavicular lymph nodes. |
| **M Distant Metastasis** | |
| MO | No (known) distant metastasis. |
| M1 | Distant metastasis present. |

Once the T, N, and M status is determined, the patient may be placed into one of seven stage groupings (Table 22–3). Stage I is now made up of patients with either T1 or T2 disease without lymph node or distant metastatic disease (Fig. 22–4). Stage II consists of patients with T1 or T2 disease and either ipsilateral lobar or hilar lymph node metastases (Fig. 22–5). Stage IIIA is made up of those patients with either T3 or N2 disease, or both (Fig. 22–6), and stage IIIB consists of those patients with either T4 or N3 disease (Fig. 22–7). Stage IV is composed of those patients with any known distant metastases (M1).

Although these stage groupings reflect the therapeutic and prognostic features of the various patient groups more appropriately than did the previous AJC stage groupings, some problems still remain. One is that patients with T1 N0 M0 disease have a better prognosis than that of those with T2 N0 M0 disease (approximately 70% vs 60% 5-year survival, respectively).[4] It would be better if these two groups were separated. Second, many patients with N2 disease (those with gross lymph node involvement on roentgenograms of the chest and approximately 80–90% of those with unsuspected but with positive biopsy of mediastinal lymph nodes on preoperative mediastinal exploration) have initially nonresectable disease but unfortunately are grouped in stage IIIA, which is supposed to represent those patients with extravisceral pleural extension that is thought to be completely resectable for cure. However, with the advent of neoadjuvant therapy for both stage IIIA and stage IIIB disease, this may be of lesser import in the future.[29–32] Nonetheless, this latter staging problem needs to be addressed by further refinement of the staging system. However, the new International System represents an overall improvement and should be accepted by those dealing with the problem of lung cancer.

In the histologic subset of patients with small cell carcinoma of the lung, the T, N, and M designations and the respective stage groupings are not generally used. Instead, most investigators working with this subgroup of patients divide the extent of the disease process into localized or extensive disease categories only.[33] The first designation, localized disease, is used to denote those patients in whom the disease is confined to the ipsilateral hemithorax with or without ipsilateral supraclavicular lymph node involvement; pleural effusion may be present. The second category, extensive disease, is used to identify those in whom the disease has spread elsewhere beyond the ipsilateral hemithorax. In the vast majority of patients with small cell carcinoma, these broad categories have been found to be sufficient for therapeutic and prognostic necessities. However, a very small number of patients in the localized disease category are best further subdivided by the International T, N, and M staging system into those who have very limited disease (stages I and limited stage IIIA, non-N2 disease), since such patients may well be candidates for surgical resection in addition to the standard chemotherapeutic regimens.

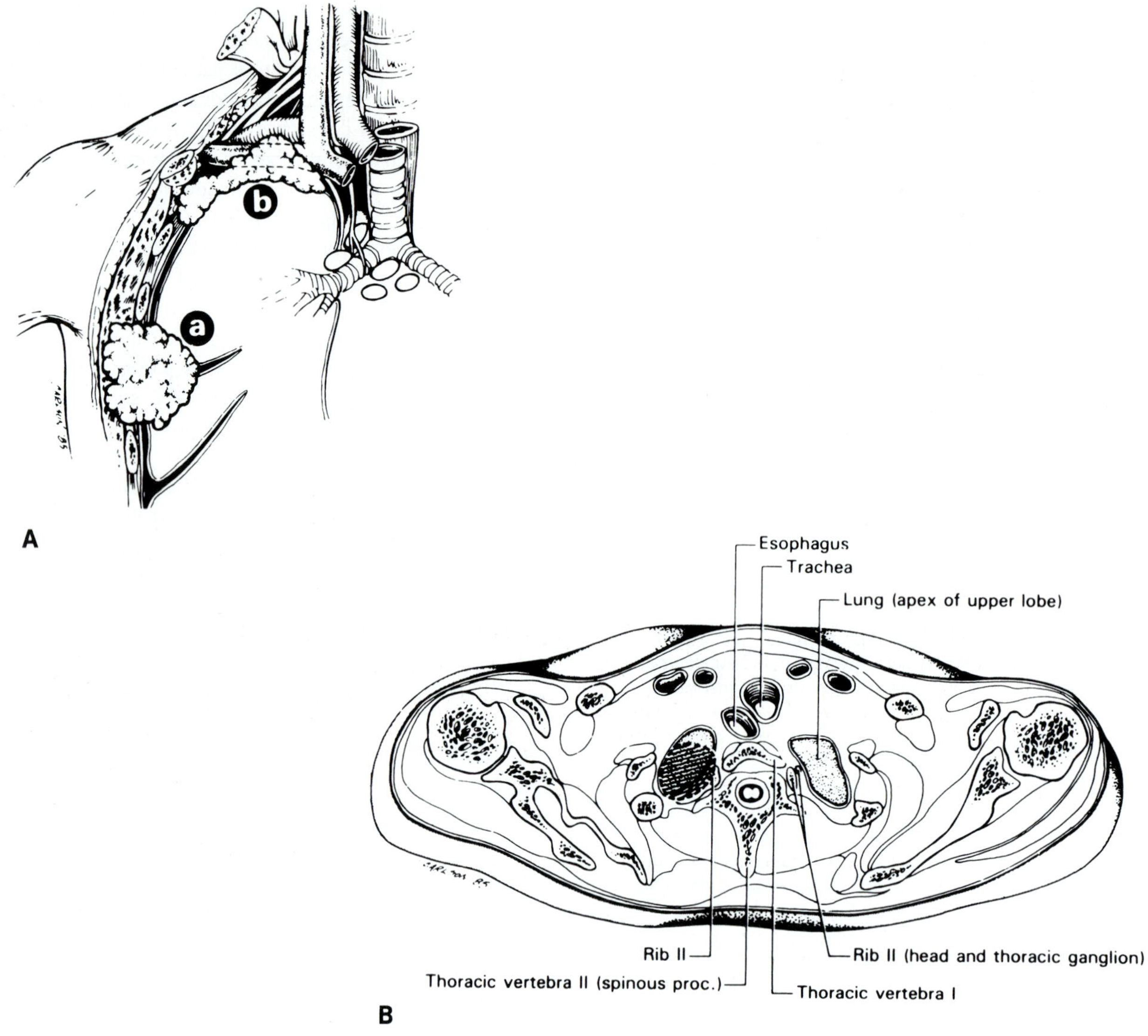


**Figure 22–2. A.** T3: A tumor of any size with direct extension into the (a) chest wall (b) including superior sulcus tumors. **B.** T3: Superior sulcus tumor with no involvement of the vertebral body. *(From Mountain CF: A new international staging system for lung cancer. Chest 89:225S, 1986, with permission.)*

## STAGING VALUE OF THE CLINICAL PRESENTATION

In order to determine the T, N, and M status of patients with carcinoma of the lung and to place the patients in the appropriate stage categories, the clinical presentation of the patient affords the initial indication of the possible extent of the disease process. The vast majority of patients (approximately 90–95%) with carcinoma of the lung are symptomatic at the time of presentation. The remaining patients are identified primarily by the incidental discovery of a pulmonary lesion on a routine roentgenogram of the chest. The number of patients in this category appears to be increasing, at least in most surgical series. A smaller number of carcinomas of the lung are identified by a positive sputum cytology in an asymptomatic individual with a normal roentgenogram of the chest undergoing a screening evaluation. This finding is termed an occult lung carcinoma.

In the Mayo Lung Project[34] conducted to evaluate the efficacy of lung cancer screening in a high-risk population, 91 patients with unsuspected lung cancer were initially identified. Of these "prevalent" cases, 59 were discovered by roentgenograms of the chest, 17 occult tumors by sputum examination, and 15 by both examinations. In those patients subsequently found to develop lung cancer, examination of roentgenograms of the chest detected six times as many new cancers as did sputum cytology.

The asymptomatic patients in whom the disease is identified initially by roentgenographic or sputum examinations generally have relatively early disease, whereas the symptomatic patient may have either early or late disease. In the Mayo Project, 54% of the "prevalent" cases under-

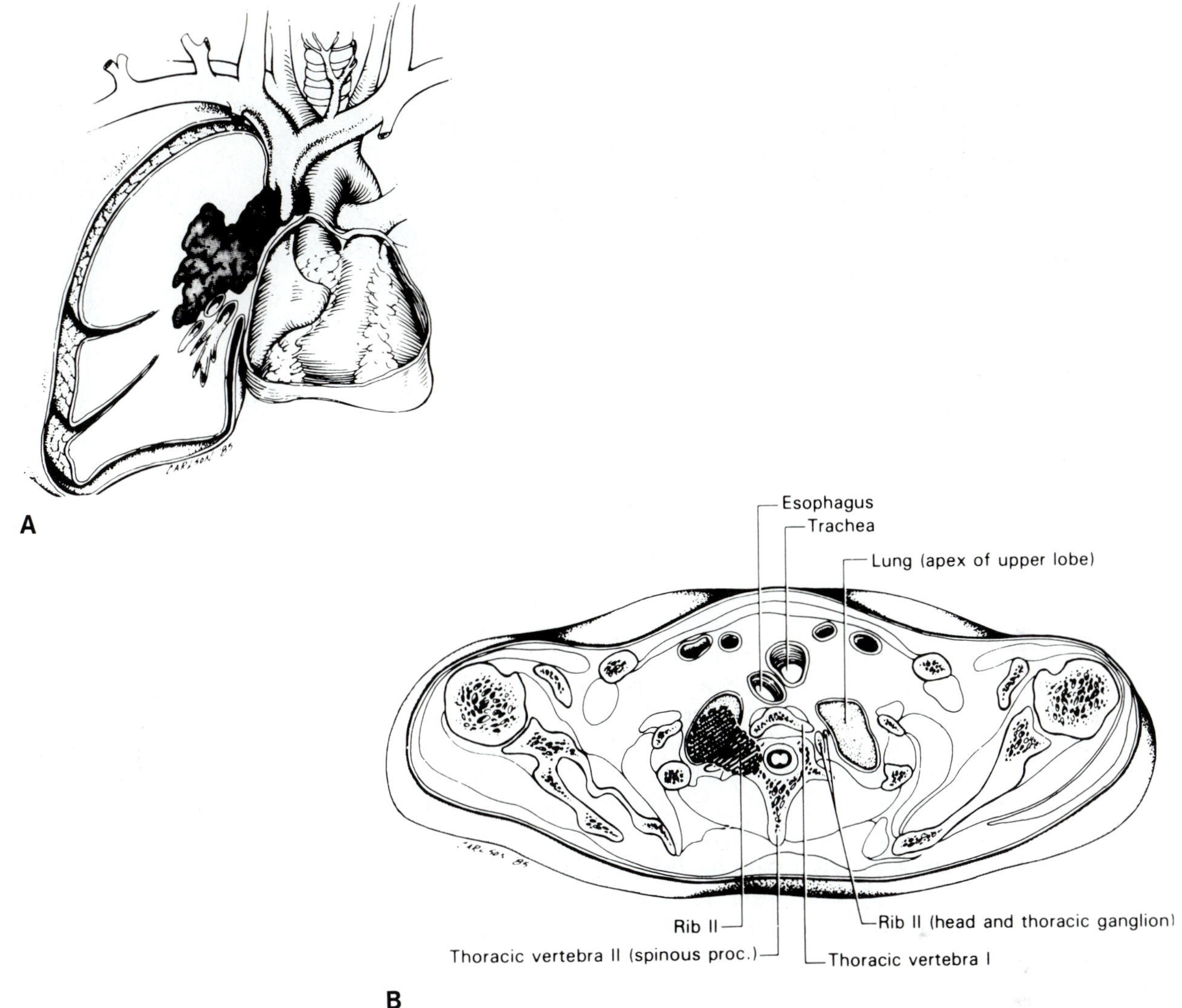


**Figure 22–3. A.** T4: Superior vena cava syndrome—tumor involving great vessels. **B.** T4: Tumor invading vertebral body—unresectable, produces Pancoast's syndrome. *(From Mountain CF: A new international staging system for lung cancer. Chest 89:225S, 1986, with permission.)*

**TABLE 22–3. STAGE GROUPING OF TNM SUBSETS**

| | | | |
|---|---|---|---|
| Occult carcinoma | TX | N0 | M0 |
| Stage 0 | TIS | Carcinoma in situ | |
| Stage I | T1 | N0 | M0 |
| | T2 | N0 | M0 |
| Stage II | T1 | N1 | M0 |
| | T2 | N1 | M0 |
| Stage IIIA | T3 | N0 | M0 |
| | T3 | N1 | M0 |
| | T1–3 | N2 | M0 |
| Stage IIIB | Any T | N3 | M0 |
| | T4 | Any N | M0 |
| Stage IV | Any T | Any N | M1 |

went resection for cure, whereas in symptomatic patients usually less than 25% can be managed by resection.

The symptoms and signs of a lung tumor are categorized as bronchopulmonary, extrapulmonary intrathoracic, extrathoracic metastatic, extrathoracic nonmetastatic, and miscellaneous.[35] Many of these symptoms and signs may be sufficient to initially stage the patient clinically.

*Bronchopulmonary* symptoms consist of cough, hemoptysis, respiratory infection, and, occasionally, dull chest pain, wheezing, and stridor. These symptoms are due to the presence of the tumor within the lung causing irritation, ulceration, or obstruction of a bronchus, with or without infection in the parenchyma distal to the lesion. These features by themselves are of no help in suggesting the T stage of the tumor.

*Extrapulmonary intrathoracic* symptoms are due to either direct extension of the tumor beyond the visceral

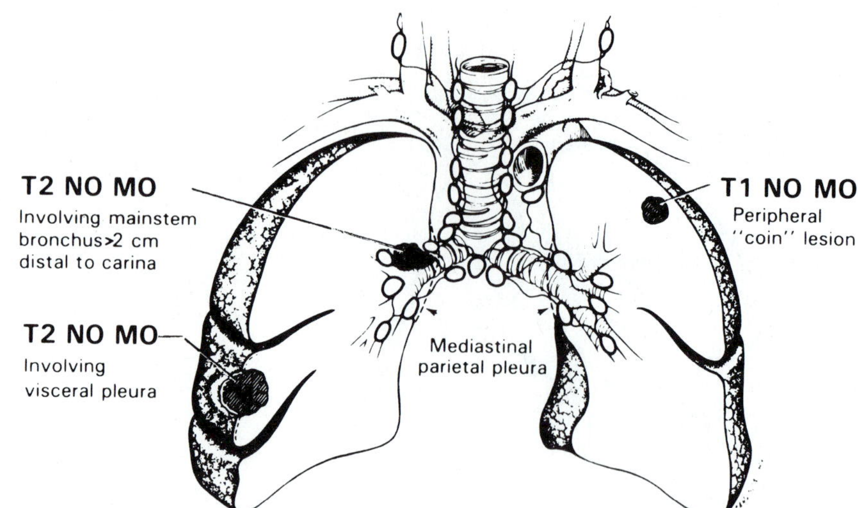


**Figure 22–4.** Stage lung carcinoma with no lymph node involvement. *(From Mountain CF: A new international staging system for lung cancer. Chest 89:225S, 1986, with permission.)*

pleural envelope, its metastatic spread to mediastinal lymph nodes, or the presence of a malignant pleural effusion. The signs and symptoms may be chest-wall pain, hoarseness, superior vena cava syndrome, shortness of breath due to pleural effusion or phrenic nerve paralysis, dysphagia, pain in the upper extremity, or Horner's syndrome, among others. These manifestations may be due either to a T3 or T4 lesion or to N2 involvement and automatically place the patient into one of the stage III categories.

*Extrathoracic metastatic* symptoms are all those related to the spread of the tumor to distant sites; the liver, brain, contralateral lung, adrenal, skeletal system, and kidney are common sites of involvement. Any such spread, once it is confirmed, represents M1 disease and places the patient into the stage IV category.

*Extrathoracic nonmetastatic* symptoms consist of metabolic, neuromuscular, skeletal, dermatologic, vascular, and hematologic findings (Table 22–4). Approximately 2% of patients with lung carcinoma seek medical advice because of such symptoms and signs, although a greater number will have the paraneoplastic features when these are sought for. None of these manifestations is specific, and each may occur in association with other malignant lesions.

The majority of the metabolic manifestations are the result of the secretion of endocrine or endocrinelike substances by the tumor. At times, some of these syndromes may be produced by tumors that are still resectable, but, unfortunately, most are found in association with small cell carcinomas (Table 22–5).

Cushing's syndrome occurs most often in patients with small cell carcinoma. These patients differ from those with classic Cushing's syndrome. Essentially, these differences consist of reversal of the sex ratio, older age incidence, prominence of hypokalemic alkalosis, fewer physical stigmas of typical Cushing's syndrome, and a more rapid, fulminating clinical course. Significant amounts of adrenocorticotrophic hormone (ACTH) have been demonstrated in the tumor tissue and blood of these patients. Studies utilizing small cell cancer cell lines suggest that the tumor cells secrete ACTH precursor peptides (pro-ACTH) and pro-opi-

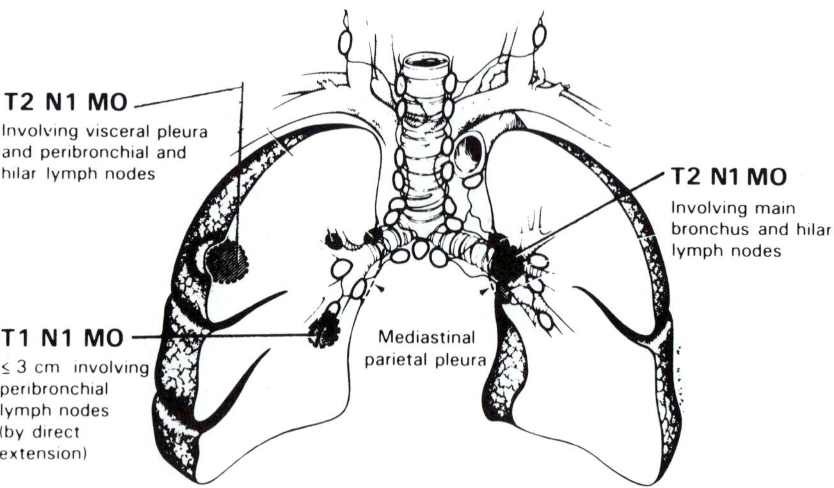


**Figure 22–5.** Stage II lung carcinoma with intrapulmonary and/or hilar nodes involved. *(From Mountain CF: A new international staging system for lung cancer. Chest 89:225S, 1986, with permission.)*

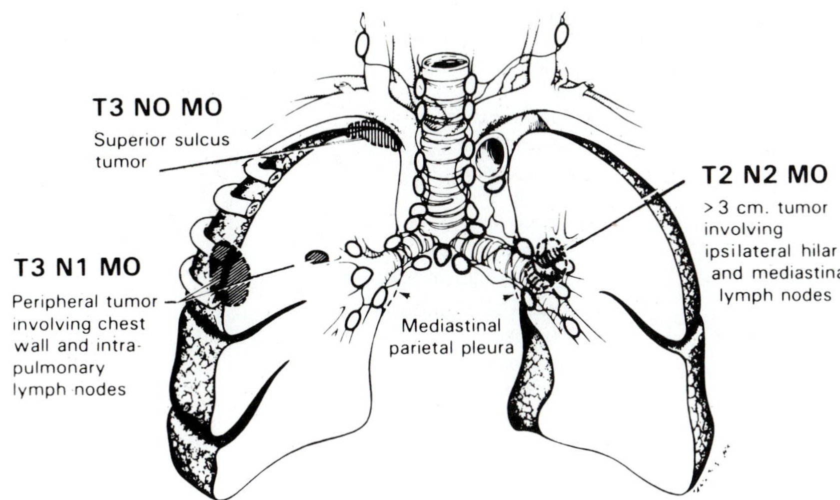


**Figure 22–6.** Stage IIIA lung carcinoma. *(From Mountain CF: A new international staging system for lung cancer. Chest 89:225S, 1986, with permission.)*

omelanocortia (POMC) and not ACTH per se.[36] By physiologic, physiochemical, and immunochemical tests, the ectopic ACTH is indistinguishable from the normal hormone, although the tumors have physiologic autonomy, since high-dose dexamethasone fails to suppress the levels of end products of ACTH in the urine.

Excessive antidiuretic hormone production (arginine vasopressin) also is seen, most often in patients with small cell tumors. Hyponatremia is reported to be present to some degree in one third of the patients with this type of tumor. Positive immunoassay of an arginine-vasopressin-like material has been reported in these patients. Elevated levels of atrial natriuretic peptide (ANP) have also been noted in these patients.[37] The symptoms are those of water intoxication with anorexia, nausea, and vomiting accompanied by increasing severe neurologic complications. Hypotonicity of the plasma, hyponatremia, persistent renal sodium loss, relative hypertonicity of the urine, absence of clinical evidence of fluid depletion, and normal renal and adrenal function may be the presenting features.

Hypercalcemia is a frequent complication of malignant disease, and, although it often results from bony metastases, it may be caused by excessive secretion of a polypeptide, parathyroid hormone-related protein (PTHrP), similar to parathyroid hormone, by the tumor. An accompanying hypophosphatemia frequently is found. Most of the tumors that are associated with hypercalcemia are the squamous cell type. Clinically, the patient may have somnolence and mental changes as well as anorexia, vomiting, and weight loss. Frequently, the tumor may be resectable, and excision of the tumor will result in a reversal of the abnormal calcium levels in the blood.

Ectopic gonadotropin production is found rarely in association with carcinoma of the lung. There have been a number of male patients with tender gynecomastia, often associated with hypertrophic pulmonary osteoarthropathy,

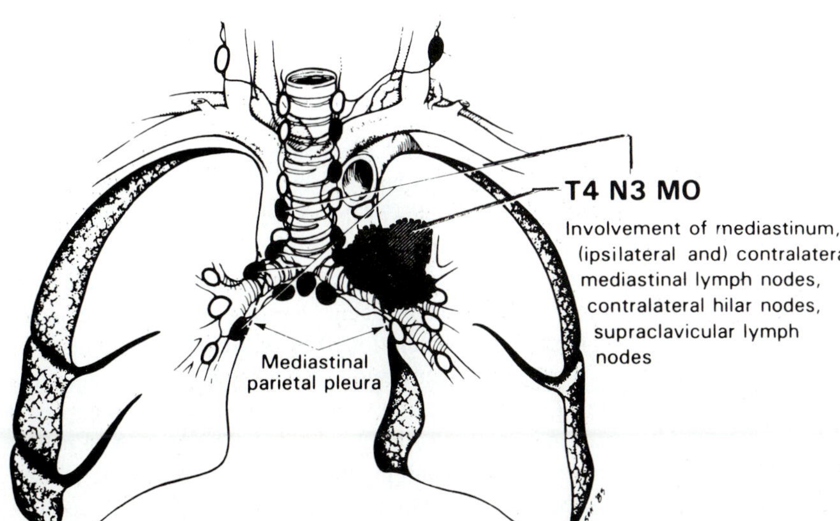


**Figure 22–7.** Stage IIIB lung carcinoma. *(From Mountain CF: A new international staging system for lung cancer. Chest 89, 225S, 1986, with permission.)*

**TABLE 22–4. PARANEOPLASTIC SYNDROMES IN LUNG CANCER PATIENTS**

**Metabolic**
- Hypercalcemia
- Cushing's syndrome
- Inappropriate antidiuretic hormone production
  - Carcinoid syndrome
- Gynecomastia
- Hypercalcitonemia
- Elevated growth hormone level
- Elevated prolactin, follicle-stimulating hormone, luteinizing hormone levels
- Hypoglycemia
- Hyperthyroidism

**Neurologic**
- Encephalopathy
- Subacute cerebellar degeneration
- Peripheral neuropathy
- Polymyositis
- Autonomic neuropathy
- Lambert-Eaton syndrome
- Opsoclonus and myoclonus

**Skeletal**
- Clubbing
- Pulmonary hypertrophic osteoarthropathy

**Hematologic**
- Anemia
- Leukemoid reactions
- Thrombocytosis
- Thrombocytopenia
- Eosinophilia
- Pure red cell aplasia
- Leukoerythroblastosis
- Disseminated intravascular coagulation

**Cutaneous and Muscular**
- Hyperkeratosis
- Dermatomyositis
- Acanthosis nigricans
- Hyperpigmentation
- Erythema gyratum repens
- Hypertrichosis lanuginosa acquisita

**Other**
- Nephrotic syndrome
- Hypouricemia
- Secretion of vasoactive intestinal peptide with diarrhea
- Hyperamylasemia
- Anorexia-cachexia

*From Shields TW: Presentation, diagnosis and staging of bronchial carcinoma and of the asymptomatic solitary pulmonary nodule. In Shields TW (ed): General Thoracic Surgery, 4th ed. Philadelphia, Lea & Febiger, 1994, with permission.*

in whom production of gonadotropin has been documented. As in patients with hypercalcemia, some of the tumors associated with ectopic gonadotropin production may be resectable. The histologic appearance of these tumors resembles undifferentiated large cell carcinoma. Adenocarcinomas also are known to produce human chorionic gonadotropin in tissue culture.

Other hormone levels may be affected in lung cancer patients. Elevated levels of calcitonin have been documented. Its production occurs mostly in small cell tumors. Increased levels of growth hormone may be seen in patients with lung cancer of all types.

The carcinomatous neuromyopathies are the most frequent extrathoracic, nonmetastatic manifestations of carcinoma of the lung. If specifically looked for, one or more types of neuromyopathy may be found in approximately 15% of the patients. These findings may be found in patients with all cell types (56% small cell carcinoma, 22% squamous cell carcinoma, 16% anaplastic tumor, and 5% adenocarcinoma).[38]

**TABLE 22–5. FREQUENCY OF PARANEOPLASTIC ENDOCRINE SYNDROMES RELATIVE TO CELL TYPE OF LUNG CANCER**

| | Small Cell | Adeno/Large Cell | Squamous Cell |
|---|---|---|---|
| Cushing's syndrome | +++ | +/– | +/– |
| SIADH[a] | ++++ | +/– | +/– |
| Tumor hypercalcemia | + | + | ++++ |
| Gynecomastia | ++ | + | +/– |

[a]Syndrome of inappropriate antidiuretic hormone.
*(From Shields TW: Presentation, diagnosis and staging of bronchial carcinoma and of the asymptomatic solitary pulmonary nodule. In Shields TW (ed): General Thoracic Surgery, 4th ed. Philadelphia, Lea & Febiger, 1994, with permission.)*

Carcinomatous myopathies are the most common syndromes encountered. The two types seen are the myasthenic-like syndrome and polymyositis. The former (the Lambert-Eaton syndrome) is probably a defect of neuromuscular conduction and is seen in patients with small cell cancer. The voltage-gated calcium channels of the peripheral cholinergic nerve terminals are believed to be the target of antibodies formed in association with the tumor. The differentiation from true myasthenia can be determined by distinct differences in electrophysiologic changes between the two conditions.[39] Also, 75% of patients with the Lambert-Eaton syndrome and a primary lung cancer will be seropositive by radioimmunoassay that detects antibodies that react with the calcium channel components extracted from small cell lung cancer cells.[40] Clinically, the syndrome is characterized by weakness and marked fatigability of the proximally located muscles of the extremities, particularly those of the pelvic girdle and thighs. The features of the polymyositis are similar to those of the myasthenic syndrome, except that muscular wasting is more prominent, and a primary degeneration of the muscle fibers occurs.

Peripleural neuropathy, encephalomyopathy, subacute cerebellar degeneration, and rarely visual paraneoplastic syndromes may also be recognized. The cause and pathogenesis of these neuromyopathies are unclear. The current hypothesis is that they arise as autoimmune or altered immune responses to substances produced by the tumor cells.

The recognition and differentiation of these neuromyopathies from metastatic lesions are important, since resection of a non-small cell lung tumor may be possible.

The most frequent peripheral sign of lung carcinoma is clubbing of the fingers, which, at times, is associated with generalized hypertrophic pulmonary osteoarthropathy. In this latter syndrome, the periosteal proliferation and new bone formation seen at the ends of the long bones may occur before other symptoms of the lung lesion are manifested. Bone pain, hydroarthrosis, fever, and night sweats are the common manifestations. The cause remains unknown. The incidence of hypertrophic pulmonary osteoarthropathy in patients with carcinoma of the lung has been reported to be from 2% to 12%. Hypertrophic pulmonary osteoarthropathy is not found in patients with small cell tumors, but its incidence in patients with the other three major cell types is equally distributed. The presence of these findings does not denote per se nonresectability of the tumor.

Other nonmetastatic symptoms may be seen with any cell type. It is to be emphasized that the presence of the extrathoracic nonmetastatic syndromes is not dependent upon the T, N, or M status of the lesion. In those patients with non-small cell tumors, many of the tumors are resectable.

Miscellaneous nonspecific symptoms such as weight loss (especially >10–15% of the patient's normal weight), weakness, anorexia, lassitude, and malaise do not denote any stage per se, but as a general rule their presence suggests a poor functional status and, thus, a poor prognosis for the patient.

## SPECIAL LABORATORY STUDIES—TUMOR MARKERS

A variety of substances, including the aforementioned hormonelike substances, are produced in excess in patients with carcinoma of the lung (Table 22–6). The hormonal substances, particularly "big" ACTH and oncofetal carcinoembryonic antigen (CEA) as well as the products associated with increased cell turnover ($\beta_2$-microglobulin and other polyamines), have been identified in many patients with non-small cell tumors. These substances have been studied as to their value in the diagnosis of patients with lung carcinoma.[41,42] Unfortunately, the levels in themselves are not diagnostic since these substances may be elevated by other nonspecific causes. Increased levels of these substances are frequently found in smokers and particularly in those with chronic lung disease.

Tumor biomarker production is more common in small cell carcinomas; among the biomarkers are bombesin, neuron-specific enolase, creatinine kinase, calcitonin, and other peptides.[43] The levels of these markers are related frequently to the stage of the disease. Also, the identification of these substances may aid in differentiating the "classic" oat cell and intermediate cell types from the more aggressive variant form; the latter type produces less of these substances as a rule (Table 22–7).

**TABLE 22–6. PEPTIDE HORMONES PRODUCED BY LUNG CANCER**

| |
|---|
| ACTH[a]—pro ACTH |
| Arginine vasopressin[a] |
| Parathyroid hormone |
| Parathyroid hormone-related protein |
| Vasoactive intestinal polypeptide[a] |
| Melanocyte-simulating hormone[a] |
| β-Human chorionic gonadotropin[a] |
| Atrial natriuretic peptide |
| Transforming growth factors a and b |
| Interleukin-1a |
| Granulocyte-colony-stimulating factor |
| Gastin-releasing peptide—Bombesin |
| Somatostatin |
| Growth hormone |
| Calcitonin |
| Physalemin |
| Neuron-specific enolase |
| Neurophysin |
| β-Endorphin |
| Neurotensin |
| Glucagon |

[a]Hormones that produce documented paraneoplastic syndromes.

*(Adapted from Richardson GE, Johnson BE: Paraneoplastic syndromes in lung cancer. Curr Opin Oncol 4:323, 1992, with permission.)*

Various tumor oncogenes including the *K-ras* oncogene mutation[44] and overproduction of *HER-2/neu* (*C-erb B-2*, p 185 neu) oncogene[45] have been identified in varying percentages of patients with adenocarcinoma, and, although of some prognostic value, they are not important in the staging process. The same is true of p53 tumor suppressor gene mutations in patients with non-small cell lung cancer.[46] *C-myc* proto-oncogenes are amplified or overexpressed without amplification in over 80% of small cell tumors. Those patients with amplification have a poorer prognosis than the patients without amplification.[47]

## INITIAL DIAGNOSTIC EVALUATION

Standard posterior-anterior and lateral roentgenograms of the chest and the usual laboratory examinations constitute

**TABLE 22–7. BIOCHEMICAL CHARACTERISTICS OF CLASSIC v. VARIANT CELL LINES OF SMALL CELL LUNG CANCER**

| Neuroendocrine Markers | Classic Cell Line | Variant Cell Line |
|---|---|---|
| L-Dopa decarboxylase | ++++ | – |
| Bombesin | ++++ | – |
| Neuron-specific enolase | ++++ | + |
| Creatine kinase BB | ++++ | ++++ |

the first diagnostic steps in the staging process. Sputum cytology and bronchoscopy normally should follow as the second steps, except CT should precede the bronchoscopy as previously noted in patients initially believed to be surgical candidates.

Roentgenographic examination consisting of standard roentgenograms of the chest are abnormal in 98% of the patients. It has been estimated that by the time a tumor is recognized on roentgenogram of the chest, it has completed three fourths of its natural history. Moreover, the roentgenographic abnormality frequently antedates the first symptoms or signs of the disease by 7 or more months.[48] The early and frequently unrecognized findings are a small homogeneous (nodular lesion) or nonhomogeneous density (linear-shaped lesion), infiltration along the course of a blood vessel, a segmental consolidation, subtle enlargement of a hilus, segmental or lobar obstructive emphysema (a rare finding), or a segmental atelectasis.[49] It is to be noted that the limit of visibility of a solitary lesion is one of 0.7 cm in size, and, in most instances, rarely is a lesion recognized until it is at least 1 cm in size.[50]

The usual finding on the roentgenogram may be classified as hilar, pulmonary parenchymal, and intrathoracic extrapulmonary. In the older literature, hilar abnormality, alone or associated with other findings, was present in 41% of patients; obstructive pneumonitis, collapse, or consolidation in 41%; and a parenchymal mass of varying sizes in 42%. Various extrapulmonary intrathoracic manifestations were observed in 11% (mediastinal widening and pleural effusion being the more common findings). At present a peripheral nodular mass is reported to be the most common roentgenographic presentation.[51,52] Parenchymal changes due to obstruction and to infection are observed much less often than formerly recorded (Table 22–8). Unusual roentgenographic manifestations may include a thin-walled cystic cavity, eccentric calcification in a peripheral nodule, and occurrence of bilateral solitary nodules. The latter may occur in 1% of all lung cancer patients and may represent synchronous primary tumors or a primary and a single pulmonary metastasis. Satellite tumor nodules may be observed in approximately 1% of patients.

**TABLE 22–8. ROENTGENOGRAPHIC FINDINGS IN 200 PATIENTS WITH LUNG CANCER**

| | % |
|---|---|
| Tumor in the periphery of the lung | 39.5 |
| Hilar tumor | 19.5 |
| Atelectasis | 13.5 |
| Pleural effusion | 7.0 |
| Hilar invasion | 5.0 |
| Normal | 4.0 |
| Infiltrative shadow in the periphery | 3.0 |
| Other | 8.5 |

*(Adapted from Hayata Y (ed): Lung Cancer Diagnosis, Tokyo, Igaku-Shoin, 1982, with permission.)*

Cell type may influence the roentgenographic presentation.[53] The characteristic finding in each cell may be briefly noted.

Squamous cell carcinoma is commonly associated with findings of obstructive pneumonitis, collapse, or consolidation. A hilar abnormality is also often present. Approximately one third of the squamous cell tumors appear as a peripheral mass. Formerly, two thirds of these were usually larger than 4 cm, but at present small lesions are more frequently seen. Cavitation is more common in the larger peripheral squamous cell carcinomas than in other lung carcinomas and occurs in up to 20% of the patients with squamous cell tumors.

Adenocarcinomas are most often peripheral masses and frequently smaller than 3 cm, although larger peripheral lesions may still be observed. Cavitation is rare. A hilar abnormality appears to be more common than in the past, but an obstructive parenchymal lesion is noted infrequently. A subtype of adenocarcinoma, bronchioalveolar carcinoma frequently presents as a solitary peripheral nodule and represents approximately 35% of all peripheral masses. It may present as a localized area of pneumonic infiltrate of varying extent (the presence of an air bronchogram in the area is common) or less often as multiple unilateral or bilateral coalescent multinodular infiltrates.

Large cell undifferentiated carcinomas are most likely to be peripheral lesions (approximately 60%), and two thirds of these are larger than 4 cm. Cavitation occurs in about 6% of these peripheral lesions. A hilar abnormality and parenchymal changes are each present in association with about one third of these tumors. Ten percent of the patients with this type of tumor have obvious mediastinal widening.

Small cell undifferentiated tumors appear primarily as hilar abnormalities (78%). These are associated with mediastinal widening in many of the patients. A parenchymal obstructive lesion occurs in slightly less than two fifths of the patients and a peripheral mass in less than one third, the majority (three fourths) of these peripheral lesions being <4 cm in size; the peripheral lesion is frequently associated with hilar or mediastinal enlargement.

The roentgenogram may suggest with fair accuracy the T status, especially for peripheral T1 or T2 lesions (Fig. 22–8), but it is generally unhelpful in determining the final pathologic status of a central lesion (clinical T2 lesion) (Fig. 22–9). As a rule, extension of the local tumor beyond the visceral pleural envelope (T3 or T4 disease) cannot be discerned on the standard films, although the presence of a pleural effusion suggests the possibility of the presence of T4 disease.

Enlargement of the hilus may suggest N1 disease (Fig. 22–10), but such involvement is interpreted incorrectly in over a third of the patients. The interpretation of the mediastinum on the standard roentgenograms of the chest for the presence or absence of mediastinal lymph node involvement is also unreliable except in two specific instances.

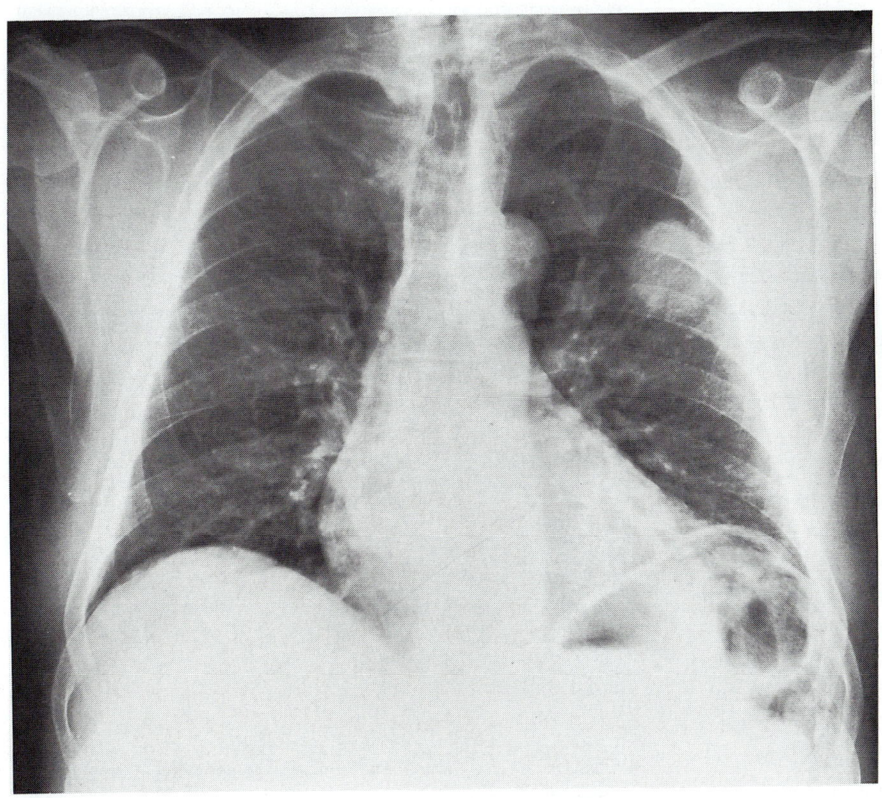

**Figure 22–8.** Peripherally located T2 lung carcinoma. Mediastinal and hilar lymph nodes negative.

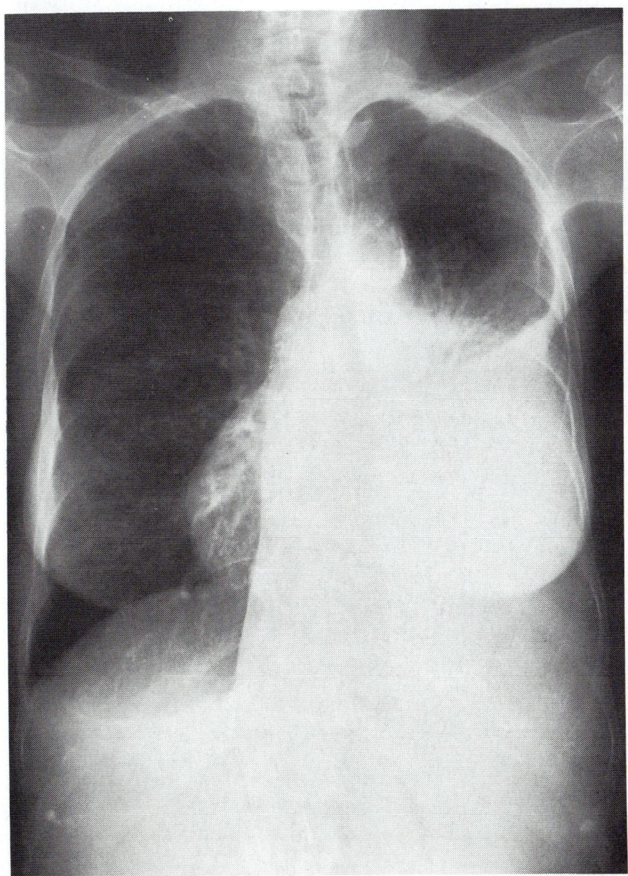

**Figure 22–9.** Central tumor of left lower bronchus with atelectasis of left lower lobe.

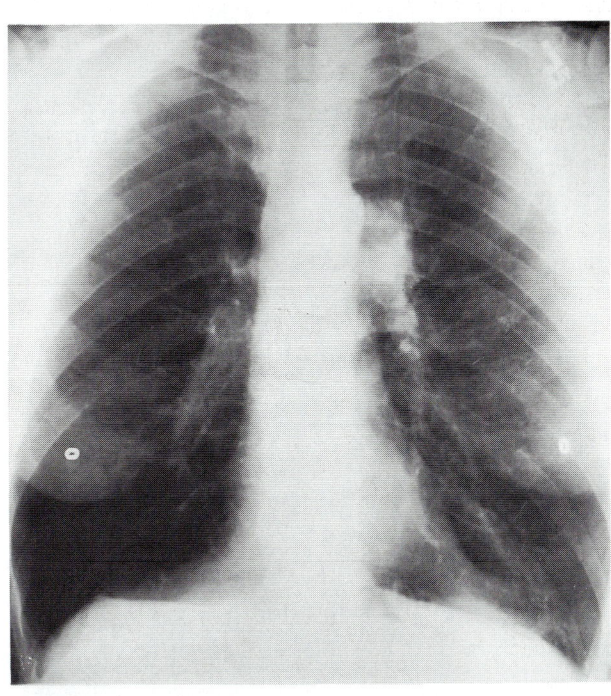

**Figure 22–10.** Central lung carcinoma presenting as an enlarged hilar shadow. *(From Shields TW: The use of mediastinoscopy in lung cancer: The dilemma of mediastinal lymph nodes. In Kittle CF, Current Controversies in Thoracic Surgery. Philadelphia, Saunders, 1986, p 145, with permission.)*

First, when the patient has a peripheral lesion and the hilar shadow and mediastinal shadow are normal, the absence of N2 involvement may be predicted in approximately 90–95% of these patients (Fig. 22–11).[54] Second, when the mediastinal shadow is grossly abnormal (Fig. 22–12), N2 or even N3 disease is present in almost all such patients, and biopsy of the mediastinal lymph nodes only is required to establish its presence. Otherwise, when the hilus is enlarged, or the mediastinum is suspiciously abnormal or if either structure is obscured by the tumor or associated parenchymal disease (Fig. 22–13), the standard roentgenogram is of no value in predicting which patient has N2 involvement (which is present in as many as a third of such patients). In these cases, additional studies, as will be discussed, must be carried out.

Elevation of the diaphragm may be observed. This may be indicative only of volume loss in the lung from atelectasis but may be due to hemidiaphragmatic paralysis caused by tumor involvement of the phrenic nerve. To verify paralysis, however, a sniff test observed during fluoroscopy is required; paradoxical motion of the involved leaf of the diaphragm confirms the presence of paralysis. Rib invasion may be identified in some patients with severe chest wall pain (T3 disease) (Fig. 22–14), and vertebral body or other bony metastasis as well as contralateral pulmonary metastases (M1 disease) may be seen occasionally on the initial films of the chest.

Laboratory examinations are generally nonspecific. Abnormal liver function studies, particularly an elevated alkaline phosphatase level, may be suggestive of possible

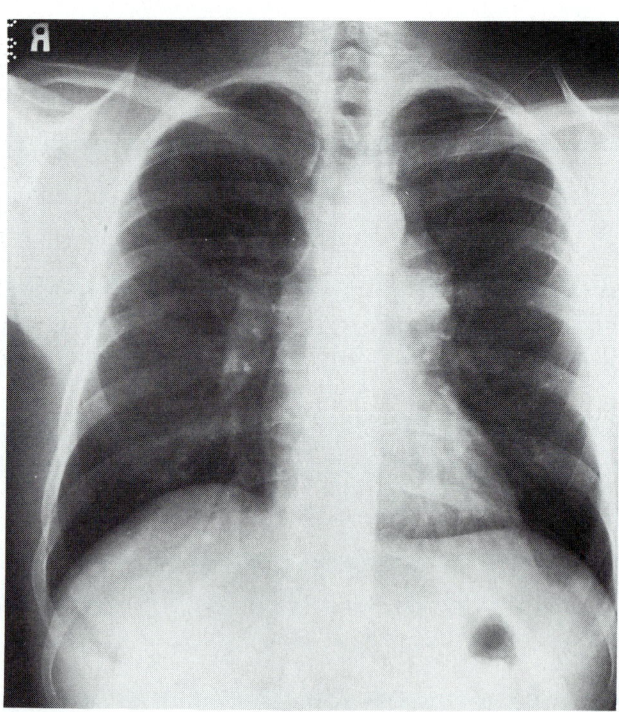

**Figure 22–12.** Grossly abnormal mediastinal shadow. No indication for CT examination. Lymph nodes positive for tumor on mediastinoscopy.

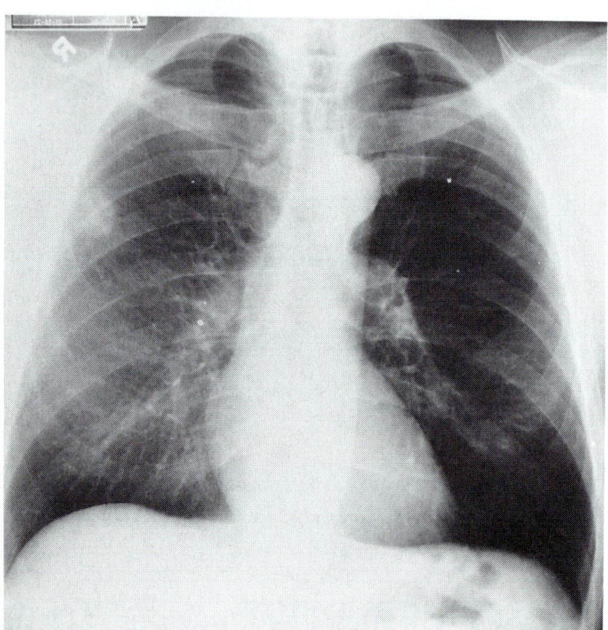

**Figure 22–11.** Peripherally located T1 tumor with normal hilar and mediastinal shadows. No preoperative mediastinal exploration. Lymph nodes negative for tumor at thoracotomy.

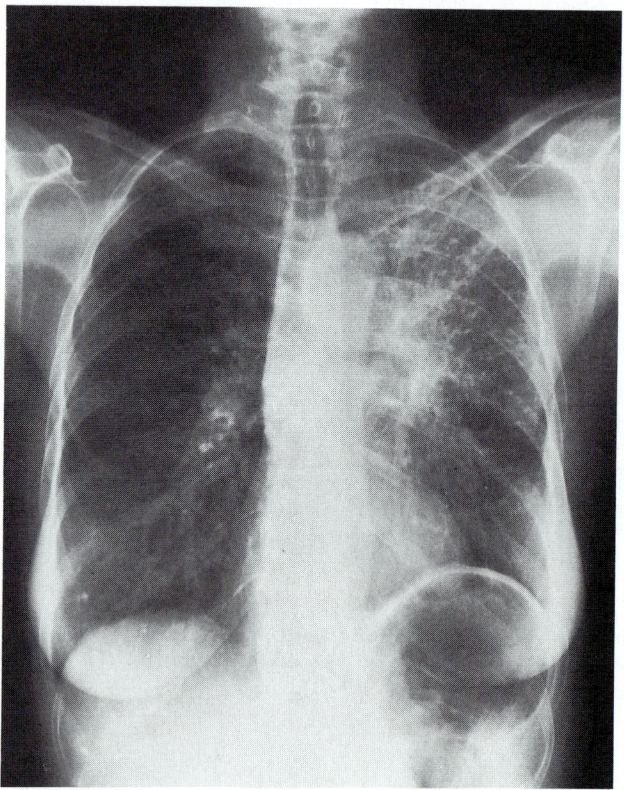

**Figure 22–13.** Indeterminate hilar and mediastinal shadows. Areas obscured by overlying parenchymal disease in left upper lobe. CT examination indicated prior to any mediastinal exploration.

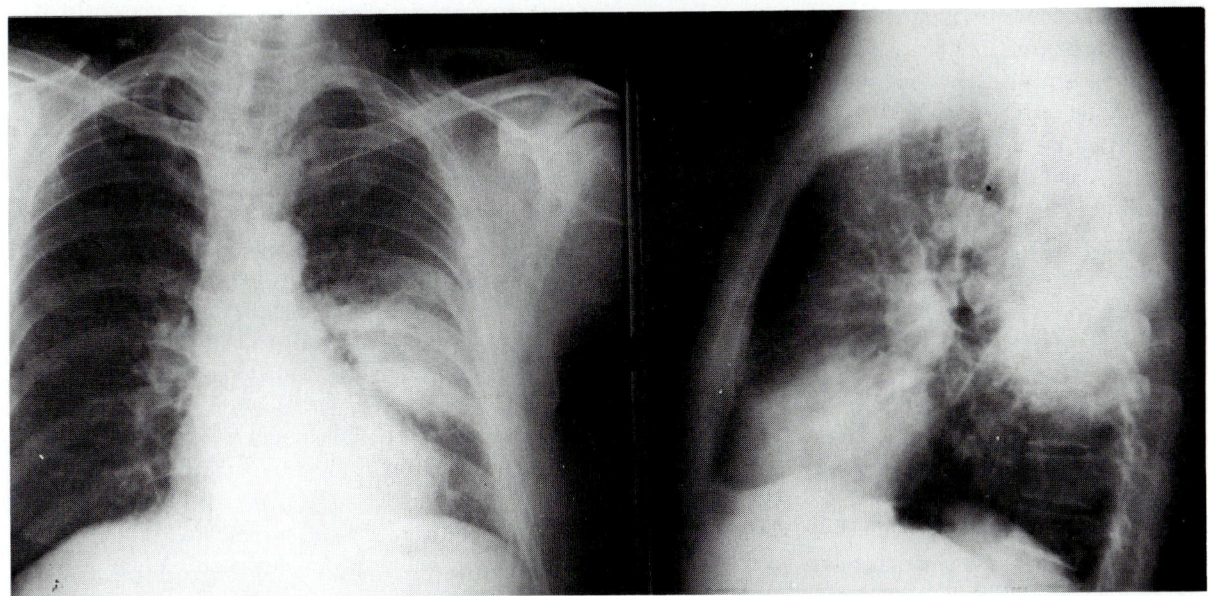

A

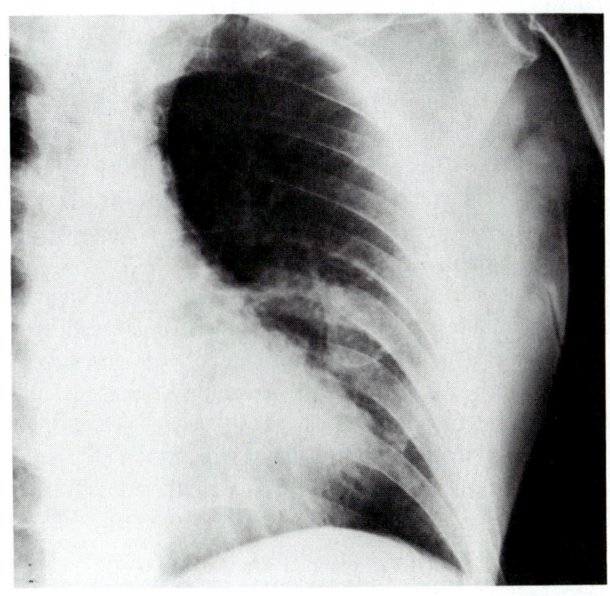

B

**Figure 22–14.** **A.** Peripherally located pulmonary tumor. **B.** Erosion of 7th rib evident, roentgenographic T3 lesion.

metastatic involvement of that organ. Specific imaging studies of the liver to rule in or out metastatic involvement is then indicated. Elevated serum calcium levels may be present. This may be a manifestation of metastases to the skeleton or may be the result of PTHrP polypeptide secretion by the tumor as noted previously.

Bronchoscopic examination is a required step in the staging process in almost all patients with carcinoma of the lung. Bronchoscopy may identify the site of the tumor and identify its distance from the tracheal carina and its presence or absence at an orifice of a lobar bronchus.

When the tumor is within 2 cm of the tracheal carina, the lesion is by definition a T3 lesion. When it is present at the site of a lobar orifice, it is a T2 lesion regardless of its size. When the lobar orifice is free of disease and the tumor is distal to it, the primary tumor is either a T1 or T2 lesion depending upon its size. Enlargement of the tracheal carina or fixation of either main stem bronchus or of the bronchus intermedius on the right suggests the presence of N2 disease. Of course, bronchoscopy permits biopsy of the lesion when it is within reach of the endoscope.

Once these initial studies are completed, it may be necessary to obtain further noninvasive as well as invasive studies to define the extent of the patient's disease; this is particularly true in those patients with non-small cell carcinomas thought to have resectable disease (stages I, II, and IIIA) as well as in those patients who may be candidates for radical irradiation (stages IIIA and IIIB) or are candidates for initial neoadjuvant therapy to be followed by possible resection (stages IIIA and IIIB). Those patients with evident distant metastases need only confirmation of such disease, and any further extensive evaluation is unnecessary.

## SPECIAL ROENTGENOGRAPHIC STUDIES

Standard anterior-posterior tomography is indicated infrequently, and, except for the evaluation of the tracheal air column in a few patients or to initially evaluate a small peripheral lung nodule,[8] this roentgenographic study is of little value in the staging processes in patients with carcinoma of the lung. Calcification per se in a peripheral nodule is not diagnostic of benign disease, and an eccentrically placed area of calcification may be seen in some peripheral carcinomas (5%). However, a central core of calcification, laminar rings of calcification, or a "popcorn" distribution of calcification within a peripheral lesion denote benignancy of the nodule.[52] Last, it is to be noted that standard tomograms reveal little reliable information relative to the status of either N1 or N2 involvement.

Contrast studies of the esophagus are indicated in any patient with dysphagia. Also, a barium swallow may aid in the identification of enlarged posterior subcarinal lymph nodes by revealing a filling defect in the barium column in the region of the tracheal carina. When such a defect is identified, the lymph nodes should be sampled for the presence of tumor by a fine-needle transbronchoscopic aspiration. When tumor is present, it is indicative of nonresectable N2 disease.

Bronchography is rarely indicated in the evaluation of lung tumors. Some, however, believe it continues to be useful in tumors that cannot be fully assessed by fiber-optic bronchoscopy. The positive findings consist of obstruction and stenosis of the distal bronchial lumen or displacement of the bronchial tree in the vicinity of the peripheral lesion.[55]

Angiography is indicated rarely for the evaluation of possible involvement of the ipsilateral main stem pulmonary artery when there is extensive hilar disease. Nonresectability of the tumor is present in over 90% of patients when there is involvement within 1.5 cm of the origin of the artery on the left and just proximal to the takeoff of the truncus anterior on the right. Involvement of the pulmonary veins as they enter the pericardium or involvement of the superior vena cava or either innominate vein usually precludes resection (T4 disease).[56]

Involvement of the azygos system as demonstrated by azygography likewise denotes nonresectability. However, this special examination is indicated infrequently, if at all, at present.

## COMPUTED TOMOGRAPHY

CT examination of the chest and upper abdomen has become a standard diagnostic procedure in patients with carcinoma of the lung. Its greatest contribution in the staging process is the evaluation of the possible enlargement of lymph nodes in the superior mediastinum (Fig. 22–15). Local invasion may also be recognized by encirclement of vascular structures, by direct invasion of vertebral bodies, and by the demonstration of unsuspected pleural effusion. Chest-wall or mediastinal invasion or involvement of other adjacent structures that may abut a tumor is poorly demonstrated by CT,[57] although on occasion extension through the chest wall may be demonstrated (Fig. 22–16). Enlargement of inferior mediastinal nodes (paraesophageal and pulmonary ligament lymph nodes) is not identified by this examination. Moreover, CT scan will frequently fail to identify enlarged lymph nodes in the subcarinal or in the aortic window area. Modest enlargement of subdiaphragmatic lymph nodes also are not identified by CT exam of the upper abdomen. However, examination of the upper abdomen as part of an indicated chest CT may reveal occult metastases to the liver or to an adrenal gland. Occult liver metastases may be present in 3–6.5% in asymptomatic patients with normal liver function studies, and occult adrenal metastases in 3% to over 7% of patients thought to have only local chest disease.[58] The possibility of occult adrenal metastases is increased with the extent of the disease process within the chest, i.e., the presence of N2 disease increases the likelihood of its presence.

Last, the use of high-resolution CT to evaluate solitary peripheral nodules has been suggested. An increased density [a high hounsfield unit (HU) number] of a peripheral lesion supports its benignancy, since this represents the presence of microcalcifications, which are not present in a malignant lesion. In the original investigation of this technique, a lesion with an HU of >164 was considered to be

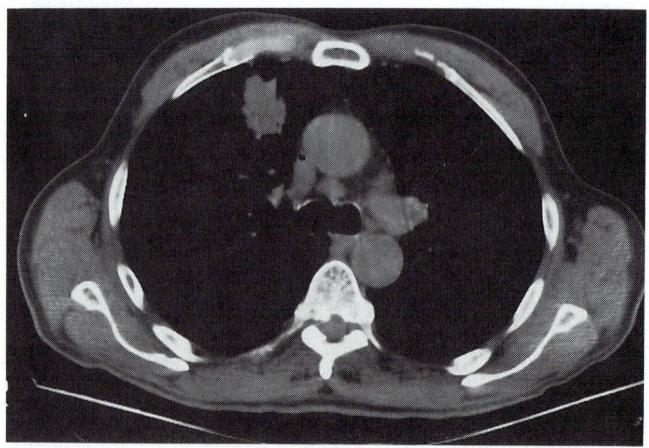

**Figure 22–15.** CT scan showing peripherally located tumor on the right with an enlarged pretracheal node just above the carina. Mediastinoscopy revealed metastatic tumor in the enlarged node.

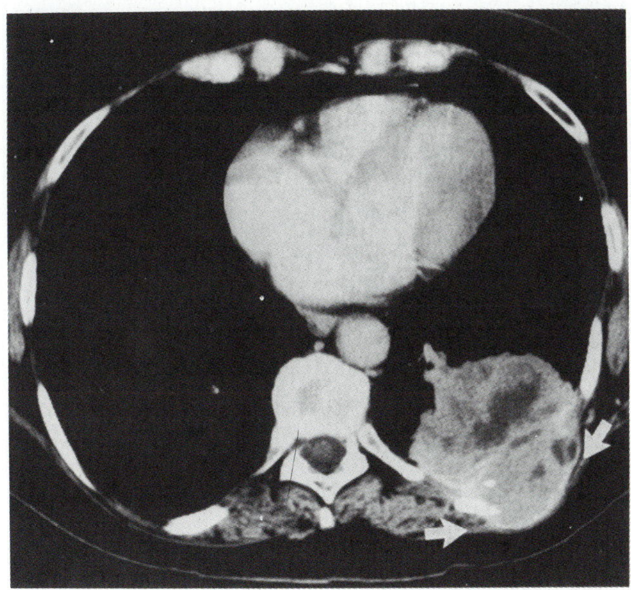

**Figure 22–16.** Chest-wall invasion: CT scan shows necrotic mass with extension through the rib cage. *(From Klein JS, Webb WR: The radiologic staging of lung cancer. J Thorac Imaging 7:29, 1991, with permission.)*

benign, and one with a lesser unit member could or could not be malignant.[59] Unfortunately, many centers were not able to reproduce these findings. However, with the development of new generations of scanners and the use of a standard reference phantom, most centers are now able to duplicate similar findings.

As noted, however, the most valuable contribution of CT examination is in the evaluation of the superior mediastinal lymph nodes. With the use of contrast infusion, enlargement of the paratracheal, right superior tracheobronchial, left anterior, subaortic, and subcarinal lymph nodes may be recognized. In the author's own experience, this is less reliable for evaluation of the subaortic and subcarinal lymph nodes than in the other aforementioned areas. It is considered by many that a lymph node visualized on CT that is <1 cm in size will have a low incidence of involvement by metastatic disease. In one series, the incidence was 7%.[60] Another series has shown that in patients with squamous cell tumor, the incidence of metastatic involvement in normal-sized nodes is less than is that in patients with adenocarcinoma.[61] Moreover, the presence of multiple small nodes (<1 cm in size) in patients with adenocarcinoma suggests an even greater possibility of metastatic disease being present. Lymph nodes 1 cm or greater in size are involved by tumor in 55–65% of instances. Since lymph nodes may be enlarged only by inflammatory changes in 35–45% of instances, all enlarged nodes need to be biopsied to confirm the presence or absence of tumor involvement. The identification of an enlarged lymph node on CT should not be accepted as proof that metastatic disease is present. This is particularly true in patients with squamous cell tumors. Nodes >3 cm in size are almost always involved by tumor, but biopsy or needle aspiration, likewise, is indicated to prove its presence (see Chapter 8).

## MAGNETIC RESONANCE IMAGING

At present, magnetic resonance imaging (MRI) yields approximately the same information as does the CT examination, although it is of more value in identifying vascular and mediastinal invasion than is CT (Fig. 22–17).[62,63] It is of special value when the use of contrast material is contraindicated in the patient, which lessens the value of the CT exam. At times MRI may reveal extension of the tumor through the chest wall when the CT examination has been indeterminant (Fig. 22–18). Its use also permits the obtainment of sagittal and coronal views that may, in specific instances, reveal extension of the disease process beyond the confines of the thorax.[64] Its use is particularly helpful in the evaluation of superior sulcus tumors as to their extent and the possible involvement of the brachial plexus (Fig. 22–19). Likewise, it may delineate vertebral body invasion as well as detection of spinal canal invasion.

## ULTRASONOGRAPHY

Ultrasound has been used in many institutions for the detection of pleural effusion and for the guidance for biopsy of peripheral lung or mediastinal masses. With the development of transesophageal endoscopic ultrasonography, it has become possible to identify lymph nodes in the inferior por-

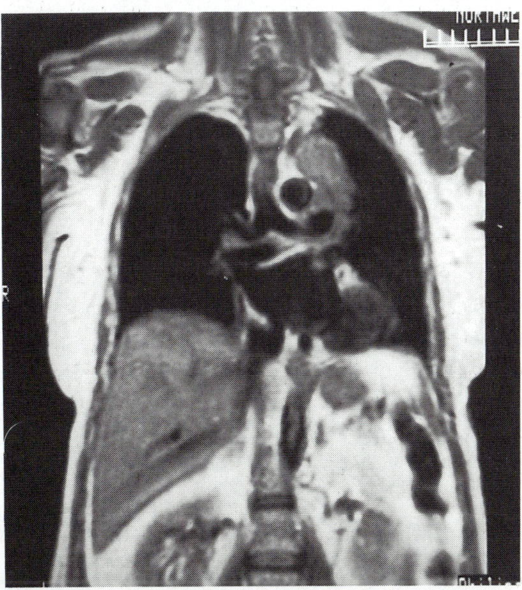

**Figure 22–17.** MRI: Frontal view revealing local invasion about the great vessels on the left.

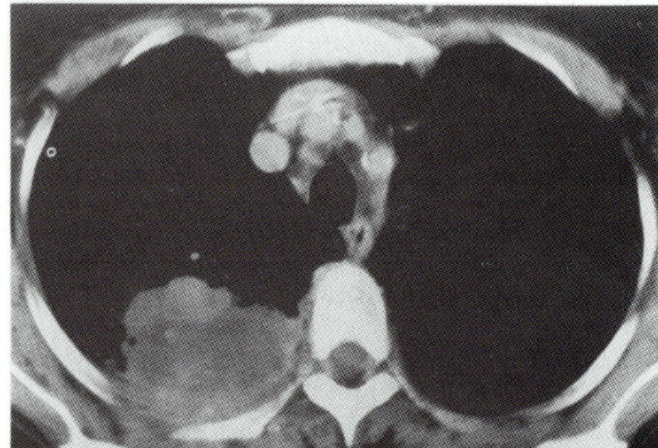

A

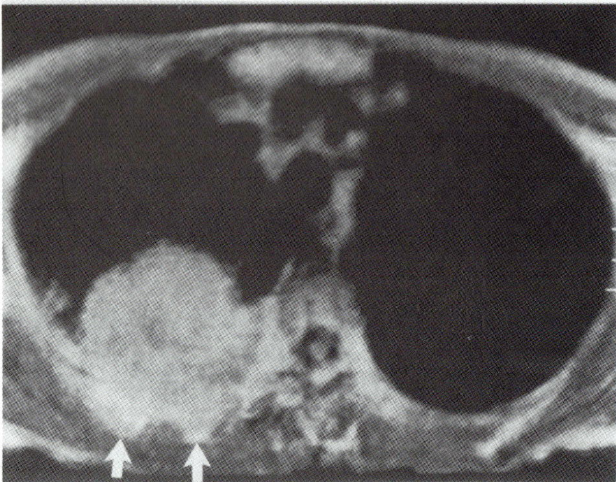

B

Figure 22–18. Chest-wall invasion: **A.** CT scan shows extensive pleural contact of tumor and obtuse angles at the posterior pleural surface. **B.** Axial MR scan shows tumor extending into posterior chest wall (arrows). *(From Klein JS, Webb WR: The radiologic staging of lung cancer. J Thorac Imaging 7:29, 1991, with permission.)*

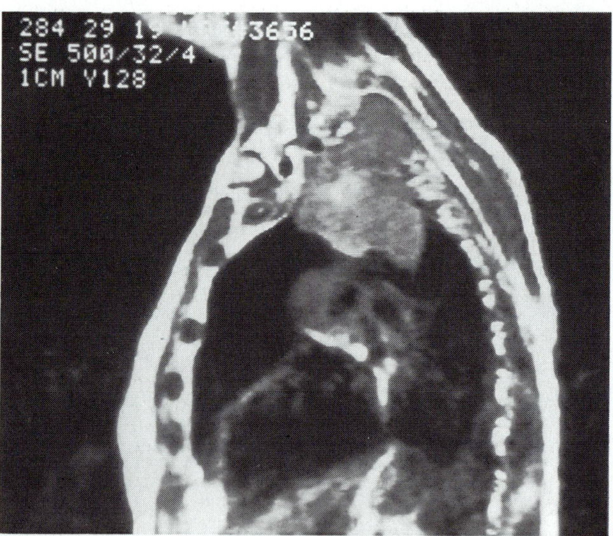


**Figure 22–19.** MRI: Lateral view revealing extrathoracic growth of a superior sulcus tumor. *(Used by courtesy of Martin F. McKneally.)*

tion of the mediastinum (subcarinal, paraesophageal, and pulmonary ligament lymph nodes) that cannot be evaluated by CT scan.[65] Also, this technique frequently may detect enlarged nodes in the aortopulmonary window that were not identified by CT scan (Fig. 22–20).[66] Although this examination has yet to become popular, the potential value of its use in conjunction with the CT scan in the preoperative noninvasive evaluation of mediastinal lymph nodes in selected patients appears self-evident.

## PHOTON EMISSION TOMOGRAPHIC IMAGING

Photon emission tomography (PET) using various radiolabeled monoclonal antibodies[67] and glucose analogue 2-[F-18-fluro-2-deoxy-D-glucose] (FDG)[68,69] has been studied as to its value in differentiating malignant from benign lung lesions and as to its possible role in evaluating the presence of metastatic tumor in the mediastinal lymph nodes. PET has also been reported with the use of [$^{11}$C] L-methionine by Japanese investigators,[70] but the use of [$^{11}$C] L-methionine has been somewhat less discriminating than either the use of FDG or radiolabeled monoclonal antibodies. The efficacy of the use of FDG is based on the high rate of glycolysis in tumors as contrasted with a lesser rate in nonmalignant lesions. However, crossover with active inflammatory lesions such as active aspergillosis, active tuberculosis, and lung abscesses does occur. Nonetheless, several recent studies have shown a high rate of positive studies (high rate of uptake) in patients with malignant solitary peripheral nodules compared with a very low uptake in nonmalignant nodules. In one report, PET-FDG scans correctly identified 44 of 47 malignant nodules, and there were only 3 false-positive findings in 14 granulomas and 1 organizing pneumonia.[69] However, the evaluation of the mediastinal lymph nodes for the presence of metastatic involvement by the various techniques of PET has been less successful and appears to have no better results than those obtained by CT examination.

## RADIONUCLIDE STUDIES

Radionuclide studies of the brain, liver, and skeleton are indicated only when symptoms, signs, or abnormal laboratory findings of possible involvement are present. Routine radionuclide scans in asymptomatic patients are of too low a yield to be indicated.[71–73]

Specifically, the use of a radionuclide bone scan in asymptomatic elderly patients with clinical stage I and II

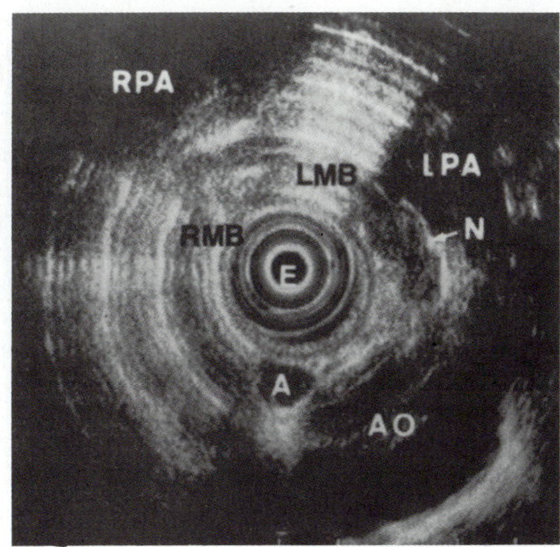


A

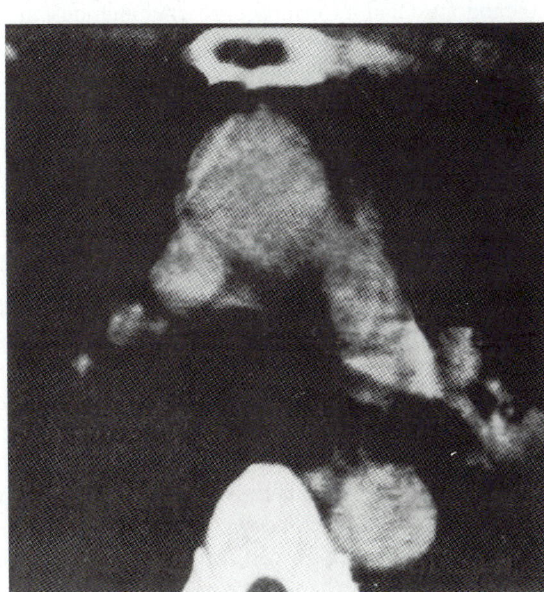

B

**Figure 22–20.** Metastatic lymph nodes in the left tracheobronchial area as shown by transesophageal endoscopic ultrasound examination (**A**), whereas CT scan (**B**) does not reveal any nodes at the same level. AR = aorta; LMB = left main bronchus; LPA = left pulmonary artery; N = lymph node with clear lobulated contours highly suggestive of metastases; RMB = right main bronchus; RPA = right pulmonary artery. *(From Kondo D, Imaizumi M, Abe T, et al: Endoscopic ultrasound examination for mediastinal lymph node metastases of lung cancer. Chest 98:586, 1990, with permission.)*

non-small cell carcinoma is frequently misleading because of a high false-positive yield. This may be well over 10%, and the time and effort needed to disprove the presence of metastatic disease is excessive. In this patient subgroup, a true positive yield is only in the range of 2–4% at most. However, in patients with advanced stage IIIA (nonresectable N2 disease) and stage IIIB disease and who may be candidates for radical irradiation or neoadjuvant therapy, a routine bone scan and an upper abdominal CT scan may advance the stage grouping to stage IV and negate the use of a neoadjuvant approach or the value of intensive local radiation therapy to the chest in this patient subgroup. It is to be noted that CT examinations of the upper abdomen and brain have supplanted the radionuclide scans of these sites in most institutions.

Since the brain is the frequent site of first failure, particularly in patients with adenocarcinoma,[74–77] there is some enthusiasm for routine screening with CT examination of MRI of this site in patients with T2 N0, stage II, and stage IIIA disease of this latter cell type. Also, it has been suggested that metastases to the brain from an adenocarcinoma are not stage related, and, thus, CT scan or MRI should be done in all potential surgical patients with adenocarcinoma.[78] However, other workers report that in asymptomatic patients with resectable adenocarcinoma, cranial metastasis is seen by and large only in patients with stage III disease, particularly in those with known N2 disease.[79,80] Thus, one should be selective in the evaluation of the brain even in patients with adenocarcinoma.

Gallium 67 scanning of the mediastinum for the identification of lymph nodes possibly involved by metastatic disease is carried out in some clinics.[81] However, most have abandoned this study, since CT of the superior mediastinum, as noted, is very satisfactory in identifying lymph nodes 1 cm or greater in size, which in the majority of instances may be involved by metastatic disease.

In patients with symptoms or signs suggestive of involvement of distant metastatic sites, the use of radionuclide scans or CT examinations is indicated to demonstrate the presence of metastatic disease. Even though only one organ system may be suspect for involvement, all three areas—brain, skeleton, and upper abdomen—should be evaluated in this situation. Tissue confirmation of a positive scan finding is necessary in most instances by the appropriate biopsy technique.

Radionuclide perfusion and ventilation scans play an important role in the evaluation of patients with poor ventilatory function who are potential candidates for operation. This subject will be discussed subsequently.

## LYMPH NODE BIOPSY

Palpable lymph nodes in either supraclavicular area must be biopsied either by an open technique or by needle aspiration. The presence of metastatic tumor denotes N3 disease. The biopsy of nonpalpable nodes, the so-called scalene lymph node biopsy, is not indicated, since the yield is too low and more satisfactory information is gained by mediastinal lymph node biopsy.

The superior mediastinal lymph nodes may be evaluated by either mediastinoscopy or by mediastinotomy (the Chamberlain procedure).[82] The latter procedure is most useful in patients with suspicious lymph nodes in the aortic pulmonary window or in the anterior mediastinal lymph node group (usually in patients with left upper lobe tumors).[83] The other superior lymph node groups including the anterior subcarinal lymph nodes are readily accessible by mediastinoscopy. A technique to extend the range of mediastinoscopy (extended cervical mediastinoscopy) to visualize and enable biopsy of the anterior and subaortic lymph nodes has been suggested,[84–86] but most surgeons have either employed the Chamberlain procedure or more recently a left-sided VATS approach for the evaluation of the lymph nodes in these areas. A number of surgeons have reported that the investigation of the aortic pulmonary (subaortic) and anterior mediastinal lymph node groups can be carried out more effectively by a left-sided VATS approach rather than by the Chamberlain procedure.[26,87–89] On the right side, VATS has also been successfully used to evaluate enlarged periazygos and posteriorly located subcarinal lymph nodes that at times are difficult to evaluate by the standard cervical mediastinoscopy. The ipsilateral pulmonary ligament lymph nodes may also be evaluated during the VATS procedure. The selection of the appropriate procedure should be based on the location of the suspicious lymph nodes on the CT exam in the individual patient. It should be noted that prior to or in conjunction with a Chamberlain procedure or a VATS approach to investigate enlarged aortic pulmonary window or paraaortic nodes, that a standard cervical mediastinoscopy should also be done.

Some surgical groups believe that all patients with potentially resectable lung carcinoma should undergo a prethoracotomy mediastinal exploration.[88–93] With this policy, approximately a quarter of the patients with potentially resectable non-small cell lung cancer will be found to have metastatic disease in one or more superior mediastinal or anterior subcarinal lymph node groups (Table 22–9). Despite the relatively high yield of positive results, a false-negative result will occur in approximately 10% of the patients who undergo a mediastinoscopy. A false-negative result is even higher (33%) in selected patients with early small cell lung cancer who are believed to be potential surgical candidates. Of patients with metastatically involved lymph nodes identified by prethoracotomy mediastinal exploration, 80–90% will have nonresectable disease. (These patients may be considered for neoadjuvant therapy followed by resection.) Such metastatic involvement is characterized by a contralateral location of the involved lymph node (N3 disease), a high ipsilateral paratracheal position of the lymph node, extracapsular extension of the tumor with fixation of the lymph node to adjacent structures, and involvement of multiple nodal stations. In addition, a variable number of patients will be found to have small cell lung cancer that had not been diagnosed prior to the mediastinal exploration. The remaining 10–20% of patients with nodal metastasis may be considered for possible surgical resection; the metastatic involvement is characterized by low ipsilateral paratracheal, superior tracheobronchial, subaortic, or subcarinal location of the involved lymph node; absence of fixation; disease confined to within the capsule of the lymph node; and involvement of only one or, at most, two nodal stations.[89,94–96]

In contrast to this philosophy, other groups will proceed to an exploratory thoracotomy without a prethoracotomy mediastinal exploration in all patients whose roentgenograms and bronchoscopic examinations are not suggestive of mediastinal disease.[97] When enlarged mediastinal nodes are evident by CT examination, thoracotomy may still be recommended by some without a prethoracotomy exploration.[98] With either course of action, a large number of patients will be found to have N2 disease at thoracotomy, and, under such circumstances, curative resections can be carried out in only approximately 50% of patients with this N2 disease. However, in those patients without roentgenographic or CT evidence of enlarged mediastinal lymph nodes, especially those with clinical stage I disease, complete resection can be accomplished in 61–95% of the patients (Table 22–10).

A more selective approach has been practiced by many groups.[54,99,100] Even though I do not believe a CT scan is necessary in patients with a peripheral T1 lesion and normal hilar and mediastinal shadows are present on the roentgenogram, in reality, a CT scan is routinely obtained in all patients. When the mediastinal lymph nodes are <1 cm in size (except in the presence of multiple small lymph nodes in patients with adenocarcinoma), no further evaluation of the mediastinal lymph nodes is done preoperatively. Even when metastatic nodal disease is present in this subset of patients, a complete, potentially curative resection can be carried out in most patients. When the nodes are 1 cm or greater in size, mediastinal exploration is carried out by mediastinoscopy, combined with either a mediastinotomy or a

**TABLE 22–9. ROUTINE PREOPERATIVE MEDIASTINOSCOPY**

| | | Positive Yield—% | | | |
|---|---|---|---|---|---|
| **Author** | **Year** | **Stage I** | **Stage II** | **Stage III** | **Total** |
| Yoshimatsu[95] | 1975 | 12 | 36 | 66 | 49 |
| Maassen[92] | 1985 | 11 | 24 | 71 | 36 |
| Coughlin et al[93a] | 1985 | 15 (T1) | 26 (T2) | 41 (T3) | 27 |

[a]Clinical stage not recorded; % is for T status only.

**TABLE 22–10. RESECTION OF N2 LESIONS BY PRETREATMENT CLINICAL STAGE**

| | | Number Explored and Found to Have N2 Disease | Complete Resection | % |
|---|---|---|---|---|
| Stage I | T1 N0 M0 | 22 | 21 | 95 |
| | T2 N0 M0 | 44 | 27 | 61 |
| Stage II | T1 N1 M0 | 2 | 2 | 100 |
| | T2 N1 M0 | 11 | 7 | 63 |
| Stage III | T3 N0 M0 | 35 | 9 | 26 |
| | T3 N1 M0 | 2 | 0 | 0 |
| **Total** | | 116 | 66 | 57 |

*(Adapted from Martini N et al: J Thorac Cardiovasc Surg 80:390, 1980, with permission.)*

VATS approach as necessary. In approximately 55–65% or more of such patients, the lymph nodes are found to be positive, i.e., involved by metastatic disease. The criteria for subsequent thoracotomy in the patients with positive lymph nodes are the same as noted previously in the aforementioned discussion on routine mediastinal exploration (see Chapter 11).

## NEEDLE BIOPSY

The role of fine-needle biopsy in the diagnosis and staging of carcinoma of the lung is variable. Routine percutaneous needle biopsy of peripheral lesions is done in many institutions. However, except for the probability of establishing a prethoracotomy diagnosis in 85–95% of the malignant peripheral lesions, it adds nothing to the staging process. In patients with lesions abutting the chest wall, with symptoms of chest-wall pain, or findings of erosion of an adjacent rib, the biopsy will yield evidence of a T3 lesion. Its use is particularly recommended in the evaluation of patients with lesions in the superior sulcus region.

Needle biopsy of an enlarged mediastinal lymph node may establish an N2 status. When a biopsy of the pleura in a patient with an ipsilateral pleural effusion is positive, it categorizes the lesion as T4. It is to be noted that even in the absence of either a positive pleural fluid cytology or a positive needle biopsy of the pleura, approximately 95% of such patients will have a malignant effusion (T4) or extensive local disease (T4 or N2), which will preclude definitive resection.

Needle biopsy or open biopsy or suspected metastatic sites is indicated to confirm the presence of M1 disease. This is especially true of a liver or adrenal mass discovered on upper abdominal CT or by radionuclide studies of symptomatic organ systems. Needle bone marrow aspiration and biopsy are indicated in all patients with small cell cancer who are thought to have only local disease, since metastatic disease will be found in over 40%, which places the patients in the extensive disease category.

## ROUTINE VIDEO-ASSISTED SURGICAL STAGING PRIOR TO THORACOTOMY

It has been suggested by some surgeons that video-assisted surgical exploration of the hemithorax be done selectively or even perhaps routinely prior to thoracotomy. The selective use may be for the evaluation of inaccessible lymph node stations as noted or for the determination of re-

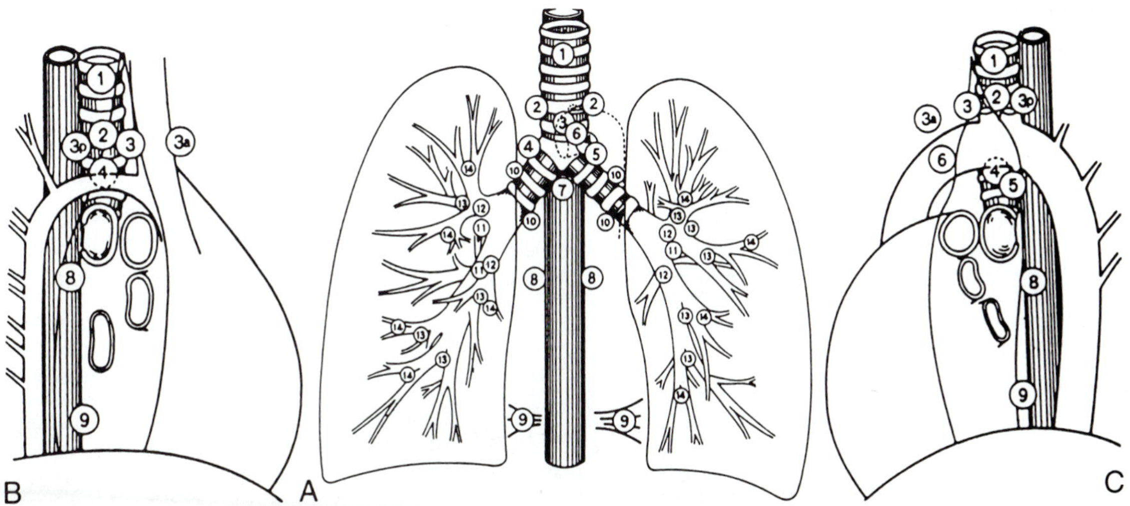


**Figure 22–21.** Naruke map of mediastinal and bronchopulmonary lymph node stations. **A.** Frontal view. **B.** Right lateral view. **C.** Left lateral view. See Table 22–11 for designations of numbered lymph node stations. *(From Naruke T, Suemasu K, Ishikawa S: Lymph node mapping and curability of various levels of metastasis in resected lung cancer. J Thorac Cardiovasc Surg 76:832, 1978, with permission.)*

**TABLE 22–11. DEFINITIONS OF REGIONAL NODE STATIONS IN THE NARUKE MAP**

| Station | Definition |
|---|---|
| 1 | Superior mediastinal or highest mediastinal—these nodes are present along the upper one third of the trachea within the thorax, the lower level of which is at the upper border of the brachiocephalic vein as it crosses in front of the trachea. |
| 2 | Paratracheal—these nodes are located between station 1 and station 2 on the lateral sides of the trachea. |
| 3 | These nodes are separated into 3 groups: pretracheal (3), retrotracheal (3p), and anterior tracheal (3a); these latter nodes are present in the anterior (prevascular) compartment and lie on the anterior aspect of the brachiocephalic vein and the upper portion of the superior vena cava. |
| 4 | Superior tracheal bronchial—these lymph nodes are located at or close to the obtuse angle between the trachea and either main stem bronchus. The nodes on the right are in the obtuse angle level with and beneath the azygos vein. Those on the left are medial to the subaortic nodes. |
| 5 | Subaortic—these nodes lie in the aortopulmonary window adjacent to the ligamentum arteriosum. |
| 6 | Paraaortic—these nodes are located in the anterolateral wall of the ascending aorta and aortic arch anterior to the left vagus nerve. |
| 7 | Inferior tracheobronchial or subcarinal—these nodes are located just beneath the point where the trachea divides into the two main stem bronchi. |
| 8 | Paraesophageal—these nodes are just caudad to the level of the tracheal bifurcation and are adjacent to the esophagus. |
| 9 | Pulmonary ligament—these nodes lie within the pulmonary ligament and are present on the posterior wall and edge of the inferior pulmonary vein as well as extend down to the diaphragm. |
| 10 | Hilar—these nodes are just distal to the trachea and extend along the length of either main stem bronchus. |
| 11 | Interlobar—these nodes are present in between the lobar bronchi. |
| 12 | Lobar—nodes present around a lobar bronchus. |
| 13 | Segmental—nodes located along a segmental bronchus. |
| 14 | Subsegmental and parenchymal—nodes present around a subsegment bronchus or distal in the lung parenchyma. |

*(From Naruke T: Mediastinal lymph node dissection. In Shields TW (ed): General Thoracic Surgery, 4th ed. Philadelphia, Lea and Febiger 1994, p 469, with permission.)*

**TABLE 22–12. DEFINITIONS OF REGIONAL NODE STATIONS IN AMERICAN THORACIC SOCIETY MAP**

| Station | Definition |
|---|---|
| 2R | Right upper paratracheal (suprainnominate) nodes to the right of the midline of the trachea between the intersection of the caudal margin of the innominate artery with the trachea and the apex of the lung (includes highest R mediastinal node). (Radiologist may use the same caudal margin as in 2L.) |
| 2L | Left upper paratracheal (supraaortic) nodes: nodes to the left of the midline of the trachea between the top of the aortic arch and the apex of the lung (includes highest L mediastinal node). |
| 4R | Right lower paratracheal nodes: nodes to the right of the midline of the trachea between the cephalic border of the azygos vein and the intersection of the caudal margin of the brachiocephalic artery with the right side of the trachea (includes some pretracheal and paracaval nodes). (Radiologists may use the same cephalic margin as in 4L.) |
| 4L | Left lower paratracheal nodes: nodes to the left of the midline of the trachea between the top of the aortic arch and the level of the carina, medial to the ligamentum arteriosum (includes some pretracheal and paracaval nodes). (Radiologists may use the same cephalic margin as in 4L.) |
| 5 | Aortopulmonary nodes: subaortic and paraaortic nodes, lateral to the ligamentum arteriosum or the aorta or left pulmonary artery, proximal to the first branch of the left pulmonary artery. |
| 6 | Anterior mediastinal nodes: nodes anterior to the ascending aorta or the innominate artery (includes some pretracheal and preaortic nodes). |
| 7 | Subcarinal nodes: nodes arising caudal to the carina of the trachea but not associated with the lower lobe bronchi or arteries within the lung. |
| 8 | Paraesophageal nodes: nodes dorsal to the posterior wall of the trachea and to the right or left of the midline of the esophagus (includes retrotracheal, but not subcarinal nodes). |
| 9 | Right or left pulmonary ligament nodes: nodes within the right or left pulmonary ligament. |
| 10R | Right tracheobronchial nodes: nodes to the right of the midline of the trachea from the level of the cephalic border of the azygos vein to the origin of the right upper lobe bronchus. |
| 10L | Left peribronchial nodes: nodes to the left of the midline of the trachea between the carina and the left upper lobe bronchus, later to the ligamentum arteriosum. |
| 11 | Intrapulmonary nodes: nodes removed in the right or left lung specimen plus those distal to the main stem bronchi or secondary carina (includes interlobar, lobar, and segmental nodes). |

*(From American Thoracic Society: Clinical staging of primary lung cancer. Am Rev Respir Dis 127:659, 1983; with permission.)*

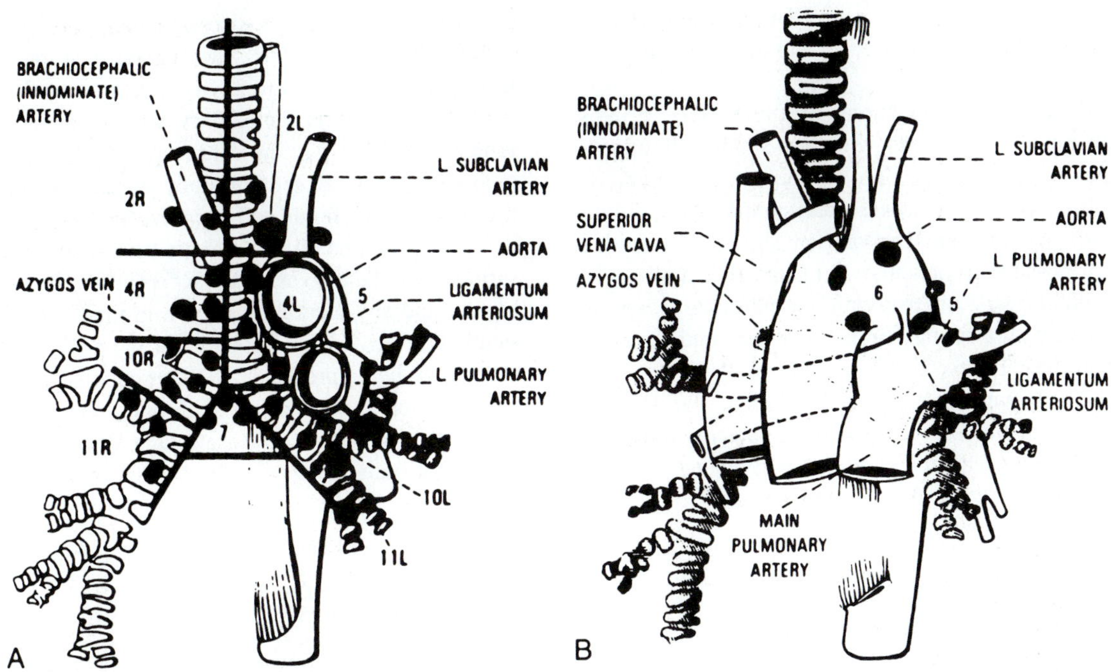


**Figure 22–22.** American Thoracic Society lymph node map: **A.** Frontal view with aorta, superior vena cava, and pulmonary arteries removed to reveal the trachea and main stem bronchi. **B.** Frontal view with vascular structures intact. See Table 22–12 for designations of numbered lymph node stations. *(From Tisi GM, Friedman PJ, Peters RM, et al: Clinical staging of primary lung cancer. Am Rev Respir Dis 127:659, 1983, with permission.)*

sectability of tumors that are questionable on CT or MRI.[101] Routine use may be helpful in ruling out pleural metastases that are not accompanied with a pleural effusion, and in one study the incidence of this finding was slightly >4%.[102] This latter incidence is higher than has been normally experienced, and in most series unsuspected pleural metastasis is in the range of 1–2%.[103] Thus, at present the routine use of VATS prior to thoracotomy can be questioned.

## PLEURAL LAVAGE

It has been suggested by several investigators that routine pleural lavage, at the time of thoracotomy, even in the absence of evidence of pleural effusion or pleural seeding be done, since the presence of positive tumor cell cytology advances the patients to a potentially more advanced stage category (prognostically to at least a stage IIIA and possibly to a stage IV [Japanese] level).[104,105] Whether or not this is confirmed or becomes accepted practice is not yet determined.

## COMPLETION OF THE STAGING PROCESS

With the completion of one or more of the various staging procedures in the appropriate sequence, it will be found that approximately one fourth of the patients with non-small cell

**TABLE 22–13. POSTSURGICAL SURVIVAL ACCORDING TO TNM CLASSIFICATION**

| | Mountain[a] | | Naruke[b] | |
|---|---|---|---|---|
| TNM Subset | No. Patients | 5-Year Survival (%) | No. Patients | 5-Year Survival (%) |
| T1N0M0 | 429 | 68.5 | 245 | 75.5 |
| T2N0M0 | 436 | 59.0 | 241 | 57.0 |
| T1N1M0 | 67 | 54.1 | 66 | 52.5 |
| T2N1M0 | 250 | 40.0 | 153 | 40.0 |
| T3N0M0 | 57 | 44.2 | 106 | 33.3 |
| T3N1M0 | 29 | 17.6 | 85 | 39.0 |
| Any N2M0 | 168 | 28.8 | 368 | 15.1 |

[a]*(From Mountain CF: A new international staging system for lung cancer. Chest 89:225S–233S, 1986, with permission).*
[b]*(From Naruke T, Goya T, Tsuchiya R, et al: Prognosis and survival in resected lung carcinoma based on the new international staging system. J Thorac Cardiovasc Surg 96:440–447, 1988, with permission.)*

carcinoma will have stage I, II, or IIIA disease. Another quarter will have stage IIIB disease, and the remaining one half will have stage IV disease.

The therapeutic implications of these stage groups have been noted. In patients with non-small cell tumors with clinical stage I, II, or IIIA without grossly involved mediastinal lymph node disease, a resectability rate of over 95% should be achieved. Exploration should be avoided when at all possible in patients with stage IIIB disease. In patients with stage IV disease with one possible exception (i.e., a patient with a solitary brain metastasis and a stage I or II primary lesion), resection is contraindicated.

In patients with small cell carcinoma, the role of surgery is as yet unresolved. However, there is evidence that resection plus chemotherapy in early stage disease (stage I disease and even in some patients with stage IIIA-non-N2 disease) may be of benefit.[106–111]

## POSTTHORACOTOMY STAGING

Final staging of the patient's disease is completed by the pathologic examination of the resected specimen and the evaluation of the ipsilateral mediastinal lymph nodes (either removed by sampling of each mediastinal lymph node station or preferably by a systematic ipsilateral lymph node dissection). The location of the lymph nodes should be recorded by either the Naruke map (Fig. 22–21, Table 22–11)[112] or by the American Thoracic Society map (Fig. 22–22, Table 22–12.[113] Unfortunately, in the latter, mediastinal stations 10R and 10L include some lymph nodes that can be argued to be hilar in location; this may or may not have some influence (more favorable) on the prognosis when these nodes are included as mediastinal nodes. The resected margins should be checked for the presence of tumor. The presence of satellite nodules (considered as stage IIIA disease, although the Japanese refer to their presence as intrapulmonary metastasis, i.e., M1—stage IV disease) should be noted. Resections should be considered as incomplete only if known biopsy proven gross or microscopic disease has been left in the hemithorax.[114]

The final pathologic stage may be used as the major guide as to the approximate prognosis of the patient (Table 22–13).[4,115] It should be noted that each stage group is composed of a heterogeneous population so that other factors such as cell type, size of the lesion, sex of the patient, number of sites of lymph node involvement as well as the presence of the *K-ras* oncogene mutation and *HER-$^2$/neu* oncogenes overexpression and p53 tumor suppressor gene mutation may all variously affect the patient's prognosis.

## FUNCTIONAL STATUS

Determination of the performance status of the patients with small cell lung carcinoma is of great importance. The performance status is a discrete measure of the patient's ambulatory nature. This may be defined on a 10-point Karnofsky scale (Table 22–14) or a 5-point Zubrod scale. Any patient who is ambulatory less than one half of the time and requires nursing care responds poorly to any regimen of therapy. Except in study circumstances, such patients probably should only receive palliative care. In patients with non-small cell tumors, the vast majority of the surgical candidates have a performance status of 90 or higher, and any marked reduction in their functional status should be viewed with suspicion for the possibility of distant metastases being present. Like their counterparts with small cell carcinoma, the patients with non-small cell carcinoma and distant metastatic disease (stage IV) who have a poor functional status are not candidates for aggressive therapy.

**TABLE 22–14. KARNOFSKY SCALE OF PERFORMANCE STATUS**

| Condition | Percentage | Comments |
|---|---|---|
| **A:** Able to carry on normal activity and to work. No special care is needed. | 100 | Normal, no complaints, no evidence of disease |
| | 90 | Able to carry on normal activity, minor signs or symptoms of disease |
| | 80 | Normal activity with effort, some signs or symptoms of disease |
| **B:** Unable to work. Able to live at home, care for most personal needs. A varying degree of assistance is needed. | 70 | Cares for self, but unable to carry on normal activity or to do active work |
| | 60 | Requires occasional assistance, but is able to care for most of his needs |
| | 50 | Requires considerable assistance and frequent medical care |
| **C:** Unable to care for self. Requires equivalent of institutional or hospital care. Disease may be progressing rapidly. | 40 | Disabled, requires special care and assistance |
| | 30 | Severely disabled, hospitalization indicated although death not imminent |
| | 20 | Hospitalization necessary, very sick, active supportive treatment necessary |
| | 10 | Moribund, fatal processes progressing rapidly |
| | 0 | Dead |

In patients with potentially resectable disease non-small cell carcinoma, the physiologic status of the cardiovascular and respiratory systems must be evaluated in an attempt to determine whether or not the patient may tolerate (risk evaluation) the contemplated operative procedure. The specific cardiac and pulmonary function studies are discussed elsewhere in the text (see Chap. 1). The evaluation of the ventilatory and cardiac status should be done in a stepwise fashion, reserving the more sophisticated tests for those patients in whom the functional status is border-

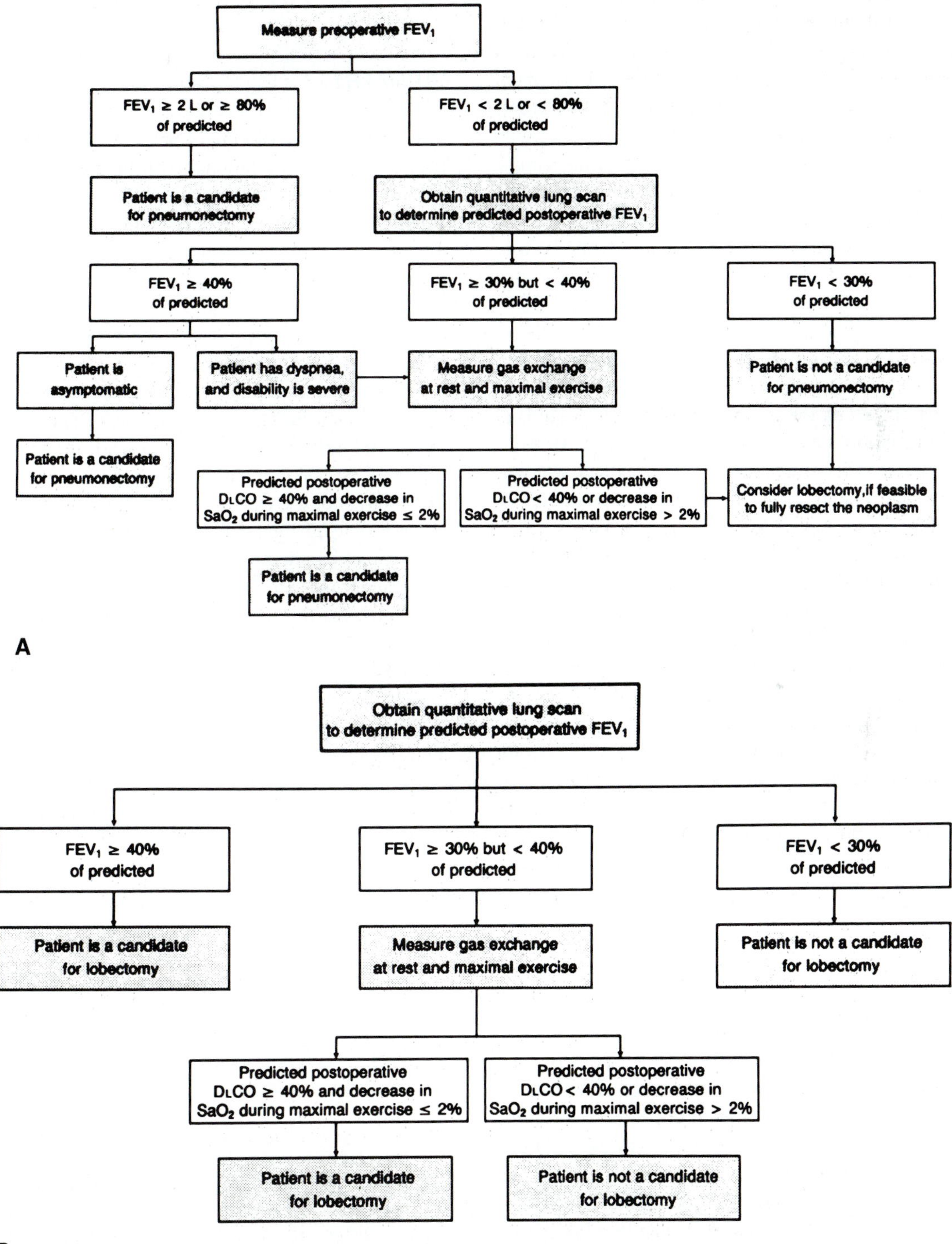


**Figure 22–23.** **A.** Assessing the suitability of pneumonectomy in patients with lung cancer. $FEV_1$ = forced expiratory volume in 1 second, DLCO = carbon monoxide-diffusing capacity, $SaO_2$ = arterial oxygen saturation. **B.** Assessing the suitability of lobectomy in patients with lung cancer. *(From Arroliga AC, Buzaid AC, Matthay RA: Which patients can safely undergo lung resection? J Respir Dis 12:1080–1086, 1991, with permission.)*

line.[116–118] Moreover, it must be emphasized that the physiologic test results must be viewed in the light of the patient's overall functional status, the roentgenographic features of the patient's disease, the presence of comorbid conditions, and the extent of the contemplated surgical resection.

It is believed by some that the possible eventuality of a pneumonectomy should be functionally considered in all potential surgical candidates.[119] This realistically only becomes rarely necessary in a patient in whom the planned procedure was not initially considered to necessitate complete removal of the lung.

There is no single set of values for the various pulmonary function studies, blood gas determinations or maximum oxygen consumption with exercise that may be used to determine whether or not the risks of resection are too high. However, a preoperative $FEV_1$ of 40% or less of predicted normal, a predicted postoperative $FEV_1$ below 30% of normal, an MVV <45–50% of normal, a DLCO <40%, a $PCO_2$ >45 mm Hg, and a peak oxygen consumption ($VO_2$ peak) <10 mL/kg per minute generally precludes any surgical consideration. When the results of these various studies predict moderate impairment the determination of the predicted postoperative $FEV_1$ by radiospiromatic methodology for tolerance of a pneumonectomy or a lesser resection is appropriate for risk evaluation in most patients (Fig. 22–23A,B).[120] However, it has become apparent that the determination of maximum oxygen consumption during exercise may be of even greater value in risk evaluation in functionally poor candidates.[121–123] Not only does this study predict the risk of the possibility of a postoperative death, but it also predicts the risk of postoperative complications, which the standard pulmonary ventilatory functions do not.[124] A $VO_2$ peak <10 mL/kg per minute predicts both high mortality and morbidity rates. A $VO_2$ peak ≤15 mL/kg per minute predicts a lesser mortality rate but still a high complication rate, whereas a $VO_2$ peak ≥15 (especially above 20 mL/kg per minute) predicts a near-zero mortality and a minimum morbidity rate.

The cardiac status may be initially evaluated by the patient's history and standard electrocardiograms. When either is abnormal, a stress test is indicated, and even at times a thallium-201 scan to evaluate myocardial perfusion may need to be done. When either of these are abnormal, a coronary angiogram should be obtained to determine if a correctable lesion is present. When a correctable abnormality is uncovered, the appropriate cardiac procedure should precede (occasionally may accompany) the necessary pulmonary resection.[125,126]

The cardiac risk factors that may contraindicate resection are a recent myocardial infarction, uncontrolled heart failure, or an uncontrollable arrhythmia. Generally, 3 months should be permitted to elapse after an infarct prior to thoracotomy. This time period can be shortened if adequate myocardial function can be ascertained by a dipyridamole 201 thallium (T1) scan or 201Tl echocardiography. Intensive hemodynamic monitoring is required postoperatively. With such a regimen, a reinfarction rate of only 5.7% after noncardiac surgery within the first 3 months of the initial infarction has been reported.[127] Unfortunately with reinfarction, the mortality rate is high, particularly when the episode occurs within 48 hours of the procedure.[128,129]

## SUMMARY

The diagnosis and staging of patients are essential phases of the management of patients with lung cancer. At the completion of the "staging process," the cell type of the tumor should be known (not necessary per se in patients with an asymptomatic peripheral nodule), the extent of the disease should be determined as well as possible, and the functional status and physiologic status (for proposed surgical candidates) should have been established. With this information in hand, the appropriate therapeutic course may be recommended and a meaningful prognosis be assigned.

When the patient is a surgical candidate, and exploration and definitive resection are carried out, the T and N status of the lesion must be changed as necessary to reflect the findings of the examination of the resected lung and the removed mediastinal nodes. The patients who have undergone resection should be classified by the pathologic (postsurgical) T and N designations. In doing so the patient can be assigned to the appropriate stage group for the proper determination of his or her prognosis. Also important is that the pathologic stage classification, along with the final histologic cell type, may permit the surgeon to recommend appropriate adjuvant therapy when such is available. When an adjuvant therapy is still experimental, the patient can be entered into a suitable, prospective, randomized adjuvant trial that may be under investigation for the patient's stage of disease.

## REFERENCES

1. Carlens E: Mediastinoscopy: A method for inspection and tissue biopsy of the superior mediastinum. *Chest* **36**:343, 1959
2. Denoix PF: Enquete permanent dans les anticancereux. *Bull Inst Nat Hyg* (Paris) **1**:70, 1964
3. Beahrs OH, Myers MH (eds): *The Manual for Staging Cancer.* American Joint Committee on Cancer. Philadelphia, Lippincott, 1973
4. Mountain CF: A new international staging system for lung cancer. *Chest* **89**:225S–235S, 1986
5. Hyde L, Yee J, Wilson R, Patno ME: Cell type and natural history of lung cancer. *JAMA* **193**:52, 1965
6. Oswald NC, Hinson KFW, Canti G, Miller AB: The diagnosis of primary lung cancer with special references to sputum cytology. *Thorax* **26**:623, 1971
7. Kato H: Sputum cytology diagnosis. In Hayata Y (ed): *Lung Cancer Diagnosis.* Tokyo, Igaku-Shoin, 1982, p 85
8. Karsell PR, McDougall JC: Diagnostic tests for lung cancer. *Mayo Clin Proc* **68**:288–296, 1993

9. Fennesy JJ: Bronchial brushing and transbronchial forceps biopsy in the diagnosis of pulmonary lesions. *Dis Chest* **53:**377, 1968
10. Hattori S, Matsuda M: TV brushing method for early diagnosis of small peripheral lung cancer. In Deeley TJ (ed): *Carcinoma of the Bronchus.* New York, Appleton-Century-Crofts, 1971, p 53
11. Faber LP, Monson DO, Amato JJ, Jensik RJ: Flexible fiberoptic bronchoscopy. *Ann Thorac Surg* **16:**163, 1973
12. Hayashi T: Brushing cytology in lung cancer detection. In Hayata Y (ed): *Lung Cancer Diagnosis.* Tokyo, Igaku-Shoin, 1982, p 120
13 Martini N, Zamen MB, Melamed MR: Early diagnosis of carcinoma of the lung. In Roth JA, Ruckdeschel JC, Weisenburger TH (eds): *Thoracic Oncology.* Philadelphia, Saunders, 1989, p 133
14 Payne WS, Bernatz PE, Pairolero PC, et al: Localization and treatment of radiographically occult lung cancer. In Delarue NC, Eschapasse H (eds): *Lung Cancer.* Philadelphia, Saunders, 1985, p 80
15. Lam S, MacAulay C, Jung J, et al: Detection of dysplasia and carcinoma in-situ cancer using a lung imaging fluorescence endoscope (LIFE) device. *J Thorac Cardiovasc Surg* **105:**729, 1993
16. Tockman MS, Gupta PK, Myers JD, et al: Sensitive and specific monoclonal antibody recognition of human lung cancer antigen on preserved sputum cells: A new approach to early lung cancer detection. *J Clin Oncol* **6:**1685, 1988
17. Tockman MS, Gupta PK, Pressman NJ, Mulshine JL: Considerations in bringing a cancer biomarker to clinical application. *Cancer Res* **52**(suppl):2711S, 1992
18. Roth JA: Advances in cellular and molecular biology of non small cell lung cancer. In Roth JA, Cox JD, Hong WK: *Lung Cancer.* Boston, Blackwell Scientific Publications, 1993, pp 85–104
19. Oho K: Fiberoptic bronchoscopy. In Hayata Y (ed): *Lung Cancer Diagnosis.* Tokyo, Igaku-Shoin, 1982, p 120
20. Sagel SS, Ferguson TB, Forrest JV, et al: Percutaneous transthoracic aspiration needle biopsy. *Ann Thorac Surg* **26:**399, 1978
21 Mark JBD, Marlin SI, Castellino RA: The role of bronchoscopy and needle aspiration in the diagnosis of peripheral lung masses. *J Thorac Cardiovasc Surg* **76:**266, 1978
22. Calhoun P, Feldman PS, Armstrong P, et al: The clinical outcome of needle aspirations of the lung when cancer is not diagnosed. *Ann Thorac Surg* **41:**592, 1986
23. Landreneau RJ, et al: Thoracoscopic resection of 85 pulmonary lesions. *Ann Thorac Surg* **54:**415, 1992
24. Shenk DA, Strollo PJ, Pickard JS, et al: Utility of the Wang 18-gauge transbronchial histology needle in the staging of bronchogenic carcinoma. *Chest* **96:**272, 1989
25. Harrow EM, Oldenburg FA, Lingenfelter MS, et al: Transbronchial needle aspiration in clinical practice. A five-year experience. *Chest* **96:**1268, 1989
26. Krasna MJ, Mack MJ: *Atlas of Thorascopic Surgery.* St. Louis, Quality Medical Publishing, 1944
27. McCarthy WJ, Christ ML, Fry WA: Intraoperative fine needle aspiration biopsy of thoracic lesions. *Ann Thorac Surg* **30:**24, 1980
28. Mountain CF: Lung cancer staging classification. *Clin Chest Med* **14:**43, 1993
29. Rusch VW, Albain KS, Crawley J, et al: Successful surgical resection of both stages IIIa and IIIb non small cell cancer after intensive preoperative chemotherapy: A Southwest Oncology Group trial. Presented at the 72nd Annual Meeting of the American Association for Thoracic Surgery; April 29, 1992; Los Angeles
30. Rusch VW, Albain KS, Crawley J, et al: Neoadjuvant therapy for Stage IIIb non-small cell lung cancer. Presented at the Annual Meeting of the Society of Thoracic Surgeons; January 1994; New Orleans
31. Strauss GM, Langer MP, Elias AD, et al: Multi-modality treatment of stage IIIa non-small cell lung carcinoma: A critical review of the literature and strategies for future research. *J Clin Oncol* **10:**829–838, 1992
32. Yashar J, Weitberg AB, Glicksman AS, et al: Preoperative chemotherapy and radiation therapy for stage IIIa carcinoma of the lung. *Ann Thorac Surg* **53:**445–448, 1992
33. Feld R, Payne D, Shepherd FA: Small cell lung cancer. In Shields TW (ed): *General Thoracic Surgery,* 4th ed. Philadelphia, Lea and Febiger, 1994, p 1241
34. Fontana RS, Sanderson DR: Screening for lung cancer: A progress report. In Mountain CF, Carr DR (eds): *Lung Cancer, Current Status and Prospects for the Future.* Austin, Texas, University of Texas Press, 1986, p 51
35. Shields TW: Presentation, diagnosis and staging of bronchial carcinoma and of the asymptomatic solitary pulmonary nodule. In Shields TW (ed): *General Thoracic Surgery,* 4th ed. Philadelphia, Lea and Febiger, 1994, p 1122
36. Stewart MF, Crosby SR, Gibson S, et al: Small cell lung cancer cell lines secrete predominantly ACTH precursor peptides not ACTH. *Br J Cancer* **60:**20, 1989
37. Cogan E, Debieve MF, Pepersack T, et al: High plasma levels of atrial natriuretic factor in SIADH (letter). *N Engl J Med* **314:**1258, 1986
38. Morton DL, Itabashi HH, Grimes OF: Nonmetastatic neurological complications of bronchogenic carcinoma. *J Thorac Cardiovasc Surg* **51:**14, 1966
39. Lambert EH, Eaton LM, Rooke ED: Defect of neuromuscular conduction associated with malignant neoplasms (abstract). *Am J Physiol* **187:**612, 1956
40. Lennon VA, Lambert EH: Autoantibodies bind solubilized calcium channel-to-conotoxin complexes from small cell lung carcinoma: a diagnostic aid for Lambert-Eaton myasthenic syndrome. *Mayo Clin Proc* **64:**1498, 1989
41. Yalow RS, Eastridge CE, Higgins G Jr, Wolf J: Plasma and tumor ACTH in carcinoma of the lung. *Cancer* **44:**1789, 1979
42. Vincent RG, Chu TM, Lane WW, et al: Carcinoembryonic antigen as a monitor of successful surgical resection in 130 patients with carcinoma of the lung. In Muggia F, Rozencweig M (eds): *Lung Cancer: Progress in Therapeutic Research.* New York, Raven, 1979, p 191
43. Carney DN, Broder L, Edelstein M, et al: Experimental studies of the biology of human small cell lung cancer. *Cancer Treat Rep* **67:**27, 1983
44. Rodenhuis S, Slebas RJC: Clinical significance of ras oncogene activation in human lung cancer. *Cancer Research* **52** (suppl): 2665s–2669s, 1992
45. Tateiski M, Ishida T, Mitsudomi T, et al: Prognostic value of c-erbB-2 protein expression in human lung adenocarcinoma and squamous cell carcinoma. Eur J Cancer **27:**1372, 1991
46. Horio Y, Takahashi T, Kuroishi T, et al: Prognostic significance of p53 mutations and 3p deletions in primary resected non-small cell lung cancer. *Cancer Res* **54:**1, 1993
47. Johnson BE, Ihde DC, Makuch RW: *myc* family oncogene amplification in tumor cell lines established from small cell lung cancer patients and its relationship to clinical course. *J Clin Invest* **79:**1629, 1987
48. Rigler LG: A roentgen study of the evolution of carcinoma of the lung. *J Thorac Cardiovasc Surg* **34:**283, 1957
49. Rigler LG: The earliest roentgenographic signs of carcinoma of the lung. *JAMA* **195:**655, 1966
50. Spratt JS Jr, Ter-Pogossian M, Long RTL: The detection and growth of intrathoracic neoplasms: The lower limits of radiographic distinction of the antemortem size, the duration, and the pattern of growth as determined by direct measuration of tumor diameters from random thoracic roentgenograms. *Arch Surg* **86:**283, 1963
51. Amemia R, Oho K: X-ray diagnosis of lung cancer. In Hayata Y (ed): *Lung Cancer Diagnosis.* Tokyo, Igaku-Shoin, 1982, p 4
52. Swett HA, Nagel JS, Sostman HD: Imaging methods in primary lung carcinoma. *Clin Chest Med* **3:**331, 1982
53. Byrd RB, Carr DT, Miller WE, et al: Radiographic abnormalities in carcinoma of the lung as related to histological cell type. *Thorax* **24:**573, 1969
54. Backer CL, Shields TW, Lockhart CG, et al: Selective preoperative

evaluation for possible N2 disease in carcinoma of the lung. *J Thorac Cardiovasc Surg* **93:**337, 1987

55. Osada H: Bronchography. In Hayata Y (ed): *Lung Cancer Diagnosis.* Tokyo, Igaku-Shoin, 1982, p 68
56. Sanders DE, DeLarue NC, Lau G: Angiography as a means of determining resectability of primary lung cancer. *AJR* **87:**884, 1962
57. Glazer GM: Radiologic staging of lung cancer using CT and MRI. *Chest* **96:**44S, 1990
58. Pagani JJ: Non-small cell lung carcinoma adrenal metastases: Computed tomography and percutaneous needle biopsy in their diagnosis. *Cancer* **53:**1058, 1984
59. Siegelman SS, Zerhouni EA, Leo FP, et al: CT of the solitary pulmonary nodule. *AJR* **134:**1, 1980
60. Gross DH, Glazer GM, Orringer MB, et al: Bronchogenic carcinoma metastatic to normal-sized lymph nodes: Frequency and significance. *Radiology* **166:**71, 1988
61. Izbicki RJ, Thetter O, Karg O, et al: Accuracy of computed tomographic scan and surgical assessment for staging of bronchial carcinoma: a prospective study. *J Thorac Cardiovasc Surg* **104:**413, 1992
62. Webb WR: Magnetic resonance imaging of the chest. *Curr Opin Radiol* **1:**40, 1989
63. Webb WR, Gatsonis C, Zerhouni EA, et al: CT and MR imaging in staging non-small cell bronchogenic carcinoma: Report of the Radiologic Diagnostic Oncology Group. *Radiology* **178:**705, 1991
64. Gamsu G: Magnetic resonance imaging in lung cancer. *Chest* **89:**242S, 1986
65. Kondo D, Imaizumi M, Abe T, et al: Endoscopic ultrasound examination for mediastinal lymph node metastases of lung cancer. *Chest* **98:**586–593, 1990
66. Lee N, Inoue K, Yamamoto R, Kinoshita H, et al: Patterns of internal echoes in lymph nodes in the diagnosis of lung cancer metastasis. *World J Surg* **16:**986, 1992
67. Rusch V, Macapinlac H, Heelan R, et al: NR-LU-10 monoclonal antibody scanning. *J Thorac Cardiovasc Surg* **106:**200, 1993
68. Gupta NC, Frank AR, Dewan NA, et al: Solitary pulmonary nodules: detection of malignancy with PET with 2-[F-18]-fluoro-2-deoxy-P-glucose. *Radiology* **184:**441, 1992
69. Scott W, Schwabe J, Gupta N, et al: PET-FDG imaging: detection of malignancy in lung tumors and mediastinal lymph nodes. Presented at the 30th Annual Meeting of the Society of Thoracic Surgeons; January 31, 1994; New Orleans.
70. Kubota K, Matsuzawa T, Fujiwara T: Differential diagnosis of solitary pulmonary nodules with position emission tomography using [$^{11}$C]L-Methionine. *J Comput Assist Tomogr* **12:**794, 1988
71. Ramsdell JW, Peters RM, Taylor AT Jr, et al: Multiorgan scans for staging lung cancer. *J Thorac Cardiovasc Surg* **73:**653, 1977
72. Ichinose Y, Hara N, Ohta M, et al: Preoperative examination to detect distant metastasis is not advocated for asymptomatic patients with stage 1 and 2 non-small cell lung cancer. *Chest* **96:**1104, 1989
73. Little AG, Stitik FP: Clinical staging of patients with non-small cell lung cancer. *Chest* **97:**1431–1438, 1990
74. Feld R, Rubinstein LV, Weisenberger TH, et al: Sites of recurrence in resected Stage I non-small cell lung cancer: A guide for future studies. *J Clin Oncol* **2:**1352, 1984
75. Mountain CF, McMurtrey MF, Frazier OH, et al: Present status of postoperative adjuvant therapy for lung cancer. *Cancer Bull* **32:**108, 1980
76. Immerman SC, Vanecko RM, Fry WA, et al: Site of recurrence in patients with Stages I and II carcinoma of the lung resected for cure. *Ann Thorac Surg* **32:**23, 1981
77. Ludwig Lung Cancer Study Group: Patterns of failure in patients with resected stage I and II non-small cell carcinoma of the lung. *Ann Surg* 205:67, 1987
78. Salvatierra A, Baamonde C, Llamas JM, et al: Extrathoracic staging of bronchogenic carcinoma. *Chest* **97:**1052–1058, 1990
79. Salbeck R, Grau HC, Artmann H: Cerebral tumor staging in bronchial carcinoma by computed tomography. *Cancer* **66:**2007–2011, 1990
80. Kormans P, Bradshaw JR, Jeyasingham K: Preoperative computed tomography of the brain in non-small cell bronchial carcinoma. *Thorax* **47:**106–108, 1992
81. DeMeester TR, Bekerman C, Joseph JG, et al: Gallium-67 scanning for carcinoma of the lung. *J Thorac Cardiovasc Surg* **72:**699, 1976
82. Shields TW: The use of mediastinoscopy in lung cancer: The dilemma of mediastinal lymph nodes. In Kittle CF (ed): *Current Controversies in Thoracic Surgery.* Philadelphia, Saunders, 1986, p 145
83. Jolly PC, Hill LD III, Lawless PA, West TL: Parasternal mediastinotomy and mediastinoscopy—Adjuncts in the diagnosis of chest disease. *J Thorac Cardiovasc Surg* **66:**549, 1973
84. Ginsberg RJ, Rice TW, Goldberg M, et al: Extended cervical mediastinoscopy—A single staging procedure for bronchogenic carcinoma of the left upper lobe. *J Thorac Cardiovasc Surg* **94:**673, 1987
85. Ginsberg RJ: The role of preoperative surgical staging in left upper lobe tumors. *Ann Thorac Surg* **57:**526, 1994
86. Lopez L, Varela A, Friexnet J, et al: Extended cervical mediastinoscopy: Prospective study of 50 cases. *Ann Thorac Surg* **57:**555, 1994
87. Landreneau RJ, Hazelrigg SR, Mack MJ, et al: Thoracoscopic mediastinal lymph node sampling: Useful for mediastinal lymph node stations inaccessible by cervical mediastinoscopy. *J Thorac Cardiovasc Surg* **106:**554, 1993
88. Lewis RL, Caccavalo RJ, Sisler GE, Mackenzie JW: One hundred consecutive patients undergoing video-assisted thoracic operations. *Ann Thorac Surg* **54:**421, 1992
89. Sugarbaker DJ, Strauss GM: Advances in surgical staging and therapy of non-small cell lung cancer. *Semin Oncol* **20:**163, 1993
90. Pearson FG, DeLarue NC, Ilves R, et al: Significance of positive superior mediastinal nodes identified at mediastinoscopy in patients with resectable cancer of the lung. *J Thorac Cardiovasc Surg* **83:**1, 1982
91. Sarin CL, Nohl-Oser HC: Mediastinoscopy. *Thorax* **24:**585, 1969
92. Maassen W: Accuracy of mediastinoscopy. In DeLarue NC, Eschapasse H (eds): *International Trends in General Thoracic Surgery,* Vol 1. *Lung Cancer.* Philadelphia, Saunders, 1985, p 42
93. Coughlin M, Deslauriers J, Beaulieu M, et al: Role of mediastinoscopy in pretreatment staging of patients with primary lung cancer. *Ann Thorac Surg* 40:556, 1985
94. Patterson GA, Ginsberg RJ, Poon Y, et al: A prospective evolution of magnetic resonance imaging, computed tomography and mediastoscopy in the preoperative assessment of mediastinal node status in bronchogenic carcinoma. *J Thorac Cardiovasc Surg* **94:**679, 1987
95. Yoshimatsu H: Mediastinal lymph nodes involvement in the patients classified in Stage I. Quoted in Hayata Y (ed): *Lung Cancer Diagnosis.* Tokyo, Igaku-Shoin, 1982, p 250
96. Patterson GA, Piazza D, Pearson FG, et al: Significance of metastatic disease in subaortic lymph nodes. *Ann Thorac Surg* **43:**155, 1987
97. Martini N, Flehinger BJ, Zaman MB, Beattie EJ Jr: Results of resection in non-oat cell carcinoma of the lung with mediastinal lymph node metastases. *Ann Surg* **198:**386, 1983
98. Watanabe Y, Shimizu J, Oda M, et al: Aggressive surgical intervention in N2 non-small cell cancer of the lung. *Ann Thorac Surg* **51:**256–261, 1991
99. Lewis JW Jr, Pearlberg JL, Beute GH, et al: Can computed tomography of the chest stage lung cancer? Yes and no. *Ann Thorac Surg* **49:**591–596, 1990
100. Daly BDT, Mueller JD, Faling LJ, et al: N2 lung cancer: Outcome in patients with false negative chest CT scans. *J Thorac Cardiovasc Surg* **105:**904, 1993
101. Reed CE: Commentary: Lymph node dissection and staging. In Krasna MJ, Mack JM (eds): *Atlas of Thoracoscopic Surgery.* St. Louis, Quality Medical Publishing, 1994, p 195

102. Wain JC: Video-assisted thoracoscopy and the staging of lung cancer. *Ann Thorac Surg* **56:**776, 1993
103. Raviaro GC, Varoli F, Rebuffat C, et al: Videothorascopic approach for lung cancer: staging and treatment. In Motta G (ed): *Lung Cancer, Frontiers in Science and Treatment.* Genoa, Italy, G Motta Publ, 1994, p 325
104. Buhr J, Berghauser KH, Morr H, et al: Tumor cells in intraoperative pleural lavage: An indicator for poor prognosis of bronchogenic carcinoma. *Cancer* **65:**1801–1804, 1990
105. Okumura M, Ohshima S, Kotake Y, et al: Intraoperative pleural lavage cytology in lung cancer patients. *Ann Thorac Surg* **51:**599–604, 1991
106. Shields TW, Higgins GA Jr, Matthews MJ, Keehn RJ: Surgical resection in the management of small cell carcinoma of the lung. *J Thorac Cardiovasc Surg* **84:**481, 1982
107. Meyer JA: Surgical resection as an adjunct to chemotherapy for small cell carcinoma of the lung. In Bates M (ed): *Bronchial Carcinoma.* Berlin, Heidelberg, Springer-Verlag, 1984, p 177
108. Meyer JA: Five-year survival in treated stage I and II small cell carcinoma of the lung. *Ann Thorac Surg* **42:**668, 1986
109. Ohta M, Hara N, Ichinose Y, et al: The role of surgical resection in the management of small cell carcinoma of the lung. *Jpn J Clin Oncol* **16:** 289, 1986
110. Karrer K, Shields TW, Denck H, et al: The importance of surgery and multimodality treatment for small cell bronchial carcinoma. *J Thorac Cardiovasc Surg* **97:**168, 1989
111. Ichinose Y, Hara N, Ohta M, et al: Comparison between resected and irradiated small cell lung cancer in patients stages I through IIIa. *Ann Thorac Surg* **53:**95, 1992
112. Naruke T, Suemasu K, Ishikawa S: Lymph node mapping and curability of various levels of metastasis in resected lung cancer. *J Thorac Cardiovasc Surg* **76:**832, 1978
113. Tisi GM, Friedman PJ, Peters RM, et al: Clinical staging of primary lung cancer. *Am Rev Respir Dis* **127:**659, 1983
114. Shields TW: The incomplete resection. *Ann Thorac Surg* **47:**487–488, 1989
115. Naruke T, Goya T, Tsuchiya R, et al: Prognosis and survival in resected lung carcinoma based on the new international staging system. *J Thorac Cardiovasc Surg* **96:**440–447, 1988
116. Olsen GN, Block J, Tobias JA: Prediction of postpneumonectomy function using quantitative macroaggregate lung scanning. *Chest* **66:**13, 1974
117. Ali MK, Mountain CF, Ewer MS, et al: Predicting loss of pulmonary function after pulmonary resection for bronchogenic carcinoma. *Chest* **77:**337, 1980
118. Ali MK, Ewer MS, Morice RC, Mountain CF: Physiological evaluation of the patient with lung cancer. Annual Clinical Conference on Cancer, Vol 28. In Mountain CF, Carr DR (eds): *Lung Cancer: Current Status and Prospects for the Future.* Houston, The University of Texas System Cancer Center, 1986, p 99
119. Olsen GN: Pulmonary physiologic assessment of operative risk. In Shields TW (ed): *General Thoracic Surgery,* 4th ed. Philadelphia, Lea & Febiger, 1994, p 279
120. Arroliga AC, Buzaid AC, Matthy RA: Which patients can safely undergo lung resection? *J Respir Dis* **12:**1080, 1991
121. Morice RC, Peters EJ, Ryan MB, et al: Exercise testing in the evaluation of patients at high risk for complications from lung resection. *Chest* **101:**356, 1992
122. Bechard D, Wetstein L: Assessment of exercise consumption: a preoperative criterion for lung resection. *Ann Thorac Surg* **44:**344–349, 1987
123. Walsh GL, Morice RC, Putnam JB, et al: Resection of lung cancer is justified in high-risk patients selected by exercise oxygen consumption. Presented at the 30th Annual Meeting of the Society of Thoracic Surgeons; February 1, 1994; New Orleans
124. Smith TP, Kinasewitz GT, Tucker WY, et al: Exercise capacity as a predictor of post-thoracotomy morbidity. *Am Rev Respir Dis* **129:**730, 1984
125. Piehler JM, Trastek VF, Pairolero PC, et al: Concomitant cardiac and pulmonary operations. *J Thorac Cardiovasc Surg* **90:**662, 1985
126. Miller DL, Orszulak TA, Pairolero PC, et al: Combined operation for lung cancer and cardiac disease. Presented at Annual Meeting of the Society of Thoracic Surgeons; January 1994; New Orleans
127. Rao TH, Jacobs KH, Err EL: Re-infarction following anesthesia in patients with myocardial infarction. *Anesthesiology* **59:**449, 1983
128. Steen PA, Tinker JH, Tarhan S: Myocardial infarction after anesthesia and surgery. *JAMA* **239:**2566–2570, 1978
129. Tarhan S, Moffit EA, Taylor WF, et al: Myocardial infarction after general anesthesia. *JAMA* **220:**1451–1454, 1972

CHAPTER

# 23

# Surgical Treatment of Lung Carcinoma

Michael Burt, Nael Martini, and Robert J. Ginsberg

According to data published by the American Cancer Society, carcinoma of the lung in the United States remains both the second most common cancer (prostate carcinoma being first) and the leading cause of death from cancer in men, accounting for 33% of cancer related deaths.[1] Historically, for women, the most common cause of cancer death was breast carcinoma, but since 1985 this has changed. The most common cause of cancer death in women is now lung carcinoma and accounts for 23% of the deaths from cancer, with breast cancer accounting for 18%.[1]

Overall, the cure rate of lung carcinoma is low, with approximately 10–13% of patients alive at 5 years.[1] The American Cancer Society predicts 172,000 new cases for 1994 (100,000 men, 72,000 women). In addition, it is predicted that 153,000 people will die of lung cancer in the United States in 1994 (94,000 men, 59,000 women).

Treatment of lung carcinoma is decided after comprehensive staging. (See Chap. 22.) Except for small cell carcinoma, surgery is accepted as the most effective therapy for lung carcinoma.[2–4]

Although Milton Anthony was probably the first to deliberately open the chest in 1821 without tracheal intubation, it was not until 1909, when Meltzer and Auer introduced intratracheal anesthesia, that the positive pressure exerted by thoracotomy could be controlled effectively.[5]

In 1933, Graham and Singer[6] performed the first successful pneumonectomy for lung carcinoma. In that report they reviewed the experience reported in the literature with pulmonary resection for carcinoma and found that all patients (n = 11) who had undergone pneumonectomy had died. Apparently there were six patients who had undergone lesser resections who had survived 1 or more years following resection. It is of historical interest to quote the surgical technique from Graham and Singer's article:

> At the operation, however, which was performed April 5, with intratracheal anesthesia of nitrous oxide and oxygen, it was found that the carcinoma extended so closely to the bronchus of the lower lobe that it was impossible to save the latter bronchus. Moreover, there were many nodules in the upper portion of the lower lobe about which uncertainty existed as to whether they were tumor tissue or areas of inflammation. Finally, also the interlobar fissure was not complete. For all these reasons it was decided to remove the entire lung. The adhesions between the lower lobe, chest wall and diaphragm were separated without great difficulty. A small rubber catheter was tied tightly around the hilus as close to the trachea as possible. Crushing clamps were placed on the hilus below the catheter and the lung was cut off with an electric cautery knife. The open end of the left main bronchus was carefully cauterized with the actual cautery as far up as the catheter would permit in order to destroy the mucous membrane thoroughly. A transfixing double ligature of number 2 chromic catgut was tied around the stump just distal to the catheter and the latter was then removed. No bleeding occurred. Another transfixing ligature of number 2 chromic catgut was placed where the catheter had been. The stump of the pulmonary artery was then ligated separately with catgut, and seven radon seeds of 1.5 millicuries each were inserted into various parts of the stump. Several enlarged tracheobronchial

glands were removed from the mediastinum, and seven ribs from the third to the ninth, inclusive, were removed from the transverse process of the spine to the anterior axillary line. The ribs were removed for the purpose of allowing the soft tissues of the chest wall to collapse against the bronchial stump and therefore to obliterate as much as possible the pleural cavity. The first and second ribs were not removed at this time merely because it was desired not to do too much operating at once. Nevertheless, it was felt that there would be some danger of the development of an empyema in the upper part of the pleural cavity because of the failure to obliterate that space. The wound was closed tightly, but provision for drainage was made by the use of an air-tight catheter brought out through a stab wound.

Dr. Graham's patient, Dr. Gilmore, continued to practice medicine for 24 years after his surgery and died March 6, 1963.

After this report, other surgeons began to perform pneumonectomy as the operation of choice for lung carcinoma. In 1950, Churchill et al[7] proposed that lobectomy for carcinoma of the lung was as effective for cure and safer than pneumonectomy.[8] Today, the surgical treatment of carcinoma includes many types of pulmonary resections, tailored to both the malignant process with its anatomic extent and the patient's physiologic status. Lobectomy is the procedure of choice when the disease is limited to a lobe or a lobar bronchus.[7,9] When the tumor is in the main bronchus or pulmonary hilus, or crosses lobar fissures, pneumonectomy becomes necessary in order to encompass all disease and obtain clear margins of resection.

An elective segmentectomy or wedge resection has been advocated for small, early peripheral carcinomas of the lung.[10,11] Jensik et al[12] performed 168 segmental resections on patients with peripheral stage I bronchogenic carcinoma from 1957 to 1978. The actuarial survival was 53% at 5 years. Forty-five patients had died of their disease at the time of reporting, and in 16 of the 45 (36%), there was local recurrence in the same lobe or the mediastinum. (See Chap. 25.)

Table 23–1 lists six studies evaluating lesser resections (segmentectomy or wedge resection) in patients with stage I non-small cell lung cancer. Five of the studies were retrospective in nature,[12–16] but the study by Ginsberg and Rubinstein (for the Lung Cancer Study Group)[17] was a randomized comparison of lobectomy vs. a lesser pulmonary resection. The locoregional recurrence rate in the five retrospective series ranged from 4.4% to 22.7% and from 4.9% to 11.5% for lesser resection vs. lobectomy, respectively. The Lung Cancer Study Group trial randomized 247 patients to undergo lobectomy vs. segmentectomy or wedge resection. As listed in Table 23–1, the group having a lesser resection had a significantly increased locoregional recurrence rate compared with the group having lobectomy. This increased rate of recurrence translated into a decreased survival at 5 years for those undergoing a lesser resection compared with lobectomy.

Therefore, we suggest that wedge resection may be adequate for the elderly or for patients with limited cardiopulmonary reserve, for whom thoracotomy alone poses a serious risk. However, such a procedure is not recommended for good-risk patients because of the high incidence of local tumor recurrence and shorter survival time that it entails for a group of patients with potentially curable lesions.

The role of video-assisted thoracoscopic surgery (VATS) in patients with resectable disease is controversial. Although there are a number of series demonstrating the feasibility of VATS[18–22] pulmonary resection in patients with non-small cell lung carcinoma, the efficacy of VATS vs. thoracotomy for pulmonary resection awaits the results of randomized trials. (See Chap. 12B.)

Whatever type of pulmonary resection is selected for an individual, one cannot stress enough the importance of a complete resection in the surgical treatment of non-small cell carcinoma of the lung.

The outlook for patients undergoing an incomplete resection is dismal. Shields[23] reported 221 patients undergoing incomplete resection for bronchogenic carcinoma and divided the residual disease as: (1) mediastinal tissues (T4), (2) mediastinal lymph nodes, (3) parietal pleura or chest wall, and (4) bronchial stump. The overall survival reported in this series was 26% at 1 year, 8.5% at 3 years, and 4% at 5 years. All 5-year survivors had squamous cell carcinoma with a positive bronchial margin. There is a negative impact on survival whether the bronchial stump residual tumor is mucosal[24] or extramucosal.[24,25]

In order to be complete, a mediastinal lymph node dis-

**TABLE 23–1. STAGE I NON-SMALL CELL LUNG CANCER: LOBECTOMY VS. SEGMENTECTOMY OR WEDGE RESECTION**

| | n | | Local Recurrence | | 5-year Survival | |
|---|---|---|---|---|---|---|
| **Series** | ***Segment/Lobe*** | | ***Segment/Lobe*** | | ***Segment/Lobe*** | |
| Jensik et al[12] | 168 | N/A | 9.5% | N/A | 53% | N/A |
| Hoffman et al[13] | 33 | 112 | N/A | N/A | 26% | 25% |
| McCormack et al[14] | 53 | N/A | 19.3% | N/A | 33% | N/A |
| Read et al[15] | 113 | 131 | 4.4% | 11.5% | N/A | N/A |
| Warren et al[16] | 68 | 105 | 22.7% | 4.9% | 47% | 65% |
| Ginsberg et al[17] | 122 | 125 | 17.2% | 6.4% | 50% | 68% |

section becomes an integral part of the operation, since this affords the most accurate method of assessing nodal involvement, which is crucial to accurate surgical and, more importantly, pathologic staging.[26]

We routinely perform a mediastinal lymph node dissection in all patients with resectable lung tumors and record the results on our mediastinal lymph node map (Fig. 23–1). This data is updated after pathologic results are available. A potentially curative resection is defined by us as resection of the primary tumor plus a systematic dissection of all accessible mediastinal lymph nodes. At completion of the procedure, there should be no tumor left behind, and all margins of resection must be microscopically clear of tumor. The technique of mediastinal lymph node dissection, as we perform it, is relatively simple.

There are three mediastinal lymph node compartments amenable to exploration and dissection: (1) the superior mediastinal or paratracheal compartment on the right side, (2) the aortico-pulmonary window on the left, and (3) the subcarinal and inferior mediastinal compartment on both right and left.

On the right side, the superior mediastinal lymph node compartment is that contained between the trachea and superior vena cava from the level of the pulmonary artery to the right innominate artery and right recurrent laryngeal nerve. This compartment is exposed by incising the mediastinal pleura above the azygos vein. The pleura is reflected, and the fat pad with all its nodes is gently dissected away from the vena cava, trachea, and underlying ascending arch of the aorta. The vagus nerve and azygos vein are protected and spared. An en bloc dissection of all visible and palpable nodes is readily feasible in this compartment. It is possible also to free the paratracheal bed on either side through this exposure, and any lymph nodes in the left paratracheal region are thus detected and removed.

The anterior mediastinum (anterior to the superior

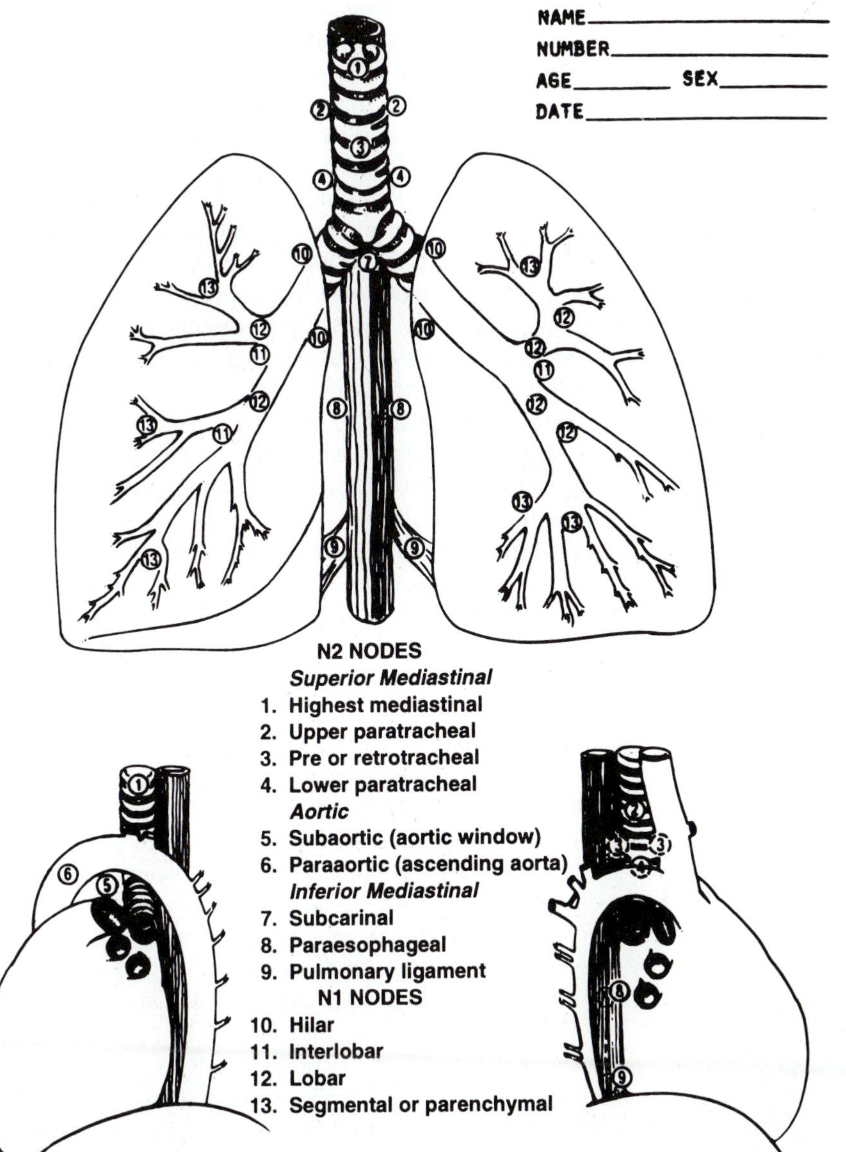


**Figure 23–1.** Lymph node map used to record location of peribronchial, hilar, and mediastinal lymph nodes during pulmonary resection and mediastinal lymph node dissection.

vena cava) is not routinely included in the dissection. Palpable nodes in this region, when present, are surgically excised without a formal dissection pattern being followed.

To gain access to the inferior mediastinal compartment, the posterior mediastinal pleura is incised from the level of the main stem bronchus to the inferior pulmonary ligament exposing the subcarinal, paraesophageal, and inferior pulmonary lymph nodes. Adequate excision of these node-bearing areas is possible with direct visualization of the tracheal bifurcation, the opposite bronchus, and the pericardium.

On the left side, access to nodes in the supra-aortic compartment and superior mediastinum is extremely limited, except for what may be palpable between the phrenic nerve and the vagus nerve. In this compartment, nodes are simply sampled without a formal dissection. Nodes in the aortico-pulmonary window are those found between the left main pulmonary artery and the arch of the aorta, from the recurrent laryngeal nerve to the phrenic nerve. These are routinely excised during a left pulmonary resection. The nodes in the subcarinal region and inferior mediastinum are also removed in a manner similar to that described for right-sided lesions. The posterior mediastinal pleura is opened from the lower border of the left main bronchus to the inferior pulmonary ligament, anterior to the descending aorta. By following the inferior border of the main bronchus, and by gently retracting the descending aorta and esophagus, access to and dissection of the subcarinal lymph nodes is readily possible. Dissection of the lower paraesophageal and inferior mediastinal lymph nodes at the pulmonary ligament pose no problem.

A complete mediastinal lymph node dissection and not mere sampling is thus possible, the advantages of which are a more accurate assessment of nodal involvement and more favorable long-term survival. It is important to point out that no morbidity is incurred by including a node dissection at the time of thoracotomy. The additional 15–30 minutes necessary to perform a formal dissection has not adversely affected the intraoperative or postoperative course of these patients.

## SURGICAL TREATMENT OF OCCULT (TX N0 M0) NON-SMALL CELL LUNG CARCINOMA

Few patients are found to have lung carcinoma before it becomes radiographically apparent. These patients represent 1.5% of our clinical case experience in primary lung cancer at Memorial Hospital.[27] These are individuals who participate in early lung cancer detection programs and submit sputum cytologic examinations on a routine basis, or patients who present to institutions with hemoptysis in the absence of any abnormal findings on routine chest roentgenograms. Occult carcinomas presenting in this fashion need a careful investigation to localize the site of the cancer. The fact that the patient has a normal chest roentgenogram and a positive sputum cytology does not necessarily indicate that the patient has lung carcinoma, let alone an early lung carcinoma.[28] A careful head and neck examination is essential. In our experience, patients who present with a positive sputum cytology in the absence of radiologic findings are noted to have a carcinoma in the head and neck region in one out of three instances. If the head and neck examination is normal, then a careful diagnostic bronchoscopy is performed. With the use of the modern fiber-optic bronchoscope, it has become possible to extend the inspection of the tracheobronchial tree from the main stem and lobar bronchi to segmental and subsegmental bronchi. By this method alone with careful and diligent inspection of the tracheobronchial tree in patients with radiologically occult carcinomas, one can usually identify the site of the lung carcinoma. If the lesion is located centrally in a main or a lobar bronchus, it is readily visualized and a biopsy easily obtained. However, in many instances the tracheobronchial tree appears entirely normal at bronchoscopy. In these instances, a meticulous sampling of each segmental bronchus by endobronchial brushing and cytologic analysis becomes necessary. Careful attention to detail to avoid cross-contamination has resulted in localizing these peripheral tumors in nearly all instances. Following localization, the treatment of choice for a radiologically occult carcinoma of the lung is surgical extirpation of the primary tumor by lobectomy or pneumonectomy. Since most occult carcinomas are relatively central in position, lesser resections usually are not possible. Unfortunately, despite early detection and localization, one out of three patients presenting with radiologically occult carcinomas are found at operation to have advanced disease with lymphatic metastases or extension to parietal pleura and mediastinum.[28]

The detection of radiologically occult lung carcinoma is uncommon. The case yields from lung cancer screening programs directed at detecting this presumably earliest stage of disease have been extremely low. Of 10,040 male cigarette smokers 45 years of age or older screened in our own prospective study of early lung cancer detection, all were evaluated by chest radiography, and half were randomized for additional sputum cytologic analysis, the so-called dual screening group. For the entire screened population, 53 confirmed lung cancers were found, a yield of 0.5%. Of these, 23 were detected in the roentgenogram-only group and 30 in the dual screen group.[29] Of 4968 patients in the dual screen group, 7 cases of proven radiographically occult lung carcinoma in the in situ or microinvasive stage were detected, a yield of less than 0.2%. Nationwide, less than half of 1% of all lung cancers seen are detected in the radiographically occult stage. Over the past 35 years at Memorial Sloan-Kettering Cancer Center, we have been able to accumulate 65 patients with radiographically occult carcinomas of the lung. Ninety percent of these have been epidermoid carcinomas. Few were adenocarcinomas, and to date we have not observed a small cell carcinoma at a radiologically occult stage. Fiber-optic bronchoscopy localized these lesions in nearly all instances.

More sophisticated techniques of in vivo fluorescent staining of mucosal malignancy with hematoporphyrin derivative may further enhance the sensitivity and specificity of bronchoscopic localization. Parenterally administered hematoporphyrin derivative has been shown to be taken up selectively by malignant endobronchial cells, which can then be visualized bronchoscopically by laser-stimulated fluorescence. This technique has proven helpful in identifying and localizing occult malignancy that is not apparent at routine bronchoscopy.[30] This method allows detection of carcinoma in situ together with atypical squamous metaplasia.

A newer method of bronchoscopic fluorescence imaging that depends on tissue autofluorescence and does not require injection of hematoporphyrin has been described.[31] The imaging system allows the detection of dysplasia and carcinoma in situ with greater sensitivity than routine light bronchoscopy.

Photodynamic therapy using transbronchoscopic laser-induced photoexcitation of hematoporphyrin derivative had been shown effective in early studies of Hayata et al[32] in eradicating occult endobronchial lung cancer. More recent studies have demonstrated a 64–85% complete response rate in patients with T1 or T1 N0 non-small cell lung carcinoma treated with photodynamic therapy.[33,34] Three-year survival ranged from 50% to 70%, with or without external beam radiation therapy.[33,34]

The treatment of choice of radiologically occult lung carcinoma is surgical resection. The median survival of these patients is very long and presently holds at 9 years. Importantly, we have not observed a single case of recurrence of the original lung carcinoma following resection of a radiographically occult stage I lung cancer, despite periods of follow-up extending to 25 years. Unfortunately, the risk of developing other carcinomas in this group of patients remains a threat to long-term survival. In our experience, 45% of these patients develop new carcinomas, the majority of which are new airway carcinomas. It is essential, therefore, that a continued surveillance of these patients be carried out at 6–12-month intervals indefinitely.

## SURGICAL TREATMENT OF STAGE I (T1 N0 M0, T2 N0 M0) NON-SMALL CELL LUNG CARCINOMA

The true incidence of patients that present with lung carcinoma as stage I cannot be easily determined. However, approximately 20% of patients referred to our center are in this stage.[34a] This includes patients whose tumors (1) are 3 cm or less in greatest dimension, surrounded by lung or visceral pleura, and without extension proximal to a lobar bronchus (T1); or (2) are >3 cm in greatest diameter, or a tumor of any size that invades visceral pleura or has associated atelectasis extending to the hilum, and is >2 cm distal to carina (T2); and (3) have no nodal or distant metastases (N0 M0). Patients presenting as such should be meticulously staged, both pre- and intraoperatively. Preoperative staging includes a thorough history, physical examination, blood chemistries (to include SGOT, alkaline phosphatase, and LDH), chest x-ray, and chest and upper abdominal computed tomography (CT) (to include liver and adrenal glands). Controversy exists over the need for routine preoperative bone and brain scans without signs or symptoms referable to these organ systems. Data would suggest that without clinical evidence of involvement, routine brain and bone scans are not necessary.[34b] (See Chap. 22.) In the opinion of the authors, the frequency of detecting metastatic disease in otherwise operable patients with lung carcinoma has been underestimated.[34b] Intraoperative staging would include a systematic lymph node dissection. Surgical resections would include lobectomy, bilobectomy, or pneumonectomy. In patients with limited pulmonary reserve, segmentectomy or wedge resection, although suboptimal, may be considered.

For patients with clinical stage I non-small cell lung cancer who are physiologically able to tolerate the planned pulmonary resection (Chaps. 1–3), surgery has become the gold standard. Prior to 1986, the TNM classification system included T1 N1 tumors in stage I, along with T1 N0 and T2 N0 tumors. Therefore, older series reporting the results of surgical resection for stage I non-small cell lung cancer included patients with N1 nodes, and the overall survival figures were subsequently lower. The results of resection for patients with stage I (T1 N0 or T2 N0) non-small cell lung cancer in four series are listed in Table 23–2. In these series, lobectomy or pneumonectomy was performed in 89–100% of the patients, with pneumonectomy comprising only 4–7% of operations in the two large series.[35,38] In the series from our institution[38] and that of Ichinose et al,[37] a formal mediastinal lymph node dissection (MLND) was performed in 94–100% of patients. The operative mortality in the two later reports[37,38] ranged from 0% to 2.3%. The 5-year survival for patients with T1 N0 non-small cell lung cancer ranged from 63% to 85%. The report from Schultze et al[36] reported the lowest 5-year survival in T1 N0 patients and probably reflects the fact that an MLND was not reported; therefore, their series may have included occult N2 patients. The 5-year survival for patients with T2 N0 tumors who underwent an MLND was 67–68%.[37,38] In the Memorial Sloan-Kettering Cancer Center experience, the survival of T1 N0 patients was significantly greater than T2 N0 (Fig. 23–2). Overall, for patients with pathologic stage I non-small cell lung cancer undergoing resection (including an MLND), the 5-year survival is 75%.[38]

**TABLE 23–2. RESULTS OF RESECTION IN PATIENTS WITH STAGE I NON-SMALL CELL LUNG CANCER**

| Series | Year | N | n | | Lobectomy or Pneumonectomy | MLND | Postoperative Mortality | Effect of Histology | 5-Year Survival | | |
|---|---|---|---|---|---|---|---|---|---|---|---|
| | | | *T1N0* | *T2N0* | | | | | *T1N0* | *T2N0* | *Overall* |
| Mayo[35] | 1981 | 461 | 225 | 236 | 96% | NR | 2.2% | NS | 80% | 62% | NR |
| Schultze et al[36] | 1983 | 110 | 49 | 61 | 100% | NR | 7.8% | NS | 63% | 50% | NR |
| Ichinose et al[37] | 1993 | 151 | 71 | 80 | 96% | 100% | 0% | NS | 85% | 67% | NR |
| MSKCC[38] | 1994 | 598 | 291 | 307 | 89% | 94% | 2.3% | NS | 82% | 68% | 75% |

NS = not significant; NR = not reported; MSKCC = Memorial Sloan-Kettering Cancer Center; MLND = mediastinal lymph node direction.

In the four series listed in Table 23–2, histology was not a significant prognostic factor for survival. In most series, age, sex, pleural involvement, or grade were not significant prognostic factors.[35,38] In the study of Ichinose et al,[37] grade and deoxyribonucleic acid (DNA) ploidy were significant prognostic factors in a multivariate analysis.

Although the results of surgical resection for patients with stage I lung carcinoma are favorable, it is imperative that careful follow-up be maintained, since recurrent cancer or a new lung primary may develop in as many as 39% of patients, as documented by the Mayo Clinic series.[39] These researchers found that of 346 patients with postsurgical stage I lung carcinoma (an old TNM classification that included 18 patients with T1 N1 M0) followed from 5 to 10.8 years, 39% would develop recurrent cancer. Of these, 75 (56%) were distant metastases, 25 (18%) were locoregional recurrence, and 35 (20%) were new primary lung carcinomas. The pattern of recurrence was markedly different depending on the cell type (Table 23–3), with distant metastases more common in adenocarcinoma (including large cell carcinoma) and new primary lung cancers more common in alveolar cell carcinoma.

In a recent report from our institution of 598 patients undergoing resection for stage I non-small cell lung cancer, 27% developed a recurrence.[38] Of the 159 patients who developed a recurrence, 60% did so within 2 years and 91% within 5 years. Nine percent developed a recurrence more than 5 years after resection. In our series, histology did not influence the pattern of recurrence, with 28% being locoregional and 72% being distant (with or without loco-regional recurrence). Thirty-four percent developed a second primary. The new cancers were in the lung in 33%, breast in 16%, head and neck in 13%, colon/rectum in 8%, bladder in 7%, and other sites less commonly.

It is recommended, therefore, that all patients be followed after treatment with periodic chest radiography and clinical evaluation at 3-month intervals the first year, at 4-month intervals the second year, and at 6-month intervals thereafter. Routine sputum cytology after resection is not routinely warranted.[40,41]

Since the survival of stage I non-small cell lung carcinoma, adequately staged by mediastinal lymph node evaluation, has been demonstrated to be from 82% to 85% for T1 tumors and from 67% to 68% for T2 tumors,[37,38] adjuvant

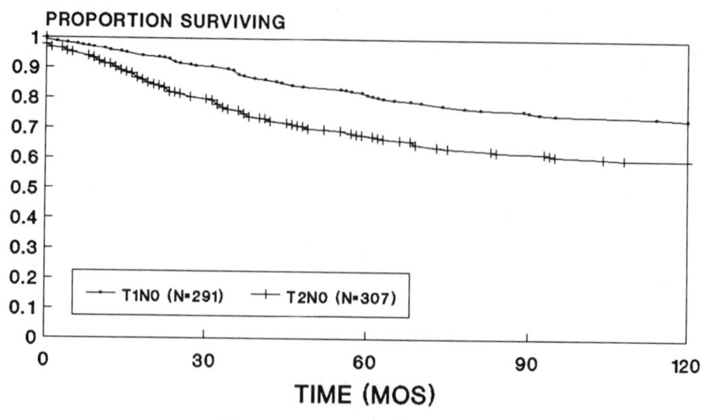


**Figure 23–2.** Survival of 598 patients with stage I (T1 N0 M0, T2 N0 M0) non-small cell lung carcinoma following complete resection.

**TABLE 23-3. PATTERNS OF RECURRENCE AFTER SURGICAL RESECTION IN STAGE I LUNG CANCER: DIFFERENCES IN CELL TYPE**

| | % | | |
|---|---|---|---|
| | *Loco-regional Recurrence* | *Distant Metastases* | *New Primary* |
| Adenocarcinoma (n = 150) (includes large cell) | 18 | 71 | 10 |
| Squamous cell carcinoma (n = 155) | 23 | 49 | 28 |
| Bronchoalveolar cell carcinoma (n = 47) | 6 | 29 | 65 |

*(Adapted from Pairolero PC, Williams DE, Bergstralh EJ, et al: Postsurgical stage I bronchogenic carcinoma: Morbid implications of recurrent disease. Ann Thorac Surg 38:331–338, 1984.)*

therapy does not appear warranted at this time. Although preliminary evidence that immunotherapy appeared to prolong survival in patients with stage I non-small cell lung carcinoma,[42] these results were not confirmed by a multicenter, randomized trial.[43]

At this point in time, until more effective and less toxic agents are identified, we do not recommend adjuvant antineoplastic therapy in patients with completed resected stage I lung carcinoma. Chemoprevention, on the other hand, appears to benefit this group of patients. After the initial randomized trial demonstrated a significant decrease in second primaries in patients receiving isotretinoin (synthetic retinoid) after resection of squamous cell carcinoma of the head and neck compared with placebo,[43a] investigators have been interested in chemoprevention for patients with resected early stage non-small cell lung cancer. Pastorino et al[43b] have recently reported 307 patients with completely resected stage I non-small cell lung cancer randomized to retinol palmitate (vitamin A, 300,000 IU, orally, daily for 12 months) vs. no treatment.[43b] There was a significant decrease in second primary tumors in the group receiving vitamin A (12% treated vs. 18% untreated). The commonest new primary cancer arose in lung (61% in treated, 64% in untreated patients). These early data are extremely important; however, they need to be corroborated by larger randomized trials currently in progress.

## SURGICAL TREATMENT OF STAGE II (T1 N1 M0, T2 N1 M0) NON-SMALL CELL LUNG CARCINOMA

Approximately 10% of patients will present with stage II non-small cell lung carcinoma.[34a] These are patients with primary tumors confined to the lung and >2 cm distal to carina, as defined in the previous section, with metastases to peribronchial or ipsilateral hilar lymph nodes. Again, as with stage I lung carcinomas, surgical resection can be accomplished by lobectomy, bilobectomy, or pneumonectomy, accompanied by a mediastinal lymph node dissection. Lesser pulmonary resections are reserved for patients whose preoperative pulmonary evaluation deems them unsuitable for lobectomy. Since the older system of staging included T1 N1 as stage I and T2 N1 as stage II, data concerning results of surgical resection in the new stage II (T1 N1 M0, T2 N1 M0) as a group are sparse. Shields et al[44] were the first to suggest in 1980 that T1 N1 lesions be classified with T2 N1 lesions as stage II. We agreed with this new stage grouping and published our initial experience with resected T1 N1 and T2 N1 non-small cell lung cancer in 1983.[45]

For patients with clinical T1 N1 or T2 N1 non-small cell lung cancer and who can tolerate the planned resection, surgery has become the accepted standard. Table 23–4 lists the results of resection in stage II non-small cell lung cancer of four series from 1986 to 1994. The overall survival in completely resected stage II non-small cell lung cancer ranges from 39% to 49%. The survival of patients with completely resected T1 N1 and T2 N1 tumors ranges from 40% to 54% and 38% to 40%, respectively, and is illustrated by the results from Memorial Sloan-Kettering Cancer Center (Fig. 23–3).

A multivariate analysis of prognostic factors in 214 patients from our institution revealed that increasing size of the primary tumor and increasing number of N1 nodes with metastases impacted negatively on survival.[48] Age, sex, pleural involvement, and histology were not independent predictors of survival. The study of Yano et al[49] also did not demonstrate a survival difference for different histologies. In addition, this study demonstrated a significant decrease in survival for patients with hilar nodes positive for metastases compared with those with lobar nodes positive.

**TABLE 23-4. RESULTS OF RESECTION IN PATIENTS WITH STAGE II NON-SMALL CELL LUNG CANCER**

| | | | n | | 5-Year Survival | | |
|---|---|---|---|---|---|---|---|
| **Series** | **Year** | **n** | ***T1 N1*** | ***T2 N1*** | ***T1 N1*** | ***T2 N1*** | ***Overall*** |
| Mountain et al[46] | 1986 | 317 | 67 | 250 | 54% | 40% | NR |
| Naruke et al[47] | 1988 | 219 | 66 | 153 | 52% | 38% | 43% |
| Martini et al[48] | 1992 | 214 | 35 | 179 | 40% | 38% | 39% |
| Yano et al[a49] | 1994 | 78 | 19 | 56 | NR | NR | 49% |

NR = not reported.
[a]Three patients had a T3 tumor.

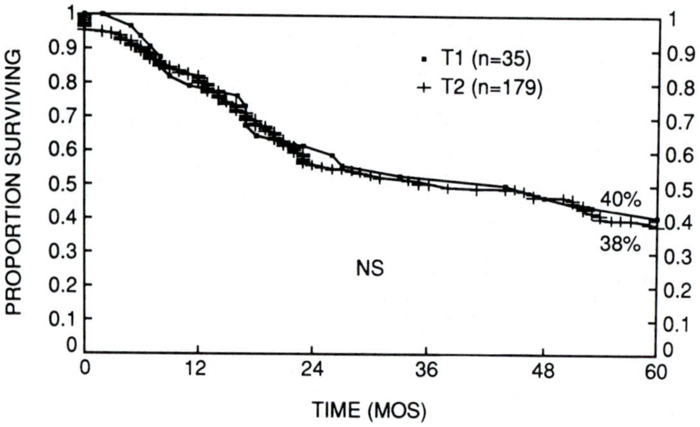

**Figure 23–3.** Survival of 214 patients with stage II (T1 N1 M0, T2 N1 M0) non-small cell lung carcinoma following complete resection.

Similar survival patterns have been obtained with surgical resection by the Lung Cancer Study Group[50] for stage II carcinoma carefully staged intraoperatively by lymph node sampling. Their findings concerning histology were somewhat different from Martini et al[48] and Yano et al.[49] They found histology to be a prognostic factor, with squamous cell carcinoma having a more favorable prognosis for both T1 N1 and T2 N1 lesions (Table 23–5). The Ludwig Lung Cancer Study Group has also found similar survival patters in patients with T1 N1 M0 and T2 N1 M0 carcinoma.[51]

Recurrence, both loco-regional and distant, after adequate resection for stage II lung carcinoma has been amply documented. In the study of Martini et al,[48] the loco-regional and distant recurrence rate was 55%, with 21% of the recurrences being loco-regional and 79% being distant. Of the 90 patients with distant metastases, 47% had brain metastases. In this study, as in others,[51–53] the histologic cell type influenced the site where failure ultimately recurred (Table 23–6). As seen, adenocarcinoma tends to recur distally more often, while squamous cell carcinoma tends to recur locally more frequently in postsurgical stage II lung carcinoma patients.

Since the overall survival of completely resected stage II patients is only 40–50%, adjuvant therapy has been suggested in patients with stage II non-small cell carcinoma; however, its role and the type of adjuvant to use remain unclear due to the small number of patients seen at this stage of the disease.

**TABLE 23–5. FIVE-YEAR SURVIVAL IN STAGE II NON-SMALL CELL LUNG CARCINOMA BY HISTOLOGIC CELL TYPE**

| | % | | |
|---|---|---|---|
| | *Squamous cell carcinoma (%)* | *Adenocarcinoma (%)* | *P* **value** |
| T1 N1 M0 | 75 | 52 | 0.04 |
| T2 N1 M0 | 53 | 25 | 0.01 |

*(Adapted from Holmes EC: Treatment of stage II lung cancer (T1 N1 and T2 N1). Surg Clin North Am 67:945–949, 1987.)*

Postoperative immunotherapy has not demonstrated a significant impact on survival.[54] Two large randomized trials of preoperative radiation therapy for patients with resectable non-small cell lung cancer of all operable stages have demonstrated no benefit.[55,56] A randomized trial of postoperative radiation therapy by the Lung Cancer Study Group (LCSG) in completed resected stage II and III squamous cell carcinoma significantly reduced the loco-regional recurrence rate in the group receiving radiation, but it had no impact on survival.[57] One very small randomized trial of preoperative cisplatin, cyclophosphamide, and vindesine in patients with stage I, II, and III non-small cell lung cancer demonstrated no significant impact on survival.[58] The LCSG performed a randomized trial of postoperative cytoxan, adriamycin, and cisplatin (CAP) vs. no treatment in 283 patients with T1 N1 or T2 N0 non-small cell lung cancer and demonstrated no overall survival advantage of postoperative CAP chemotherapy.[59] Two large Veterans Administration trials evaluating cytoxan and/or methotrexate,

**TABLE 23–6. SITES OF RECURRENCE BY HISTOLOGY AFTER CURATIVE RESECTION IN PATIENTS WITH STAGE II NON-SMALL CELL LUNG CANCER**

| Variable | Overall | Squamous Carcinoma | Adenocarcinoma |
|---|---|---|---|
| No Recurrence | 93 (45)[a] | 49 (53) | 44 (39) |
| Recurrence | 114 (55) | 44 (47) | 70 (61) |
| Local/Regional | 24 (21) | 15 (34) | 9 (13) |
| Distant | 90 (79) | 29 (64) | 61 (87) |
| Brain | 42 | 10 | 32 |
| Bone | 19 | 10 | 9 |
| Lung | 16 | 4 | 12 |
| Liver | 13 | 4 | 9 |
| Other | 12 | 4 | 8 |
| Subtotal | 207 | 93 | 114 |
| Postop Deaths | 7 | 5 | 2 |
| **Total** | **214** | **98** | **116** |

[a]Numbers in parentheses are percentages, excluding postoperative deaths.
*(Adapted from Martini N, Burt ME, Bains MS, et al: Survival after resection of stage II non-small cell cancer. Ann Thorac Surg 54:460–466, 1992.)*

or CCNU and hydroxyurea after curative resection of stage I, II, or III non-small cell lung cancer demonstrated no benefit.[60,61] At this point in time, adjuvant therapy cannot be recommended for patients completely resected for stage II non-small cell lung cancer. Newer clinical trials of adjuvant therapy are desperately needed for this stage of disease.

## SURGICAL TREATMENT OF STAGE III NON-SMALL CELL LUNG CARCINOMA

Probably the two most important aspects of the new international staging system for non-small cell carcinoma of the lung are (1) creating a new category, stage IV, for patients with metastatic (M1) disease; and (2) dividing stage III patients into a group who may be offered surgical intervention (IIIA) and a group where surgical treatment should be considered only under special circumstances or in a protocol setting (IIIB). The two subdivisions of stage III will be discussed separately.

### Surgical Treatment of Stage IIIA (T3 N0–1 M0, T1–3, N2 M0) Non-Small Cell Lung Carcinoma

Stage IIIA patients include those with limited, circumscribed extrapulmonary extension of the primary tumor (T3) and/or metastases confined to ipsilateral mediastinal or subcarinal lymph nodes (N2).

#### *Surgical Treatment of T3 (Chest Wall Invasion) Non-Small Cell Lung Carcinoma (Exclusive of superior sulcus tumors; see Chap. 24)*

Although the majority of lung carcinomas are confined to the chest cavity, approximately 5% will invade parietal pleura and chest wall.[62] The operative approach to patients with carcinomas invading parietal pleura or chest wall includes:

1. pulmonary resection (pneumonectomy, bilobectomy, lobectomy, segmentectomy, or wedge resection as indicated by location and extent of the tumor in lung or bronchus.
2. the affected soft tissue (parietal pleura or intercostal muscles) or skeletal (rib) resection.
3. mediastinal lymph node dissection.
4. chest-wall reconstruction.

As far as the extent of soft tissue and bony chest-wall resection, no doubt exists that if the tumor extends past the parietal pleura into chest wall, en bloc resection of the bony chest wall should be done. The resection should encompass all areas of tumor invasion by a minimum of several centimeters.[63]

When a peripheral carcinoma is fixed to the parietal pleura, some investigators recommend an extrapleural dissection,[62,64] and some recommend an en bloc chest-wall resection.[65,66] One approach that has yielded acceptable results[62] is that if the parietal pleural attachment is discovered at thoracotomy, a trial of extrapleural dissection is attempted. If a tumor-free plane is readily achieved, an extrapleural resection is performed. If any resistance is encountered during the extrapleural approach, dissection is stopped, and en bloc resection of chest wall and lung is undertaken. By utilizing this approach, more than 88% of tumors invading only parietal pleura can be resected.[62]

As far as reconstruction of a chest-wall defect is concerned, a separate section in this book (Chap. 34) and an excellent review by McCormack et al[67] describe in detail the various methods available for chest-wall reconstruction. A small skeletal defect need not be repaired, except for cosmetic reasons. A posterior defect, which will be covered by scapula, need not be repaired even if it is 5–7 cm in diameter. Because the scapula covers the defect, no physical deformity exists, and no flail chest results postoperatively.

When reconstruction is indicated, many materials have been used (Table 23–7). We prefer the marlex mesh-methylmethacrylate method described in detail in the review by McCormack et al.[67] Basically, the method involves outlining the skeletal defect on a sheet of marlex mesh. Methylmethacrylate is then mixed and spread over the marlex mesh to within 1 cm of the outlined defect. A second sheet of marlex mesh is placed over this to form the sandwich. While the methylmethacrylate is hardening, it can be molded to the contour needed. After hardening, the free edge of marlex is sutured to the edge of the skeletal defect with heavy, nonabsorbable suture. If a large, soft-tissue defect exists over the marlex-methylmethacrylate sandwich, a myocutaneous flap or free flap may be utilized. For this, the expertise of the plastic surgeon is often called upon.

The overall operative mortality in modern series ranges from 4% to 12%.[62–66,68] The overall 5-year survival

**TABLE 23–7. METHODS OF RECONSTRUCTION FOLLOWING RESECTION OF LUNG CARCINOMA INVADING THE CHEST WALL**

| | |
|---|---|
| Autogenous | Bone<br>Ribs-whole or split<br>Fascia lata<br>Muscle |
| Composite | Fascia lata with bone chips<br>Fascia lata with bone graft |
| Alloplastic materials | Solid plates or strips of metal, Lucite, or fiber glass |
| Synthetics | Tantalum<br>Stainless steel<br>Tetrafluoroethylene (Teflon)<br>Nylon<br>Polypropylene<br>Gore-Tex |
| Composite synthetic | Marlex mesh and methyl methacrylate |

*(Adapted from McCormack PM, Bains MS, Martini N, et al: Methods of skeletal reconstruction following resection of lung carcinoma invading chest wall. Surg Clin North AM 67:979–986, 1987.)*

in five modern series reviewed was remarkably similar and ranged from 26% to 40% (Table 23–8).

In the report by McCaughan et al,[62] 125 patients underwent operation for non-small cell carcinoma of the lung invading chest wall. Superior sulcus tumors were excluded from this report. The overall operative mortality in this series was 4%. Survival was determined by three factors: (1) complete vs. incomplete resection, (2) presence or absence of lymph node metastases, and (3) parietal pleural vs. chest-wall involvement. Complete resection was performed in 62% of the patients with a 5-year actuarial survival of 40% (Fig. 23–4). In those patients with a complete resection, the presence of lymph node metastases (N1 or N2) decreased the 5-year survival from 56% (no lymph node metastases) to 21% (N1 or N2) (Fig. 23–5). This detrimental impact on survival has also been observed by Albertucci et al,[65] who reported 42%, 32%, and 0% 5-year survival in patients with N0, N1, and N2 nodal diseases, respectively. Other authors had noted a similar phenomenon.[66,69] The depth of invasion also appears to affect survival with a 5-year survival of 48% in those with parietal pleura only involved vs. 16% in those with chest-wall involvement.

The benefit of adjuvant radiation therapy in patients with chest involvement has not been demonstrated in a controlled randomized study. In a retrospective review, however, Patterson et al[69] have demonstrated a 5-year survival of 56% in 13 irradiated patients vs. 30% in 22 nonirradiated patients. Whether this finding would be corroborated by a randomized trial is questioned.

The most important prognostic factor in patients with a non-small cell lung cancer invading chest wall is whether a complete resection can be performed. This is emphasized by the fact that in the series of McCaughan et al,[62] the median survival of 48 patients unable to have complete resection was 9 months, and there were no 3-year survivors. This contrasts markedly to the survival in those patients with complete resection, except in patients with mediastinal lymph node metastases, as also demonstrated by Ratto et al.[70]

In summary, all patients with non-small cell lung carcinoma directly invading parietal pleura and chest wall should undergo thoracotomy, provided (1) there are no distant metastases, (2) the patient's cardiopulmonary status allows operation, and (3) there is no preoperative evidence of extensive mediastinal lymph node metastases. At thoracotomy, a complete resection will be possible in the majority, with subsequent prognosis dependent on lymph node status as noted earlier.

**TABLE 23–8. RESULTS OF RESECTION OF BRONCHOGENIC CARCINOMA INVOLVING CHEST WALL**

| | | | % | |
|---|---|---|---|---|
| Series | Year | n | *Postoperative Mortality* | *5-Year Survival* |
| Patterson et al[69] | 1982 | 35 | 8.5 | 38 |
| Trastek et al[64] | 1984 | 73 | 12.3 | 40 |
| McCaughan et al[62] | 1985 | 125 | 4.0 | 40 |
| Allen et al[66] | 1991 | 52 | 3.8 | 26 |
| Albertucci et al[65] | 1992 | 37 | 10.8 | 30 |

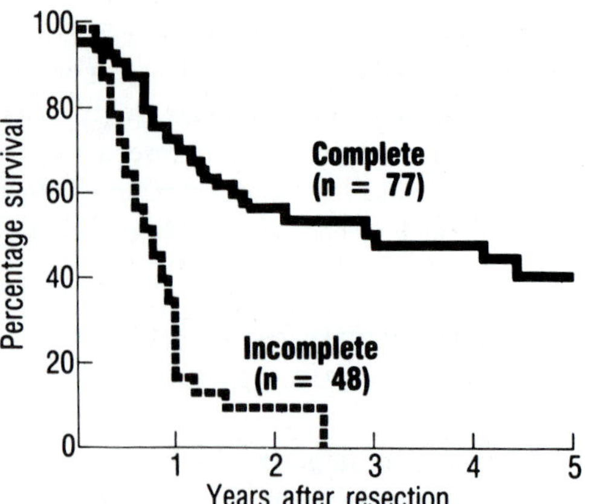


**Figure 23–4.** Survival of 125 patients with T3 (chest wall) non-small cell lung carcinoma following complete or incomplete resection.

### *Surgical Treatment of T3 (Proximity to Carina) Non-Small Cell Lung Carcinoma*

An endobronchial carcinoma within 2 cm of the carina is considered a T3 lesion. Operations designed to afford resection in this circumstance include (1) pneumonectomy, (2) sleeve lobectomy, and (3) sleeve pneumonectomy.

The most important diagnostic procedure in evaluating patients with non-small cell lung cancer in proximity to the carina is bronchoscopy. Thoracic surgeons must be able to appreciate the gross and subtle findings, such as submucosal spread, at bronchoscopy to be able to select candidates for sleeve resection as well as pneumonectomy. Although preoperative selection is important, much of the

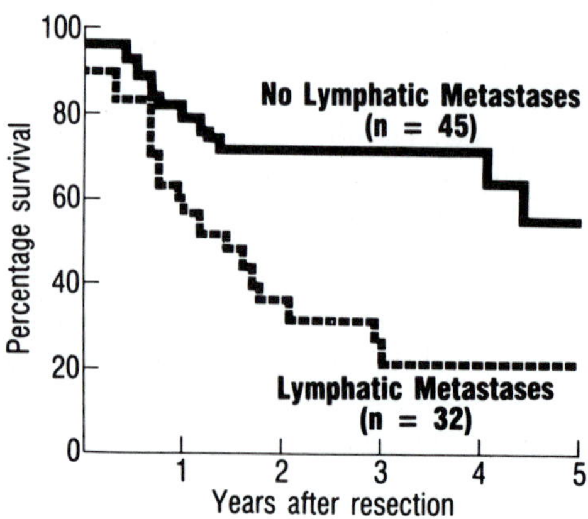


**Figure 23–5.** Survival of 77 patients with T3 (chest wall) non-small cell lung carcinoma following complete resection and analyzed for the presence or absence of lymph node (N1 or N2) metastases.

decision to proceed with resection depends on the intraoperative evaluation. If peribronchial tumor or lymph node involvement at the planned resection site is identified, sleeve resection must be considered.

Sleeve lobectomy has yielded satisfactory survival rates and acceptable operative mortality (Table 23–9). In fact, the operative mortality has been comparable in sleeve lobectomy when compared with pneumonectomy. Operative mortality rates for sleeve lobectomy are in the range of 0–8%[71–76] and compare favorably with the 6% reported for pneumonectomy.[77]

Survival following sleeve lobectomy for non-small cell lung carcinoma is dependent on the stage of disease. Faber[78] has reviewed the experience with sleeve lobectomy at the Rush-Presbyterian-St. Luke's Medical Center, and data abstracted from this experience is presented in Table 23–10 and demonstrates that survival following sleeve resection, as in other pulmonary resections, is determined by pathologic stage. This finding has also been recently corroborated by Mehran et al,[75] who found that increasing nodal status and stage significantly impacted negatively on survival.

The indication for sleeve pneumonectomy is a bulky central tumor in proximity to or involving the carina or tracheobronchial angle.[78] Even after careful preoperative and intraoperative selection, Faber[78] reported an overall operative mortality of 27% in 37 patients. The major complication in this series was anastomotic dehiscence, which carried a mortality of 100%. The overall survival at 5 years in this group of 37 patients was 16%.

Table 23–11 lists the data from three other reports of sleeve pneumonectomy for bronchogenic carcinoma. The poor survival is documented by the report of Dartevelle et al,[80] but the operative mortality appears to be decreasing over time.

### *Surgical Treatment of N2 Disease (Mediastinal Lymph Node Metastases) in Patients with Non-Small Cell Lung Carcinoma*

Patients presenting with metastases to ipsilateral mediastinal and/or subcarinal lymph nodes (N2) represent approximately 45% of those with non-small cell lung carcinoma.[3]

**TABLE 23–10. SURVIVAL FOLLOWING SLEEVE LOBECTOMY FOR NON-SMALL CELL LUNG CARCINOMA**

| Stage | N | 5-Year Survival (%) |
|---|---|---|
| I | 69 | 38 |
| II | 24 | 20 |
| III | 18 | 15 |

*(Adapted from Faber LP: Results of surgical treatment of stage III lung carcinoma with carinal proximity. The role of sleeve lobectomy versus pneumonectomy and the role of sleeve pneumonectomy. Surg Clin North Am 67:1001–1014, 1987.)*

There are those who subscribe to the notion that the presence of N2 disease is a contraindication to attempts at locoregional control with resection, with or without adjuvant chemotherapy and/or radiation therapy, and utilize mediastinoscopy to exclude these patients from a surgical approach. Others utilize mediastinoscopy to select those patients with N2 disease that might benefit from a surgical approach.[82–84] For this group of patients, Pearson[85] has recently suggested the following guidelines to exclude those patients from surgery who are found at mediastinoscopy to have metastases to mediastinal lymph nodes:

1. presence of contralateral nodal disease
2. extranodal extension
3. high paratracheal nodal disease

There are reports in the literature describing 5-year survival rates for patients with N2 disease undergoing resection (and postoperative radiation therapy) without preoperative mediastinoscopy in the range of 20–30% in both earlier, retrospective[86–89] and later prospective[90] studies.

When discussing surgery for N2 disease, one must realize that in most series reported, the denominator (the total number of patients presenting with N2 disease) is not discussed. In our series, which spanned 1974–1981, 1598 patients with non-small cell lung cancer were seen; 706 (44%) were determined to have mediastinal lymph node metastases. Of these, 404 (57%) were considered to have operable tumors, but only 151 cases were completely resectable (37% of all thoracotomies for N2 and 21% of all N2 cases). Complete resection entailed removal of the primary tumor

**TABLE 23–9. SLEEVE LOBECTOMY: MORTALITY AND 5-YEAR SURVIVAL**

| | | % | |
|---|---|---|---|
| Series | N | *Operative Mortality (%)* | *5-Year Survival (%)* |
| Faber et al[71] | 101 | 2.0 | 30 |
| Bennett et al[72] | 80 | 7.5 | 34 |
| Van Den Bosch et al[73] | 50 | 8.0 | 41 |
| DesLauriers et al[74] | 72 | 0 | 64 |
| Mehran et al[75] | 142 | 2.1 | 46 |

**TABLE 23–11. RESULTS OF SLEEVE PNEUMONECTOMY FOR BRONCHOGENIC CARCINOMA**

| | | | % | |
|---|---|---|---|---|
| Series | Year | n | *Operative Mortality* | *5-Year Survival* |
| DesLauriers et al[79] | 1979 | 16 | 31 | NR |
| Faber[78] | 1987 | 37 | 27 | 16 |
| Dartevelle et al[80] | 1988 | 55 | 11 | 23 |
| Roviaro et al[81] | 1994 | 28 | 4 | NR |

NR = not reported.

and all accessible mediastinal lymph nodes, with no residual disease left behind. Postoperative radiation to the mediastinum was used in 90% of patients.

Mediastinoscopy was not routinely performed as part of staging before thoracotomy. Clinical determination of N2 disease was based largely on roentgenographic and bronchoscopic findings. Patients with a normal-appearing mediastinum on routine chest roentgenograms and a normal carina at bronchoscopy without compression or distortion of the trachea or main bronchi were classified as having N0 or N1 disease. Patients with abnormal mediastinum on chest roentgenograms suggestive of N2 disease, as well as those with findings at bronchoscopy suggestive of N2 disease, were considered to have clinically manifested N2 disease. Some of these cases were histologically documented by mediastinoscopy or bronchoscopic biopsies.

Of 404 patients surgically explored, 225 were classified as having N0 or N1 disease, and of these, 119 (53%) had complete resection. On the other hand, 179 patients had clinically manifest N2 disease, and 32 of these (18%) had complete resection. Of those 151 patients having complete resection, the male to female ratio was 1.3:1.0, age ranged from 37 to 78 years (median 60), 46 had epidermoid carcinoma, 94 adenocarcinoma, and 11 large cell carcinoma. Clinical staging of the 151 completely resected patients demonstrated that 86 were thought to be stage I, 18 stage II, and 47 stage III. Extent of resection in these patients included lobectomy in 119 (79%), pneumonectomy in 26 (17%), and wedge resection or segmentectomy in 6 (4%).

Pathologic staging in this group revealed 42 patients (28%) with T1 N2 M0, 76 (50%) in T2 N2 M0, and 33 (22%) T3 N2 M0. Interestingly, although N1 disease was found in most patients, 41 (27%) did not have N1 involvement, suggesting that skip metastases from primary tumor to mediastinal nodes, bypassing the peribronchial and hilar nodes, do occur.

The overall 5-year survival in this group of 151 patients undergoing complete resection with N2 disease was 30% (Fig. 23–6). There was no significant difference in survival between patients with epidermoid carcinoma (30%) and those with adenocarcinoma (32%). Survival was related to the size and extent of the tumor. In those with T1 tumors, 5-year survival was 46%, T2 27%, and T3 14% (Fig. 23–7).

Survival was also compared in patients in whom N2 status was clinically apparent preoperatively without benefit of mediastinoscopy and in those with clinical N0 or N1 disease (Fig. 23–8). Patients presenting with radiologic or endoscopy evidence of N2 disease had a poorer survival. Survivals at 3 and 5 years in patients with clinical N0 or N1 disease were 47% and 37%, respectively, compared with 9% at 3 and 5 years in patients whose N2 disease was clinically apparent before thoracotomy. This difference was statistically significant ($P = .0002$).

Although the size of involved node(s) did not influence survival, the number of nodes affected survival. Patients with a single involved N2 node had a much better prognosis than those with multiple nodal involvement, either at one level or multiple levels (Fig. 23–9). Survival by

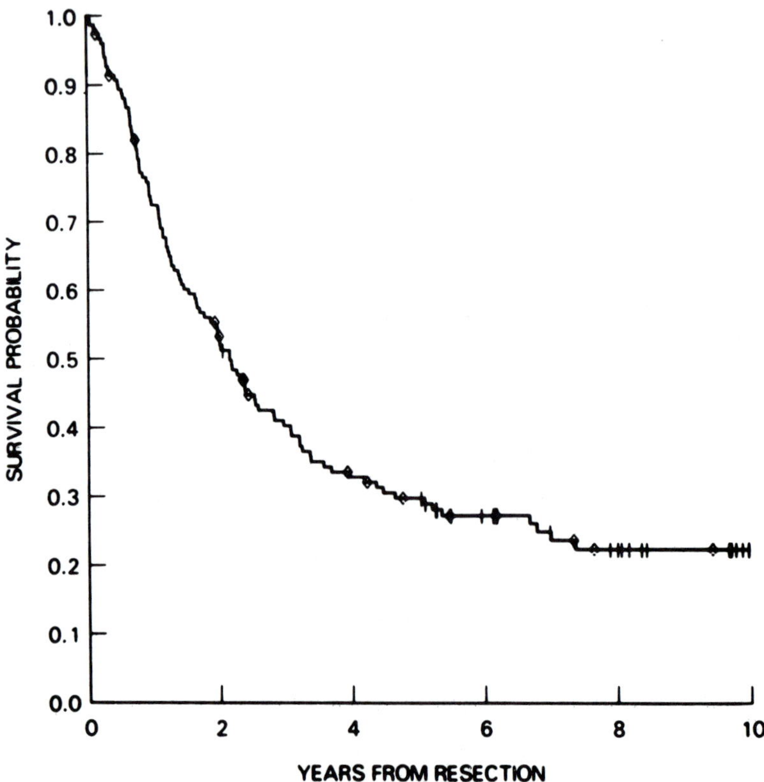


**Figure 23–6.** Survival of 151 patients with N2 non-small cell lung carcinoma following complete resection.

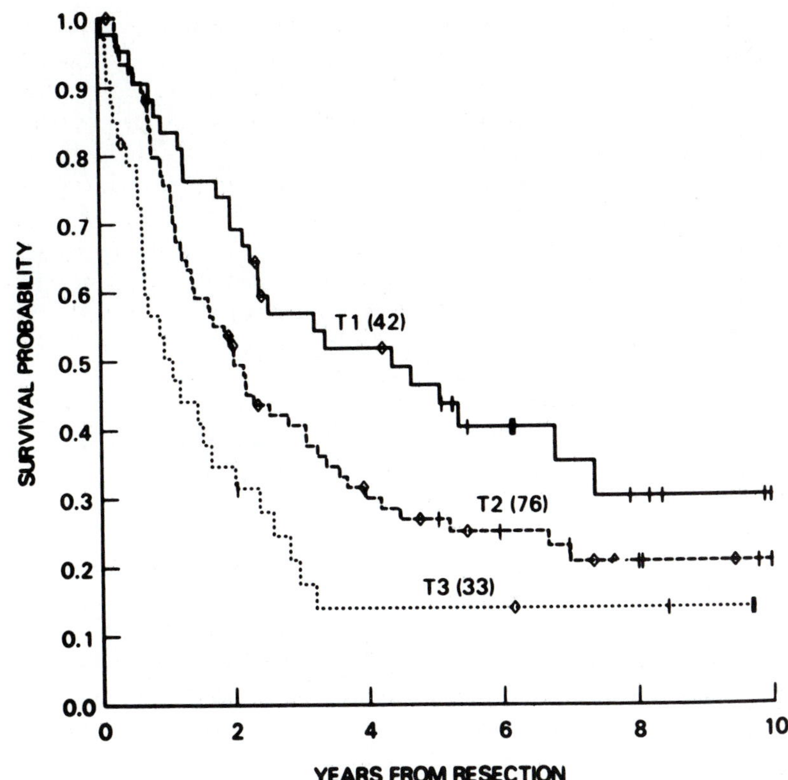


**Figure 23–7.** Survival of 151 patients with N2 non-small cell lung carcinoma following complete resection and analyzed by size and extent of tumor (T1, T2, or T3).

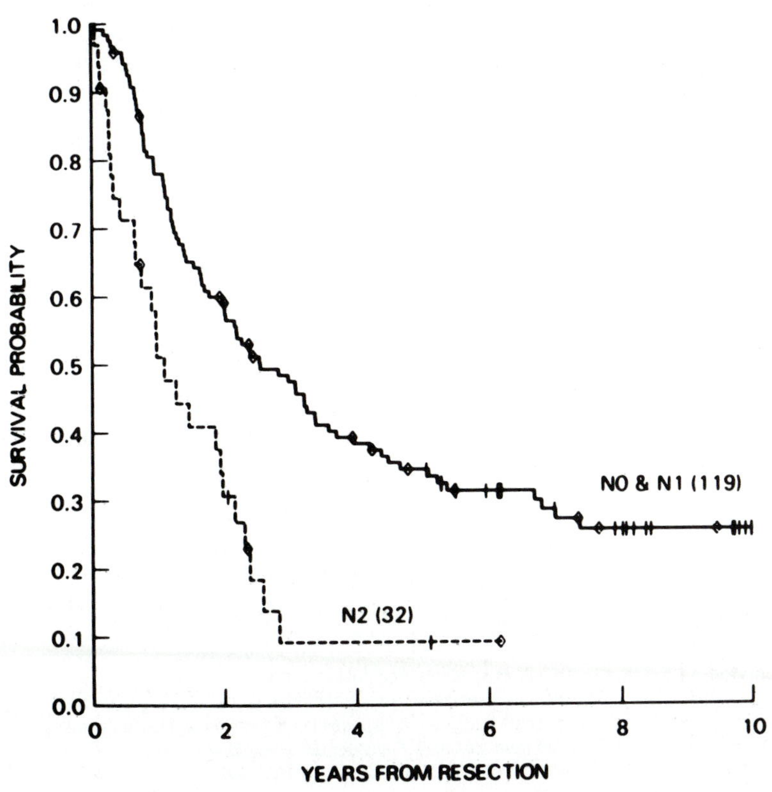


**Figure 23–8.** Survival of 151 patients with N2 non-small cell lung carcinoma following complete resection and analyzed by clinical stage presentation (N0 plus N1 vs. N2).

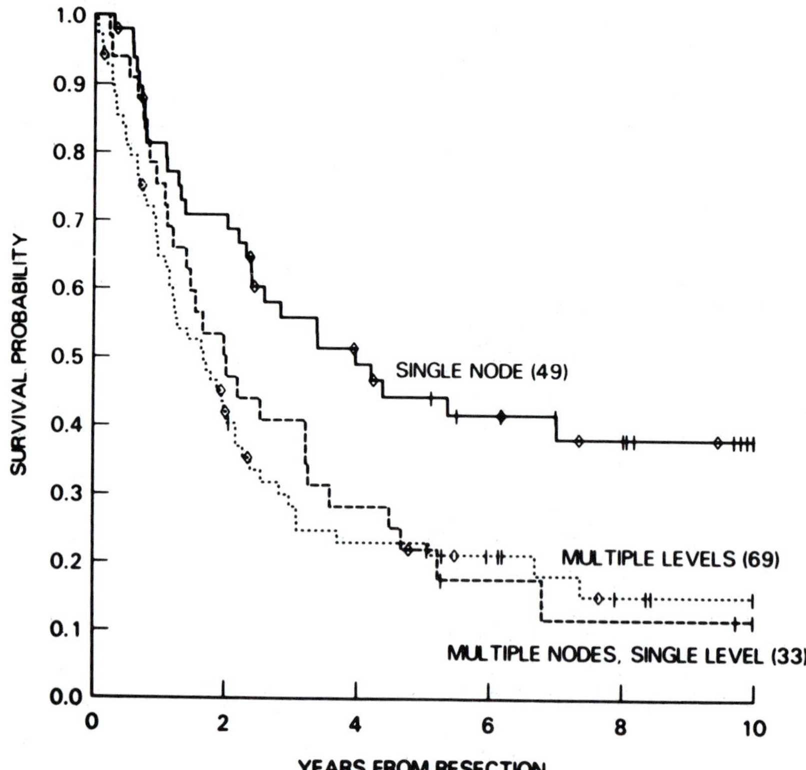


**Figure 23–9.** Survival of 151 patients with N2 non-small cell lung carcinoma following complete resection and analyzed by single vs. multiple nodes involved and by level of involved nodes.

level of involved nodes was also calculated. There were 37 patients with N2 disease in upper paratracheal nodes (levels 1 and 2), and their 5-year survival was 20%. In those who did not have positive nodes at these levels, survival was 32% ($P = .13$). Also, 49 patients had subcarinal lymph node involvement (level 7) and 102 did not; the 5-year survivals were 22% and 33%, respectively ($P = .16$). Survival following resection in patients with N2 disease in the aorticopulmonary window was 35% at 5 years. In essence, prolonged survival was observed with nodal involvement in any of the major mediastinal compartments.

Although the overall 5-year survival following complete resection was 30%, 73% of patients developed recurrent disease (Table 23–12). Loco-regional recurrence rate was only 20% of those patients that recurred when surgery and radiation therapy were combined; however, distant recurrences were found in 80% of those that recurred. Of those that recurred, 80% of the patients with adenocarcinoma and 87% with epidermoid carcinoma did so within 2 years after therapy.

The results of other reports evaluating the role of surgery in patients with N2 non-small cell lung cancer are listed in Table 23–13 and for the most part agree with our results. The postoperative mortality ranged from 1.3% to 10%, with a median of 4.4% in the 2076 patients reported. The 5-year survival ranged from a low of 7% to 34% in the 13 series. A very important point is apparent when one is analyzing results of surgery for N2 non-small cell lung cancer, the manner in which the N2 disease was documented. When N2 disease was unsuspected, either by computed tomography (CT) and/or mediastinoscopy, but discovered after a curative resection, the 5-year survival was significantly higher than those patients who went to thoracotomy with preoperative documentation of N2 disease.

The role of adjuvant therapy in patients with stage IIIA non-small cell lung carcinoma is becoming clearer as more centers report the results of controlled clinical trials. The Lung Cancer Study Group has reported their results with

**TABLE 23–12. SITES OF RECURRENCE ACCORDING TO HISTOLOGY IN PATIENTS WITH RESECTED N2 LUNG CARCINOMA**

| | Adenocarcinoma | Large Cell Carcinoma | Epidermoid Carcinoma |
|---|---|---|---|
| Total no. patients | 92[a] | 11 | 46 |
| Total recurrences[b] | 71 (77) | 10 (91) | 30 (65) |
| Local | 4 (6) | 1 (10) | 2 (7) |
| Regional | 10 (14) | 3 (30) | 4 (13) |
| Distant | 57 (80) | 6 (60) | 24 (80) |
| Brain | 20 | 2 | 8 |
| Bone | 7 | 2 | 6 |
| Liver | 5 | 1 | 1 |
| Lung | 9 | 1 | 4 |
| Other | 5 | — | 2 |
| Multiple | 7[c] | — | 1 |
| Unknown | 4 | — | 2 |

[a]Two additional patients died postoperatively.
[b]Numbers in parentheses are percentages.
[c]Two patients had brain metastases in addition to recurrence in other sites.
*(Adapted from Martini N, Flehinger BJ: The role of surgery in N2 lung cancer. Surg Clin North Am 67:1037–1049, 1987.)*

**TABLE 23–13. RESULTS OF RESECTION IN PATIENTS WITH NON-SMALL CELL LUNG CANCER WITH N2 DISEASE**

| | | | | % | | | |
|---|---|---|---|---|---|---|---|
| Series | Year | n | Suspected Preoperatively | *Postoperative Mortality* | *5-Year Survival* | Intent | Detection of N2 |
| Smith et al[88] | 1978 | 56 | No | 2.8 | NR | Curative | NR |
| Pearson et al[85] | 1982 | 62 | No | NR | 24 | Curative | Mediastinoscopy |
| | | 79 | Yes | NR | 9 | Curative | Mediastinoscopy |
| Kirsch et al[86] | 1982 | 136 | No | 4.4 | 21 | Curative | NR |
| Martini et al[90–92] | 1983 | 104 | No | 1.3 | 34 | Curative | Chest x-ray, bronchoscopy |
| | | 47 | Yes | 1.3 | 9 | Curative | Chest x-ray, bronchoscopy |
| Naruke et al[93] | 1988 | 426 | NR | 3.8 | 14 | All | NR |
| Watanabe et al[94] | 1991 | 47 | No | 2.1 | 20 | All | CT |
| | | 190 | Yes | 2.1 | 16 | All | CT |
| Cybulsky et al[95] | 1992 | 61 | No | 7.2 | 17 | All | CT |
| | | 63 | Yes | 7.2 | 7 | All | CT |
| VanKlaveren et al[95] | 1993 | 32 | No | 10.0 | 10 | Curative | Mediastinoscopy |
| Conill et al[97] | 1993 | 113 | No | 3.5 | 12 | Curative | NR |
| Daly et al[98] | 1993 | 37 | No | NS | 28 | Curative | CT |
| Mountain et al[99] | 1994 | 307 | NR | 5.2 | 31 | Curative | NR |
| Goldstraw et al[100] | 1994 | 149 | No | 5.4 | 20 | Curative | CT |
| Miller et al[101] | 1994 | 167 | No | 4.8 | 24 | Curative | Chest x-ray or CT |

NR = not reported; All = all resections included (i.e., incomplete and complete); CT = chest computed tomography.

adjuvant therapy in stage II and III non-small cell lung cancer.[102] An updated report in patients with stage II and III epidermoid lung carcinoma randomized to postoperative adjuvant radiation therapy vs. no adjuvant therapy demonstrated that there was no survival advantage in those receiving radiotherapy.[57] There was, however, a significant decrease in loco-regional recurrence rates in those receiving adjuvant radiotherapy. The same group also randomized patients with stage II and III adenocarcinoma and large cell carcinoma of lung to receive postoperative immunotherapy (bacillus Calmette-Guerin plus levamisole) vs. chemotherapy (cytoxan, adriamycin, and cisplatin).[103] Although overall survival was similar in both groups, those that received chemotherapy had a significant increase in disease free survival. Approximately 44% of the patients in this study were stage II, and 56% stage III, of which 84% were N2. Two randomized trials of postoperative chemotherapy in completely resected stage III non-small cell lung cancer have been reported, and the results are listed in Table 23–14. Neither trial demonstrated a significant difference in survival between the two treatment arms.

We had previously reported the results of a prospective evaluation of preoperative chemotherapy (cisplatin and vindesine with or without mitomycin C) in 41 patients with non-small cell lung carcinoma who were operable, but for clinically evident N2 disease (as demonstrated by chest x-ray and/or bronchoscopy).[106] We recently updated our series, which now includes 136 patients with histologically documented N2 non-small cell lung cancer receiving preoperative chemotherapy (mitomycin, vinblastine, cisplatin).[107] Following chemotherapy, 77% had a major radiographic response, which was complete in 10%. One hundred fourteen patients were explored with thoracotomy, and 78% had complete resection of disease. Of those having a complete resection, 19 (21%) had no microscopic evidence of disease in the resected specimen. Survival at 5 years from diagnosis was 17% for all patients and 26% for those who had a complete resection.

To date, there have been many one-arm phase I and II trials of preoperative chemotherapy with or without radiation therapy in patients with stage IIIA disease. Most series report results very similar to our own and are critically analyzed in the recent reviews of Strauss et al,[108] Ginsberg,[109] and Shephard.[110]

There have been three randomized trials of preoperative chemotherapy plus surgery vs. surgery alone for patients with stage IIIA non-small cell lung cancer, and the results of these trials are listed in Table 23–15. The trials of

**TABLE 23–14. POSTOPERATIVE CHEMOTHERAPY IN PATIENTS WITH STAGE III NON-SMALL CELL LUNG CANCER: RANDOMIZED TRIALS**

| Series | Group | n | N2 (%) | CDDP | 5-Year Survival (%) |
|---|---|---|---|---|---|
| Ohta et al[104] | Surgery | 91 | 67 | N/A | 41 |
| | Surgery + VP | 90 | 90 | 80 mg/M2 | 35 |
| Pisters et al[105] | Surgery + RT | 36 | 100 | NA | 44 |
| | Surgery + VP + RT | 36 | 100 | 120 mg/M2 | 31 |

CDDP = cisplatin; VP = vindesine + Cisplatin; RT = radiation therapy; N/A = not applicable.

**TABLE 23–15. RANDOMIZED TRIALS OF PREOPERATIVE CHEMOTHERAPY IN PATIENTS WITH STAGE IIIA NON-SMALL CELL LUNG CANCER**

| Series | Year | Group | n | N2 (%) | CDDP | Survival | |
|---|---|---|---|---|---|---|---|
| | | | | | | *3 Year (%)* | *Median* |
| Pass et al[111] | 1992 | Surgery + RT | 14 | 100 | N/A | 15 | 16 mo |
| | | Surgery + EP | 13 | 100 | 80 mg/M2 | 47 | 29 mo |
| Roth et al[112] | 1994 | Surgery | 32 | 69 | N/A | 15 | 11 mo |
| | | Surgery + CEP | 28 | 71 | 100 mg/M2 | 56 | 64 mo |
| Rossell et al[113] | 1994 | Surgery | 30 | 63 | N/A | 0 | 8 mo |
| | | Surgery + MIP | 30 | 83 | 50 mg/M2 | 30 | 26 mo |

CDDP = cisplatin; RT = radiation therapy; EP = etoposide + platinum; CEP = cytoxan + etoposide + platinum; MIP = mitomycin + ifosfamide + platinum; N/A = not applicable.

Roth et al[112] and Rossell et al[113] demonstrated a significant increase in survival in the group given preoperative chemotherapy compared with the group receiving surgery alone. The three trials reported similar treatment mortality (0–6%) and response rates (approximately 60%). The resectability rate in the Pass et al and Rossell et al trials were 85–90%, but only 31–39% in the Roth et al trial.

In summary, it appears from the current literature that patients with documented N2 non-small cell lung cancer should be offered preoperative chemotherapy in controlled clinical trials. Although the data indicate that preoperative chemotherapy plus surgery offers a survival advantage over surgery alone, a comparison between induction chemotherapy followed by surgery or high-dose radiation therapy has not been done. With data indicating that induction chemotherapy followed by radiation is superior to radiation alone in stage III non-small cell lung cancer,[114] the question arises, What is the best local therapy for patients after induction chemotherapy?

## Surgical Treatment of Stage IIIB Non-Small Cell Lung Carcinoma

### *Surgical Treatment of T4 (Pleural Effusion) Non-Small Cell Lung Carcinoma*

Although the new international staging system classifies malignant pleural effusion as T4 and notes that most pleural effusions associated with lung cancer are malignant, there are a few patients with cytologically negative fluid that is nonbloody and not an exudate. If these three criteria are met, the effusion is judged not secondary to the tumor and classified as T1, T2, or T3, with the effusion being excluded as a staging element. Although the number of patients that would fall into this category is small, determining this possibility has great prognostic implications in the care of these patients.

Data concerning the results of therapy in patients with cytologically negative, ipsilateral pleural effusion associated with carcinoma of the lung are sparse. In a study from the Mayo Clinic,[115] 66 of 73 patients (90%) with ipsilateral, cytologically negative pleural effusion underwent thoracotomy. Of these, only four patients (6%) were able to have a complete resection. These four patients, however, were long-term survivors.

When patients present with otherwise operable, non-small cell lung carcinoma and an ipsilateral pleural effusion, a careful evaluation of the character of that effusion is warranted. Thoracentesis should be the initial procedure. If the fluid is not an exudate, nonbloody and cytologically negative, then perhaps thoracoscopy should be considered.[116]

In a recent review,[117] thoracoscopy has been demonstrated to yield a diagnosis in approximately 94% of patients presenting with pleural effusion (Table 23–16). At the time of thoracoscopy, careful inspection of the visceral and parietal pleura may reveal areas of pleural metastases, which can be easily biopsied. If thoracoscopic directed biopsy of pleural lesion reveals metastatic disease, the diagnostic workup is complete and the patient classified as T4 and inoperable.

If thoracoscopy does not reveal evidence of pleural metastases, then a patient previously classified as T4 may indeed have T1, T2, or T3 disease and be an operable candidate. Again, the number of patients who may potentially benefit from this added diagnostic procedure may be small, approximately 6% of patients with cytology negative, ipsilateral pleural effusions, but gratifying results at the time of thoracotomy may be found.[115]

Patients with cytologically positive pleural effusion as-

**TABLE 23–16. DIAGNOSTIC ACCURACY OF THORACOSCOPY IN PLEURAL EFFUSION**

| Series | n | Diagnostic Yield (%) |
|---|---|---|
| Weissberg et al[118] | 113 | 96 |
| De Camp et al[119] | 121 | 94 |
| Oldenberg et al[120] | 32 | 88 |
| Canto et al[121] | 172 | 95 |
| **Total** | **438** | **94** |

*(Adapted from Thomas P: Thoracoscopy: An old procedure revisited. In: Kittle CF (ed): Current Controversies in Thoracic Surgery. Philadelphia, Saunders, 1986, pp 101–106.)*

sociated with lung carcinoma have a particularly poor prognosis. The median survival in this group is 6–9 months with negligible 5-year survival.[122] Therapy is directed at improving symptoms by controlling the effusion. Tube thoracoscopy is performed with drainage of the effusion. If the lung re-expands, then chemical pleurodesis can be done and will be successful in approximately 80% of patients.[123]

If the lung does not re-expand to allow visceral and parietal pleura to coapt, then attempts at chemical pleurodesis will fail. Decortication and subtotal pleurectomy may be indicated in this situation, if the patient can tolerate the procedure and has a life expectancy measured in months rather than weeks.[124] In addition, this procedure may be indicated in patients who have recurrent pleural effusions after successful chemical pleurodesis or in whom repeated attempts to perform chemical pleurodesis have failed.

### *Surgical Treatment of T4 (Mediastinum) Non-Small Cell Lung Carcinoma*

Patients presenting pre- or intra-operatively with non-small cell lung carcinoma of any size and invading the mediastinal structures (heart, great vessels, trachea, esophagus, vertebral body, or carina) are considered T4 tumors in the new TNM staging system. Although considered by most to be inoperable (if diagnosed preoperatively) or unresectable (if found at thoracotomy), the data are sparse concerning the role of surgery in these patients. On the basis of retrospective reviews of small numbers of patients, some authors have advocated an aggressive surgical approach to localized non-small cell lung carcinoma invading mediastinal pleura and contained structures.[64,125,126]

We reviewed 225 consecutive patients undergoing operation for non-small cell lung carcinoma with pathologically confirmed mediastinal invasion at our institution in an attempt to evaluate the role of surgery in these patients.[127] This group was derived from two clinical groups: (1) 196 patients with clinical mediastinal invasion, of which 152 underwent operation with 137 patients (90%) having pathologic mediastinal invasion and 15 (10%) having pathologic T1 or T2 tumor; and (2) 88 patients operated on for T1 or T2 tumors, but demonstrating mediastinal invasion at the time of surgery. Clinical and pathologic characteristics of these 225 patients are listed in Table 23–17. As noted, the majority of patients (61%) demonstrated mediastinal lymph node metastases. The most common mediastinal structures invaded were pulmonary artery, pericardium, pulmonary vein, aorta, and superior vena cava, and approximately 50% of patients demonstrated multiple sites of involvement.

Four modes of intraoperative therapy were utilized: (1) complete resection (22%), (2) incomplete resection (pulmonary and/or nodal) with brachytherapy to residual disease utilizing iodine-125 interstitial implantation or iridium-192 afterloading (15%), (3) brachytherapy alone (44%), and (4) incomplete or no resection without brachytherapy (19%). The majority of patients underwent some form of adjuvant therapy; including preoperative chemotherapy (4%), preoperative radiotherapy (9%), postoperative chemotherapy (20%), or postoperative radiotherapy (70%).

**TABLE 23–17. CHARACTERISTICS OF OPERATED PATIENTS WITH PRIMARY MEDIASTINAL INVASION BY NON-SMALL CELL LUNG CARCINOMA**

| Characteristics | Operated Patients |
|---|---|
| Number | 225 |
| Median age at diagnosis (y) | 59 |
| Male:Female ratio | 2.3:1 |
| Histology (%) | |
| Epidermoid carcinoma | 53 |
| Adenocarcinoma | 41 |
| Large cell carcinoma | 5 |
| Other | 2 |
| Side of disease (%) | |
| Right | 55 |
| Left | 45 |
| Pathologic nodal status (%) | |
| N0 | 25 |
| N1 | 13 |
| N2 | 61 |
| Clinical T3 (%) | 61 |
| Mediastinal structures involved[a] (%) | |
| Pulmonary artery | 37 |
| Pericardium | 25 |
| Pulmonary vein | 23 |
| Aorta | 19 |
| Superior vena cava | 18 |
| Phrenic nerve | 13 |
| Unspecified | 9 |
| Esophagus | 7 |
| Recurrent laryngeal nerve | 6 |
| Myocardium (atrium) | 3 |
| Adjuvant therapy (%) | |
| Preoperative chemotherapy | 4 |
| Preoperative radiotherapy | 9 |
| Postoperative chemotherapy | 20 |
| Postoperative radiotherapy | 70 |

[a]Of 225 patients, 107 had multiple sites of mediastinal involvement.
*(Adapted from Burt ME, Pomerantz AH, Bains MS, et al: Results of surgical treatment of stage III lung cancer invading mediastinum. Surg Clin North Am 67:987–1000, 1987.)*

A brief description of the techniques of brachytherapy in the treatment of unresectable (either for anatomic or physiologic reasons) non-small cell lung carcinoma (primary or nodal disease) will be presented. However, the reader is referred to the atlas of Hilaris et al[128] for an in-depth review of brachytherapy.

Brachytherapy consists of implantation of a radioactive source either directly into tumor (permanent) or in juxtaposition (temporary). Permanent implants can be utilized for both primary or nodal residual or unresectable disease. It requires measuring the tumor volume to be treated (with calipers), calculation of the dose required to treat this volume, and direct implantation of iodine-125 into the tumor by hollow, stainless-steel needles with a special applicator.

Temporary implantation is utilized for chest-wall, diaphragmatic, or small mediastinal nodal disease. It consists of placement of several small flexible plastic catheters along the area to be treated, suturing the catheters in place with absorbable sutures, and then bringing the catheters through the chest wall. Sources of iridium-192 are inserted through these catheters and left in place until the calculated dose is delivered, and then both the iridium-192 sources and catheters are removed. Interstitial brachytherapy is used in patients with unresectable disease because it allows delivery of a higher dose than external radiation alone, the treatment is precisely localized and readily adaptable to tumor shape, the dose falls rapidly outside the implanted volume, and thus damage to normal tissues is less than external radiation.

The overall mortality rate for patients undergoing operation for mediastinal invasion was 2.7%, and the postoperative complication rate was 13%.

Overall survival for these 225 patients was 22% at 2 years, 13% at 3 years, and 7% at 5 years (Fig. 23–10). Of the 120 patients with epidermoid carcinoma, and the 91 with adenocarcinoma, 5-year survival was identical: 7%. (There were no 5-year survivors among the 14 patients with large cell carcinoma.) Survival by treatment modality is displayed in Table 23–18. There appears to be a survival advantage in patients treated by complete resection and incomplete resection plus brachytherapy compared with incomplete resection or no resection and brachytherapy alone.

Macchiarini et al[129] have recently reported their experience with 23 patients treated with induction chemotherapy with or without radiation for T4 non-small cell lung cancer.[129] Their postoperative mortality was 9%, with a 3-year survival of 54%.

In general, patients with mediastinal invasion have a poor prognosis when treated operatively, with overall 5-year survival being 7%. At this time, patients with mediastinal invasion should not undergo operation alone, but adjuvant therapy, to increase resectability, with possible downstaging of disease, should be considered in this group of patients.

## SURGICAL TREATMENT OF STAGE IV (T1–4, N0–2, M1) NON-SMALL CELL LUNG CARCINOMA

Stage IV non-small cell lung carcinoma includes patients with distant metastatic disease (M1). In discussing the role of surgery in patients with distant metastases, the single brain metastasis appears the only area studied well enough, with results satisfactory enough, to be acceptable for attempted resection.[129a]

The incidence of solitary brain metastasis from non-small cell lung carcinoma in autopsy series varies from 27% to 48%.[130–132] From the onset of symptoms, various authors have reported the average survival without treatment to be from less than 1 month[130] to 6 months.[133] With such a dismal prognosis, resection of a single brain metastasis with or without radiation therapy has been advocated by many authors in patients presenting with a single brain metastasis as the only site of metastatic disease, with otherwise operable lung carcinoma.[129,133]

Operative mortality rates of 2–44% have recently been reported, with survival rates averaging 2.6 to 12 months following craniotomy.[129]

Mandell et al[134] have reported their experience with

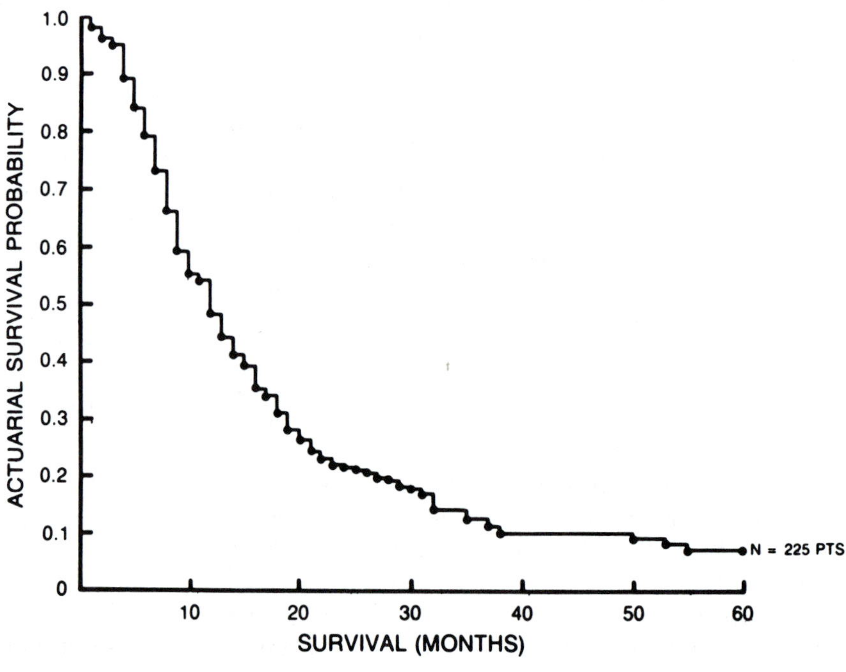


**Figure 23–10.** Survival of 225 patients with mediastinal invasion undergoing surgical treatment.

**TABLE 23–18. NON-SMALL CELL CARCINOMA OF LUNG WITH MEDIASTINAL INVASION: SURVIVAL BY MODE OF THERAPY**

| | | | % | | |
|---|---|---|---|---|---|
| | N | Median months | *2-Year* | *3-Year* | *5-Year* |
| Complete resection | 49 | 17 | 29 | 21 | 9 |
| Incomplete resection and brachytherapy | 33 | 12 | 30 | 22 | 22 |
| Brachytherapy alone | 101 | 11 | 21 | 9 | 0 |
| Incomplete or no resection | 42 | 8 | 9 | 0 | 0 |
| Unoperated | 44 | 8 | 10 | 0 | 0 |

*(Adapted from Burt ME, Pomerantz AH, Bains MS, et al: Results of surgical treatment of stage III lung cancer invading mediastinum. Surg Clin North Am 67:987–1000, 1987.)*

104 patients treated with single brain metastasis from non-small cell lung carcinoma. Thirty-five patients were treated with surgical resection and radiation therapy and 69 with radiation therapy alone. There was a significant difference in survival between the treatment groups with a median survival of 16 months vs. 4 months for those treated with surgery plus radiotherapy vs. radiotherapy alone, respectively. Although the difference in survival was significantly different, interpretation must be tempered by the fact that this is a retrospective review, and selection bias may have contributed more to the difference in survival than the two treatments.

We recently reported our experience with 185 patients undergoing resection of brain metastases from non-small cell lung cancer.[135] The overall survival rate was 13% at 5 years, with a median survival of 14 months. For patients presenting with a synchronous brain metastasis and otherwise operable loco-regional disease, resection of the brain metastasis and the loco-regional disease translated into a significant prolongation in survival compared with those whose loco-regional disease was treated with chemotherapy and/or radiation therapy.

Recently, Patchell et al[136] reported a randomized trial of resection plus whole brain radiation vs. whole brain radiation (WBRT) alone for patients with brain metastasis (non-small cell lung cancer composed 70–80%). This trial confirmed the survival advantage of surgery plus WBRT (median 9.2 months) vs. WBRT alone (median 3.4 months) ($P < 0.01$). In addition, this study demonstrated that recurrence at the primary brain site was significantly less and that patients remain functionally independent significantly longer in the surgical group compared with the WBRT-alone group.

Because of these data, we currently recommend resection of the brain metastasis from non-small cell lung cancer if it is solitary and the patient's life expectancy is otherwise favorable.

If the brain lesion is detected after pulmonary resection, then craniotomy is indicated. If brain and lung present synchronously, and if both the thoracic and neurosurgeon deem their respective lesions potentially, completely resectable, then craniotomy is performed first with thoracotomy shortly afterward.[137]

The need for postoperative radiation therapy after resection of single metastasis from non-small cell carcinoma has been routinely performed in the past, but it is currently being questioned in favor of focal radiotherapy or no radiation therapy.[135] This controversy awaits the results of appropriate clinical trials.

## THE PROBLEMS OF SURGICAL THERAPY FOR SMALL CELL CARCINOMA

For the most part, small cell carcinoma of lung is not a surgical disease. Most patients present with mediastinal adenopathy easily recognized on chest x-ray, and diagnosis in this situation is usually made by bronchoscopic or percutaneous fine-needle biopsy. Once the diagnosis is established, and an extent of disease workup (including bone marrow biopsy) has been completed, treatment consists of chemotherapy and radiotherapy for most patients.

Surgery may be indicated in a small percentage of patients with small cell carcinoma. For the most part, this situation occurs intraoperatively when a patient is explored for presumed non-small cell carcinoma and a diagnosis of small cell carcinoma is made at operation. If, at thoracotomy, a diagnosis of stage I small cell carcinoma is made, complete resection should be attempted. Higgins et al[138] have described four long-term survivors of 11 patients in this situation. Shields et al[139] reviewed their experience with 132 patients undergoing "curative" resection for small cell carcinoma, which represented 4.7% of all curative resections for lung carcinoma in the Veteran's Administration Surgical Oncology Group. Fifty-four percent also received chemotherapy. Table 23–19 lists the 5-year survival in those patients. The 5-year survival rates in patients with stage I disease are such that if an intraoperative diagnosis of small cell carcinoma is made, resection is indicated. Although the data are limited, we recommend postoperative chemotherapy in this situation. In carefully staged preoperative patients, we would also recommend resection with

**TABLE 23–19. FIVE-YEAR SURVIVAL IN 132 PATIENTS WITH SMALL CELL CARCINOMA RESECTED FOR "CURE"**

| TNM | N | 5-year survival (%) |
|---|---|---|
| T1 N0 M0 | 26 | 60 |
| T1 N1 M0 | 16 | 31 |
| T2 N0 M0 | 23 | 28 |
| T2 N1 M0 | 39 | 9 |
| T3/N2 | 28 | 4 |

*(Adapted from Shields TW, Higgins GA, Matthews MJ, et al: Surgical resection in the management of small cell carcinoma of the lung. J Thorac Cardiothorac Surg 84:481–488.)*

postoperative chemotherapy. This recommendation is supported by the data of Meyer[140] and Shepherd et al.[141] Patients presenting with stage II or III small cell carcinoma of the lung should not undergo resection unless done so in a protocol setting. These patients are best served by chemotherapy and radiation.

## SUMMARY: SURGICAL TREATMENT OF NON-SMALL CELL LUNG CARCINOMA

It is clearly evident that there are subsets of patients with advanced non-small cell lung carcinoma that benefit from surgery or surgery combined with radiation and/or chemotherapy. One subset of patients has been identified as tumors extending to chest wall that can be completely resected. It is also noted that nearly 45% of all lung carcinoma presents with mediastinal lymph node metastases and that 20% of this large group of patients is amenable to surgical resection despite the presence of these metastases.[90] This represents a total of nearly 10% of all non-small cell lung carcinomas presenting to treatment. In patients with stage I lung carcinoma, treatment by resection currently holds an 82% 5-year survival for the small tumors (T1) and 68% for the larger ones (T2).[35–38] Hence, stage I carcinoma of lung treated by resection has clearly a very favorable prognosis with two out of three patients anticipated to remain alive and well many years hence. In patients with N1 disease, a 50% 5-year survival is also attainable by surgical resection, but adjuvant therapy needs to be explored in this group of patients to enhance the control both locally and distally in those patients who fail treatment.[46–49]

From 1973 to 1980, a total of 1493 patients were seen at Memorial Sloan-Kettering Cancer Center for management of their lung carcinomas. Thoracotomy for control of their tumor was offered to 961 patients or 64% of the patients; 18% of these were 70 years or older and the male/female ratio was 2 to 1. Of these nearly 1000 thoracotomies for primary lung carcinoma, despite the liberal surgical indications presented, only 20 postoperative deaths were noted, an operative mortality of 2%.[142] Proper case selection and careful preoperative and perioperative management are necessary to minimize complications. We have identified high-risk groups to be (1) patients over 70 years of age in whom a major resection is being considered, (2) patients with cardiovascular disease, and (3) patients with severely restricted pulmonary reserve regardless of their age. To minimize complications, a lesser resection may be considered in the elderly and in all physiologically compromised persons who present an increased risk for surgery.

Assuming these precautions, we continue vigorously and confidently to promote operative intervention combined, where indicated, with appropriate adjuvant therapy as the means of cure or palliation for non-small cell lung cancer. Indeed, in our retrospective 23-year experience, for those treated patients with primary lung carcinoma who most closely reach an operational definition of cure, i.e., 10-year disease-free survival without death from original disease, less than 3% were treated by means excluding surgery.[143] Thus, to deny thoracotomy to a clinically operable patient with stage I, stage II, or specified subsets of localized stage III non-small cell lung carcinoma, is, in our opinion, to capitulate to the disease.

## REFERENCES


1. Boring CC, Squires TS, Tong T, Montgomery S: Ca-A *Cancer J Clin* **44:**7–26, 1994
2. Kirsch MM, Rotman H, Agenta L, et al: Carcinoma of the lung: Results of treatment over ten years. *Ann Thorac Surg* **21:**371–377, 1976
3. Martini N, Bains MS, McCormack P, et al: Surgical treatment of non-small cell carcinoma of the lung: The Memorial Sloan-Kettering Experience. In Hoogstraten B, Addis BJ, Hansen HH, Martini N, Spiro SG (eds): *Lung Tumors: Lung, Mediastinum, Pleura, and Chest Wall.* New York, Springer-Verlag, 1988, pp 111–132
4. Mountain CF: Therapy of stage I and stage II non-small cell lung cancer. *Semin Oncol* **10:**71–80, 1983
5. Brewer LA III: The first pneumonectomy: Historical notes. *J Thorac Cardiovasc Surg* **88:**810–826, 1984
6. Graham EA, Singer JJ: Successful removal of an entire lung for carcinoma of the bronchus. *JAMA* **101:**1371–1374, 1933
7. Churchill ED, Sweet RH, Soutter L, et al: The surgical management of carcinoma of the lung. *J Thorac Surg* **20:**349–365, 1950
8. Baue AE, Evarts A: Graham and the first pneumonectomy. *JAMA* **251:**261–264, 1984
9. Beattie EJ Jr: The surgical treatment of lung tumors. Pneumonectomy or lobectomy. *Surgery* **42:**1124–1128, 1957
10. Le Roux BT: Management of bronchial carcinoma by segmental resection. *Thorax* **27:**70–75, 1972
11. Jensik RJ, Faber LP, Milloy FS, et al: Segmental resection for lung cancer. Fifteen year experience. *J Thorac Cardiovasc Surg* **66:**563–568, 1973
12. Jensik RJ, Faber LP, Kittle CF: Segmental resection for bronchogenic carcinoma. *Ann Thorac Surg* **28:**475–480, 1979
13. Hoffman TH, Ransdell HT: Comparison of lobectomy and wedge resection for carcinoma of the lung. *J Thorac Cardiovasc Surg* **79:**211–217, 1980
14. McCormack PM, Martini N: Primary lung carcinoma. Results with conservative resection in treatment. *N Y State J Med* **80:**612–616, 1980
15. Read RC, Ysder G, Schaeffer RC: Survival after conservative resection for T1 N1 M1 non-small cell lung cancer. *Ann Thorac Surg* **49:**391–400, 1990
16. Warren WH, Faber LP: Segmentectomy versus lobectomy in patients with stage I pulmonary carcinoma: Five year survival and patterns of intrathoracic recurrence. *J Thorac Cardiovasc Surg* **107:**1087–1094, 1994
17. Ginsberg RJ, Rubinstein L, for the Lung Cancer Study Group: A randomized comparative trial of lobectomy versus limited resections for patients with T1 N0 non-small cell lung cancer. *Lung Cancer* **7:**83, 1991
18. Lewis RJ, Caccavale RJ, Sisler GE, MacKenzie JW: Video-assisted thoracic surgical resection of malignant lung tumors. *J Thorac Cardiovasc Surg* **104:**1679–1687, 1992
19. Kirby TJ, Mack MJ, Landreneau RJ, Rice TW: Initial experience with video-assisted thoracoscopic lobectomy. *Ann Thorac Surg* **56:**1248–1253, 1993
20. Walker WS, Carnochan FM, Pugh GC: Thoracoscopic pulmonary

lobectomy: Early operative experience and preliminary clinical results. *J Thorac Cardiovasc Surg* **106:**1111–1117, 1993

21. Shennib HAF, Landreneau R, Mulder DS, Mack M: Video-assisted thoracoscopic wedge resection of T1 lung cancer in high risk patients. *Ann Surg* **218:**555–560, 1993
22. McKenna RJ: Lobectomy by video-assisted thoracic surgery with mediastinal node sampling for lung cancer. *J Thorac Cardiovasc Surg* **107:**879–882, 1994
23. Shields TW: The fate of patients after incomplete resection of bronchial carcinoma. *Surg Gynecol Obstet* **139:**569–572, 1974
24. Liewald F, Hatz RA, Dienemann H, Sinder-Plassmann L: Importance of microscopic residual disease at the bronchial margin after resections for non-small cell carcinoma of the lung. *J Thorac Cardiovasc Surg* **104:**408–412, 1992
25. Kaiser LR, Fleshner P, Keller S, Martini N: Significance of extramucosal residual tumor at the bronchial resection margin. *Ann Thorac Surg* **47:**265–269, 1989
26. Cahan WG, Watson WL, Pool JL: Radical pneumonectomy. *J Thorac Cardiovasc Surg* **22:**449–473, 1951
27. Martini N, Beattie EJ Jr: Current view in primary pulmonary cancer. *Int Adv Surg Oncol* **3:**275–287, 1980
28. Martini N, Melamed MR: Occult carcinomas of the lung. *Ann Thorac Surg* **30:**215–223, 1980
29. Flehinger BJ, Melamed MR, Zaman MB, et al: Early lung cancer detection, results of the initial (prevalence) radiologic and cytologic screening in the Memorial Sloan-Kettering Study. *Am Rev Respir Dis* **130:**555–560, 1984
30. Cortese DA, Kinsey JH, Woolner LB, et al: Hematoporphyrin derivative in the detection and localization of radiographically occult lung cancer. *Am Rev Respir Dis* **126:**1087–1088, 1982
31. Lam S, MacAuley C, Hung J, et al: Detection of dysplesia and carcinoma in situ with a lung imaging fluorescence endoscope device. *J Thorac Cardiovasc Surg* **105:**1035–1040, 1993
32. Hyata Y, Kato H, Konaka C, et al: Photoradiation therapy with hematoporphyrin derivative in early stage I lung cancer. *Chest* **86:**169–177, 1984
33. Imamura S, Kusunoki Y, Takifuji N, et al: Photodynamic therapy and/or external beam radiation therapy for roentgenologically occult lung cancer. *Cancer* **73:**1608–1614, 1994
34. Furuse K, Fukuoka M, Kato H, et al: A prospective phase II study on photodynamic therapy with photofrin II for centrally located early-stage lung cancer. *J Clin Oncol* **11:**1852–1857, 1993

34a. Martini N: Preoperative staging and surgery for non-small cell lung cancer. In Aisner J (ed): *Lung Cancer.* New York, Churchill Livingstone, 1985, pp 101–130

34b. Ransdell JW, Peters RM, Taylor AT, et al: Multi-organ scans for staging lung cancer. Correlation with clinical evaluation. *J Thorac Cardiovasc Surg* **73:**653–659, 1977

35. Williams DE, Pairolero PC, Davis CS, et al: Survival of patients surgically treated for stage I lung cancer. *J Thorac Cardiovasc Surg* **82:**70–76, 1981
36. Schultze S, Holm-Bentzen M, Hoier-Madsen K, Olesen A: Results of surgical treatment for lung cancer. *Scand J Thor Cardiovasc Surg* **17:**61–64, 1983
37. Ichinose Y, Hara N, Ohta M, et al: Is T factor of the TNM staging system a predominant prognostic factor in pathologic stage I non-small cell lung cancer? A multivariate prognostic factor analyses of 151 patients. *J Thorac Cardiovasc Surg* **106:**90–94, 1993
38. Martini N, Bains MS, et al: Incidence of local recurrence and secondary primary tumors in resected stage I lung cancer. *J Thorac Cardiovasc Surg.* **109:**120–129, 1994
39. Pairolero PC, Williams DE, Bergstralh EJ, et al: Postsurgical stage I bronchogenic carcinoma: Morbid implications of recurrent disease. *Ann Thorac Surg* **38:**331–338, 1984
40. NCI Cooperative Early Lung Cancer Detection Program: Results of initial screen (prevalence) summary and conclusions. *Am Rev Respir Dis* **130:**565–570, 1984
41. Melamed MR, Flehinger BJ, Zaman MB, et al: Screening for early lung cancer: Results of the Memorial Sloan-Kettering Study in New York. *Chest* **81:**44–53, 1984
42. McKneally MF, Maver C, Kausel HW: Regional immunotherapy of lung cancer with intrapleural BCG. *Lancet* **1:**377–379, 1976
43. Mountain CF, Gail MH: Surgical adjuvant intrapleural BCG treatment for stage I non-small cell lung cancer. Preliminary report of the National Cancer Institute Lung Cancer Study Group. *J Thorac Cardiovasc Surg* **82:**649–657, 1981

43a. Hong WK, Lippman JM, Itri L, et al: Prevention of second primary tumors with isotretinoin in squamous cell carcinoma of the head and neck. *N Engl J Med* **323:**789–796, 1990

43b. Pastorino V, Infante M, Maioli M, et al: Adjuvant treatment of stage I lung cancer with high-dose vitamin A. *J Clin Oncol* **11:** 1206–1212, 1993

44. Shields TW, Humphrey EW, Matthews M, Eastridge CE, Keehan BS: Pathological stage grouping of patients with resected carcinoma of the lung. *J Thorac Cardiovasc Surg* **80:**400–405, 1980
45. Martini N, Flehinger BJ, Nagasaki F, Hart B: Prognostic significance of N1 disease in carcinoma of the lung. *J Thorac Cardiovasc Surg* **86:**646–653, 1983
46. Mountain CF: A new international staging system for lung cancer. *Chest* **89:**2255–2335, 1986
47. Naruke T, Goya T, Tsuchiya R, Suemasu K: Prognosis and survival in resected lung carcinoma based on the new international staging system. *J Thorac Cardiovasc Surg* **96:**440–447, 1988
48. Martini N, Burt ME, Bains MS, et al: Survival after resection of stage II non-small cell lung cancer. *Ann Thorac Surg* **54:**460–466, 1992
49. Yano T, Yokoyama H, Inoue T, et al: Surgical results and prognostic factors of pathologic N1 disease in non-small cell carcinoma of the lung: Significance of N1 level: Lobar or hilar nodes. *J Thorac Cardiovasc Surg* **107:**1398–1402, 1994
50. Holmes EC: Treatment of stage II lung cancer (T1 N1 and T2 N1). *Surg Clinic North Am* **67:**945–949, 1987
51. Ludwig Lung Cancer Study Group: Patterns of failure in patients with resected stage I and stage II non-small cell carcinoma of the lung. *Ann Surg* **205:**67–71, 1987
52. Feld R, Rubinstein LV, Weisenburger TH: Sites of recurrence of resected stage I non-small cell lung cancer. *J Clin Oncol* **2:**1352–1358, 1984
53. Immerman SC, Vanecko RM, Fry WA, et al: Site of recurrence in patients with stages I and II carcinoma of the lung resected for cure. *Ann Thorac Surg* **32:**23–27, 1981
54. Ludwig Lung Cancer Study Group: Adverse effect of intrapleural Corynebacterium parvum as adjuvant therapy in resected stage I and II non-small cell carcinoma of the lung. *J Thorac Cardiovasc Surg* **89:**842–847, 1985
55. Warram J: Preoperative irradiation of cancer of the lung: Final report of a therapeutic trial: A collaborative study. *Cancer* **36:**914–925, 1975
56. Shields TW: Preoperative radiation therapy in the treatment of bronchial carcinoma. *Cancer* **30:**1386–1394, 1972
57. The Lung Cancer Study Group: Effects of postoperative mediastinal radiation on completely resected stage II and III epidermoid cancer of the lung. *N Engl J Med* **315:**1377–1381, 1986
58. Dantzenberg B, Benichou J, Allard P, et al: Failure of the perioperative PCV neoadjuvant polychemotherapy in resectable bronchogenic non-small cell carcinoma. *Cancer* **65:**2435–2441, 1990
59. Lung Cancer Study Group: Preliminary report of a clinical trial comparing post-adjuvant chemotherapy vs. no therapy for T1 N1, T2 N0 non-small cell lung cancer. *Lung Cancer* **4:**A160, 1988
60. Shields TW, Humphrey EW, Eastridge CE, Keehn RJ: Adjuvant cancer chemotherapy after resection of carcinoma of the lung. *Cancer* **40:**2057–2062, 1977
61. Shields TW, Higgins GA, Humphrey EW, et al: Prolonged intermittent adjuvant chemotherapy with CCNV and hydroxyurea after resection of carcinoma of the lung. *Cancer* **50:**1713–1721, 1982

62. McCaughan BC, Martini N, Bains MS, McCormack PM: Chest wall invasion in carcinoma of the lung. *J Thorac Cardiovasc Surg* **89:**836–841, 1985
63. Pairolero PC, Trastek VF, Payne WS: Treatment of bronchogenic carcinoma with chest wall invasion. *Surg Clin North Am* **67:**959–964, 1987
64. Trastek VF, Pairolero PC, et al: En bloc (non-chest wall) resection for bronchogenic carcinoma with parietal fixation. *J Thorac Cardiovasc Surg* **87:**352–358, 1984
65. Albertucci M, DeMeester TR, Rothberg M, et al: Surgery and the management of peripheral lung tumors adherent to the parietal pleura. *J Thorac Cardiovasc Surg* **103:**8–13, 1992
66. Allen MS, Mathisen DJ, Grillo HC, et al: Bronchogenic carcinoma with chest wall invasion. *Ann Thorac Surg* **51:**948–951, 1991
67. McCormack PM, Bains MS, Martini N, et al: Methods of skeletal reconstruction following resection of lung carcinoma invading chest wall. *Surg Clin North Am* **67:**979–986, 1987
68. Piehler JM, Pairolero PC, Weiland LH, et al: Bronchogenic carcinoma with chest wall invasion: Factors affecting survival following en bloc resection. *Ann Thorac Surg* **34:**684–691, 1982
69. Patterson GA, Ilves R, Ginsberg RJ, et al: The value of adjuvant radiotherapy in pulmonary and chest wall resection for bronchogenic carcinoma. *Ann Thorac Surg* **34:**692–697, 1982
70. Ratto GB, Piacenza G, Frola C, et al: Chest wall involvement by lung cancer: Computed tomographic detection and results of operation. *Ann Thorac Surg* **51:**182–188, 1991
71. Faber LP, Jensik RJ, Kittle CF: Results of sleeve lobectomy for bronchogenic carcinoma in 101 patients. *Ann Thorac Surg* **37:** 279–285, 1984
72. Bennett WF, Smith RA: A twenty-year analysis of the results of sleeve resection for primary bronchogenic carcinoma. *J Thorac Cardiovasc Surg* **76:**840–845, 1978
73. Van Den Bosch JNN, Bergstein PGN, Laros CD, et al: Lobectomy with sleeve resection in the treatment of tumors of the bronchus. *Chest* **80:**154–157, 1981
74. DesLauriers J, Gaulin P, Beaulieu N, et al: Long-term clinical and functional results of sleeve lobectomy for primary lung cancer. *J Thorac Cardiovasc Surg* **91:**871–879, 1986
75. Mehran RJ, Deslauriers J, Piraux M, et al: Survival related to nodal status after sleeve resection for lung cancer. *J Thorac Cardiovasc Surg* **107:**576–583, 1994
76. Lowe JE, Bridgman AH, Sabiston DC: The role of bronchoplastic procedures in the surgical management of benign and malignant pulmonary lesions. *J Thorac Cardiovasc Surg* **83:**227–234, 1982
77. Ginsberg RJ, Hill LD, Egan RT, et al: Modern thirty-day operative mortality for surgical resections in lung cancer. *J Thorac Cardiovasc Surg* **86:**654–658, 1983
78. Faber LP: Results of surgical treatment of stage III lung carcinoma with carinal proximity. The role of sleeve lobectomy versus pneumonectomy and the role of sleeve pneumonectomy. *Surg Clin North Am* **67:**1001–1014, 1987
79. Deslauriers J, Beaulieu M, Benazera A, McClish A: Sleeve pneumonectomy for bronchogenic carcinoma. *Ann Thorac Surg* **28:**465–474, 1979
80. Dartevelle PG, Khalite J, Chapelier A: Tracheal sleeve pneumonectomy for bronchogenic carcinoma: Report of 55 cases. *Ann Thorac Surg* **46:**68–72, 1988
81. Roviaro GC, Varoli F, Rebuffat C, et al: Tracheal sleeve pneumonectomy for bronchogenic carcinoma. *J Thorac Cardiovasc Surg* **107:**13–18, 1994
82. Coughlin N, DesLauriers J, Beaulieu N, et al: Role of mediastinoscopy in pretreatment staging of patients with primary lung cancer. *Ann Thorac Surg* **40:**556–560, 1985
83. Patterson GA, Piazza D, Pearson FG, et al: Significance of metastatic disease in subaortic lymph nodes. *Ann Thorac Surg* **43:**155–159, 1987
84. Pearson FG, Delarue NC, Ilves R, et al: Significance of positive superior mediastinal nodes identified at mediastinoscopy in patient with resectable cancer of the lung. *J Thorac Cardiovasc Surg* **83:**1–11, 1982
85. Pearson FG: Mediastinal adenopathy. The N2 lesion. In Delarue NC, Eschapasse H (eds): *International Trends in General Thoracic Surgery,* Vol. VI. Philadelphia, Saunders, 1985, pp 104–107
86. Kirsh MM, Sloan H: Mediastinal metastases in bronchogenic carcinoma: Influence of post-operative irradiation, cell type, and location. *Ann Thorac Surg* **33:**459–464, 1982
87. Naruke T, Suemasu K, Ishikawa S: Lymph node mapping and curability at various levels of metastasis in resected lung cancer. *J Thorac Cardiovasc Surg* **76:**832–839, 1978
88. Abbey-Smith R: The importance of mediastinal lymph node invasion by pulmonary carcinoma in selection of patients for resection. *Ann Thorac Surg* **25:**5–11, 1978
89. Mountain CF: The biological operability of stage III non-small cell lung cancer. *Ann Thorac Surg* **40:**60–64, 1985
90. Martini N, Flehinger BJ, Zaman MB, Beattie EJ Jr: Results of resection in non-oat cell carcinoma of the lung with mediastinal lymph node metastases. *Ann Surg* **198:**386–397, 1983
91. Martini N, Flehinger BJ, Zaman MB, Beattie EJ Jr: Prospective study of 445 lung carcinoma with mediastinal lymph node metastases. *J Thorac Cardiovasc Surg* **80:**390–397, 1980
92. Martini N, Flehinger BJ: The role of surgery in N2 lung cancer. *Surg Clin North Am* **67:**1037–1049, 1987
93. Naruke T, Goya T, Tsuchiya R, Suemasu K: The importance of surgery to non-small cell carcinoma of lung with mediastinal lymph node metastases. *Ann Thorac Surg* **46:**603–610, 1988
94. Watanabe Y, Shimizu J, Oda M, et al: Aggressive surgical intervention in N2 non-small cell cancer of the lung. *Ann Thorac Surg* **51:**253–261, 1991
95. Cybulsky IJ, Lanza LA, Ryan B, et al: Prognostic significance of computed tomography in resected N2 lung cancer. *Ann Thorac Surg* **54:**533–537, 1992
96. van Klaveren RJ, Festen J, Otten HJAM, et al: Prognosis of unsuspected but completely resectable N2 non-small cell lung cancer. *Ann Thorac Surg* **56:**300–304, 1993
97. Conill C, Astudillo J, Verger E: Prognostic significance of metastases to mediastinal lymph node levels in resected non-small cell lung carcinoma. *Cancer* **72:**1199–1202, 1993
98. Daly BDT, Mueller JD, Faling LJ, et al: N2 lung cancer: Outcome in patients with false-negative computed tomographic scans of the chest. *J Thorac Cardiovasc Surg* **105:**904–911, 1993
99. Mountain CF: Surgery for stage IIIa-N2 non-small cell lung cancer. *Cancer* **73:**7589–7598, 1994
100. Goldstraw P, Mannam GC, Kaplan DK, Michail P: Surgical management of non-small cell lung cancer with ipsilateral mediastinal node metastasis (N2 disease). *J Thorac Cardiovasc Surg* **107:**19–28, 1994
101. Miller DL, McManus KG, Allen MS, et al: Results of surgical resection in patients with N2 non-small cell lung cancer. *Ann Thorac Surg* **57:**1095–1101, 1994
102. The Lung Cancer Study Group: A randomized comparison of the effects of adjuvant therapy in resected stages II and III non-small cell carcinoma of the lung. *Ann Surg* **202:**335–341, 1985
103. Holmes EC, Gail N: Surgical adjuvant therapy for stage II and III adenocarcinoma and large-cell undifferentiated carcinoma. *J Clin Oncol* **4:**710–715, 1986
104. Ohta M, Tsuchiya R, Shimoyama M, et al: Adjuvant chemotherapy for completely resected stage III non-small cell lung cancer. *J Thorac Cardiovasc Surg* **106:**703–708, 1993
105. Pisters KMW, Kris MG, Grella RJ, et al: Randomized trial comparing postoperative chemotherapy with vindesine and cisplatin plus thoracic irradiation with irradiation alone in stage III (N2) non-small cell lung cancer. *J Surg Oncol.* In press.
106. Martini N, Kris MG, Gralla RJ, et al: The effects of preoperative chemotherapy on the resectability of non-small cell lung carcinoma

with mediastinal lymph node metastases (N2 M0). *Ann Thorac Surg* **45**:370–379, 1988

107. Martini N, Kris MG, Flehinger BJ, et al: Preoperative chemotherapy for stage IIIa (N2) lung cancer: The Sloan-Kettering Experience with 136 patients. *Ann Thorac Surg* **55**:1365–1374, 1993
108. Strauss GM, Langer MP, Elias A, Skavin AT, Sugarbaker D: Multimodality treatment of stage IIIA non-small cell lung carcinoma: A critical review of the literature and strategies for future research. *J Clin Oncol* **10**:829–838, 1992
109. Ginsberg RJ: Multimodality therapy for stage IIIA (N2) lung cancer: An overview. *Chest* **103**:3565–3595, 1993
110. Shephard FA: Induction chemotherapy for locally advanced non-small cell lung cancer. *Ann Thorac Surg* **55**:1585–1592, 1993
111. Pass HI, Pogrebriak HW, Steinberg SM, et al: Randomized trial of neoadjuvant therapy for lung cancer: Interim analysis. *Ann Thorac Surg* **53**:992–998, 1992
112. Roth JA, Fossela F, Kowaki R, et al: A randomized trial comparing perioperative chemotherapy and surgery with surgery alone in resectable stage IIIA non-small cell lung cancer. *J Natl Cancer Inst* **86**:673–680, 1994
113. Rossell R, Gomez-Codina J, Campo C, et al: A randomized trial comparing preoperative chemotherapy plus surgery with surgery alone in patients with non-small cell lung cancer. *N Engl J Med* **330**:153–158, 1994
114. Dillman RO, Seagren SL, Propert KR, et al: A randomized trial of induction chemotherapy plus high dose radiation versus radiation alone in stage III non-small cell lung cancer. *N Engl J Med* **323**:940–945, 1990
115. Decker DA, Dines PE, Payne WS, et al: The significance of cytologically negative pleural effusion in bronchogenic carcinoma. *Chest* **74**:640–642, 1978
116. Boutin C, Viallat JR, Cargnino P, et al: Thoracoscopy in malignant pleural effusions. *Am Rev Respir Dis* **124**:588–592, 1981
117. Thomas P: Thoracoscopy: An old procedure revisited. In Kittle CF (ed): *Current Controversies in Thoracic Surgery.* Philadelphia, Saunders, 1986, pp 101–106
118. Weissberg D, Kaufman M, Zurkowski Z: Pleuroscopy in patients with pleural effusions and pleural masses. *Ann Thorac Surg* **29**:205–208, 1980
119. DeCamp PT, Moreley PW, Scott MC, Hatch HB Jr: Diagnostic thorascopy. *Ann Thorac Surg* **16**:79–84, 1973
120. Oldenburg FA, Newhouse MT: Thoracoscopy: A safe, accurate procedure using the rigid thoracoscope and local anesthesia. *Chest* **75**:45–50, 1979
121. Canto A, Blasco E, Casillas N, et al: Thoracoscopy in the diagnosis of pleural effusion. *Thorax* **32**:550–554, 1977
122. Martini N, McCormack P: Therapy of stage III (non-metastatic disease). *Semin Surg Oncol* **10**:95–110, 1983
123. Austen EH, Flye MW: The treatment of recurrent malignant pleural effusion. *Ann Thorac Surg* **28**:190–203, 1979
124. Martini N, Bains MS, Beattie EJ Jr: Indications for pleurectomy in malignant effusion. *Cancer* **35**:734–738, 1975
125. Levett JM, Darakjian HE, DeMeester TR, et al: Bronchogenic carcinoma located in the aortic window. The importance of the primary lesion as a determinant of survival. *J Thorac Cardiovasc Surg* **83**:551–562, 1982
126. Yoshimura H, Kazama S, Asari H, et al: Lung cancer involving the superior vena cava: Pneumonectomy with concomitant partial resection of superior vena cava. *J Thorac Cardiovasc Surg* **77**:83–86, 1979
127. Burt ME, Pomerantz AH, Bains MS, et al: Results of surgical treatment of stage III lung cancer invading mediastinum. *Surg Clin North Am* **67**:987–1000, 1987
128. Hilaris BS, Nori D, Anderson LL: *An Atlas of Brachytherapy.* New York, MacMillan, 1988
129. Macchiarini P, Chapelier AR, Monnet I, et al: Extended operations after induction therapy for stage IIIb (T4) non-small cell lung cancer. *Ann Thorac Surg* **57**:966–973, 1994

129a. Magilligan DJ Jr: Treatment of lung cancer metastatic to the brain. *Surg Clin North Am* **67**:1073–1080, 1987

130. Richard P, McKissock W: Intracranial metastases. *Br Med J* **1**:15–18, 1963
131. Galluzzi S, Payne PM: Brain metastasis from primary bronchial carcinoma: A statistical study of 741 necropsies. *Biol J Cancer* **10**:408–414, 1956
132. Deeley TJ, Price-Edwards JM: Radiotherapy in the management of cerebral secondaries from bronchial carcinoma. *Lancet* **1**: 1209–1213, 1968
133. Knights EM Jr: Metastatic tumors of the brain and their relation to primary and secondary pulmonary cancer. *Cancer* **7**:259–264, 1954
134. Mandell L, Hilaris BS, Sullivan M, et al: The treatment of single brain metastasis from non-oat cell lung carcinoma. Surgery and radiation versus radiation therapy alone. *Cancer* **58**:641–649, 1986
135. Burt M, Wronski M, Arbit E, Galicich J, Ginsberg R: Solitary brain metastasis from non-small cell lung cancer: Results of therapy. *J Thorac Cardiovasc Surg* **103**:399–411, 1992
136. Patchell RA, Tibbs PA, Walsh JW, et al: A randomized trial of surgery in the treatment of single metastases to the brain. *N Engl J Med* **322**:494–500, 1990
137. Sundaresan N, Galicich JH: Surgical treatment of brain metastasis. Clinical and computerized tomography evaluation of the results of treatment. *Cancer* **55**:1382–1388, 1985
138. Higgins GA, Shields TW, Kuhn RJ: The solitary pulmonary nodule. *Arch Surg* **10**:570–575, 1975
139. Shields TW, Higgins GA, Matthews MJ, et al: Surgical resection in the management of small cell carcinoma of the lung. *J Thorac Cardiovasc Surg* **84**:481–488, 1982
140. Meyer JA: Effect of histologically verified TNM stage on disease central in treated small cell carcinoma of the lung. *Cancer* **55**:1747–1752, 1985
141. Shepherd FA, Ginsberg RJ, Evans WK, et al: Reduction in local recurrence and improved survival in surgically treated patients with small cell lung cancer. *J Thorac Cardiovasc Surg* **86**:498–506, 1983
142. Nagasaki F, Flehinger BJ, Martini N: Complications of surgery in the treatment of carcinoma of the lung. *Chest* **82**:25–29, 1982
143. Temeck BK, Flehinger BJ, Martini N: A retrospective analysis of 10 year survivors from carcinoma of the lung. *Cancer* **53**:1405–1408, 1984

CHAPTER

# 24

# Superior Sulcus Tumors

Joseph S. McLaughlin

A superior sulcus tumor is a bronchiogenic carcinoma located in the extreme apex of the lung that invades the pleura and adjacent structures and produces classic signs and symptoms.

## HISTORIC PERSPECTIVE

Although described by Edwin Hare[1] in 1838, the syndrome generally bears the name of Henry Pancoast[2] because of his clear description of the findings in seven patients in 1932. Prior to 1950 the condition was uniformly fatal; most patients died in agony from bony and brachial plexus invasion.[3] Operation was not considered feasible, and irradiation was considered ineffective. Chardack and MacCallum[4] are credited with the first successful en bloc resection of the tumor including the right upper lobe; the first and second ribs; and brachial plexus roots, T1, C8, and C7. Haas and associates[5] in 1954 reported significant tumor sensitivity to high-dosage irradiation and demonstrated a decrease in what had been intractable pain. Shaw, Paulson, and Kee[6] in their landmark report in the *Annals of Surgery* in 1960 described the successful use of preoperative irradiation followed by en bloc resection in 18 patients, a treatment scheme that continues to be the standard by which others are judged.

## THE SYNDROME

Edwin Hare, a house surgeon at the Staford County General Infirmary, wrote to the *London Medical Gazette* in 1838 to describe a patient who presented with pain and parasthesia along the distribution of the ulnar nerve in association with a mass in the neck (Fig. 24–1). The patient had ptosis, pupillary constriction, and anhidrosis (Horner's syndrome). Later he developed paraplegia and urinary retention and died. Hare performed an autopsy and found a tumor invading the brachial plexus, the cervical sympathetics, the vagus and phrenic nerves, the carotid artery, and the vertebral bodies.

In 1924 Pancoast[7] described the clinical and x-ray finding in three patients with "apical chest tumors." In 1932 the then professor of radiology at the University of Pennsylvania presented the now famous Chairman's address to the Section of Radiology at the 83rd Annual Session of the American Medical Association entitled "Superior Pulmonary Sulcus Tumor—Tumor Characterized by Pain, Horner's Syndrome, Destruction of Bone and Atrophy of Hand Muscles." His patients totaled seven. He described a "sharply defined shadow in the apex of the thorax, destruction of one or all three of the upper ribs in their posterior aspects and the adjacent transverse processes and sometimes slight vertebral body erosion." He described the characteristic pain, Horner's syndrome, and wasting of the muscles of the hand. He coined the term *superior sulcus* to describe the location of the tumor, presumably referring to the groove in the apex of the lung made by the subclavian artery. He wrongly believed that the tumor arose from embryonic rests, but he indicated that a better understanding of the histopathology could change this opinion. Parenthetically, in 1932 Tobias[8] of Buenos Aires, writing in Spanish in the *Revista Medica Latino-Americana,* clearly defined the syndrome and attributed its cause to bronchiogenic carcinoma.

Paulson,[9] whose personal experience with this condition is unparalleled, has documented the symptomatology. The presenting symptom most frequently cited is pain localized to the shoulder. With time the pain, which becomes unremitting, spreads to the medial area of the scapula and extends along the ulnar nerve distribution of the arm to involve the elbow (T1 distribution) and the medial forearm and hand (C8 distribution) (Fig. 24–2). In Zipoyn's[10] series

**TUMOR IMPLICATING THE NERVES OF THE LEFT SIDE**

TUMOR INVOLVING CERTAIN NERVES

*To the Editor of the Medical Gazette.*

*Sir,*

If you are of opinion that the points connected with physiology and pathology in the following case, render it worthy of a place in your very valuable publication, I shall be much obliged to you to give it insertion.

I am, sir, your obedient servant.

EDW. SELLECK HARE, M.R.C.S.

House-Surgeon to the Stafford County General Infirmary

September 11, 1838.

Thomas Willetts, aged 40, married, of an unhealthy complexion, was admitted to the Infirmary, under the care of Dr. Knight, on the 8th of last June. He had been attacked a month before with pain, tingling and numbness along the course of the ulnar nerve of the left arm, which was most severe at the elbow, where there had also been some swelling and redness. There was, besides, pain through the left shoulder, extending across the chest to the opposite side, and upwards to the left eye and teeth of that side; also a sense of pulsation in different parts of the body, and sleepless nights. The tongue was clean, appetite good, no cough, or physical sign of pulmonary disease, and the secretions were all natural.

**Figure 24–1.** Reproduction of Dr. Hare's letter to the editor of the *Medical Gazette* and the initial paragraph of the report of a patient with a superior sulcus tumor.

of 37 patients, 34 were treated for cervical osteoarthritis or bursitis for an average of 6 months prior to diagnosis. Many patients when first seen will support their elbow with the uninvolved hand to relieve the pain. Examination reveals atrophy of the muscles of the hand and loss of the triceps tendon reflex. With tumor growth, the sympathetic chain is involved with the production of Horner's syndrome. Rib and vertebral involvement increases the pain. In the University of Maryland series of 73 patients, many with far advanced lesions, 25% had palpable supraclavicular nodes or masses, 23% had significant weight loss, and 5% had superior vena cava syndrome. Recurrent nerve and phrenic paralysis was present in 10% and 5% respectively, and paraplegia occurred in 5%.[11] Important in this spectrum of signs and symptoms is the frequently mild nature or absence of pulmonary symptoms early in the course of the disease.

## PATHOLOGY

It is clear that epithelial cell bronchiogenic carcinoma is the usual cause of the syndrome (Table 24–1). Most often the tumor is squamous cell, but large cell and adenocarcinoma taken together are as common. Small cell carcinoma is rare in this location. Other tumors, both primary and metastatic, and fungal and other infections have been reported but are anecdotal.[12–15]

It has been stated that the classic syndrome is produced by a low-grade or slow-growing squamous cell carci-

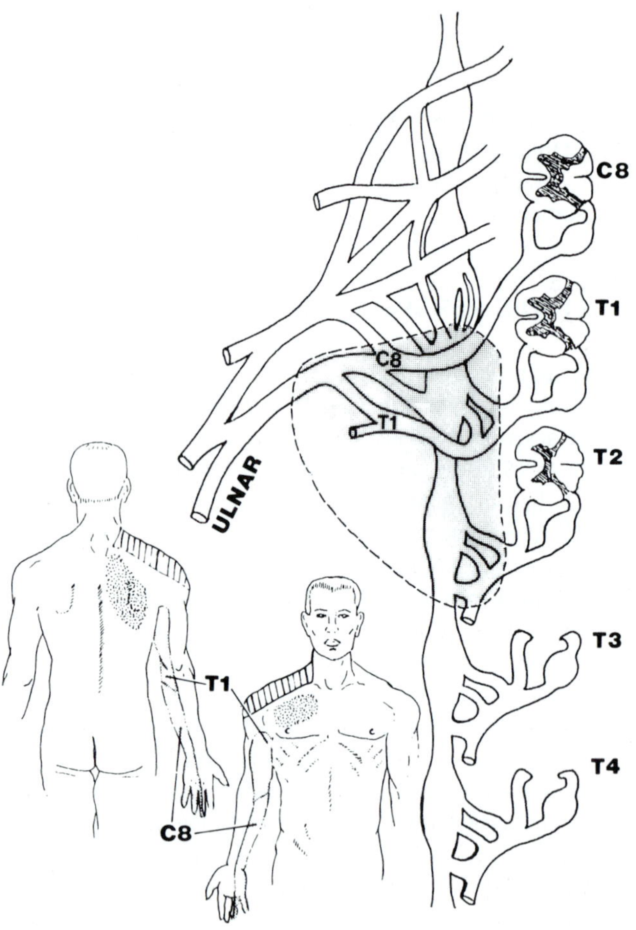


**Figure 24–2.** Neural structures at the thoracic inlet involved by direct extension of a carcinoma in the superior pulmonary sulcus. The shaded area indicates the region of potential involvement, typically including C8, T1, and T2 nerve roots; the lower trunk of the brachial plexus; and the sympathetic chain. The dermatomes of C8 and T1 are illustrated, as well as the regions of referred pain in the scapular and pectoral regions (mediated through afferent pain fibers of the sympathetic trunk and ganglia). *(Modified from Paulson DL: Carcinomas in the superior pulmonary sulcus. J Thorac Cardiovasc Surg 70:1095, 1975, with permission.)*

**TABLE 24–1. CELLULAR CLASSIFICATION**

| | | Percent | | | |
|---|---|---|---|---|---|
| **Author** | **Ref No** | ***Squamous*** | ***Large*** | ***Adeno*** | ***Small*** |
| Paulson | 9 | 45 | 33 | 17 | |
| Attar et al[a] | 11 | 47 | | 20 | |
| Kowaki et al | 33 | 25 | 6 | 54 | 2 |
| Hilaris et al | 35 | 51 | 49[b] | | |

[a]Undifferentiated, 18%; undetermined, 15%.
[b]Combined large cell and adenocarcinoma.

noma. One can argue this view. It may well be that the tumor produces symptoms early in its course simply because it arises adjacent to and early on invades structures that call attention to its presence.

## DIAGNOSIS AND STAGING

Paulson indicates that clinical and chest x-ray findings are diagnostic in 95% of patients. Transcervical needle biopsy was introduced by McGoon[16] in 1964 and was modified by others to include fluoroscopic, sonographic, and computed tomography (CT) guidance. Paulson et al[17] reported a 95% success rate in obtaining a cellular diagnosis, and CT-guided fine-needle biopsy using cytologic techniques has emerged as the standard for reaching a pretreatment diagnosis.

By definition Pancoast tumors are classified T3, since they invade the chest wall. If their location is posterior, they involve the stellate ganglion and the posterior aspect of the upper ribs and extend upward to involve the brachial plexus and medially to involve the transverse processes and vertebral bodies. If the location is anterior, the anterior portion of the first rib, the anterior scalene muscle, the subclavian vessels, and the phrenic nerve are involved.[18] Once mediastinal and cervical invasion has taken place, these tumors are classified as T4. Brachial plexus, stellate ganglion, rib, and transverse process involvement do not rule out the potential for resection. More ominous is involvement of the subclavian artery, but even in this circumstance resection is possible particularly if only the adventitia is involved. Partial vertebral body resection has been carried out, and it is suggested that one quarter of the vertebral body can be removed without significantly compromising the structural integrity of the column.[6] Once mediastinal invasion including vertebral foramina, vagus nerve, and vena cava involvement takes place, these tumors rarely are cured by resection.

Nodal involvement is the key to potential curability once resectability is established. Characteristically, lymph node spread occurs relatively late in the course of these cancers. Thus, in most surgical series N0 status is common. In Paulson's series of 131 patients, 49 were considered inoperable at the time of presentation because of distant metastases, local extent of the tumor, or concurrent disease states and advanced age. Three refused operation. All of these patients died within 2 years. Seventy-nine patients (60%) came to operation following preoperative irradiation, and 78 were resected (Fig. 24–3). Seventeen patients had lymph node metastases; none survived 2 years. In contrast, 44% of patients without nodal metastases survived 5 years.

The Memorial Sloan-Kettering Cancer Center series is similar.[19] Of 129 patients who underwent thoracotomy, 87 (67%) were status N0, and 19 were status N2; 23 were status N3 because of supraclavicular node involvement but had negative mediastinal nodes. The median survival for the 109 patients with negative mediastinal nodes was 20 months and the 5-year survival, 29%. For the 19 patients with positive mediastinal nodes, the median survival was 9 months, and only 10% lived 5 years.

Komaki[20] reported a series of 85 previously untreated patients seen at the M.D. Anderson Cancer Center between 1977 and 1987. The series is weighted toward irradiation therapy, i.e., only 25 patients were surgically treated. Forty-three patients were classified as stage IIIA, and 42 were classified as Stage IIIB. Sixteen patients classified as Stage IIIA underwent surgical therapy, whereas only nine patients

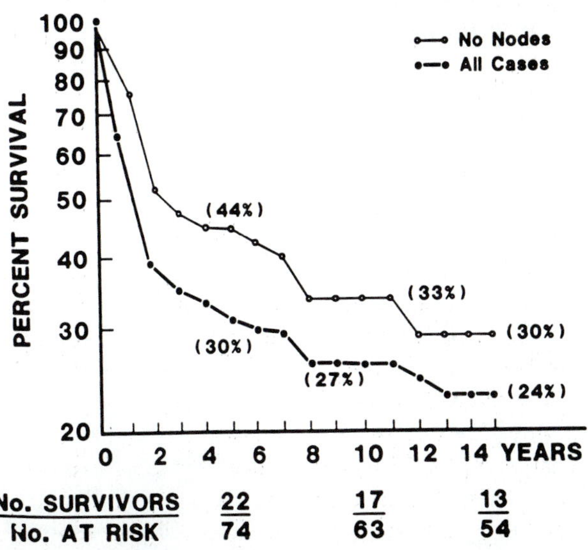


**Figure 24–3.** Paulson's series of 131 patients with observed 5-, 10-, and 15-year survival in 78 patients following preoperative irradiation and resection. None of 17 patients with lymph node involvement survived 2 years.

classified as IIIB underwent surgery, a statistically significant difference. When surgery was part of the treatment, 52% (13/25) of patients lived 2+ years compared with 22% (13/60) when surgery was not part of the treatment. High-performance status as judged by the Karnofsky Performance Scale, less than 5% weight loss, and lack of direct extension into the vertebral bodies were highly significant factors for better survival.

## RADIOLOGIC EVALUATION

Initially the tumor may be obscure and present as a small homogenous cap at the apex of the lung that may resemble pleural thickening (Fig. 24–4). More often a mass is identified clouding the lung markings above the clavicle that contrasts to the clarity of the opposite apex (Fig. 24–5A). Bone destruction of the posterior aspects of the first, second, and, at times, the third rib may be apparent (Fig. 24–6A,B). The tumor shadow may extend medially toward the mediastinum, and later the hilum and upper mediastinum are involved and enlarged by metastatic invasion. This area of the chest may not be defined, and bone destruction may not be identified by routine chest x-ray studies. Apical lordotic views or tomograms more clearly define this area, but these techniques now are replaced by computed tomography (CT).[21]

Computed tomography has become the advanced standard in the radiologic diagnosis of chest disorders and is of great value in the diagnosis and preoperative staging of superiors sulcus tumors (Fig. 24–7). CT can identify involvement and invasion of the brachial plexus, the chest wall, and the adjacent mediastinal structures including the vertebral bodies, the vena cava, the trachea and the esophagus. Contrast CT gives information of subclavian vein and artery involvement and at times delineates adjacency from invasion. Therefore, CT is extremely useful in determining resectability.

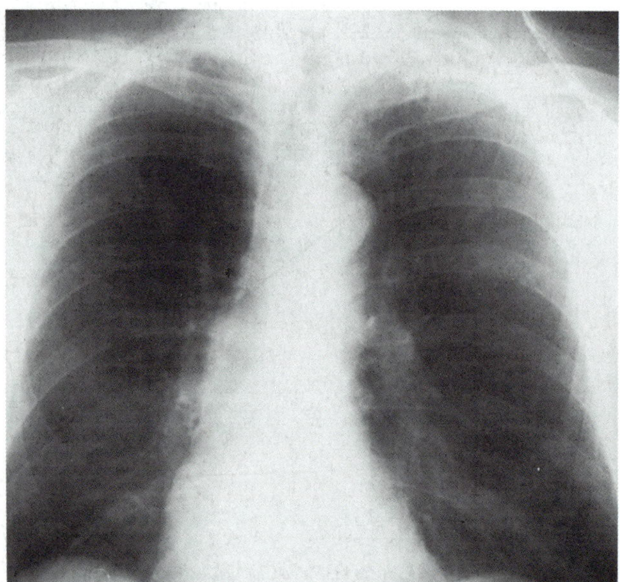

**Figure 24–4.** Carcinoma of the superior sulcus mimicking apical "pleural thickening."

CT has proven to be of considerable value in determining mediastinal node metastases from bronchiogenic carcinoma.[22–24] Nodal involvement is the major determinate of survival in surgically resected patients. Lymph nodes <1 cm are most often benign but may be positive in up to 30% of patients. Lymph nodes >1 cm are often malignant, but false positive values of up to 40% are reported. Mediastinoscopy is indicated in those patients who are going to be denied curative therapy because of enlarged lymph nodes only.

Magnetic resonance imaging (MRI) is reported to be more accurate than CT in determining invasion of cervical structures and the vertebral bodies and particularly the foramina (Fig. 24–8A,B). It has no advantage over CT in delineating the lung and its structure. Heelan and his associates[25] prospectively compared the correlation between clinical symptoms and the surgical specimen with the findings on CT and MRI interpreted independently and blindly by diagnostic radiologists. Thin-section coronal and sagittal T1-weighted MRI images correlated with the patient's symptoms with significantly more accuracy than did CT scanning (0.94 accuracy with MRI vs 0.63 with CT), and MRI is recommended to delineate the extent of cervical invasion prior to resection and is becoming routine in the preoperative evaluation.

## PREOPERATIVE EVALUATION

The history, the physical examination, and the chest x-ray are diagnostic in most cases; CT-guided thin-needle biopsy should provide a tissue diagnosis. Appropriate blood chemistry studies give evidence of bony or liver metastases. Since brain, liver, adrenal, and bone metastasis are common, CT evaluation of the brain and upper abdomen and bone scans are indicated. Cardiac evaluation and pulmonary function studies are routinely performed.

Bronchoscopy is carried out to evaluate the status of the tracheal bronchial tree. Since these are peripheral tumors, they are rarely seen, but Attar et al[11] noted that cytology may be positive in up to 30% of cases. Other authors have confirmed this relatively low yield.

## TREATMENT

Robert Shaw and his partners Donald Paulson and John Kee were premier thoracic surgeons in Dallas in 1956 when they were presented with a patient with a Pancoast's tumor. The patient was thought to be incurable and was referred for irradiation therapy; 3000 cGy was administered, and, remarkably, the tumor shrunk by half, and the patient's pain dra-

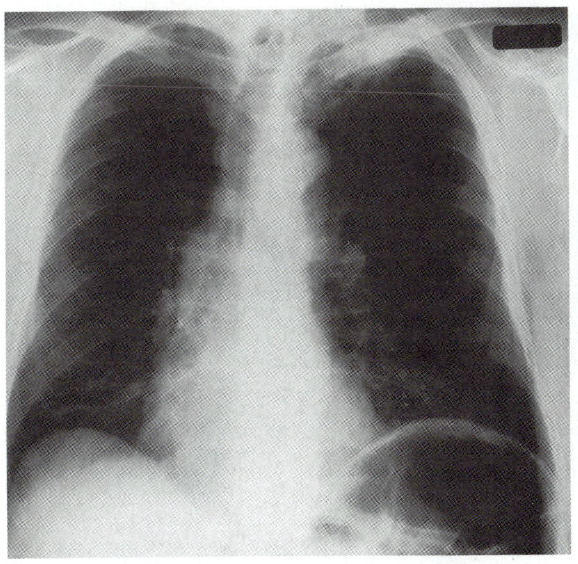

A

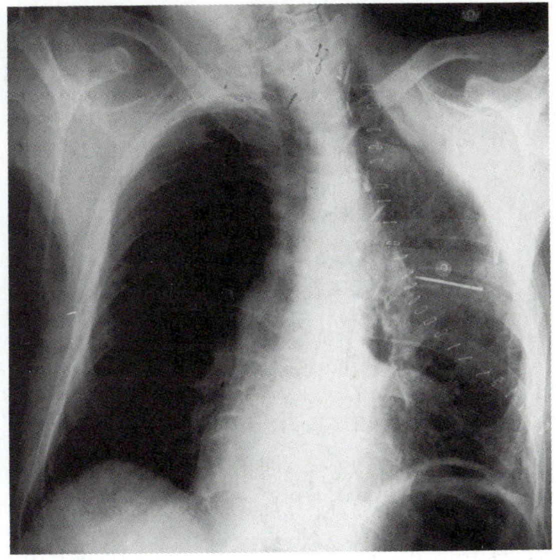

B

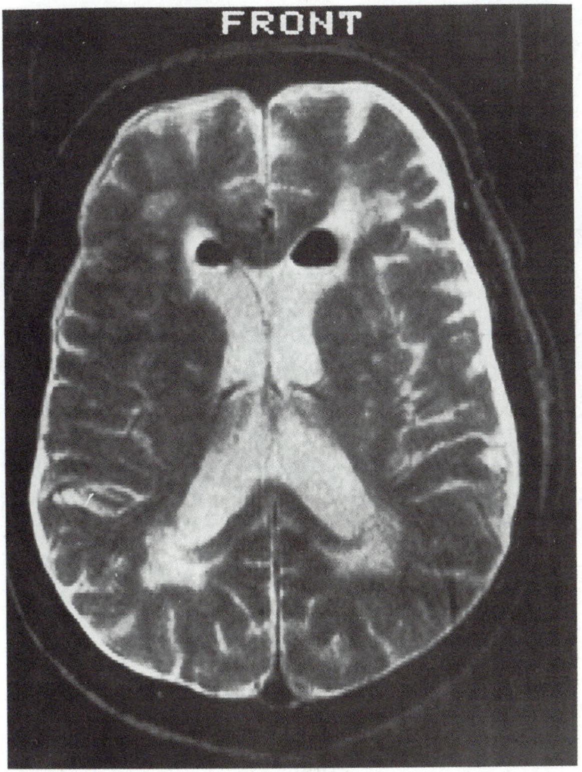


C

**Figure 24–5. A.** Left apex is "clouded" by a superior sulcus tumor. Note the clarity of the right apex above the clavicle. **B.** Chest roentgenogram following enbloc resection of left upper lobe, chest wall, and related structures. **C.** Spinal fluid leak and severe headaches led to MRI, which revealed air in the lateral ventricles. Patient treated by chest tube drainage and antibiotics with resolution of drainage in 4 days.

matically improved. This was the era of thoracoplasty, and these skilled surgeons had no difficulty in combining chest wall resection and lobectomy to radically remove the tumor and the surrounding structures en bloc. Shaw[26] in 1984 reported that this patient was alive 27 years later. Paulson[9] updated the series, which included 131 patients in 1985. Forty-nine patients (38%) were deemed inoperable upon presentation, and three patients refused operation. All 52 patients died within 2 years. Seventy-nine patients completed preoperative irradiation therapy, and 78 underwent radical resection. There were two deaths (2.6%). The 5-year survival was 31%, the 10-year survival was 26%, and the 15-year survival was 22%. Forty-four percent of patients without nodal involvement survived 5 years, 33% survived 10 years, and 30% survived 15 years. No patient who survived 5 years died of recurrent lung cancer. In contrast, only 3 of 17 patients with nodal involvement survived 1 year, and none survived 2 years. Quality of life was excel-

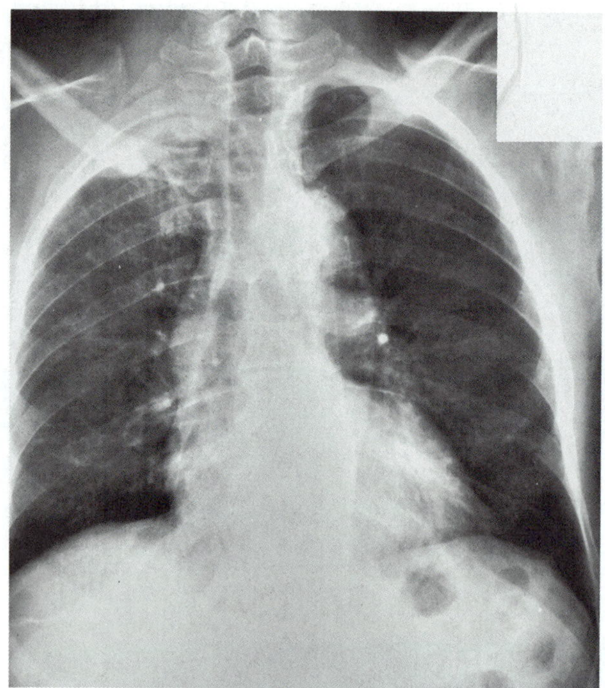

A

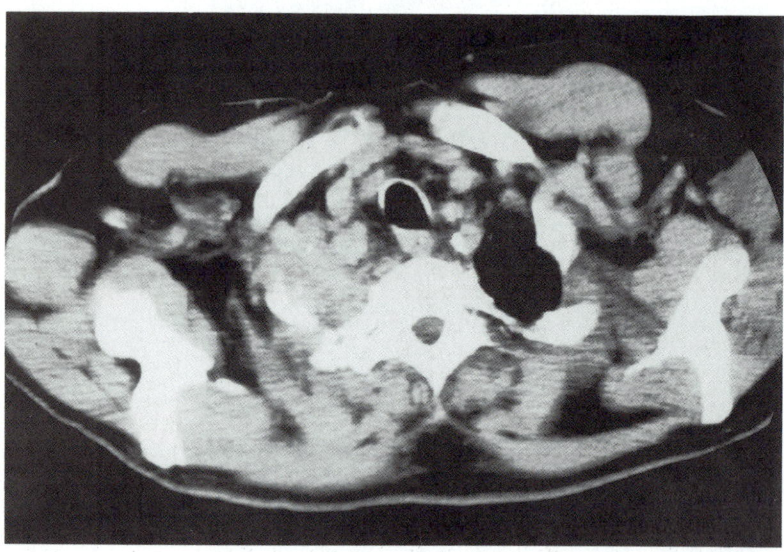

B

**Figure 24–6. A.** Carcinoma of superior sulcus with clouding of the apex and destruction of the first rib. **B.** CT scan filmed on mediastinal windows demonstrates apical mass, vertebral body adjacency, and first-rib involvement.

lent in survivors but was poor in those who died within 3 years because of local recurrence and distant metastasis with accompanying pain and debility. Similar experience has been reported by a number of authors.[27–31]

## OPERATIVE MANAGEMENT

### The Posterior Approach[6,9]

The patient is appropriately monitored for a major thoracic procedure. This includes radial artery cannulation and Swan-Ganz catheterization or a triple-lumen catheter inserted on the side opposite the tumor. Ventilation is carried out through a double-lumen endotracheal tube.

The patient is positioned in the lateral decubitus position with the arm forward and mobile. Cleansing and draping must allow wide access to the lower neck, back, axilla, and chest.

The incision is begun high in the back midway between the spinous process of the second or third vertebrae and the spine of the scapula (Fig. 24–9A,B). The incision is contoured caudally parallel to the medial border of the scapula and is curved forward approximately 2 cm below the tip of the scapula to the anterior axillary line or slightly beyond. The subcutaneous tissues, the latissimus dorsi, the

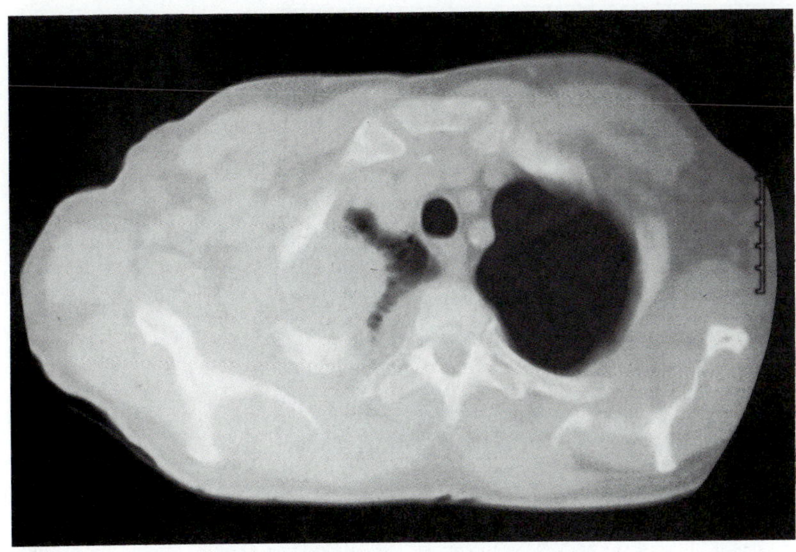

**Figure 24–7.** CT scan filmed on bone windows shows spiculation of tumor reaching to vena cava and subclavian artery and destroying ribs.

lower part of the trapezius, and the rhomboid major muscles are divided in the skin incision plane. The superior portion of the trapezius and the levator scapulae should be preserved; division is not necessary for exposure, and they are important structures for shoulder stabilization.

The scapula is elevated anteriorly and superiorly, and the serratus anterior attachments to the upper ribs are divided. This provides excellent exposure of the apex of the rib cage.

The serratus posterior superior muscle is divided at its attachments to the upper four ribs. The lumbodorsal fascia is incised longitudinally and elevated from the ribs and their transverse processes. The dorsal ligaments and muscles between the upper three ribs and their transverse processes are divided at this time, or this step may be delayed until the ability to resect is assured. If the tumor does not involve the transverse processes, only rib resection is necessary.

The pleural cavity is entered through the third or fourth intercostal space depending upon radiologic identification of rib involvement. Entry should be well anterior of tumor invasion of the chest wall. The intercostal muscle and its neurovascular bundle is preserved for later use.

Ribs two and three and at times four are divided well anterior to the tumor. The first rib is divided at the costochondral junction. Downward traction allows identification and protection of the subclavian vein and artery and division of the scalenus anterior and medius muscles at their attachment to the first rib or higher if invaded by tumor. The lower trunk of the brachial plexus lies posterior to these vascular structures. It is formed by the joining of nerve roots C8 and T1. T2 joins later to form the intercostobrachial nerve. If the patient has a history of pain radiating to the hand, C8 probably is involved, and division of the entire trunk that includes the ulnar nerve distal to the tumor is indicated. If there is any doubt of C8 involvement, this step is deferred, since it is possible to separate the upper and lower portions of the trunk if only the lower portion is invaded.

Attention is directed posteriorly. The transverse process of the lower most rib to be resected is denuded and divided with rib shears flush with the vertebral body. The rib cage flap and its attached transverse process can be elevated to expose and allow clipping and division of the intercostal vessels and nerve. Care must be taken not to retract the nerve roots during this process.

This procedure is repeated upward to the first rib. The posterior scalenus muscle attachments and other ligamentous structures to this rib are divided. The large first intercostal nerve and its accompanying vessels lie beneath. The dura may extend along this nerve root, and spinal fluid leakage is a possibility. Again, care must be taken not to place undue tension on this structure as it is divided. Nerve T8 lies above and is divided if involved. If not involved, it is traced distally, and only the lower portion of the combined trunk is included in the resection.

Dissection of the tumor from the subclavian artery usually can be accomplished in the subadventitial plane. Because of its course, the internal mammary artery may require ligation and division but usually is sufficiently medial and can be preserved. The thyrocervical trunk may be sacrificed if invaded. Resection and grafting rarely are indicated but can be accomplished. Ribbed Gortex grafts #6 or #8 are appropriate. The remaining fascial structures and the stellate ganglion are divided, freeing the tumor and chest wall from above.

If necessary, the tumor is dissected from the vertebral bodies with an osteotome. Preoperative MRI should determine the extent of involvement of the vertebrae. Operation is not indicated if invasion is more than superficial or if the foramina are involved. Approximately one quarter of a vertebral body can be removed without reducing structural integrity. Bleeding from cancellous bone is controlled with hemostatic materials. The foramina must not be packed because of the possibility of transverse myelitis. Bleeding can be controlled by gentle pressure and by specific-point, low-voltage coagulation outside of the canal.

Remaining is a pulmonary resection of appropriate magnitude. Most authors prefer lobectomy, but satisfactory

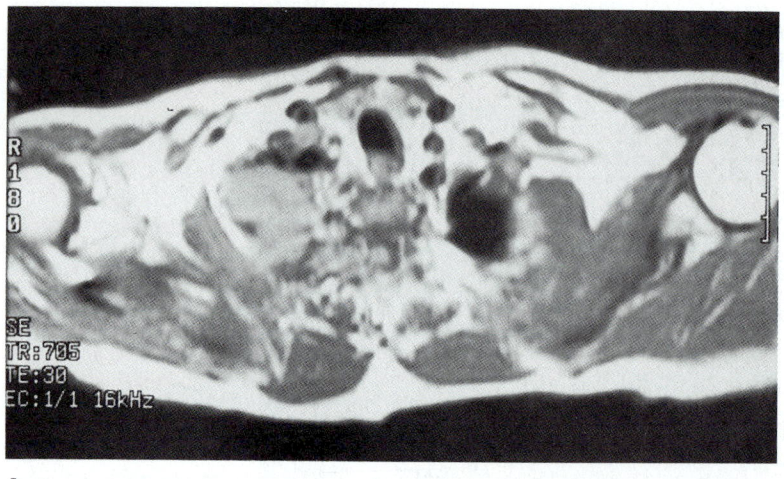


A

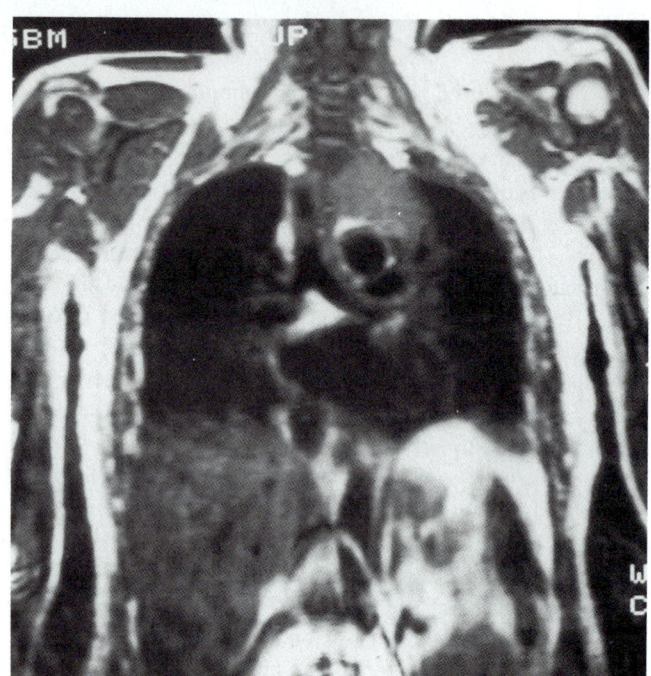

B

**Figure 24–8.** **A.** MRI: T1-spin echo axial image show apical tumor with vascular and vertebral body invasion. **B.** MRI: T1-spin echo coronal image shows apical tumor involving subclavian artery, brachial plexus, and vertebral bodies.

results have been obtained from segmental resection. Since lobectomy has the better chance of removing involved lymphatics, this seems the better procedure and can be performed readily through the defect produced by the chest wall excision.

Closure is not difficult. The defect for the most part is posterior and is obliterated by the scapula and its muscular attachments. Consideration has been given to suture of the posterior serratus to the uppermost rib and to the use of plastic mesh to close the defect—neither has gained much favor. Two chest tubes are inserted, one in the apex, but away from the vessels and one in the posterior gutter. Absorbable sutures are used for closure.

Mortality from resection has approximated 3%. Morbidity is that from pulmonary and chest wall resection and those unique occurrences from the procedure. Atelectasis is common with chest wall resection and requires constant surveillance and attention to pulmonary toilet. Bronchoscopy is frequently required. Chest wall pain is severe but is reduced significantly by epidural analgesia. Air leaks usually are nonconsequential; however, air leaks in association with spinal fluid leakage may lead to pneumoencephally, which results in severe headaches (Fig. 24–5C) Paulson reported five instances of spinal cord leakage, two of which led to meningitis. With proper chest tube drainage, most spinal cord leaks will stop, but rarely muscle plasty is required. When spinal cord leakage is identified intraoperatively, the foramina should not be packed with hemostatic material, but rather an intercostal muscle flap should be placed over the area. There is, of course, loss of neurologic function from resection of nerves. This is reasonably well tolerated, and the defect is not so severe if the eighth cervical nerve can be preserved. Horner's syndrome is common as a presenting sign and symptom complex and is present

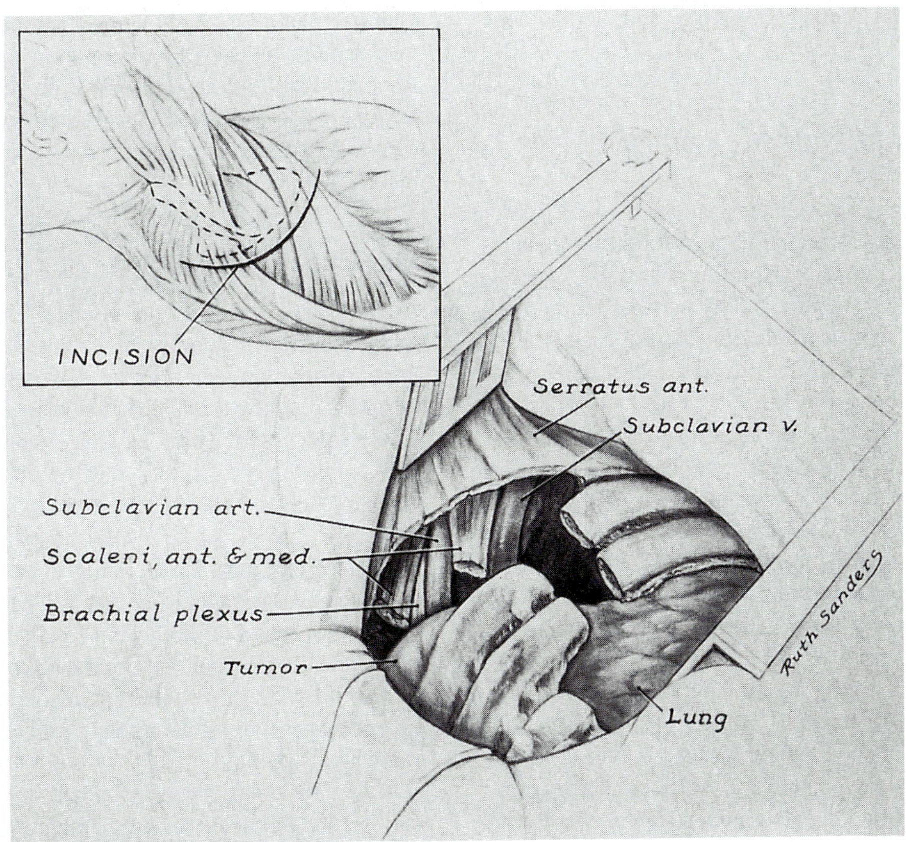


**A**

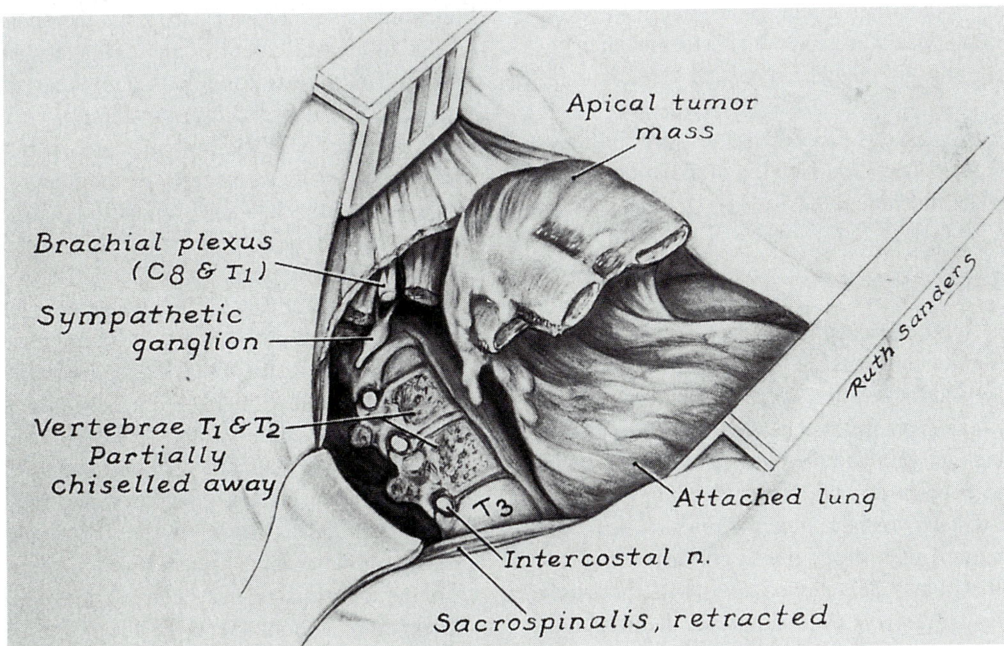


**B**

**Figure 24–9. A.** Incision and anterior exposure for extended en bloc resection of a carcinoma in the right superior pulmonary sulcus. The first three ribs are divided anteriorly; the muscular attachments to the first and second ribs are separated, and the subclavian vessels and brachial plexus are exposed. *(From Shaw RR, Paulson DL, Kee JL Jr: Treatment of the superior sulcus tumor by irradiation followed by resection. Ann Surg 154:29, 1961, with permission.)* **B.** Posterior aspect of en bloc resection of the chest wall and tumor, together with the lower root of the brachial plexus, the sympathetic chain, intercostal nerves, and parts of vertebrae. *(From Shaw RR, Paulson DL, Kee JL Jr: Treatment of the superior sulcus tumor by irradiation followed by resection. Ann Surg 154:29, 1961, with permission.)*

postoperatively from stellate ganglion and sympathetic trunk resection.

## ANTERIOR TRANSCERVICAL APPROACH

Philippe Dartevelle and associates[18] at the Hôpital Marie-Lannelougue of the Paris-Sud University describe an anterior transcervical approach to the thoracic outlet used to resect superior sulcus tumors in 29 patients from 1980 through 1991. Preoperative irradiation was not used.

It has long been recognized that cervical structures invaded by these tumors are difficult to expose and deal with through the classic posterior thoracotomy. The anterior cervical approach gives excellent exposure of the area and facilitates resection of these tumors and reconstruction of the vascular structures (Fig. 24–10A–D). Combined with the posterior approach in two thirds of patients, a more complete resection can be carried out.

The patient is positioned supine with the neck extended and the head turned away from the operative side. The incision extends along the anterior border of the sternocleidomastoid muscle and is curved below the medial half of the clavicle. The sternocleidomastoid muscle is detached from the clavicle, and the myocutaneous flap formed is dissected free and rotated laterally and superiorly, exposing the cervical area. The scalene fat pad is examined for nodal metastasis and dissected. The superior mediastinum is assessed, and the cervical extent of the tumor is determined. If resection appears possible, the costoclavicular ligament is divided, and the medial half of the clavicle is removed.

Dartevelle divides the procedure into three phases: (1) dissection of the veins, (2) dissection of the arteries, and (3) dissection of the brachial plexus.

### Dissection of the Veins

The jugular and subclavian veins are freed from the surrounding tissues and their branches ligated and divided. The jugular vein is divided above the junction with the subclavian vein. This maneuver gives access to the posterior aspect of the subclavian vein and the thoracic duct and vertebral vein. If the subclavian vein is invaded, it is divided proximally and distally to the tumor for removal with the specimen. The tumor may invade the origin of the innominate vein, which also may be removed along with the specimen. On the left, the thoracic duct should be identified and ligated. This dissection exposes the cupula of the thorax.

### Dissection of the Arteries

The subclavian artery is exposed and isolated following division of the anterior scalene muscle. The phrenic nerve should be preserved during these maneuvers unless it is invaded by tumor, in which case it is sacrificed. The subadventitial plane is sought and developed if possible. This may require division of the internal mammary artery, the thyrocervical trunk, and at times the vertebral artery. If the tumor invades the vessel, a portion may be resected and continuity reestablished by primary anastomosis or by graft reconstruction.

### Dissection of the Nerves

Attention is directed to the brachial plexus. The extent of tumor invasion is determined. Exposure may be excellent if the tumor is more anterior and dissection is readily accomplished from lateral branches to the medial trunk and roots. If necessary and if possible, nerve roots C8 and T1 are divided proximally. This step may be difficult from the anterior approach and may best be carried out through the thoracotomy.

The trunk beyond the tumor is isolated and is divided or tagged for later identification and partial or complete division. The vertebral bodies are easily exposed, and, when necessary, the tumor is separated with the osteotome. Dartevelle believes vertebral invasion is a contraindication to operation. The stellate ganglion and the sympathetic chain are divided.

The first and second ribs are divided anteriorly and may be divided posteriorly by extending the incision in the delto-pectoral grove for additional exposure. Division of the medial scalene muscle facilitates the removal of the ribs either at this time or later during the thoracotomy approach.

If the tumor extent is predominately anterior or anterior and lateral, it is possible to completely remove it and a portion of the lung through the anterior cervical approach. Once the anterior portion of ribs one and two are removed, excellent exposure of the apex of the lung for stapler resection is achieved. For those tumors that are posterior or medial and abut or invade the vertebrae, a posterior thoracotomy usually is necessary to complete the resection.

The major advantage of the anterior approach is the ability to deal with invasion of the subclavian vein and artery and related structures. It is not an effective approach to those tumors that invade the posterior aspects of the ribs and their transverse processes, the stellate ganglion and sympathetic chain and the vertebral bodies, and which produce the classic Pancoast-Tobias syndrome. Dartevelle indicates that as experience with this technique has been gained, more extensive resection of the chest wall with posterior tumor excision has been carried out with excellent success and without the need for posterior thoracotomy. The time required to perform this procedure particularly when combined with thoracotomy is a major disadvantage. Phrenic paralysis is a hazard. Results in this highly select group of patients have been impressive. Twenty-five of 29 patients (86%) were treated with postoperative irradiation, and 11 of those received adjunctive chemotherapy. Fifty percent have survived 2 years, and 31% have survived 5 years.

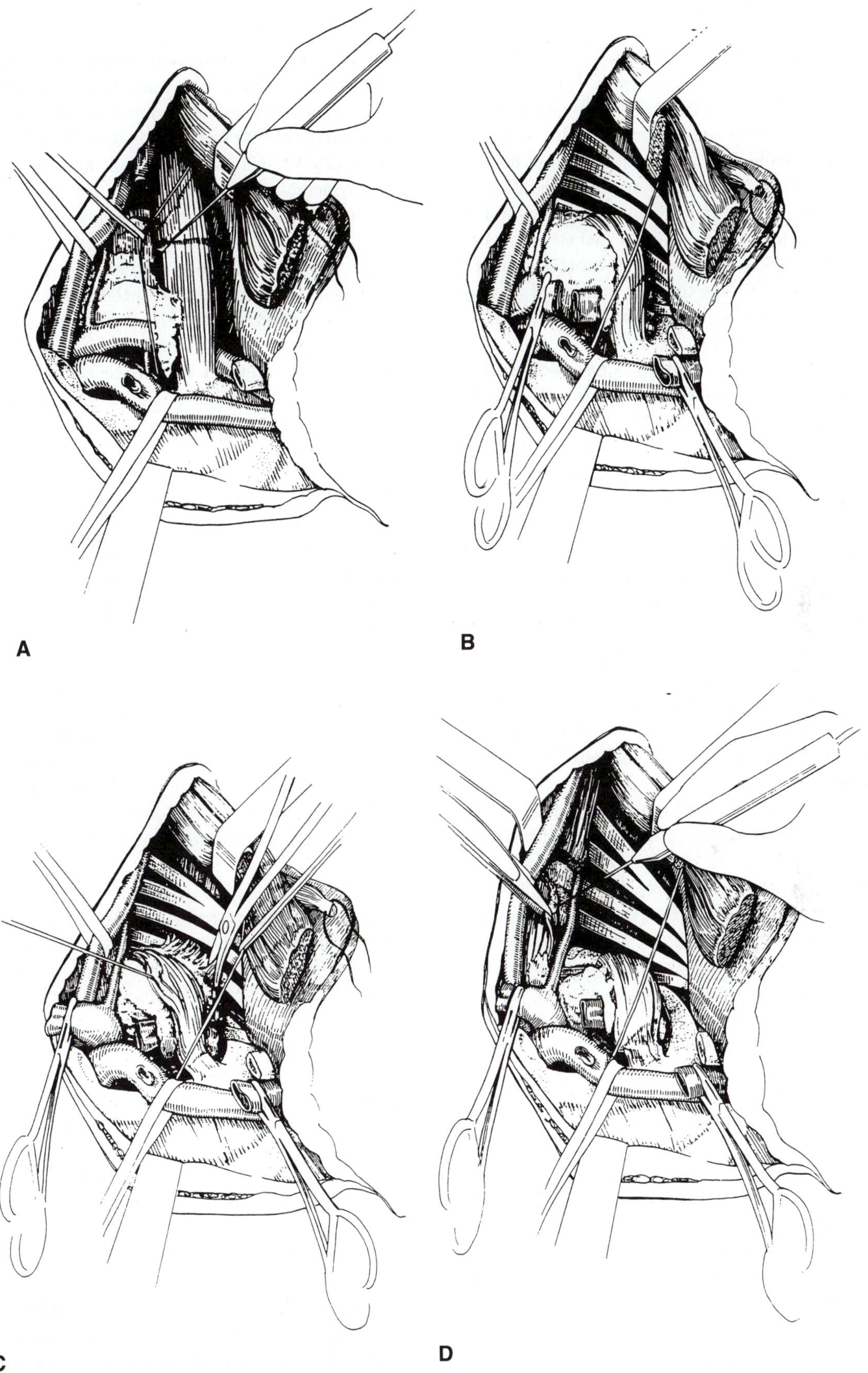


**Figure 24–10.** **A.** Exposure of subclavian artery after division of insertion of anterior scalenus muscle on first rib. **B.** Subclavian artery can be freed from tumor by dividing all collateral branches (vertebral artery is generally preserved if not invaded), and, if involved, it can be divided proximally and distally. **C.** The spread of tumor to brachial plexus requires an "out-in side" neurolysis if upper nerve roots are involved or a resection of T-1 if lower trunk or nerve roots are involved. **D.** Vertebral artery can be freed from tumor, prevertebral muscles detached from vertebral bodies, and both stellate ganglion and sympathetic chain isolated and eventually resected. *(From Dartevelle PG, Chapelier AR, Macchiarini P, et al: Anterior transcervical-thoracic approach for radical resection of lung tumors invading the thoracic inlet. J Thorac Cardiovasc Surg 105:1025–1034, 1993.)*

## RADIATION THERAPY

Pancoast reported that radiation therapy was not effective in the treatment of superior sulcus tumors. This belief undoubtedly related to the imprecise methodology of the time. Haas and associates in 1954 clearly demonstrated the value of therapy using high-dosage irradiation over a wide field. Patients treated with a 23-MeV betatron had an average survival of 32.4 months compared with 7.5 months in patients treated by conventional x-ray therapy. Pain relief was consistent, but complication rates were high because of the extremely high dosages used.

Subsequently, a number of authors have demonstrated the effectiveness of high-dosage radiotherapy. Kowaki and colleagues at the Medical College of Wisconsin reported 36 patients treated by external irradiation only between 1963 and 1977.[32] Between 1978 and 1983, an additional 32 patients were evaluated.[33] Sixty-five of the 68 patients had a histologic diagnosis. Fifty-five patients presented with pain in the shoulder, arm, or chest; 20 had evidence of mediastinal node involvement; and 14 had evidence of rib or vertebral body erosion. Ten patients had stage II disease T1 or T2, N1, M0 but either refused surgery or had medical reasons for inoperability.

All but five patients were treated by supervoltage photon external irradiation. The medium dose was 6000 cGy in 30 fractions over 6 weeks. Computed tomography of the thorax was routinely used for treatment planning and assessment from 1979 on.

Relief of pain was achieved in 91% of patients. Seven of 10 patients with bony metastasis recalcified their lesions. Disease-free survival was 65%, 38%, 25%, and 15% at 12, 24, 36, and 48 months, respectively. No patient survived longer than 24 months if the primary tumor was not controlled. The most common site of recurrence was the brain with 23 patients (34%) suffering cerebral metastasis. Prophylactic cerebral radiotherapy may be justified if local control is achieved particularly if the histologic diagnosis is adeno- or large-cell carcinoma.

## PREOPERATIVE IRRADIATION

Many reports, including those of Shaw and Paulson, demonstrate the efficacy of preoperative irradiation therapy.[27–34] Hilaris et al[35] reported the results of treatment of Pancoast tumors at the Memorial Sloan-Kettering Cancer Center. Survival of 82 patients who received preoperative irradiation and 46 patients who did not were compared by multivariate analysis. Those patients with negative mediastinal nodes who received preoperative irradiation had a 34% 5-year survival rate compared with 21% for those not treated. Patients with positive mediastinal nodes had a better prognosis when treated than those not treated: 15% vs. 8% 5-year survival.

Ginsberg et al[36] updated this series through 1991 paying particular attention to intraoperative brachytherapy. Only those patients who came to thoracotomy were analyzed. One hundred and twenty-six patients underwent thoracotomy, and 100 were resected; 117 received pre- and/or postoperative external beam radiation, and 102 received brachytherapy. Sixty-nine (56%) had complete resection, 49 of whom received brachytherapy. The 5-year survival was 41%. Lobectomy was performed in 22 patients, and a large wedge resection was performed in 47. The 5-year survival rate for lobectomy was 60% compared to 33% for wedge resection, figures that approach statistical significance ($P = .06$). Intraoperative brachytherapy had no influence on loco-regional recurrence or survival in patients with completely resected tumors. The overall survival in 55 patients with no or incomplete resection was 9%. Brachytherapy was carried out in 53. Survival was the same whether no or incomplete resection was performed.

Several adverse prognostic factors were identified. These included Horner's syndrome (4 of 30 surviving 5 years), N2 disease (0 of 21 surviving 5 years), and N3 supraclavicular disease (1 of 7 surviving 5 years). In patients with vertebral body invasion (T4 disease), only 2 of 22 survived 5 years and both were among the 14 patients undergoing complete resection of the vertebral component.

This series indicates that complete resection (specifically lobectomy) in those patients treated with preoperative irradiation is the most important prognostic sign. Furthermore, some patients in whom no or incomplete resection is performed can be cured by irradiation and brachytherapy. Of interest are the similar cure rates noted by Kowaki et al[32] and by Van Houtte[37] in patients treated for cure with external irradiation.

It appears that if a patient does not have a resectable tumor as determined by CT scan or MRI, external irradiation is in order. Brachytherapy may be of value in those patients who are explored and in whom only incomplete resection can be accomplished, but the evidence is not compelling.

## POSTOPERATIVE IRRADIATION

The value of postoperative irradiation is unclear, but this modality is used with great frequency and is an integral part of many treatment schemes for lung cancer, including superior sulcus tumors. The University of Maryland series reported by Attar et al[11] is unique. Five patients with T3 and M0 disease underwent extended resection only. Four had N0 disease, and one had N1 disease. The patient with N1 disease died of metastasis at 10 months. One patient died at 3 years of undetermined cause. There were three survivors at 2.6 years, 7.5 years, and 9.5 years. These results in this small segment of a larger series raises the question: Is postoperative irradiation of value when complete resection is carried out? There are no comparable series, but one can draw inferences from the literature.

Van Houtte and colleagues[38] conducted a controlled clinical study comparing patients with lung cancer who underwent complete resection and were found to have no lymphatic metastasis and no tumor beyond the lungs. These patients were randomized to receive 6000 cGy over 6 weeks or no irradiation therapy. The surgery-only group had a 43% 5-year survival compared with 24% survival in the group treated with radiation. These results strongly suggest that postoperative irradiation is not indicated for patients in whom complete resection is carried out and in whom negative nodes are found.

Green et al,[39] Kirsch et al,[40] and Chung et al[41] in retrospective studies demonstrated a statistically significant benefit from postoperative irradiation in patients in whom nodal metastasis was identified.

The report by the Lung Cancer Study Group indicates that there is no survival benefit from postoperative radiotherapy in completely resected patients with nodal metastasis from squamous cell cancer.[42] However, postoperative radiation did significantly decrease the incidence of local (intrathoracic) recurrence. In the Memorial series reported by Ginsberg, postoperative irradiation following immediate operation and brachytherapy was as effective as preoperative irradiation and brachytherapy in achieving complete resection, loco-regional control, and ultimate curability. Dartevelle believes that preoperative irradiation is unnecessary when using the anterior transcervical thoracic approach but routinely prescribes postoperative irradiation "because of the fear of late local relapse." He notes that a majority of patients suffer systemic relapse and suggests that effective chemotherapy would be more important in the long term.

Shahian et al[43] and Ellis report 18 patients treated by preoperative irradiation and en bloc operation. Fourteen were treated with additional irradiation postoperatively because of positive nodes and/or residual tumor at the margins of the resections. No deaths accompanied operation, and 56% of the patients lived 5 years. These authors suggest that the use of postoperative irradiation in patients with residual tumor achieve results comparable to those in whom margins are clear.

## CHEMOTHERAPY AND INDUCTION THERAPY

There are no series of comparable groups of patients treated with or without chemotherapy, but many surgeons in recent years indicate the use of chemotherapy in combination with radiotherapy and/or surgical resection in the treatment of Pancoasts' tumor. Ginsberg et al[36] notes that 10 patients in the Memorial series who were treated preoperatively with platinum-based chemotherapy fared poorly, with no long-term disease-free survivors. Dartevelle suggests that chemotherapy is important but gives no data on its use. We have adopted a protocol of induction therapy that combines preoperative chemotherapy with cisplatin and 5-fluorouracil with preoperative radiotherapy and radical resection based upon the encouraging results with this type of treatment modality in other invasive lung cancers.[44–46] Whether this is the proper course is speculative, but methods based upon results in well-conducted trials of similar if not exact entities seem appropriate for a disease with such devastating consequences.

## SUMMARY

Pancoast's tumor usually is an epithelial bronchogenic carcinoma of the extreme apex of the lung that invades the adjacent structures. The presenting symptom is pain that may become devastating.

Treatment by preoperative irradiation and radical en bloc resection has produced the best results. The anterior transcervical-thoracic approach has added a new dimension for dealing with subclavian vessel and brachial plexus involvement. High-voltage irradiation is effective in relieving pain and may cure patients not suitable for operation, but it has not proven nearly so effective as combination therapy including surgery.

Methodologies using combinations of irradiation, chemotherapy, and operation, adopted from treatment schemes for other lung and similar cancers, currently are being applied.

## REFERENCES


1. Hare ES: Tumor involving certain nerves. *London Med Gas* **1**:16–18, 1838
2. Pancoast HK: Superior pulmonary sulcus tumor. *JAMA* **99:** 1391–1396, 1932
3. Walker JE: Superior sulcus pulmonary tumors (Pancoast syndrome). *J Med Assoc Ga* **35**:364–365, 1946
4. Chardack WM, MacCallum JD: Pancoast syndrome due to bronchogenic carcinoma: Successful surgical removal and postoperative irradiation. *J Thorac Surg* **25**:402–412, 1953
5. Haas LL, Harvey RA, Langer SS: Radiation management of otherwise hopeless thoracic neoplasms. *JAMA* **154**:323–326, 1954
6. Shaw RR, Paulson DL, Kee JL: Treatment of the superior sulcus tumor by irradiation followed by resection. *Ann Surg* **154**:29–40, 1961
7. Pancoast HK: Importance of careful roentgenray investigation of apical chest tumors. *JAMA* **83**:1407–1411, 1924
8. Tobias JW: Sindrome apico-costo-vertebral dolorosa por tumor, apexiano. Su valor diagnostico en el cancer primitivo pulmonar. *Rev Med Lat Am* **19**:1522–1556, 1932
9. Paulson DL: Technical considerations in stage III disease: The "superior sulcus" lesion. In Delarue NC, Eschapasse H (eds): *International Trends in General Thoracic Surgery,* Vol I. Philadelphia, Saunders, 1985, pp 121–133.
10. Ziporyn T: Upper body pain: Possible tipoff to Pancoast tumor. *JAMA* **246**:1759–1763, 1981
11. Attar S, Miller JE, Satterfield J, et al: Pancoast's tumor: Irradiation or surgery? *Ann Thorac Surg* **28**:578–586, 1979
12. Johnson DH, Hainsworth JD, Greco FA: Pancoast's syndrome and small cell lung cancer. *Chest* **82**:602–606, 1982

13. Eiben C, Indihan FJ, Hunter SW: Thoracic actinomyocosis mimicking the Pancoast syndrome. *Minn Med* **66:**541–544, 1983
14. Chen KTK, Padmanabhan A: Pancoast syndrome caused by extramedullary plasmacytoma. *J Surg Oncol* **24:**117–118, 1983
15. Chong KM, Lennox SC, Sheppard MN: Primary hemangiopericytoma presenting as a Pancoast tumor. *Ann Thorac Surg* **55:**518–519, 1993
16. McGoon DC: Transcervical technique for removal of specimen from superior sulcus tumor for pathologic study. *Ann Surg* **159:**407–410, 1964
17. Paulson DL, Weed TE, Rian RL: Cervical approach for percutaneous needle biopsy of Pancoast tumors. *Ann Thorac Surg* **39:**586–587, 1985
18. Dartevelle PG, Chapelier AR, Macchiarini P, et al: Anterior transcervical-thoracic approach for radical resection of lung tumors invading the thoracic inlet. *J Thorac Cardiovasc Surg* **105:**1025–1034, 1993
19. Hilaris BS, Martini N, Luomanen RKJ, et al: The value of preoperative radiation therapy in apical cancer of the lung. *Surg Clin North Am* **54:**831–840, 1974
20. Kowaki R, Mountain CF, Holbert JM et al: Superior sulcus tumors: Treatment selection and results for 85 patients without metastasis (MO) at presentation. *Int J Radiat Oncol Biol Phys* **19:**31–36, 1990
21. Webb WR, Jeffrey RB, Godwin JD: Thoracic computed tomography in superior sulcus tumors. *J Computed Assist Tomogr* **5:**361–365, 1981
22. Breyer RH, Karstaedt N, Mills SA, et al: Computed tomography for evaluation of mediastinal lymph nodes in lung cancer: Correlation with surgical staging. *Ann Thorac Surg* **38:**215–220, 1984
23. Libshitz HI: CT of mediastinal lymph nodes in lung cancer: Is there a "state of the art"? (editorial). *AJR A J Roentgenol* **141:**1081–1085, 1983
24. Glazer GM, Orringer MB, Gross BH, et al: The mediastinum in non-small cell lung cancer: CT-surgical correlation. *AJR Am J Roetgenol* **142:**1101–1105, 1984
25. Heelan RT, Demas BE, Caravelli JF et al: Superior sulcus tumor: CT and MR imaging. *Radiology* **170:**637–641, 1989
26. Shaw RR: Pancoast's tumor. *Ann Thorac Surg* **37:**343–344, 1984
27. Miller JI, Mansour KA, Hatcher CR: Carcinoma of the superior pulmonary sulcus. *Ann Thorac Surg* **28:**44–47, 1979
28. Kirsh MN, Dickerman R, Fayos J, et al: Value of chest wall resection in the treatment of superior sulcus tumors of the lung. *Ann Thorac Surg* **15:**339–346, 1973
29. Wright CD, Moncure AC, Shepard JO, et al: Superior sulcus lung tumors. *J Thorac Cardiovasc Surg* **94:**69–74, 1987
30. Sartori F, Rea F, Calabro F, et al: Carcinoma of the superior pulmonary sulcus: Results of irradiation and radical resection. *J Thorac Cardiovasc Surg* **104:**679–683, 1992
31. Mathisen DJ, Grillo HC, Wright CD, et al: Superior sulcus tumors: Results of combined treatment (irradiation and radical resection). *J Thorac Cardiovasc Surg* **94:**69–74, 1987
32. Kowaki R, Roh J, Cox J, et al. Superior sulcus tumors: Results of irradiation of 36 patients. *Cancer* **48:**1563–1568, 1981
33. Grover FL, Kowaki R: Superior sulcus tumors. In: Roth JA, Ruckdeschel JC, Weisenberger TH (eds): *Thoracic Oncology.* Philadelphia, Saunders, 1994
34. Fuller DB, Chambers JS: Superior sulcus tumors: Combined modality *Ann Thorac Surg* **57:**1133–1139, 1994
35. Hilaris BS, Martini N, Wong GY, Dattatreyudu N: Treatment of superior sulcus tumor (Pancoast tumor). *Surg Clin North Am* **67:**965–977, 1987
36. Ginsberg RJ, Martini N, Zaman M, et al: The influence of surgical resection and intraoperative brachytherapy in the management of superior sulcus tumor. *Ann Thorac Surg* **57:**1440–1445, 1994
37. Van Houtte P, MacLennan I, Poulter C, et al: External radiation in the management of superior sulcus tumor. *Cancer* **54:**223–227, 1984
38. Van Houtte P, Rocmans P, Smets P, et al: Post operative radiation therapy in lung cancer: A controlled trial after resection of curative design. *Int J Radiat Oncol Biol Phys* **6:**983–986, 1980
39. Green N, Kurohara SS, George FW III, et al: Postresection irradiation for primary lung cancer. *Radiology* **116:**405–407, 1975
40. Kirsch MM, Sloan H: Mediastinal metastases in bronchogenic carcinoma: Influence of postoperative irradiation, cell type, and location. *Ann Thorac Surg* **33:**459–463, 1982
41. Chung CK, Stryker JA, O'Neill M Jr, et al: Evaluation of adjuvant postoperative radiotherapy for lung cancer. *Int J Radiat Oncol Biol Phys* **8:**1877–1880, 1982
42. The Lung Cancer Study Group: Effects of postoperative mediastinal radiation on completely resected stage II and stage III epidermoid cancer of the lung. *N Engl J Med* **315:**1377–1381, 1986
43. Shahian DM, Neptune WB, Ellis FH: Pancoast tumors: Improved survival with preoperative and postoperative radiotherapy. *Ann Thorac Surg* **43:**32–38, 1987
44. Martini N, Kris MG, Flehinger BJ, et al: Preoperative chemotherapy for stage IIIa (N2) lung cancer: The Sloan-Kettering experience with 136 patients. *Ann Thorac Surg* **55:**1365–1374, 1993
45. Rusch VW, Albain KS, Crowley JJ, et al: Surgical resection of stage IIIA and stage IIIB non-small cell lung cancer after concurrent induction chemoradiotherapy: A Southwest Oncology Group Trial. *J Thorac Cardiovasc Surg* **105:**97–106, 1993
47. Faber LP, Kittle CF, Warren WH, et al. Preoperative chemotherapy and irradiation for stage III non-small cell lung cancer. *Ann Thorac Surg* **47:**669–677, 1989

CHAPTER

# 25

# Limited Pulmonary Resection

Jonathan Somers and L. Penfield Faber

Any pulmonary resection in which less than a complete lobe is removed is properly termed a *limited pulmonary resection.* The two procedures best fitting this definition are segmentectomy and wedge resection. A segmentectomy is an anatomic pulmonary resection of the pulmonary artery, vein, bronchus, and parenchyma of a particular segment of the lung. Alternatively, a wedge resection is a nonanatomic removal of a portion of lung parenchyma that may or may not traverse segmental planes. These two procedures are currently used in the treatment and diagnosis of a variety of disease processes including bacterial and fungal infections, tuberculosis, and bronchiectasis. They are also used for the resection of primary lung cancers, second and third primary lung cancers, and tumors metastatic to the lung when conservation of lung tissue is important. Limited pulmonary resection for early-stage primary bronchogenic carcinoma in noncompromised patients remains controversial, and thoracic surgeons must be aware of the stated advantages and disadvantages.

## HISTORICAL ASPECTS

At approximately the same time Graham and Singer[1] performed the first successful pneumonectomy for bronchogenic carcinoma using the mass ligation technique, a variety of lesser pulmonary resections were also in use. The procedures were done mostly for inflammatory disease. In 1939 Churchill and Belsey[2] described 44 resections of the lingula in connection with left lower lobectomy for bronchiectasis. In this era of mass ligation, it is interesting to note that the author's described technique of segmentectomy included individual ligation of the bronchus, pulmonary artery, and vein. These authors stated that "the bronchopulmonary segment may replace the lobe as the surgical unit of the lung." In 1942 Kent and Blades[3] detailed the technical steps necessary to accomplish a lobectomy. Five years later, Overholt and Langer[4] described segmental resection for bronchiectasis, and shortly after this, Chamberlain et al[5] reported 300 segmentectomies for tuberculosis.

Although many felt that limited resection was acceptable treatment for diseases of inflammatory or infectious nature, there was resistance to the concept that segmentectomy would be applicable to a pulmonary malignancy. Reinhoff[6] stated in 1944 that "the only efficacious method for treatment of pulmonary carcinoma is by surgical removal of the entire organ together with the regional lymphatic nodes." Ochsner and DeBakey[7] also stated that "treatment of pulmonary malignancy consists of total extirpation of the involved lung." As technical familiarity with the hilar structures became more widespread, thoracic surgeons would occasionally apply the techniques of segmentectomy to primary and secondary malignancies. Review of Overholt et al's[8] report on a 42-year experience with resection of primary cancer of the lung reveals that a small percentage of resections from 1932 to 1944 were segmentectomies. In 1956 Thomas[9] reported on three patients with carcinoma of the lung who had segmental resection and he described the advantages of a conservative resection. In 1963 Rasmussen et al[10] reported on 17 patients who had a limited resection for lung cancer; the sole criterion for this procedure was the poor clinical status of the patient. Similarly, poor cardiopulmonary reserve and advanced age were the criteria used for patient selection in a series of 18 patients reported by Bonril-Roberts and Clagett.[11] Although the limited resection had gained some acceptance as a treatment for metastatic cancers,[12,13] few accepted it as a treatment for primary bronchogenic carcinoma.

In 1972 LeRoux[14] described 17 patients with primary lung cancer managed by segmental resection, and he noted that the time of survival and pattern of recurrence was no different from those managed by a more extensive resection. In 1973 Jensik et al[15] described 123 patients who were treated with segmental resection for bronchogenic carcinoma, many of whom survived for 5 to 10 years. Over the past two decades, there have been many additional reports of both segmental and wedge resections for primary bronchogenic carcinoma,[16–24] and the role of these procedures in the treatment of lung cancer is becoming better understood.

## INDICATIONS FOR LIMITED RESECTION

The limited pulmonary resection is currently used for a variety of infectious and neoplastic diseases. While the indications are clear and widely accepted for benign processes, they are less clear for primary, secondary, and metastatic malignancies.

Consideration for a limited resection begins with the history. Decreased exercise capability, smoking history, bronchitis, and use of bronchodilators and steroids are all indicators of a decreased pulmonary reserve. Symptoms of angina pectoris, the occurrence of a prior myocardial infarction, age, prior pulmonary resection, and general physical well-being are also factors that must be considered when one is selecting the appropriate procedure for an individual patient.

On chest x-ray, a small peripheral lesion alerts the surgeon to the possibility of limited resection. The computed tomography (CT) scan allows clinical staging and confirms the solitary, peripheral location and depicts the presence or absence of enlarged regional lymph nodes (Fig. 25–1). The

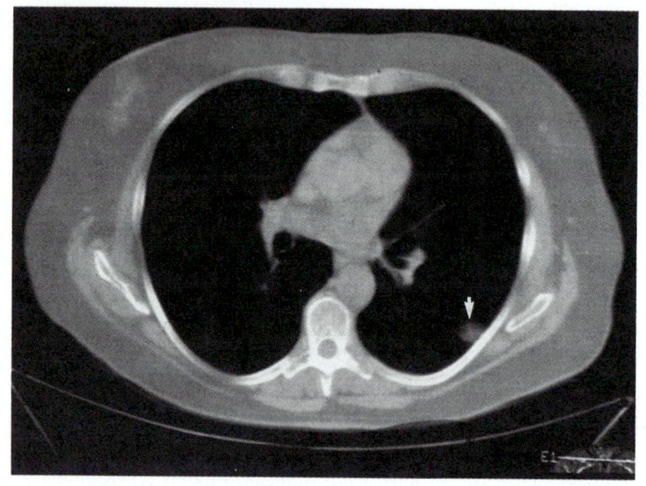

**A**

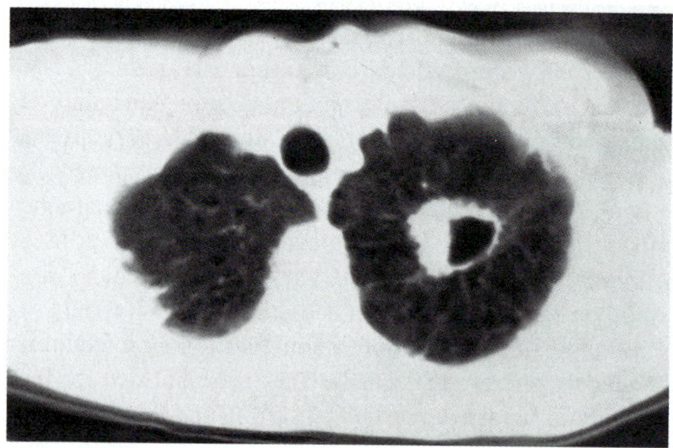

**B**

**C**

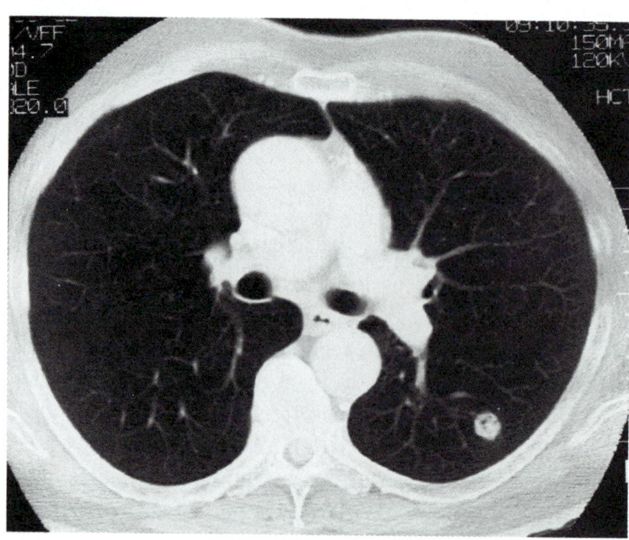

**D**

**Figure 25–1.** CT scans of four different lung cancers having a limited resection: (**A**): superior segmentectomy. (**B**): apico-posterior segmentectomy. (**C**): anterior segmentectomy. (**D**): superior segmentectomy.

major and minors fissures can frequently be identified on the CT scan, and when the lesion is correlated with the known anatomic boundaries of the pulmonary segments, it can be determined whether a segmental or wedge resection is feasible. Centrally located lesions usually, but not always, require lobectomy. More than one segment of a lobe can be removed to accomplish an adequate resection. Lymph nodes >1 cm in diameter in the mediastinum on CT scan are evaluated by mediastinoscopy. Nodal metastasis is a relative contraindication for limited pulmonary resection since lobar node dissection is limited with segmentectomy. Rarely, segmentectomy in conjunction with adjuvant therapy may be considered in this situation if lobectomy is clearly contraindicated because of high risk.

Fiberoptic bronchoscopy is done prior to every planned segmentectomy, despite the fact that a diagnosis of cancer is made infrequently by brushing or transbronchial biopsy. Segmental anatomy is noted, and a synchronous second primary cancer is ruled out. The procedure is usually done following intubation and must prior to thoracotomy.

Screening spirometry should be carried out if there is any dyspnea on exertion, long smoking history, treatment for asthma, or cardiac problems. Arterial blood gases are obtained if spirometry places the patient in a moderate or high-risk group (Table 25–1). Pulmonary function values and arterial blood gas results that would indicate the need for consideration of a limited pulmonary resection are discussed in detail in Chapter 1. While various criteria for determining inoperability have been published,[25–29] few have specifically addressed the issue of criteria for the use of limited resection. Miller et al[26] concluded that "the minimum criteria for elective wedge or segmental resection are a maximum voluntary ventilation of 35–45% of the predicted, a forced expiratory volume in 1 second of 0.6 L min, and a mean forced expiratory flow of 0.6 L. Using these values as the criteria of inoperability; wedge, segmental or open biopsy was carried out in 248 patients with 1 postoperative mortality (0.4%). He then expanded his original report in reporting 32 patients who had a limited pulmonary resection and marked impairment of pulmonary function.[28] These patients all had an $FEV_1$ ≦1 L, forced expiratory flow ≤0.6 L, and a maximum voluntary ventilation under 40% of predicted. There were no operative deaths in this group of 10 segmentectomies and 22 wide-wedge resections. Bechard and Weststein[29] stated that the lower limit of the $FEV_1$ if 0.9 L for wedge or segmental resection.

**TABLE 25–1. INTERPRETATION OF SPIROMETRY IN RELATION TO RISK OF ANY OPERATIVE PROCEDURE**

| | High Risk | Moderate Risk | Low Risk |
|---|---|---|---|
| Vital capacity | <1.85 L | 1.85–3.0 L | >4.0 L |
| First second forced vital capacity | <1.2 L | 1.2–3.0 L | >3.2 L |
| Maximum voluntary ventilation | <28 L/min | >30 <80 L/min | >80 L/min |
| Maximum midexpiratory flow | <1 L/sec | >1.0 <2.0 L/s | >2.0 L/s |

*(From Peters RM: Identification, assessment and management of surgical patients with chronic respiratory disease. In Greenfield LJ (ed):* Problems in General Surgery, *Vol 1. Philadelphia, Lippincott, 1984, pp 432–444, with permission.)*

Radionuclide scanning has proven to be more predictable of postoperative residual lung function in patients undergoing pneumonectomy rather than those of limited resection. Ali et al[30] determined that lung scanning to predict postoperative function was inaccurate when the resection was limited to two segments or less. Quantitative lung scanning is currently not effective in determining resectability for a small peripheral lung cancer.

Pulmonary function tests alone do not necessarily make a patient inoperable. There are other clinical factors that must be evaluated to permit the clinician to make a sound judgment as to whether the patient should have a resection. Marginal pulmonary function may permit a limited resection, but when coupled with a poorly functioning myocardium, thoracotomy is contraindicated. A history of cardiac ischemia or prior myocardial infarction would indicate the need for further testing including thallium-201 stress test and even coronary angiography. Other factors to consider strongly in a patient with marginal pulmonary function are mental status, obesity, nutritional status, and renal dysfunction. No single piece of information renders the patient inoperable for a limited resection. Sound clinical judgment is required to correlate all of the pulmonary function data in association with the other listed factors to reach the final decision of operability.

## Second Primary

A thoracotomy and pulmonary resection for primary bronchogenic carcinoma decreases pulmonary function to varying degrees depending upon the amount of lung tissue resected and the final loss of chest wall and pulmonary compliance. A second lung resection must therefore fully encompass the pathology, yet preserve as much lung as possible.

Autopsy studies have revealed a 3.5%–14% incidence of multiple primary tumors in the lung, and clinical studies have established the incidence of second primary lung cancers.[31–35] The criteria that we have used to determine a second primary lung cancer include different histologic cell type from the first lung cancer, location of the new lesion in the contralateral lung or different ipsilateral lobe in the presence of synchronous bilateral tumors, and a prolonged interval between resections.[36,37] The length of this interval is controversial. Screening for a primary tumor elsewhere is of obvious importance in defining this group of patients.

In our experience, segmentectomy has played a significant role in the management of the patient with a second primary lung cancer (Fig. 25–2). Over a 28-year period, we have operated on 106 patients with either a second or third resection for a new lung cancer; 62% (66/106) of these resections were segmentectomies. The mortality rate for the group undergoing segmentectomy was 6.6% (4/66) and 8.5% (9/106) overall. A similar percentage (9/14) undergoing third resection had segmentectomy (Table 25–2). Eleven of the patients with secondary pulmonary carcinomas had synchronous lung primaries, and the remaining 95 had metachronous primaries. In the group of 95 patients with metachronous lung cancers, the probability of a patient being tumor-free was 50% at 3 years and 28% at 5 years. The mean interval between the first and second resection was 49 months. The probability of 5-year survival for this group of patients having metachronous cancers was 35%, and the 10-year probability of survival was 22%. Results have been discouraging in our group of synchronous tumors, since there have been no long-term survivors. Conversely, Ferguson et al[34] reported a 2-year survival rate of 60% and a median survival time of 27 months in synchronous stage 1 lung cancers.

Limited resection must also be considered when one is contemplating staged bilateral thoracotomies for synchronous primaries. Ferguson et al[34] reported on 17 synchronous bilateral primary lung cancers and 11 unilateral lesions. Nineteen patients had resection of both pulmonary lesions, and segmentectomy (or wedge resection) played a significant role in accomplishing these procedures without mortality.

When one is considering a resection in a patient following a prior pneumonectomy, limited resection is of paramount importance.[38] Careful clinical staging to determine the feasibility of complete resection and physiologic testing to determine operability are required. We have performed 9 segmentectomies and 11 wedge resections on patients who have had prior pneumonectomies for bronchogenic carcinoma. The time interval has varied from 4 months to 16 years between the two resections, and the operative morality was 5% (1/20). Four patients (20%) have survived 5 years following the second resection.

Surgical resection remains the therapy of choice for patients with second and third primary bronchogenic carcinoma. Limited resection is usually required in this situation to minimize postoperative morbidity and mortality. However, conservation of lung tissue must not compromise a cancer operation, and more extensive resection may be indicated if cardiopulmonary function will permit. Pulmonary resection after a prior pneumonectomy is feasible, and a limited resection is of the essence in this instance.

## Age

Patients over the age of 70 frequently are afflicted by cardiac disease, chronic obstructive pulmonary disease, diabetes, renal impairment, or other major medical problems. All of these factors place the elderly patient at increased risk following thoracotomy and pulmonary resection. Breyer et al[39] reviewed the data from five centers on patients over the age of 70 having a resection for lung carci-

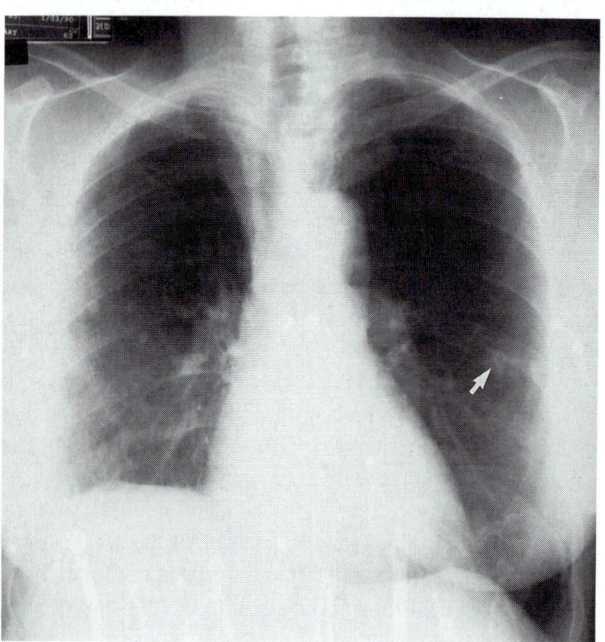

A

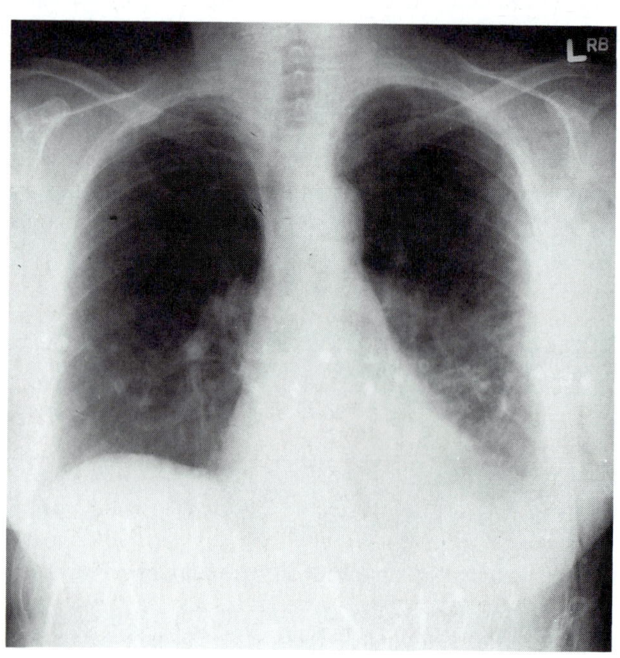

B

**Figure 25–2. A.** A second primary lung cancer in a 63-year-old female who had a right upper lobectomy 5 years previously. **B.** Postoperative film on day 6 after lingulectomy.

**TABLE 25–2. SURGICAL PROCEDURES PERFORMED AT FIRST, SECOND, AND THIRD OPERATIONS**

| Procedures | Resections | | |
|---|---|---|---|
| | *First* | *Second* | *Third* |
| Segmentectomy | 31 | 66 | 9 |
| Lobectomy | 47 | 14 | — |
| Sleeve lobectomy | 8 | 1 | — |
| Pneumonectomy | 19 | — | — |
| Carinal resection | 1 | — | — |
| Completion lobectomy | — | 6 | 2 |
| Completion pneumonectomy | — | 16 | 2 |
| Tracheal resection | — | 1 | — |
| Sternotomy, bilateral | — | 2 | — |
| Unresectable | — | — | 1 |
| Total | 106 | 106 | 14 |

noma. The mortality for this group was 17.2% (53/308). Berggren et al[40] reported 82 patients, 70 years of age or over who underwent lobectomy, bilobectomy, or pneumonectomy for bronchogenic carcinoma, and the reported hospital mortality was 15.9%. It is interesting to note that none of these patients had a limited pulmonary resection. Keagy et al[41] reported an operative mortality of 2.3% in 43 patients age 70 years or older who underwent pulmonary resection for bronchogenic carcinoma. They attributed these impressive results to improved postoperative management and newer anesthetic techniques. There were 5 limited resections in this group of 32 resections.

Breyer et al[39] reviewed our experience with patients over the age of 70 that had pulmonary resection for primary lung cancer. The mortality of the 150 patients undergoing pulmonary resection for carcinomas was 4% (6/150). Multiple logistic regression analysis revealed that age, sex, and a history of prior myocardial infarction were not associated with an increased risk of major complication or death. However, of most important significance, it was found that the amount of lung tissue removed, a history of congestive heart failure and a history of previous pulmonary resection were all related to an increased risk of major complication or death. The incidence of major complications was significantly less in the patients undergoing wedge or segmental resection than in those undergoing lobectomy or pneumonectomy. A limited resection was also directly related to a decreased mortality in this group of patients, since 52 had a segmentectomy, and operative mortality in this group was 2% (1/52). Weiss[42] reported a 5-year survival rate of 13% for pneumonectomy; 21% for lobectomy, and, significantly, 42% for segmentectomy. The higher probability of survival in the segmentectomy patients is related to the fact that these were primarily stage I lesions. A lung sparing procedure must be considered for the older patient with early stage lung cancer, since it is associated with fewer postoperative complications and a lesser morality than either lobectomy or pneumonectomy (Fig. 25–3).

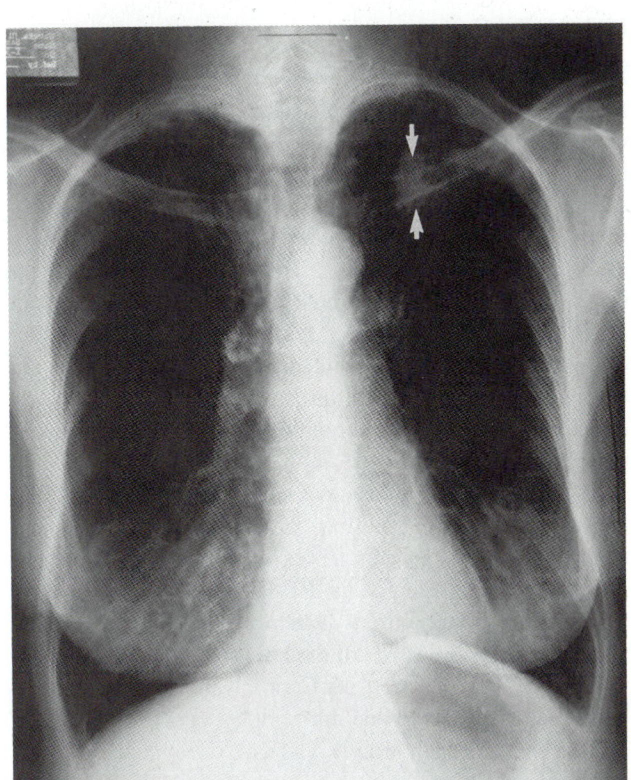

A

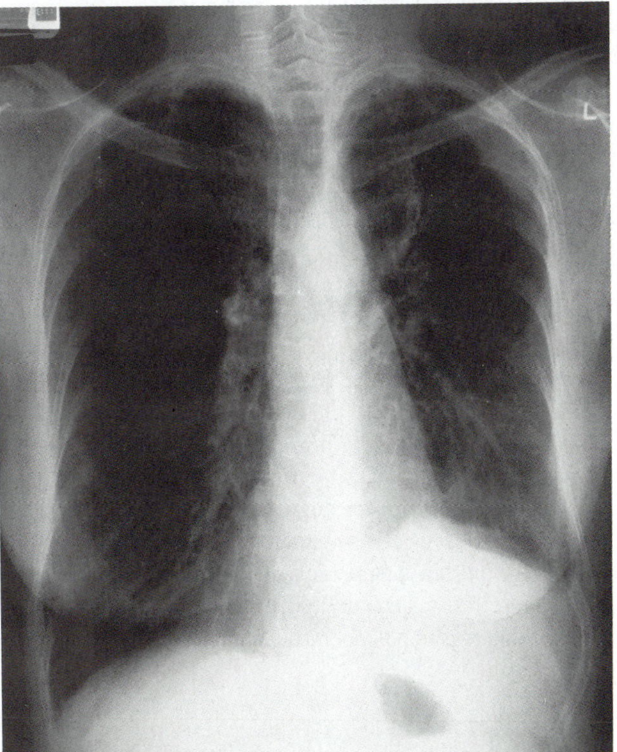

B

**Figure 25–3.** **A.** Chest x-ray of a vigorous and well-motivated 69-year-old female. CT scan is depicted in Figure 1B. $FEV_1$ is 0.72 L (39%), and MVV is 26 L (33%). **B.** Postoperative chest x-ray following apico-posterior segmentectomy.

### Metastatic Cancer

Surgical resection is frequently indicated for metastatic tumors to the lung, and the recent development of effective chemotherapeutic agents for certain bone and soft-tissue malignancies has further broadened the indications for resection of pulmonary metastases. For multiple reasons, a limited resection is the procedure of choice for pulmonary metastases. Metastatic lesions are often multifocal occurring in separate lobes or in both lungs, and the patients are often severely debilitated. Furthermore, many of the chemotherapeutic agents used are potentially harmful to the lung. Frequently, second, third, or even fourth thoracotomies and resections are required (particularly for metastatic sarcomas).

Because most metastatic lesions are blood-borne and, hence, peripheral in location, the majority of lesions are best removed with a wedge resection. However, this type of resection can be dangerous for lesions located near the hilum. Median sternotomy is helpful for bilateral lesions, although posterior lesions of the left lower lobe are difficult to resect by this approach. McCormick and Martini[43] report an overall 5-year survival for solitary of 25% metastatic disease and 15% for multiple lesions.

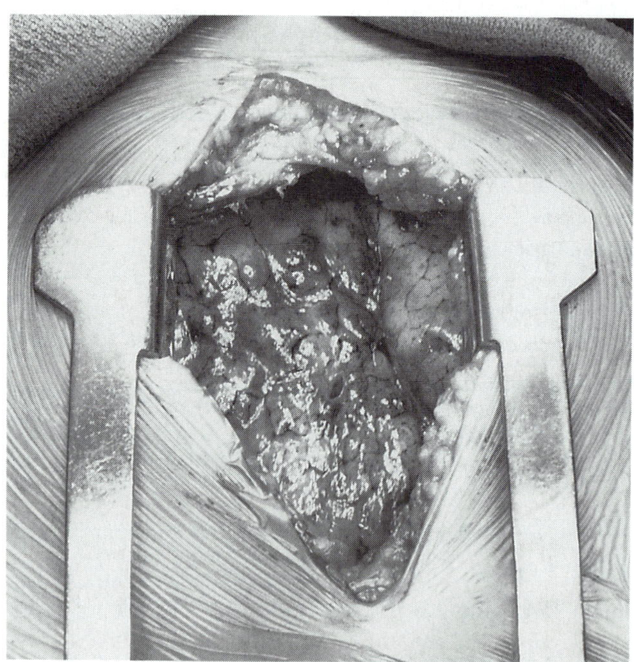

**Figure 25–4.** Lateral incision through the fifth intercostal space for a planned segmentectomy. Head of the patient is to the left.

## TECHNIQUE OF LIMITED RESECTION

Bronchoscopy is always carried out prior to a segmentectomy or wedge resection to alert the surgeon to any variation in segmental anatomy and also to be certain that the cancer does not involve the segmental orifice, which would negate the limited resection. The bronchoscopy can be performed as a separate procedure on an outpatient basis or at the time of thoracotomy. Preparation for one-lung anesthesia is carried out, and this can be accomplished with a long, single-lumen endotracheal tube or with a double-lumen endotracheal tube. One-lung anesthesia enhances exposure for a possible larger resection if required along with a complete mediastinal lymph node dissection. The latter should always be accomplished with a limited resection for proper staging.

A lateral incision through the fourth and fifth intercostal spaces is used for planned limited resection (Fig. 25–4). The posterolateral incision is not used, since it requires more operative time to open and close and is associated with increased postoperative pain.

### Segmentectomy

The surgeon must be totally familiar with segmental anatomy prior to embarking on this type of resection. Overholt and Langer[44] have superbly depicted this technique. There can be variation of size and location of the pulmonary artery, vein, and bronchus to each and every segment. The presence of an anomalous fissure is helpful and often occurs at the superior portion of the lingula, where the variation may range from a slight indentation to a complete separation to almost delineate a left middle lobe. There may be indentation to varying degrees at the base of the superior segment of the right or left lower lobe and at the inferior portion of the lower lobes separating the medial basal segment from the other basal segments.[14]

The pulmonary artery supply to the left upper lobe is not constant, and careful dissection is always required to precisely determine which artery goes to which segment. The posterior segmental artery to the right upper lobe is not constant and, on occasion, may not be present. The pulmonary artery to the posterior segment of either upper lobe may arise from the branch to the superior segment of the lower lobe, and, in this instance, it is necessary to preserve the arterial supply to the segment that is not being removed. The pulmonary artery branch to the lingula may occasionally arise as the first branch off the main pulmonary artery and proceed just anterior to the upper lobe bronchus to the lingula. Whenever the lingular artery is not found in the major fissure, it must be looked for anteriorly. Venous drainage of the segment has less variations, but each segmental vein is carefully dissected free, and only a minimum number of veins are removed with the specimen.

Segments commonly resected on the right are the anterior, apical, and posterior segments of the right upper lobe; the posterior segment of the right upper lobe and superior segment of the right lower lobe in continuity; and the four basal segments of the right lower lobe in one unit. Individual basilar segments of the lower lobe can be resected, but this procedure requires careful technique to be certain that the vascular or bronchial supply to the remaining basal segments is not compromised. Segmental resections of the left lung include the apico-posterior, anterior, and lingular segments of the left upper lobe; superior, anteromedial basal segment of the left lower lobe; and the basal segments of the left lower lobe. The left upper lobe frequently has a bifurcating bronchus and segmentectomy of the superior division of the left upper lobe includes the apico-posterior and anterior segments. The lingula is synonymously referred to as the inferior division of the left upper lobe. The inferior segment of the lingula can be separately resected as well. The posterior segment of the left upper lobe and superior segment of the left lower lobe can be resected as a unit when a tumor crosses the major fissure posteriorly. Resection of the lateral and posterior basal segments of the left lower lobe is technically difficult and is reserved for those patients with very marginal function (Fig. 25–5).

After the chest is opened, a very careful assessment of the location of the tumor and the hilar structures is carried out. The tumor is ideally <3 cm in diameter, located at the periphery of the lobe, and is in the central portion of a segment or segments. Lobar and mediastinal lymph nodes are carefully palpated for evidence of metastatic carcinoma. Any suspicious node is removed and sent for frozen section analysis, and, if carcinoma is present, segmental resection is extremely unlikely to result in cure. It may be necessary to carry out a segmentectomy or wedge resection in association with a lymph node dissection if the pulmonary status of the patient will not permit lobectomy. The tumor mass may be located in close proximity to the intersegmental plane,

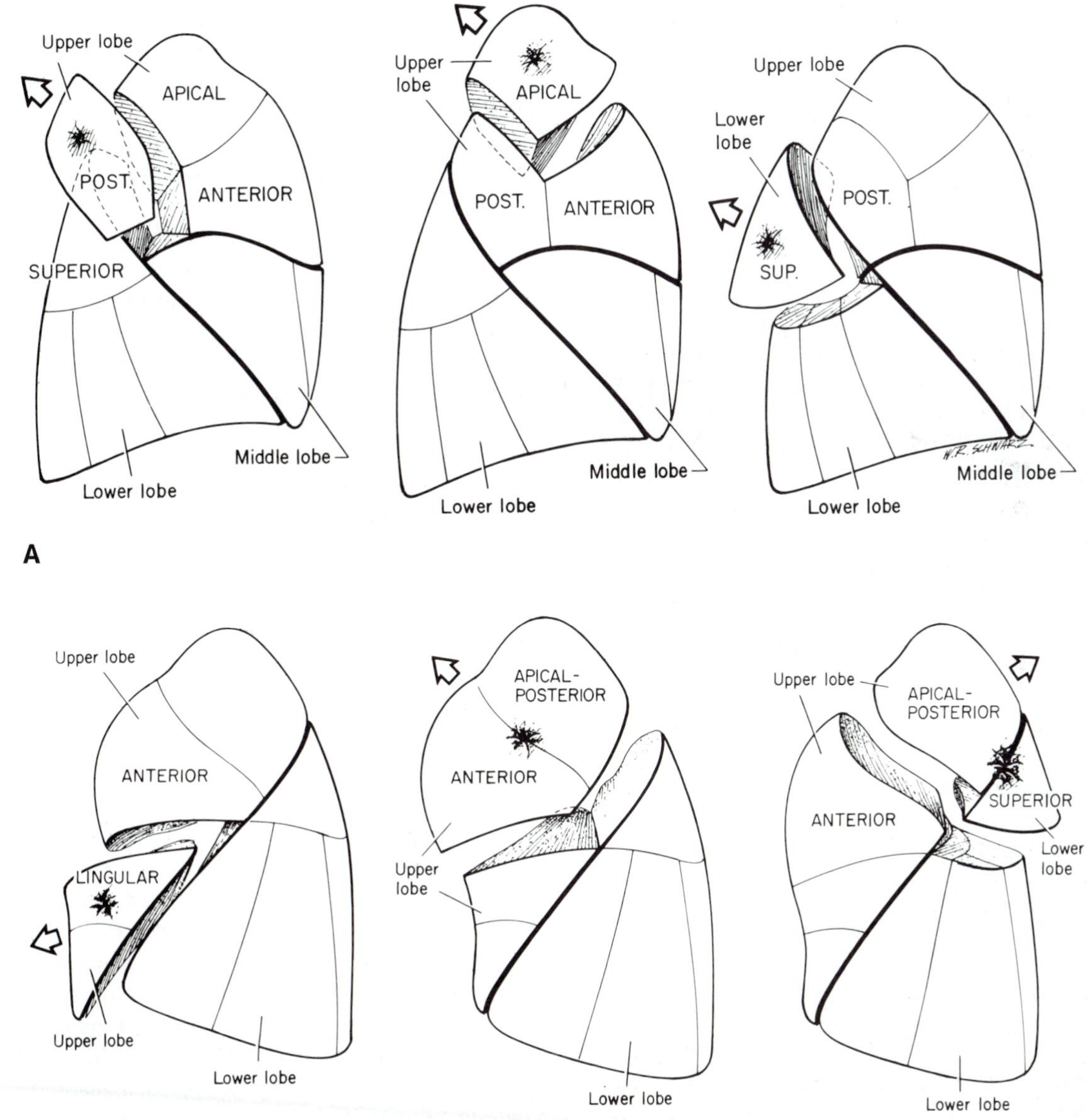


**Figure 25–5.** Various types of segmentectomies that can be done.

and, in this instance, lobectomy becomes the operation of choice, or two adjacent segments can be removed to ensure an adequate parenchymal margin of resection. These types of resections would include the apico-posterior segments of the right upper lobe in continuity, the superior division of the left upper lobe, the inferior division of the left upper lobe, and all basal segments of either lower lobe.

Frequently, a tissue diagnosis has not been established prior to the thoracotomy, and the surgeon is unsure as to whether he or she is dealing with benign or malignant disease. It is inappropriate to carry out an incisional biopsy of the pulmonary nodule, since seeding of the operative field with cancer cells may occur. Diagnosis of the nodule can be established by two methods. One is to do a wedge resection and have the pathologist perform a frozen section analysis of the tumor. If cancer is identified, an anatomic segmentectomy can then be accomplished, encompassing all margins of the wedge resection. Our recommended technique is to perform needle aspiration cytology of the tumor as described by Fry[45] (Fig. 25–6). Close to 100% reliability in the diagnosis of cancer is achieved with this technique. The cytopathologist must be experienced in reading the smears and must also be familiar with the rapid staining technique so that significant operating room delay does not occur.

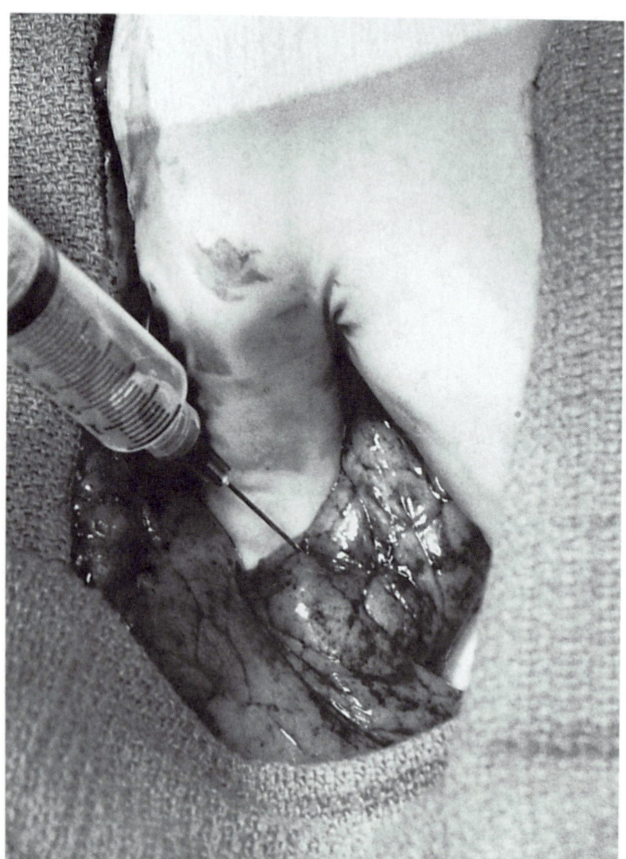

**Figure 25–6.** Needle aspiration of lung nodule for cytologic examination.

Once a diagnosis of cancer is established, the proper resection is then carried out.

The dissection begins with identification of the pulmonary artery to the segment to be removed, and it is ligated and transected. The segmental bronchus lies in close proximity to the pulmonary artery, and it is freed of adventitial tissue and bronchial lymph nodes. At this point in the dissection, it is necessary to remove routinely a segmental and/or lobar lymph node and sent it to pathology for frozen section analysis. The presence of microscopic nodal metasis requires that a decision be made either to complete the segmentectomy because of poor cardiopulmonary function or proceed with lobectomy and enhanced lymphadenectomy.

Temporary occlusion of the segmental bronchus to verify anatomic segmental boundaries by differential atelectasis is ineffective, since collateral ventilation from the adjacent segment or lobe will inflate the segment of the clamped bronchus. The bronchus can be transected and closed with either the stapling technique or with interrupted fine absorbable sutures. The 3.5-mm, leg-length staple is used for segmental bronchial closure. If there is difficulty in placing the stapling instrument around the bronchus due to close proximity of adjacent hilar structures, the suture technique should be used.

The pulmonary vein defines the peripheral boundary of the segment, and unnecessary resection of adjacent pulmonary veins will result in postoperative venous engorgement of the adjacent lung tissue. Frequently, the segment to be removed is adjacent to a minor or major fissure that is incomplete, and the fissure is easily separated by one application of the stapling instrument.

Following division of the hilar structures, it is necessary to remove the segment(s) along the intersegmental plane anatomically delineated by the pulmonary vein. It is our preference to complete the segmentectomy with the lung inflated, rather than deflated with one-lung anesthesia, since excessive lung tissue is not removed and the proper segmental plane is more readily identified. Traction is placed on a right-angle clamp holding the bronchus and pulmonary artery, and the segmental plane is developed along its venous tributaries. As gentle traction is placed on the clamp, the thumb and forefinger of the other hand are rolled over the remaining lung parenchyma to develop the segmental plane of dissection. Small intersegmental bronchi and vessels are individually transected and ligated to permit the continued separation of the segment. Some prefer the use of a sponge to accomplish this aspect of the dissection. When the visceral pleural surface is reached, it is transected, and the segment is removed.

During the development of the intersegmental plane, it is important that continued attention is directed toward achieving an adequate margin of parenchymal resection beyond the tumor. Following completion of the segmentectomy, the parenchymal margin is carefully inspected to be certain that an adequate margin has been achieved. After removal of the segment, the lung becomes atelectatic, and the margin may appear in close proximity to the tumor. However, if the surgeon felt that the margin was adequate while the lung was inflated, then most likely an adequate resection has been accomplished.

A lap sponge is used to apply pressure for several minutes to the raw surface of the residual lung tissue to provide hemostasis. The remaining lung is then carefully inspected for bleeding points that are cauterized, and small bronchi are individually ligated or transfixed. Sterile saline is used to detect any major bubbling from the raw surface, and this technique is repeated several times to be certain that all significant air leaks are closed. It is important to achieve good hemostasis, since a postoperative hematoma or hemothorax can be a major complication.

A second method of completing the intersegmental parenchymal plane is to use the GIA stapler in one or two applications (Fig. 25–7). Stapling of the lung is the last step with this technique of resection and is carried out only after the pulmonary artery and bronchus have been transected in the usual fashion (Fig. 25–8). The veins draining the seg-

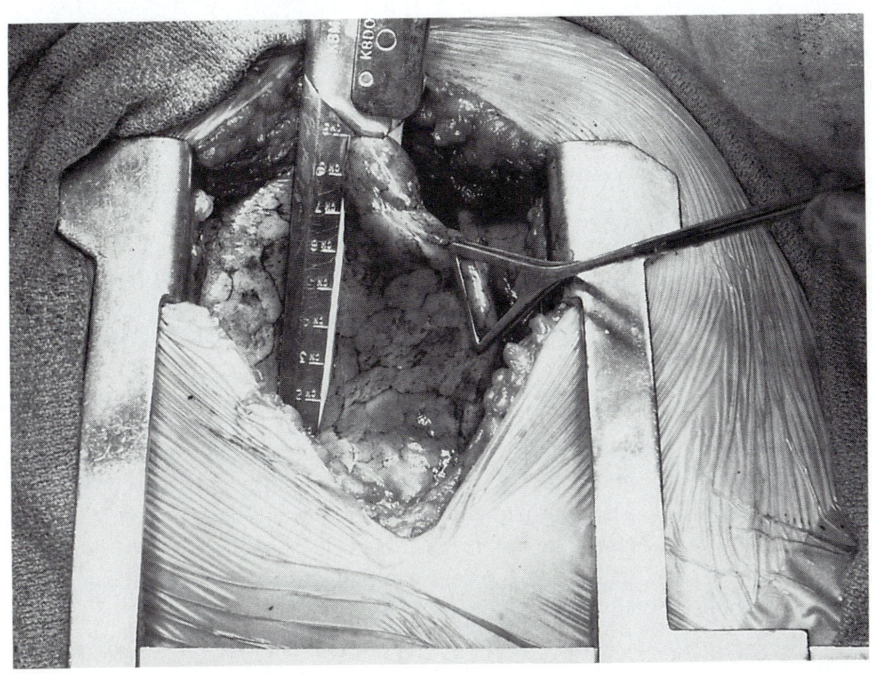

A

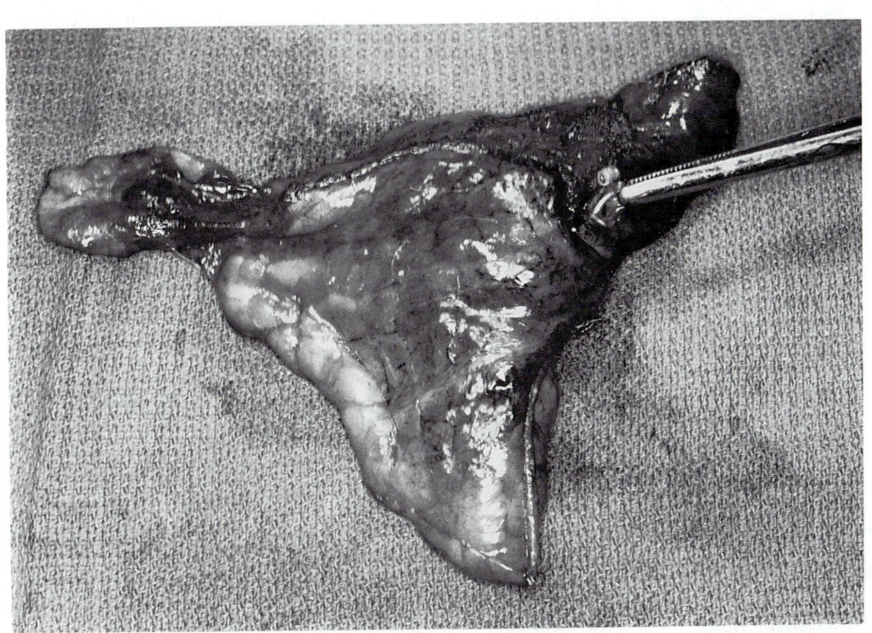

B

**Figure 25–7. A.** First application of GIA 90-mm stapler for lingulectomy. **B.** Resected segment with bronchus held by forceps.

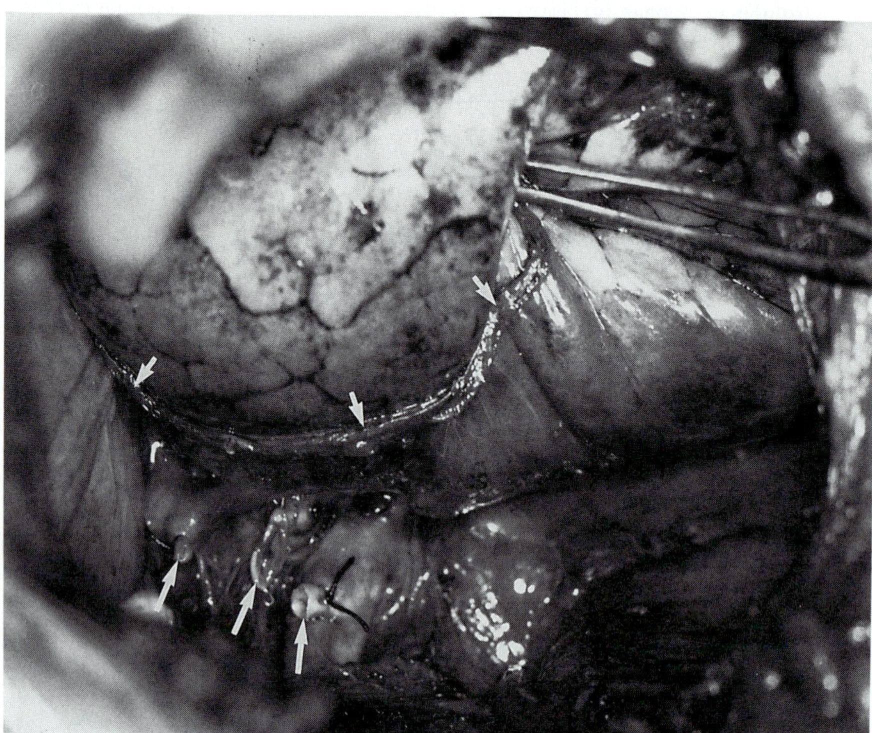

**Figure 25–8.** Lung staple line and bronchus, artery and vein depicted by arrows.

ment can be individually ligated or included in the staple line. The staple line must be carefully inspected for adequacy of closure, and any defects are closed with interrupted absorbable sutures. If there is any question about the integrity of the staple line in emphysematous lung, the entire closure should be reinforced with a running absorbable suture. The use of staples has decreased the incidence of prolonged postoperative air leaks and, when properly applied, can be quite effective.

There are several ways to manage the raw surface of the remaining lung tissue to minimize postoperative air leaks, and the surgeon should be familiar with them all (Fig. 25–9). It may be appropriate to approximate the edges of the visceral pleura with interrupted absorbable tissues, and this technique is particularly applicable following a posterior or apical segmentectomy of the right upper lobe and an anterior segmentectomy of the left upper lobe. Adequate hemostasis is very important, since a postoperative hematoma in the approximated lung can result in hemoptysis or the development of a lung abscess.

A raw segmental surface can be approximated to the surface of the adjacent lobe along a fissure and is accomplished by the use of several interrupted absorbable sutures. This technique utilizes the intralobar visceral pleural surface of the normal lobe to serve as the pleural surface for the denuded segmental surface. Following apico-posterior segmentectomy of the left upper lobe, clockwise rotation of the remaining lingula and anterior segment approximates the raw surface to the superior segment of the lower lobe. After superior segmentectomy of either lower lobe, the denuded superior aspect of the basilar segments is approximated to the intralobar pleural surface of the upper lobe. The approximation technique results in a lung that can be considered as reconstituted. It is small size but has essentially the same configuration and is less prone to prolonged air leak.

A large, broad-based pleural flap can be effectively cover the remaining raw segmental surface and is used when the parenchymal air leaks appear to be excessive. The flap must not hinder expansion of the lung and should cover the entire segmental surface. Absorbable interrupted sutures through the visceral pleura are used to anchor the flap in place. Chest tube placement is critical in order to minimize postoperative complications, and the anterior tube must be placed to the apex and well anterior to evacuate all of the air and permit full expansion of the lung. The basal tube is inserted dependently and posteriorly to evacuate blood and fluid. Suction at 20 cm of water pressure is begun in the operating room and usually maintained until the air leak stops.

## Wedge Resection

In contrast to segmentectomy, wedge excisions consist of a nonanatomic resection of a peripheral portion of lung tissue that includes the tumor nodule. There are various techniques that can be utilized for wedge resection; they include the stapling; cautery excision; and the clamp, cut, and sew methods. Wedge resection can be accomplished with the lung inflated or deflated by one-lung anesthesia. We prefer the lung to be inflated when the wedge resection is done to

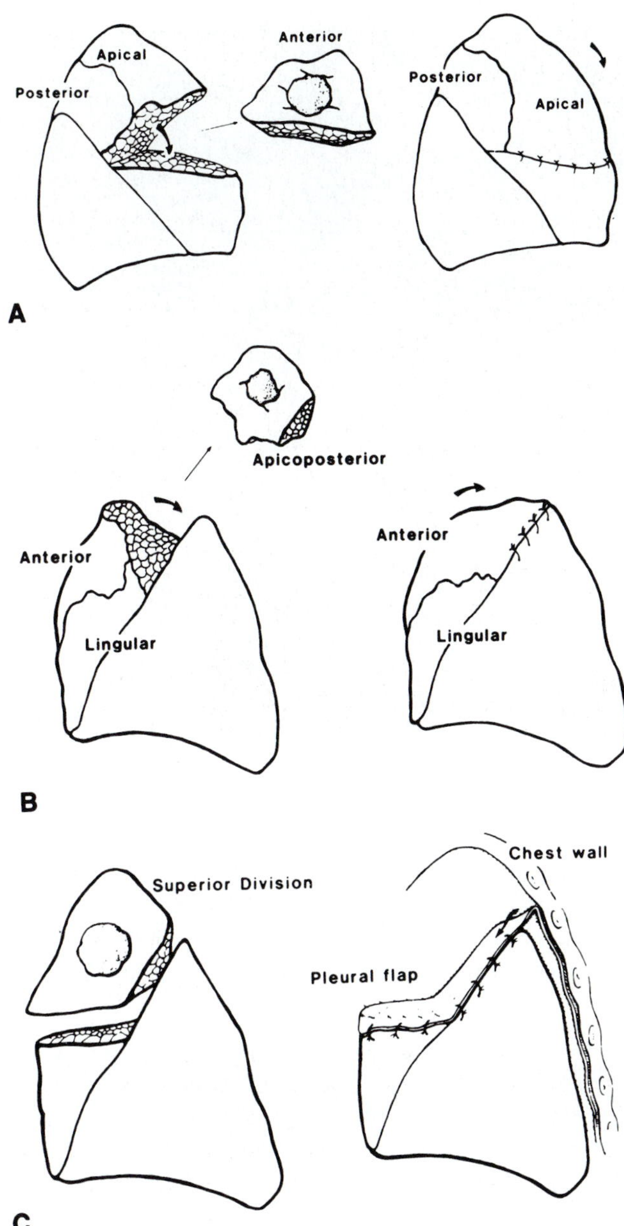


**Figure 25–9.** Methods of managing the raw surface of a segmentectomy.

ensure a more precise resection with minimal removal of lung tissue. This latter point is particularly true when metastatic carcinomas are excised. It is technically simpler to carry out the wedge resection with the lung collapsed, but the surgeon must be certain that an excessive amount of lung tissue is not removed.

The stapling technique is fast and simple, and two applications of the GIA stapler carry out the classic wedge resection (Fig. 25–10). A stapler can also be placed in a linear fashion along the edge of the lobe to resect a peripheral tumor.

On occasion, the tumor nodule is located on the surface in a more central location of the lobe. In this instance, it is not possible to place a stapler into the depths of the parenchyma, and the cautery technique of excision is recommended. A V-shaped portion of lung tissue is removed by cautery excision with a 2-cm margin beyond the edges of the tumor. Bleeding can be troublesome with this technique, but individual vessels are cauterized and suture ligated as they are encountered, and larger bronchi are suture transfixed. The surface of the lung is reapproximated by using interrupted absorbable sutures through the visceral pleura. It is not possible to approximate the raw edges of the deeper lung tissue, since the sutures will pull out and cause more bleeding. Precise hemostasis is necessary to minimize the postoperative complication of intraparenchymal hematoma, and it is not unusual to see a hematoma on the early postoperative chest x-ray that will clear in 2–3 months' time. The cautery technique also works well for lesions on the edge of the lobe and for small metastatic nodules (Fig. 25–11).

Occluding clamps can be placed on each side of a peripheral lesion, and the wedge of lung tissue is excised along the edges of the occluding clamps. A running mattress suture is then placed proximal to the clamps, and, after the clamps are removed, a running over and over suture is placed to close the defect in the lung.

Wedge resection can also be performed by using the technique of video-assisted thoracic surgery (VATS). Technical concerns when one is using this technique include margin adequacy, regional lymph node sampling, or resection and localization of deep-seated lesions. Information regarding this approach is available in Chapter 12.

## COMPLICATIONS

Table 25–3 outlines the expected complications that follow limited resection. Prolonged air leak (one that is present 7 days or longer after the resection) is the most common major complication following segmentectomy. This problem has been minimized by the technique of stapled transection of the intersegmental plane. Prolonged air leak is rare after wedge resection, since the edges of the lung are stapled or suturedmated tightly.

Air leaks are minimized by achieving full expansion of the lung. A persistent air leak and space complication usually relates to failure of the lung to expand adequately or incomplete closure of a subsegmental bronchus at the time of the resection. Proper chest tube placement, vigorous postoperative pulmonary care, adequate pain control, incentive spirometry, induced coughing, bedside bronchoscopy, nasotracheal aspiration, humidification, and mini-tracheostomy are all key factors in achieving maximal lung expansion and preventing air leaks. Pain is limited both by the use of a limited incision (via a lateral fourth or fifth intercostal incision) and continuous epidural anesthesia.[52] Chest tube suction at 20 cm of water pressure is begun in the operating room and is maintained for a minimum of 7 days if the air

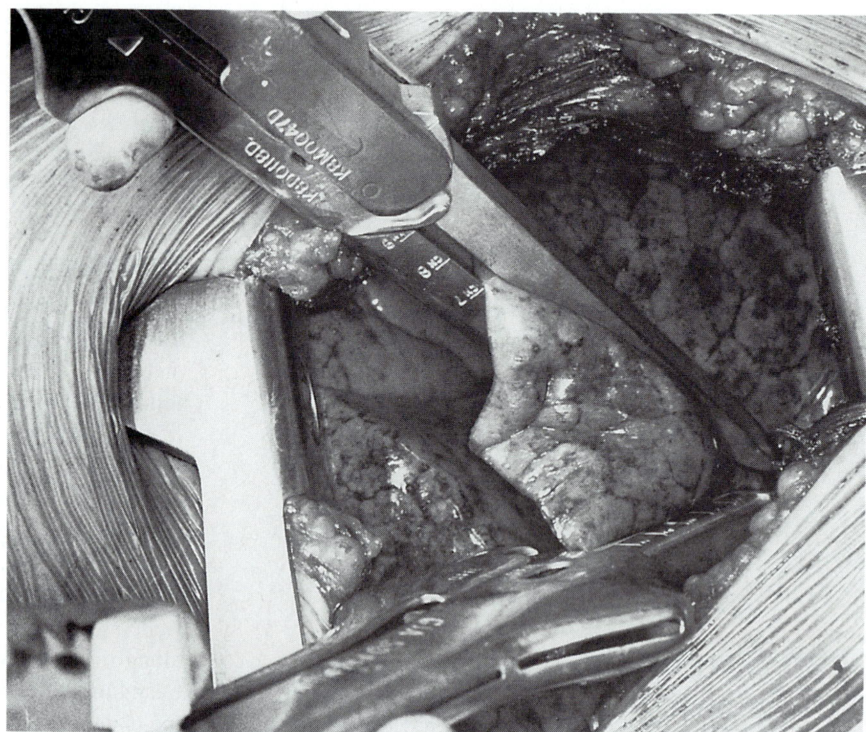

**Figure 25–10.** Stapling technique for wedge resections. Two instruments are placed for illustrative purposes.

leak persists. If the air leaks persists to 12–14 days, suction is usually discontinued. If a pleural space does not develop or enlarge, the tube can be connected to a one-way valve, and the patient is discharged from the hospital. The valve is tested for air leak at weekly intervals, and, since most small alveolar leaks will close fairly rapidly, the tube can be usually removed in 2–3 weeks. A benign or noninfected pleural space will obliterate in several weeks. (Pneumoperitoneum can be helpful to elevate the diaphragm and assist in space obliteration; however, it must be used in the first few days after surgery to achieve satisfactory results, or the lung will have been fixed in place by intrapleural adhesions.) If an in-

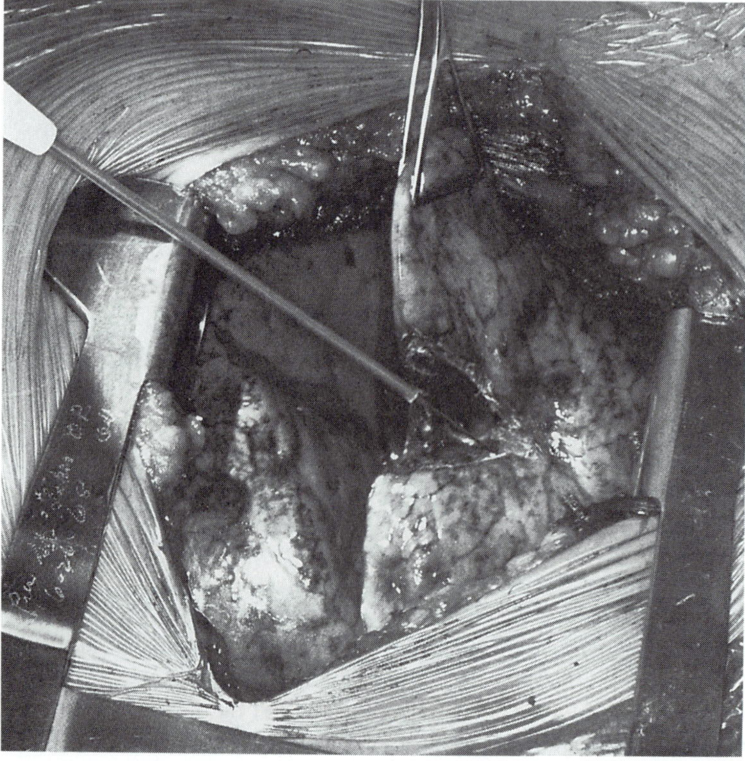

**Figure 25–11.** Cautery wedge excision of a pulmonary nodule.

**TABLE 25–3. COMPLICATION: STAGES I AND II (348 PATIENTS)**

| | |
|---|---|
| Air leak over 7 days | 34 |
| Reinsert chest tube | 12 |
| Reoperation for air leak | 7 |
| Tracheostomy | 6 |
| Empyema | 5 |
| Hemorrhage | 5 |
| Additional resection | 3 |

**TABLE 25–4. PATIENT GROUPS—LIMITED RESECTION**

| | No. |
|---|---|
| Previous resection | 82 |
| Carcinoma Stages III–IV | 137 |
| Carcinoma Stages I–II | 348 |
| Total | 567 |

fection does develop in the space, open tube drainage is carried out, and the empyema is then treated in standard fashion. If the air leak persists through the valve longer than 4 weeks after discharge from the hospital, the patient has a fistula, and the tube is converted to open drainage. A small empyema space and fistula will obliterate over a time frame of several weeks, and the tube is slowly backed out at weekly intervals. A large infected space that does not progressively obliterate will require thoracoplasty or myoplasty for closure.

Empyema and open tube drainage following limited resection occur infrequently. Thoracoplasty and myoplasty are practically never required in this setting, since only a small portion of lung has been removed. Similarly, bleeding is distinctly unusual after limited resection. Most bleeding complications are related to either an unligated bronchial artery at the hilum, a transected intercostal vessel, or coagulopathy.

## CLINICAL EXPERIENCE

Our most recent review includes 567 patients who have undergone a limited resection for bronchogenic carcinoma, 547 of whom had anatomic segmentectomies and 20 of whom had wedge resections. We prefer an anatomic resection for lung cancer; wedge resection is only employed when the patient's condition is tenuous and the location of the lesion is favorable. The age of the patients in this review ranged from 29 to 87 years, and 30% were over the age of 70.

Limited resection has been used in three basic groups of patients: (1) those with a prior resection for bronchogenic carcinoma (n = 82), (2) patients with a stage III or IV carcinoma, and (n = 137), (3) stage I or stage II primary bronchogenic carcinoma as determined by surgical-pathologic findings (n = 348) (Table 25–4). The operative resections accomplished prior to segmentectomy are depicted in Figure 25–12. Prior resections of significance included pneumonectomy in 20 and sleeve lobectomy in 4.

There have been 137 patients considered to have a stage III or stage IV bronchogenic carcinoma by virtue of extension into the chest wall, mediastinum or diaphragm, or brain metastasis. A limited resection was used in this latter group of patients who were found to have synchronous primary bronchogenic carcinoma and solitary brain metastasis. The superior sulcus tumor is frequently treated preoperatively with radiation, and, as the tumor mass decreases in size, a small amount of tumor or fibrosis may remain at the apex of the lung. An apico-posterior segmentectomy in conjunction with resection of the first and second ribs can provide adequate margins. The limited resection in this instance must be accompanied by documentation that regional lymph nodes are free of any evidence of metastatic

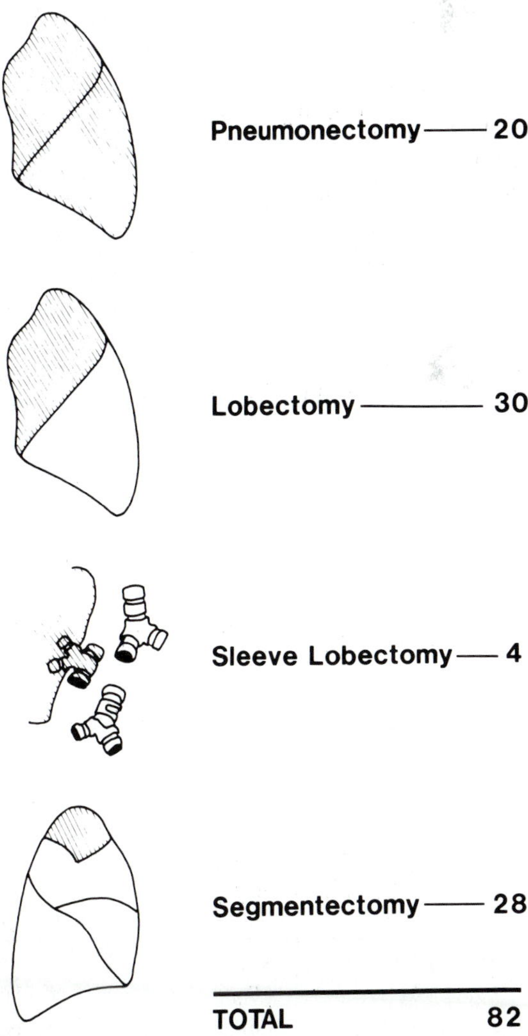


**Figure 25–12.** Resections done prior to limited resection.

carcinoma. We have applied neoadjuvant chemotherapy and/or radiation to peripheral lesions of the lung that have invaded the chest wall, and, in this instance, a limited resection in continuity with chest-wall resection can be carried out. The incidence of the limited resection for stage IIIA bronchogenic carcinoma has been decreasing in our more recent experience and is now only rarely utilized for the superior sulcus resection. Early in our series of patients, we participated in a randomized study of preoperative radiation, and many of the segmentectomies were from this group of patients.

There have been 348 limited resections done for stage I and II primary bronchogenic carcinoma. These patients had a more favorable pathologic condition in that there was no previous cancer history and the tumors were small. In over 90% of patients with peripheral lesions, the regional lymph nodes were benign. The tumor sites for the stage I and stage II primary carcinoma resections are shown in Table 25–5. The most frequently performed resection of the left upper lobe was removal of the superior division, principally because the tumor involved two or more segments and was often located deep within the parenchyma. The remainder of the resections of the left upper lobe were of the lingula, anterior and apico-posterior segments. Left lower lobe resections were of the superior segment, while basilar resections consisted of either single, multiple, or all of the entire basilar group. When tumor extended across the major fissure, eight patients had a portion of the contiguous lobes excised. The right upper lobe was involved in 97 procedures, and the anterior segment was the one most frequently resected. The apical and posterior segments were also resected singularly or as a combined unit. Two operations were done on the middle lobe, one a medial and one a lateral segmentectomy that were accomplished because of severely compromised pulmonary reserve. There were 48 lower lobe resections, the most common of which was removal of the superior segment of the lower lobe. There were seven examples of tumor extension across the fissure with removal of superior and posterior segments in continuity.

Table 25–6 shows the pathologic analysis according to the size of the tumors and the status of lymph nodes for all patients undergoing limited resection for stage I and II carcinoma. Approximately 75% of the lesions were under 3 cm in diameter, and positive lymph nodes were identified in 26

**TABLE 25–5. LOCATION OF TUMORS—STAGES I AND II CARCINOMA**

| | Lung | |
|---|---|---|
| | ***Left*** | ***Right*** |
| Middle lobe | — | 2 |
| Lower lobe | 38 | 48 |
| Across fissure | 8 | 8 |
| Totals | 193 | 155 |

**TABLE 25–6. TUMOR CHARACTERISTICS**

| | No. of Patients |
|---|---|
| Size | |
| T1—3 cm or less | 260 |
| T2—>3 cm | 84 |
| No residual tumor | 4 |
| Total | 348 |
| Nodal metastases | |
| Negative—N0 | 322 |
| Positive—N1 | 26 |
| Total | 348 |

specimens. The four patients that did not have residual microscopic tumor were part of the group that had been selectively randomized for preoperative radiation. The histologic distribution of the resected primary cancer shows 51% (176/348) are adenocarcinoma and 31% (108/348) are squamous (Table 25–7).

The morality data is seen in Table 25–8 and substantiates the true efficacy of a conservative pulmonary resection. The overall mortality for the 567 resections is 2.3% (13/567) and for the patient's undergoing a previous resection, 4.8% (4/82). There was one death in a patient having a limited resection after prior pneumonectomy. The lowest mortality has been achieved in the group undergoing a resection for the first time for a primary lung cancer, and this mortality rate is 1.1% (4/348).

## RESULTS

Survival in our limited resection series is dependent upon the categorization of each clinical group. The first group consists of those patients that have had a prior resection, and the second resection was for a first or second primary or possible metastasis. In this group of 82 patients, a current actuarial survival analysis reveals a 33% survival at 5 years and an 18% survival at 10 years following the second resection.

The group of patients with stage III cancer have a significantly lower survival rate. Life table analysis currently

**TABLE 25–7. HISTOLOGY—STAGES I AND II CARCINOMA**

| Cell Type | Patients | % |
|---|---|---|
| Adenocarcinoma | 176 | 51 |
| Squamous cell | 108 | 31 |
| Undifferentiated | 32 | 9 |
| Small cell | 10 | 3 |
| Bronchoalveolar | 22 | 6 |
| Total | 348 | 100 |

**TABLE 25–8. OPERATIVE MORTALITY**

| | Patients | Mortality | % |
|---|---|---|---|
| Previous resection | 82 | 4 | 4.8 |
| Stage III/IV carcinoma | 137 | 5 | 3.6 |
| Stage I/II carcinoma | 348 | 4 | 1.1 |
| Totals | 567 | 13 | 2.3 |

reveals a cumulative survival of 10% at 5 years. Many of these patients had preoperative radiation or preoperative radiation in combination with chemotherapy, and it is not possible to provide an acute assessment of the merit of a limited resection in stage III bronchogenic carcinoma.

A life table analysis of our 296 patients with stage I or II disease done in 1986[41] revealed a survival of 52% at 5 years, 31% at 10 years, and 11% at 15 years (Fig. 25–13). This is compared with our initial report in 1973,[15] when we reported an actuarial 5-year survival of 56%. Analysis has not been accomplished comparing the stage I and II patients; the number of wedge resections is too small for comparison purposes. The analysis of our data includes all operative deaths as well as the death of a patient from any cause.

## WEDGE RESECTION

The majority of published results of wedge resections involve a small number of cases. However, Errett et al[17] evaluated 197 patients with a stage I non-small cell carcinoma. There were 100 wedge resections and 97 lobectomies. The 30-day operative mortality for wedge resection was 3% (3/100) and 2.1% (2/97) for lobectomy. Actuarial 2-year survival was 72% in the wedge group and 74% in the lobectomy group. There was no reported difference in local recurrence. They concluded that the results of wedge resection can be favorable compared with those for lobectomy for stage I lung cancer. Hoffman and Ransdell[16] reported on 33 patients who had a wedge resection for stage I lung cancer without operative mortality. However, four patients had synchronous brain metastasis, and the 5-year survival rate for those patients at risk was 26%. Local recurrence was not evaluated, and mediastinal lymph nodes were only sampled if they were abnormal to palpation. McCormick and Martini[43] reported a 19.3% recurrence rate in 53 patients undergoing a limited resection. In this group, there were 48 wedge resections and eight segmentectomies. Actuarial survival at 5 years was 33%. Miller and Hatcher[28] reported on 32 patients who underwent a limited resection (wedge 22, seg 10) because of significant compromise in pulmonary function. There was one operative death, and a 5-year actuarial survival of 31% was noted.

## CONTROVERSIES

Both segmentectomy and lobectomy have been proposed as the procedures of choice for stage I carcinoma of the lung.[19–24] To be considered an operation of choice and not one of compromise, limited resection should have similar long-term survival and recurrence rates when compared with lobectomy. Martini and Beattie[46] established the benchmark when they reported on 91 lobectomies for stage I lung cancer. The actuarial 5-year survival rate at 1 year was 93% and 85% at 3 years. Martini and Beattie stated that "any resection less extensive than lobectomy decreases the

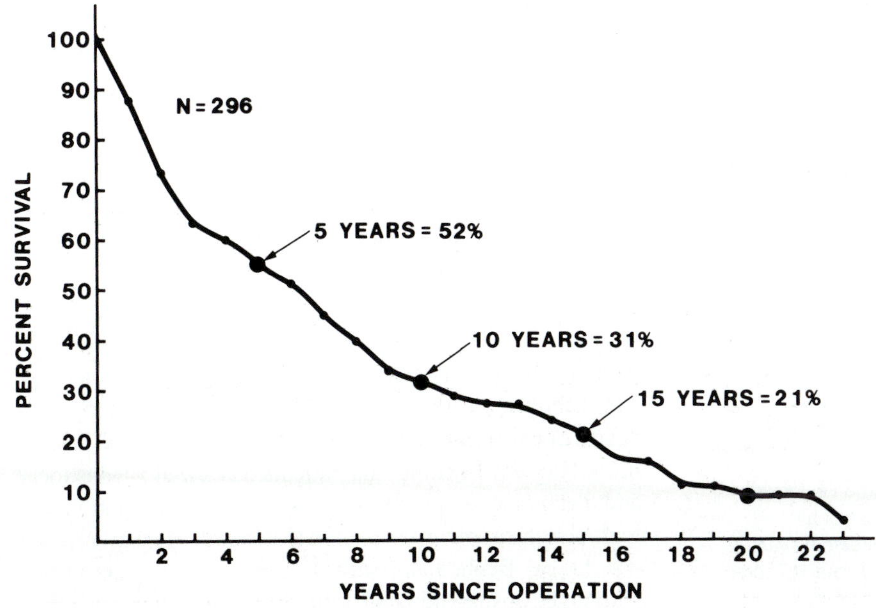


**Figure 25–13.** Life table analysis of 296 limited resections for primary stage I and II bronchogenic carcinoma.

chance of long term survival." Read et al[47] analyzed 244 patients who underwent lobectomy (131) or segmentectomy/wedge (113) for T1 N0 M0 bronchogenic carcinoma. In the limited resection group, 107 patients had segmental resection. The results of conservative resection showed no statistically significant difference from that of lobectomy. When survival data was calculated using only deaths as a result of the initial lesion, the Kaplan-Meier survival for the limited resection group of patients (107 segmentectomies, 6 wedge) was approximately 82% at 5 years compared with 73% for the lobectomy group. Mortality for the limited resection group of patients was 3.5% (4/113).

We recently analyzed 169 patients who either underwent a primary segmental resection or lobectomy for stage I lung cancer (T1 N0, T2 N0) operated on from 1980 to 1988.[18] All patients were followed for 5 years. No survival advantage of lobectomy over segmental resection was noted for patients with tumors 3.0 cm in diameter or smaller, but a survival advantage was apparent for patients undergoing lobectomy for tumors larger than 3.0 cm. Actual survival for the 66 patients who underwent segmental resection for a stage I lung cancer at 5 years was 53%. The actual 5-year survival of the 103 patients undergoing lobectomy with the identical cancer stage in the same time period was 64% ($P$ = 0.35) (Fig. 25–14).

Preliminary data from the Lung Cancer Study Group prospective randomized trial comparing lobectomy with a limited resection of segmentectomy or adequate wedge resection for T1 N0 primary lung cancers demonstrated no significant difference between the two groups in the overall death rate or the cancer death rate.[19]

Williams et al[48] reported on the survival of patients surgically treated for stage I lung cancer. There were 30 patients who had N1 lesions, and the probability of survival at 5 years for 495 patients was 56%. If only lung cancer deaths were considered and mortalities were eliminated, the 5-year probability of survival was 69%. In this group there were 22 patients who had a limited resection (segmentectomy/wedge), and the 5-year probability of survival was 70% for T1 N0 lesions and 50% for T2 N0 lesions. This analysis included all causes of death and was not significantly different from the survival rate for patients undergoing lobectomy.

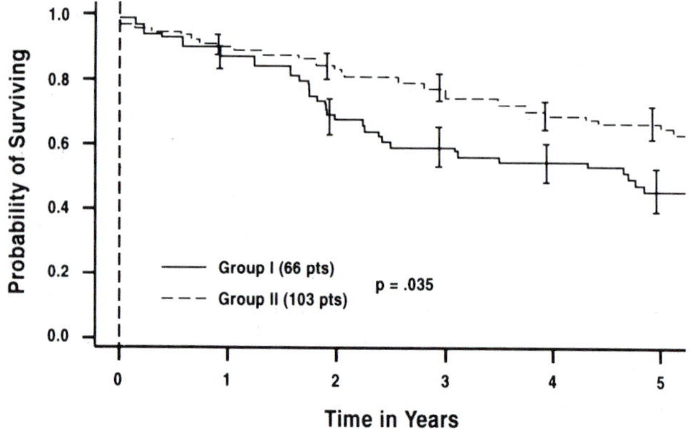


**Figure 25–14.** Kaplan-Meier survival plot for segmentectomies (group I) and lobectomies (group II) with carcinomas of all diameters *(From: Warren WH, Faber LP: Segmentectomy versus lobectomy in patients with stage I pulmonary carcinoma. J Thorac Cardiovasc Surg 107:1087–1094, 1994, with permission.)*

Statistics for long-term survival following resection for stage I lung cancer do vary. There are no reports that compare with those of Martini and Beattie.[46] Review of the many articles on this subject indicate that probability of survival varies from 55%–70% and that long-term survival comparing segmentectomy with lobectomy favors lobectomy.

Locoregional recurrence of the cancer is always a possibility when a limited resection is carried out. There is a great deal of variation in the reported incidence of local recurrence following segmentectomy or wedge resections, and this relates to a lack of a uniform definition for local recurrence. The initial question that arises is whether the new cancer is a recurrence or a second primary. Our criteria for the definition of a second primary lung cancer has included a tumor-free interval of 24 months and the new tumor to be located in a separate and distinct ipsilateral lobe.[37] A similar definition would define that the second lesion be outside the area anatomically contiguous to the previous lung cancer and its regional lymphatics. However, others feel that if the cancer appears in the ipsilateral chest in any location or at any time interval, it is a locoregional recurrence. These differences in definition can account for variances in statistical reporting.

The Lung Cancer Study Group[19] has reported a statistically significant ($P$ = .02) increase in the recurrence rate associated with limited resection. There were 8 locoregional recurrences in 123 patients undergoing lobectomy for T1 N0 lung cancer (6.5%) and 12 local recurrences in 84 patients undergoing segmentectomy or wedge resection (14.2%).

Warren's recent analysis of our data comparing 66 segmentectomies vs. 103 lobectomies for stage I (T1–2 N0) disease revealed that the incidence of the development of a second ipsilateral cancer at any postoperative time interval was 22.7% (15/66) in the segmental resections and 4.9% (5/103) in the lobectomies (Tables 25–9 and 25–10). This prevalence decreased to 13.6% (segments) vs. 3.9% (lobes) if local recurrence was defined as lesions occurring within 2 years of resection.[18]

Pairolero et al[33] reported on recurrent disease in 346 patients who underwent resection for a non-small cell stage I bronchogenic carcinoma and were followed from 5 to 10 years. Local recurrence developed in only 7.2% of the entire group, but 14 additional patients had simultaneous local and distant metastasis. If the 14 patients are added to the 25 with only local recurrence, then the overall local recurrence was 11.3%. Bennett and Smith[49] noted a 40% recurrent rate within the ipsilateral lung following segmentectomy. The

**TABLE 25–9. SITES OF INTRATHORACIC RECURRENT CARCINOMA—GROUP I (66 PATIENTS) AND GROUP II (103 PATIENTS)**

| | Ipsilateral Recurrences | Bilateral Recurrences | Contralateral Recurrences |
|---|---|---|---|
| Group I (segmentectomy) | 15/66 (22.7%) | 1/66 (1.5%) | 3/66 (4.5%) |
| Group II (lobectomy) | 5/103 (4.9%) | 1/103 (1.0%) | 3/103 (2.9%) |

*(From Warren WH, Faber LP: Segmentectomy versus lobectomy in patients with Stage I pulmonary carcinoma. J Thorac Cardiovasc Surg 107:1087–1094, 1994, with permission.)*

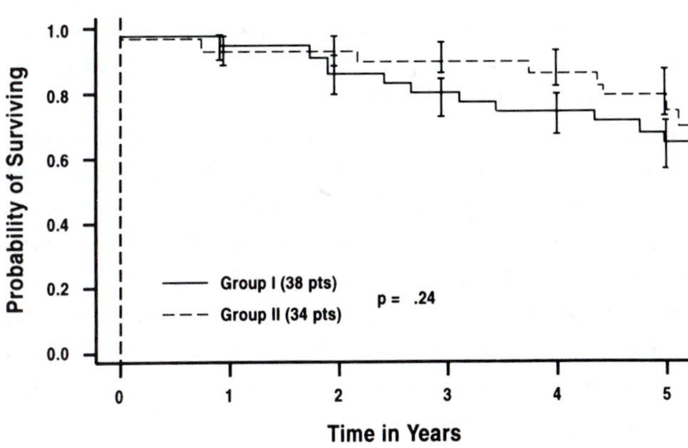


**Figure 25–15.** Kaplan-Meier Survival plot for segmentectomy (group I) and lobectomy (group II) with carcinomas ≤2 cm in diameter. *(From Warren WH, Faber LP: Segmentectomy versus lobectomy in patients with Stage I pulmonary carcinoma. J Thorac Cardiovasc Surg 107:1087–1094, 1994, with permission.)*

data of Read et al[47] in contrast, demonstrated an 11.5% (15/131) local recurrence rate in patients undergoing lobectomy and a 4.4% (5/113) in those undergoing segmentectomy. The explanation for these variances remains elusive and possibly relates to different definitions of local recurrence.

Size of the primary lesion affects long-term survival. Survival is enhanced when the lesion is <2.0 cm in diameter and is worsened by tumors >3 cm. Stair et al[50] and Read et al[47] demonstrated a significantly improved survival in patients whose lesion was <2 cm in diameter. Our recent data also indicated improved survival for those patients having a lesion <2 cm in diameter with no statistical difference in survival for the smaller lesion when lobectomy and segmentectomy were compared[48] (Fig. 25–15). The Lung Cancer Study Group only dealt with lesions <3 cm in diameter. Pairolero et al's review[28] of 346 patients with postsurgical stage I bronchogenic carcinoma revealed that probability of survival after resection for a T1 N0 cancer was 70% compared with 58.2% for the patients with T2 N0 lesions ($P$ = 0.12).

Propensity for recurrence tends to favor adenocarcinoma, but, again, the literature is at variance. Pairolero et al[33] noted that the percent of local recurrence did not differ in the various histologic groups. An earlier report of the Lung Cancer Study Group[51] identified a postoperative cancer recurrence in 107 of 572 resected patients with T1 N0 non-small cell lung cancer. Local and distant recurrence was more frequent and higher in the nonsquamous group with local recurrence at 8.6%. Read et al[47] noted that squamous histology carried a more favorable long-term prognosis than did tumors of nonsquamous histology. Nonsquamous tumors that grossly communicated with a segmental or subsegmental bronchus carried a significantly worse prognosis than squamous lesions of similar location ($P$ = 0.007). However, the Lung Cancer Study Group[51] found no significant difference in death or recurrence rate when histologies were compared. Analysis of our recent data for the histologic types in our stage I patients shows no statistical difference in survival between squamous and nonsquamous cancer.[18]

**TABLE 25–10. RELATIVE RISK OF LOCAL/REGIONAL RECURRENCE IN GROUP I AND GROUP II ACCORDING TO TUMOR DIAMETER**

| Tumor Diameter (cm) | Group I (segmentectomy) (%) | Group II (lobectomy) (%) |
|---|---|---|
| <2.0 | 9/38 (24) | 2/34 (6) |
| 2.1–3.0 | 3/13 (23) | 1/10 (10) |
| >3.0 | 3/15 (20) | 3/59 (5) |

*(From Warren WH, Faber LP: Segmentectomy versus lobectomy in patients with Stage I pulmonary carcinoma. J Thorac Cardiovasc Surg 107:1087–1094, 1994, with permission.)*

## THE DILEMMA

The planned surgical resection for each and every patient must be individualized. The magnitude of the resection is guided by the patient's general and cardiophysiologic status, clinical stage of the cancer, and associated disease entities. Only patients with clinical stage I cancers are possible candidates for a curative limited resection. However, the trend of data indicates that it may not be an operation of choice in the low-risk patient. Ginsburg and Rubinstein[19] have stated that "limited resection, either wedge or segmentectomy, cannot be recommended as a resection of choice for T1 N0 M0 lung cancer." While this may well be true for patients who are able to tolerate a lobectomy, there is no question that limited resection is indicated for patients with marginal cardiopulmonary function, since mortality is lower and approximate long-term survival is achieved.

When one chooses a type of limited resection, segmentectomy is preferred over wedge resection for several reasons: First, pulmonary lymphatics drain centrally in a segmental anatomic plane and are accordingly removed with segmentectomy. Second, during segmentectomy, regional lymph nodes can be resected when the segmental artery and bronchus are exposed; mediastinal lymphadenectomy can be performed at the same time. Last, parenchymal margins of resection are more clearly identified during anatomic resection, and a longer length of bronchus is removed eliminating the possibility for local bronchial recurrence. These factors all negate the wedge resection as a planned curative procedure for primary lung cancer. It remains to be seen whether localized parenchymal radiation following wedge resection will be of benefit.

Lesions <2 cm in diameter and those of squamous histology offer better long-term prognosis for a limited resection. Wedge resection, though not ideal, is more justifiable in this situation. It remains to be proven whether wedge resection accomplished by the open technique or by video-assisted technique provides the same long-term results as either segmentectomy or lobectomy. Currently, these methods are not procedures of choice for primary lung cancer. Segmentectomy remains the operation of choice for the compromised patient with early-stage lung cancer.

## REFERENCES


1. Graham EA, Singer JJ: Successful removal of an entire lung for carcinoma of the bronchus. *JAMA* **101:**1371–1374, 1993
2. Churchill ED, Belsey R: Segmental pneumonectomy in bronchiectasis. *Ann Surg* **109:**481–499, 1939
3. Kent EM, Blades B: The anatomic approach to pulmonary resection. *Ann Surg* **116:**783–794, 1942
4. Overholt RH, Langer L: A new technique for pulmonary segmental resection. Its application in the treatment of bronchiectasis. *Surg Gynecol Obstet* **84:**257–268, 1947
5. Chamberlain JM, Story CF, Klopstock R, et al: Segmental resection for pulmonary tuberculosis (300 cases). *J Thorac Surg* **26:**471, 1953
6. Reinhoff WF: The present status of the surgical treatment of primary carcinoma of the lung. *JAMA* **126:**1123–1128, 1944
7. Ochsner A, DeBakey M: Primary pulmonary malignancy treatment by total pneumonectomy. *Surg Gynecol Obstet* **68:**435–451, 1939
8. Overholt RH, Neptune WB, Ashraf M: Primary cancer of the lung—42 year experience. *Ann Thorac Surg* **20:**511–519, 1975
9. Thomas CP: Conservative resection of the bronchial tree. *J R. Coll Surg Edinb* **1:**169–186, 1956
10. Rasmussen RA, Basinger CE, Harrison RW, et al: Choice of operation in the treatment of bronchogenic carcinoma. (A review of 813 cases of which 209 were treated by resection). *Dis Chest* **46:**190–197, 1964
11. Bonfils-Roberts EA, Clagett OT: Contemporary indications for pulmonary segment resections. *J Thorac Cardiovasc Surg* **63:**433–438, 1972
12. Clagett OT, Wollner LB: Surgical treatment of solitary metastatic pulmonary lesion. *Med Clin North Am* **48:**939–943, 1964
13. Thomford NB, Woolner LB, Clagett OT: The surgical treatment of metastatic tumors of the lung. *J Thorac Cardiovasc Surg* **49:**357–363, 1965
14. LeRoux TT: Management of bronchial carcinoma by segmental resection. *Thorax* **27:**70–74, 1972
15. Jensik RJ, Faber LP, Milloy FJ, Monson DO: Segmental resection for lung cancer. *J Thorac Cardiovasc Surg* **66:**563–572, 1973
16. Hoffman TH, Ransdell HT: Comparison of lobectomy and wedge resection for carcinoma of the lung. *J Thorac Cardiovasc Surg* **79:**211–217, 1980
17. Errett LE, Wilson J, Chiu RCT, et al: Wedge resection as an alternative procedure for peripheral bronchogenic carcinomas in poor risk patients. *J Thorac Cardiovasc Surg* **90:**656–661, 1985
18. Warren WH, Faber LP: Segmentectomy versus lobectomy in patients in stage I pulmonary carcinoma: Five year survival and patterns of intrathoracic recurrence. *J Thorac Cardiovasc Surg* **107:**1087–1094, 1994
19. Ginsburg RJ, Rubinstein L: A randomized comparative trial of lobectomy versus segmentectomy for patients with T1 N0 non SCLA lung cancer. *Lung Cancer* **7**(suppl): 83A, 1991
20. Errett LE, Wilson J, Chiu RCJ, et al: Wedge resection as an alternative procedure for peripheral bronchogenic carcinomas in poor risk patients. *J Thorac Cardiovasc Surg* **90:**656, 1987
21. Jensik RJ: Mini resection of small peripheral carcinomas of the lung. *Surg Clin North Am* **67:**951, 1987
22. Crabbe MM, Patrissi GA, Fontenelle LJ: Minimal resection for bronchogenic carcinoma. Should this be standard therapy? *Chest* **95:**968, 1989
23. Crabbe MM, Patrissi GA, Fontenelle LJ: Minimal resection for bronchogenic carcinoma. An update. *Chest* **99:**1421, 1991
24. Macchiarini P, Fontanini G, Hardin JM, et al: Most peripheral node-negative, non-small cell lung cancers have low proliferative rates and no intra-tumoral and peri-tumoral blood and lymphatic vessel invasion. Rationale for treatment with wedge resection alone. *J Thorac Cardiovasc Surg* **104:**892, 1992
25. Peters RM: Identification assessment and management of surgical patients with chronic respiratory disease. In Greenfield LV (ed): *Problems in General Surgery,* Vol 1. Philadelphia, Lippincott, pp 432–444, 1984
26. Miller JI, Grossman GD, Hatcher CR: Pulmonary function test criteria for operability and pulmonary resection. *Surg Gynecol Obstet* **153:**893–895, 1981
27. Schwaber JR: Evaluation of respiratory status in surgical patients. *Surg Clin North Am* **50:**673, 1970
28. Miller JI, Hatcher CR: Limited resection of bronchogenic carcinoma in the patient with marked impairment of pulmonary function. *Ann Thorac Surg* **44:**340–343, 1987
29. Bechard D, Wetstein L: Assessment of exercise oxygen consumption as preoperative criterion for lung resection. *Ann Thorac Surg* **44:**344–349, 1987
30. Ali MK, Mountain CG, Ewer MS, Johnston D, Haynie TP: Predicting loss of pulmonary function after pulmonary resection for bronchogenic carcinoma. *Chest* **77:**337–342, 1980
31. Auerbqach O, Stout AO, Hammond EC, Garfinel L: Multiple primary bronchial carcinomas. *Cancer* **20:**699–705, 1967
32. Salerno TA, Munro DD, Blundell PE, Chiu RJC: Second primary bronchogenic carcinoma. Life-table analysis of surgical treatment. *Ann Thorac Surg* **27:**3–6, 1979
33. Pairolero PC, Williams DE, Bergstrath EJ, et al: Post-surgical stage I bronchogenic carcinoma: Morbid implications of recurrent disease. *Ann Thorac Surg* **38:**331–338, 1984
34. Ferguson MD, DeMeester TR, DesLauriers J, Little AG, et al: Diagnosis and management of synchronous lung cancers. *J Thorac Cardiovasc Surg* **89:**378–385, 1985
35. Temeck BK, Flehinger BJ, Martini N: A retrospective analysis of 10 year survivors from carcinoma of the lung. *Cancer* **53:**1405–1408, 1984
36. Mathisen DJ, Jensik RJ, Faber LP, Kittle CF: Survival following resection for second and third primary lung cancers. *J Thorac Cardiovasc Surg* **88:**502–510, 1984
37. Faber LP: Resection for second and third primary lung cancer. *Semin Surg Oncol* **9:**135, 1993
38. Kittle CF, Faber LP, Jensik RJ, Warren WH: Pulmonary resection in patients after pneumonectomy. *Ann Thorac Surg* **40:**294–299, 1985

39. Breyer RH, Zippe C, Pharr WF, et al: Thoracotomy in patients over age seventy years: Ten year experience. *J Thorac Cardiovasc Surg* **81:**187–193, 1981
40. Berggren H, Ekroth R, Malmber R, et al: Hospital mortality and long-term survival in relation to preoperative function in elderly patients with bronchogenic carcinoma. *Ann Thorac Surg* **38:**633–636, 1984
41. Keagy BA, Pharr WF, Bowles RE, et al: A review of morbidity and mortality in elderly patients undergoing pulmonary resection. *Am Surg* **50:**213–216, 1984
42. Weiss W: Operative mortality and five year survival rates in patients with bronchogenic carcinoma. *Am J Surg* **128:**799–804, 1974
43. McCormick P, Martini N: Secondary tumors in the lung. In Shield TW (ed.): *General Thoracic Surgery,* Philadelphia, Lea & Febiger, 1989, pp 951–959
44. Overholt RH, Langer L: The technique of pulmonary resection. Springfield, Illinois, Charles C Thomas, 1949
45. Fry WA: Needle biopsy for the diagnosis of intrathoracic lesions: Transthoracic needle biopsy. In Kittle CF (ed.): *Current Controversies in Thoracic Surgery,* Saunders, Philadelphia, 1986, pp 87–91
46. Martini N, Beattie EJ Jr: Results of surgical treatment in stage I lung cancer. *J Thorac Cardiovasc Surg* **74:**499, 1977
47. Read RC, Yoder G, Schaeffer RC: Survival after conservative resection for T1 N0 M0 non-small cell lung cancer. *Ann Thorac Surg* **49:**391, 1990
48. Williams EE, Pairolero PD, Davis CS, et al: Survival of patients surgically treated for stage I lung cancer. *J Thorac Cardiovasc Surg* **82:**70–76, 1981
49. Bennett WF, Smith RA: Segmental resection for bronchogenic carcinoma: A surgical alternative for the compromised patient. *Ann Thorac Surg* **27:**169–172, 1978
50. Stair JM, Womble J, Schaefer RF, Read RC: Segmental pulmonary resection for cancer. *Am J Surg* **150:**659–664,1985
51. Thomas P, Rubinstein L: Lung cancer study group: Cancer recurrence after resection: T1 N0 non-small cell lung cancer. *Ann Thorac Surg* **49:**242, 1990
52. El-Baz NM, Faber LP, Jensik RJ: Continuous epidural infusion of morphine for treatment of pain after thoracic surgery: A new technique. *Anesth Analg* **63:**757,1984

CHAPTER

# 26

# Bronchoplastic Techniques for Lung Resection

Richard N. Gates and Paul F. Waters

## HISTORICAL PERSPECTIVE

Bronchoplastic procedures were initially developed in the late 1940s to preserve lung parenchyma while removing benign proximal bronchial lesions. Price-Thomas[1] and D'Abreau and MacHale[2] were the first to report approaches to both main stem bronchi for the treatment of such tumors. Gebauer[3] demonstrated that the technique was applicable to proximal bronchial stenosis caused by tuberculosis. Thus, the early 1950s ushered in the era of bronchoplastic procedures for the treatment of benign proximal lesions of the bronchus.

Allison[4] performed the first bronchoplastic resection for lung carcinoma in 1952. However, the general consensus favoring radical cancer operations at that time limited initial enthusiasm for this "conservative" approach to lung cancer surgery. With time, the principles of surgical oncology were developed and the role of bronchoplastic procedures in the treatment of lung carcinoma elucidated. The indications for bronchoplastic procedures as well as the surgical technique and its results have been well documented in the literature.[5–23]

Recent refinements in vascular surgical technique have allowed for pulmonary artery sleeve resections to be combined with bronchoplastic resections.[19,22,24] Combining these procedures has expanded the indications for lung conserving operations in the treatment of lung carcinoma. The pioneering work of the Toronto Lung Transplant Group has led to the clinical reality of successful lung transplantation.[25] This has fortuitously resulted in a tremendous amount of research regarding bronchial physiology and healing. Much of this work is applicable to bronchoplastic procedures and has greatly advanced the field.

## DIAGNOSIS

Accurate preoperative and intraoperative diagnosis and staging of lesions where bronchoplastic resections are planned is critical. While the surgeon's goal is preservation of lung tissue, this must never be achieved at the expense of a compromised procedure. Preoperative evaluation should include a careful history and physical exam, blood laboratories, pulmonary function studies, chest x-ray, computed tomography (CT) scan, bronchoscopy, and occasionally magnet resource imaging (MRI) or angiography.

Particular attention should be paid to the chest x-ray with regard to an enlarged mediastinum with tracheal compromise. The presence of a postobstructive process should be carefully sought. Computed tomography should be performed with IV contrast to assist in the evaluation of invasion of mediastinal structures or the perihilar vasculature. The CT scan should not be used to stage mediastinal lymph nodes. All patients with carcinoma and anticipated resection should undergo mediastinoscopy or parasternal mediastinal exploration with pathologic lymph node sampling prior to or at the time of the definitive procedure. The inability of CT scanning or gross surgical inspection to accurately stage lung carcinoma is well documented.[26–30] The importance of proper staging can not be overemphasized in the era of neoadjuvant clinical trials for stages IIIa and IIIb bronchogenic carcinoma.

Bronchoscopy is essential to evaluate the technical feasibility of a bronchoplastic resection. The extent of a primary endobronchial lesion should be carefully defined and the operative strategy planned. For malignant lesions, multiple biopsies of adjacent normal appearing mucosa should be performed to rule out submucosal tumor extension. On occasion the CT scan will suggest vascular involvement of a tumor where a bronchoplastic resection is planned. In such cases an MRI scan may better define the local vascular anatomy and assist in planning the operation.[31,32]

At the time of definitive surgery, preoperative evaluation and staging should be confirmed. Once this is done, the final decision to perform the bronchoplastic procedure is made. The resected specimen should be expediently delivered to the pathology laboratory for intraoperative confirmation of histologically negative proximal and distal margins. Should margins be identified as positive, further resection is indicated as pulmonary function allows. Improved survival with tumor-free margins is expected in such cases. This is particularly true when the final pathologic staging reveals stage I or II disease.[33]

## INDICATIONS

Bronchoplastic procedures are performed either with or without associated parenchymal lung resection. In practice, the only bronchoplastic resections performed without associated lung resections are those for the left main stem bronchus or carina. Benign lesions or small isolated T3 carcinomas may be resected from the long left main bronchus without loss of lung parenchyma (Fig. 26–1). In general, sleeve resections can be divided into those performed for benign disease and those performed for carcinoma. For carcinoma, resections fall into three broad categories (Fig. 26–2): (1) isolated tumor at the lobar orifice, (2) tumor of the main bronchus or infiltration of the main bronchus by contiguous involved lymph nodes, or (3) peripheral primary tumor with infiltration of the lobar orifice or main bronchus with involved lymph nodes. For benign lesions, resections fall into two categories (Fig. 26–3): (1) tumor residing at the lobar orifice, and (2) tumor within the main bronchus.

Whenever technically feasible, benign bronchial lesions should be resected using bronchoplastic techniques. For the most common benign endobronchial lesion, the typical carcinoid tumor, this is generally possible. The prognosis of a patient with a typical carcinoid tumor undergoing a bronchoplastic resection vs. a standard resection is identical regardless of lymph node status as long as a complete resection is achieved.[34] In both cases 10-year tumor-related survival approaches 100%. Thus, when possible, a bronchoplastic procedure and regional lymphadenectomy should be performed. Atypical carcinoids behave similarly to well-differentiated non-small cell carcinoma and should be surgically managed as such.[35] Tuberculous bronchial stenosis represents another indication for bronchoplastic procedures in benign disease.[36] While relatively rare, the incidence of this tuberculosis related complication may be on the rise in the United States. More uncommonly, foreign body or post-traumatic strictures may occur that are resistant to dilatation and subsequently require bronchoplastic resections.

When determining the appropriateness of a bronchoplastic resection, patients are best considered in two groups: those with and those without adequate pulmonary reserve to undergo a pneumonectomy. We generally feel that patients with an $FEV_1$ of 2 L or greater and a maximum voluntary ventilation of >50% of predicted are candidates for pneumonectomy.[37,38] When $FEV_1$ is <2 L, a split lung study may be helpful in predicting postoperative $FEV_1$. If this prediction is 800 mL or greater following resection, than pneumonectomy is usually acceptable. If a patient fails

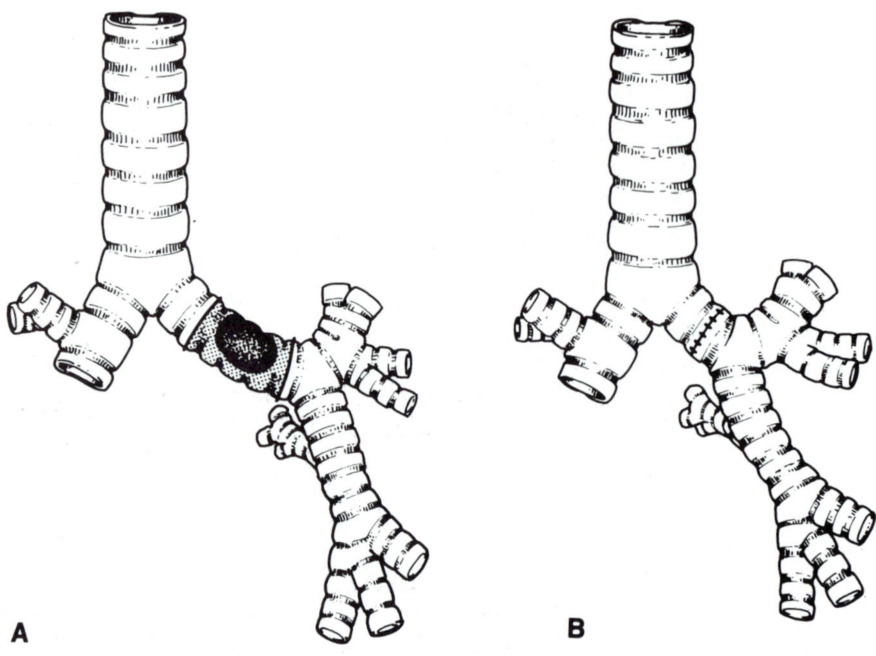


**Figure 26–1.** Left main stem bronchus resection for benign lesions or small T3, N0, M0 carcinomas.

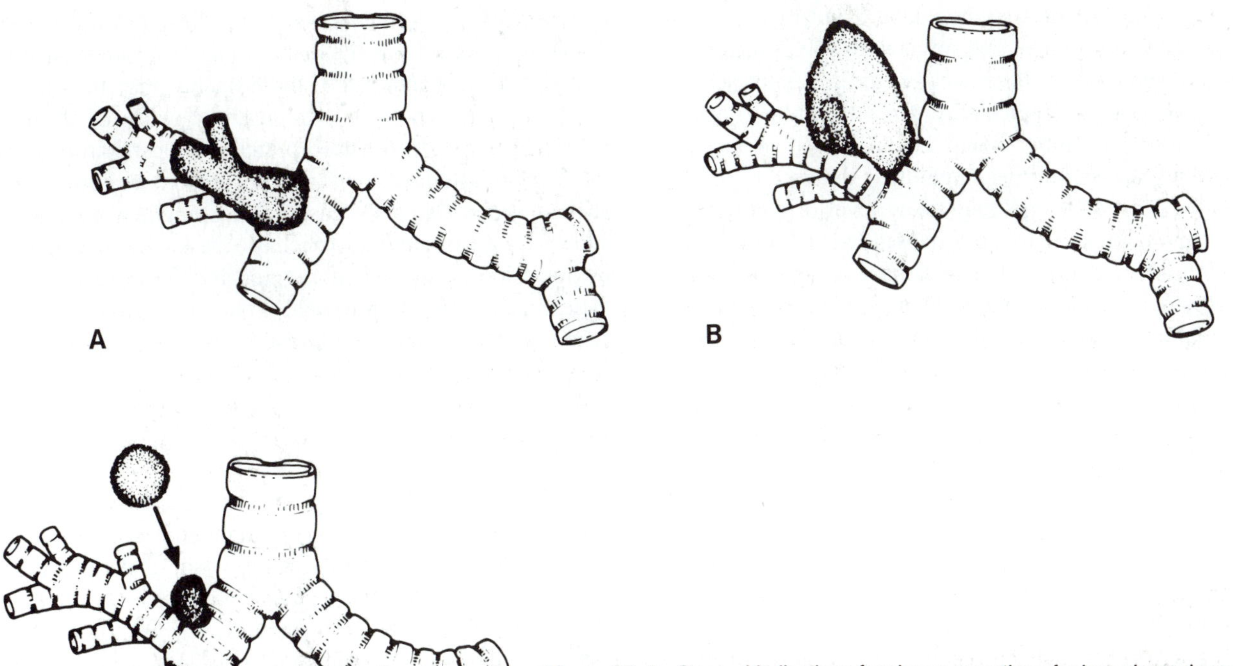


Figure 26–2. General indications for sleeve resections for bronchogenic carcinoma. A. Isolated tumor at the lobar orifice. B. Tumor of the main bronchus or infiltration of the main bronchus by contiguous involved lymph nodes. C. Peripheral tumor with infiltration of the lobar orifice or main bronchus with involved lymph nodes.

these criteria, then a sleeve resection is the patient's only operative alternative. In such instances, sleeve resection should be undertaken only after careful evaluation demonstrates negative N2 lymph nodes and a high probability that a histologically negative resection margin can be obtained.

For patients with pulmonary function adequate to tolerate pneumonectomy, some controversy arises as to when to perform a sleeve resection. Generally, we perform a sleeve resection in such patients when the tumor is amenable to a right upper lobe, left upper lobe, right middle lobe, or right bilobe sleeve resection. Other technically feasible but rather uncommon sleeve resections are reserved for patients with inadequate pulmonary reserve in whom pneumonectomy is contraindicated. As will be seen, morbidity and mortality for the aforementioned sleeve resections are low. Thus, the use of a sleeve resection for such patients appears to be prudent in light of the anticipated advantage in postoperative pulmonary function these patients can expect. Further, a conservative sleeve lobectomy may allow the patient to undergo a future pulmonary resection should the need arise. Contralateral second primary lung carcinomas have been reported to occur in patients having undergone sleeve resection with an incidence of 7.6% and a mean interval between sleeve operation and second tumor of 54 months (range 6–197).[39] Finally, in the era of neoadjuvant radiation and chemotherapy, one should be aware of the preoperative radiation dosage. Poor bronchial healing after bronchoplastic procedures may occur when a preoperative clinical fraction exceeds 36 Gy.[40] This should be considered a relative but not absolute contraindication to a sleeve resection.

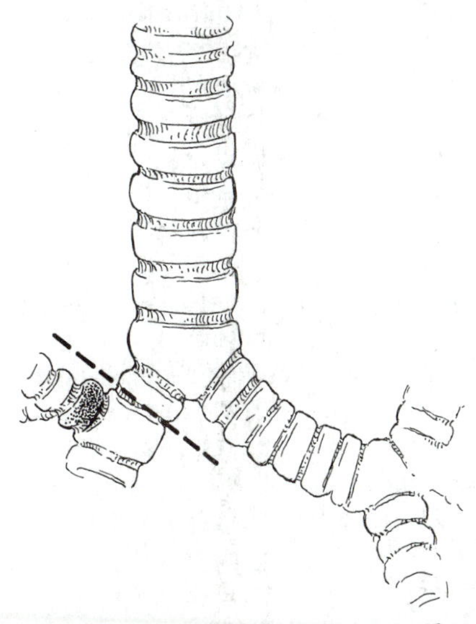

Figure 26–3. General indications for sleeve resection in benign bronchogenic lesions include tumor within the main bronchus and tumor residing at the lobar orifice as seen here.

## SURGICAL TECHNIQUE

The development of double-lumen endotracheal tubes has greatly advanced the anesthetic management of thoracic surgical patients. Their use should be standard for most bronchoplastic procedures. The surgeon as well as the anesthesiologist should bronchoscopically confirm endotracheal tube position prior to thoracotomy. Once the chest is open, the position of the tube should be confirmed manually. Should hypoxia occur during single-lung ventilation, this is frequently relieved by applying a low level of continuous positive airway pressure to the collapsed lung. If immediate extubation is not done at the conclusion of the operation, the double-lumen tube should be changed to a single-lumen tube of sufficient caliber to allow for diagnostic and therapeutic bronchoscopy.

There are several technical principles that should be followed when one performs bronchoplastic procedures. Bronchial healing is dependent upon an intact vascular supply. Excessive skeletonization of the main bronchus and branch bronchi should be avoided. Only involved lymph nodes and bronchi should be excised. Avoiding unnecessary dissection preserves bronchial arteries and enhances anastomotic healing. In addition, minimal dissection promotes effective mucociliary function in the postoperative period.[41] The bronchial suture line should be without tension. Division of the inferior pulmonary ligament is frequently all that is required here. For cases requiring further length, mobilization of the carina is helpful. This should be done in the anterior and posterior planes to avoid devascularization of the trachea itself.

The bronchial anastomosis is predicated on careful tissue to tissue apposition. The open bronchial ends should be divided smoothly so that no incomplete cartilaginous rings are present. Since there is a gradual diminution in bronchial size distal from the carina, bronchoplastic procedures frequently lend themselves to the anastomotic technique of "telescoping" (Fig. 26–4). Here, the smaller distal bronchial segment is brought up into the lumen of the larger proximal segment. The membranous portion of the bronchus should be sewn first with sutures placed to allow them to be tied within the bronchus as the distal bronchus is telescoped in. The cartilaginous portion of the bronchus may then be sutured with the knots placed on the outside of the new bronchial lumen.[42] We have preferred to perform this single-layer anastomosis with an absorbable braided suture such as Vicryl®. In some cases telescoping may not be possible because of similar bronchial size or the potential for compression of a distal subsegmental bronchi that may be "telescoped" into the proximal bronchus. When this is the case, a careful direct end-to-end anastomosis using interrupted suture technique should be used. As with bronchial stumps, the anastomosis is tested for an air leak by submersion in saline during a valsalva with 40 cm of water pressure.

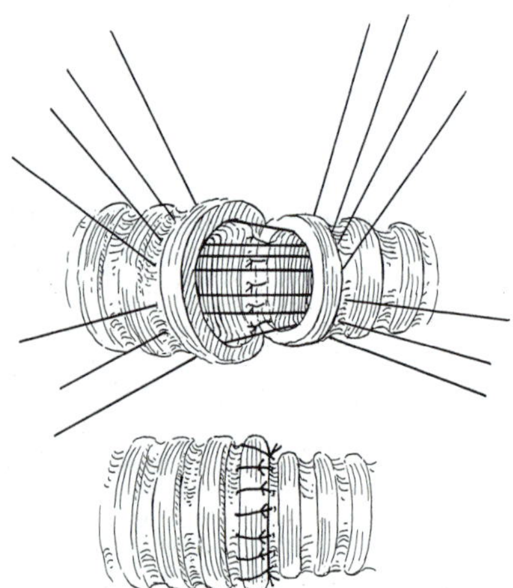

**Figure 26–4.** The anastomotic technique of "telescoping" the bronchus. The distal segment of bronchus is brought up into the lumen of the proximal segment.

"Wrapping" of bronchial anastomoses is controversial. Early canine models of lung transplantation demonstrated a positive effect on bronchial healing when omentopexy was used.[43,44] Thus, most lung transplant centers used some form of anastomotic reinforcement during the 1980s. However, the confounding variable of high-dose steroids and its negative impact upon bronchial healing soon became clear.[45] With changes in immunosuppressive protocols, many centers were able to achieve low and comparable rates of anastomotic complications without the use of anastomotic wraps.[42,46] In the 1990s most centers do not routinely wrap the bronchial anastomosis following lung transplantation. For nonimmunosuppressed patients undergoing uncomplicated sleeve resections, wraps probably afford no extra protection from anastomotic complications.[47,48] Thus, we do not routinely use them in these clinical settings. For complicated sleeve resections where previous radiation therapy or where ongoing infection may be present, a bronchial wrap based on the omentum, pericardial fat pad, or intercostal musculature may be used. When a pulmonary artery sleeve resection is performed a vascularized tissue pedicle should probably be placed between the reconstructed artery and bronchus as a precaution.

After completion of the bronchoplastic procedure, the lung should be re-expanded and examined for ventilation and the potential for torsion assessed. Fine sutures may be used to stabilize lobes to one another or the chest wall. Immediate bronchoscopic examination of the anastomosis should be performed at the conclusion of the procedure.

Sleeve resections of the right or left upper lobe represent the vast majority of bronchoplastic resections (Fig. 26–5). These procedures are best performed through a posterolateral thoracotomy. However, both may be done through an anterior-lateral thoracotomy or median sternotomy if unusual circumstances dictate this approach. Sleeve resections involving the lower lobes should be approached through a posterolateral thoracotomy. Regarding the left upper lobe sleeve, the left main stem bronchus may be visualized by mobilization and anterior retraction of the left main pulmonary artery. This is facilitated by dividing the ligamentum arteriosum and freeing the arch aorta. The

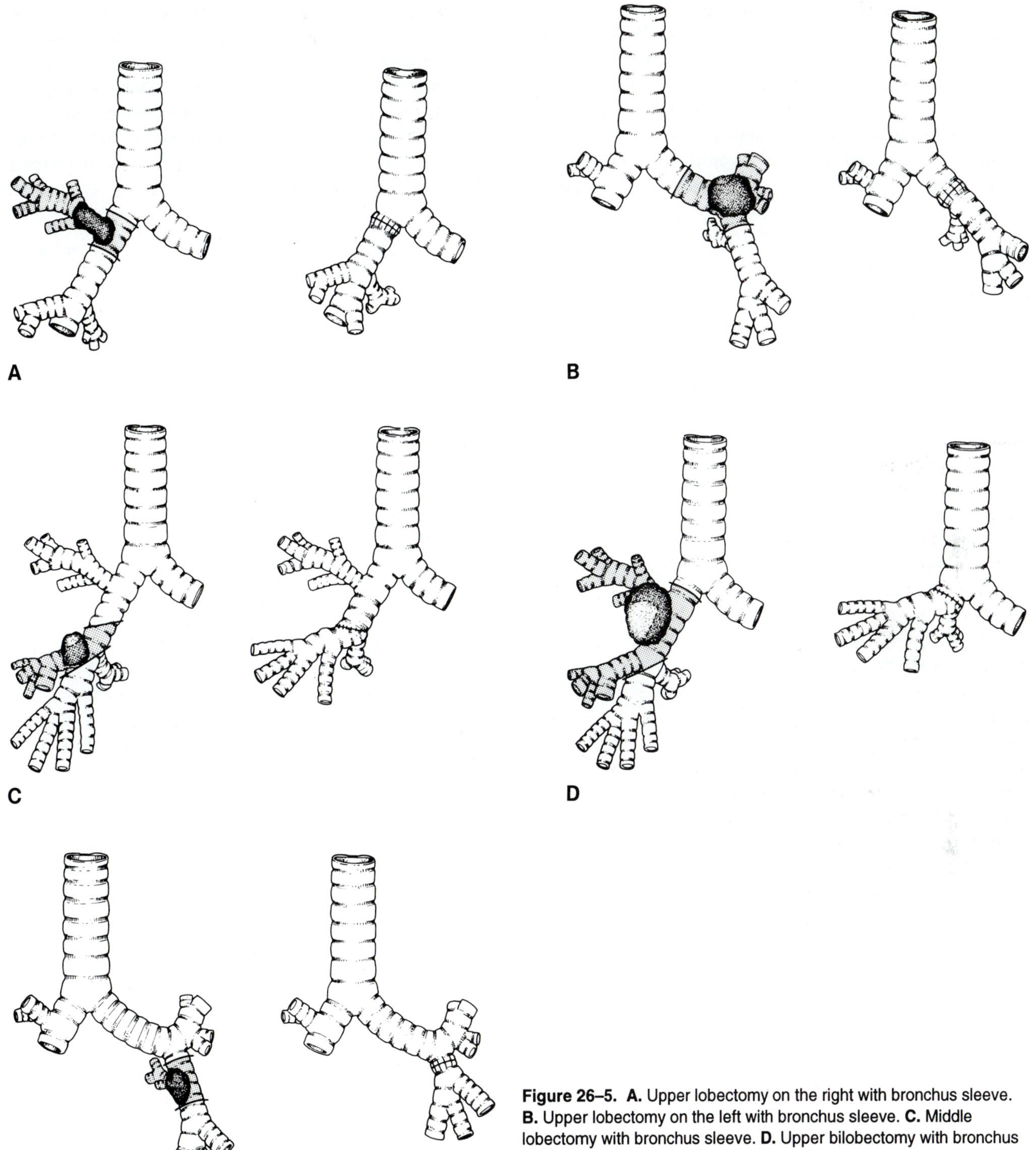


**Figure 26–5. A.** Upper lobectomy on the right with bronchus sleeve. **B.** Upper lobectomy on the left with bronchus sleeve. **C.** Middle lobectomy with bronchus sleeve. **D.** Upper bilobectomy with bronchus sleeve. **E.** Resection of the apical lower lobe segment on the left with bronchus sleeve.

trachea and right main stem bronchus are dissected in the anterior and posterior plane to achieve even greater mobility of the left main stem bronchus if necessary. For the right upper-lobe sleeve resection, the azygous vein is transected giving excellent exposure of the proximal right main stem bronchus. The bronchus intermedius is then exposed to reveal the takeoff of the middle lobe bronchus and the bronchus to the superior segment of the lower lobe. This allows for careful inspection of the distal resection line. Uncommonly, an upper lobe orifice tumor may extend anterior-inferior and require an upper and middle bilobectomy (Fig. 26–5). Upper-lobe orifice tumors that have spread posterior-inferior to involve the superior segment of the lower lobe should be managed by pneumonectomy. Small tumors of the right middle-lobe orifice may occasionally be managed by sleeve middle lobectomy (Fig. 26–5). However, this is uncommon, since the superior segment bronchus frequently is in the way.

A variety of other innovative but uncommon sleeve resections has been described and applied (Fig. 26–6). These resections have greater bronchial reconstruction angulation as well as size mismatch. Great care must be taken to avoid kinking or compression of the pulmonary artery in these cases. At times, pulmonary artery resection and reconstruction may need to be applied. We have reserved the use of these uncommon sleeve resections for patients with inadequate pulmonary function to tolerate pneumonectomy.

Advances in vascular technique and an increased appreciation of the segmental anatomy of the pulmonary artery have recently allowed for tangential or circum-

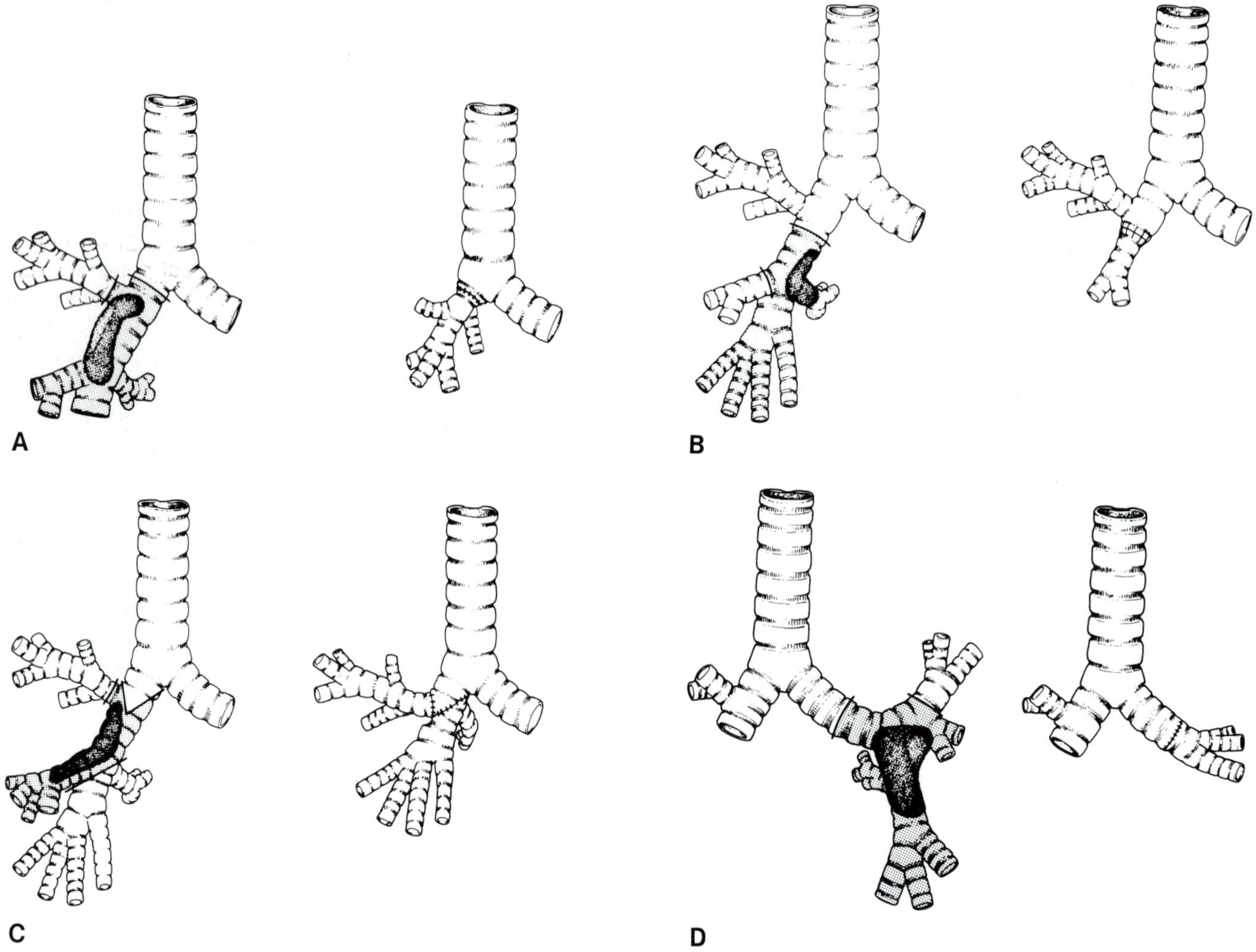

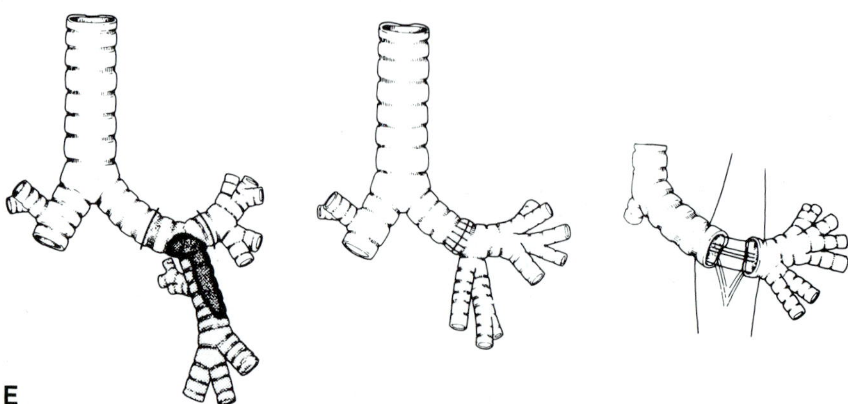


**Figure 26–6.** Uncommon bronchoplastic resections. **A.** Sleeve right middle and lower bilobectomy. **B.** Sleeve right lower lobectomy for tumor at the lower lobe superior segment bronchial orifice. **C.** Sleeve right middle lobectomy for a lateral tumor extending from the middle lobe orifice to the carina of the upper lobe. **D.** Lower lobectomy on the left with bronchus sleeve. **E.** Sleeve left lower lobectomy and lingulectomy for lower-lobe tumors that also involve the lingular bronchus.

ferential sleeve resection of the pulmonary artery to be performed in conjunction with bronchoplastic resections.[19,22,24,32,49] The vast majority of circumferential pulmonary artery sleeve resections are performed in association with left upper lobe sleeve resections (Fig. 26–7). Tangential resection of the involved artery is preferred only if involvement is minimal and the resulting repair does little to narrow the arterial lumen. Otherwise, circumferential resection with end-to-end anastomosis is indicated. As for bronchial anastomoses, the absence of tension upon the arterial repair is of paramount importance. If this cannot be achieved primarily, then a Goretex® or pericardial tube interposition graft can be used. Arterial reconstruction should be carried out after lobectomy and bronchoplasty. This allows for an accurate assessment of the position to be resected and reconstructed pulmonary artery. Careful intrapericardial proximal control as well as distal intralobar control of the left or right pulmonary artery is mandatory. Alternatively, distal control can be achieved at the level of the pulmonary veins. As mentioned previously, a vascularized pedicle should be placed between the pulmonary artery suture line and the reconstructed bronchus to help avoid a broncho-arterial fistulae. Care must be taken not to interpose too much tissue or the pulmonary artery may become compromised.

## POSTOPERATIVE CARE

After completion of the sleeve resection, bronchoscopy is performed in the operating room to inspect the anastomosis and to clear secretions. Depending upon the patient's general health and pulmonary function, extubation may be carried out in the operating room or subsequently. In patients who remain intubated overnight, a morning bronchoscopy to clear mucous and clotted blood is performed prior to extubation. Gentle and frequent endotracheal suctioning with a soft-tip catheter is recommended during mechanical ventilation. Once extubated, it is imperative that vigorous chest physiotherapy be practiced. This should include inhalational therapy, chest percussion and drainage, incentive spirometry, and early ambulation. Patients who develop significant atelectasis or demonstrate poor ability to clear secretions should undergo frequent therapeutic bronchoscopy and may be considered for early tracheostomy to facilitate pulmonary toilet.

Approximately 1 week after surgery, a follow-up bronchoscopy is performed. At this time the anastomosis may be graded in three general categories: (1) no evidence of ischemia, healthy mucosa with normal healing; (2) mild ischemia with some mucosal sloughing but preserved structure; (3) or frank ischemia with mucosal necrosis and impending or partial/complete dehiscence. Patients in the first category generally do exceedingly well in both the short and long term. Patients in the second category generally do well in the early postoperative period but may develop subsequent stenosis due to stricture or excessive granulation tissue. As such, these patients need frequent bronchoscopic follow-up and careful monitoring of their pulmonary function tests (PFTs) as outpatients. Excessive granulation tissue has recently been successfully treated with laser ablation. Strictures can be treated by stenting[50,51] or initially by dilation.[52,53] For patients in the third category, overall results are poor. In healthy patients who can

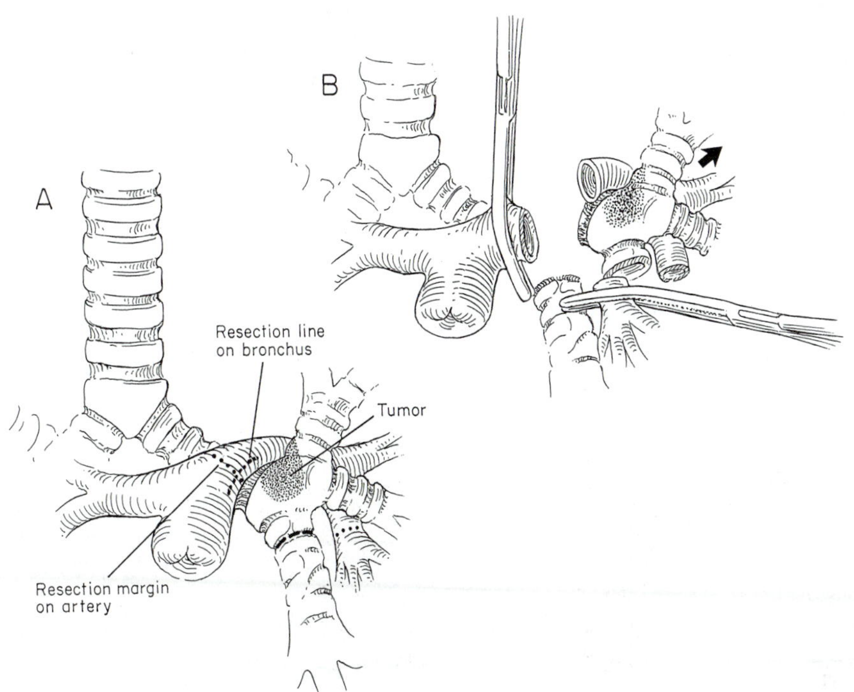


**Figure 26–7.** Combined left upper lobe sleeve resection and pulmonary artery sleeve resection.

tolerate completion pneumonectomy, this should be undertaken without delay. In patients who cannot tolerate pneumonectomy, the situation is more difficult. In extubated patients with a small area of dehiscence, conservative drainage and supportive care may be successful. Consideration to perform a delayed anastomotic wrap with a muscle-based flap should be considered. In patients with complete dehiscence who cannot tolerate pneumonectomy, salvage regardless of therapy is rare.

All patients should be carefully monitored for the development of a bronchopleural fistula. Subtle changes in temperature, heart rate, respiratory rate, sputum production, and mental status many indicate early sepsis secondary to a fistula. Such patients should be carefully evaluated with a physical exam, white blood cell count, arterial blood gas, chest x-ray, and bronchoscopy if the index of suspicion is high. In cases where pulmonary artery sleeve resection or tangential excision has been performed, partial or complete arterial thrombosis may occur. Both these complications tend to occur in the early postoperative period. Complete thrombosis of the right or left pulmonary artery presents similar to a massive pulmonary artery embolus with an acute and dramatic deterioration. The diagnosis can generally be made on clinical grounds with the aid of a chest x-ray demonstrating poor vascular markings. If time is available, the diagnosis can be confirmed by perfusion scanning or angiography. These patients should be promptly treated with completion pneumonectomy.

## RESULTS

Early mortality after bronchoplastic resection is quite variable and has ranged between 0% and 12%[12–14,16–19,21–23] (Table 26–1). These figures are similar to the reported early mortality of 6.2% for pneumonectomy and 2.9% for lobectomy reported by the Lung Cancer Study Group.[54] Major morbidity ranges between 2.5% and 14%.[12,16,18,21–23] Common postoperative complications include bronchopleural fistula in 0%–8%[1,2–14,16–19,21,23] anastomotic local recurrence in 5–25%,[12,13,16–19,22,23] empyema, cicatrical stricture, excessive granulation tissue at the anastomosis, and pneumonia. The management of bronchopleural fistulas has been previously discussed. Local recurrence may rarely be treated with re-sleeve resection but generally requires completion pneumonectomy. Management of cicatrical stricture and excessive granulation tissue is as previously described. The observed mortality rate of 0–12% for bronchoplastic procedures is in the same range as that for pneumonectomy. Thus, the procedure should be offered to all appropriate candidates without fear of increased morbidity or mortality.

Overall actuarial 5-year survival for patients with carcinoma has ranged around 30–50%. For stage I it has been between 36% and 71%, for stage II between 18% and 55%, and for stage III between 0% and 30%.[12–14,16–19,21,23] These survival rates are comparable with those of patients undergoing standard resections for lung carcinoma where anticipated stage I, II, and III 5-year survival is approximately 55%, 32%, and 15%, respectively.[55] Thus, with appropriate selection and surgical technique, bronchoplastic procedures for lung carcinoma do not compromise survival.

Results for vascular sleeve resections and combined bronchovascular sleeve procedures are similar although the experience within the literature is smaller. Early mortality for isolated vascular sleeve procedures is reported between 0% and 8%. For combined bronchovascular operations, it is between 0% and 13%[19,22,24,32,49] (Table 26–2). Vogt-Moykopf et al[19] have demonstrated a 35% 5-year survival for stage I and II disease.

Complications that may occur are arterial thrombosis, local recurrence, bronchovascular fistula, and others seen with isolated bronchoplastic procedures. Acute arterial thrombosis is sudden in presentation and requires emergency pneumonectomy. Local recurrence is best treated by completion pneumonectomy as well. Bronchovascular fis-

**TABLE 26–1. BRONCHOPLASTY RESULTS**

| Author(s) | Year/N | Early Mortality (%) | Percent: *BP Fistula* | Percent: *Local Recurrence* |
|---|---|---|---|---|
| Bennett and Abbey-Smith | 1978/96 | 8 | 2 | 25 |
| Shaw and Luke | 1979/100 | 8 | 1 | 5 |
| Ungar et al | 1982/261 | 7 | 2 | NA |
| Fermin et al | 1983/90 | 1 | 0 | 5 |
| Faber et al | 1984/101 | 2 | 7 | 9 |
| Deslauriers et al | 1986/72 | 0 | 0 | 16 |
| Vogt-Moykopf et al | 1986/399 | 12 | 8 | 16 |
| Watanabe et al | 1990/79 | 1 | 0 | NA |
| Maggi et al | 1993/73 | 4 | NA | 8 |
| Mehran et al | 1994/142 | 2 | 1 | 23 |

NA, not available.

**TABLE 26–2. ANGIOPLASTIC AND BRONCHOVASCULAR MORTALITY**

| | Percent | |
|---|---|---|
| Author (Year) | *Angioplastic* | *Bronchovascular* |
| Belli et al (1985) | | 9 (n = 6) |
| Vogt-Moykopf et al (1986) | 8 ( n = 51) | 13 (n = 29) |
| Maggi et al (1993) | 6 (n = 18) | 0 (n = 4) |
| Reed et al (1993) | | 0 (n = 6) |
| Rendina et al (1993) | | 0 (n = 10) |

tulas present with sudden massive hemoptysis and are generally fatal. Early recognition with endobronchial occlusion and emergency pneumonectomy may salvage an occasional patient.

Bronchoplastic and bronchovascular procedures lead to a significant improvement in postoperative pulmonary function when compared to pneumonectomy.[56] This is achieved without additional morbidity, mortality, or decrease in long-term survival. The benefit of these procedures in terms of quality of life is difficult to measure but easy for the patient to appreciate. Therefore, when following appropriate patient selection, bronchoplastic and bronchovascular procedures should be performed without hesitation.

## REFERENCES


1. Price-Thomas C: Concerning resection of the bronchial tree. *J R Coll Surg Edinb* **1–2:**169–186, 1956
2. D'Abreau AL, MacHale SJ: Bronchial "adenoma" treated by local resection and reconstruction of the left main bronchus. *Br J Surg* **39:**355–357, 1952
3. Gebauer PW: Bronchial resection and anastomosis. *J Thorac Surg* **26:**241–260, 1953
4. Allison PR: Course of thoracic surgery in Groningen. Quoted by Jones PW. *Ann R Coll Surg Engl* **25:**20–38, 1959
5. Paulson DL, Shaw RR: Bronchial anastomosis and bronchoplastic procedures in the interest of preservation of the lung. *J Thor Cardiovasc Surg* **29:**238–259, 1955
6. Johnston JB, Jones PH: The treatment of bronchial carcinoma by lobectomy and sleeve resection of the bronchus. *Thorax* **14:**48–54, 1959
7. Price-Thomas C: Lobectomy with sleeve resection. *Thorax* **15:**9–11, 1960
8. MacHale SJ: Carcinoma of the bronchus: Survival following conservative resection. *Thorax* **21:**343–346, 1966
9. Paulsen DL, Urschel HC, McNamara JJ, Shaw RR: Bronchoplastic procedures for bronchogenic carcinoma. *J Thorac Cardiovasc Surg* **59:**38–48, 1970
10. Jensik RJ, Faber LP, Milloy FJ, Amato JJ: Sleeve lobectomy for carcinoma. *J Thorac Cardiovasc Surg* **64:**400–412, 1972
11. Naruke T, Yoneyama T, Ogata T, Suemasu K: Bronchoplastic procedures for lung cancer. *J Thorac Cardiovasc Surg* **73:**927–935, 1977
12. Bennett WF, Abbey-Smith R: A twenty-year analysis of the results of sleeve resection for primary bronchogenic carcinoma. *J Thorac Cardiovasc Surg* **76:**840–845, 1978
13. Shaw KM, Luke DA: Lobectomy with sleeve resection of the bronchus for malignant disease of the lung and the influence of the suture material used for the bronchial repair. *J Thorac Cardiovasc Surg* **27:**325–329, 1979
14. Ungar I, Gyeney I, Scherer E, Szarvas I: Sleeve lobectomy: An alternative to pneumonectomy in the treatment of bronchial carcinoma. *J Thorac Cardiovasc Surg* **29:**41–46, 1982
15. Lowe JE, Bridgman AH, Sabiston DC: The role of bronchoplastic procedures in the surgical management of benign and malignant pulmonary lesions. *J Thorac Cardiovasc Surg* **83:**227–334, 1982
16. Fermin RK, Azariades M, Lennox SC, et al: Sleeve lobectomy (lobectomy and bronchoplasty) for bronchial carcinoma. *Ann Thorac Surg* **35:**442–449, 1983
17. Faber LP, Jensik RJ, Kittle CF: Results of sleeve lobectomy for bronchogenic carcinoma in 101 patients. *Ann Thorac Surg* **37:**279–284, 1984
18. Deslauriers J, Graulin P, Beaulieu M: Long-term clinical and functional results of sleeve resection for primary lung cancer. *J Thorac Cardiovasc Surg* **92:**871–879, 1986
19. Vogt-Moykopf I, Fritz T, Meyer G, et al: Bronchoplastic and angioplastic operations in bronchial carcinoma: Long-term results of a retrospective analysis for 1973–1983. *Int Surg* **71:**211–220, 1986
20. Frist WH, Mathisen DJ, Hilgenberg AD, Grillo HC: Bronchial sleeve resection with and without pulmonary resection. *J Thorac Cardiovasc Surg* **93:**350–357, 1987
21. Watanabe Y, Shimizu J, Oda M, et al: Results in 104 patients undergoing bronchoplastic procedures for bronchial lesions. *Ann Thorac Surg* **50:**607–614, 1990
22. Maggi G, Casadio C, Pischedda F, et al: Bronchoplastic and angioplastic techniques in the treatment of bronchogenic carcinoma. *Ann Thorac Surg* **55:**1501–1507, 1993
23. Mehran RJ, Deslauriers J, Piraux M, et al: Survival related to nodal status after sleeve resection for lung cancer. *J Thorac Cardiovasc Surg* **107:**576–583, 1994
24. Belli L, Meroni A, Rondinara G, et al: Bronchoplastic procedures and pulmonary artery reconstruction in the treatment of bronchogenic carcinoma. *J Thorac Cardiovasc Surg* **90:**167–171, 1985
25. Cooper JD. Lung transplantation. *Ann Thorac Surg* **47:**28–44, 1989
26. Patterson GA, Ginsberg RJ, Pon PY, et al: A prospective evaluation of magnetic resonance imaging, computed tomography, and mediastinoscopy in the pre-operative assessment of mediastinal node status in bronchogenic carcinoma. *J Thorac Cardiovasc Surg* **94:**679–684, 1987
27. Gephardt GN, Rice TW: Utility of frozen section evaluation of lymph nodes in the staging of bronchogenic carcinoma at mediastinoscopy and thoracotomy. *J Thorac Cardiovasc Surg* **100:**853–859, 1990
28. Gross BH, Glazer GM, Orringer MB, et al: Bronchogenic carcinoma metastatic to normal sized lymph nodes: frequency and significance. *Radiology* **166:**71–74, 1988
29. Whittlesey DN: Prospective computed tomographic scanning in the staging of bronchogenic cancer. *J Thorac Cardiovasc Surg* **95:**976–982, 1988
30. Izbicki JR, Thetter O, Karg O, et al: Accuracy of computed tomographic scan and surgical assessment for staging of bronchial carcinoma. *J Thorac Cardiovasc Surg* **104:**413–420, 1992
31. Kesler KA, Conces DJ, Heimansohn DA, et al: Assessing the feasibility of bronchoplastic surgery with magnetic resonance imaging. *Ann Thorac Surg* **52:**145–147, 1991
32. Rendina EA, Venuta F, Ciriaco P, et al: Bronchovascular sleeve resection: Technique, perioperative management, prevention, and treatment of complications. *J Thorac Cardiovasc Surg* **106:**73–79, 1993
33. Liewald F, Hatz RA, Dienemann H, et al: Importance of microscopic residual disease at the bronchial margin after resection for non-small cell carcinoma of the lung. *J Thorac Cardiovasc Surg* **104:**408–412, 1992
34. Schreurs AJM, Westermann CJJ, van den Bosch JMM, et al: A twenty-five-year follow-up of ninety-three resected typical carcinoid tumors of the lung. *J Thorac Cardiovasc Surg* **104:**1470–1475, 1992

35. Rea F, Binda R, Spreafico G, et al: Bronchial carcinoids: A review of 60 patients. *Ann Thorac Surg* **47:**412–414, 1989
36. Kato R, Kakizaki T, Hangai N, et al: Bronchoplastic procedures for tuberculous bronchial stenosis. *J Thorac Cardiovasc Surg* **106:** 1118–1121, 1993
37. Olsen GN, Block AJ: Pulmonary function testing in evaluations for pneumonectomy. *Hosp Pract* **9:**137–141, 1973
38. Miller JI: Physiologic evaluation of pulmonary function in the candidate for lung resection. *J Thorac Cardiovasc Surg* **105:**347–352, 1993
39. Van Schil PEY, de la Riviere AB, Knaepen PJ, et al: Second primary lung cancer after bronchial sleeve resection. *J Thorac Cardiovasc Surg* **104:**1451–1455, 1992
40. Inui K, Takahashi Y, Hasegawa S, et al: Effect of pre-operative irradiation on wound healing after bronchial anastomosis in mongrel dogs. *J Thorac Cardiovasc Surg* **106:**1059–1064, 1993
41. Paul A, Marelli D, Shennib H, et al: Mucociliary function in autotransplanted, allotransplanted, and sleeve resected lungs. *J Thorac Cardiovasc Surg* **98:**523–528, 1989
42. Calhoon JH, Grover FL, Gibbons WJ, et al: Single lung transplantation—alternative indications and technique. *J Thorac Cardiovasc Surg* **101:**816–825, 1991
43. Lima O, Goldberg M, Peters WJ, et al: Bronchial omentopexy in canine lung transplantation. *J Thorac Cardiovasc Surg* **83:**418–421, 1982
44. Turrentine MW, Kesler KA, Wright CD, et al: Effect of omental, intercostal, and internal mammary artery pedicle wraps on bronchial healing. *Ann Thorac Surg* **49:**574–579, 1990
45. Goldberg M, Lima O, Morgan E, et al: A comparison between cyclosporin A and methylprednisone plus azathioprine on bronchial healing following canine lung allotransplantation. *J Thorac Cardiovasc Surg* **85:**821–826, 1983
46. Auteri J, Jeevanandam V, Sanchez J, et al: Normal bronchial healing without bronchial wrapping in canine lung transplantation. *Ann Thorac Surg* **53:**80–84, 1992
47. Faber LP: Results of surgical treatment of stage III lung carcinoma with carinal proximity: The role of sleeve lobectomy versus pneumonectomy and the role of sleeve pneumonectomy. *Surg Clin North Am* **67:**1001–1014, 1987
48. LoCicero J, Massad M, Obav J, et al: Short-term and long-term results of experimental wrapping techniques for bronchial anastomosis. *J Thorac Cardiovasc Surg* **103:**763–766, 1992
49. Reed RC, Ziomek S, Ranval TJ, et al: Pulmonary artery sleeve resection for abutting left upper lobe lesions. *Ann Thorac Surg* **55:** 850–854, 1993
50. Cooper JD, Pearson FG, Patterson GA, et al: Use of silastic stents in the management of airway problems. *Ann Thorac Surg* **47:**371–378, 1989
51. Wallace MJ, Charnsangavej C, Ozawa K, et al: Tracheobronchial tree expandable metallic stents used in experimental and clinical applications. *Radiology* **158:**309–312, 1986
52. Cohen MD, Weber TR, Rao CC: Balloon dilatation of tracheal and broncheal stenosis. *AJR* **142:**477–478, 1984
53. Nakamura K, Terada N, Ohi M, et al: Tuberculous stenosis: Treatment with balloon bronchoplasty. *AJR* **157:**1187–1188, 1992
54. Ginsberg RJ, Hill LD, Eagan RT, et al: Modern thirty-day operative mortality for surgical resections in lung cancer. *J Thorac Cardiovasc Surg* **86:**654–658, 1983
55. Humphrey EW, Smart CR, Winchester DP, et al: National survey of the pattern of care for carcinoma of the lung. *J Thorac Cardiovasc Surg* **100:**837–843, 1990
56. Weisel RD, Cooper JD, Delarue NC, et al: Sleeve lobectomy for carcinoma of the lung. *J Thorac Cardiovasc Surg* **78:**839–849, 1979

CHAPTER

# 27

# Multimodality Therapy of Carcinoma of the Lung

## *Irradiation, Chemotherapy, and Immunotherapy*

E. Carmack Holmes and Steven D. Colquhoun

### INTRODUCTION

Present therapy for lung cancer remains based on the three standard forms of treatment available for any cancer: surgery, chemotherapy, and radiation therapy. Chemotherapy has unfortunately not had the impact that it has on other solid tumors such as breast cancer, testicular cancer, and sarcomas. Fortunately, newer combinations of chemotherapeutic agents and treatment schedules are giving higher response rates. While radiation therapy is a very effective palliative tool, the combination of surgery and radiation therapy remains controversial. Surgery is the only curative modality. Unfortunately, curative surgery is applicable to only a small percentage of patients with lung cancer. For this reason, efforts are now being directed toward developing surgical adjunctive therapy to improve postoperative survival. To this end, considerable effort has been directed towards the evaluation of combining surgery, radiation therapy, and chemotherapy. Immunosuppression has been shown to be a common feature of patients with lung cancer,[1,2] but attempts to demonstrate therapeutic efficacy of immunotherapy have not been successful.[3]

In the United States 172,000 patients develop lung cancer annually[4]; 50% of these (86,000) will have disease confined to the thorax without clinical evidence of dissemination (Fig. 27–1). Approximately 30% will have stage I disease, which is potentially curable by surgery alone, and 30% will have more advanced local disease, some of whom can be resected surgically but with a low expectation of cure. The rest will have either technically unresectable disease or resectable disease with a low cure rate. It is this population of patients, numbering about 86,000 annually, that potentially would benefit from combination therapy, including chemotherapy, surgery, and radiation therapy. An improvement in the cure rate of these patients would have a major impact on cancer mortality statistics.

For purposes of discussing treatment options, a distinction is made between small cell carcinoma and the other forms, collectively referred to as non-small cell carcinomas. Small cell carcinoma is particularly aggressive and tends to be disseminated at the time of diagnosis. Only about 25% of patients with small cell carcinoma will have disease confined to the thorax at the time of their presentation.[5] In this chapter, the treatment of small cell carcinoma will be considered apart from the treatment of non-small cell carcinoma of the lung (NSCLC).

Until recently, studies evaluating combinations of surgery, chemotherapy, and radiation therapy have been very disappointing. There have been a number of problems with these previous trials that may, in part, explain their failure: (1) Many trials involved single-agent chemotherapy, in which the agent was only marginally effective or not effective at all. (2) In many of the trials involving chemotherapy, the doses were inadequate for maximal ef-

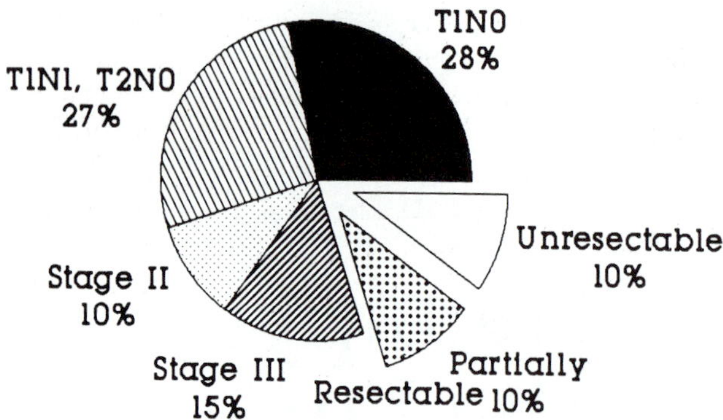


**Figure 27–1.** Distribution of stages within patients who present with lung cancer clinically localized to the thorax; 70,000 cases annually.

fect. (3) In the majority of trials, studies were neither randomized nor stratified for important risk factors such as cell type, nodal involvement, performance status, age, and other important prognostic variables. (4) In most of these previous trials, careful intraoperative staging was not performed, so it is impossible to determine whether the patient had stage I, II, or, in some cases, stage III disease. Also in the design of surgical adjuvant trials, it is important to know the patterns of recurrence in patients with different stages of lung cancer and different histologic types. Much of this information, especially in regards to NSCLC, was not known just a few years ago. Now, as a result of studies such as those of the Lung Cancer Study Group (LCSG), the first site of recurrence in most patients with resected non-small cell carcinoma of the lung can be predicted with considerable accuracy.[6] Therefore, it is important to pay careful attention to the staging of lung cancer and also to the patterns of recurrence when one is discussing the surgical adjuvant therapy of lung cancer.

## STAGE AND SURVIVAL

The staging system for lung cancer has traditionally employed the TNM system. (See also Chap. 22.) In the original classification (Table 27–1), N1 disease referred to metastasis to the lymph nodes in the hilar area or the bronchopulmonary area, and N2 disease represented metastasis to mediastinal lymph nodes, including subcarinal lymph nodes. In this system stage I disease was T1N0, T2N0, and T1N1; stage II was T2N1. Stage III represented a very heterogeneous group of tumors, including tumors that were operable, tumors that were inoperable, and even tumors that had widely metastasized. This original classification has been changed, in part because of the heterogeneity of survival within stage I, since the T1N1 subset tends to behave more like stage II (T2N1) disease. In addition, the heterogeneity within stage III was found to be confusing and not sufficiently precise for modern-day management.

A new international staging system has recently been proposed and accepted by oncologists worldwide.[7] This system retains the useful components of the past TNM system but has redefined stage I and stage II disease, as well as the subsets of stage III disease (Table 27–2). In this new system, stage I represents T1N0 and T2N0, whereas T1N1 disease has been placed in the stage II category along with T2N1. An additional node group, N3, has been added, which represents metastasis to the contralateral mediastinal lymph nodes, contralateral hilar nodes, or supraclavicular lymph nodes. In addition, a new classification has been added, T4, which describes a tumor of any size with invasion of the mediastinum or involving the heart, great vessels, trachea, esophagus, vertebral body, carina, or malignant pleural effusion. As can be seen in Table 27–2, stage III has now been divided into three separate categories: stage IIIa; stage IIIb, representing advanced local disease; and stage IV, reserved for patients with dissemination beyond the thorax. This new staging system will be used in the future. However, the survival information that is currently available is based on the old staging classification, which will be used throughout this chapter.

Many studies have attempted to correlate survival following surgery with the TNM classification. Unfortunately, most of these studies did not employ careful intraoperative staging techniques; therefore, the results are not reliable. However, several groups have performed careful intraoperative staging, and, therefore, reliable information has now

**TABLE 27–1. STAGE GROUPING OF TNM SUBSETS IN THE INITIAL SYSTEM OF LUNG CANCER STAGING**

| | Stage Grouping | | |
|---|---|---|---|
| Stage I | T1 | N0 | M0 |
| | T2 | N0 | M0 |
| | T1 | N1 | M0 |
| Stage II | T2 | N1 | M0 |
| Stage III | Any T3 | Any N2 | Any M1 |

**TABLE 27–2. STAGE GROUPING OF TNM SUBSETS IN THE NEW SYSTEM OF LUNG CANCER STAGING**

| | Stage Grouping | | |
|---|---|---|---|
| Occult carcinoma | TX | N0 | M0 |
| Stage 0 | TIS | Carcinoma in situ | |
| Stage I | T1 | N0 | M0 |
| | T2 | N0 | M0 |
| Stage II | T1 | N1 | M0 |
| | T2 | N1 | M0 |
| Stage IIIA | T3 | N0 | M0 |
| | T3 | N1 | M0 |
| | T1–T3 | N2 | M0 |
| Stage IIIB | Any T | N3 | M0 |
| | T4 | Any N | M0 |
| Stage IV | Any T | Any N | M1 |

become available relating TNM classification and histologic type and patterns of recurrence. At the time of thoracotomy, all thoracic surgeons should perform intraoperative staging. Sampling of paratracheal nodes, carinal nodes, hilar nodes, and bronchopulmonary nodes should be performed. Using these careful intraoperative staging techniques, the Lung Cancer Study Group has performed a careful analysis of approximately 1000 patients who have undergone surgical resection, intraoperative staging, and careful clinical follow-up (Table 27–3).[8] These studies show excellent survival with T1N0 disease. Survival diminishes with more advanced subsets of stage I disease and within stage II disease. A significant observation is that patients with adenocarcinoma do worse than patients with squamous cell carcinoma in most of these categories. Perhaps the most controversial aspect of these studies relates to the survival of patients with N2 disease. The somewhat surprising survival in patients with N2 disease indicates that, again, there is a great deal of heterogeneity within the N2 subsets. The difference in survival between squamous and nonsquamous disease becomes most apparent when there is nodal involvement. It is important to recognize the rather high survival in patients with squamous carcinoma who have N1 disease and small primary tumors (T1). As Martini and Pearson have pointed out, the extent of lymph node involvement is an important determinant of survival. Pearson[9] showed that patients who had mediastinal lymph node involvement determined by mediastinoscopy had a worse survival than did patients in whom mediastinoscopy was negative but who at thoracotomy were found to have N2 disease. For instance, in the completely resected squamous cell tumors, the 5-year survival rate was 34% in those patients who were mediastinoscopy-negative and 18% in the patients who were mediastinoscopy-positive. These observations are supported by those of Martini et al[10] in which patients who had N2 disease not apparent preoperatively but discovered only at the time of thoracotomy had a much better survival than those who had clinical evidence of mediastinal involvement. In addition, patients with microscopic lymph node involvement have better survival than those with macroscopic disease, and those patients who had multilevel mediastinal disease did not have as good a survival as those with minimal disease. Therefore, it is clear that mediastinal lymph node involvement is not a contraindication to surgical resection. Survival with mediastinal lymph node involvement depends on the number of nodes involved, the location of these nodes, and the extent to which the involved nodes are occupied by tumor.[11]

**TABLE 27–3. FOUR-YEAR POSTOPERATIVE SURVIVAL BY TNM**

| Classification | Survivors of Squamous Carcinoma, %; *N* = 549 | Survivors of Adenocarcinoma, %; *N* = 572 |
|---|---|---|
| Stage I | | |
| T1 NO | 83 | 69 (*P* = .02) |
| T2 NO | 64 | 57 |
| T1 N1 | 75 | 52 (*P* = .04) |
| Stage II | | |
| T2 N1 | 53 | 25 (*P* < .01) |
| Stage III | | |
| T3 NO | 37 | 21 |
| N2 | 46 | 35 |

*(From Mountain CF et al: J Surg Oncol 35:147–156, 1987, with permission.)*

## NON-SMALL CELL CARCINOMA

With an understanding of the nature and importance of accurate staging in non-small cell lung cancer, it becomes possible to discuss the problems faced in its treatment. With data based on careful intraoperative nodal sampling and careful clinical follow-up, one can predict with some degree of accuracy the failure rate in the various T and N subsets. Such longitudinal studies have given valuable information regarding the patterns of recurrence in patients with resected non-small cell carcinoma, indicating that in general the first recurrence is a systemic one.[6,12,13] However, there are striking differences between the different histologies. For instance, local recurrence is more common in patients with squamous carcinoma, whereas the brain is a more frequent site of first recurrence in patients with adenocarcinoma and large cell undifferentiated carcinoma.[13] This kind of information is also very useful in selecting the proper adjuvant therapy. Patients at high risk for local recurrence following resection would perhaps benefit from local postoperative radiation therapy, and those at risk for brain recurrences would perhaps benefit from therapy directed to the central nervous system. With these important considerations in mind, we will consider the rationale for and the current status of surgical adjuvant therapy in non-small cell lung cancer.

### Chemotherapy for Non-Small Cell Lung Cancer

Chemotherapy for non-small cell lung cancer has not been as effective as chemotherapy in many other solid tumors. However, more recently, combination chemotherapy regimens, especially those containing cisplatin, have shown improved response rates in patients with advanced disease.[14–17] As in other situations, the response rates are much higher in patients with good performance status and smaller tumor burdens, and response rates in patients who have disease localized to the thorax are much higher than in those with metastatic disease beyond the thorax.[18–22] Response rates of up to 60% in advanced localized disease have been reported.[22] This suggests that local tumor reduction with surgery or radiation therapy would yield an even greater response to systemic chemotherapy. Given that systemic relapse far exceeds local recurrence in lung cancer, the ultimate solution to the problem of lung cancer will require a systemic therapy capable of obliterating microscopic metastatic disease. It is obvious, then, that systemic adjuvant chemotherapy may well hold the key to prolonging the disease-free interval and survival in patients with resectable lung cancer. Local modalities such as radiation therapy can be quite useful in controlling recurrences in those situations where local recurrence is likely, but effective systemic therapy is essential.

## SURGICAL ADJUVANT THERAPY

### Randomized Trials

The advent of more effective systemic chemotherapy has led to a renewed interest in the evaluation of surgical adjuvant therapy. These interventions have employed (1) systemic chemotherapy following surgical resection, either alone or in combination with radiation therapy, or (2) preoperative chemotherapy and/or radiation followed by surgery.

The efficacy of surgical adjuvant therapy in patients with several solid tumor types is well known. These include pediatric tumors such as Wilms' tumors and childhood rhabdomyosarcoma as well as breast cancer, testicular cancer, and osteosarcoma. In the past 20 years, numerous studies have also been performed evaluating chemotherapy following surgery for lung cancer. Unfortunately, most of these studies were not properly controlled for important prognostic variables such as nodal status and histology. However, these early pioneering studies are of important historical significance. Shields et al reviewed the experience of the Veterans Administration with surgical adjuvant chemotherapy in 417 resected patients.[23] In this series of studies, various combinations of postoperative chemotherapy were employed. There was no improvement in survival in the group receiving chemotherapy.

More recently, the Lung Cancer Study Group initiated a series of prospective randomized trials in patients with stage II and IIIA resectable lung cancer. These studies include a detailed analysis of the pathology of the resected cancer, relevance of staging to survival, patterns of recurrence, surgical mortality and morbidity, and the role of multimodality therapy in resectable lung cancer. In one study the Lung Cancer Study Group evaluated patients with completely resected stage II and stage III adenocarcinoma and large-cell undifferentiated carcinoma of the lung.[12] At that time, the literature indicated that the median disease-free survival in such patients was 6–7 months. As with all Lung Cancer Study Group's studies, careful intraoperative staging was an absolute requirement before patients could be entered into the study. All patients were required to have intraoperative nodal sampling of the paratracheal, carinal, hilar, and bronchopulmonary lymph nodes. Following surgery and pathologic staging, patients were randomized to receive adjuvant chemotherapy consisting of cytoxan, adriamycin, and cisplatin (CAP) or postoperative immunotherapy consisting of intrapleural Bacillus Calmette-Guerin (BCG) and leviamosol. A total of 130 patients were randomized into this study. Ninety percent of the patients had positive lymph nodes and, therefore, had IIIA disease. The patients receiving chemotherapy had a significantly longer time to recurrence than patients receiving the immunotherapy (Fig. 27–2). The treatment difference was statistically significant (log rank analysis $P = .032$). This study represented the first documentation of a beneficial effect of adjuvant systemic chemotherapy in patients with resected lung cancer. The Lung Cancer Study Group also performed a study evaluating postoperative chemotherapy and radiation therapy in resected non-small-lung cancer in patients with microscopic residual disease or extensive lymph node involvement at the time of surgery.[24] All patients underwent careful intraoperative staging at the time of surgery and were randomized postoperatively to receive chemotherapy plus radiation therapy or radiation therapy alone. The chemotherapy was cytoxan, adriamycin, and cisplatin. One hundred and sixty-four patients were randomized into the study with a balanced distribution of prognostic factors between the treatment groups. There were significantly fewer recurrences in the chemotherapy group ($P = .002$) (Fig. 27–3). Figure 27–4 shows the improved disease-free survival in patients receiving chemotherapy with squamous histology ($P = .045$), and Figure 27–5 shows a significant improvement in disease-free survival in patients with adenocarcinoma treated with chemotherapy ($P = .013$). Therefore, the combination of chemotherapy and radiation therapy significantly prolonged the disease-free interval in these patients when compared with a match control group receiving radiation therapy alone.

Recently, two additional randomized trials have evaluated perioperative adjuvant therapy in patients with resectable IIIA non-small cell lung cancer.[25,26] In these studies, higher doses of cisplatin were used when compared

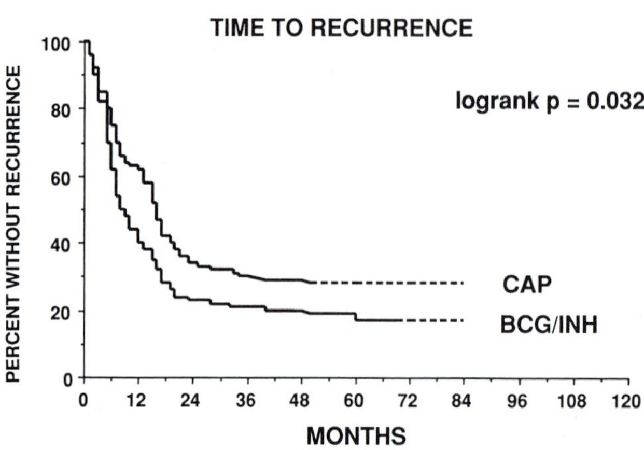


**Figure 27–2.** Time to recurrence in stage IIIA completely resected patients in The Lung Cancer Study Group Trial. The Chemotherapy (CAP) Group had a significant prolongation in disease-free survival.

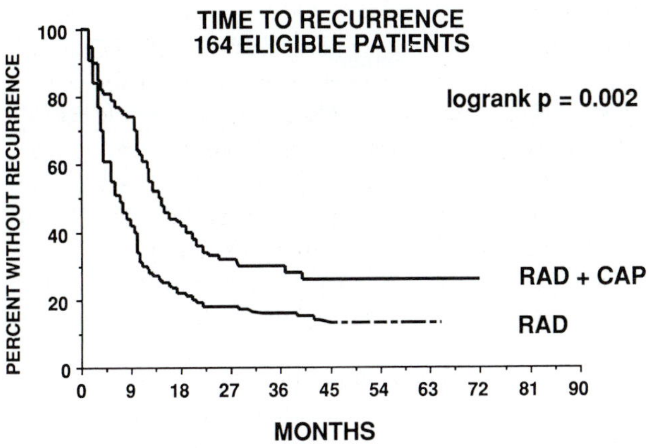


**Figure 27–3.** Time to recurrence in all patients with resected IIIA disease in The Lung Cancer Study Group trial evaluating past operative radiation alone or radiation plus chemotherapy (CAP).

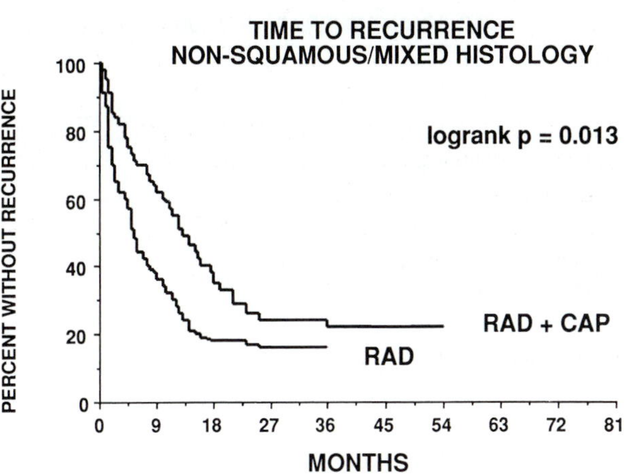


**Figure 27–5.** Time to recurrence in resected IIIA nonsquamous histology in the same trial as Figures 27–3 and 27–4.

with the Lung Cancer Study Group studies. The M.D. Anderson Group compared surgery alone to surgery with pre- and postoperative cytoxan, etoposide, and cisplatin. All patients had resectable IIIA lung cancer. A statistically significant difference in overall survival between the two treatment groups was observed (Table 27–4). The estimated median survival in the chemotherapy group was 64 months compared with 11 months in the surgery-alone group ($P$ = .008). Similar results were reported by Rosell et al[25] from Spain. In this study, stage IIIA non-small cell lung cancer patients were randomized to receive three cycles of preoperative MIC chemotherapy (mitomycin-C, ifosfamide, and cisplatin) or surgery alone. All patients received postoperative radiation therapy. The median survival was 26 months in the chemotherapy group and 8 months in the surgery-alone group ($P$ = .001).

Thus, four randomized phase III trials in resectable stage IIIA lung cancer have shown statistically significant improvement in patients receiving perioperative chemotherapy.

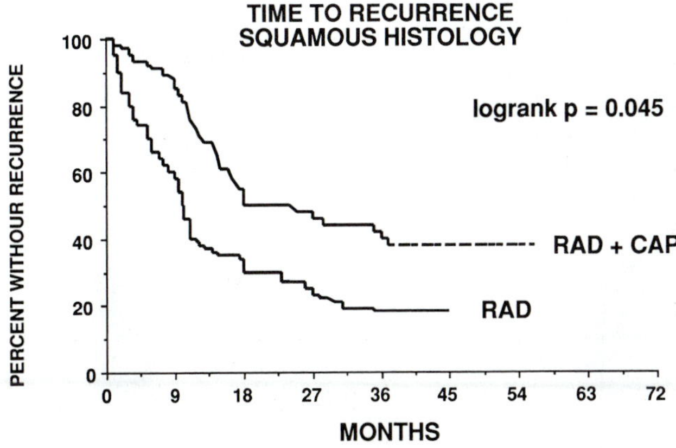


**Figure 27–4.** Time to recurrence in patients with resected IIIA squamous histology in the same trial as Figure 27–3.

## Nonrandomized Trials

During the past several years, there has been considerable interest in the use of chemotherapy prior to surgical resection in patients with various grades of stage IIIA and IIIB lung cancer. Many phase II studies have been performed and evaluated the response to therapy and resectability. None of these trials have been randomized, and the survival benefit is difficult to judge. Some studies have included patients with disease felt to be so extensive that it was technically unresectable. In others, patients with chest wall involvement and negative regional nodes have been included, and, in others, the only criteria was the presence or absence of mediastinal lymph node involvement. Thus, it is not possible to compare the results of these various studies. However, preoperative chemotherapy alone or in combination with radiation therapy gives high clinical response rates in disease confined to the thorax. In addition, the histologic complete response rates are 20–25%.

The Memorial Sloan-Kettering group evaluated preoperative chemotherapy alone in stage IIIA lung cancer.[27] These patients received two to three cycles of MVP (mitomycin, vindesine, and cisplatin) chemotherapy. All patients had clinical N2 disease defined as bulky mediastinal lymph node metastasis. The overall response rate to chemotherapy was 77%, and 65% of the patients underwent a complete resection. The overall survival was 28% at 3 years, 17% at 5 years, with a median survival of 19 months. Patients who had a complete resection had a better survival than those undergoing incomplete resection. Other groups have employed a combination of chemotherapy and radiation therapy. These studies have sought to exploit the known synergism between 5FU (fluorouracil) and radiation therapy as well as the possible synergism between cisplatin and radiation therapy.[28–30] These studies have been performed by a variety of different groups including the Lung Cancer Study Group, the Southwest Oncology Group, and the group at Rush Presbyterian Medical Center in Chicago. In some of

**TABLE 27–4. ADJUVANT THERAPY IN STAGE IIIA NSCLC[a]**

| | | Percent | | |
|---|---|---|---|---|
| | Median Survival (mo)[b] | *Response Rate* | *Resectability* | *Operative Mortality* |
| Surgery and chemotherapy | 64 | 35 | 61 | 3 |
| Surgery alone | 11 | — | 66 | 6 |

[a]Roth et al
[b]$P = .008$.

these studies, patients had extensive IIIA and IIIB disease that was felt by the surgeon to be unresectable. In others, there was a wider diversity of IIIA disease. In some instances, the purpose of the preoperative therapy was to stage the tumor down and convert unresectable patients to resectable ones. The results of all these studies have been remarkably similar. Response rates to chemotherapy have varied between 50% and 70%. Median survivals have varied between 15 and 20 months with complete resectability rates of 60%. Complete histologic clearance of all tumor has also been seen in 20–25% of the patients entered in these studies. Figures 27–6 and 27–7 are examples of typical chemical response to preoperative neoadjuvant therapy.

These studies evaluating preoperative or induction surgical adjuvant therapy indicate that high response rates can be obtained in patients with advanced disease localized to the thorax. In addition, those who respond to the therapy frequently undergo complete resection with very low operative morbidity. Although preoperative therapy of this kind can cause a significant increase in the difficulty of surgical dissection, the postoperative morbidity and mortality has been quite acceptable. Although the survival in certain subsets of patients is impressive, the question still remains as to whether the addition of surgery to chemotherapy and radiation therapy in these patients actually prolongs overall survival. A phase III randomized trial is currently being performed by the Southwest Oncology Group in which patients with stage IIIA lung cancer who are considered unresectable are being randomized to receive chemotherapy plus radiation therapy with or without surgery. Hopefully, this prospectively randomized phase III trial will give some important answers in regard to the role of surgery in patients with extensive IIIA disease.

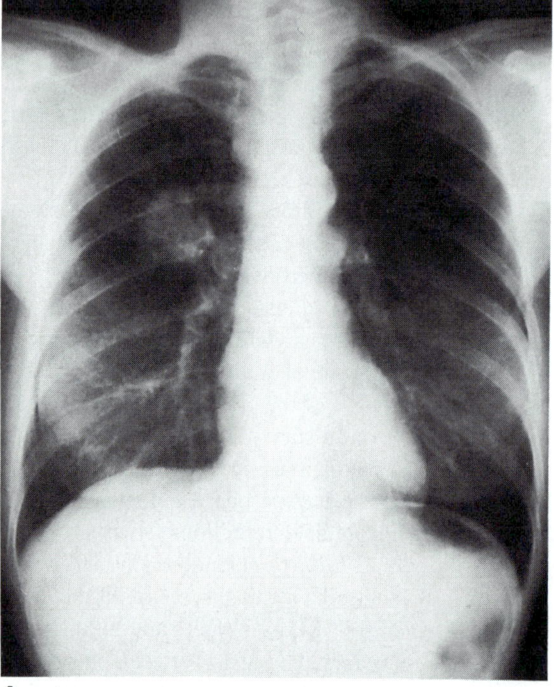

A

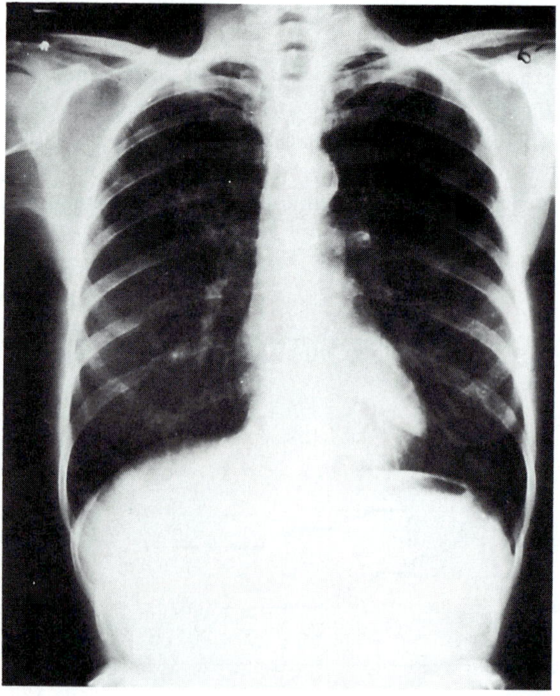

B

**Figure 27–6. A.** Large cell undifferentiated lung cancer in the right upper lobe with extensive mediastinal metastases. **B.** Marked tumor reduction following preoperative treatment with 5-FU, cisplatin, and radiation therapy.

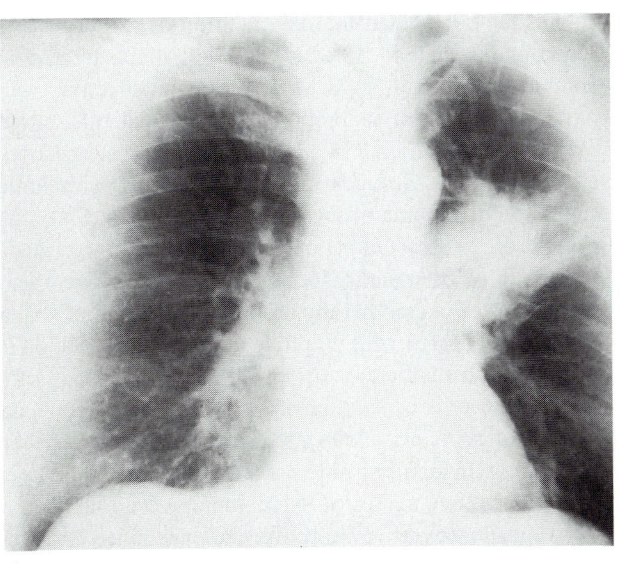
A

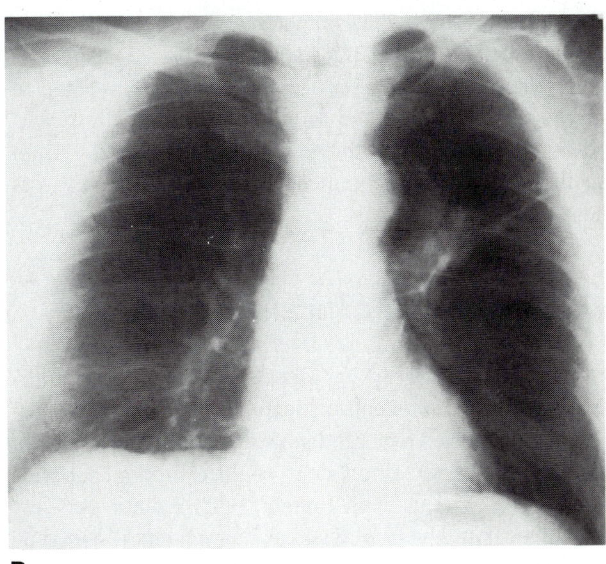
B

**Figure 27–7. A.** Unresectable adenocarcinoma localized to the thorax. **B.** Following treatment with preoperative radiation therapy and CAP chemotherapy.

## Radiation Therapy

### *General Considerations*

In general, radiation therapy is an effective modality for treatment of patients with lung cancer. It is effective in palliating symptoms arising in the thorax, such as pain, hemoptysis, and bronchial obstruction. It is also very effective in controlling painful bony metastases. Although radiation therapy is an effective local or locoregional modality, most patients with lung cancer die because of disseminated disease. On the other hand, local control is obviously necessary if patients are to be cured.

Many studies have evaluated preoperative and postoperative radiation therapy for patients with lung cancer, including two large randomized trials looking at preoperative radiation therapy. The Veterans Administration Collaborative Study randomly assigned 331 patients to receive 4000–5000 cGy preoperatively. Although 25% of the patients had no recognizable tumor in the resected specimen, survival was not significantly increased.[31] In another randomized trial using 4000 cGy preoperatively, postoperative complications, such as bronchopleural fistula, were more frequent in the group receiving preoperative radiation therapy, and survival was not prolonged.[32] Although no prospective randomized trials have evaluated preoperative radiation therapy for patients with superior sulcus tumors, a number of retrospective studies suggest that it is effective in this setting, and preoperative radiation therapy is used fairly routinely for such patients.[33] Several studies, most of which have been retrospective, have evaluated postoperative radiation therapy in patients with lung cancer. Some studies have suggested that radiation is effective for patients with squamous disease but not for patients with adenocarcinoma,[34] whereas other studies have suggested the reverse.[35] The Lung Cancer Study Group recently completed a prospective randomized trial in which patients with stage II and resectable stage III squamous carcinoma were randomly assigned to receive 5000 cGy postoperative radiation therapy or no further treatment. Although survival was not significantly prolonged in the group receiving radiation therapy, there were essentially no local recurrences in this group, whereas about 35% of the recurrences in the nonirradiated group were local. Radiation therapy was thus extremely effective in controlling local recurrence, but this effect did not translate into a significant prolongation in survival.[13]

Our recommendations for the management of patients with resected non-small cell cancer are as follows:

- *Stage I disease:* The treatment of stage I NSCLC is surgical resection of the primary tumor accompanied by careful intraoperative staging of the intrapulmonary, hilar, and ipsilateral mediastinal lymph nodes. This therapy is curative in more than 60–70% of patients with pathologic stage I disease.
- *Stage II disease:* Patients with positive intrapulmonary or hilar lymph nodes at the time of surgical resection (N1 disease) are at increased risk of recurrence compared to patients with stage I disease. Although 40–50% of these patients are potentially cured, the increased risk of recurrence is sufficiently high to warrant experimental postoperative therapy in properly controlled trials.
- *Stage III disease:* The management of this group of patients is difficult and will be heavily influenced by the skill and experience of the thoracic surgeon. In general, if possible, surgical resection is indicated. Preoperative

chemotherapy and radiation therapy may convert many of the unresectable stage IIIA patients to resectable. Radiation therapy will prevent local recurrence in resected squamous disease. There is mounting compelling evidence that patients with *resectable* IIIA benefit from chemotherapy. We recommend it in this subset of A patients.

## SMALL-CELL LUNG CANCER

For many years surgery has been considered contraindicated in patients with small-cell carcinoma (SCC). This position was supported by a randomized study in Great Britain that reported that radiation therapy yielded survival superior to surgery in patients with limited SCC.[36] Until very recently this position was accepted as dogma, and it was generally conceded that patients with SCC of the lung were not candidates for surgical resection under any circumstance. However, reports over the past several years have challenged this position. One study, from the Veterans Administration Cooperative Group, indicated that an overall 5-year survival of 23% can be obtained in patients with small cell carcinoma of the lung undergoing surgery.[37] The 5-year survival in this study ranged from 3.6% in patients with N2 disease to 60% in patients with T1N0 disease (Table 27–5). This report, as well as others, has led to a reassessment of the role of surgery in patients with SCC of the lung.[38,39] The development of better chemotherapy for small cell carcinoma of the lung has also encouraged a reappraisal of surgery in this disease. Response rates to chemotherapy are frequently in excess of 75% in patients with small cell carcinoma of the lung limited to the thorax. Indeed, 2-year survivals of 20% in patients treated with chemotherapy and radiation therapy alone have been reported. However, many patients with limited SCC of the lung who are treated with chemotherapy and radiation therapy alone develop local recurrences, with up to 50% of these patients having a local recurrence as their first site of recurrence.[40] Since local recurrence is a major problem in these patients, the role of surgery is currently being re-evaluated as a means of local control. In this setting, surgery is adjunctive to the chemotherapy. Several nonrandomized studies have indicated that the addition of surgery will essentially eliminate local recurrences in patients treated with combination therapy.[41,42] More recent prospective studies have indicated that in properly selected patients, surgery may well be beneficial. In one study by the Eastern Cooperative Oncology Group,[43] 20 of 37 patients with limited small cell carcinoma of the lung were resected. Sixty-three percent of the resected patients are still alive with a median follow-up of 24 months. In this study patients were given two cycles of chemotherapy preoperatively, and postoperatively were treated with prophylactic cranial irradiation and additional chemotherapy. As in other studies, some of the resected specimens no longer contained small-cell carcinoma, but contained elements of non-small cell carcinoma of the lung. In another study patients were treated preoperatively with three cycles of chemotherapy with an 84% objective response rate. Twenty-five patients underwent thoracotomy; four were found to be unresectable. Forty-eight percent of the patients were alive at 3–5 years following surgery. The best results were in those patients who had no evidence of small cell carcinoma of the lung in the resected specimen. The resected patients received an additional three cycles of chemotherapy postoperatively. Four of the 21 patients undergoing resection had no evidence of histologically viable tumor in the specimen. These authors concluded that long-term survival appeared to be largely restricted to those patients with either minimal or no evidence of viable small cell lung cancer at the time of surgery. However, the survival of the entire group, including responders and nonresponders, was not improved.[44]

The studies to date allow the following conclusions: (1) Preoperative chemotherapy does not increase surgical morbidity or mortality. (2) Surgery in combination with chemotherapy and/or radiation therapy increases local control. (3) Of the resected specimens, 20–30% either have no viable tumor or have non-small cell cancer in the specimen. (4) No prospective randomized studies have been performed evaluating the role of surgery in patients with limited small cell carcinoma of the lung. Such a prospective randomized study is currently under way by the Lung Cancer Study Group but has not yet been completed.

Based on current information, the following recommendations can be offered: (1) Stage I patients should have surgery, followed by chemotherapy and prophylactic cranial irradiation. (2) At least four cycles of preoperative chemotherapy should be given in order to maximize the effect. (3) The role of surgery in patients with stage II and stage III limited small cell carcinoma of the lung remains controversial and awaits the results of prospective randomized trials.

**TABLE 27–5. SURGERY IN SMALL-CELL LUNG CANCER (*N* = 132)**

| Stage | 5-Year Survival, % |
|---|---|
| T1N0 | 60 |
| T1N1 | 31 |
| T2N0 | 28 |
| T2N1 | 9 |
| T3 or T2 | 3.6 |
| | (overall 23%) |

*(From TW Shields, Higgins GA, Mathew MJ, et al: J Thorac Cardiovasc Surg 84:481–488, 1982, with permission.)*

## REFERENCES

1. Holmes EC, Golub SH: Immunologic defects in lung cancer patients. *J Thorac Cardiovasc Surg* **71**:161–168, 1976
2. Giuliano AE, Rangel DM, Golub SH, et al: Serum-mediated immunosuppression in lung cancer. *Cancer* **43**:917–924, 1979

3. Mountain CM, Gail MH, The Lung Cancer Study Group: Surgical adjuvant intrapleural BCG treatment for stage I non-small cell lung cancer. *J Thorac Cardiovasc Surg* **82**:649–657, 1981
4. Boring CC, Squires TS, Tong T, Montgomery S. Cancer statistics, 1994. *Cancer.* **44**:7–26, 1994
5. Van Houtte P, Salazar OM, Phillips CE, et al: Lung cancer. In *Clinical Oncology: A Multidisciplinary Approach,* 6th ed. New York, American Cancer Society, 1983, pp 142–153
6. Feld R, Rubinstein LV, Weisenburger TH, The Lung Cancer Study Group: Sites of recurrence in resected stage I non-small cell lung cancer: A guide for future studies. *J Clin Oncol* **2**:1352–1357, 1984
7. Mountain CF: A new international staging system for lung cancer. *Chest* **89**(suppl): 225S–233S, 1986
8. Mountain CF, Lukeman JM, Hammar SP, et al: Lung cancer classification: The relationship of disease extent and cell type to survival in a clinical trials population. *J Surg Oncol* **35**:147–156, 1987
9. Pearson FG: Lung cancer—The past twenty-five years. *Chest* **89**(suppl):200S–205S, 1986
10. Martini N, Flehinger BJ, Zaman MB, et al: Results of resection in non-oat cell carcinoma of the lung with mediastinal lymph node metastases. *Ann Surg* **198**:386–397, 1983
11. Thomas PA, Piantadosi S, Mountain CF: The Lung Cancer Study Group: Should subcarinal lymph nodes be routinely examined in patients with non-small cell lung cancer? *J Thorac Cardiovasc Surg* **95**:883–887, 1988
12. Holmes EC, Gail M, The Lung Cancer Study Group: Surgical adjuvant therapy for stage II and stage III adenocarcinoma and large-cell undifferentiated carcinoma. *J Clin Oncol* **4**:710–715, 1986
13. Weisenburger TH, Gail M, The Lung Cancer Study Group: Effects of postoperative mediastinal radiation on completely resected stage II and stage III epidermoid carcinoma of the lung. *N Engl J Med* **315**:1377–1381, 1986
14. Gralla RJ, Ephraim S, Cosper MD, et al: Cis-platinum and vindesine combination chemotherapy for advanced carcinoma of the lung: A randomized trial. *Ann Intern Med* **95**:414–420, 1981
15. Eagan RT, Frytak S, Creagan JN, et al: Phase II study of cyclophosphamide, Adriamycin and cis-platinum in patients with adenocarcinoma and large cell carcinoma of the lung. *Cancer Treat Rep* **63**:1589–1591, 1979
16. Lad TE, Nelson RB, Ulrich D, et al: Immediate versus postponed combination chemotherapy (CAMP) for unresectable non-small cell lung cancer: A randomized trial. *Cancer Treat Rep* **65**:973–978, 1981
17. Evans WK, Feld R, DeBaer G, et al: Cyclophosphamide, doxorubicin and cis-platinum in the treatment of non-small cell bronchogenic carcinoma. *Cancer Treat Rep* **65**:947–954, 1981
18. Longeval A, Klastersky J: Combination chemotherapy with cis-platinum and etoposide in bronchogenic squamous cell carcinoma and adenocarcinoma: A study for the EORTC Lung Cancer Working Party (Belgium). *Cancer* **50**:1751–1756, 1982
19. Fram R, Skarin A, Balikian J, et al: Combination chemotherapy followed by radiation therapy in patients with regional stage III unresectable non-small cell cancer. *Cancer Treat Rep* **69**:587–590, 1985
20. Wagner H Jr, Ruckdeschel J, Bonomi P, et al: Treatment of locally advanced non-small cell lung cancer (NSCLC) with Mitomycin C, Vinblastine and cis-DDP (MVP) followed by radiation therapy: An ECOG pilot study. *Proc Am Soc Clin Oncol* **4**:183 (abst C–716), 1985
21. Bonomi P, Sandler S, Bushy J, et al: Adjuvant chemotherapy in locally advanced squamous cell bronchogenic carcinoma. *Proc Am Soc Clin Oncol* **3**:228 (abst C–892), 1984
22. Kris MG, Gralla RG, Martini N, et al: Trial of preoperative Cisplatin plus vinca alkaloid chemotherapy in non-small cell lung cancer (NSCLC) patients with clinically apparent, ipsilateral, mediastinal lymph node metastases. *Proc Am Soc Clin Oncol* **6**:177 (abst C–697), 1987
23. Shields TW, Humphrey EW, Eastridge CE, Keehn RJ: Adjuvant cancer chemotherapy after resection of carcinoma of the lung. *Cancer* **40**:2057–2062, 1977
24. Lad T, Rubinstein L, Sadeghi A, The Lung Cancer Study Group: The benefit of adjuvant treatment for resected locally advanced non-small cell lung cancer. *J Clin Oncol* **6**:9–17, 1988
25. Rosell R, Gomez-Codina J, Camps C: A randomized trial comparing preoperative chemotherapy plus surgery with surgery alone in patients with non-small cell lung cancer. *N Engl J Med* **330**:153–158, 1994
26. Roth JA, Fossella F, Komaki R, et al: A randomized trial comparing perioperative chemotherapy and surgery with surgery alone in resectable stage III non-small cell lung cancer. *J Natl Cancer Inst* **86**:673–680, 1994
27. Martin N, Kris MG, Flehinger BJ, et al: Preoperative chemotherapy for stage III A (N2) lung cancer: The Sloan-Kettering Experience with 136 patients. *Ann Thorac Surg* **55**:1365–1374, 1993
28. Rusch VW, Albain KS, Crowley JJ, et al: Surgical resection of stage III A and stage III B non-small cell lung cancer after concurrent induction chemoradiotherapy: A Southwest Oncology Group Trial. *J Thorac Cardiovasc Surg* **105**:97–106, 1993
29. Weiden PL, Piantidosi S, for the Lung Cancer Study Group: Preoperative chemotherapy and radiation therapy in stage III non-small cell lung cancer: A phase II study of the lung cancer study group. *J Natl Cancer Inst* **83**:366–372, 1991
30. Faber LP, Kittle CF, Warren WH, et al: Preoperative chemotherapy and irradiation for stage III non-small cell lung cancer. *Ann Thorac Surg* **47**:669–77, 1989
31. Shields TM, Higgins GA, Lawton R, et al: Preoperative x-ray therapy as an adjunct in the treatment of bronchogenic carcinoma. *J Thorac Cardiovasc Surg* **59**:49–55, 1970
32. Committee for Radiation Therapy Studies: Preoperative irradiation of cancer of the lung. *Cancer* **23**:219–226, 1969
33. Anderson TM, Moy PM, Holmes EC: Factors affecting survival in superior sulcus tumors. *J Clin Oncol* **4**:1598–1603, 1986
34. Choi NCH, Grillo H, Gardiello M, et al: Basis for new strategies in postoperative radiotherapy of bronchogenic carcinoma. *Int J Radiat Oncol Biol Phys* **6**:31–35, 1980
35. Kirsh MV, Sloan H: Mediastinal metastases in bronchogenic carcinoma: Influence of postoperative irradiation, cell type and location. *Ann Thorac Surg* **5**:459–463, 1982
36. Fox W, Scadding JG: Medical Research Council comparative trial of surgery and radiation therapy for primary treatment of small-celled or oat-celled carcinoma of the bronchus: Ten-year follow-up. *Lancet* **2**:63–65, 1973
37. Shields TW, Higgins GA Jr, Matthews MJ, et al: Surgical resection in the management of small cell carcinoma of the lung. *J Thorac Cardiovasc Surg* **84**:481–488, 1982
38. Meyer JA, Parker FB: Small cell carcinoma of the lung (collective review). *Ann Thorac Surg* **30**:602–609, 1980
39. Meyer JA, Comis RL, Ginsberg SJ, et al: The prospect of disease control by surgery combined with chemotherapy in stage I and stage II small cell carcinoma of the lung. *Ann Thorac Surg* **36**:37–41, 1983
40. Perez CA, Einhorn L, Oldham RK, et al, The Southeastern Cancer Study Group: Randomized trial of radiotherapy to the thorax in limited small cell carcinoma of the lung treated with multiagent chemotherapy and elective brain irradiation: A preliminary report. *J Clin Oncol* **2**:1200–1208, 1984
41. Shepherd FA, Ginsberg RJ, Feld R, et al: Reduction in local recurrence and improved survival in surgically treated patients with small cell lung cancer. *J Thorac Cardiovasc Surg* **86**:498–506, 1983
42. Prager RL, Roster JM, Hainsworth JD, et al: The feasibility of "adjuvant surgery" in limited small cell carcinoma: A prospective evaluation. *Ann Thorac Surg* **38**:622–626, 1984
43. Baker RR, Ettinger DS, Ruckdeschel JD, et al: The role of surgery in the management of selected patients with small cell carcinoma of the lung. *J Clin Oncol* **5**:697–702, 1987
44. Williams CJ, McMillan I, Lea R, et al: Surgery after initial chemotherapy for localized small cell carcinoma of the lung. *J Clin Oncol* **5**:1579–1588, 1987

CHAPTER

# 28

# Indications for Resection of Pulmonary Metastases

Pauline W. Chen and Harvey I. Pass

## INTRODUCTION

Pulmonary metastases are the second most common form of metastatic disease for all histologies[1] and as such are an integral part of thoracic surgery. While controversy exists regarding an aggressive approach, up to 20% of cases found to have metastatic disease at autopsy have only pulmonary disease.[2] Moreover, in certain histologies, such as soft-tissue sarcomas, the lungs are the most frequent site of first recurrence,[3] and systemic therapy affects pulmonary disease in less than 30% of these patients.[4] Improved survival has been documented in those sarcoma patients who could be completely resected compared with those who could not be rendered free of disease. The thoracic surgeon thus plays a fundamental part in the treatment of and issues surrounding pulmonary metastases.

## HISTORY

The history of treatment of pulmonary metastases corresponds to the evolution in thoracic surgery and anesthetic techniques. Initial reports were anecdotal in nature. In 1882, Weinlechner performed the first pulmonary metastatectomy, resecting the metastatic deposit en bloc with his patient's chest wall sarcoma.[5] Krolein, 2 years later, excised a pulmonary nodule during the resection of a chest wall sarcoma. In 1926 Divis performed the first isolated metastatectomy, resecting a right lower-lobe metastasis; the procedure was performed for the first time in the United States by Torek[6] in 1930.

Metastatectomy gained credibility in the early part of this century with the first documented long-term survivor. Barney and Churchill,[7] having resected a solitary renal adenocarcinoma metastasis to the lung, documented a 23-year survival. The patient ultimately expired from coronary artery disease. Additionally, Alexander and Haight[8] in 1947 reported cures in three out of their six patients who underwent metastatectomy.

While those results clearly piqued the interests of surgeons, more rigorous examination of the role of pulmonary metastatectomy did not take place until the 1950s and 1960s with increasing sophistication of surgical and anesthetic techniques. Thomford et al,[9] Martini et al,[10] and Morton et al[11] produced comparable postthoracotomy survival rates for those patients undergoing resection of pulmonary metastases. The call for a more aggressive approach to lung metastases had begun, and its importance in extending survival rates of oncologic patients had become increasingly obvious.

## PATHOGENESIS

Multiple mechanisms are postulated to play a role in the development of pulmonary metastases: hematogenous dissemination, endobronchial metastases, lymphangitic spread, bronchial artery dissemination, and spread from transbronchial aspirations. Pulmonary disease from extrathoracic sites most commonly arises from hematogenous dissemination.[12] Tumor emboli are released from the primary or other sites of disease.[13,14] While most of these clumps of released tumor are destroyed, others escape filtration by the pulmonary capillary bed and become seeds of metastatic disease. Liotta et al[15] showed a direct correlation between the number and size of tumor emboli with the development of pulmonary disease in the animal model. Evidence of these tumor emboli can be seen radiographically filling pulmonary capillaries and are occasionally confused with other diffuse infiltrative processes seen on chest radiographs such as infection or edema.[16] Development of pulmonary metastases from these tumor emboli can be shown to correlate with the size and growth rate of the primary site and duration of observation.[15]

Endobronchial metastases also play a part in the development of pulmonary disease. These lesions most frequently involve renal cell and breast carcinomas, while colon and thyroid cancers are less commonly involved. Endobronchial metastases usually arise from direct metastasis to the bronchus or from a parenchymal or mediastinal lymph node metastasis with direct bronchial extension.[17,18]

Lymphangitic spread is usually borne of hematogenous metastases extending from capillaries to lymphatics. These metastases occasionally arise secondary to retrograde lymphatic spread from abdominal nodal groups to hilar and mediastinal nodes. Bronchial arterial spread and spread from transbronchial aspirations are also at times responsible for the development of pulmonary metastases.[17–19]

## PATIENT EVALUATION

The appearance of intrathoracic lesions in the setting of an extrathoracic neoplasm poses a difficult clinical dilemma. While the onset of multiple lesions is usually unequivocal evidence for metastatic disease, the appearance of a solitary nodule is less straightforward. The histology of the primary site usually offers some insight. In the setting of a primary melanoma, sarcoma, or highly anaplastic carcinoma, a new pulmonary lesion almost always represents metastatic disease. The solitary pulmonary lesion is more likely to be a second primary neoplasm if the patient's primary was a squamous carcinoma; it could be either a metastasis or a new primary if the original cancer was an adenocarcinoma.[20]

### Signs and Symptoms

Only 1–15% of patients with pulmonary metastases become symptomatic. Given the peripheral or subpleural locations of these lesions, patients rarely develop symptoms prior to diagnosis. When symptoms do occur, patients will commonly complain of dyspnea, cough, wheezing, hemoptysis, or chest pain. The indolent development of dyspnea can be attributed to endobronchial obstruction, parenchymal replacement, pleural effusion, or lymphatic invasion. The acute onset of dyspnea may be secondary either to hemorrhage into a lesion or into the pleural space, or it may be due to pneumothorax. While the mechanism of pneumothorax associated with metastases is unclear, it is postulated to be due to tumor necrosis or erosion into a bronchus, or formation of a bullous lesion that eventually ruptures.[14]

*Endobronchial lesions* can also cause dyspnea, as well as hemoptysis, necessitating bronchoscopic examination. *Lymphangitic carcinomatosis*, seen most frequently in carcinomas of the stomach, breast, prostate, and pancreas, produces debilitating symptoms out of proportion to radiologic findings. These patients may exhibit progressive dyspnea, cough, and subacute cor pulmonale, while radiographs may only reveal an increase in the linear background pattern of the lung fields.[19,21] *Chest pain* is a most ominous symptom, which reflects the development of discontinuous parietal pleural metastases.

### Roentgenographic Examination

Patients diagnosed with an extrathoracic malignant neoplasm should obtain posteroanterior and lateral chest radiographs at the time of resection of the primary neoplasm and during subsequent follow-up. Other studies such as computed tomography (CT) of the chest and magnetic resonance imaging (MRI) may be obtained as well. While the initial radiographic exams serve as a baseline for future exams, they also aid in defining other comorbid thoracic disease. As a starting point in a patient's follow-up, these initial studies also serve as a standard to which future serial studies can be compared.[12]

### Roentgenographic Appearance

The topography of a lung metastasis reflects the pathophysiology of dissemination. The vast majority of metastases are found in the peripheral one third of the lung fields, most often at the lung bases. This distribution corresponds to hematogenous spread via the flow through the pulmonary circulation.[12] An exception to this pattern is choriocarcinoma, which has a greater distribution of metastases to the posterior portion of the upper lobes, which is attributed to metastatic seeding during curettage while the patient is in Trendelenburg position.[22,23] Pulmonary metastases from any histology do not appear to affect one lobe or to lateralize preferentially.[24,25]

Pulmonary metastases most commonly present as well-circumscribed spherical nodules, unassociated with linear densities.[3] While those lesions that have radiographic evidence of invasion into surrounding parenchyma tend to be primary lung cancers, metastatic lesions are sharply demarcated.[14] Occasionally, they appear in a "hairy" or "star" configuration, thus mimicking bronchopneumonia or infection.[14,24] Those lesions in the pleura can take on a distinctive pattern, appearing as pleural studs.[24] The size of pulmonary metastases can vary greatly and is a manifestation of disease chronicity.

Other characteristics, such as cavitation, calcification, lobar collapse, and bullous changes, can be seen in radiologic studies of pulmonary metastases. Cavitation is sometimes noted in sarcoma and carcinoma metastases and may appear more frequently in patients undergoing chemotherapy.[14] Calcification can be seen most commonly in metastatic osteosarcoma; occasionally in metastatic chondrosarcoma; and more rarely in synovial cell sarcoma, thyroid carcinoma, ovarian carcinoma, and mucinous carcinomas arising from the gastrointestinal tract. Chemotherapy and radiation may also result in calcification.[13,26–28] Endobronchial involvement, which presents in 2–28% of patients with pulmonary metastatic disease, can also present with lobar collapse. Bullous changes, as mentioned earlier as a reason for pneumothorax, may sometimes be the harbinger of metastatic disease in patients with sarcoma.[29]

### *Computed Tomography*

Since 1978, CT has evolved into the gold standard for evaluation of pulmonary metastases. In multiple studies, CT has effectively replaced conventional chest radiography and linear tomography as the most reliable noninvasive diagnostic procedure.[3,30–34] In chest CT scans, pulmonary metastases are usually well circumscribed and marked by the absence of a "twinkling star sign," which is caused by the radial artifacts of pulmonary vasculature.[35] Compared with more conventional techniques, pleural and subpleural lesions can be more easily detected with the CT scanner. In fact, with the addition of contrast enhancement, CT can surpass conventional techniques by up to a factor of $10^3$.

CT, however, remains costly and rarely detects lung lesions <3 mm in diameter. Occasionally, larger lesions will be missed, and central lesions can be obscured by pulmonary vasculature. Nodules adjacent to the diaphragm or lung apices can be missed because of the tangential relationship of CT scan cuts to those structures. Lesions as large as 1.5 cm have been missed, presumably secondary to nodule movement caused by respiratory excursion and variations.[36] With the advent of the faster helical CT scanners and their ability to obtain numerous sections during a single breath hold, newer generation CT scanners are able to reconstruct sections as necessary as well as generate three-dimensional images. The potential of these helical CT scanners in the imaging of pulmonary metastases will no doubt further refine sensitivity and specificity as they evolve.

CT can not only detect new nodules but also define the disease's natural history through serial exams. Isolated scans give little information in regards to a new lesion; however, by plotting a lesion against the cumulative information afforded by serial studies, CT scans can afford a high predictive value.[3] Questionable lesions can be followed with as frequent as 2–3-month interval scans to document any changes that would justify surgical intervention.

Patients with primary tumors that are likely to metastasize first to the lung, as well as those patients for whom aggressive resection is contemplated, should undergo chest CT scans at initial presentation as a baseline study or as part of the preoperative evaluation. In those cases where multiple nodules are seen on plain radiographs at initial presentation, CT scans are useful for documentation of response to therapy; follow-up can usually be maintained with chest radiographs.

For those patients whose primary histology metastasizes initially to extra-thoracic sites, those sites are usually evaluated prior to obtaining a chest CT scan. In those histologies that metastasize first to the liver, chest CT scans can be foregone if the patient's liver CT scans are negative and if there is no clinical or laboratory evidence of hepatic metastasis. With a negative bone scan in patients with tumors likely to metastasize to bone, a CT scan of the chest can be obtained if plain chest radiographs reveal abnormalities.[12]

Intervals between CT scans depend on histology as well. In those histologies where the probability of lung metastases is high, scans should be obtained frequently. Soft tissue and osteogenic sarcomas, e.g., are most likely to metastasize within 2 years of initial diagnosis; chest CT scans every 3 months in sarcoma patients are recommended.[3,37]

### *Magnetic Resonance Imaging*

The role of magnetic resonance imaging (MRI) is still being explored. Given the significant ionizing radiation dose per chest CT scan (0.5–2.0 rad or 5–20 mGy) and the frequency of screening required for patients with those histologies prone to pulmonary metastases, MRI presents a theoretical advantage, particularly in younger patients. In a recent trial conducted at the National Cancer Institute, MRI was found to be as sensitive as CT scan and significantly more sensitive than conventional chest radiography. Moreover, the use of gadopentetate dimeglumine contrast and the short-time inversion recovery (STIR) images, which have additive $T_1$- and $T_2$ weighted characteristics, increase the MRI's discriminating abilities.[38] However, more work needs to be conducted before the MRI's role in the evaluation and follow-up of patients with pulmonary metastases is finalized.

### *Invasive Diagnostic Procedures Exclusive of Thoracotomy*

In certain patients with lung nodules of unknown histology, documentation of metastatic disease has a major impact on therapy of the primary tumor. Other patients are unable to tolerate thoracotomy but require histologic verification for further management. In these subgroups of patients, other, more invasive diagnostic maneuvers exclusive of thoracotomy may be necessary.

Patients with an associated pleural effusion should undergo thoracentesis and cytologic examination. Sputum cytology and bronchoscopy are of limited value in diagnosing pulmonary metastases. Notable findings were documented in only 5% of sputum cytologic examinations and 10% of bronchoscopies in one series of patients with documented pulmonary metastases.[39] Bronchoscopy, however, is crucial for verification of endobronchial metastases and their evaluation for possible surgical intervention.

Fine-needle aspiration is of limited use in the diagnosis of pulmonary metastases. Any patient with a nodule favorable for resection and who can tolerate thoracotomy should undergo surgical intervention. Fine-needle aspiration biopsies may be a viable alternative for those patients unable to tolerate thoracotomy and who need histologic verification for further treatment.[12] One series of 123 patients revealed that 14.6% of metastatic nodules would be missed, and 1.6% would be diagnosed with fine-needle aspiration. However, 83.8% of patients undergoing fine-needle aspiration had a histologically correct diagnosis made.[40] Detection of metastatic melanoma,[41] breast cancer, gastrointestinal cancers, soft-tissue sarcomas, and germinal tumors using fine-needle aspiration biopsies has been documented.[42–46] Complications from this procedure include air leaks into the pleura (27.2%) necessitating tube thoracostomy in 4–5% of patients, transient hemoptysis (2–5%), and air embolism (0.07%). Seeding of the needle tract, while of theoretical and anecdotal concern, is rare and is prevented by puncturing the tumor at a site where a distance of at least 4 cm exists between the tumor surface and pleura.[45,47]

Video-assisted thoracoscopic surgery (VATS) is becoming increasingly popular in the diagnosis and treatment of pulmonary metastases and is controversial. For diagnosis, VATS has been shown to be virtually 100% sensitive and 100% specific. Complications are rare and include atelectasis (1.2%), pneumonia (0.8%), and air leak for more than 1 week (1.6%). VATS allows more rapid patient recovery, and the average hospital stay in one study was 2.4 days.[48–51] For those nodules that are too small or too far from the pleural surface to be visualized intraoperatively, a two-staged procedure analogous to needle localization for breast biopsies can be performed. CT-guided hookwires can be used for localization, thus permitting thoracoscopic excision.[52]

VATS has also been used to assist the traditional approach of median sternotomy. By visualizing the retrocardiac left lower lobe, VATS offers increased exposure in the setting of a median sternotomy.[53] However, the role of VATS alone in metastatectomies with curative intent remains controversial. The benefits of VATS metastatectomy include reduced cost, shorter hospital stay, and more rapid institution of therapy for the primary tumor. Anesthetic time required for thoracoscopic resection decreases with the surgeon's experience.[54] However, the completeness of pulmonary resections using VATS remains to be demonstrated. VATS precludes bimanual palpations of the lungs for lesions not visualized by CT scan or on the surface, thus limiting the surgeon to finger palpation. Moreover, CT scans, especially the more conventional nonhelical type, can underestimate the number of nodules in up to 28% of patients, thus seriously hindering a complete resection.[55] At this time, VATS seems, therefore, to be most applicable as a diagnostic procedure.[56]

## EVALUATION FOR SURGICAL RESECTION

Several criteria exist for evaluating the suitability of a patient to undergo surgical resection for pulmonary metastases[12,57,58] (Table 28–1). As few as one third of patients with metastatic disease will meet these criteria,[59] and only a portion of these patients will be cured of their disease.

Thus, prior to resection, these patients require an extensive functional and staging workup. Depending upon the patient's primary site and histology, extensive radiologic, radionuclide, and endoscopic evaluation must be performed. In those patients requiring multiple wedge resections or lobectomy, pulmonary reserve must be thoroughly evaluated. Pulmonary function testing can be used to predict adequate postoperative ventilatory reserve. In general, a patient with an $FEV_1$ of 800–1000 mL will not need prolonged respiratory support postmetastatectomy.[12,57] Quantitative ventilation perfusion scanning can be used to determine postresection $FEV_1$.[60] In those patients previously exposed to bleomycin with resultant pulmonary fibrosis and those patients in reoperative settings, careful workup of pulmonary reserve is essential.

Cardiac reserve must also be adequately assessed to determine whether a patient can safely tolerate thoracotomy and lung resection. Prior chemotherapy with doxorubicin (Adriamycin) can cause significant left ventricular dysfunction, particularly in those patients who have received cumulative doses >500 mg/m$^2$ body surface. Radionuclide cineangiography can be used at rest and during exercise to assess clinical or subclinical evidence of doxorubicin-induced cardiomyopathy.[61–63]

### Prognostic Factors

Despite a plethora of studies, no universal criteria predict long-term survival in patients who undergo resection of pulmonary metastases. While those basic criteria that dictate patient selection remain important, little agreement can be found among the myriad studies reporting on prognostic factors for long-term survival. Studies have focused on radiographic findings and facets of tumor biology such as

**TABLE 28–1. PATIENT SELECTION CRITERIA**

1. Local control of the primary tumor or potential for control should metastatectomy be performed first.
2. Absence of metastases to other nonpulmonary sites.
3. Adequate pulmonary function to tolerate resection.
4. Radiologic evidence consistent with metastases.
5. Pulmonary metastatic disease that can be completely resected.
6. Lack of any other effective therapy.

doubling time, disease-free interval, and histology, with little agreement. The most frequently examined factors are resectability, number of metastases resected, preoperative studies, disease-free interval, tumor doubling time, nodal status, and adjuvant chemotherapy.

### Resectability

Complete resectability of pulmonary metastases from sarcoma,[64–66] osteogenic sarcoma,[66,67] carcinoma,[68] and other histologies[69–71] has been shown to have some significance in prognosis. Resectability, given differing philosophies of thoracic surgeons and the limitations of preoperative studies, is determined at operation. A patient is deemed unresectable if there is involvement beyond the visceral envelope, as in pleural and diaphragmatic involvement, pleural effusion histologically positive for malignancy, lymph node involvement, or discontinuous pericardial involvement. Poor patient pulmonary reserve can also limit resectability.[12] In selected patients, extended resection to include the chest wall or other thoracic structures may achieve long-term survival[72] and, thus, alter more conservative definitions of resectability. Completeness of resection is perhaps the only prognostic factor upon which there is some agreement.

### Number of Metastases Resected

Earlier studies seemed to indicate that prognosis correlated with numbers of metastases resected, worsening as the number increased.[64] More recent studies in patients with metastatic sarcomas have found no correlation between number of nodules resected and long-term survival. In osteogenic[67,73,74] and Ewing's[75] sarcomas, resection of three to five or more nodules was associated with a significantly poorer prognosis than less than three to five nodules. Colon cancer had a significantly poorer prognosis with greater than one nodule. No significant difference attributable to nodule number could be found in breast cancer.[76]

### Preoperative Studies

Given the disparity that can occur between preoperative and intraoperative counts, the number of nodules on preoperative radiographic studies has debatable significance as a prognostic factor. Often, preoperative radiographic studies will underestimate the number of nodules resected by as much as a factor of 8.

Studies examining the significance of number of nodules on preoperative studies have only been reviewed osteogenic and soft tissue sarcomas. Putnam et al[64] found significantly improved survival in those patients with four or fewer nodules on preoperative conventional lung tomograms. In a more recent evaluation of National Cancer Institute sarcoma patients, those with six or more nodules on chest CT scan had significantly decreased survival.[66]

### Disease-free Interval

In osteogenic and soft-tissue sarcomas, disease-free interval is generally believed to influence the long-term outcome of metastatectomy.[64,66,68,77] Disease-free interval is defined as the time from primary tumor resection until the appearance of pulmonary metastases. A notable exception is Pastorini's study of 56 patients in which no benefit was seen in longer disease-free intervals.[65] Prognosis after metastatectomy in Ewing's sarcoma[75] and colon cancer[78] appear not to be affected by disease-free interval; conversely, breast cancer metastatectomy patients had a better prognosis if their disease-free interval was >1 year.[76] Of note, only 46% of patients with synchronous metastases in soft-tissue sarcomas had resectable metastases.[64] In those who were completely resected, however, no difference in survival could be found when compared with patients with metachronous metastases. Similar findings have been shown in Ewing's sarcoma,[75] carcinoma,[68] and renal cell cancer.[79]

### Tumor Doubling Time

While tumor doubling time would theoretically seem to be of significance in prognosis, practical application renders this factor far less useful. Several studies have shown tumor doubling time to have a significant correlation with survival, i.e., a short tumor doubling time is associated with decreased survival after metastatectomy.[72,80] However, the prudence of waiting to measure tumor doubling time is questionable. In those patients where an unclear radiologic picture or clinical history draw the diagnosis of metastasis into question, serial CT examinations may be in order. Given the body of data on prolonged survival in properly selected patients with pulmonary metastases, delaying surgery to document doubling time is unnecessary.

### Nodal Status

Because patients are considered eligible for metastatectomy only in the absence of mediastinal disease, nodal status has been rarely analyzed. However, nodal involvement in one study of patients with sarcoma and in another study of patients with varying histology show significantly poorer prognosis in those patients with nodal involvement.[64,80]

### Adjuvant Chemotherapy

No randomized studies are available examining the effect of adjuvant or neoadjuvant chemotherapy for pulmonary metastatectomy. At the National Cancer Institute, Jablons et al[66] noted no difference in the survival rates of those patients who received postthoracotomy chemotherapy vs. those who did not. At M.D. Anderson, preoperative chemotherapy for patients with pulmonary metastases from soft-tissue sarcomas did not appear to be a significant prognostic factor.[81]

### Other Variables

Other variables examined include laterality or bilaterality of disease, age, and gender. In the setting of a soft tissue sarcoma metastases, laterality appears to have little effect on prognosis in those patients completely resected. Age or gender of the patient does not appear to correlate with survival.[12]

## SURGICAL RESECTION

### Technique

The technique of pulmonary metastatectomy has been generally standardized, involving either a median sternotomy or a lateral thoracotomy approach. After the patient is intubated with a double-lumen endotracheal tube (which allows selective complete lung collapse), the surgeon meticulously explores the thoracic cavity. Abnormal lesions are then resected while the lung is inflated, thus preserving as much lung function as possible while providing adequate margins. Peripheral lesions can be surrounded by or positioned in the cut-out portion of Duvall lung clamps. For those lesions requiring more extensive resection, segmentectomy or lobectomy may be required.[12] The most desirable operative approach for metastatic disease, if possible, is median sternotomy.[65,66,82] By using this approach, both lungs can be simultaneously palpated, allowing the surgeon to find metastases not detected by preoperative radiographic studies. If a large number of nodules on one side necessitates formal resection, concomitant exploration of the contralateral lung allows the surgeon to assess the complete pulmonary picture prior to deeming a situation resectable or unresectable. Moreover, with wide mediastinal exposure, complete lung collapse facilitated by the double-lumen endotracheal tube, placement of posterior packs, and elevation of the lung using lung clamps, this approach can facilitate almost any procedure, even more extended resections. Left lower lobectomies are slightly more difficult using this approach but can be performed. One study has proposed the use of VATS to assist in this slightly more difficult location.[53] In the setting of postoperative patient comfort and rehabilitation, the avoidance of staged thoracotomies is also advantageous.[12] In sum, there are no differences in morbidity, mortality, or long-term survival when the two approaches are compared.[25]

Previous sternal irradiation constitutes an absolute contraindication to a median sternotomy, given poor wound healing. Relative contraindications include obesity, central staple line recurrences, and posteromedial chest wall disease. Large posterior or central lesions, particularly in the left upper lobe or the need for possible sleeve type resection may render a thoracotomy more advantageous to perform.[82]

Bilateral anterior thoracotomies with transverse sternotomy (clamshell) or unilateral thoracotomy with partial or complete median sternotomy (hemi-clamshell) have recently been proposed for pulmonary metastatectomy. These approaches facilitate exploration of lower lobe disease and hemithoracic extension of mediastinal disease, in addition to allowing exposure of the mediastinum, pericardium, pleura, and lung.[83] Further work needs to be done in the area of alternate approaches.

### Newer Techniques Currently Under Study

Recent studies have proposed the use of Neodymium: Yttrium-Aluminum-Garnet (Nd:YAG) lasers.[84,85] The YAG laser does not require a bloodless field, has deep pulmonary parenchymal penetration, and can seal blood and air leaks. Theoretically, the deeper thermal penetration enhances margins. However, the YAG laser's use appears to require increased operative time, hospital staff, and duration of chest tube suction.[86] The ultimate effects on long-term survival have yet to be documented.

The use of the ultrasonic aspirator in pulmonary metastatic disease is still experimental. The ultrasonic vibrations of the titanium tip lyse the lung while leaving blood vessels and bronchi intact. Clips or suture ligatures can then be used to control these structures. In the study by Verazin et al[87] of 18 patients who underwent pulmonary metastatectomy with ultrasonic aspirator, three patients had prolonged air leaks, one of whom required decortication.[87] Further studies need to be conducted on this technique.

Isolated lung perfusion with chemotherapeutic agents is also under study as a possible mode of treatment for pulmonary metastases. The prevalence of pulmonary disease despite systemic therapy, particularly in histologies such as soft-tissue sarcomas where overall response rate is less than 30%, has provided the impetus to explore loco-regional therapy. Theoretically, the delivery of high concentrations of chemotherapy into the pulmonary system while excluding the systemic circuit would increase the efficacy of these agents. The earliest papers, which concentrated on technique and pharmacokinetics, emerged in the late 1950s and early 1960s.[88] Johnston et al[89] explored bilateral isolated lung perfusion in the early 1980s in a canine model. More recent studies have perfected the technique, refined the knowledge on pharmacokinetics, and examined toxicity in the animal model. Weksler et al[90] perfused rats injected with methylcholanthrene-induced sarcoma cells with doxorubicin or saline. Twenty-one days after perfusion, there was complete clearance of macro- and microscopic evidence of tumor in those animals perfused with doxorubicin compared with massive tumor replacement in those perfused with saline. Human trials have begun at the National Cancer Institute, where a phase I trial is underway using interferon, tumor necrosis factor, and hyperthermia in humans.

### Reoperation

An aggressive approach to recurrent pulmonary metastases has been evaluated in several institutions.[91–93] While the role of reoperative metastatectomies is unclear in most histologies, there appears to be some long-term survival benefit in reresecting pulmonary metastases from soft-tissue sarcomas. In a retrospective study of patients with soft-tissue sarcomas, 43 patients had two or more thoracic explorations for metastatic disease. In 89 reoperations, operative mortality was 0%, and 31 of 43 patients were rendered free of disease at reoperation with a median survival of 25 months compared with 10 months in patients deemed unresectable at second operation. Median sternotomy was used up to four times in a single patient with subsequent resections utilizing thoracotomy. Other than disease-free interval greater than 18 months and resectability, no other factors in univariate analysis predicted long-term survival after reoperation.[91]

In a similar study from M.D. Anderson, 34 patients underwent re-resection. The only factor that predicted longer survival after re-resection was the resection of a single metastasis. Those patients with two or more recurrent nodules had a median survival of only 14 months.[93]

**TABLE 28–2. OSTEOGENIC SARCOMA**

| Author(s) (yr) | No. Patients | 5-Year Survival (%) Unless Otherwise Indicated |
|---|---|---|
| Giritsky et al[98] (1978) | 12 | 38 (3 y) |
| Telander et al[95] (1978) | 28 | 57 (4 y) |
| Burgers et al[97] (1980) | 6 | 60 |
| Morrow et al[102] (1980) | 11 | 36 |
| Putnam et al[67] (1983) | 39 | 40 |
| Mountain et al[69] (1984) | 56 | 51 |
| Vogt-Moykopf et al[68] (1988) | 41 | 33 (3 y) |
| DiLorenzo and Collin[118] (1988) | 10 | 50 |
| Roberts et al[103] (1989) | 16 | 23 |
| Carter et al[99] (1991) | 25 | 20 |

*(From Pass HI: Treatment of metastatic cancer to the lung. In deVita V, Hellman S, Rosenberg S (eds): Principles and Practice of Oncology. Philadelphia: Lippincott, 1993, p 2198, with permission.)*

## SPECIFIC HISTOLOGIES

### Osteogenic Sarcoma

Five-year survival in patients treated by amputation alone prior to an aggressive approach to pulmonary disease were as low as 17%,[94] with most patients succumbing to pulmonary dissemination. With adjuvant or neoadjuvant chemotherapy and more aggressive surgical resection, the salvage rate more than doubled in some studies. Telander et al[95] at the Mayo Clinic documented a 5-year survival rate as 23% from 1946 to 1974 vs. one of 57% in the time period from 1974 to 1977. Pastorini et al[96] had 3-year survivals of 20% from 1970 to 1983, which increased to 46% from 1984 to 1988.

While the individual contributions of aggressive surgical resection and of chemotherapy are impossible to evaluate, their coupling has changed salvage rates for patients with osteogenic sarcoma, justifying the use of metastatectomies in their care.[68,96–101] The 5-year survival rates for these patients is now generally accepted to be 35–40%[12] (Table 28–2).

### Soft-tissue Sarcoma

Most soft-tissue sarcomas metastases occur within the first 2 years of initial diagnosis, and most occur in the lung. An aggressive approach to metastases has pushed the 5-year survival rate to as high as 33% in multiple studies[64–66] (Table 28–3). Factors correlating with survival include disease-free interval, ability to render the patient free of disease at operation, and possibly the number of nodules found in preoperative studies. In the most recent study of those patients at the National Cancer Institute, the number of metastases resected had no correlation with survival in patients rendered completely free of disease.[66] Thus, the only limiting factor regarding resection is sufficient lung function and reserve.

### Urinary Tract

In patients with renal cell cancer, approximately half will present with metachronous or synchronous pulmonary metastases.[79] Resecting the metastases results in varying 5-year survival rates, ranging from 13% to 50%, and in median survivals of 23–33 months[68,69,79,102,103] (Table 28–4). Because many of these patients' survivals are analyzed in studies combining their results with other histologies, the contribution of those patients with renal cell cancer is difficult to analyze. Pogrebniak analyzed 23 such patients from the National Cancer Institute experience (1985–1991). Most of the resected patients had received IL-2 based immunotherapy, thus making it difficult to differentiate the relative efficacy of surgery vs. immunotherapy.[104] How-

**TABLE 28–3. SOFT-TISSUE SARCOMA**

| Author(s) (y) | No. Patients | 5-Year Survival (%) Unless Otherwise Indicated |
|---|---|---|
| Martini et al[119] (1978) | 409 | 15–25 |
| Creagan et al[77] (1979) | 112 | 29 |
| Putnam et al[64] (1984) | 63 | 30 (3 y) |
| Mountain et al[69] (1984) | 49 | 33 |
| Vogt-Moykopf et al[68] (1988) | 56 | 33 |
| Jablons et al[66] (1989) | 68 | 33 |
| Pastorini et al[96] (1990) | 72 | 50 (3 y) |
| Lanza et al[81] (1991) | 24 | 22 |
| Casson et al[93] (1991) | 58 | 26 |

*(From Pass HI: Treatment of metastatic cancer to the lung. In DeVita V, Hellman S, Rosenberg S (eds): Principles and Practice of Oncology. Philadelphia, Lippincott, 1993; p 2198, with permission.)*

TABLE 28–4. URINARY TRACT

| Author(s) (y) | No. Patients | 5-Year Survival (%) Unless Otherwise Indicated |
|---|---|---|
| Morrow et al[102] (1980) | 30 | 24 |
| Mountain et al[69] (1984) | 20 | 54 |
| Vogt-Moykopf et al[68] (1988) | 42 | 42 |
| Roberts et al[103] (1989) | 33 | 24 |
| diSilverio et al[120] (1991) | 20 | 35 |
| Pogrebniak et al[79] (1992) | 23 | 43 mo (mean) |

*(From Pass HI: Treatment of metastatic cancer to the lung. In DeVita V, Hellman S, Rosenberg S (eds): Principles and Practice of Oncology. Philadelphia, Lippincott, 1993, p 2198, with permission.)*

ever, patients who underwent complete resection of metastatic disease had a significantly longer survival (mean 49 months) compared with those patients who had had incomplete resections (median 16 months). Overall, mean survival for all patients was 43 months. Survival post-metastatectomy had no correlation with number of nodules on preoperative tomograms, number of nodules resected, or disease-free interval.[79]

## Testicular Cancer

Nonseminomatous germ cell tumors of the testes are exquisitely sensitive to chemotherapy. Frequently, only benign teratomas are found in these patients following a course of chemotherapy.[68–70,102,105] These patients become candidates for thoracotomy when there is no response or partial response followed by recurrence to chemotherapy, markers begin to rise in the setting of no chemotherapeutic options, or when cytoreductive surgery is necessary to determine if viable tumor exists[12] (Table 28–5). Because of the frequent coupling of retroperitoneal and metastatic pulmonary disease, a recent paper advocates one-stage median sternotomy and retroperitoneal lymph node dissection.[106] The role of salvage chemotherapy after thoracotomy is still under investigation.[107]

## Head and Neck

The lung is the first site of recurrence for all head and neck cancers, save for lip, tonsil, and adenoid cancers.[12] Moreover, given common risk factors, this patient population is at high risk for second primary lung cancers. Thus, resection becomes more pressing in these patients in order to evaluate new nodules. Five-year survival rates approach 44% for these patients[68,102] (Table 28–5).

Finley et al,[108] in their retrospective study of 58 patients, found improved long-term survival in patients with only one malignant pulmonary nodule, locoregional control of the primary, and disease-free interval 1 year.

TABLE 28–5. OTHER HISTOLOGIES

| Author(s) (y) | No. Patients | 5-Year Survival (%) Unless Otherwise Indicated |
|---|---|---|
| Breast | | |
| Wright et al[113] (1982) | 18 | 27 |
| Mountain et al[69] (1984) | 30 | 27 |
| Lanza et al[76] (1987) | 37 | 50 |
| Staren et al[122] (1992) | 33 | 35 |
| Head and neck | | |
| Mountain et al[69] (1984) | 48 | 41 |
| Vogt-Moykopf et al[68] (1988) | 12 | 44 |
| Finley et al[108] (1992) | 7 | 43 |
| Uterine-cervical | | |
| Mountain et al[69] (1984) | 22 | 8 |
| Seki et al[123] (1992) | 32 | 52 |
| Testicular | | |
| Mountain et al[69] (1984) | 20 | 54 |
| Vogt-Moykopf et al[68] (1988) | 12 | 44 |
| Venn et al[70] (1989) | 42 | 84 |

*(From Pass HI: Treatment of metastatic cancer to the lung. In DeVita V, Hellman S, Rosenberg S (eds): Principles and Practice of Oncology. Philadelphia, Lippincott, 1993, p 2199, with permission.)*

## Colorectal

Only 1% of patients with colorectal cancers will present with isolated pulmonary metastases as a first site of recurrence. However, the lung is the most frequent site of extra-abdominal metastases.[109] Five-year survival rates in these patients vary widely according to study, ranging from 13% to 61%[12,69,102,103,110] (Table 28–6). The largest series of patients (139 patients) quotes a 5-year survival rate of 31%.[76] Control of the primary site is generally agreed upon as an important prognostic factor,[76,110,111] and some studies advocate reresection in selected patients with recurrent pulmonary metastases.[76,112]

TABLE 28–6. COLON AND RECTAL

| Author(s) (y) | No. Patients | 5-Year Survival (%) Unless Otherwise Indicated |
|---|---|---|
| Cahan[117] (1974) | 31 | 31 |
| McCormack and Attiyeh[121] (1979) | 35 | 22 |
| Morrow et al[102] (1980) | 16 | 13 |
| Mountain et al[69] (1984) | 28 | 28 |
| Roberts et al[103] (1989) | 13 | 23 |
| Mori et al[112] (1993) | 35 | 38 |
| McAfee et al[78] (1992) | 139 | 30 |
| Saclarides et al[110] (1993) | 23 | 16 |

*(From Pass HI: Treatment of metastatic cancer to the lung. In DeVita V, Hellman S, Rosenberg S (eds): Principles and Practice of Oncology. Philadelphia, Lippincott, 1993, p 2198, with permission.)*

**TABLE 28–7. MELANOMA**

| Author(s) (y) | No. Patients | 5-Year Survival (%) Unless Otherwise Indicated |
|---|---|---|
| Cahan[117] (1973) | 12 | 33 |
| Dahlback et al[116] (1980) | 8 | 7 mo (median) |
| Morrow et al[102] (1980) | 12 | 12 |
| Mountain et al[69] (1984) | 58 | 13 mo (median) |
| Pogrebniak et al[115] (1988) | 33 | 13 mo (median) |

*(From Pass HI: Treatment of metastatic cancer to the lung. In DeVita V, Hellman S, Rosenberg S (eds): Principles and Practice of Oncology. Philadelphia, Lippincott, 1993, p 2199, with permission.)*

### Breast

The efficacy of metastatectomy in breast cancer patients has not been clearly established, despite the fact that approximately one fifth of patients will die of isolated but potentially resectable lung metastases. Five-year survival rates range from 27% to 50%[77,102,113] (Table 28–5). However, the individual contributions of surgery and adjuvant therapy are unclear. A recent study showed a 5-year survival rate of 36% in those who underwent complete resection but those patients that were incompletely resected had a 5-year survival rate of 42%.[114]

### Melanoma

A recent retrospective review of 49 melanoma patients who underwent pulmonary metastatectomy revealed a median survival of 13 months.[115] These unrewarding findings are corroborated in other studies[69,102,116,117] (Table 28–7). The National Cancer Institute study found no correlation between survival and Clark's level, disease-free interval, lymph node status, or number of nodules found on preoperative studies. Despite these dismal numbers, 16 patients were found to have benign disease even in the face of documentation of a new nodule in 13 of these patients.[115] For this reason alone, thoracic exploration may be indicated in order to rule out benign disease. However, given the unfavorable natural history and multiplicity of nodules, melanoma is not a favorable histology for metastatectomy.

## SUMMARY

Surgery continues to be important in treatment for pulmonary metastases. While sufficient evidence exists in certain histologies to warrant a highly aggressive approach, work on newer treatments and diagnostic methods continues to evolve. At the National Cancer Institute, a phase I trial is exploring isolated lung perfusion with tumor necrosis factor, interferon, and hyperthermia in humans. As clinicians and scientists, thoracic surgeons can uniquely integrate these facets in the delivery of care; as such, pulmonary metastases remain an important part of thoracic surgery.

## REFERENCES


1. Willis RA: Secondary tumors of the lung. In: *The Spread of Tumors in the Human Body.* London: Butterworths, 1973, pp 167–174
2. Viadana E, Irwin D, Bross J, et al: Cascade spread of blood-borne metastases in solid and non-solid cancers of humans. In: Weiss L, and Gilbert H (eds): *Pulmonary Metastasis.* Boston, GK Hall, 1978, pp 143–167
3. Pass HI, Dwyer A, Makuch R, et al: Detection of pulmonary metastases in patients with osteogenic and soft tissue sarcoma: The superiority of CT scan compared to conventional linear tomograms using dynamic analysis. *J Clin Oncol* **3:**1261–1265, 1985
4. Baciewicz FA, Arrendondo M, Chaudhuri B, et al: Pharmacokinetics and toxicity of isolated perfusion of lung with Doxorubicin. *J Surg Res* **50:**124–128, 1991
5. van Dongen JA, van Slooten EA: The surgical treatment of pulmonary metastases. *Cancer Treat Rep* **5:**29–48, 1978
6. Torek F: Removal of metastatic carcinoma of the lung and mediastinum: Suggestions as to technique. *Arch Surg* **21:**1416–1424, 1930
7. Barney JD, Churchill ED: Adeno-carcinoma of the kidney with metastasis to the lungs treated by pulmonary resection. *J Urol* **42:**269–276, 1939
8. Alexander J, Haight C: Pulmonary resection for solitary metastatic sarcomas and carcinomas. *Surg Gynecol Obstet* **85:**129–135, 1947
9. Thomford NR, Wodner LB, Clagett OT. The surgical treatment of metastatic tumors in the lungs. *J Thorac Cardiovasc Surg* **49:**357–363, 1965
10. Martini N, Huvos AG, Mike V, et al: Multiple pulmonary resections in the treatment of osteogenic sarcoma. *Ann Thorac Surg* **12:**271–280, 1971
11. Morton DL, Joseph WL, Ketcham AS, et al: Surgical resection and adjunctive immunotherapy for selected patients with multiple pulmonary metastases. *Ann Surg* **178:**360–365, 1973
12. Pass HI: Treatment of metastatic cancer to the lung. In DeVita V, Hellman S, Rosenberg S (eds): *Principles and Practice of Oncology.* Philadelphia, Lippincott, 1993, pp 2186–2200
13. Muller KM, Respondek M: Pulmonary metastases: Pathological anatomy. *Lung* **168:**1137–1144, 1990
14. Libshitz HI, North LB: Pulmonary metastases. *Radiol Clin North Am* **20:**437–451, 1982
15. Liotta LA, Kleinerman J, Saidel GM: The significance of hematogenous tumor cell clumps in the metastatic process. *Cancer Res* **36:**889–894, 1976
16. Dwyer AJ, Reichert CM, Wollering EA, et al: Diffuse pulmonary metastasis in melanoma: Radiographic-pathologic correlation. *AJR* **143:**983–984, 1984
17. Berg HK, Petrelli NJ, Herrera L, et al: Endobronchial metastasis from colorectal carcinoma. *Dis Colon Rectum* **27:**745–748, 1984
18. Shapshay SM, Strom MS: Tracheobronchial obstruction from metastatic distant malignancies. *Ann Otol Rhinol Laryngol* **91:** 648–651, 1982
19. Janower ML, Blennerhassett JB: Lymphangitic spread of metastatic cancer to the lung. *Radiology* **101:**267–273, 1971
20. Cahan WG, Shah JP, Castro EB: Benign solitary lung lesions in patients with cancer. *Ann Surg* **187:**241–244, 1978
21. Schwarz MI, Waddell LC, Dombeck DH, et al: Prolonged survival in lymphangitic carcinomatosis. *Ann Intern Med* **71:**779–783, 1969
22. Hendin AS: Gestational trophoblastic tumors metastatic to the lung. *Cancer* **53:**58–61, 1984
23. Wagner D: Trophoblastic cells in the bloodstream in normal and abnormal pregnancy. *Acta Cytol* **12:**137–139, 1968

24. Crow J, Slavin G, Kreel L: Pulmonary metastasis: A pathologic and radiologic study. *Cancer* **46:**2595–2602, 1981
25. Roth JA, Pass HI, Wesley MN, et al: Comparison of median sternotomy and thoracotomy for resection of pulmonary metastasis in patients with adult soft-tissue sarcomas. *Ann Thorac Surg* **42:**134–138, 1986
26. Rosenfield AT, Sanders RC, Custer LE: Widespread calcified metastases from adenocarcinoma of the jejunum. *Am J Dig Dis* **20:**990–994, 1975
27. Panella J, Mintzer RA: Multiple calcified pulmonary nodules in an elderly man. *JAMA* **244:**2559–2560, 1980
28. Zollikofer C, Castaneda-Zuniga W, Stenlund R, et al: Lung metastases from synovial sarcoma simulating granulomas. *AJR* **135:** 161–163, 1980
29. Sarno RC, Carter BL: Bullous change by CT heralding metastatic sarcoma. *Comput Radiol* **9:**115–120, 1985
30. Kreel L: Computed tomography of the thorax. *Radiol Clin North Am* **16:**575–584, 1978
31. Cohen M, Grosfeld J, Baehner R, et al: Lung CT for detection of metastases: Solid tissue neoplasms in children. *AJR* **139:**895–898, 1982
32. Piekarski J-D, Schlumberger M, LeClere J, et al: Chest computed tomography (CT) in patients with micronodular lung metastases of differentiated thyroid carcinoma. *Int J Radiat Oncol Biol Phys* **11:**1023–1027, 1985
33. Lund G, Heilo A: Computed tomography of pulmonary metastases. *Acta Radiol* **23:**617–620, 1982
34. Sones PJ, Torres WE, Colvin RS, et al: Effectiveness of CT in evaluating intrathoracic masses. *AJR* **139:**469–475, 1982
35. Kuhns LR, Borlaza G: The "Twinkling Star" sign; An aid in differentiating pulmonary vessels from pulmonary nodules on computed tomograms. *Radiology* **135:**763–764, 1980
36. Krudy AG, Doppman JL, Herdt JR: Failure to detect a 1.5 centimeter lung nodule by chest computed tomography. *J Comput Assist Tomogr* **6:**1178–1180, 1983
37. Chiles C, Ravin CE: Intrathoracic metastasis from an extrathoracic malignancy: A radiographic approach to patient evaluation. *Radiol Clin North Am* **23:**427–438, 1985
38. Feuerstein IM, Jicha DL, Pass HI, et al: Pulmonary metastases: MRI imaging with surgical correlation—A prospective study. *Radiology* **182:**123–129, 1992
39. Vincent RG, Choksi LB, Takita H, et al: Surgical resection of the solitary pulmonary metastases. In: Weiss L, Gilbert HA (eds): *Pulmonary Metastases.* Boston, GK Hall, 1978, p 224
40. Johnston WW: Percutaneous fine needle aspiration biopsy of the lung: A study of 1,015 patients. *Acta Cytol* **28:**218–224, 1984
41. Poellein S, Rothenberg J, Penkava RR: Metastatic malignant melanoma in the lung. *Arch Pathol Lab Med* **106:**119–120, 1982
42. Pilotti S, Rilke F, Gribauldi G, et al: Transthoracic fine needle aspiration biopsy in pulmonary lesions. *Acta Cytol* **28:**225–232, 1984
43. Nieberg RK: Fine needle aspiration cytology of alveolar soft parts sarcoma. *Acta Cytol* **28:**198–202, 1984
44. Nguyen G-K, Jeannot A: Cytopathologic aspects of pulmonary metastasis of malignant fibrous histiocytoma, myxoid variant. *Acta Cytol* **26:**349–353, 1982
45. Crosby JH, Kager B, Hoeg K: Transthoracic fine needle aspiration. *Cancer* **56:**2504–2507, 1985
46. Silverman JF, Weaver MD, Gardner N, et al: Aspiration biopsy cytology of malignant schwannoma metastatic to the lung. *Acta Cytol* **29:**15–18, 1985
47. Nordenstrom BE: Technical aspects of obtaining cellular material from lesions deep in the lung. *Acta Cytol* **28:**233–242, 1984
48. Mack MJ, Hazelrigg SR, Landreneau RJ, et al: Thoracoscopy for the diagnosis of the indeterminate solitary pulmonary nodule. *Ann Thorac Surg* **56:**825–832, 1993
49. Bonniot J-P A, Homasson J-P D, Roden SL, et al: Pleural and lung cryobiopsies during thoracoscopy. *Chest* **95:**492–493, 1989
50. Lewis RJ, Caccavale RJ, Sisler GE: Special report: Video-endoscopic thoracic surgery. *N J Med* **88:**473–474, 1991
51. Page RD, Jeffrey RR, Donnelly RJ: Thoracoscopy: A review of 121 consecutive surgical procedures. *Ann Thorac Surg* **48:**66–68, 1989
52. Shah RM, Spirn PW, Salazar AM, et al: Localization of peripheral pulmonary nodules for thoracoscopic excision: Value of CT-guided wire placement. *AJR* **161:**279–283, 1993
53. Hazelrigg SR, Naunheim K, Auer JE, et al: Combined median sternotomy and video-assisted thoracoscopic resection of pulmonary metastases. *Chest* **104:**956–958, 1993
54. Dowling RD, Ferson PF, Landreneau RJ: Thoracoscopic resection of pulmonary metastases. *Chest* **102:**1450–1454, 1992
55. McCormack PM, Ginsberg KB, Bains MS, et al: Accuracy of lung imaging in metastases with implication for the role of thoracoscopy. *Ann Thorac Surg* **56:**863–866, 1993
56. Dowling RD, Keenan RJ, Ferson PF, et al: Video-assisted thoracoscopic resection of pulmonary metastases. *Ann Thorac Surg* **56:**772–775, 1993
57. Matthay RA, Arrolica AL: Resection of pulmonary metastases. *Am Rev Respir Dis* **148:**1691–1696, 1993
58. Todd TR: Pulmonary metastatectomy; Current indications for removing lung metastases. *Chest* **103:**401s–403s, 1993
59. Shepherd MP: Endobronchial metastatic disease. *Thorax* **37:**362–365, 1982
60. Boysen PG, Block J, Olsen GN, et al: Prospective evaluation for pneumonectomy using the $^{99m}$technetium quantitative perfusion lung scan. *Chest* **72:**422–425, 1977
61. Dresdale A, Bonow RO, Wesley R, et al: Prospective evaluation of Doxorubicin-induced cardiomyopathy resulting from postsurgical adjuvant treatment of patients with soft tissue sarcomas. *Cancer* **52:**51–60, 1983
62. Mason JW, Brustow MR, Billingham ME, et al: Invasive and noninvasive methods of assessing Adriamycin-induced cardiotoxic effects in man: Superiority of histopathologic assessment using endomyocardial biopsy. *Cancer Treat Rep* **62:**857–864, 1978
63. Gottidiener JS, Mathisen DJ, Borer JS, et al: Doxorubicin cardiotoxicity: Assessment of late left ventricular dysfunction by radionuclide cineangiography. *Ann Intern Med* **84:**430–435, 1981
64. Putnam JB, Roth JA, Wesley MN, et al: Analysis of prognostic factors in patients undergoing resection of pulmonary metastases from soft tissue sarcomas. *J Thorac Cardiovasc Surg* **87:**260–268, 1984
65. Pastorini U, Valente M, Gaspirini M, et al: Median sternotomy and multiple lung resections for metastatic sarcomas. *Eur J Cardiothorac Surg* **4:**477–482, 1990
66. Jablons D, Steinberg SM, Roth J, et al: Metastatectomy for soft tissue sarcoma. *J Thorac Cardiovasc Surg* **97:**695–705, 1989
67. Putnam JB, Roth JA, Weley MN, et al: Survival following aggressive resection of pulmonary metastases from osteogenic sarcoma: Analysis of prognostic factors. *Ann Thorac Surg* **36:**516–523, 1983
68. Vogt-Moykopf I, Buzelbruck H, Merkle NM, et al: Results of surgical treatment of pulmonary metastases. *Eur J Cardiothorac Surg* **2:**224–232, 1988
69. Mountain CF, McMurtrey MJ, Hermes KE: Surgery for pulmonary metastasis: A 20-year experience. *Ann Thorac Surg* **38:**323–329, 1984
70. Venn GE, Sarin S, Goldstraw P: Survival following pulmonary metastatectomy. *Eur J Cardiothorac Surg* **3:**105–110, 1989
71. Putnam JB, Suell DM, Natarajan G. Extended resection of pulmonary metastases: Is the risk justified? *Ann Thorac Surg* **55:** 1440–1446, 1993
72. Joseph WL, Morton DL, Adkins PC: Prognostic significance of tumor doubling time in evaluating operability in pulmonary metastatic disease. *J Thorac Cardiovasc Surg* **61:**23–31, 1971
73. Casson AG, Putnam JB, Natarajan G: Five-year survival after pul-

monary metastatectomy for adult soft tissue sarcoma. *Cancer* **69:**662–668, 1992

74. Meyer WH, Schell MJ, Kumar APM: Thoracotomy for pulmonary metastatic osteosarcoma. *Cancer* **59:**374–379, 1987
75. Lanza LA, Miser JS, Pass HI, et al: The role of resection in the treatment of pulmonary metastases from Ewing's sarcoma. *J Thorac Cardiovasc Surg* **94:**181–187, 1987
76. Lanza LA, Natarajan G, Roth JA: Long-term survival after resection of pulmonary metastases from carcinoma of the breast. *Ann Thorac Surg* **54:**244–248, 1992
77. Creagan ET, Fleming TR, Edmonson JH, et al: Pulmonary resection for metastatic nonosteogenic sarcoma. *Cancer* **44:**1908–1912, 1979
78. McAfee MK, Allen MS, Trastek VF, et al: Colorectal lung metastases: Results of surgical excision. *Ann Thorac Surg* **53:**780–786, 1992
79. Pogrebniak HW, Haas G, Linehan WM, et al: Renal cell carcinoma: Resection of solitary and multiple metastases. *Ann Thorac Surg* **54:**33–38, 1992
80. Takita H, Edgerton F, Karakousis C, et al: Surgical management of metastases to the lung. *Surg Gynecol Obstet* **152:**191–194, 1981
81. Lanza LA, Putnam JB, Benjamin RS, et al: Response to chemotherapy does not predict survival after resection of sarcomatous pulmonary metastases. *Ann Thorac Surg* **51:**219–224, 1991
82. Pogrebniak HW, Pass HI: Initial and reoperative pulmonary metastatectomy: Indications, technique, and results. *Semin Surg Oncol* **9:**142–149, 1993
83. Bains MS, Ginsberg RJ, Jones WG, et al: The clamshell incision: An improved approach to bilateral pulmonary and mediastinal tumors. Presented at the Society of Thoracic Surgeons meeting; January 31–February 2, 1994.
84. Harvey JC, Lee K, Beattie EJ: Utility of the Neodymium: Yttrium-Aluminum-Garnet (Nd: YAG) laser for extensive pulmonary metastatectomy. *J Surg Oncol* **54:**175–179, 1993
85. Fanta J, Koutecky J, Rehak F: Use of the Nd: YAG laser in the surgical treatment of lung metastases in children. *Pediatr Hemat Oncol* **8:**375–377, 1991
86. Branscheid D, Krysa S, Wollkopf G, et al: Does Nd: YAG laser extend the indications for resection of pulmonary metastases? *Eur J Cardiothorac Surg* **6:**590–597, 1992
87. Verazin GT, Regal A-M, Antkowiak JG, et al: Ultrasonic surgical aspirator for lung resection. *Ann Thorac Surg* **52:**787–790, 1991
88. Jacobs JK, Flexner JM, Scott HW: Selective isolated perfusion of the right or left lung. *J Thorac Cardiovasc Surg* **42:**546–552, 1961
89. Johnston MR, Christensen CW, Minchin RF, et al: Isolated total lung perfusion as a means to depiver organ-specific chemotherapy: Long-term studies in animals. *Surgery* **98:**35–44, 1985
90. Weksler B, Lenert J, Ng B, et al: Isolated single lung perfusion with doxorubicin is effective in eradicating soft tissue sarcoma lung metastases in a rat model. *J Thorac Cardiovasc Surg* **107:**50–54, 1994
91. Pogrebniak HW, Roth JA, Steinberg SM, et al: Reoperative pulmonary resection in patients with metastatic soft tissue sarcoma. *Ann Thorac Surg* **52:**197–203, 1991
92. Rizzoni WE, Pass HI, Weley MN, et al: Reoperative pulmonary metastatectomies for patients with adult soft tissue sarcomas. *Ann Thorac Surg* **121:**1248–1252, 1986
93. Casson AG, Putnam JB, Natarajan G, et al: Efficacy of pulmonary metastatectomy for recurrent soft tissue sarcoma. *J Surg Oncol* **47:**1–4, 1991
94. Marcove RC, Mike V, Hajek JV, et al: Osteogenic sarcoma under the age of 21: A review of 145 operative cases. *J Bone Joint Surg* **52:**411–421, 1970
95. Telander RL, Pairolero PC, Pritchard DJ, et al: Resection of pulmonary metastatic osteogenic sarcoma in children. *Surgery* **84:**335–340, 1978
96. Pastorini U, Valente M, Santoro A, et al: Results of salvage surgery for metastatic sarcomas. *Ann Oncol* **1:**269–273, 1990
97. Burgers JMV, Breur K, van Dobbenburgh OA, et al: Role of metastatectomy without chemotherapy in the management of osteosarcoma in children. *Cancer* **45:**1664–1668, 1980
98. Giritsky AS, Etcubanas E, Mark JBD: Pulmonary resection in children with metastatic osteogenic sarcoma. *J Thorac Cardiovasc Surg* **75:**354–361, 1978
99. Carter SR, Grimer RJ, Sneath RS, et al: Results of thoracotomy in osteogenic sarcoma with pulmonary metastases. *Thorax* **46:** 727–731, 1991
100. Snyder CL, Saltzman DA, Ferrel KL, et al: A new approach to the resection of pulmonary osteosarcoma metastases; Results of aggressive metastatectomy. *Clin Orthopaed Rel Research* **270:**247–253, 1991
101. Skinner KA, Eilber FR, Holmes EC, et al: Surgical treatment and chemotherapy for pulmonary metastases from osteosarcoma. *Arch Surg* **127:**1065–1071, 1992
102. Morrow CE, Vassilopoulos PP, Grage TB: Surgical resection for metastatic neoplasms of the lung: Experience at the University of Minnesota Hospitals. *Cancer* **45:**2981–2985, 1980
103. Roberts DG, Lepore V, Cardillo G, et al: Long-term follow-up of operative treatment for pulmonary metastases. *Eur J Cardiothorac Surg* **3:**292–296, 1989
104. Sherry RM, Pass HI, Rosenberg SA, et al: Surgical resection of metastatic renal cell carcinoma and melanoma after response to interleukin-2-based immunotherapy. *Cancer* **69:**1850–1855, 1992
105. Carsky S, Ondrus D, Schnorrer M, et al: Germ cell testicular tumors with lung metastases: Chemotherapy and surgical treatment. *Int Urol Nephrol* **24:**305–311, 1992
106. Mandelbaum I, Yaw PB, Einhorn LH, et al: The importance of one-stage median sternotomy and retroperitoneal node dissection in disseminated testicular cancer. *Ann Thorac Surg* **36:**524–527, 1983
107. Steyerberg EW, Keizer HJ, Zwartendijk J, et al: Prognosis after resection of residual masses following chemotherapy for metastatic nonseminomatous testicular cancer; A multivariate analysis. *Br J Cancer* **68:**195–200, 1993
108. Finley RK, Verazin GT, Driscoll DL, et al: Results of surgical resection of pulmonary metastases of squamous cell carcinoma of the head and neck. *Am J Surg* **164:**594–598, 1992
109. Turk PS, Wanebo HJ: Results of surgical treatment of nonhepatic recurrence of colorectal carcinoma. *Cancer* **71:**4267–4277, 1993
110. Saclarides TJ, Krueger BL, Szeluga DJ, et al: Thoracotomy for colon and rectal cancer metastases. *Dis Colon Rectum* **36:**425–429, 1993
111. Yano T, Hara N, Ichinose Y, et al: Results of pulmonary resection of metastatic colorectal cancer and its application. *J Thorac Cardiovasc Surg* **106:**875–879, 1993
112. Mori M, Tomoda H, Ishida T, et al: Surgical resection of metastatic colorectal cancer and its application. *J Thorac Cardiovasc Surg* **106:**875–879, 1993
113. Wright JO, Brandt B, Ehrenhaft JL: Results of pulmonary resection for metastatic lesions. *J Thorac Cardiovasc Surg* **83:**94–99, 1982
114. McDonald ML, Deschamps C, Ilstrup DM, et al: Pulmonary resection for metastatic breast cancer. Abstract from poster program presented at the meeting of the Society of Thoracic Surgeons; January 31–February 2, 1994.
115. Pogrebniak HW, Stovroff M, Roth JA, et al: Resection of pulmonary metastases from malignant melanoma: Results of a 16-year experience. *Ann Thorac Surg* **46:**20–23, 1988
116. Dahlback O, Hafstrom L, Jonsson P-E, et al: Lung resection for metastatic melanoma. *Clin Oncol* **6:**15–20, 1980
117. Cahan WG: Excision of melanoma metastases to lung: Problems in diagnosis and management. *Ann Surg* **178:**703–709, 1973
118. DiLorenzo M, Collin P-P: Pulmonary metastases in children: Results of surgical treatment. *J Pediatr Surg* **23:**762–765, 1988
119. Martini N, McCormack PM, Bains MS, et al: Surgery for solitary

and multiple pulmonary metastases. *N Y J Med* Sept: 1711–1713, 1978

120. diSilverio F, Facciolo F, D'Eramo G, et al: Surgery of pulmonary metastases from renal and bladder carcinoma. *Scand J Urol Nephrol Suppl* **138:**215–218, 1991
121. McCormack PM, Attiyeh FF: Resected pulmonary metastases from colorectal cancer. *Dis Colon Rectum* **22:**553–556, 1979
122. Staren E, Salerno C, Rongrone A, et al: Pulmonary resection from metastatic breast cancer. *Arch Surg* **127:**1282–1284, 1992
123. Seki M, Nakagawa K, Tsuchiya S, et al: Surgical treatment of pulmonary metastases from uterine cervical cancer. *J Thorac Cardiovasc Surg* **104:**876–881, 1992

CHAPTER

29

# Lung Transplantation

R. Sudhir Sundaresan and G. A. Patterson

## INTRODUCTION AND HISTORICAL PERSPECTIVE

There has been an exponential increase in the utilization of lung transplantation as a treatment for end-stage lung disease. The first human lung transplant was performed by Dr. James Hardy at the University of Mississippi in 1963. This patient died 18 days later. In the ensuing two decades, some 44 lung transplants were performed around the world with no real success. Most of these transplants were performed on debilitated patients as "rescue" attempts after they became ventilator-dependent. Most recipients succumbed to either failure of bronchial anastomotic healing and/or the development of multiple system failure. The first successful lung transplant associated with prolonged survival was accomplished by the Toronto Lung Transplant Group in 1983. The patient received a single lung transplant for idiopathic pulmonary fibrosis and survived for over 6 years before succumbing to complications secondary to renal failure. Subsequently, there has been tremendous innovation in strategies for recipient and donor selection, lung preservation methods, immunosuppression, and operative techniques, leading to the establishment of successful lung transplant programs worldwide with highly satisfactory early and medium-term results. Whereas technical and preservation difficulties and problems with bronchial anastomotic healing formerly hindered success in lung transplantation, these now appear to have been largely overcome. Acute rejection is usually readily controlled and rarely causes major morbidity. However, chronic lung allograft rejection is the main factor limiting prolonged survival. This chapter provides an overview of the preoperative evaluation as well as the intra- and postoperative management of the lung transplant patient. Pertinent aspects of donor selection criteria and organ preservation will also be covered, as well as the approach to commonly encountered postoperative problems.

## PATHOPHYSIOLOGY OF END-STAGE LUNG DISEASE

The following clinical conditions constitute the majority indications for lung transplantation:

1. Obstructive lung disease
   - Chronic obstructive pulmonary disease (COPD)
   - Alpha 1 antitrypsin deficiency emphysema
2. Cystic fibrosis (CF)
3. Restrictive lung disease
   - Idiopathic pulmonary fibrosis (IPF)
4. Pulmonary hypertension
   - Primary pulmonary hypertension (PPH)
   - Eisenmenger's syndrome

A number of "miscellaneous" conditions have also been treated by lung transplantation. Examples include sarcoidosis, lymphangiomyomatosis, pulmonary fibrosis from prior chemo- or radiotherapy, idiopathic bronchiectasis, and repeat lung transplantations. The end-stage pathophysiology of these clinical entities has been summarized recently by Triantafillou and Heerdt[1] and by Trulock.[2]

Obstructive lung disease is estimated to affect 10 million Americans, and COPD has been the fifth leading cause of death in the United States since the late 1970s.[3] Emphysema is the most common obstructive disorder requiring lung transplantation. An important subtype of emphysema is that related to alpha-1 antitrypsin deficiency. This is a congenital disease in which there is a lack of protection against neutrophil elastase in the distal airways. The prevalence of homozygosity for the type Z variant is estimated at

1 in 1500 to 1 in 5000; these patients progress to severe bullous emphysema in their fourth or fifth decades of life. Functionally, obstructive lung disease is characterized by a chronic elevation in airway resistance. There is a decrease in expiratory flow rates ($FEV_1$, FVC, and ratio of $FEV_1$/FVC) and air trapping (increased total lung capacity [TLC] and functional residual capacity [FRC]). There is also a tendency for somewhat regional involvement of the lung, often with the formation of discrete bullae. This is particularly true in patients with alpha-1 antitrypsin deficiency who typically have a basilar pattern of destruction in contrast to the apical predominant destruction characteristic of chronic obstructive pulmonary disease (Fig. 29–1). Clinically, patients with end-stage obstructive lung disease are dyspneic, orthopneic, and have tremendously hyperexpanded chests. They usually have abnormal blood gases, notable for hypoxemia. Most patients requiring transplantation are dependent on supplemental oxygen especially at exercise. Hypercarbia is also commonly observed. Multicenter trials have identified *age* and the *degree of airways obstruction* (as reflected by the baseline postbronchodilator $FEV_1$) as the best prognostic factors. Both the IPPB and the NOTT trials showed that in patients under the age of 65 without hypoxemia, there is an 80% 2-year survival when the $FEV_1$ is less than 30% of predicted, and that uncorrected hypoxemia worsens the prognosis considerably.[4]

Cystic fibrosis (CF) is an inherited disease with an incidence of 1 in 2000 live births in the United States. It is the most common cause of end-stage obstructive lung disease in the first three decades of life.[5] Functionally, this disease affects all exocrine glands. In the lung, the excessive amount of thick viscid secretions along with poor ciliary clearance lead to mucous plugging and chronic pulmonary sepsis (with bronchiectasis), which are accompanied by obstructive physiology (decreased $FEV_1$ and FVC, increased TLC and FRC) and eventually impaired gas exchange (hypoxemia, hypercapnia). Therapeutic advances have dramatically improved the outlook for CF patients, but the majority of patients die of respiratory failure in the third or fourth decade of life.[6] Clinically, cystic fibrosis patients tend to be small, malnourished, and hypoxemic; display digital clubbing; and have copious amounts of pulmonary secretions. It is not uncommon that they have sustained (and even undergone prior thoracic operations for) complications of their disease, including pneumothorax and/or massive hemoptysis.

Idiopathic pulmonary fibrosis (IPF) is the most common restrictive lung disease requiring lung transplantation. In this disease, excessive interstitial deposition of collagen results in a significant loss of pulmonary compliance, associated with diminished lung volumes and expiratory flow rates, but usually with preservation of the $FEV_1$/FVC ratio.

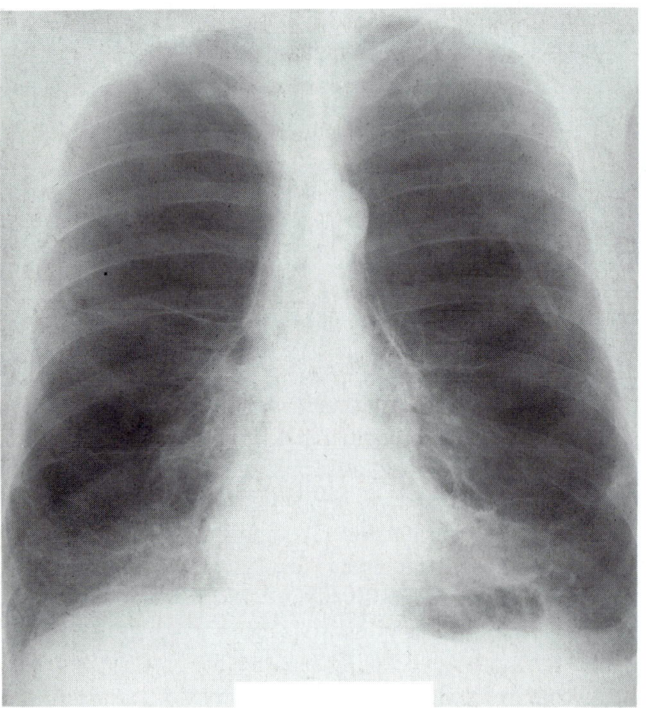

A

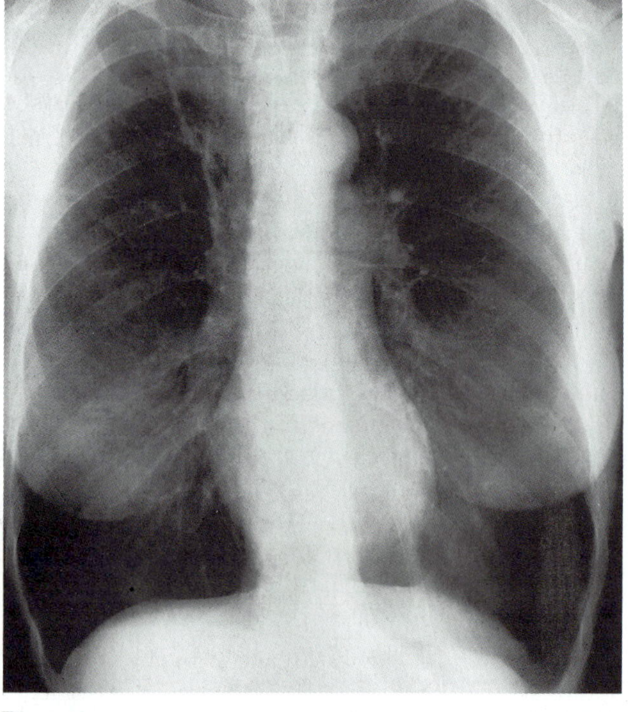

B

**Figure 29–1. A.** A posteroanterior chest roentgenogram in a patient suffering from emphysema due to chronic obstructive lung disease. Marked hyperinflation is apparent. The bilateral upper lung zone destruction is typical of these patients. *(From Pearson FG et al: Thoracic Surgery/Esophageal Surgery. New York, Churchill Livingstone, 1995, with permission.)* **B.** A posteroanterior chest roentgenogram from a patient with emphysema due to alpha-1 anti-trypsin deficiency. Once again, significant hyperinflation is noted with widened intercostal spaces and flattened diaphragms. However, as is typically the case in alpha-1 anti-trypsin deficiency, the lower lung zones are most affected.

Another key feature is a reduction in the diffusing capacity. The fibrotic process also eventually obliterates pulmonary vessels resulting in secondary pulmonary hypertension. Clinically, such patients are dyspneic and orthopneic, display digital clubbing, and require supplemental oxygen. There is considerable evidence that the median survival for these patients is <5 years from the time of diagnosis.[7]

Primary pulmonary hypertension (PPH) is the most common form of pulmonary hypertension requiring lung transplantation. It is an idiopathic process affecting the small pulmonary arteries leading to luminal obliteration and a sustained elevation in pulmonary vascular resistance and right ventricular afterload. It tends to affect young individuals, more often females. The National Institutes of Health PPH registry has characterized the clinical course of this disease.[8] The estimated median patient survival is 2.8 years, with a 1-year survival of 68% and a 5-year survival of 34%. Mortality in PPH has been found to correlate with central venous pressure >10 mm Hg, mean pulmonary artery pressure >60 mm Hg, and cardiac index <2 L/min.[8] In PPH, pulmonary mechanics (and hence, expiratory flow rates) are normal. Therefore, PPH patients can appear relatively normal clinically, unless they develop overt right ventricular failure or a right to left shunt (Eisenmenger's physiology), in which case they may display hypoxemia, cyanosis, ascites, and peripheral edema. Medical therapy is notoriously ineffective. Calcium channel blockers may decrease pulmonary vasculature resistance. Some patients will benefit from continuous infusion of prostacyclin.

## RECIPIENT SELECTION

The crucial questions are, *Which patients* with severe end-stage lung disease should be transplanted? and *What is the ideal timing* of the transplant procedure? Unfortunately, these questions cannot always be answered exactly. The general principle followed is to choose patients who are ill enough to require the transplant, but who are well enough to undergo the procedure with acceptable mortality and morbidity.[9] Information useful in trying to make this determination includes knowledge about the natural history and prognosis in the above disease categories; observation of trends in each given patient (as reflected by their subjective impression of quality of life, along with objective evaluation of functional status by means of physiologic parameters); and, finally, by the documentation of life-threatening events, which may force the transplant to be performed earlier. On the basis of this information, one can subjectively determine an appropriate survival probability for the patient given their underlying disease, and compare this with the survival probability after undergoing a lung transplant, which can be gleaned from registry data.[10] It is important to take into account the length of time a patient might wait for a suitable donor after they are placed on the active transplant list. In our program, the current median waiting time is 9–12 months.

General guidelines for selecting recipients for lung transplantation are presented in Table 29–1 and probably do not differ substantially from the general guidelines in other organ transplantations. Contraindications to lung transplantation are shown in Table 29–2. Guidelines for the timing of referral of patients with the common forms of end-stage lung disease treated by transplantation at the Washington University Medical Center have been summarized by Trulock[2] and are shown in Table 29–3.

It is important to ensure that there are no other treatment options available that might avoid or even delay the need for transplantation. The recent development of bilateral volume reduction surgery for emphysema[11] has enabled us to apply successfully that option in a number of patients who had been on our transplant list. Not only does this strategy avoid the perils of transplantation but it also enables use of a precious donor supply in patients with no other option.

## PREOPERATIVE EVALUATION AND MANAGEMENT OF POTENTIAL LUNG TRANSPLANT RECIPIENTS

### Preoperative Evaluation for Lung Transplantation

Evaluation occurs in a "stepwise" manner. The initial patient referral is often achieved by telephone call or letter. It is important that all medical records, x-rays, computed tomography (CT), etc., be made available for the initial screening. If this initial review and screening are satisfactory, a formal evaluation takes place at the lung transplant center. The scheme for evaluation of potential recipients[2] is shown in Table 29–4. All of the resultant data is then reviewed by a multidisciplinary recipient selection team, allowing a decision to be rendered as to whether or not the patient is a suitable candidate for lung transplantation, ac-

**TABLE 29–1. RECIPIENT SELECTION: GENERAL GUIDELINES**

| |
|---|
| Clinically and physiologically severe lung disease |
| Limited life expectancy (12–24 months) |
| "Other" medical or surgical treatment ineffective/unavailable/inappropriate, and prognosis poor without lung transplant |
| Ambulatory with rehabilitation potential |
| Satisfactory nutritional status |
| Appropriate "mental" state |
| Satisfactory psychosocial profile and good "support system" |
| Comprehend and accept procedure/results/complications/future implications |
| Well-motivated and compliant with treatment |
| Adequate financial resources for medications and follow-up |
| Absence of any contraindications |

**TABLE 29–2. CONTRAINDICATIONS TO LUNG TRANSPLANTATION**

| Absolute | Relative |
|---|---|
| Acutely ill/unstable | Systemic diseases, possibly with involvement of nonpulmonary vital organs (renal, hepatic, etc.) |
| Significant disease of other organ systems, especially: cardiac, renal, hepatic, CNS | Cardiac disease (coronary artery disease, ventricular dysfunction) |
| Uncontrolled sepsis (pulmonary/other) | Ongoing high-dose steroids |
| Uncontrolled neoplasm | Age >65 years |
| Still smoking | Unsatisfactory nutritional status (obesity/cachexia) |
| Psychologic/Social problems, including drug/alcohol abuse | Osteoporosis |
| Noncompliant with treatment | Major prior cardiac/thoracic operation |
| Inadequate resources | |

cording to the criteria already summarized. Once accepted for transplantation and placed on the active waiting list, potential recipients are required to relocate within 6–9 months to the transplant center along with their support person. Patients with emphysema, pulmonary fibrosis or septic lung disease must also participate regularly in a rigorous cardiopulmonary rehabilitation program. This results in a definite increase in strength and exercise tolerance. Patients with pulmonary vascular disease are excused from this requirement because of the risk of sudden death with exercise.

**TABLE 29–3. GUIDELINES FOR TIMING REFERRAL FOR LUNG TRANSPLANTATION**

- Chronic obstructive pulmonary disease and antitrypsin deficiency emphysema
  - Postbronchodilator $FEV_1 < 30\%$ predicted
  - Resting hypoxia ($Po_2 < 55–60$ mm Hg)
  - Hypercapnia
  - Significant secondary pulmonary hypertension
  - Clinical course
    - Determine rate of decline of $FEV_1$
    - Life-threatening exacerbations
- Cystic fibrosis
  - Postbronchodilator $FEV_1 < 30\%$ predicted
  - Resting hypoxia ($Po_2 < 55$ mm Hg)
  - Hypercapnia
  - Clinical course: extremely important
    - Increasing frequency and severity of exacerbations
    - Weight loss
  - Controversial issues regarding acceptability for transplantation
    - Colonization with panresistant *Pseudomonas* species, *Aspergillus*, or mycobacteria
    - Liver disease
- Idiopathic pulmonary fibrosis
  - VC, TLC < 60% predicted
  - Resting hypoxia
  - Significant secondary pulmonary hypertension
  - Clinical, radiologic, physiologic score > 60 after 6 months of therapy
- Primary pulmonary hypertension
  - NYHA class III or IV
  - Mean right atrial pressure ≥ 10 mm Hg
  - Mean pulmonary arterial pressure ≥ 50 mm Hg
  - Cardiac index ≤ 2.5 L/min per square meter

**TABLE 29–4. SCHEME FOR EVALUATION OF POTENTIAL RECIPIENTS**

- Medical history and physical examination
- Chest radiograph, electrocardiogram, and routine blood tests
- Other laboratory tests
  - ABO blood type
  - HLA type and panel of reactive antibodies (PRA)
  - Serologic tests for hepatitis A, B, and C; human immunodeficiency virus; cytomegalovirus
- Pulmonary studies
  - Standard pulmonary function tests and arterial blood gases
  - Quantitative ventilation-perfusion lung scan
  - Cardiopulmonary exercise test
  - CT of chest[a]
- Cardiovascular studies
  - Radionuclide ventriculography
  - Doppler echocardiography (with saline contrast[a])
  - Right-heart catheterization
  - Left-heart catheterization with coronary angiography[a]
  - Transesophageal echocardiography[a]
- Rehabilitation assessment
  - Six-minute walk test
  - Determination of supplemental oxygen requirements (rest and exercise)
- Psychosocial evaluation
- Nutritional assessment
- Additional appropriate studies to determine the status of any other medical problems

[a] *In selected patients as indicated.*

## Choice of Transplant Procedure

### *Obstructive Lung Disease*

Both single and bilateral lung transplantation can be successfully used to treat end-stage obstructive lung disease.[12,13] In the early days of lung transplantation, hyperinflation of the native lung associated with contralateral mediastinal shift, crowding of the graft, and ventilation/perfusion imbalance was frequently observed following single-lung transplant. However, these problems can be minimized by oversizing the donor to the recipient and by paying attention to proper technique of preservation so as to minimize reperfusion injury and its attendant decrease in compliance. In general, single-lung transplantation (SLT) is reserved for those emphysema patients that are older (over age 55), who might represent a "high risk," who have had prior surgery on one side, and/or in whom there is a significant difference in lung function between the two sides (as judged by preoperative ventilation and perfusion nuclear scintigraphy) (Fig. 29–2). Bilateral lung transplantation

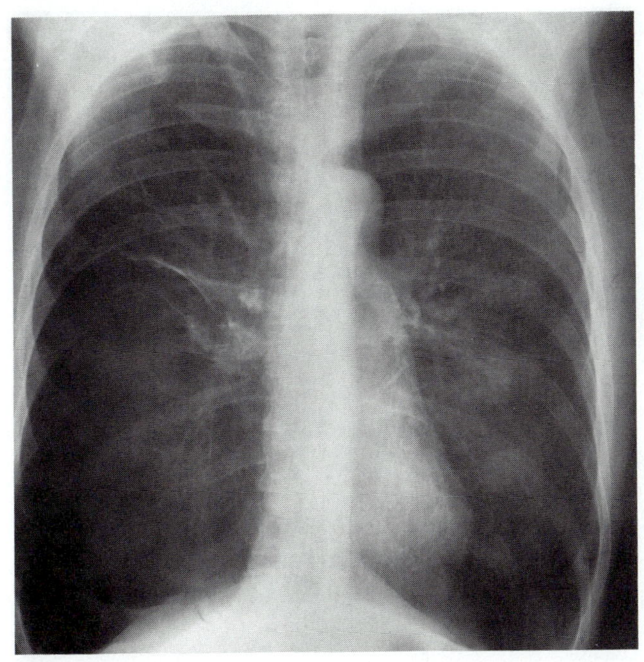

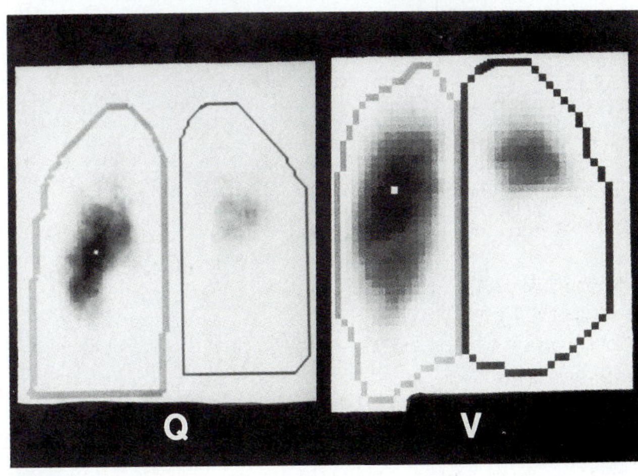


A B

**Figure 29–2. A.** A posteroanterior chest roentgenogram in a patient suffering from alpha-1 anti-trypsin deficiency. **B.** Posterior perfusion (Q) ventilation (V) nuclear scintigraphy images from the same patient. Note the predominance of perfusion and ventilation to the left lung with marked reduction of perfusion and ventilation to the right side, particularly the right base, as a result of the marked bullous disease at the right base.

(BLT) is utilized to treat younger emphysema patients, who may have severe bilateral disease, and/or as a strategy to treat large recipients using small donor lungs.

### *Cystic Fibrosis*

Patients with cystic fibrosis or other sepsis lung disease must undergo BLT (Fig. 29–3). An SLT procedure would expose the graft to the risk of infection from the native lung. SLT and contralateral native lung pneumonectomy would expose the empty pleural space to the risk of post-pneumonectomy empyema and bronchopleural fistula.

### *Idiopathic Pulmonary Fibrosis*

SLT is theoretically ideal in treating IPF, since the diminished compliance and elevated pulmonary vascular resistance of the native lung favor both ventilation and perfusion of the allograft, respectively (Fig. 29–4). Bilateral lung transplantation has been employed occasionally when the recipient is a large individual, especially if the fibrotic process is associated with normal lung volumes.

### *Primary Pulmonary Hypertension*

The ideal operation for PPH is still a matter of controversy. The traditional operation consisted of a combined heart-lung transplantation[14]; however, the scarcity of donor organs has led us to employ SLT with excellent results (Fig. 29–5). Patients with PPH are a challenge to manage postoperatively, due to the fact that virtually all of cardiac output is directed to the allograft, despite having relatively equal distribution of ventilation between the lungs. This can be a particular problem if there is a serious allograft reperfusion injury and resultant allograft edema. Another problem with employing SLT to treat PPH is that any significant late graft problem (e.g., CMV pneumonitis or chronic rejection) leads to very severe functional V/Q mismatch, which often proves fatal. For this reason, several experienced programs have advocated bilateral lung transplantation as the preferred option in these patients (Fig. 29–6). It is possible that bilateral lung transplantation will provide these patients more functional reserve in the long term.

## Timing of Transplantation

As already mentioned, lung transplantation is not considered as an option until the patient's life expectancy is estimated to be between 12 and 24 months. The scarcity of suitable donors along with the exponential increase in lung transplant activity nationwide has prolonged the average waiting period. Statistics from the United Network for Organ Sharing (UNOS) for 1992[15] showed that only about 30% of the patients on the active waiting list would receive a donor organ during that year and that the average wait for a lung transplant in the United States is 13.5 months. One of the potential consequences of this longer wait is that patients on the active waiting list can undergo functional deterioration and may even ultimately require ventilatory sup-

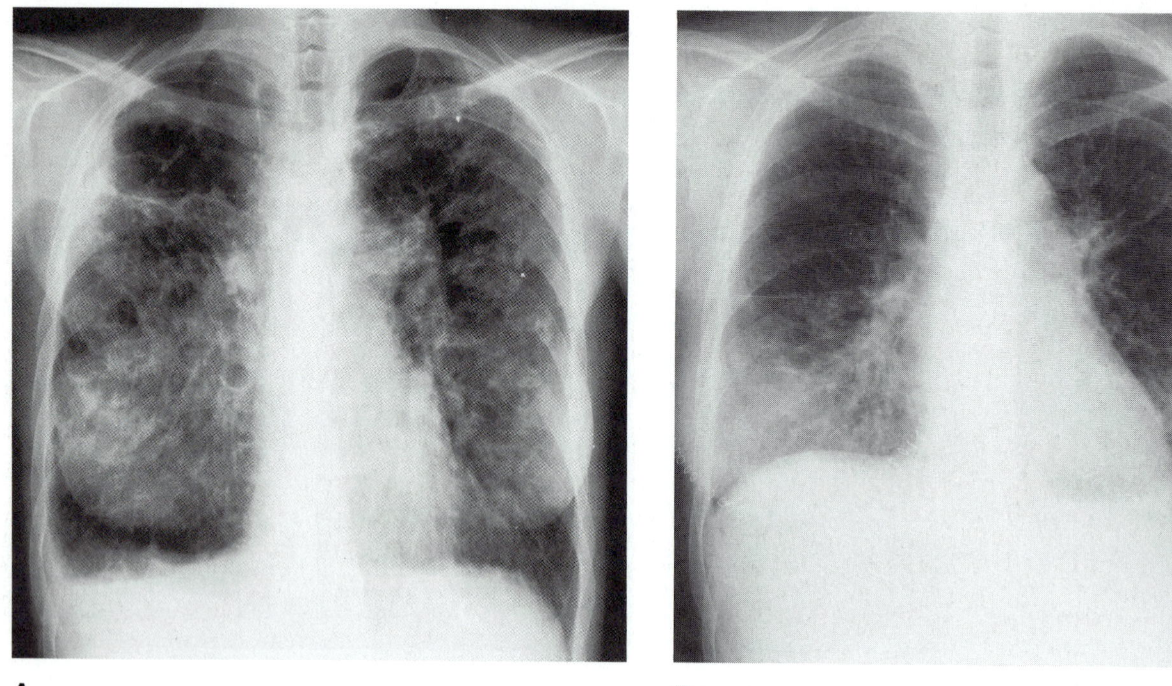

A B

**Figure 29–3. A.** Preoperative posteroanterior chest roentgenogram taken in a patient suffering from cystic fibrosis. Note the marked bilateral hyperinflation with cystic destruction of both lungs. *(From Pearson FG et al: Thoracic Surgery/Esophageal Surgery. New York, Churchill Livingstone, 1995, with permission.)* **B.** Postoperative posteroanterior chest roentgenogram in the same patient following bilateral sequential single-lung transplant. Note the return of normal chest contour. *(From Pearson FG et al: Thoracic Surgery/Esophageal Surgery, New York, Churchill Livingstone, 1995, with permission.)*

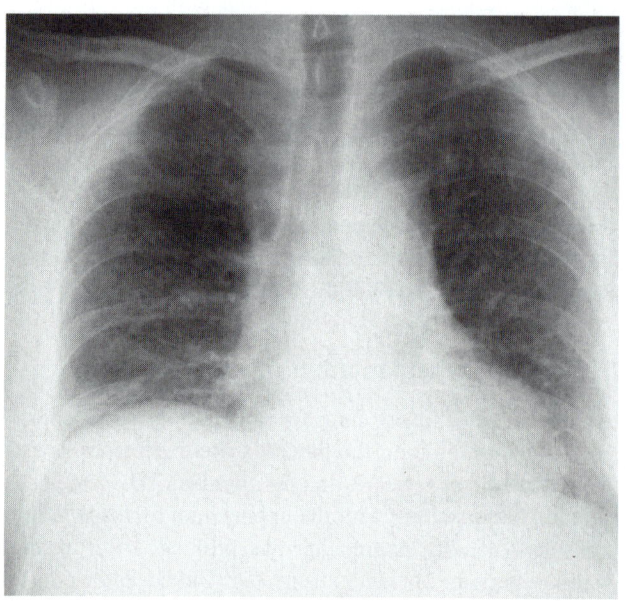

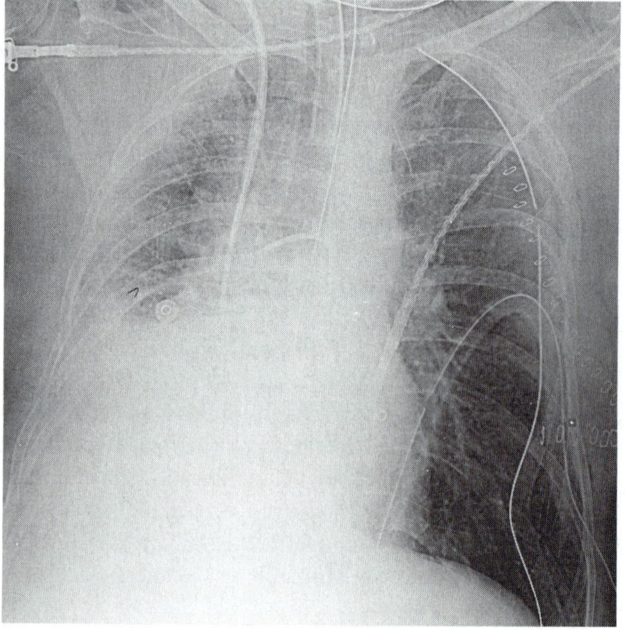

A B

**Figure 29–4. A.** Preoperative posteroanterior chest roentgenogram in a patient suffering from idiopathic pulmonary fibrosis. Note the diffuse interstitial markings and small lung volumes. *(From Pearson FG et al: Thoracic Surgery/Esophageal Surgery, New York, Churchill Livingstone, 1995, with permission.)* **B.** Postoperative PA portable chest roentgenogram in the same patient immediately following left single-lung transplant. With replacement of an oversized left-lung allograft, the mediastinum has been shifted to the right. *(From Pearson FG et al: Thoracic Surgery/Esophageal Surgery, New York, Churchill Livingstone, 1995, with permission.)*

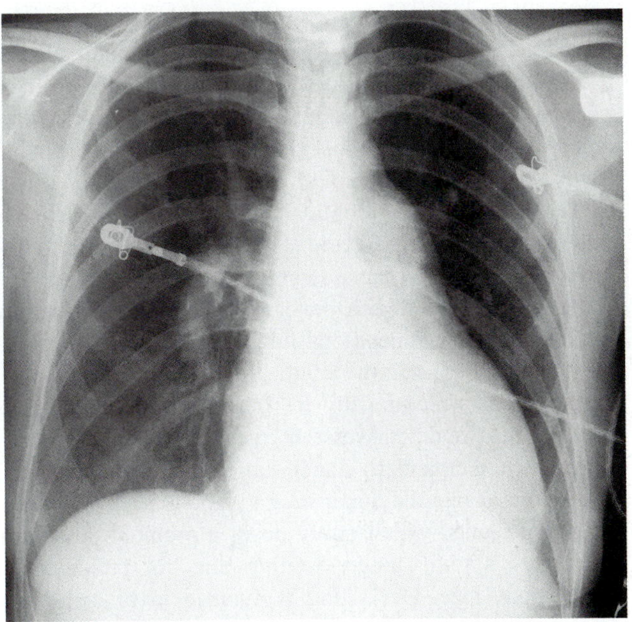

A

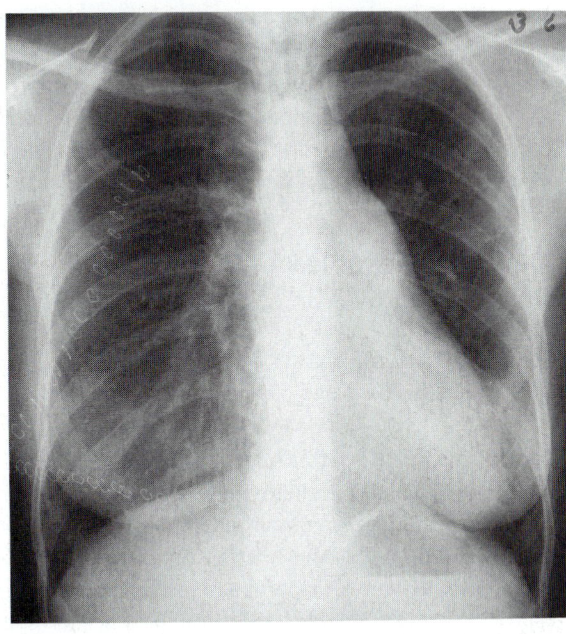

B

**Figure 29–5. A.** Preoperative posteroanterior chest roentgenogram in a patient suffering from ASD-Eisenmenger's syndrome. Note the tremendous enlargement of the right ventricle and both pulmonary arteries. *(From Pearson FG et al: Thoracic Surgery/Esophageal Surgery, New York, Churchill Livingstone, 1995, with permission.)* **B.** Posteroanterior chest roentgenogram in the same patient 2 weeks following right single-lung transplantation. Note the dramatic reduction in right ventricular and pulmonary arterial size. The relative lack of perfusion to the native lung is apparent from the absence of vascular markings on the left side. *(From Pearson FG et al: Thoracic Surgery/Esophageal Surgery, New York, Churchill Livingstone, 1995, with permission.)*

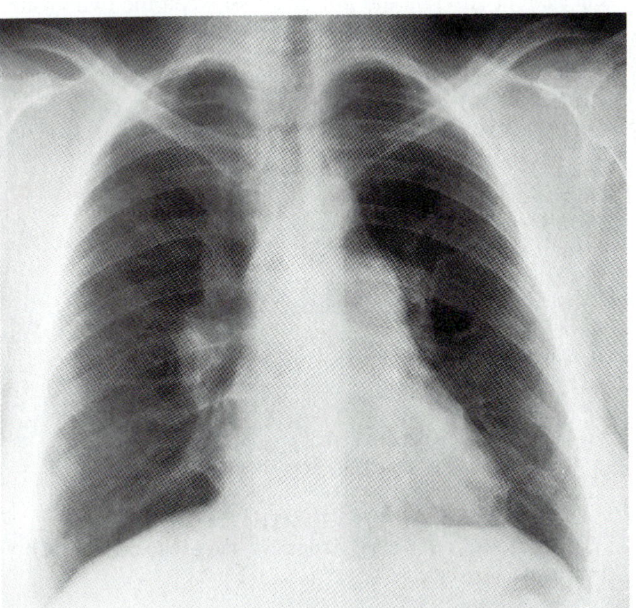

A

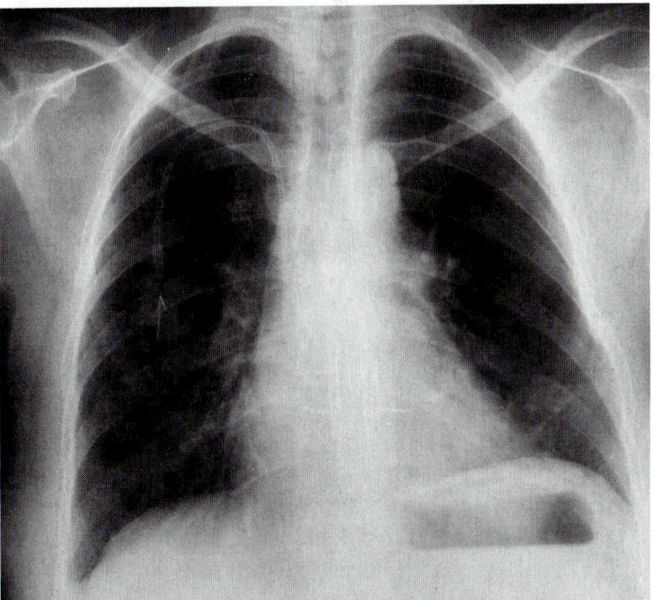

B

**Figure 29–6. A.** Preoperative posteroanterior chest roentgenogram in a female patient suffering from primary pulmonary hypertension. Note the marked increase in right ventricular and pulmonary arterial size. **B.** Postoperative posteroanterior chest roentgenogram in the same patient following bilateral sequential single-lung transplantation. The cardiac silhouette is decreased in size as is the diameter of both pulmonary arteries consistent with a marked reduction in pulmonary artery pressure. The patient suffered a traction injury to the left phrenic nerve and has a left diaphragmatic paralysis as a result.

port. Inevitably, some patients will die while waiting, the risk of which is highest with PPH, IPF, and CF and lowest with COPD.[2] Therefore, earlier referral of patients for consideration of lung transplantation may be appropriate so that they can be activated on the waiting list earlier to compensate for the somewhat longer wait.

## "Other" Important Issues

### Age Guidelines

There is no absolute cut-off, but the approximate limits are age 55 years for BLT and 65 years for SLT.

### Ventilatory Support While Waiting

Initially mechanical ventilation was regarded as an absolute contraindication to lung transplantation. In keeping with this, we still do not accept referrals for lung transplantation in patients in whom the problem is ventilator-dependent respiratory failure. However several patients have undergone successful lung transplantation after developing respiratory failure during their wait for a suitable donor.[16]

### Corticosteroid Therapy

This was also traditionally regarded as a contraindication to lung transplantation on the basis of early data from experimental canine autotransplants showing it to have a prejudicial effect on bronchial anastomotic healing.[17] An obvious logistic problem is that many patients with end-stage lung disease (especially COPD and IPF) are treated with steroids, and attempts to wean such patients off these agents completely prior to lung transplantation can be associated with considerable subjective and objective deterioration. There is now a moderate clinical experience with lung transplantation in patients taking corticosteroids, and available data suggest that (1) low-dose prednisone (<0.2 mg/kg per day) does not increase the risk of airway complications,[18] and (2) low-dose steroids may actually enhance early bronchial circulation in the allograft.[19]

### Prior Surgery

Early in lung transplantation, this was considered a relative contraindication. The main concerns were related to the increased complexity, the prolonged operating time, and the excess bleeding, all of which would lead to a higher mortality and morbidity. These concerns were especially prominent in CF patients who are known to have severe pleural adhesions. A number of modifications in transplant technique have decreased the bleeding associated with the transplant procedure, so that prior surgery is generally not considered a contraindication.

## Criteria for Donor Lung Suitability

Only 20–25% of multiple-organ donors have lungs that satisfy the traditional rigorous donor criteria making them suitable for transplantation. Unfortunately, less than half of these are identified as lung donors. This shortage of suitable donor lungs is the main impediment to more widespread application of lung transplantation. Most lung transplant centers recognize the traditional criteria of donor lung suitability that were recently summarized by us[20] and are presented in Table 29–5. The preliminary criteria must be satisfied initially, after which a retrieval team is sent to the donor hospital to permit a final assessment to be carried out.

Size match between donor and recipient is based on predicted lung volumes (total lung capacity, TLC; vital capacity, VC), based on the height, sex, and age of the donor and recipient. Occasionally we make use of vertical lung measurement and transverse thoracic diameter to suitably size match recipient to donor lungs. We deliberately attempt to oversize the donor lung by about 20% for single-lung transplants, which rarely poses a problem other than creating a slightly longer waiting time for recipients of larger body size. Oversizing is avoided in bilateral lung transplants so as to facilitate recipient chest closure.

A number of strategies have recently ensued to overcome the donor lung scarcity. These include the following:

(1) Use of "marginal" donor lungs (i.e., donor lungs failing to meet all of the traditional criteria). We recently performed a retrospective analysis of a consecutive series of lung transplants and compared the outcome of recipients receiving "ideal" donor lungs with those who received "marginal" donor lungs. A number of recipient parameters including Aa gradient (immediately and at 24 hours), days spent on the ventilator, 30-day operative mortality, and current patient survival did not differ between the two groups, confirming our notion that under carefully selected circum-

**TABLE 29–5. TRADITIONAL CRITERIA FOR DONOR LUNG SUITABILITY**

- Preliminary
  - Age <55 years
  - ABO compatibility
  - Chest roentgenogram
    - Clear
    - Allows estimate of size match
  - History
    - Smoking ≤20 pack-years
    - No significant trauma (blunt, penetrating)
    - No aspiration/sepsis
    - Gram stain and culture data if prolonged intubation
    - No prior cardiac/pulmonary operation
  - Oxygenation
    - Arterial oxygen tension ≥300 mm Hg, on inspired oxygen fraction of 1.0, 5 cm $H_2O$ positive end-expiratory pressure
  - Adequate size match
- Final assessment
  - Chest roentgenogram shows no unfavorable changes
  - Oxygenation has not deteriorated
  - Bronchoscopy shows no aspiration or mass
  - Visual/manual assessment
    - Parenchyma satisfactory
    - No adhesions or masses
    - Further evaluation of trauma

stances, use of marginal donor lungs does not compromise successful outcome of lung transplantation.[21] Careful judgment must obviously be exercised in these circumstances, and we do not compromise on donor lung quality in single-lung transplantation for primary pulmonary hypertension.

(2) Unilateral lung assessment. Occasionally a donor is identified to have unsatisfactory gas exchange, yet the dysfunction is confined to one lung by radiographic and bronchoscopic evaluation. There is good evidence from the Toronto Lung Transplant Group[22] that in these circumstances, a unilateral lung assessment (accomplished by the use of a double-lumen endotracheal tube and pulmonary artery clamping, to isolate ventilation and perfusion to the uninjured lung) can accurately identify suitable single-lung grafts that can be used with very satisfactory results.

(3) Living related donors. Recently, the group at University of Southern California has described a technique whereby a right and left lower lobe are extracted from two different adults and then used as separate single lung allografts in a related pediatric cystic fibrosis recipient.[23] This group has reported the use of this highly innovative approach in transplanting seven cystic fibrosis patients with excellent results.

## TECHNIQUE OF LUNG PRESERVATION AND EXTRACTION

### Current Technique of Lung Preservation

In the Washington University Lung Transplant Program, we currently accomplish lung preservation using techniques shared by most other centers. This is achieved by bolus administration of prostaglandin E-1 before inflow occlusion and cross-clamp; pulmonary artery flush using 3 L of cold (4°C) Euro Collins solution; extraction of the lungs semi-inflated with 100% oxygen; transportation of the grafts under hypothermic conditions (0–1°C); and, finally, protection during implantation by topical cooling with ice slush.

The rationale for this approach is based on laboratory evidence that:

1. prostaglandin E-1 exerts a variety of beneficial effects apart from pulmonary vasodilatation.[24]
2. lung grafts appear to be capable of utilizing alveolar oxygen during the preservation interval to maintain a low level of aerobic metabolism until reperfusion.[25]

Using preservation methods similar to that described earlier, we have demonstrated satisfactory lung function after ischemic intervals as long as 24 hours in a canine left lung allotransplant model.[26]

### Technique of Donor Lung Extraction

This topic was recently the subject of a detailed description by our group.[20] The procedure is performed through median sternotomy, extended inferiorly to the pubis to permit extraction of the abdominal organs. The three basic components of the thoracic dissection are:

1. venous inflow: The intrapericardial superior and inferior vena cavae (SVC, IVC) are isolated, and the SVC is encircled with heavy silk ligatures.
2. arterial: The ascending aorta and main pulmonary artery (PA) are separated from one another and encircled with umbilical tapes.
3. airway: The posterior pericardium (between the aorta and SVC) is incised, exposing the distal trachea.

On completion of the thoracic and abdominal dissection, the patient is heparinized to permit cannulation, which can be performed by all teams simultaneously, or in a sequential fashion, as long as the donor maintains a stable condition. A cardioplegia cannula is inserted in the ascending aorta, and the common pulmonary artery is cannulated at its bifurcation. Occasionally, the interatrial groove must be developed so as to increase the amount of left atrial cuff on the right pulmonary veins. Flushing of the thoracic grafts is accomplished as follows:

1. bolus administration of PGE-1 (500 µg).
2. inflow occlusion (ligation of the SVC and clamping of the IVC).
3. venting of the right heart (by transecting the IVC above the clamp, which necessitates a prior request to the abdominal team to cannulate the abdominal segment of the IVC, so that their effluent flush can drain off the table).
4. cross-clamping the ascending aorta and administration of cardioplegia.
5. amputating the tip of the left atrial appendage to allow the lung flush to be started.
6. flooding the chest with iced saline and maintaining gentle manual ventilation of the lungs with 100% percent oxygen during the flush.

On completion of the flush, the heart is extracted first. All cannulae are removed, the cavae and ascending aorta are transected, and the distal common PA is transected starting at the cannulation site. The left atrial incision is made last; it is best accomplished by the surgeon on the left side of the table (Fig. 29–7). This dissection is started near the left inferior pulmonary vein, then taken around superiorly and inferiorly until complete, leaving a small rim of atrial muscle around the orifices of all four pulmonary veins.

Finally, the lung grafts are extracted en bloc by:

1. digitally encircling the trachea and dividing it between two applications of the TA-30 stapling device.
2. division of the esophagus superiorly and inferiorly by sequential application of the A stapler.
3. transection of the descending thoracic aorta.

In this fashion, the double lung block is freed up from the thoracic spine, leaving the aorta and esophagus attached

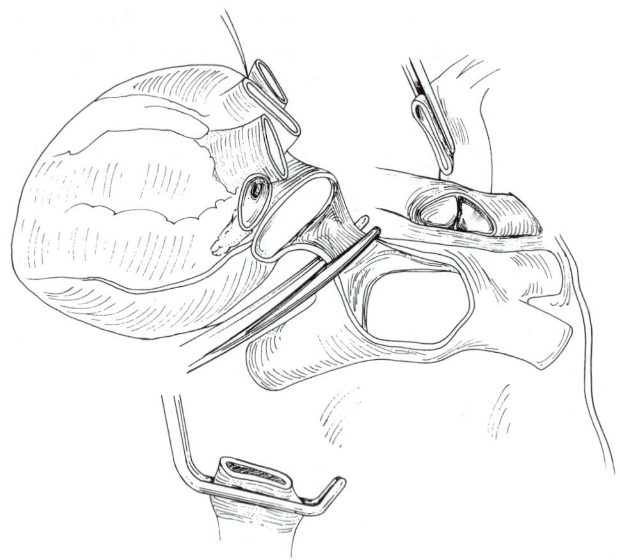

**Figure 29–7.** The ascending aortic is divided. The main pulmonary artery has been transected at its bifurcation. The heart is retracted upward and to the right to enable safe division of the left atrium, leaving suitable atrial cuffs on both cardiac and lung allografts. *(From Shields TW: General Thoracic Surgery, 4th ed. Baltimore, Williams & Wilkins, 1994, with permission.)*

so as to minimize the chance of any extraction injury to the airway or pulmonary artery. The double lung block is triple-bagged and transported in an ice chest. If the two lungs are to be used at different centers, they can be separated rapidly at this point by dividing the posterior pericardium, the middle of the left atrium, the pulmonary artery (at its bifurcation), the residual mediastinal tissue, and finally by dividing the proximal left main bronchus between two applications of the TA-30 stapling instrument (Fig. 29–8).

## THE LUNG TRANSPLANTATION PROCEDURE

### Anesthetic Considerations

The important anesthetic considerations pertaining to lung transplantation have been well summarized recently by Triantafillou.[27] The important principal is that a proper appreciation of the underlying pathophysiology and details unique to each patient will allow the approach to be individualized in each case (including careful titration of anesthetic drugs, fluid administration, ventilatory management, and use of cardiopulmonary bypass when necessary). This approach is far more likely to achieve a successful outcome than rigid adherence to a strict protocol.

Data from the preoperative evaluation (especially left and right heart catheterization, V/Q scans, radionuclide and echocardiography studies) are reviewed by the anesthesiologist prior to the transplant. Right ventricular function is one of the most important considerations, since it is often affected by the underlying pulmonary disease. Careful intraoperative monitoring of right ventricular function is the main determinant of the necessity for pharmacologic, ventilatory, and circulatory support alternatives.

Routine intraoperative monitoring of the lung transplant recipient includes urine output, temperature, electrocardiogram (ECG), pulse oximetry, and systemic arterial and pulmonary arterial pressure. In addition, we employ continuous mixed venous oxygen saturation ($Svo_2$) monitoring, a two-dimensional transesophageal echocardiography probe, and a mass spectrometer. In most patients, an epidural catheter is inserted prior to induction of anesthesia for postoperative pain management. A left-sided double-lumen tube is used for virtually all lung transplants. In cystic fibrosis patients, a regular endotracheal tube is used ini-

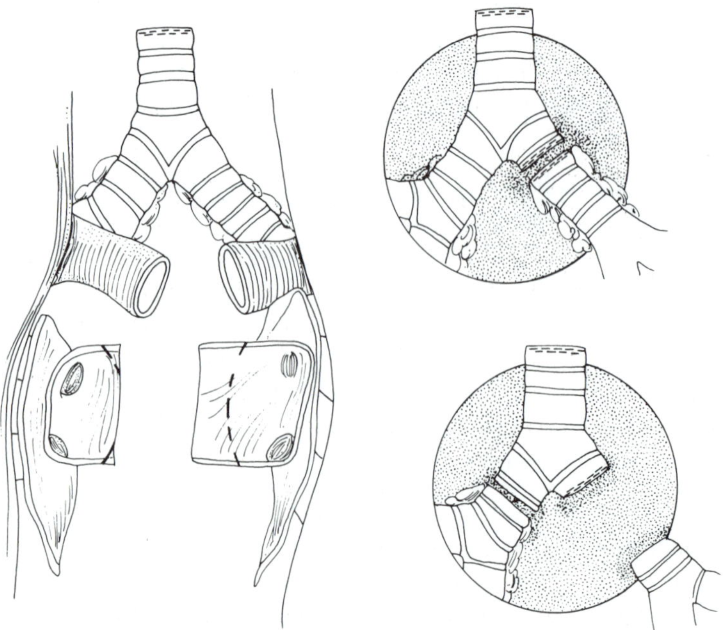

**Figure 29–8.** The donor pericardium and left atrium are divided with the left atrium further trimmed (dotted lines). The airway is transected and kept sealed using a GIA stapling device across the proximal left main stem bronchus. The donor airway is further revised for implantation as shown at bottom right. *(From Shields TW: General Thoracic Surgery, 4th ed. Baltimore, Williams & Wilkins, 1994, with permission.)*

tially to facilitate a thorough bronchoscopy and aspiration of all purulent airway secretions. It is then replaced with a left endobronchial tube. In some small individuals (who cannot accommodate a double-lumen tube), a standard endotracheal tube along with a bronchial blocking catheter may be used. Another alternative used commonly in pediatric lung transplantation is a single-lumen endotracheal tube and cardiopulmonary bypass.

Intraoperative ventilatory management can be challenging, particularly in patients with COPD. In single-lung transplantation for emphysema, the risk of rupturing a bleb or bulla in the dependent lung leading to tension pneumothorax must always be kept in mind. A more common reason for cardiovascular instability after anesthesia induction in COPD patients is the increased intrathoracic pressure caused by air trapping under positive pressure ventilation. If insufficient exhalation time is allowed, a situation analogous to "pulmonary tamponade" can occur. This pathophysiologic change is easily recognized using transesophageal echocardiography. Careful tailoring of ventilatory management will usually achieve optimum gas exchange with minimum hemodynamic consequences. In patients with obstructive lung disease, the use of moderately low tidal volumes (8–10 mL/kg), increased respiratory rate (15–20 breaths per minute), and a high peak inspiratory flow assuring a sufficiently long expiratory time (inspiratory:expiratory ratio usually 1:5) will work satisfactorily. The hemodynamic instability accompanying this ventilatory disturbance can also be managed by appropriate fluid administration and use of a mixed adrenergic agent. Despite all these attempts, a moderate degree of hypercapnia may have to be accepted in exchange for hemodynamic stability. Manual ventilation is another option in managing severe ventilatory problems. Other common causes of ventilatory insufficiency include migration of the endobronchial tube and, in patients with septic lung disease, accumulation of purulent secretions in the contralateral lung. A careful check for tube placement and frequent suctioning are necessary to rule out these possibilities. Ultimately, if the patient remains unstable despite all of these maneuvers, cardiopulmonary bypass should be instituted promptly so as to complete the procedure safely under controlled circumstances.

The patient is maintained on $FIO_2$ equal to 1.0 intraoperatively until the transplantation is completed. Hypoxemia during one-lung ventilation can be managed by the application of oxygen insufflation, continuous positive airways pressure (CPAP), or intermittent ventilation of the nondependent lung. Clamping of the ipsilateral pulmonary artery will, in general, immediately abolish the shunt and associated hypoxemia. For patients with septic lung disease, frequent airway toilet may be needed to maintain patency of the airways and sufficient oxygenation.

Cardiopulmonary bypass (CPB) is routinely used for all transplants for pulmonary vascular disease and is instituted prior to extraction of the recipient lung. CPB is almost never required in single-lung transplantation for emphysema, but is occasionally required for single-lung transplants for IPF, especially if there is associated secondary pulmonary hypertension. In bilateral sequential lung transplantation, allograft dysfunction is sometimes noted after reperfusion of the first lung being implanted, resulting in unsatisfactory gas exchange and/or hemodynamics upon clamping of the pulmonary artery of the remaining native lung. In the majority of cases, appropriate fluid administration, use of inotropic agents and pulmonary vasodilators (mainly PGE1), and control of acidosis will ameliorate this problem successfully, but in about 10–20% of bilateral lung transplants, CPB is required to facilitate the implantation of the second lung.

## Technique of Lung Transplantation

### *Incision and Approach*

Single-lung transplantation is accomplished through a posterolateral thoracotomy. For patients with Eisenmenger's syndrome, a median sternotomy can be used to accomplish cardiac repair along with right single-lung transplantation. When the thoracotomy approach is used, the ipsilateral groin is always prepped and draped within the field, so that femoral cannulation can be performed if required. Bilateral lung transplantation is now accomplished through the bilateral transverse thoracosternotomy incision ("clam shell" approach) by using the fifth intercostal space for emphysema patients and the fourth intercostal space for cystic fibrosis recipients. This incision first used for bilateral sequential single-lung transplantation by the Washington University Group[28] has effectively replaced sternotomy for procedures requiring bilateral lung replacement. The exposure provided is far superior to that afforded by median sternotomy.[29]

### *Choice of Side*

One consideration in single-lung transplantation is to try to avoid the side of a prior thoracotomy or pleurodesis if possible. Otherwise, in single-lung transplantation for obstructive or restrictive lung disease, the approach is to transplant the side with the least function demonstrated by preoperative quantitative ventilation-perfusion lung scanning. In single-lung transplantation for primary pulmonary hypertension, the approach is to transplant the side with the best function so as to minimize postoperative V/Q mismatching. Bilateral lung replacement is accomplished by using a bilateral sequential single-lung technique, in which the side with the least function is transplanted first. If there is no discrepancy between the sides, then our approach is to reimplant the right lung first.

### *Cannulation for Cardiopulmonary Bypass*

General criteria for the use of cardiopulmonary bypass in lung transplantation have already been summarized in the earlier section dealing with anesthetic management. When CPB is required in single-lung transplantation, cannulation is usually performed in the chest. In right single-lung transplants, this involves cannulating the right atrium and the ascending aorta, whereas in left single-lung transplantation, the common pulmonary artery and descending thoracic aorta may be used. Alternatively, femoral cannulation can also be employed in left single-lung transplants. In bilateral lung transplants, standard cannulation techniques utilize the right atrial appendage and ascending aorta.

### *Conduct of the Operation*

For all lung transplants in patients with pulmonary vascular disease, the patient must be placed on cardiopulmonary bypass prior to any significant manipulation of the heart or lungs. In patients with primary pulmonary hypertension and severe hypoxemia, it is necessary to rule out the presence of a patent foramen ovale. These are usually identified during the evaluation. However, a transesophageal echocardiogram bubble study is performed after anesthesia induction. If a patent foramen ovale, significant enough to require closure, is identified, then closure is performed immediately after institution of cardiopulmonary bypass. Subsequently, the right lung is excised and the allograft implanted. A similar order is followed in Eisenmenger's syndrome, i.e., the patient is first placed on cardiopulmonary bypass, following which the cardiac defect is repaired. Then pneumonectomy is performed, and the allograft is implanted. In bilateral lung transplantation for primary pulmonary hypertension, the patient is first placed on cardiopulmonary bypass, after which both native lungs are excised. The allografts are then inserted in a bilateral sequential fashion.

Aside from lung transplants for pulmonary vascular disease, cardiopulmonary bypass is used in a selective fashion. In single-lung transplantation, after initial dissection of hilar vessels, the ipsilateral pulmonary artery is temporarily occluded. The patient is then carefully observed, with attention paid to the pulmonary artery pressure and also right ventricular function, as judged by transesophageal echocardiography. If PA occlusion is well tolerated, then pneumonectomy is performed, followed by implantation of the graft. In bilateral lung transplantation, cardiopulmonary bypass is rarely necessary at the start of the operation, and the necessity usually arises after implantation of the first allograft. At this point, the PA to the remaining native lung is temporarily occluded. Once again, if this results in unsatisfactory oxygenation, hemodynamics, and/or right ventricular function, which are refractory to the measures described earlier, then CPB is utilized to facilitate excision of the native lung and implantation of the second graft. In the majority of cases, the bilateral sequential technique can be employed without the need for CPB.

### *Technique of Lung Implantation*

We continue to use a technique that is a modification of that originally described by Cooper and colleagues.[30] The recipient pneumonectomy is started after the lung is collapsed, followed by division of the pulmonary ligament. The PA and its first branch are then dissected, which allows temporary PA occlusion to be performed. If this is tolerated satisfactorily, then the first branch of the PA is divided between ligatures, and the remainder of the arterial trunk is divided between vascular staple lines. Pulmonary venous tributaries are divided between ligatures peripherally, near the hilum of the lung, with the venous stumps left as long as possible. Both pulmonary veins are also fully mobilized intrapericardially. Finally, the main bronchus is transected (Fig. 29–9). On the right, this division is made just proximal to the right upper lobe takeoff, and on the left side, one or two rings above the left main bronchial bifurcation. In patients with end-stage lung disease, the bronchial circulation can be hypertrophied, and it is imperative to secure adequate hemostasis around the bronchus and in the subcarinal space prior to implantation.

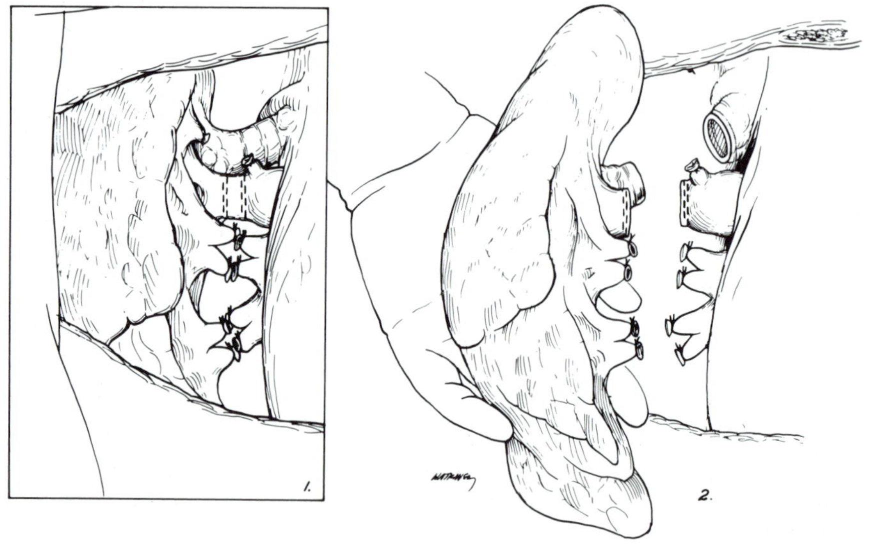


**Figure 29–9.** Excision of the native right lung. The pulmonary artery is stapled beyond its first upper lobe branch. The pulmonary veins are divided between ligatures and the bronchus is transected to just proximal to the upper lobe orifice. *(From Shields TW: General Thoracic Surgery, 4th ed. Baltimore, Williams & Wilkins, 1994, with permission.)*

Topical cooling of the graft during implantation is critical: It is accomplished by wrapping the allograft in a gauge sponge soaked in ice slush. The bronchial anastomosis is performed first (Fig. 29–10), using a continuous 4-0 monofilament absorbable suture to approximate the membranous portion. We now approximate the donor and recipient cartilaginous arches using a telescoping or intussuscepting technique. We use interrupted figure-of-eight or horizontal mattress sutures of a similar suture material, so that the smaller bronchus telescopes by about one cartilaginous ring within the larger bronchus. The use of simple interrupted sutures to perform an end-to-end anastomosis, as originally described, is used only for small-caliber donor and recipient bronchi. We generally approximate the loose peribronchial nodal tissue around the donor and recipient bronchi to cover the bronchial anastomosis. Bronchial omentopexy is no longer employed. We perform the PA anastomosis next by applying a vascular clamp centrally on the recipient artery and then trimming the donor and recipient arteries to appropriate lengths. An end-to-end anastomosis is then created by using a continuous 5-0 monofilament nonabsorbable suture interrupted at two sites. The left atrial anastomosis is performed last, after application of a Statinsky clamp centrally on the recipient left atrium. A large recipient atrial cuff is created by excising the pulmonary vein stumps and trimming them appropriately. The anastomosis is then created using a continuous 4-0 monofilament nonabsorbable suture, which is also interrupted at two sites around the anastomosis (Fig. 29–11). Before we restore perfusion to the graft, 500–1000 mg of methylprednisolone is administered. Gentle manual ventilation of the graft is commenced, and then the graft is de-aired both antegrade (by temporarily releasing the PA clamp) and retrograde (by temporarily releasing the left atrial clamp). At this point, the suture line at the left atrial anastomosis is tied, and full perfusion is restored to the graft, ending the ischemic interval. Two chest drains are inserted in the pleural space, and a standard closure is performed. Finally, the double-lumen endotracheal tube is exchanged for a regular single-lumen tube. Fiber-optic bronchoscopy is carried out through the tube to verify that the donor bronchial mucosa is pink and viable, and to aspirate any blood and secretions from the donor and recipient airways.

The early success of the Toronto Lung Transplant Group was based heavily on a meticulous approach to the bronchial anastomosis. On the basis of early experimental studies, they judged high-dose corticosteroids to be harmful to bronchial anastomotic healing[17] and, therefore, never used these agents perioperatively. Their technique consisted of simple interrupted sutures to produce an end-to-end anastomosis and routine use of bronchial omentopexy, both to promote anastomotic healing as well as to contain the leak should an anastomotic dehiscence occur. More recent experimental data, obtained from a porcine lung allograft model, have shown that the perioperative use of steroids actually appears to increase bronchial blood flow when added to a standard immunosuppressive regimen consisting of cyclosporin and azathioprine.[19] In clinical lung transplantation, the San Antonio group were responsible for popularizing the telescoping technique of bronchial anastomosis as

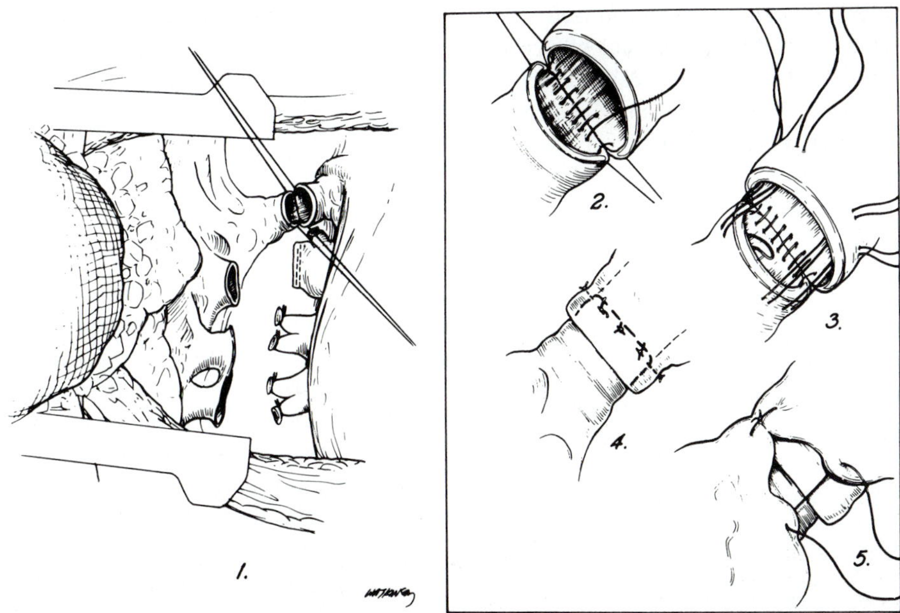


**Figure 29–10.** A right bronchus anastomosis is depicted with the lung cooled by topical crushed ice. The membranous wall is opposed first. The cartilaginous wall is intussuscepted, in this case, donor into recipient bronchus, one cartilaginous ring. Peribronchial nodal tissue covers the anastomosis. *(From Shields TW: General Thoracic Surgery, 4th ed. Baltimore, Williams & Wilkins, 1994, with permission.)*

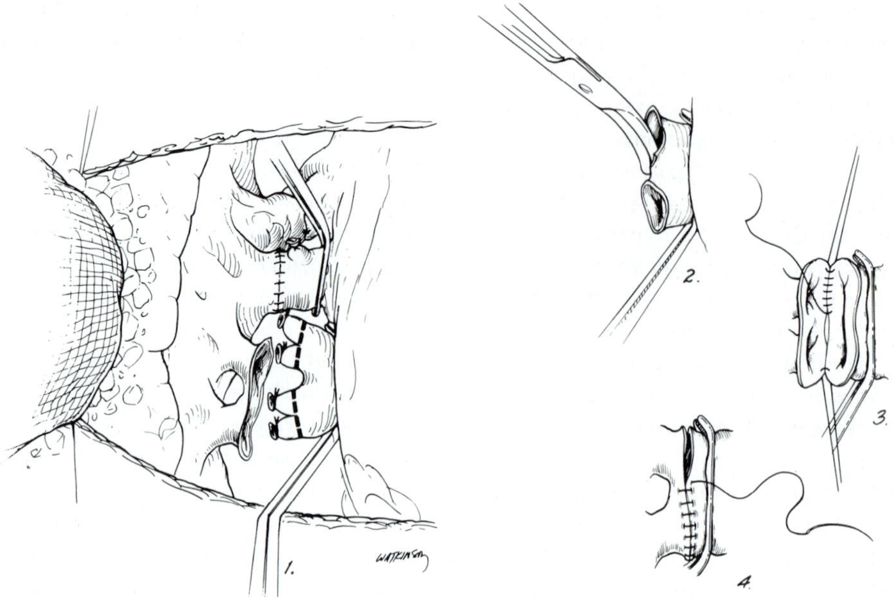


**Figure 29–11.** A central left atrial clamp is in place while the vein stumps are amputated and the bridge of atrial muscle is divided. A 4-0 polypropylene suture is used to complete the anastomosis. *(From Shields TW: General Thoracic Surgery, 4th ed. Baltimore, Williams & Wilkins, 1994, with permission.)*

described earlier.[18] Their approach has been to use figure-of-eight or horizontal mattress sutures to intussuscept the smaller bronchus into the larger one by one cartilaginous ring. This technique appears to provide greater security for the cartilaginous portion of the airway. The San Antonio group has not routinely provided coverage for the bronchial anastomosis (and in particular, has not used omentopexy). Perioperative corticosteroids were routinely utilized. Yet they have not observed any significant incidence of airway complications associated with this approach. A recent retrospective study between the Washington University Lung Transplant Program and that at the University of Toronto also compared their respective approaches to bronchial anastomosis and subsequent management.[31] A series of patients at Washington University, undergoing end-to-end anastomosis with routine omentopexy and no perioperative corticosteroids, were compared to a series of patients at the University of Toronto who underwent telescoping anastomoses covered with local tissue and no omentopexy, along with routine perioperative corticosteroid use. No significant difference in the incidence of airway anastomotic problems were noted between these groups,[31] and, therefore, most centers now favor the latter approach.

## POSTOPERATIVE MANAGEMENT

The strategies discussed in this section reflect the biases of the Washington University Lung Transplant Program.

### Monitoring Utilized in the Intensive Care Unit

All lung transplant patients are admitted postoperatively to the intensive care unit, where monitoring includes the following: electrocardiogram, oximetric evaluation of oxygen saturation (both arterial and mixed venous), and continuous monitoring of systemic and pulmonary arterial pressures. All patients undergo quantitative perfusion lung scanning immediately posttransplantation, to document the percentage of overall pulmonary blood flow to the graft (in cases of single-lung transplantation), or to document the distribution between the two sides following bilateral lung transplantation.

### Pain Control

Pain relief is achieved effectively with the use of an epidural catheter. This is placed preoperatively in virtually all patients, except those who are anticoagulated, or in patients with pulmonary vascular disease, in whom systemic heparinization and cardiopulmonary bypass are mandatory. In these cases, when the epidural catheter is not placed preoperatively, it is placed as soon after the transplant as possible. After several days the epidural catheter is removed, and patient-controlled analgesia (PCA) is initiated as soon as the patient can cooperate.

### Ventilation

Ventilatory management varies with the type of transplantation. In single-lung transplantation for emphysema, no positive end-expiratory pressure (PEEP) is utilized, to avoid distention of the overly compliant native lung. Conversely, in single-lung transplantation for PPH, we deliberately employ 10 cm of water PEEP for at least 36 hours, since we believe that this minimizes the development of edema in the allograft. In bilateral lung transplantation or in single-lung transplants for IPF, standard ventilatory parameters are used, with 5–10 cm of water PEEP.

Optimal oxygenation is achieved by minimizing fluid administration, careful use of diuretics and PEEP, and aggressive utilization of chest physiotherapy and frequent bronchoscopies.

The approach to weaning and extubation is also somewhat variable. In single-lung transplantation for IPF and emphysema and in bilateral lung transplants, we favor early weaning and extubation. In our experience, the median duration of ventilation is 2–3 days, and in very straightforward cases, some patients have been extubated within 24 hours of the procedure. In single-lung transplantation for PPH, the patients are maintained sedated, paralyzed, and, therefore, on full ventilatory support for at least 36 hours posttransplantation. This is performed to avoid the development of pulmonary hypertensive crises.

## Postural Drainage and Physiotherapy

This is important to achieve maximum secretion clearance and early weaning and extubation. Single-lung transplant recipients are maintained in the lateral position with the allograft side "up" for the first 24 hours. Bilateral lung transplant recipients are maintained supine as much as possible in the first 12 hours, then rotated from side to side as tolerated. Physiotherapy consists of vigorous chest percussion and postural drainage and includes early mobilization of the patient after extubation. These aggressive maneuvers are withheld for the first 36 hours in single-lung recipients for PPH.

## Hemodynamics

Most patients are maintained on low-dose dopamine infusion (1–3 μg/kg per minute) for the first 24–48 hours so as to promote diuresis. We also tend to utilize prostaglandin E1 infusion (at a dose between 10 and 100ng/kg per minute) to control the pulmonary artery pressures and pulmonary vascular resistance. Recently, inhaled nitric oxide (at 40–80 parts per million) has been found to be useful in decreasing pulmonary artery pressures and improving oxygenation in patients with early allograft dysfunction.[32]

## Bronchoscopy

Bronchoscopy is useful for clearance of airway secretions, inspection of the integrity of the anastomosis, and obtaining washings to guide antimicrobial therapy. Bronchoscopy is performed in the operating room at the end of the transplantation, then on the first postoperative day and again immediately prior to extubation, and also whenever indicated by the clinical situation.

## Pleural Drainage

We insert two drains in each pleural space at the time of transplantation. In general, we have had an aggressive policy toward early removal of these drains, as soon as there is no evident air leak and when fluid drainage is minimal.

## Nutrition

Intravenous alimentation is started within 24 hours of the transplantation. In most patients, an oral diet is started within 5–7 days of the procedure, but if prolonged ventilatory support will be required, then IV alimentation is stopped, and a feeding tube is inserted to provide enteric feeding.

## Infection Control

### *Antibiotic Prophylaxis*

In patients with chronic septic lung disease (e.g., cystic fibrosis), initial antibiotics are directed at the recipient's organisms, based on preoperative culture and sensitivity data.

Otherwise, in most cases, initial antibiotic prophylaxis is guided by donor specimens (washings obtained during the donor bronchoscopy, as well as swabs from the donor bronchus at the time of implantation) and swabs from the recipient bronchus at the time of recipient pneumonectomy. If no organisms are identified in these specimens, then we use cefazolin 1 g IV q8hrs for at least 3 or 4 days.

If gram-positive organisms are identified, we use Vancomycin 1 g q12hs. If gram-negative organisms are seen, we use ceftazidime 1–2 g IV q8hs. However, if there is progression of pulmonary infiltrates despite use of intravenous Ceftazidime, then we convert this to Imipenem 500 mg IV q6hs.

### *Documented Bacterial Infections*

Treatment here is based on culture and sensitivity data.

### *Herpes Simplex Prophylaxis*

We utilize acyclovir 200 mg bid for at least 2 years after the transplantation.

### *Pneumocystis Carina Prophylaxis*

This is achieved with Septra-DS, one tablet orally twice a day on Monday, Wednesday, and Friday after oral intake starts.

### *Oropharyngeal Candida Prophylaxis*

We utilize nystatin 500,000 U in the form of a mouthwash qid.

### *CMV Prophylaxis*

We attempt to match donor and recipient CMV serology. CMV infection occurs routinely and is most severe in CMV negative recipients receiving CMV positive donors. Therefore, we employ CMV prophylaxis when a CMV-positive graft is implanted into a CMV-negative recipient. Our current CMV prophylaxis regimen begins on day 14 and consists of ganciclovir 5 mg/kg IV bid for 3 weeks, followed by ganciclovir 5 mg/kg IV od for 8–9 weeks and ganciclovir 5 mg/kg IV three times weekly for 4 weeks.

### Immunosuppression

Most programs use a "triple-drug" protocol that combines cyclosporine, azathioprine, and corticosteroids. The protocol followed currently at Washington University is:

1. Pretransplant: Azathioprine 2 mg/kg IV
2. Posttransplant
   - Cyclosporine 3–5 mg/h IV, later converted to an oral dose (bid). (Cyclosporine dose is adjusted based on the level as determined by a whole blood immunoassay.)
   - Azathioprine 2 mg/kg intravenously daily (initially), later converted to 2 mg/kg orally daily.
   - Steroids: Methylprednisolone 500–1000 mg IV before reperfusion,—then 0.5 mg/kg IV daily, × 4 days —convert to prednisone—0.5 mg/kg orally daily for 3 months, tapered to 15 mg PO daily at 1 year
   - Antithymocyte globulin (ATGAM, Upjohn, Kalamazoo, Michigan) 15 mg/kg IV over 8–24 hours for 1 week (usually from the 1st to 8th postoperative days).

## FOLLOW-UP STRATEGIES AND PROCEDURES REQUIRED IN LUNG TRANSPLANT RECIPIENTS

### Surveillance

Lung transplant recipients have an ongoing risk of acute and chronic rejection as well as septic complications. A description of the common pathologic entities arising in these patients, along with an approach to their diagnosis and management, is given in the next section. Therefore, an approach to routine surveillance (i.e., monitoring of the clinically and physiogically stable patient) seems appropriate. Different lung transplant centers vary in their approach to surveillance, but the fundamental components include:

### *Clinical Follow-up*

Patients are encouraged to report any untoward symptoms early. In our program, following hospital discharge, patients reside in our area and are followed in our postoperative follow-up clinic for 3 months before returning to their home community. Once there they return to the care of the referring pulmonologist, ensuring that close contact and dialogue with our program is maintained.

### *Pulmonary Function Tests*

We have tended to focus mainly on the $FEV_1$. The recommendations of the International Society for Heart and Lung Transplantation in 1993[33] are that spirometry in lung transplant patients should be performed with equipment conforming to American Thoracic Society standards, without prior bronchodilator therapy, and ideally monthly in the first year posttransplantation. This would allow a baseline value of the $FEV_1$ (the average of the two previous highest consecutive measurements taken 3–6 weeks apart) to be established. This baseline value may of course continue to increase with time. Significant allograft dysfunction would then be based on a fractional decline in the $FEV_1$ relative to this baseline value. At the Washington University Lung Transplant Program, spirometry is carried out weekly in the first 3 months, then monthly between 3 and 12 months posttransplantation, and then every 1–3 months beyond 1 year.[34] Other centers have advocated the use of small, easily affordable home spirometers to monitor graft function at home.[35] These devices are useful for the early detection of downward trends in the $FEV_1$.

### *Chest Radiograph*

Chest radiographs are obtained on a schedule similar to that for pulmonary function testing, and, of course, whenever clinically indicated. Chest CT scanning is not routinely done for surveillance, but it can be obtained if clinical, radiographic, or bronchoscopic findings suggest the occurrence of an intrathoracic complication following the transplantation, such as bronchial dehiscence, pleural effusion, or empyema.

### *Fiber-optic Bronchoscopy (FOB) with Transbronchial Lung Biopsy (TBLB)*

At the Washington University Lung Transplant Program, fiber-optic bronchoscopy is performed liberally in the early postoperative period as already summarized earlier under "postoperative management." Subsequently, surveillance bronchoscopies with transbronchial biopsy are performed at 3–4 weeks postoperatively, at around 3 months, at around 6 months, then at 1 year, and then annually thereafter.[36] Transbronchial biopsy is also performed for clinical indications including symptoms (dyspnea, cough), signs (fever, adventitious chest sounds), the presence of radiographic infiltrates, and the finding of declining spirometry and/or oxygenation. At our program, FOB is performed with topical anesthesia and IV sedation, with an endotracheal tube inserted over the fiber-optic bronchoscope. TBLB is obtained by using fluoroscopic guidance with a 2-mm fenestrated biopsy forcep. If there is a discrete infiltrate, the majority of biopsies are taken there, with a few being taken from uninvolved areas. If there is a diffuse infiltrate or a relatively normal chest radiograph, then biopsies are obtained from all available bronchopulmonary segments. In bilateral lung transplant recipients, biopsies are taken from only one lung. An average of 10 TBLB are obtained per procedure. Our practice for handling the specimens has been to send them in formaldehyde for routine hematoxylin and eosin (H and E) staining. Gomori methenamine silver stains are routinely obtained to detect the presence of fungi or *Pneumocystis carinii,* and acid fast staining is routinely done to detect the presence of mycobacteria. Additionally, immunoperoxidase staining (for detection of CMV infection), and connective tissue stains (for detection of *Bronchiolitis obliterans*) are obtained if clinically indicated.

### Open-Lung Biopsy

Occasionally patients present with clinical and physiologic deterioration in whom fiber-optic bronchoscopy with TBLB is performed but is inconclusive. Under these circumstances, open-lung biopsy has occasionally been necessary to clarify the underlying pathology (especially in documenting the presence of *Bronchiolitis obliterans*).

### Drainage of Septic Collections

Pigtail catheters can be inserted into loculated fluid pockets under CT control by interventional radiologists. Open window (rib resection) thoracostomy has also occasionally been necessary for open drainage of loculated empyema cavities.

### Procedures Related to Airway Stent Placement and Manipulation

This will be discussed later under management of bronchial anastomotic complications.

## CLINICAL-PATHOLOGIC ENTITIES ENCOUNTERED IN THE LUNG TRANSPLANT RECIPIENT

### Acute Rejection

Lung allografts may be more prone to acute rejection than other solid organ allografts. A number of factors have been speculated upon as possibly providing a basis for this presumption, including the following: the large size of the lung allograft (thereby providing a large "antigenic inoculum"); the fact that the lung contains large populations of immunologically active cells (including macrophages, dendritic cells, and T and B lymphocytes); the fact that the lung accommodates virtually the entire cardiac output; and the fact that the lung is constantly exposed to environmental (inhaled) pathogens, with the ensuing inflammatory process resulting in release of cytokines such as interferon gamma, leading to subsequent up-regulation of MHC antigen expression.

A detailed description of the pathogenesis of lung allograft rejection is beyond the scope of this chapter, but it is believed to arise from a similar cascade of cellular and molecular events as in other solid organ allografts. Alloantigen presentation in the context of MHC molecules ultimately results in the generation of cytotoxic T lymphocytes (CTL), which then affect direct lysis of graft cells, including the vascular endothelium and also the parenchymal cells of the graft.

Acute lung allograft rejection is a frequent clinical problem, although the actual prevalence is unknown since only some episodes are proven histologically, whereas many episodes are identified and treated simply on clinical grounds. Lung transplant recipients are susceptible to acute rejection anytime between within 3–5 days of the transplant to several years later, but the risk seems to decrease with time. In our experience, virtually all patients have at least one acute rejection episode in the first 3–4 weeks posttransplantation. The Papworth Group in Cambridge has reported on its findings in heart-lung transplant recipients, using only histologically proven acute rejection episodes.[37] Sixty percent of these recipients experience acute rejection in the first month, and over 60% of all acute rejection episodes were found to occur within the first 3 months after heart-lung transplantation.

Acute lung allograft rejection has various manifestations, and unfortunately none are truly specific for rejection. The manifestations early after lung transplantation (within the first month) can also differ substantially from those in the late phase (i.e., several months or even years after the transplant). In the first weeks after lung transplantation, the first indication of acute rejection may simply be that the patient has malaise. Frequently patients will complain of mild dyspnea. They may experience fever (more than 0.5°C above previous stable baseline), a drop in oxygenation ($Po_2$ dropping by more than 10 mm Hg below previous stable baseline), a slight drop in spirometry ($FEV_1$ dropping by more than 10% from previous stable baseline), and the chest radiograph may show a new or changing infiltrate (in particular, a hilar or basal haziness). The main differential diagnosis in the early postoperative period includes acute rejection, bacterial sepsis, and pulmonary edema (resulting either from reperfusion injury or from iatrogenic fluid overload). In the late posttransplantation period, a similar constellation of clinical features may be noted, but the chest x-ray is often not abnormal. At this stage, the main differential diagnosis is between acute rejection, CMV infection, and chronic allograft rejection.

The clinical picture described earlier usually raises the suspicion of acute rejection, and steps must be taken to rule out an infection in the graft. Not uncommonly, such episodes are identified and then treated on clinical grounds only, so that the diagnosis of acute rejection is ascertained only in retrospect, after one observes the appropriate response to treatment (Fig. 29–12). However, it appears that the best approach for diagnosing acute rejection is by fiberoptic bronchoscopy with TBLB. Bronchoalveolar lavage (BAL) is usually done concomitant to TBLB, but it is useful mainly in identifying infection within the graft. The utility of transbronchial lung biopsy in diagnosing acute lung allograft rejection in heart-lung transplant recipients is well established, with a sensitivity of 84% and specificity of 100%.[38]

The key histologic finding in acute lung allograft rejection is that of perivascular mononuclear cellular infiltrates (Fig. 29–13). The lung rejection study group of the International Society for Heart and Lung Transplantation formulated a classification system to standardize the nomenclature in heart and lung rejection.[39] The pertinent features of their classification system appear in Table 29–6. In addition to establishing guidelines for differentiating acute and chronic lung allograft rejection, this scheme also permits grading of the severity of acute rejection (with grades A1–A4 ranging from minimal to severe acute rejection) based on the frequency, density, and distribution of these mononuclear infiltrates.[39]

Our approach to the management of acute lung allograft rejection at Washington University has recently been summarized by Trulock[34] and is similar to that followed by most lung transplant programs. The basic components include:

1. High-dose corticosteroids. This is usually given in the form of an intravenous bolus of methylprednisolone, 500–1000 mg daily for 3 days. This will usually reverse most acute rejection episodes.
2. An increase in the maintenance prednisone dose to 1 mg/kg per day, then tapering back to the previous dose over 2–3 weeks. This approach has been found to be useful in treating severe acute rejection episodes, especially if the oral prednisone dose has been drastically diminished or actually discontinued.
3. In unusual acute rejection episodes refractory to steroids, options include the use of OKT3 monoclonal antibody (5 mg/day for 10–14 days), or Anti-thymocyte globulin (ATGAM, 10–20 mg/kg per day for 10–14 days).

Successful treatment of acute rejection episodes as described above will generally effect improvement in the clinical, radiographic, histologic, and physiologic parameters. Despite this, however, several investigators have furnished evidence to suggest that repeated or severe early acute rejection episodes predispose the lung transplant recipient to the later development of chronic lung rejection/bronchiolitis obliterans.[40]

## CMV Infection

Clinically significant CMV infection in lung transplant recipients occurs with variable incidence. The clinical mani-

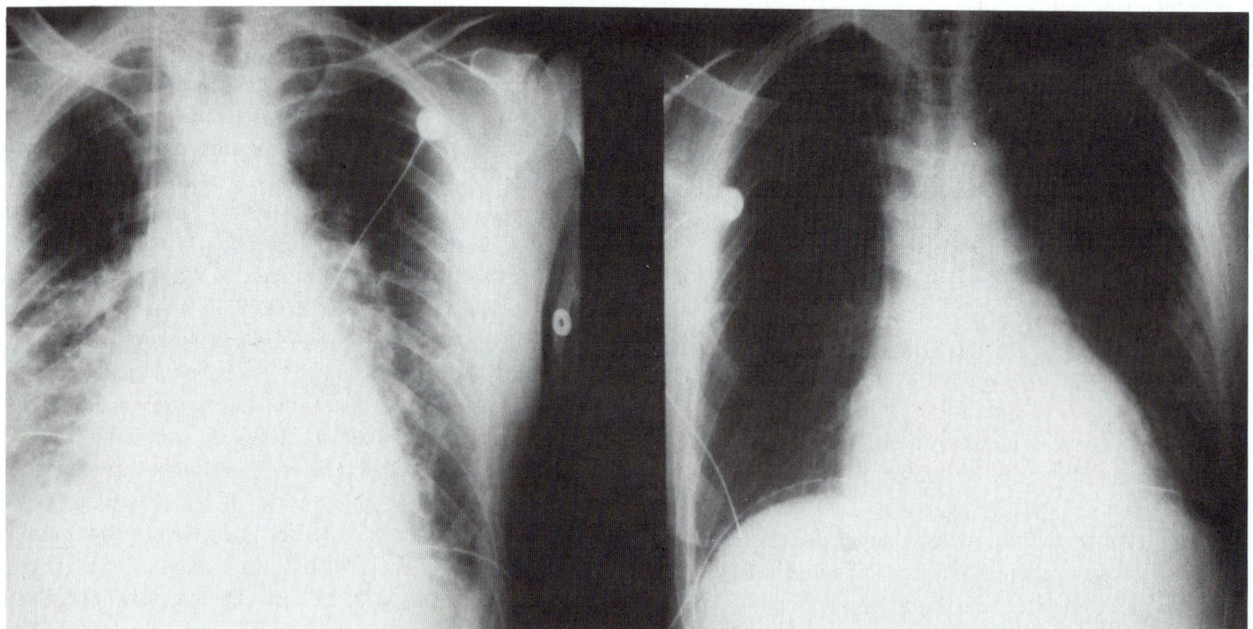

**Figure 29–12.** Posteroanterior chest radiograph from a patient 7 days after bilateral sequential single lung transplantation. On the left, an x-ray from the morning of the seventh postoperative day showing diffuse bilateral infiltrates. A clinical diagnosis of rejection was made and the patient received methylprednisolone 1 g by IV bolus. Shown on the right is a chest x-ray taken 8 hours later. Note the dramatic improvement in infiltrates consistent with the typical response of acute rejection to steroid bolus therapy. *(From Shields TW: General Thoracic Surgery, 4th ed. Baltimore, Williams & Wilkins, 1994, with permission.)*

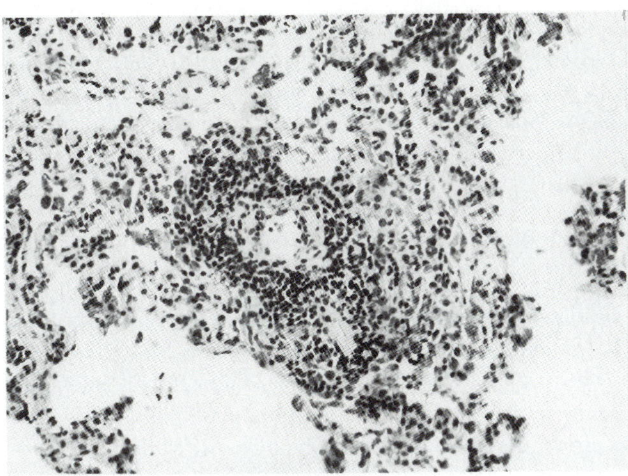

**Figure 29–13.** A photomicrograph of a transbronchial biopsy specimen showing typical early (A1b) rejection. Isolated perivascular cuffs of lymphocytes are noted. *(From Shields TW: General Thoracic Surgery, 4th ed. Baltimore, Williams & Wilkins, 1994, with permission.)*

**TABLE 29–6. WORKING FORMULATION FOR CLASSIFICATION AND GRADING OF PULMONARY REJECTION**

A. Acute rejection
   0. Grade 0—No significant abnormality
   1. Grade 1—Minimal acute rejection
      a. With evidence of bronchiolar inflammation
      b. Without evidence of bronchiolar inflammation
      c. With large airway inflammation
      d. No bronchioles are present
   2. Grade 2—Mild acute rejection
      a. With evidence of bronchiolar inflammation
      b. Without evidence of bronchiolar inflammation
      c. With large airway inflammation
      d. No bronchioles to evaluate
   3. Grade 3—Moderate acute rejection
      a. With evidence of bronchiolar inflammation
      b. Without evidence of bronchiolar inflammation
      c. With large airway inflammation
      d. No bronchioles to evaluate
   4. Grade 4—Severe acute rejection
      a. With evidence of bronchiolar inflammation
      b. Without evidence of bronchiolar inflammation
      c. With large airway inflammation
      d. No bronchioles to evaluate
B. Active airway damage without scarring
   1. Lymphocytic bronchitis
   2. Lymphocytic bronchiolitis
C. Chronic airway rejection
   1. Bronchiolitis obliterans—subtotal
      a. Active
      b. Inactive
   2. Bronchiolitis obliterans—total
      a. Active
      b. Inactive
D. Chronic vascular rejection
E. Vasculitis

festations can mimic those of acute rejection and include a subjective worsening of respiratory status, fever, new or changing infiltrates on chest radiograph, and possibly a lymphocytosis.[41] Once again, an important diagnostic maneuver in differentiating CMV infection from acute rejection is fiber-optic bronchoscopy with transbronchial lung biopsy. Trulock[36] reported the sensitivity of transbronchial lung biopsy to be 91% for the diagnosis of CMV pneumonia. The basis for the pathologic diagnosis is the presence of characteristic intracellular inclusions on H and E stains and/or a positive immunoperoxidase stain.

Our approach to CMV prophylaxis has already been summarized. Clinical CMV infections in lung transplant patients can affect a variety of anatomic sites (in particular the GI tract) apart from the lung allograft. Our treatment of documented CMV in lung allograft recipients consists of gancyclovir 5 mg/kg IV for 2–3 weeks.

CMV infection in lung transplant recipients carries major significance. The Pittsburgh group have reported that CMV pneumonitis was responsible for the death of 16% of their heart-lung transplant recipients and that follow-up of survivors of CMV infection revealed that 90% developed bronchiolitis obliterans.[41]

## Chronic Lung Allograft Rejection/Bronchiolitis Obliterans Syndrome

With the achievement of considerably better early survival in clinical lung transplantation, the entity of obliterative bronchiolitis became recognized as perhaps the main impediment to prolonged survival. Obliterative bronchiolitis (OB) is an inflammatory disorder of the small airways (leading to obstruction and destruction of pulmonary bronchioles) and was first described in the lung transplant population in 1984.[42] It was originally felt that OB affected about 25–30% of patients surviving more than 3 months beyond their heart-lung transplant. With increasing clinical experience, OB is also being recognized after isolated single- and bilateral-lung transplantation, and it appears to have no predilection for age, sex, or indication for transplantation. A recent retrospective review of our lung transplant experience showed that OB appears to exhibit considerable latency (taking an average of 15 months until onset) and that if followed for a sufficient time interval, its prevalence is as high as 50%.[43]

This syndrome of chronic lung allograft dysfunction is associated with characteristic clinical, functional, and histologic changes. Clinically the patient generally complains of dry or productive cough and dyspnea that is refractory to bronchodilators, along with generalized and progressive respiratory difficulty. The predominant functional abnormality is airflow obstruction, as evidenced by serial decline in the $FEV_1$. In this regard, OB has been likened to chronic obstructive pulmonary disease, except that the progression of the airflow obstruction occurs over several months, instead of being drawn out over many years. The characteristic histologic correlate of this form of graft dysfunction is obliterative bronchiolitis, which consists of dense fibrosis and scar tissue that obliterates the bronchiolar wall and lumen, bronchiectatic widening of the peripheral as well as central bronchi, mucus plugging of the airways, and some degree of interstitial fibrosis in the surrounding lung parenchyma (Fig. 29–14).

A recent meeting of representative members of the International Society for Heart and Lung Transplantation was held for the purpose of developing a clinically applicable classification and staging system for chronic lung allograft rejection. In the ensuing report,[33] this group proposed the use of the term *bronchiolitis obliterans syndrome* (BOS) to connote this graft dysfunction secondary to progressive airway disease for which there is no specific identifiable etiology. This terminology was based on recognition of the fact that the clinical and functional aspects of chronic lung rejection are usually, but not always, coexistent with the histologic hallmark (OB). A number of theories regarding the pathogenesis of BOS have been put forth and suggest an immunologic basis for BOS, leading to the prevalent (but unproven) presumption that BOS is a manifestation of chronic lung allograft rejection.

To date, the fibrosis resulting from BOS is irreversible, and, thus, there is no satisfactory treatment for established BOS. Since the true pathogenesis of BOS is unknown, the usual treatment in most centers has been empiric and consists of augmented immunosuppression[44] similar to that described earlier for acute lung rejection. A few patients will stabilize with augmented immunosuppression. Most afflicted patients experience a steady progression of the disease and often succumb to it, or to opportunistic infections induced by the augmented immunosuppression. Repeat transplantation has been attempted in some centers for severe BOS with far less success than primary lung transplantation.[10] Hence, a strong research effort to elucidate the etiology and pathogenesis of BOS is vital if any hope of effective prophylactic or therapeutic intervention is to be entertained.

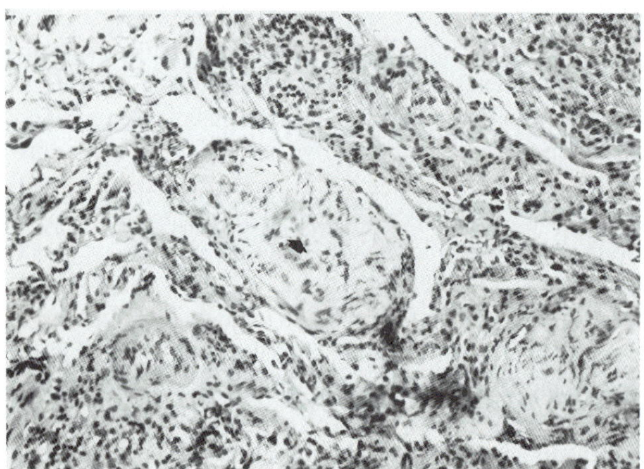

**Figure 29–14.** A photomicrograph of a transbronchial biopsy specimen reveals the typical findings of bronchiolitis obliterans thought to result from chronic rejection. Mature fibrous obliteration of the bronchiolar lumen is evident (arrow). *(From Shields TW: General Thoracic Surgery, 4th ed. Baltimore, Williams & Wilkins, 1994, with permission.)*

## Bronchial Anastomotic Complications

These were formerly very frequent and one of the main impediments to progress in the field of lung transplantation. Their incidence is now dramatically decreased, for a variety of reasons that have already been enumerated, including better graft preservation (thereby maintaining superior microcirculation in the graft and better preservation of collateral flow to the bronchial arteries), better techniques of airway anastomosis (including the telescoping method), and the early routine use of corticosteroids perioperatively.

In the majority of cases, failure of bronchial anastomotic healing represents an ischemic complication of the airway, and it can create a spectrum of different clinical presentations. The least serious form consists of patchy zones of necrosis of the donor airway mucosa; this is a common finding and usually carries no significance. The more serious variety consists of ischemic necrosis at the suture line, the severity of which will vary according to the degree of anastomotic dehiscence that has occurred there. Early posttransplantation, this form may manifest either with air leak or with features of sepsis arising due to the associated mediastinal collection. If extensive dehiscence occurs, a massive air leak may result, and, rarely, fistulization can occur between the pulmonary artery and bronchial anastomosis. The usual late sequelae of this complication are strictures or the development of a malacic segment in the bronchus. At this late stage, the patient may present with new onset of dyspnea, stridor, or wheeze.

Workup of airway anastomotic complications begins with an appropriate recognition of the suggestive clinical signs. Proper documentation and evaluation is then achieved by chest radiograph, fiber-optic bronchoscopy, and chest CT scanning (to document the presence of any mediastinal pathology, such as air or fluid collections).

In the acute phase of an anastomotic dehiscence, the most important priority is to achieve adequate drainage, either by chest tube, by percutaneous drainage using CT control, or even by performing mediastinoscopy to provide transcervical drainage. Once adequate drainage has been achieved, the majority of airway anastomotic complications can be handled by conservative means. In the intermediate phase, periodic rigid bronchoscopy for debridement and dilatation of the airway may become necessary. We have not found laser therapy useful, since we believe from our own experience and that of others that excessive damage especially to the critically important donor lobar bronchi is frequently produced, making a difficult stricture impossible to manage conservatively. Finally, when a mature stricture results, silastic endobronchial stents are inserted over a rigid bronchoscope and can be utilized to maintain airway patency. In general, stent therapy of proximal right main bronchial strictures is a satisfactory option. However, the presence of long strictures or strictures located distally in the left main bronchus are much less favorable lesions for stent placement. While satisfactorily positioned stents result in a dramatic improvement in lung function,[45] they are also prone to complications. They may migrate out of position, necessitating bronchoscopic replacement. Mucus plugging can be obviated by inhalational therapy with N-aceytylcysteine (Mucomyst). Finally, granulation tissue can overgrow either end of the stent. This is the one circumstance when we have found Nd:YAG laser fulguration useful.

When used in the treatment of rigid strictures, the stents can often be removed after about 1 year, when the airway has achieved sufficient rigidity and a satisfactory caliber around the stent. However, when used for bronchomalacia, the stents must be retained permanently. Such malacic strictures can be effectively managed by placement of wire mesh stents without fear of the wire of the stents becoming embedded in the airway wall. Most airway complications can be treated conservatively, with a combination of drainage followed later by bronchoscopic dilatation and/or stent placement.

Schafers and colleagues[46] have recently reported a successful experience in a small number of patients with bronchial strictures who underwent bronchoplasty. Retransplantation is an option but in general is reserved as the last resort.

## RESULTS OF LUNG TRANSPLANTATION

Until recently, "success" in lung transplantation tended to be based upon hospital survival rates. In recent years, indications have expanded, techniques have been refined, and early results have steadily improved.[47,48] We recently reported on the results of 131 consecutive lung transplants performed at our institution and documented a 92% hospital survival rate.[48] Therefore, we must now, in addition to analyzing early survival, critically evaluate the long-term survival rates and also the functional results following lung transplantation. Data are now available to provide "medium-term" actuarial survival curves for 2–3 years posttransplantation in the various patient subsets (Fig. 29–15).

### Survival Trends

The St. Louis International Lung Transplant Registry is a voluntary international registry maintained by Dr. Joel D. Cooper. It contains survival and other clinical data and, as of the September 1994 update, represents a cumulative experience of over 2700 lung transplants from more than 121 lung transplant programs worldwide. Actuarial survival data for the reported international experience is shown in Figure 29–16. One-year survival for all patients is 70%, and a sufficient number of recipients have survived 5 years to determine a 5-year survival of 43%. The 3-year actuarial survival by the type of transplant (shown in Fig. 29–17) shows a slight (but not significant) survival advantage for patients undergoing bilateral compared to single-lung replacement. Three-year actuarial survival by diagnosis is shown in Figure 29–18 and does not differ substantially between the different groups. The long-term results of lung transplantation may be expected to continue to improve in the future, since the vast majority of reported transplants (about 90%) was recorded over the past 4 years,[10] many from new centers that are still gathering experience.

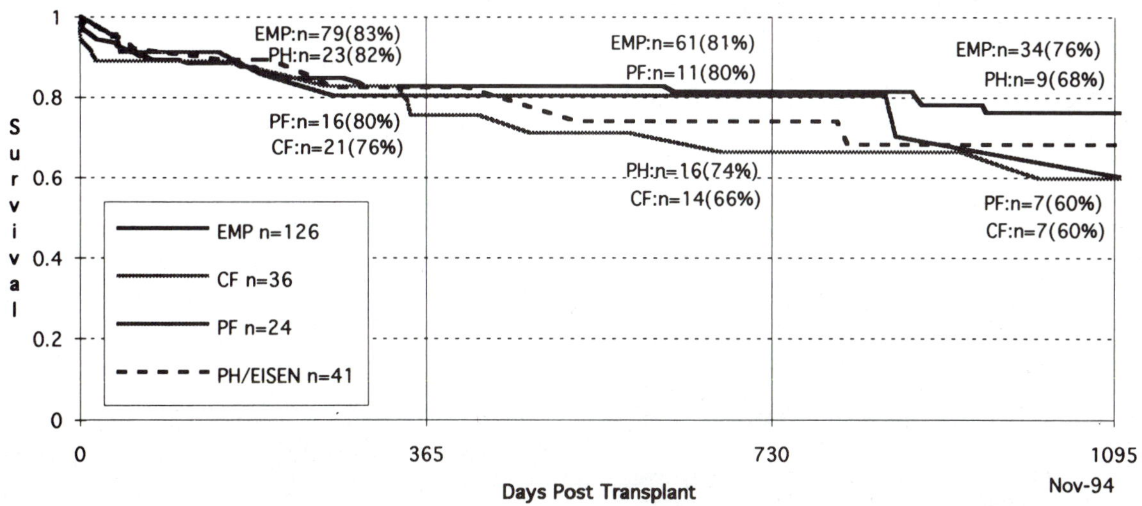


**Figure 29–15.** Three-year actuarial survival from the Washington University (Barnes Hospital) lung transplant program by disease. As in many programs, patients with emphysema seem to have a somewhat better long-term prognosis than patients suffering from pulmonary fibrosis and cystic fibrosis.

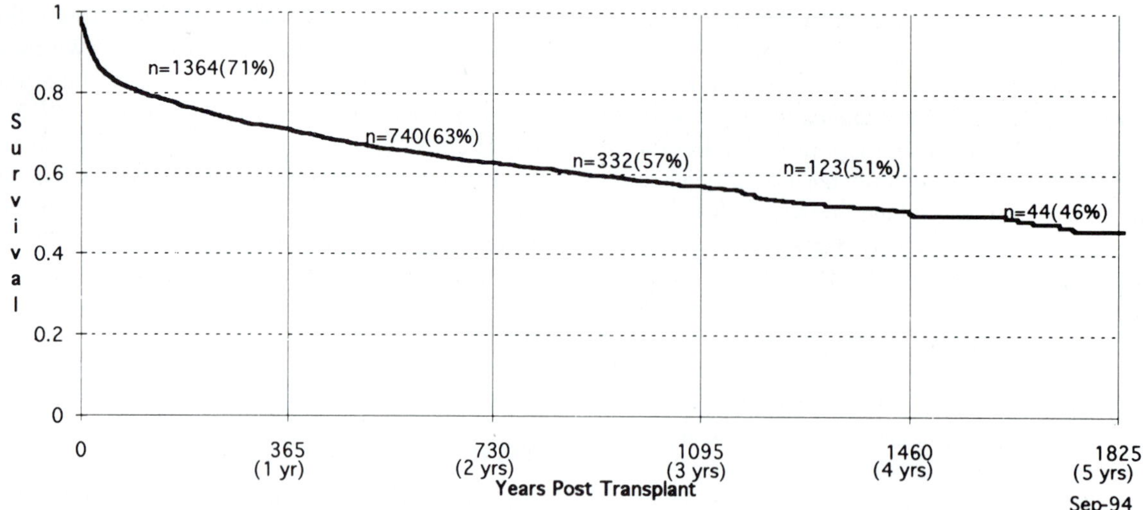


**Figure 29–16.** Overall 5-year actuarial survival from all cases reported to the St. Louis International Lung Transplant Registry.

## Functional Results

In general, the functional result and outcome of lung transplantation have been excellent and sustained in all of the diagnostic groups. Two recently published reports have analyzed the functional outcome in single- and bilateral lung transplantation for emphysema.[12,13] In the University of Toronto report,[12] 3-month posttransplantation data were compared to preoperative data for single-lung and bilateral lung recipients, whereas we at Washington University[13] compared 2-month posttransplantation to preoperative data between these two groups. Both studies documented a significant improvement in $FEV_1$, arterial blood gas parameters, and distance covered in the 6-minute walk test. However, both studies documented that the improvement in $FEV_1$ and arterial oxygen tension were significantly better after bilateral lung replacement than after single-lung replacement.[12,13] The Toronto study also showed superior performance in the 6-minute walk test after bilateral lung replacement.[12] However, the Washington University study showed a higher incidence of complications in the bilateral lung transplant group. These were mainly cardiovascular complications (supraventricular arrhythmias), but they also included airway anastomotic complications and pneumothoraces. Therefore, it appears that both SLT and BLT are suitable operations for emphysema, both in terms of actuarial survival and functional improvement. BLT is a longer, more complex operation with a higher perioperative com-

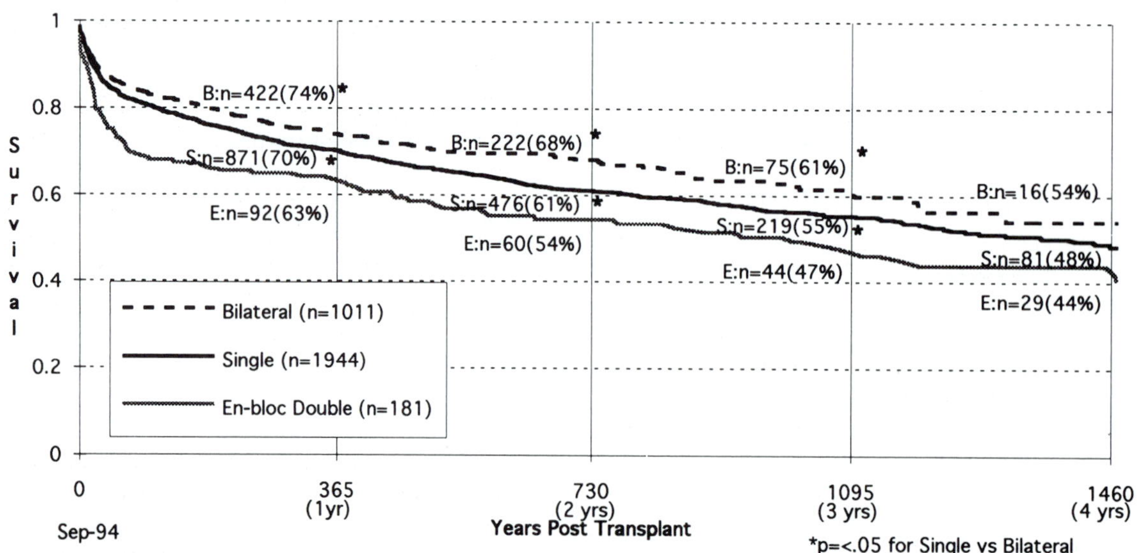


**Figure 29–17.** Actuarial survival curves from the St. Louis International Lung Transplant Registry by transplant type. Bilateral sequential single-lung transplants seem to have a slightly better long-term prognosis than do patients receiving single-lung allografts. The high early operative mortality of en bloc double-lung transplantation accounts for the overall reduced survival in that patient group.

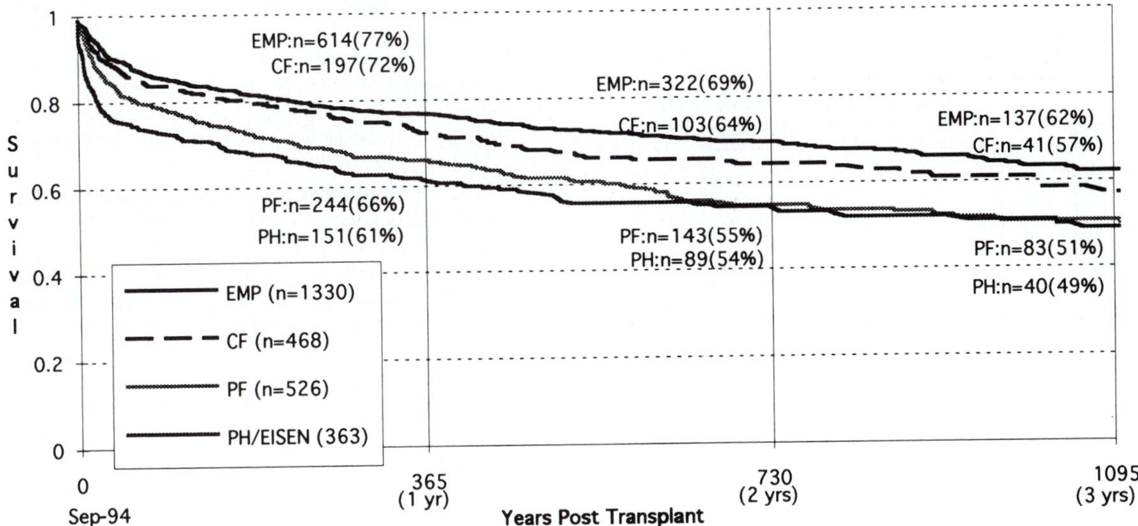


**Figure 29–18.** Three-year actuarial survival from the St. Louis International Lung Transplant Registry by disease. As in the Washington University program, patients with emphysema have a superior long-term prognosis. However, contrary to our own experience, in the international experience patients with pulmonary hypertension have a lower survival overall.

plication rate, but which provides a significantly better improvement in physiologic parameters ($FEV_1$, $PaO_2$) and in functional status (performance in 6-minute walk test). Furthermore, BLT provides more functional reserve in the event of a serious late graft complication (i.e., chronic allograft rejection). Two obvious advantages of single-lung transplantation are that it is a shorter, simpler, less complicated operation, as well as the fact that it achieves more transplants from the same number of donors. Ultimately, the optimal transplant procedure in obstructive lung disease is not yet resolved. We currently tend to offer SLT to patients over the age of 60 and/or who might otherwise represent a "high risk" and BLT to most emphysema patients under the age of 50–55.

Pasque and colleagues[49] reported the initial Washington University experience with single-lung transplantation for pulmonary vascular disease. They reported on seven patients undergoing right single-lung transplantation for pulmonary hypertension, two of whom had simultaneous closure of atrial septal defects. All patients had severely compromised right ventricular function preoperatively, yet there was no operative mortality in this group. Right ventricular functional recovery was excellent, as evaluated by a number of parameters: At 13 weeks, PA systolic pressure decreased to 29 ± 6 mm Hg (from 92 ± 7 mm Hg preoperatively), CVP decreased to 1 ± 2 mm Hg (from 10 ± 6 mm Hg preoperatively), and pulmonary vascular resistance index decreased to 232 ± 73 dyne • s • $cm^{-9}$ (from 1924 ± 663 preoperatively). At 17 weeks, right ventricular ejection fraction improved to 51 ± 11% (from 22 ± 15%), and quantitative perfusion lung scanning showed 89 ± 7% of total pulmonary blood flow being directed to the allograft. Finally, all patients were in New York Heart Association Class I or II postoperatively, whereas all had been in NYHA Class III or IV preoperatively.

Since that report, longer follow-up of more than 30 patients undergoing single lung transplantation for pulmonary vascular disease has shown that:

1. The dramatic improvement (decrease in pulmonary vascular resistance and improvement in right ventricular function) documented in the early report is actually sustained to as long as 3 years' follow-up.
2. Despite the resultant ventilation-perfusion imbalance, functional status is markedly improved in these patients. There is no subjective dyspnea or limitation of exercise tolerance related to dead space ventilation of the native lung.

These findings, along with the technical simplicity of the operation (resulting in a very acceptable mortality and morbidity), coupled with the fact that it makes more optimal use of donor organs, make single-lung transplantation an attractive option for patients with pulmonary vascular disease. However, BOS affects up to 50% of these recipients and, as it progresses, will cause a gradual decline in ventilation to the hyperperfused allograft. This is extremely poorly tolerated and, hence, mandates consideration of other technical options, primarily bilateral lung transplantation.

The ideal transplant procedure for cystic fibrosis is a subject of some controversy. Bilateral sequential lung transplantation provides excellent results.[50] Indeed, Egan and his associates[51] have recently reported the largest single institution experience with bilateral lung transplantation for patients with cystic fibrosis. There were no operative deaths (a remarkable accomplishment) and, as has been reported

**TABLE 29–7. CAUSES OF TRANSPLANT RECIPIENT DEATHS: DEATHS OCCURRING AFTER 90 DAYS POSTTRANSPLANT (n = 407)**

| Causes of Death | n | % of Deaths >90 Days | % of Total Transplants |
|---|---|---|---|
| Infection (other than CMV) | 117 | 29 | 4 |
| BO/Rejection | 112 | 28 | 4 |
| Malignancy | 26 | 6 | <1 |
| Respiratory failure | 26 | 6 | <1 |
| CMV | 18 | 4 | <1 |
| Hemorrhage | 8 | 2 | <1 |
| Heart failure | 9 | 2 | <1 |
| Other | 84 | 21 | 3 |

*CMV = cytomegalovirus.*

previously, functional results were outstanding. However, the Papworth and Harefield groups continue to advocate heart lung transplantation with domino procedure whenever possible.[52]

Pulmonary fibrosis, the condition for which isolated lung transplantation was first successfully employed, represents a minority condition in most lung transplant programs. However, the functional results of single-lung transplantation are excellent. Indeed, the longest surviving lung transplant recipient received a right single-lung transplant for IPF almost 7 years ago and continues to do well.

## Causes of Late Death

Table 29–7 lists the major causes of death in lung transplant recipients occurring more than 90 days posttransplantation; these data are derived from the January 1994 update of the International Registry and represent the international experience. Although bronchiolitis obliterans is listed as the second leading cause of death (at 28% of all late fatalities), the majority of fatal septic episodes and lymphoproliferative malignancies arise in turn as a consequence of the heightened immunosuppression used to treat this entity. Therefore, it is quite clear that the development of BOS in lung transplant recipients is the main factor limiting long-term survival (directly or indirectly) and that the achievement of a better understanding of the immunologic and molecular mechanisms of this process is the main challenge facing clinical lung transplantation today.

## REFERENCES


1. Triantafillou AN, Heerdt PM: Lung transplantation. *Int Anesthesiol Clin* **29**:87–109, 1991
2. Trulock EP: Recipient selection. *Chest Surg Clin North Am* **3**:1–18, 1993
3. Feinleib M, Rosenberg HM, Collins JG, et al. Trends in COPD morbidity and mortality in the United States. *Am Rev Respir Dis* **140**:S9–S18, 1989
4. Anthonisen NR: Prognosis in chronic obstructive pulmonary disease: Results from multicenter clinical trials. *Am Rev Respir Dis* **140**: 595–599, 1989
5. Holsclaw DS: Cystic fibrosis: Overview and pulmonary aspects in young adults. *Clin Chest Med* **1**:407–421, 1980
6. Kerem E, Reisman J, Corey M, Canney GJ, Levison H: Prediction of mortality in patients with cystic fibrosis. *N Engl J Med* **326**: 1187–1191, 1992
7. Hay JG, Turner-Warwick M: Interstitial pulmonary fibrosis. In: Murray JF, Nadel JA (eds). *Textbook of Respiratory Medicine*. Philadelphia, Saunders, 1988, pp 1445–1461
8. D'Alonzo GE, Barst RJ, Ayres SM, et al: Survival in patients with primary pulmonary hypertension: Results from a National Prospective Registry. *Ann Intern Med* **115**:343–349, 1991
9. Marshall SE, Kramer MR, Lewiston NJ, et al: Selection and evaluation of recipients for heart-lung and lung transplantation. *Chest* **98**:1488–1494, 1990
10. Pohl MS: St. Louis International Lung Transplant Registry Results. In: Patterson GA, Couraud L (eds). *Current Topics in General Thoracic Surgery: Lung Transplantation,* 1995, vol. 3, pp 455–465. Amsterdam, Elsevier.
11. Cooper JD, Trulock EP, Triantafillou AN, et al. Bilateral pneumectomy (volume reduction) for chronic obstructive pulmonary disease. *J Thorac Cardiovasc Surg*. In press.
12. Patterson GA, Maurer JA, Williams TJ, et al: Comparison of outcomes of double and single lung transplantation for obstructive lung disease. *J Thorac Cardiovasc Surg* **101**:623–632, 1991
13. Low DE, Trulock EP, Kaiser LR, et al: Morbidity, mortality, and early results of single vs. bilateral lung transplantation for emphysema. *J Thorac Cardiovasc Surg* **103**:1119–1126, 1992
14. Reitz BA, Wallwork J, Hunt SA, et al: Heart-lung transplantation. Successful therapy for patients with pulmonary vascular disease. *N Engl J Med* **306**:557–564, 1982
15. UNOS Update, September 1993.
16. Low DE, Trulock EP, Kaiser LR, et al: Lung transplantation of ventilator dependent patients. *Chest* **101**:8–11, 1992
17. Lima O, Cooper JD, Peters WJ, et al: Effects of methyl prednisolone and azathioprine on bronchial healing following lung autotransplantation. *J Thorac Cardiovasc Surg* **83**:418–421, 1982
18. Calhoon JH, Grover FL, Gibbons WJ, et al: Single lung transplantation: Alternative indications and technique. *J Thorac Cardiovasc Surg* **101**:816–825, 1991
19. Inui K, Schafers HJ, Aoki M, et al: Bronchial circulation after experimental lung transplantation. The effect of long-term administration of prednisolone. *J Thorac Cardiovasc Surg* **105**:474–479, 1993
20. Sundaresan S, Trachiotis GD, Aoe M, et al: Donor lung procurement: Assessment and operative technique. *Ann Thorac Surg* **56**:1409–1413, 1993
21. Sundaresan S, Semenkovich J, Ochoa L, et al: Successful outcome of lung transplantation is not compromised by the use of marginal donor lungs. *J Thorac Cardiovasc Surg*. In press.
22. Puskas JD, Winton TL, Miller JD, et al: Unilateral donor lung dysfunction does not preclude successful contralateral single lung transplantation. *J Thorac Cardiovasc Surg* **103**:1015–1018, 1992
23. Cohen RG, Barr ML, Schenkel FA, et al: Living-related donor lobectomy for bilateral lobar transplantation in patients with cystic fibrosis. *Ann Thorac Surg* **57**:1423–1428, 1994
24. Novick RJ, Reid KR, Denning L, et al: Prolonged preservation of canine lung allografts: The role of prostaglandins. *Ann Thorac Surg* **51**:853–859, 1991
25. Date H, Matsumura A, Manchester JK, et al: Changes in alveolar oxygen and carbon dioxide concentrations and oxygen consumption during lung preservation: The maintenance of aerobic metabolism during lung preservation. *J Thorac Cardiovasc Surg* **105**:492–501, 1993
26. Date H, Matsumura A, Manchester JK, et al: Evaluation of lung metabolism during successful twenty-four-hour canine lung preservation. *J Thorac Cardiovasc Surg* **105**:480–491, 1993

27. Triantafillou AN: Anesthetic considerations. *Chest Surg Clin North Am* **3:**49–73, 1993
28. Pasque MK, Cooper JD, Kaiser LR, et al: Improved technique for bilateral lung transplantation: Rationale and initial clinical experience. *Ann Thorac Surg* **49:**785–791, 1990
29. Patterson GA, Cooper JD, Goldman B, et al: Technique of successful clinical double-lung transplantation. *Ann Thorac Surg* **45:**626–633, 1988
30. Cooper JD, Pearson FG, Patterson GA, et al: Technique of successful lung transplantation in humans. *J Thorac Cardiovasc Surg* **93:** 173–181, 1987
31. Miller JD, de Hoyos A, University of Toronto and Washington University Lung Transplant Programs: An evaluation of the role of omentopexy and of early perioperative corticosteroid administration in clinical lung transplantation. *J Thorac Cardiovasc Surg* **105:** 247–252, 1993
32. Okabayashi K, Triantafillou AN, Yamashita M, et al: Inhaled nitric oxide reduces lung allograft reperfusion injury. *Surgical Forum* **45:**276–278, 1994.
33. Cooper JD, Billingham M, Egan T, et al: A working formulation for the standardization of nomenclature and for clinical staging of chronic dysfunction in lung allografts. *J Heart Lung Transplant* **12:**713–716, 1993
34. Trulock EP: Management of lung transplant rejection. *Chest* **103:**1566–1576, 1993
35. Otulana BA, Higenbottam T, Ferrari L, et al: The use of home spirometry in detecting acute lung rejection and infection following heart-lung transplantation. *Chest* **97:**353–357, 1990
36. Trulock EP, Ettinger NA, Brunt EM, et al: The role of transbronchial lung biopsy in the treatment of lung transplant recipients. An analysis of 200 consecutive procedures. *Chest* **102:**1049–1054, 1992
37. Hutter JA, Despins P, Higenbottam T, et al: Heart-lung transplantation: better use of resources. *Am J Med* **85:**4–11, 1988
38. Higenbottam T, Stewart S, Penketh A, Wallwork J: Transbronchial lung biopsy for the diagnosis of rejection in heart-lung transplant patients. *Transplantation* **46:**532–539, 1988
39. Yousem SA, Berry GJ, Brunt EM, et al: A working formulation for the standardization of nomenclature in the diagnosis of heart and lung rejection: Lung Rejection Study Group. *J Heart Transplant* **9:**593–601, 1990
40. Yousem SA, Dauber JA, Keenan R, et al: Does histologic rejection in lung allografts predict the development of bronchiolitis obliterans? *Transplantation* **52:**306–309, 1991
41. Zeevi A, Ukhis ME, Spichty KJ, et al: Proliferation of cytomegalovirus-primed lymphocytes in bronchoalveolar lavages from lung transplant patients. *Transplantation* **54:**635–639, 1992
42. Burke CM, Theodore J, Dawkins KD, et al: Post transplant obliterative bronchiolitis and other late lung sequelae in human heart-lung transplantation. *Chest* **86:**824–829, 1984
43. Sundaresan S, Trulock EP, Cooper, et al: Prevalence and outcome of bronchiolitis obliterans syndrome after lung transplantation. Accepted abstract. Society of Thoracic Surgeons.
44. Paradis IL, Duncan SR, Dauber JH, et al: Effect of augmented immunosuppression on human chronic lung allograft rejection. *Am Rev Respir Dis* **145:**A705, 1992
45. Schafers HJ, Haydock DA, Cooper JD: The prevalence and management of bronchial anastomotic complications in lung transplantation. *J Thorac Cardiovasc Surg* **101:**1044–1052, 1991
46. Schafers HJ, Schafer CM, Zink C, et al: Surgical treatment of airway complications after lung transplantation. *J Thorac Cardiovasc Surg* **107:**1476–1480, 1994
47. de Hoyos AL, Patterson GA, Maurer JR, et al: Pulmonary transplantation. Early and late results. *J Thorac Cardiovasc Surg* **103:** 295–306, 1992
48. Cooper JD, Patterson GA, Trulock EP, et al: Results of single and bilateral lung transplantation in 131 consecutive recipients. *J Thorac Cardiovasc Surg* **107:**460–471, 1994
49. Pasque MK, Trulock EP, Kaiser LR, Cooper JD: Single lung transplantation for pulmonary hypertension. Three-month hemodynamic follow-up. *Circulation* **84:**2275–2279, 1991
50. Ramirez JC, Patterson GA, Winton T, et al: Bilateral lung transplantation for cystic fibrosis. *J Thorac Cardiovasc Surg* **103:**287–294, 1992
51. Egan TM, Detterbeck FC, Mill MR, et al: Improved results of lung transplantation for patients with cystic fibrosis. *J Thorac Cardiovasc Surg.* **109:**224–235, 1995.
52. Oaks TE, Aravot D, Dennis C, et al: Domino heart transplantation: The Papworth experience. *J Heart Lung Transplant* **13:**433–437, 1994

# CHAPTER 30

# Benign and Malignant Disorders of the Pleura

Joseph LoCicero, III

Except for primary pleural mesothelioma, virtually all pleural space pathology is secondary to one of two pathogenic mechanisms: (1) a breach in the integrity of the pleural membrane with contamination of the space by foreign substances such as air, blood, chyle or purulent material; and (2) an imbalance in the dynamic equilibrium of the pleura with fluid accumulation.

## BASIC CONSIDERATIONS

### Anatomy of the Pleura

#### *Gross Anatomy*

The pleural is a serous membrane originating from the internal coelom.[1] The parietal segment covers the inner surface of the ribs, diaphragm, and mediastinum, while the visceral pleura begins at the pulmonary hilus contiguous with the parietal pleura and covers all lung surfaces, including the fissures. The two pleural leaflets are separated by a virtual space lubricated by minimal amounts of pleural fluid. This arrangement provides efficient mechanical coupling between the passive elastic lung and the dynamic chest wall.

#### *Histology*

The actual pleural lining is a monolayer of mesothelial cells resting over a basement membrane. These flat mesothelial cells have the potential to perform several functions including fluid reabsorption (pinocytosis), phagocytosis of foreign materials, formation of collagen and elastin, and biochemical functions such as plasminogen activation. Electron microscopy demonstrates microvilli within the cell membrane that are important in allowing sliding of the pleural leaflets.

Beneath the basement membrane of the visceral pleura, there is a layer of loose connective tissue directly attached to the interlobar septae. This fibroelastic network helps to distribute the mechanical forces generated by the bony thorax.

#### *Blood Supply*

The blood supply of the parietal pleura is exclusively systemic. The costal pleura is supplied by intercostal arteries and branches from the internal thoracic arteries, while the mediastinal pleura is vascularized by bronchial upper diaphragmatic and internal thoracic arteries. The blood supply to the pleural dome comes from the subclavian arteries. For the most part, venous drainage goes into the peribronchial veins. In contrast, the visceral pleura is vascularized by both systemic (bronchial arteries) and pulmonary circulations. The venous drainage goes to the pulmonary venous system.

#### *Lymphatic Drainage*

The pleural surfaces are located at the boundary of two different lymphatic systems. In the subpleural space of the visceral pleura, large lymphatic capillaries form a mesh network that drains into the pulmonary lymphatic system. These capillaries are more abundant over the lower lobes and are connected to the deep pulmonary plexus located into the interlobular and peribronchial spaces.

The lymphatic drainage of the parietal pleura is more elaborate with direct communications between the pleural space and the parietal pleural lymphatic channels. These communications known as stomata are 2–6 μm in diameter and predominate over the lower portions of the mediastinum, diaphragm, and chest wall. They have endoluminal valves and drain into a network of submesothelial lymphatic lacunae. Over the costal pleura, these collecting vessels form parallel to the ribs to reach the internal thoracic node chain anteriorly and the intercostal nodal chain posteriorly. At the diaphragm, the drainage goes to the retrosternal, mediastinal, and celiac nodes. These trans-diaphragmatic anastomoses allow for the passage of fluid and foreign particles from the peritoneal cavity into the pleural space.

### *Innervation*

The visceral pleura is devoid of somatic innervation. In contrast, the parietal pleura is innervated through a rich network of somatic, sympathetic, and parasympathetic fibers. At the chest wall, these fibers travel through the intercostal nerves. Pain stimuli at the diaphragm are transmitted through the phrenic nerve.

## Physiology of the Pleural Space

### *Mechanics*

The respiratory system can be schematically represented as two elastic structures: the lung and the thorax.[2] These elastic structures are coupled in series (Fig. 30–1). Both of these structures pull in opposite directions with resulting pressures described by the following equation:

$$P_{RS} = P_L + P_W,$$

where $P_{RS}$ represents pressure of the respiratory system, $P_L$ represents transpulmonary pressure developed in the lung, and $P_W$ equals transthoracic pressure developed in the chest wall. The measurable pressures at the boundary of these structures are the alveolar ($P_{ALV}$), pleural ($P_{PL}$), and barometric ($P_{BAR}$) pressures. The pleural pressure is equal to the difference between the alveolar and transpulmonary pressures as shown in the following equations:

$$P_L = P_{ALV} - P_{PL}$$
$$P_{PL} = P_{ALV} - P_{AL}.$$

In static conditions where $P_{ALV}$ is equal to zero, the equation simplifies to:

$$P_{PL} = -P_L.$$

This equation indicates that the static pressure-volume curve of the lung as shown in Fig. 30–2 is representative of pleural pressures.

The pleural pressure is negative essentially at all points during the breathing cycle. At the level of functional residual capacity, $P_{PL}$ equals –2 to –5 cm $H_2O$ in the sitting position. As lung volume increased during inspiration, the pleural pressure becomes more negative reaching –25 to –35 cm $H_2O$ at full inspiration. In physiologic conditions, the pleural pressure is not uniform throughout the pleural space. It is more negative at the apex (–8 cm $H_2O$) than at the base (–2 cm $H_2O$). This vertical pleural pressure gradient is largely the effect of gravity acting upon the deformable lung in the more rigid chest wall.

Measurement of pleural pressure has been difficult in the past. Now several machines are available to facilitate in the measurement of pulmonary mechanics. These systems utilize an esophageal catheter. A specialized nasogastric tube with a balloon is placed into the esophagus at 40 cm from the incisors. The balloon is about 10 cm long. It is initially filled with 8 mL of air, then all but 0.5–1.5 mL is extracted. The catheter is attached to the pressure transducer. Pressure measurements are esophageal pressure below the

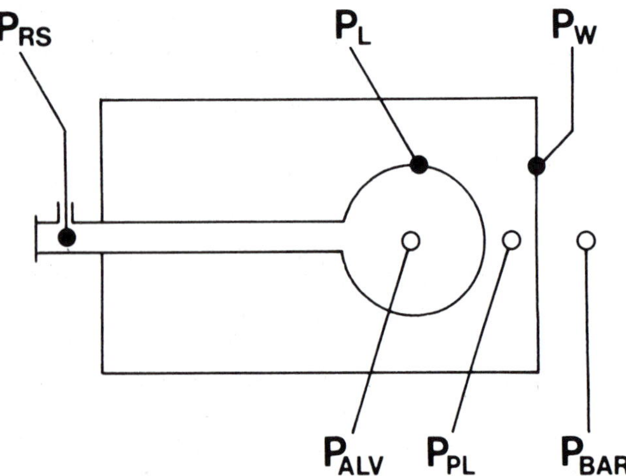


**Figure 30–1.** Mechanical representation of the respiratory system. $P_{RS}$ is total respiratory system pressure; $P_L$, lung pressure; $P_W$, chest wall pressure; $P_{ALV}$, alveolar pressure; $P_{PL}$, pleural pressure; $P_{BAR}$, barometric pressure.

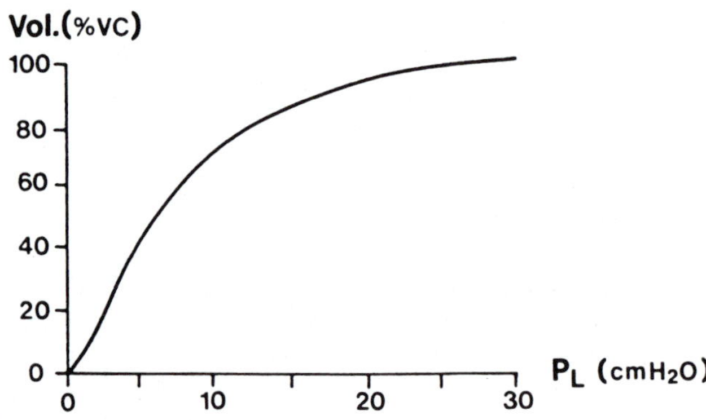


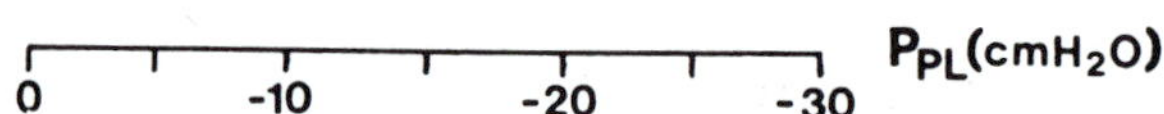


**Figure 30–2.** Static pressure–volume curve of the lung. VC is vital capacity; $P_L$, lung pressure; $P_{PL}$, pleural pressure.

trachea. These track pleural pressure accurately. To get the pleural pressure precisely, airway pressure is measured simultaneously. Pleural pressure is the difference between airway pressure and esophageal pressure.

### *Pressure Changes in Disease*

Several known factors can change pleural pressure. For example, an increase in lung elastic recoil, which in turn decreases the pleural pressure, is seen with interstitial disease, pulmonary edema, atelectasis, or postpulmonary resection. An increase in airway resistance as seen in chronic obstructive lung disease, bronchial stricture, or partially obstructed endotracheal tube results in more negative intrapleural pressure during inspiration.

### *Fluid Movements*

Although pleural pressures are constantly negative, only a small amount of fluid (8–10 mL) is normally present in the pleural space (Table 30–1). Pleural fluid is continuously produced and reabsorbed. However, the rate of turnover is controversial. In humans the reported absorption rates range from 200 to 1000 mL in 24 hours.

In the pleural space the hydrostatic pressure is approximately –5 cm $H_2O$. The oncotic pressure, which corresponds to a protein content of 10 g/L, is 4 cm $H_2O$. Since the parietal pleura is entirely tributary to the systemic circulation, the capillary hydrostatic pressure is high at 26 cm $H_2O$, while the oncotic pressure equals 29 cm $H_2O$ with normal blood protein contents. The net balance of 8 cm $H_2O$ positive pressure favors fluid movement toward the pleural space (Fig. 30–3).

Because of its venous drainage into the pulmonary circulation, the visceral pleural capillary hydrostatic pressure of 12 cm $H_2O$ is lower than that of the parietal pleura. However, other pressure parameters are constant. This results in an effective pressure gradient of –6 cm $H_2O$, which allows the visceral pleura to reabsorb the fluid secreted by the parietal pleura.

The lymphatic system, particularly that of the parietal pleura plays an important role in the reabsorption of excess pleural fluid and proteins. For example, fluid filtration by the Starling equation would tend to concentrate proteins in the pleural fluid. But, because of parietal pleural lymphatic reabsorption of protein, this does not occur.

**TABLE 30–1. COMPOSITION OF NORMAL PLEURAL FLUID**

| | | |
|---|---|---|
| Volume: | 0.1–0.2 mL/kg | |
| Protein: | 10–20 g/L | |
| Albumin: | 50–70% | |
| Glucose: | As in plasma | |
| LDH: | ≤50% of plasma level | |
| Cells/mm$^3$: | 1000–5000 | |
| Mesothelial cells: | | 3–70% |
| Monocytes: | | 30–70% |
| Lymphocytes: | | 2–30% |
| Granulocytes: | | 10% |
| pH: | >7.60 | |

## INVESTIGATION OF THE PLEURAL SPACE

### Radiologic Evaluation

Roentgenograms of the chest remain the best first-line evaluation of the pleura. Plain roentgenograms are sufficient for pneumothorax and occasionally point to the cause of symptoms and to the etiology of pleural effusions. Shifts in the mediastinum can be diagnosed. Often other findings such as atelectasis, pneumonia, and sometimes bronchial occlusion can be discerned by this simple study. Computed tomography (CT) scans can be of help in delineating parenchymal pathology but are not very sensitive in determining pleural pathology. A magnetic resonance imaging (MRI) scan may be more helpful in evaluating tumors of the chest wall that may involve the pleura.

### Thoracentesis

For pleural effusions, thoracentesis is the least invasive and often the simplest diagnostic tool in the diagnosis of pleural diseases.[3] It may be performed in the outpatient setting with a minimum of morbidity. It will differentiate between a transudate (most often benign) and an exudate (infection or malignancy) and may establish the diagnosis.

Many detailed descriptions of thoracentesis are available. Basically, a point low in the effusion is chosen by examination of the patient and the chest x-ray. This point is preferably in the ninth or tenth interspace posteriorly for a freely movable nonloculated pleural effusion. After sterile preparation and installation of a local anesthetic, a 14- or 16-gauge needle and catheter are slowly inserted above the superior border of the rib aspirating during entry. When fluid returns, the catheter is advanced and the needle retracted. A three-way stop clock facilitates the extraction of up to 1500 mL of fluid at one time.

Fluid obtained at thoracentesis should routinely be sent for hematocrit, red and white cell count, differential cell count, fluid, pH, specific gravity, total protein, lactate dehydrogenase, glucose, amylase, and specialized examination such as cytologic examination for malignancy and microbiologic stains and cultures to include the aerobic and anaerobic bacteria, fungus, and tuberculosis. Special tests such as cholesterol and triglycerides or examination for vegetable fibers may be sent when there is a high degree of suspicion for chylothorax or esophageal perforation, respectively.

In experienced hands, complications should be in the range of 1–3%.[3] Potential complications include pneumothorax, hemothorax, infection, reexpansion pulmonary edema, and hypovolemia.

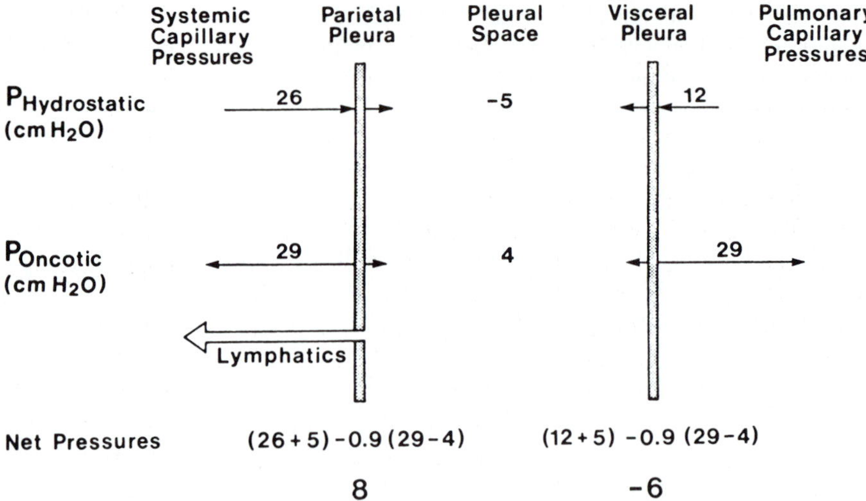


**Figure 30–3.** Fluid movement through the pleural space. Note that resulting pressures favor the formation of fluid at the level of the parietal pleura and its resorption through the visceral pleura.

### Pleural Biopsy

Needle biopsy of the pleura often accompanied thoracentesis in the past.[4] These nonspecific biopsies could enhance the diagnostic capabilities of a thoracentesis but just as often added only to the potential for complications. Lack of experience and rudimentary equipment lead to nondiagnostic biopsies yielding more chest-wall muscle and little pleura on microscopic examination. This technique, while still used occasionally, has been supplanted by the use of modern thoracoscopy.

### Thoracoscopy

Alternatively known as video-assisted thoracic surgery, thoracoscopy today has become a versatile tool. Coupling older technology with video cameras and using specifically designed equipment has sparked a resurgence in its use. It remains an excellent tool for the diagnosis and treatment of pleural diseases, which was its original application.[5] The specifics of techniques are discussed in Chapter 12.

## MANAGEMENT OF PLEURAL DISEASES

### Pneumothorax

Air entry in the pleural space always follows a breach in the continuity of the visceral pleural whether it occurs spontaneously or following trauma (Table 30–2).

#### *Primary Spontaneous Pneumothorax*

Predominately in young, healthy males, primary spontaneous pneumothorax is usually due to intrapleural rupture of a peripheral lung bleb. The pathogenesis of these blebs is unknown but seem to occur more frequently in tall, thin individuals. Theories include (1) rapid growth rate of the lung relative to the pulmonary vasculature during development, which might cause secondary bleb formation; and (2) higher transpulmonary pressures at the apex of tall individuals causing increased alveolar distending pressures.[6]

Acute pleuritic chest pain is the predominant symptom of acute pneumothorax, which may subside within 12–24 hours of onset. Physical exertion is unrelated to the occurrence of pneumothoraces. Although the extent of lung collapse is best quantified by measuring the air space defect on volume constructed CT scans, this is infrequently done and is too costly. Percentages are often assigned with little knowledge of the radiographic anatomy of the chest.[7] When one is referring to a pneumothorax, it is often best to describe it in nonspecific terms such as minimal, small, moderate, large, total, and tension pneumothorax.

**Management During the First Episode.** Patients with a small pneumothorax and minimal symptoms can be observed. Kircher and Swart[8] have shown that in such cases, air reabsorption is relatively constant at a rate of 50–75 mL/day. The gas in the pneumothorax is composed of atmospheric air. The major components and approximate percentages are nitrogen (79%), oxygen (21%), and carbon dioxide (0.05%). The carbon dioxide diffuses immediately into the surrounding tissues. The oxygen is absorbed within

**TABLE 30–2. CLASSIFICATION OF PNEUMOTHORAX**

Spontaneous pneumothorax
- Primary (no identifiable pathology)
- Secondary (chronic obstructive lung disease)
- Catamenial
- Neonatal

Traumatic pneumothorax
- Blunt or penetrating thoracic injuries
- Iatrogenic: mechanical ventilation, monitoring techniques, minor diagnostic procedures, postoperative

Diagnostic pneumothorax

short order through the lung. It is the remaining nitrogen that is absorbed slowly. Some have advocated supplemental oxygen in hopes of displacing the nitrogen with varying reports of success.

Activities should be restricted in these patients for at least 2–3 days. Indications for closed-tube drainage include a moderate-sized (>25%) pneumothorax on the first radiograph, tension pneumothorax, disease in the contralateral lung, significant persisting symptoms, or progression of the pneumothorax on successive radiographs.

Tension pneumothorax (Fig. 30–4) may require immediate life-saving action because the mediastinum shifts to the contralateral side interfering with ventilation, venous return, and cardiac output. When this diagnosis is suspected, immediate placement of a large-bore catheter is indicated even without radiographic confirmation. Once the tension is relieved, the subsequent management is similar to that of patients with uncomplicated episodes.

The presence of a pleural effusion is reported in 15–20% of patients with spontaneous pneumothorax, but significant hemothoraces (>500 mL) are uncommon. In the latter cases, the bleeding is usually arterial and secondary to a torn adhesion between the visceral and parietal pleura. The onset of hemothorax is often insidious, and the diagnosis can be further delayed if a small anterior drainage tube was initially used to evacuate the space. Grossman[9] has shown that intrapleural blood may induce a chemical pleuritis, which in turn may reduce the risk of recurrence.

Most air leaks have either sealed when the pleural space is drained or will do so within 12–24 hours following tube drainage. In approximately 3–4% of patients, however, a bronchopleural fistula will persist after drainage. Operative management should be considered in patients whose air leaks persist for >5–7 days (Table 30–3). Some have advocated even an earlier approach in order to decrease length of stay and time away from work. In other cases, the lung will only partially re-expand despite proper tube placement and adequate suction. A large bronchopleural fistula and/or trapped lung are the usual factors responsible for this problem. Management may require surgical intervention for direct closure of the fistula and/or lung decortication.

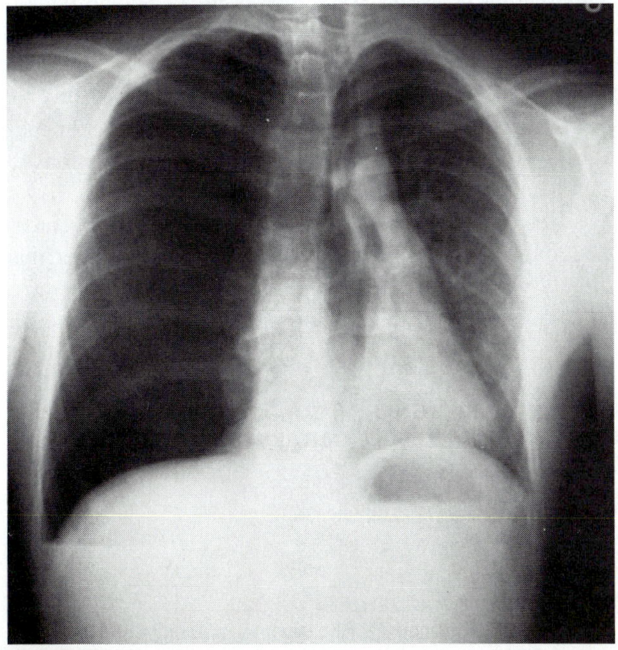

**Figure 30–4.** Tension pneumothorax. PA chest radiograph of a 19-year-old man with spontaneous right-sided spontaneous tension pneumothorax.

Bilateral spontaneous pneumothoraces are rare. Bilateral drainage is often necessary in the acute phase. Asynchronous bilateral pneumothoraces are much common and account for 5–10% of all cases. Surgical fixation of at least one side is indicated in these patients to prevent total pulmonary collapse, if there is a bilateral simultaneous recurrence.

In pregnant women, treatment should be conservative with avoidance of radiographs and surgery. It is also important that the obstetrician be notified of the possibility that a pneumothorax may occur during the trauma of delivery.

Finally, surgical intervention is indicated at the first episode in patients with large bullae, significant contralateral lung disease, or pneumonectomy; patients living in isolated areas; or patients with an occupation where a recurrence would be a significant hazard, such as airline personnel and deep sea divers.

**Principals of Tube Drainage.** The preferred site of insertion is the third or fourth intercostal space anterior axillary line. This site is not only more cosmetically acceptable (no obvious scar or danger of tube placement through breast tissue), but also the technique of insertion is easier (no chest-wall muscles to traverse) and is safer (no danger of puncturing the internal mammary artery). These tubes are directed anteriorly. An alternative placement would be a standard posterolateral tube in the fifth interspace. The technique for chest tube insertion is described in Chapter 6.

So and Yu[10] suggested that leaving the tube for a period of at least 3–4 days may induce a local inflammatory reaction that would lower the chances of recurrence. This concept is supported by the observation of Mills and Baisch[11] that there were fewer recurrences in patients

**TABLE 30–3. INDICATIONS FOR SURGICAL INTERVENTION FOR FIRST-EPISODE PNEUMOTHORAX**

| Indication |
|---|
| Persistent bronchopleural fistula (> 4 days) |
| Bilateral pneumothoraces |
| Failure to re-expand lung |
| Significant contralateral lung disease |
| Contralateral pneumectomy |
| Specialized occupation (pilot, diver) |
| Isolation from medical care |

whose oral temperature reached 38.5° developed a leukocytosis of 12,000 cells/mm$^3$ or had radiologic evidence of pleural thickening over the apex. One-way flutter valves, such as the Heimlich, enable the pleural space to be evacuated without the use of a water seal system, and outpatient management is safe, efficient, and economical.[12]

**Management of Recurrence.** About 20% of patients develop a recurrent pneumothorax, but Gobbel and associates[13] reported an increased risk in patients who have had more than one previous episode. Seventy-five percent of recurrences are ipsilateral, and most often recur within 2 years of the first episode. Risk factors include chronic obstructive lung disease, air leak for more than 48 hours during the first episode, and a large air cyst seen on chest x-ray (Table 30–4).

When a surgical procedure is required, two principles are important: removal of the offending blebs and production of pleural symphysis. The operation may be performed by axillary thoracotomy or by the video-assisted approach. The axillary thoracotomy is done through the third interspace. Almost invariably, small blebs can be seen at the apex of the lung. These are excised with a stapling device. The parietal pleura is then abraded or stripped from the endothoracic fascia starting at the level of the incision and up to the apex. A chest tube is left at the apex of the pleural space. The operation can usually be completed within 30 minutes.

The reported results for mechanical abrasion have been consistently good and have the advantage of preserving an extrapleural plane should a thoracotomy be required at a later time.[14] By doing a parietal pleurectomy, one creates an inflammatory surface with which secondary adhesions to the visceral pleura will form. Gaensler[15] noted that parietal pleurectomy produces uniform adhesions between the pleura and endothoracic fascia. He first recommended this procedure in patients with diffuse lung disease and for those with no demonstrable lesion at the time of thoracotomy. Deslauriers et al[16] described parietal pleurectomy as the operation offering the best chance to achieve permanent pleurodesis.

The average postoperative in-hospital stay for thoracotomy is 3–5 days. Most patients are able to return to normal activities within 4–6 weeks. For the video-assisted thoracic surgery procedure, most patients stay in the hospital 1–3 days and usually fully recover by 2 weeks.

Sterile talc and doxycycline (1 gram in 50 mL of 50% Dextrose in water) are the only agents still in use for chemical pleurodesis. Their main problems are their toxicity, the nonuniformity of pleural adhesions, and the variability of results. Despite these objections, experience in debilitated patients suggests that it may be effective as first-line therapy, and the American Thoracic Society has listed it as an important first-line therapy.[17] The use of talc in younger patients, particularly those with cystic fibrosis, should be discouraged, since these patients may require lung transplantation at a later date. Talc causes highly vascularized adhesions making transplantation nearly impossible to perform.

**TABLE 30–4. RISK FACTORS FOR RECURRENCE**

| | |
|---|---|
| More than one previous episode | Chronic obstructive lung disease |
| Air leak for more than 48 h during first episode | Large cysts seen on x-ray |
| (?) Nonoperative management of first episode (VS tube drainage) | |
| (?) Tube drainage for only 24 h during first episode (VS 3–4 days) | |
| (?) Leucocytosis >12,000; temp. >101°F during first episode | |

### *Secondary Spontaneous Pneumothorax*

Secondary spontaneous pneumothoraces occur predominantly in older people with documented pulmonary disease.[18] Most of these patients have chronic obstructive lung disease, although secondary pneumothoraces can also be seen in association with a variety of other pulmonary pathologies (Table 30–5). In contrast to primary pneumothoraces, the predominant presenting symptom is severe shortness of breath, which may progress to lung failure. Chest pain is almost never an important feature of the clinical presentation. All patients with secondary pneumothorax should initially be treated by intercostal tube drainage. These patients often have prolonged air leak. But because of significant operative risks, tube drainage should be considered for a longer period of time than in patients with primary pneumothorax. Virtually all air leaks will stop if the pleural space is adequately drained, if the lung is fully expanded and if the attending physician is patient. For individuals with moderate or severe emphysema, indications remain the same as those of primary pneumothorax.

The recurrence rate after one episode of secondary pneumothorax is 50%.[19] This is considerably higher than patients with primary pneumothorax. When the operative risk is satisfactory, these patients should have operative fix-

**TABLE 30–5. PULMONARY DISORDERS OFTEN ASSOCIATED WITH SECONDARY PNEUMOTHORAX**

Chronic obstructive lung disease

Tuberculosis, active or inactive

Catamenial

Miscellaneous disorders:

- Congenital: cystic fibrosis
- Endobronchial obstruction: neoplasm, foreign body
- Infection: pneumonia, lung abscess
- Diffuse disease: fibrosis, collagen, or interstitial disease
- Asthma

ation. If the operative risk is prohibitive, pleural symphysis may be accomplished with chemical sclerosants.

## Thoracic Empyema

Thoracic empyema is defined as a purulent pleural effusion or an effusion with positive bacteriologic cultures. By contrast, parapneumonic effusions are sterile collections associated with bacterial pneumonia, lung abscess, or bronchiectasis.[20] Graham and Bell[21] described the basic principles of empyema management 70 years ago that still apply today: adequate drainage of the empyema cavity with careful avoidance of pneumothorax in the early stages and early sterilization and obliteration of the infected space.

### *Pathogenesis*

While the normal pleural space is resistant to infection, the abnormal space, such as one contaminated with blood or fluid, is highly susceptible to empyema formation (Table 30–6).

Most empyemas are the result of bacterial suppuration in organs contiguous with the pleural space. The lung is the most common.[22,23] In such cases, empyema occurs by direct bacterial contamination across the visceral pleura or by free intrapleural rupture of microscopic lung abscesses into the space. Most, if not all, primary empyemas originate by contamination of a subclinical parapneumonic process (Fig. 30–5). Other potential sources of infection should be evaluated carefully when the cause of empyema is unclear, including infections in the deep posterior region of the neck, esophageal perforation, and, more infrequently, infections of the chest wall or thoracic spine. Empyema secondary to infected mediastinal nodes is a highly unusual event.

Although subphrenic abscesses can occasionally contaminate the pleural space through direct transdiaphragmatic erosion, most effusions associated with these abscesses are sterile exudates. Direct inoculation of the pleural space may occur more commonly today during minor thoracic interventions such as thoracentesis, chest tube insertion, or percutaneous drainage of perihepatic, hepatic, or biliary abscesses.

**TABLE 30–6. PATHOGENESIS OF THORACIC EMPYEMAS**

**Primary infection of the pleural space (0%)**
**Secondary infection of the pleural space (100%)**
- Contamination from a source contiguous to the pleural space (60%)
  - Lung
  - Mediastinum (esophagus, nodes)
  - Deep cervical
  - Chest wall and spine
  - Subphrenic, paracolic abscesses
- Direct innoculation in the pleural space (35–40%)
  - Minor diagnostic procedures
  - Postoperative infection
  - Penetrating chest injuries
- Hematogenous seeding in the pleural space (<1%)
  - Late postpneumonectomy empyema

Virtually all posttraumatic empyemas are associated with one of two risk factors: penetration of the chest wall or presence of a hemothorax. In the first instance, empyema formation is the result of organic foreign material that is carried into the pleural space.[24] In the second instance, the hemothorax becomes secondarily infected, usually due to contamination from the chest tube or from adjacent infected lung. It has been shown that hemopneumothorax is more likely to become infected secondarily than a pneumothorax or a hemothorax alone.[25] In rare instances, traumatic empyemas will follow blunt esophageal rupture or acute diaphragmatic hernia with bowel strangulation and/or necrosis.

Other than the unusual event of late postpneumonectomy empyema, there is very little evidence that hematogenous bacterial seeding of the pleural space occurs.

### *Stages of Disease*

Three distinct stages are indicative of disease progression within the pleural space.

The preempyema phase (stage I) is often called a parapneumonic effusion. There is considerable swelling of the pleural membranes with outpouring of exudative fluid. Fibrin is deposited over all surfaces, but the material is not thickened enough to prevent complete reexpansion of the lung once the space is emptied.

In the fibrinopurulent phase (stage II), bacterial invasion is added to this inflammatory process. There are heavy fibrin deposits over all of the pleural surfaces, and some degree of lung entrapment occurs. The pleural fluid has a positive bacteriology or becomes grossly purulent.

During the chronic phase (stage III), there is massive ingrowth of fibroblasts and neocapillaries. The lung is imprisoned within a thick fibroptic peel and is virtually functionless. It can no longer expand even if the space is emptied.

Although complications may occur at any time, they are more likely to develop during the chronic phase of the disease. Empyema necessitatis (Fig. 30–6) is characterized by the dissection of pus through the soft tissues of the chest wall eventually eroding through the skin. More rarely seen complications include rib or spine osteomyelitis, pericarditis, mediastinal abscess formation, or transdiaphragmatic rupture of the empyema into the peritoneal cavity.

### *Diagnosis*

The possibility of empyema should always be raised in the presence of an acute illness with an associated pleural effusion. Typical symptoms such as fever or local tenderness are often present. LeRoux et al[26] noted that empyemas are nearly always posterior and lateral and that most extend to the diaphragm early in the acute phase. Radiologically,

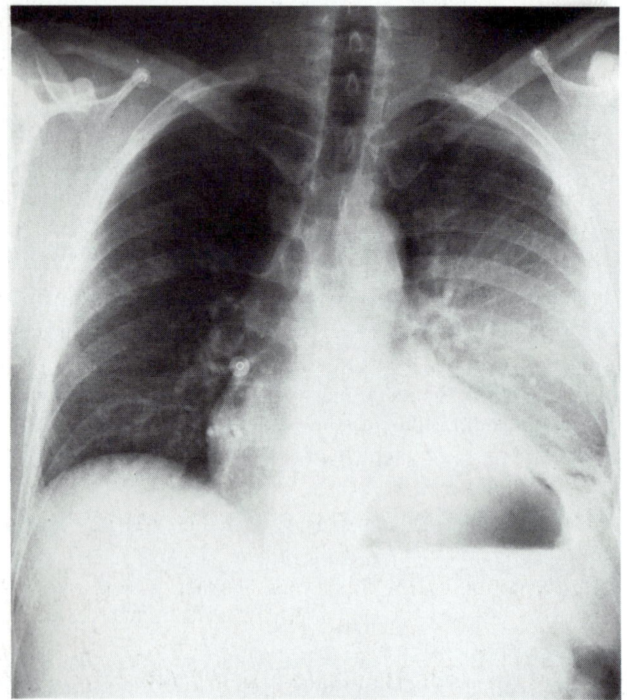

A

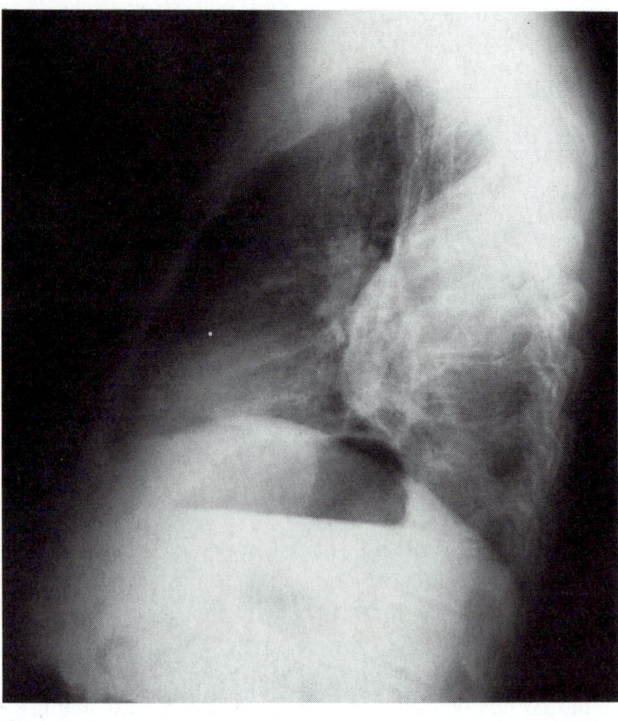

B

**Figure 30–5.** Empyema secondary to pyogenic pneumonia. PA **(A)** and lateral **(B)** chest radiograph of a 53-year-old patient with parapneumonic empyema. Note the typical image of a posteriorly located inverted D-spaced density.

theclassic image is that of a posteriorly located, inverted D-shaped density seen on the lateral chest film.

The initial step in evaluation is to document the presence of fluid in the pleural space. This is best accomplished by ultrasonography, which can distinguish between pleural fluid and parenchymal consultation or pleural thickening. Once the presence of fluid has been confirmed, thoracentesis should be carried out.

Orringer[27] noted that gross appearance and odor of the pleural fluid are among the most significant items of information obtainable by thoracentesis. Thin fluid, even with positive bacteriology, may respond to selective antibiotics and therapeutic thoracentesis.

The aspirated fluid should be sent for Gram's stain, aerobic and anaerobic cultures, and antibiotic sensitivity. Studies have shown that penicillin-resistant *Staphycoccus aureus,* gram-negative bacteria, and anaerobic organisms are the most common agents found in empyemas. Bartlett and associates[28] found that 76% of empyema patients had either anaerobic bacteria alone or in combination with aerobic bacteria. A more recent survey performed by Alfageme and colleagues[29] noted only a 31% anaerobic participation. They also noted 43% of all empyemas were polymicrobial, averaging 2.63 kinds of organisms per infection.

Pleural effusions with low fluid pH (<7), low glucose, (<50 mg/dL), and high LDH contents (>1000 IU/L) should be drained because these parameters indicate a complex effusion and/or an impending empyema.[20,30] These changes can be discerned before organisms are found on gram stain or culture. Physiologically, these values are explained by an increase in leukocyte activity and acid production in the pleural fluid. Patients who are immunocompromised may not have these findings in the pleural fluid, yet should be treated aggressively.

### *Management of Empyema*

Four basic principles apply to the management of all forms of empyema: (1) drainage of the collection, (2) obliteration of the space, (3) investigation and treatment of the underlying infection, (4) treatment of the associated intercurrent medical conditions. In stage I this can often be accomplished by the use of nonoperative interventions (Table 30–7). Stage II may require thoracoscopy or thoracotomy with empyemectomy and/or decortication. Less invasive measures such as thoracentesis or tube thoracostomy may play a role in special circumstances. Stage III mature empyema nearly always requires a surgical procedure, particularly to achieve obliteration of the empyema space. These techniques will be considered in order of complexity.

**Thoracentesis.** Although it is of limited use, thoracentesis with complete evacuation of the pleural space may be effective in early free flowing parapneumonic effusions (stage I disease).[31] This technique, along with antibiotics, is often the best therapy in children or in patients deemed incapable of coping with a chest tube. Such patients must be followed

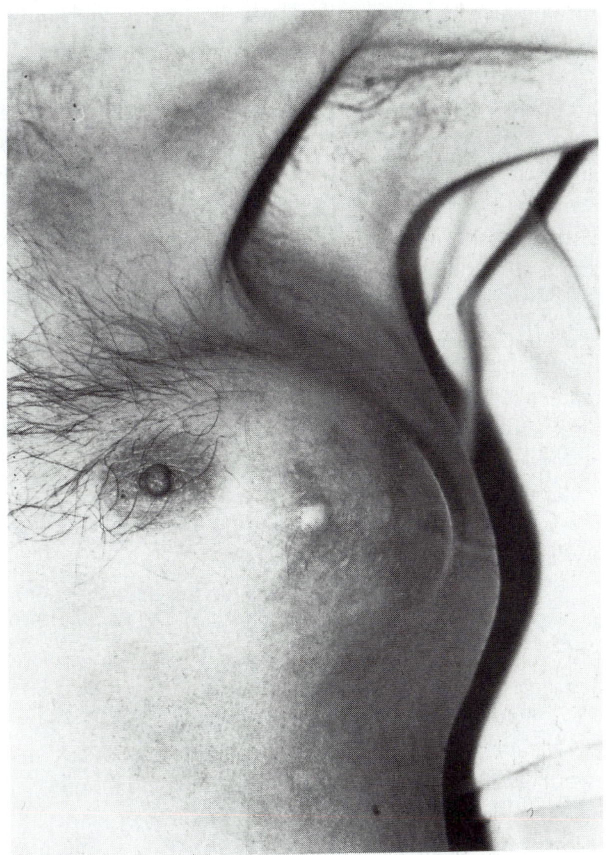

**Figure 30–6.** Empyema necessitatis. Photograph of a 54-year-old man with empyema necessitatis eroding through the soft tissues of the chest wall.

closely with frequent (at least every other day) chest radiographs to monitor the hemithorax for reaccumulation of fluid. Repeat thoracentesis is often not successful, and more aggressive measures may be required.

**Tube Drainage.** Closed tube thoracostomy is currently the most common management of empyema management.[32] Even in cases of late stage II and early stage III empyemas, it is appropriate as a first step to drain the purulent collection and stabilize the patient. Since the fluid is likely to be thick and full of protein, it is best to choose a large-caliber tube, such as a 32 French or larger. It should be placed low and directed posteriorly in the chest to establish dependent drainage. If radiographs such as decubitus films suggest that the fluid is loculated, tubes should be placed near the inferior border of the collection. Ultrasonography is helpful in delineating this location. Digital exploration should always be performed to assess the stage of the empyema and to break up early loculations within the fluid.

**TABLE 30–7. PRINCIPLES OF EMPYEMA MANAGEMENT**

| |
|---|
| Complete drainage of purulent collection |
| Obliteration of empyema space |
| Investigation and treatment of underlying infection |
| Management of associated conditions |

The primary goal of tube drainage is prompt removal of the empyema fluid with expansion of the lung. The tube should be initially attached to suction and, if the lung expands, left in place until the patient is afebrile for 48 hours and the drainage falls to below 50 mL/day. After the initial 48 hours, suction is not as important, and the tube may be placed on water seal or attached to a one-way valve and a drainage bag to allow the patient to ambulate.

Image-guided catheter drainage of empyemas has met with limited successes, and isolated reports continue to appear in the literature.[33,34] This technique seems to work in highly selected patients and should be reserved for those cases where the patient is severely debilitated, has multiple medical problems, or there is a small isolated pocket in an area anatomically difficult to drain with a larger tube.

**Decortication.** Late stage II and stage III empyemas are always associated with a fibrin coating over the visceral pleura. This thick covering becomes firm and does not permit the pliable lung to re-expand. If left alone, this becomes infiltrated with fibroblasts that form a dense scar intimately attached to the lung. The goal of decortication is to peel away this deposit and allow the lung to re-expand, satisfying the second principal of empyema management. Many centers now advocate an early aggressive approach to empyemas as soon as it is evident that tube thoracostomy is ineffective.[35,36] Successful management using decortication will often decrease hospital stay and improve pulmonary function sooner than conservative management. Initial operative approach may be thoracoscopy or open thoracotomy.[37,38] In general, the approach should be adjusted so that the empyema cavity may be entered directly. This usually means an incision between the fifth and eighth interspace. The loose material is evacuated and the parenchymal peel inspected. A thick firm fibrous covering may be difficult to remove without severe parenchymal damage. One should incise the covering and attempt to enter the plane between the abnormal tissue and the visceral pleura. Often visceral pleura is intimately attached and must be stripped away along with the fibrin. Enough of this deposit must be removed to allow complete re-expansion of the lung. The parietal pleura may also need to be stripped to remove a large amount of purulent material. Particular attention should be directed at the diaphragm, which can be trapped in the same process, preventing normal function. If the rind is too adherent to allow safe removal without significant damage to the underlying lung, other strategies such as open drainage, thoracoplasty, or muscle interpositions should be considered.

**Open Drainage.** Often at the time of chest tube placement and discovery of a space problem, a determination can be made about the potential effectiveness of decortication. In cases where decortication may be too hazardous, open drainage may be the best approach.[39,40] This may be accomplished by either tube drainage or rib resection.

If the chest tube is in a dependent portion (inferior and/or posterior at the border of the empyema), it may be used as the open drainage tube. If it is not, another tube should be placed. The tube should be disconnected from closed suction apparatus and covered with a sterile gauze pad. A chest roentgenogram obtained several hours later should confirm that no pneumothorax has occurred. Once this is established, the tube may be attached to a collection bag or cut to fit a customized stoma drainage bag.

For large or unusually located collections such as posterior cavities, open drainage is best established by rib resection (Fig. 30–7). We prefer to resect approximately 10 cm of two ribs with preservation of the intercostal bundles. The incision is made in the interspace between the two ribs, and periosteal removal of the ribs is accomplished. The skin is then sewn to the thickened pleura to "marsupialize" the opening (Fig. 30–8). The advantage of such a drainage procedure is that the patient's incision becomes painless within a few days, and the hole is large enough to allow easy inspection and mechanical debridement. The patient or the family can then be taught to use a hand-held shower head to irrigate this space.

With either method, progress is slow, but healing will usually occur within 3–6 months. The operative opening will contract and eventually leave the patient with only a small cosmetic defect.

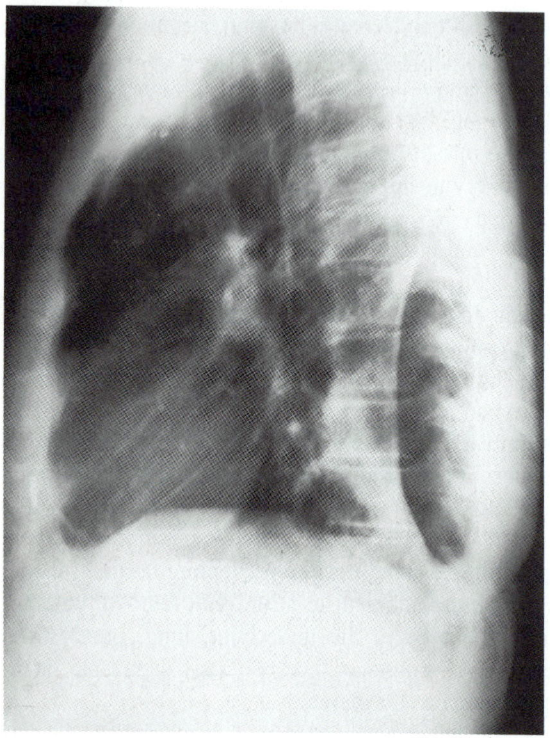

**Figure 30–7.** Lateral radiograph of patient with a posterior-loculated empyema following coronary artery bypass grafting. This was treated with open drainage. Note the markedly thickened visceral pleural peel on the empyema cavity.

**Complex Management.** Both because of the widespread use of outpatient antibiotics and the desire of patients and primary care physicians to withhold consultations, there seems to be a rise in the number of patients presenting with late stage III empyema. These patients may have diverse symptoms such as shortness of breath related to decreased vital capacity or chest-wall pain related to empyema necessitatis. They may or may not present with fever or systemic signs of bacteremia. In these individuals, preoperative assessment will point to the maturity of the fibrothorax. Chronicity alone may give a clue to the maturity of the fibrothorax. Patients whose pleural symptoms are over 4 weeks old are more likely to have a dense fibrothorax. This corresponds with the fibroblast ingrowth and fibrosis phase of wound healing.

A CT scan may be helpful in showing the loculated nature of the empyema. These signs include a cavity filled with a substance of multiple densities. The borders are often hyperdense indicating a thick, solid, and possibly fibrous layer against the lung.

Patients with complex, mature empyemas still must have the purulent material removed, but obliteration of the space by decortication may be impossible or dangerous. Other means must be found. If the space is in the upper chest or involves the apex of the lung, a thoracoplasty may be the best solution. This is described in Chapter 31. If the space is in the lower chest or associated with a bronchopleural fistula, a muscle transposition may work best. This is also described in Chapter 31. In special cases such as postpneumonectomy empyema, an intermediate step known as a Clagett procedure may provide long lasting results.

Clagett and Geraci[41] in 1963 reported a technique of space sterilization for a postpneumonectomy empyema. In this technique, an open-window thoracostomy is done. The space is irrigated daily for 4–8 weeks. When the space is considered clean and sterile, the patient is given a general anesthetic, and the window is closed in layers. Prior to closure of the window, the space is filled with antibiotic solution. Reported success rate with this procedure has varied over the years.[42,43] The best results are in patients without a bronchopleural fistula. When a fistula is present, the success rate is very low, in the range of 5–10%.

**Lytic Agents.** With the surging emphasis on less invasive techniques, interest in the use of lytic agents instilled within the pleural cavity again are being considered. Introduced in 1950 by Tillet and Sherry,[44] this treatment lost favor because these early preparations lacked purity and antibiotics and surgical techniques improved. Within the last few years, several small series have reported limited success in dissolution of the loculations and presumably the pleural fibrotic peel.[45,46] Streptokinase is the best agent and is used

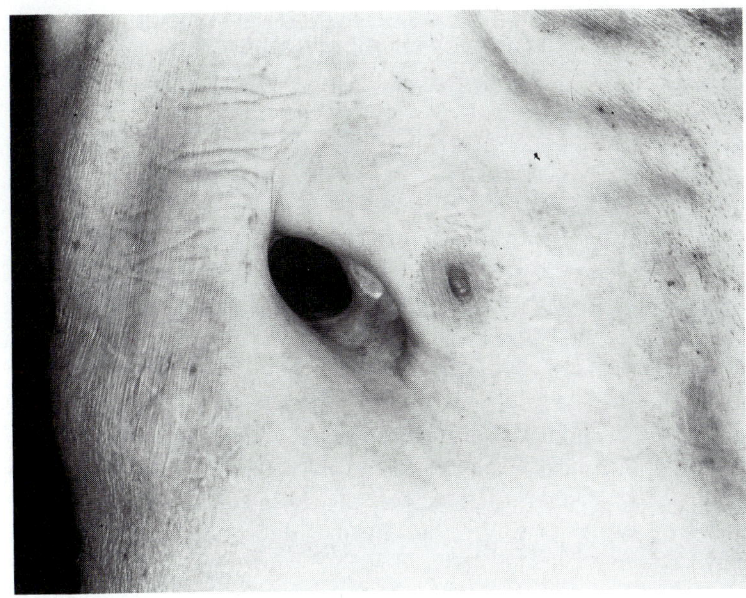

**Figure 30–8.** Management of chronic empyema, open-window thoracostomy. Photograph of a patient with an open thoracic window created for drainage of a postpneumonectomy empyema.

in a mixture of 250,000 U with 100 mL of normal saline. This is instilled through the chest tube, which is clamped for several hours. This process is repeated daily for up to 2 weeks. This can be done with minimal systemic absorption or toxity. Success rates in the selected series can be as high as 90%.[46]

**Outcome.** As a rule, the earlier the empyema is recognized and treated, the better the results. For all stages, mortality rate may be as high as 10% in healthy patients and 50% in elderly or debilitated patients.[47]

## Pleural Neoplasms

### *Malignant Pleural Effusion*

Of all pleural effusions seen at a general hospital, 20–50% are malignant.[48] Most of these are associated with advanced lung or breast cancers. Malignant effusions occasionally can be secondary to pleural metastasis from ovarian, genitourinary, or gastrointestinal primary malignancies. Much less common are effusions from mesotheliomas, metastatic sarcomas, or lymphomas. Malignant effusions quite often are the first indication of a malignancy.[49]

**Pathophysiology.** Malignant effusions are always secondary to a disturbance in the dynamic equilibrium between production and reabsorption of pleural fluid. Local inflammation and increased capillary permeability are associated with tumor implants. This increases fluid transudation. Lymphatic obstruction with cancer often impairs reabsorption. When the pulmonary vein is obstructed, the gradient between the visceral and parietal pleura disappears, also contributing to effusion.

Paraneoplastic effusions are associated with malignancies but do not contain malignant cells. Most are due to lymphatic obstruction causing decreased absorption or are sympathetic effusions in response to obstructive atelectasis.

**Fluid Characteristics.** The gross appearance of malignant pleural fluid is nonspecific. Nearly all malignant effusions are exudates with high protein and LDH contents (Table 30–8). Bloody effusion strongly suggests an underlying malignancy. Light and Ball[50] noted that amylase levels >160 U may suggest an underlying primary bronchogenic cancer.

The presumptive diagnosis of malignant pleural effusion must always be substantiated by the cytologic and/or histopathologic data. Salyer and colleagues[51] noted that the combination of cytology and pleural biopsy will establish the diagnosis in up to 90% of patients. Thoracoscopy is indicated when studies of the pleural fluid and needle pleural biopsies have not confirmed the diagnosis. In fact, thoracoscopy has rapidly becoming the procedure of choice for simultaneous diagnosis and management. It can establish the diagnosis in 95% of cases.

**TABLE 30–8. CHARACTERISTICS OF PLEURAL FLUID IN MALIGNANT EFFUSIONS**

| | |
|---|---|
| Gross appearance: | Often nonspecific<br>Can be bloody or milky |
| Biochemistry: | Exudate with high protein (>3 g/dL) and LDH (>200 U) contents<br>Low pH (<7.3) and glucose (<60 mg/dL)<br>High amylase (>160 U) |
| Pathology: | Positive cytology and histology |
| Miscellaneous: | Positive chromosomal examination<br>High CEA (>20 mg/dL) content |

**Management.** The overall plan should take into account the site and histology of the primary tumor, the symptomatology of the patient, and the overall medical status of the individual. Expected length of survival is also important in determination of the therapy. The goal of therapy should always be permanent symptom relief with a minimum of morbidity, particularly in those patients with short life expectancies.

Although, cure would be the ideal therapeutic option, this is not always possible or desirable. Many of these patients are debilitated or have significant impairment secondary to metastatic disease elsewhere. Under these circumstances, palliation is the pragmatic goal. The definition of palliation is relief of symptoms. In terms of pleural effusions, this is relatively easy to measure. Nearly all of these patients experience dyspnea, often at rest. Some experience chest pain. Complete and permanent removal of the effusion will give the optimal result. However, since parenchymal involvement may also produce a decrease in vital capacity, some patients with this associated problem may not experience complete return to normalcy. Whatever therapy is chosen, the quality of life should be maintained or improved. For any complicated procedure, there should be minimal morbidity and hospitalization. Postprocedure follow-up likewise should require minimal intensity.

Several therapeutic options are available: (1) pleurectomy, (2) mechanical pleurodesis, (3) talc poudrage, (4) pleuroperitoneal shunt, and (5) tube thoracostomy and sclerosis.

The most invasive method would be pleurectomy. Although quite effective, significant metastatic pleural involvement often leads to major blood loss and moderate-to-severe pain caused by the thoracotomy.

At the other end of the spectrum are tube thoracostomy and chemical sclerosis. Because these chemical agents work best at high concentrations, tubes are traditionally left until the daily output decreases below an arbitrary number between 3 and 5 mL/kg per day. This time interval varies from patient to patient and may require as little as 1 day or as long as 2 weeks. Since these agents work by producing an intense pleural reaction that eventually results in visceral and parietal fusion, apposition of these two surfaces is essential. Thus, after installation of the sclerosing agent, tubes usually remain in place for an additional 48 hours. Although shorter regimens are used, this gives the best chance for adequate pleurodesis. This leads to a hospital stay of a minimum of 5 days.

The agents available for sclerosis have varying success rates (Table 30–9). The range of success among the sclerosing agents is great.[52] In some cases, agents are no longer available for use, such as tetracycline. Other agents have significant side effects making them less desirable. Webb and colleagues[53] described a method of instilling talc suspension through the chest tube that gave excellent short-term results. Daniel and colleagues[54] have recently reported a similar series using thoracoscopy. Five grams of talc should be suspended in 100 mL of saline. Sterile talc is not presently available in the United States; our protocol is to dry and sterilize the talc in widemouthed jars suitable for crimp tops. Vials are filled with 5-g aliquots of asbestos free talc and sterilized at 150° for 4 hours. All jars except one are closed. The talc from that jar undergoes microbiologic and pyrogen testing. The batch should be rechecked quarterly for sterility. The mixture must be agitated just prior to installation to ensure that the talc enters the chest and does not stay in the syringe. The chest tube should be clamped for 1–2 hours to allow the talc to distribute and settle out in the chest. Although this has a reasonable success rate, photographs from the report of Webb et al[53] demonstrate that the talc may clump, leading to accumulation of fluid in loculated spaces.

**TABLE 30–9. MALIGNANT PLEURAL EFFUSIONS: SUCCESS RATE OF CHEMICAL SCLEROSANTS**

| | % | |
|---|---|---|
| Agent | Success Range | Mean |
| Quinacrine | 64–100 | 86 |
| Mustard | 7–85 | 44 |
| Radioisotopes | 28–80 | 56 |
| Bleomycin | 60–85 | 71 |
| Tetracycline | 25–100 | 69 |
| Talc | 72–100 | 96 |

Pleuroperitoneal shunts have been proposed as an alternative therapeutic method in the continued management of patients with malignant pleural effusion.[55] However, patient compliance is low, since the reservoir chamber is only 2 mL, and the patients must pump the shunt a minimum of 400 times per day.

Video-assisted procedures offer an excellent alternative to these approaches.[56] They can be performed with a shorter hospital stay, which eliminates the up-front waiting period for the fluid to decrease in amount. They can be performed under local or general anesthesia. All of the pleural fluid can be completely drained and the pleural cavity inspected for adhesions. By lysing adhesions, the surgeon can eliminate loculated pockets of fluid. Pleurodesis may then be accomplished by with a wide variety of methods, including pleurectomy, mechanical pleural abrasion, and talc poudrage. All of these methods have been performed using the video-assisted technique.

### Mesothelioma

Mesotheliomas are uncommon mesodermal neoplasms classified into three main tumor groups: (1) benign localized mesotheliomas, (2) malignant localized or fibrous sarcomatous mesotheliomas, and (3) malignant epithelial or diffuse mesotheliomas.

**Benign Localized Mesotheliomas.** Although recognized over a century ago, benign localized mesotheliomas have a confusing terminology.[57] Synonymous names include fibrous mesotheliomas, pleural fibroma, and localized fibrous mesotheliomas.

In contrast to the diffuse variety, benign localized mesotheliomas are unassociated with asbestos exposure.[58] They are usually asymptomatic and detected on routine chest radiographs. Extrathoracic manifestations such as pulmonary osteoarthropathy, fever, or hyperglycemia occur in one third of patients. These peraneoplastic syndromes are strong indicators of benignancy. Most benign localized mesotheliomas arise from the visceral pleura and are well-encapsulated dedunculated masses (Fig. 30–9). Unless the resection is incomplete, surgical removal is always curative.[59]

**Malignant Localized Mesotheliomas.** Twenty percent of all primary malignant pleural tumors are localized. They often present as symptomatic masses and may be difficult to differentiate from primary chest-wall neoplasms. Proper management of such tumors must include wide enbloc excision of all involved tissue including lung, chest wall, soft tissues, and skin, wherever necessary. When surgical resection is incomplete, the prognosis is poor.[60] Adjuvant therapy, such as external beam radiation or interstitial implantation of radioisotopes, is of little value.

**Malignant Diffuse Mesotheliomas.** The reported incidence of diffuse malignant mesotheliomas ranges from 0.8 to 2.1 new cases/million per year. The association between malignant diffuse mesothelioma and asbestos exposure was first suggested by Wagner and colleagues,[61] who observed a large number of cases in South Africa in asbestos mine workers. They noted that the latent period between exposure and tumor development averaged 20 years. They also showed that the intensity of exposure may be more important than its duration. Other than direct exposure to asbestos fibers, there is some evidence that mesotheliomas are more common among people living in areas surrounding asbestos plants and in relatives of asbestos workers. Although smoking is not a risk factor for mesothelioma, it does contribute to diminishing the patient's overall condition.

### *Diagnosis and Staging*

The majority of malignant mesothelioma patients are middle-aged men presenting with pleuritic chest pain and/or shortness of breath. Most have a clear history of asbestos exposure. Chest roentgenograms will show pleural effusion and pleural thickening often associated with calcifications (Fig. 30–10).

Because pleural fluid cytology is difficult to interpret, the diagnosis of diffuse mesothelioma should always be substantiated by larger biopsy specimens. Special stains, immunohistochemical techniques, and electron microscopy must be requested routinely on these specimens.

Malignant mesothelioma encompasses three main types: epithelial type accounting for 50% of all mesotheliomas, mesenchymal (16%), and mixed (34%).[62] The epithelial type is most often confused with adenocarcinoma. Extensive investigations comparing mesothelioma with metastatic adenocarcinoma now make it relatively easier to separate these two entities. Both stain positive for periodic schiff stain, but mesothelioma digested with diastose become negative while adenocarcinomas remain positive. The major difference on immunohistochemical staining. Adenocarcinomas differentially stain positive for CEA, B72.3, Lew M1, 44-36A, and 624A12, while mesotheliomas are

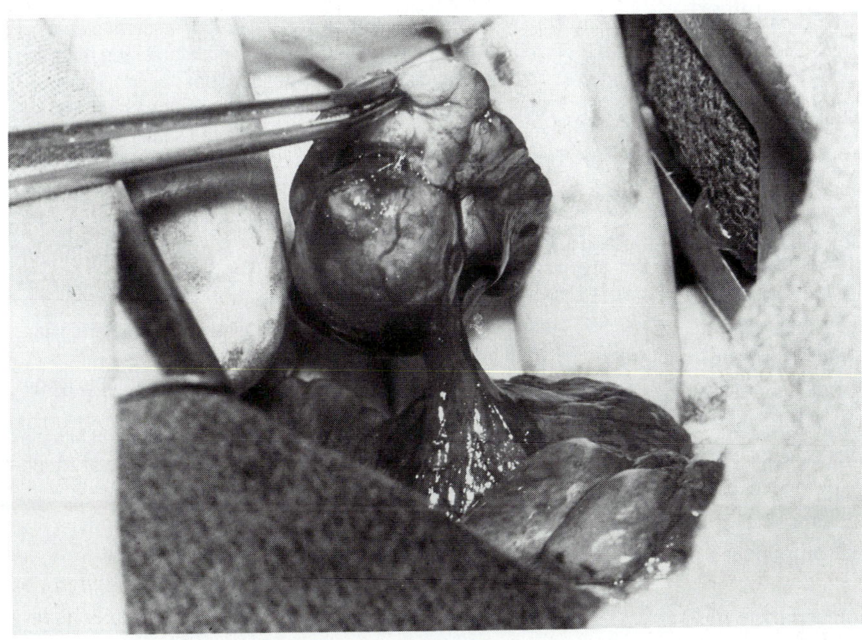

**Figure 30–9.** Benign localized fibrous mesothelioma. Operative photograph showing a typically well-encapsulated and lobulated benign pleural neoplasm. Note that the tumor originates from the visceral pleura (left upper lobe).

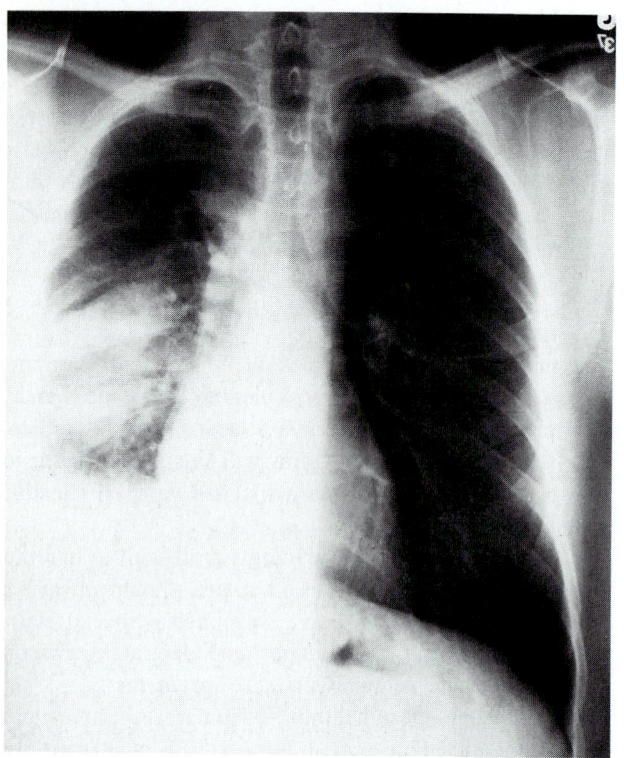

A

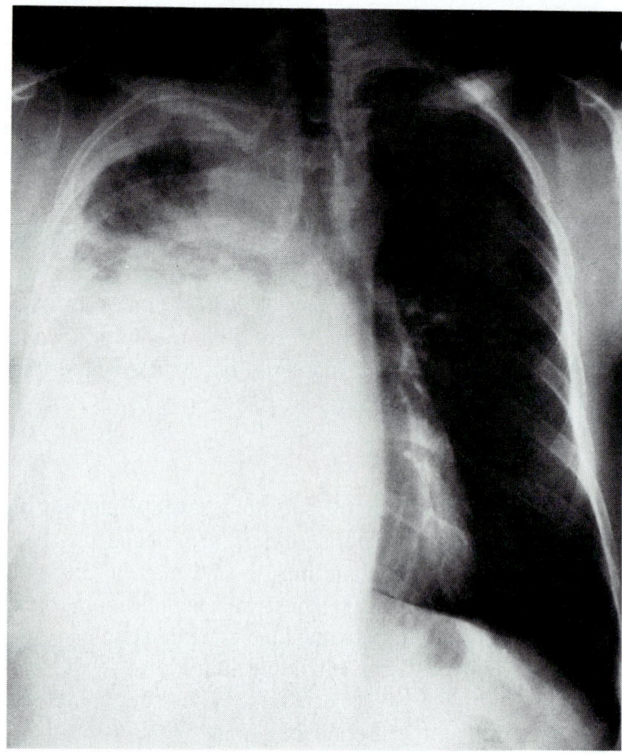

B

**Figure 30–10.** Diffuse mesothelioma. **A.** PA chest radiograph of a 23-year-old patient with diffuse mesothelioma presenting as pleural thickening. **B.** Chest radiograph taken 6 months later and showing considerable progression of the disease.

positive for MS, a human mesothelioma cell line.[63] Electron microscopy may also be helpful. Mesotheliomas have longer microvilli and more prominent desmosomes than adenocarcinomas. They also have a different distribution of intracellular organelles.

As with other cancers, staging has become an important issue in mesothelioma. Tables 30–10 and 30–11 list the American Cancer Society staging schema.[64] Stage I denotes limited stage disease, while stages II–IV denote extensive or metastatic disease.

### *Therapy*

The median survival of patients with a diagnosis of diffuse malignant mesothelioma is 6–14 months, with most patients ultimately dying of local complications rather than distant disease. Accepted therapeutic modalities range from supportive care only to pleurectomy with or without radical extrapleural pneumonectomy.

Because all reported treatment modalities are not very satisfactory, many physicians believe that supportive care remains the best form of therapy. One of the most useful techniques has been sclerosis for the effusion component of the disease.

Subtotal pleurectomy with gross tumor removal has

**TABLE 30–10. PLEURAL MESOTHELIOMA TNM CLASSIFICATION**

| | |
|---|---|
| **Primary Tumor (T)** | |
| T1 | Tumor limited to ipsilateral parietal and/or visceral pleura |
| T2 | Tumor invades any of the following: ipsilateral lung, endothoracic fascia, diaphragm, or pericardium |
| T3 | Tumor invades any of the following: ipsilateral chest wall muscle, ribs, or mediastinal organs or tissues |
| T4 | Tumor directly extends to any of the following: contralateral pleura, lung, peritoneum, intra-abdominal organs, or cervical tissues |
| **Regional Lymph Nodes (N)** | |
| NX | Regional lymph nodes cannot be assessed |
| N0 | No regional lymph node metastasis |
| N1 | Metastasis in ipsilateral peribronchial and/or ipsilateral hilar lymph nodes, including direct extension |
| N2 | Metastasis in ipsilateral mediastinal and/or subcarinal lymph node(s) |
| N3 | Metastasis in contralateral mediastinal, contralateral hilar, ipsilateral or contralateral scalene, or supraclavicular lymph node(s) |
| **Distant Metastasis (M)** | |
| MX | Distant metastasis cannot be assessed |
| M0 | No evidence of distant metastasis |
| M1 | Distant metastasis |

**TABLE 30–11. PLEURAL MESOTHELIOMA: STAGE GROUPING**

| | | | |
|---|---|---|---|
| Stage I | T1 | N0 | M0 |
| | T2 | N0 | M0 |
| Stage II | T1 | N1 | M0 |
| | T2 | N1 | M0 |
| Stage III | T1 | N2 | M0 |
| | T2 | N2 | M0 |
| | T3 | N0 | M0 |
| | T3 | N1 | M0 |
| | T3 | N2 | M0 |
| Stage IV | Any T | N3 | M0 |
| | T4 | Any N | M0 |
| | Any T | Any N | M1 |

been promoted by Memorial Sloan-Kettering Cancer Center.[65] The operation can be done with a low operative mortality and has the advantage of preserving the lung and diaphragm. In addition, it nearly always controls the recurrence of pleural effusions. Residual disease over the diaphragm is treated with radioisotope implants and external beam radiation given 4–6 weeks postoperatively. With these modalities, McCormick and Martini[59] have been able to extend the 1-year survival to 60% and the median survival to 21 months. Rusch[66] has added intrapleural chemotherapy with similar encouraging results.

Radical surgery in the form of extrapleural pneumonectomy was first recommended by Eiselberg[67] in 1992. This procedure involved en bloc removal of the parietal pleura and its contents, including the lung, the mediastinal pleura, the pericardium, and the diaphragm. The diaphragm and pericardium must be reconstructed with synthetic material. Table 30–12 gives the results for pneumonectomy for malignant mesothelioma.[68–71] Until the recent series, the results have been dismal with a high operative mortality rate and the low long-term survival rate. Sugarbaker and associates[71] have limited the operative mortality and have a seeming improvement in 2-year survival but note that patients with stage II or more advanced disease have a significantly low survival rate.

Despite the availability of new techniques, such as megavoltage beam radiation and computerized dosimetry, complete eradication of the tumor is nearly impossible, and survival rates have yet to be documented.[72]

The role of adjuvant chemotherapy remains unclear. Earlier reports on the use of doxorubicin as a single agent raised some hope, but subsequent reports did not confirm those encouraging early results.[73,74] New and innovative approaches are being pioneered at the National Institutes of Health by Pass and colleagues,[75,76] who are evaluating adjuvantive photodynamic therapy and gene manipulation.

## Chylothorax

Obstruction of the thoracic duct or injury to this structure can cause chylothorax. This condition is rare but remains a treatable condition.

### *Anatomy of the Thoracic Duct*

The thoracic duct originates in the abdomen as a single efferent trunk of the cisterna chyli, a lymphatic dilation located anterior to the vertebral bodies of the last thoracic and first two lumbar vertebras.[77] It ascends into the right posterior mediastinum through the aortic hiatus of the diaphragm. It then extends extrapleurally along the vertebral column between the azygos vein and the descending aorta and behind the esophagus. At approximately the tracheal bifurcation, it crosses the midline to the left, where it is located behind the aortic arch and to the left of the esophagus. After entering the neck, it arches laterally at the seventh cervical vertebra and then downward in front of the scalenus anticus muscle, where it enters the venous system at the junction of the jugular and left subclavian veins.

The thoracic duct anatomy as described is only present in about half of the population. The most common variation is a double system originating from the cisternia chyli. Another variation includes multiple ducts at the diaphragmatic hiatus. The right thoracic duct is a short trunk collecting lymph from the right side of the head and neck, right upper extremity, and right side of the superior mediastinum through bronchial mediastinal trunks. It empties into the venous system at the junction of the right internal jugular and subclavian veins.

### *Physiology*

**Mechanics of Lymph Flow.** The upward flow of chyle is maintained by several factors: (1) transdiaphragmatic pressure gradient with the positive pressure abdomen and the negative pressure chest, (2) increased intraabdominal ductal pressure produced by fat or water intake and bowel peristal-

**TABLE 30–12. RESULTS OF EXTRAPLEURAL PNEUMONECTOMY FOR MALIGNANT MESOTHELIOMA**

| | | | % | | |
|---|---|---|---|---|---|
| **Author** | **Year** | **No. Patients** | ***Operative Mortality*** | ***2-Year Survival*** | ***5-Year Survival*** |
| Bamler[68] | 1974 | 17 | 23 | 35 | |
| Butchart[69] | 1976 | 29 | 31 | 10 | 3.5 |
| DaValle et al[70] | 1986 | 33 | 9 | 24 | 6 |
| Sugarbaker et al[71] | 1993 | 32 | 6 | 50 | |

sis, and (3) autonomous contraction of the thoracic duct for suctionlike effects of blood flow in the large upper thoracic and cervical veins.[78] Other factors such as pulsations from adjacent arteries may also play a role.

Multiple intraductal valves prevent backflow of chyle. These valves are found throughout the length of the duct, but exact locations are inconsistent. They appear to be more competent in the upper portion of the duct.

In the normal individual, 1500–2500 mL of chyle flows through the system per day. After ingestion of a fatty meal, the flow rate may rise to 200 mL/h.

**Composition of Chyle.** Chyle is an odorless, milky-white alkaline substance. Because nearly 60–70% of all ingested fat enters the intestinal lacteals and is transported to the thoracic duct, the triglyceride content of chyle is high and varies between 0.4 and 6 g/dL. Microscopic fat globules can easily be seen if chyle is collected after a meal and the emulsification stained with sudan III dye.

Total protein content of the thoracic lymph is also high with concentrations between 1 and 7 g/dL. The albumin/globulin ratio is 3:1. The white blood cell count varies between 2000 and 20,000 cells/mm$^3$, and 90% of these cells are T-cell lymphocytes. The remainder of the cells are usually eosinophils.

The specific gravity of chyle is at or greater than 1.012. Other constituents of chyle include sugar, urea, enzymes, and electrolytes in about the same concentration as blood.

### *Etiology and Pathogenesis of Chylothorax*

**Congenital Chylothorax.** Although called congenital, most chylothoraces found at birth are due to birth trauma (Table 30–13). Robinson[79] reported three such patients who had difficult forceps delivery. By contrast, chylothoraces occurring in young children are usually related to congenital abnormalities of the chyliferous channels, the cisternia chyli, or the thoracic duct itself. In some of these cases, they may be associated with chylopericardium or chyloperitoneum.

**Traumatic Chylothorax.** Injury to the thoracic duct or one of its tributaries is the most common cause of chylothorax. This usually occurs during intrathoracic surgery. Typically, it occurs following surgery on the thoracic aorta or the great arteries for congenital problems. It also may occur following mobilization of the esophagus. The incidence remains low in the range of 0.3–0.5% of cardiothoracic procedures.[80] Most extensive types of surgeries, such as radical esophagectomy or mediastinal exenteration, increase the incidence. Chylothoraces secondary to blunt thoracic injuries are uncommon. They are almost always associated with vertebral fractures or hyperextension injuries of the spine.

**Nontraumatic Chylothorax.** A multitude of disease processes may result in chylothorax. These include malignancies involving mediastinal nodes such as lymphoma or carcinoma, radiation fibrosis of the mediastinum, or local inflammatory reactions.[81] Chylothorax develops through an interaction of several factors.[82] The thoracic duct can be obstructed along its course either from within or by extrinsic compression. This obstruction, most commonly seen in malignancies, leads to increased intraductal pressure that can be followed by lymph transudation from the main duct or one of its tributaries. Direct neoplastic extension into the thoracic duct can also disrupt its wall and create a direct fistula. Patients who have chylous ascites may develop chylothorax by transdiaphragmatic leak of fluid.[82]

Several cases of chylothorax have been reported in association with superior vena cava thrombosis secondary to central venous catheters. In such cases, the thoracic duct is obstructed at its junction to the venous system, which results in an increase in ductal pressure causing lymph transudation.

### *Diagnosis of Chylothorax*

The clinical manifestations of chylothorax are those of pleural effusion. When the fluid is drained by thoracentesis, it rapidly reaccumulates and may even present under some tension (Fig. 30–11). Clinical manifestations also may be related to the underlying disease process or to progressive

**TABLE 30–13. PATHOGENESIS OF CHYLOTHORAX**

| Classification | Etiology | Pathogenesis |
|---|---|---|
| Congential | Birth injury<br>Congenital fistula | 1. Direct leakage from thoracic duct |
| | Malformation of lymphatics | 2. Leakage from dilated collateral pathways |
| Acquired, traumatic | Postoperative<br>Blunt trauma<br>Penetrating trauma | 3. Tear in thoracic duct |
| Acquired, nontraumatic | Neoplastic<br>Nonneoplastic | 4. Ductal compression with increase intraductal pressure and secondary transudation |
| | | 5. Disruption of ductal lumen integrity |
| | | 6. Increased shearing forces on the duct |
| | | 7. Transdiaphragmatic leakage of chyle |
| Superior vena cava obstruction | Intravenous catheters | 8. Increase in intraductal pressure with secondary rupture |

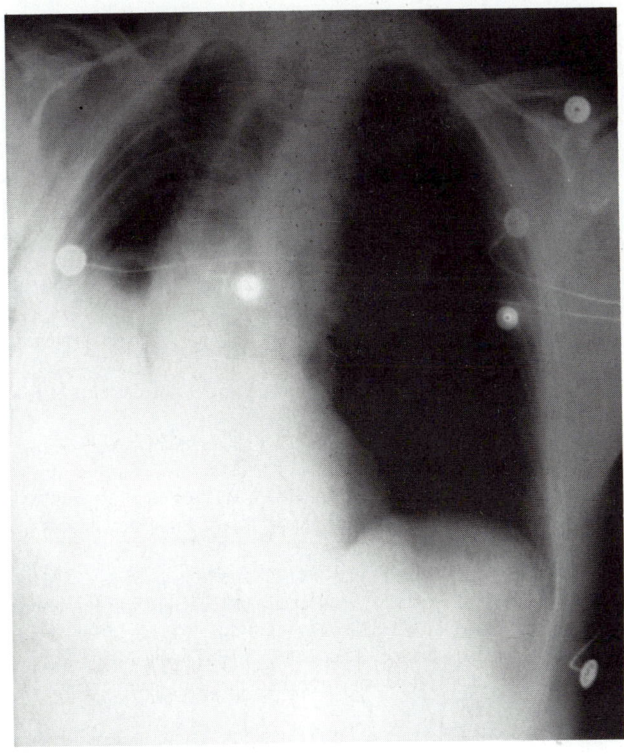

A

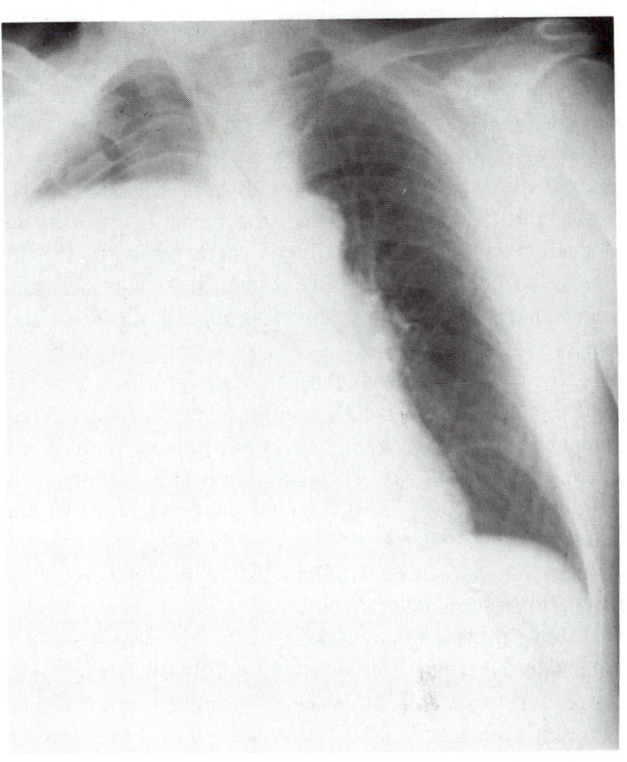

B

**Figure 30–11. A.** PA radiograph done 2 days after right pneumonectomy and showing normal mediastinal shift to the right. **B.** Five days later, the chest x-ray shows mediastinal shift to the left secondary to the rapid intrapleural accumulation of chyle.

loss of fat, protein, fluid, and white cells. In long-standing chyle leaks, these losses can be extreme and lead to dehydration and weight loss.

The diagnosis of chylothorax is usually made by analysis of the fluid. The most common test now is microscopic evaluation searching for chylomicrons. In addition, clearing of the fat by shaking the chyle with ether (1–2 mL) and staining of fat globules with Sudan III stain may be helpful. Standard contrast lymphangiography or nuclear lymphangiography with technicium 99 are now rarely used.

True chyle must be distinguished from pseudochyle. Pseudochyle is a liquid resembling chyle that can be seen as a result of pleural tumor or chronic infections. Pseudochyle has a gross milky appearance as does chyle but has a low triglyceride level and has a specific gravity < 1.012. It contains less protein and lymphocytes. The milky appearance of pseudochyle is due to cholesterol crystals.

### *Management*

Although opinions differ as to the ideal management, most authors agree that, at least initially, the management should be nonoperative.[83,84] Maloney and Spencer[83] noted that conservative management with nutritional support and repeated thoracenteses resulted in spontaneous closure in 11 of 13 patients.

Once the diagnosis of chylothorax is confirmed, the pleural space should be drained and dietary management begun. There are now oral preparations containing medium chain triglycerides. The triglycerides are directly absorbed into the portal system rather than through the intestinal lymphatics. By doing so, they reduce the lymph flow through the duct. Although this is helpful, the lymph flow remains fairly high. Eventually most patients must be started on total parenteral nutrition.

Nontraumatic chylothoraces often may be managed nonoperatively. Selle et al[85] noted that most idiopathic cases in neonates responded well to thoracentesis. When patients present with widespread mediastinal involvement with carcinoma, radiation therapy has been reported to be of some value. These patients may also benefit from chemical pleurodesis.

The treatment of traumatic chylothorax is most often surgical. In the adult, conservative management should be abandoned if the chyle leak is greater than 1 L/day for 7 days or if the leak persists for more than 2 weeks. If the chylothorax has occurred after an esophageal resection or pneumonectomy, reoperation should be done earlier. In children, surgery is usually indicated when the drainage is greater than 100 mL/day per year of age for more than 2–3 weeks.[85] In all instances, exploration should be done without delay when the lung appears to be trapped or when the nutritional complications begin to manifest themselves.[79]

There are two currently acceptable techniques for closing a thoracic duct fistula: direct ligation of the fistula and subdiaphragmatic duct ligation. In the first instance, thoracotomy or thoracoscopy is done on the side of effusion. Location of the fistula may be facilitated by the administration of heavy cream. This will increase the flow rate. Dyes such as methylene blue are not of much help, because they tend to stain all of the surrounding tissues once given. Once the fistula it is oversewn or ligated, the repair is checked by manually hyperinflating the lungs for a period of 30–45 seconds. If the fistula cannot be found, Bessone et al[86] recommended partial pleurectomy and tube drainage of the pleural space.

The second approach consists of thoracic duct ligation at the diaphragmatic level. Since the first description of the technique by Lamson[87] in 1948, it has been recommended by multiple authors.[85,88] The operation is best done through a right thoracotomy. The procedure involves ligation of the duct itself and often mass ligature of all tissue between the azygous vein and the aorta at the diaphragmatic hiatus. This latter technique is helpful in patients with accessory ducts. In a series by Patterson and associates,[88] ligation achieved immediate cessation of drainage in four of five cases.

## REFERENCES


1. Gray SW, Skandalakis JE: Development of the pleura. In Chretien J, Bignon J, Hirsch A: *The Pleura in Health and Disease.* New York, Marcel Dekker, 1985, p 1
2. Thews G: Pulmonary respiration. In Schmidt RF, Thews G: *Human Physiology.* New York, Springer, 1983, p 456
3. Bartter T, Mayo PD, Pratter MR, et al: Lower rates and higher yield for thoracentesis when performed by experienced operators. *Chest* **103:**187, 1993
4. Cugel DW: Thoracentesis and pleural biopsy. *Chest Surg Clin North Am* **2:**649, 1992
5. Rusch VW, Mountain C: Thoracoscopy under regional anesthesia for the diagnosis and management of pleural disease. *Am J Surg* **154:**274, 1987
6. Withers JN, Fishback ME, Kiehl PV, et al: Spontaneous pneumothorax/Suggested etiology and comparison of treatment methods. *Am J Surg* **108:**772, 1964
7. Jenkinson SG: Pneumothorax. *Clin Chest Med* **6:**153, 1985
8. Kircher LT, Swart RL: Spontaneous pneumothorax and its treatment. *Ann Thorac Surg* **22:**163, 1976
9. Grossman LA: Recurrent bilateral spontaneous pneumothorax treated with artificial hemothorax. *Ann Int Med* **39:**1303, 1953
10. So S, Uy D: Catheter drainage of spontaneous pneumothorax: Suction or no suction, early or late removal? *Thorax* **37:**46, 1982
11. Mills B, Baisch BF: Spontaneous pneumothorax, a series of 400 cases. *Ann Thorac Surg* **1:**286, 1965
12. Mercier C, Page A, Berdant A, et al: Out-patient management of intercostal tube drainage in Spontaneous pneumothorax. *Ann Thorac Surg* **22:**163, 1976
13. Gobbel NG, Rhea WG, Nelson IA, Daniel RA: Spontaneous pneumothorax. *J Thorac Cardiovasc Surg* **46:**331, 1963
14. Clagett OT: The management of spontaneous pneumothorax. *J Thorac Cardiovasc Surg* **55:**761, 1968
15. Gaensler EA: Parietal pleurectomy for recurrent spontaneous pneumothorax. *Surg Gynecol Obstet* **102:**293, 1956
16. Deslauriers J, Beaulieu B, Despres JP, et al: Transaxillary pleurectomy for treatment of spontaneous pneumothorax. *Ann Thorac Surg* **30:**569, 1980
17. Light RA: Management of spontaneous pneumothorax. *Am Rev Resp Dis* **148:**245, 1993
18. Lichter I: Long term follow-up of planned treatment of spontaneous pneumothorax. *Thorax* **29:**32, 1974
19. Dines DE, Clagett OT, Payne WS: Spontaneous pneumothorax in emphysema. *Mayo Clin Proc* **45:**481, 1970
20. Light RW: Parapneumonic effusions and empyema. *Semin Respir Med* **9:**37, 1987
21. Graham EA, Bell RD: Open pneumothorax: Its relation to the treatment of acute empyema. *Am J Med Sci* **156:**839, 1918
22. Light RW: Management of parapneumonic effusions. *Arch Inst Med* **141:**1339, 1981
23. Light RW, Girar WM, Jenkinson SG, George RB: Parapneumonic effusions. *Am J Med* **69:**507, 1980
24. Thurer RJ, Palatioanos GM: Surgical aspects of the pleural space. *Semin Respir Med* **9:**98, 1987
25. Ogilivie AG: Final results in traumatic hemothorax: A report of 230 cases. *Thorax* **5:**116, 1950
26. Le Roux BT, Mohlala ML, Odfell JA, Whitton ID: Suppurative disease of the lung and pleural space, Part I: Empyema thoraces and lung abscess. *Curr Probl Surg* **23**:1–86, 1986
27. Orringer MB: Thoracic empyema: Back to basics. *Chest* **93:**901,1988
28. Bartlett JG, Gorbach SL, Thadepalli H, Finegold SM: Bacteriology of empyema. *Lancet* **1:**338, 1974
29. Alfageme I, Munoz F, Pena N, et al: Empyema of the thorax in adults: Etiology, microbiologic findings and management. *Chest* **103:**839, 1993
30. Houston MC: Pleural fluid pH: Diagnostic, therapeutic and prognostic value. *Am J Surg* **154:**333, 1987
31. Strange C, Sahn SA: Management of the parapneumonic pleural effusions and empyema. Infectious disease. *Clin North Am* **5:**539, 1991
32. Mandal AK, Thadepalli H: Treatment of the spontaneous bacterial empyema thoraces. *J Thorac Cardiovasc Surg* **94:**414, 1987
33. Kerr A, Vasudevan VP, Powell S, et al: Percutaneous catheter drainage for acute empyema: improved cure rate using CAT scan, fluoroscopy and pig tail drainage catheters. *N Y State J Med* **91:**4, 1991
34. Lee MJ, Saini S, Brink JA, et al: Interventional radiology of the pleural space: management of thoracic empyema with image guided catheter drainage. *Semin Intervent Radiol* **8:**29, 1991
35. Vanway C, Narrod J, Hopeman A: The role of early limited thoracotomy in the treatment of empyema. *J Thorac Cardiovasc Surg* **96:** 436, 1988
36. Muskett A, Burton N, Karwande SV, et al: Management of refractory empyema with early decortication. *Am J Surg* **156:**529, 1988
37. Ridley PD, Baimbridge MV: Thoracoscopic debridement and pleural irrigation and management of empyema thoraces. *Ann Thorac Surg* **51:**461, 1991
38. Ferguson MK: Thoracoscopy for empyema, bronchopleural fistula and chylothorax. *Ann Thorac Surg* **56:**644, 1993
39. Weissberg D: Empyema and broncho-pleural fistula. Experience with open window thoracostomy. *Chest* **82:**447, 1982
40. Bayes AJ, Wilson JAS, Chiu RCJ, et al: Clagett open-window thoracostomy in patients with empyema who had and had not undergone pneumonectomy. *Can J Surg* **30:**329, 1987
41. Clagett OT, Geraci JE: A procedure for the management of postpneumonectomy empyema. *J Thorac Cardiovasc Surg* **45:**141, 1963
42. Stafford EG, Clagett OT: Postpneumonectomy empyema. Neomycin installations and definitive closure. *J Thorac Cardiovasc Surg* **63:**771, 1972
43. Goldstraw P: Treatment of post pneumonectomy empyema. The case for fenestration. *Thorax* **34:**740, 1979
44. Tillett WS, Sherry S: The effect in patients of streptococcal fibrinolysin (Streptokinase) and streptococcal deoxyribonuclease on fibrinous, purulent and sanguineous pleural exudations. *J Clin Invest* **28:**173, 1949
45. Aye RW, Froese DP, Hill LD: Use of purified streptokinase and empyema hemothorax. *Am J Surg* **161:**561, 1991

46. Robinson LA, Moulton AL, Fleming WH, et al: Intrapleural fibrinolytic treatments of multiloculated thoracic empyemas. *Ann Thor Surg* **57**:803, 1994
47. Ashbaugh DG: Empyema thoraces: Factors influencing morbidity and mortality. *Chest* **99**:1162, 1991
48. Hausheer FH, Yarbro JW: Diagnosis and treatment of malignant pleural effusion. *Semin Oncol* **12**:54, 1985
49. Sahn SA: Malignant pleural effusions. *Semin Respir Med* **9**:43, 1987
50. Light RW, Ball WC: Glucose and amylase in pleural effusions. *JAMA* **225**:257, 1973
51. Salyer WR, Eggleston JC, Erozan YS: Efficacy of pleural needle biopsy and pleural fluid cytopathology in the diagnosis of malignant neoplasm involving the pleura. *Chest* **67**:536, 1975
52. Hausheer FF, Yarbro JW: Diagnosis and management of malignant pleural effusions. *Sem Oncol* **12**:54, 1985
53. Webb WR, Ozmen V, Moulder BV, et al: Iodized talc pleurodesis for the treatment of pleural effusions. *J Thorac Cardiovasc Surg* **103**:881, 1992
54. Daniel TM, Tribble CG, Rogers BM: Thoracoscopy and talc poudrage for pneumothoraces and effusions. *Ann Thorac Surg* **50**:186, 1990
55. Little AG, Kadowaki MH, Ferguson MK, et al: Pleural peritoneal shunting: Alternative therapy for pleural effusions. *Ann Surg* **208**:443, 1988
56. LoCicero J: Thoracoscopic management of malignant pleural effusion. *Ann Thorac Surg* **56**:641, 1993
57. Wagner E: Das tuberkelahnliche Lymphadenom (der cytogene oder reticulierte Tuberkel). *Arch Heilk (Leipzig)* **11**:497, 1870
58. Briselli M, Mark EJ, Dickersin GR: Solitary fibrous tumors of the pleura: Eight new cases and review of 360 cases in the literature. *Cancer* **47**:2678, 1981
59. McCormack PM, Nagasaki F, Hilaris BS, Martini N: Surgical treatment of pleural mesothelioma. *J Thorac Cardiovasc Surg* **84**:834, 1982
60. Martini N, McCormack PJ, Bains MS, et al: Pleural mesothelioma. *Ann Thorac Surg* **43**:363, 1978
61. Wagner JC, Sleggs CA, Marchand P: Diffuse pleural mesothelioma and asbestos exposure in the North Western Cape Province. *Br J Int Med* **17**:260, 1960
62. Hillerdal G: Malignant mesothelioma. 1982: Review of 4710 published cases. *Br J Dis Chest* **77**:321, 1983
63. Hsu SM, Hsu PL, Zhao X, et al: Establishment of human mesothelioma cell lines (MS–1,2) in the production of a monoclonal antibody (antiMS) with diagnostic and therapeutic potential. *Can Res* **48**:5228, 1988
64. Beahrs OH, Henson DE, Hutter RVP, et al: *Manual for Staging of Cancer,* 3rd Ed. Philadelphia, Lippincott, 1988
65. Martini N, Bains MS, Beattie EJ Jr: Indications for pleurectomy in malignant effusion. *Cancer* **35**:734, 1975
66. Rusch VW: Pleurectomy and a decortication and adjuvant therapy for malignant mesothelioma. *Chest* **103**:(suppl 4) 382S, 1993
67. Eiselberg AV: IM Protokoll der Gesellschaft der Artze in Wien. *Wien Klin Wochenschr* 509, 1992
68. Bamler KJ, Maassen W: Uber die Verteilung der benignen und malignen Pleuratumoren im Krankengut einer lungenchirurgischen Klinik mit besonderer Beruksichtingung des malignen Pleuramesothelioms und seiner radikalen Behandlung einschliesslich der Ergebnisse des Zwerchfellerstzes mit konservierter dura mater. *Thorax Chirurgie* **22**:386, 1974
69. Butchart EG, Ashcroft T, Barnsley WC, Holden MP: Pleurapneumonectomy in the management of diffuse malignant mesothelioma of the pleura. Experience with 29 patients. *Thorax* **31**:15, 1976
70. DaValle MJ, Faber LP, Kittle CF, et al: Extrapleural pneumonectomy for diffuse, malignant mesothelioma. *Ann Thorac Surg* **42**:612, 1986
71. Sugarbaker DJ, Mentzer SJ, DeCamp M, et al: Extrapleural pneumonectomy in the setting of multimodality approach to malignant mesothelioma. *Chest* **103**(suppl 4):377, 1993
72. Vogelzang NJ, Schultz SM, Iannucci AM, et al: Malignant mesothelioma. The University of Minnesota experience. *Cancer* **53**:377, 1984
73. Kucuksu N, Thomas W, Ezdinli EZ: Chemotherapy of malignant diffuse mesothelioma. *Cancer* **37**:1265, 1976
74. Harvey VJ, Slevin ML, Ponder BA, et al: Chemotherapy of diffuse malignant mesothelioma. Phase 11 trials of single-agent 5-fluorouracil and adriamycin. *Cancer* **54**:961, 1984
75. Pogrebniak HW, Lubensky IA, Pass HI: Differential expression of platelet derived growth factor beta in malignant mesothelioma: A clue to future therapies? *Surg Oncol* **2**:235, 1993
76. Tochner ZA, Pass HI, Smith PD, et al: Intrathoracic photodynamic therapy: A canine normal tissue tolerance study in early clinical experience. *Lasers Surg Med* **14**:118, 1994
77. Allen L: The lymphatic system and spleen. In Anson BJ: Morris' Human Anatomy, 12th ed. New York, McGraw Hill, 1966, p 859
78. Witleb E: Functions of the vascular system. In Schmidt RF, Thews G: *Human Physiology.* New York, Springer-Verlag, 1983, p 421
79. Robinson CLN: The management of chylothorax. Collective review. *Ann Thorac Surg* **39**:90, 1985
80. Cevese PG, Vecchioni R, D'Amico DF, et al: Postoperative chylothorax. *J Thorac Cardiovasc Surg* **69**:966, 1975
81. Mark JBD: Discussion of Milswon JW. et al: Chylothorax: An assessment of current surgical management. *J Thorac Cardiovasc Surg* **89**:221, 1985
82. Strausser JL, Flye MW: Management of nontraumatic chylothorax. *Ann Thorac Surg* **31**:520, 1981
83. Maloney JV, Spencer FC: The nonoperative treatment of traumatic chylothorax. *Surgery* **40**:121, 1956
84. Hashim SA, Roholt HB, Babayan VK, et al: Treatment of chyluria and chylothorax with medium chain triglyceride. *N Engl J Med* **270**:756, 1964
85. Selle JG, Snyder WH, Schreiber JT: Chylothorax: Indications for surgery. *Ann Surg* **177**:245, 1973
86. Bessone LN, Ferguson TB, Burford TH: Chylothorax. *Ann Thorac Surg* **12**:527, 1971
87. Lampson RS: Traumatic chylothorax. *J Thorac Surg* **17**:778, 1948
88. Patterson GA, Todd TRJ, Delarue NC, et al: Supradiaphragmatic ligation of the thoracic duct in intractable chylous fistula. *Ann Thorac Surg* **32**:44, 1981

CHAPTER

# 31

# Pleural Space Problems and Thoracoplasty

Watts R. Webb and Lynn H. Harrison, Jr.

Thoracic surgery as a specialty had its beginnings in the surgical treatment of pulmonary tuberculosis and its pleural space problems. Although the development of effective chemotherapy had almost eliminated the need for surgical treatment of tuberculosis and pleural space problems, with the recent resurgence of tuberculosis in the immune-suppressed patient, the thoracic surgeon today continues to be presented with difficult problems in management of both tuberculous and nontuberculous chronic empyema cavities. This chapter will review the lessons learned from the surgical treatment of tuberculosis and the developing guidelines for present-day management of pleural space problems.

## HISTORICAL BACKGROUND

The observation that nature attempted to heal tuberculosis by isolating and collapsing the involved portion of lung led to collapse therapy for tuberculosis.[1] This began with using sandbags and positioning the patient with the diseased side down. Costal excursions could be reduced further by intercostal neurectomy and transection of the accessory muscles of respiration (scalenotomy). The phrenic nerve was cut or crushed (1911). Air was introduced into the pleural space (pneumothorax) and into the peritoneal space (pneumoperitoneum) to create long-term and presumably reversible collapse. Because adhesions frequently limited the degree of pulmonary collapse with pneumothorax, intrapleural pneumonolysis (Jacobaeus, 1913) was performed with the cautery through a thoracoscope and became the antecedent of modern thoracoscopy. Further surgical techniques had to be developed because empyema frequently occurred when the lung failed to re-expand after discontinuance of the pneumothorax.

### Thoracoplasty for Tuberculosis

The evolution of thoracoplasty began with de Cerenville (1885), who resected short lengths of two or more ribs anteriorly to collapse the chest wall over apical disease. Schede[2] in 1890 described a thoracoplasty primarily for localized empyema that included not only multiple ribs but also the parietal pleura, periosteum, intercostal muscles, and intercostal neurovascular bundles. This allowed for collapse of the chest wall when the parietal pleura was rigid. The procedure was mutilating, and the sacrifice of intercostal nerves resulted in cutaneous anesthesia and paresthesias of the abdominal wall. It left a poorly protected heart and an unstable chest wall with a large, open wound requiring long periods of packing before healing was complete. Even with aggressive efforts at physical therapy, the patients often had restricted motion of the shoulder and limited use of the ipsilateral arm.

Brauer and Friedrich (1907) resected full lengths of the second through the ninth ribs, including the periosteum and intercostal muscles, in an attempt to mimic the collapse obtained by pneumothorax. This single-stage decostalization produced massive instability of the chest wall and carried a mortality rate of 40%. Gourdet (1912) obtained good results in treating nontuberculous empyema with relatively short resections of several ribs in the paravertebral gutter. This provided collapse with a lower mortality than the more radical thoracoplasties. Wilms applied this concept to the management of tuberculosis in 1911.[1]

These various approaches ultimately evolved into the classical three-stage thoracoplasty described by Alexander[3] in 1937. The ribs were removed from the vertebral laminae forward. To permit stiffening of the periosteal beds, 2–3 weeks were allowed between stages. The periosteum was left in situ so that new bone formation would ensure long-term collapse of the diseased lung (Fig. 31–1). This procedure resulted in a 75–80% rate of sputum conversion and cavity closure[4] even without chemotherapy.

### Plombage for Tuberculosis

Because both the conventional thoracoplasty and the Schede thoracoplasty were debilitating and cosmetically unacceptable, extrapleural paraffin plombage[5] was introduced in the 1950s as a less mutilating form of collapse therapy. Various materials (blood, plastic balls, polyethylene sponges, wax) were placed extrapleurally between the lung and the ribs (Fig. 31–2). Alternatively, the periosteum was stripped from the ribs and collapsed with the intercostal muscles and neurovascular bundles by placing the plombage between the ribs and the periosteum and intercostal muscles. This extraperiosteal plombage had fewer complications than the extrapleural site. These operations provided good, selective collapse that could be accomplished in one stage. They offered freedom from postoperative paradoxical thoracic motion, little or no interference with efficient cough and expectoration of secretions, and almost no deformity of the chest wall. Pulmonary function following plombage was better than that following a conventional thoracoplasty of similar extent,[6] and postoperative recovery was faster. In patients who had positive sputum, plombage resulted in sputum conversion and control of the tuberculosis in 60% of patients.[5] Many of the materials used for plombage was complicated by tuberculous or nontuberculous infections. In one series, however, 150 formalinized polyvinyl alcohol sponges (Ivalon) were used in 144 consecutive patients.[7] Eighty-five of these were for plombage, and the remaining 65 were performed concomitant with or following pulmonary resections. Only three became infected, and none of these was tuberculous. Infected sponges were easily removed and the ribs resected in a conversion thoracoplasty with early healing. The Ivalon plombage ultimately was abandoned because the osteoplastic thoracoplasty became recognized as a better alternative.

## OSTEOPLASTIC THORACOPLASTY

In 1954 Bjork[8] described an osteoplastic thoracoplasty that in essence had all the advantages of the plombage thoracoplasty without the disadvantages. The posterior ends of the upper ribs are resected in increasing lengths back to the tip of the transverse processes that are left intact. A short segment of the first rib could be resected, or preferably the periosteum could be reflected from its inferior surface. In the original description, the intercostal bundles were divided posteriorly, but frequently this could be avoided. An apicolysis is performed, and the apical pleura is reflected down to the aortic arch or the azygos vein or as low as desired. The periosteum, intercostal muscle, and/or pleura are sutured to the mediastinal structures to prevent escape of the apex of the lung superiorly (Fig. 31–3). The ribs are reflected down, and the posterior ends are fixed with wire to the uppermost intact rib. This procedure can be safely performed at the time of a pulmonary resection because of the immediate complete stability of the chest wall. For many, this remains the technique of choice for a tailoring thoracoplasty to reduce the size of the hemithorax after an extensive pulmonary resection.

Surgical intervention of tuberculosis drastically declined after the development of effective antituberculosis chemotherapy. Tuberculosis was diagnosed at an earlier stage, and the complications of the disease occurred much less frequently. Before this happened, however, the surgical treatment of tuberculosis had catapulted thoracic surgery into prominence.

## PLEURAL SPACE PROBLEMS

Acute thoracic empyema is usually an extension of a pulmonary infection. Persistence of the empyema usually implies one of the following conditions: inadequate drainage,

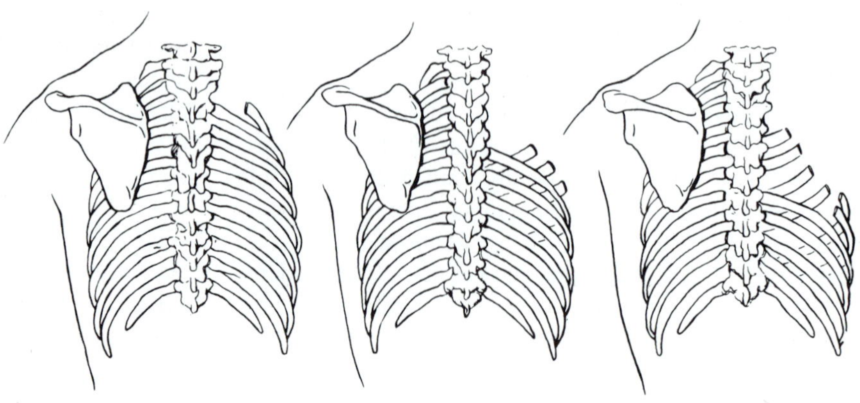

**Figure 31–1.** The classical three-stage thoracoplasty as described by Alexander.

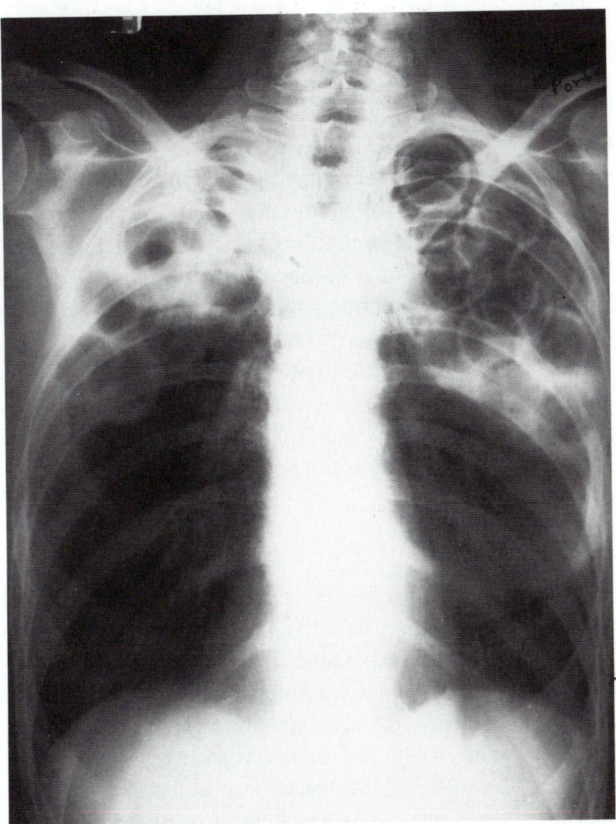

Figure 31–2. Chest x-ray after a plombage, with plastic balls seen at the apex of the right chest.

chronic pulmonary disease (such as tuberculosis, fungus, or neoplasm), immune suppression, or a foreign body within the pleural space. A chronic organizing empyema is extremely morbid, can be very difficult to eradicate, and has a significant mortality rate. Treatment of a thoracic empyema requires control of the pulmonary process (infection, neoplasm), control of the infecting organisms in the cavity by dependent drainage and antibiotics, closure of a bronchopleural fistula if one is present, and obliteration of the dead space.

The pathologic response of the empyema may be divided into three phases,[9] which gradually merge one into the other. The first phase is exudative. There is immediate outpouring of thin fluid of relatively low cellular content, and re-expansion of the lung is readily achieved. The second phase is fibrinopurulent. This stage is characterized by large quantities of frank pus and deposition of fibrin covering both the visceral and parietal pleurae. Progressive loculation and formation of a limiting membrane begins to fix the lung so it becomes progressively less expandable. The third phase is organizing. This stage is characterized by a very thick exudate and a thick inelastic "peel" on both the visceral and parietal pleural surfaces demonstrable by the aspirating needle or by roentgenologic techniques.

## Tube Thoracostomy

Adequate dependent drainage of an acute exudative empyema can be provided by a chest tube with closed water sealed drainage and suction. However, if the tube is positioned improperly or if the collection has progressed to a stage in which the material has become semisolid (fibrinopurulent), the drainage will be incomplete. Also, simple drainage is less likely to be effective for treatment of postoperative empyema or empyema in patients who have associated serious illnesses (such as alcohol abuse, immunosuppression, or chronic pulmonary disease).[10,11]

Between 10 days and 2 weeks after insertion of the tube, the walls of the empyema cavity are usually adherent to the lateral chest wall so that the lung cannot collapse and the chest tube can be converted to open drainage. This open drainage is used for debilitated patients whose physiologic status precludes a more aggressive approach to treatment of the empyema space. Open drainage is often unsatisfactory,

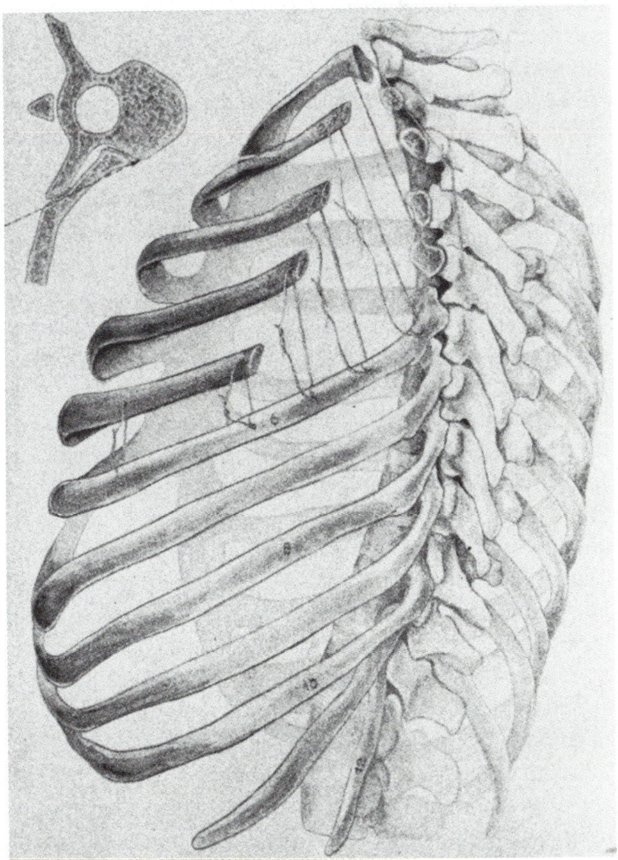

**Figure 31–3.** Osteoplastic thoracoplasty as described by Bjork resects increasing portions of the posterior segments of the ribs. These are folded down and wired to the lowest rib (six in this illustration). This forms a solid bony chest wall, and, if the first rib is left intact, there is minimal deformity. *(From Bjork VO: Thoracoplasty: A new osteoplastic technique. J Thorac Surg 28:194–211, 1954, with permission.)*

because obliteration of the pleural space may occur slowly and the tube may be required for many months, years, or indefinitely. The tube needs to be changed frequently as it is difficult to secure to the skin for prolonged periods of time, and the patient finds it most unpleasant.

## Eloesser Flap

The Eloesser flap[12] was devised to provide tubeless drainage of a loculated space within the pleural cavity or the entire pleural space for a postpneumonectomy empyema. The procedure, as originally conceived by Eloesser, was designed to produce a one-way valve allowing pus to egress but not allowing the ingress of air, thus maintaining the pleural negative pressure while allowing drainage of the pleural space without a tube. The procedure made a U-shaped skin incision producing a skin flap that was based toward the patient's head. A segment of rib was resected over the most dependent portion of the empyema cavity. The skin flap was folded into the opening and sutured to the pleura so that the drainage site through the chest wall was lined by skin on the upper half of the tract. The flap of skin was supposed to produce a one-way valve effect without an inlying tube.

Currently, when long-term drainage of an empyema cavity is desired, the term *Eloesser flap* is often used, but the procedure carried out is considerably different from that described by Eloesser.[13] The Eloesser flap has evolved into an operation of marsupialization in which skin flaps are inverted into the tract and sutured to the pleura around the entire circumference of the tract. There is no attempt to produce a one-way valve to prevent pneumothorax. Therefore, the lung adjacent to the cavity must be adherent to the chest wall.

An "Eloesser flap" is created by removing segments of two ribs (Fig. 31–4) and suturing the skin to the pleura. Any loculations should be broken and fibrinous debris removed. The wound is packed to debride the empyema space and to keep the tract open until the pleural space is obliterated. The packing should be changed daily with wet-to-dry dressings using saline or Dakin's solution. Within a few weeks, the cavity is well debrided and contains only clean granulation tissue. However, it takes many months until the cavity is obliterated by the granulation tissue and may take years in an immunocompromised patient or one with a postpneumonectomy empyema. In many of these patients, a thoracoplasty and/or muscle flaps can be used to obliterate the cavity and attain early healing.

## Clagett Procedure

In 1963 Clagett and Geraci[14] described a two-stage procedure for treatment of chronic empyema spaces. Initially, open drainage is created, and the empyema cavity is irrigated daily with half-strength Dakin's solution for 6–8 weeks. When the cavity is lined by clean, healthy granulation tissue, the sinus tract is excised, the chest wall is closed in layers, and the pleural space is filled with 0.25% neomycin solution in normal saline. This procedure has a success rate of 25–60%[15,16] and can be repeated after a failed procedure with a 60% success rate.[15] The pleura absorbs significant amounts of neomycin so that serum levels associated with nephrotoxicity and respiratory suppression may result if high concentrations of neomycin are used.[16] A less toxic antibiotic may be chosen based upon culture and sensitivity of a specimen from the pleural space. The Clagett procedure alone is not effective in patients with bronchopleural fistulae or patients with tuberculosis, because the latter have an increased risk of recurrent empyema, recurrent tuberculosis, or superimposed infection with *Aspergillus* in the residual cavity.[17]

## Thoracoscopy

There has been a progressively enlarging experience with thoracoscopy to break loculations, debride the empyema cavity, and establish dependent drainage. The chest is irrigated with saline and an antibiotic solution through a small apical chest tube and is drained through a larger, basilar chest tube. The chest tubes are removed after three consecutive sterile cultures. Braimbridge[18] reported excellent success with this method. The few failures occurred in patients with malignancies or total empyema of the chest cavity, where the apex of the lung is fixed and is separated significantly from the chest wall. In early cases, a fairly effective decortication can be accomplished. Once the peel has become thick and well organized, decortication is much more effectively done by open thoracotomy.

## Decortication

The key to restoring good health to a patient with a thoracic empyema is thorough cavitary debridement with removal of all pus and necrotic tissue and re-expansion of healthy lung to fill the pleural space. Controlling any residual pulmonary disease and removing any constricting tissue that prevents full expansion are, therefore, important considerations. As Thomas Burford used to say, "As the lung goes, so goes the pleura." Recent trends are toward more aggressive use of decortication in the treatment of pleural empyema, especially in immunocompromised patients.[19]

Decortication can be performed alone or at the time of pulmonary resection. Chest tubes are inserted and placed on suction. If the lung is healthy and fully without air leak or significant drainage, the tubes may be removed in a few days. If, on the other hand, an air leak or drainage persists, the tubes are left on suction for 2 or 3 weeks, at which time the pleural surfaces usually are well adherent. The tubes then can be converted to open drainage and gradually shortened in increments over the next few weeks until completely removed.

Decortication has also proved extremely successful in

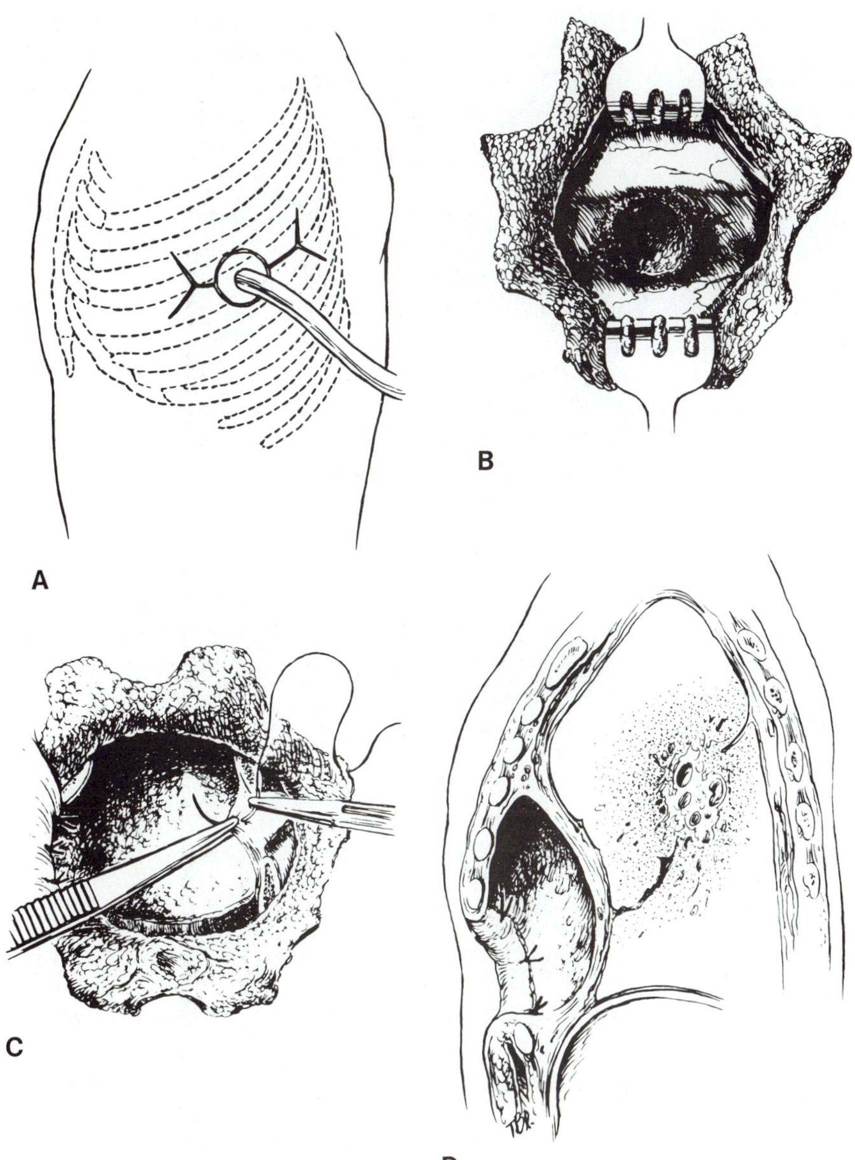


**Figure 31–4.** The modified Eloesser flap involves **(A)** removal of the chest tube tract and carrying the incision down to the ribs. **B.** Two ribs and the intervening intercostal muscle are removed. **C.** The skin is sutured to the pleura to create long-term, dependently located drainage for the cavity **(D)**.

children. Gustafson et al[20] decorticated 10 children for a refractory symptomatic empyema because of extensive pleural involvement or limitation of lung expansion. Two of the 10 had a concomitant lobectomy, and all had complete removal of the visceral and parietal peels with excellent long-term results.

## Thoracoplasty

If the lung will not expand to the chest wall, then collapse therapy can bring the chest wall to the lung or mediastinum. There are three basic types of thoracoplasty. The *conventional* thoracoplasty (Alexander type) involves the subperiosteal, extrapleural, posterolateral resection of sufficient ribs to obliterate the intrathoracic space (Fig. 31–1). The procedure is generally performed in stages, because one-stage resection of 10 ribs produces severe flail. The *tailoring* thoracoplasty is a lesser procedure involving resection of enough ribs to reduce the thoracic volume when it is anticipated that insufficient lung tissue will remain to fill the pleural space following a pulmonary resection. The *Schede* thoracoplasty is resection of not only ribs but also intercostal muscles, endothoracic fascia, and parietal pleura, so that only the skin and extrathoracic muscles remain to collapse onto the residual lung or lung space. The original Schede operation is mutilating, and there are better alternative modifications. Horrigas and Snow,[21] e.g., found that a modified Schede thoracoplasty was effective in 13 patients in closing infected pleural spaces. Eleven of these patients had bronchopleural fistulas that were successfully closed by concomitant use of extrathoracic muscle flaps.

Alexander[3] promulgated the following principles for the safe application of the conventional thoracoplasty while

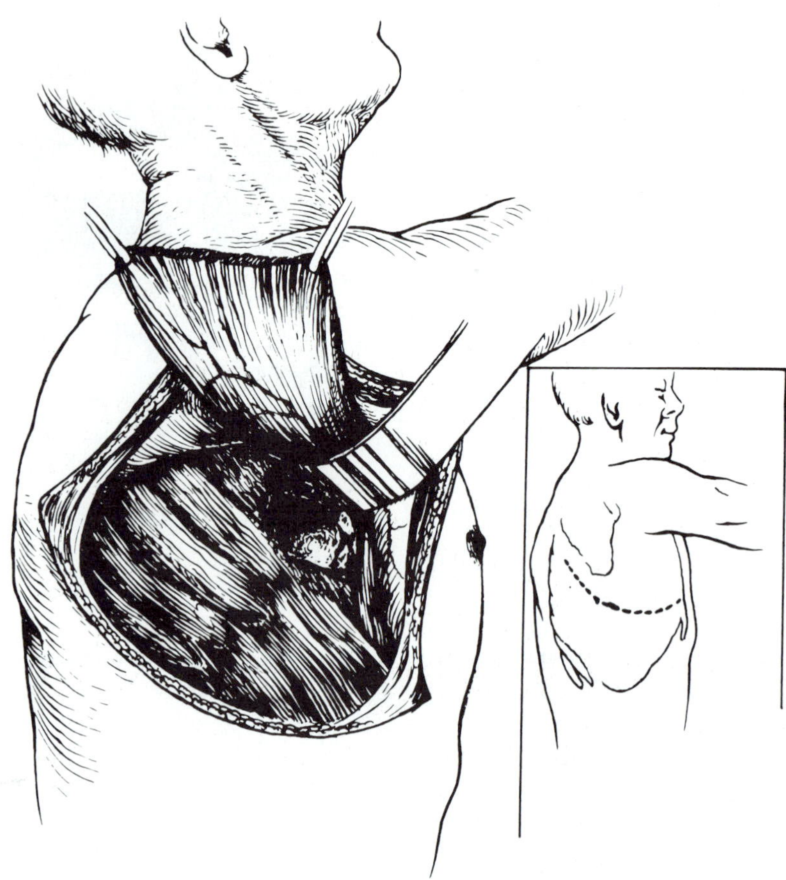

**Figure 31–5.** Through a standard thoracotomy incision (inset), the latissimus dorsi muscle is mobilized and transposed into the pleural cavity through the bed of the second or third rib.

accomplishing its goal of obliterating the space within the thoracic cavity:

1. The procedure should be done in stages limited in extent to the ability of the patient to withstand the operation, but performed in rapid enough succession that immobility does not occur between stages.
2. The first rib should be resected to allow collapse of the apex of the chest cavity. However, this is no longer regarded as necessary, as periosteal stripping of only the undersurface of this rib will allow the apex to collapse and better preserve chest contours.
3. The posterior extent of the resection should include portions of the transverse processes.
4. Sparing or sloping resection of the anterior portion of the lower ribs will minimize deformity and enhance the structural integrity needed for preservation of pulmonary function.

Thoracoplasty does obliterate the intrathoracic space very successfully and permanently controls the empyema. It also often closes a bronchopleural fistula or enables it to be closed more easily by another surgical procedure (such as muscle transposition). The overall success rate of thoracoplasty in eliminating thoracic space problems is 73%.[17] The major disadvantage of an extensive thoracoplasty is the disability that occurs postoperatively. All patients who undergo a thoracoplasty should have physical therapy postoperatively to promote shoulder mobility. Despite this, these patients frequently get a "frozen shoulder" that results in a minimally functional arm, which is especially devastating when this occurs to the dominant arm. A thoracoplasty usually is now performed only when other procedures have failed or cannot be performed. Occasionally, a decorticated lung does not expand to fill the thoracic cage. Iioka and associates[22] described a one-stage operation designed to encourage the trapped lung to re-expand gradually. Through a posterolateral skin incision, the pyofibrinous necrotic tissues are thoroughly evacuated. The visceral peel overlying the collapsed lung is removed to facilitate expansion. If the decorticated lung does not fill the pleural cavity, subperiosteal stripping of the ribs allows the parietal wall, consisting of parietal pleura, periosteum, and intercostal muscle, to collapse onto the surface of the lung. This parietal wall is usually thick and fibrinous, so curettage or parietal pleurectomy may be necessary to make it pliable. The pleura is closed watertight, a chest tube is placed in the space between the lung and the parietal wall. The space between the parietal wall and the ribs fills with serous fluid, which is gradually resorbed with re-expansion of the lung. This procedure was successful in 60 of 65 patients.[22] This is a modification of thoraco-mediastinal plication described in 1961 by Andrews[23] who also sutured the pleuro musculoperiosteal wall to the mediastinal or visceral pleura.

Fungal empyema may be particularly difficult to eradicate, especially if active infection or cavitation remains in the residual lung. Utley[24] used a one-stage completion pneumonectomy and modified eight-rib thoracoplasty in these patients with fungal cavities in the lung, fungal empyema, and bronchopleural fistulas. The intercostal bundles were sutured to the bronchial stump as reinforcement. Antibiotics and antifungal irrigations were used postoperatively through the chest tube, which was left in place 6–8 weeks. All wounds healed primarily with long-term good results.

## Muscle Transposition

Although plombage is now of only historic significance, the concept of filling the pleural space led to the transposition of chest wall muscles into a chronic empyema cavity.[25–28] Muscle is an ideal tissue to place in a contaminated space, because it obliterates the space, and its rich blood supply not only resists infection but helps to control it.[26,27] The latissimus dorsi, pectoralis major, pectoralis minor, serratus anterior, and rectus abdominis muscles and the omentum can be rotated singly or in combination to obliterate any size residual pleural space.[28,29] The choice is based upon the surgeon's preference, the size of the pleural space, and whether a muscle has been previously divided at thoracotomy.

Generally, a 5-cm segment of the second rib is removed to provide adequate entrance for the muscle into the pleural space (Fig. 31–5). The origin, insertion, and all other attachments of the muscles to the chest wall, other than a single, dominant blood supply, are divided. The nerves should also be preserved, because the muscles atrophy without innervation. Various muscles can be transposed to reach any intrathoracic location.

The latissimus dorsi is a triangularly shaped muscle that covers the lower back from the seventh thoracic vertebra to the sacrum. The muscle originates from a broad aponeurosis that attaches to all the spinous processes caudal to T6. The predominant blood supply is from subscapular branches of the axillary artery.

The rectus abdominis is a thick, flat band of muscle arising from the anterior surface of the fifth, sixth, and seventh costal cartilages and the xiphoid process. Three to five tendinous insertions cross the muscle and adhere to the anterior rectus sheath. The dual blood supply is from the superior epigastric artery (the continuation of the internal mammary artery) and the inferior epigastric artery (from the external iliac artery).

The pectoralis major muscle fibers originate from the medial clavicle, the sternocostal junction, and external oblique aponeurosis at its junction with the rectus fascia, and insert on the lateral lip of the intertubercular sulcus of the humerus. The dominant blood supply is the pectoral branch of the thoracoacromial artery, which arises from the axillary artery 2 cm medial and 2 cm caudal to the coracoid process of the scapula. When the muscle is mobilized with preservation of this artery, it can reach the upper half of the pleural space or the main stem bronchus. The muscle can also be mobilized with preservation of the perforating branches of the internal mammary artery while sacrificing the pectoral branch of the thoracoacromial artery. In this way, the muscle can be rotated into the mediastinum after sternal debridement for mediastinitis.

The serratus anterior arises from the side of the chest to insert on the vertebral margin of the scapula. Its dominant blood supply is the lateral thoracic artery from the second part of the axillary artery.

The omentum offers a variable amount of tissue supplied by the gastroepiploic arcade.

All flaps are prepared by cutting all attachments of the flap except the nerves and blood supply upon which it is based. The latissimus, pectoralis, and serratus muscles can cover a bronchopleural fistula or fill an upper thoracic space. When one is covering a bronchopleural fistula, the muscle is sutured over the bronchial stump and mediastinum with absorbable sutures. The patients should be ventilated with as low positive pressure as possible and removed from the ventilator as soon as feasible, because the positive pressure tends to disrupt the bronchial closure. The rectus abdominis muscle can fill a space in the anterior or inferior chest, while the omentum can reach any location in the chest.

The transposition of these muscles results in minimal functional disability of an upper extremity. As an alternative to the Clagett procedure, this approach offers an 88% success rate in controlling postpneumonectomy empyema.[26–28] In the presence of a bronchopleural fistula, use of a muscle flap to close the fistula at the time of the first-stage open drainage has been extremely successful.[28,30] Later, the second stage can be done when the pleural cavity is clear and the fistula definitely closed.

An interesting new development is the use of intrathoracic free flaps using microvascular techniques to transfer distant muscle flaps into the thoracic activity. The microvascular anastomosis is performed extrathoracically with excellent revascularization success and closure of bronchial fistulas.[30]

## Muscle-Sparing Thoracotomy Incision

Because muscle flaps are being used with increasing frequency for many different purposes, the thoracic surgeon should consider a thoracotomy incision that spares the major muscles of the chest wall. Often the latissimus muscle does not need to be cut at all. The serratus fibers are separated only for a distance of 2 in. from the border of the latissimus muscle to the origin on the underlying rib. Care should be taken to preserve the neurovascular bundle for the serratus, which lies on its superficial surface just posterior to the anterior border of the latissimus. The intercostal muscles are then cut from the transverse process to the internal mammary artery. The muscle spacing incision is particularly desirable in infants and children to avoid major structural deformities with growth.[31]

This incision offers excellent exposure for all types of lung resections, including segmentectomy, sleeve resection, and intrapericardial pneumonectomy. Contraindications include tumors invading the ribs, Pancoast tumors, very large tumors (>10 cm), and repeat thoracotomies.

## GUIDELINES FOR TREATMENT OF A THORACIC PATIENT WITH A CHRONIC EMPYEMA CAVITY

1. As soon as the diagnosis of acute empyema is made, closed chest tube drainage is performed.
2. If the patient remains toxic or if the empyema is incompletely drained, thoracoscopy with lysis of adhesions and additional tube placement under videoscopic control is undertaken. This is especially advisable for immunocompromised patients. If the empyema is in the fibrinopurulent or organizing phase, open decortication is employed.
3. If the patient is not physiologically able to tolerate a decortication, an Eloesser flap may be performed. The patient is instructed regarding outpatient care of the wound, including irrigation of the cavity provided there is no bronchopleural fistula. In a few weeks, when the cavity is clean, obliteration of the pleural space may be facilitated by muscle transposition.
4. Thoracoplasty is now very infrequently used. Muscle transposition offers an alternative treatment that is much less debilitating, though at times the two may be combined.
5. Postpneumonectomy empyema is initially managed with a chest tube and open-window thoracotomy (the Clagget procedure). After the cavity is cleaned by irrigation and drainage, the sterilized space may be allowed to remain (the second stage of the Clagget procedure). If needed, the space can be obliterated by muscle transposition. If a bronchopleural fistula is present, muscle transposition is the treatment of choice, because it controls the fistula and obliterates the space. Here, again, it may need to be combined with a partial thoracoplasty.

## REFERENCES


1. Langston HT, Barker WL: Pleuropulmonary tuberculosis. In DB Effler (ed): *Blade's Surgical Disease of the Chest,* 4th Ed. St. Louis, Mosby, 1978, pp 299–303
2. Schede M: Die Behandlung der Empyeme. *Verhandl Cong innere Med Wiesbaden* **9:**41, 1890
3. Alexander J: *The Collapse Therapy of Pulmonary Tuberculosis.* Springfield, Illinois, Thomas, 1937
4. Kergin FG: An operation for chronic pleural empyema. *J Thorac Surg* **26:**430, 1953
5. Fox RT, Lees WM, Shields TW, Iwa T: Extraperiosteal paraffin plombage thoracoplasty. One to nine year follow-up of 785 operations. *J Thorac Cardiovasc Surg* **44:**371–384, 1962
6. Gaensler EA, Strieder JW: Progressive changes in pulmonary function after pneumonectomy: The influence of thoracoplasty, pneumothorax, oleothorax, and plastic sponge plombage on the side of pneumonectomy. *J Thorac Surg* **22:**1–34, 1951
7. Allan MB, Jr, Webb WR: The Use of a plastic sponge (Ivalon) in operative procedures for pulmonary tuberculosis. *J Thorac Surg* **34:**21–35, 1957
8. Bjork VO: Thoracoplasty: A new osteoplastic technique. *J Thorac Surg* **28:**194–211, 1954
9. Webb WR, Andrews NC, Parker EF, et al: Management of nontuberculous empyema. *Am Rev Resp Dis* **85:**935–936, 1962
10. Fishman NH, Ellertson DG: Early pleural decortication for thoracic empyema in immunosuppressed patients. *J Thorac Cardiovasc Surg* **74:**537–541, 1977
11. Lemmer JH, Botham MJ, Orringer MG: Modern management of adult thoracic empyema. *J Thorac Cardiovasc Surg* **90:**849–855, 1985
12. Eloesser L: An operation for tuberculous empyema. *Surg Gynecol Obstet* **60:**1096–1097, 1935
13. Hurvitz RJ, Tucker BL: The Eloesser flap: Past and present. *J Thorac Cardiovasc Surg* **93:**958–961, 1986
14. Clagett OT, Geraci JE: A procedure for the management of post pneumonectomy empyema. *J Thorac Cardiovasc Surg* **45:**141–145, 1963
15. Stafford EG, Clagett OT: Postpneumonectomy empyema: Neomycin instillation and definitive closure. *J Thorac Cardiovasc Surg* **63:**771–775, 1972
16. Meakins JL, Allard J: Neomycin absorption following Clagett procedure for postpneumonectomy empyema. *Ann Thorac Surg* **29:**32–35, 1980
17. Hopkins RA, Ungerleider RM, Staub EW, Young WG Jr: The modern use of thoracoplasty. *J Thorac Surg* **40:**181–187, 1985
18. Braimbridge M: Discussion of Lemmer JH, Botham MJ, Orringer MH: Modern management of adult thoracic empyema. *J Thorac Cardiovasc Surg* **90:**853, 1985
19. Emerson JD, Borvchow IB, Baichoff GR, et al: Empyema. *J Thorac Cardiovasc Surg* **62:**967, 1971
20. Gustafson RA, Murray GF, Ward HE, Hill RC: Role of lung of decortication in symptomatic empyemas in children. *Ann Thorac Surg* **49:**940–947, 1990
21. Horrigas TP, Snow NJ: Thoracoplasty: Current application to the infected pleural space. *Ann Thorac Surg* **50:**695–699, 1990
22. Iioka S, Sawamura K, Mori T, et al: Surgical treatment of chronic empyema: A new one-stage operation. *J Thorac Cardiovasc Surg* **74:**409–417, 1985
23. Andrews NC: Thoraco-mediastinal plication (a surgical technique for chronic empyema). *J Thorac Lung* **6:**809, 1961
24. Utley JR: Completion pneumonectomy and thoracoplasty for bronchopleural fistula and fungal empyema. *Ann Thorac Surg* **55:** 672–676, 1993
25. Hankins JR, Miller JE, McLaughlin JS: The use of chest wall muscle flaps to close bronchopleural fistulas: Experience with 21 patients. *Ann Thorac Surg* **25:**491–499, 1978
26. Miller JI, Mansour KA, Nahai F, et al: Single-stage complete muscle flap closure of the postpneumonectomy empyema space: A new method and possible solution to a disturbing complication. *Ann Thorac Surg* **38:**227–231, 1984
27. Cicero R, del Vecchyo C, Porter JK, Carreno J: Open window thoracostomy and plastic surgery with muscle flaps in the treatment of chronic empyema. *Chest* **89:**374–377, 1986

28. Pairolero PC, Arnold PG, Pichler JM: Intrathoracic transposition of extrathoracic skeletal muscle. *J Thorac Cardiovasc Surg* **86:** 809–817, 1983
29. Pairolero PC, Arnold PG, Trastek VF, Meland NB, Kay PP: Postpneumonectomy empyema. The role of intrathoracic muscle transposition. *J Thorac Cardiovasc Surg* **99:**958–966, 1990
30. Hammond DC, Fisher J, Meland NB: Intrathoracic free flaps. *Plast Reconstr Surg* **91:**1259–1264, 1993
31. Soucy P, Bass J, Evans M: The muscle-sparing thoracotomy in infants and children. *J Pediatr Surg* **26:**1323–1325, 1991

CHAPTER

32

# Thoracic Outlet Syndromes

Harold C. Urschel, Jr.

## INTRODUCTION AND HISTORICAL BACKGROUND

*Thoracic outlet syndrome* (TOS), a term coined by Rob and Standover,[1] refers to compression of the subclavian vessels and brachial plexus at the superior aperture of the chest. It was previously designated according to presumed etiologies as scalenus anticus, costoclavicular, hyperabduction, cervical rib, and first thoracic rib syndromes. These syndromes are similar, and the compression mechanism is often difficult to identify. Most compressive factors operate against the first rib (Fig. 32–1).[2,3]

Until 1927 a cervical rib was commonly thought to be the cause of symptoms of this syndrome. Galen and Vesalius first described the presence of a cervical rib.[4] Hunauld, who published an article in 1742, is credited by Keen[5] as being the first to describe the importance of the cervical rib. In 1818 Cooper treated symptoms of cervical rib with some success (cited by Adson and Coffey[6]), and in 1861 Coote[7] did the first cervical rib removal. Sir James Paget[8] in 1875 in London and von Schroetter[9] in 1884 in Vienna described the syndrome of thrombosis of the axillary-subclavian vein, which bears their names. Halsted[10] stimulated interest in dilation of the subclavian artery distal to cervical ribs, and Law[11] reported the role of adventitious ligaments in the cervical rib syndrome. Naffziger and Grant[12] and Ochsner and associates[13] popularized division of the scalenus anticus muscle. Falconer and Weddell[14] and Brintnall and associates[15] incriminated the costoclavicular membrane in the production of neurovascular compression. In 1945 Wright[16] described the hyperabduction syndrome with compression in the costoclavicular area by the tendon of the pectoralis minor. Rosati and Lord[17] added claviculectomy to anterior exploration, scalenotomy, cervical rib resection (when one was present), and section of the pectoralis minor and subclavian muscles, as well as the minor and subclavian muscles, and the costoclavicular membrane. The role of the first rib in causing neurovascular compression was recognized by Bramwell[18] in 1903. Murphy[19] is credited with the first resection of the first rib and in 1910 reported a collective review of 112 articles related to compression from the cervical ribs.[20] Brinckner and Milch[21,22] and Telford and associates[23] (1937, 1948) suggested that the first rib was the culprit. Clagett[2] emphasized first rib resection through a posterior thoracoplasty approach to relieve neurovascular compression. In 1962 Falconer and Li[24] reported the anterior approach for first rib resection, whereas Roos[25] and Roos and Owens[26] introduced the transaxillary route for first rib resection. Caldwell et al[27] introduced the method of measuring motor conduction velocities across the thoracic outlet in diagnosing thoracic outlet syndrome. Urschel and associates[28,29] popularized reoperation for recurrent thoracic outlet syndrome.

## SURGICAL ANATOMY

At the superior aperture of the thorax, the subclavian vessels and the brachial plexus traverse the cervicoaxillary canal to reach the upper extremity (Fig. 32–2). The cervicoaxillary canal is divided by the first rib into two sections: the proximal one, composed of the costoclavicular space, and the distal one, composed of the axilla. The proximal division is more critical for neurovascular compression. It is bounded superiorly by the clavicle, inferiorly by the first rib, anteromedially by the costoclavicular ligament, and posterolaterally by the scalenus medius muscle and the long thoracic nerve. The scalenus anticus muscle, which inserts on the scalene tubercle of the first rib, divides the costoclavicular space into two compartments: the anterior one

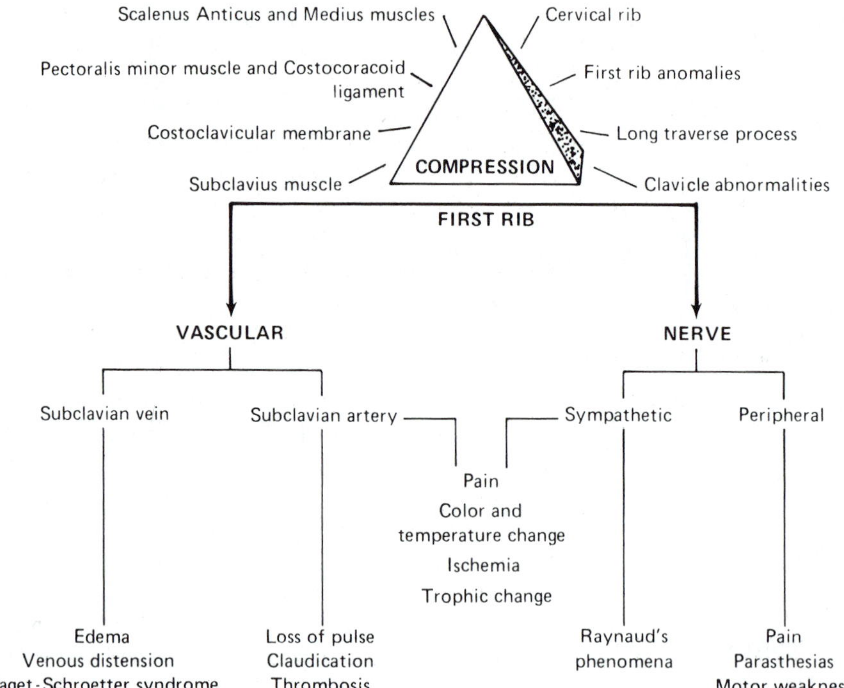


**Figure 32–1.** Thoracic outlet syndrome. Schematic drawing illustrating the relationship of the neurovascular bundle to scalene muscles, first rib, costoclavicular ligament, and subclavius muscle. *(From Urschel, Razzuk: Surg Annual. New York, Appleton-Century-Crofts, 1973, p 234, with permission.)*

containing the subclavian vein and the posterior one containing the subclavian artery and the brachial plexus. This compartment bounded by the scalenus anticus anteriorly, the scalenus medius posteriorly, and the first rib inferiorly, is called the scalene triangle.

## FUNCTIONAL ANATOMY

The cervicoaxillary canal, particularly its proximal segment, the costoclavicular space, normally has ample room for passage of the neurovascular bundle. Narrowing of this

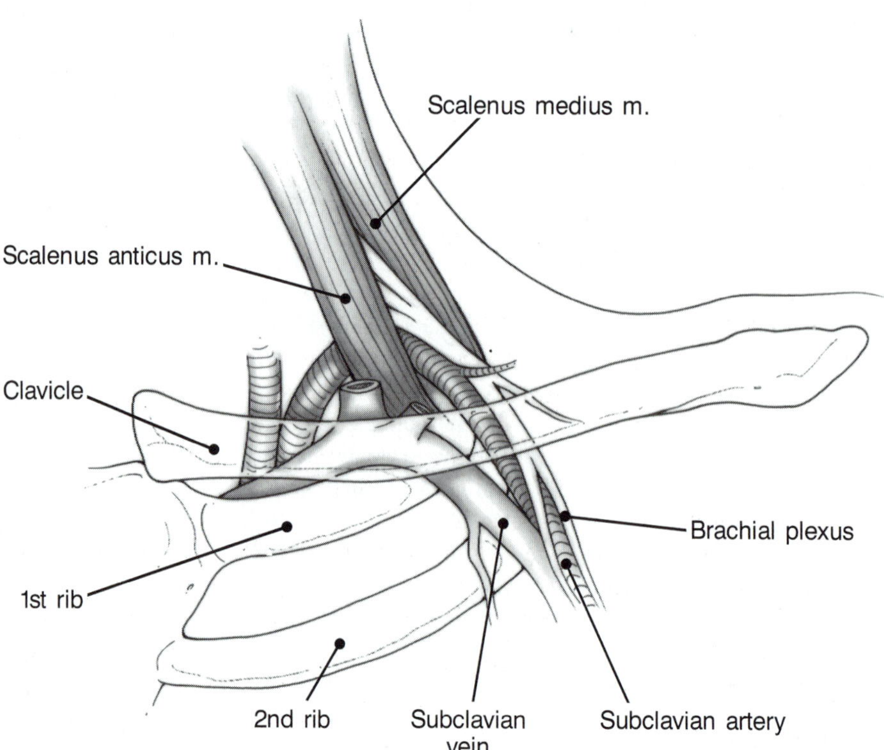


**Figure 32–2.** Relationship of the neurovascular bundle to the scalenus muscles, clavicle, and first rib.

space occurs during functional maneuvers. It narrows during abduction of the arm because the clavicle rotates backward toward the first rib and the insertion of the scalenus anticus muscle. In hyperabduction, the neurovascular bundle is pulled around the pectoralis minor tendon, the coracoid process and the head of the humerus; the coracoid process tilts downward and exaggerates the tension on the bundle. The sternoclavicular joint, which ordinarily forms an angle of 15–20 degrees, forms a smaller angle when the outer end of the clavicle descends as in drooping of the shoulders in poor posture, and narrowing of the costoclavicular space may occur.[17] During normal inspiration, the scalenus anticus muscle raises the first rib and narrows the costoclavicular space. In cases of severe emphysema or excessive muscular development in young adults, this muscle may cause an abnormal lift of the first rib.

The subclavian artery and brachial plexus traverse the scalene triangle on the first rib. This triangle is 1.2 cm at its base and approximately 6.7 cm in height. Anatomic variations may narrow the superior angle of the triangle, cause impingement on the upper components of the brachial plexus, and produce the upper type of scalenus anticus syndrome that involves the trunk containing elements of C5 and C6. If the base of the triangle is raised, compression of the subclavian artery and the trunks containing components of C7, C8, and T1 results in the lower type of scalenus anticus syndrome. Both types have been described by Swank and Simeone.[30]

## COMPRESSION FACTORS

Many factors may cause compression at the thoracic outlet, but the basic factor is deranged anatomy, to which congenital, traumatic, and, occasionally, atherosclerotic factors may contribute (Table 32–1).[17] Bony abnormalities are present in approximately 30% of patients, either as a cervical rib, a bifid first rib, fusion of the first and second ribs, clavicular deformities, or previous thoracoplasties.[31] These abnormalities can be seen on a chest x-ray, but special views of the lower cervical spine may be required in some cases of cervical ribs.

**TABLE 32–1. FACTORS THAT CAUSE COMPRESSION OF THE NEUROVASCULAR BUNDLE AT THE THORACIC OUTLET**

| Congenital | Traumatic |
|---|---|
| Cervical rib | Fracture of clavicle or first rib |
| Adventitious fibrous bands | Dislocation of head of humerus[15] |
| Bifid clavicle or first rib | Crushing injury to upper thorax |
| Exostosis of clavicle and first rib | Sudden muscular shoulder girdle efforts |
| Rudimentary first thoracic rib | Cervical spondylosis |
| Scalene muscles (anterior, middle, or minimus) | |
| Enlarged transverse process of C7 | |
| Omohyoid muscle | |

The double-crush hypothesis reported by Upton and McComas in 1973[32] states that a proximal source of nerve compression will render the distal nerve segment more susceptible to a second site of compression. These authors hypothesized that one site alone would not cause a clinical disturbance but that the summation of two sites would produce symptoms. This hypothesis is directly applicable to brachial plexus compression in that several anatomical structures may compress the brachial plexus, each of which on their own would not be enough to cause symptoms. The association between carpal and cubital tunnel syndromes and TOS is supported by this double-crush hypothesis. In our workmen's compensation patients with TOS, all had clinical evidence of either carpal or cubital tunnel syndrome as well. Twenty-four percent of patients had electrical evidence of carpal and cubital tunnel syndrome.

With an increase in jobs requiring repetitive activity (assembly lines, keyboarding), a cumulative trauma disorder or repetitive stress disorder is now recognized. This disorder relates to multilevel nerve compression. Specific anatomical structures and particular positions of the extremity will increase the pressure around the nerve and ultimately produce symptomatic nerve compression. If the wrist is in other than a neutral position, pressures increase around the median nerve in the carpal tunnel; elbow flexion produces increased pressure around the ulnar nerve in the cubital tunnel, and elevation of the arms overhead increases pressure around the lower trunk of the brachial plexus. Patients with cumulative trauma disorders will frequently have bilateral multilevel nerve compression. Hand surgeons who are trained to focus on the distal portion of the extremity are encouraged to evaluate their patients for concomitant TOS. Similarly, thoracic surgeons treating patients with TOS will find a significant association between TOS and carpal and cubital tunnel syndromes. We now recognize that both upper extremities work together as one unit and that problems in one extremity can soon be associated with complaints in the opposite extremity secondary to compensation by overuse. Physicians recognize that pathology at an ankle joint can eventually result in pathology at the contralateral hip joint. The patient should be evaluated for pathology at all points in the "circle"—wrist, elbow, shoulder, and neck.

## SYMPTOMS AND SIGNS

The symptoms of TOS depend on whether the nerves, blood vessels, or both are compressed. Neurogenic manifestations are more frequent than vascular ones. Symptoms consist of pain and paresthesias, which are present in approximately 95% of cases, and motor weakness and occasionally atrophy of hypothenar and interosseous muscles, which is the ulnar type of atrophy, in approximately 10%. The symptoms occur most commonly in areas supplied by the ulnar nerve, including the medial aspects of the arm and hand, the fifth finger, and the lateral aspects of the fourth finger. The onset of pain is usually insidious and commonly involves the neck, shoulder, arm, and hand. The pain and paresthesias may be precipitated by strenuous exercises or sustained physical efforts with the arm in abduction and the neck in hyperextension. Symptoms may be initiated by sleeping with arms abducted and hands clasped behind the neck. Trauma to the upper extremities or the cervical spine may be a precipitating factor. Physical examination may be noncontributory. Objective physical findings when present usually consist of hypesthesia along the medial aspect of the forearm and hand. Atrophy, when evident, is usually described in the hypothenar and interosseous muscles with clawing of the fourth and fifth fingers. In the upper type of TOS, in which components of C5–6 are compressed, pain is usually in the deltoid area and the lateral aspect of the arm. The presence of this pain requires exclusion of a herniated cervical disk.[17] Entrapment of C7 and C8 components that contribute to the median nerve produces symptoms in the index and sometimes middle fingers. Components of C5, C6, C7, C8, and T1 can be compressed by a cervical rib and produce symptoms of various degrees in the distribution of these nerves.

In some patients, the pain is atypical, involving the anterior chest wall or parascapular area, it is termed *pseudoangina* because it simulates angina pectoris. These patients may have normal coronary arteriograms but decreased ulnar nerve conduction velocities to 48 m/s and less, strongly suggesting the TOS. Shoulder, arm, and hand symptoms that usually provide the clue for a TOS may be absent or minimal compared with the severity of the chest pain. The diagnosis of thoracic outlet syndrome is frequently overlooked, with patients committed to becoming "cardiac cripples" without an appropriate diagnosis. They may develop severe depression when told that their coronary arteries are normal and there is no etiology for their pain.[33]

Arterial compression produces coldness, weakness, easy fatigability of the arm and hand, and pain that is usually diffuse.[28,31] Raynaud's phenomenon is noted in approximately 7.5% of patients with TOS. Unlike Raynaud's disease, which is usually bilateral and symmetric and elicited by cold or emotion, Raynaud's phenomenon in neurovascular compression is usually unilateral and is more likely to be precipitated by hyperabduction of the involved arm, turning the head, or carrying heavy objects. Sensitivity to cold may be present. Sudden onset of cold and blanching of one or more fingers may be followed by cyanosis and persistent rubor. Vascular compression symptoms may be a precursor of arterial thrombosis.[17] Arterial occlusion, usually of the subclavian artery, is manifested by persistent coldness, cyanosis, or pallor of the fingers and, in some instances, ulceration or gangrene. Palpation in the parascapular area may reveal a prominent pulsation, which indicates poststenotic dilation or aneurysm of the subclavian artery. Less frequently, the symptoms are those of venous obstruction or occlusion, commonly recognized as "effort thrombosis" or Paget-Schroetter syndrome.[34] This results in edema, discoloration of the arm, distention of the superficial veins of the limb and shoulder, and aches and pains. In some patients the condition is observed upon waking; in others it follows sustained efforts with the arm in abduction. Sudden backward and downward bracing of the shoulders or heavy lifting or strenuous physical activity involving the arm may constrict the vein and initiate venospasm, with or without subsequent thrombosis. There is usually moderate tenderness over the axillary vein and a cordlike structure may be felt that corresponds to the course of the vein. The acute symptoms may subside in a few weeks or days as the collateral circulation develops. Recurrence follows if collateral circulation is inadequate.[17]

Physical findings are more common in patients with primarily vascular rather than neural compression. Loss or diminution of the radial pulse and reproduction of symptoms can be elicited by the three classical maneuvers—the Adson or scalene test,[6] the costoclavicular test, and the hyperabduction test.[27]

## DIAGNOSIS

The diagnosis of TOS depends upon the history, physical and neurologic examination, films of the chest and cervical spine, an electromyogram (EMG), and ulnar nerve conduction velocity (UNCV). In some cases with atypical manifestations, other diagnostic procedures such as cervical myelography, arteriography,[35] or phlebography[36] should be considered. A detailed history and physical and neurologic examinations can often result in a tentative diagnosis of neurovascular compression. This diagnosis is strengthened when one or more of the classic maneuvers is positive and is confirmed by decreased UNCV.[3]

### Clinical Maneuvers

Loss or decrease of radial pulses and reproduction of symptoms can be elicited by three maneuvers: (1) Adson or scalene test[6]—This tightens the anterior and middle scalene muscles and decreases the space magnifying any preexisting compression of the subclavian artery and brachial plexus. The patient is instructed to take and hold a deep breath, extend the neck fully, and turn the head toward the side. Obliteration or decrease of the radial pulse suggests compression.[17,28] (2) Costoclavicular test (military position)—The shoulders are drawn downward and backward. This maneuver narrows the costoclavicular space by approximating the clavicle to the first rib and compressing the neurovascular bundle. Changes in the radial pulse and production of symptoms indicate compression. (3) Hyperabduction test—When the arm is hyperabducted to 180 degrees, the neurovascular bundle is pulled around the pectoralis minor tendon, the coracoid process, and the head of the humerus. If the radial pulse is decreased, compression should be suspected.

## RADIOGRAPHIC FINDINGS

Films of the chest and cervical spine help to reveal bony abnormalities, particularly cervical ribs and degenerative changes. If osteophytic changes and intervertebral space narrowing are present, a cervical computed tomographic (CT) scan or magnetic resonance imaging (MRI) should be done to rule out bony encroachment and narrowing of the spinal canal or intervertebral foramina.

## ELECTRODIAGNOSTIC TESTING

### Sensory Testing

Just as the histopathology of chronic nerve compression spans a broad spectrum, so will the patient's clinical findings. Initially, patients may be asymptomatic at rest. Only with positional or pressure provocative maneuvers will they become symptomatic. With time, patients may develop subtle sensory abnormalities that can only be detected by measuring the threshold of the system using vibratory or pressure threshold measurements. Eventually, with nerve injury and loss of fibers, loss of two points discrimination will develop.

Provocative tests are used to elicit symptoms from a patient who is asymptomatic at rest. These include percussion of the nerve (Tinel's sign) and pressure and positional provocative tests. In patients with TOS, these tests will be performed at the common nerve entrapment sites in the upper extremity (carpal tunnel, median nerve in the forearm, cubital tunnel, and brachial plexus). The examiner percusses over the nerve with four to six taps and the presence or absence of a tingling sensation within the distribution of that nerve is recorded. Movement and pressure provocative tests are held for a total of 60 seconds and are considered positive if paresthesia, numbness, or pain occurs in the appropriate nerve distribution. Provocative movement tests include arm elevation, elbow flexion, and wrist flexion (Phalen's sign). The pressure provocative tests include direct pressure with the examiner's thumb or fingertips on the brachial plexus, the ulnar nerve in the cubital tunnel, and the median nerve in the forearm proximal to the carpal tunnel. A rest period of a minute between each test allows return to the asymptomatic state.

The threshold of the rapidly adapting fiber receptor system can be assessed qualitatively with a tuning fork and quantitatively with a vibrometer. The "wrong end" of a 256-cps tuning fork is held against the skin. This end of the tuning fork is used in order to provide adequate amplitude for perception of the stimulus. A fixed-frequency (120 cps), varying-amplitude Vibratron II (Sensortek, Clifton, New Jersey) will quantify the threshold of the quickly adapting fibers. The vibrating portion of the Vibratron II is placed against the skin, and the smallest stimulus perceived is identified as the baseline vibration threshold and recorded in microns of motion. (Variable frequency, variable amplitude vibrometers are also available that provide a "vibrogram" of the patient's response to a number of frequencies of vibration. Since the higher frequencies of vibration are the most sensitive to nerve compression, such an instrument is of great interest in evaluating TOS patients.)

Pressure thresholds can be assessed quantitatively by using Semmes-Weinstein monofilaments. These nylon monofilaments are applied perpendicular to the cutaneous surface, and pressure is increased until bending of the monofilament is observed. These probes are of increasing weight with the lightest monofilament marked 1.65 and the heaviest marked 6.65. The number of the probe on the filament represents the logarithm of 10 times the force in 0.1 mg required to bow the monofilament. The number of the lightest probe that will elicit a perception and localization of pressure is recorded.

Assessment of innervation density indicates the number of receptors. Innervation density of slowly adapting receptors is measured by a static two-point discrimination test and the innervation density of the quickly adapting receptors is measured using a moving two-point discrimination test. Moving and static two-point discrimination (M2PD, S2PD) is assessed using a Disk-criminator T.M. (P.O. Box 16392, Baltimore MD, 20210). M2PD is assessed by slowly moving the prongs of the Disk-criminator longitudinally with just enough pressure to elicit a response. The subject is then asked to identify if one or two prongs is felt. The smallest spacing the subject is able to identify correctly in two of three trials is recorded in millimeters. A simple analogy helps to describe and understand the concept between innervation density, threshold, and the tests used to measure sensibility.

### Somatosensory Potential

Somatosensory-evoked potentials have been suggested in the diagnosis of TOS to deal with the proximal location of the compressive problem. Machleder et al[37] demonstrated in a group of 80 TOS patients that 74% had abnormal SSEPs.[37] Similarly, Yiannikas and Walsh[38] found SSEPs to be useful in the diagnosis. By contrast, Borg et al[39] found SSEPs to be abnormal only in patients with positive clinical signs. Both Borg et al and Machleder et al stressed the dynamic nature of this compressive neuropathy by suggesting SSEP assessment in neutral and then stressed positions.

### Nerve Conduction Velocities

This test is used widely in the differential diagnosis of arm pain, tingling, and numbness with or without motor weakness of the hand. Such symptoms may result from compression at various sites: in the spine; at the thoracic outlet; around the elbow, where it causes ulnar nerve palsy; or on the flexor aspects of the wrist, where it produces carpal tunnel syndrome. Conduction velocities of the ulnar, median, radial, and musculocutaneous nerves can be measured reliably.[40,41] Caldwell and associates[27] improved the technique of measuring ulnar nerve conduction velocity.

Electromyography and conduction velocities of each upper extremity are done with the Meditron 201 AD or 312 or the TECA-3 electromyograph; a coaxial cable with three needles or surface electrodes are used to record muscle action potentials in the hypothenar or first dorsal interosseous muscle, which appear on the fluorescent screen. Electromyography is usually normal in TOS.

Conduction velocity is determined by the Drusen-Caldwell technique[27] with the arm fully extended at the elbow and in about 20 degrees of abduction at the shoulder to stimulate over the course of the ulnar nerve. The nerve is stimulated at four points—supraclavicular fossa, middle upper arm, below the elbow, and at the wrist (Fig. 32–3)[28]—by a unit that imparts an electrical stimulus of 350 V that is approximately equal to 300 V with the patient's load with a skin resistance of 5000 Ω. Supramaximal stimulation is used at all points to obtain maximal response. The duration of the stimulus is 0.2 ms, except for muscular individuals, for whom it is 0.5 ms. Time of stimulation, conduction delay, and muscle response appear on the TECA screen; time markers occur each millisecond on the sweep. The latency period from the four points to the recording electrode in milliseconds is obtained from the TECA digital recorder or calculated from the tracing on the screen. The distance in millimeters between two adjacent sites of stimulation is measured with steel tape. The velocities in meters per second are calculated by subtracting the distal latency from the proximal latency and dividing the distance between two points of stimulation by the latency difference.

$$\text{Velocity (m/s)} = \frac{\text{distance between two adjacent stimulation points (mm)}}{\text{difference in latency (ms)}}$$

Normal values of UNCV are 72 m/s or above across the thoracic outlet; 55 m/s or above around the elbow; and 59 m/s or above in the forearm.[27] Wrist delay is 2.5–3.5 m/s. Decreased velocity in a segment or increased delay at the wrist indicates either compression, injury, neuropathy, or neurologic disorders. Decreased velocity across the outlet is consistent with TOS. Decreased velocity around the elbow signifies ulnar nerve entrapment or neuropathy. Increased delay at the wrist indicates carpal tunnel syndrome. The clinical picture of TOS correlates fairly well with the conduction velocity across the outlet. Any value less than 70 m/s indicates neurovascular compression. Compression is called slight at 66–69 m/s, mild at 60–65 m/s, moderate at 55–59 m/s, and severe when the velocity is 54 m/s or below.

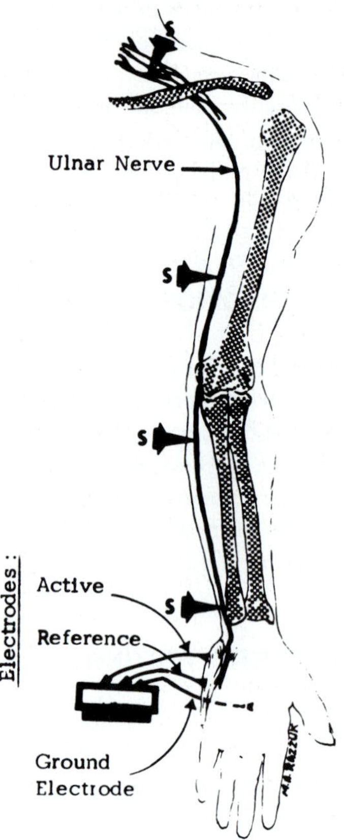


**Figure 32–3.** Ulnar nerve stimulation points (**S**) in the supraclavicular fossa (over the trunks of the plexus), above the elbow, below the elbow, and at the wrist.

## ANGIOGRAPHY

Simple clinical observations usually suffice to determine the degree of vascular impairment in the upper extremity. Peripheral angiography[42,43] is indicated in some cases, as in the presence of a paraclavicular pulsating mass, the absence of radial pulse, or the presence of supraclavicular or infraclavicular bruits. Retrograde or antegrade arteriograms of the subclavian and brachial arteries to demonstrate or localize the pathology should be obtained. In cases of venous stenosis or obstruction, as in Paget-Schroetter syndrome, phlebograms are used to determine the extent of thrombosis and the status of the collateral circulation.

## DIFFERENTIAL DIAGNOSIS

The thoracic outlet syndrome should be differentiated from various neurologic, vascular, cardiac, pulmonary, and esophageal conditions (Table 32–2).[17,28]

Neurologic causes of pain in the shoulder and arm are more difficult to recognize and may arise from the spine, brachial plexus, or peripheral nerves. A common cause of upper extremity pain is a herniated cervical intervertebral disk, which almost invariably occurs between the fifth and sixth or the sixth and seventh vertebrae and produces characteristic symptoms. Onset of pain and stiffness of the neck is variable. The pain radiates along the medial border of the scapula into the shoulder, occasionally into the anterior chest wall, and down the lateral aspect of the arm, at times into the fingers. Numbness and paresthesias in the fingers may be present. The segmental distribution of pain is a prominent feature. A herniated disk between C5 and C6 vertebrae compresses the C6 nerve root, causing pain or numbness primarily in the thumb and to a lesser extent in the index finger. The biceps muscle and the radial wrist extensor are weak, and the reflex of the biceps muscle is reduced or abolished. A herniated disk between the C6 and C7 vertebrae, which compresses the C7 nerve root, produces pain or numbness in the index finger and weakness of index finger flexion and ulnar wrist extension; the triceps muscle is weak, and its reflex is reduced or abolished. Any of these herniated disks may cause numbness along the ulnar border of the arm and hand due to spasm of the scalenus anticus muscle. Rarely, pain and paresthesias in the ulnar distribution may be related to herniation between the C7 and T1 vertebrae, which causes compression of the C8 nerve root. Compression of the latter nerve root produces weakness of intrinsic hand muscles.[43] Although rupture of the fifth and sixth disks produces hypesthesia in this area, only rupture of the seventh disk produces pain down the medial aspect of the arm.[17] The diagnosis of a ruptured cervical disk is based primarily on the history and physical findings; lateral films of the cervical spine reveal loss or reversal of cervical curvature with the apex of the reversal of curvature at the level of the disk involved. Electromyography can localize the site and extent of the nerve root irritation. When a herniated disk is suspected, cervical myelography should be done to confirm the diagnosis.

Another condition that causes upper extremity pain is cervical spondylosis, a degenerative disease of the intervertebral disk and the adjacent vertebral margin that causes spur formation and the production of ridges into the spinal canal or intervertebral foramina. Films and a computed tomography (CT) or magnetic resonance imaging (MRI)[44] scan of the cervical spine and electromyography help in making the diagnosis of this condition.

Several arterial and venous conditions can be confused with thoracic outlet syndrome; the differentiation can often be made clinically.

In patients who present with chest pain alone, it is important to suspect the thoracic outlet syndrome in addition to angina pectoris. Exercise stress testing and coronary angiography will exclude coronary artery disease.

**TABLE 32–2. DIFFERENTIATION OF THORACIC OUTLET SYNDROME FROM OTHER CONDITIONS**

| | |
|---|---|
| **Cervical Spine** | |
| Ruptured intervertebral disk | Osteoarthritis |
| | Spinal cord tumors |
| **Peripheral Nerves** | |
| Entrapment neuropathy | Medical neuropathies |
| Carpal tunnel—median nerve | Trauma |
| Ulnar nerve—elbow | Tumor |
| Radial nerve | |
| **Brachial Plexus** | |
| Superior sulcus tumor | |
| Trauma—postural palsy | |
| Several arterial and venous conditions can be confused with thoracic outlet syndrome. However, the differentiation can often be made clinically. These conditions include: | |
| **Arterial** | |
| Arteriosclerosis | Embolism |
| Aneurysm | Functional |
| Occlusive disease | Raynaud's disease |
| Thromboangiitis obliterans | |
| **Venous** | |
| Thrombophlebitis | |
| Mediastinal venous obstruction | Reflex vasomotor dystrophy |
| Malignant | Causalgia |
| Benign | Vasculitis, collagen disease |

## THERAPY

Initial management in the majority of patients with TOS is nonoperative. Patients are taught that overhead activity aggravates their symptoms. Modifications in their job or even job change is attempted. Work that requires overhead activity, heavy lifting, repetitive motions, or use of vibratory tools will aggravate TOS and mitigate against a good long-term surgical result. Rest periods with the arms down are recommended periodically during the day. Patients who tend to sleep with the arms above their head will aggravate TOS; sleeping with elbows flexed will aggravate cubital tunnel syndrome. Resting wrist splints at night to maintain the wrist in a neutral position and soft elbow pads to cushion the ulnar nerve and block elbow flexion are recommended.

### Physical Therapy

Many of the symptoms of TOS are a consequence of muscle imbalance in the cervicothoracic region. A relaxed forward posture with the head anteriorly displaced related to the thorax will result in a shortening of the flexor muscles, weakness of the extensor muscles, and subsequent loss of the cervical lordosis. We follow McKenzie's approach and recognize three factors that predispose to pain in this region: faulty posture, an increased frequency of flexion, and loss of extension.[45] Exercises are recommended to increase neck retraction and correct the cervical lordosis. In addition to posture abnormalities, muscle imbalance is addressed. Muscular assessment will identify muscle imbalance patterns (weakness vs. tightness) and identify the presence of referred pain pattern via trigger points. Muscle imbalance occurs when some muscles become tight while others become weak. Janda[46] described a proximal crossed syndrome in the upper extremity in patients with TOS in which the pectoralis major and minor, upper trapezius, scalene, and sternocleidomastoid muscles become tight. Weakness occurs in the scapular stabilizers including the middle and lower trapezius, rhomboid, and serratus anterior muscles. Tightness of the scalene muscles is recognized as a major contributor to nerve compression of the brachial plexus. Muscles that exhibit a decreased range of motion or strength can be evaluated for the presence of a hyperirritable fossa (myofacial trigger points). Patient with very tight and tender scalenes may benefit from local anesthetic block of the scalene muscles at their insertion at the first rib. Travell and Simons[47] have described a technique in the treatment of trigger points including Stretch and Spray with Fluorimethane.® With a decrease in the irritability of the lesion, more aggressive stretching can be implemented including hold-relaxed techniques (maximal contraction followed by maximal relaxation). Once control of pain and a range of movement are achieved, then a progressive strengthening program will be instituted. This will be directed toward the scapular stabilizers, the upper back, and posture muscles of the cervical spine (middle and lower trapezius, rhomboids, and serratus anterior). During these strengthening exercises, the stretching and range of movement program will be maintained. A successful, conservative physical therapy program for TOS will require that patients incorporate these exercises into their daily routines and become responsible for their programs.

Similarly, a soft cervical collar made from two roles of stockinette stuffed with soft gauze pads can be used. Abnormal posture patterns are demonstrated to the patients, and efforts are made to correct these. Obesity and hypertrophic breasts will aggravate TOS, and weight loss plans are recommended. Occasionally breast reduction is indicated.

Patients with TOS should be given physiotherapy when the diagnosis is made, including heat massages, active neck exercises, stretching of the scalenus muscles, strengthening of the upper trapezius muscle, and posture instruction. Because sagging of the shoulder girdle, which is common among the middle-aged, is a major etiologic factor in this syndrome, many patients with less severe cases are improved by strengthening the shoulder girdle and improving posture.[43]

Most patients with TOS who have ulnar nerve conduction velocities of more than 60 m/s improve with conservative management. If the conduction velocity is below that level, most patients, despite physiotherapy, will remain symptomatic, and surgical resection of the first rib and correction of other bony abnormalities may be needed. If symptoms continue after physiotherapy, and conduction velocity shows slight or no improvement or regression, resection of the first rib and cervical rib, when present, should be considered. Claggett[2] popularized the high posterior thoracoplasty approach for first rib resection, Falconer and Li[24] emphasized the anterior approach, and Roos[25] introduced the transaxillary route.

## SURGICAL MANAGEMENT AND TECHNIQUES

Several routes have been described to remove the first rib: posterior,[48] transaxillary,[25] supraclavicular,[24] infraclavicular, transthoracic, and through the bed of the resected clavicle.[49]

### Supraclavicular Approach

The supraclavicular approach releases soft-tissue compressive structures in the interscalene position of the brachial plexus. The lower trunk and root of C8 and T1 can be completely identified and protected while the most posterior aspect of the first rib is resected under direct vision. A cervical rib or prolonged transverse processes is easily removed from this supraclavicular approach. The incision site is shown in Figure 32–4 and the exposure schematically depicted in the drawing in Figure 32–5. Loupe magnification (4.5 ×), microbipolar cautery and a portable nerve stimulator (Concept 2, Clearwater, Florida) are used. A sandbag is placed between the scapulae, and the neck is extended to the nonoperative side. Long-acting paralytic agents are avoided.

An incision in a neck crease parallel 2 cm above the clavicle is made. The supraclavicular nerves are identified just beneath the platysma and mobilized for vessel loop retraction. The omohyoid is divided, and the supraclavicular

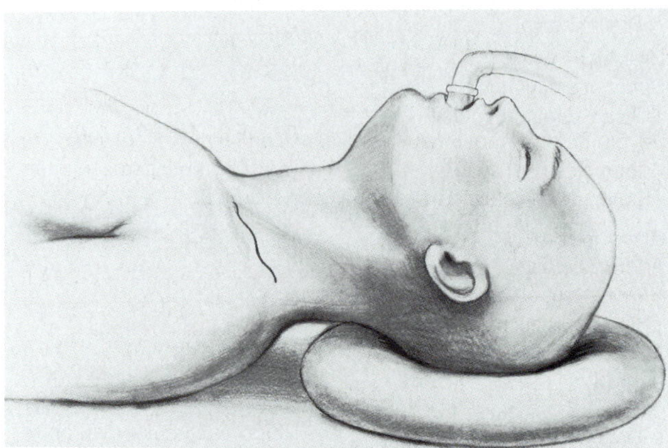

**Figure 32–4.** The patient is postioned with the head and neck extended. A supraclavicular incision is used.

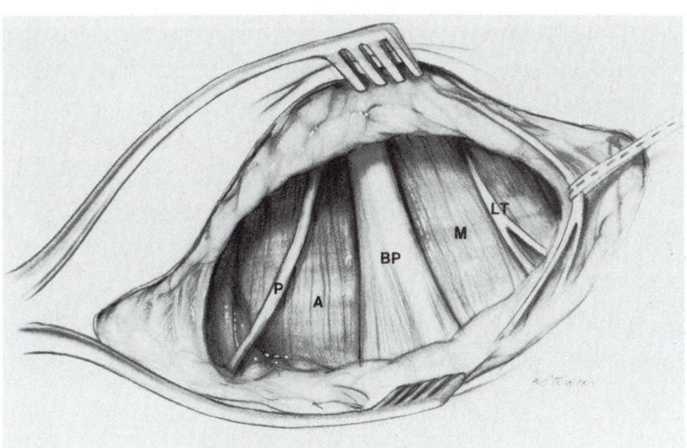


**Figure 32–5.** A schematic drawing of the exposure shows the phrenic nerve (P), brachial plexus (BP), long thoracic nerve (LT), and anterior (A) and middle (M) scalene muscles.

fat pad is elevated. The scalene muscles and the brachial plexus are then easily palpated. The lateral portion of the clavicular head of the sternocleidomastoid[3] is divided and repaired later. The phrenic nerve is seen on the anterior surface of the anterior scalene muscle. The long thoracic nerve is noted on the posterior aspect of the middle scalene muscle. The anterior scalene muscle is divided from the first rib. The subclavian artery is immediately behind this. An umbilical tape is placed around the subclavian artery. The phrenic nerve is avoided and not mobilized. The upper, middle, and lower trunks of the brachial plexus are easily seen and gently mobilized. The middle scalene muscle is now divided from the first rib. It has a broad attachment to the first rib, and care is taken to avoid injury to the long thoracic nerve. The long thoracic nerve may have multiple branches and may come through and posterior to the middle scalene muscle. With division of the middle scalene muscle, the brachial plexus is easily visualized and mobilized. The lower trunk and the C8 and T1 roots are identified above and below the first rib. Congenital bands and thickening in Sibson's fascia are divided. The first rib is encircled and divided where easily visible with bone-cutting instruments. The posterior segment of the rib is removed back to its spinal attachments with rongeurs. A fine elevator is used to separate the soft-tissue attachments to the first rib. The posterior edge of the first rib is grasped firmly with a rongeur. With a rocking and twisting motion, the posterior aspect of the first rib is removed so that the cartilaginous articular facets with the costal vertebral and costal transverse joints are removed. The anterior portion of the first rib is removed. A cervical rib or long transverse process will be removed similiarly. As described by Luoma and Nelems,[50] we open the pleura facilitating postoperative draining into the chest cavity rather than allowing fluid to collect in the operative site around the brachial plexus. When the pleura is opened, the intercostobrachial nerve, which is noted on the dome of the pleura, is protected. The wound is closed in a subcuticular fashion, and a simple suction drain is utilized after wound closure and maximal inflation of the lungs by the anesthetist.

## Transaxillary Approach

The transaxillary route is an expedient approach for complete removal of the first rib without the need for major muscle division without the need for retraction of the brachial plexus, as in the supraclavicular approach[24]; and without the difficulty of removing the posterior segment of the rib, as in the infraclavicular approach. This approach shortens the postoperative disability and provides better cosmetic results than the anterior and posterior approaches.

The patient is placed in the lateral position with the involved extremity abducted to 90 degrees by traction straps wrapped around the forearm and attached to an overhead pulley. An appropriate weight, usually 3 lb, is used to maintain this position without undue traction (Fig. 32–6).[28] A transverse incision is made in the axilla below the hairline between the pectoralis major and the latissimus dorsi muscles and deepened to the external thoracic fascia (Fig. 32–7). The intercostobrachial cutaneous nerve, which passes from the chest wall to the subcutaneous tissue in the center of the operative field, is protected.

The dissection is extended cephalad along the external thoracic fascia to the first rib. With gentle dissection, the neurovascular bundle and its relation to the first rib and both scalenus muscles are clearly outlined to avoid injury (Fig. 32–8).

The insertion of the scalenus anticus muscle is identified, skeletonized, and divided (Fig. 32–9). The first rib is dissected subperiosteally with a periosteal elevator and separated carefully from the underlying pleura to avoid a pneumothorax. A segment of the middle portion of the rib is resected, followed by subperiosteal dissection and resection of the anterior portion of the rib at the costochondral junction. After the costoclavicular ligament is cut, the posterior segment of the rib is similarly dissected subperiosteally and resected in fragments, including the articulation with the transverse process; the neck; and the head with a long, special double-action pituitary rongeur. It is preferable to remove the first rib entirely, because a residual portion, particularly if long, will cause recurrence of symptoms. The scalenus medius muscle should not be cut from its insertion on the second rib but rather stripped with a periosteal elevator to avoid injury to the long thoracic nerve that lies on its posterior margin. The eighth cervical and first thoracic nerve roots may be seen at this point. If a cervical rib is present, its anterior portion, which usually articulates with the first rib, should be resected at a point when the middle portion of the first rib is removed. The remaining segment of the cervical rib should be removed after removal of the posterior segment of the first rib. The wound is drained, and only the subcutaneous tissues and skin require closure, because no muscles have been divided. The patient is encouraged to use the arm for self-care but to avoid heavy lifting

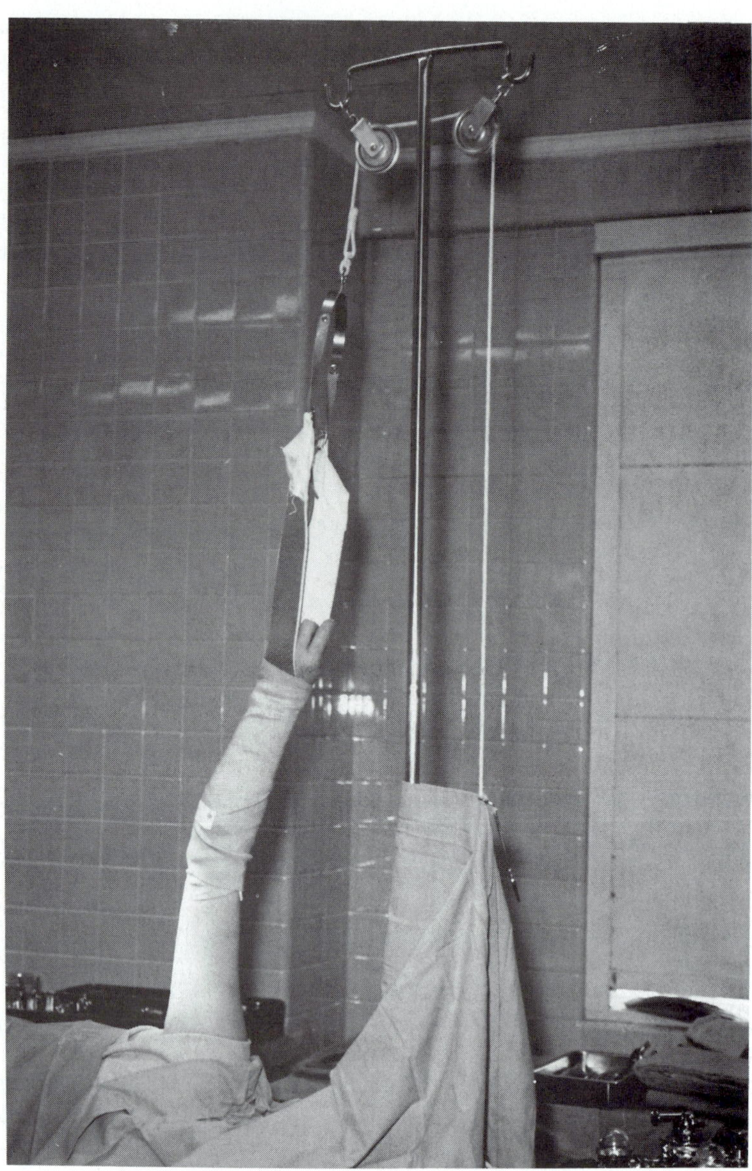

**Figure 32–6.** Transaxillary resection of first rib. The arm, which is abducted to 90 degrees by traction straps on the forearm, is attached to an overhead pulley. *(From Urschel, Razzuk: Surgery of the Chest. Philadelphia, Saunders, 1983, p 449, with permission.)*

until at least 3 months after the operation. Cervical muscle stretching should be started at the end of the first week, and gentle exercising of the arm can be started at the end of the third week after operation.

## Paget-Schroetter Syndrome (Effort Thrombosis)

"Effort" thrombosis of the axillary-subclavian vein is usually secondary to unusual exertion or excessive use of the arm in addition to the presence of one or more compressive elements.[36,51,52]

The thrombosis is caused by trauma[53] or unusual occupations requiring repetitive muscular activity (professional athletes, linotype operators, painters, and beauticians.) Cold and trauma such as carrying skis over the shoulder may increase this possibility,[54] as may increased thrombogenicity. For many years, therapy consisted of elevation of the arm and anticoagulants with subsequent return to work. If symptoms recurred, the patient was considered for a first-rib resection, with or without thrombectomy[55] as well as resection of the scalenus anterior muscle and removal of any other compressive element in the thoracic outlet, such as a cervical rib or abnormal bands.[56–59]

In patients treated conservatively with elevation and Coumadin, Adams and DeWeese[36] found a 12% incidence of pulmonary embolism. Occasional venous distention occurred in 18% of patients and late residual arm symptoms of swelling, pain, and superficial thrombophlebitis were noted in 68% of the patients (postphlebitic syndrome). Phlegmasia cerulean dolens was present in one patient.

Recent availability of thrombolytic agents,[60–62] combined with prompt surgical decompression of the compressive elements in the thoracic outlet,[63] have reduced morbidity and the necessity for thrombectomy and have

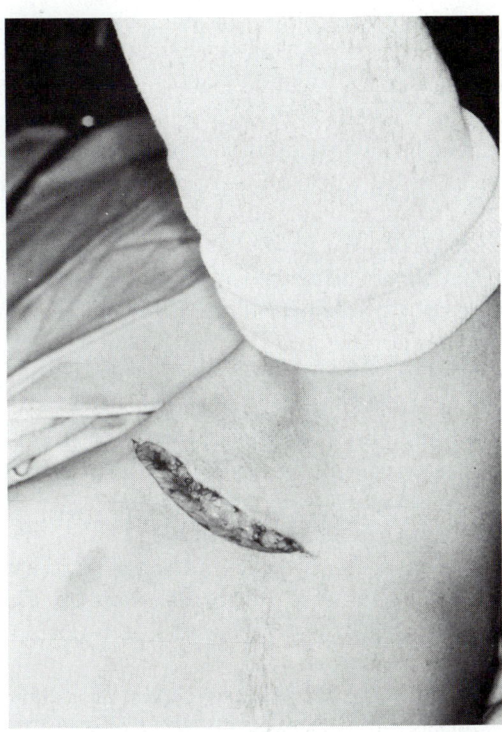

**Figure 32–7.** A transverse incision is made below the hairline between pectoralis major and latissimus dorsi muscle and is carried to the chest wall.

substantially improved clinical results, including the ability to return to work.[34] An advantage of urokinase over streptokinase is its direct action on the thrombosis distal to the catheter (a local thrombolytic effect).[64–66] Streptokinase produces systemic effects with potential complications. Heparin after a thrombolytic agent followed by surgical in-

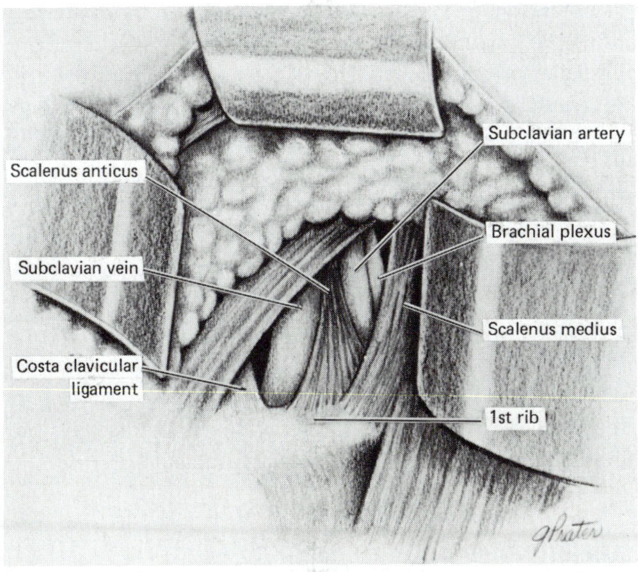


**Figure 32–8.** Exposure of the neurovascular bundle and the first rib.

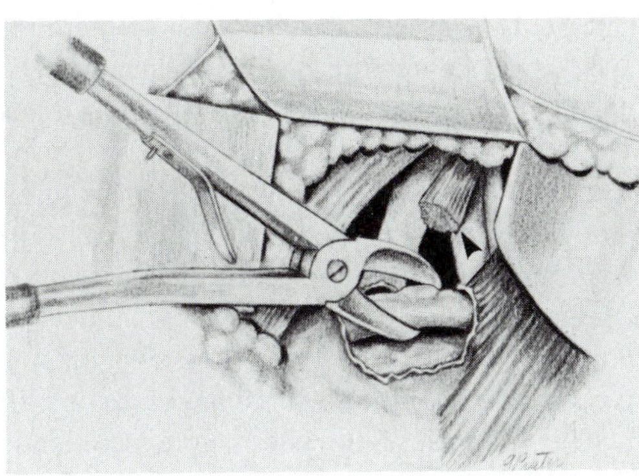

**Figure 32–9.** The scalenus anticus (arrow) is severed, and the first rib is separated from the periosteum and divided at that point.

tervention is another advantage. Some of the long-term disability was related to the morbidity from a thrombectomy as well as recurrent thrombosis.[59,67,68]

The natural history of Paget-Schroetter syndrome suggests moderate morbidity[69,70] with conservative treatment alone. Bypass with vein or other conduits has limited application.[71–73] Causes other than thoracic outlet syndrome must be treated individually.[74] Intermittent obstruction of the subclavian vein[75] can lead to thrombosis, and decompression should be employed prophylactically.

## REOPERATION FOR RECURRENT TOS

Complete extirpation of the first rib relieves symptoms in patients with TOS not relieved by physiotherapy. In the surgically treated patients, 10% develop various degrees of shoulder, arm, and hand pain and paresthesias that are usually mild and short-lasting and respond well to a brief course of physiotherapy and muscle relaxants. In a few patients (1.6%), symptoms persist or become progressively more severe and often involve a wider area of distribution because of entrapment of the intermediate trunk in addition to the lower trunk and C8 and T1 nerve roots. Symptoms may recur 1 month to 7 years after rib resection; in most patients they recur within the first 3 months. Symptoms consist of an aching or burning type of pain, often associated with paresthesias, involving the neck, shoulder, parascapular area, anterior chest wall, arm, and hand. Vascular lesions are uncommon and consist of minor causalgia and an occasional injury of the subclavian artery with subsequent false aneurysm formation caused by the sharp edge of a remaining posterior stump of an incompletely resected first rib. Recurrence is diagnosed on the basis of history, physical examination, and decreased nerve conduction velocity across the outlet. Diagnostic evaluation should also include thorough neurologic evaluation, chest and cervical spine films, cervical myelography, and subclavian artery angiography, when indicated.

There are two groups of patients who require reoperation. There is pseudorecurrence in patients who did not have relief after the initial operation in whom the second rib was mistakenly resected, leaving a rudimentary first rib. True recurrence occurs in patients whose symptoms were relieved after the first operation but who have a significant segment of the first rib remaining with scar formation around the brachial plexus. Physiotherapy should be given to all patients with symptoms of neurovascular compression after first rib resection. If the symptoms persist and the conduction velocity remains below normal, reoperation is indicated. This is done with a posterior thoracoplasty incision to better expose the nerve roots, brachial plexus, and subclavian artery and vein. This reduces the danger of injury to these structures. This incision provides a wider field for resection of any bony abnormalities or fibrous bands and allows extensive neurolysis of the nerve roots and brachial plexus. This is not always possible with the limited transaxillary exposure. The supraclavicular approach is inadequate for reoperation.

The technique includes a high thoracoplasty incision that extends from 3 cm above the angle of the scapula, halfway between the angle of the scapula and the spinous processes, and caudad 5 cm from the angle of the scapula. The trapezius and rhomboid muscles are divided. The scapula is retracted from the chest wall by making a subperiosteal incision over the fourth rib. The posterior superior serratus muscle is divided and the sacrospinalis muscle retracted medially. The first rib remnant and cervical rib remnant, if present, are removed subperiosteally, and the regenerated periosteum is removed. In the authors' experience, most regenerated ribs occur from the end of an unresected rib segment rather than from periosteum, although the latter is possible. To reduce the incidence of bony regeneration, it is important in the initial operation to remove the first rib totally in all patients.

If there is excessive scarring, it may be prudent to do the sympathectomy initially.[76–78] A 1-in. segment of the second rib is resected posteriorly to locate the sympathetic ganglion. This way the first thoracic nerve may be easier to locate below rather than through the scar. The T1, T2, and T3 thoracic ganglia are removed. Care is taken to avoid damage to the C8 ganglion (upper aspect of the stellate ganglion), which would produce a Horner's syndrome.[76,77]

Neurolysis of the nerve root and brachial plexus is done with the help of a nerve stimulator and is carried down to but not into the nerve sheath. Neurolysis is extended peripherally over the brachial plexus as far as any scarring persists. Excessive neurolysis is not good. Opening of the nerve sheath produces more scarring than it relieves.

The subclavian artery and vein are released if symptoms suggests the need for this. The scalenus medius muscle is divided. After meticulous hemostasis, a large, round Jackson-Pratt drain is placed close to but not touching the brachial plexus and is brought out through the subscapular space via a stab wound into the axilla. Methylprednisolone acetate (Depo-Medrol; 80 mg) is left in the area of the nerve plexus, but the patient is not given systemic steroids unless keloid formation has occurred. The wound is closed in layers with interrupted heavy vicryl sutures to provide adequate strength, and the arm is kept in a sling and used gently for the first 3 months. Range-of-motion exercises are done to prevent shoulder limitation, but overactivity is avoided to minimize excessive scar formation.

When the problem is vascular and involves false or mycotic aneurysms, a bypass graft is interposed from the innominate or carotid artery proximally, through a separate tunnel distally, to the brachial artery. The graft is usually done with the saphenous vein, although other conduits may be used. The arteries supplying and leaving the infected aneurysm are ligated. Subsequently, the aneurysm is resected by a transaxillary approach with no fear of bleeding or ischemia of the arm.

The sympathectomy relieves chest wall pain that resembles angina pectoris, esophageal disease, or even a tumor in the lung by denervating the deep fibers that accompany the arteries and bone.

The results of reoperation are good if an accurate diagnosis is made and the proper procedure is used.[78,79] More than 800 patients have been followed up for 6 months to 15 years. All patients improved initially after reoperation, and in 79% the improvement was maintained for more than 5 years. In 14% of the patients, symptoms were managed with physiotherapy; 7% required a second reoperation, in every case because of rescarring. There were no deaths, and only one patient had an infection that required drainage.

## SUMMARY

Thoracic outlet syndrome is recognized in approximately 8% of the population. Its manifestations may be neurologic, vascular, or both, depending on the component of the neurovascular bundle predominantly compressed. The diagnosis is made by UNCV. Treatment is initially conservative, but persistence of significant symptoms is an indication for first-rib resection. This occurs in approximately 5% of patients with diagnosed thoracic outlet syndromes. Primary resection is done preferably through the transaxillary approach along with removal of a cervical rib if present. Symptoms of various degrees may recur after first-rib resection in approximately 10% of patients.[80] Most of the patients improve with physiotherapy, and only 1.6% require reoperation. Reoperation for recurrent symptoms is done through a high posterior thoracoplasty incision.

## REFERENCES

1. Rob CG, Standover A: Arterial occlusion complicating thoracic outlet compression syndrome. *Br Med J* **2**:709, 1958

2. Clagett OT: Presidential address: Research and prosearch. *J Thorac Cardiovasc Surg* **44:**153, 1962
3. Urschel HC Jr, Razzuk MA, Wood RE, Paulson DL: Objective diagnosis (ulnar nerve conduction velocity) and current therapy of the thoracic outlet syndrome. *Ann Thorac Surg* **12:**608, 1971
4. Borchardt M: Symptomatologie und therapie der Halsrippen. *Berl Klin Worhenschr* **38:**1265, 1901
5. Keen WW: The symptomatology, diagnosis and surgical treatment of cervical ribs. *Am J Sci* **133:**173, 1907
6. Adson AW, Coffey JR: Cervical rib: A method of anterior approach for relief of symptoms by division of the scalenus anticus. *Ann Surg* **85:**839, 1927
7. Coote H: Pressure on the axillary vessels and nerve by an exostosis from a cervical rib; interference with the circulation of the arm; removal of the rib and exostosis, recovery. *Med Times Gaz* **2:**108, 1861
8. Paget J: *Clinical Lectures and Essays.* London, Longmans Green, 1875
9. von Schroetter L, Erkankungen der Gefossl. In: Nathnogel J (ed): *Handbuch der Pathologie und Therapie.* Wein, Holder, 1884
10. Halsted WS: An experimental study of circumscribed dilation of an artery immediately distal to a partially occluding band, and its bearing on the dilation of the subclavian artery observed in certain cases of cervical rib. *J Exp Med* **24:**271, 1916
11. Law AA: Adventitious ligaments simulating cervical ribs. *Ann Surg* **72:**497, 1920
12. Naffziger HC, Grant WT: Neuritis of the brachial plexus—mechanical in origin: The scalenus syndrome. *Surg Gynecol Obstet* **67:**722, 1928
13. Ochsner A, Gage M, DeBakey M: Scalenous anticus (Naffziger) syndrome. *Am J Surg* **28:**699, 1935
14. Falconer MA, Weddell G: Costoclavicular compression of the subclavian artery and vein: Relation to scalenus syndrome. *Lancet* **2:**539, 1943
15. Brintnall ES, Hyndman OR, Van Allen WM: Costoclavicular compression associated with cervical rib. *Ann Surg* **144:**921, 1956
16. Wright IS: The neurovascular syndrome produced by hyperabduction of the arm. *Am Heart J* **29:**1, 1945
17. Rosati LM, Lord JW: Neurovascular compression syndromes of the shoulder girdle. *Modern Surgical Monographs.* New York, Grune and Stratton, 1961
18. Bramwell E: Lesion of the first dorsal nerve root. *Rev Neurol Psychiatry* **1:**236, 1903
19. Murphy T: Brachial neuritis caused by pressure of first rib. *Aust Med J* **15:**582, 1910
20. Murphy T: *Aus Med J* **15:**582, 1910; as cited by Brickner WM, Milch H (ref 21).
21. Brickner WM, Milch H: First dorsal vertebra stimulating cervical rib by mal development or by pressure symptoms. *Surg Gynecol Obstet* **40:**38, 1925
22. Brickner WM: Brachial plexus pressure by the normal first rib. *Ann Surg* **85:**L858, 1927
23. Telford ED, Mottershead S: Pressure of the cervicobrachial junction. *J Bone Joint Surg (Am)* **30:**249, 1948
24. Falconer MA, Li FWP: Resection of the first rib in costoclavicular compression of the brachial plexus. Lancet **1:**59, 1962
25. Roos DB: Transaxillary approach for first rib resection to relieve thoracic outlet syndrome. *Ann Surg* **163:**354, 1966
26. Roos DB, Owens JC: Thoracic outlet syndrome. *Arch Surg* **93:**71, 1996
27. Caldwell JW, Crane CR, Drusen EM: Nerve conduction studies in the diagnosis of the thoracic outlet syndrome. *South Med J* **64:**210, 1971
28. Urschel HC Jr, Razzuk MA: Current management of thoracic outlet syndrome. *N Engl J Med* **286:**21, 1972
29. Urschel HC Jr, Razzuk MA, Albers JE, et al: Re-operation for recurrent thoracic outlet syndrome. *Ann Thorac Surg* **21:**19, 1976
30. Swank WL, Simeone FA: The scalenous anticus syndrome. *Arch Neurol Psychiatr* **51:**432, 1944
31. Urschel HC Jr, Paulson DL, McNamara JJ: Thoracic outlet syndrome. *Ann Thorac Surg* **6:**1, 1968
32. Upton ARM, McComas AJ: The double crush in nerve entrapment syndromes. *Lancet* **2:**359–362, 1973
33. Urschel HC Jr, Razzuk MA: Thoracic outlet syndrome. In: Shields TW (ed): *General Thoracic Surgery,* 2nd ed. Lea & Febiger, Philadelphia, 1983
34. Urschel HC, Razzuk MA: Pagett-Schroetter syndrome effort thrombosis: Axillary-subclavian vein thrombosis. *Ann Thorac Surg* **52:**1217–1221, 1991
35. Rosenberg JC: Arteriography demonstration of compression syndromes of the thoracic outlet. *South Med J* **59:**400, 1966
36. Adams JT, DeWeese JA: "Effort" thrombosis of the axillary and subclavian veins. *J Trauma* **11:**923–930, 1971
37. Machleder HI, Moll F, Nuwer M, et al: Somatosensory evoked potential in the assessment of thoracic outlet compression syndrome. *J Vasc Surg* **6:**177, 1987
38. Yiannikas C, Walsh JC: Somatosensory evoked responses in the diagnosis of thoracic outlet syndrome. *J Neurol Neurosurg Psychiatry* **46:**234–240, 1983
39. Borg K, Edstrom L, Lindblom U: "Numbed finger"—an overview and a proposal for a survey. *Lakartidningen* **80:**5076–5080, 1983
40. Razzuk MA, Krusen EM, Caldwell JW, Urschel HC Jr: The clinical value and technique of measuring nerve conduction velocities for thoracic outlet syndrome. In Greep JC, Lemmen HAJ, Roos DB, Urschel HC Jr (eds): *Pain in Shoulder and Arm,* The Hague/Boston/London, Martinus Nijhoff, 1979
41. Jebsen RH: Motor conduction velocities in the median and ulnar nerves. *Arch Phys Med* **48:**185, 1967
42. Lang EK: Roentgenographic diagnosis of the neurovascular compression syndromes. *Adiology* **79:**58, 1962
43. Krusen EM: Cervical pain syndromes. *Arch Phys Med* **49:**376, 1968
44. Rapoport S, Blair DN, McCarthy SM, et al: Brachial plexus: Correlation of MR imaging and CT pathologic findings. *Radiology* **167:**161–169, 1988
45. Mackinnon SE, Dellon AL: *Surgery of the Peripheral Nerve.* New York, Thieme Medical Publishers, 1988
46. Janda V: Muscles and cervicogenic pain syndromes. In Grant R (ed): *Clinics in Physical Therapy, Physical Therapy of the Cervical and Thoracic Spine,* New York, Churchill Livingstone, 1988
47. Travell JG, Simons DG: Myofascial pain and dysfunction. In: *The Trigger Point Manual.* Baltimore/London, Williams & Wilkins, 1983
48. Martinez NS: Posterior first rib resection for total thoracic outlet syndrome decompression. *Contemp Surg* **15:**13, 1979
49. Lord JW, Urschel HC: Total claviculectomy. *Surg Rounds* **1:**17–27, 1988
50. Luoma A, Nelems B: *Thoracic Outlet Syndrome Thoracic Surgery Perspective,* Saunders, Neurosurgical Clinics of North America, 1991, pp 187–226
51. Johnston KW: Neurovascular conditions involving the upper extremity. In: Rutherford RB (ed): Vascular Surgery, 3rd ed. Philadelphia, Saunders, 1989, pp 801–898
52. Aziz K, Straenley CJ, Whelan TJ: Effort-related axilla-subclavian vein thrombosis. *Am J Surg* **152:**57–61, 1986
53. Cikrit DF, Dalsing MC, Bryand BJ, et al: An experience with upper-extremity vascular trauma. *Am J Surg* **160:**229–233, 1990
54. Daskalakis E, Bouhoutsos J: Subclavian and axillary vein compression of musculoskeletal origin. *Br J Surg* **67:**573–576, 1980
55. DeWeese JA, Adams JT, Gaiser DI: Subclavian venous thrombectomy. *Circulation* **16**(suppl 2):158–170, 1970
56. Prescott SM, Tikoff G: Deep venous thrombosis of the upper extremity: A reappraisal. *Circulation* **59:**350–357, 1979
57. Roos D: Thoracic outlet nerve compression. In: Rutherford RB (ed): *Vascular Surgery,* 3rd ed. Philadelphia, Saunders, 1989, pp 858–875
58. Inahara T: Surgical treatment of "effort" thrombosis of the axillary and subclavian veins. *Am Surg* **34:**479–483, 1968

59. Campbell BE, Chandler JG, Tegtmeyer CJ: Axillary, subclavian and brachycephalic vein obstruction. *Surgery* **82:**816–826, 1977
60. Sundqvist SB, Hedner U, Kullenberg KHE, et al: Deep venous thrombosis of the arm: a study of coagulation and fibrinolysis. *Br Med J* **283:**265–267, 1981
61. Rubenstein M, Greger WP: Successful streptokinase therapy for catheter induced subclavian vein thrombosis. *Arch Intern Med* **140:**1370–1371, 1980
62. Zimmerman R, Marl H, Harenberg J, et al: Urokinase therapy of subclavian axillary vein thrombosis. *Klin Wochenschr* **59:**851–857, 1981
63. Taylor LM, McAllister WR, Dennis DL, et al: Thrombolytic therapy followed by first rib resection for spontaneous subclavian vein thrombosis. *Am J Surg* **149:**644–647, 1985
64. Becker GJ, Holden RW, Robe FE, et al: Local thrombolytic therapy for subclavian and axillary vein thrombosis. *Radiology* **149:**419–423, 1983
65. Drury EM, Trout HH, Giordono JM, et al: Lytic therapy in the treatment of axillary and subclavian vein thrombosis. *J Vasc Surg* **2:**821–829, 1984
66. Eisenbud DE, Brener BJ, Shoenfeld R, et al: Treatment of acute vascular occlusions with intra-arterial urokinase. *Am J Surg* **160:**160–165, 1990
67. Drapanas T, Curran W: Thrombectomy in the treatment of "effort" thrombosis of the axillary and subclavian veins. *J Trauma* **6:**107–116, 1966
68. Painter TD, Karpf M: Deep venous thrombosis of the upper extremity: 5 years experience at a university hospital. *Angiology* **35:**743–752, 1984
69. Tilney NL, Griffiths HFG, Edwards EA: Natural history of major venous thrombosis of the upper extremity. *Arch Surg* **101:**792–796, 1970
70. Coon WW, Willis PW: Thrombosis of axillary subclavian veins. *Arch Surg* **94:**657–663, 1966
71. Hansen B, Feins RS, Detman DE: Simple extra-anatomic jugular vein bypass for subclavian vein thrombosis. *J Vasc Surg* **2:**291–299, 1985
72. Hashmonai M, Schramek A, Farbstein J: Cephalic vein cross-over bypass for subclavian vein thrombosis: A case report. *Surgery* **80:**563–564, 1976
73. Jacobson JH, Haimov M: Venous revascularization of the arm: Report of three cases. *Surgery* **81:**599–604, 1977
74. Loring WE: Venous thrombosis in the upper extremity as a complication of myocardial failure. *Am J Med* **27:**397–410, 1952
75. McLaughlin CW, Popma AM: Intermittent obstruction of the subclavian vein. *JAMA* **113:**1960–1968, 1939
76. Palumbo LT: Anterior transthoracic approach for upper extremity thoracic sympathectomy. *Arch Surg* **72:**L659, 1956
77. Palumbo LT: Upper dorsal sympathectomy without Homer's syndrome. *Arch Surg* **71:**743, 1955
78. Urschel HC Jr, Razzuk MA: Posterior thoracic sympathectomy. In Malt RA (ed): *Surgical Techniques Illustrated: A Comparative Atlas.,* Philadelphia, Saunders, 1985
79. Urschel HC Jr: *Re-operation for Thoracic Outlet Syndrome. International Trends in General Thoracic Surgery,* Vol II. St. Louis, Mosby, 1986
80. Urschel HC Jr, Razzuk MA: The failed operation for thoracic outlet syndrome: The difficulty of diagnosis and management. *Ann Thorac Surg* **42:**523–528, 1986

# CHAPTER 33

# Chest Wall Abnormalities

Eric W. Fonkalsrud

A variety of malformations of the chest wall may be identified in infancy and early childhood. The most common are the pectus escavatum and pectus carinatum anomalies. Sternal clefts and a variety of developmental abnormalities involving the ribs, costal cartilages, and spine are less common.

## SKELETAL ANOMALIES

Various deviations from the normal pattern of 12 symmetric ribs occasionally occur. One or more ribs may be completely absent or only partially developed. A rib may bifurcate, and one component articulate with a somewhat hypoplastic adjacent rib or fuse with it. If the costal defects are extensive, they may cause moderate to severe cosmetic and/or functional abnormalities. Severe fusion can lead to progressive kyphoscoliosis, or it may cause serious compression of the lungs with resultant ventilatory disturbance (Fig. 33–1). An extreme form of narrow and rigid thorax with multiple cartilaginous anomalies in which the patient progresses to death through respiratory insufficiency has been termed *asphyxiating thoracic dystrophy of the newborn* or Jeune's disease. Infants with severe fusion anomalies may require prolonged respiratory assistance; often they have associated cardiac anomalies and other systemic anomalies that result in high mortality. Attempts at surgical correction have generally been unsuccessful, since volume increase provided by surgical reconstruction does not improve respiratory insufficiency. These infants experience recurrent pneumonias that lead to interstitial fibrosis and eventually pulmonary hypertension, which causes death in infancy or early childhood. Spinal defects, such as hemivertebrae, are commonly associated with costal abnormalities.

*Sprengel's deformity* is an anomaly in which the scapula is hypoplastic and fixed in an elevated position to the vertebral column by fibrous bands, cartilage, or bone. Movement of the ipsilateral shoulder is thereby limited. Winging of the scapula, typically present in this anomaly, can also result from traumatic or operative injury to the long thoracic nerve.

Anomalies of the ribs and sternum, particularly the pectus defects, commonly occur in patients with Marfan's syndrome and in association with certain congenital heart defects. The combination of absence of the pectoralis major and minor muscles, ipsilateral breast hypoplasia, and absence of segments of two to four ribs characterizes *Poland's syndrome,* a variant of the pectus abnormalities.[1] Patients with this syndrome require rib grafts from the contralateral thorax to stabilize the chest wall during early childhood, followed by muscle flap transfer and eventually breast reconstruction during adolescence (Fig. 33–2A,B). Absence of the pectoralis muscle may occur as an isolated defect.

*Supernumerary ribs* are usually located in the cervical region and rarely cause symptoms. In rare cases, an extra rib may arise in the midthoracic level and cause pain by pressure on adjacent intercostal nerves; rib resection is curative.

## CONGENITAL ANOMALIES OF THE STERNUM AND COSTAL CARTILAGES

### Sternal Clefts

The embryonic sternum appears before the second month of intrauterine development as bilaterally paired condensations of mesenchyme, at first independent of the ribs, which eventually become cartilaginous.[2] The cartilage bars migrate steadily toward the midline and fuse, following which the sternum divides transversely into three segments, or

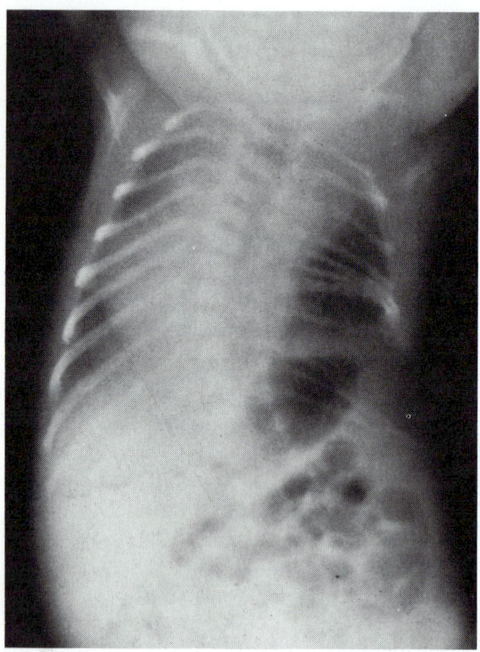

**Figure 33–1.** Neonate with extensive rib fusion, scoliosis, displacement of mediastinal structures, and severe respiratory distress.

sternebrae: the manubrium, the gladiolus (or body), and the xiphoid. This complex process is closely related to the descent and muscularization of the septum transversum of the diaphragm and the closure of the pericardial sac.

Failure of the embryonic sternal bars to meet and fuse in the midline leads to the development of a *sternal cleft,* known as *bifid sternum* or *congenital sternal fissure.* A simple cleft of the sternum may occur unassociated with other major anomalies. When associated with the heart's being positioned outside the chest wall, it is known as *ectopia cordis.* A ventricular septal defect is almost invariably present, and there may be an associated atrial septal defect, as well as pulmonary stenosis.[3] In the most extreme form *(pentalogy of Cantrell)* the cleft involves the lower sternum and is associated with ectopia cordis, a ventral diaphragmatic defect, a midline abdominal defect or omphalocele, a defect of the pericardium allowing communication with the peritoneal cavity, and a cardiac anomaly.

Most sternal clefts involve the manubrium and extend inferiorly to encompass varying amounts of the sternal gladiolus. Approximately half of isolated clefts extend inferiorly to the level of the fourth or fifth rib; one fourth go down to the xiphoid, and the remainder are total. Partial simple clefts have been superior in location in almost all cases. When inferior clefts occur, they are usually associated with the pentalogy of Cantrell. The configuration of the superior defect varies from that of a broad U, occasionally 2–5 cm across, which is usually seen in partial clefts, to a narrow V shape that most often occurs when the cleft extends to the xiphoid. When the sternal cleft is broad, the heart can often be seen to pulsate through the skin, suggesting the term *partial ectopia cordis.* True ectopia cordis, however, should be reserved for those rare cases in which the heart is situated outside the thorax.

When the defect is confined to the sternum and is covered with skin, surgical repair may often be elective. When repair is carried out during the first 2 years of life, a satisfactory closure of the sternal cleft can usually be obtained without grafting by surgically completing the cleft and then freshening the edges of the defect. The two sides may then be approximated with interrupted nonabsorbable sutures in most cases.[4] Undue tension on the suture line and underlying heart may be avoided by making oblique relaxing incisions in the upper three costal cartilages bilaterally.[5] In patients in whom the sternal cleft is associated with defects of the pericardium, anterior diaphragm, and abdominal wall, early surgical repair is obligatory, employing a midline tho-

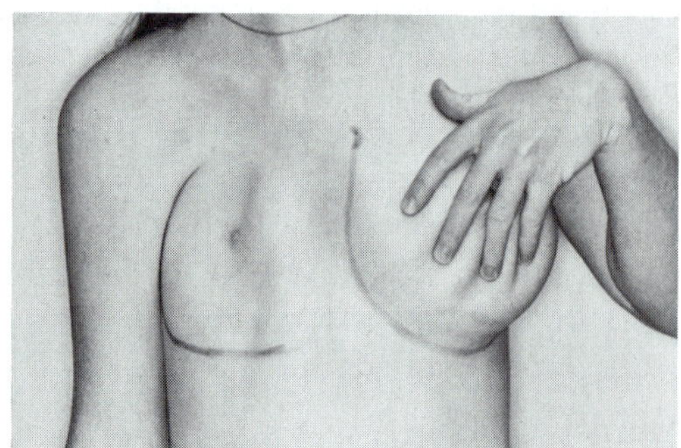

A

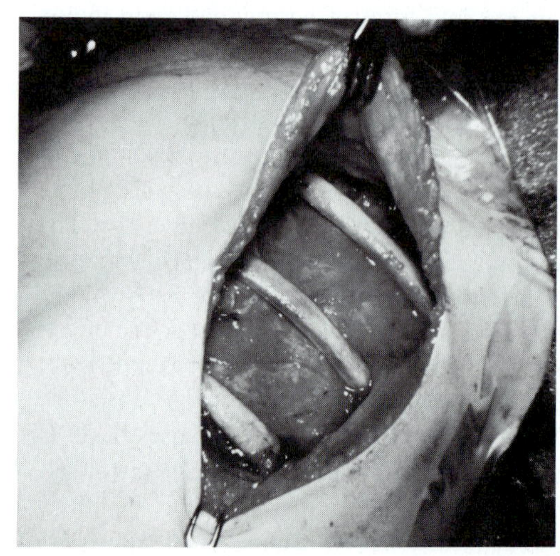

B

**Figure 33–2. A.** Poland's syndrome in a 17-year-old girl, showing absence of segments of sternomastoid muscles. **B.** Free rib grafts placed across the skeletal defect and wired to the sternum medially and ribs

racoabdominal incision. The pericardium is repaired, the diaphragm attached anteriorly, the sternal bars brought together in the midline, and the diastasis recti corrected, by utilizing large flaps of rectus fascia or autogenous fascia lata if necessary.[3,6] Repair in early infancy is generally recommended if the patient is healthy enough to tolerate the procedure. Increase in the size of the defect can occur during the first few months of life. With age, the chest wall becomes somewhat more rigid and loses its flexibility for repair.

Whereas complete ectopia cordis is generally incompatible with life, thoracoabdominal ectopia with a distal sternal cleft has a better prognosis. Several patients have survived into adulthood with or without surgical repair but with correction of the associated omphalocele.[7]

## PECTUS EXCAVATUM

*Pectus excavatum,* or *funnel chest,* is a congenital anomaly of the anterior thorax characterized by a prominent posterior curvature of the body of the sternum, usually involving its lower one half to two thirds, with its deepest point just cephalad to the junction with the xiphoid. The lower costal cartilages bend posteriorly to form a depression, the lateral borders of which usually are angled more sharply than the superior and inferior portions of the deformity. Asymmetric deformities are common with the concavity somewhat deeper on the right and the sternum rotated slightly to the right. The most common configuration is a symmetric depression involving the lower half of the sternum extending laterally almost to the costochondral junctions, with outward bowing of the lower costal cartilages over the abdomen to give a "potbelly" appearance. The upper chest wall characteristically has a decreased anteroposterior diameter.

The pathogenesis of pectus deformities remains unclear, but there is no relation to the development of rickets. It has been postulated that a band of tissue retracts the sternum posteriorly; however, this concept is supported neither by operative findings nor by the therapeutic ineffectiveness of simple retrosternal dissection. More recently it has been postulated that the deformity results from unbalanced growth in the costochondral regions. This theory further explains the occasional asymmetric appearance, the frequent association of other defects of osteogenesis and chondrogenesis, and the existence of a completely opposite type of deformity, pectus carinatum. The involved cartilages are often fused, bizarrely deformed, or rotated. Resected cartilage segments occasionally show a disorderly arrangement of cartilage cells, perichondritis, and areas of aseptic necrosis. Resected cartilage segments occasionally show a disorderly arrangement of cartilage cells, perichondritis, and areas of aseptic necrosis.

Pectus excavatum is inherited through either parent, although not clearly as a recessive trait (Fig. 33–3). The

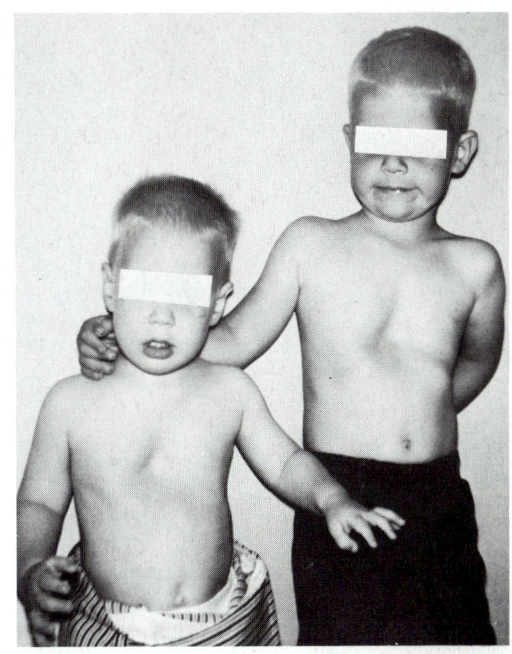

**Figure 33–3.** Brothers with pectus excavatum deformities.

anomaly is believed to occur in as many as 1 in 400 births, but is uncommon in blacks and Hispanics. Other malformations may coexist—especially musculoskeletal anomalies, including scoliosis, which occurs in approximately 20% of cases, clubfoot, syndactylism, Marfan's syndrome, and Klippel-Feil syndrome. Usually the deformity is apparent soon after birth, progresses during early childhood, and becomes even more pronounced in early adolescence. Deep inspiration tends to accentuate the deformity. Regression rarely occurs spontaneously.

Symptoms are uncommon during early childhood, apart from a shy awareness of the abnormality and a typical unwillingness to expose the chest while one is swimming or taking part in other athletic activities. Easy fatigability and decreased stamina and endurance often become apparent during early adolescence when the child becomes involved in competitive sports. When the deformity is moderate to severe, the heart is considerably displaced into the left chest, and pulmonary expansion during inspiration is moderately confined[8] (Fig. 33–4). There is an appreciable incidence of chronic bronchitis, asthma, and occasional bronchiectasis, particularly in adolescents. Most of these patients have an asthenic habitus, poor posture, and a relaxed protuberant abdomen. The xiphoid may be bifid, twisted, or displaced to one side.

Several methods of quantifying the severity of anterior chest deformities have been proposed, although none has been widely accepted. Most include some measurement of the distance between the sternum and the spine as a primary consideration. The use of transverse and anterior–posterior measurements obtained from computerized axial tomograms of the chest is an accurate method; however, it is

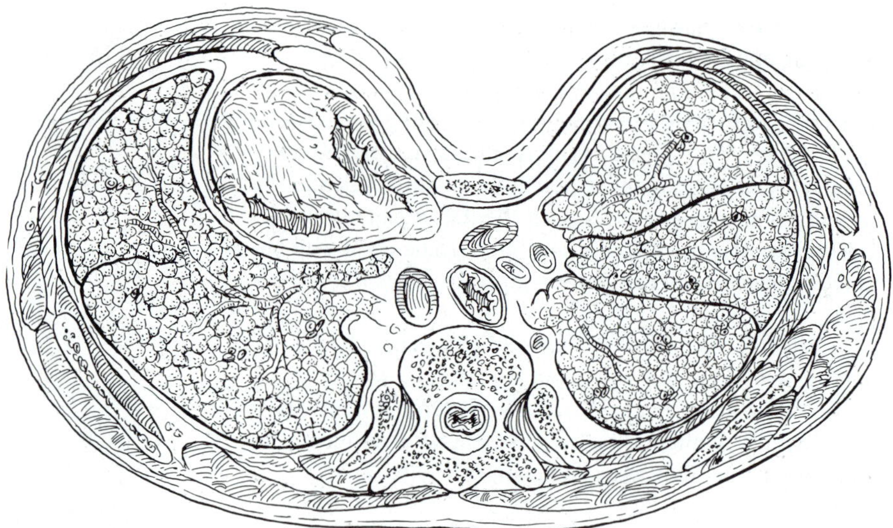

**Figure 33–4.** Cross section of chest in a patient with pectus excavatum, showing displacement of heart into left hemithorax by depressed sternum.

costly and in our experience is rarely necessary. The severity of the deformity may also be measured by a depression index on a scale of 1–10, as defined by Welch.[9] For purposes of comparison, the distance between the anterior sternum and the anterior spine should be measured at the level of the manubrium and also at the maximal lower sternal depression, as noted on lateral chest roentgenograms (Fig. 33–5). Moiré phototopography may indicate the severity of the depression with striking contrast. Standard chest x-rays usually show the heart to be displaced varying degrees into the left chest.

Echocardiographic abnormalities are common, often showing right axis deviation and depressed ST segments; mitral valve prolapse may also be demonstrated, particularly in patients with Marfan's syndrome. A functional systolic cardiac murmur is often present along the upper left sternal border, possibly due to partial pulmonary outflow compression. Angiocardiograms show compression of the right ventricular outflow tract. This compression is reflected physiologically in right heart catheterization pressures and pressure waves, similar to those with constrictive pericarditis.

Conventional pulmonary function tests while at rest are almost always within normal limits or borderline in children with pectus excavatum, but it is difficult to obtain valid measurements in young patients. Beiser and associates[10] showed that six children with mild to moderate deformities studied with right heart catheterization while awake and at rest had a normal cardiac index. A decrease in cardiac output and stroke volume during intense upright exercise occurred in each of these children, which contrasted with normal patients of comparable age. After surgical repair, the cardiac output during intense upright exercise increased by an average of 38% in half the patients, and the hemodynamic response to mild exercise changed toward normal.

Studies by Cahill and associates[11] using the cycle ergometer to evaluate exercise performance in children of various ages, both before and after pectus repair, have shown a significant improvement in maximal voluntary ventilation. Exercise performances were improved as measured both by total exercise time and by maximal oxygen consumption. After repair, the patients showed a lower heart rate and higher minute ventilation compared with preoperative values. These observations support the hypothesis

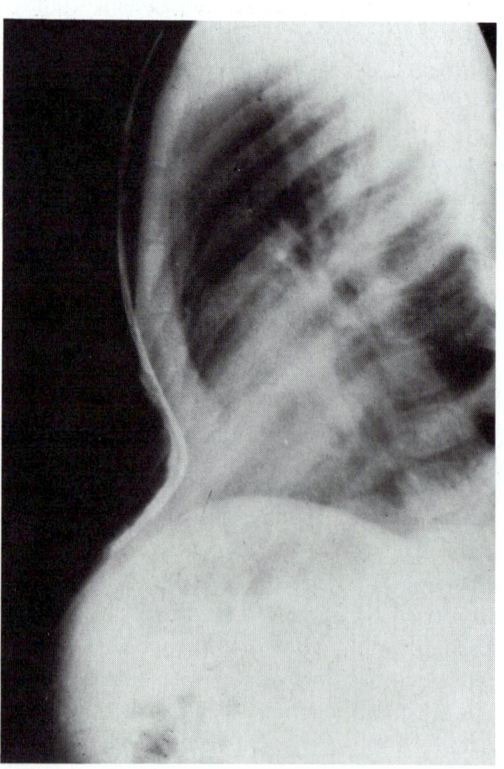

**Figure 33–5.** Lateral chest radiograph with barium paste on skin in a 9-year-old boy with pectus excavatum, showing compression of the heart.

that both the restricted cardiac stroke volume and the increased work of breathing that have been reported in pectus excavatum patients can be ameliorated by operative repair of the anomaly. Thus, although the excavatum deformity is cosmetically unattractive, the major indication for surgical repair is physiologic.[12] There are no studies that indicate that breathing exercises or weight lifting ameliorate the defect of its effects; weight lifting may adversely effect patients with Marfan's syndrome.

## TREATMENT

Inasmuch as almost all young children with pectus excavatum deformities are asymptomatic, the selection of patients for surgical correction requires good clinical judgment. Children with moderate or severe depression of the sternum should undergo surgical repair at approximately 3–5 years of age under optimal circumstances. Because repair can be performed far more readily at this age than in adolescence or later in life, only the mild deformities unlikely ever to require repair are not treated during this period. The risk of anesthesia is minimal, and the long-term cosmetic and functional results are optimal, if repair is performed between the third and fifth years.

The first surgical treatment of pectus excavatum was reported by Sauerbruch[13] in 1931. Current surgical repair of pectus excavatum encompasses various modifications of the original procedure described by Brown[14] and modified by Ravitch.[15] In 1958, Welch[16] recommended total preservation of the perichondrial sheaths and intercostal muscle bundles, anterior sternal wedge osteotomy, and anterior suture fixation of the sternum at the osteotomy site without internal stabilization. Maintenance of the elevated sternum in the corrected position by external traction has almost universally been abandoned in favor of various methods of internal fixation.

The preferred operative technique uses general endotracheal anesthesia, with the patient in the supine position and the arms abducted slightly. A transverse submammary incision is preferred to the previously recommended vertical incision, for cosmetic reasons. The incision is arched slightly cephalad in the midportion to provide good exposure to the upper sternum (Fig. 33–6). Cutaneous and pectoralis muscle flaps are elevated to expose the depressed portion of the sternum and the abnormal costal cartilages. The lower four or five costal cartilages (depending on the length and severity of the anomaly) are resected, and the perichondrial sheaths are kept as nearly intact as is feasible (Fig. 33–7). Electrocautery helps minimize blood loss. The xiphoid is divided from its attachment to the sternum, and the mediastinal structures are bluntly dissected free from the undersurface of the sternum (Fig. 33–8). The attachments of the costal cartilages and intercostal muscles to the sternum are divided by electrocautery, freeing the entire lower portion of the sternum. A transverse wedge osteotomy is performed through the anterior table of the sternum at the level of the cephalad transition from the normal to the depressed sternum (Fig. 33–9). The posterior table of the sternum is partially fractured, and the lower sternum is then elevated to the desired position, where it is secured with interrupted nonabsorbable sutures through the anterior table of the sternum.[17] Care is taken to maintain a good blood supply to the lower sternum and to avoid complete transection at the site of the transverse osteotomy, to prevent necrosis of the distal segment.

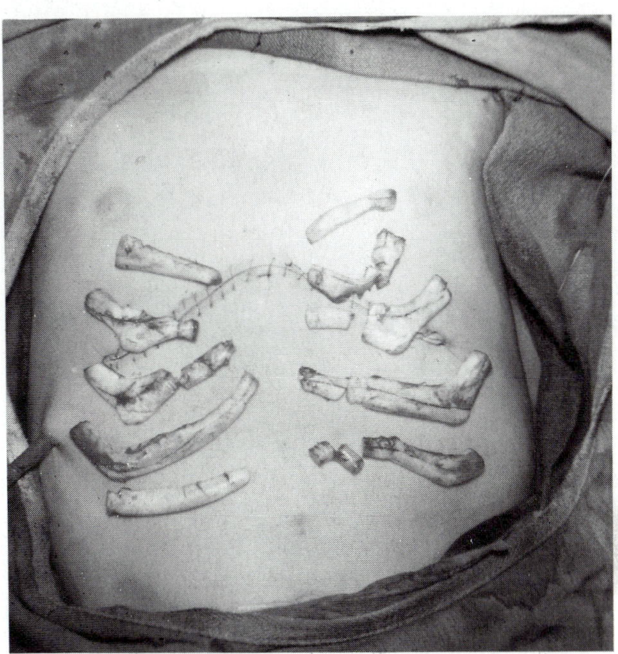

**Figure 33–6.** Through a transverse incision across the anterior chest with slight upward curvature in the midportion, skin flaps are elevated, and the pectoralis and rectus muscles are mobilized from the lower anterior chest. The lower four to five costal cartilages are resected subperiosteally.

In young children (<3 years of age) we prefer to approximate the perichondrial sheath of the lowermost ribs posterior to the sternum, to provide a table of support[18] (Fig. 33–10). The remaining perichondrial sheaths and intercostal muscles are then reattached to the side of the sternum, and the xiphoid is reattached to the lower end (Fig. 33–10). The wound is drained through the right pleural space for approximately 24 hours. In patients >4 years of age, a stainless steel support bar is placed transversely across the anterior chest, where it is attached on each side to the rib just lateral to the costochondral junction at such a level that the inferiormost portion of the sternum is given support (Fig. 33–11). The bar is secured in place with wire sutures placed through the ribs. Patients in whom extensive costal cartilage resection has been performed and a long segment of sternum mobilized inferior to the transverse osteotomy will experience considerable posterior leverage (in contrast to most young children) and will frequently develop recurrent depression unless a support bar is used. The

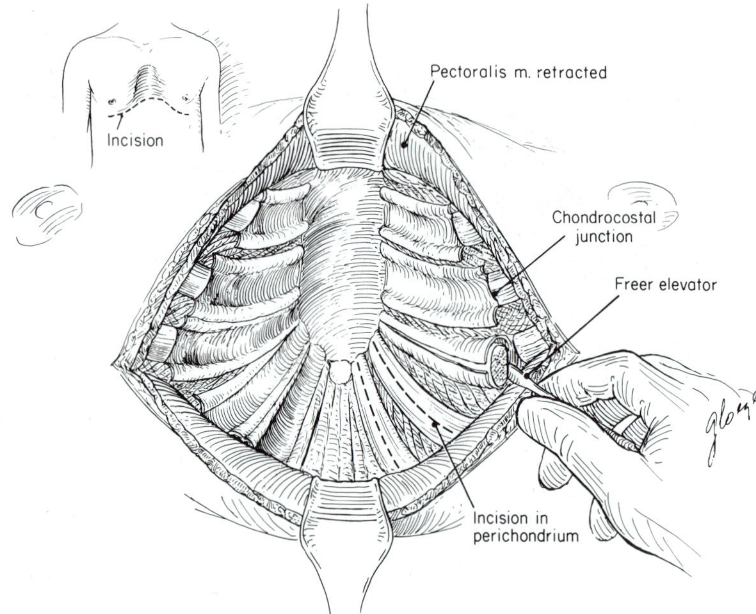


**Figure 33–7.** Standard incision used for repair of pectus excavatum deformities. Costal cartilage segments have been resected subperiosteally from sternum to costochondral junctions laterally.

sternal support bar is generally removed within 5–6 months postoperation, under general anesthesia, on an outpatient basis. A variety of malleable metallic wires[19] and metal strips[20]—even pieces of autogenous rib—have been used by some other authors to provide sternal support. The muscle closure is shown in Figure 33–12.

Entering the pleura on one side of the chest, usually

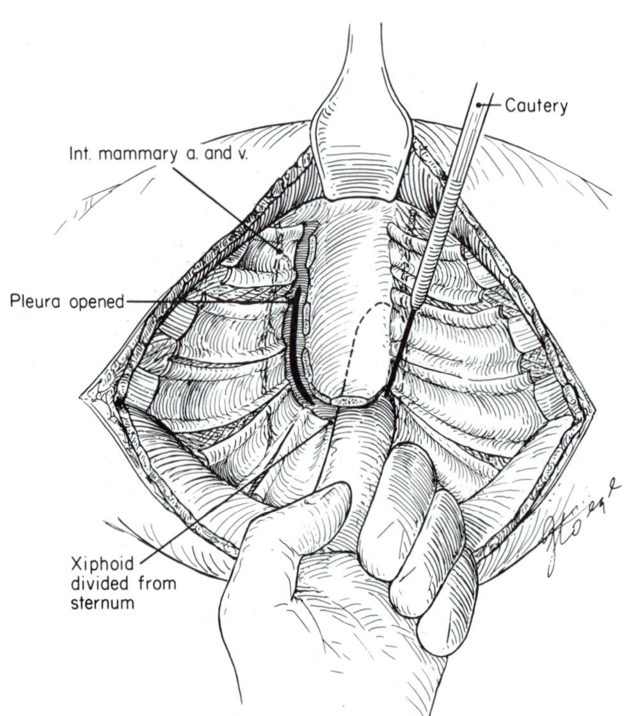


**Figure 33–8.** The xiphoid, intercostal muscles and perichondrial sheaths are detached from the lower sternum with electrocautery.

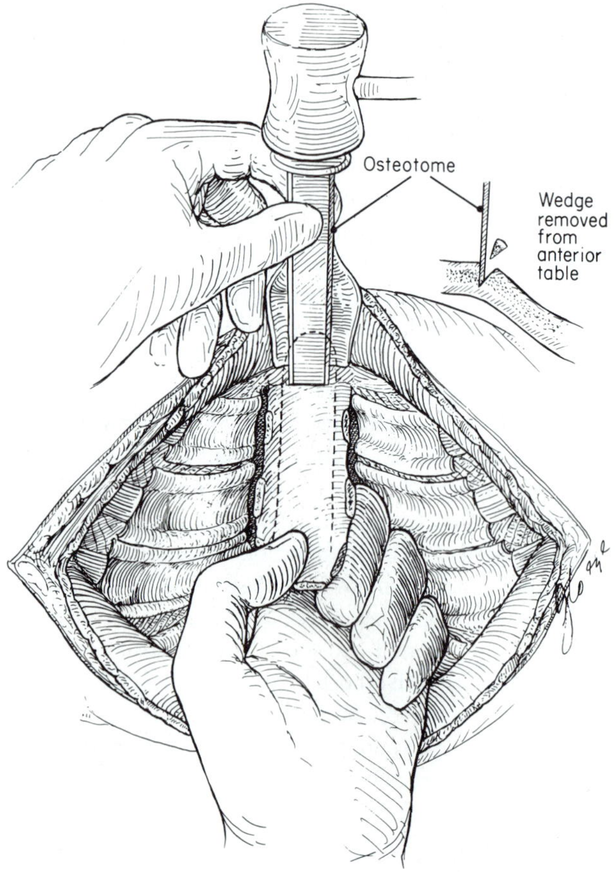


**Figure 33–9.** A transverse wedge osteotomy is made through the anterior table of the sternum at the superiormost level where posterior depression begins.

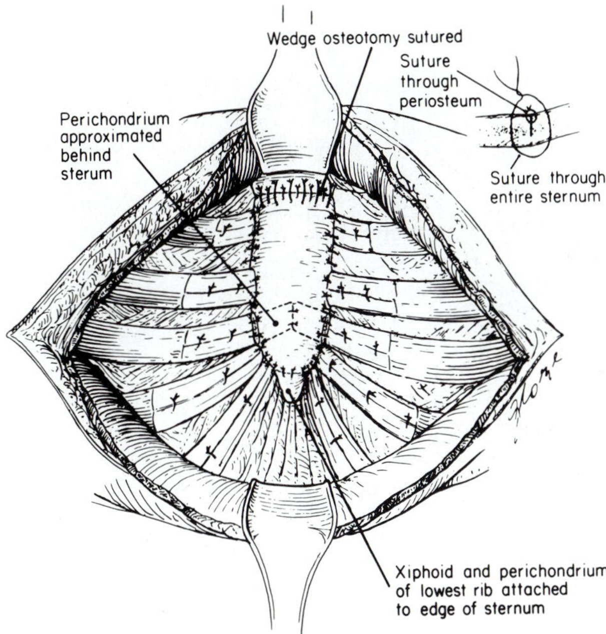


**Figure 33–10.** Reconstruction of anterior chest in children <4 years of age showing perichondrial sheaths sutured together below the lower sternum for support, instead of steel strut. Full thickness sutures are placed across the sternal osteotomy.

the right, has minimal significance as long as it is recognized and appropriately drained with a small chest tube. We prefer to allow mediastinal fluid to drain into the right pleural cavity for easy tube drainage or absorption. Frequent deep inspirations are encouraged during the early postoperative period to minimize the risk of atelectasis. Antibiotics are given preoperatively and postoperatively for approximately 1 week; wound infections and/or chondritis are uncommon. Blood transfusions are very rarely required. Hospitalization longer than 3–4 days postoperation is rarely necessary regardless of the patient's age. The chest should be protected from direct trauma for 4–6 weeks, after which it becomes very solid.

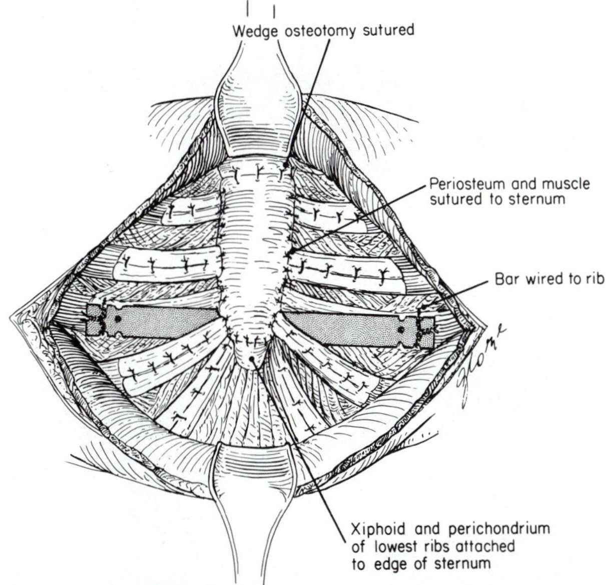


**Figure 33–11.** After gentle fracture of the posterior table of the sternum without displacement, the osteotomy is closed with nonabsorbable sutures. The xiphoid and perichondrial sheaths are sutured back to the sternum. A stainless-steel strut is sutured to the fifth rib bilaterally to provide support to the lower tip of the sternum.

Periosteal regeneration of new cartilage or bone is usually complete within 2 months after operation and provides a rigid support for the chest wall. Since the pectoralis muscles are reconstructed after elevation from the anterior chest wall during the repair, extensive physical activity using the pectoralis muscles should be deferred for at least 8–10 weeks postoperatively. Although there is a slight tendency for pectus excavatum deformities to recur during adolescence, this has happened in fewer than 2% of our patients when autogenous or prosthetic sternal supports were used during the repair[21] (Fig. 33–13A,B). Occasionally, however, a patient develops a protrusion of one or more costal cartilages slightly superior to the level of resection years after the operation. Recurrent pain or severe cosmetic deformity may warrant subperiostal resection of such involved cartilages at a later time, usually in midadolescence. There should be virtually no mortality associated with repair of pectus excavatum or carinatum deformities.

The very high frequency of improvement in respiratory symptoms, exercise tolerance, and endurance as well as cosmetic appearance following repair of 275 patients in our clinical experience supports the view that children with severe pectus deformities should undergo repair at an early age.[21–23] Routine use of substernal support, with minimal pre- and postoperative testing, has provided excellent clinical results at low cost.

## PECTUS CARINATUM

Protrusion deformities of the anterior chest wall (*pigeon breast,* or *chicken breast*) are approximately 10 times less common than depression deformities.[24] Associated disorders, including congenital heart disease, Marfanoid habitus, scoliosis, kyphosis, and musculoskeletal defects, are more frequent than in patients with excavatum. The deformity is often mild or almost imperceptible in early childhood and becomes increasingly prominent in early adolescence.

The anomaly is believed to stem from an overgrowth of costal cartilages, with forward buckling and secondary deforming pressure on the gladiolus and xiphoid process. The carinatum deformities are more variable than the excavatum anomalies. Two principal types are recognized. One is termed *chondromanubrial,* in which the protuberance is maximal in the upper portion of the sternum and the gladiolus, or lower end, is directed posteriorly so that an apparent saucerization-type depression is evident. The second and more common form, termed *chondrogladiolar,* has the

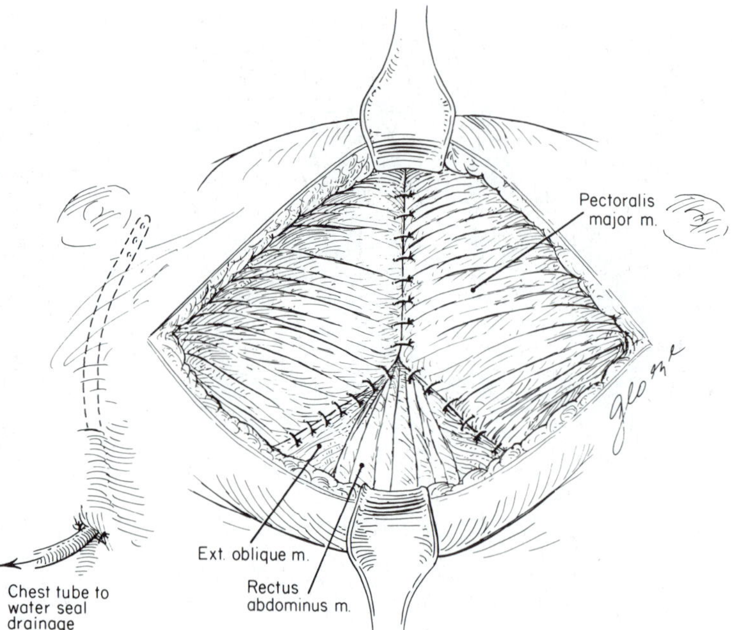


**Figure 33–12.** Closure of the pectoralis and rectus muscles over the bony thorax after repair of pectus excavatum. After opening of the pleura, wound drainage is routinely performed through a right chest tube for 36 hours.

greatest prominence in the lower portion, or xiphisternum.[25] Minor forms of protrusion anomalies occur with moderate frequency in which one, or occasionally two costal cartilages may buckle outward at the level of the manubrium, but without sternal deformity.

Pectus carinatum tends to produce a rigid chest with increased anteroposterior diameter locked into a position of nearly full inspiration (Fig. 33–14). Respiratory efforts are inefficient, being accomplished largely by the diaphragm and accessory muscles of respiration. There may be gradual loss of lung compliance, progressive emphysema, and superimposed pulmonary infection. The incidence of asthma is higher in patients with carinatum than in those with excavatum deformities. Some type of chest deformity occurs in other family members in approximately one third of cases.

Considerable variation in surgical treatment is necessary because of the diversity of carinatum deformities.[26,27] The same exposure is used as for excavatum deformities, with resection of the more severely involved costal cartilages, leaving the perichondrium intact. The transverse os-

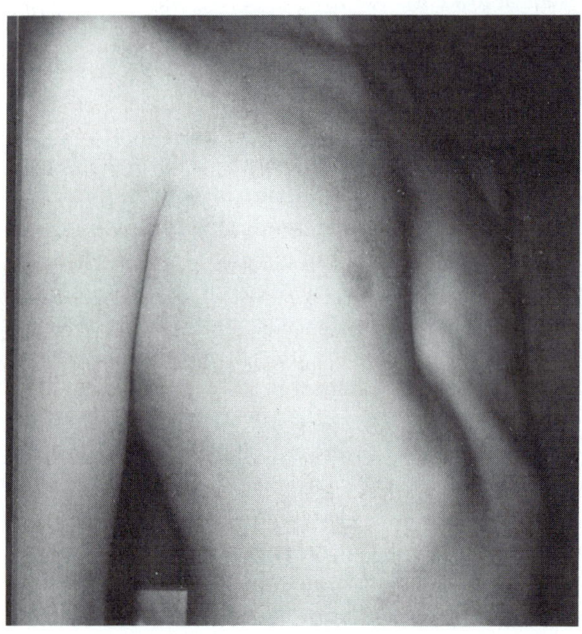

A

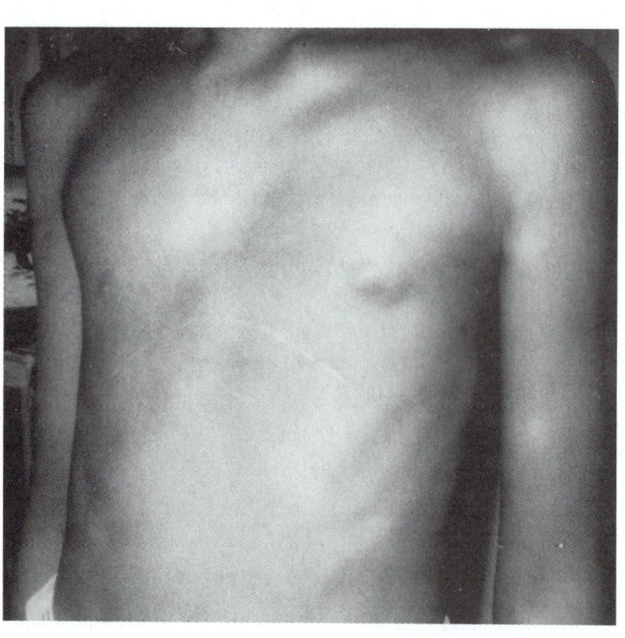

B

**Figure 33–13. A.** Seven-year-old boy with pectus excavatum deformity. **B.** Appearance of same boy 10 months postoperation.

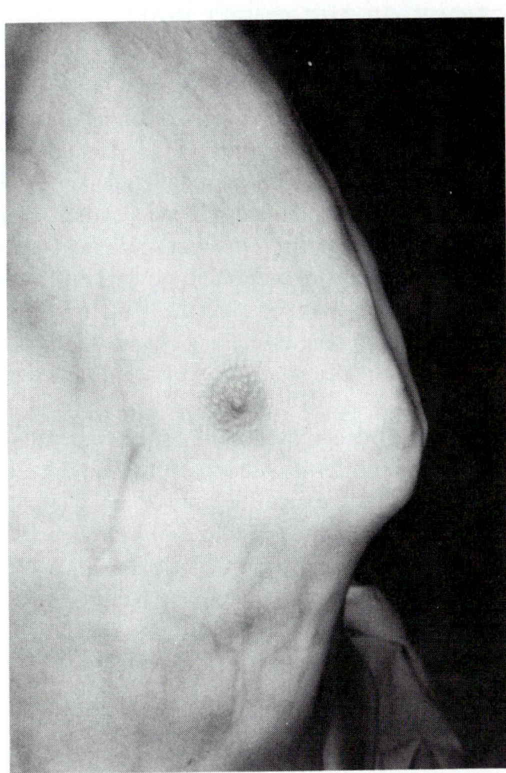

**Figure 33–14.** Severe pectus carinatum deformity of the anterior chest in 17-year-old boy.

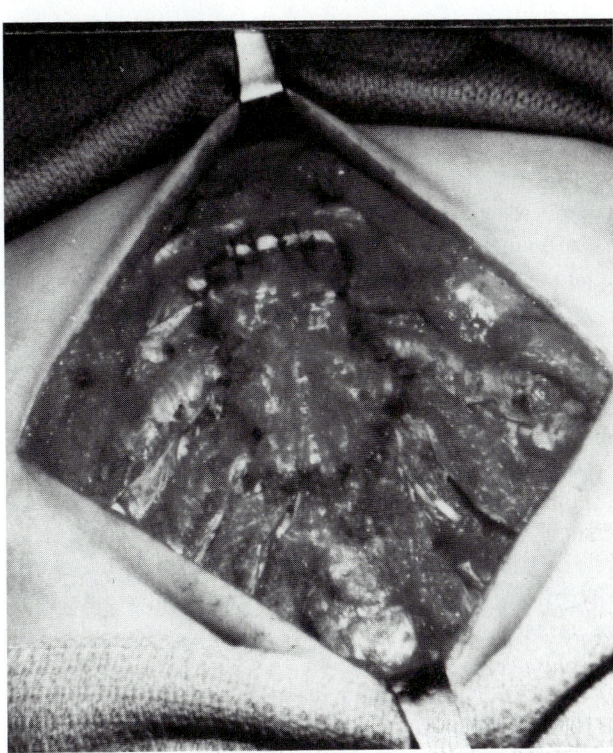

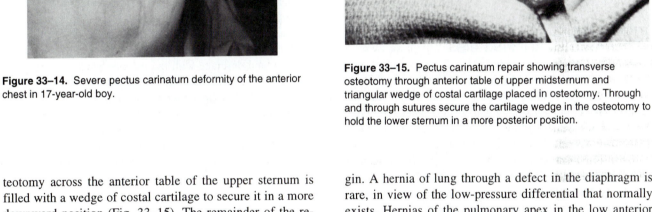

**Figure 33–15.** Pectus carinatum repair showing transverse osteotomy through anterior table of upper midsternum and triangular wedge of costal cartilage placed in osteotomy. Through and through sutures secure the cartilage wedge in the osteotomy to hold the lower sternum in a more posterior position.

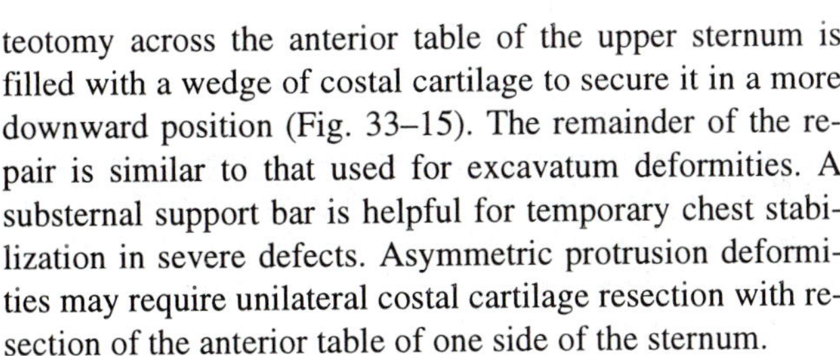

teotomy across the anterior table of the upper sternum is filled with a wedge of costal cartilage to secure it in a more downward position (Fig. 33–15). The remainder of the repair is similar to that used for excavatum deformities. A substernal support bar is helpful for temporary chest stabilization in severe defects. Asymmetric protrusion deformities may require unilateral costal cartilage resection with resection of the anterior table of one side of the sternum.

Complications after surgical repair of carinatum deformities are rare and resemble those experienced in patients with depression anomalies. The long-term results following surgery are often more dramatic than those after excavatum repair. Several patients with asthma or emphysema-like symptoms have shown marked clinical improvement. Operations in which the lower end of the sternum is completely reversed are more likely to be followed by avascular sternal necrosis.

## PNEUMONOCELE—HERNIA OF THE LUNG

A *pneumonocele* is a hernia of pulmonary tissue outside the normal pleural boundaries that may involve the costal parietes, the superior anterior mediastinum, or the diaphragm and may be of spontaneous, traumatic, or postoperative origin. A hernia of lung through a defect in the diaphragm is rare, in view of the low-pressure differential that normally exists. Hernias of the pulmonary apex in the low anterior neck at the suprasternal notch, or laterally from beneath the clavicles, are occasionally seen in patients afflicted with chronic bronchitis and obstructive emphysema, and as an occupational complication of glassblowers and of musicians who play wind instruments. A congenital or acquired weakness of the endothoracic fascia and its apical condensations (Sibson's fascia) allows the overdistending lung to insinuate itself into the neck, exaggerating the normal rise of the apical pleura medial to the scalenus muscles. A soft, nontender, crepitant swelling appears in the supraclavicular fossa of one or both sides; this enlarges and becomes tense with forced expiration.

Costal (parietal) pneumonocele is the most common variety. When spontaneous, it is usually situated parasternally or paravertebrally, where the intercostal muscles are incomplete. After costochondral dislocations and multiple rib fractures, and not infrequently after thoracotomy, a pulmonary hernia may be discovered early or late. In posttraumatic cases, a tear of the parietal pleura and laceration of intercostal structures provide a path for egress of lung, aided by the stress of coughing and the hydraulic effect of concomitant pleural effusion.

Oblique chest x-rays tangential to the defect may demonstrate the herniation as it increases in size during forced expiration, but standard chest x-rays often fail to reveal the lesion. Posttraumatic pneumonoceles situated in the lower third of the chest may be associated with diaphragmatic lacerations and herniated abdominal viscera, complicating the diagnosis and the surgical treatment. A large pulmonary hernia may interfere somewhat with ventilation mechanics, but most are asymptomatic.

Occasionally surgery is necessary because of the patient's occupation or because of the size of the lesion, which may produce some discomfort and limitation of physical activity. Surgical repair should be deferred for 4–6 months after healing of the original wound, especially if infection has intervened. Smaller defects may be repaired by turning flaps of perichondrium and periosteum from adjacent ribs and approximating these with nonabsorbable sutures. Larger defects may require mobilization of adjacent ribs by osteotomy. Marlex mesh or autogenous fascia may be used to bridge extensive defects.

## STERNOCHONDRAL AND COSTOCHONDRAL SEPARATIONS—SLIPPING RIBS

The sternochondral articulations of the second to the seventh ribs are true joints, lined with synovial membranes that tend to resorb and eventually disappear in later life. These joints are subject, therefore, to arthritic changes, direct or hematogenous infections, and, occasionally, traumatic separations. While a definite history of acute external trauma is rare, recurrent cough, heavy lifting, and violent embracing may play etiologic roles. Separation and dislocation may take place also at the costochondral junction, where no joint space exists, and the demarcation between cartilage and bone is irregular. The cartilages of the lower ribs may be congenitally distorted, twisted, and angulated so that encroachment on the neighboring ribs or cartilages may occur during forced respirations and postural changes.

Symptoms usually occur in adults with intermittent, occasionally sharp, pain localized to a specific area or radiating along intercostal nerve distributions. There may be tenderness over the involved joint or rib tip, unusual mobility of the rib in response to deep pressure, and a palpable click during manipulation. Chronic gastrointestinal disease may be suspected when the pain follows a lower intercostal nerve into the abdominal wall.

Radiographs are usually of little diagnostic help, since the cartilages are not radio-opaque. The differential diagnosis includes intercostal neuritis associated with malunited rib fracture, chronic osteomyelitis and chondritis, and neoplasms of ribs and cartilage. If relief of pain and disability is not obtained by rest, splinting of the ribs, local heat, and intercostal nerve block, the area should be explored and the suspected cartilage excised for histologic evaluation.

## INFECTIONS OF THE CHEST WALL

Infections of the soft tissues are commonly observed in young patients with systemic illness, such as diabetes and blood dyscrasias, in those undergoing chemotherapy for malignancy, in patients with immunodeficiency disorders, and in certain other conditions. Carbuncles have a predilection for the skin of the posterior neck and trunk. A neglected empyema that has drained spontaneously through an intercostal space may involve the soft tissues secondarily. Acute and chronic infections of the chest wall may follow needle aspiration of a pulmonary abscess or empyema.

Two types of deep chest wall abscess warrant special consideration. *Subpectoral abscess* results from infection in the upper extremity, the anterior ribs, or, occasionally, the breast. *Hemolytic streptococci* and *Staphylococcus aureus* are the usual causative organisms. The patient is acutely ill, febrile, and uncomfortable. There is a visible and palpable fullness in the subclavicular and pectoral regions. The skin may be reddened and edematous. Movement of the shoulder is painful, especially during abduction and external rotation. There may be deep tenderness and swelling in the axilla itself. Treatment consists of appropriate antibiotic therapy and drainage with the incision placed at the lateral border of the pectoralis major, employing Silastic suction catheters. Follow-up x-rays of the ribs and sternum should be obtained.

*Subscapular abscess,* under the internal surface of the scapula and the attached serratus muscle, develops spontaneously or as the result of direct extension from osteomyelitis of the scapula or subscapular bursitis. After a posterolateral thoracotomy or upper thoracoplasty, a hematoma may localize and become infected, causing limitation of motion in the shoulder and a prominence of the scapular border medially. The diagnosis is established by aspiration, using a large-bore needle inserted at the vertebral border of the scapula. If pus is encountered, it should be drained independently and antibiotics given. The ribs, pleura, or lung must be evaluated as a possible primary septic focus. If the exudate is originally sterile, a tuberculous or mycotic etiology should be considered.

## INFECTIONS OF THE RIBS AND STERNUM

*Osteomyelitis* involving the bony thorax is likely to be a sequela of direct wounds and comminuted fractures, producing devitalized osseous fragments. Tuberculous or mycotic infection may involve ribs by direct extension from an infected lung or pleura, but serious osteomyelitis rarely develops in rib stumps after open drainage of purulent empyema, providing there is no residual devitalized bone.

Hematogenous osteomyelitis tends to involve the anterior end of the ribs near the costochondral junction or the posterior portion at the angle.[28] The suppurative process may break through the periosteum into the surrounding soft tissues of the chest wall, but the pleural space is rarely involved except in granulomatous disease. Pyogenic osteomyelitis of the sternum is usually caused by wound infection complicating median sternotomy, the most frequent causative organisms being staphylococci and gram-negative bacilli.

Acute osteomyelitis produces fever, severe local pain, tenderness, swelling of the surrounding soft tissues, and drainage of purulent material after a tract is established. In chronic cases, the systemic manifestations may be minimal. Failure of the chest wound to heal or the reappearance of external drainage after a period of quiescence and apparent closure signals a lingering infection. Often the costal infection is a minor part of the more significant inflammatory process in the pleural cavity. Routine x-rays may be of little value in detecting acute cases and assessing chondritis. Laminograms and/or ultrasound or computed tomography (CT) scans help to establish the diagnosis.

Appropriate antibiotics may succeed in curing acute osteomyelitis. Refractory infections and those with radiographic changes indicating chronicity suggest that the osteomyelitic segment should be excised back to normal rib or cartilage whenever possible.

*Chondritis* may be of hematogenous or local origin. Cartilage is a relatively avascular tissue that resists infection poorly. Nonabsorbable multifilament suture material placed through cartilage creates an easy route for entry of organisms unless aseptic technique is meticulous. Chondritis and osteomyelitis of chronic character are occasionally caused by tuberculosis, *Brucella* species, or *Salmonella typhosa.* Appropriate chemotherapeutic medications should be administered when the diagnosis involves any of these organisms. Chondritis in any of the upper five cartilages can be managed by resecting the individual cartilage from the sternum to normal rib laterally. Because lower costal cartilages tend to fuse, a more extensive extirpation is sometimes required.[29]

*Tietze's disease* is a syndrome of uncertain etiology, possibly infectious, characterized by an insidious onset of swelling in a costal cartilage (usually the second), followed by local pain and tenderness.[30] Most patients are in the third to fifth decades, some with a history of antecedent upper respiratory tract infection. A sharply localized tenderness and swelling over one or more of the costal cartilages, with no inflammatory reaction in the overlying skin, is usually present. X-rays are normal, and routine laboratory tests are negative. Excision of the involved cartilages may be warranted when pain is severe and prolonged, and when persistence of swelling suggests a chronic chondritis or possible malignant neoplasm. Resection of the cartilage is followed by complete relief of symptoms. However, this is a benign and ordinarily self-limited disease, requiring no specific treatment in most cases. Excised cartilage in such patients rarely shows abnormalities.

## REFERENCES


1. Ravitch MM: Poland's syndrome. In Ravitch MM (ed): *Congenital Deformities of the Chest Wall and Their Operative Correction.* Philadelphia, Saunders, 1977, pp 233–271
2. Hanson FB: The ontogeny and phylogeny of the sternum. *Am J Anat* **26:**41, 1919
3. Cantrell JR, Haller JA, Ravitch MM: A syndrome of congenital defects involving the abdominal wall, sternum, diaphragm, pericardium and heart. *Surg Gynecol Obstet* **107:**602, 1958
4. Longino LA, Jewett TC Jr: Congenital bifid sternum. *Surgery* **38:**610, 1955
5. Sabiston DC: The surgical management of congenital bifid sternum with partial ectopia cordis. *J Thorac Surg* **35:**118, 1959
6. Haller JA, Cantrell JR: Diagnosis and surgical correction of combined congenital defects of supraumbilical abdominal wall, lower sternum and diaphragm. *J Thorac Cardiovasc Surg* **51:**286, 1966
7. Major JW: Thoracoabdominal ectopia cordis. Report of a case successfully treated by surgery. *J Thorac Surg* **26:**309, 1953
8. Ravitch MM: Pectus excavatum and heart failure. *Surgery* **30:**178, 1951
9. Welch KJ: Chest wall deformities. In Holder TH, Ashcraft K (eds): *Pediatric Surgery.* Philadelphia, Saunders, 1980, pp 162–182
10. Beiser GD, Epstein SE, Stampfer M, et al: Impairment of cardiac function in patients with pectus excavatum, with improvement after operative correction. *N Engl J Med* **287:**267, 1972
11. Cahill JL, Lees GM, Robertson HT: A summary of preoperative and postoperative respiratory performance in patients undergoing pectus excavatum and carinatum repair. *J Pediatr Surg* **19:**430, 1984
12. Shamberger RC, Welch KJ: Cardiopulmonary function in pectus excavatum. *Surg Gynecol Obstet* **166:**383, 1988
13. Sauerbruch F: Operative beseitigung der angeborenen trichterbrust. *Deutsch Z Chir* **234:**760, 1931
14. Brown AL: Pectus excavatum (funnel chest). *J Thorac Surg* **9:**164, 1939
15. Ravitch MM: The operative treatment of pectus excavatum. *Ann Surg* **129:**429, 1949
16. Welch KJ: Satisfactory surgical correction of pectus excavatum deformity in childhood: A limited opportunity. *J Thorac Surg* **36:**697, 1958
17. Ravitch MM: Technical problems in the operative correction of pectus excavatum. *Ann Surg* **162:**29, 1965
18. Fonkalsrud EW, Follette D, Sarwat AK: Pectus excavatum repair using autologous perichondrium for sternal support. *Arch Surg* **113:**1433, 1978
19. Rehbin F, Wernicke HH: The operative treatment of funnel chest. *Arch Dis Child* **32:**5, 1957
20. Adkins PC, Blades B: A stainless steel strut for correction of pectus excavatum. *Surg Gynecol Obstet* **113:**111, 1961
21. Fonkalsrud EW, Salman T, Guo W, et al: Repair of pectus deformities with sternal support. *J Thorac Cardiovasc Surg* **107:**37, 1994
22. Humphreys GH II, Jaretzki A III: Pectus excavatum, late results with and without operation. *J Thorac Cardiovasc Surg* **80:**686, 1980
23. Haller JA, Scherer LR, Turner CS, et al: Evolving management of pectus excavatum based on a single institutional experience of 664 patients. *Ann Surg* **209:**578, 1989
24. Robicsek S, Sanger PW, Taylor FH, et al: The surgical treatment of chondrosternal prominence (pectus carinatum). *J Thorac Cardiovasc Surg* **45:**691, 1963
25. Brodkin HA: Pigeon breast—congenital chondrosternal prominence. *Arch Surg* **77:**261, 1958

26. Ravitch MM: Pectus carinatum. In Ravitch MM (ed): *Congenital Deformities of the Chest Wall and Their Operative Correction.* Philadelphia, Saunders, 1977, pp 206–332
27. Shamberger RC, Welch KJ: Surgical correction of pectus carinatum. *J Pediatr Surg* **22:**48, 1987
28. Brock R: Osteomyelitis of the rib. *Guys Hosp Rep* **106:**156, 1957
29. Wilcox RE: Chondritis with associated osteomyelitis. *J Thorac Cardiovasc Surg* **49:**210, 1965
30. Teitze A: Uber eine eigenartgie Häufung von Fallen mit Dystrohpie der Rippenknorpel. *Berl Klin Wochenschr* **58:**829, 1921

CHAPTER

# 34

# Chest Wall Tumors

Patricia M. McCormack

## BACKGROUND

Chest wall reconstruction has presented a challenge to surgeons since Parham's[1] first description of a thoracic resection in 1898.

Control of ventilation is important to a successful outcome. Fell[2] and O'Dwyer[3] contributed significantly in this early age of anesthesia.

Over the next several decades, advances in endotracheal ventilation allowed pulmonary resections to be safely performed. Graham and Singer[4] described the first pneumonectomy in 1933.

In chest wall tumors requiring resection of the skeletal structures, however, postoperative complications ensued when a "flail chest" resulted and respiratory insufficiency led to prolonged ventilatory support—or death.

Efforts to avoid such outcomes led to the use of various replacements to reconstruct the defect and restore adequate respiration.

Autogenous materials have included fascia lata in 1947 by Watson and James,[5] large cutaneous flaps as described by Maier,[6] and rib grafts used by Bisgard and Swenson.[7]

The myocutaneous flaps used extensively today were first described by Campbell[8] in 1950. He used the latissimus dorsi muscle with immediate skin grafting. It took another 20 years for this excellent contribution to be adapted extensively.

The 1950s and 1960s marked increasing interest in this problem and papers by Blades and Jones,[9] Converse et al,[10] Myre and Kirklin,[11] Rees and Converse,[12] Starzynski et al,[13] Martini et al,[14] and Le Roux[15] each added refinements of techniques to conquer a formidable problem.

In 1963, the use of transposed omentum to supply a vascular bed was detailed by Kiricuta.[16] Thus, all elements were in place for the arrival of synthetic materials that would revolutionize the reconstruction of a chest-wall defect.

The tedium and multiple incisions needed for autogenous rib and fascia lata grafts are disadvantages. The steel plates, strips, and bands were nonpliable, foreign bodies with added complications of erosion and extrusion.

The synthetic meshes and solid patches are readily available and allow for immediate dependable reconstruction of the rigid chest wall.[17–22] Replacement of the soft tissues by various myocutaneous flaps, as well as the use of transplanted omentum when it is needed, have been described eloquently by many authors.

State-of-the-art surgery for chest wall tumors today calls for complete resection, reconstruction of rigid and soft-tissue components with omentum, if needed, and a hospital stay of 6–10 days with no dependence on a respirator.

Chest wall tumors are rare. Malignant chest wall tumors account for only 5% of all thoracic malignancies.

From 1963 to 1983, at Memorial Sloan-Kettering Cancer Center, 317 malignancies in chest wall were resected (Table 34–1). In this review we have defined chest neoplasms to be those benign and malignant tumors arising in the chest wall (83), and primary (127) or metastatic (107) tumors of the lung that extend into or invade the chest wall. No primary mediastinal tumors are included.

## PRESENTATION

Nearly 75% of these tumors are found by the patients as a painless mass. Bone tumors cause pain as they expand the cortex and periosteum or when the destruction of cortical bone leads to a pathologic fracture. This occurs in half of bone tumor cases. We have noted that metastatic tumors to the bony thorax present symptomatically earlier than primary tumors in the same area. We believe this is due to the

**TABLE 34–1. MALIGNANT TUMORS OF THE CHEST WALL, 1963–1983**

| Type | Number |
|---|---|
| Primary carcinoma of lung | 127 |
| Metastatic carcinoma | 71 |
| Sarcoma-primary | 83 |
| Sarcoma-metastatic | 38 |
| Total | 317 |

increased doubling time of most metastases as compared with primary tumors.

Tumors of the cartilaginous ribs are most often initially seen on chest x-rays. Since the advent of the computerized scanner, small asymptomatic tumors are being diagnosed both in soft tissue and in bone before they are large enough to present symptoms.

## DIAGNOSIS

The approach to a chest wall tumor is made in two steps. First, the size and invasiveness is determined, followed by the histology.

Computed tomography (CT) scanning has greatly enhanced our ability to distinguish whether a lesion is cystic or solid and to demonstrate bony invasion. Magnetic resonance imaging (MRI) has the additional advantage of outlining all vascular structures and imaging in the sagittal and coronal planes as well as the transverse. Spinal invasion and great vessel involvement may be delineated by this technique. It must be remembered, however, that neither technique has proven infallible, so if doubt exists, exploration is indicated. Plane tomography has been supplemented by these new techniques where they are available. In lesions 5 cm or smaller, when complete resection will not be mutilating, an excisional biopsy is the preferred procedure.

In larger tumors, a core needle biopsy or an incisional biopsy is done first. Care must be taken to plan the biopsy incision in such a way that the subsequent excision can readily encompass the biopsy scar. Upon receipt of the final pathologic report, a definitive treatment plan is made.

## BENIGN TUMORS

These tumors can originate in the skin and in soft or bony tissues, as shown in Table 34–2. None of these are included in our present review of 317 cases; they are mentioned here for completeness.

Cutaneous *nevi* include the junctional nevus. This pigmented lesion is distinguished from a melanoma on pathologic grounds. It should be completely excised, with adequate margins.

*Lipomas* can occur wherever there are fat cells. They are extremely common tumors that form well-circumscribed, thinly encapsulated tumors of mature adipose tissue. Spindle cell variants occur in the shoulder area, while hibernomas are found on the chest wall and interscapular region. Some lipomas are situated deeper and may infiltrate a muscle. These require a wider excision and may recur.[23] Clinical diagnosis is usually sufficient for this slowly enlarging, freely movable subcutaneous mass. Resection is indicated only for cosmetic purposes or when doubt exists as to the true nature of the lesion.

**TABLE 34–2. BENIGN TUMORS OF THE CHEST WALL**

| |
|---|
| Superficial soft tissue |
| Skin nevus |
| Lipoma |
| Lymphangioma |
| Hemangioma |
| Deep soft tissue |
| Fibroma |
| Rhabdomyoma |
| Neurofibroma |
| Desmoid tumor |
| Bone and cartilage |
| Fibrous dysplasia |
| Chondroma |
| Osteochondroma |

*Lymphangiomas* become a tumor of the thorax only when they extend inferiorly from their more common site of origin in the neck. Such tumors are poorly circumscribed. They may become large and present in the thoracic inlet. Complete excision will preclude recurrence (Fig. 34–1).

*Hemangiomas* may present on the skin or in the subcutaneous layers. Superficial hemangiomas (so-called birthmarks) are treated only when cosmetically indicated. Cavernous hemangiomas and arteriovenous malformations will

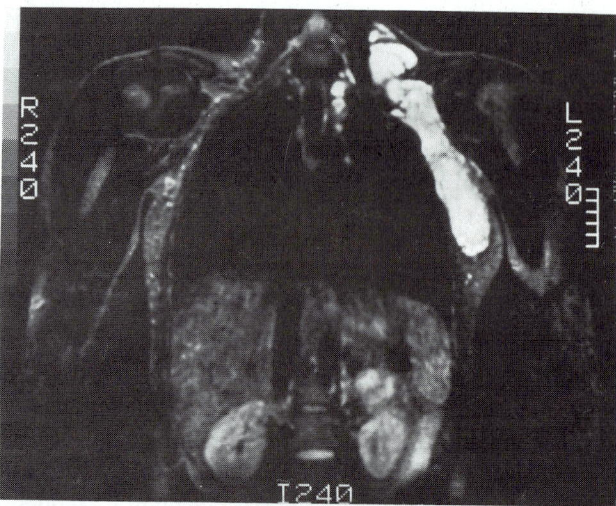


**Figure 34–1.** Lymphangioma. Sagittal MRI scan showing the mass extending from above the clavicle to the lower thorax.

cause increasing problems as they become larger; they should be excised when contraindications to surgery are minimal.[24] There is one type that involves the trunk in 35% of cases and is difficult to differentiate from a sarcoma on histology.[25]

## DEEP SOFT-TISSUE TUMORS

*Fibroma* is a rare chest-wall tumor that usually presents as a slowly growing mass near a joint, but it can also occur anywhere in the soft tissue. The indolent growth and lack of infiltration make the diagnosis apparent on clinical grounds. Resection is indicated only for treating symptoms or for cosmetic reasons.

*Rhabdomyoma* is a very rare benign counterpart of an equally rare muscle malignancy. It presents as a mass arising in a muscle. A slow growth pattern indicates a benign tumor. A biopsy should be done to confirm this. The tumor should be removed if it interferes with the function of the muscle involved or if its size makes it cosmetically displeasing. The excision must include the entire tumor to prevent local recurrence.

*Neurofibroma* can occur as an isolated lesion, but usually these tumors are multiple and associated with von Recklinghausen's multiple neurofibromatosis. Although most lesions are benign, malignant degeneration can occur. When new symptoms appear—an enlarging mass or pain—excision is recommended (Fig. 34–2). Needle biopsy may miss the significant spot, so excisional biopsy should be done. When these tumors occur near the vertebral body, the presence of a "dumbbell" tumor with extension into the spinal canal must be documented by CT or MRI scan. If present, neurosurgical consultation is needed for combined resection.

*Desmoid tumors* arise from the deep fascia and con-

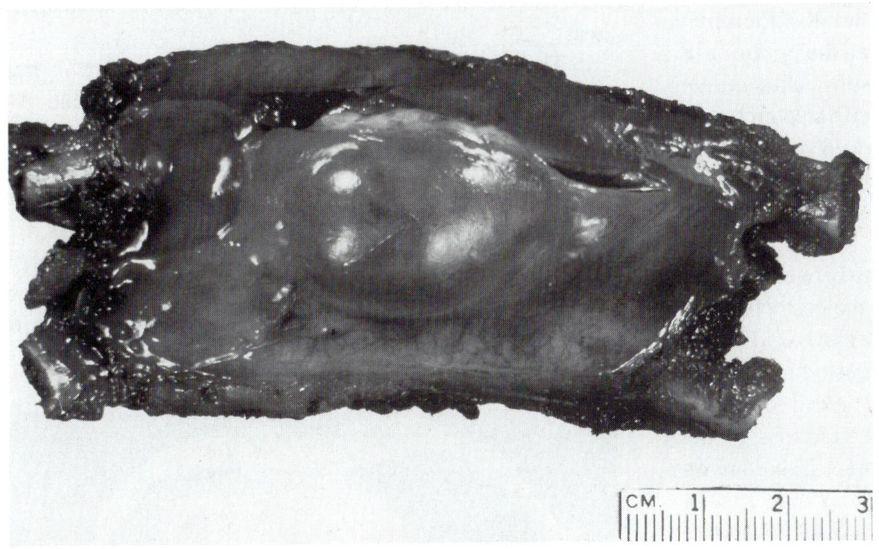


A

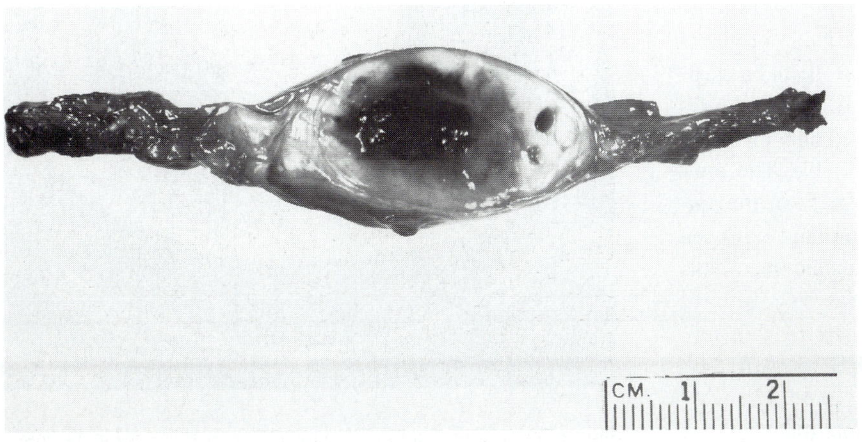


B

**Figure 34–2.** Neurofibroma. **A.** Pleural surface of specimen filling the intercostal space. **B.** Cut surface demonstrating the pattern of growth of this benign lesion.

nective tissue of muscle; the chest wall is a favorite site for this lesion. Because of the local invasion capability of these tumors, some pathologists and clinicians do not consider them benign but rather think of them as low-grade fibrosarcomas. They present as slowly enlarging masses that frequently involve the shoulder girdle. Pain due to pressure on surrounding structures is often a presenting symptom. Desmoid tumors occur most commonly on the anterolateral chest wall. Their low-grade malignant potential reflects the slow rate of growth. They have not been reported to metastasize. The potential for local recurrence is very high. Their growth pattern shows infiltration of bony, neural, and vascular structures. They recur locally, despite wide margins that are microscopically free of tumor. Treatment is extensive local resection.[26] External beam radiation therapy and local brachytherapy are recommended after adequate excision, to control recurrence.[27]

## BONE AND CARTILAGE TUMORS

*Fibrous dysplasia* causes 30% of benign tumors of chest wall. This is the most common tumor of the ribs. Presentation is usually a slow, painless expansion on the posterior or lateral aspect of a rib. Pain occurs when sufficient enlargement stretches the periosteum or when the rib fractures. The natural history of this tumor is of continued growth with pain and deformity. Malignant change is very unusual. Prompt excision is recommended. Complete excision of the tumor is curative.

*Chondroma* usually occurs in patients between 20 and 40 years of age. It can arise in the ribs at the costochondral junction or in the sternum. Growth is very slow. Radiologically, the appearance is of a medullary mass whose expansion thins the bony cortex. Clinically, according to the description by Marcove and Huvos[28] of chondromas of the ribs, a lesion <4 cm in size is a benign tumor. There are no other clear indications to separate this from a malignant counterpart. Biopsy often does not give a clear differentiation. Therefore, these tumors should be treated as malignancies, with complete resection including adequate margins.

*Osteochondroma* and *osteoblastoma* are very rare. They have a characteristic growth pattern: They originate from the bony cortex of the rib and have a stalk and a cartilaginous covering over the tumor mass. Growth may be directed inward, in which case they are detected only on x-ray. If growth is directed outward, a mass is palpable. These tumors have been reported to become malignant in rare instances. Recurrences after complete excision have not been reported. Complete excision is the recommended treatment.

## MALIGNANT TUMORS OF THE CHEST WALL

Table 34–3 lists the various malignant tumors that can arise on the chest wall. Malignancies of skin alone usually are melanomas; they are not included as distinct chest wall entities. Occasionally, a *basal cell tumor* will recur and require chest-wall resection for control. Figure 34–3 shows a CT scan demonstrating an infiltrating locally destructive basal cell carcinoma. Figure 34–4 shows the resected specimen.

**TABLE 34–3. MALIGNANT TUMORS OF THE CHEST WALL**

| |
|---|
| Soft tissue |
| Malignant melanoma |
| Liposarcoma |
| Lymphangiosarcoma |
| Basal cell carcinoma |
| Fibrosarcoma |
| Rhabdomyosarcoma |
| Neurofibrosarcoma |
| Bone and cartilage |
| Chondrosarcoma |
| Osteogenic sarcoma |
| Ewing's sarcoma |
| Myeloma |
| Primary carcinoma of the lung/metastatic tumors |
| Sarcomas |
| Carcinomas |

The *malignant liposarcoma* is rare in the thoracic area. Resection with clear margins is effective treatment. *Angiosarcoma* can occur in a lymphedematous arm secondary to chest wall and/or axillary radiotherapy.[29] Figure 34–5 illustrates an example of this malignancy that required partial excision of the sternum and bilateral ribs to encompass it.

*Fibrosarcoma, rhabdomyosarcoma,* and *neurofibrosarcoma,* when occurring on the chest wall, are similar to these tumors arising elsewhere. A painful, rapidly growing

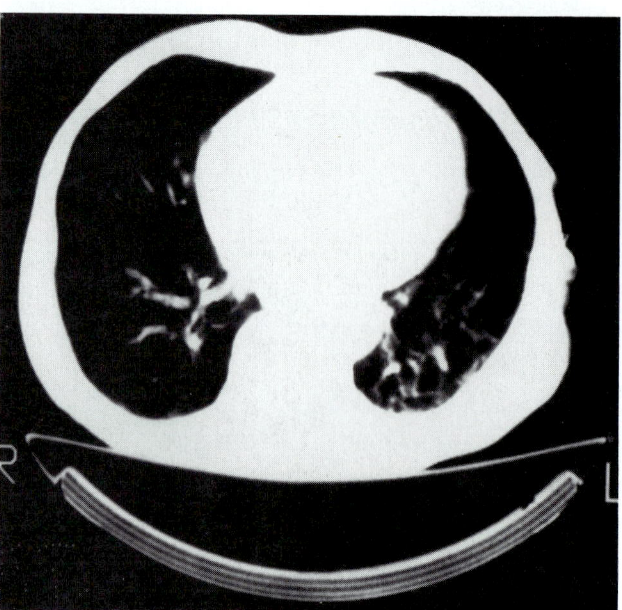


**Figure 34–3.** Basal cell carcinoma. CT scan showing destructive lesion of the left lateral chest wall.

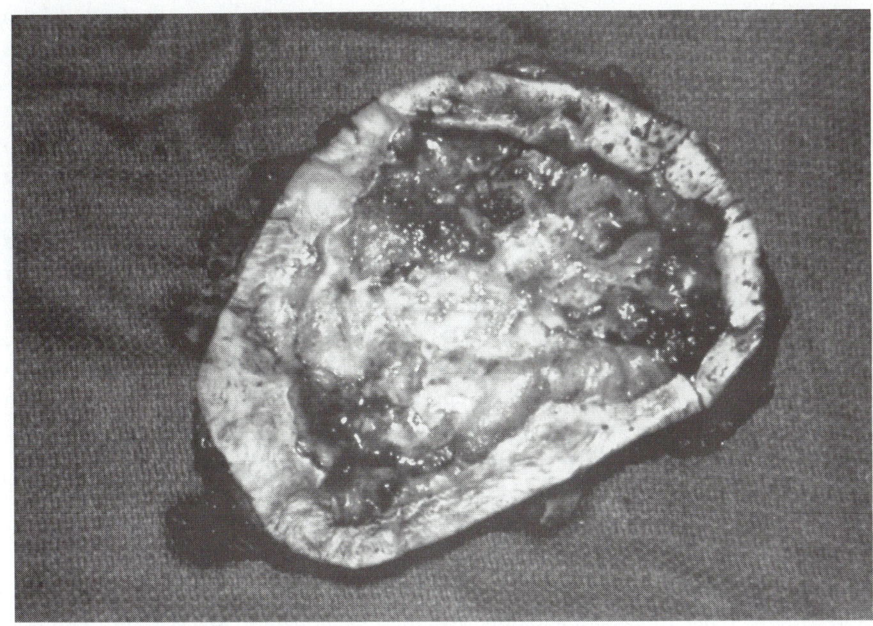

**Figure 34–4.** Resected basal cell carcinoma specimen.

mass is characteristic. Complete resection following diagnosis is the best treatment. Less-than-complete resection results in recurrence. Wide resection is recommended.[30] Incision placement depends on the presence of skin invasion by the tumor. If the skin is uninvaded, a linear incision is placed to allow development of skin flaps adequate for removal of the entire soft-tissue tumor with clear margins. Muscle dissection en bloc with the malignant tumor is similar to the technique used in resecting any sarcoma. The dissection should be done so that the tumor is never visualized or entered during its removal. If this means removing a portion of the rigid chest wall to obtain a free deep margin, this should be done. This technique and reconstruction techniques are described later.

As in similar tumors of extrathoracic origin, the age group varies, peaking at 40, with no sex advantage.

## MALIGNANT TUMOR OF BONE AND CARTILAGE

*Chondrosarcoma* is the most common malignant tumor of both the sternum and the entire chest wall. It affects the anterior, rather than posterior, costal junctions, so it occurs

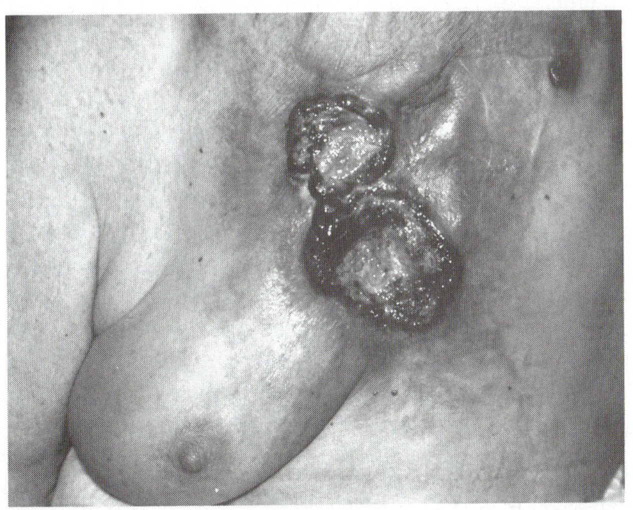

A

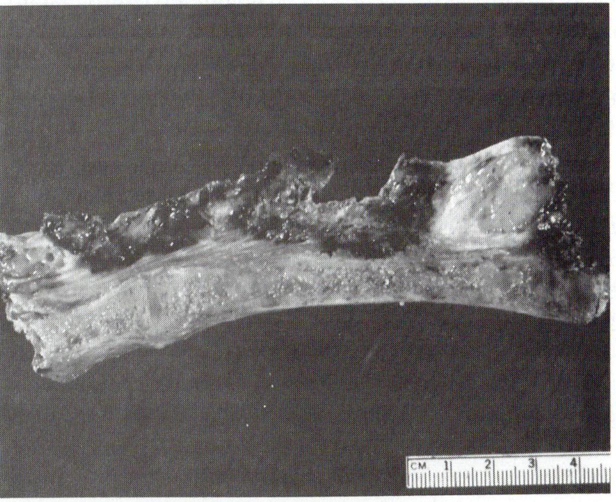


B

**Figure 34–5. A.** Angiosarcoma arising from lymphedematous chest wall following forequarter amputation for the same tumor. **B.** Destruction of bone by tumor.

predominantly on the front of the chest. As a slowly growing tumor, it arises from contiguous structures and can reach a large size. The x-ray will show a tumor mass with destruction of the bony cortex.

Histologic grading is of prognostic significance. Grade I tumors portend good survival, while grades II and III carry a more grim prognosis and higher rates of metastatic disease, local recurrence, and death.[30]

Treatment is excision of all tumor with a wide margin of normal tissue (5-cm margins with one normal rib above and below, and adequate sternal margins). The manubrium or xiphoid may be retained if the tumor has not crossed these anatomic junctions. When indicated, the entire sternum may be excised. Reconstruction techniques are described later. The Mayo Clinic reported 96 patients with chondrosarcoma of the thorax. The 10-year actuarial survival rate (Kaplan/Meier method) was 96% for widely resected tumors (recurrence rate 14%), 65% for tumors with limited resection (recurrence rate 60%), and 14% for those resected for palliation only.[23] Marcove and Huvos[28] reported on 27 patients with chondrosarcoma of the ribs. Local excision resulted in prompt local recurrence. They emphasized the importance of histologic grading and noted that sudden increase in size indicated a change to a more malignant grade. In his series they showed the following: grade I (13 patients), 10 alive 3–10 years, 3 dead of disease 2–12 years; grade II (7 patients), 6 dead of disease 1–7 years, 1 alive 18 months; and grade III (7 patients), 6 dead of disease 1–4 years, 1 no evident disease 19 years after resection. They stressed also that adequate resection meant taking, with the tumor, the underlying pleura, a normal rib above the tumor, and a normal rib below it.[28]

*Osteogenic sarcoma* usually occurs in the long bones of young adults. Less often it is found in the ribs. The natural history is of a tumor with greater virulence and earlier hematogenous spread than chondrosarcoma. The prognosis is correspondingly poorer. The lungs are the almost exclusive site of early metastases. Plain x-rays or CT scans are required before definitive treatment can be planned. Osteogenic sarcoma responds to both chemotherapy and radiotherapy. At present, in the case of local disease only, radical surgical resection is carried out. Chemotherapy is given for micrometastases after the wound has healed. If there is simultaneous diagnosis of the primary tumor and lung metastases, chemotherapy is given as first treatment. Chemotherapy consists of vincristine, Adriamycin, and high-dose methotrexate, as described by Marcove and Rosen.[31] They used this regimen preoperatively initially. Chemotherapy is also used when there is failure due to distant metastases. Results show a survival rate of 15–25% with combination surgery and chemotherapy. Where there has been no evidence of new tumor and/or a response of all visible tumor following several cycles of therapy, surgical resection of all tumor is then carried out. If a major resection is needed for the primary tumor, we choose to resect the pulmonary metastasis first. If the metastatic disease is found to be unresectable, then the primary tumor is usually treated by a method other than a major resection. When all disease has been resected from the lungs, the primary tumor is then excised.

*Ewing's sarcoma* is a rare chest-wall neoplasm. It presents as a rapidly expanding tender mass and is seen most often in adolescent males. Systemic symptoms of malaise, fever, and leukocytosis are common. Early metastases are common, both to other bones and to lungs. Local control for this tumor can be achieved with surgery or radiotherapy. However, because of the prevalence of distant metastases, the importance of adding chemotherapy should be considered an integral part of the treatment. This will improve the long-term prognosis. Multiple-agent therapy is recommended. Chan et al[32] use actinomycin, vincristine, cyclophosphamide, and Adriamycin. Zucker et al[33] use vincristine, cyclophosphamide, Adriamycin, and procarbazine in combination.

*Myelomatous tumors* in the ribs are usually only one manifestation of the generalized disease of multiple myeloma. This tumor accounts for 20% of the malignant neoplasms of the thorax and is usually found in males aged 60–70 years. These tumorous deposits are distributed throughout the skeleton. Confirmation of the diagnosis is made by Bence Jones proteinuria, immunoelectrophoresis, or bone marrow biopsy. Treatment is by chemotherapy, combined with radiotherapy when indicated for painful lesions. A solitary myelomalike tumor very rarely occurs without the systemic disease. This is usually termed a *plasmacytoma* pathologically, and it should be excised.[24,34]

## PRIMARY LUNG TUMORS

Primary lung tumors invade the chest wall in 5% of all cases reported. Such cases are staged as T3 tumors by the staging criteria of the American Joint Committee on Cancer.[35] Prognostic criteria of vital importance in these cases are status of mediastinal lymph nodes, status of distant metastases, and location of tumor with reference to the spine and mediastinum. In a report from Memorial Sloan-Kettering Cancer Center, results of a 10-year period (1974–1983) showed 1252 patients seen for lung cancer, excluding Pancoast's tumors. In this report, 233 patients had small-cell carcinomas, and 125 patients had neoplasms that invaded the rigid thorax. These patients had no extrathoracic metastatic tumor and were medically fit. Table 34–4 illustrates the depth of chest wall invasion in these patients. Fourteen patients had no pulmonary resection and were treated intraoperatively with brachytherapy, using iodine 125 implants. This was supplemented after surgery with external radiotherapy; 7 months was the median survival for these patients.

The remaining 111 patients underwent resection of lung and contiguous involved chest wall. Sixty-six patients required parietal pleural excision alone to encompass all

**TABLE 34–4. DEPTH OF CHEST WALL INVASION IN LUNG CANCER, 1974–1983**

| Number of Patients (N = 125) | Depth of Invasion |
|---|---|
| 70 | Pleura |
| 43 | Pleura + intercostal muscle + rib |
| 12 | Pleura + intercostal muscle + spine |

tumor, while 45 patients had resection of the rigid chest wall in continuity with the lung. From one to five rib segments were removed. Two thirds of these patients had reconstruction of the skeletal defect. The remaining defects were <5 cm or were located under the scapula so that reconstruction was unnecessary. The only operative death was due to bronchopneumonia following en bloc right upper lobectomy with parietal resection of four ribs. Marlex mesh was used for reconstructing the defect, and a flail was not demonstrated postoperatively.

Complete resection was possible in 62% of these patients. Survival results are shown in Table 34–5.[36]

These statistics are similar to those of Piehler et al[37] in treating these tumors. There is some controversy concerning the extent of resection needed for tumor invasion beyond the visceral pleura. Several authors believe that full thickness chest wall resection is needed in every case. They report a 75% survival rate in 22 patients with rib resection and 28% for those patients who had a parietal pleurectomy only.[37,38]

The surgical technique we advocate is to begin an extrapleural dissection at a distance from the site of invasion. If the parietal pleura separates easily from the intercostal structures, we have found that microscopic invasion is limited to the parietal pleura. Resection of this pleura en bloc with the lung tumor is sufficient.[39]

If resistance is met during the finger dissection, invasion into the intercostal muscle is present; in that event, a full-thickness chest wall resection is carried out. One normal rib above and below the area, plus a 5-cm margin on the involved rib, is outlined. Intercostal neurovascular structures are identified and secured, and the involved chest wall is excised. The pulmonary resection is then carried out in the usual manner, and the lung and chest wall tumor are removed en bloc. A mediastinal lymph node dissection is then carried out to surgically stage the tumor. Survival using this technique is shown in Table 34–5.

**TABLE 34–5. SURVIVAL IN RESECTION OF LUNG CANCER WITH CHEST WALL INVASION**

| Chest Wall Invasion | 5-Year Survival (%) |
|---|---|
| All with complete resection | 40 |
| Negative regional lymph nodes | 56 |
| Positive regional lymph nodes | 21 |
| Tumor confined to parietal pleura | 48 (CR, 77)[a] |
| Negative lymph nodes | 62 |
| Tumor invading ribs | 16 (CR, 53)[a] |
| Negative nodes | 35 |

[a]*CR, complete resection.*

Complete resection of these tumors is essential. When this is not possible, median survival is only 9 months. Even microscopically positive margins treated with postoperative radiation therapy did not alter this outcome, since all patients die of their disease in 12 months. Patterson et al[40] report an improved survival with adjunctive radiation, but the study was not randomized.

Invasion of the spine precludes complete resectability; in the 12 patients in our series with invasion of the spine, median survival was 10 months. In such cases, it can afford considerable palliation to resect all tumor and reconstruct the spine.[41]

## MAMMARY CARCINOMAS

Mammary carcinoma remains the most common malignant tumor in women. A small percentage of these tumors involve the chest wall. Recurrence following resection or radiation, very large or deeply situated tumors, or metastases to the internal mammary lymph nodes chain necessitates presentation of these tumors to the thoracic surgeon. Of our 317 chest wall resections for malignancy from 1963 through 1983, 29 (13%) were for tumors of mammary origin. Twelve of these patients were resected at the time of the first recurrence subsequent to primary therapy. Eight patients had two recurrences each, and the remaining nine patients from three to six each, before chest-wall resection was done. The techniques of resection are identical, and many resections include the sternum to obtain clear surgical margins. Proximity to the thoracic inlet increases the likelihood of involvement of the subclavian artery or vein. MRI scans have proven useful to indicate vascular involvement so that appropriate planning can be made preoperatively (Fig. 34–6). Survival results in this group of patients are directly related to the stage of the breast neoplasm. Of the 29 patients completely resected, 11 are free of disease for a median time of 51 months; 8 survived a median of 48 months with recurrent or residual disease; and 10 lived a median of 13 months before succumbing to their cancer.[42]

## METASTATIC TUMORS OF THE CHEST WALL

### Carcinomas

When there is widespread metastatic disease throughout the body, this very frequently involves the chest wall. This occurs mostly in ribs, but soft tissues also harbor tumors. These present no surgical problem, since systemic therapy is used. However, in the case of a solitary metastasis to the chest wall, because systemic therapy has little effect, a resection is almost always indicated (Fig. 34–7). A needle

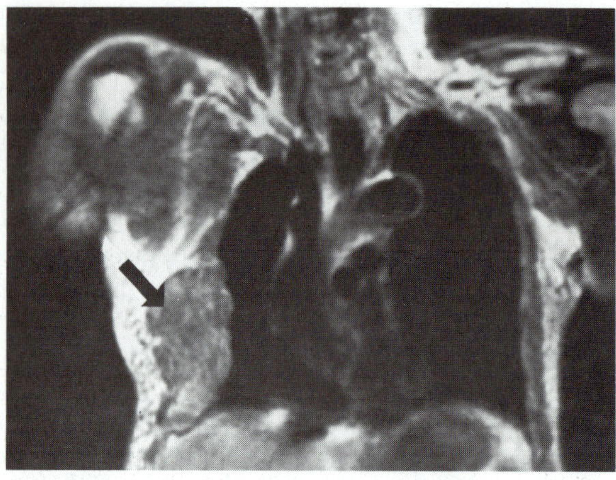

**Figure 34–6.** Mammary carcinoma. MRI scan illustrating the clarity with which vascular structures are visualized. This tumor invades the right lateral chest wall (*arrow*).

biopsy confirms the diagnosis. A complete search for other metastases is carried out. If none are found, excision should be done. From 1963 to 1983, the most frequent metastatic carcinoma we have seen has been from a mammary primary, followed by renal, colon, and salivary gland tumors. Survival is related to stage of disease, but we have seen 16 5-year survivors (Table 34–6).

Metastatic *sarcoma* to the chest wall is the least common type of malignant tumor involving the thorax. These sarcomas comprise just 11% (36/317) of the chest-wall tumors over the 20-year period 1963–1982. A needle biopsy should confirm the sarcoma diagnosis. When the patient has a known primary sarcoma, a diligent search for other disease must yield no other tumor sites before a chest wall resection is done. Again, as in the metastatic carcinomas, the ultimate prognosis depends on the disease stage. We have seven 5-year survivors in this group.

## SURGICAL TECHNIQUES

Guidelines to follow when one is resecting tumors include a 2- to 3-cm clear margin of soft tissue and a normal rib above and below the tumor, with a 5-cm clear rib margin. Violation of the tumor should be avoided and a full-thickness chest wall resection carried out, including parietal pleura. Contiguous structures invaded by the tumor should also be removed when possible. Included with the surgical specimen should be one normal myofascial plane below the skin. However, overlying skin should always be taken if it is adherent to the tumor or if it is the site of a previous biopsy (Fig. 34–8).

Tumors near the thoracic inlet pose anatomic problems; proximity to neurovascular structures requires careful planning. Involvement of the shoulder girdle may require a forequarter amputation, with chest-wall incontinuity, to eradicate the tumor. Tumors arising low in the lateral rib cage may require resection of the involved diaphragm. Reconstruction may be completed by direct closure, or a Gor-Tex patch, which is impermeable to air and liquids, may be used to restore the barrier between the pleural and peritoneal cavities.

Radiation therapy should also be considered in the planning of overall treatment for chest wall tumors.[43] Intraoperative application, by using brachytherapy techniques[44] for implantation, or by afterloading utilizing radioactive sources for microscopically positive margins in areas where further resection is not possible, has been proven successful. Radiation therapy following excision of desmoid tumors is also recommended to decrease local recurrence.

## PROSTHESIS CONSTRUCTION

When surgical margins have been declared free of tumor, chest tubes are placed in the routine fashion. Reconstruction is then planned. For a lesion <5 cm, several choices are available. If the defect is bony only, no replacement may be needed. If one is desired, mesh alone, or a small Gor-Tex patch, is sufficient. If soft-tissue replacement is also needed, a myocutaneous flap or advancement flaps can be used with or without mesh.

In larger defects, several choices for replacement of the rigid chest wall are readily available: Marlex mesh, usually doubled if used alone, or a Gor-Tex patch. Either choice is trimmed to size and sutured to the wall of the defect with full-thickness interrupted sutures.

Methyl methacrylate can be added to the Marlex mesh to make a composite that can be molded to match the body's contour and provide excellent cosmetic results. A "pattern" of the prosthesis is made by laying a clean gauze over the surgical defect and gently pressing it against the cut edge (Fig. 34–9). A layer of Marlex mesh is laid on top of this pattern. Methyl methacrylate is next mixed thoroughly, in the container provided, until it becomes thick enough to spread over the Marlex mesh. The pattern is filled in within 0.5 cm of the edge with a thin layer. The second piece of mesh is placed on the methacrylate to complete the "sandwich" (Fig. 34–10). This is then placed, for hardening, over an appropriately shaped object to enable the prosthesis to assume the needed contour. If the adjacent chest wall is used to provide this contour, then a protective pad must be placed under the "sandwich," since it reaches 140°F as it hardens and may cause a severe burn. When hardened, the mesh is trimmed to size and sutured around the bony edge of the defect. The suture is heavy and nonabsorbable (Fig. 34–11).

If desired, a second method allows replacement of sternum alone. A layer of mesh is sutured to the underside of the surgical defect. After the methacrylate is mixed, a small portion is placed in an Asepto syringe while it is still

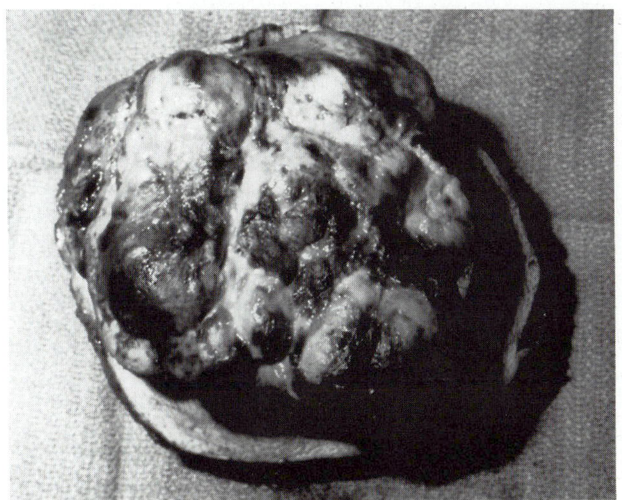

A

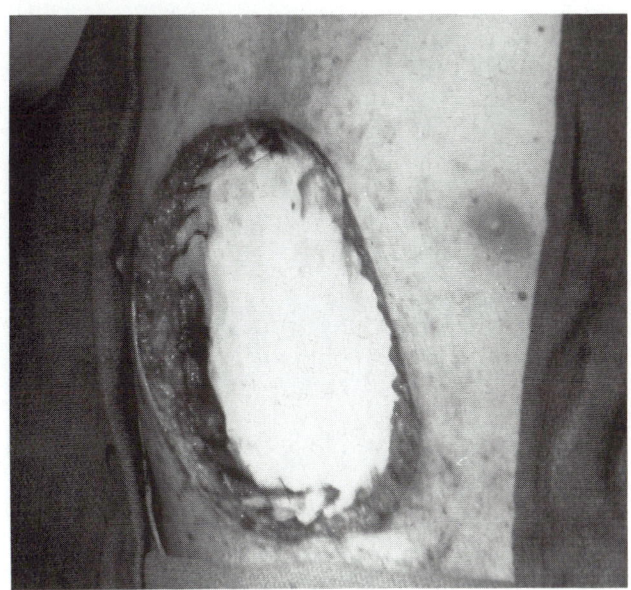

B

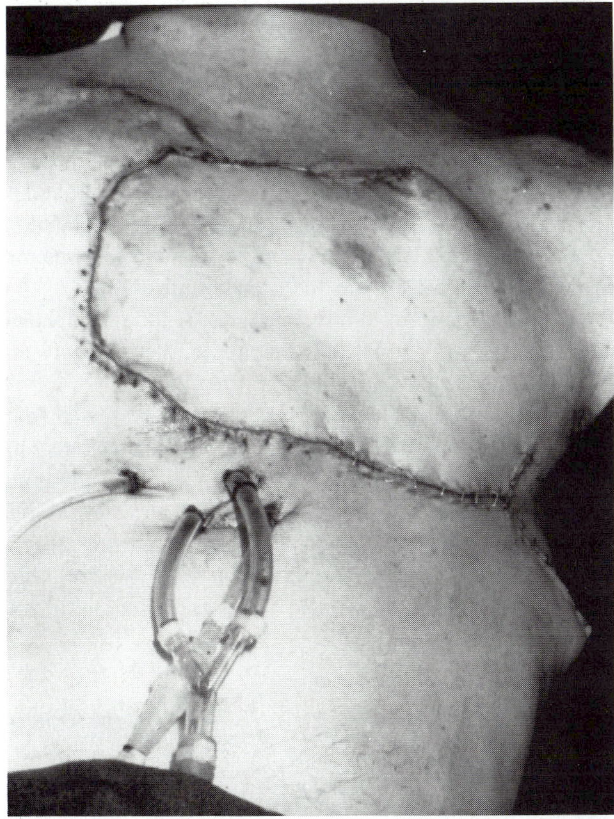

C

**Figure 34–7. A.** Metastatic renal cell tumor that grew to a size of 10 cm in the sternum. **B.** Reconstruction in place. **C.** Lateral skin flap raised to cover the defect.

quite thin and injected into the marrow cavity of the remaining sternum. The rest of the methacrylate is then molded to the shape of the resected bone. This hardens and is solidly fused with the residual sternum. A second layer of mesh is then sutured onto the top of the defect.

The Gor-Tex patch is impermeable and makes an excellent replacement for the diaphragm. It is not incorporated with body tissues, becomes lax with time, and is considerably more expensive than the meshes.[45] Marlex mesh is incorporated by the body tissues and retains its shape. It has been proven to be stronger than surrounding ribs in the case of trauma.

The omentum can be advanced whenever it is judged useful according to the techniques described later in this chapter. It is usually placed between the synthetic prosthesis and the myocutaneous flap.

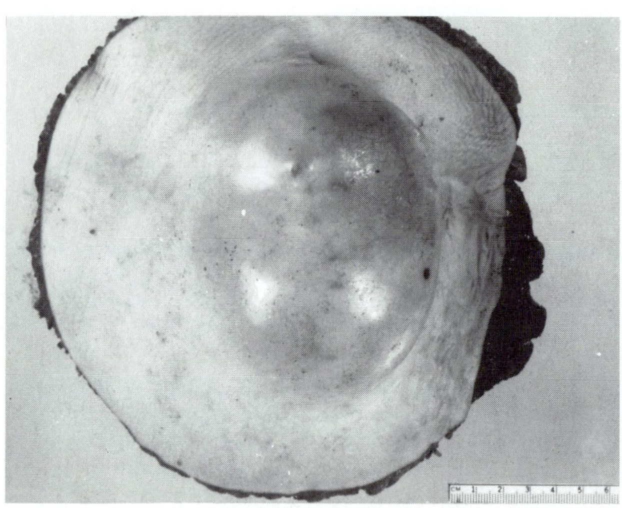

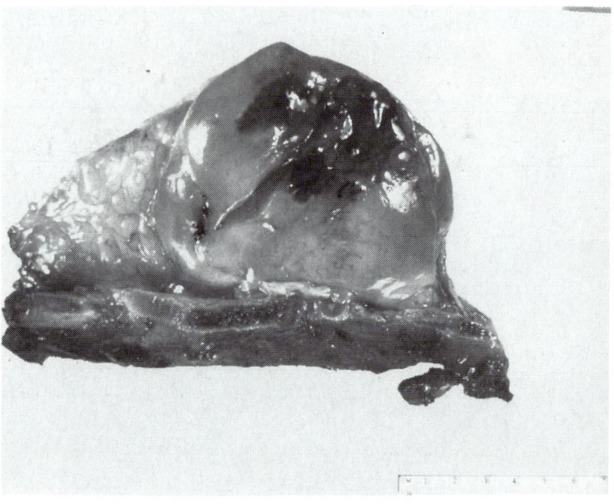

A B

**Figure 34–8. A.** Adequate surgical soft-tissue margin around a tumor. **B.** The complete chest wall must be included in the resection, because of tumor encroachment into ribs.

## SOFT-TISSUE REPLACEMENT

When a soft-tissue and/or skin defect is present, the plastic surgeon needs to plan replacement strategy preoperatively. Patient positioning and draping techniques need to be considered. A detailed discussion with the patient is necessary.[45,46]

The basic graft types used are (1) split-thickness skin grafts, based on omentum; (2) delayed flaps; (3) myocutaneous flaps; and (4) the free flap. The opposite breast can be used for soft-tissue coverage when the cosmetic result is not paramount.

The greater omentum can also be used.[47] This option has two major indications: an infected recipient site, or the need for a base for a split-thickness skin graft. The approach to harvest the omentum can be through the original site if it is located near the diaphragm. When the resection is in the area of the lower sternum or anterior chest wall, a tunnel can be made into the peritoneal cavity. When there has been no prior abdominal surgery, the omentum can be grasped and gently brought into the excision site.[48]

In instances of prior abdominal surgery, or when there is a need for the omentum to reach the thoracic inlet, a separate midline incision is made below the xiphoid process. The transverse colon with attached omentum is brought intothe wound. The arterial supply of the omentum comes from the arcade formed by the right and left gastroepiploic arteries (Fig. 34–12). A right, a middle, and a left omental artery and vein arise from the arcade and descend in the vertical direction to form a second arcade at the distal edge. Either the right or the left gastroepiploic artery can sustain the entire omentum as a pedicle or a free flap.

To raise a pedicle flap, the omentum is dissected from the transverse colon and the greater curvature of the stomach. Selection of the pedicle artery is made, and the other artery is divided. The distribution of the omental arteries dictates how further incisions are made to increase the length of the omentum to reach the excision site (Fig. 34–13). A tunnel is then made under the intervening soft

**TABLE 34–6. MALIGNANT TUMORS OF THE CHEST WALL (1963–1983)**

| | 5-Year Survivors |
|---|---|
| Primary carcinoma | 40/127 |
| Metastatic carcinoma | 16/71 |
| Primary sarcoma | 22/83 |
| Metastatic sarcoma | 7/36 |
| Total | 85/317 |

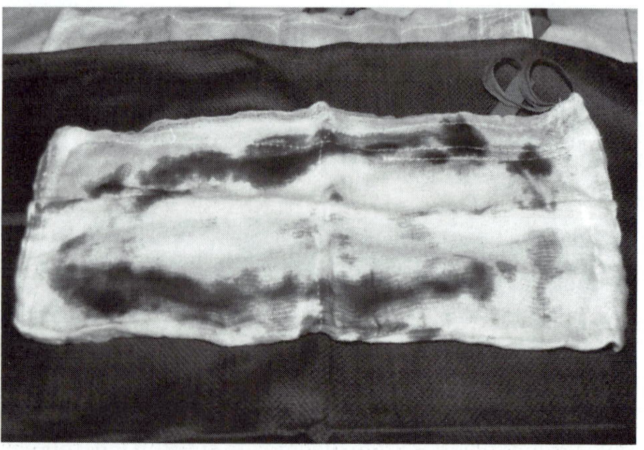

**Figure 34–9.** Pattern for reconstructive prosthesis made by laying clean gauze on surgical margin.

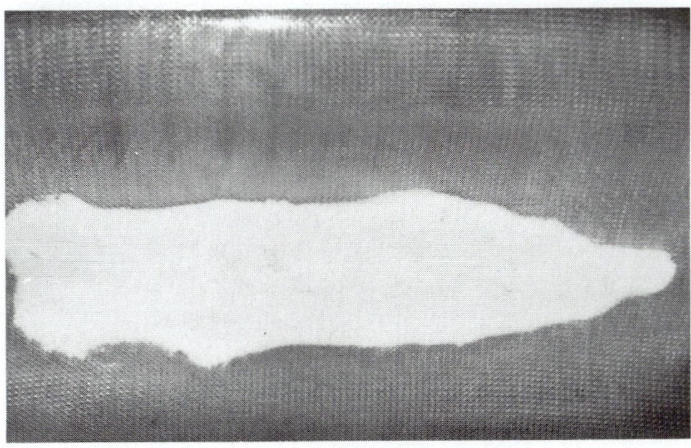

Figure 34–10. Completed "sandwich" of prosthesis.

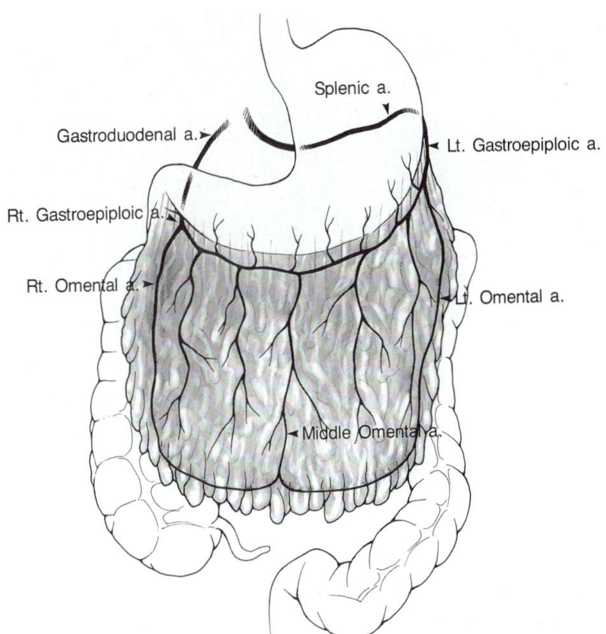


Figure 34–12. Blood supply of the omentum.

tissue, and the omentum is delivered and sutured into place at the defect. The laparotomy incision is closed around the pedicle, with care taken to prevent strangulation and avoid an incisional hernia (Fig. 34–14).

When the omentum is to be used as a free flap, the recipient artery and vein are prepared. The omentum is then harvested with the donor vascular pedicle prepared and brought to the excision site. One team closes the abdominal incision, while the microvascular surgeons proceed with the anastomoses at the excision site. A split-thickness skin graft can then be prepared and sutured to the skin and omentum at the excision site, or an alternate local skin flap can be raised for coverage.

A "delayed flap" is one constructed of the full subcutaneous tissue as well as skin. A random donor area is selected for transfer and "delayed" over a 3-week period by interrupting blood supply progressively from three sides and forcing one end to be the "supply pedicle." After 3 weeks, the flap is transferred based on the donor site pedicle. This is severed when the graft has established viability at the excision site. While this procedure is passable, the delay and multiple operations make it less than optimal.

A deltopectoral flap (Fig. 34–15) was used extensively for anterior chest wall defects until about 20 years ago. It has been supplanted by the myocutaneous flap and, in specific instances, the free flap.

For the most part, three myocutaneous flaps are used in chest wall reconstruction: latissimus dorsi, pectoralis major, and rectus abdominis. Table 34–7 lists the important anatomic aspects of each muscle flap. The site of the defect and the availability of blood supply dictate the choice of

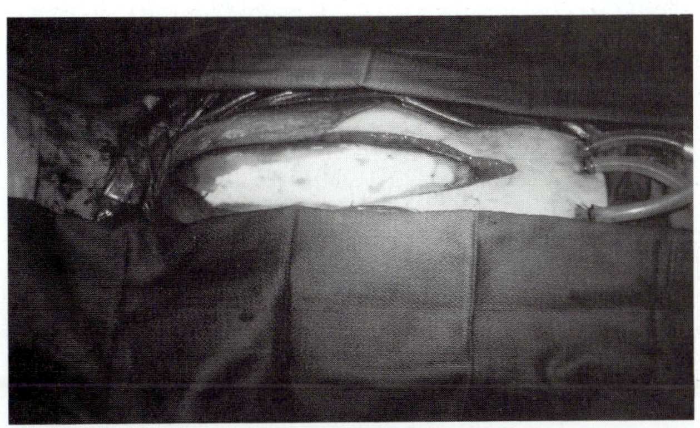

Figure 34–11. "Sandwich" sutured into place to fill defect of excised sternum.

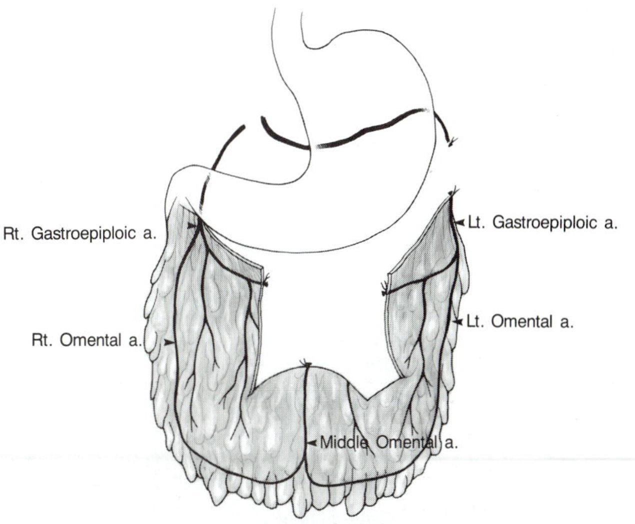


Figure 34–13. Omentum dissected for transfer.

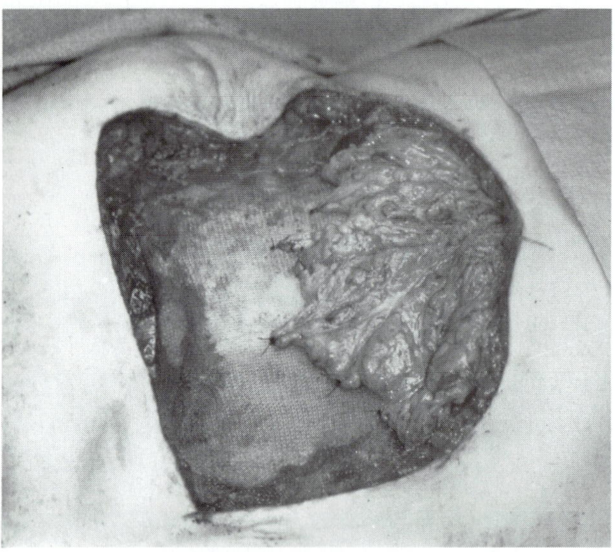

**Figure 34–14.** Omentum brought up and sutured onto top of sternal reconstruction. This protects the distal tip of the Bakamjian flap used to cover this defect.

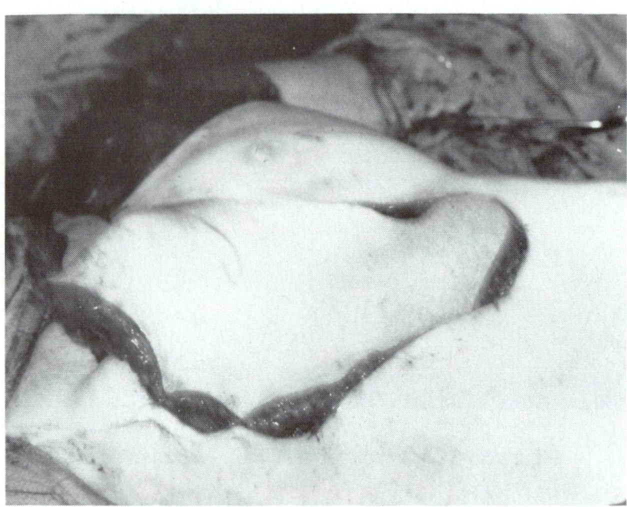

**Figure 34–15.** Deltopectoral flap transferred from left shoulder to cover surgical defect.

flap. Figure 34–16A–C illustrates the respective areas these flaps can cover.

Positioning and draping of the patient on the table must accommodate both the excision of the tumor and the soft-tissue reconstruction.[48]

If the latissimus dorsi muscle is to be used, the patient is prepped and draped in full lateral position, with the arm draped free. A donor site for a split-thickness skin graft must also be planned. When the patient is fully draped, the table can be turned as near horizontal as possible while the tumor is resected and the rigid replacement secured in place. Subsequently, the table is returned to the lateral position; the size of the skin paddle needed is now known, and the muscle is freed, with the skin in place. A tunnel is then created under the axillary fold, and the myocutaneous flap is delivered to the operative site and sutured to the skin edge of the defect (Fig. 34–17). The donor site skin is closed primarily, if possible. If necessary, a split-thickness skin graft is used.

When a pectoralis major or rectus abdominis muscle flap is to be used, the patient can remain supine for both surgical procedures.[49,50]

## FREE FLAPS

For chest-wall defects, a myocutaneous pedicle flap is the first choice for reconstruction, because it gives the best result consistently and can be done safely by the general plastic surgeon with standard equipment.

When there is no local flap that can fill the particular need—because of prior radiation therapy, or previous incisions that have severed arterial supply, or because the size and site of the defect place it beyond the reach of a local pedicle flap—a free flap can be used.

Specialized personnel and equipment are necessary for this microvascular surgery. The plastic surgeon trained in this subspecialty will select the appropriate muscle and skin paddle needed to cover the defect. Hidalgo et al[51] describe in excellent detail the selection process and techniques. The

**TABLE 34–7. MYOCUTANEOUS FLAPS**

| Muscle | Origin | Insertion | Blood Supply |
|---|---|---|---|
| Latissimus dorsi | Spine T6–L5<br>Crest of ilium<br>Lower 4 ribs | Lesser tubercle of humerus | Thoracodorsal |
| Pectoralis major | Clavicle<br>Sternum<br>Aponeurosis of external oblique muscle | Greater tubercle of humerus | Pecotral branch of thoracoacromial<br>Internal mammary<br>Lateral thoracic |
| Rectus abdominis | Crest of pelvis | 5,6,7 costal cartilages | Superior epigastric<br>Inferior epigastric |

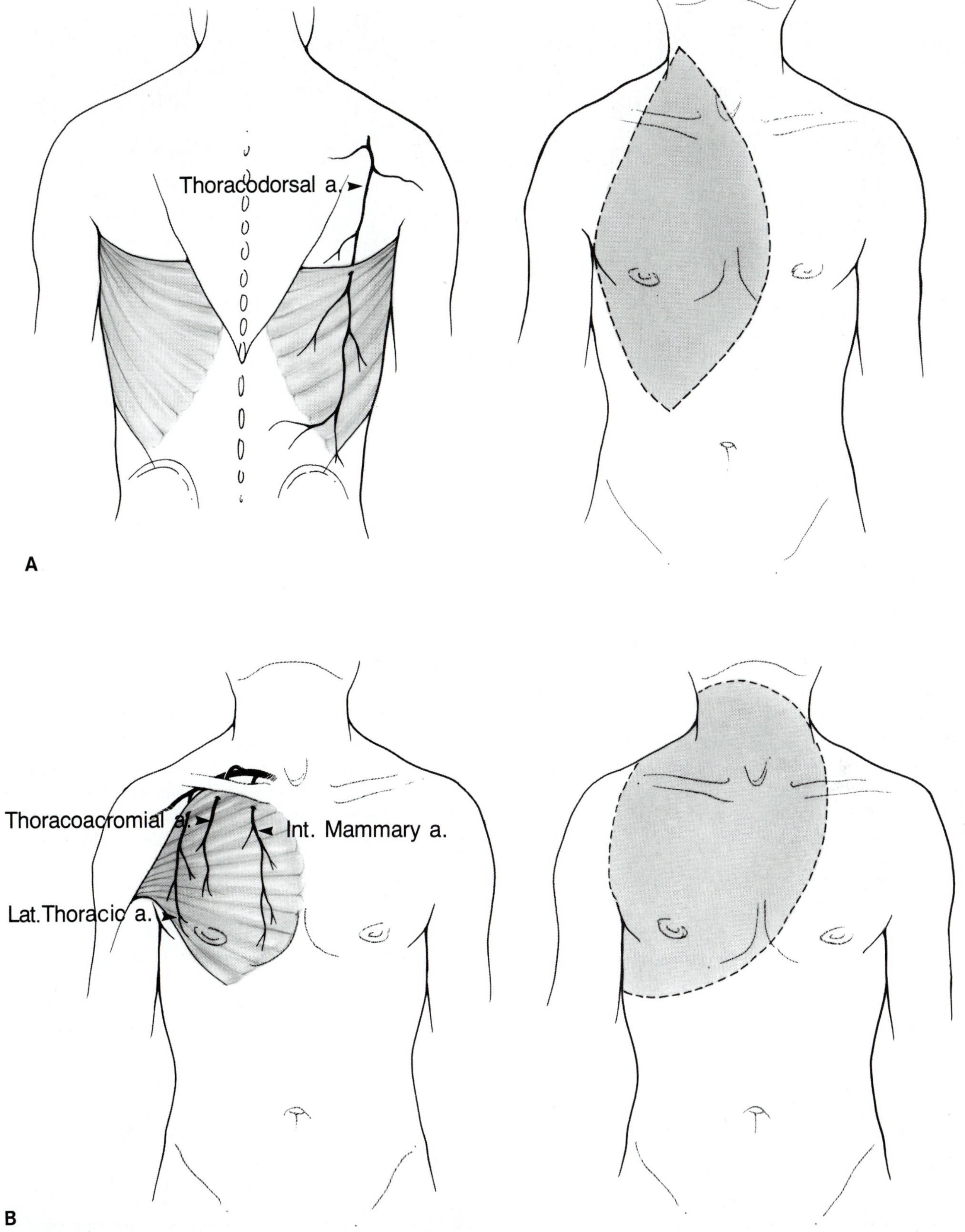


**Figure 34–16.** **A.** Latissimus dorsi muscle—blood supply and coverage area. **B.** Pectoralis major muscle—blood supply and coverage area. *(Continued.)*

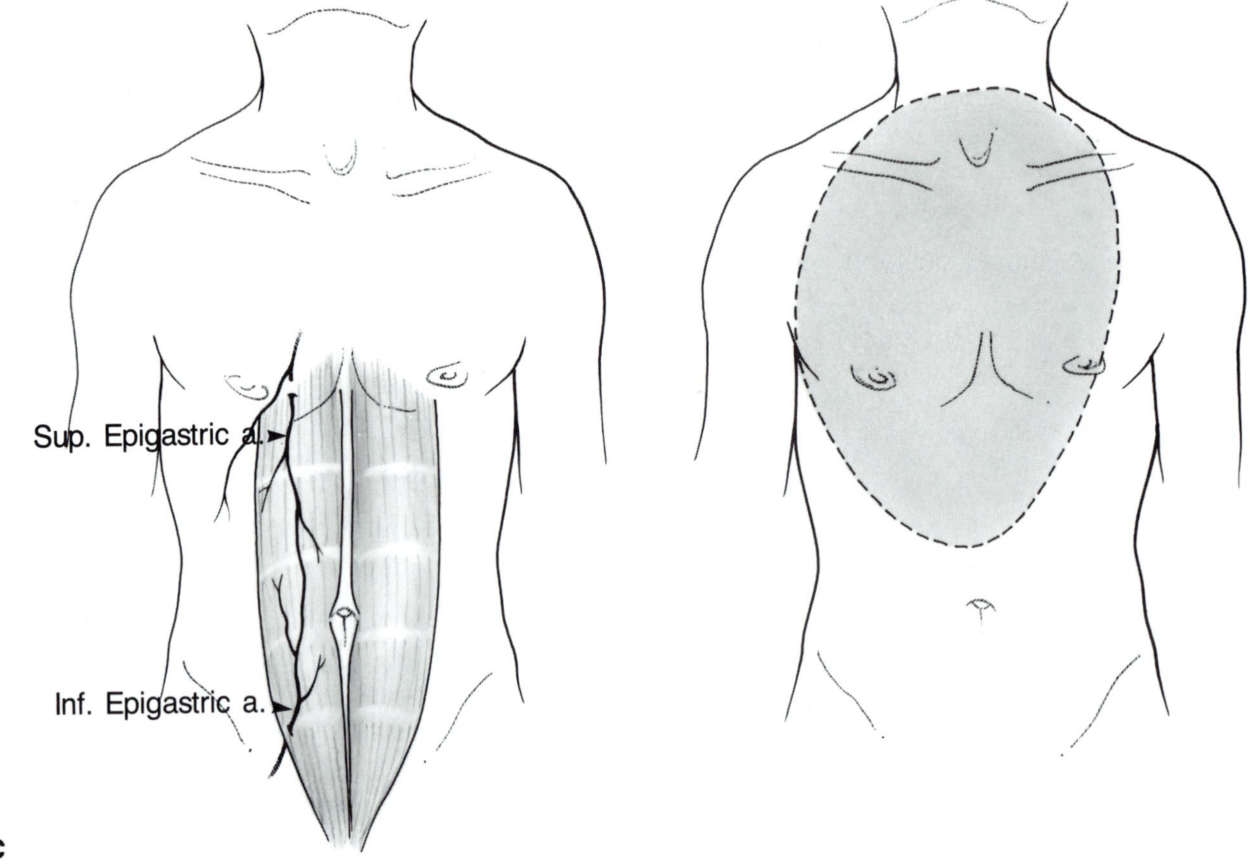


**Figure 34–16.** *(Continued.)* **C.** Rectus abdominis muscle—blood supply and coverage area.

recipient artery and vein are prepared and the donor free flap brought to the operative site. Anastomosis of the donor and recipient artery(s) and vein(s) is performed under the microscope. In skilled hands the results are excellent, with a success rate over 90%.

## RESULTS

In the analysis of survival data in malignant chest-wall tumors, two major considerations merit attention. First, removal of a fungating, painful, or bleeding tumor mass will give the patient an improved quality of survival, although it may not prolong life. A second group of patients, in whom symptoms are directly related to compression or invasion of lung or neurovascular structures, will show marked improvement in symptoms and well-being with resection of these tumors. Results in these cases are not measured by survival rates but by survival quality of life.

All benign tumors are resected for cure. Long-term survival is achieved with a wide excision of the tumor. Persistent disease and local recurrence are the consequences of incomplete resection. Prior to the use of the technique described here, a lesser resection was the norm because of the postoperative problems of flail and prolonged need for respirator support. Since the development of the rigid "sandwich," every patient but one in our series was extubated in the immediate postoperative period without difficulty. That patient had a long-standing, low-grade chondrosarcoma of the sternum and clavicles compressing the trachea. The pa-

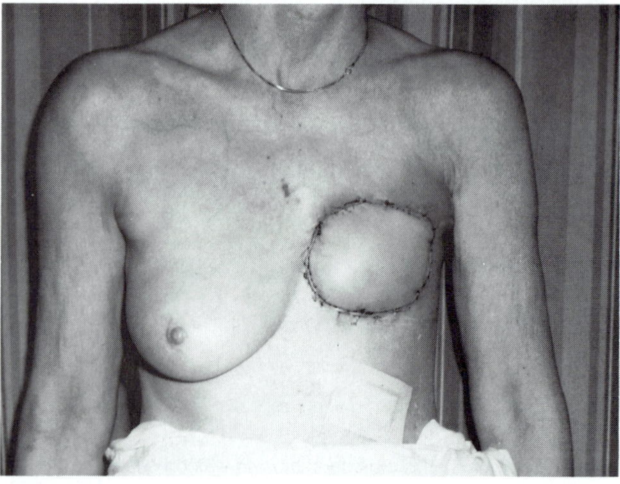

**Figure 34–17.** Latissimus dorsi myocutaneous flap used to replace soft-tissue deficit.

tient did not have flail chest but rather a tracheomalacia, which required intubation for 48 hours postanesthesia.

Of the patients in our series with soft-tissue sarcoma of the chest wall, 55% (65/119) are alive without disease, and 22% (22/83) are alive for more than 5 years following resection.

It is important that the surgeon feel confident about the reconstruction of bony defects resulting from surgical resection. If this confidence is present, an adequate margin will be taken, and persistence of tumor or local recurrence will not be a problem. The availability of materials needed for the reconstruction, and the ease of constructing and inserting the custom-made prosthesis, supplies the basis for this confidence and ensures an improved cure rate for these tumors.

## REFERENCES


1. Parham FW: Thoracic resection for tumors growing from the bony wall of the chest. *Trans Surg Gynecol Assoc* **11**:223–363, 1898
2. Fell GE: Forced respiration. *JAMA* **16**:325–330, 1891
3. O'Dwyer J: Fifty cases of croup in private practice treated by intubation of the larynx with a description of the method and the dangers incident thereto. *Med Rec* **32**:557–571, 1887
4. Graham EA, Singer JJ: Successful removal of an entire lung for carcinoma of the bronchus. *JAMA* **101**:1371–1374, 1933
5. Watson WL, James AG. Fascia lata grafts for chest wall defects. *J Thorac Surg* **16**:399–406, 1947
6. Maier HC: Surgical management of large defects of the thoracic wall. *Surgery* **22**:169–178, 1947
7. Bisgard JD, Swenson SA Jr: Tumors of the sternum. *Arch Surg* **56**:570–577, 1948
8. Campbell DA: Reconstruction of the anterior thoracic wall. *J Thorac Surg* **19**:456–461, 1950
9. Blades B, Paul JS: Chest wall tumors. *Ann Surg* **131**:976–983, 1950
10. Converse JM, Campbell RM, Watson WL: Repair of large radiation ulcers situated over the heart and the brain. *Ann Surg* **133**:95–103, 1951
11. Myre TT, Kirklin JW: Resection of tumors of the sternum. *Ann Surg* **144**:1023–1028, 1956
12. Rees TD, Converse JM: Surgical reconstruction of defects of the thoracic wall. *Surg Gynecol Obstet* **121**:1066–1072, 1965
13. Starzynski TE, Snyderman RK, Beattie EJ Jr: Problems of major chest wall reconstruction. *Plast Reconstr Surg* **44**:525–535, 1969
14. Martini N, Starzynski TE, Beattie EJ Jr: Problems in chest wall resection. *Surg Clin North Am* **49**:313–322, 1969
15. Le Roux BT: Maintenance of chest wall stability. *Thorax* **19**:397–405, 1964
16. Kiricuta I: L'emploi au grand epiploon dans le chirugi du sein cancereux. *Prese Med* **71**:15–17, 1963
17. Eschpasse H, Gaillard J, Faurnial G, et al: Utilisation de prostheses en resine acrylique pour la réparation des vastes pertes de substance de la parou thoracique. *Acta Chir Belg* **76**:281–285, 1977
18. Graham J, Usher FC, Perry JL, Barkley HT: Marlex mesh as a prosthesis in the repair of thoracic wall defects. *Ann Surg* **151**:469–479, 1960
19. Jurkiewicz MJ, Arnold PG: The omentum: An account of its use in the reconstruction of the chest wall. *Ann Surg* **185**:548–554, 1977
20. McCormack P, Bains MS, Beattie EJ Jr, Martini N: New trends in skeletal reconstruction after resection of chest wall tumors. *Ann Thorac Surg* **31**:45–52, 1981
21. Ramming KP, Holmes EC, Zarem HA, et al: Surgical management and reconstruction of extensive chest wall malignancies. *Am J Surg* **144**:146–151, 1982
22. Arnold PG, Pairolero PC: Chest wall reconstruction: Experience with 100 consecutive patients. *Ann Surg* **199**:725–732, 1984
23. Addis BJ: Pathology of tumors of the pleura and chest wall. In Hoogstraten B, et al (eds): *Lung Tumors*. New York, Springer-Verlag, 1988, p 205
24. Threlkel JB, Adkins RB: Primary chest wall tumors. *Ann Thorac Surg* **11**:450, 1971
25. Allan PW, Enzinger FM: Hemangioma of skeletal muscle. *Cancer* **29**:8, 1972
26. Baffi RR, Didolkar MS, Bakamjian V: Reconstruction of sternal and abdominal wall defects in a case of desmoid tumor. *J Thorac Cardiovasc Surg* **74**:105, 1977
27. Martini N, McCormack PM, Bains MS: Chest wall tumors: Clinical results of treatment. In Grillo HC, Eschapasse H (eds): *International Trends in General Thoracic Surgery*. Philadelphia, Saunders, 1977
28. Marcove RC, Huvos AG: Cartilaginous tumors of the ribs. *Cancer* **27**:794, 1971
29. Watkins E, Gerard FP: Malignant tumors involving chest wall. *J Thorac Cardiovasc Surg* **39**:117, 1960
30. Teitelbaum SL: Tumors of the chest wall. *Surg Gynecol Obstet* **129**:1050, 1969
31. Marcove R, Rosen G: En bloc resections for osteogenic sarcoma. *Cancer* **45**:3040, 1980
32. Chan R, Sutow W, Lindberg R, et al: Management and results of localized Ewing's sarcoma. *Cancer* **43**:1001, 1979
33. Zucker J, Henry-Amar M, Sarrazin D, et al: Intensive septemic chemotherapy in localized Ewing's sarcoma in childhood. A historical trial. *Cancer* **52**:415, 1983
34. Burt M, Karpeh M, Ukoha O, et al: Medical tumors of the chest wall. *J Thorac Cardiovasc Surg* **105**:89–96, 1993
35. American Joint Committee on Cancer: *Manual for Staging of Cancer*, 2nd Ed. Philadelphia, Lippincott, 1983, p 99
36. McCaughan BC, Martini N, Bains MS, McCormack PM: Chest wall invasion of carcinoma of the lung: Therapeutics and prognostic implications. *J Thorac Cardiovasc Surg* **51**:417, 1966
37. Piehler JM, Pairolero PC, Weeland LH, et al: Bronchogenic carcinoma with chest wall invasion: Factors affecting survival following en-bloc resection. *Ann Thorac Surg* **34**:684, 1982
38. Grillo HC, Greenberg JJ, Wilkins EW Jr: Resection of bronchogenic carcinoma involving thoracic wall. *J Thorac Cardiovasc Surg* **51**:417, 1966
39. McCormack PM, Bains MS, Beattie EJ Jr, Martini N: New trends in skeletal reconstruction after resection of chest wall tumors. *Ann Thorac Surg* **31**:45, 1981
40. Patterson GA, Ilves R, Ginsberg RJ, Cooper JD, Todd TRJ, Pearson FG: The value of adjuvant radiotherapy in pulmonary and chest wall resection for bronchogenic carcinoma. *Ann Thorac Surg* **34**:692, 1982
41. Sundaresan N, Bains MS, McCormack PM: Surgical treatment of spinal cord compression in patients with lung cancer. *Neurosurgery* **16**:350, 1985
42. McCormack PM, Bains MS, Burt ME, et al: Locally recurrent mammary carcinoma failing multimodality therapy. A solution. *Arch Surg* **124**:158–161, 1989
43. Tobias SL: Radiotherapy of mediastinal and chest wall tumors. In Hoogstraten B, et al (eds): *Lung Tumors*, New York, Springer Verlag, 1988
44. Hilaris B, Nori D, Beattie EJ Jr, Martini N: Value of perioperative brachytherapy in the management of non-oat cell carcinoma of the lung. *Int J Radiat Oncol Biol Phys* **9**:1161, 1983
45. Arnold PG, Pairolero PC: Use of pectoralis major muscle flaps to repair defects of the anterior chest wall. *Plast Reconstr Surg* **63**:205, 1979
46. Arnold PG, Pairolero PC: Chest wall reconstruction: Experience with 100 consecutive patients. *Ann Surg* **199**:725, 1984

47. Jacobs EQ, Hoffman S, et al: Reconstruction of a large chest wall defect using greater omentum. *Arch Surg* **113:**886, 1978
48. Hidalgo DA : Omentum free flaps. In Shaw WW, Hidalgo DA (eds): *Microsurgery in Trauma.* New York, Futura, 1987
49. Seyfer AE, Graeber GM, Wind GG: *Atlas of Chest Wall Reconstruction.* Rockville, Maryland, Aspen Press, 1986
50. Seyfer AE, Graeber GM: The use of latissimus dorsi and pectoralis major myocutaneous flaps in chest wall reconstruction. *Contemp Surg* **22:**29, 1983
51. Hidalgo DA, Bermant MA, Keller A, Shaw WW: Basic principles. In Shaw WW, Hidalgo DA (eds): *Microsurgery in Trauma.* New York, Futura, 1987

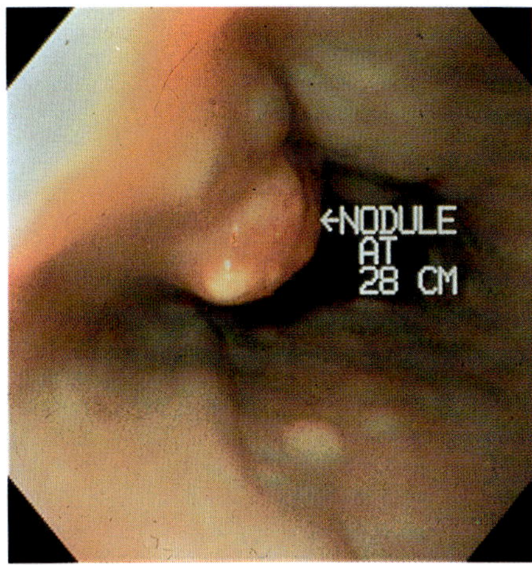


**Figure 9–4.** A squamous cell carcinoma of the upper midthoracic esophagus with intramural metastases.

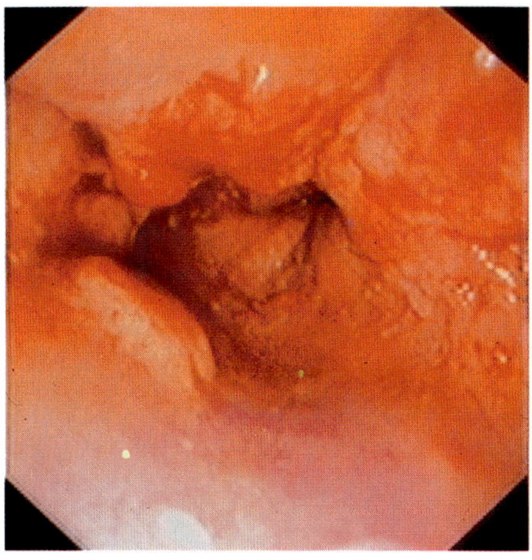

**Figure 9–5.** An adenocarcinoma arising in a Barrett's esophagus.

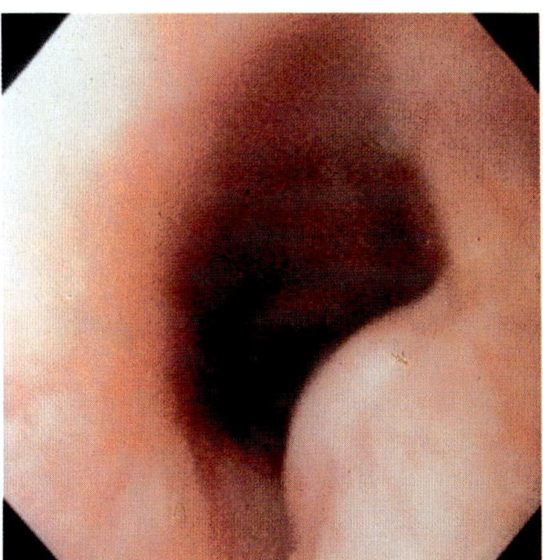

**Figure 9–12.** A leiomyoma of the upper thoracic esophagus.

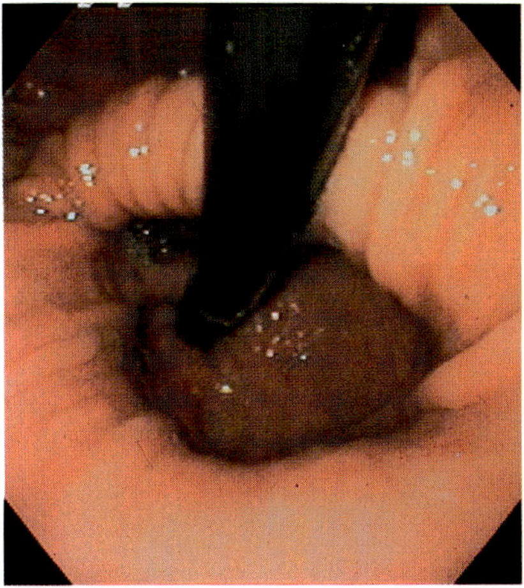

**Figure 9–14.** A retroflexed view from the gastric cardia of a type I hiatal hernia.

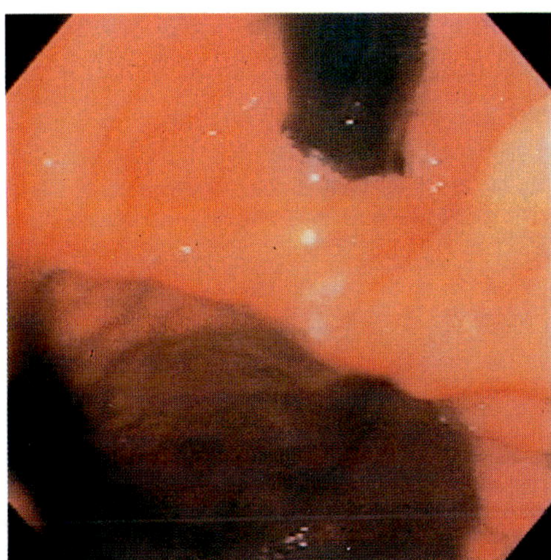

**Figure 9–15.** A retroflexed view from the gastric cardia of a type II hiatal hernia.

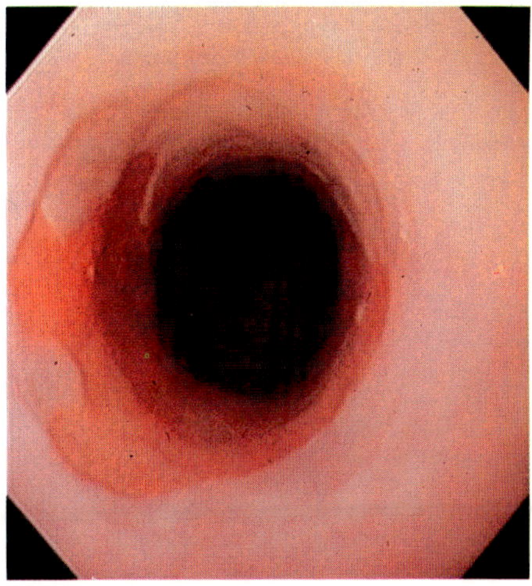

**Figure 9–16.** Barrett's esophagus. The squamocolumnar junction is seen in the midthoracic esophagus.

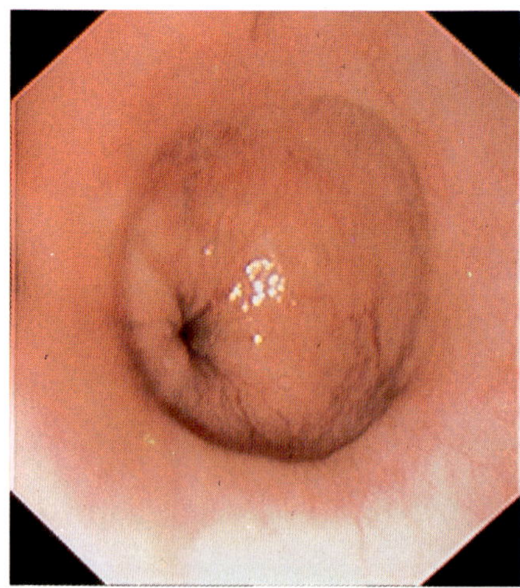

**Figure 9–17.** The lower, dilated esophagus of achalasia

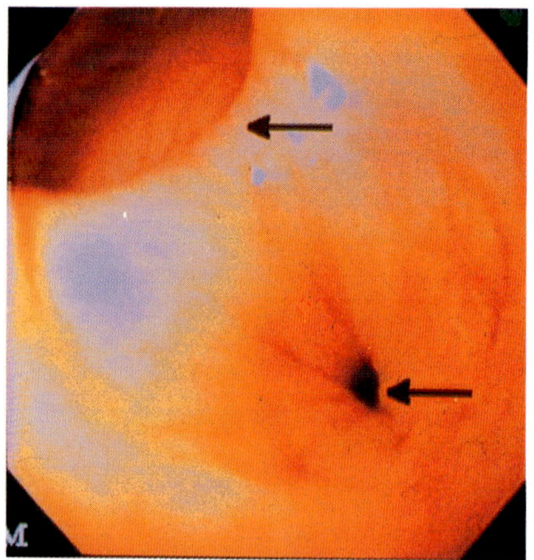

**Figure 9–18.** A epiphrenic diverticulum (upper arrow) and the dilated terminal esophagus of achalasia (lower arrow).

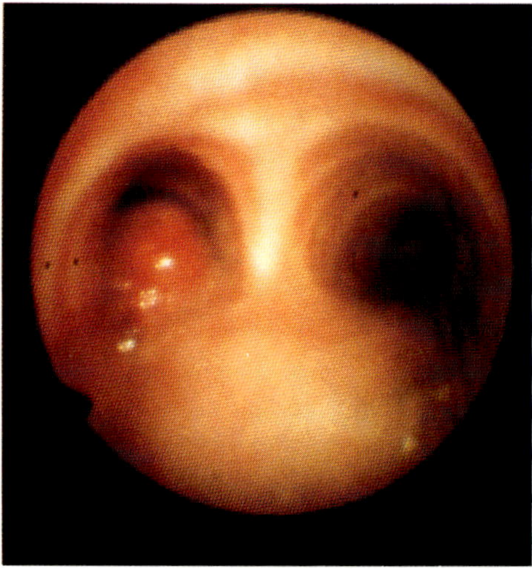

**Figure 21–8A.** *Bronchial carcinoid* (KCC I). Typical tumor in left mainstem bronchus seen by bronchoscopy.

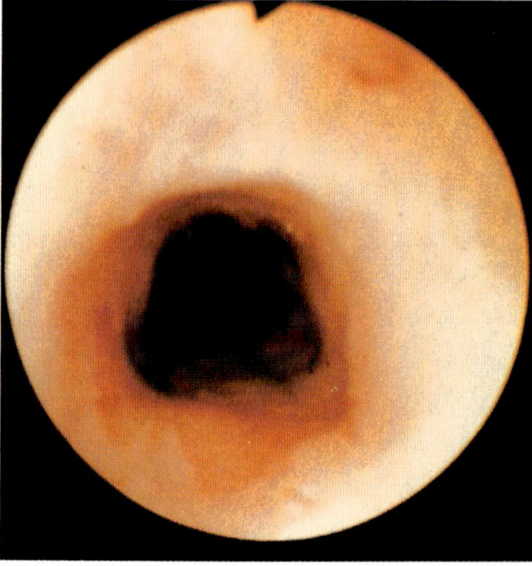

**Figure 43–4.** Barrett's esophagus is identified at endoscopy by an irregular squamocolumnar junction within the tubular esophagus. The columnar mucosa has a feathery red appearance.

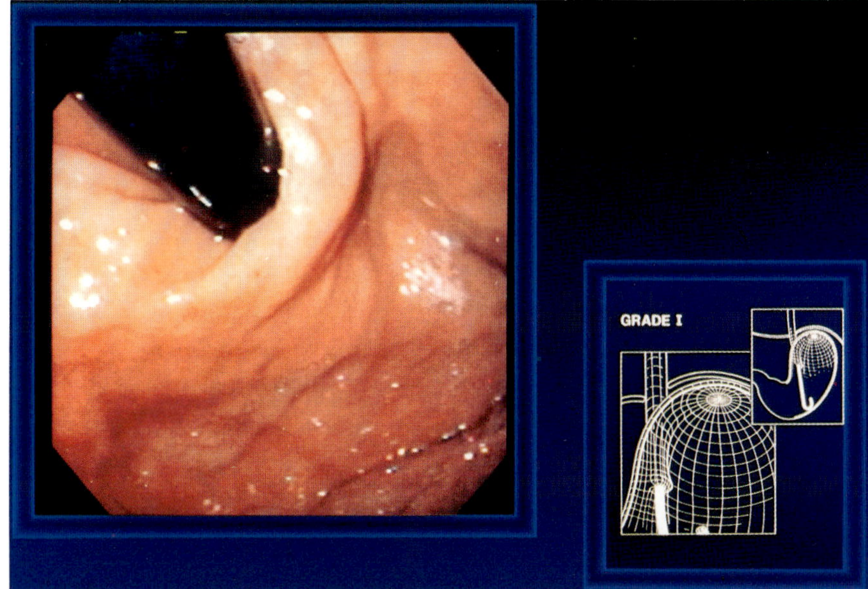


**Figure 45–3.** The grade I GEV is a normal valve. It is a musculomucosal fold that adheres the retroflexed endoscope through all phases of respiration; it opens for swallowing but closes promptly.

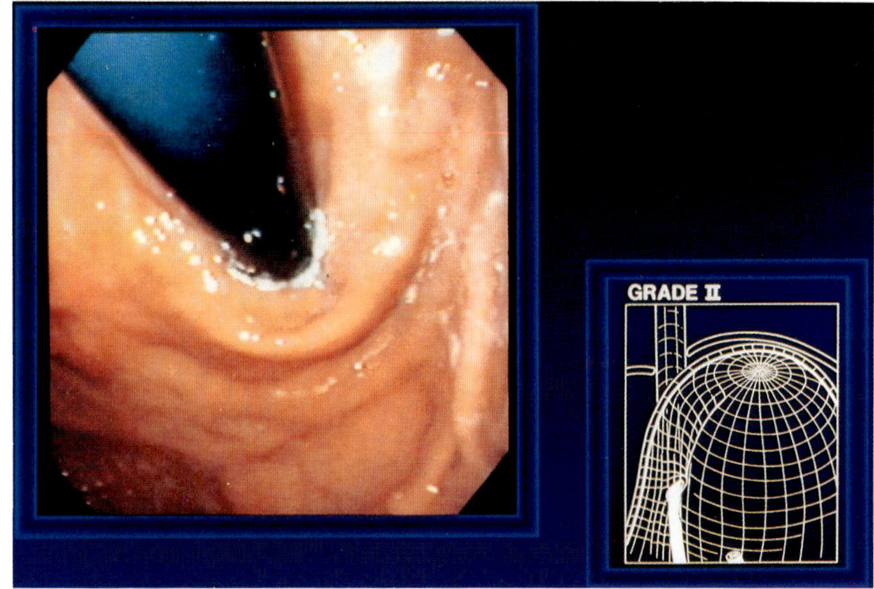


**Figure 45–4.** Grade II GEV, slightly less well defined but still opens for swallowing, closes promptly, and does not allow reflux.

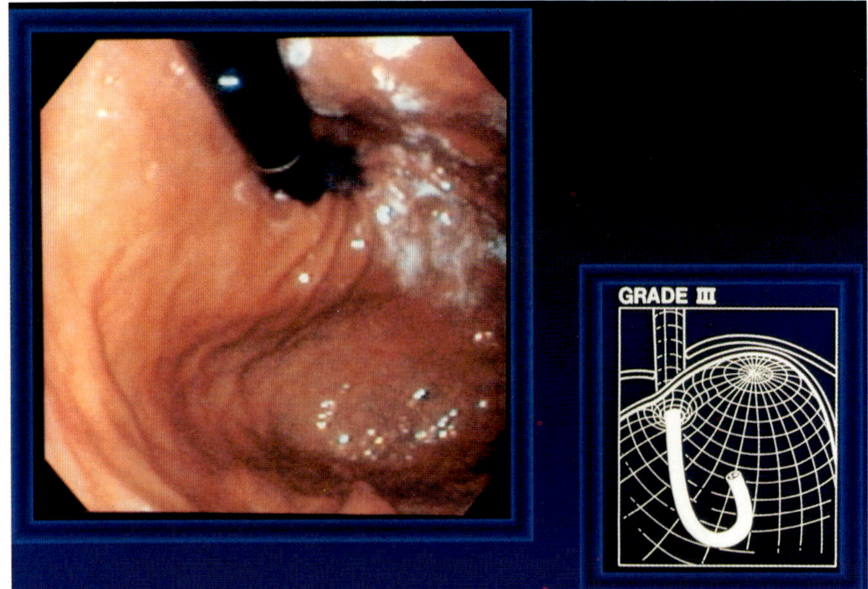


**Figure 45–5.** Grade III valve opens frequently, closes poorly, is poorly defined, and may be associated with a hiatal hernia.

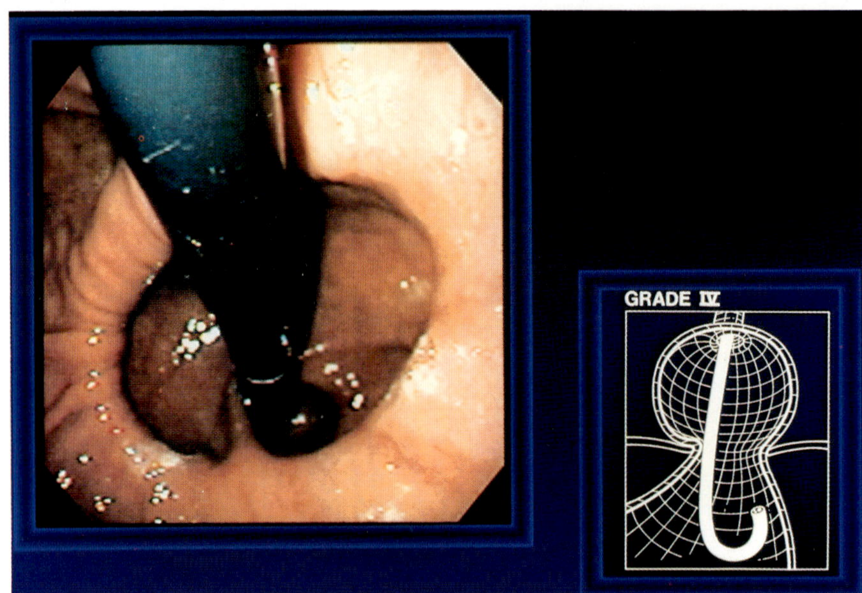


**Figure 45–6.** In patients with a grade IV valve, there is no definable mucosal fold, and the esophagus remains open most of the time it is viewed. A hiatal hernia is invariably present.

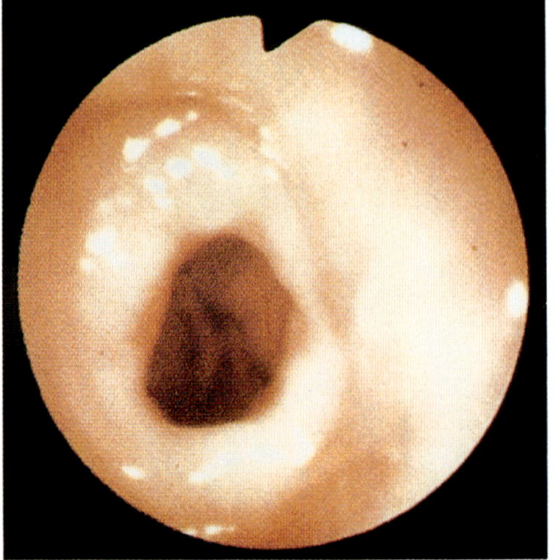

**Figure 47–3.** Endoscopic photograph shows a fibrotic stricture, which represents the end stage of continued reflux and chronic esophagitis.

CHAPTER

35

# The Diaphragm

## *Developmental, Traumatic, and Neoplastic Disorders*

Thomas R. Weber, Thomas F. Tracy, Jr., and Mark L. Silen

### HISTORY

Many early descriptions of congenital and acquired diaphragmatic defects have been appreciated for centuries. In 1579 Ambrose Pare described autopsy findings in two patients suffering sequelae of traumatic diaphragmatic rupture.[1] Before 1700 Bonet[2] described a congenital form of diaphragmatic hernia. Subsequently, Petit further differentiated the congenital from the acquired hernias. Giovanni Morgagni completed his monograph on diaphragmatic hernia in 1769. The typical posterolateral congenital diaphragmatic hernia is most commonly associated with Vincent Bochdalek,[3] who discussed it in 1848, although he was clearly not the first to describe the defect. In 1853 Bowditch[4] first reported the antemortem diagnosis of diaphragmatic rupture in the English literature, and somewhat later, in 1886, Riolfi reduced prolapsed omentum and repaired a diaphragm laceration.[5] Successful treatment of a congenital defect followed shortly thereafter in 1901, when Aue[6] completed closure of a posterolateral left-sided diaphragmatic defect in a 9-year-old boy. It was not until 1946 that Robert Gross[7] reported the first successful correction of a congenital diaphragmatic hernia in a newborn infant. Within a few years his series had grown to 63 children, and the modern era of diaphragmatic surgery had begun.[8]

### EMBRYOLOGY

The development of the diaphragm is a complex process taking place between the fourth and eighth weeks of fetal development. The large central portion of the diaphragm is formed from the septum transversum. This mesodermal tissue between the developing heart and liver fuses ventrally, but it leaves large posterolateral defects known as the pleuroperitoneal canals. These spaces are particularly important to the development of the lungs. Early lung expansion into the surrounding mesenchyme helps to form bilateral folds. By about the seventh week, these fuse with the septum transversum forming bilateral pleuroperitoneal membranes, thus dividing the thoracic and abdominal cavities. Additional myoblasts from cervical segments 3, 4, and 5 then penetrate the membranes and form the muscular part of the diaphragm. The development of the lung cavity also helps define a short mesentery of the esophagus that contributes to the development of the diaphragmatic crura and the most dorsal portion of the diaphragm.[9,10]

The completed diaphragm therefore is a fusion of the following important structures: (1) the septum transversum forming the central tendon; (2) bilateral pleuroperitoneal membranes, which are reinforced by striated muscle components; and (3) the mesentery of the esophagus forming crural and dorsal structures. It is easy to imagine that incomplete or absent fusion of the pleuroperitoneal folds would lead to a posterolateral diaphragm defect. If such a defect is present in the 9th or 10th week, it may be filled with intestinal contents that are returning into the abdomen proper during that stage of development. Further investigation will allow a fuller understanding of this complex process.

## ANATOMY

The diaphragm is a broad musculofascial sheet. The central tendinous portion underlies the pericardium and the medial portions of the lungs. The peripheral muscular portion radiates centrally from the sternum, the ribs, and the lumbar vertebrae. The diaphragm is commonly illustrated in two dimensions, as a curved line; it should more properly be thought of as a dome (Fig. 35–1). The diaphragm moves dramatically, reaching the level of the fifth rib during expiration and flattening at the lower chest margin during full inspiration. The sternal portion of the diaphragm arises as two bands from the back of the xiphoid process. The costal portion is attached to the cartilage and bone of the lower six ribs. The lumbar segment arises as two crura from the arcuate ligament overlying the psoas and quadratus lumborum muscles at the level of the first lumbar vertebra.

There are three major openings in the diaphragm, although one, the aortic hiatus, is technically an opening behind the diaphragm rather than in it (Fig. 35–2). The aorta, the thoracic duct, and often the azygos vein traverse this posterior opening. The musculotendinous crura arising from the lumbar vertebrae define the esophageal hiatus. Generally the right crus splits to encircle the esophagus, although there is sometimes a contribution from the left crus. The opening is located anterior and slightly to the left of the aortic hiatus, while the vena cava foramen is found even more anterior and to the right. This opening in the central tendinous portion of the diaphragm contains the vena cava, major lymphatics, and often branches of the right phrenic nerve. Much smaller openings allow passage of the splanchnic nerves through the crura posteriorly and the internal mammary vessels anteriorly as they become the superior epigastric vessels.

Arteries from many sources nourish the diaphragm. The inferior phrenic arteries, which arise from either the celiac trunk or directly from the aorta, are the main supply to the abdominal side. The superior surface is supplied from the thoracic aorta, internal mammary, and the lower intercostal arteries. The pericardiacophrenic artery accompanies the phrenic nerve and contributes additional blood supply.[11]

The phrenic nerves are the only motor nerves to the diaphragm. They arise from the cervical plexus with contributions from C-3, 4, and 5 and divide at the surface of the diaphragm into three branches: sternal, anterolateral, and posterior. Each nerve ramifies primarily on the abdominal surface of the diaphragm, often in association with branches of the inferior phrenic artery.[12]

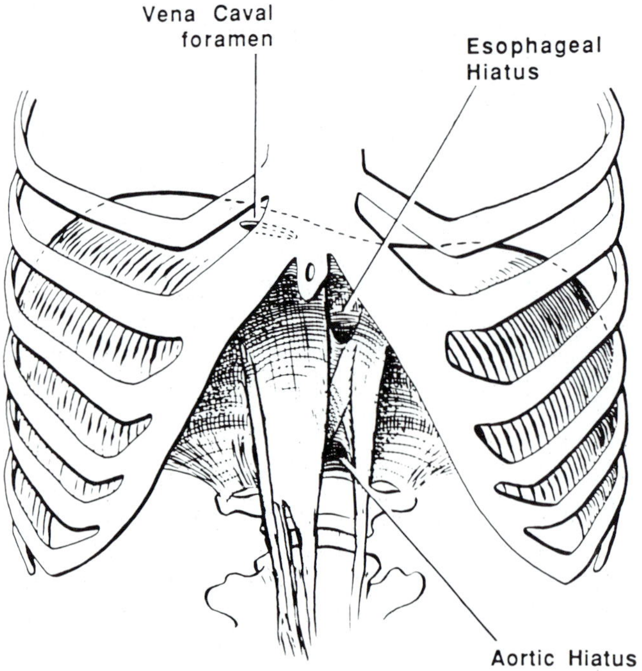

Vena Caval foramen

Esophageal Hiatus

Aortic Hiatus

Figure 35–1. Frontal view of the diaphragm, emphasizing its dome shape. The three major openings are located at slightly different levels.

## DIAPHRAGMATIC HERNIAS

Diaphragmatic hernias include (1) posterolateral hernias of Bochdalek, (2) subcostal anterior hernias of Morgagni, (3) esophageal hernias, and (4) acquired hernias due to diaphragmatic rupture. This chapter will discuss congenital and traumatic hernias. Hiatal hernias will be discussed in Chapters 42 and 48.

## CONGENITAL DIAPHRAGMATIC HERNIA OF BOCHDALEK

Herniation of abdominal contents through a diaphragmatic hernia of Bochdalek occurs in approximately 1 in 4000 live births.[13] The defect, which may vary considerably in size, is posterolateral and affects the left hemi-diaphragm in approximately 85% of cases. Left-sided hernias usually contain the stomach and spleen, small and large intestine, and often the left lobe of the liver. Right-sided hernias often contain the right lobe of the liver as well as portions of small and large intestine. A true hernia sac is present in only about 10% of cases. More commonly, the abdominal contents lie free in the pleural space. The compressed lung on the affected side is always hypoplastic. Few bronchial

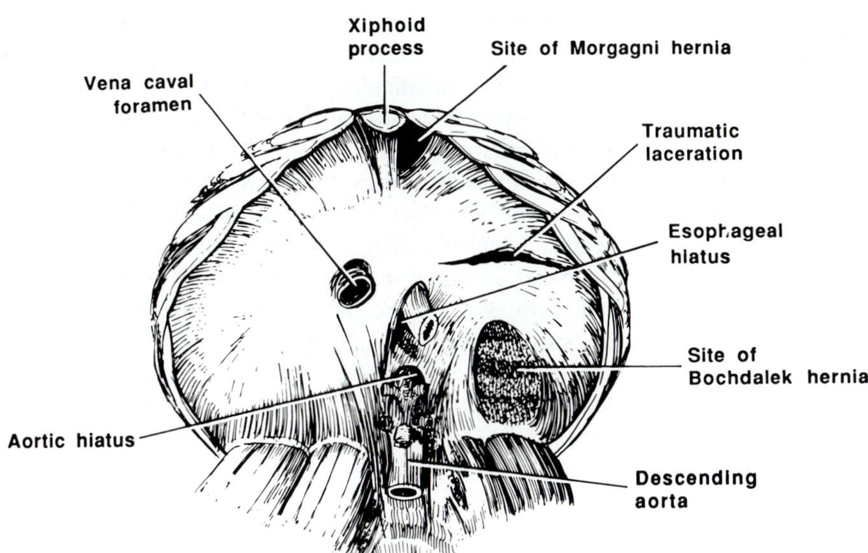


**Figure 35–2.** View of the undersurface of the diaphragm, showing the normal openings. Typical locations of the most common hernias are also depicted.

branches lead to few alveoli, and the pulmonary vasculature is also abnormal.[14,15] The mediastinum shifts away from the hernia, and the crowded contralateral lung is also compromised in its development although to a lesser degree.

Two important elements contribute to the pathophysiology of this condition: (1) inadequate ventilation and (2) pulmonary hypertension. Some babies are born with such severe pulmonary hypoplasia that there is inadequate gas exchange surface in the lungs to support life. Other infants clearly have adequate gas exchange initially, but as they swallow air, the gut in the thorax distends causing increased mediastinal shift and compression of both lungs. In babies with marginal reserve, this sequence of events can be lethal. As important as these factors are, however, it is not pulmonary hypoplasia alone that causes death. Many babies can be adequately ventilated initially but later decompensate with severe hypoxemia. Autopsy studies show unpredictable correlations between lung size and mortality.[16]

Pulmonary hypertension becomes the major life-threatening condition for many babies with congenital diaphragmatic hernias. Because this condition mimics normal fetal circulation, it has been termed *persistent fetal circulation* (PFC). This syndrome may be seen in otherwise normal babies but is commonly associated with diaphragmatic hernia.[17,18] Normal fetal circulation is characterized by pulmonary hypertension with pulmonary arterial blood $PO_2$ of 20 mm of mercury. The complex and dramatic transition to normal physiology after birth is incompletely understood. Changes in arterial and alveolar oxygen tensions and a changing milieu of endogenous vasoactive compounds modulate this transition. Babies with congenital diaphragmatic hernia are often particularly susceptible to the stimuli causing pulmonary hypertension. The most important of these are acidosis and hypoxemia.[19] Changes in cardiac output and the balance between systemic and pulmonary resistance are also important. Severe pulmonary hypertension is marked by right to left shunting through the persistent foramen ovale and the patent ductus arteriosus.[20]

Careful anatomic studies have revealed abnormalities in the muscle of the pulmonary artery walls. Normally, muscle is found in the walls of the branching pulmonary arteries out to the terminal bronchioles. In some infants with diaphragmatic hernia, muscle in the arteries extends throughout the respiratory bronchioles and into the alveoli.[21] This increased distribution as well as increased thickness of the muscle is associated with pulmonary hypertension. When a significant amount of blood is being shunted away from the lungs, a vicious cycle is established. Hypoxemia worsens, and in turn, anaerobic metabolism causes more serious acidosis. These events stimulate increased pulmonary hypertension, and the cycle continues (Fig. 35–3). This spiral of deterioration is highly lethal.

Recent experimental studies[22] have suggested that surfactant deficiency may also be present in newborns with congenital diaphragmatic hernia. These early studies have led to the clinical use of surfactant in these newborns, with encouraging results.[23] Further confirmation of these initial results will hopefully come with a controlled trial.

## Clinical Presentation and Diagnosis

The signs and symptoms of diaphragmatic hernia result from a variable degree of respiratory compromise. Some babies are in severe distress from the time of their first breath while others develop difficulty much later. About three fourths of patients present with some difficulty in the first few hours of life. Dyspnea and tachycardia are common, and cyanosis can also develop. Breath sounds are absent on the affected side. Occasionally bowel sounds can be heard in the thorax. The mediastinum is shifted away from

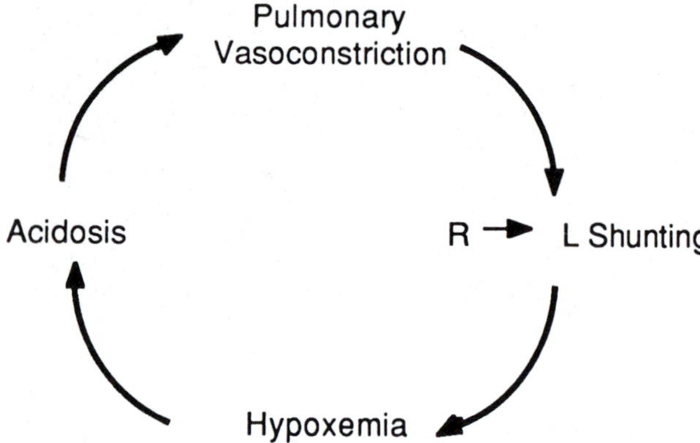


**Figure 35–3.** The vicious circle of pulmonary hypertension. Hypercarbia may also contribute to acidosis, further fueling this dangerous cycle.

the defect causing tracheal deviation and lateral displacement of the heart impulse. The abdomen is almost always strikingly scaphoid.

The diagnosis is generally confirmed by a chest x-ray, which characteristically shows abdominal contents in the chest with mediastinal deviation away from the affected side (Figs. 35–4, 35–5). The differential diagnosis includes congenital cystic adenomatoid malformation, other cystic diseases of the lung, eventration of the diaphragm, and *Staphylococcal* pneumonia with pneumatocele formation in older patients. Simple passage of a gastric tube will often confirm the stomach's location in the chest. Ultrasound or contrast studies of the gastrointestinal tract are rarely necessary. Routine ultrasound during pregnancy has allowed diagnosis of this condition prenatally.[24] Occasionally, the diagnosis is not made until the child is several weeks, months, or even years of age (Fig. 35–6). These patients may present with a variety of respiratory symptoms. Sometimes the presentation is that of a bowel obstruction, when the intestinal tract, often the colon, becomes obstructed in the chest.

Other serious anomalies may coexist with diaphragmatic hernias. All of the babies have pulmonary hypoplasia and intestinal malrotation. Congenital heart disease, central nervous system abnormalities, and other serious lesions including trisomy 13 and 18 are seen with increased frequency.[25,26]

### Preoperative Risk Factors

Babies with congenital diaphragmatic hernia generally fall into three groups. Those in the first group present late or with very mild symptoms. They are not likely to develop pulmonary hypertension and have a very high survival rate. A second group presents with advanced pulmonary failure at birth. These babies have severe bilateral pulmonary hypoplasia and refractory pulmonary hypertension. Despite vigorous therapy, these patients do not survive. An intermediate group presents with significant distress, but their underlying condition still offers a chance for survival.

If these groups could be accurately identified, appropriate therapy could be tailored to each group's needs. Although several factors are known to be associated with in-

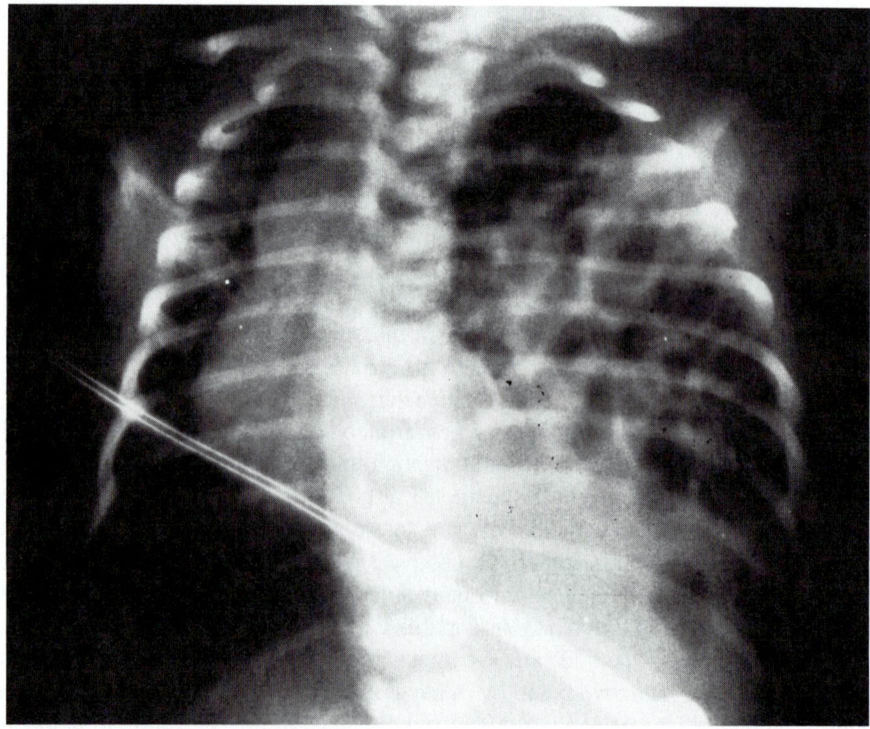

**Figure 35–4.** Initial film of a newborn in respiratory distress, prior to endotracheal intubation. The left hemithorax is filled with a bowel gas pattern. Mediastinal structures are deviated well to the right. Tracheal deviation is an important sign to identify on initial radiographs.

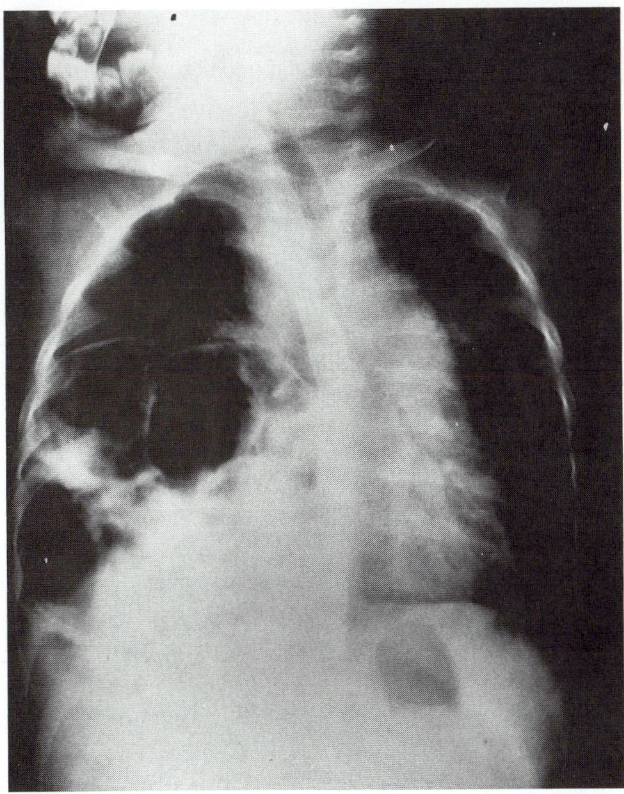

**Figure 35–5.** Right-sided Bochdalek hernia containing liver and some bowel. Often right-sided hernias contain less bowel than left-sided defects.

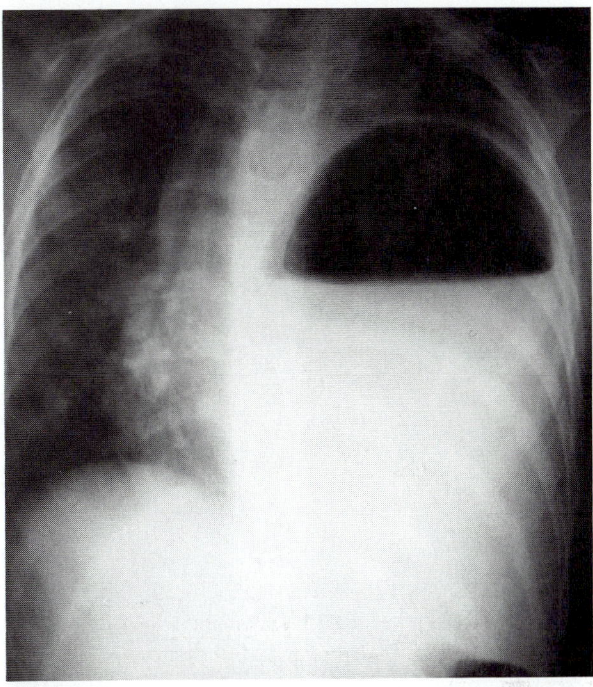

**Figure 35–6.** This 3-year-old presented with the acute onset of respiratory distress. She had been well previously. A left-sided Bochdalek hernia was suspected; at operation the stomach and spleen were reduced from the chest and the posterolateral defect closed.

creased mortality, there continues to be some overlap among these three groups. It has been difficult therefore, to adopt new treatment strategies on the basis of these predictive factors.

Arterial blood gas determinations have been important in predicting mortality. The pH and $P_{CO_2}$ have each been helpful. In Mishalany's series, an admission pH of greater than 7.2 predicted 100% survival, but only 11% survived if the pH was <7.0.[27] This acid-base alteration was mostly due to $CO_2$ retention. Boix-Ochoa's early experience showed uniform survival when the $P_{CO_2}$ could be normalized with mechanical ventilation. Babies who remained hypercarbic died.[28] A more recent study showed a 100% survival in infants with a $P_{CO_2}$ <35 mm of mercury compared with only 33% survival when the $P_{CO_2}$ was >50 mm of mercury.[29] It is even more useful to look at these parameters when correlated with a measure of the patient's ventilation. Babies clearly have more severe respiratory failure when very high ventilator settings are required to lower the $P_{CO_2}$. Bohn has suggested using the ventilatory index (mean airway pressure × respiratory rate) to further quantify this situation. Babies with the highest risk required a ventilatory index >1000 to normalize the $P_{CO_2}$. He documented a 100% survival in 15 babies achieving preoperative preductal $P_{CO_2}$ <40 with ventilatory indices <1000. When higher ventilatory parameters had to be used, only 22% of 28 babies survived.[30]

Various measures of oxygenation have also shown correlation with survival. One such measure is the alveolar-arterial oxygen difference ($A\text{-}aDO_2$). With the infant breathing 100% oxygen, and if one assumes the respiratory quotient is equal to one, the sea level $A\text{-}a\ DO_2 = 740 - PaO_2 - PaCO_2 - 47$. Although no absolute criteria have been established to differentiate survivors from nonsurvivors, most survivors have A-a $DO_2$'s significantly less than 300, while nonsurvivors generally exhibit values of 300 to over 600.[30]

## Preoperative Care

Once the diagnosis of congenital diaphragmatic hernia is established, a nasogastric tube should be placed to minimize the accumulation of gas in the bowel. If assisted ventilation is needed, the baby should have endotracheal intubation, since mask ventilation contributes to gaseous distention of the bowel. Monitoring of arterial blood gases is essential. Insertion of an umbilical artery line allows monitoring of postductal arterial blood gases (Fig. 35–7). Preductal blood gas determinations through a right radial artery line are recommended. The use of IV pulmonary

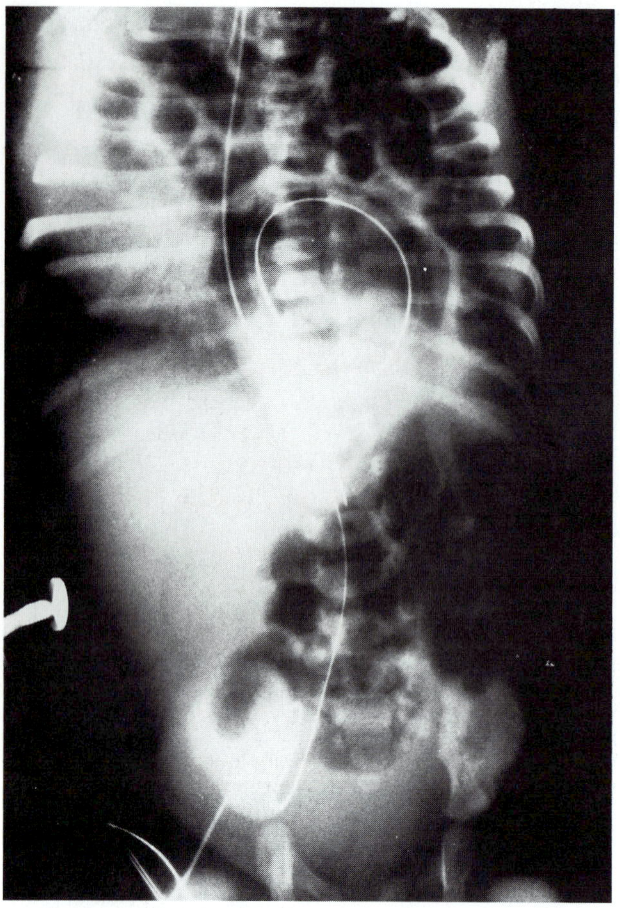

**Figure 35–7.** A catheter has been introduced through the right umbilical artery and advanced into the aorta. The ideal location of the catheter tip is between vertebrae L3 and L4. The diagnosis of a congenital diaphragmatic hernia is easily confirmed by the coiled nasogastric tube in the left chest. Bowel contents have herniated well across the midline to the right of the trachea. The scaphoid nature of the abdomen is evident.

vasodilators preoperatively has enjoyed only variable success.[31,32] Hyperventilation is desirable to prevent hypercarbia and acidosis, both of which stimulate pulmonary hypertension. Although not always successful, ventilatory rates in excess of 100/min may be necessary. Infants should be ventilated on 100% oxygen initially, and sedated and paralyzed if necessary. These patients are at risk of pneumothorax, a grave complication that must be quickly diagnosed and treated if clinical deterioration occurs. Until recently, most felt that the period of initial resuscitation should be short and that the infant should be prepared for operation with dispatch. Recent studies suggest that pulmonary function, rather than improving, actually deteriorates for several hours following operation.[33] This has led to interest in initial nonsurgical treatment of certain infants. Such preoperative stabilization might include the use of extracorporeal membrane oxygenation (ECMO—described later).[34]

## Operative Repair

Intraoperative monitoring should include an arterial line and continuous oximetry as well as the capability to measure endtidal $Co_2$. A subcostal incision gives excellent exposure, and the herniated viscera can usually be easily withdrawn from the pleural cavity. When a hernia sac is present, it should be excised and the ipsilateral lung inspected. This lung is generally quite hypoplastic, appearing as a "nubbin" in the upper thorax, and no attempt should be made to inflate it. The posterior and medial extent of the defect is quite variable. Frequently, the posterior peritoneum cephalad to the adrenal must be incised to identify the diaphragm remnant. Often a significant segment of muscle can be unrolled in this location. An ipsilateral chest tube is placed under direct vision, and the defect is then closed using interrupted 3-0 nonabsorbable horizontal mattress sutures. When no posterior rim is present, sutures can be placed around the ribs posteriorly. Very large defects may be impossible to close primarily. A variety of prosthetics have been suggested including Marlex and Silastic. We presently prefer a patch of Gortex for this closure, having used it successfully in numerous infants who survived with the help of pre- and postoperative ECMO.

Following repair, the abdomen is thoroughly but quickly examined. No attempt is made to correct malrotation. The abdominal wall is stretched manually to accommodate the intestinal contents. Usually all layers of the abdomen can be closed, but if it is determined that a tight closure will compromise the bowel or respiratory excursion, only the skin is closed. The resulting ventral hernia can be repaired later. A transthoracic repair has been advocated by some, and it is especially useful for right-sided hernias. Others prefer the abdominal approach for both right and left hernias.

## Postoperative Care

Successful postoperative care centers around the avoidance of, and treatment of, pulmonary hypertension. These infants are extremely precarious in the first few days of life. Often an initial 4–12-hour period of postoperative stability, the so-called honeymoon period,[35] is followed by clinical deterioration marked by increasing pulmonary hypertension. Certain protective measures are available that may modify or prevent this sequence.

Continuous monitoring is extremely important (Fig. 35–8). Transcutaneous monitoring of $Po_2$ and $Pco_2$ provides an easy means to detect early hypercarbia or hypoxemia. Oximetry may be used to follow oxygen saturations. The initial $Po_2$ should be kept above 100 mm Hg. Meticulous attention to ventilation is paramount. Hyperventilation should be used as necessary to maintain the $Pco_2$ below 40 mm Hg. Any degree of metabolic acidosis should be vigorously treated. Special attention must be paid to all chest tubes. The tube on the ipsilateral side is generally placed to

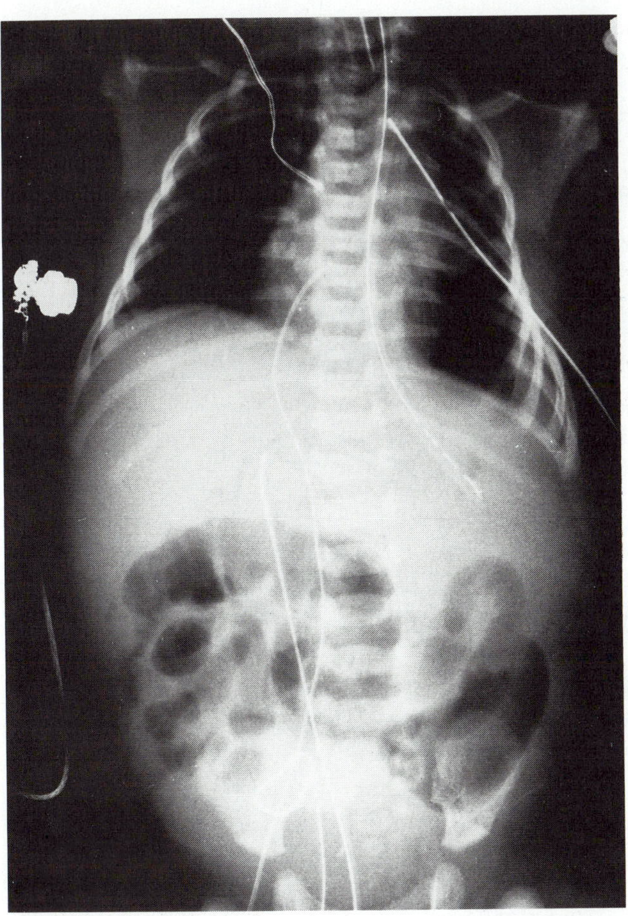

**Figure 35–8.** Umbilical vessel cannulation may not be completely satisfactory for monitoring purposes. This baby has had repair of a left-sided Bochdalek hernia. The umbilical artery catheter has not advanced well into the aorta. Arterial spasm around the catheter may not allow reliable arterial sampling. The umbilical venous line is lodged in the intrahepatic portal system; it cannot be advanced into the atrium, and it should not be used for infusion of hypertonic solutions or inotropic agents. A right atrial line for central venous pressure monitoring has subsequently been introduced through the right greater saphenous vein at the groin.

underwater seal only, but several centimeters of suction may be necessary to avoid rapid shifts of the mediastinum that might cause hyperexpansion or compression of either lung. Contralateral pneumothorax is such a highly lethal complication that consideration should be given to placing a contralateral chest tube prophylactically when high-pressure ventilation is being used. Weaning from the ventilator should be done very slowly and carefully during the first few postoperative days. Muscle paralysis is important for full control of ventilation.

A variety of IV vasodilators have been used to abort or reverse pulmonary hypertension. Initial enthusiasm for this seemingly attractive therapy has waned. The usefulness of any single agent has been unpredictable. Unfortunately, no one agent has been found that acts specifically on the pulmonary vasculature. Available drugs simultaneously lower systemic vascular resistance, and at times these effects may predominate and actually worsen right-to-left shunting. In addition, these agents are less effective in the face of acidosis and hypoxemia. The many IV agents that have been used to treat pulmonary hypertension include tolazoline, isoproterenol, chlorpromazine, nitroglycerine, nitroprusside, and acetylcholine. Of these, tolazoline has been the most widely used. Since this drug has a potent effect on the systemic circulation as well, volume resuscitation is often necessary prior to its use. Frequently, concurrent use of an inotropic agent, either dopamine or dobutamine, is required to prevent systemic hypotension. Tolazoline is usually begun as a bolus of 1–2 mg/kg IV and followed with a drip of 1–2 mg/kg/h.[36,37] Cardiac output must be maximized. Central venous pressure monitoring can be helpful in guiding volume infusion. Noninvasive estimates of cardiac output have also proved useful.

The use of inhaled nitric oxide in newborns with pulmonary hypertension has received enthusiastic support, following initial promising reports.[38] Although the use of this agent in newborns with diaphragmatic hernias is somewhat limited, it appears that nitric oxide is a potent pulmonary vasodilator with little systemic response when used as an inhaled agent. However, dose, frequency of administration, and safety and efficacy of long-term use remain important questions to be resolved with future studies.

Despite the most diligent therapy, severe pulmonary hypertension may persist. Until recently, these infants all died. Attempts to salvage such desperately ill babies have included two new modalities: high-frequency ventilation (HFV) and extracorporeal membrane oxygenation (ECMO). High-frequency ventilation is a ventilator technique using very high ventilatory frequencies. Rates from 200 to 2000 cycles/min have been used. Gas transport results from augmented diffusion rather than the bulk flow of gases. It is particularly useful in lowering $PCO_2$ values, and generally the mean airway pressure can be lowered as well. These effects are attractive in patients with pulmonary hypoplasia and pulmonary hypertension since $CO_2$ retention is common, and high ventilator pressures exacerbate pulmonary hypertension. Thus far, HFV has been used infrequently and with little success in congenital diaphragmatic hernia; however, as experience grows it may prove useful.[39]

Extracorporeal membrane oxygenation is becoming a standard adjunct in the care of selected neonates with congenital diaphragmatic hernia. ECMO can immediately reverse the effects of pulmonary hypertension. Acidosis and hypoxemia, the most potent stimuli for continued pulmonary hypertension, are easily treated. In addition, ECMO allows marked reduction of airway pressures and inspired oxygen concentrations, both of which are detrimental to the delicate neonatal lung. The cardiac support supplied by partial bypass may also be useful. Arteriovenous or veno-venous technique is used with cannulation through the common carotid artery and/or the internal jugular vein in the neck (Figs. 35–9, 35–10).

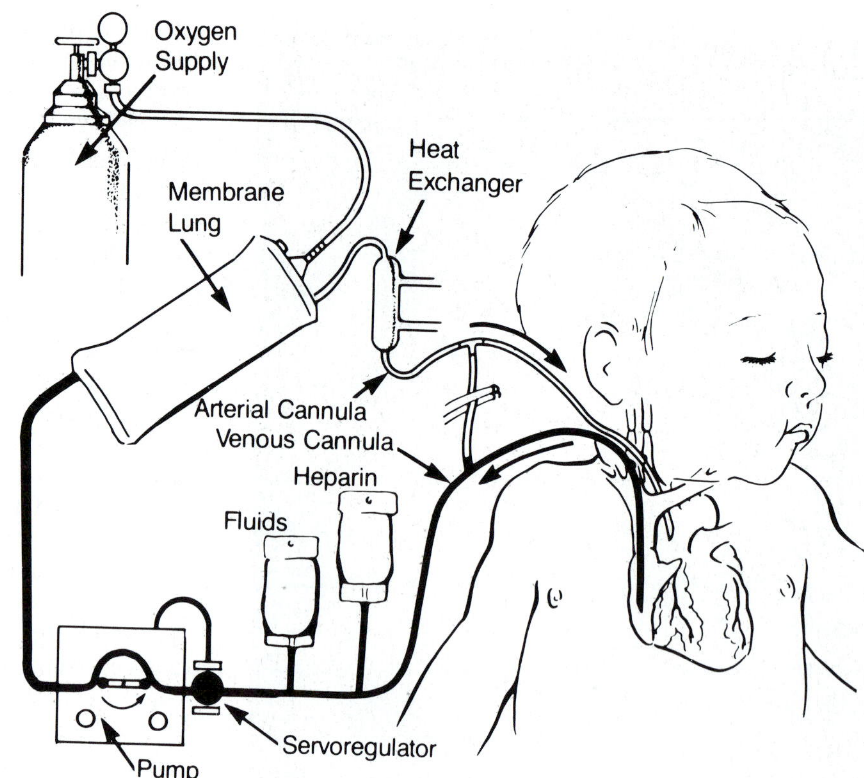


**Figure 35–9.** Extracorporeal membrane oxygenation (ECMO). The basic elements of the ECMO circuit are depicted. The common carotid artery and internal jugular vein are cannulated by using local anesthesia and muscle paralysis.

A report from the neonatal ECMO central registry describes the outcome of 93 infants with congenital diaphragmatic hernia requiring ECMO. This group of patients deteriorated postoperatively, and all were expected to die. Fifty-eight percent survived ECMO and were discharged.[40] This appears to be a significant advance in the treatment of these babies, although the experience of individual centers has been varied. Some series have been disappointing,[41] while others have shown increased overall survival.[42,43] Indications for the use of ECMO are still under discussion. Some centers require that a baby must have had a $Po_2$ of >100 at some time during his life to be eligible for the therapy. Others have used ECMO in all babies failing conventional therapy and have some survivors even from very high-risk groups. More information on patients' selection factors will be forthcoming as centers using different criteria accumulate more experience.

## Results

Most series of diaphragmatic hernia infants who require ventilation within the first day of life report an overall survival of about 50%. When one is comparing results from various groups, it is important to examine differences in patient populations. Infants who develop no early respiratory distress rarely die from this disease. Clearly a series treating a higher percentage of babies in distress within the first few hours would be expected to have fewer survivors. Some series report recent survival of 75–80%.[43,44,45]

Congenital diaphragmatic hernia is still a highly lethal condition. The true mortality in unselected patients appears to be approximately 80%. This was suggested by a study using prenatal ultrasound[46] and confirmed recently by an autopsy study from a single hospital.[47] As many as one third of these babies are stillborn. Virtually all of the stillborn babies have lethal associated nonpulmonary anomalies, as do a significant percentage of those live-born. There is presently no hope for improving mortality in these groups. Progress must come by salvaging the very difficult babies with marginal lung volumes and pulmonary hypertension.

Recently, in utero repair of diaphragmatic hernia has been attempted, with limited success.[48] These technical accomplishments, thus far attempted at only one maternal-fetal center, have demonstrated that repair can be completed and the fetus allowed to further grow and develop in utero. Persistent questions regarding appropriate timing, patient selection, maternal safety and management of complications, and operative refinements have limited the enthusiasm and applicability of this approach. Whether this becomes standard therapy in the future for selected cases of diaphragmatic hernia remains to be seen.

It is noteworthy and encouraging that babies who survive the neonatal period do quite well. They continue to grow more alveoli for about the first 7 years of life. Subtle changes may persist on pulmonary function testing, but the children have good exercise tolerance and lead essentially normal lives.[49,50]

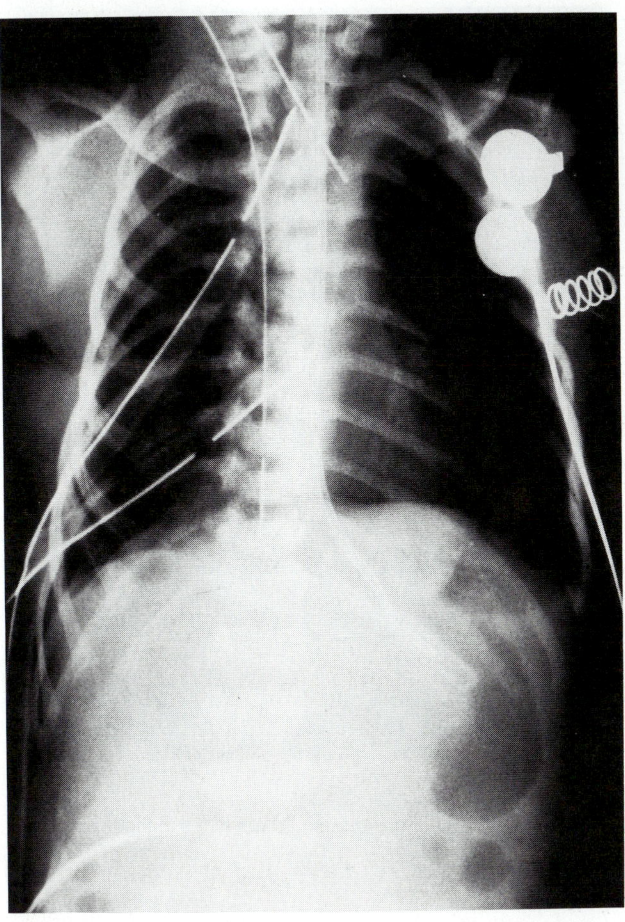

**Figure 35–10.** Repair of this right-sided Bochdalek hernia was followed by a brief "honeymoon period." In the face of severe pulmonary hypertension and progressive hypoxemia, the baby was placed on ECMO. The two ECMO cannulae can be seen entering through the neck. The arterial catheter is positioned into the aortic arch and the venous cannula is advanced well into the right atrium. This boy's pulmonary hypertension resolved, and he was successfully weaned from ECMO and from the ventilator.

## FORAMEN OF MORGAGNI HERNIA

Herniation through the substernal foramen of Morgagni can occur at three sites. Two short muscular bands extend from the anterior central diaphragm tendon to the posterior xiphoid process, and a potential space exists between them. Just lateral to these bands are triangular openings in the diaphragm that enclose the superior epigastric arteries and veins, and lymphatics. These spaces also contain fat and areolar tissue, and they are potential points of herniation as well because of their lack of rigidity.

Herniation of viscera (colon, stomach, small bowel) occurs most commonly toward the right side but occasionally can lie directly behind the sternum or even into the pericardium. A peritoneal sac is virtually always present and should be excised during the repair. The symptoms of Morgagni hernia vary from none to feelings of mild to moderate substernal pressure or pain, or severe pain if incarceration or strangulation occur. Hematemesis may develop from mucosal venous congestion if the stomach is contained in the hernia.

The diagnosis of Morgagni hernia is suggested by plain chest x-ray, showing an enlarged cardiac silhouette or an air-fluid level. Barium contrast studies can confirm the presence of stomach or colon within the hernia. Peritoneography can also be used to make the diagnosis (Fig. 35–11).

These defects are most easily repaired through an abdominal approach. An upper midline incision allows reduction of the viscera, excision of the peritoneal sac, and repair of the defect. Frequently repair requires suturing of the tendinous portion of the diaphragm to the underside of the sternum. Large defects should be closed with a prosthetic patch to avoid phrenic nerve entrapment from widely placed sutures. Recurrence is extremely unusual in these cases.[51]

## TRAUMATIC HERNIA

Traumatic diaphragmatic hernias can be produced by penetrating or blunt thoracoabdominal trauma. This diagnosis needs to be entertained in any severe trauma of the lower chest or upper abdomen. The condition is frequently overlooked, leading to pulmonary problems or the formation of a chronic hernia. Associated injuries are very common[52] and may distract the surgeon from careful examination of the diaphragm.

Diaphragm rupture in blunt trauma is uncommon. Usually a burst-type injury causes radial lacerations of the central tendon of the diaphragm. Approximately 80–90% occur in the left hemi-diaphragm, since the liver provides the right hemi-diaphragm with an element of protection from direct forces.[53] The incidence of diaphragmatic ruptures with blunt trauma is generally considered to be 1–3%.

The path of any projectile or stab wound in the area of the diaphragm must be followed carefully. Since the diaphragm is dome-shaped, it may be injured in more than one place by a single penetration. Any wound between the fourth intercostal space and the umbilicus may potentially injure the diaphragm. Right-sided lacerations may be missed because of tamponade by the underlying liver.[55]

Symptoms are due primarily to associated injuries. The diaphragmatic rupture itself may cause a degree of respiratory distress as the hemithorax accumulates effusion or is compromised with bowel contents. Sometimes mediastinal shift will be significant. If a herniated viscus sustains concomitant injury, intestinal spillage may occur in the pleural space.

The diagnosis is usually suggested by chest x-ray. The stomach is often seen in an abnormally high position, and sometimes other hollow organs are noted in the chest. The course of the nasogastric tube may be seen entering the left chest, confirming the diagnosis. If there is no immediate visceral herniation, the diagnosis may be missed (Fig.

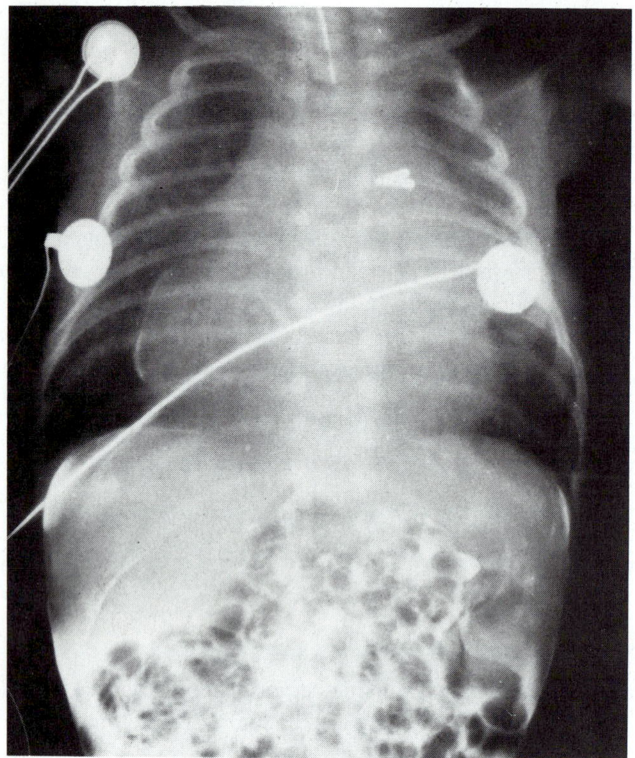


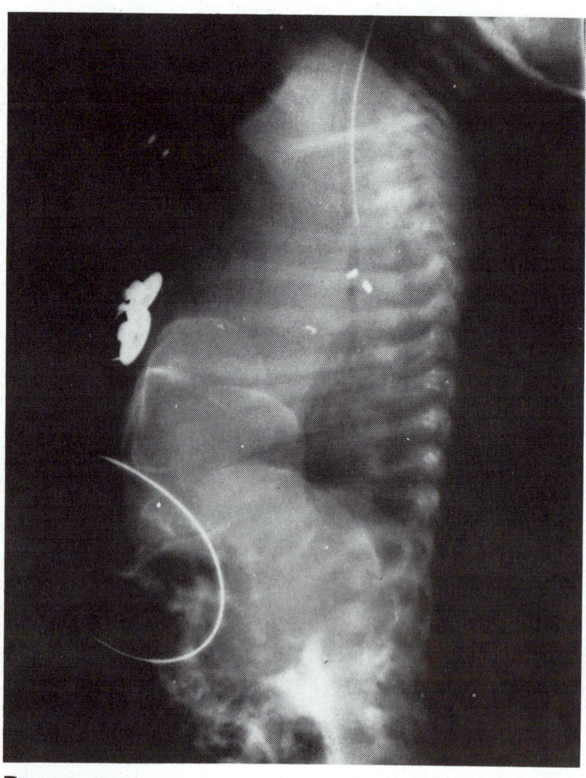


**Figure 35–11. A.** Contrast peritoneogram outlining a right-sided Morgagni hernia. **B.** Lateral x-ray showing bowel loops in the anterior hernia sac.

35–12). Subsequent herniation and effusion formation will often cause respiratory distress. Traumatic hernias are frequently misdiagnosed as loculated hemopneumothorax leading to the erroneous use of chest tubes. Sonography may also contribute to the diagnosis of traumatic diaphragmatic hernia. Barium studies of the intestine or colon are often helpful in diagnosis of chronic hernias.

If the defect is recognized acutely, repair should be undertaken. Abdominal exploration usually offers the best exposure. Associated injuries can be recognized and repaired, and the diaphragmatic defect can be exposed adequately. A single-layer closure of interrupted nonabsorbable sutures has been used successfully. Some surgeons prefer a two-layer closure. A chest tube should be placed for temporary drainage.

Chronic hernias can be managed electively, unless they present with signs of acute intestinal obstruction. Often the colon or a portion of the stomach is herniated into the chest. After proper preparation, these can be approached either transabdominally or transthoracically. The thoracic approach allows better access to multiple adhesions that often involve the intestine and the pulmonary parenchyma. Primary repair of the diaphragm is usually possible, but prosthetic patches can be employed when necessary. There should be a very small incidence of recurrent herniation following repair. The mortality associated with diaphragmatic injury is often quoted as 10–15%. This is largely due to associated injuries but is occasionally a consequence of complications from a missed diagnosis.

## Eventration

The term *diaphragmatic eventration* is most often used to describe elevation of part or all of the hemidiaphragm. Some authors restrict the term to congenital abnormalities of the diaphragm not associated with phrenic nerve paralysis. More commonly, however, the term encompasses both congenital and acquired abnormalities that result in marked weakness and elevation of a portion of diaphragm. The acquired condition results from unilateral phrenic nerve paralysis. The most common causes are birth trauma, injury during cervical or thoracic operations, invasion by tumors, or some pleural or pulmonary infections. The congenital form exhibits marked thinning of the diaphragm with poor or absent muscle development between the pleura and peritoneum. Migration of abdominal contents into the thorax interferes with lung development in a less pronounced but similar manner to a congenital diaphragmatic hernia. Differentiating an eventration from a Bochdalek hernia with an intact sac may be difficult.

Most small eventrations are asymptomatic. Infants are more likely to be symptomatic from an eventration than older children, and sometimes they will exhibit marked respiratory insufficiency. The diaphragm will often move in a

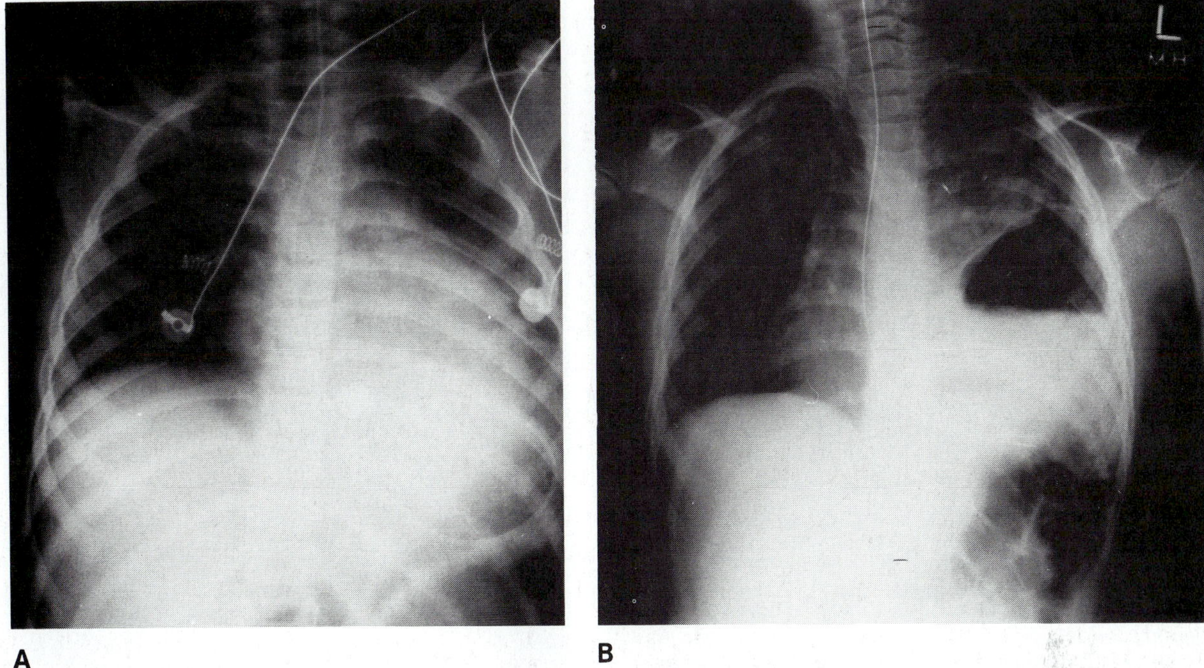


**Figure 35–12.** Traumatic diaphragmatic rupture: This 5-year-old was involved in an automobile accident. **A.** Initial x-ray shows a small amount of haziness at the left base. No rib fractures were identified. The nasogastric tube can be seen coiled in the normal position. The patient initially did well but 2 days later was noted to have decreased breath sounds on the left. **B.** Repeat x-ray clearly shows herniation of the stomach into the left chest. Abdominal exploration revealed a sizable diaphragmatic laceration. Reduction of the herniated stomach and spleen and laceration closure was followed by an uneventful recovery.

paradoxical fashion, especially when the eventration is due to phrenic nerve paralysis. Since the baby's mediastinum is very mobile, it may exhibit a to-and-fro flutter that severely inhibits gas exchange. Sometimes the only symptoms are wheezing or dyspnea on exertion. Gastrointestinal symptoms such as postprandial fullness and dysphagia have been described and are probably related to the abnormal position of the stomach and esophagus under a left eventration.

The diagnosis of eventration of the diaphragm can usually be made by examining PA and lateral chest x-rays (Figs. 35–13, 35–14). Fluoroscopy can document abnormal or paradoxical movement of the hemidiaphragm. Ultrasonography can give similar information and also identify the location of solid organs such as the liver, which typically bulge up under a right-sided eventration. It will help differentiate the condition from subpulmonic pleural conditions or primary hepatic abnormalities.

Small asymptomatic eventrations require no treatment. Operative plication of the eventration should be performed if the patient is symptomatic. A very large eventration should also be plicated even if the patient is asymptomatic. This is especially true in infants, since the abnormal position of the diaphragm will further compromise future lung development.

The eventration is generally best approached through the sixth or seventh interspace. Several nonabsorbable sutures are used to plicate the flaccid diaphragm from anterior to posterior, with careful avoidance of the phrenic nerve branches. The plication should return the diaphragm to its normal position. Since many of these defects exhibit a thin membrane anteriorly with better diaphragmatic muscle posteriorly, the muscle can be brought forward and fixed to the costal margin with permanent sutures. In such circumstances, the thinned-out diaphragm need not be excised. An abdominal approach has been suggested especially for bilateral eventrations, but separate thoracotomies performed a few weeks apart are favored by most.

Significant improvement in respiratory function is usually seen immediately, particularly in infants.[57] Older subjects with long-standing eventration may show less improvement in pulmonary function following repair.[58]

## Tumors of the Diaphragm

Primary tumors of the diaphragm are exceedingly rare. Benign lesions are somewhat more common than malignant tumors. Simple cysts have been described as well as lipomas, fibromas, and neurogenic tumors.[59] Malignant tumors of the diaphragm include fibrosarcoma and rare vascular or muscular sarcomas. Most commonly, the diaphragm is invaded secondarily by a malignant tumor from surrounding structures. Benign neoplasms are usually asymptomatic; they are frequently discovered incidentally on chest x-ray. Invasive malignancies often exhibit symptoms related to their primary organ of origin. While plain x-rays may be

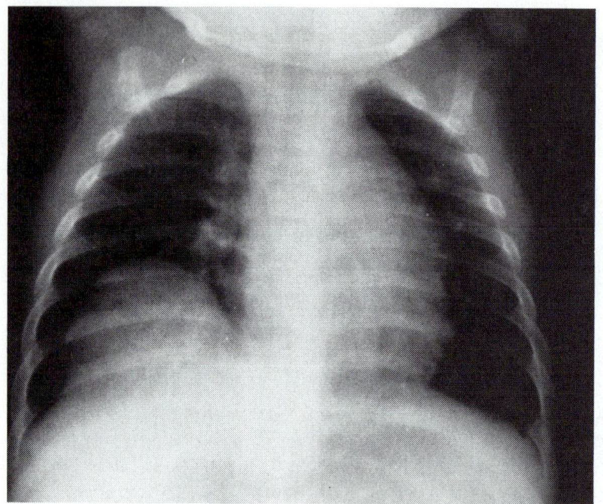

A

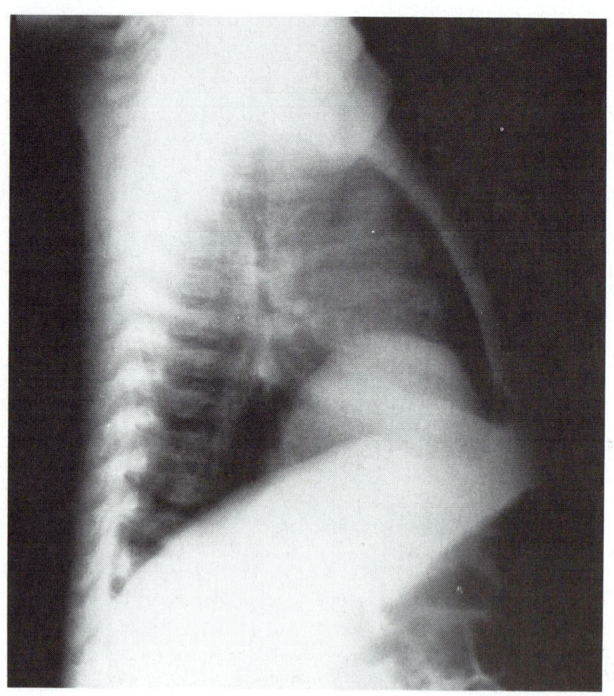

B

**Figure 35–13. A,B.** X-rays showing a sizable eventration of the diaphragm in a 2-month-old boy. He was minimally symptomatic. As is often the case, the anterior portion of the diaphragm is affected.

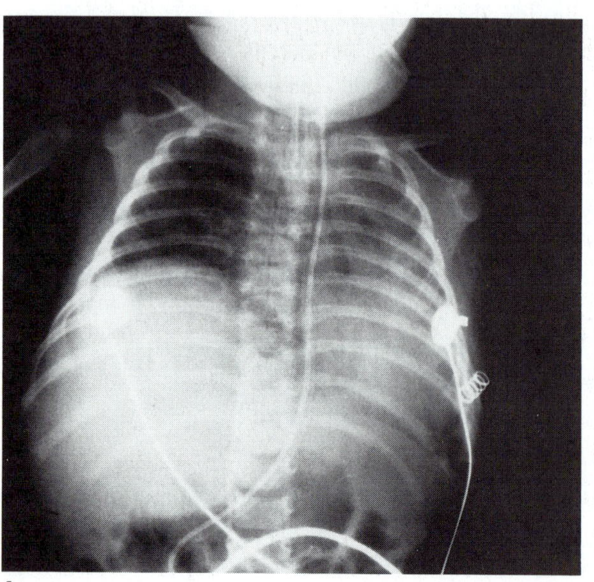

A

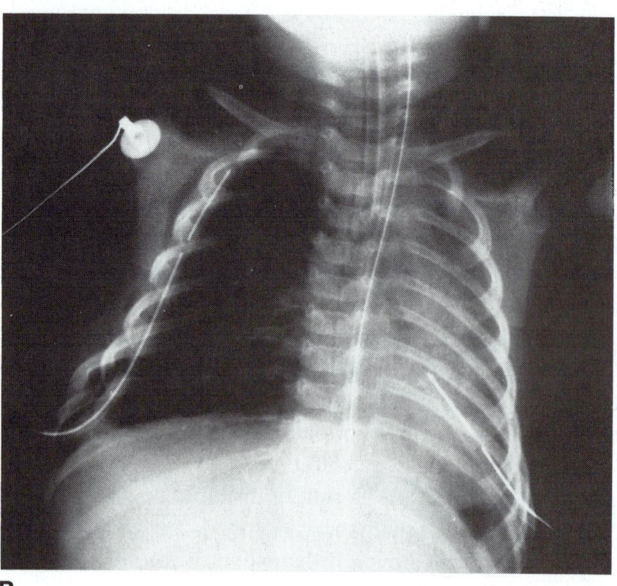

B

**Figure 35–14. A.** Marked eventration of the right hemidiaphragm can easily be seen in this x-ray. This baby's left-sided Bochdalek hernia was repaired at another hospital; following clinical deterioration, she was transferred to us for ECMO. After successful removal from ECMO, a central catheter extravasated TPN into the right chest. She subsequently developed progressive elevation of the right hemidiaphragm from phrenic nerve paresis. **B.** This x-ray shows flattening of the right hemidiaphragm following plication of the eventration. A small, recurrent left-sided diaphragmatic hernia was repaired at the same time. The patient survived a long hospitalization and is doing well at home.

abnormal, anatomic detail is more accurately imaged with computed tomography (CT) scanning.

Whenever possible, the tumor should be excised with direct suture closure of the defect. If a chest wall excision is also required or extensive removal of the diaphragm is necessary, closure of the defect will require a prosthetic patch or muscle flap.

## REFERENCES


1. Paré A: Oeuvres completes, VO1, 2 Malaigne JF (Ed.) Paris, Bailliere, 1840, pp 94–100
2. Bonet T: De Suffocations. Obsevatic XL1 Suffocatio excitata a tenuium intestorum vulnus diaphgramatis in thoracem ingestu Selpulchretum sive anatomia procteia et cadaveribus morbo denatus. Geneva, 1679
3. Bochdalek VA: Einige Betrachtungen uber die Entstehung des angeborenen Zwerchfellbruches. Als Bietrag zur pathologischen Anatomie der Hernien. *Vierteljahrsschrift Praky Heilkund* **3:**89, 1848
4. Bowditch HI: Diaphragmatic hernia. *Buffalo Med J* **9:**1–39, 66–94, 1853
5. Hedblom CA: Diaphragmatic hernia. *JAMA* **85:**947–953, 1925
6. Aue O: Ober angeborene Zwerchfellhernien. *Deutsch Chir* **160:**14, 1920
7. Gross RE: Congenital hernia of the diaphragm. *Am J Dis Child* **71:**579, 1946
8. Gross RE: Congenital hernia of the diaphragm. In *Surgery of Infancy and Childhood.* Philadelphia, Saunders, 1953, p 428
9. Bremer JL: The diaphragm and diaphragmatic hernia. *Arch Pathol* **36:**539–549, 1943
10. Iritani I: Experimental study on embryogenesis of congenital diaphragmatic hernia. *Anat Embryol* **169:**133–139, 1984
11. Woodburne RT: *Essentials of Human Anatomy.* New York, Oxford University Press, 1969, pp 278–280
12. Woodburne RT: *Essentials of Human Anatomy.* New York, Oxford University Press, 1969, pp 441–447
13. Stauffer UG, Rickham PP: Congenital diaphragmatic hernia and eventration of the diaphragm. In Rickham PP, Lister J, Irvings JM (eds): *Neonatal Surgery.* London, Butterworth, 1978, pp 163–178
14. Boyden EA: The structure of compressed lungs in congenital diaphragmatic hernia. *Am J Anat* **134:**497, 1972
15. Levin DL: Morphologic analysis of the pulmonary vascular bed in congenital left-sided diaphragmatic hernia. *J Pediatr* **92:**805, 1978
16. Reale FR, Esterly JR: Pulmonary hypoplasia: A morphometric study of infants with diaphragmatic hernia, anencephaly, and renal malformations. *Pediatrics* **51:**91–96, 1973
17. Fox WW, Duara S: Persistent pulmonary hypertension in the neonate: Diagnosis and management. *J Pediatr* **103:**505, 1983
18. Shochat SJ: Pulmonary vascular pathology in congenital diaphragmatic hernia. *Pediatr Surg Int* **2:**331–335, 1987
19. Peckham GJ, Fox WW: Physiologic factors affecting pulmonary artery pressure in infants with persistent pulmonary hypertension. *J Pediatr* **93:**1005, 1978
20. Murdock AI, Burrington JB, Swyer, PR: Alveolar to arterial oxygen tension difference and venous admixture in newly born infants with congenital diaphragmatic herniation through the foramen of Bochdalek. *Biol Neonate* **17:**161–172, 1971
21. Reid LM: Pathological changes in humans. In: Sandor GGS, Macnab AJ, Rastogi RB (eds). *Persistent Fetal Circulation.* Mt. Kisco, NY Futura Media Services, 1984, p 37
22. Glick PL, Stannard V, Leach C, et al: Pathophysiology of congenital diaphragmatic hernia II: The fetal lamb CDH model is surfactant deficient. *J Pediatr Surg* **27:**382, 1992
23. Glick PL, Leach C, Besner G: Pathophysiology of congenital diaphragmatic hernia III: Exogenous surfactant therapy for the high risk neonate with CDH. *J Pediatr Surg* **27:**866, 1992
24. Bell MJ, Ternberg JL: Antenatal diagnosis of diaphragmatic hernia. *Pediatrics* **60:**738, 1977
25. Greenwood RD, Rosenthal A, Nadas AS: Cardiovascular abnormalities associated with congenital diaphragmatic hernia. *Pediatrics* **57:**92, 1976
26. Puri P, Gorman F: Lethal nonpulmonary anomalies associated with congenital diaphragmatic hernia: Implications for early intrauterine surgery. *J Pediatr Surg* **19:**29, 1984
27. Mishalany HG, Nakkada K, Woolley MM: Congenital diaphragmatic hernias: Eleven years experience. *Arch Surg* **114:**1118–1123, 1979
28. Boix-Ochoa J, Peguero G, Seijo G, et al: Acid-base balance and blood gases in prognosis and therapy of congenital diaphragmatic hernia. *J Pediatr Surg* **19:**49–57, 1974
29. Ruff SJ, Campbell JR, Harrison MW, Campbell TJ: Pediatric diaphragmatic hernias. *Am J Surg* **139:**641–645, 1980
30. Bohn, D: Blood gas and ventilatory parameters in predicting survival in congenital diaphragmatic hernia. *Pediatr Surg Int* **2:**336–340, 1987
31. Ein SH, Barker G: The pharmacological treatment of the newborn diaphragmatic hernia—update 1987. *Pediatr Surg Int* **2:**341–345, 1987
32. Stevens DC, Schreiner RL, Bull MJ, et al: An analysis of tolazoline therapy in the critically ill neonate. *J Pediatr Surg* **15:**964, 1980
33. Sakai H, Tamura M, Bohn DJ, et al: The effect of surgical repair on respiratory mechanics in congenital diaphragmatic hernia. *J Pediatr* **111:**432–438, 1987
34. Connors RH, Tracy T, Bailey PV et al: Congenital diaphragmatic hernia repair on ECMO. *J Pediatr Surg* **25:**1043, 1990
35. Collins DL, Pomerance JJ, Travis KW, et al: A new approach to congenital posterolateral diaphragmatic hernia. *J Pediatr Surg* **12:**149, 1977
36. Bloss RS, Turmen T, Beardmore HE, at al: Tolazoline therapy for persistent pulmonary hypertension after congenital diaphragmatic hernia repair. *J Pediatr* **97:**984, 1980
37. Levy FJ, Rosenthal A, Freed MD, et al: Persistent pulmonary hypertension in a newborn with congenital diaphragmatic hernia: Successful management with tolazoline. *Pediatrics* **60:**740, 1977
38. Kinsella JP, Abman SH. Inhalation nitric oxide therapy for persistent pulmonary hypertension of the newborn. *Pediatrics* **91:**997, 1993
39. Karl R, Ballantine TVN, Snider MT: High-frequency ventilation at rates 375 to 1,800 cycles per minute in four neonates with congenital diaphragmatic hernia. *J Pediatr Surg* **18:**822, 1983
40. Langham MR, Krummel TM, Bartlett RH, et al: Mortality with extracorporeal membrane oxygenation following repair of congenital diaphragmatic hernia in 93 infants. *J Pediatr Surg 22:*1150–1154, 1987
41. Vacanti JP, O'Rourke PP, Lillehei CW, et al: The cardiopulmonary consequences of high-risk congenital diaphragmatic hernia. *Pediatr Surg Int* **3:**1–5, 1988
42. Heaton JF, Redmond CR, Graves ED, et al: Congenital diaphragmatic hernia. *Pediatr Surg Int* **3:**6–10, 1988
43. Weber, TR, Connors RH, Pennington DG, et al: Neonatal diaphragmatic hernia: Am improving outlook with extracorporeal membrane oxygenation. *Arch Surg* **122:**615–618, 1987
44. Hansen J, James S, Burrington J, Whitfield J: The decreasing incidence of pneumothorax and improving survival of infants with congenital diaphragmatic hernia. *J Pediatr Surg* **19:**385–388, 1984
45. Bailey PV, Connors RH, Tracy TF, et al: A critical analysis of extracorporeal membrane oxygenation for congenital diaphragmatic hernia. *Surgery* **106:**611, 1989
46. Adzick NS, Harrison MR, Glick PL, et al: Diaphragmatic hernia in the fetus: Prenatal diagnosis and outcome in 94 cases. *J Pediatr Surg* **20:**357–361, 1985
47. Puri P, Gorman WA: Natural history of congenital diaphragmatic hernia: implications of management. *Pediatr Surg Int* **2:**327–330, 1987
48. Harrison M, Adzick S, Flake A, et al: Correction of congenital di-

aphragmatic hernia in utero VI. Hard-earned lessons. *J Pediatr Surg* **28:**1411, 1993
49. Reid IS, Hutcherson RJ: Long-term follow-up of patients with congenital diaphragmatic hernia. *J Pediatr Surg* **11:**939, 1976
50. Wohl ME, Griscom NT, Strieder DJ, et al: The lung following repair of congenital diaphragmatic hernia. *J Pediatr* **90:**405, 1977
51. Thomas TV: Subcostosternal diaphragmatic hernia. *J Thorac Cardiovasc Surg* **63:**180, 1970
52. Hood RM: Traumatic diaphragmatic hernia. *Ann Thorac Surg* **12:**311, 1971
53. Pomerantz M, Rodgers BM, Sabiston DC Jr: Traumatic diaphragmatic hernia. *Surgery* **64:**529, 1968
54. Brearly S, Tubbs N: Rupture of the diaphragm in blunt injuries of the trunk. *Injury* **12:**480, 1980
55. Payne JH, Yellin AZ: Traumatic diaphragmatic hernia. *Arch Surg* **117:**18, 1982
56. Haller JO, Schneider M, Kussner EG, et al: Sonographic evaluations of the chest in infants and children. *Am J Roentgenol* **134:**1019, 1980
57. Symbas PN, Hatcher CR Jr, Waldo W: Diaphragmatic eventration in infancy and childhood. *Ann Thorac Surg* **24:**113, 1977
58. Varpela E, Laustela EV, Viljaneu A: Acquired eventration of diaphragm: Results of surgery. *Ann Chir Gynecol* **66:**284, 1977
59. Olafsso G, Ransling A, Olen O: Primary tumors of the diaphragm. *Chest* **59:**568, 1971

CHAPTER

# 36

# The Diaphragm

## *Dysfunction and Induced Pacing*

John A. Elefteriades and Debra E. Weese-Mayer

### STRUCTURE AND FUNCTION

Although life may be sustained without the diaphragm by means of the accessory muscles of respiration—the external and internal intercostal, abdominal, scalene, and sternocleidomastoid muscles—the quality of life is greatly improved with competent function of the diaphragm. The diaphragm is a versatile structure, having both voluntary and involuntary control centers, that moves air at the rate demanded by voluntary command or metabolic necessity. Muscle fibers of the diaphragm are of three types: fatigue-resistant slow-twitch high oxidative fibers (Type I, 55 ± 5% of fibers); intermediate fatigue-resistant fast-twitch high oxidative fibers (Type IIA, 21 ± 6% of fibers); and fatigue-prone fast-twitch low oxidative high glycolytic fibers (Type IIB, 24 ± 3% of fibers).[1] The fast-twitch easily fatigued and slow-twitch fatigue-resistant fibers prepare the diaphragm for the wide range of energy requirements during routine and extraordinary activities.

The diaphragm is a musculofibrous sheet that separates the abdominal and thoracic cavities with two components: a dome-shaped muscle mass that arises from the thoracic cage and the upper lumbar vertebrae and a large central tendon. The muscle mass comprises two embryologic, anatomic, and functionally distinct parts—costal and crural—with different segmental innerventions and fiber compositions.[2,3] The thin and ribbon-like costal muscle inserts on the ribs and sternum. The crural muscle, which is thicker, inserts on the lumbar vertebrae in a complex criss-cross configuration to accommodate the hiatus of the esophagus and aorta (Fig. 36–1).

The diaphragm is innervated by the phrenic nerves, which arise from the third, fourth, and fifth cervical segments of the spinal cord. Motoneurons supply and proprioceptic neurons innervate the diaphragmatic muscle. Sensory neurons also innervate the diaphragmatic pleural and peritoneal surfaces. Motoneurons predominate and have a discharge impulse frequency from the brain to the diaphragm muscle that ranges from 10 to 30 Hz.

Stimulation of the costal and of the crural portions of the diaphragm has different actions on the chest wall.[4,5] Contraction of the costal portion causes the diaphragm to flatten, displacing the abdominal viscera downward. The increased abdominal pressure exerts an outward inspiratory force on the lower rib cage. The upward pull of the costal diaphragm during inspiration also causes the lower ribs to lift, enlarging the thoracic cavity. Contraction of the crural part causes only downward displacement of the diaphragm.

### (ACQUIRED) PARALYSIS OF THE DIAPHRAGM

Paralysis of the diaphragm, caused by injury to the phrenic nerve or by primary neuromuscular disorders, may be partial or complete, temporary or permanent, and involve one or both nerves. The peripheral components of the nerve, the lower motoneurons, or the central components, the upper motoneurons, may be involved. Paralysis of the diaphragm produces a restrictive ventilatory impairment (reduction in vital capacity, forced expiratory volume, and transdiaphragmatic pressure gradient)[6] and an increase in ventilation-perfusion mismatch. Unilateral paralysis reduces ventilatory

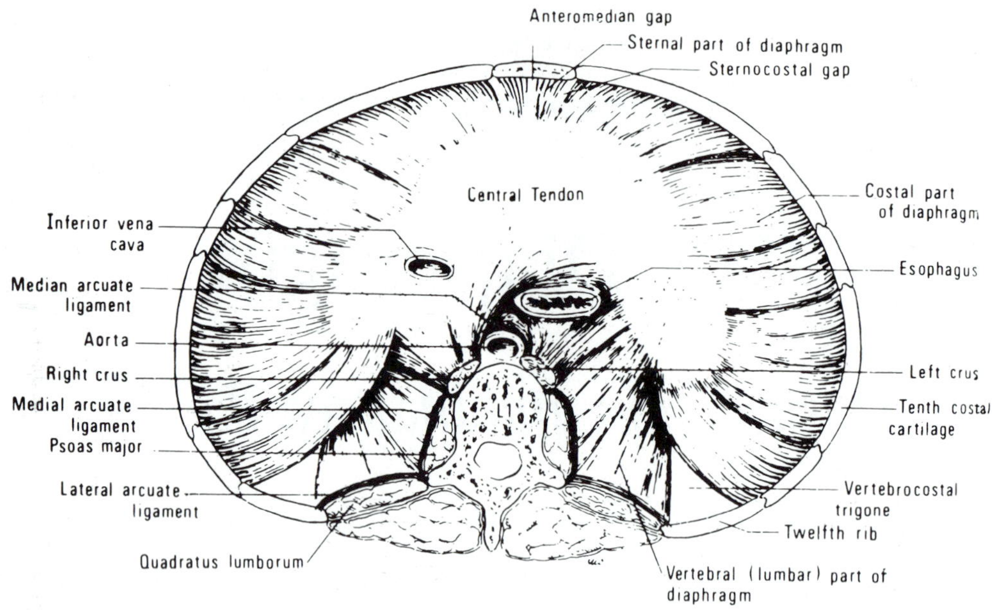


**Figure 36–1.** The anatomy of the human diaphragm as seen from below. *(From Osmond DG: Functional anatomy of the chest wall. In Roussos C, Macklem PT [eds]: The Thorax, Part A, in Lenfant C [ed]: Lung Biology in Health and Disease, vol 29. New York, Marcel Dekker, 1985, p 222, with permission.)*

function in older children and adults by about 25%, which usually is well tolerated. In contrast, in infants and young children it causes severe respiratory embarrassment.[7] Bilateral paralysis is far more disabling, resulting in a 60% reduction in respiratory function.[8] Bilateral paralysis of the diaphragm may produce failure of spontaneous respiration, necessitating mechanical ventilation; on occasion, spontaneous ventilation, by means of accessory muscles, may suffice, but with a marked propensity for respiratory infection.[3]

Paralysis of the diaphragm can be categorized as idiopathic, posttraumatic, and other. Lower motoneuron disease is discussed separately from upper motoneuron disease.

## Lower Motoneuron Disease

### *Idiopathic Paralysis of the Diaphragm*

Paralysis for which no cause can be identified is usually unilateral but can be bilateral.[9,10] The typical clinical features of unilateral paralysis are mild to moderate dyspnea, accentuated in the supine position, with cough and chest pain, separately or simultaneously. There may have been a cold or an undiagnosed febrile illness, or a minor injury to the neck or shoulder that cannot be correlated with the paralysis. Symptoms may be abrupt in onset and cause considerable disability. Inward movement of the abdomen on inspiration, most apparent in the supine position, suggests paralysis of the diaphragm. Patients have a preference for sleeping sitting up. In infants, inward movement on the affected side is accentuated in the lateral decubitus position and with the affected side up.[7] Computed tomography (CT) of the neck and mediastinum should rule out organic lesions (lung or mediastinal tumors) compressing the phrenic nerves.[11] That a paralyzed diaphragm may be found incidentally during a routine physical examination or on a chest radiograph suggests some people may have asymptomatic unilateral paralysis that is not diagnosed.

With unilateral diaphragmatic paralysis elevation of the hemidiaphragm is seen on a chest radiograph. At fluoroscopy, on voluntary inspiration in the supine position, the diaphragm moves paradoxically on the paralyzed side. When the patient is erect, the diaphragm may move downward passively during inspiration, giving a false impression of normalcy. A positive sniff test—rapid upward movement of the diaphragm when a patient in the supine position sniffs briskly—suggests paralysis. Transcutaneous electrical stimulation of the phrenic nerves in the neck shows diminished or absent response of the diaphragm or prolongation of conduction time, which is indicative of lower motoneuron injury or disease.[12] This test also detects return of function.

Diabetic neuropathy affecting the phrenic nerve may be the cause of otherwise unexplained diaphragmatic paralysis.[13] Local expression in the phrenic nerve of a more generalized neuropathic process may be a cause of otherwise idiopathic unilateral phrenic nerve paralysis.[14]

### *Posttraumatic Paralysis of the Diaphragm*

The most common cause of paralysis of the diaphragm is injury to the phrenic nerves during a cardiac operation.

The nerves may be injured directly by dissection or by electrocautery, especially near the superior vena cava on the right and the aortic arch on the left, where the nerves come anteriorly. During redo operations, trauma to the phrenic nerves at these locations may occur even in expert hands. The left phrenic nerve may be injured during dissection of the upper portion of the pedicle of the left internal mammary artery. We ask the anesthesiologist to avoid complete neuromuscular blockade when both mammary arteries are being harvested, to avoid the catastrophe of bilateral phrenic nerve injury; diaphragmatic twitch indicates that the dissection is approaching the phrenic nerve.

During cardiac operations, ice-cold solutions or slush placed in the pericardial sac to reduce myocardial metabolism may lead to diaphragmatic paralysis. One, usually the left, or both phrenic nerves may be affected.[15] The diagnosis can generally be made at the bedside when respiratory failure recurs on removal of mechanical ventilation.[7,15]

Paralysis of the diaphragm is reported to occur after 6.3–26% of open heart operations.[16–19] The reported incidence actually depends on the definition; abnormal chest radiographic appearance of the diaphragm is seen in 84% of patients, abnormal diaphragmatic motion by echo in 46%, and abnormal phrenic nerve conduction study in 26%.[19] Many cases are relatively minor and go unrecognized.

Recent reviews of phrenic nerve injury following cardiac surgery have demonstrated a number of important factors.[15,17,18,20–23] Elimination of slush or use of an insulating pad greatly decreases the incidence of diaphragmatic paralysis.[22] (Fig. 36–2). Sparing the pericardiophrenic artery, a high medial branch of the internal mammary artery, during mobilization of the mammary pedicle decreased phrenic nerve ischemia in an animal model[23]; such ischemia may well play an important role in clinic phrenic nerve dysfunction. Most cases of unilateral paralysis from intraoperative cold injury resolve in 3–6 months.

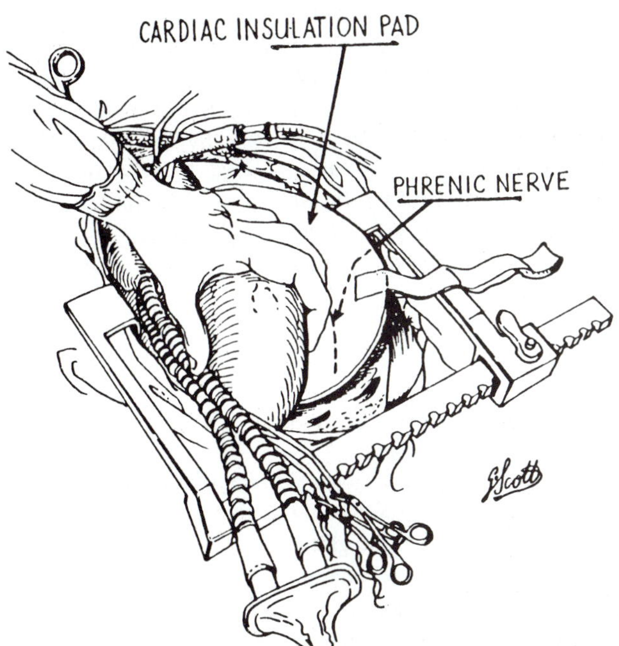


**Figure 36–2.** Application of cardiac insulation pad behind left ventricle to protect phrenic nerve from cold solution in percardial sac. *(From Wheeler WE, Rubis LJ, Jones CW, Harrah JD: Etiology and prevention of topical cardiac hypothermia induced phrenic nerve injury and left lower lobe atelectasis during cardiac surgery. Chest 88:680, 1985, with permission.)*

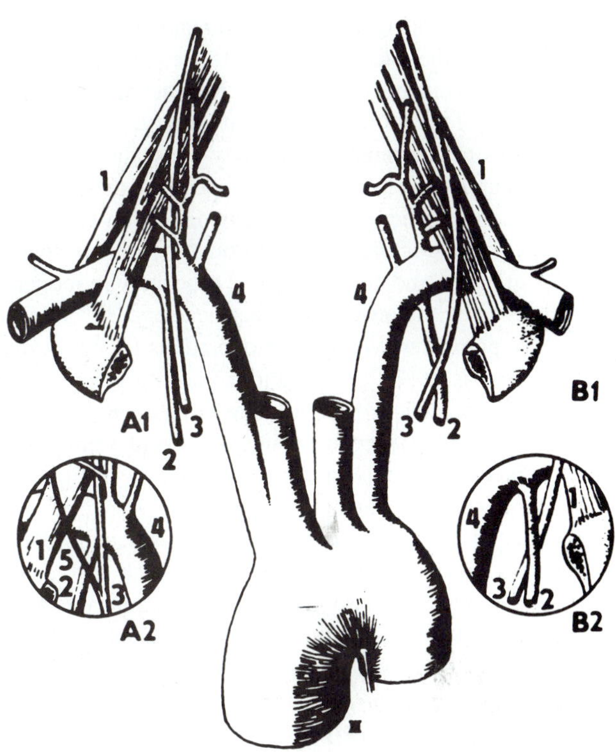


**Figure 36–3.** Anatomy of the interrelations between the phrenic nerves and the internal mammary arteries. **Insets:** Anatomic variants. 1 = scalenus muscle; 2 = internal mammary artery; 3 = phrenic nerve; 4 = subclavian artery; 5 = accessory branch of phrenic nerve. *(From Setina M, Cerny S, Grim M, Pirk J: Anatomical interrelation between the phrenic nerve and the internal mammary artery as seen by the surgeon. J Cardiovasc Surg (Torino) 1993 34(6):499–502.)*

The devastating phenomenon of bilateral phrenic nerve injury following a cardiac operation does occur[24–26] and requires positive-pressure ventilation for prolonged periods. Fortunately, function usually returns even after many months of mechanical ventilation.

Occult diaphragmatic dysfunction related to phrenic nerve injury can be identified quite commonly in patients who have unexplained failure to wean from mechanical ventilation after cardiac operations.[27] These patients have a high incidence of complications and death related to respiratory problems.

The anatomy of the phrenic nerve and the origin of the internal mammary artery have implications regarding mammary artery harvesting[28,29] (Fig. 36–3). The phrenic nerve enters the chest between the subclavian artery and vein (anterior to the subclavian artery). On the left, the nerve enters the chest lateral to the mammary artery and crosses the artery obliquely to its pericardial position. The nerve may pass anterior or posterior to the mammary artery in crossing it medially. On the right, the nerve remains medial to and runs parallel to the artery on its way to the pericardium. Injuries can be avoided by attention to these details during the mobilization of the proximal mammary artery.

Injuries to the phrenic nerve may occur during operations for congenital heart disease, especially the Blalock-Taussig shunt procedure.[30–32] Unless dissection to expose the underlying structures is meticulous, the phrenic nerve may be stretched and compressed or, especially in reoperations, injured by the heat of the electrocautery.[33,34] The incidence of phrenic nerve injury in operations for congenital heart disease is 10%.[35,36] A right thoracotomy appears to increase the incidence.[37] Even unilateral phrenic nerve injury is a very serious problem in infants and young children. It predisposes the patient to ventilatory difficulties, ventilator dependence, and even death.[36]

Injury to the phrenic nerve is seen in noncardiovascular procedures during dissections in the neck and mediastinum. An unusual cause of phrenic nerve injury is accidental needle puncture during placement of a subclavian or jugular vein catheter or electrode.[33,38–40]

### *Other Causes of Paralysis of the Diaphragm*

External trauma to the phrenic nerve (motor vehicle collisions, falls, gunshot wounds, birth injuries) and compression or invasion of the nerve by adjacent abnormal organic structures may cause diaphragmatic paralysis. Chiropractic neck manipulation may cause bilateral phrenic nerve injury.[41,42] Bronchogenic carcinoma, thymoma, calcified or caseous tuberculous lymph nodes, other tumors arising in the neck or mediastinum, and osteophytes in the vertebral root canals have been incriminated.

### *Treatment of Lower Motoneuron Disease*

Unless complications arise, idiopathic or traumatic unilateral paralysis is usually well tolerated and is treated conservatively. Dyspnea occurs, especially with exercise, but improves with time. Exercising the accessory muscles of respiration is helpful. Function returns after idiopathic disease in only about 9% of patients. Patients who have had posttraumatic disease, including those who have undergone open heart operations, may recover adequate pulmonary function to allow normal activities within a few weeks. A large number, however, have shown residual paralysis for more than a year.[15,16,34]

Electrical stimulation of the nonconductive lower motoneurons is not effective. Plication should be considered in an adult if symptoms are disabling, if there is recurring atelectasis of the lower lobe, and if there is no evidence of recovery in 12 months.[29,30] When paralysis is secondary to compression and the compressing agent can be removed, mechanical ventilation is provided for as long as required. Recovery from temporary compression can be expected in a few weeks or months but may take much longer.[13] The purpose of plication is to lower the paralyzed diaphragm, relieve the upward pressure on the lower lobe, and prevent paradoxic motion. Through a lateral thoracotomy,[43,44] the redundant diaphragm is reduced in size by means of suture imbrication or, if redundancy is excessive, by means of excision of the central portion with reapproximation of the edges with strong nonabsorbable sutures. In adults disabled from diaphragmatic paralysis, plication was followed by marked symptomatic improvement.[44] Evidence from studies of animals has shown that plication produces beneficial effects on the mechanics of respiration.[45]

Successful reinnervation of the diaphragm has been accomplished in a number of patients by prompt anastomosis of peripheral components of the phrenic nerve severed at operation[46]; by interposition of a graft where anastomosis of the severed phrenic nerve was not possible[47]; and, in animals, by anastomosis of the distal segment of the severed phrenic nerve to a viable peripheral nerve with intact central communication.[48] Electrical stimulation of the distal end of a severed phrenic nerve is ineffective after several weeks,[49] as nerve degeneration and muscle atrophy occur, as with other peripheral nerve-muscle groups.

The simplest test to monitor recovery of phrenic nerve and diaphragmatic function after injury is percutaneous electrical stimulation of the nerve and fluoroscopic observation of diaphragmatic motion. Ultrasound has been helpful in difficult cases.[50,51]

### Upper Motoneuron Disease

Diaphragmatic paralysis also is caused by destruction of the upper motoneurons. The brain stem and upper cervical spinal cord may be invaded by an organic lesion or may suffer iatrogenic injury from the treatment of a congenital or acquired lesion. Central alveolar hypoventilation syndrome may result. Central alveolar hypoventilation also may occur in children on an idiopathic basis. If the condition does not resolve spontaneously or in response to therapy, pacing the diaphragm by electric stimulation of the lower motoneurons in the phrenic nerve, if viable, is the treatment of choice.

## HICCUP (SINGULTUS)

Hiccup is characterized by episodes of discrete, involuntary, spasmodic contraction of the diaphragm that terminate abruptly in closure of the glottis. Rarely lasting more than a few minutes without an ongoing cause, hiccup is one of the most frequent disorders of muscular function. Hiccup apparently serves no useful purpose and its exact pathogenesis is an enigma. Participation of the accessory muscles of respiration and the diaphragm[52,53] supports the concept of a hiccup center in the brain stem. The discrete burst of activity of the inspiratory muscles occurs synchronously in both hemidiaphragms and the external intercostal muscles. Hiccup does not intrinsically impair ventilation as one might expect; in fact, if the effect of closure of the glottis is prevented by tracheostomy, spasmodic contractions of the diaphragm produce hyperventilation.[54]

Clinical observation has implicated, among other possible causes, a lesion in the lateral medullary area of the brain stem (Wallenberg's syndrome), infection, tumor, multiple sclerosis, local irritation of the diaphragm or phrenic nerve, uremia, and diabetes mellitus.[55,56] Repeated episodes of hiccup may accompany a small hiatal hernia.

Though the common brief form of hiccup is not debilitating, occasionally hiccup is long lasting and intractable, its episodes persisting for months, even years, with relief coming only during sleep, if at all—a condition known as *hoquet diabolique*.[56] Characteristically the person awakens in the morning breathing normally, then about an hour later, usually soon after eating, begins to hiccup. The spasmodic contractions continue, at first in slow cadence, then after a short time at a rate of 20–30 per minute, without relief throughout the day. After the patient falls asleep and sleep deepens (stages 3 and 4), the spasms stop. The sequence is repeated the following day and each day thereafter for a week or so. Then, for no apparent reason, the episode terminates, only to return as before in several days or weeks. Hiccup persisting for long periods leads to anxiety, exhaustion, anorexia, loss of weight, and insomnia, which eventually may become life-threatening.

### Treatment

Popular remedies to treat hiccup include drinking fluids, especially carbonated beverages, chewing granulated sugar, and placing an ice cube on the base of the tongue. The most effective simple remedy is local irritation of the posterior pharynx by insertion of a digit or soft rubber catheter or a pliable plastic rod (Goncz JH, personal communication, 1984) through the mouth. Pharyngeal massage may be effective because it stimulates a neural plexus, interrupting the afferent arc of the hiccup, most likely served by the vagus nerve.[56]

When hiccup persists, the cause is sought with sophisticated imaging techniques to examine the brain stem and diaphragm. Antispasmodic medications have been tried, such as valproic acid by mouth to tolerance,[57] chlorpromazine, as a single IV bolus of 50 mg,[58] metoclopramide, 10 mg by mouth qid,[54] and carbamazepine, 200 mg tid.[58] Ephedrine, up to 10 mg IV, has been successful when hiccup has occurred during anesthetization.[59] Before administration of any antispasmodic drug, however, conditions that might be worsened by such medication must be ruled out.

To stop persistently intractable hiccup, that is, hiccup unresponsive to medical treatment and intrapharyngeal or intraesophageal manipulation, several measures have been suggested. Immobilization of the diaphragm by ablation of both phrenic nerves would probably result in respiratory failure; thus this radical procedure is contraindicated. Another approach is to immobilize the diaphragm with controlled tetanic electrical stimulation of both phrenic nerves—a special application of the techniques of diaphragmatic pacing discussed below. Glenn has had experience with this technique.[60] A diaphragmatic pacemaker is implanted surgically, as for other indications. The current delivered to the nerve is limited to that which substantially reduces diaphragmatic excursions, as observed at fluoroscopy, without discomfort. No effort is made to immobilize the diaphragm completely. Stimulation is strictly limited to 8 hours a day for no more than 5 days consecutively followed by at least 2 days without stimulation. Stimulation is discontinued during eating and sleeping.

Ventilation during tetanic stimulation of the diaphragm is maintained by the accessory muscles and residual diaphragmatic contractions, and possibly by the tetanic contractions themselves.

Tetanic stimulation is an unphysiologic approach to treating hiccup and is recommended only in extreme cases in which symptoms are life-threatening and the only alternative method of control is bilateral phrenic nerve paralysis. A logical approach to hiccup control is blockage of the efferent impulse to the diaphragm. Development of an asymmetric two-electrode cuff well suited for application of collision block of peripheral nerve transmission has therapeutic implications for the control of intractable hiccup.[61]

## PACING OF THE DIAPHRAGM

### History

Use of electrical stimulation of the phrenic nerve to induce contraction of the diaphragm and induce artificial ventilation dates back to a suggestion by Hufeland in 1783 in his doctoral dissertation entitled "The Use of Electricity in Asphyxia."[62] Talonen reviewed the historical background of diaphragmatic pacing.[63] In 1818, Ure demonstrated the feasibility of electrical stimulation of the phrenic nerve in a "freshly hung criminal." Patterson reports, "The success of it was truly wonderful. Full . . . breathing instantly commenced. The chest heaved and fell; the belly was protruded and again collapsed, with the relaxing and retiring diaphragm"[64] (Fig. 36–4). In the 1800s, electrical stimulation of the phrenic nerve was popularized by Duchenne de Boulogne[65] and Beard and Rockwell[66] as a technique for cardiopulmonary resuscitation. Duchenne stated, "It is apparent from all my experiments on men and on animals, alive and dead, that stimulation of the phrenic nerve by electrical current can produce contraction of the diaphragm." In 1927, Isreal used transcutaneous stimulation of the phrenic nerves for ventilation of apneic newborns.[67] In the 1950s, Sarnoff et al used electrophrenic respiration extensively for the treatment of patients with polio.[68]

Over the last two decades, the father of modern diaphragmatic pacing, Dr. William Glenn, has proved, in a large series of patients cared for at Yale University, that di-

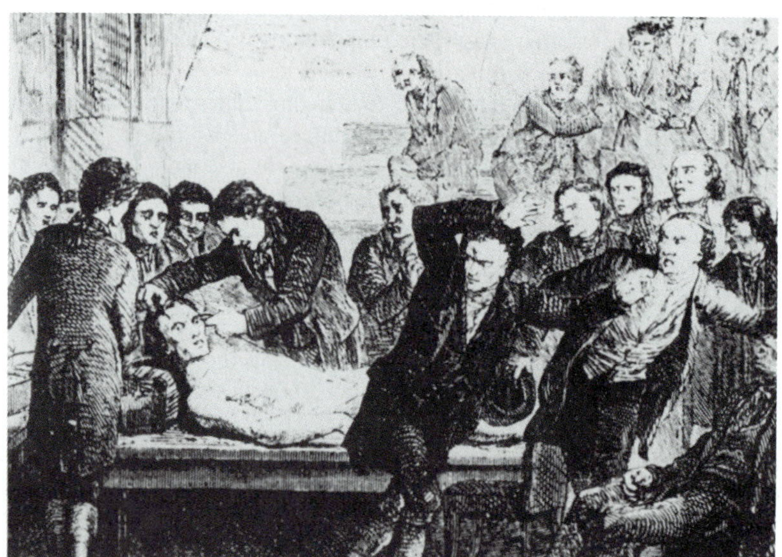

**Figure 36–4.** Ure's induction of artificial respiration (Glascow, 1818) by galvanic stimulation of the left phrenic nerve in a "freshly hung criminal." *(From Ure A: An account of some experiments made on the body of a criminal immediately after execution, with physiological and practical observations. J Sci Arts (Lond) 6:283, 1819.)*

aphragmatic pacing is an effective and clinically useful modality. This led to organized programs for diaphragmatic pacing at a number of other centers in the United States and abroad. Now nearly 1000 patients worldwide have been treated by diaphragmatic pacing.[69]

## Indications

Pacing of the diaphragm is an accepted form of ventilatory support in two clinical settings: central alveolar ventilation (or sleep apnea, in which respiratory drive is deficient) and spinal cord injury (most commonly quadriplegia, in which, although the drive for respiration exists, injury to the spinal cord itself prevents the transmission of stimuli to the phrenic nerves). These two indications account for most clinical cases of diaphragmatic pacing.

Diaphragmatic pacing has been used for chronic obstructive pulmonary disease (COPD) to preserve ventilation despite suppression of the hypoxic drive by oxygen administration.[70] Diaphragmatic pacing may, however, have a more important role in COPD than currently appreciated, as discussed later.

Diaphragmatic pacing is not indicated when the phrenic nerve is dysfunctional (traumatic injury, iatrogenic injury, tumor, neuropathy syndromes), when the muscular apparatus of breathing is dysfunctional (myasthenia gravis, muscular dystrophies), and in advanced primary disease of the pulmonary parenchyma, or obstructive sleep apnea syndromes. Figure 36–5 shows the appropriate and inappropriate circumstances for diaphragmatic pacing.

### *Central Alveolar Hypoventilation*

The various sleep apnea syndromes are still not fully characterized, and miscommunication and confusion persist.[71] The most basic distinction is between obstructive and central sleep apnea. In obstructive sleep apnea, the upper airway closes during inspiration, preventing ventilation; respiratory drive is normal, and respiratory muscle activity is preserved. The brain tells the muscles to breathe, but anatomic closure of the upper airway prevents exchange of air. Obstructive apnea can be caused by tumors of the pharynx, abnormal morphology of the pharynx (including enlarged tonsils and adenoids, macroglossia, and micrognathia), obesity, or simply an exaggerated relaxation of the pharyngeal musculature with sleep. In central sleep apnea, there is a failure of respiratory drive, with no respiratory muscle activity. The brain does not tell the muscles to breathe; the response to hypoxia and hypercapnea is diminished. Central hypoventilation is not usually caused by disease of the cerebral cortex. It is usually the medullary respiratory control center that is affected, by tumor, infection (encephalitis), stroke, or trauma (including iatrogenic injury). Idiopathic cases may represent dysfunction of the medullary chemoreceptors for hypoxia and hypercarbia.

The blunted response to hypoxia and hypercapnia that characterizes central sleep apnea also prevails during the day in many if not most patients, although voluntary contribution to ventilation during the day increases minute volume to a certain extent. Thus, the term *central hypoventilation* is a better descriptor than sleep apnea. The term *Ondine's curse* has been used to describe this condition. Ondine was a mythologic water spirit who appears in modern times in a play by Giraudoux. Ondine's husband was cursed to stop breathing whenever he fell asleep.

People with central hypoventilation often, but not always, have a characteristic pickwickian habitus. Chronic hypoxia and hypercapnia, as well as the fragmented sleep pattern itself, lead to daytime somnolence. Over time, chronic hypoxia may lead, by means of hypoxic vasoconstriction and pulmonary hypertension, to right heart failure.

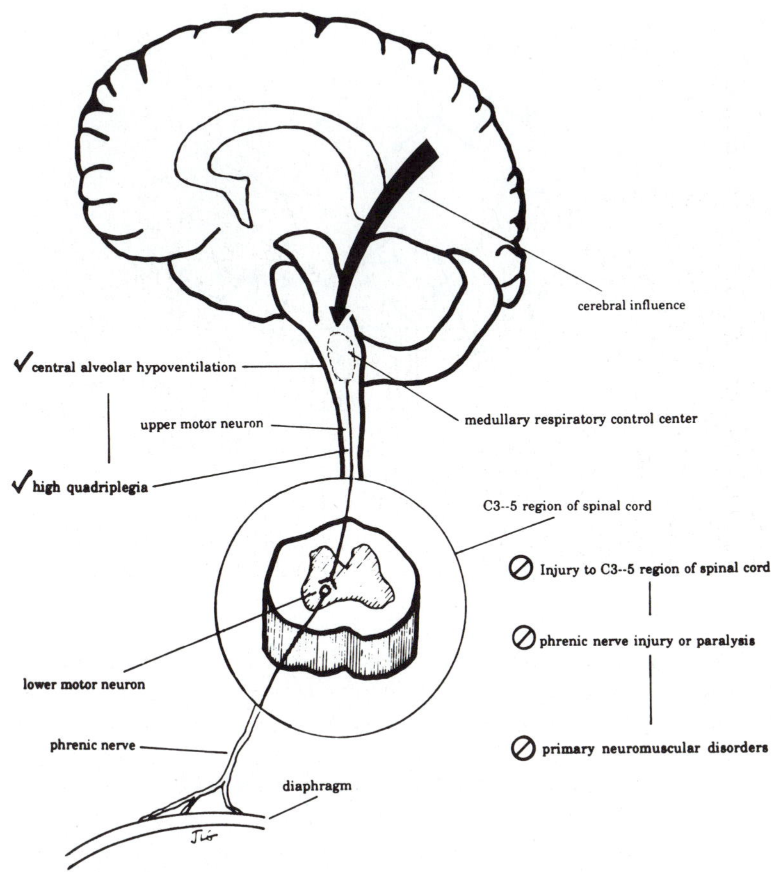


**Figure 36–5.** Areas of respiratory control system appropriate or inappropriate for diaphragm pacing. The (involuntary) medullary respiratory control center is subject to a degree of cerebral (voluntary) influence. The upper motor neurons of the phrenic system have their cell bodies in the medullary respiratory control center. The axons of the upper motor neurons synapse in the spinal cord with the lower motor neurons at the level of C3–C5. The phrenic nerve proper is composed of the axons of those lower motor neurons. Check marks indicate appropriate indications for diaphragmatic pacing. International *verboten* symbols indicate inappropriate indications. *(From Shields TW: General Thoracic Surgery, 4th ed. Baltimore, Williams & Wilkins, 1994, with permission.)*

Adequacy of respiratory drive can be assessed in terms of the ventilatory response to hypercapnia or hypoxia (Fig. 36–6). Ventilation should increase linearly as $PCO_2$ increases. Ventilation should increase linearly as oxygen saturation falls (or exponentially as $PO_2$ falls). Primary weakness of the muscles of respiration can give intermediate responses but is usually easily diagnosed by the standard spirometric tests of pulmonary function. Our own policy is to perform a 24-hour respiratory control study with hourly assessment of asleep-awake status, end-tidal carbon dioxide level, and oxygen saturation. A characteristic pattern in central hypoventilation (Fig. 36–7) is severe nighttime hypoventilation with mild daytime hypercarbia.

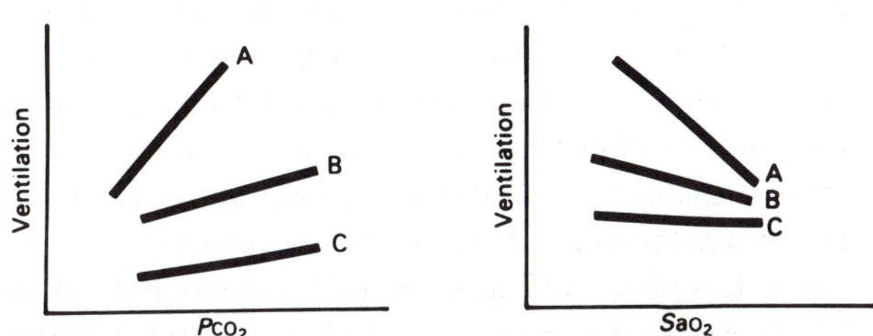


**Figure 36–6.** The ventilatory response to hypercapnia and hypoxia. **A.** Normal. **B.** Patients with chest wall disorders. **C.** Central hypoventilation. *(From Schneerson J: Disorders of ventilation. Oxford, England, Blackwell, 1988, Chap 6, with permission.)*

Central alveolar hypoventilation is well-treated by diaphragmatic pacing. The lack of respiratory drive is compensated by the artificially induced ventilation.

### *Quadriplegia*

The lower motor neurons of the phrenic nerve are located in the spinal cord at the level of C3, C4, and C5. Quadriplegia at levels below this range does not disrupt respiration. Quadriplegia involving the C3, C4, and C5 levels may disrupt respiration to a degree that depends on the actual damage to the lower motor neurons of the phrenic nerve. To the extent these neurons are damaged, the phrenic nerve becomes dysfunctional. Diaphragmatic pacing cannot overcome this damage. Quadriplegia at the C2–3 level or higher does not damage the phrenic nerve motor neurons; quadriplegia at these levels does, however, impair or eliminate spontaneous ventilation by disrupting the tracts that lead from the medullary respiratory control center to the spinal cord. The accessory muscles of respiration—intercostals (T1–12), abdominals (T7–L1), and pelvic muscles (L1–S2)—are denervated by these spinal cord lesions. Only the sternocleidomastoid and trapezius muscles, innervated by the spinal accessory nerve (cranial nerve XI), remain

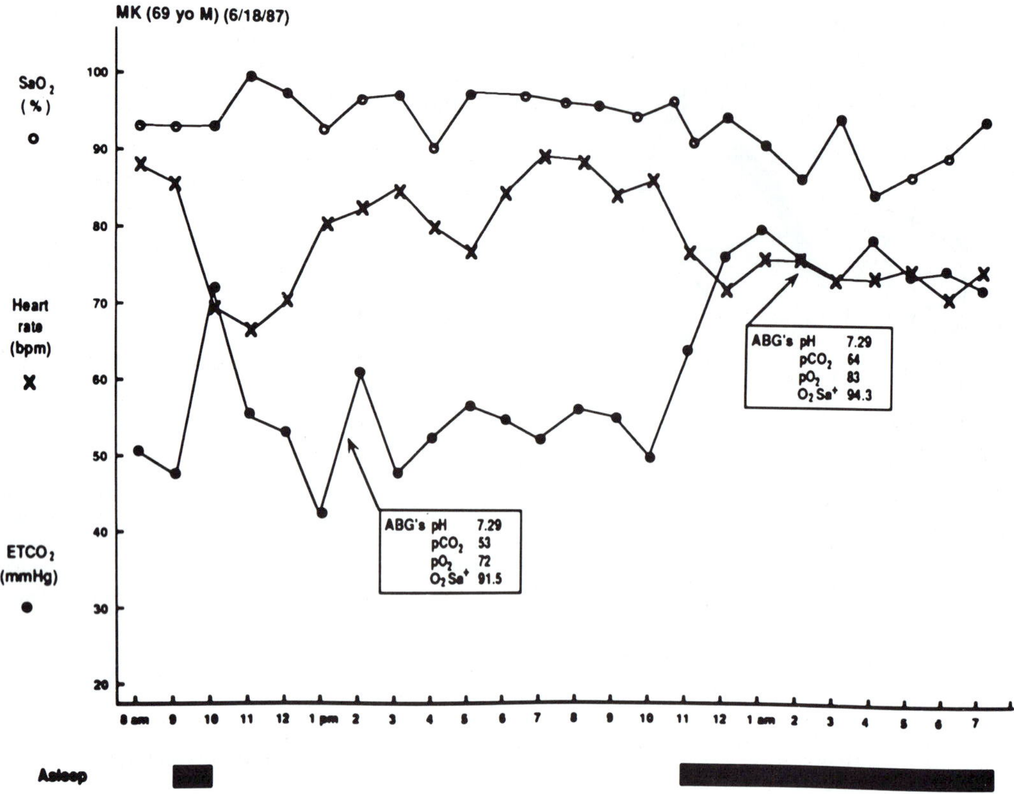


**Figure 36–7.** Twenty-four hour respiratory control study (preoperative) in a patient with central hypoventilation. Carbon dioxide is abnormally high throughout the 24-hour period, rises to 69 mm Hg during a morning nap, and is very high throughout the night's sleep (peaking at 78 mm Hg at 1 A.M.). Oxygen saturation falls to 83% at 4 A.M., reflecting critically low tidal volume from severe hypoventilation. *(From Shields TW: General Thoracic Surgery, 4th ed. Baltimore, Williams & Wilkins, 1994, with permission.)*

functional with quadriplegia at the C2–3 level or higher. Respiratory paralysis from high quadriplegia is correctable by diaphragmatic pacing. The neurologic findings that distinguish high quadriplegia (C2–3 or higher) are shown in Figure 36–8. In general, in high quadriplegia, sensation is intact only to the clavicles and motor function is disrupted from the deltoid muscle and below.

Whitehead et al[72] provide one of the best current overall references on high quadriplegia. With increased public awareness of cardiopulmonary resuscitation techniques, improved emergency care delivery systems, widespread availability of positive pressure ventilation, and improved long-term respiratory care, many more patients are surviving accidents that cause quadriplegia. The yearly incidence of spinal cord injury in the United States has been estimated at 30–35 per million population, or about 6000–7000 cases per year. The number of patients with spinal cord injury currently alive is estimated at 200,000. Most injuries are from motor vehicle collisions, diving accidents, gunshot wounds, falls, and iatrogenic injuries. Developmental and vascular abnormalities, infarctions, and transverse myelitis also produce quadriplegia.

When a patient with high quadriplegia manifests respiratory paralysis and the phrenic nerve is found to be intact by percutaneous testing, diaphragmatic pacing is indicated if the patient's overall status allows.

## Prerequisites

### *Phrenic Nerve Function*

We receive many calls on a regular basis inquiring about diaphragmatic pacing for patients with primary phrenic nerve dysfunction from tumor, mass, trauma, iatrogenic injury, especially reoperations on the heart, or idiopathic causes. Unfortunately, current practice cannot offer effective treatment for these patients. Pacing of the diaphragm requires an intact phrenic nerve. The intact nerve is stimulated and in turn produces contraction of the diaphragm.

Experimental studies of direct stimulation of the diaphragm have been conducted,[73] but these techniques have not been generally applied clinically. Even these direct approaches to diaphragmatic stimulation probably rely on stimulation of the radicles of the phrenic nerve as it divides in the central portions of the diaphragm. Unlike cardiac muscle, the diaphragm is not an electrical syncitium that propagates an electrical impulse throughout the muscle. Furthermore, even if direct stimulation proves feasible, with

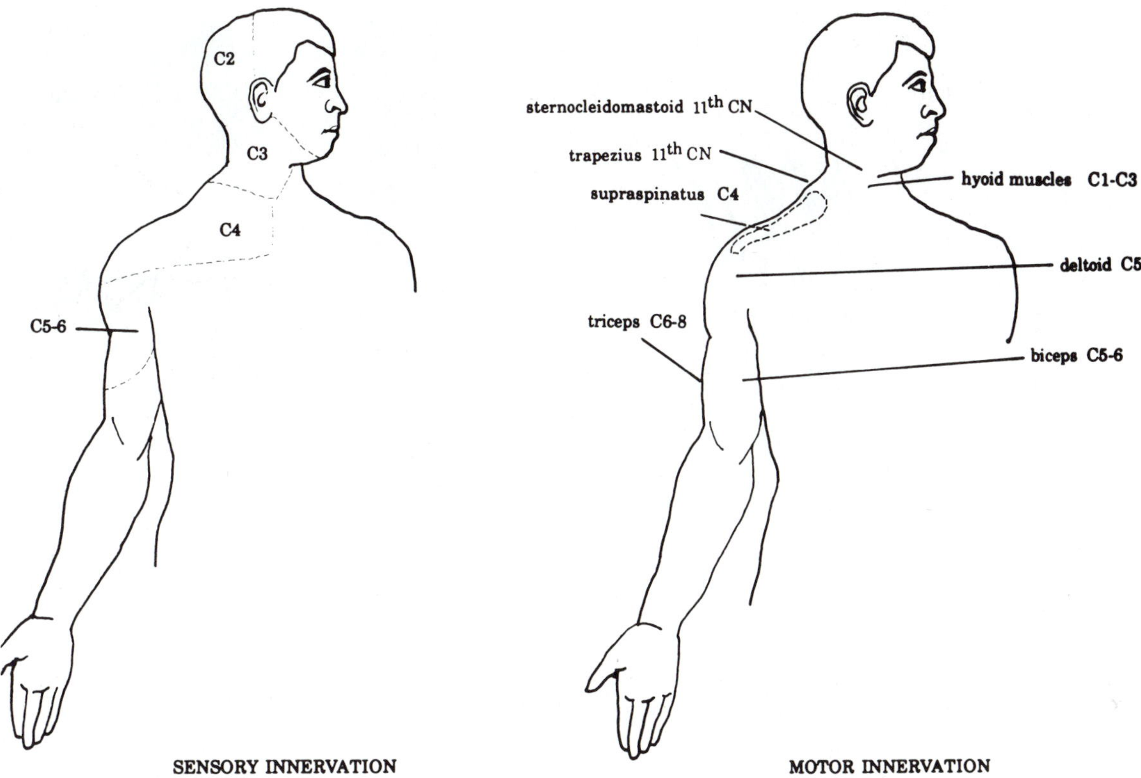


**Figure 36–8.** Sensory and motor findings that allow discrimination of high quadriplegia. Quadriplegia at C2–3 or higher is well treated by diaphragmatic pacing. *(From Shields TW: General Thoracic Surgery, 4th ed. Baltimore, Williams & Wilkins, 1994, with permission.)*

phrenic nerve injury, atrophy of the denervated muscle likely interferes with effective diaphragmatic contraction. Thus, there is no cure for injury to the phrenic nerve.

Because an intact phrenic nerve is essential for diaphragmatic pacing, testing the status of the nerve assumes paramount importance. Sarnoff[74] and Shaw (from Glenn's team)[12] described the technique for transcutaneous testing of phrenic nerve conduction (Fig. 36–9). The technique is similar to electromyelography (EMG) or any nerve conduction test. A thimble electrode facilitates testing the phrenic nerve. The motor point is located medial to the lateral edge of the clavicular head of the sternocleidomastoid muscle. The thimble electrode pushes the sternocleidomastoid medially and directs the current posteriorly. Presence or absence of diaphragmatic contraction is observed. Intact conduction produces a dramatic and easily recognized contraction of the diaphragm. Measurement of the muscle action potential of the diaphragm, phrenic nerve conduction time (normal for adults, 7.5–10 msec), and fluoroscopy can be used. We find simple clinical inspection to be adequate. Failure to elicit a strong diaphragmatic contraction almost invariably indicates lack of viability of the phrenic nerve. In rare cases, the nerve cannot be stimulated percutaneously. If pacing is deemed critical, surgical exploration and direct stimulation of the nerve are pursued.

With spinal cord injury, it is common to have some improvement in phrenic nerve function over time. A patient initially dependent on a respirator may become capable of breathing spontaneously. For this reason, we wait at least 3 months after injury before accepting a patient into the pacing program. It usually takes this much time for recovery from injury to other organ systems and institution of effective respiratory, bowel, bladder, and skin protection and physical and psychologic rehabilitation, which is essential in the patient's future.

In some cases of injury lower than C3 that involve the C3–C5 areas where the cell bodies of the phrenic nerve are located, the phrenic nerves may be partially injured but still viable. Pacing may be indicated in some of these patients, although benefit may be limited. The decision must be considered with great care.

### Pulmonary Function

It is essential for diaphragmatic pacing that the ability of the lungs to oxygenate and ventilate be well preserved. Pacing cannot compensate for severe restrictive or obstructive lung disease. In most patients who undergo pacing, measured pulmonary function tests are normal or near normal.

### Chest Wall Configuration

Major deformities of the chest wall contraindicate pacing by interfering with ventilatory function.

### Diaphragm Function

The diaphragmatic muscle must be inherently sound. A primary muscular disorder is not appropriate for pacing. In

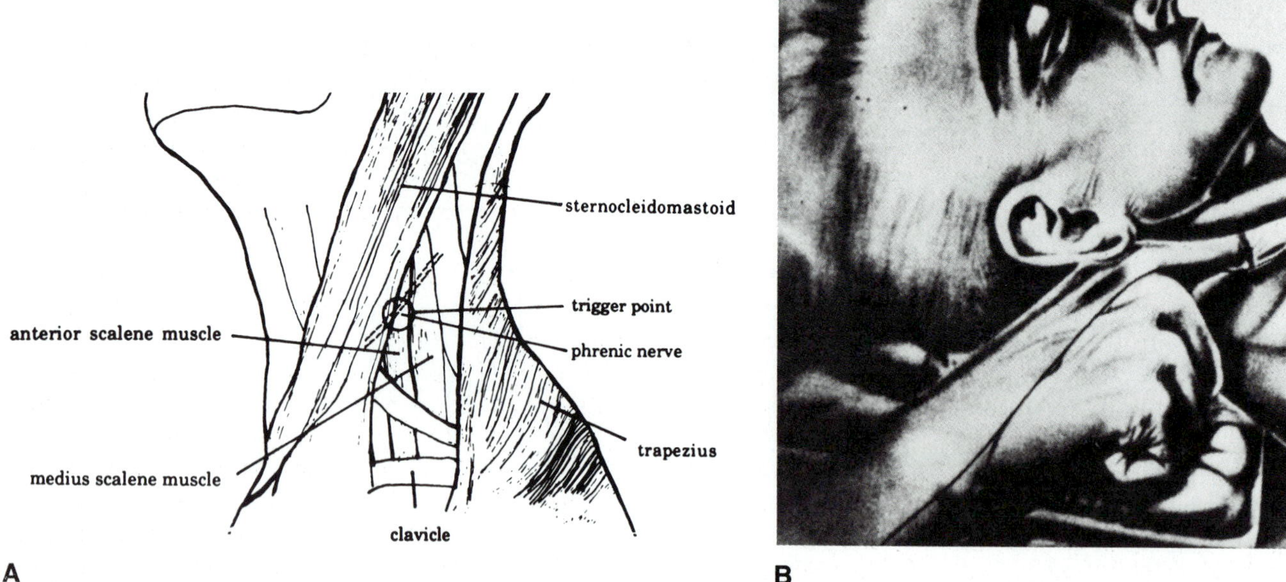


**Figure 36–9.** Testing for viability of the phrenic nerve by percutaneous electrical stimulation. **A.** The trigger point at the border of the clavicular head of the sternocleidomastoid muscle where the phrenic nerve is accessible to stimulation as it crosses the scalene muscles. **B.** Application of the thimble electrode. *(From Sarnoff SJ, et al: Electrophrenic respiration. VII. The motor point of the phrenic nerve in relation to external stimulation. Surg Gynecol Obstet 93:190–196, 1975.)*

central hypoventilation, we demonstrate at least a 5-cm excursion of the diaphragm with voluntary breathing before we attempt diaphragmatic pacing. In quadriplegic patients, a brisk downward deflection of the diaphragm with percutaneous stimulation of the phrenic nerve is sought. The atrophy of disuse of the diaphragm in quadriplegia can be corrected by gradual conditioning.

### *Psychosocial Factors*

Diaphragmatic pacing is not appropriate when the injury producing quadriplegia also results in permanent cortical injury and impaired cognitive capacity. Aside from important issues of health care allocation, brain damage prevents appreciation of many of the benefits of diaphragmatic pacing. For both patients with central hypoventilation and those with quadriplegia, an attentive and supportive family is essential to success.

## Techniques

### *Pulse-train Stimulation*

A cardiac pacemaker delivers a single stimulus, which produces a contraction of the entire heart, the electrical syncytium of the ventricular muscle. Skeletal muscles, including the diaphragm, behave differently. A single stimulus produces an ineffective contraction. A train of stimuli (Fig. 36–10) are required to produce a summated contraction that is mechanically effective. The pulse train stimulation has the following critical electrical parameters: rate (the overall number of pulse trains delivered per minute, corresponding, in diaphragmatic pacing, to the respiratory rate); amplitude (voltage of each stimulus in the train); frequency (in Hz, representing the timing of stimuli with a pulse train); current (in milliamperes); pulse width (the length of time that each stimulus is maintained); and pulse train duration (the

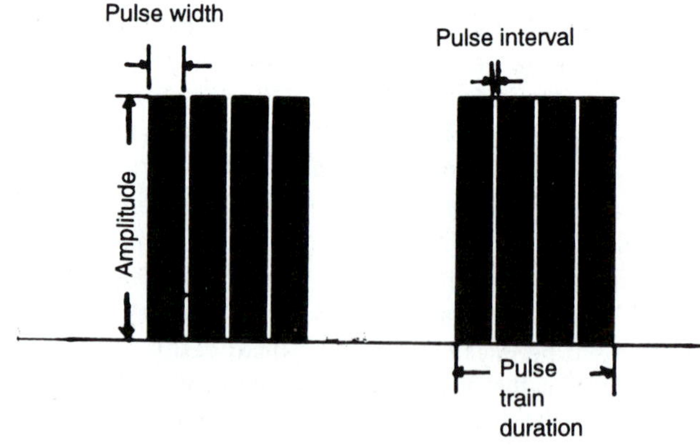


**Figure 36–10.** Pulse train stimulation. *(From Shields TW: General Thoracic Surgery, 4th ed. Baltimore, Williams & Wilkins, 1994, with permission.)*
Characteristics describing pulse train stimulation are as follows:
*rate* (bpm): overall number of pulse trains delivered per minute;
*amplitude* (V): voltage of each stimulus in pulse train;
*pulse width* (ms): duration of an individual pulse;
*pulse interval* (ms): duration between pulses in a train;
*frequency* (Hz): timing of stimuli with a pulse train [frequency (Hz) = 1000/pulse interval]; and
*pulse train duration* (ms): overall duration of one train of pulses.

length of time that the pulses continue at the prescribed frequency, corresponding, in diaphragmatic pacing, to the inspiration duration.) The frequency can also be expressed by its inverse, the pulse interval (i.e., frequency (Hz) = 1000 msec/pulse interval, so that 40 msec corresponds to 25 Hz, 90 msec to 11.1 Hz, 110 msec to 9.1 Hz, etc.). The elicited muscle contraction lasts only for the duration of the pulse train.

Stimulation of the diaphragm or other skeletal muscle by pulse trains over time results in an orderly sequence of histologic, ultrastructural, and biochemical changes.[75,76] Vascular supply increases, enzyme patterns change, and mitochondrial capacity increases. These changes reflect transformation from a mixture of fast (glycolytic) and slow (oxidative) muscle fibers to exclusively slow fibers. The transition to oxidative fibers allows sustained mechanical work. No nondiaphragmatic skeletal muscle is able to sustain mechanical work continuously without such conditioning (for example, no one can do push-ups 24 hours a day, day after day). Although in its normal function the diaphragm works 24 hours a day, the pattern of recruitment of individual nerve fascicles and motor units (tens to hundreds of muscle fibers per axon) is such that many motor units are dormant during an individual breath, allowing metabolic recovery. With the pulse train stimulation of diaphragmatic pacing, most or all nerve fascicles and all muscle groups are stimulated maximally during each breath, necessitating the adaptive changes described. In addition, in quadriplegia the diaphragm has often atrophied from disuse during mechanical ventilation and must be gradually restored to a functional state.

### Apparatus

The generator for diaphragmatic pacing remains outside the body (Fig. 36–11). A table model, about the size of a clock radio, and a portable model, about the size of a personal cassette player are available. The output from the generator is carried to an antenna, the coil of which is taped securely to the patient's skin over the receiver site. The implanted receiver, about the size and shape of a pocket watch, lies under the skin over the flat portion of the lower anterolateral ribcage. The antenna transmits a signal by radiofrequency to the implanted receiver, which generates, by means of inductive coupling, a stimulating signal. The receiver stimulates the phrenic nerve by means of an electrode placed under the nerve. Despite the external position of the generator and the inductive coupling arrangement for transmission of the signal to the body, the system is reliable and easy to use.

The electrode is a half-cuff or 180° model developed at Yale for diaphragmatic pacing (Fig. 36–12) and subsequently used in other applications. We prefer not to surround the nerve circumferentially because of potential for entrapment and encircling cicatrix (Fig. 36–13). In a detailed study of the thoracodorsal nerve, we found no disadvantage in terms of the adequacy of stimulation by a 180° compared with a 360° electrode.[77]

### Commercial Devices

There is currently only one manufacturer of diaphragm pacemakers approved for clinical use in the United States (Avery Laboratories, Glen Cove, NY). The early model (I107A) has been well tested in the clinical situation but has exhibited premature receiver failure due to deficiencies in hermetic sealing. This problem has led to a need for frequent receiver changes.[78] The later model (I110A) is borrowed from a pain control application. Although approved for diaphragmatic use, this device remains unproved for life-sustaining application. In our laboratory we have demonstrated an uncoupling of the external antenna from the subcutaneously implanted receiver with only small displacements (1–2 cm) of the magnitude commonly expected in clinical practice. We are currently gaining experience with a device manufactured in Finland (Atrotec OY, Tampere, Finland), which is approved for clinical investigation. Early experience has been favorable.

Low volume of implantation and low profit potential has limited the development of equipment, which has lagged behind that of cardiac pacemakers. Development of a fully implantable system, as in cardiac pacing, would be an important advance. The feasibility of such a system has been demonstrated in the laboratory at Yale.[79] The requirement for pulse train stimulation complicates design characteristics beyond those for cardiac pacing. Rate-responsive diaphragmatic pacing in which sensor-based feedback technology is used, as in modern cardiac pacing, is an exciting possibility for the future.

### Surgical Procedure

Initially many implants of the electrode were done in the neck. We now implant the electrode in the chest, because in some patients accessory radicles (originating below the C3–5 level) join the phrenic nerve late and would not be stimulated by an electrode in the neck[80] (Fig. 36–14).

A minithoracotomy is done anteriorly in the second or third intercostal space (Fig. 36–15). The pectoral muscle is split in the direction of its fibers. The internal mammary artery and vein are divided to avoid disruption during spreading of the interspace. A flat spot is identified on the mediastinum above the heart where the phrenic nerve is accessible and where the electrode can sit comfortably. Extreme care is taken in handling the nerve—injury is disastrous. The mediastinal pleura is incised parallel to the nerve and several millimeters away from the nerve and its nutrient vessels; this is done anterior and posterior to the nerve. The electrode is slipped atraumatically behind the mobilized phrenic structures, so that the phrenic bundle rests inside the half-cuff platinum contact of the electrode. Minor oozing from the artery or vein that accompanies the nerve is not treated, because it stops spontaneously and cautery could injure nerve fibers. The Silastic (polymeric silicone) por-

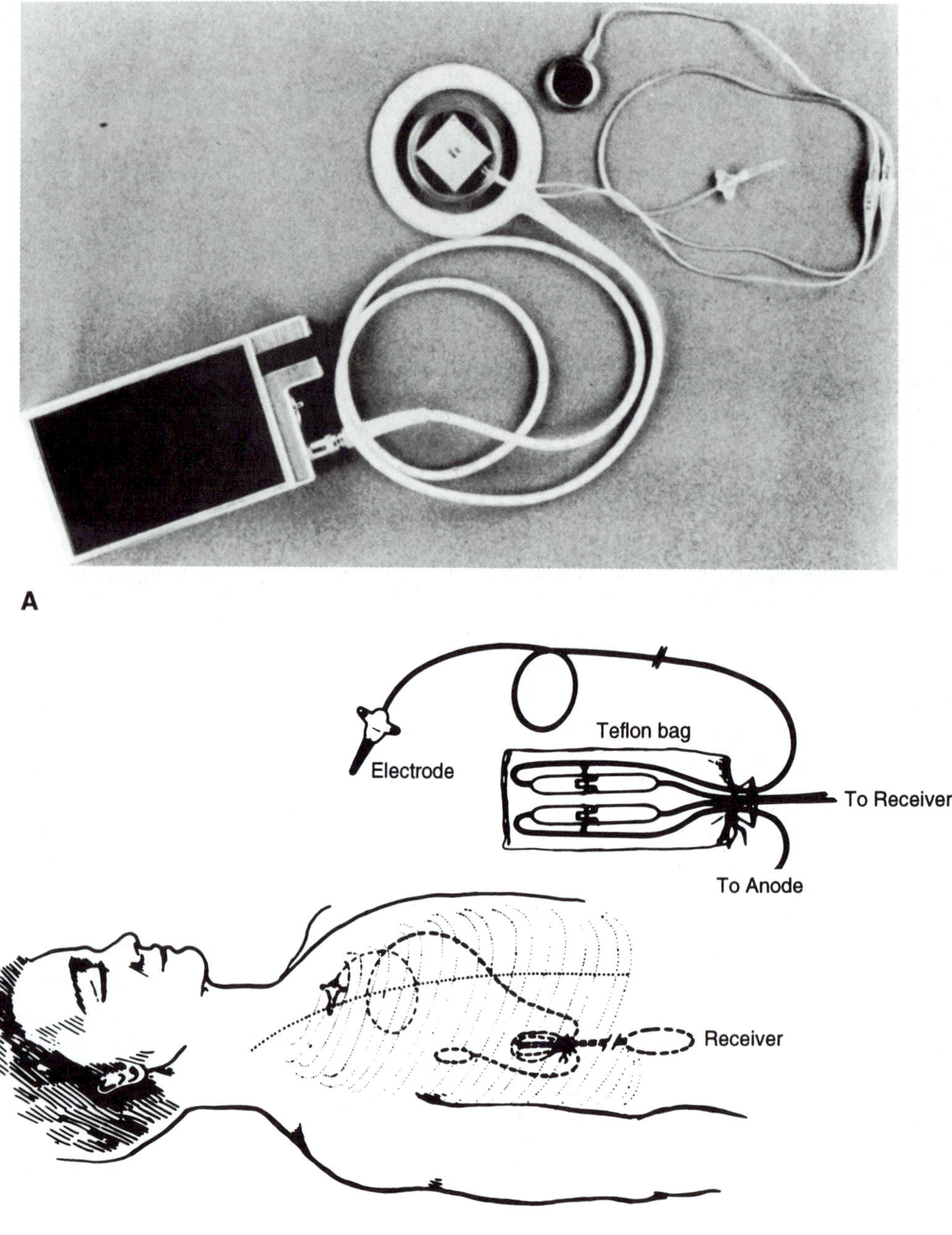


**Figure 36–11.** The apparatus for diaphragmatic pacing. **A.** The hardware: transmitter, external antenna, implantable receiver, and phrenic nerve electrode. The transmitter remains outside the body, as does the antenna, which is taped securely to the skin over the implanted receiver. **B.** Equipment in place in patient. Phrenic nerve electrode is placed at the level of the upper thorax. The implanted receiver is situated over a flat portion of the lower chest wall. *(From Shields TW: General Thoracic Surgery, 4th ed. Baltimore, Williams & Wilkins, 1994, with permission.)*

tions of the electrode are secured to the pleura that overlies the mediastinum. Perfect lie of the electrode must be obtained, with no distortion or traction on the nerve. Distortion or traction could result in injury to or dysfunction of the nerve. With careful technique, we have not seen an iatrogenic injury to or dysfunction of the nerve in many years, although this has been common in centers with limited experience.[81]

The end of the electrode is passed through the chest wall (atraumatically in a chest tube carrier) into a pocket made through a separate incision over a flat portion of the anterolateral lower rib cage. Some redundant wire is looped gently on the surface of the lung within the thorax. Three separate subpockets are made, one for the receiver, one for the indifferent electrode (the "can" is not the indifferent electrode, unlike the arrangement with unipolar cardiac pacemakers), and the junction box (the connection between the receiver and the wires from the nerve electrode and the indifferent electrode). The junction box and excess wire

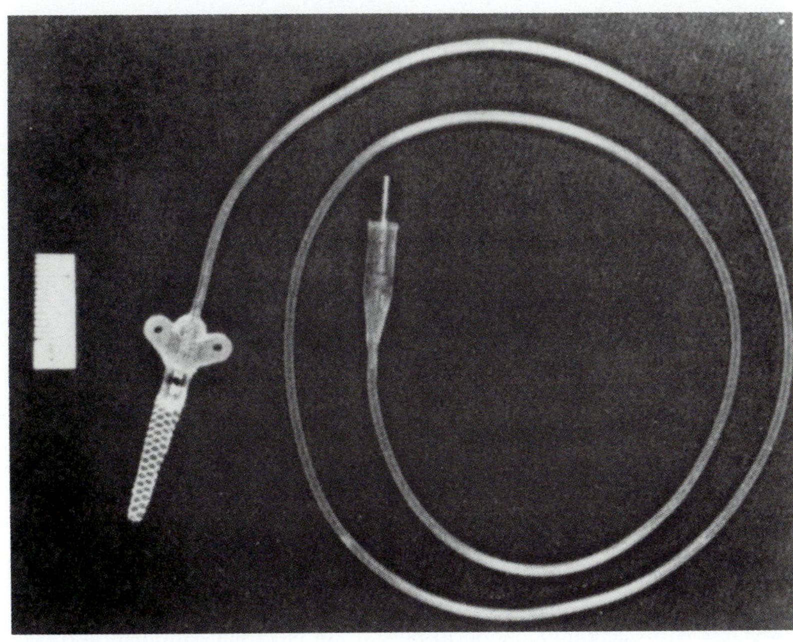

**Figure 36–12.** Detail of 180° phrenic nerve electrode. *(From Shields TW: General Thoracic Surgery, 4th ed. Baltimore, Williams & Wilkins, 1994, with permission.)*

lengths are secured inside a Teflon (polytetrafluoroethylene) bag; the wires are very fine, much more so than cardiac pacing wires, and inclusion in the Teflon bag facilitates safe access at the time of receiver change. It is essential that the copper coil on the receiver and the metal plate of the indifferent electrode face outward, away from the body. This optimizes communication between the external antenna and the receiver and avoids stimulation of chest wall muscles. The subpockets are closed tightly, because the position of the components must be very stable. As with any subcutaneous implantation of foreign bodies, the incision is kept away from the implanted hardware to prevent pressure on the incision, improper healing, or extrusion.

A test of the system is conducted with a sterile antenna passed to an off-table transmitter to confirm function before undraping. Excellent contraction of the diaphragm with pacing should be confirmed. Threshold should be 1.0–2.0 mA. Failure to pace or a high threshold requires re-evaluation of connections, wires, and lead position, and exclusion of extraneous tissue in the half-cuff electrode.

We use prophylactic antibiotics to prevent infection, which would be disastrous if the nerve were involved. The right and left implantations are done about 2 weeks apart.

### *Electrical and Ventilatory Settings*

Inspiration duration (1.3 sec) and pulse width (150 μsec) are preset at the factory. Inspiration duration can be adjusted to 0.6 sec for children. Respiratory rate is selected individually for each patient. For bilateral pacing in adults, we aim for 6–10 breaths per minute. For unilateral pacing, higher rates are required, usually 12–14 breaths per minute.

Current is set according to fluoroscopic testing with

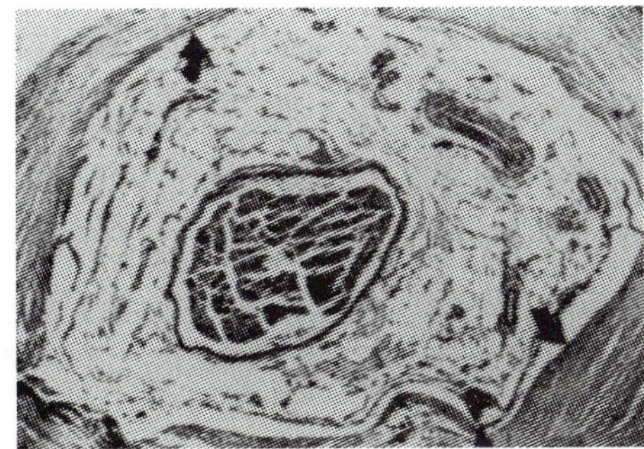

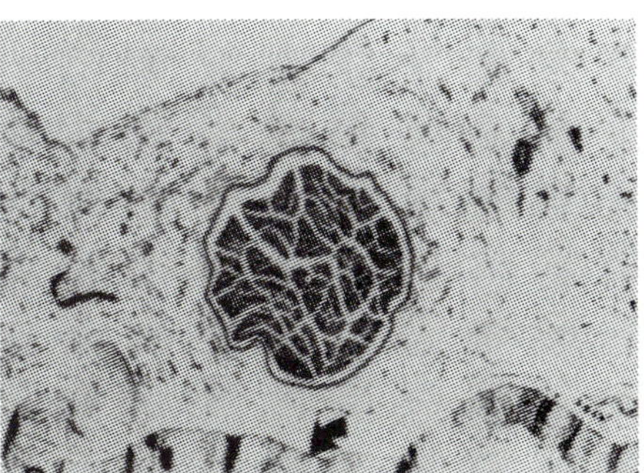

**Figure 36–13.** Histologic section of phrenic nerve after long-term stimulation with a 360° electrode (**left**) and a 180° electrode (**right**) (hematoxylin and eosin stain, × 39.) Note circumferential fibrous cicatrix that occurred with 360° electrode only. 180° electrode elicits only a band of fibrous tissue on side facing the nerve. Although both nerve fascicles are normal, the potential for damage with the 360° configuration is suggested. *(From Kim JH, et al: Light and electron microscopic studies of phrenic nerves after long-term electrical stimulation. J Neurosurg 58:85, 1980, with permission.)*

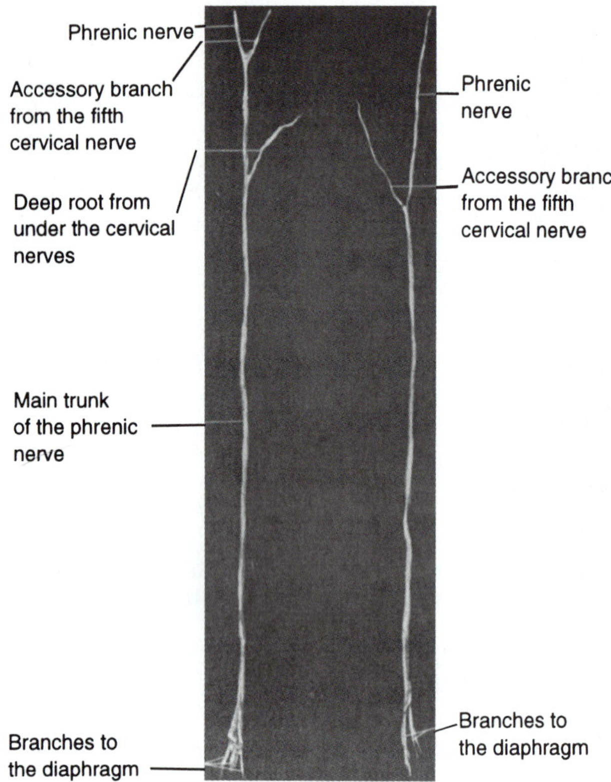


**Figure 36–14.** Phrenic nerves removed with exeresis. This was practiced in the early 20th century in the treatment of apical tuberculosis. To completely paralyze the diaphragm, surgeons found it necessary to remove all branches of the phrenic nerve. This they accomplished by avulsing the nerves in the neck. The *nebenphrenicus* is probably the branch of the fifth cervical nerve, the so-called accessory branch, shown here joining the other branches at a high level on the right side and a low level on the left. On the left side, such a branch would probably not be stimulated by an electrode placed in a cervical location. The specimen from the right side illustrates a branch from the lower cervical cord joining the main trunk. This branch certainly would be missed by stimulation from a cervical location. *(From Glenn WWL, Sairenji H: Diaphragm pacing in the treatment of chronic ventilatory insufficiency. In Roussos C, Macklem PT [eds]: Thorax, Part B. New York, Marcel Dekker, 1985 p 1434.)*

the patient in the supine position conducted before institution of pacing and at intervals thereafter. A standardized radiographic system is used that can be reproduced from time to time and from patient to patient. A ruler with lead numerals 1 through 12 is placed behind the patient with the 1 at the dome of the diaphragm. With the x-ray distance kept constant at 30 cm, reproducible readings result. In our standard fluoroscopic test, we first determine maximum voluntary descent of each diaphragm (for patients with central hypoventilation; patients with quadriplegia usually are not capable of spontaneous diaphragmatic motion). Movement of 8–10 cm is usual for adults. Subsequently, testing of paced ventilation is conducted to determine threshold current (that current which produces a just-discernible contraction of the diaphragm) and current for maximal excursion. The maximal descent of the diaphragm by pacing is recorded for future comparison. For clinical conduct of pacing, the current is set just above the current for maximal excursion.

### *Conduct of Pacing*

Pacing can be done unilaterally, bilaterally on alternate sides (usually at 12-hour intervals), or bilaterally simultaneously. Although unilateral pacing may suffice for selected patients, especially in central alveolar hypoventilation, our preference since the introduction of conditioning to low-frequency stimulation has been for bilateral pacing, usually aiming for 24-hour continuous stimulation.

Pacing is not begun until 2 weeks after the implantations. We found that earlier pacing leads to pleural effusion, possibly from disruption of immature adhesions by the strong diaphragmatic contraction.

A program of gradual conditioning is used to restore diaphragms atrophied by disuse (quadriplegia) and allows accommodation to pulse-train electrical stimulation (quadriplegia and central alveolar hypoventilation). This adaptation takes weeks to months. For patients with quadriplegia, pacing is begun at 15 minutes per waking hour and gradually increased to 30 minutes. The pacing period is gradually increased, each pacing period followed by an equal period of rest on the ventilator. When the pacing period reaches 12 hours, the rest period is gradually and progressively shortened until full-time pacing is achieved. Changes in pacing period are made about every 7–14 days depending on patient tolerance. With increases in pacing period, the frequency of stimuli in the pulse train is decreased progressively (usually to about 7.1 Hz), to minimize diaphragmatic fatigue and allow longer pacing periods. Concurrently, the number of respirations is decreased progressively to the minimum number for adequate ventilation (usually 7–8 breaths per min in adults), again to decrease fatigue. (To maintain adequacy of ventilation in patients with quadriplegia when they sit, a snug abdominal binder is applied, and respiratory rate is increased by 1 breath per minute.) The conditioning phase usually requires 3–6 months, longer with quadriplegia patients. Patients with central hypoventilation can be advanced more quickly, because their diaphragms are not atrophied.

Tidal volume, minute ventilation, end-tidal partial pressure of carbon dioxide ($PCO_2$), and oxygen saturation are monitored regularly, at the beginning and end of each pacing period, and hourly during pacing. Monitoring is done noninvasively with oxygen saturation and carbon dioxide monitors, and the results are correlated periodically with arterial blood-gas values.

A fall in tidal volume and a rise in carbon dioxide is evidence of diaphragmatic fatigue, unless there is a correctable pulmonary problem. The patient is rested on mechanical ventilation at least overnight, and pacing is resumed with a shorter pacing period.

In patients with central hypoventilation who require

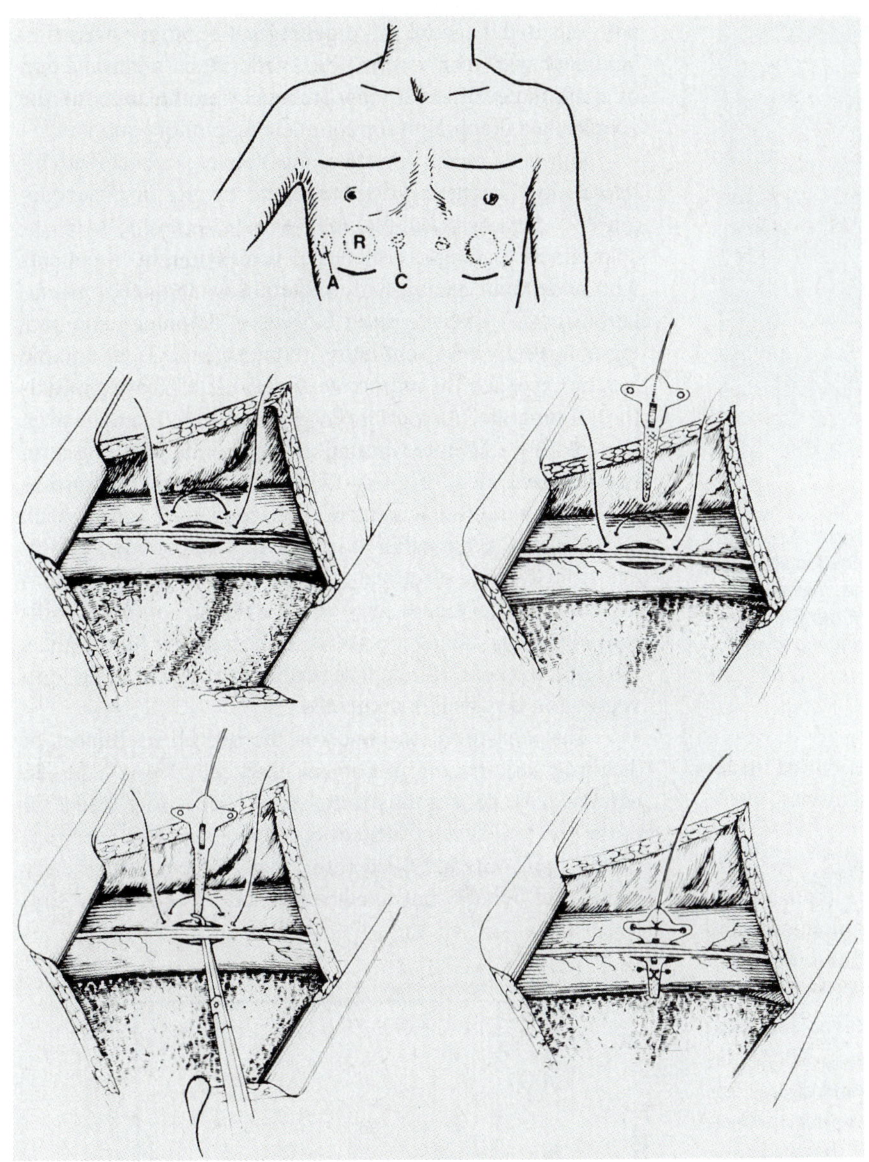


**Figure 36–15.** Transthoracic approach to the phrenic nerves for diaphragmatic pacing. **Top.** Incisions in the second interspace for nerve access. Incisions at costal margin for implantation of receiver (**R**), anode plate (**A**), and connectors (**C**). **Middle and bottom.** Sequential steps in implantation of 180° electrode behind the phrenic nerve.

only part-time (nocturnal) ventilation, the schedule can be implemented immediately and fully, because the period off pacing is adequate to prevent diaphragmatic fatigue. For this part-time pacing, high-frequency pacing (20–25 Hz; pulse interval, 40–50 msec) suffices.

### Aftercare

The operation to place the pacemaker is straightforward, but unlike a cardiac pacemaker, the device cannot be turned on and the patient discharged. Careful monitoring during adaptation is required. Even after hospital discharge, concerted and knowledgeable care is essential. Temporary stresses (infection, intercurrent illness, operations related to cutaneous, urologic, or orthopedic complications of quadriplegia) can tax the reserve of diaphragmatic pacing, which does not automatically adjust to increased respiratory requirements, and lead to the need for positive pressure ventilation. Once positive pressure ventilation is begun, without involvement of the original diaphragmatic pacing center, mechanical ventilation is perpetuated as a crutch.

### Tracheostomy

The care of all patients with diaphragmatic pacing is made safer and easier with permanent tracheostomy. Pacing can produce upper airway obstruction by extremely vigorous diaphragmatic contraction combined with lack of coordination with the phasic muscles of the upper airway. For this reason, we ask patients to leave the stoma open during sleep. Periodic dysfunction of the system may occur, and the tracheostomy provides a secure access for positive pressure ventilation during such times.

Once full-time ventilation is achieved and secure, we substitute a Teflon tracheal button (Fig. 36–16) for the conventional tracheostomy tube. This device maintains the airway but has the advantages of better cosmetics (hardly visible when in place), normal speech, and reduced tracheal

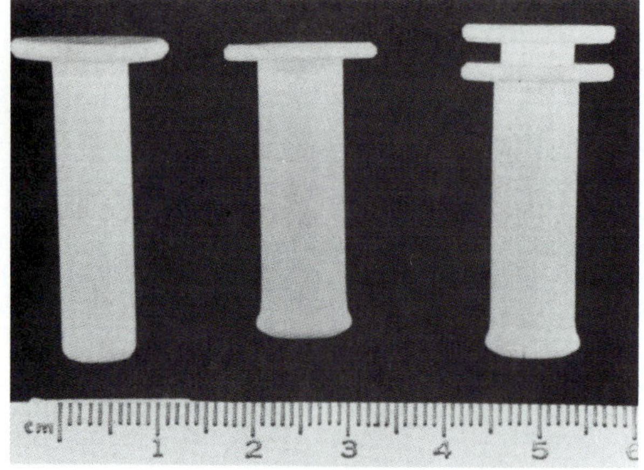


**Figure 36–16.** The tracheal button used to replace the tracheostomy tube. **Left.** Inner plug. **Middle.** Open tube. **Right.** The two components assembled together. The flange of the button sits flush with the skin when the button is in place in the stoma, maintaining patency indefinitely but being minimally apparent. *(From Glenn WWL, et al: Long-term ventilatory support by diaphragm pacing in quadriplegia. Ann Surg 183:566, 1976.)*

irritation and injury. The inner plug of the button is removed during sleep to assure an unobstructed airway.

### *Pacing in Infants and Young Children*

Hunt, Brouillette, and Weese-Mayer[81–85] and their associates clarified characteristics specific to pacing in infants and young children. Their experience with 32 patients with predominantly congenital central hypoventilation demonstrates that pacing is effective (22 of 32 patients survived and most were rehabilitated adequately to return home). These authors established that pacing of one diaphragm is poorly tolerated (excess mediastinal motion), that a shorter inspiration duration (0.6 sec) is more efficient, and that full-time bilateral pacing in infants or young children is not feasible. For pacing during sleep, a rate of 16 breaths per minute is used; the rate is increased to 18–25 breaths per minute for pacing during waking hours. The difference in tolerance for duration of pacing compared with the situation in adults has been attributed to immaturity of the musculoskeletal apparatus for breathing.[86] By the age of 8–10 years, goals and techniques of pacing approximate those for adults. These patients use oxygen saturation and end-tidal carbon dioxide monitoring at home after hospital discharge for continued quantitative assessment of adequacy of oxygenation and ventilation during the diaphragmatic pacing regimen.

## Results

Effectiveness of diaphragmatic pacing has been demonstrated conclusively since 1970, when Glenn et al first achieved total ventilatory support of a quadriplegic patient with complete respiratory paralysis.[87] This required alternate-side pacing—bilateral high-frequency ventilation was not tolerated because of diaphragmatic fatigue. Another landmark was achieved in 1980, with Glenn's introduction of continuous bilateral, low-frequency stimulation of the conditioned diaphragm for complete respiratory support.[88]

Our most recent review of the Yale experience with bilateral, low-frequency diaphragmatic pacing in quadriplegia[89,90] demonstrated the long-term effectiveness of diaphragmatic pacing as a means of ventilation. In 14 patients who underwent pacing with bilateral low-frequency stimulation for 2–10 years (mean 6.5 years) diaphragmatic pacing completely met ventilatory requirements. Tidal volume met or exceeded the requirements calculated from the Radford nomogram.[91] Arterial blood gases were maintained in normal range. Minute ventilation was maintained long-term without decrement (Fig. 36–17). Pacing parameters (threshold and maximum) remained unchanged over time, which was evidence against theoretic concerns[92] about nerve damage from chronic electrical stimulation. The limited pathologic material available showed no evidence of any significant histologic damage to nerve, diaphragm, or lungs. Thus, the effectiveness of diaphragmatic pacing for long-term ventilation was well documented.

The next question concerns the overall usefulness of diaphragmatic pacing in clinical practice.[81,93] At Yale, 86 patients have undergone pacing since 1966. More than 93% of the patients have benefited. In 38 patients (44%) the ventilatory goal was achieved fully. Partial success (clinically significant benefit, but another method of ventilatory sup-

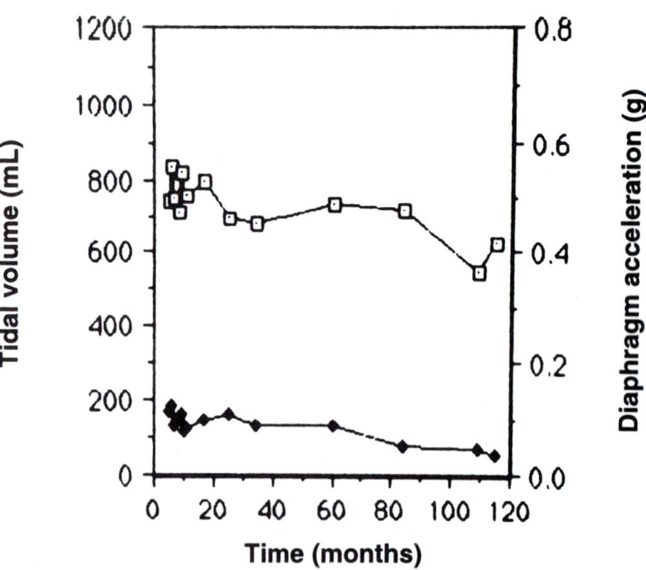


**Figure 36–17.** Ten-year assessment of tidal volume and diaphragmatic acceleration in a patient with quadriplegia. (Open squares denote tidal volume and closed diamonds denote diaphragmatic acceleration.) Tidal volume is well-maintained over time. Diaphragmatic acceleration remains at the desired low levels as well, signifying that the conditioned state of the diaphragmatic muscle is maintained (with conditioning to oxidative metabolism, fibers become slow twitch). *(From Shields TW: General Thoracic Surgery, 4th ed. Baltimore, Williams & Wilkins, 1994, with permission.)*

port also required) was obtained in another 42 patients (49%). Pacing-related complications (overpacing, underpacing, and phrenic nerve injury, which are avoidable by current techniques) occurred in 8 of 86 patients (9.3%). After the recognition of the benefits of bilateral, low-frequency stimulation, the treatment of a number of patients, including some with central alevolar hypoventilation, was converted to this modality after pacing for variable periods on one side at a time.

Glenn et al reviewed the worldwide experience with diaphragm pacing.[81] Four hundred seventy-seven patients underwent implantation of a diaphragmatic pacemaker. Detailed analysis was confined to 165 patients from six major centers for whom complete data were available. Preoperative transcutaneous phrenic nerve stimulation in the neck was a reliable predictor of phrenic nerve viability. Pacing was applied during sleep only in 46% of patients, part-time night or day or both in 15%, and full-time in 27%. Eleven percent of patients did not undergo pacing for long periods of time. Compromised function of the phrenic nerve deemed related to the procedure or electrode was seen in 13% of patients. The incidence of nerve injury or dysfunction was lowest with a half-cuff electrode placed in the chest (3.7%). We have not seen this complication in the last 12 years at Yale; thoracic implantation of a half-cuff electrode is our preferred approach. Infection occurred in 4.5% of surgical procedures. The overall success of diaphragmatic pacing in meeting ventilatory needs was complete success, 47%; clinically significant ventilatory support, 36%; failure or minimal support, 17%. Fifty-nine percent of the patients were alive at the time of follow-up studies.

Another important question is whether diaphragmatic pacing produces better results than other therapeutic modalities. In particular, it can be asked whether diaphragmatic pacing improves clinical status or life-expectancy in central hypoventilation or in high quadriplegia. In central hypoventilation, without pacing, progressive respiratory deterioration is common. Death from hypoventilation may occur. Patients who do survive have sequelae of prolonged hypoventilation and hypoxia, including permanent cerebral dysfunction and cor pulmonale. No effective medical treatment of central hypoventilation is known. Positive pressure ventilation, either intermittently or continuously, is the only alternative for life-threatening hypoventilation. Treatment of central hypoventilation by positive pressure ventilation seems to impinge on quality of life, but direct comparison with diaphragmatic pacing has not been done. Likewise, it would seem that diaphragmatic pacing would prolong life and forestall complications, but no controlled comparative studies exist.

With quadriplegia as well no controlled comparative studies of pacing as opposed to mechanical ventilation have been performed. Such studies would require multi-institutional organization, given the relatively small numbers of patients treated by pacing. In the absence of controlled studies, some inferences can be drawn. Other centers have reported positive experiences.[63,94–97] Carter et al compared their experience over 17 years in treating patients with spinal cord injuries with mechanical ventilation (19 patients) or diaphragmatic pacing (18 patients).[98] Overall mortality was not statistically significantly different—a 39% survival rate with pacing as opposed to 32% with mechanical ventilation. The most recent review from that same group points more strongly to a survival advantage for the patients who undergo diaphragmatic pacing.[99] Our data[89,90] on continuous, bilateral, low-frequency stimulation in quadriplegia shows an excellent survival rate—100% at 9 years among patients who completed a pacing protocol. This exceeds the 63% 9-year survival rate expected from the data of Carter et al on mechanical ventilation.

### Advantages of Diaphragmatic Pacing

Diaphragmatic pacing offers a number of advantages over positive pressure ventilation.[69,98,100,101]

1. *Increased independence.* First and foremost is the increased independence afforded by freedom from a ventilator. Patients with central hypoventilation can walk and those with quadriplegia can travel to school or work. The portable units are about the size and shape of the telemetric transmitters for monitoring heart rate and rhythm. Recently a patient with hypoventilation came to Yale requiring 24-hour positive pressure ventilation in an intensive care unit. After successful institution in 24-hour bilateral diaphragmatic pacing, he was discharged fully ambulatory and able to return to work full time. Many other pacing patients travel regularly for work, school, or pleasure.
2. *Improved speech.* With diaphragmatic pacing, the tracheostomy tube is replaced by a tracheal button. This restores a closed and unobstructed airway. Normal speech is again possible; the movement of air during expiration provides the substrate for speech. For patients incapacitated by high quadriplegia, restoration of speech is tantamount to liberation from isolation.
3. *Avoidance of tracheal injury.* The problems of long-term intubation of the trachea—stenosis, malacia, esophageal fistula, and chronic infection—are common, serious, life-threatening, and often impossible to correct. These problems are eliminated with diaphragmatic pacing. The tracheal button is noninjurious and nonirritating.
4. *Physiologic negative pressure ventilation.* Unlike mechanical ventilation, diaphragmatic pacing allows negative pressure inspiration, the normal inspiratory mechanism of the body. Troublesome recurrent lower lobe atelectasis, so common in patients who undergo long-term positive pressure ventilation, virtually disappears when diaphragmatic pacing is instituted.
5. *Avoidance of sudden death due to ventilator problems.* Sudden death due to tracheostomy occlusion or dis-

lodgment, disconnection of the ventilator tubing, primary malfunction of the ventilator, or power loss is a common terminal event in patients on a positive pressure ventilator. Patients with quadriplegia, especially, cannot correct such problems because of their immobility. If no attendant is immediately available, the patient may die. Diaphragmatic pacing eliminates the risk of these problems.

6. *Possibility of improvement in life expectancy.* Although conclusive data from controlled studies are not available, our experience suggests that diaphragmatic pacing improves survival over that expected with mechanical ventilation.

## Goals

### *Technical Improvement in Stimulating Apparatus*

A fully implantable diaphragmatic pacing system would constitute an important advance. Current systems are asynchronous with respect to the native respiratory pattern. Development of a demand-type unit is certainly feasible. Furthermore, as with sensor-based cardiac pacemakers, a physiologically responsive system for diaphragmatic pacing that increases rate with increasing respiratory requirement would clearly be feasible. The small number of diaphragmatic pacemakers used each year has limited profit potential, so commercial investment has been limited. Improved pacing systems for the diaphragm may emerge as a byproduct of the intensive investigation of pacing of skeletal muscle for cardiac support.[102] Current systems for diaphragm pacing do not incorporate alarms. Pulse oximetry may be an easy and effective approach to detect malfunctions or other serious problems with ventilation in the diaphragm pacing patient.[103]

### *Comparative Clinical Trials*

Direct comparison of diaphragmatic pacing with other modalities in both central hypoventilation and quadriplegia is necessary. In central hypoventilation, comparison with medical management and mechanical ventilation can be carried out. In quadriplegia, no medical management is feasible for patients with apnea; comparison would necessarily be with mechanical ventilation. Collaborative studies involving multiple institutions would be required for reliable conclusions.

## ACKNOWLEDGMENT

Appreciation is expressed to Dr. William W. L. Glenn, Charles W. Ohse Professor Emeritus of Surgery at Yale University, the father of diaphragmatic pacing, who taught and continues to teach the art of diaphragmatic pacing to the clinical team at Yale University and who was primary author of the chapter on diaphragmatic pacing in the earlier edition of this book.

## REFERENCES

1. Lieberman DA, Faulkner JA, Craig AB Jr, Maxwell LC: Performance and histochemical composition of guinea pig and human diaphragm. *J Appl Physiol* **34**:233, 1973
2. DeTroyer A, Sampson M, Sigrist S, Macklem PT: Action of costal and crural parts of the diaphragm on the rib cage in dog. *J Appl Physiol* **53**:30, 1982
3. Rochester DF: The diaphragm: Contractile properties and fatigue. *J Clin Invest* **75**:1397, 1985
4. Osmond DG: Functional anatomy of the chest wall. In Roussos C, Macklem PT (eds): *The Thorax,* Part A. In Lenfant C (ed): *Lung Biology in Health and Disease,* Vol 29. New York, Marcel Dekker, 1985, pp 199–233
5. Edwards RHT, Faulkner JA: Structure and functions of the respiratory muscle. In Roussos C, Macklem PT (eds): *The Thorax,* Part A. In Lenfant C (ed): *Lung Biology in Health and Disease,* vol 29. New York, Marcel Dekker, 1985, pp 297–326
6. Newson-Davis J, Goldman M, Loh L, Casson M: Diaphragm function and alveolar hypoventilation. *Q J Med* **45**:87, 1976
7. Robotham JL: A physiological approach to hemidiaphragm paralysis. *Crit Care Med* **7**:563, 1979
8. Wang CS, Josenhaus WT: Contribution of the diaphragmatic/abdominal displacement to ventilation in supine man. *J Appl Physiol* **31**:576, 1971
9. Camfferman F, Bogaard JM, Van de Meche FGA, Hilvering C: Idiopathic bilateral diaphragm paralysis. *Eur J Respir Dis* **67**:65, 1985
10. Celli BR, Rassulo J, Corral R: Ventilatory muscle dysfunction in patients with bilateral idiopathic diaphragmatic paralysis: Reversal by intermittent external negative pressure ventilation. *Am Rev Respir Dis* **136**:1276, 1987
11. Shin MS, Ho KJ: Computed tomography evaluation of the pathologic lesion for idiopathic diaphragmatic paralysis. *J Comput Assist Tomogr* **6**:257, 1982
12. Shaw RK,Glenn WWL, Hogan JF, Phelps ML: Electrophysiological evaluation of phrenic nerve function in candidates for diaphragm pacing. *J Neurosurg* **53**:345, 1980
13. White JE, Bullock RE, Hudgson P, et al: Phrenic neuropathy in association with diabetes. *Diabetes Med* **9**(10):954–956, 1992
14. Laguent A, Ellie E, Saintarailles J, et al: Unilateral diaphragmatic paralysis: An electrophysiologic study. *J Neurol Neurosurg Psychiatry* **55**(4):316–318, 1992
15. Brown KA, Hoffstein V, Byrick RJ: Bedside diagnosis of bilateral diaphragmatic paralysis in a ventilatory dependent patient after open-heart surgery. *Anesth Analg* **64**:1208, 1985
16. Dajee A, Pellegrini J, Cooper G, Karlson K: Phrenic nerve palsy after topical cardiac hypothermia. *Int Surg* **68**:345, 1983
17. Esposito RA, Spencer FC: The effect of pericardial insulation on hypothermic phrenic nerve injury during open heart surgery. *Ann Thorac Surg* **43**:303, 1987
18. Wheeler WE, Rubis LJ, Jones CW, Harrah JD: Etiology and prevention of topical cardiac hypothermia-induced phrenic nerve injury and left lower lobe atelectasis during cardiac surgery. *Chest* **88**:680, 1985
19. DeVita MA, Robinson LR, Rehder J, et al: Incidence and natural history of phrenic neuropathy occurring during open heart surgery. *Chest* **103**(3):850–6, 1993
20. Laub GW, Muralidharan S, Chen C, et al: Phrenic nerve injury: A prospective study. *Chest* **100**(2):376–9, 1991
21. Avila JM, Peiffert B, Maureira JJ, et al: Reduction in the incidence of postoperative diaphragmatic paralysis by using a phrenic nerve protector. *Ann Chir* **45**(8):689–91, 1991

22. Efthimiou J, Butler J, Woodham C, et al: Diaphragm paralysis following cardiac surgery: Role of phrenic nerve cold injury. *Ann Thorac Surg* **52**(4):1005–8, 1991
23. O'Brien JW, Johnson SH, VanSteys SJ, et al: Effects of left internal mammary artery dissection on phrenic nerve perfusion and function. *Ann Thorac Surg* **52**(2):182–8, 1991
24. Werner RA, Geiringer SR: Bilateral phrenic nerve palsy associated with open-heart surgery. *Arch Phys Med Rehabil* **71**(12):100–2, 1990
25. Olopade CO, Staats BA: Time course of recovery from frostbitten phrenic nerve after coronary artery bypass graft surgery. *Chest* **99**(5):1112–5, 1991
26. Gordon PC, Bateman ED, Linton DM: Bilateral phrenic nerve palsy following cardiac surgery in a diabetic patient. *Anaesth Intensive Care* **20**(4):511–4, 1992
27. Diehl JL, Lofaso F, Deleuze P, et al: Clinically relevant diaphragmatic dysfunction after cardiac operations. *J Thorac Cardiovasc Surg* **107**(2):487–98, 1994
28. Setina M, Cerny S, Grim M, Pirk J: Anatomical interrelation between the phrenic nerve and the internal mammary artery as seen by the surgeon. *J Cardiovasc Surg (Torino)* **34**(6):499–502, 1993
29. Henriques-Pino J, Mendiola-Lagunas E, Prates JC: Origin of the internal thoracic artery and its relationship to the phrenic nerves. *Surg Radiol Anat* **15**(1):31–4, 1993
30. Lynn AM, Jenkins JG, Edmonds JF, Burns JE: Diaphragmatic paralysis after pediatric surgery: A retrospective analysis of 34 cases. *Crit Care Med* **11**:280, 1982
31. Stewart S, Alexson C, Manning J: Bilateral phrenic nerve paralysis after the Mustard procedure: Experience with four cases and recommendations for management. *J Thorac Cardiovasc Surg* **92**:138, 1986
32. Watanabe T, Trusler GA, Williams WG, et al: Phrenic nerve paralysis after pediatric surgery. *J Thorac Cardiovasc Surg* **94**:383, 1987
33. Mickell JJ, Oh KS, Siewers RD, et al: Clinical implications of postoperative unilateral phrenic nerve paralysis. *J Thorac Cardiovasc Surg* **76**:297, 1978
34. Sivak ED, Razau M, Groves LK, Loop FD: Long-term management of diaphragmatic paralysis complicating prosthetic valve replacement. *Crit Care Med* **11**:438, 1983
35. Mok Q, Ross-Russell R, Mulvey D, et al: Phrenic nerve injury in infants and children undergoing cardiac surgery. *Br Heart J* **65**(5):287–92, 1991
36. Russell RI, Mulvey D, Laroche C, et al: Bedside assessment of phrenic nerve function in infants and children. *J Thorac Cardiovasc Surg* **101**(1):143–7, 1991
37. Helps BA, Ross-Russell RI, Dicks-Mireau C, Elliot MJ: Phrenic nerve damage via a right thoracotomy in older children with secundum ASD. *Ann Thorac Surg* **56**(2):328–30, 1993
38. Lam DS, Ramos AD, Platzker AC, et al: Paralysis of diaphragm complicating venous alimentation. *Am J Dis Chest* **135**:382, 1981
39. Vest JV, Pereira M, Senior RM: Phrenic nerve injury associated with venipuncture of the internal jugular vein. *Chest* **78**:777, 1980
40. Armengaud MH, Trevoux-Paul J, Boucherie JC, Cousin MT: Diaphragmatic paralysis after puncture of the internal jugular vein. *Ann Fr Anesth Reanim* **10**(1):77–80, 1991
41. Pandit A, Kalra S, Woodcock A: An unusual cause of bilateral diaphragmatic paralysis. *Thorax* **47**(3):201, 1992
42. Tolge C, Iyer V, McConnell J: Phrenic nerve palsy accompanying chiropractic manipulation of the neck. *South Med J* **86**(6):688–90, 1993
43. Marcos JJ, Grover FL, Trinkle JK: Paralyzed diaphragm: Effect of plication on respiratory mechanics. *J Surg Res* **16**:523, 1974
44. Wright CD, Williams JG, Ogilvie CM, Donnelly RJ: Results of diaphragmatic plication for unilateral diaphragmatic paralysis. *J Thorac Cardiovasc Surg* **90**:195, 1985
45. Takeda S, Nakahara K, Fujii Y, et al: Effects of diaphragm plication for phrenic nerve paralysis on respiratory mechanics and diaphragm function. *Nippon Geka Gakkai Zasshi* **92**(9):1367–70, 1991
46. Brouillette RT, Hahn YS, Noah ZL, et al: Successful reinnervation of the diaphragm after phrenic nerve transection. *J Pediatr Surg* **21**:63, 1986
47. Merav AD, Attai LA, Condit DD: Successful repair of a transected phrenic nerve with restoration of diaphragmatic function. *Chest* **84**:642, 1983
48. Krieger AJ, Danetz I, Wu SZ, et al: Electrophrenic respiration following anastomosis of phrenic with brachial nerve in the cat. *J Neurosurg* **59**:262, 1983
49. Johnson V, Eiseman B: Reinforcement of ventilation with electrophrenic pacing of the paralyzed diaphragm. *J Thorac Cardiovasc Surg* **62**:651, 1971
50. Ambler R, Gruenwald S, John E: Ultrasound monitoring of diaphragm activity in bilateral diaphragmatic paralysis. *Arch Dis Child* **60**:170, 1985
51. McCauley RG, Labid KB: Diaphragmatic paralysis evaluated by phrenic nerve stimulation during fluoroscopy or real-time ultrasound. *Radiology* **153**:33, 1984
52. Newsom-Davis J: An experimental study of hiccup. *Brain* **93**:851, 1970
53. Nathan MD, Leshner RT, Keller AP Jr: Intractable hiccups (singultus). *Laryngoscope* **90**:1612, 1980
54. Samuels L: Hiccup: A ten year review of anatomy, etiology, and treatment. *Can Med Assoc J* **67**:315, 1952
55. Currier RD, Giles CL, DeJong RN: Some comments on Wallenberg's lateral medullary syndrome. *Trans Am Neurol Assoc* **85**:36, 1960
56. McFarling DA, Susac JO: Hoquet diabolique: Intractable hiccups as a manifestation of multiple sclerosis. *Neurology* **29**:797, 1979
57. Jacobson PL, Messenheimer JA, Farmer TW: Treatment of intractable hiccups with valproic acid. *Neurology* **29**:797, 1979
58. Williamson BW, MacIntyre IM: Management of intractable hiccups. *Br Med J* **2**:501, 1977
59. Sohn VZ, Conrad LJ, Katz R: Hiccup and ephedrine. *Can Anesth Soc J* **25**:431, 1978
60. Glenn WWL, Elefteriades JE: The diaphragm: Dysfunction and induced pacing. In Baue AE, Geha AS, Hammond GL, et al (eds): *Glenn's Thoracic and Cardiovascular Surgery,* 5th ed. Norwalk, Connecticut, Appleton & Lange, 1991, pp 531–568
61. Sweeney JD, Mortimer JT: An asymmetric two electrode cuff for generation of unidirectional propagated action potentials. *IEEE Trans Biomed Eng* 33:541, 1986
62. Hufeland CW: Usum uis electriciae in asphyxia experimentis illustratum. Dissertatio Inauguralis Medica, Göttingen, Germany, 1783
63. Talonen P: A more natural approach to nerve stimulation in electrophrenic respiration. Doctoral Thesis. Tampere University of Technology. Tampere, Finland, 1990
64. Patterson FLM: The Clydesdale experiments: An early attempt at resuscitation. *Scott Med J* **31**:050–052, 1986
65. Duchenne GBA: De l'ectrisation localisee et de son application a la pathologie et a le therapeutique par courant induits et par courants galvaniques interrompus et continus par le Dr. Duchenne. Paris, Balliere, 1872
66. Beard GM, Rockwell AD: A practical treatise on the medical and surgical uses electricity. New York, William Wood, 1878, pp 664–6
67. Isreal F: Uber die Wiederbelebung scheintoter Neugeborener mit Hilfe des elektrischen Stroms. *Z Geburtshilfe Perinatal* **91**:601–22, 1927
68. Sarnoff SJ, Maloney JV, Sarnoff LC, et al: Electrophrenic respiration in acute bulbar poliomyelitis. *JAMA.* **143**:1383–90, 1950
69. Maxon J, Shneerson JM: Diaphragmatic Pacing. *Am Rev Respir Dis* **148**:533–36, 1993
70. Glenn WWL, Gee BL, Schachter EN: Diaphragm pacing: Application to a patient with chronic obstructive pulmonary disease. *J Thoracic Cardiovasc Surg* **75**:273, 1978
71. Shneerson J: Sleep apnoeas. In: *Disorders of Ventilation.* Oxford, England, Blackwell Scientific, 1988, Chap 6

72. Whitehead GG, Carter RE, Charlifue SW, et al: A collaborative study of high quadriplegia. Grant Report, U.S. Department of Education, Rehabilitation Research and Demonstrations: Field Initiated Research. 1985 (Contract: Gayle Whiteneck, PhD, Craig Hospital, Englewood, Colorado)
73. Peterson DK, Nochomovitz M, DiMarco AF, et al: Intramuscular electrical activation of the phrenic nerve. *IEEE Trans Biomed Eng* **33:**342–51, 1986
74. Sarnoff SJ, Sarnoff LC, Whittenberger JL, et al: Electrophrenic respiration. VII. The motor point of the phrenic nerve in relation to external stimulation. *Surg Gynecol Obstet* **93:**190–5, 1951
75. Salmons S, Hendriksson J: The adaptive response of skeletal muscle to increased use. *Muscle Nerve* **4:**94–98, 1981
76. Mannion JD, Stephenson LW: Potential uses of skeletal muscle for myocardial assistance. *Surg Clin North Am* **65:**679–87, 1985
77. Letsou GV, Hogan JF, Lee P, et al: Comparison of 180-degree and 360-degree skeletal muscle nerve cuff electrodes. *Ann Thorac Surg* **54:**925–931, 1992
78. Weese-Mayer DE, Morrow AS, Brouillette RT, et al: Diaphragm pacing in infants and children: A life-table analysis of implanted components. *Am Rev Respir Dis* **139:**974–979, 1989
79. Hogan JF, Holcomb WG, Glenn WWL: A programmable, totally implantable, battery-powered diaphragm pacemaker: Design characteristics. In Saha S (ed): *Proceedings of the Fourth New England Bioengineering Conference.* Elmsford, NY, Pergamon, 1976, pp 221–223
80. Kelly WD: Phrenic nerve paralysis: Special consideration of the accessory nerve. *J Thorac Surg* **19:**923, 1950
81. Glenn WWL, Brouillette RT, Bezalel D, et al: Fundamental considerations in pacing of the diaphragm for chronic ventilatory insufficiency: A multi-center study. *Pace* **11:**2121–2122, 1988
82. Hunt CE, Matalon SV, Thompson TR, et al: Central hypoventilation syndrome: Experience with bilateral phrenic nerve pacing in 3 neonates. *Am Rev Respir Dis* **118:**23, 1978
83. Brouillette RT, Ilbalvi MN, Klemka-Walden L, et al: Stimulus parameters for phrenic nerve pacing in infants and children. *Pediatr Pulmonol* **4:**33, 1988
84. Weese-Mayer DE, Silvestri JM, Menzies LJ, et al: Congenital central hypoventilation syndrome: Diagnosis, management, and long-term outcome in thirty-two children. *J Pediatr* **120:**381–387, 1992
85. Weese-Mayer DE, Hunt CE, Brouillette RT, Silvestri JM: Diaphragm pacing in infants and children. *J Pediatr* **120:**1–8, 1992
86. Motoyama EK: Pulmonary mechanics during early postnatal years. *Pediatr Res* **11:**220–223, 1977
87. Glenn WWL, Holcomb WG, McLaughlin AJ, et al: Ventilatory support in a quadriplegic patient with radiofrequency electrophrenic respiration. *N Engl J Med* **286:**513, 1972
88. Glenn WWL, Hogan JF, Loke JSO, et al: Ventilatory support by pacing of the conditioned diaphragm in quadriplegia. *N Engl J Med* **310:**1150, 1984
89. Elefteriades JA, Hogan JF, Handler A, Loke JA: Long-term follow-up of bilateral pacing of the diaphragm in quadriplegia. *N Engl J Med* **326:**1433–1434, 1992
90. Elefteriades JA, Hogan JF, Handler A, Kim Y: Long-term follow-up of bilateral pacing of the conditioned diaphragm in quadriplegia. Submitted for publication
91. Radford EP, Ferris BG, Kriete BC: Clinical use of a nomogram to estimate proper ventilation during artificial respiration. *N Engl J Med* **251:**877–884, 1954
92. McCreery DB, Agnew WF: Mechanisms of stimulation-induced neural damage and their relation to guidelines for safe stimulation. In Agnew WF, McCreery DB (eds): *Neural Prostheses: Fundamental Studies.* Englewood Cliffs, New Jersey, Prentice-Hall, 1990, pp 297–313
93. Glenn WWL, et al: Twenty years of experience in phrenic nerve stimulation to pace the diaphragm. *Pace* **9:**780, 1986
94. Mayr W, Bijak, Girsch W, et al: Multichannel stimulation of phrenic nerves by epineural electrodes: Clinical experience and future developments. *ASAIO J* **39:**M729–M735, 1993
95. Brule JF, Leriche B, Normand J, et al: Phrenic nerve stimulation in respiratory paralysis after spinal cord injuries. *Neurochirurgie* **37:**127–32, 1991
96. Nakajima K, Sharkey PC: Electrophrenic respiration in patients with cranio-cervical trauma. *Stereotact Funct Neurosurg* **54:**233–36, 1990
97. Carter RE: Respiratory aspects of spinal cord injury management. *Paraplegia* **25:**262–266, 1987
98. Carter RE: Comparative study of electrophrenic nerve stimulation and mechanical ventilation in traumatic spinal cord injury. *Paraplegia* **25:**86–91, 1987
99. Carter RE: Experience with ventilator dependent patients. *Paraplegia* **31:**150–153, 1993
100. Elefteriades JA: Discussion of Miller JI, Farmer JA, Stuart W, Apple D. Phrenic nerve pacing in quadriplegia. *J Thorac Cardiovasc Surg* **99:**35–40, 1990
101. Tibbals J: Diaphragmatic pacing: An alternative to long-term mechanical ventilation. *Anesth Intensive Care* **19**(4):597–601, 1991
102. Higgins R, Letsou G, Detmer W, et al: Accessory skeletal muscle ventricles for circulatory support: Early experience with SMV's in continuity with the circulation. *Basic Appl Myol* **1:**89–94, 1991
103. Marzocchi M, Brouillette RT, Weese-Mayer DE, et al: Comparison of transthoracic impedance/heart rate monitoring and pulse oximetry for patients using diaphragm pacemakers. *Pediatr Pulmonol* **8:**29–32, 1990

CHAPTER

# 37

# The Mediastinum


Malcolm M. DeCamp, Jr,
Scott J. Swanson,
and David J. Sugarbaker


The mediastinum is strategically located between both pleural spaces. It extends from the neck to the diaphragm. It is traversed by the aerodigestive tract, the great vessels of the arterial, venous, and lymphatic circulation, and the autonomic nervous system. In addition to these organs, the mediastinum also contains cells that arise from the pharyngeal pouches, neural crest, and urogenital ridges in embryonic life. Because of the central location of the mediastinum and the diverse collection of organs close to it, an immense variety of benign and malignant mass lesions of the mediastinum come to the attention of thoracic surgeons. In many patients, resection offers the best chance of cure after an accurate tissue diagnosis is made. Many of these mass lesions arise from the heart, aorta, lungs, or esophagus or represent lymphatic extension of granulomatous disease or metastases from other carcinomas. These are important possibilities to be considered in the differential diagnosis of any mediastinal mass. Because they are more common, lesions of the heart, aorta, lungs, and esophagus are discussed extensively in other chapters. Our focus is primary neoplasms and cysts of the other mediastinal structures. Although none of these entities is singularly common, a systematic approach to the localization, diagnosis, staging (when indicated), and resection (when appropriate) of these lesions is proposed.

## HISTORY

A colorful history surrounds many of the surgically relevant mediastinal lesions. The extension of a goiter into the anterosuperior mediastinum was first described in 1749.[1] The initial experience with successful resections were in Germany in the early to middle 19th century.[2,3] This experience was followed by a sentinel report in 1901 of 1000 thyroidectomies by Kocher.[4] In that report, Kocher describes special techniques for extirpating substernal goiters.

Churchill is credited with the initial recognition of ectopic parathyroid glands within the mediastinum that produce primary hyperparathyroidism. Bauer and Federman[5] recounted their resection of an adenoma through a sternotomy in 1932. In a review involving more than 6100 patients who underwent parathyroidectomy, Creswell and Wells[6] reported that 121 patients (2%) required sternotomy for resection of a mediastinal gland.

Cystic malformations of the aerodigestive tract were first described in the North American literature in 1929. That year Mixter and Clifford[7] described a bronchogenic cyst that presented as a subcarinal mass.

The evolution of surgery of the thymus has a fascinating history. The symptom complex of ptosis, dysarthria, and weakness was described by several German clinicians in the late 19th century. In 1885, Jolly[8] unified the cluster of findings and called the disease *myasthenia gravis pseudoparalytica.* The syndrome was correlated with thymic disease in 1901 in a joint report by Lacquer and Weigert[9]. The autoimmune aspect of the pathophysiology of this disease would wait some 70 years until Almon et al[10] described circulating autoantibodies to the acetylcholine receptor (AchR) at the neuromuscular junction. The first report of the successful resection of a thymic mass in the treatment of the disease is credited to Blalock, who performed the resection in 1936.[11] By 1944 Blalock was promoting transsternal resection for myasthenia gravis (MG) in patients with and those without suspected thymoma.[12] Because of excessive operative mortality with the transsternal approach and with the introduction of mediastinoscopy by Carlens in 1959,[13] the transcervical approach became preferred for patients with nonthymomatous MG. As anesthetic and critical care techniques evolved, the mortality for each of these surgical approaches approached zero, and both are acceptable today.

## ANATOMY

A precise understanding of the anatomy of the mediastinum is critical for the localization, safe biopsy, and potential extirpation of any primary mediastinal mass. To facilitate discussion and to provide a framework for reviewing the literature, a somewhat arbitrary division of the mediastinum into anterior (includes superior), middle, and posterior (includes costovertebral sulci) regions is proposed. As various lesions enlarge they may either displace adjacent organs into other regions or directly invade other zones. Precise anatomic barriers are not surgically relevant.

The anterior mediastinum extends from the manubrium and the first ribs inferiorly to the diaphragm. The anterior border is the posterior sternal table, which extends posteriorly to the pericardium and innominate vein. Contained within this region are the thymus, aortic arch vessels, and associated lymph nodes. Because of the common embryologic origin of parathyroid tissue and thymus, parathyroid glands may be found in this region of the mediastinum. Thyroid masses may also enlarge and present as substernal, anterior-superior mediastinal lesions.

The middle mediastinum extends only as superior as the pericardial reflection. Above this, the anterior mediastinum directly apposes the posterior compartment. The middle region extends inferiorly to the diaphragm and posteriorly to the anterior border of the spine. As such, this region contains the heart and intrapericardial ascending aorta, pericardium, trachea and associated lymph nodes, and both pulmonary hila. The superior vena cava (SVC) also is in the middle mediastinum. Pathologic conditions that affect this vessel may originate in either the anterior or middle mediastinum. They are discussed in the separate section on SVC syndrome.

The posterior mediastinum extends from the superior aspect of the first thoracic vertebral body inferiorly to the diaphragm. Anteriorly the border is the ventral aspect of the vertebral bodies, which extends posteriorly to the articulation with each rib. This incorporates the costovertebral sulci and includes segmental nerve roots and the sympathetic chain. Additional structures comprising the posterior compartment are the esophagus, vagus nerves, thoracic duct, azygous vein, and descending aorta.

## EPIDEMIOLOGY AND INCIDENCE

Because the causes of mediastinal neoplasms are diverse, true incidence and prevalence data are lacking. What is remarkable is the stability over decades of the histologic mix of the various lesions. Table 37–1 recounts the largest reported series in each of the last five decades.[14–18] Neurogenic tumors and thymic neoplasms comprise a steady 30–40% of all lesions in each series. The variations likely represent heterogenous cohorts with regard to age, because neurogenic tumors predominate in the pediatric age group.[15,18]

Tumor location varies according to age. This pediatric–adult dichotomy in terms of anatomy of mediastinal masses is depicted in Table 37–2.[18] Lesions of the posterior mediastinum dominate pediatric series, and masses in the anterior mediastinum are more common when only adults are considered. If all mediastinal lesions are considered in a pediatric series, neurogenic tumors that arise in the posterior mediastinum are most common. These neoplasms account for one third to one half of all pediatric mediastinal masses. Most are neuroblastomas, a malignant neoplasm most common among children 3 years of age and younger. The second most common malignant neoplasm in the pediatric population is lymphoma, which is usually found in the anterior mediastinum. These tumors are more common in the adolescent years. Germ cell tumors are the second most common anterior mediastinal mass in children. Fortunately more than two thirds of these lesions are benign teratomas.

**TABLE 37–1. HISTOLOGIC COMPOSITION OF MEDIASTINAL MASSES REPORTED OVER 5 DECADES[a]**

| Histologic Composition | Sabiston and Scott[14] (n = 101) 1952 | Heimberger et al[15] (n = 92) 1963 | Benjamin et al[16] (n = 209) 1972 | Davis et al[17] (n = 400) 1986 | Azanow et al[18] (n = 257) 1993 |
|---|---|---|---|---|---|
| Neurogenic | 20 | 21 | 23 | 14 | 18 |
| Thymic | 17 | 10 | 16 | 17 | 25 |
| Lymphoma | 11 | 9 | 15 | 15 | 17 |
| Germ cell | 9 | 10 | 13 | 10 | 11 |
| Mesenchymal | 1 | 4 | 11 | 6 | 2 |
| Endocrine | 2 | 8 | 11 | 3 | 4 |
| Cyst | 17 | 24 | 9 | 25 | 18 |

[a]Numbers are percentage of occurrence of the histologic composition in each series. A category of other lesions provides an additional percentage to equal 100%.

**TABLE 37–2. LOCATION OF PRIMARY MEDIASTINAL MASSES IN ADULTS AND CHILDREN[a]**

| Location | Adult (n = 195) | Pediatric (n = 62) |
|---|---|---|
| Anterior | 65 | 38 |
| Middle | 10 | 10 |
| Posterior | 25 | 52 |

[a]Numbers are percentage of masses in the area.
*(Based on Azanow KS, et al: Primary mediastinal masses: A comparison of adult and pediatric populations. J Thorac Cardiovasc Surg 106:67, 1993.)*

**TABLE 37–4. ANTERIOR MEDIASTINAL MASSES IN ADULTS (n = 827)**

| Type of Tumor | Percentage |
|---|---|
| Thymic | 46 |
| Lymphoma | 24 |
| Germ cell | 15 |
| Endocrine | 15 |

*(Data from Refs. 18, 23–28.)*

Thymic masses are unusual in children. They are most likely to be a benign cyst or simple thymic hyperplasia. Resection may be necessary because of symptoms or for the confirmation of a benign histologic diagnosis. Other pediatric lesions comprise cysts of pericardial or aerodigestive origin and mesenchymal lesions of vascular or areolar tissue. Nearly all these tumors are benign. The spectrum of pediatric masses that affect the anterior mediastinum is depicted in Table 37–3.[18–22]

Series of adults show their own characteristic histologic profile.[18,23–28] Anterior compartment lesions predominate with thymic neoplasms leading the list (Table 37–4). Adult series are comprised of fewer posterior lesions. This reflects the less frequent discovery of neurogenic lesions in the adult population. In addition, when a neurogenic lesion is discovered it is invariably benign. Thymoma is the most common neoplasm of the thymus and may be associated with MG. Lymphomas are the second most common of the anterior mediastinal masses in adults, with primary germ cell tumors in the mediastinum ranking third. A variety of endocrine lesions rounds out the most common neoplasms in adults.

Despite differences between children and adults in terms of location and histologic features of mediastinal masses, one disturbing characteristic is common to both groups. The incidence of malignancy in any of the mediastinal masses is increasing. Azanow et al[18] reviewed two groups of patients—one between 1940 and 1960 and a second from 1960 to the mid 1980s. The incidence of malignancy of mediastinal masses in children increased from 7% in the earlier cohort to 47% in the later years. Similarly, malignancy was found in 25% of lesions in adults in the earlier series and was found in nearly 50% of mediastinal lesions seen in the latter two decades. Another series reported by Cohen et al corroborated this observation.[29] Cohen et al found a significant increase in malignant lesions when they compared posterior mediastinal lesions detected before 1970 (1 in 35) with those found in the period from 1970 to 1989 (12 in 42). This held true for anterior mediastinal masses. The malignancy rate went from 13 of 42 masses (31%) before 1970 to 53 of 89 masses (60%) in the most recent cohort. Whether this finding is due to more sophisticated diagnostic methods or a true increase in malignancy is unclear; the trend remains disturbing.

**TABLE 37–3. ANTERIOR MEDIASTINAL MASSES IN CHILDREN (n = 204)**

| Type | Percentage |
|---|---|
| Lymphoma | 41 |
| Germ cell | 23 |
| Thymus | 21 |
| Mesenchymal | 15 |

*(Data from Refs. 18–22.)*

## SYMPTOMS AND SIGNS

Symptoms at the time of diagnosis of the mediastinal lesion are present in 48–62% of patients.[17,18,29] The percentage of symptomatic lesions in children is slightly higher, ranging from 58 to 78%.[18,29] The most common symptoms are chest pain, dyspnea, and cough. The presence of any symptom usually suggests a malignant lesion, but pain suggests frank invasion by the tumor. A logistic regression analysis performed by Cohen et al[29] found the presence of symptoms, anterior location of the tumor, and large tumor size to be associated with histologic findings of malignancy. In that analysis patient age, sex, race, size, and laboratory data were not predictive of malignancy.

Despite the reported association between symptoms and malignancy, studies continue to show an increasing cohort of patients with asymptomatic malignant disease.[17] Several explanations have been promoted, including the increased availability of thoracic imaging, including computed tomography (CT), in general medical practice; the use of screening chest radiographs, especially in military personnel; and the increase in prevalence of lymphomas in most series. Therefore, although the presence of symptoms remains ominous, their absence is hardly reassuring.

Other less frequently reported symptoms referable to mediastinal masses include dysphagia, hoarseness, Horner's syndrome, SVC syndrome, palpitations, malaise, weakness, and weight loss. In addition, physical findings, including adenopathy, distended neck veins, plethora, and hyperreflexia, may be seen. Neurogenic lesions may encroach on the spinal canal, giving signs of cord compression. Systemic syndromes are the hallmark of endocrine processes, which include hyperthyroidism or hyperparathyroidism. Paroxysmal malignant hypertension suggests pheochromocytoma and may be seen with some other pediatric neurogenic tumors. Thymomatous MG may be associated with hypogammaglobulinemia, arthralgias, and red cell aplasia. Rare mesenchymal lesions such as mesothelioma and fibrosarcoma are known to produce an insulin-like substance, leading to hypoglycemia.

## DIAGNOSTIC APPROACH

### Blood Work

Serum chemistries and hematologic evaluations provide information adjunctive to that obtained with the imaging and biopsy techniques discussed herein. Because mediastinal lesions are so diverse, screening is impractical. Characteristic laboratory findings support a specific diagnosis and may focus the diagnostic evaluation, whereas clinical suspicions based on images and symptoms may suggest certain corroborative assays of blood or bodily fluids.

Perhaps the most useful indication for serologic examination in the evaluation of an anterior mediastinal mass occurs with suspected germ cell tumors. The histologic features and treatment of and prognosis for germ cell tumors are tightly linked to the levels of β-human chorionic gonadotropin (HCG) and α-fetoprotein (AFP) in the blood. These substances serve as markers of malignancy and can be used to evaluate the efficacy of therapy. Absence of these markers supports a diagnosis of seminoma or a benign lesion such as a mature teratoma.

### Conventional Radiography

Nearly all mediastinal lesions are found on posteroanterior and lateral chest radiographs. Harris et al[30] found this to be true in 97% of patients referred to a thoracic surgeon. These simple studies provide valuable information with regard to size and location of the mass and the presence and pattern of calcification. Plain tomography and fluoroscopy have been supplanted by cross-sectional imaging techniques. A barium esophagram is essential if the lesion is associated with or believed to be of esophageal origin. Myelography may be helpful in detecting some posterior masses when dural extension is a consideration.

### Computed Tomography

Many clinicians believe CT of the chest is indicated for all patients with a suspected mediastinal mass. This modality clarifies the position of the mass and its relation to neighboring organs. The pattern of calcification is more clearly defined, as are the shape of the lesion and the distinctness of the margins. The presence or absence of distinct tissue planes can be seen, and the density of the mass can be measured. Refinements in technique have allowed the administration of IV and intrathecal contrast material to further define the relationship between a mass lesion and vascular or neural structures.

CT sometimes may obviate the need for additional diagnostic tests or biopsy. Some lesions have a characteristic CT appearance, which leads directly to resection or simple observation.[31] Examples include aneurysms of the aorta or great vessels, mediastinal lipomatosis, a prominent pericardial fat pad, pericardial cysts, and diaphragmatic hernias of the foramen of Morgagni.

In other situations, CT delineates the most expeditious route for biopsy and may dramatically alter the surgical plan. Central lesions may be better approached with mediastinoscopy, a Wang needle, or thoracoscopy. Anterior or posterior masses are amenable to fine-needle or core-needle sampling. As such, CT is a road map for the radiologist or surgeon performing the biopsy.

In addition to providing information regarding the mass lesion, CT also defines the effect of each lesion on surrounding structures. For example, bulky anterior mediastinal masses near the thoracic inlet may lead to extensive tracheal displacement or compression. Shamberger et al[32] have developed guidelines quantitated with CT to assist in the surgical and anesthetic techniques used to safely obtain a tissue diagnosis for these patients.

### Magnetic Resonance Imaging

Magnetic resonance imaging (MRI) is useful in the evaluation of some mediastinal masses. The increased cost incurred must be weighed against the valuable information this imaging modality can add. Unlike CT, MRI is superior in its ability to image not only the axial plane but also the coronal and sagittal planes. Because of this, it may be better in defining involvement by a mediastinal mass with the brachial plexus, neural foramina, diaphragm, and other mediastinal soft-tissue planes. CT remains superior for detecting bony destruction. MRI is excellent for imaging blood vessels and obviates the need for iodinated IV contrast material.[33] MRI is becoming the cross-sectional imaging modality of choice in the evaluation of neurogenic lesions, suspected vascular anomalies, and processes that involve the aortic arch and its branches[34]

### Angiography

Once the standard of reference for vascular imaging, arteriography is being replaced by contrast-enhanced CT and by MRI. These techniques are noninvasive and supply added information regarding contiguous structures. Because there is risk to the patient with arteriography, this modality should be reserved for the rare instance in which more precise delineation of endovascular anatomy is required.

## Ultrasonography

Sonographic evaluation of the chest is limited by the poor conductivity of the lungs. Cystic structures near the neck or diaphragm may be imaged with this technique and sampling of their contents facilitated. Pediatric experience exceeds that in adults because children have a thinner chest wall and larger mediastinum–to–pleural space ratio. Endoscopic ultrasonography has emerged as a valuable diagnostic and staging tool for evaluating abnormalities of the esophagus.[35]

## Radionuclide Studies

Radionuclide scanning is useful in the evaluation of only a fraction of mediastinal masses. Technetium or iodine scanning may help define the substernal extent of a thyroid mass. Gallium scanning has been useful in the staging and follow-up of tumors with known avidity for this nuclide. These tumors include lymphomas and certain nonseminomatous germ cell lesions. Finally, scanning with $^{131}$I-metaiodobenzylguanidine ($^{131}$I-MIBG) has been useful in locating extra-adrenal paraganglionic tumors, including mediastinal pheochromocytomas.[36]

## Biopsy

### *Fine-Needle Aspiration and Core-Needle Biopsy*

The percutaneous approach to obtaining tissue from a mediastinal mass allows an outpatient diagnosis to be made without the expense incurred in the operating room. In addition, patients deemed poor candidates for anesthesia can still have a diagnosis made and may be candidates for nonoperative therapies. CT or ultrasound is used to guide the needle. Fine-needle samples yield cytologic samples that may not allow a diagnosis, whereas core needle provides a histologic specimen. Electron microscopy and immunohistochemical staining allow pathologists to provide more accurate diagnoses with small specimens. Bressler and Kirkham[37] reported 100% success in achieving a diagnosis using fine-needle aspirates of anterior and posterior mediastinal lesions and a 75% diagnostic yield for middle mediastinal masses. The pneumothorax rate was only 6%. Sonographically guided aspiration has a reported diagnostic yield of 84% as long as the lesion can be imaged.[38] A transsternal needle approach with zero pneumothoraces has been reported. The technique requires a great deal of sedation and appears cumbersome.[39] Bronchoscopy with a Wang-needle aspirate by way of a transtracheal or transbronchial approach may be useful for difficult-to-reach middle mediastinal lesions.

### *Mediastinoscopy or Thoracoscopy*

Certain lesions, especially lymphomas, require large tissue samples for precise definition of cytologic subtypes, which may dictate individualized chemotherapy. In these situations general anesthesia is warranted to allow a minimally invasive surgical approach to biopsy. The choice of cervical or anterior mediastinoscopy depends on the anatomic location of the mass. Both are preferable to thoracoscopy because they can be performed on an outpatient basis.[40,41] Thoracoscopy is an excellent approach to other inaccessible posterior lesions or for the restaging of anterior lesions on which biopsies have already been performed.[41]

### *Sternotomy or Thoracotomy*

With the availability of cross-sectional imaging, interventional radiologists, and the judicious application of mediastinoscopy and video thoracoscopy, an accurate diagnosis should be achievable for any mediastinal mass. The morbidity of a sternotomy or thoracotomy should therefore be reserved for the therapeutic arena, in which the goal of complete resection justifies the larger incision.

# ANTERIOR MEDIASTINAL MASSES

## Thymoma

Thymoma is a neoplasm that originates from thymic epithelial cells. It is the most common primary neoplasm of the mediastinum, accounting for about 15% of all mediastinal masses.[17] Unlike that of other thoracic tumors, the clinical course of thymoma is rather indolent, perhaps because of the bland cytologic nature of the cells. Surgery is the mainstay of treatment, except in rare cases of widespread dissemination apparent at the time of presentation. In advanced stages radiation therapy and chemotherapy have useful adjunctive roles.

### *Clinical Presentation and Diagnosis*

Patients with thymoma are between 40 and 60 years of age and are equally likely to be male or female. They usually have no symptoms, but 25% describe vague chest problems. The diagnosis is often based on a serendipitous radiologic finding or evaluation of one of the parathymic syndromes. These include MG, which is discussed later in this chapter, red cell aplasia, and hypoglobulinemia, as well as a number of other syndromes.[42] Aside from MG, the syndromes, although mentioned frequently, are quite rare. Red cell aplasia portends a poor prognosis.

The diagnosis of thymoma depends on obtaining tissue. Findings of fine-needle aspiration biopsy may be definitive when an experienced cytopathologist performs the histologic examination. However, differentiation between entities such as lymphoma and thymoma can be difficult without a substantial aliquot of tissue.[43] Acquisition of a large sample can be facilitated with a small anterior mediastinotomy. It is crucial to determine if there is any compromise of the airway (Fig. 37–1), particularly when consideration is given to the anesthetic technique to be used for surgical procedure.

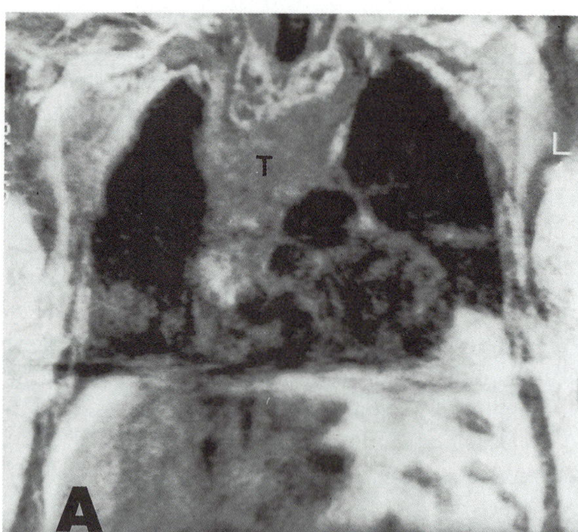


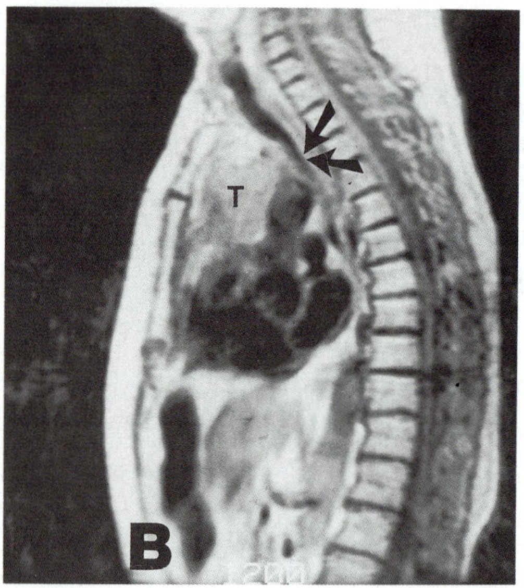


**Figure 37–1. A.** Coronal MRI of an invasive thymoma (T) that involves both thymic lobes effacing the right atrium and extending into the neck. **B.** Sagittal MRI of the same lesion demonstrates tracheal compression (arrows).

There are various ways to characterize thymomas. Traditionally tumors have been classified on the basis of the proportion of lymphocytes present relative to the population of epithelial or spindle cells. Kirchen and Muller-Hermelink[44] proposed a different classification system based on whether the tumor cells appear more like thymic medullary or thymic cortical cells. In this schema, thymic carcinoma is included toward the cortical thymoma end of the spectrum. Medullary thymomas tend to be less aggressive. Cortical thymomas and thymic carcinomas, however, can show metastatic involvement or local invasion[44] (Fig 37–1). The diagnosis of thymic carcinoma is based on the exclusion of another primary lesion such as carcinoma of the lung.[45]

The major factor in determining the biologic behavior of thymomas and in determining their prognosis is their clinical stage. Stage I and II lesions have either an intact capsule or local invasion into surrounding tissues, including pleura or pericardium. Stage III thymomas have associated gross invasion of structures such as the lung, pericardium, or aorta (Fig. 37–1). Stage IV lesions have associated disseminated disease (IV-A denotes intrathoracic dissemination, IV-B denotes extrathoracic dissemination).

### Treatment

Surgical excision is the treatment of choice for thymomas when evidence of widespread dissemination is not present. If there is concern that a complete excision cannot be accomplished, there may be a role for neoadjuvant treatment before exploration.[46] The preferred approach is median sternotomy. Posterolateral thoracotomy may be preferable if there is a need to control the pulmonary hilum because of the bulk of the tumor. The cornerstone of treatment of this lesion is complete surgical excision, which can be achieved approximately 90% of the time.[47] For tumors that cannot be completely removed at the time of operation, there appears to be a role for radiation therapy to improve local control. Cisplatin-based combination chemotherapy may be beneficial in cases of widespread disease.[48,49] The most common sites of recurrence are the lung, pleura, and mediastinum; the most common distant site is bone. For recurrent tumors re-excision should be considered in addition to both chemotherapy and radiation therapy.[50]

Results may be broken down on basis of tumor stage. The 10-year survival rate is 85–100% for stage I disease, 60–84% for stage II disease, 21–77% for stage III disease, and 26–47% for stage IV-A tumors.[42]

## Myasthenia Gravis

The first clinical description of MG was made by Thomas Willis, of Oxford, in 1672 in his book on the physiology and pathology of disease, *De Anima Brutorum.*[51] Willis described a "spurious Palsie," in which the afflicted persons "in the morning are able to walk firmly, to fling about their Arms hither and thither, or to take up any heavy thing" but before noon "they are scarce able to move Hand or Foot."[52] Since that time many variations of these descriptions and clinical scenarios have been observed. Although MG is still an incompletely understood syndrome, much has been learned since those early descriptions, including an association of the disease with antibodies to AchR.

### Epidemiology and Pathology

MG is a relatively rare neuromuscular disorder with a prevalence of 0.5–14.2 per 100,000 population, a rate that has been on the rise over the past 40 years.[53,54] This trend has been attributed to an increase in the life spans of patients with MG because of an improvement in treatment over this time. The disease is more common in women (female-to-male ratio, 2:1). An accepted generalization is that MG affects young women and old men. A more accurate description is that the disease occurs at a higher rate in the first few decades of life in women, but the incidence in the last half of life is approximately equal in men and women.[55]

The pathogenic process in MG consists of autoantibodies binding to AchR followed by attachment of complement factors. Next, complement-mediated end-plate destruction and transient cellular infiltration of the neuromuscular junction take place. With this, neuromuscular transmission begins to fail and symptoms related to fatigue and weakness develop. Last, the cellular infiltrate disappears and the end-plate structure degenerates with subsequent continued denervation and reinnervation.[56] Despite these observations, the exact relationship between the clinical course of MG and these AchR antibodies is not clear. For example, there may be striking clinical improvement with thymectomy without any change in the level of AchR antibodies.[57] It would appear that MG is an autoimmune process, but what triggers or sustains the weakness syndrome remains to be elucidated.

The relation between the thymus gland and MG is interesting. Seventy percent of patients with MG have thymic lymphoid hyperplasia, 10% have neoplastic thymoma, and the other 20% show thymic atrophy.[58] The hyperplasia is of the lymphoid or follicular type, which contains activated germinal centers. The mechanism of hyperplasia is unknown. The degree of hyperplasia and atrophy does not seem to correlate with the severity of the disease. In 1939, Blalock et al showed improvement of MG with thymectomy;[11] since that time the operation has been a mainstay of treatment.

### *Clinical Presentation*

MG is a disease of neuromuscular transmission and as such presents with muscle weakness. More than one muscle group usually is involved. Symptoms are more prominent with repetitive activity; a period of rest leads to improvement. The muscles innervated by the cranial nerves are involved more often than the other muscles and at an earlier point in the disease. Patients with MG, therefore, have prominent ptosis, ophthalmoplegia, dysarthria, and dysphagia.[59] Muscles of mastication can become so weak that patients are unable to close their jaws. The clinical course of MG is unpredictable. MG can remain quiescent for a long time and then accelerate or have a steady, progressive decline. Involvement of the respiratory muscles tends to bode poorly because ventilation and clearance of secretions become serious problems. Pregnancy can temporarily relieve or worsen the course of the disease, particularly in the postpartum period.[60] The classification is a descriptive one that differentiates between purely ocular involvement and generalized muscle weakness. In the latter, differentiation is made between a mild or moderate course as opposed to a more severe course based on either a rapid or extensive presentation of symptoms. Patients with fulminant disease tend to have a worse outcome than others.[61] Diagnosis is based on consistent clinical features and can be confirmed by various tests. Jolly, in 1885, coined the term *myasthenia gravis pseudoparalytica* and in the same article described the classic fatiguing response to repetitive electrical nerve stimulation now known as the Jolly test.[8] More commonly, a Tensilon test is performed. In the test IV administration of edrophonium (Tensilon), a short-acting anticholinesterase, leads to marked, immediate improvement in most patients with MG.

### *Treatment*

Thirty years ago, one fourth of patients with MG died of the disease. Current treatment strategies provide a reasonably normal life expectancy for patients.[62] The specific treatment plan depends on the clinical situation. There is still controversy about the optimal combination of drugs and the decision for and the timing of surgical intervention.

**Cholinesterase Inhibitors.** Cholinesterase inhibitors improve muscle weakness because they increase the amount of acetylcholine available. However, because they do not affect AchR antibodies, these agents do not change the course of the disease. Pyridostigmine bromide has a longer duration of action and is, therefore, preferred over neostigmine bromide. These drugs can be given orally, intranasally, or by nebulizer and should be used only in the minimum dose necessary to achieve an effect. There is controversy whether these agents can damage the neuromuscular junction with chronic use. The side effects mostly involve the gastrointestinal tract. They include nausea, vomiting, cramping and diarrhea. Bradycardia and psychosis (bromism as a result of overdosage of pyridostigmine bromide) are uncommon.

**Immunosuppressive Drugs, Including Corticosteroids.** Prednisone leads to marked improvement or remission in 80% of patients with MG within 6–8 weeks of initiation of treatment. Thirty percent of patients experience some worsening (within 3 weeks), which can last for approximately 1 week. For this reason, patients must be monitored very carefully during the beginning of steroid administration.[62] Overall, prednisone is a very effective treatment of MG. The use of prednisone must be balanced against the risk of chronic steroid use. If prednisone cannot be discontinued over time, other therapies, particularly thymectomy, should be considered. Immunosuppressive agents such as azathioprine, cyclosporine, and cyclophosphamide may produce marked and sustained improvement in patients with MG, particularly those who have not responded to prednisone or thymectomy. In addition to the risk of immunosuppression, the cost, the delay in onset of effect, and the requirement for chronic administration must be considered.

**Plasma Exchange.** Plasmapheresis is an extremely effective form of acute treatment of MG. The technique is particularly useful when a dramatic and rapid response is necessary, as with impending myasthenic crisis or to minimize perioperative morbidity and mortality at the time of thymectomy. Plasmapheresis works by removing pathogenic circulating substances from the blood, such as AchR antibodies, complement, and immune complexes, although the correlation with a decrease in AchR antibodies titers is variable. The effects last anywhere from several weeks to 1 or 2 months. The disadvantages relate to the risk of chronic central venous access and the cost of replacing the lost proteins and plasma components.

**Thymectomy.** Although there are still no controlled trials documenting the benefit of thymectomy in MG, most neurologists recommend thymectomy as the cornerstone of treatment.[62] Kirschner[63] classified the indications for thymectomy in MG on the basis of presence or absence of a thymoma. If there is no thymoma and if symptoms are completely or almost completely controlled by cholinesterase inhibitors or if the symptoms are only ocular, surgical therapy may be deferred. In most other circumstances thymectomy is the procedure of choice, because it achieves a good or complete response in 85% of patients and can be performed with minimal morbidity and mortality.[64] Of note, thymectomy should not be performed on an emergency basis. The crisis should be managed nonoperatively (usually by plasmapheresis) because the risks of surgical intervention in this setting outweigh the benefits. If a thymoma is present, Kirschner points out that the operation should be performed as soon as symptoms can be controlled.[63] These patients may need prolonged ventilatory support because their MG symptoms may be more difficult to control in the postoperative period. Mild MG also may become exacerbated after the thymoma is removed. A reoperation should be considered if there is a suspicion of incomplete resection, if a patient's disease is clinically difficult to manage, or if there is a recurrence of a thymoma, whether or not symptoms of MG have recurred. Similarly, if there is residual thymoma after radiation therapy or chemotherapy, resection should be performed.

The technique of surgical resection is controversial. The traditional approach involves a median sternotomy with resection of all thymic tissue. However, there are advocates of a transcervical technique. This is thought to be less painful than a sternotomy but still provides adequate exposure that does not compromise the resection.[65] More recently, the use of thoracoscopy has been suggested as a less invasive technique that may allow an adequate resection.[66] If a thymoma is present, exposure through a median sternotomy is essential; all extensions of thymic tissue and areas of contiguous spread as well as localized satellite lesions should be resected.[67]

The results of thymectomy for MG are variable. Most reports suggest a drug-free remission rate of 10–20% and an otherwise complete remission rate of 30–40%. Another twenty-five percent of patients experience dramatic improvement. A small percentage of patients are worse after the operation, or a recurrence develops after improvement.[68,69] Factors associated with an improved outcome include young age, female sex, short period of preoperative symptoms, hyperplastic gland, and lack of need for preoperative immunosuppressive agents or steroids.

## Lymphomas

### *Incidence*

Mediastinal lymphoma usually presents as a component of a more diffuse systemic process. However, primary mediastinal lymphoma occurs approximately 10% of the time. In a study that examined mediastinal lesions over an extended period of time at a tertiary medical center, lymphomas represented 14% of these masses.[17] Over approximately 60 years, this fraction has remained stable. Of masses in the anterosuperior mediastinum, thymomas accounted for 30% and lymphomas were the second most frequent at 20%. Cysts were the most common lesion in the middle mediastinum while again lymphomas were second, at 20%.[17] Only rarely are lymphomas found in the posterior mediastinum. In the aforementioned series, non-Hodgkin's lymphomas were somewhat more common than Hodgkin's lymphomas, although other reports suggest that there is a preponderance of Hodgkin's lymphoma.[70] The difference can probably be accounted for by the age of the presenting population. Hodgkin's lymphoma has a peak incidence in the third and fourth decade of life, whereas non-Hodgkin's lymphoma occurs evenly throughout the first five decades of life. The nodular sclerosing type of Hodgkin's lymphoma was the most common form of Hodgkin's lymphoma seen in both studies. Among patients with non-Hodgkin's lymphoma, histiocytic, lymphoblastic, and lymphocytic subtypes were seen with a similar frequency.

### *Presentation and Diagnosis*

Most patients experience chest heaviness or discomfort and a cough. A variable number have shortness of breath as a result of airway or lung compression (Fig. 37–2) or from an effusion in either the pleural or the pericardial space. Symptoms are almost always present when the disease is bulky (more than one third of the lateral chest wall diameter). in this group of patients, SVC syndrome may be seen in addition to the aforementioned symptoms.[71] All symptoms and particularly the presence of SVC syndrome are more common in the pediatric age group, perhaps as a result of bulkier disease relative to the space available. Patients with lymphoma may experience nonspecific B-type symptoms

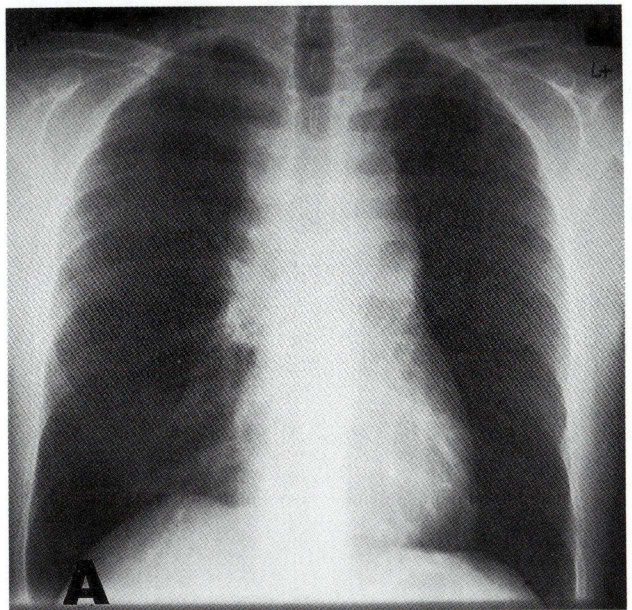


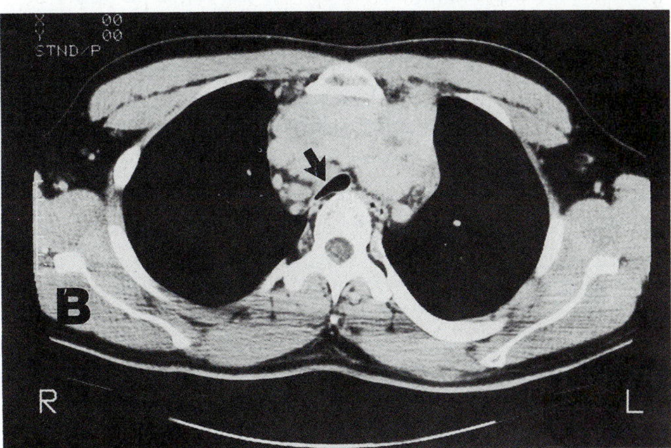


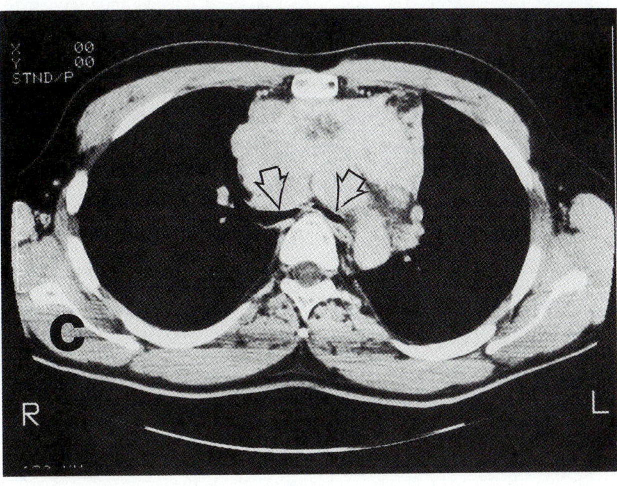


**Figure 37–2. A.** Frontal radiograph showing widened mediastinum in a 23-year old man with non-Hodgkin's lymphoma. **B.** CT scan showing the heterogenous anterior tumor mass with marked tracheal compression (solid arrow). **C.** CT scan demonstrates extent of mass compressing both mainstem bronchi (open arrows).

including fevers, night sweats, and weight loss in addition to symptoms related to the mass.

When one suspects a lymphoma in the mediastinum, an accurate tissue diagnosis is crucial. Fine-needle aspiration generally does not provide a large enough specimen for a diagnosis that includes the cell type.[72] When one is considering lymphoma in the differential diagnosis of a mediastinal mass, evaluation for more easily accessible nodal tissue should be carried out. A bone marrow biopsy should be performed if it would make the need to biopsy mediastinal tissue unnecessary. In addition, although there are no specific serum markers for lymphoma, serum lactic dehydrogenase and alkaline phosphatase levels should be measured. These levels, if elevated, help focus the investigation. When tissue from the mass is necessary, one of several surgical approaches can be undertaken depending on the anatomic relations of the mass in question. Mediastinoscopy (cervical or anterior), anterior mediastinotomy, median sternotomy, or thoracotomy can be used to evaluate, perform a biopsy, or remove the mass in question. Not infrequently it is difficult to differentiate between a lymphoma and an unusual thymoma or a frozen section of an isolated anterior mediastinal mass. If the mass cannot easily be removed, attempts at extirpation should be delayed until a final diagnosis has been made. Even in the setting of a SVC syndrome, tissue can almost always be obtained before therapy is begun if local anesthesia or careful general anesthesia is used during the biopsy.

### *Treatment*

Lymphoma, even if isolated to the mediastinum, is best treated nonsurgically. Mediastinal lymphomas are treated in a similar manner to treatment of lymphomas found elsewhere in the body. Cell type and stage determine what combination of radiation therapy and chemotherapy should be used. In general, T-cell lymphomas are treated with chemotherapy whereas B-cell tumors are treated with both radiation therapy and chemotherapy. Lymphomas confined to the mediastinum are stage I or II lesions and usually are treated with only radiation therapy. If the tumor is bulky or involves surrounding extranodal tissue, chemotherapy in addition to radiation therapy increases the disease-free survival rate from less than 50% to more than 80% 10 years after treatment.[73] Overall, there has been improvement in the survival rate for mediastinal Hodgkin's lymphoma over the past 60 years from 15% to 75%.[17] Unfortunately, there has not been a corresponding increase in the survival rate among patients with non-Hodgkin's lymphoma, whose survival still remains poor. Surgical intervention, other than for diagnosis, has not been an important part of the treatment plan in lymphoma of the mediastinum. There are, however, instances in which it is important. If there is a residual or recurrent mass after otherwise successful treatment, an operation is indicated to determine the nature of the mass. In children, though, these masses are usually thymic hyperplasia and can be treated with steroids. Residual masses in patients with non-Hodgkin's lymphoma after multimodality therapy may resolve without intervention.[70] Finally, if at the time of biopsy the entire mass can be readily excised, this should be done because it simplifies the local component of the treatment regimen.

### *Castleman's Disease*

Castleman's disease, or angiofollicular lymph node hyperplasia, is a poorly understood lymphoproliferative disorder. In discussions of mediastinal masses it is mentioned because it can present as isolated mediastinal lymphadenopathy. There are two forms of this entity. The hyaline vascular type is more common. It tends to be slow growing and occurs asymptomatically in patients with localized disease. The plasma cell type is less common, tends to be multifocal, and presents with vague symptoms of weight loss, malaise, and fever.[74] Neither of these is a surgical disease; however, they may be encountered in the course of evaluation of a mediastinal mass. There are reports of malignant transformation of this process, which, when it occurs, is more common in the multicentric plasma cell type.[74] Therefore, if a lesion consistent with Castleman's disease is encountered at the time of biopsy, the lesion should be removed in its entirety. If this is not feasable, close clinical follow-up is recommended.

## Germ Cell Tumors

Primary germ cell tumors that arise in extragonadal sites are uncommon in people of all ages. They represent 3% of germ cell tumors in adults and only 7% of germ cell tumors in children.[75] In children primary germ cell tumors present most commonly as sacrococcygeal masses in the newborn. In adults they can be found in the retroperitoneum or pineal gland, although the mediastinum is the most common location, accounting for 50–70% of all extragonadal primary tumors.[76] Germ cell tumors are the third most common anterior mediastinal mass in adults. In children, in whom thymic masses are rare, germ cell tumors account for one fourth of lesions and are second only to lymphomas in the etiology of anterior mediastinal disease.[26,77]

Current experimental evidence suggests the cells responsible for these tumors are derived from germinal cell rests that migrated to the mediastinum from the urogenital ridge in embryologic life.[75,78] Authors of autopsy studies argue against the metastatic tumor theory because less than 5% of patients who die with presumed mediastinal primary germ cell tumors were found to have any testicular disease.[79] Nevertheless, it is important to exclude a gonadal primary lesion with a physical examination and scrotal ultrasonography whenever a mediastinal germ cell lesion is diagnosed. The staging implication of these findings dictates considerable differences for prognosis and treatment.

In pediatric series, mediastinal germ cell tumors present at all ages, equally divided between boys and girls. Whereas in adults benign germ cell tumors are equally distributed between the sexes, more than 90% of malignant tumors arise in men in their third decade of life.

Benign teratoma, or dermoid cysts, represents the most commonly diagnosed mediastinal germ cell tumor (Fig. 37–3). This histologic composition accounts for up to 70% of childhood mediastinal germ cell tumors and is seen 60% of the time in adult series. Seminoma is the predominant malignant lesion, constituting nearly half the malignant cell cohort. Malignant teratoma, also known as teratocarcinoma, is the next most common tumor, followed by the relatively rare primary yolk sac tumors, endodermal sinus carcinoma, choriocarcinoma, and embryonal cell carcinoma. Mixed malignant lesions are frequently seen and behave biologically according to their most malignant component.[80–82]

### *Mediastinal Teratoma*

The true incidence of mediastinal teratoma is unknown. Less than half of lesions resected have a premonitory symptom. Calcification of some degree is present on plain radiographs in 20–30% of patients with benign teratoma[83] (Fig. 37–3). These tumors contain elements of ectodermal, endodermal, and mesodermal origin, some of which may be immature. Fortunately, with mediastinal teratomas, even the immature elements display no tendency toward malignant degeneration.

Because of this benign behavior, the treatment of mediastinal teratoma is surgical resection. There is no role for adjunctive radiation therapy or chemotherapy. Involvement of or adherence to adjacent structures may necessitate an en bloc resection. The largest reported series is from the Mayo Clinic; 64 of 69 patients enjoyed long-term survival, and there were no reports of recurrence.[84]

### *Seminoma*

The histology of mediastinal seminoma is identical to its testicular counterpart. It is, therefore, required that all pa-

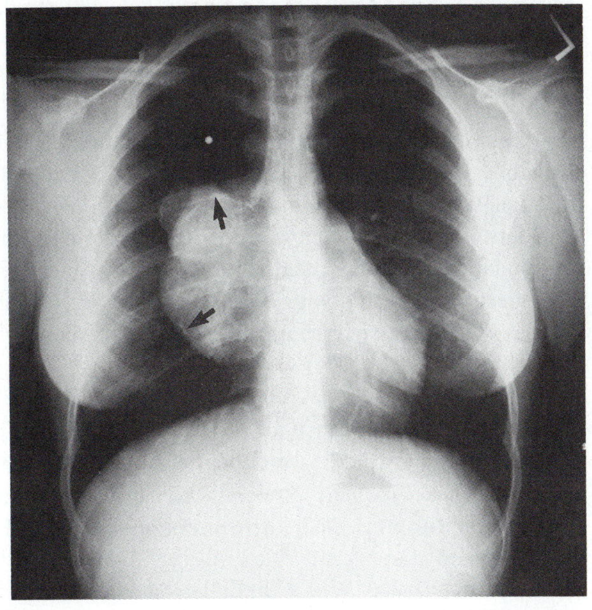


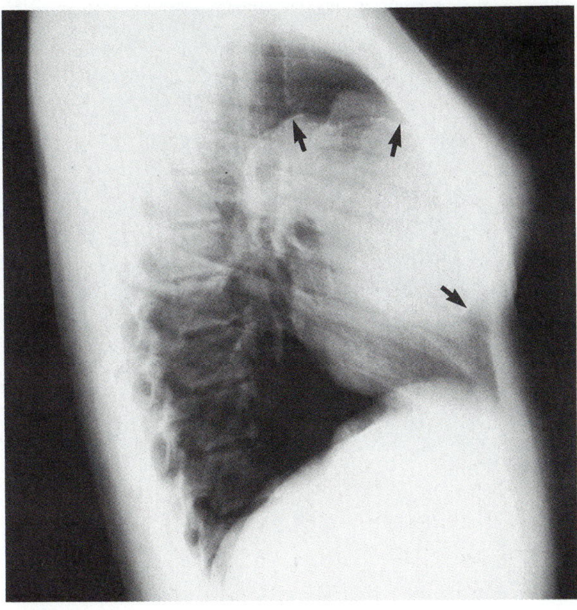


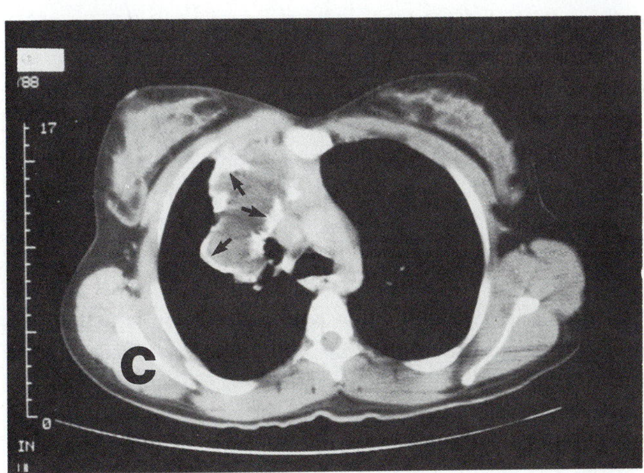


**Figure 37–3.** Frontal **A.** and lateral **B.** radiographs showing a benign mediastinal teratoma (arrows). Note the peripheral calcium (arrows) and the cystic nature of this lesion on CT scan **C.**

tients with biopsy-proved mediastinal seminoma undergo careful staging with a scrotal examination and sonogram, measurement of serum tumor markers, and CT evaluation of the abdomen and retroperitoneum. Any evidence of tumor below the diaphragm suggests advanced or systemic disease. As many as 10% of patients with pure seminoma may have mild (<100 mIU/mL) elevation in HCG level.[75] Any elevation in AFP level, however, suggests a mixed tumor. The presence of extrathoracic disease or any elevation in AFP level mandates the use of induction chemotherapy in the management of mediastinal seminoma.

The therapy for pure seminoma that originates in the mediastinum is predominantly nonsurgical. Traditionally viewed as curable with radiation therapy alone, mediastinal seminomas managed with local therapy by Jain et al[85] were brought into remission only 50% of the time. This is in direct contrast to the use of cisplatin based chemotherapy, which resulted in a durable complete remission rate of 88–100%.[85,86] Our current recommendations are to use chemotherapy initially for bulky disease and radiation therapy for limited lesions. After induction chemotherapy, patients with residual disease 3 cm or larger on radiographs (Fig. 37–4) should undergo resection for detection of persistent, viable tumor. This finding may dictate the need for adjuvant chemotherapy or thoracic irradiation.[87]

### *Mediastinal Nonseminomatous Germ Cell Tumors*

Measurement of the serum tumor markers (AFP and HCG) are extremely valuable in the diagnosis and management of mediastinal nonseminomatous germ cell tumors (MNSGCT). It provides prognostic information and often dictates the therapeutic modality most likely to benefit the patient. The most common tumor marker in patients with MNSGCT is AFP. It is elevated in 80% of patients. Thirty percent of

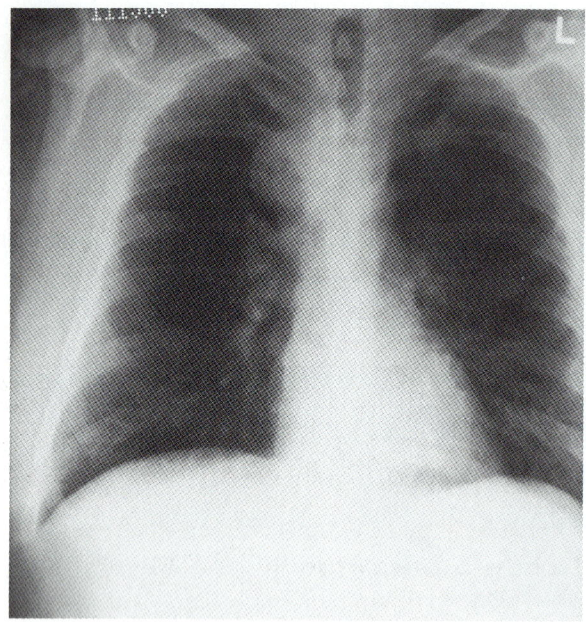


**Figure 37–4.** Frontal radiogaph of residual germ cell tumor in the right paratracheal region after induction chemotherapy.

tumors elaborate detectable HCG as well. Most important, remission is accompanied by normalization of both markers, whereas relapse is signaled by recurrent elevation.[75]

Combination chemotherapy with surgical intervention in selected cases of MNSGCT has resulted in improved survival for patients with the disease. Unlike for most solid tumors, durable remissions are possible even after failed first- and second-line chemotherapy. Unfortunately MNSGCT have a poorer prognosis than their testicular cousins. They appear to be more chemotherapy-resistant and may degenerate into non–germ cell malignant tumors such as leukemia, sarcoma, or carcinoma.[88] Historical survival with surgery and non–cisplatin-based chemotherapy was a meager 3%. Cisplatin-containing regimens have produced a 50–58% long-term survival rate in patients with MNSGCT.[75,81] Autologous bone marrow transplantation and other innovative strategies, including growth factor and stem cell support, are allowing further dose-intensive protocols, which may improve the rate of remission.

Surgical resection has been reserved for patients with residual masses seen on radiographs after successful induction therapy signaled by the normalization of all serum tumor markers (Fig. 37–4). Histologic findings in resected specimens are scar, necrosis, or mature teratomatous elements.[89] Extirpation may also be considered in selected cases of relapse if remote disease is carefully excluded and the lesion appears technically resectable. Because these patients invariably are young and given the active investigative atmosphere regarding novel systemic therapies, an aggressive surgical stance is warranted in multimodality therapy for MNSGCT.

## MIDDLE MEDIASTINAL MASSES

### Mediastinal Cysts

A variety of cystic masses come to the attention of thoracic surgeons. Collectively they comprise almost 20% of all mediastinal masses.[23] Though they may arise in all anatomic locations within the mediastinum, most cysts are of foregut origin and begin in the middle mediastinum. Anteriorly located lesions include thymic cysts and dermoid cysts or teratomas. The latter are discussed in the section on germ cell tumors.

#### *Cysts of Foregut Origin*

Three subtypes of foregut cystic malformations warrant discussion. These include bronchogenic cysts, esophageal cysts or duplications, and neuroenteric cysts. Often bronchogenic and esophageal lesions are considered jointly as enterogenous cysts. When these lesions have associated vertebral anomalies, they are considered neuroenteric cysts.

#### *Bronchogenic Cysts*

These lesions are the most common mediastinal cystic mass, accounting for 60% of all such lesions in a 40-year experience reported from the Mayo Clinic.[23] The most common mediastinal location is the subcarinal region (Fig. 37–5) although many lesions are found invested by pulmonary parenchyma. The latter tend to produce more symptoms and may rarely communicate with the bronchial tree. Symptoms are present in as many as two thirds of these cysts and are related to compression of adjoining structures and obstruction of the distal lung, which produces cough and infection.[90,91] In pediatric series, symptoms are the rule. Bronchogenic cysts make up only 13% of congenital cystic foregut lesions diagnosed in children.[92] The diagnosis is supported by plain radiography and CT.[93]

The treatment options for bronchogenic cysts range from observation to aspiration to resection. Symptomatic lesions clearly require resection.[94] Historically this involved thoracotomy, though videothoracoscopy has been applied successfully to these diseases.[95] Series reported from both the Massachusetts General Hospital[96] and the Cleveland Clinic[91] advocate resection even for asymptomatic lesions. Both institutions noted a tendency for symptoms to develop over time. In addition both series noted increased perioperative complications for resection of symptomatic lesions. These data suggest that waiting for symptoms before resection leads to increased operative risk. Partial resection may occasionally be necessary because of cyst adherence to vital structures. In this situation, recurrences are reported and often require repeat intervention.[97] Aspiration for the confirmation of a benign diagnosis and for the instillation of a sclerosant (ethanol or bleomycin) has been reported, though long-term follow-up data are lacking.[90,98] This may be a useful therapy for patients deemed not suitable for surgery. Finally, case reports

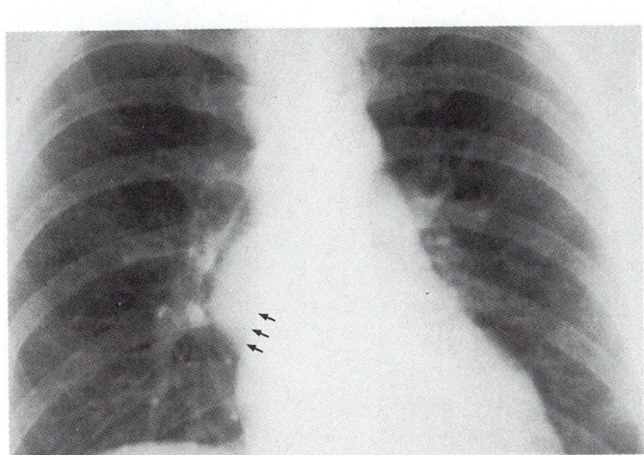

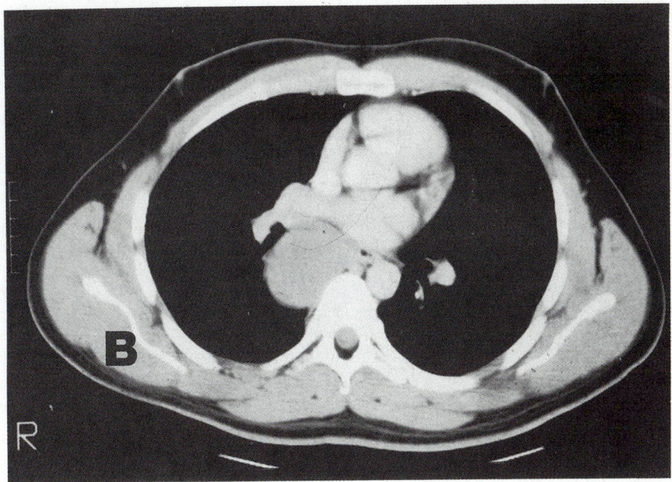


A

**Figure 37–5. A.** Frontal radiogaph showing a mass in the right hilum. The right heart border is preserved (arrows). **B.** CT scan of same lesion shows it to be a bronchogenic cyst in the subcarinal space.

of associated malignancy lend some credence to the concept of complete resection.[99]

### *Esophageal Cysts*

Though similar to bronchogenic cysts, esophageal cysts are lined with some form of gastrointestinal epithelium. The most common histologic feature is a stratified squamous lining that links the cyst with its esophageal origin. Acid-secreting gastric mucosa has been described. Most of these cysts are found in children and are associated with other alimentary tract duplications, though 25% remain asymptomatic only to be diagnosed in the adult years. Most are found along the lower third of the thoracic esophagus with a 2:1 predilection for the right chest.[100] The advent of endoscopic ultrasonography has facilitated the accurate diagnosis of these duplications,[35] though resection remains the therapy of choice. Just as with bronchogenic lesions, esophageal cysts are prone to become infected. Because of associated gastric mucosa, they may also spontaneously hemorrhage. Resection may leave defects in the esophageal musculature or mucosa. These defects must be meticulously repaired. We advocate buttressing the repair with a locally derived flap of vascularized tissue, such as the pericardial fat pad, pleura, or intercostal muscle.

### *Neuroenteric Cysts*

Neuroenteric cysts are rare, accounting for only 5–10% of foregut lesions.[101] They are always associated with a vertebral anomaly. The spectrum of bony problems includes fused or hemivertebrae. The vertebral anomaly is commonly cephalad to the cyst as the esophagus descends during fetal development.[102] Most lesions present in infancy with respiratory or neurologic findings. Resection through a thoracotomy is the optimal therapy. Careful imaging, including the selective use of MRI[93] to exclude extension into the neural foramen or spinal canal or the association of a meningocele, is important. Such findings require a staged approach to resection in which a posterior neurosurgical procedure precedes resection of the mediastinal component.[103]

### *Miscellaneous Cysts*

**Thymic Cysts.** Thymic cysts are rare cystic derivatives of the pharyngeal pouches. They are universally benign but must be differentiated from cystic degeneration of thymomas or other more worrisome pathologic conditions. As patients age, the cyst itself may degenerate and develop a thickened, calcified capsule with heterogenous fluid within it (Fig. 37–6). In this stage, the cyst may be confused with a teratoma. Excision either by means of thoracoscopy or sternotomy is curative and excludes other histologic diagnoses.[104]

**Pericardial Cysts.** These simple cystic lesions are commonly found at the cardiophrenic angles. They must be differentiated from prominent fat pads or Morgagni hernias. This differentiation is easily accomplished with CT, which allows analysis of the density of the cyst fluid.[31,105] The cysts are characteristically filled with a clear serous fluid; hence their other name, *spring water cysts.* Characteristic lesions can be aspirated and followed clinically. Resection is indicated for changes in radiographic appearance over time or for symptoms. There is no reported malignant potential.

**Rare Cysts.** Cysts of the thoracic duct have been reported. As expected, the lesions contained chyle. Therapy was simple excision.[106] Pancreatic pseudocysts have presented in the mediastinum but are best treated by internal drainage of their subdiaphragmatic component.[107] Some lesions defy

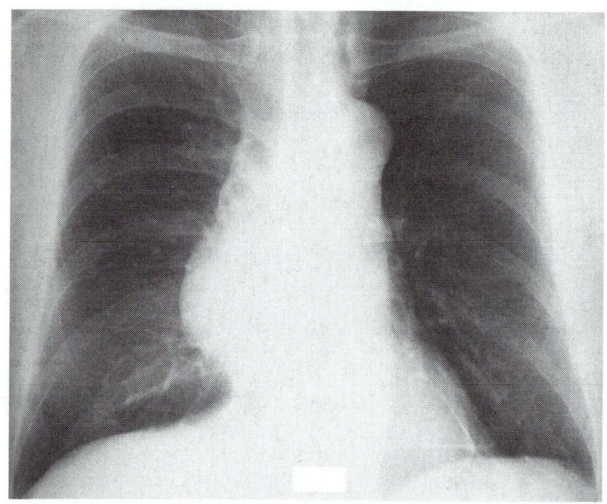


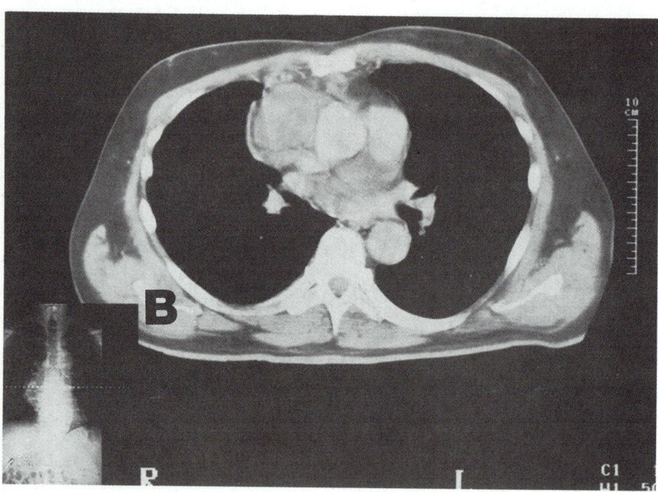


**Figure 37–6. A.** Frontal radiograph shows a mass obscuring the right heart border. **B.** CT image shows mass that at resection was found to be a thymic cyst.

histologic classification and contain bland fluid without the suggestion of the origin of the cyst. Such lesions are best labeled *nonspecific mediastinal cysts.*

## POSTERIOR MEDIASTINAL MASSES

### Neurogenic Tumors

Neurogenic tumors are one of the most common neoplasms of the mediastinum. When all age groups are considered, these tumors are the most frequently encountered mediastinal mass, accounting for 20–35% of all lesions. In an adult population, the incidence falls to about 15%.[17] Neurogenic tumors are predominantly located in the posterior mediastinum. The tumors are derived from embryonic neural crest cells that originate from the nerve sheaths, the spinal ganglia, or the sympathetic and parasympathetic components of the autonomic nervous system. Neurilemmomas, or schwannomas, and neurofibromas arise from the nerve sheath. Ganglioneuromas, ganglioneuroblastomas, and neuroblastomas originate from the sympathetic ganglia. Tumors originating from the paraganglionic system include pheochromocytomas (chromaffin) and chemodectomas (nonchromaffin). Finally, there are tumors of peripheral neuroectodermal origin that when malignant are referred to as *Askin tumors* .

#### *Diagnosis*

Mediastinal neurogenic tumors present as asymptomatic lesions in the posterior mediastinum on chest radiographs or as a result of excessive hormone production by the rare intrathoracic pheochromocytoma. On occasion the tumor grows to such a size or is located in such a way that it causes compressive symptoms. These features can be related to the associated nerve root or to neighboring vital structures in the chest, such as the trachea, esophagus, or spinal cord. Malignant forms of these lesions tend to present with symptoms. In addition to pheochromocytoma, neuroblastomas are hormonally active and can be detected with measurement of catecholamines or their breakdown products (vanillylmandelic acid, VMA) in the urine.[108] As a result, these tumors have related symptoms such as diarrhea, cramping, and hypertension. Thoracic CT or MRI can be used to secure the diagnosis of a posterior mediastinal mass and to assess the relation between the mass and associated structures such as the esophagus, aorta, and spinal cord,[109,110] an important point in planning a surgical procedure. Further studies to document metastatic disease are performed on a patient-by-patient basis.

#### *Nerve Sheath Tumors*

Tumors originating from the nerve sheath account for 40–60% of all mediastinal neurogenic neoplasms. They are slow growing and have a peak incidence in the third and fourth decades of life. Typically symptoms are not present, but symptoms are common in patients with malignant tumors. When present, symptoms are usually the result of pressure on surrounding structures, which leads to pain involving the associated nerve trunk. More than 75% of nerve sheath tumors are neurilemmomas that appear firm and tan or translucent and well encapsulated (Fig. 37–7). One fourth are neurofibromas. Thirty percent of patients with neurofibromas have von Recklinghausen's neurofibromatosis.[111] Neurofibromas are also tan but are more friable and histologically more disordered than neurilemmomas. These neoplasms are infrequently malignant (neurogenic sarcomas); a patient history of neurofibromatosis or older age increases this probability. Nerve sheath tumors also can have extension through the intervertebral foramen, giving them a

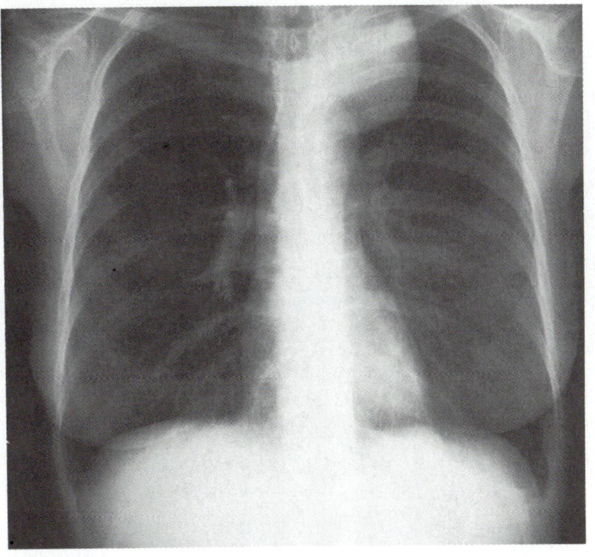

A

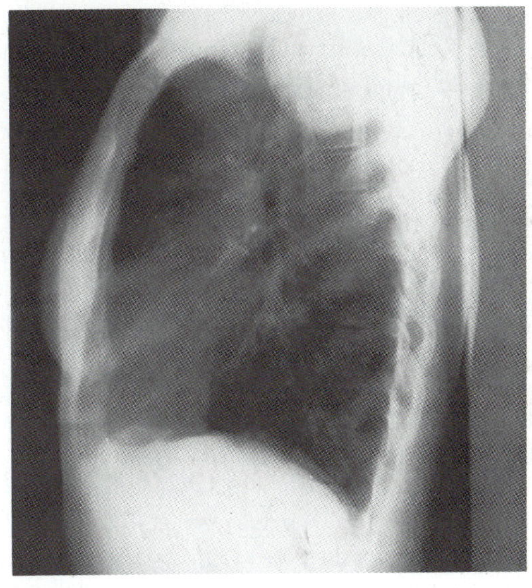

B

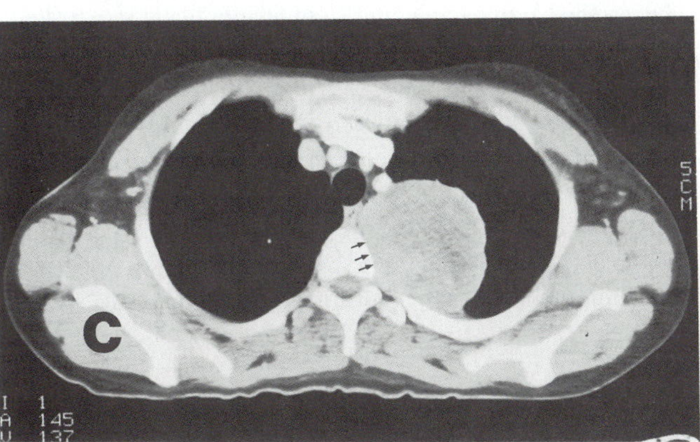


**Figure 37–7.** Frontal **A.** and lateral **B.** radiographs showing smooth-bordered posterior mediastinal mass. **C.** CT scan shows a solid mass abutting but not invading the spine (arrows). This lesion was found to be a benign schwannoma at histologic examination.

dumbbell-shaped appearance. This has importance in terms of surgical approach and, therefore, must not be overlooked.[109]

### *Tumors of the Autonomic Nervous System*

Tumors that originate from sympathetic ganglion cells make up about one third to one half of mediastinal neurogenic lesions. A spectrum exists from benign to malignant within this group. Ganglioneuromas are benign, ganglioneuroblastoma are mixed, and neuroblastomas are malignant. The latter two lesions tend to occur in the pediatric population.[112] Ganglioneuromas and ganglioneuroblastomas are encapsulated and associated with a dense stroma, whereas neuroblastomas rarely have a capsule and are quite cellular with less differentiation.[113] Twenty percent of all neuroblastomas present within the thorax, with a median age at presentation of 11 months.[108]

### *Paraganglionic Tumors*

Paragangliomas tend to occur in two distinct places within the chest. They are associated with the aorticosympathetic paraganglia in the costovertebral sulcus and with the region of the aortic body in the middle mediastinum. They are quite rare and account for a small percentage of thoracic neurogenic tumors.[114] Tumors of the aortic body, or chemodectomas, have an equal distribution in both sexes and tend to occur in young adults. The most useful information with respect to prognosis is gained at the time of operation, when the local aggressiveness can be determined and the completeness of resection gauged. Aortic body paragangliomas may have a higher incidence of residual disease than chemodectomas in other locations because of a larger tumor size at the time of diagnosis or involvement of surrounding vital structures, which makes complete removal hazardous.[114] Metastatic disease is reported to occur 6–30% of the time depending on the length of the follow-up periods. Aorticosympathetic paragangliomas or mediastinal pheochromocytomas tend to occur in middle-aged men. They secrete catecholamines but with a lower frequency than their intra-abdominal counterparts. The malignant potential of these tumors is higher in the extra-adrenal position. As with other mediastinal tumors, the diagnosis of malignancy is best made on clinical grounds at the time of the surgical procedure. These two types of paragangliomas have similar histologic features. They show an organoid arrangement of chief cells with a reticulum network and a well-vascularized stroma.[114]

### *Treatment*

A posterior mediastinal mass is most likely a neurogenic tumor and should be removed. Rarely does a lesion not require surgical intervention. Attempts at closed biopsy may be harmful given the location of these lesions. The essential aspect of therapy is complete surgical excision, which is best approached through a posterolateral thoracotomy except when there is an intraspinal component to the tumor ("dumbbell" tumor). In this case a combined strategy with the neurosurgical team is indicated. The tumor is approached either with the patient in the thoracotomy position with a vertical extension over the vertebral column[115] or with the patient in the prone position.[116] Some surgeons advocate a thoracoscopic approach for uncomplicated neurogenic tumors.[117] Paragangliomas of the aortic body may be optimally resected through a median sternotomy. On occasion the tumors can adhere to the myocardium or great vessels, necessitating cardiopulmonary bypass to allow excision.

Prognosis depends on completeness of resection whether the lesion is benign or malignant. The benign entities tend to correlate with an excellent patient survival rate (>75% at 5 years) when resection is complete.[111] Of the malignant tumors, neuroblastomas are the most common and do well with surgical excision and postoperative multimodality therapy. One report gave an 88% 4-year actuarial survival rate.[108] Malignant schwannomas tend to have a poor patient prognosis whether or not therapy is aggressive.[111]

## SUPERIOR VENA CAVA SYNDROME

The SVC syndrome was originally described by William Hunter in 1757.[118] The causes of the obstruction that leads to the characteristic symptoms and physical findings of SVC syndrome have shifted from a benign granulomatous process, reported by McIntire and Sykes in 1949,[119] to a clinical entity currently associated in 90% of cases with malignant neoplasms.[120,121] Untreated, the syndrome has a fatal outcome in 6–7 months. Simple medical measures may lead to symptomatic improvement, though definitive therapy often involves the use of thoracic irradiation or combination chemotherapy. Surgical intervention other than for diagnostic purposes remains controversial, though in selected patients it may provide long-term palliation.

The pathogenesis of SVC syndrome is multifactorial. The SVC is a thin-walled vein abutted by several more solid structures, including the trachea and right main stem bronchus with associated lymph nodes, the aorta, the pulmonary artery, and the pericardium. The SVC is subject to compression or invasion by pathologic conditions that affect any of these adjacent mediastinal structures. The increasing long-term use of life-sustaining, endovascular catheters for chemotherapy, antibiotics, hyperalimentation, or dialysis and IV devices for cardiac pacing and defibrillation has created a third or iatrogenic cause of SVC syndrome.[122] These cases are manifest primarily by SVC thrombosis without extrinsic disease. Treatment of these patients is often challenging. Although removal of the foreign body may be necessary for effective therapy, the catheter or device may be essential to maintain life.

Most extrinsic disease that leads to SVC syndrome begins in the right paratracheal space or right pulmonary hilum. Symptoms are dictated by the rapidity with which obstruction occurs and the availability of collateral channels. Patency of the azygous vein is critical. SVC obstruction cephalad to the azygocaval junction results in upper extremity and chest wall collateral flow to the residual SVC and right atrium through the azygous arch. Obstruction between the azygous vein and right atrium leads to retrograde azygous blood flow with collaterals draining into the inferior vena cava and back to the right heart. More severe problems arise as intraluminal thrombus forms and is propagated by venous stasis into caval tributaries. Upper body venous hypertension impedes lymph drainage from the head, neck, and arms, leading to lymphedema. Venous hypertension may result in excessive thoracic duct pressures, precipitating leaks and resulting in the chylothoraces.

### Symptoms and Signs

Swelling of the face, neck, and arms, dyspnea, or orthopnea and cough are the most common symptoms of SVC obstruction. Distended and tortuous veins over the chest wall, neck, and head along with plethora and cyanosis of the face and lips constitute the usual physical findings. If the syndrome has evolved slowly, it may be asymptomatic. Patients with symptoms suggesting cerebral edema (changes in mental status, vertigo, seizures) or laryngeal edema (hoarseness or stridor) have a poor prognosis. Emergency intervention is required. Parish et al from the Mayo Clinic found an average survival time of only 6 weeks if these patients did not undergo decompression.[121]

### Malignant Causes

Malignant disease of the thorax occurs in 90% of patients with SVC syndrome.[123] Lung cancer accounts for 67–82% of cases.[120,121,124] Two thirds of lung cancers are of non-small cell histologic type, and the others are small cell carcinomas. Bulky lymphomas arising in the anterior mediastinum and extending posteriorly are the second most common malignant lesion. Metastases from extrathoracic sites complete this list of malignant causes of SVC obstruction.

## Benign Causes

Series reported from the Cleveland Clinic[125] and Mayo Clinic[121] highlight the benign causes of SVC syndrome. Both institutions describe a chronic, granulomatous, fibrosing mediastinitis in most cases. *Histoplasma capsulatum* is the most common organism identified by culture, special stains, or complement-fixation titers, but it was present in only 20% of patients in one study.[126] *Blastomyces* has been implicated as another precipitating organism.[127] Tuberculosis, *Nocardia* infection, syphilis, actinomycosis, sarcoid tumors, and radiation therapy have all been associated with benign SVC syndromes. Any of these stimuli apparently may initiate a granulomatous response with subsequent immune reactions characterized by a desmoplastic response and excessive collagen deposition in the mediastinal soft tissues.

## Diagnosis

The diagnosis of SVC syndrome begins with recognition of the aforementioned symptoms and signs related to upper body venous hypertension. SVC obstruction appears as a widened mediastinum on plain radiographs[128] and can be confirmed with contrast-enhanced CT or MRI.[129] Radionuclide scanning confirms the obstruction but provides limited useful anatomic data. CT demonstrates the presence and pattern of collaterals. Venography is invasive, requires large volumes of IV contrast material, and provides little additional information.

A tissue diagnosis is desirable in all cases. Fine-needle aspirates using CT- or ultrasound-guided techniques have yielded a specific diagnosis in as many as 83% of cases.[130] Open biopsy by means of either mediastinoscopy or mediastinotomy can be safely accomplished. The risks of dissecting through engorged mediastinal collaterals should be weighed carefully against the need to have a histologic sample. Suspected lymphoma is an example in which a cell-type specific diagnosis may require such intervention.

## Treatment

The treatment of SVC syndrome depends on cause and prognosis. Simple supportive measures such as elevation of the head, supplemental oxygen, diuretics, and steroids may improve symptoms.[131] Strategies for relief of obstruction may involve radiation therapy, chemotherapy, or surgery.

Thoracic irradiation is the modality most commonly used to treat SVC syndrome. The field commonly includes the tumor along with hilar, mediastinal, and supraclavicular nodes. Fractions of greater than 3–4 Gy/day are recommended to a total dose of 30–40 Gy. The worst toxicity is dysphagia.[131] A 90% response rate can be expected,[123] though relapses are common. This therapy remains valuable, however, because some patients derive long-term benefit. As many as 10% of patients with bronchogenic carcinoma at some time have SVC syndrome. Perez et al noted that 10% of these patients were alive 2.5 years after primary radiation therapy to relieve their obstruction.[124]

Chemotherapy is a reasonable alternative for lesions known to be sensitive to specific agents. Small-cell carcinoma[132] and lymphoma[133] are the leading examples. Patients may see relief of symptoms within 1 week, though both lesions are prone to relapse. Radiation therapy given as an adjunct after successful induction chemotherapy may prolong symptom-free survival for these patients.

Surgical approaches to SVC obstruction have included decompression, thrombectomy, caval replacement, and bypass. The use of percutaneously placed endovascular stents has been described.[134] Decompression of fibrosing mediastinitis by resection or evacuation of the granulomatous process has been detailed by Ferguson and Burford.[135] This may be expected to relieve SVC symptoms in the absence of intraluminal thrombosis. Thrombectomy is a reasonable approach for catheter-induced acute obstruction. Success depends on early operative intervention, removal of the foreign body, and long-term anticoagulation. Thrombolytic therapy is an arguable nonsurgical alternative, though the potential risk of embolization of lysing clot into the pulmonary circulation remains undefined.

Replacement or bypass of the obstructed vena cava is a substantial surgical challenge. A variety of conduits have been used with variable results. Early experience with Dacron polyester conduits was plagued by graft thrombosis.[136] Other investigators[137,138] noted success with the use of externally reinforced, expanded polytetrafluoroethylene grafts. Doty et al[139] had the largest experience using autogenous tissue. They used a composite vein graft constructed from longitudinally split saphenous vein sutured in a spiral manner around a 10- to 15-mm stent. Grafts made in this manner can be placed in the bed of the resected SVC or used as bypass conduits from the brachiocephalic venous branches to the right atrial appendage. Patency rate is reported to be 78% with as many as 15 years of follow-up.[120]

All authors described careful patient selection when replacement or bypass of the SVC was considered. Candidates should have clinically significant upper body venous hypertension without a mass lesion involving the thoracic inlet. For benign fibrosing mediastinitis, a waiting period of 6–12 months from the onset of symptoms is warranted to allow for collateral formation, which obviates the need for surgical intervention. Patients with malignant disease in which cure is unlikely and palliation is the goal, patients with rapid onset of symptoms, or those in whom symptoms are severe and life-threatening (laryngeal or cerebral edema) are candidates for replacement or bypass. In this highly selected subgroup, palliative decompression may extend survival beyond the expected 6 weeks seen without treatments.[120]

TABLE 37–5. MESENCHYMAL TUMORS OF THE MEDIASTINUM

| Tissue of Origin | Presentation | Treatment and Prognosis |
|---|---|---|
| **Adipose Tissue** | | |
| Lipoma | Common, benign,<br>Anterior mediastinum<br>Encapsulated | Surgery<br>Good prognosis |
| Liposarcoma | Rare, malignant, symptomatic<br>Pain and respiratory distress | Surgery and radiation therapy<br>Poor prognosis |
| **Fibrous Tissue** | | |
| Fibroma | Benign, encapsulated<br>Becomes large, symptomatic<br>May transform to sarcoma | Surgery<br>Good prognosis |
| Fibrosarcoma | Malignant<br>Cough, pain, and dyspnea<br>Hypoglycemia | Unresectable<br>Poor prognosis<br>Chemo- and radiation therapy not helpful |
| **Blood Vessel** | | |
| Hemangioma | Rare, 25–33% malignant<br>Multifocal, may bleed<br>More common in children<br>Anterior and posterior mediastinum | Surgery, but difficult<br>Recurrence rare |
| Hemangiopericytoma | Rare, benign and malignant<br>Originates from pericapillary arterioles | Surgery<br>Doxorubicin if malignant<br>Course variable |
| **Lymph Vessel** | | |
| Lymphangioma<br>(Cystic hygroma) | Benign<br>Neck or mediastinal origin<br>Common in children<br>Tends to grow and infiltrate | Surgery, but difficult<br>Recurrence rare<br>If chylothorax, give postoperative low-dose radiation therapy |

*(From King RM, et al: Primary mediastinal tumors: A follow-up study of 208 patients. J Pediatr Surg 17:512, 1982.)*

## MESENCHYMAL TUMORS OF THE MEDIASTINUM

Primary mesenchymal tumors of the mediastinum are rare. They make up 6% of mediastinal masses[17,23] and are malignant more than 50% of the time. Both incidence and malignancy rate are increased in a pediatric population to 10% and 85%, respectively.[140] The presentation of these lesions is variable. When malignant, these tumors tend to be associated with symptoms. The classification of these lesions has always been difficult because they do not fit neatly into an anatomic location or originate from the same structure. Table 37–5[141] outlines the most common of these rare tumors.

Other sporadic mesenchymal tumors of the mediastinum include thymolipoma, thymoliposarcoma, hemangioendothelioma, leiomyoma, leiomyosarcoma, mesenchymoma, and localized fibrous tumors. These should be dealt with on an individual basis; experience with them is quite limited.

## REFERENCES


1. Haller A: *Disputationes Anatomicae Selectae.* Gottingen, Vandenhoeck 1749, p 96
2. Billroth T: Geschwulster der Schiddr use. *Chir Klin Zuruch* 1869, p 67
3. Klein O: Ueber die Austrottung verschiedener uceschwulste: Besonders jener der Ohrspercheldruse und der Schelddruse. *J Chir Augen-Heilk* **120:**106, 1820
4. Kocher T: Bericht uber ein zweites tousend Kropfexcisionen. *Arch Klin Chir* **64:**454, 1901
5. Bauer W, Federman DD: Hyperparathyroidism epitomized: The case of Captain Charles E. Martell. *Metabolism* **11:**21, 1962
6. Creswell LL, Wells SA: Mediastinal masses originating in the neck. *Chest Surg Clin North Am* **2:**23, 1992
7. Mixter CG, Clifford SH: Congenital mediastinal cysts of gastrogenic and bronchogenic origin. *Ann Surg* **90:**714, 1929
8. Jolly F: Ueber myasthenia gravis pseudoparalytica. *Berl Klin Wochenschr* **32:**1–7, 1885
9. Lacquer L, Weigert C: Beitrage zur Lehyre von de Erb'schen Krankheit. I. Uber de Erb schen Krankheit (myasthenia gravis) (Lacquer). II. Pathologisch-anatomischer Beitrag zur Erb'schen Krankjheit (myasthenia gravis) (Weigert). *Zentralb Neuro* **20:**594, 1901
10. Almon RR, Andrew AG, Appel SH: Serum globulin in myasthenia gravis: Inhibition of L-Bungaroton to acetylcholine receptors. *Science* **186:**55, 1974
11. Blalock A, Mason MF, Morgan HJ, et al: Myasthenia gravis and tumors of the thymic regions: Report of a case in which the tumor was removed. *Ann Surg* **110:**544, 1939
12. Blalock A: Thymectomy in the treatment of myasthenia gravis: Report of twenty cases. *J Thorac Surg* **13:**316, 1944
13. Carlens E: Mediastinoscopy: A method for inspection and tissue biopsy in the superior mediastinum. *Dis Chest* **36:**343, 1959

14. Sabiston DC Jr, Scott HW: Primary neoplasms and cysts of the mediastinum. *Ann Surg* **136:**777, 1952
15. Heimberger IL, Battersby JS, Vellios F: Primary neoplasms of the mediastinum: A fifteen-year experience. *Arch Surg* **86:**120, 1963
16. Benjamin SP, McCormack LJ, Effler DB: Primary lymphatic tumors of the mediastinum. *Cancer* **30:**708, 1972
17. Davis RD, Oldham HN Jr, Sabiston DC Jr: Primary cysts and neoplasms of the mediastinum: Recent changes in clinical presentation, methods of diagnosis, management and results. *Ann Thorac Surg* **44:**229–37, 1987
18. Azanow KS, Pearl RH, Zurcher R, et al: Primary mediastinal masses: A comparison of adult and pediatric populations. *J Thorac Cardiovasc Surg* **106:**67–72, 1993
19. Whittaker LD, Lynn HB: Mediastinal tumors and cysts in the pediatric patient. *Surg Clin North Am* **58:**893, 1973
20. Pokomy WJ, Sherman JO: Mediastinal masses in infants and children. *J Thorac Cardiovasc Surg* **68:**869, 1974
21. Bowen RJ, Kiesewetter WB: Mediastinal masses in infants and children. *Ann Surg* **112:**1003, 1977
22. King RM, Telander RL, Smithson WA, et al: Primary mediastinal tumors in children. *J Pediatr Surg* **17:**512, 1982
23. Wychulis AR, Payne WS, Clagett OT, et al: Surgical treatment of mediastinal tumors. *J Thorac Cardiovasc Surg* **62:**379, 1971
24. Rubush JL, Gardner IC, Boyd WK, et al: Mediastinal tumors: Review of 186 cases. *J Thorac Cardiovasc Surg* **65:**216, 1973
25. Luosta R, Koikkalainen K, Jyrala A, et al: Mediastinal tumors: A follow-up study of 208 patients. *Scand J Thorac Cardiovasc Surg* **12:**258, 1978
26. Mullen B, Richardson JD: Primary anterior mediastinal tumors in children and adults. *Ann Thorac Surg* **42:**338–45, 1986
27. Ovrum E, Birkeland S: Mediastinal tumors and cysts: A review of 191 cases. *Scand J Thorac Cardiovasc Surg* **86:**727, 1983
28. Nandi P, Wong KC, Mok CK, et al: Primary mediastinal tumours: Review of 74 cases. *J R Coll Surg Edinb* **25:**460, 1980
29. Cohen AJ, Thompson L, Edwards FH, Bellamy RF: Primary cysts and tumors of the mediastinum. *Ann Thorac Surg* **41:**378–86, 1991
30. Harris GJ, Harmon PK, Trinkel JK, Grover FL: Standard biplane roentgenography is highly sensitive in documenting mediastinal masses. *Ann Thorac Surg* **44:**238, 1987
31. Pugatch RD, Faling LJ, Robbins AH, et al: CT diagnosis of benign mediastinal abnormalities. *AJR* **134:**685, 1980
32. Shamberger RC, Holzma RS, Griscow NT, et al: CT quantitation of tracheal cross-sectional area as a guide to the surgical and anesthetic management of children with anterior mediastinal masses. *J Pediatr Surg* **26:**138, 1991
33. Katz ME, Glazier HS, Siegel MJ et al: Mediastinal vessels: Postoperative evaluation with MR imaging. *Radiology* **161:**647, 1986
34. VonSchulthess GK, McMurdok, Tscholakoff D et al: Mediastinal masses: MR imaging. *Radiology* **158:**289, 1986
35. VanDam J, Rice TW, Sivak MV Jr: Endoscopic ultrasonography and endoscopically guided needle aspiration for the diagnosis of upper gastrointestinal tract frequent cysts. *Am J Gastroenterology* **87:**762–5, 1992
36. Shapiro B, Sisson J, Kalff V, et al: The location of a middle mediastinal pheochromocytoma. *J Thorac Cardiovasc Surg* **87:**814, 1984
37. Bressler EL, Kirkham JA: Mediastinal masses: Alternative approaches to CT-guided needle biopsy. *Radiology* **191:**391–6, 1994
38. Heilo A: Tumors in the mediastinum: US-guided histologic core-needle biopsy. *Radiology* **189:**143, 1993
39. D'Agostino HB, Sanchez RB, Laoide RM, et al: Anterior mediastinal lesions: Transsternal biopsy with CT guidance work in progress. *Radiology* **189:**703, 1993
40. Rendina EA, Venuta F, DeGiacomo T, et al: Comparative merits of thoracoscopy, mediastinoscopy and mediastinotomy for mediastinal biopsy. *Ann Thorac Surg* **57:**992, 1994
41. Bonadies J, D'Agostino RS, Ruskis AF, Ponn RB: Outpatient mediastinoscopy. *J Thorac Cardiovasc Surg* **106:**686, 1993
42. Morgenthaler TI, Brown LR, Colby TV, et al: Thymoma. *Mayo Clin Proc* **68:**1110–1123, 1993
43. Kohman LJ: Approach to the diagnosis and staging of mediastinal masses. *Chest* **103** (Suppl):328–330, 1993
44. Kirchen T, Muller-Hermelink HK: New approaches to the diagnosis of thymic epithelial tumors. *Prog Surg Pathol* **70:**167–189, 1989
45. Weide LG, Ulbright TM, Loehrer PJ, Williams SD: Thymic carcinoma: A distinct clinical entity responsive to chemotherapy. *Cancer* 71(4):1219–1223, 1993
46. Urgesi A, Monetti V, Ross G, et al: Role of radiation therapy in locally advanced thymoma. *Radiother Oncol* **19:**273–280, 1990
47. Nakahara K, Ohno K, Hashimoto J, et al: Thymoma: Results with complete resection and adjuvant postoperative irradiation in 141 consecutive patients. *J Thorac Cardiovasc Surg* **95:**1041–1047, 1988
48. Park HS, Shin DM, Lee JS, et al: Thymoma: A retrospective study of 87 cases. *Cancer* **73**(10):2491–2498, 1994
49. Loehrer PJ Sr, Perez CA, Roth LM, et al: Chemotherapy for advanced thymoma: Preliminary results of an intergroup study. *Ann Intern Med* **113:**520–524, 1990
50. Kirschner PA: Reoperation for thymoma: A report of 23 cases. *Ann Thorac Surg* **49:**550–554, 1990
51. Pascuzzi R: History of myasthenia gravis. *Neurol Clin North Am* **12:**231–242, 1994
52. Willis T: *De Anima Brutorum,* Oxford, 1672. (Pordage S, Transl). *Two discourses concerning the Soul of Brutes.* London, 1683
53. Treves TA, Rocca WA, Menoeghin F: Epidemiology of myasthenia Gravis. In: Anderson DW, Schoenberg DG (eds): *Neuroepidemiology: A Tribute to Bruce Schoenberg.* Boston, CRC Press, 1991, p 297
54. Phillips LH, Torner JC: Has the natural history of myasthenia gravis changed over the past 40 years? An analysis of the epidemiological literature. *Neurology* **43:** A386, 1993
55. Phillips LH: The epidemiology of myasthenia gravis. *Neurol Clin North Am* **12:**263–271, 1994
56. Maselli A: Pathophysiology of myasthenia gravis and Lambert Eaton syndrome. *Neurol Clin North Am* **12:**285–303, 1994
57. Olanow CW, Wechsler AS, Roses AD: A prospective study of thymectomy and serum acetylcholine receptor antibodies in myasthenia gravis. *Ann Surg* **196:**113, 1982
58. Castleman B, Norris EH: The pathology of the thymus gland in myasthenia gravis: A study of 35 cases. *Medicine* **28:**27, 1949
59. Hopkins LC: Clinical features of myasthenia gravis. *Neurol Clin North Am* **12:**243–261, 1994
60. Trastek VF, Shields TW: Surgery of the thymus gland. In Shields TW (ed): *General Thoracic Surgery,* 4th ed Baltimore, Williams & Wilkins, 1994, pp 1770–1801
61. Olanow CW, Wechsler AS: The surgical management of myasthenia gravis. In Sabiston Jr DC (ed): *Textbook of Surgery: The Biological Basis of Modern Surgical Practice,* 13th ed, Philadelphia, Saunders, 1986, p 2110
62. Saunders DB, Scoppetta C: The treatment of patients with myasthenia gravis. *Neurol Clin North Am* **12:**343–368, 1994
63. Kirschner PA: Myasthenia gravis and other parathymic syndromes. *Chest Surg Clin North Am* **2** (1):183–201, 1992
64. Frist WH, Thirumalai S, Doehring CB, et al: Thymectomy for the myasthenia gravis patient: Factors influencing outcome. *Ann Thorac Surg* **57:**334–8, 1994
65. Defilippi VJ, Richman DP, Ferguson MK: Transcervical thymectomy for myasthenia gravis. *Ann Thorac Surg* **57:**194–7, 1994
66. Sugarbaker DJ: Thoracoscopy in the management of anterior mediastinal masses. *Ann Thorac Surg* **56:**653–6, 1993
67. Crucitti F, Doglietto GB, Bellanone R, et al: Effects of surgical treatment in thymoma with myasthenia gravis: Our experience in 103 patients. *J Surg Oncol* **50:**43–6, 1992

68. Blossom GB, Erinstoff RM, Howells GA, et al: Thymoma for myasthenia gravis. *Arch Surg* **128**(8):855–62, 1993
69. Nussbaum MS, Rosenthal GJ, Saunders KJ, et al: Management of myasthenia gravis by extended thymectomy with anterior mediastinal disection. *Surgery* **112**(4):681–8, 1992
70. Yellin A: Lymphoproliferative diseases. *Chest Surg Clin North Am* **2**:107–120, 1992
71. Yellin A, Rosen A, Reichert N, et al: Superior vena cava syndrome: The myth—the facts. *Ann Rev Respir Dis* **14**:1114, 1990
72. Bonfiglio TA, Dvoretsky PM, Risciuli F, et al: Fine needle aspiration biopsy in the evaluation of lymphoreticular tumors of the thorax. *Acta Cytol* **29**:548, 1985
73. Hope RT, Colemain CN, Cox RS, et al: The management of state I-II Hodgkin's disease with irradiation alone or combined modality therapy: The Stanford experience. *Blood* **59**:455, 1982
74. Vasef M, Katzin WE, Mendlesohn G, Reydman M: Report of a case of localized Castleman's disease with progression to malignant lymphoma. *Am J Clin Pathol* **98**:633–636, 1992
75. Nichols CR: Mediastinal germ cell tumors: Cinical features and biologic correlates. *Chest* **99**:472–9, 1991
76. Kuhn MW, Weissbach L: Localization, incidence, diagnosis and treatment of extratesticular germ cell tumors. *Urol Int* **40**:166–72, 1985
77. Lakhoo Boyle M, Drake DP: Mediastinal teratomas: Review of 15 pediatric cases. *J Pediatr Surg* **28**:1161–4, 1993
78. Chaganti RSK, Rodriguez E, Mathew S: Origin of adult male mediastinal germ cell tumors: *Lancet* **343**:1130–2, 1994
79. Luna MA, Johnson PE: Postmortem findings in testicular tumors: In: Johnson DE (ed): *Testicular Tumors.* New York: Medical Examination, 1975
80. Knapp RH, Hurt RD, Payne WS, et al: Malignant germ cell tumors of the mediastinum. *J Thorac Cardiovasc Surg* **89**:82–9, 1985
81. Dulmet EM, Macchiavini P, Suc B, Verley JM: Germ cell tumors of the mediastinum:A 30 year experience. *Cancer* **72**:1894–901, 1993
82. Goss PE, Schwartfeger L, Blackstein ME, et al: Extragonadal germ cell tumors: A 14 year Toronto experience. *Cancer* **73**:1971–9, 1994
83. Mandelbaum I: Germ cell tumors of the mediastinum. *Chest Surg Clin North Am* **2**:203–11, 1992
84. Lewis BD, Hurt RD, Payne WS, et al: Benign teratoma of the mediastinum. *J Thorac Cardiovasc Surg* **86**: 727, 1983
85. Jain KK, Bols GJ, Bains MS, et al: The treatment of extragonadal seminoma. *J Clin Oncol* **2**:820–7, 1984
86. Loehrer PJ, Birch R, Williams SD, et al: Chemotherapy of metastatic seminoma: The Southeastern Cancer Study Group experience. *J Clin Oncol* **5**:1212–20, 1987
87. Motzer R, Bosl G, Heelan R, et al: Residual mass: An indication for further therapy in patients with advanced seminoma following systemic chemotherapy. *J Clin Oncol* **5**:1065–70, 1987
88. Nichols CR, Roth BJ, Heerema N, et al: Hematologic neoplasia associated with primary germ cell tumors. *N Engl J Med* 322:1425–29, 1990
89. Kantoff P: Surgical and medical management of germ cell tumors of the chest. *Chest* **103**:3315–3355, 1993
90. Johnston SR, Adam A, Allison DJ, et al: Recurrent respiratory obstruction from a mediastinal bronchogenic cysts. *Thorax* **47**:660–2, 1992
91. Patel SR, Meeker DP, Biscotti CV, et al: Preservation and management of bronchogenic cysts in the adult. *Chest* **106**:79–85, 1994
92. Coran AG, Drongowski R: Congenital cystic disease of the tracheobronchial tree in infants and children: Experience with 44 consecutive cases. *Arch Surg* **129**:521–7, 1994
93. Haddan MJ, Bowen A: Bronchopulmonary and neurenteric forms of frequent anomalies: Imaging for diagnosis and management. *Radiol Clin North Am* **29**:241–54, 1991
94. Bolton JW, Shahian DM: Asymptomatic bronchogenic cysts: What is the best management? *Ann Thorac Surg* **53**:1134–7, 1992
95. Hazelrigg SR, Landreneau RJ, Mack MJ, Acuff TE: Thoracoscopic resection of mediastinal cysts. *Ann Thorac Surg* **56**:659–60, 1993
96. Suen HC, Mathisen DJ, Grillo HC, et al: Surgical management and radiological characteristics of bronchogenic cysts. *Ann Thorac Surg* **55**:476–81, 1993
97. Read CA, Movont M, Varangelo R, et al: Recurrent bronchogenic cyst: An assessment for complete surgical excision. *Arch Surg* **126**:1306–8, 1991
98. Malde HM, Kedar RP, Chadda DJ: Ethanol sclerosis of a mediastinal cyst. *Can Assoc Radiol J* **44**:310–2, 1993
99. Bennheim J, Griffel B, Versano S, et al: Mediastinal leiomyosarcoma in the wall of bronchogenic cyst. *Arch Pathol Lab Med* **104**:221, 1980
100. Whitaker JA, Deffenbaugh LD, Cooke AR: Esophageal duplication cyst. *Am J Gastroenterol* **73**:329, 1980
101. Heimburger IL, Battersly JS: Primary mediastinal tumors of childhood. *J Thorac Cardiovasc Surg* **50**:92, 1965
102, D'Almeida AC, Steward DH Jr: Neuroenteric cysts: Care report and literature review. *Neurosurgery* **8**:596, 1981
103. Allen MS, Payne WS: Cystic foregut malformation in the mediastinum. *Chest Surg Clin North Am* **2**:89–106, 1992
104. Rastegar H, Arger P, Harlan AH: Evaluation and therapy of mediastinal thymic cysts. *Ann Surg* **46**:236, 1980
105. Feigin DS, Fenoglis JJ, McAllister HA, Madewell JE: Pericardial cysts: A radiologic-pathologic correlation and review. *Diagn Radiol* **125**:15, 1977
106. Okabe K, Mivra K, Konish H, et al. Thoracic duct cyst of the mediastinum: Case report. *Scand J Thorac Cardiovasc Surg* **27**:175–7, 1993
107. Furst H, Schmittenbecher PP, Dievemautt, Berger H: Mediastinal pancreatic pseudocyst. *Eur J CardioThorac Surg* **6**:46–8, 1992
108. Adams GA, Schochat SJ, Smith EI, et al: Thoracic neuroblastoma: A Pediatric Oncology Group study. *J Pediatr Surg* **28**:372–378, 1993
109. Ricci C, Rendina EA, Venuto F, et al: Diagnostic imaging and surgical treatment of dumbbell tumors of the mediastinum. *Ann Thorac Surg* **50**:586–9, 1990
110. Moon WK, Jung-Gi I, Hau MC: Malignant schwannomas of the thorax: CT findings. *J Comp Assist Tomogr* **17**(2):274–276, 1993
111. Wain JC: Neurogenic tumors of the mediastinum. *Chest Surg Clin North Am* **2**(1): 121–136, 1992
112. Joshi VV, Cantor AB, Altshuler G, et al: Age-linked prognostic categorization based on a new histologic grading system of neuroblastomas: A clinicopathologic study of 211 cases from the Pediatric Oncology Group. Cancer **8**:2197–2211, 1992
113. Zajtchuk R, Bowen TD, Seyfer AD, Brott WH. Intrathoracic ganglioneuroblastoma. *J Thorac Carciovasc Surg* **80**:605–612, 1980
114. Olson JL, Salyer WR: Mediastinal paragangliomas (aortic body tumor): A report of four cases and a review of the literature. *Cancer* **41**:2405–2412, 1978
115. Grillo HC, Ojemann RG, Scannell JG, Zervas NT: Combined approach to "dumbbell" intrathoracic and intraspinal neurogenic tumors. *Ann Thorac Surg* **36**:402, 1983
116. Alewari DE, Payne NS, Onofrio BM, et al: Dumbbell neurogenic tumors of the mediastinum. *Mayo Clin Proc* **53**:353, 1978
117. Landreneau RJ, Dowling RD, Ferson PF: Thoracoscopic resecton of a posterior mediastinal neurogenic tumor. *Chest* **102**(4):1288–90, 1992
118. Hunter W: The history of an aneurysm of the aorta with some remarks on aneurysms in general. *Med Obs Soc Phys Cond* **1**:323, 1757
119. McIntire FT, Sykes EM Jr: Obstruction of the superior vena cava: A review of the literature and report of two personal cases. *Ann Intern Med* **30**:925, 1949
120. Lochridge SK, Knibble WP, Doty DB: Obstruction of the superior vena cava. *Surgery* **85**:14, 1979

121. Parish JM, Marschke RF, Dines DE, Lee RE: Etiologic considerations in superior vena cava syndrome. *Mayo Clin Proc* **56**:407, 1981
122. Mazzetti H, Dussant A, Tentori C: Superior vena cava occlusion and/or syndrome related to pacemaker leads. *Am Heart J* **125**:831, 1993
123. Nieto AF, Doty DB: Superior vena cava obstruction: Clinical syndrome, etiology and treatment. *Curr Probl Cancer* **10**:441, 1986
124. Perez CA, Presant CA, VanAmburg A: Management of superior vena cava syndrome. *Semin Oncol* **5**:123, 1978
125. Mahajan V, Strimlan V, VanOrdstran HC, Loop FD: Benign superior vena cava syndrome. *Chest* **68**: 32, 1975
126. Dines DE, Payne WS, Bernatz PE, et al: Mediastinal granulomas and fibrosing mediastinitis. *Chest* **75**:320, 1975
127. Lagerstrom CF, Mitchell HG, Graham BS, Hammon JW Jr: Chronic fibrosing mediastinitis and superior vena caval obstruction from blastomycosis. *Ann Thorac Surg* **54**:764, 1992
128. Brown G, Husband JE: Mediastinal widening: A valuable radiographic sign of superior vena cava thrombosis. *Clin Radiol* **47**:415, 1993
129. Kim JH, Kim HS, Chung SH: CT diagnosis of superior vena cava syndrome: Importance of collateral vessels. *AJR* **161**:539, 1993
130. Ko J, Yang P, Yuan A, et al: Superior vena cava syndrome: Rapid histologic diagnosis by ultrasound guided transthoracic needle aspiration biopsy. *Am J Respir Crit Care Med* **149**:783, 1994
131. Abner A: Approach to the patient who presents with superior vena cava obstruction. *Chest* **103**:3945, 1993
132. Kane RC, Cohen MH, Brader LE et al: Superior vena cava obstruction due to small-cell anaplastic lung carcinoma. *JAMA* **235**:1717, 1976
133. Perez-Soler R, McLaughlin P, Velasquez WS, et al: Clinical features and results of management of superior vena cava syndrome secondary to lymphoma. *J Clin Oncol* **2**:260, 1984
134. Dodds GA, Harrison JK, O'Laughlin MP, et al: Relief of superior vena cava syndrome due to fibrosing mediastinitis using the palmaz stent. *Chest* **106**:315, 1994
135. Ferguson TB, Burford TH: Mediastinal granuloma: A 15 year experience. *Ann Thorac Surg* **1**:125, 1965
136. Avasthi RB, Moghissi K: Malignant obstruction of the superior vena cava and its palliation: Report of four cases. *J Thorac Cardiovasc Surg* **74**:244, 1977
137. Dartevelle PG, Chapelier AR, Pastorino V, et al: Long-term follow-up after prosthetic replacement of the superior vena cava combined with resection of mediastinal-pulmonary malignant tumors. *J Thorac Cardiovasc Surg* **102**:259, 1991
138. Moore WM Jr, Hollier LH, Pickett TK: Superior vena cava and central venous reconstruction. *Surgery* **110**:35, 1991
139. Doty DB, Doty JR, Jones KW: Bypass of superior vena cava: 15 years experience with spiral veingraft for obstruction of superior vena cava caused by benign disease. *J Thorac Cardiovasc Surg* **99**:889, 1990
140. Shields TW, Robinson PG: Mesenchymal tumors of the mediastinum. In Shields TW (ed): *Mediastinal surgery.* Philadelphia, Lea & Febiger, 1991, 272–288
141. King RM, Telander RL, Smithson WA, et al: Primary mediastinal tumors: A follow-up study of 208 patients. *J Pediatr Surg* **17**:512, 1982

CHAPTER

38

# The Trachea

## *Tracheostomy, Tumors, Strictures, Tracheomalacia, and Tracheal Resection and Reconstruction*

Douglas J. Mathisen and Hermes C. Grillo

Surgery of the trachea has evolved to encompass one of the simplest and oldest surgical techniques (tracheostomy), the very complex (repair of tracheoesophageal fistula), and areas still evolving (repair of congenital stenosis). Techniques of resection and reconstruction have evolved to allow successful single-stage repair of most tracheal abnormalities. Surgeons interested in surgery of the airway need to have an in-depth knowledge of surgical anatomy, the indications for and contraindications to surgery, methods of reconstruction, release maneuvers to reduce anastomotic tension, postoperative care, and recognition and management of complications.

### SURGICAL ANATOMY

The trachea begins at the lower border of the cricoid cartilage and is partly inset beneath the cricoid cartilage. The trachea terminates where the lateral walls of the right and left main bronchi flair out from the lower trachea. The carinal spur is useful as a landmark for the termination of the trachea, because it is clearly definable with bronchoscopy and radiography. The average trachea in adult humans measures 11 cm in length, varying roughly in proportion to the height of the person.[1] There are approximately two tracheal cartilaginous rings per centimeter of the trachea; thus, the total number of rings ranges from 18 to 22. It must be remembered that the subglottic laryngeal airway measures 1.5–2.0 cm in length before the trachea is reached. Except for some cases of congenital stenosis with circumferential rings of the trachea, the only completely circular cartilage in the upper airway is the cricoid with its broad posterior plate.

The potential for presentation of the trachea in the neck is of critical importance not only for surgical access to the trachea but also for reconstruction after resection of any length of the trachea. In young patients, particularly those who are not obese, hyperextension of the neck delivers more than 50% of the trachea into the neck.[2] In a kyphotic, aged person, particularly an obese one, the cricoid cartilage may be located at the level of the sternal notch, and even the most vigorous hyperextension may fail to deliver any of the trachea into the neck. In both the young and aged, the anatomic position of the trachea changes from an essentially subcutaneous position at the cricoid level to a prevertebral position at the carinal level. The course is thus obliquely caudad and dorsal when the patient stands erect. In kyphotic, aged patients, lateral projection becomes increasingly horizontal. The caudad extensibility and flexibility of the trachea in youth diminish with increasing age. Calcification of the cartilages also occurs with age and with injury.

The blood supply of the trachea is of special importance for resection and reconstruction of the trachea. The upper trachea is principally supplied by branches of the inferior thyroid artery.[3] The lower trachea is supplied by branches of the bronchial artery with contributions from the subclavian, highest (supreme) intercostal, internal thoracic, and innominate arteries[4] (Figs. 38–1 and 38–2). The vessels supply branches anteriorly to the trachea and posteriorly to the esophagus, arriving at the trachea through lateral pedicles of tissue. The longitudinal anastomoses between these vessels are very fine. Transverse intercartilaginous arteries branch ultimately into a submucosal capillary network (Fig. 38–3). Excessive division of the lateral tissues by circumferential dissection of the trachea can easily destroy this blood supply and thus lead to serious and sometimes disastrous complications.[5]

The anatomic relations of the recurrent nerves to the trachea and the esophagus and the point of entry of these nerves into the larynx have been well described. The close relation of the trachea to the thyroid gland also is well known. The isthmus crosses the trachea at the second and third cartilaginous rings. Intimate adherence of the medial portions of both lobes of the thyroid to the trachea is observed at this same level laterally. Because of this intimate adherence, it may become necessary to remove a lobe or sometimes the entire thyroid gland in the surgical management of a tumor in the upper trachea. Posteriorly, the esophagus has a common interface through areolar tissue with the membranous wall of the trachea. The blood supply of the esophagus and the membranous wall are intimately linked. Anteriorly, the innominate artery courses obliquely across the cartilaginous surface of the trachea. In the left lateral aspect of the trachea, the aorta arches backward across the left tracheobronchial angle where the left recurrent laryngeal nerve arrives at its place in the tracheoesophageal groove.

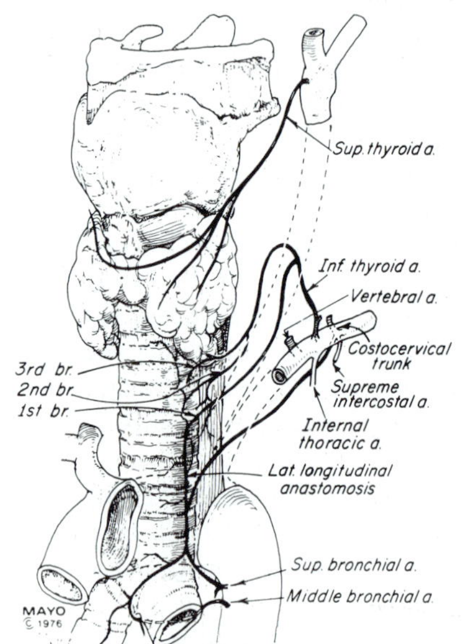


**Figure 38–1.** Left anterior view of vessels supplying the trachea. In this specimen the lateral longitudinal anastomosis links branches of the inferior thyroid, costocervical trunk, and bronchial arteries. *(From Salassa JR, et al: Ann Thorac Surg 24(2):100–107, with permission).*

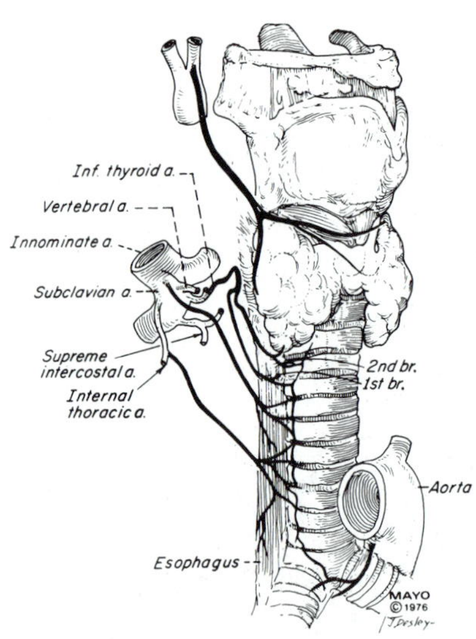


**Figure 38–2.** Right anterior view of vessels supplying the trachea. In this specimen the lateral longitudinal anastomosis links branches from the inferior thyroid, the subclavian, the internal thoracic, and the superior bronchial arteries. *(From Salassa JR, et al: Ann Thorac Surg 24(2):100–107, with permission.)*

The lymph nodes adjacent to the trachea are stations in the pathways from the lungs and mediastinum and are well known to surgeons who treat thoracic neoplasms. The lymphatic vessels of the trachea have been less well studied. Gross observations have been made of the clinical behavior of tumor metastatic from the trachea. Metastases appear to involve the most closely adjacent groups of tracheal lymph nodes. Metastases to the nodes on the opposite side from where the primary tumor lies or to the carina from lower tracheal tumors are common. More remote metastases to scalene nodes or to other cervical nodes have not often been seen.

## TRACHEOSTOMY

Tracheostomy is one of the most ancient operations and has long been used for the emergency management of upper airway obstruction. In the past two decades, tracheostomy has been used increasingly to control secretions in severely ill patients. More recently, tracheostomy has provided a route for ventilatory support in respiratory insufficiency. This increased use of tracheostomy has reawakened appreciation of the large number of serious complications that may follow the procedure. A spectrum of lesions, principally associated with use of tracheostomy for ventilatory support, has been identified.

### Indications

The occurrence of serious complications has caused critical reappraisal of the three classic indications for tracheostomy: (1) relief of upper airway obstruction; (2) control of secre-

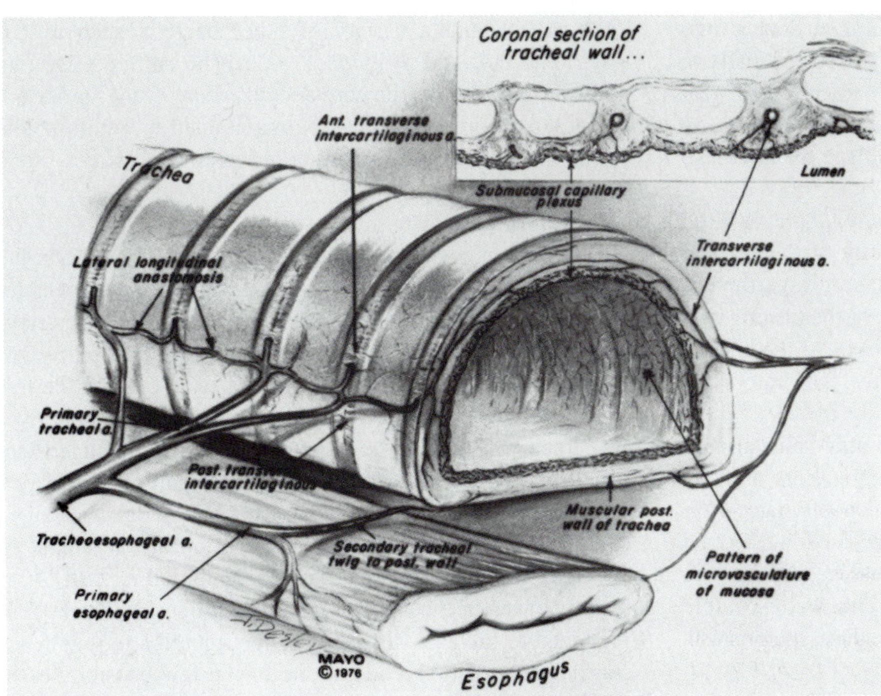


**Figure 38–3.** Tracheal microscopic blood supply. Transverse intercartilaginous arteries derived from the lateral longitudinal anastomosis penetrate the soft tissues between each cartilage to supply a rich vascular network beneath the endotracheal mucosa. *(From Salassa JR, et al: Ann Thorac Surg 24(2):100–107, with permission).*

tions; and (3) ventilatory support in respiratory failure. Tracheostomy often cannot be avoided in organic upper airway obstruction, although sometimes a tube may be slipped past an obstruction until definitive treatment is provided or a stenosis dilated with a rigid bronchoscope. Pulmonary toilet is best accomplished with humidification and pulmonary physiotherapy. Flexible bronchoscopy and minitracheostomy are used when these measures are insufficient.[6] Formal tracheotomy is therefore indicated less often for pulmonary toilet. Its primary indication is for patients with aspiration or who require mechanical ventilation.

Patients with respiratory insufficiency or impending failure are usually supported by mechanical ventilation with an endotracheal tube for varying lengths of time. If it appears that more than a day or so of support will be required, a nasotracheal tube is generally preferred for patients' comfort. There is no firm rule about the length of time an endotracheal tube may be left in place. If it becomes clear that long-term support is needed, a tracheotomy is usually performed as an elective procedure within 5–7 days. Such a plan becomes necessary because of the dangers of tube obstruction, the discomfort of a nasal or oral tube, and the considerable damage to the larynx that may result from prolonged intubation. This injury occurs especially in the posterior commissure, with damage to the arytenoid and interarytenoid area. In a prospective study of the sequelae of endotracheal intubation, Whited[7] found three reversible laryngeal stenoses and one chronic posterior stenosis in 50 patients intubated for 2–5 days, five cases of chronic laryngotracheal stenosis in 100 patients intubated for 6–10 days, and six cases of complex laryngeal stenosis in 50 patients intubated for 11–24 days. Early conversion to tracheostomy prevented these injuries. The data support a policy of conversion from endotracheal tube to tracheostomy after 7 days.

## Technique

Tracheostomy may be done with local anesthesia with the patient supine and the neck hyperextended. An anesthetist should be in attendance to maintain a clear airway, to adjust the positioning of the endotracheal tube during the procedure, and to supply oxygen or other support as needed. The procedure should be performed in the operating room, if only to maintain the most sterile conditions and to impress the operator with the need for meticulous technique. Blind tracheostomy procedures are unnecessary and are only to be condemned because of the high incidence of complications associated with them.

A horizontal incision is preferred for cosmetic reasons. Palpation of the extended neck reveals the position of the cricothyroid membrane and the cricoid cartilage below it. The incision is placed at the level of the second tracheal cartilage and carried through the platysma muscle. The strap muscles are separated vertically in the midline with minimal bleeding. The lower border of the cricoid cartilage is clearly defined, and the incision between the strap muscles and their subjacent fascia is carried down to a point below the thyroid isthmus. The isthmus is usually divided between hemostats after careful dissection beneath it in the pretracheal plane. The thyroid tissue on either side is controlled with mattress sutures.

Exact levels of the cartilaginous rings must be determined. The first cartilage must be left intact, and the opening in the trachea must be placed so that upward pressure exerted by the tube will not erode the first ring or the adjacent cricoid cartilage. The second and third cartilages (and all or part of the fourth if necessary) are incised vertically in the midline to avoid the potential danger of upward pressure by the outside of the elbow of the tube. If there is any question, it is better to incise a lower cartilage than damage a higher cartilage.

Even after centuries of tracheostomy, there is little controlled research to prove the superiority of the vertical incision over the cruciate or the horizontal incision, the excision of a disk or a segment of cartilage, or the turning of a flap. The tracheal opening probably enlarges to the size of the tube in most patients after a few days. The important point is not to make too large an opening in the tracheal wall, with a flap or not, because the flap may be destroyed or deformed. Any opening heals by cicatrization, and the larger the opening, the greater the chance for narrowing during stomal healing. If fine retractors are used in the open trachea, even a tube with a bulky low-pressure cuff may be inserted with ease with the assistance of some water-soluble lubricant. With such an elective procedure, hemostasis should be precise throughout.

Textbooks formerly indicated the site of tracheostomy to be the suprasternal notch in the extended neck. In many patients, such an approach selects a midtracheal location and places the point of potential damage from cuff injury low in the trachea. The trachea is also farther away from the cervical skin surface at this level. Further, it tends to angulate the tube. In children and in some adults, a low incision also places the inner side of the elbow of the tube close to a high innominate artery, with greater potential for erosive hemorrhage.

Once the tube has been securely seated and any attached cuff is functioning satisfactorily, the endotracheal tube is withdrawn and supportive oxygenation given through a lightweight connector attached to the tube or to its inner cannula if it is a two-part tube. The skin is loosely closed on either side of the tracheostomy tube. Sutures on either side are passed through the flange of the tracheostomy tube, fixing it securely in place, with the help of the usual tracheostomy tapes.

## Complications

Conversion of tracheostomy to a carefully performed elective procedure has largely eliminated the immediate and early complications of the procedure. The long-term complications of tracheostomy present largely in three ways: (1) sepsis, (2) hemorrhage, or (3) obstruction of the airway. Additional complications are tracheoesophageal fistula and persistence of the stoma. In general, the longer a tracheostomy is in place, especially with an inflated cuff, the greater is the chance that complications will occur.

### Sepsis

All tracheostomies are clinically contaminated, and *Staphylococcus aureus* (often a resistant strain), *Pseudomonas aeruginosa,* and a variety of other bacteria such as *Escherichia coli* and *Streptococcus* can be cultured. Despite this inevitability, sterile care and cleansing of the stoma and respiratory equipment must be maintained to minimize the possibility of invasive infection of the lower airway.

### Hemorrhage

It has been noted that the curve of the tube may erode the innominate artery and produce late hemorrhage, especially in children, in whom the trachea is small and the artery high. Massive hemorrhage also occurs from erosion by tracheostomy cuffs or even the tip of a tube through the trachea into the innominate artery as it passes obliquely over the trachea. Bleeding from granulation or more superficial tracheal erosions is more common and usually less massive. Only immediate tamponade of a major arterial leak, digitally when the leak is caused by erosion at the stoma, or with an inflated cuff when the leak is caused by cuff or tip injury lower in the trachea, and prompt surgical treatment can lead to salvage. Resection of the injured artery with suture closure of both ends is one of the few possibilities in such a contaminated field. In the small number of patients in whom this procedure has been performed successfully, neurologic problems have not appeared. The trachea requires no treatment when arterial injury has been at the stomal level. Injuries at the cuff level require resection and reconstruction.[8]

### Obstruction

Airway obstruction may occur while the tube is still in place. Cuff prolapse may occur from overdistention of the cuff and should be avoidable. If a tube with an inner cannula is used, crusts may be easily cleaned. With proper humidification, obstruction of single-lumen tubes is not commonly seen. Occasionally, obstructive granulations also form at the tip of a tube that is still in place.

Postintubation tracheal stenosis has become less of a problem with improvements in cuffs and awareness of the problem. *Every patient with signs of upper airway obstruction—wheezing or stridor, dyspnea on effort, episodes of obstruction from secretions—who has been previously intubated with either an endotracheal tube or a tracheostomy tube must be considered to have organic obstruction until proved otherwise.*

Obstructive *laryngeal lesions* from prolonged endotracheal intubation may occur at vocal cord level and consist of granulation tissue or cicatrix, particularly in the posterior commissure.[7–9] Tubes large relative to airway size especially may cause erosion at the subglottic and cricoid level with subsequent severe stenosis. Cricothyroidostomy, proposed to avoid the complications of tracheostomy, fails to eliminate cuff lesions, of course, and transfers serious stomal lesions from trachea to subglottic larynx, where surgical treatment is more difficult, less satisfactory, and often impossible.[9]

*At the stomal level,* obstruction may be due to a polypoid granuloma that forms on the healing surface of the stomal site. Narrowing and indentation at the point of cicatrization of the stoma are often seen after tracheostomy. When the stoma is large, because of an overgenerous initial operation or erosion by local infection or, most commonly, by the prying action of heavy equipment that connects the tracheostomy to the ventilator, healing may produce clinically obvious obstruction. Such stomal obstruction is usually three-sided, obstructing anteriorly and laterally, because the posterior wall is intact. Occasionally, some scarring occurs posteriorly as well. A combination of granuloma and stenosis also may produce obstruction. If the tracheostomy was placed too high, erosion of the cricoid cartilage may have occurred, with loss of substance and resultant subglottic stricture.

*At the cuff site,* pressure by the sealing cuff causes varying degrees of damage. Before the introduction of true large-volume, low-pressure cuffs, damage occurred in varying degrees in all patients in whom a cuff was inflated for more than 48 hours. In the days and weeks after insertion of the tube, erosion frequently bares numerous cartilages, leading to their fragmentation, and eventually, destruction. Occasionally, the erosion progresses anteriorly through the wall of the innominate artery or posteriorly to produce a tracheoesophageal fistula. With lesser degrees of damage, healing occurs with varying degrees of deformity and narrowing. If the tracheal wall has been deeply eroded circumferentially, a circumferential stricture occurs during healing. This may become arrested with partial closure and produce only dyspnea on effort, or it may go on to complete closure with a fatal obstructive episode. The lengths of such strictures are extremely variable, extending from 0.5 to 4 cm. Such lesions may occur with either endotracheal tubes or tracheostomy tubes, since they are caused by the cuff and not the tube. A far greater number of lesions have resulted from cuffs on tracheostomy tubes than on endotracheal tubes, since there is greater long-term exposure to tracheostomy tubes.

The tracheal cartilages *between the stoma and the cuff level* are often thinned, presumably by inflammatory changes, and this segment may become malacic. With respiratory effort, the malacic segment tends to collapse, contributing to obstruction. Granuloma may also form at the point of erosion by the *tip of the tracheostomy tube.* Children are more likely to show this lesion, since they are usually treated postoperatively without a cuff.

Although most tracheostomies close spontaneously, a large and long *persistent stoma* fails to close occasionally and requires precise surgical repair.[10] This is apt to occur in aged or debilitated patients, in patients with metabolic disease, or in those who have been exposed to steroids.

### Prevention of Tracheal Stenosis

Prevention of tracheal stenosis is of key importance. Lightweight swivel connectors have helped reduce the incidence of stomal strictures. The surgical stoma should not be excessively large in the first place.

Strictures have been associated with tubes of every material and with cuffs of varying types of materials. At cuff level, the principal preventive factor is elimination of pressure necrosis. The large-volume, low-pressure cuffs, which occlude the irregularly shaped tracheal lumen by conforming to the shape of the trachea rather than by expanding to distend and so seal the airway, may accomplish this. The introduction of such cuffs has markedly reduced the occurrence of cuff injury. However, the inextensibility of plastic materials allows conversion of most low-pressure cuffs to high-pressure cuffs if a small excess of air is introduced beyond the maximal resting volume of the unstretched cuff. Additional safeguards are direct pressure monitoring and side balloons with pop-off valves to bleed excessive air. The lesions continue to occur despite these advances.

Substitution of cricothyroidotomy for tracheotomy seems only to change the location of airway injury to a site more difficult to repair, despite the absence of complications in the experience of its original proponents.

## RADIOLOGIC EVALUATION

The primary diagnostic techniques for tracheal abnormalities are radiologic study and bronchoscopy. All too often a plain chest radiograph is considered to be normal, but on closer inspection shows an abnormality of the tracheal air column. Relatively simple radiologic techniques, without the use of contrast media, delineate tracheal abnormalities. The location of the lesion, its linear extent, extratracheal involvement, and—important to the surgeon—the amount of airway uninvolved by the process, can be determined.[11,12] In addition to standard views of the chest in various projections, centered high enough to show tracheal detail, anteroposterior filtered tracheal views of the entire airway from the larynx to the carina are obtained.[12] A lateral neck view, using soft-tissue technique with the patient swallowing and the neck hyperextended to bring the trachea up above the clavicles, is useful to define abnormalities in the upper trachea. Fluoroscopy not only demonstrates functional asymmetry of the vocal cords, if present, but may give additional information about the extent of the lesion and collapse of the airway if malacia is present. Spot radiographs usually are all that are required. In some cases, polytomography (anteroposterior and lateral views) gives additional detail, particularly of mediastinal involvement. Barium esophagography is useful to define esophageal involvement by extrinsic compression or invasion. Computed tomography (CT) offers little over conventional radiologic techniques, except to define an extratracheal component. The exact role of magnetic resonance imaging (MRI) has yet to be defined. Sagittal and coronal views, however, have been helpful in certain cases and may give more accurate detail than conventional radiographic techniques.[13]

## AIRWAY MANAGEMENT

Crucial to the management of all problems of the trachea is the ability to control the airway. Tracheal tumors and postintubation stenosis may present as emergency obstructive airway problems. Endotracheal intubation may be dangerous or even impossible, because it may lead to complete airway obstruction, especially in patients with high tracheal lesions. Simple maneuvers to elevate the head of the patient, administration of cool mist and oxygen, and careful sedation may allow control of the airway in a quasielective manner. Control is best accomplished in the operating room, where an assortment of rigid bronchoscopes, dilators, biopsy forceps, and instruments to perform emergency tracheostomy are available. Anesthesia, as in elective tracheal operations, is best accomplished with inhalation technique. It requires patience on the part of the anesthesiologist and surgeon to allow the patient to become adequately anesthetized. Induction of anesthesia deep enough to allow rigid bronchoscopy may take as long as 20 minutes. Paralyzing agents should not be used, lest there arise the lethal combination of airway obstruction and apnea.[14]

The initial evaluation should be with a rigid bronchoscope carefully inserted through the vocal cords, stopping just proximal to the level of obstruction. Rigid telescopes can be used to assess the obstruction. Most tumors, even those causing nearly total obstruction, do not restrict passage of a rigid bronchoscope. Once the status of the distal airway has been assessed, the tumor can be partially removed with biopsy forceps to determine its consistency and vascularity. For most tumors, the tip of the rigid bronchoscope can be used to core out most of the tumor. The tumor can then be grasped with biopsy forceps and removed. If bleeding ensues, the bronchoscope may be passed into the distal airway for ventilation. The bronchoscope tamponades the bleeding. Direct application of epinephrine-soaked pledgets helps control any persistent oozing. Very rarely have we had to resort to direct cauterization (with insulated electrodes) in these situations. The use of lasers has become popular in the management of malignant strictures, but we find it time consuming, expensive, and rarely advantageous when compared with bronchoscopy.

Postintubation stenosis poses a slightly different problem in airway control. Attempting to pass a large rigid bronchoscope beyond a tough, inflammatory stricture may be impossible, may result in tracheal rupture, or may cause total airway obstruction secondary to bleeding or edema. For these strictures, Jackson dilators passed through the rigid bronchoscope under direct vision and an assortment of graduated rigid bronchoscopes can be used effectively to dilate postintubation stenoses. When these tight, rigid strictures are gradually dilated, the risk of perforation and bleeding is minimized. Racemic epinephrine and steroids are often used in the first 24–48 hours to minimize postdilation edema.

It is important to understand that dilation or endotracheal removal of malignant and inflammatory strictures, whether mechanically or with laser, is only a temporary measure. In the case of inflammatory stricture, resentosis usually develops within days to weeks. The use of these techniques in emergency situations allows thorough examination of the patient and allows an elective operation. Many patients are taking high doses of steroids at the time of presentation, having been treated for refractory "asthma." When an airway is established, the steroids may be tapered and discontinued and an operation performed without the threat of impaired healing. Dilations may have to be performed repeatedly during steroid tapering.

The aforementioned maneuvers are sometimes used at the time of elective operations if the patient has presented with a stable airway. This allows assessment of the distal airway, placement of an endotracheal tube, and provision of an adequate lumen to prevent accumulation of $CO_2$ early in the procedure. At the time of tracheal resection, this tube can be pulled back or removed and a sterile cuffed endotracheal tube inserted into the distal airway. Sterile connecting tubing is passed to the anesthesiologist and connected to allow ventilation of the patient. It can be removed whenever necessary for suctioning or placement of sutures. At the conclusion of the operation, the original endotracheal tube is advanced into the distal airway and sutures tied. The patient should be breathing spontaneously at the end of the procedure, so that extubation can be performed in the operating room. High-frequency ventilation is especially useful in certain complex carinal reconstructions.

Tracheostomy may be necessary in some patients as the only way to secure control of the airway. *The tracheostomy should be placed through the most damaged portion of the trachea, allowing preservation of the maximal amount of normal trachea for subsequent reconstruction.* If tracheoscopy is being considered at the completion of tracheal resection, the opening should be placed at least two rings away from the anastomosis. The anastomosis is protected with the thyroid gland or strap muscles to avoid contamination of the suture line. This lessens the likelihood of subsequent dehiscence or stenosis. *Never* should a tracheostomy tube be placed through the anastomosis.

## TRACHEAL TUMORS

### Occurrence and Clinical Presentation

Primary tracheal tumors are rare. It is important to be aware of their behavior, however, since their very rarity makes them easy to overlook diagnostically. About two thirds of primary tracheal tumors are of two histologic types: squamous cell carcinoma and adenoid cystic carcinoma, formerly called *cylindroma.* These two types occur in about the same numbers.[15–21] The remaining third of the tumors are widely distributed in a heterogeneous group, both malignant and benign. A variety of secondary tumors involve the trachea. These include carcinomas of the larynx, thyroid, lung, and esophagus. Rarely, tumors may metastasize to the submucosa of the trachea or to the mediastinum with secondary invasion of the trachea. Thus, carcinoma of the breast and mediastinal lymphoma may invade the trachea. Incompletely removed neoplasms of the main bronchus, such as carcinoid tumors, also may invade the carina.

Tracheal tumors may present insidiously. Their most common symptoms and signs are cough (37%), hemoptysis (41%), and the signs of progressive airway obstruction, including shortness of breath on exertion (54%), wheezing and stridor (35%), and less commonly, dysphagia or hoarseness (7%). Wheezing, in particular, may cause diagnostic error. It is not commonly appreciated that wheezing may be a predominant symptom of a tracheal tumor for a prolonged period. A conventional chest radiograph usually shows clear lung fields, and on this basis the physician assumes that no organic mass lesion is present. Patients are often treated for adult-onset asthma. Hemoptysis also may not be pursued aggressively in the face of an apparently normal chest radiograph. Another presentation is with unilateral or bilateral recurrent attacks of pneumonitis. These may respond to antibiotic treatment but then recur.

Signs and symptoms vary with the type of tumor. Hemoptysis is prominent in patients with squamous cell carcinoma and usually leads to earlier diagnosis. The presence of hoarseness as an early symptom may signify advanced disease. Adenoid cystic carcinoma often presents with wheezing or stridor as a predominant symptom, leading to delay in diagnosis. Only slightly more than one fourth of these patients have hemoptysis early in the course of disease. Dyspnea, however, may be a prominent symptom. In one study[22] the mean duration of symptoms prior to diagnosis in patients with squamous cell carcinoma of the trachea was only 4 months, but with adenoid cystic carcinoma, it was 18 months. In some benign tumors or low-grade malignant tumors of the trachea, the mean duration for carriage of an incorrect diagnosis was up to 4 years. The mean duration of symptoms of miscellaneous malignant tumors was 11 months.[22]

## Diagnosis

Endoscopy is frequently the means by which a tracheal tumor is discovered in a patient who is being studied for hemoptysis of unknown origin. A high tracheal tumor may be overlooked if a flexible endoscope is passed through a previously introduced endotracheal tube or if the endoscopist is not in the habit of looking carefully at the proximal trachea. The same hazard faces endoscopists who uses a rigid bronchoscope. When a lesion is not obstructing or is of such radiologic extent that a surgical approach seems indicated in any case, endoscopy is deferred to the time of potential resection. However, when the surgical team is not trained or experienced in the management of tracheal tumors, preliminary bronchoscopy may be performed to visualize the tumor. Biopsy must be done with good judgment so that an excessively vascular tumor will not be stimulated to brisk hemorrhage. Hemorrhage in the case of a very vascular carcinoid tumor, for example, may be life-endangering or may precipitate the need for emergency surgical treatment. Biopsy of the rare hemangiomatous lesion of the trachea can be lethal. If preliminary biopsy is not done before an operation, frozen section facilities must be available. Particularly in adenoid cystic carcinoma, which is notorious for submucosal spread, biopsies of tissue a distance from the tumor may be necessary to determine resectability. Endoscopic examination of the esophagus also has a place with extensive tumors.

## Pathology

In a series of 198 patients with primary tumors of the trachea treated at the Massachusetts General Hospital between 1962 and 1989,[16] 70 had squamous cell carcinoma, 80 had adenoid cystic carcinoma, and the rest had mixed lesions. The mean age of the patients with squamous cell carcinoma was 58 years, in contrast to 43 years for those with adenoid cystic carcinoma. In the latter group, the age spread was much wider (Table 38–1).

*Squamous cell carcinoma* may be either exophytic or ulcerative. It may also be multiple and scattered over a considerable distance in the trachea. The tumor metastasizes to the regional lymph nodes and, in its more aggressive and late forms, invades mediastinal structures. In general, its progress appears to be relatively rapid in comparison with adenoid cystic carcinoma. A number of these patients have returned with a second squamous cell carcinoma of the lung or oropharynx (40% of patients who underwent resection).

*Adenoid cystic carcinoma* often has a very prolonged course of clinical symptoms, sometimes extending for

**TABLE 38–1. INCIDENCE OF PRIMARY TRACHEAL TUMORS BY AGE**

| | No. of Tumors | | |
|---|---|---|---|
| **Age (y)** | ***Squamous*** | ***Adenoid Cystic*** | ***Other*** |
| 1–10 | — | — | 4 |
| 11–19 | — | — | 8 |
| 20–29 | 1 | 13 | 11 |
| 30–39 | 1 | 16 | 9 |
| 40–49 | 9 | 19 | 5 |
| 50–59 | 29 | 15 | 6 |
| 60–69 | 24 | 13 | 4 |
| 70–79 | 6 | 5 | 1 |

*(From Grillo HC, Mathisen DJ: Ann Thorac Surg 1990;49:69–77.)*

years. After treatment, it may be many years before a recurrence is noted. Adenoid cystic carcinoma may extend over long distances submucosally in the airways and also perineurally.[20] It spreads to regional lymph nodes, although less characteristically than does squamous cell carcinoma. Although it may invade the thyroid gland or the muscular coats of the esophagus by contiguity, adenoid cystic carcinoma that has not been interfered with during an operation frequently displaces mediastinal structures before actually invading them. Metastases to the lungs are not uncommon. These may grow very slowly over a period of many years and remain asymptomatic until they are huge. Metastases to bone and other organs occur.

Among the other *malignant lesions* seen in the trachea in the series of 198 patients were 10 carcinoid tumors clearly originating in the trachea and not in the main bronchi, four mucoepidermoid carcinomas (Table 38–2), two spindle cell sarcomas, and one each of adenocarcinoma, adenosquamous, chondrosarcoma, and carcinosarcoma. The *benign lesions* consisted of neurofibroma, chondroma, chondroblastoma, leiomyoma, granular cell tumor, and hemangioma. A number of patients had several varieties of squamous papillomas. These included solitary squamous papillomas and multiple papillomatosis, either widespread or of a confluent, often verrucous, type.

**TABLE 38–2. OTHER PRIMARY TRACHEAL TUMORS**

| Type | No. of Tumors |
|---|---|
| **Benign** | |
| Squamous papilloma | |
| Multiple | 4 |
| Solitary | 1 |
| Pleomorphic adenoma | 2 |
| Granular cell tumor | 2 |
| Fibrous histiocytoma | 1 |
| Leiomyoma | 2 |
| Chondroma | 2 |
| Chondroblastoma | 1 |
| Schwannoma | 1 |
| Paraganglioma | 2 |
| Hemangioendothelioma | 1 |
| Vascular malformation | 2 |
| **Intermediate** | |
| Carcinoid | 10 |
| Mucoepidermoid | 4 |
| Plexiform neurofibroma | 1 |
| Pseudosarcoma | 1 |
| Malignant fibrous histiocytoma | 1 |
| **Malignant** | |
| Adenocarcinoma | 1 |
| Adenosquamous carcinoma | 1 |
| Small cell carcinoma | 1 |
| Atypical carcinoid | 1 |
| Melanoma | 1 |
| Chondrosarcoma | 1 |
| Spindle cell sarcoma | 2 |
| Rhabdomyosarcoma | 1 |

*(From Grillo HC, Mathisen DJ: Ann Thorac Surg 1990;49:69–77.)*

*Secondary tumors* involving the trachea have been briefly noted. Esophageal carcinoma (10 patients), in particular, may be a cause of a fistula between the esophagus and the trachea or the left main bronchus. Similarly, an occasional aggressive carcinoma of the lung resulting in a fistula as both trachea and esophagus are involved from the mediastinum. It is probable that some of the oat cell carcinomas of the trachea that have been reported[15] may have originated in the lung and invaded the trachea.

Both papillary and follicular carcinoma of the thyroid gland and mixed varieties of the two may invade the trachea primarily, usually at the level of the isthmus.[23,24] Thus, a patient initially presenting with hemoptysis may have carcinoma of the thyroid. Invasion of the trachea by thyroid carcinoma is best managed by resection with airway reconstruction. Localized extension of tumor may also require partial esophageal resection or radical resection, including laryngectomy with mediastinal tracheostomy. More commonly, invasion is seen after thyroidectomy for carcinoma in which the surgeon was aware that the tumor was shaved from the trachea. In such cases, concurrent or early resection of the involved trachea should be considered.

## Treatment

When the primary tracheal tumor is circumscribed, has not metastasized remotely, has not involved an excessive length of trachea, and has not invaded the mediastinum deeply, the best primary treatment is resection with primary reconstruction of the airway.[16,17,20,21] Considerable experience is required to make the judgment whether a tumor can be safely resected with sufficient tissue to provide a potentially curative margin and yet primarily reconstruct the airway. This is even more crucial when the tumor lies in the lower trachea or at the carinal level and when an airway has to be finally reconstructed at the time of the original operation. Particularly difficult are cases of adenoid cystic carcinoma in which after an apparently clear resection, frozen sections show microscopic tumor at the resection margins.

Both squamous cell carcinoma and adenoid cystic carcinoma of the trachea are usually responsive to irradiation, with varying long-term results.[15,16,20] In general, curative irradiation has about the same effect on squamous cell carcinoma as on carcinoma of the lung, i.e., variable palliation that lasts not much longer than 2 years with ultimate recurrence. Adenoid cystic carcinoma may respond for even longer periods, perhaps 3–7 years. (These are very general statements.) Although some investigators have advised preoperative irradiation, particularly in the management of adenoid cystic carcinoma,[20] many prefer to reserve radiation for the postoperative phase. They use radiation particularly when there are involved lymph nodes; when there is microscopic tumor in lymphatic vessels, in nerve sheaths, or at the resection margin; and when the margins appear to be too close.[16] The same approach has been applied to other primary tracheal tumors.

The total world experience in the management of tracheal tumors is small enough that it is difficult to be categorical about optimal treatment. Results to date, however, strongly indicate that the approach just described is soundly based[16,17] (Tables 38–3 to 38–5). In comparing patients with squamous cell carcinoma and adenoid cystic carcinoma treated by the vigorous protocol described with patients treated before the institution of extirpational surgery with modern techniques of resection and reconstruction, one sees that remarkable progress has been achieved. As might be expected, excellent long-term results have been obtained with benign tumors amenable to excision and also with the miscellaneous group of low-grade malignant tumors of other varieties. In general, cure has rarely been achieved when secondary tumors have been resected, except for local recurrences of carcinoid tumors at the carina. Long-term palliation, however, has been achieved with the less malignant thyroid neoplasms that invade the trachea. In a number of these patients, the ultimate cause of death was the appearance of remote metastases in bones or elsewhere in the body rather than at the local site treated for relief of airway obstruction.

In some patients in whom the larynx is extensively involved by tumor, it is not possible to salvage the organ, and laryngotracheal resection must be done. On the other hand, when only a portion of the larynx is involved, it is possible, by individually designed procedures, to salvage a functioning larynx with reconstruction of the airway.

Of the total number of tumors seen, approximately one third are clearly incurable when first seen and are not amenable to surgical resection at all. About another third can be treated with one of a variety of destructive resections, sometimes with mediastinal tracheostomies. The final third are amenable to primary resection with reconstruction of the airway[16] (Tables 38–3 and 38–4). When extirpation is not possible either because of the extent of the tumor or because of the age or medical condition of the patient, primary irradiation appears to be a reasonable palliative modality.

In some patients with adenoid cystic carcinoma that obstructs the trachea, it is probably worthwhile to perform a palliative resection if reconstruction can be done with safety, despite the presence of pulmonary metastases, because of the prolonged course these patients follow.

In a trachea acutely obstructed by tumor that cannot be removed by a primary resection because of the extent of the tumor, immediate palliation may be achieved by removing the bulk of obstructing tumor endotracheally, as described earlier. This allows the opportunity to institute radiation therapy. Removal can be done either with a morcellating biopsy forceps, the older technique, or with the application of new physical modalities, most usefully a laser for destruction of endobronchial tumor. The laser is not, however, primary treatment of most tracheal tumors, because it cannot destroy the base of the tumor without destroying the tracheal wall. It does have application, however, for multiple squamous papillomas of the trachea.

Ultimately, as a tumor recurs and laser treatment is no longer possible because of the extension of the tumor through the tracheal wall, additional palliation to prevent strangulation can sometimes be given with the judicious insertion of a silicone rubber T tube that spans the airway and allows the patient to breathe despite the presence of the tumor. Obviously, this procedure cannot be used if such a tumor extends below the carina.

Our largest experience with tracheal resection of secondary tumors invading the trachea has been with thyroid neoplasms.[24] Thirty-four patients (19 with papillary, six with follicular, four with mixed papillary and follicular, three with undifferentiated carcinoma, one with squamous, and one with carcinosarcoma) underwent resection. Twenty-seven patients underwent airway reconstruction and seven patients underwent cervicomediastinal en bloc resection with mediastinal tracheostomy. Seventeen patients had prior thyroidectomy. Ten patients who underwent airway restitution required cylindric tracheal resection, six underwent resection of the trachea with a portion of the larynx, and one underwent wedge resection. Three patients who underwent laryngotracheal resection also needed esophagectomy. Colonic reconstruction was used.

Twenty-three of the 27 patients who underwent airway reconstruction had good surgical results with speech preservation. One died of complications caused by prior irradiation and one of respiratory arrest after extubation. One of

**TABLE 38–3. PRIMARY TRACHEAL TUMORS (1962–1988)[a]**

| Procedures | Squamous | Adenoid Cystic | Other | Total | Surgical Mortality |
|---|---|---|---|---|---|
| No. of Patients | 72 | 78 | 52 | 202 | — |
| No. of Surgical Procedures | 52 (72) | 63 (81) | 45 (86) | 160 (79) | — |
| Resection and reconstruction | 43 (60) | 49 (63) | 43 (83) | 135 (67) | 6/135 (4) |
| Trachea | 33 | 21 | 29 | 83 (61) | 1/83 (1) |
| Carina | 10 | 28 | 14 | 52 (39) | 5/52 (10) |
| Laryngotracheal | 1 | 4 | 1 | 6 | 0/6 (0) |
| Staged | 2 | 6 | 1 | 9 | 5/9 (55) |
| Exploration, bypass | 6 | 4 | 0 | 10 (4) | 2/10 (20) |

[a]Numbers in parentheses are percentages.

**TABLE 38–4. RESECTION AND RECONSTRUCTION FOR TRACHEAL AND CARINAL TUMORS (PRELIMINARY RESULTS 1962–1988)**

| Diagnosis | No. of Pts. | No. of Postoperative Deaths | No. of Pts. Dead | | No. of Pts. Alive | | Not Known |
|---|---|---|---|---|---|---|---|
| | | | *Disease* | *Other* | *Disease* | *None* | |
| **Trachea** | | | | | | | |
| Adenoid cystic | 21 | 0 | 2 | 0 | 3 | 14 | 2 |
| Squamous | 33 | 1 | 7 | 2 | 0 | 19 | 4 |
| Other | 29 | 0 | 2 | 1 | 0 | 22 | 4 |
| Subtotal | 83 | 1 | 11 | 3 | 3 | 55 | 10 |
| **Carina** | | | | | | | |
| Adenoid Cystic | 28 | 3 | 2 | 2 | 0 | 19 | 2 |
| Squamous | 10 | 1 | 2 | 0 | 0 | 7 | 0 |
| Other | 14 | 1 | 1 | 0 | 0 | 10 | 2 |
| Subtotal | 52 | 5 | 5 | 2 | 0 | 36 | 4 |
| **Total** | 135 | 6 | 16 | 5 | 3 | 91 | 14 |

seven patients who underwent radical resection died in the postoperative period.

Among the patients who underwent reconstruction, 11 of 25 survivors died of their cancer 3 months to 10 years after airway reconstruction. Only two patients had tumor recurrence in the airway. The mean duration of survival among these 11 patients was 43 months. Of the six survivors in the mediastinal tracheostomy group, two died of their disease 31 months and 88 months after the operation, three died of other diseases 2–6 years after the operation, and one patient was alive without disease 16 months after resection.

Resection and primary reconstruction of the trachea invaded by carcinoma of the thyroid should be performed when technically feasible in the absence of extensive metastases. It offers prolonged palliation, avoidance of suffocation due to bleeding and obstruction, and an opportunity for cure. In carefully selected patients with massive regional involvement, radical excision with laryngectomy and esophagectomy also is appropriate.[24]

## Surgical Resection of Tracheal Tumors

The management of tracheal tumors by surgical resection represents only one general category of problems for which resection and reconstruction of the trachea are required. The problems of managing tumors are often difficult because of the unpredictability of the extent of a particular lesion.

Tracheal resection in general was limited for many years by the belief that only 2 cm of the trachea, about four rings, could be removed and the ends dependably anastomosed by primary suture.[25] This led to attempts at lateral resection that were meant to preserve some of the structure of the trachea. Subsequent patching with autogenous and foreign material and by other, more complex methods led to very limited resection of the tumor. Early recurrence and failure of healing, with resultant mediastinitis, plagued these efforts. The complications of obstruction and hemorrhage followed many attempts over decades to use various types of prosthetic materials for bridging larger defects in the trachea. Although an intussuscepting prosthesis with suturable sleeves has overcome some of these problems, the method remains unpredictable and subject to the complications described.

The application of various techniques of anatomic mobilization has allowed the resection of approximately one half of the trachea with primary reconstruction on a dependable and predictable basis.[25] Simple cervical flexion, which delivers the cervical trachea into the mediastinum, has been the most useful single maneuver for extending the resection of the trachea with primary repair. In a young person who is

**TABLE 38–5. PRIMARY TRACHEAL TUMORS**

| Tumor Type | Years Alive Without Disease | | | | | | |
|---|---|---|---|---|---|---|---|
| | 0–1 | 1–5 | 5–10 | 10–15 | 15–20 | | |
| Adenoid cystic | 7 | 13 | 9 | 1 | 4 | | |
| Squamous | 4 | 14 | 3 | 3 | 2 | | |
| | **Died with Disease at Years After Surgery** | | | | | **Mean Survival Period (mo)** | |
| | 0–1 | 1–5 | 5–10 | 10–15 | 15–20 | Surgery + Radiation | Radiation Only |
| Adenoid cystic | 0 | 1 | 1 | 1 | 1 | 113 | 24 |
| Squamous | 2 | 6 | 1 | 0 | 0 | 26 | 11 |

not obese and who has reasonably supple tissues, more than one half of the trachea may be removed with primary reconstruction. With increasing age, kyphosis, obesity, and pathologic changes, the portion of the trachea that can be removed and reconstructed becomes much less.

Suprahyoid laryngeal release is useful to gain length, especially in upper tracheal resection.[26] Various other adjunctive maneuvers have been added to increase the length of resection possible, including intrapericardial freeing of the pulmonary vessels. This technique has generally been reserved for intrathoracic approaches, although, on occasion, the maneuver has been necessary to enter the chest simply to gain length for an extended resection. When such mobilization is done, it is important to retain the bronchial blood supply. Because the left main bronchus is fixed in position, to a great degree, by the presence of the aortic arch, it is theoretically possible to divide the attachment of the left main bronchus at the carina, advance the right lung upward toward the neck after freeing the hilum, and then reimplant the left main bronchus into the bronchus intermedius. Although such reimplantation has been done after carinal resection,[16] we have avoided the use of such a radical procedure simply to gain length. The increased risk for complications, or even death, with increased complexity of the reconstruction does not seem to justify using the procedure for this purpose alone.

Critical matters in all dissections of the trachea, are the careful preservation of the lateral segmental blood supply,[25] the gentle and precise handling of all tissues, and precision of anastomosis.

Tumors of the upper portion of the trachea are usually approached through a collar incision with a vertical extension through the upper sternum if necessary. Because the extent of some tumors is not fully predictable even on preoperative radiographs and after bronchoscopy, it is generally wise to position a patient so that incisions may be extended if necessary. The incisions just described may be extended by carrying the sternal division down farther and then angling it into the right fourth interspace to add a thoracotomy to the cervical and mediastinal exposure. Tumors of the lower trachea are approached most easily through a posterolateral thoracotomy (Fig. 38–4). Laryngeal release adds no additional length for distal tracheal resection. Flexing the neck and freeing the anterior pretracheal plane have been the most helpful maneuvers to gain additional length; intrapericardial release of the pulmonary vessels also has proved helpful.

When a tumor involves the carina, various reconstructive techniques are used (Fig. 38–5). Unless the tumor is very small, it is rarely adaptable to reconstruction by approximating the right and left main bronchus to form a new carina and then attaching it to the trachea. Such suturing anchors the carina very low in the mediastinum, and if more trachea has been excised, approximation is not possible. More commonly, either the right or left main bronchus is sutured to the trachea, and a lateral anastomosis of the other bronchus to the lower portion of the tracheal wall above the initial anastomosis is performed[16,17] (Fig. 38–5). All intrathoracic anastomoses are covered with a second layer, of either pedicled pleura or pericardial fat. As in sleeve lobectomy, it is important to interpose tissue between the airway suture line and adjacent pulmonary vessels. Omentum is used only when prior irradiation is a factor.

If a recurrent laryngeal nerve is involved by tumor, the nerve is sacrificed. The nerves are usually identified and carefully saved, when possible. Local paratracheal lymph nodes are excised with the specimen when possible. Extensive lymph node dissection cannot be done, because of the possibility of destroying the blood supply to the residual portion of the trachea. In tumors high in the trachea, partial removal of the lower part of the larynx may have to be done. Individually designed procedures are necessary to preserve a functional larynx. Sometimes portions of the esophagus and other adjacent structures must be resected.

Resection is usually controlled with frozen sections to be certain that the margins are clear. Adenoid cystic carcinoma, in particular, may extend such distances that total resection of all microscopic disease is not possible, and postoperative irradiation must be administered.[16]

## TRACHEAL STRICTURES

Strictures of the trachea may result from a number of different general causes. Congenital stenoses are rare. Posttraumatic strictures occur, particularly when there has been tracheal separation. The most common type of stricture is the result of iatrogenic disease, namely, that which results from intubation, usually for ventilatory support. Infections occasionally cause stenosis of the trachea. A miscellaneous group of diseases also cause strictures or, at least, tracheal obstruction. These include amyloid disease restricted to the airway, tracheopathia osteoplastica, and a small group of truly idiopathic stenoses without a history of previous insult or infection.

### Congenital Stenosis

All forms of congenital stenosis of the trachea are rare.[27–29] The most common type seems to be an almost weblike diaphragm that occurs most commonly at the level of the cricoid cartilage.[30] Longer tracheal stenoses are less frequently seen. These have been classified into general groups, including stenosis of the entire trachea with normal larynx and main bronchi and funnel-type stenosis, in which there is a gradual narrowing to a maximum point. Funnel-type stenosis may occur in the upper, mid-, or lower trachea, involving varying portions of the trachea. Segmental stenosis is most often seen in the lower trachea, sometimes with a translocation of the main bronchus or a lobar bronchus just above the area of stenosis.[28] Segmental stenosis is also seen with pulmonary sling anomalies. Here the

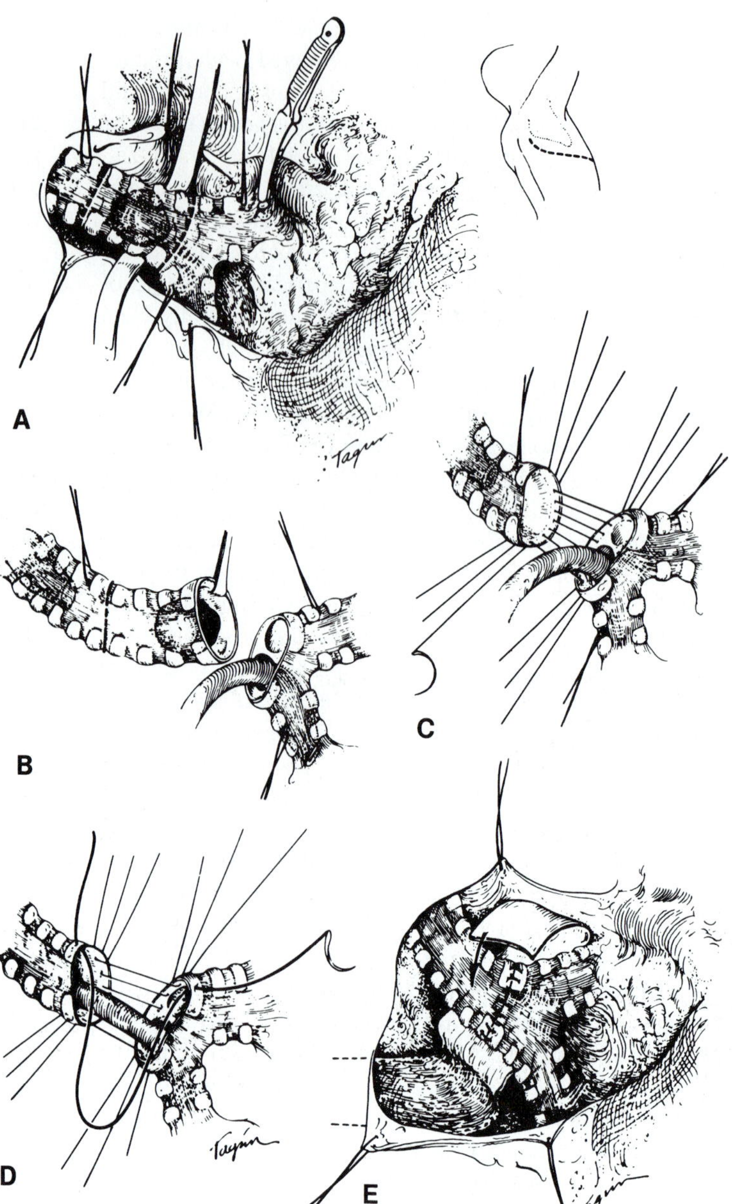


**Figure 38–4.** Reconstruction of the lower trachea. **A.** The trachea and carina have been exposed through a right posterolateral thoracotomy (fourth intercostal space or rib). If needed, the inferior pulmonary ligament may be divided and the hilum dissected to provide mobilization of the distal trachea. **B.** The trachea has been transsected below the lesion and the left lung intubated across the operative field. The right pulmonary artery may be clamped if there is evidence of shunting. **C.** Left lateral and anterior tracheal sutures are being placed. The endotracheal tube across the field may be removed intermittently for greater ease in placing sutures. **D.** A long endotracheal tube from above has now been advanced into the left main bronchus and the balance of the sutures placed on the right lateral and posterior walls. **E.** Anastomosis has been completed, and a second-layer pedicled pleural flap is being placed around the anastomosis. *(From Grillo HC: Curr Probl Surg, July 1970.)*

narrowing may be a compressive one, but in about half of patients it appears to be a true concurrent congenital anomaly of the trachea with complete cartilaginous O-shaped rings in the stenotic segment. The O-shaped rings are also seen in the other kinds of stenosis, both of the funnel type and of the other tracheal type. When one is aware of the possibility of these rings, they can be identified with bronchoscopy. Another type of stenosis accompanies a malformation of the cartilages so that they appear to be in an irregular pattern, often with half rings and segments of rings. A degree of softening is also seen with this type of lesion.

Weblike stenoses have been handled in a variety of ways, including local resection by varied techniques.[30,31] The longer stenoses often present formidable problems, since a fair segment of trachea may be involved. In a small child, resection of a long segment of trachea presents great risk for postoperative obstruction due to edema and for separation due to tension. It appears that only about one third of the trachea of most small children can be resected without risk of separation, in contrast to one half in young adults. For these reasons, it is often best to temporize and allow a child to grow before repair is done. Occasionally, a tracheostomy is absolutely necessary to tide the child over these early years.

Congenital tracheal stenosis rarely presents as an emergency airway obstruction in neonates. When it does, however, it can be a fatal problem. A neonate in this condition cannot be allowed to grow, allowing the trachea to enlarge. Dilation is impossible and T tubes are not usable. Idriss et al[29] described a promising technique of tracheo-

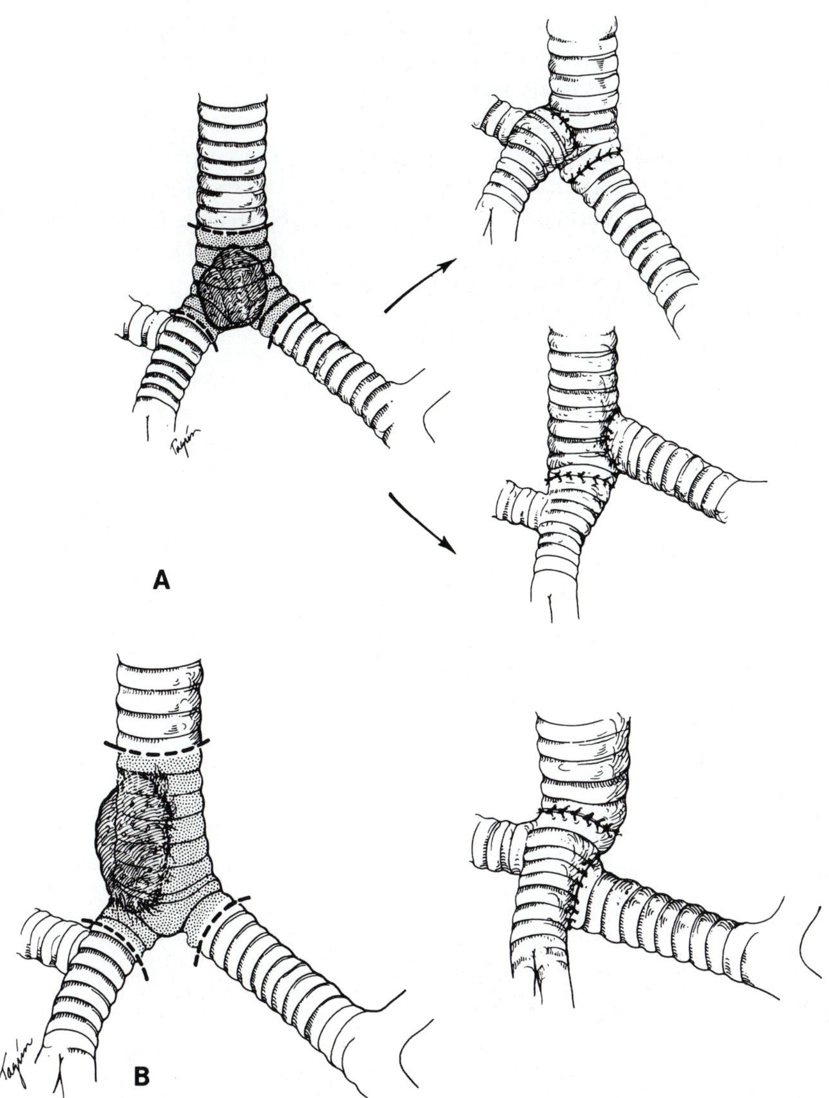


**Figure 38–5.** Modes of reconstruction after carinal resection. **A.** After carinal resection without removal of a long segment of trachea, reconstruction was done with trachea-to-bronchi end-to-end anastomosis with lateral implantation of either the right or the left main bronchus into the devolved lower trachea. **B.** Carinal resection with longer tracheal resection was repaired with direct suture of the trachea of the right main bronchus with anastomosis of the left main bronchus to the bronchus intermedius. *(From Grillo HC: Curr Probl Surg, July 1970.)*

plasty with a pericardial patch. Four infants with long congenital tracheal stenosis were operated on through a median sternotomy with extracorporeal circulation for respiratory support. The entire length of tracheal stenosis was opened anteriorly, and a rectangular pericardial patch was sutured to the edges of the trachea. All patients were extubated 7–10 days after the operation and had no symptoms at follow-up examinations 22 months after treatment.

### Slide Tracheoplasty

Tsang et al proposed slide tracheoplasty as another solution to congenital tracheal stenosis.[32] This procedure involves dividing the trachea in mid-stenosis and then opening the trachea anteriorly (midline) in the distal segment and posteriorly (midline) in the anterior segment. The two segments then slide one over the other, and an interrupted anastomosis is performed. Care must be taken to avoid interfering with the lateral blood supply. Grillo reported success in four patients using this technique.[33]

Transposition of the pulmonary artery in cases of sling has been used as a method of treatment.[34] Although this procedure may relieve compressive narrowing of the trachea with malacic change, it clearly does not correct a segmental stenosis when there are cartilaginous O-rings. In this situation, the primary treatment probably should be correction of the tracheal stenosis, with no interference with the takeoff of the elongated artery.

### Posttraumatic Stenosis

Separation of the cervical trachea may result from blunt injury to the neck. The separation may occur by avulsion of the trachea from the larynx just below the cricoid cartilage, or at a lower level. The usual mechanisms are vehicular injury, in which the neck is struck by the edge of a steering wheel or a dashboard, or sports injuries such as snowmobiling or motorcycling in which the neck is struck by an outstretched cable. When primary repair is not done, or when repair has failed, stricture results. If direct repair has not been done, a long defect appears to be present, because the trachea drops into the mediastinum when it is detached from the larynx. Careful assessment of glottic function must be made in all patients, because there is almost always either total or partial injury to the recurrent laryngeal nerve. Often this injury is permanent. It is necessary to be certain that the glottis has an adequate aperture, even if paralyzed, so that speech and breathing may be maintained. Once a glottic airway has been established by appropriate otolaryngologic procedures, e.g., cord lateralization, arytenoidectomy, or arytenoidopexy, direct repair of the stenotic segment is performed by excision of scar and reanastomosis. If the glottic aperture has been appropriately stabilized before this repair, concurrent tracheostomy is not needed, and surprisingly good vocal function is obtained. If laryngeal fracture is part of the original injury, a coordinated approach is required.

Partial or complete fracture of the mediastinal trachea may occur in conjunction with crushing sternal or anterior chest wall injuries. With massive blunt injury to the chest, usually accompanied, in adults, by fracture of multiple ribs, especially upper ribs, fracture of the lowermost portion of the trachea may occur. This fracture may occur in conjunction with a splitting injury to one or both main bronchi or as a fissure that runs upward into the membranous wall of the trachea. Because some pneumothoraces from intrathoracic tracheal lacerations respond to intubation with sealing of the injury, the tracheal lesion manifests itself later as stenosis. Usually the segment of stenosis is short and may be effectively treated by resection.

Injuries at any level may be associated with concomitant injury to the esophagus. The esophagus must be inspected very carefully by means of endoscopy and direct inspection. If an injury to the esophagus is found, it must be repaired in two layers. A strap muscle should be interposed between the esophageal suture line and the tracheal suture line to prevent subsequent tracheoesophageal fistula (Fig. 38–6).

We treated 10 patients with acute injuries and 17 with delayed traumatic laryngotracheal stenosis.[35] All 10 patients with acute injuries had an excellent airway restored with voice preservation. One of these patients required concomitant repair of an esophageal injury. Repair of delayed stenosis was successful in 16 of 17 patients. All but one patient had preservation of voice, despite the presence of vocal cord paralysis in 14 patients preoperatively. The four patients with concomitant esophageal injury underwent successful repair without development of tracheoesophageal fistula.

## Postintubation Stricture

The two principal strictures that follow intubation are located at the level of the tracheostomy stomas or at the level

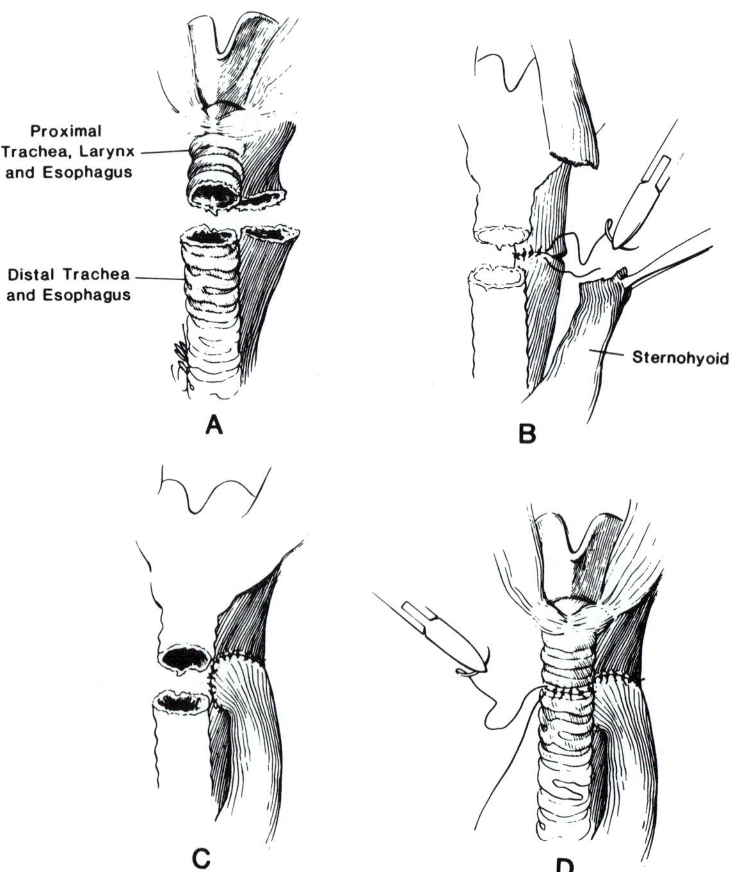


**Figure 38–6.** Repair of traumatic injury to trachea and esophagus. **A.** View of transected trachea and esophagus. **B.** Esophagus closed in two layers. **C.** Strap muscle interposed between esophagus and tracheal suture line. **D.** Completed repair.

of the tracheostomy cuff[36–38] (Figs. 38–7 and 38–8). The upper strictures usually occur in patients who are being maintained on ventilators. It may be assumed, from indirect evidence, that the cause is cicatricial healing of a stomal opening that had eroded the anterior and lateral walls of the trachea at the site of the stoma. Although this injury can be surgically abetted, and while invasive infection may also play a role, it appears to be caused most often by leverage against the stoma by the tracheostomy tube because of improperly suspended heavy equipment. It is apt to occur in a patient receiving prolonged support through a tracheostomy tube. Because the original defect was anterior and lateral, the cicatricial stenosis occurs here, producing an A-shaped stenosis as viewed through the bronchoscope with the patient supine.

In contrast, a high-pressure cuff (or a low-pressure cuff used in a high-pressure range by overinflation) produces circumferential pressure injury in the trachea. As healing occurs, circumferential stenosis results.[38,39] If erosion has been deep and has destroyed the cartilages, the resulting stenosis is not amenable to cure, even with the most prolonged stenting, since there is no normal tracheal mural architecture left. Varying degrees of depth of erosion are seen.

Cuffs on endotracheal tubes may produce stenosis. Because endotracheal tubes are usually used for the initial intubation, most patients in whom stenosis develops even after only 48 hours of ventilation have had only an endotracheal tube (Fig. 38–8B). In many such patients the injury consists of a massive cicatricial stenosis of scar tissue within the tracheal lumen, although the cartilages are not totally destroyed and may even be relatively intact. Endotracheal tubes may cause glottic stenosis and stenosis at the cricoid level, but these are not true tracheal lesions. It is important, however, to be aware of this possibility before considering repair of a tracheal lesion, because it is disastrous to perform a corrective operation on the trachea and then discover that there is an inadequately functioning glottis above it. A number of severe stenoses resulting from cricothyroidostomy have been seen in the subglottic region. High stomas in old patients with kyphosis and in whom the tube gradually erodes back through the cricoid cartilage may produce subglottic stenosis (Fig. 38–8C). A large-bore endotracheal tube may produce erosion and stenosis at the cricoid level. Repair of strictures involving the subglottic larynx is much more difficult than repair of strictures of the trachea alone.

Inflammation may cause varying degrees of thinning of cartilages in the segment between the site of a tracheal stoma and the level of a cuff stenosis below. Sometimes this area may become malacic (Fig. 38–8B). Malacia also may occur at the level of a cuff. Additional lesions that are

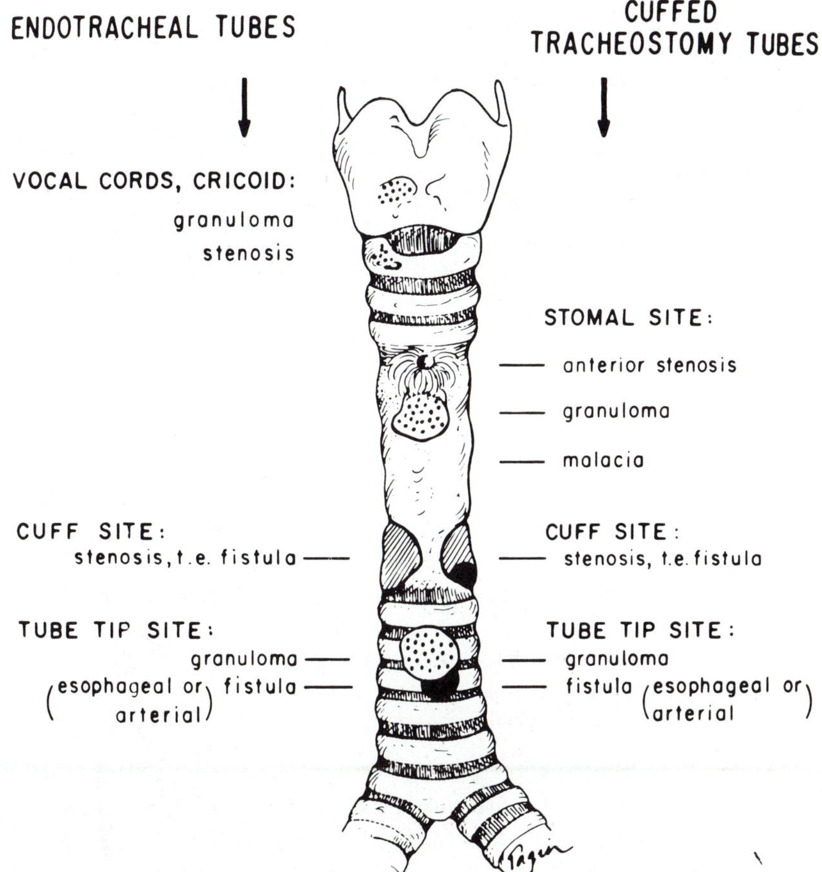


**Figure 38–7.** Locations and types of upper airway lesions evolving from injuries caused by endotracheal tubes and cuffed tracheostomy tubes. *(From Grillo HC: Curr Probl Surg, July 1970.)*

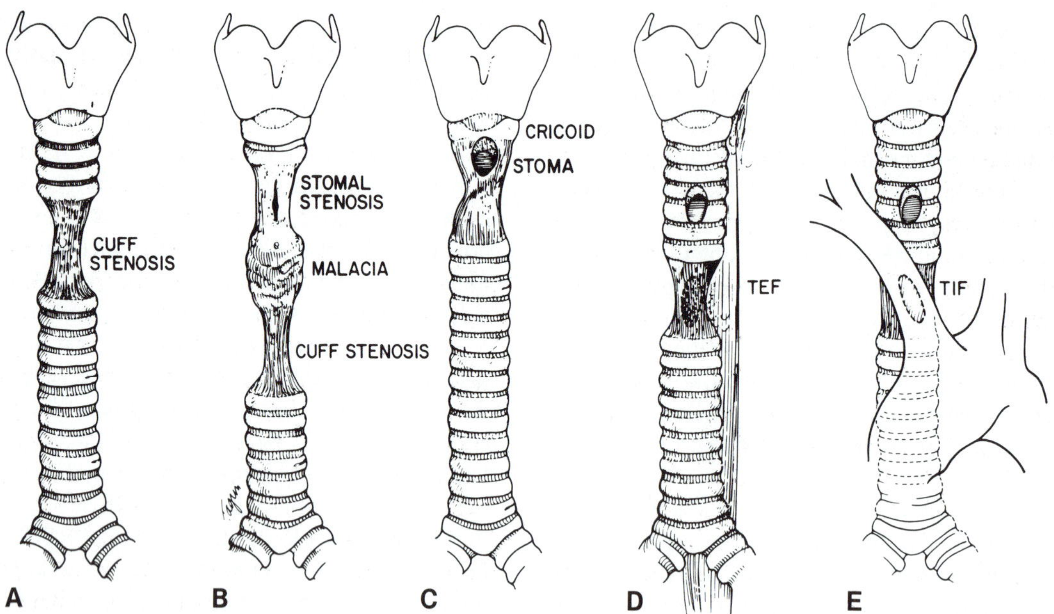


**Figure 38–8.** Principal postintubation lesions. **A.** Lesion at cuff site in a patient who has been treated with an endotracheal tube alone. The lesion is high in the trachea and is circumferential. **B.** Lesions that occur with tracheostomy tubes. At the stomal level, anterolateral stenosis is seen. At the cuff level, lower than with an endotracheal tube, circumferential cuff stenosis occurs. The segment between is often inflamed and malacic. **C.** Damage to the subglottic larynx. A high tracheostomy or one that erodes back because of the patient's anatomy may damage the inferior cricoid and produce a low subglottic stenosis as well as an upper tracheal injury. **D.** Tracheoesophageal fistula (TEF). The level of fistulization is usually where the cuff has eroded posteriorly. Occasionally, angulation of the tip of the tube may produce erosion from the tip. There is also usually severe circumferential damage at this level caused by the cuff. **E.** Tracheoinnominate fistula (TIF). A high-pressure cuff frequently rests on the trachea directly behind the innominate artery. Erosion may occur, although rarely. The more common innominate arterial injury is from a low tracheostomy in which the inner portion of the curve of the tube rests on the artery and causes direct erosion. *(From Grillo HC: J Thorac Cardiovasc Surg 78:860, 1979.)*

not truly strictures but are caused by tracheostomy tube injuries are tracheoesophageal fistula and trachea–innominate artery fistula. Tracheoesophageal fistula is seen most often in patients who have nasogastric feeding tubes in place for long periods of time in addition to an inflated cuff in the trachea (Fig. 38–8D). The pressure of these two foreign bodies acts as an erosive pincer. Anterior erosion of the tracheal wall was seen more often when high-pressure cuffs were routinely used or when the tip of a tube angulated forward. These devices sometimes caused erosion directly into the innominate artery where it crosses the trachea (Fig. 38–8E). A more common cause of innominate artery hemorrhage a tracheostomy tube so low that the tube itself rests on the elevated artery and erodes through it at the inferior margin of the stoma. Such lesions, therefore, are seen most often in children and young adults, because their tracheas are more mobile and rise up into the neck along with the innominate artery on hyperextension. These last lesions can be avoided when the tracheostomy is placed in an appropriate position at the level of the second and third tracheal rings, rather than at the sternal notch.

### Clinical Presentation

Most patients with postintubation stenosis have signs of upper airway obstruction. The patient initially reports shortness of breath on exertion. Then progressive shortness of breath occurs even at rest with wheezing and stridor. Occasionally, episodes of unilateral or bilateral pneumonitis provide a clue. Cyanosis is a very late sign. One must remember that any patient who has signs of upper airway obstruction must be considered to have an organic lesion of the trachea, particularly if he or she has undergone intubation for ventilatory support at any time in the recent past. In practice, many of these patients have been given the diagnosis of adult-onset asthma despite the record of recent intubation.

Tracheoesophageal fistula presents as suddenly far more secretions than previously noted and aspiration at attempts to swallow. Trachea–innominate artery fistula frequently gives a premonitory hemorrhage of clinically significant, but not massive, nature. Such bleeding should always be investigated with bronchoscopy to prove that one is dealing with something more than severe tracheitis. Angiography, which may show a small false aneurysm, may be of some use.

### Diagnosis

The clinical presentation and history give the presumptive diagnosis in most cases. This may be followed by simple tracheal radiographs.[40] Fluoroscopy is particularly important to be certain that the glottis is functioning adequately and, further, that there are no areas of malacia. Bronchoscopy may be performed separately in complex cases, but in simpler ones, it is done concurrently with the repair if radiologic demonstration has been adequate. A word of caution about flexible bronchoscopy with local anesthesia: *If critical airway stenosis is present, total airway obstruction may result from the bronchoscopy or secretions.* Flexible bronchoscopy should be performed in this setting only with great caution, if at all.

### Treatment

The operation for resection of benign strictures of the trachea has been so well developed and standardized that it is clearly the treatment of choice when the lesion is not excessively long and does not involve other more complex anatomic structures, such as the subglottic larynx, and when the surgeon has had reasonable experience, so that a good result may be promised.[36,37] Most tracheal strictures may be managed indefinitely by resinstituting a tracheostomy, dilating the stricture, and inserting a silicone rubber T tube (Montgomery tube; E Benson Hood Laboratories, Pembroke, Massachusetts) (Fig. 38–9).[41] With such a tube, a patient can live indefinitely, leading a fairly normal life. The tube requires changing at infrequent intervals.

We have treated 140 patients between the ages of 7 months and 95 years with either a temporary or a permanent T tube.[41] The primary diagnosis was postintubation stenosis

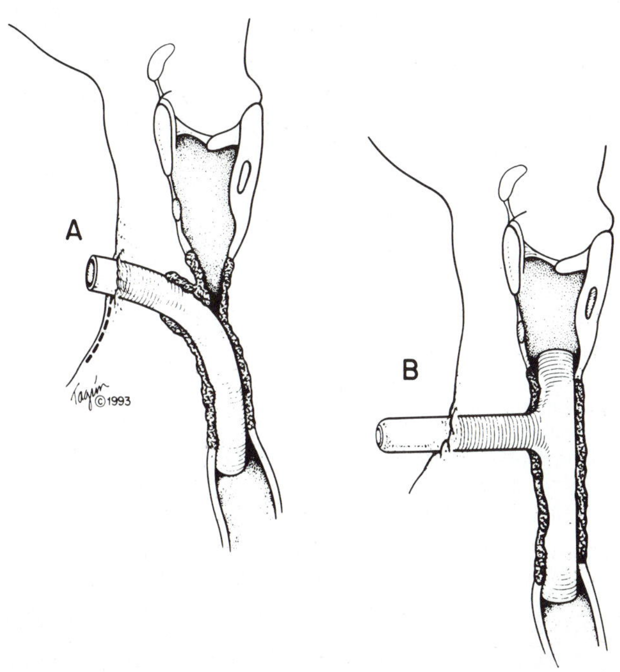


**Figure 38–9.** Straight stomal tract perpendicular to tracheal axis is important for optimal seating of T tube. **A.** Oblique tract in longstanding tracheostomy. Dotted line shows intended incision. **B.** Corrected stomal tract with T tube. *(From Gaissert HA, et al: J Thorac Cardiovasc Surg 107:600, 1994.)*

in 86 patients, burn injury in 13 patients, malignant airway tumors in 12 patients, and various other disorders in 29 patients. Placement was considered long-term in 112 patients with a duration of 1–5 years in 37 patients and more than 5 years in 12 patients. Intolerance that necessitated removal was identified in 28 patients; the intolerance was usually related to upper-limb obstruction or aspiration. The tracheal T tube restores airway patency reliably with excellent long-term results. It is the preferred management of chronic airway obstruction not amenable to surgical reconstruction.

When there is no contraindication, surgical excision and end-to-end repair is the treatment of choice. Morbidity is small, and the success rate is very high. In postintubation strictures, nearly all repairs are done through an anterior approach using a collar incision, either alone or with a vertical partial sternal division (Fig. 38–10). Dissection is kept very close to the trachea, in contrast to dissection for a tumor. This avoids injury to the recurrent laryngeal nerves. Stenoses are dilated before anesthesia is induced if they are smaller than 6 mm in diameter in order to avoid $CO_2$ retention and resultant arrhythmias. Division is usually made below a stricture (unless it is a low stricture); intubation is performed across the operative field; and the stricture is carefully dissected away from the esophagus (Fig. 38–10C). Strictures up to half the length of the trachea may be thus removed, and approximation done. In older patients or with resections of long segments of trachea, a laryngeal release may be required for additional length.[26] Tracheostomy is not used.

If the stricture involves the subglottic larynx, a single-stage repair of the lesion requires partial removal of the lower anterior subglottic larynx[9,42] (Figs. 38–11 and 38–12). If the stenosis is circumferential, the scar over the injured mucosa may be removed from the anterior surface of the cricoid plate. Appropriate tailoring of the distal segment allows repair of both these defects in a single stage, but the technique is difficult. Temporary tracheostomy is occasionally necessary in these patients.

### Results of Surgical Treatment

The results of surgical treatment of postintubation stenoses have been good. Our experience includes 503 patients who underwent tracheal resection and reconstruction from 1965 to 1992, including reoperations on patients who had undergone previous operations and patients from the earliest time when such lesions were repaired. The results included 12 deaths (3.1%), 20 treatment failures (3.9%), and 471 instances (93%) of good or satisfactory results (Table 38–6). An increasing number of our patients have undergone operations before referral.[37] Despite this factor, and the increasing complexity of cases, results have remained consistently good (Table 38–7). Laser treatment of postintubation lesions has increasingly been recognized as largely palliative. In practice, it often delays definitive treatment or complicates it.

It is extremely rare for a postintubation stenotic lesion

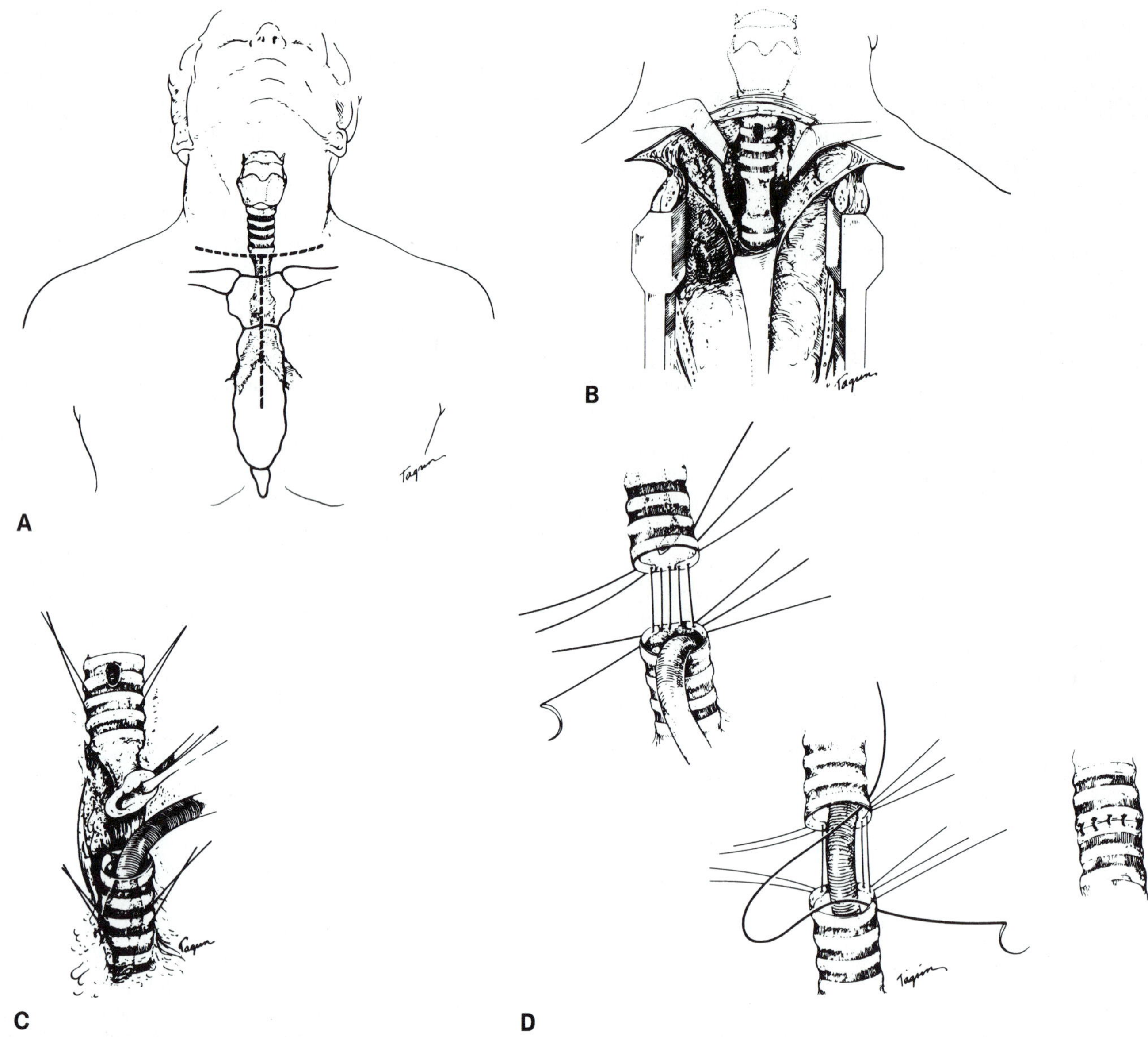


**Figure 38–10.** Reconstruction of the upper trachea. **A.** The collar incision allows exploration of the entire trachea and, in many patients, reconstruction. Division of the upper two thirds of the sternum widens the access for lower or more difficult lesions. **B.** Sternal division in this patient has made access to the lower trachea easier. Because the trachea points to the posterior, there is nothing to be gained by division of the innominate vein. The pleura is intact. **C.** The trachea has been divided below a stenotic lesion and the patient intubated directly. This allows easier dissection of a lesion that may be fused to the esophagus. **D.** The technique of anastomosis. Posterolateral sutures are placed first. The proximal tube is then advanced from above after withdrawing the tube in the distal trachea, and the anastomosis is completed. Sutures are generally tied from front to back, with all knots on the outside. The temporarily approximating lateral traction sutures are not shown, nor is the cervical flexion that removes tension. The entire trachea may be approached by way of an extension of the cervical mediastinal incision into the right fourth intercostal space. *(From Grillo HC: J Thorac Cardiovasc Surg 78:860, 1979.)*

to involve more than one half the trachea unless there has been a prior attempt at surgical intervention. If primary reconstruction cannot be performed because of the extensive involvement of the trachea, insertion of a Montgomery silicone T tube promises an excellent long-term alternative.[41] There is no indication for an open operation for insertion of a prosthesis.

Treatment of inflammatory stenosis of the upper trachea involving the subglottic larynx has yielded gratifying results.[9] We treated 80 patients by single-stage resection and reconstruction. Repair consisted of resection of the anterolateral cricoid arch in all patients plus resection of posterior laryngeal stenosis where present. The technique involves salvage of the posterior cricoid plate, appropriate resection and tailoring of the trachea, and primary anastomosis using a posterior membranous tracheal flap to resurface the bared cricoid cartilage. Among patients undergoing this procedure, there was one postoperative death from my-

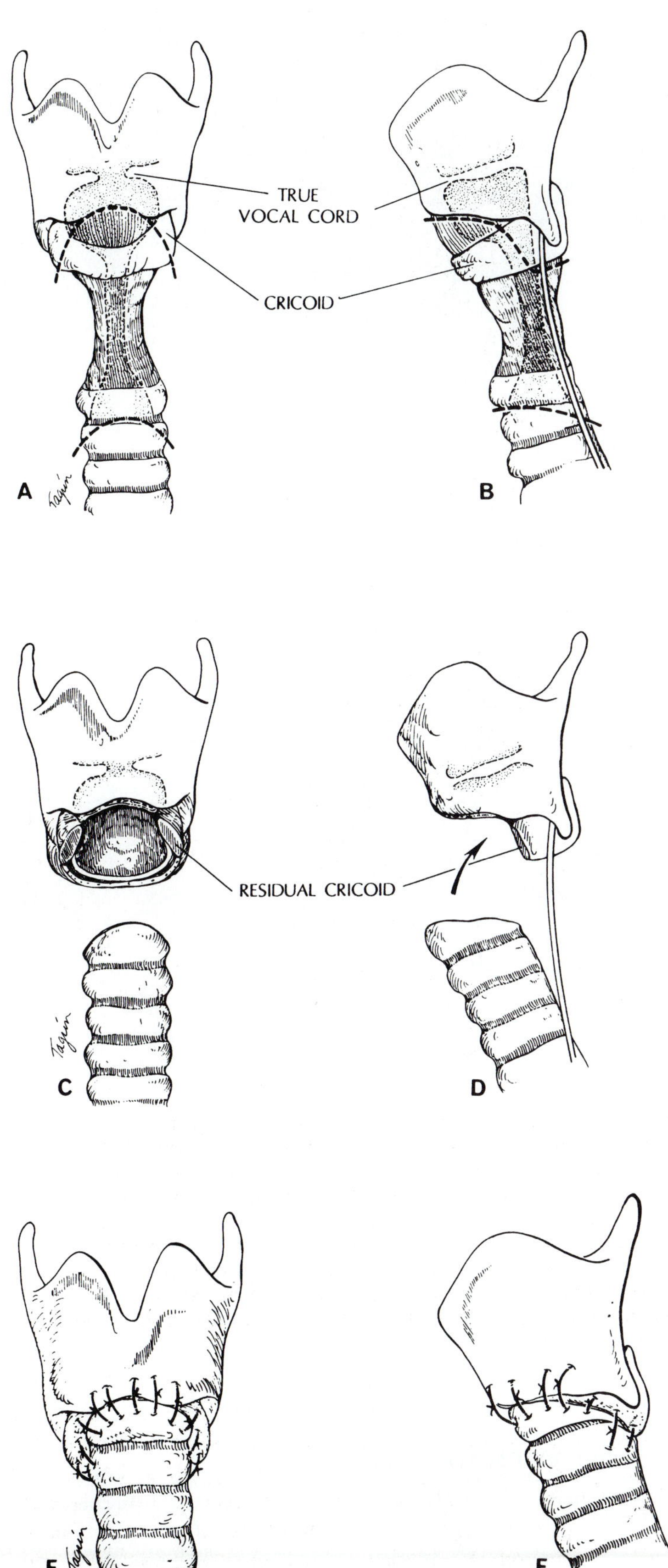


**Figure 38–11.** Operative repair of anterolateral stenosis of the subglottic larynx and upper trachea. **A.** Anteroposterior view. **B.** Lateral view. **A** and **B** show the extent of the pathologic process and the ultimate lines of transection. The stenosis extends into the subglottic larynx well above the border of the cricoid anteriorly. However, no pathologic change involves the posterior mucosal wall of the subglottic larynx or of the upper trachea. The proximal line of transection is centered in the midline just below the thyroid cartilage and swings laterally to transect the lateral lamina of the cricoid and to divide the larynx from the trachea posteriorly at the lower border of posterior cricoid lamina or cricoid plate. Inferiorly, the most proximal tracheal ring of residual trachea is cut backward to the posterior ends. **C** and **D.** Larynx and trachea after removal of the specimen. Recurrent nerves have been left intact but are not dissected out, as might be suggested by the diagrammatic representation. The mucous membrane of the larynx has been transected sharply at the same level of division as the cartilage. **E** and **F.** Anteroposterior and lateral views of the reconstruction. *(From Grillo HC: Ann Thorac Surg 33:3, 1982.)*

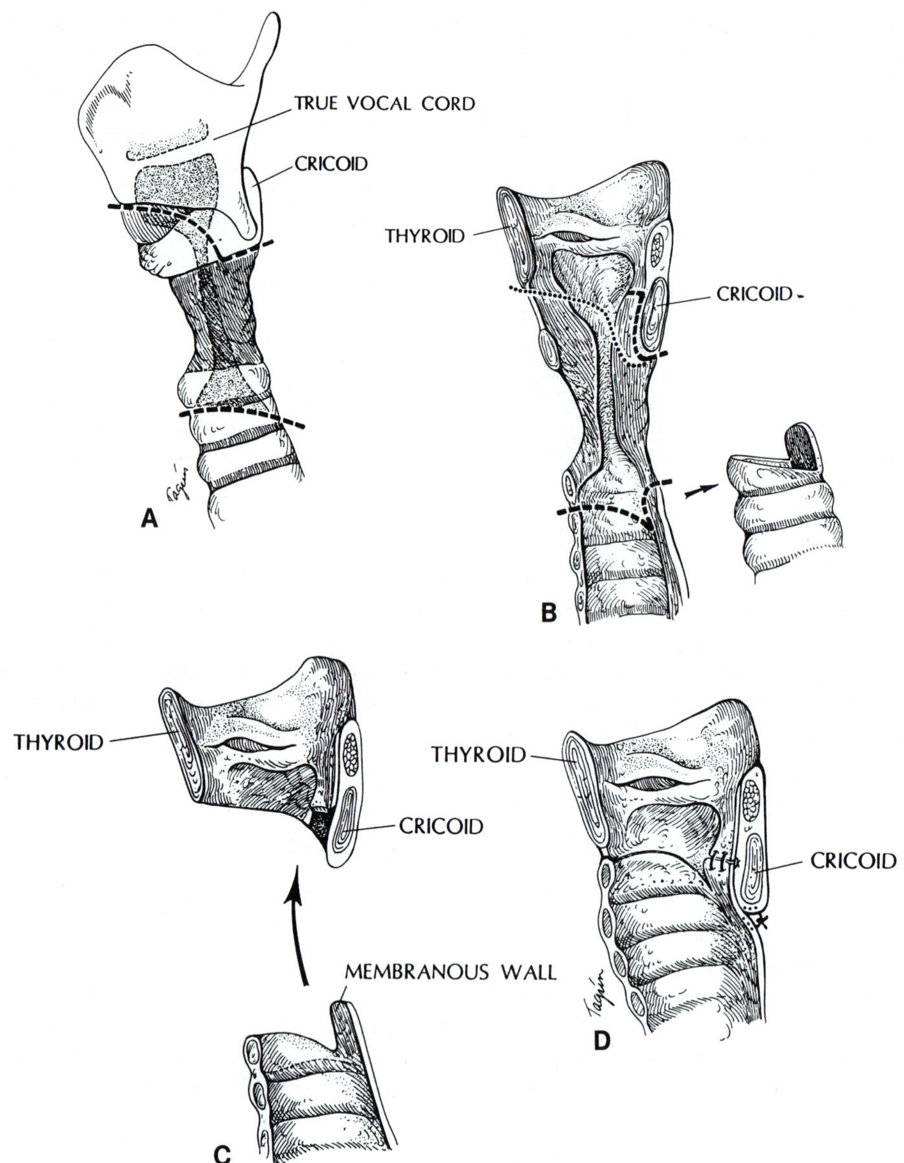


**Figure 38–12.** Resection and reconstruction of circumferential stenosis of subglottic larynx and upper trachea. **A.** External line of cartilaginous division of both larynx and trachea is same as in anterolateral stenosis. **B.** Interior view of larynx and trachea demonstrates modifications necessary when stenosis involves mucosa and submucosa just in front of posterior cricoid plate. Superior dotted line indicates external cartilaginous division of the larynx. Dashed line against anterior wall of cricoid plate indicates that the mucosa with its scarring will be cut back to within a short distance, if necessary, of the arytenoid cartilages. Inferiorly, the posterior membranous wall has been retained as a broad-based flap. **C.** Resected specimen, leaving bare area of the intraluminal portion of the lower part of the cricoid posterior lamina. The flap of membranous wall of the trachea will be fitted into this defect to provide prompt and complete mucosal coverage. **D.** Mucosa of larynx has been anastomosed to mucosa of membranous wall of trachea. External to lumen, connective tissue of membranous wall has been fixed with four sutures to inferior margin of cricoid cartilage. This assures that flap will stay firmly applied to surface. *(From Grillo HC: Ann Thorac Surg 33:3, 1982.)*

**TABLE 38–6. RESULTS OF SURGICAL TREATMENT OF POSTINTUBATION TRACHEAL STENOSIS**

| Type of Operation | No. of Patients | Good | | Satisfactory | | Failure | | Death | | Reoperation | |
|---|---|---|---|---|---|---|---|---|---|---|---|
| | | *No.* | *%* | *No.* | *%* | *No.* | *%* | *No.* | *%* | *No.* | *%* |
| Initial Operation | 503 | 427 | 84.9 | 27 | 5.3 | 19 | 3.8 | 12 | 2.4 | 18 | 3.6 |
| Reoperation | 18 | 13 | 72.2 | 4 | 22.2 | 1 | 5.6 | 0 | — | — | — |
| Overall | 503 | 440 | 87.5 | 31 | 6.2 | 20 | 3.9 | 12 | 2.4 | — | — |

**TABLE 38–7. EFFECT OF PRIOR TREATMENT ON RESULTS OF SURGICAL TREATMENT OF TRACHEAL STENOSIS**

| Treatment | Total | Good | | Satisfactory | | Failure | | Death | | Reoperation | |
|---|---|---|---|---|---|---|---|---|---|---|---|
| | | *No.* | *%* | *No.* | *%* | *No.* | *%* | *No.* | *%* | *No.* | *%* |
| Prior treatment | | | | | | | | | | | |
| T Tube | 60 | 51 | 85 | 0 | — | 3 | 5 | 2 | 3.3 | 4 | 6.7 |
| Laser | 45 | 40 | 88.9 | 1 | 2.2 | 1 | 2.2 | 0 | — | 3 | 6.7 |
| Resection and Reconstruction | 53 | 40 | 75.5 | 6 | 11.3 | 3 | 5.6 | 2 | 3.8 | 2 | 3.8 |
| Other tracheal operation | 31 | 27 | 87.1 | 1 | 3.2 | 3 | 9.7 | 0 | — | 0 | — |
| Laryngeal operation | 20 | 16 | 80 | 2 | 10 | 0 | — | 1 | 5 | 1 | 5 |
| TEF repair | 8 | 7 | 87.5 | 0 | — | 0 | — | 0 | — | 1 | 12.5 |
| No prior treatment | 342 | 295 | 86.2 | 18 | 5.3 | 12 | 3.5 | 8 | 2.3 | 9 | 2.7 |
| No prior resection and reconstruction | 450 | 387 | 86 | 21 | 4.7 | 16 | 3.6 | 10 | 2.1 | 16 | 3.6 |

TEF = tracheoesophageal fistula.

ocardial infarction. Long-term results were excellent in 18 patients, good in 48, and satisfactory in eight. Treatment failed in two patients. Three additional patients had good results at discharge but participated in the follow-up study for less than 6 months.

Management of acquired *tracheoesophageal fistula* has been controversial. We have taken a conservative approach, delaying fistula closure until the patient is weaned from mechanical ventilation.[43] A gastrostomy tube is placed to drain the stomach and eliminate possible reflux, and a jejunostomy tube is placed for feeding. Esophageal diversion is only rarely required. Most patients require concomitant resection of the injured tracheal stenosis and closure of the esophageal fistula. It is necessary to interpose viable tissue, such as strap muscle, between the two suture lines to prevent refistulization (Fig. 38–13). Only rarely can the fistula be divided and simple closure of the esophagus and trachea be accomplished (Fig. 38–14). We have treated 38 patients with acquired tracheoesophageal fistula from a variety of causes.[43] There were four deaths in the series. Two were from sepsis in patients who required mechanical ventilation after transthoracic repair of distal tracheoesophageal fistulas. The other two deaths were from an aortotracheal fistula 2 months after repair that required a T tube for malacia and tracheal separation following an extensive resection. The fistulas were successfully closed in all surviving patients. Recurrent fistulas developed in three patients but closed successfully with reoperation in two patients and drainage in one patient. Of the 34 surviving patients, 33 ate orally and 32 breathed without the need for tracheostomy.[43]

### *Reconstruction after Irradiation*

Radiation in excess of 4000 to 5000 cGy has been an absolute contraindication to airway operations, especially if given more than 1 year before the operation. The incorporation of omental wrapping with airway reconstruction has allowed tracheal resection to be successfully performed on 15 patients.[44] The vascularized pedicle of omentum is passed substernally and wrapped circumferentially around the tracheal anastomosis. There was one anastomotic dehiscence and death in a patient treated previously for lymphoma. Two patients required anastomotic stenting with T tubes. Airway operations can be cautiously considered despite previous irradiation when the omentum is used as a buttress.

### Postinfection Stenosis

A variety of specific infections can cause stenosis of the trachea. Diphtheria was notorious for producing such injuries, but it rarely is seen now. A small number of patients with a history of diphtheria in childhood have been seen with stenosis later in life. It is sometimes difficult to be certain whether the stenosis was due to tracheostomies that were established for the treatment of the diphtheria or to the diphtheria itself.

Tuberculosis can cause severe stenosis of the trachea. It appears to involve the lower trachea more often than the upper. The lesion usually begins as endobronchial tuberculosis, which, in healing, evolves to a stenosis. Most typically, the fibrosis is submucosal. An accompanying stricture of either the left or right main bronchus is also seen in such lesions—and, occasionally, one of the upper lobe bronchi as well. If the stenosis is mature and is not excessively long, resection and reconstruction may be used for definitive treatment. If there is still considerable residual inflammation, management becomes exceedingly difficult. It is, of course, difficult to treat such a patient with intubation alone because of the involvement of the carina. Otherwise, a period of watching and waiting for the inflammation to subside with chemotherapy would be the best course.

Mediastinal fibrosis may be accompanied by marked narrowing and stenosis of large segments of the trachea and bronchi.[45] It is presumed on the basis of pathologic or bacteriologic findings that some patients with mediastinal fibrosis have had histoplasmosis. Some of these patients may be amenable to surgical resection by very extensive techni-

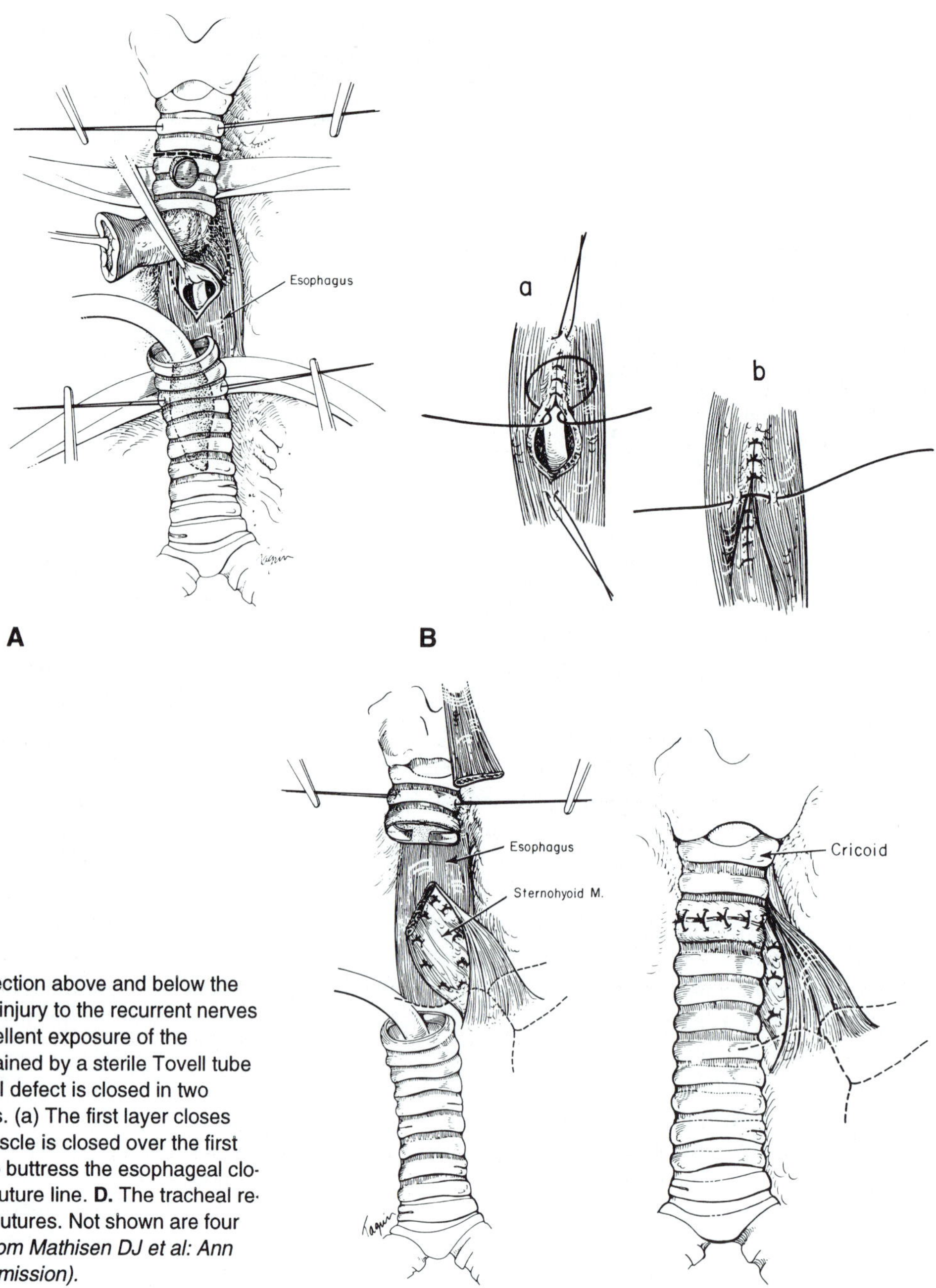


**Figure 38–13. A.** Circumferential dissection above and below the fistula is very near the trachea to avoid injury to the recurrent nerves Division of damaged trachea gives excellent exposure of the esophageal defect. Ventilation is maintained by a sterile Tovell tube in the distal trachea. **B.** The esophageal defect is closed in two layers using interrupted 4–0 silk sutures. (a) The first layer closes the esophagus. (b) The esophageal muscle is closed over the first layer. **C.** A local strap muscle is used to buttress the esophageal closure and separate it from the tracheal suture line. **D.** The tracheal repair is done with interrupted 4-0 Vicryl sutures. Not shown are four lateral traction sutures of 2-0 Vicryl. *(From Mathisen DJ et al: Ann Thorac Surg 52:759–65, 1991, with permission).*

cal maneuvers with reconstruction to save at least some of the lung tissue. In other patients the mediastinum is no massively fibrotic and the length of trachea and bronchi involved is so great that excision and reconstruction are impossible. There is no known therapy except periodic redilation or possible stenting.

Noninfectious diseases of obscure origin can cause tracheal obstruction. Examples are sarcoidosis, Wegener's granulomatosis, amyloid disease, tracheopathia osteoplastica, and idiopathic stenosis. Often the basic disease contraindicates surgical repair.

### Tracheal Stenosis After Inhalation Injury

The combined effects of inhaled irritant gases and heat in burn victims produce an intense, often transmural, inflammation of the airway further complicated by intubation. We have treated 18 such patients over a 22-year period (15 intubated).[46] Sixteen patients had sustained flame or combustion burns and two were injured by chemical agents only. The time to presentation of symptoms ranged from 0 to 4 months after the inhalation injury. Three patients underwent standard tracheal resection and reconstruction with immedi-

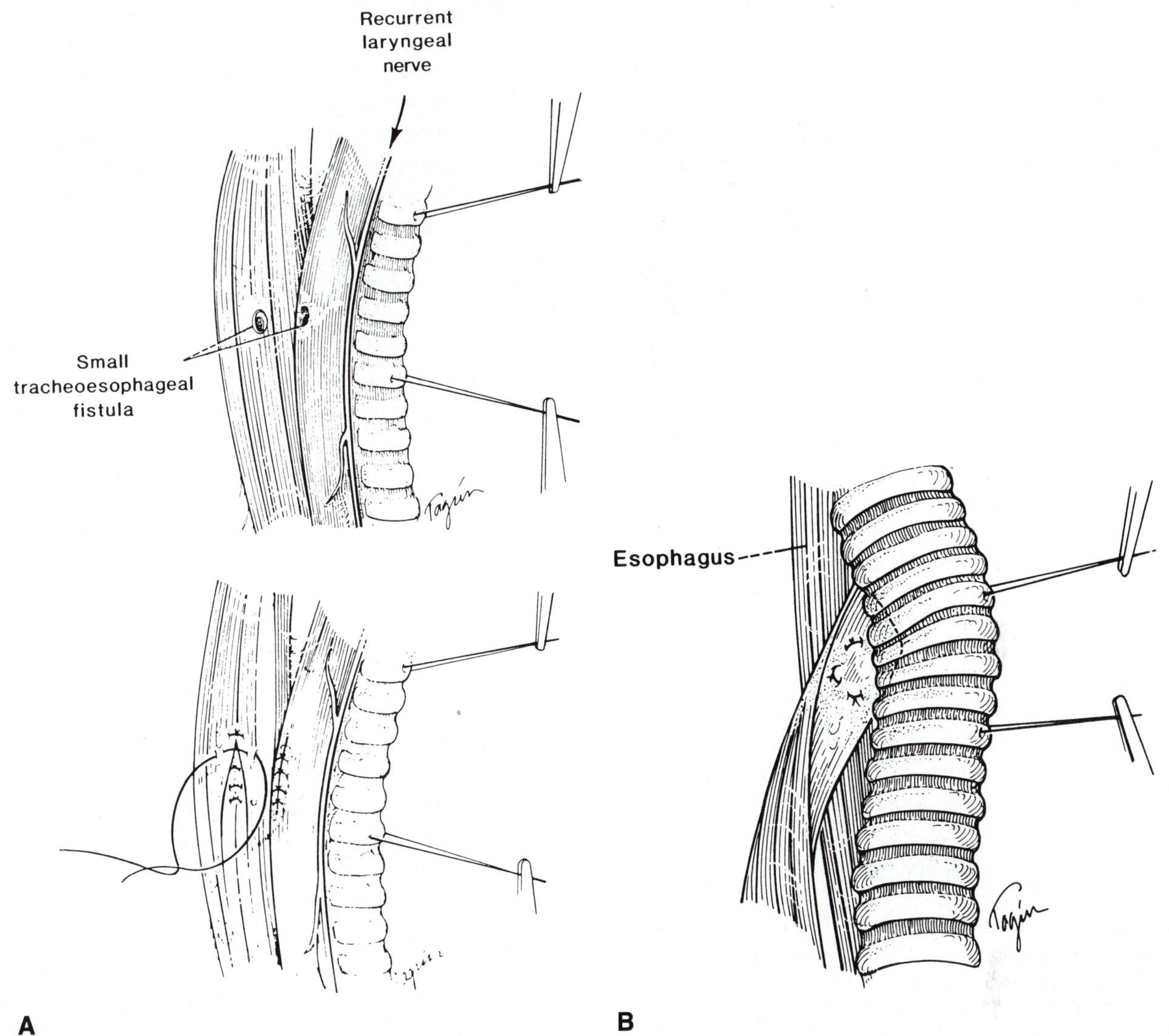


**Figure 38–14. A.** Small tracheoesophageal fistula treated by division and local repair. The recurrent nerve is elevated with the trachea. The esophagus is closed in two layers. **B.** A strap muscle is used to cover the esophageal suture line and separate it from the tracheal suture line. *(From Mathisen DJ et al: Ann Thorac Surg 52:759–65, 1991, with permission.)*

ate restenosis in two and permanent T tube in the third. Six patients underwent laryngofissure or laryngocricotracheal fissure. Stents or T tubes were removed 1–3 months later from five patients and 3 years later from one patient. T tubes were used in 15 patients (two failed because of obstruction). In the other 13 patients, the mean time the T tubes were left in place was 36 months. Follow-up findings were available for 14 patients. Five patients had permanent tracheal tubes. Nine patients did not need airway support. Five had been treated with T tube only, and four with laryngofissure and subsequent T tube. Successful outcome does not result in a normal airway. Great caution is urged in treating patients who have sustained inhalational airway injury. Strictures related to such injuries are associated with prolonged inflammation and respond best to prolonged stenting or resection and stenting of subglottic stenosis. Early tracheal resection should be avoided.

## TRACHEAL COLLAPSE

Tracheal collapse may be seen from a variety of lesions. There are many references to *congenital tracheomalacia* in the literature. Few of these cases, however, are well documented, and many have complicating factors, so the malacic changes may well have been the result of intubation. The infant trachea is composed of very fine structures, and even a small amount of injury may lead to softening of the delicate rings.

Segmental malacia is seen as a dominant lesion in a

number of patients who have had *cuff injury* to the trachea after intubation. Such a patient may have an apparently normal air column on a static radiograph. Fluoroscopic observation, however, demonstrates a segment that collapses on coughing or forced respiration.[40] Resection is the usual treatment.

Chronic *compressive lesions* may lead to collapse of the trachea. A large goiter, a cystic thymus, an aneurysm or congenital vascular malformation (e.g., a vascular ring), or an anomalous innominate artery may lead to compressive obstruction of the trachea. When the compressing lesion is excised or displaced so that pressure is no longer exerted, malacia may appear in some patients because the rings have thinned. In such patients, transient intubation may be effective. Other techniques, such as splinting with local prosthetic rings placed external to the lumen or with traction sutures pulled out over buttons placed against the cervical musculature, have been used. The problems are rare, vary greatly, and require individual solutions.

Two types of tracheal collapse are also seen with *chronic obstructive pulmonary disease.* One type consists of a softening and flattening of the trachea from front to back. When the patient coughs, the membranous wall is approximated to the cartilaginous wall, and the airway becomes obstructed, particularly in the lower half of the trachea.[47] Less commonly, in the deformity known as saber-sheath trachea (which consists of an increase in the anteroposterior dimension of the trachea with side-to-side narrowing) there rarely may be such an extreme degree of narrowing that with cough and approximation of the lateral walls of the trachea there is a considerable amount of obstruction, especially to clearance of secretions, despite the absence of malacic changes. Saber-sheath trachea involves the lower two thirds of the trachea.[48]

Various surgical procedures have been devised to correct the first type of flattening (C-type).[47] In general, these consist of pulling the corners of the cartilages together to shorten the membranous wall. Then, when the patient coughs or breathes forcefully, it is not possible for the trachea to flatten out. Saber-sheath trachea has been treated with external ring support.

*Relapsing polychrondritis,* a disease of unknown causation, leads to destruction of cartilage in many parts of the body, including the nasal septum, ears, trachea, and bronchi. Gradually, the airways soften, and the patient is subject not only to difficulty in breathing but also to recurring infections. Often the bronchi and trachea together are involved. For this reason, no effective surgical procedure has yet been devised.

*Idiopathic malacia* has been seen to develop in adults unrelated to other known disease. A few patients have undergone splinting with good results.

*Postpneumonectomy syndrome* produces compression and malacia of the junction of the trachea and the main bronchus because of extreme mediastinal shift after right-sided pneumonectomy (or left, when a right-sided aortic arch is present). Correction is very complex but has been done successfully in some patients.[49]

## COMPLICATIONS OF TRACHEAL RESECTION

In 1986, we described complications of tracheal resection covering the period from 1962 to 1982.[50] That report dealt with 86 patients who underwent resection for neoplasm (56 primary neoplasms and 30 secondary neoplasms) and 279 patients who underwent resection for postintubation injury. Complications were generally few for upper tracheal lesions. Serious complications more often followed carinal reconstruction or laryngotracheal resections without restoration of continuity.

Laryngeal edema is managed with restriction of fluid intake and administration of racemic epinephrine and a short course of steroids (24–48 hours). The edema usually regresses within 1 week. Pneumonia has been extremely rare after upper tracheal resections, because proper attention has been given to intraoperative management and to postoperative physiotherapy. All patients spend one or more days in a respiratory intensive care unit the staff of which is familiar with the management of such problems.

The most common later complication has been the formation of granulations at the suture line (Table 38–8). This is less of a problem for patients who undergo resection for tumor than for patients who have undergone tracheal reconstructions for inflammatory disease, because residual inflammation may be present in the latter patients. Granulations may usually be managed with bronchoscopic removal under light anesthesia. Often a suture is found to have worked its way into the lumen at the base of the granulations. Removal of the sutures leads to healing. In some pa-

**TABLE 38–8. COMPLICATIONS OF TRACHEAL RESECTION**

| | Reason for Resection | |
|---|---|---|
| **Complication** | ***Postintubation Lesions*** | ***Neoplasms*** |
| No. of patients | 279 | 86 |
| Granulations | 28 | 10 |
| Separation | 4 | 6 |
| Air leak only | — | 1 |
| Stenosis | | |
| Partial | 6 | 3 |
| Complete | 15 | — |
| Hemorrhage | 2 | 1 |
| Persistent stoma | 5 | — |
| Tracheoesophageal fistula | 1 | — |
| Esophagocutaneous fistula | — | 1 |
| Wound infection | 6 | — |
| Cord dysfunction | 5 | 3 |
| Aspiration | 1 | — |
| Hypoxemia | — | 1 |
| Laryngeal edema | 1 | — |
| Respiratory failure | — | 2 |
| Pneumonia | — | 2 |

*(From Grillo HC, et al: J Thorac Cardiovasc Surg 1986;91:322–328.)*

tients, multiple bronchoscopies are necessary over a period of time. The presence of granulations may be seen on radiologic images, but most often it is manifested by wheezing or minor hemoptysis. The patient must be warned in advance that these symptoms are not a cause for alarm, to avert any fear that he or she has a recurrent tumor. Triamcinolone may be injected into the base of such granulations, but there is no clear evidence supporting the efficacy of this drug. Use of absorbable Vicryl (polyglactin 910) sutures appears to prevent the problem.

Separation of the anastomosis in most patients is caused by excessive tension, which results from resecting too much trachea or failing to make adjunctive relaxing maneuvers to lessen the tension. Excessive circumferential dissection of the trachea, especially distal to the point of division, may destroy the blood supply and cause separation or stenosis. Excessive resection is more likely to occur in patients with tumors (6 of 86 patients) than in those with postintubation stenosis (4 of 279).[50] In one patient a transient air leak occurred but sealed spontaneously. Steroids have been responsible for separation in some patients. All patients who take steroids should gradually stop taking them before the operation.

Tracheal separation in the immediately postoperative period is reason to conclude there has been a serious technical error. Reoperation might be reconsidered to resuture the area and then cover it with a local muscle flap, if the area is small. If the tissues do not seem appropriate for resuturing, a tracheostomy tube may be placed across the defect, to be replaced later by a Montgomery silicone T tube. A T tube can be placed initially if a patient does not require a sealed airway. With partial restenosis, the airway that results may be tolerated and may sometimes be improved with endoscopic techniques, including laser therapy.

Injury to a recurrent nerve occurred in three patients who underwent tracheal reconstruction for neoplasms and in five who underwent reconstruction for postintubation injury. In each patient the injury was clearly the result of surgical manipulation and extensive resection.

One patient who required a repeat resection of the intrathoracic trachea, for plexiform neurofibroma involving the esophagus, had an esophagocutaneous fistula that healed spontaneously. One patient with extensive tumor involving the carina and left main bronchus underwent carinal resection and closure of the left main bronchus without removal of the left lung as described by Perelman and Koroleva.[21] The patient had severe hypoxemia and tachycardia for 3 months until the residual left lung, which had a 30% shunt, was finally removed.

Suture line leakage is extremely rare. If an airtight anastomosis without tension is achieved at the operating table, separation almost never occurs. Minimal air leakage at a suture line may occur, although this complication is exceedingly rare. Minimal leakage can be managed through suction drains, and the leak seals without further event. One patient with an end-to-end anastomosis did have leakage

**TABLE 38–9. RESULTS OF TREATMENT OF COMPLICATIONS OF TRACHEAL RESECTION PERFORMED FOR POSTINTUBATION LESIONS**

| Complication | No. | Good | Satisfactory | Failed | Death |
|---|---|---|---|---|---|
| Granulation | 28 | 24 | 4 | — | — |
| Separation | 4 | — | 2 | — | 2 |
| Restenosis | 21 | 6 | 15 | — | — |
| Malacia | 3 | 1 | — | 1 | 1 |
| Hemorrhage | 2 | 1 | — | — | 1 |
| Tracheoesophageal fistula | 1 | — | — | — | 1 |
| Vocal cord dysfunction | 5 | — | 4 | 1 | — |
| Aspiration | 1 | — | — | 1 | — |
| Wound infection | 6 | 6 | — | — | — |
| Edema | 1 | — | — | 1 | — |

*(From Grillo HC et al: J Thorac Cardiovasc Surg 1986; 91:322–328.)*

after an extended transthoracic resection in the lowermost trachea.[50] This leakage ultimately healed, with subsequent stenosis that required reoperation. Problems following carinal reconstruction are not pertinent to this discussion.

Innominate artery hemorrhage can occur after tracheal resection for tumor and end-to-end anastomosis, particularly above the carinal level. This complication should be exceedingly rare. It occurred in only one patient in more than 200 who underwent resection for benign stenosis. Careful management of the artery, as previously described, should prevent this problem.

The massive problems that can follow low mediastinal tracheostomy or extended resection, with either staged or prosthetic reconstruction, have been presented elsewhere.[16,24,25,37] The key problems are nonhealing mediastinal sepsis and erosion of the major blood vessels deep in the mediastinum. With the use of prostheses the formation of granulations with obstruction and pulmonary sepsis is too common. Late hemorrhage from vascular erosion has complicated many attempts at prosthetic replacement of the trachea. This may occur even a year or more after placement of the prosthesis.

Good results are possible if complications are handled properly. The results of management of complications are listed in Table 38–9.

## REFERENCES

1. Grillo HC, Dignan EF, Miura T: Extensive resection and reconstruction of mediastinal trachea without prosthesis or graft: An anatomical study in man. *J Thorac Cardiovasc Surg* **48**(5):741–749, 1964
2. Grillo HC: Congenital lesions, neoplasms, and injuries of the trachea. In Sabiston DC Jr, Spencer FC (eds): *Surgery of the Chest,* 5th ed. Philadelphia, Saunders, 1990, pp 335–371.
3. Miura T, Grillo HC: The contribution of the inferior thyroid artery of the blood supply of the human trachea. *Surg Gynecol Obstet* **123:**(1):99–102, 1966

4. Salassa JR, Pearson BW, Payne WS: Gross and microscopical blood supply of the trachea. *Ann Thorac Surg* **24**(2):100–107, 1977
5. Grillo HC: Tracheal blood supply. *Ann Thorac Surg* **24:**99, 1977
6. Wain JC, Mathisen DJ, Wilson D: Clinical experience with minitracheostomy. *Ann Thorac Surg* **49:**881–886, 1990
7. Whited RE: A prospective study of laryngotracheal sequelae in long-term intubation. *Laryngoscope* **94:**367–372, 1984
8. Grillo HC: Complications of tracheal operations. In Cordell AR, Ellison RG (eds): *Complications of Intrathoracic Surgery.* Boston, Little, Brown, 1979
9. Grillo HC, Mathisen DJ, Wain JC: Laryngotracheal resection and reconstruction for subglottic stenosis. *Ann Thorac Surg* **53:**54–63, 1992
10. Lawson DW, Grillo HC: Closure of a persistent tracheal stoma. *Surg Gynecol Obstet* **130:**995–998, 1970
11. Weber AL, Grillo HC: Tracheal tumors: A radiological, clinical and pathological evaluation of 84 cases. *Radiol Clin North Am* **16:**227–235, 1978
12. Momose RJ, MacMillan AS Jr: Roentgenologic investigations of the larynx and trachea. *Radiol Clin North Am* **16**(2):321–341, 1978
13. Shepard JO, McLoud TC: Imaging the airways: Computed tomography and magnetic resonance imaging. *Clin Chest Med* **12**(1):151–68, 1991
14. Wilson RS: Anesthetic management for tracheal reconstruction. In Grillo HC, Eschapasse H (eds): *International Trends in General Thoracic Surgery,* Vol 2. Philadelphia, Saunders, 1987, pp 1–18
15. Rostom AY, Morgan RL: Results of treating primary tumors of the trachea by irradiation. *Thorax* **33**(3):387–393, 1978
16. Grillo HC, Mathisen DJ: Primary tracheal tumors: Treatment and results. *Ann Thorac Surg* **49:**69–77, 1990
17. Eschapasse H: Les tumeurs trachéales primitives: Traitement chirurgical. *Rev Fr Malad Respir* **2:**425–430, 1974
18. Hajdu SI, Huvos AG, Goodner JT, et al: Carcinoma of the trachea: Clinico-pathologic study of 41 cases. *Cancer* **25:**1448, 1970
19. Houston H, Payne W, Harrison E: Primary cancers of the trachea. *Arch Surg* **2:**132, 1969
20. Pearson FC, Todd TRJ, Cooper JD: Experience with primary neoplasms of the trachea and carina. *J Thorac Cardiovasc Surg* **88:**511–518, 1984
21. Perelman M, Koroleva N: Surgery of the trachea. *World J Surg* **4:**583, 1980
22. Morgan RJ, Grillo HC: Clinical presentation of primary tracheal tumors: A frequently misdiagnosed entity. (unpublished data)
23. Ishihara T, Kikuchi K, Ikede T, et al: Resection of thyroid carcinoma infiltrating the trachea. *Thorax* **33:**378, 1978
24. Grillo HC, Suen HC, Mathisen DJ, Wain JC: Resectional management of thyroid carcinoma invading the airway. *Ann Thorac Surg* **54:**3–10, 1992
25. Grillo HC: Surgery of the trachea. *Curr Probl Surg,* July 1970
26. Montgomery WW: Suprahyoid release for tracheal anastomosis. *Arch Otol* **99**(4):255–260, 1974
27. Cantrell JP, Guild HC: Congenital stenosis of the trachea. *Am J Surg* **108:**297, 1964
28. Grillo HC: Congenital lesions, neoplasms and injuries of the trachea. In Sabiston DC Jr, Spencer FC (eds): *Gibbon's Surgery of the Chest.* Philadelphia, Saunders, 1982
29. Idriss FS, DeLeon SY, Ilbawi MN, et al: Tracheoplasty with pericardial patch for extensive tracheal stenosis in infants and children. *J Thorac Cardiovasc Surg* **88:**527–536, 1984
30. Kim SH, Hendren WH: Endoscopic resection of obstructing airway lesions of children. *J Pediatr Surg* **11:**431, 1976
31. Grillo HC, Zannini P: Management of obstructive tracheal disease in children. *J Pediatr Surg* **19:**414–416, 1984
32. Tsang V, Murday A, Gilbe C, Goldstraw P: Slide tracheoplasty for congenital funnel-shaped stenosis. *Ann Thorac Surg* **48:**632–635, 1989
33. Grillo HC: Slide tracheoplasty for long segment congenital tracheal stenosis. *Ann Thorac Surg* **58:**613–621, 1994
34. Sade RM, Rosenthal A, Fellows K, Castaneda AR: Pulmonary artery sling. *J Thorac Cardiovasc Surg* **69:**333, 1975
35. Mathisen DJ, Grillo HC: Laryngotracheal trauma. *Ann Thorac Surg* **43:**254–262, 1987
36. Grillo HC: Surgical treatment of postintubation tracheal injuries. *J Thorac Cardiovasc Surg* **78:**860, 1979
37. Grillo HC, Donahue DM, Mathisen DJ, et al: Postintubation tracheal stenosis: Treatment and Results. *J Thorac Cardiovasc Surg* **109:** 486–493, 1995
38. Andrews MJ, Pearson FG: An analysis of 59 cases of tracheal stenosis following tracheostomy with cuffed tube and assisted ventilation, with special reference to diagnosis and treatment. *Br J Surg* **60:**208, 1973
39. Cooper JD, Grillo HC: The evolution of tracheal injury due to ventilatory assistance through cuffed tubes: A pathologic study. *Ann Surg* **169:**334, 1969
40. Weber AL, Grillo HC: Tracheal stenosis: An analysis of 151 cases. *Radiol Clin North Am* **16:**291, 1978
41. Gaissert HA, Grillo HC, Mathisen DJ, Wain JC: Temporary and permanent restoration of airway continuity with the tracheal T tube. *J Thorac Cardiovasc Surg* **107:**600, 1994
42. Pearson FG, Cooper JD, Nelems JM, Van Nostrand AWP: Primary tracheal anastomosis after resection of cricoid cartilage with preservation of recurrent laryngeal nerves. *J Thorac Cardiovasc Surg* **70:**806, 1975
43. Mathisen DJ, Grillo HC, Wain JC, Hilgenberg AD: Management of acquired nonmalignant tracheoesophageal fistula. *Ann Thorac Surg* **52:**759–765, 1991
44. Muehroke DD, Grillo HC, Mathisen DJ: Reconstructive airway surgery after irradiation. *Ann Thorac Surg* **59:**14–18, 1995
45. Mathisen DJ, Grillo HC: Clinical manifestation of mediastinal fibrosis and histoplasmosis. *Ann Thorac Surg* **54:**1053–1058, 1992
46. Gaissert HA, Lofgren RH, Grillo HC: Upper airway compromise after inhalation injury. *Ann Surg* **218:**672–678, 1993
47. Herzog H, Heitz M, Keller R, Graedel E: Surgical therapy for expiratory collapse of the trachea and large bronchi. In Grillo HC, Eschapasse H (eds): *International Trends in General Thoracic Surgery,* vol 2. Philadelphia, Saunders, 1987, pp 74–90.
48. Greene RE, Lechner GL: "Saber-sheath" trachea: A clinical and functional study of marked carinal narrowing of the intrathoracic trachea. *Radiology* **115:**265, 1975
49. Grillo HC, Shepard JO, Mathisen DJ, Wain JC: Postpneumonectomy syndrome: Diagnosis, management and results. *Ann Thorac Surg* **54:**638–651, 1992
50. Grillo HC, Zannini P, Michelassi F: Complications of tracheal reconstruction: Incidence, treatment, and prevention. *J Thorac Cardiovasc Surg* **91:**322–328, 1986

# CHAPTER 39

# The Esophagus

## *Anatomy and Functional Evaluation*

Thomas J. Watson and Tom R. DeMeester

For the field of surgery to flourish, practitioners must attain a high level of understanding of the normal anatomy, physiology, and function of the organ systems. Only with such knowledge will a surgeon be able to comprehend fully the magnitude of disease processes and the spectrum of available treatment modalities, both medical and surgical. In no field of medicine is this concept more important than in the study of esophageal disorders. As gastroenterologists and other specialists continue to delineate the role of medical modalities in the management of esophageal disease, it remains for surgeons to identify the role of operative intervention in these often complex problems. The ability to recognize and diagnose potential maladies related to the esophagus and foregut and then offer a full array of treatments places surgeons in a position of leadership in the care of patients with foregut disease.

## ANATOMY

### Radiographic and Endoscopic Anatomy of the Esophagus

The esophagus begins as the continuation of the pharynx and terminates at the cardia of the stomach. With the head in its normal anatomic position, the transition from pharynx to esophagus occurs at the lower border of the sixth cervical vertebra. This corresponds topographically to the cricoid cartilage in the anterior aspect and the carotid tubercle, which is the palpable transverse process of the sixth cervical vertebra, in the lateral aspect (Fig. 39–1). Flexion and extension of the neck shift this point craniad or caudad by the length of one cervical vertebral body. After traversing the thorax and passing through the diaphragm, the esophagus terminates in the stomach at the level of the eleventh thoracic vertebra. The esophagus is firmly anchored to the cricoid cartilage at its upper end and to the diaphragm at its lower end. During deglutition, these points of fixation move craniad the distance of one cervical vertebral body.

On an anteroposterior radiograph, the esophagus lies in the midline with a deviation to the left in the lower portion of the neck and upper portion of the thorax. It returns to the midline in the midportion of the thorax near the bifurcation of the trachea (Fig. 39–2A). In the lower portion of the thorax, the esophagus again deviates to the left to pass through the diaphragmatic hiatus.

On a lateral radiograph, the esophagus follows the curve of the vertebral column, except in the lower thoracic area, where it curves anteriorly to pass through the diaphragmatic hiatus (Fig. 39–2B). This posterior curve and its terminal left anterior deviation are important in the performance of rigid esophagoscopy. The patient should be positioned to allow extension of the cervical and thoracic spine so that the rigid scope can be manipulated through this terminal arc. This region is the second most common site of iatrogenic esophageal perforation during rigid endoscopy, the first being the narrow entrance of the esophagus at the level of the cricopharyngeus.

Measurements obtained during endoscopic examination (Fig. 39–3) reveal the average distance from the incisor teeth to the cardia of the stomach to be 38–40 cm in men and 2 cm shorter in women. These distances are proportionately shorter in children. In men, the length of the esophagus from the cricopharyngeus muscle to the cardia ranges from 23 to 30 cm with an average of 25 cm. In women the range is 20–26 cm with an average of 23 cm. The distance

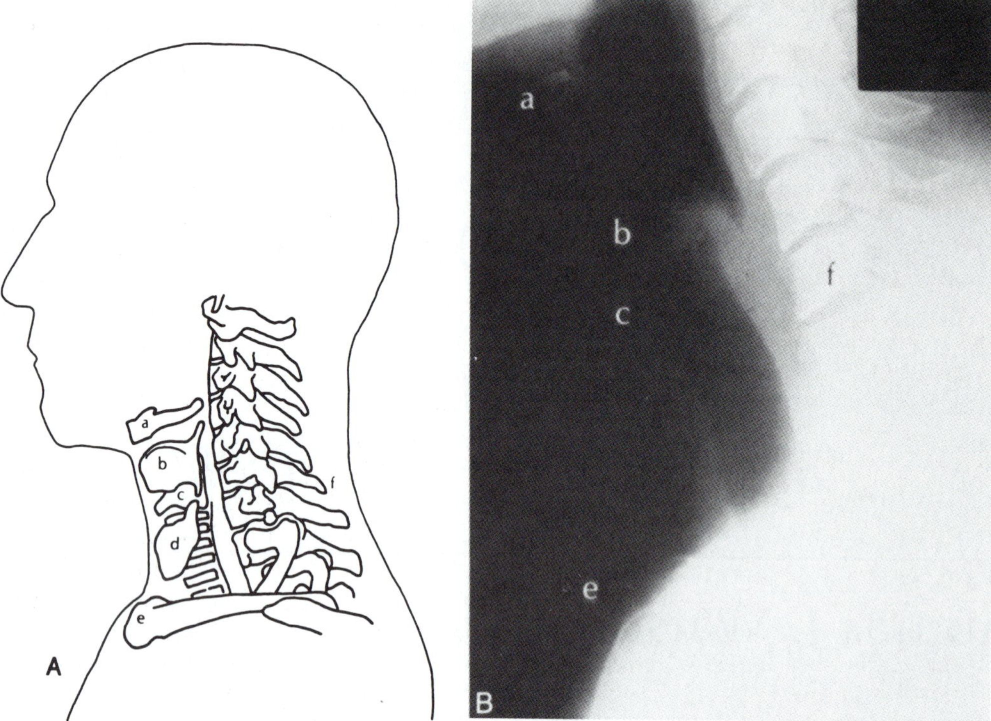


**Figure 39–1. A.** Topographic relations of the cervical esophagus. a = hyoid bone, b = thyroid cartilage, c = cricoid cartilage, d = thyroid gland, e = sternoclavicular joint, f = C6. **B.** Appearance on lateral radiograph.

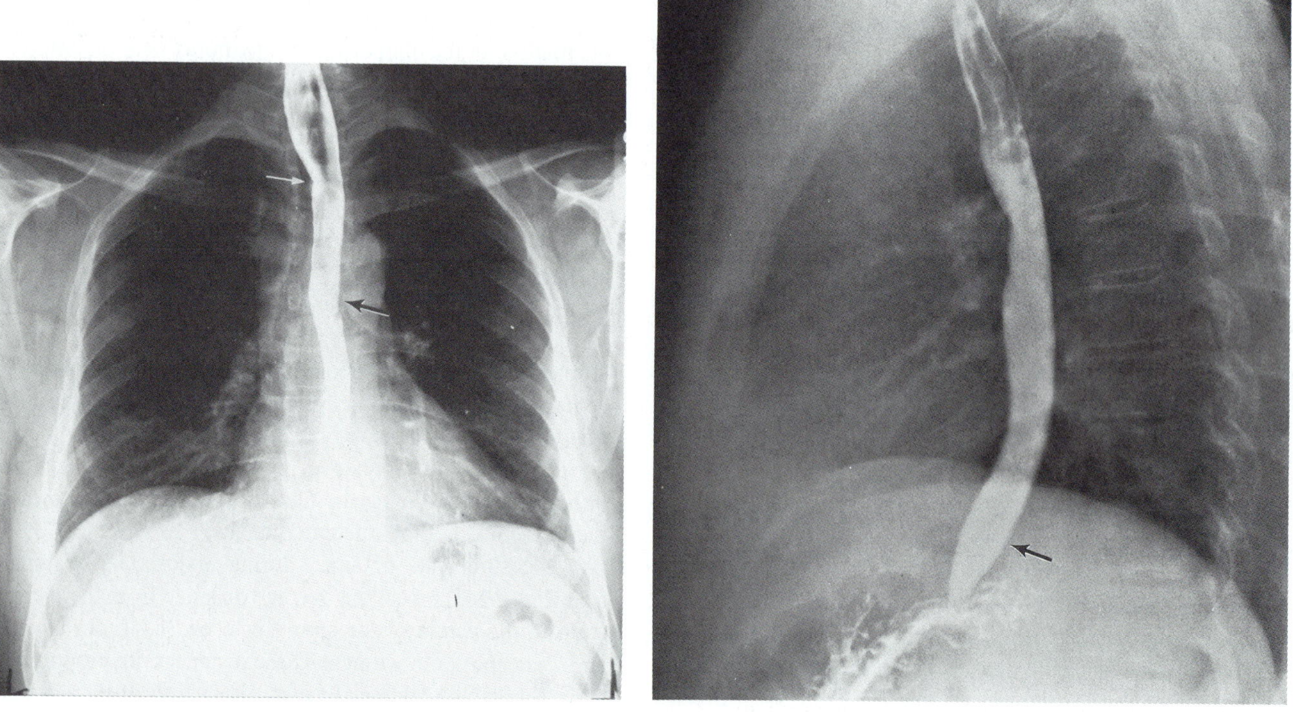


**Figure 39–2.** Barium esophagogram. **A.** Posterioanterior view. **B.** Lateral view. *White arrow* shows deviation to left. *Black arrow* shows return to midline. *Black arrow* on lateral view shows anterior deviation.

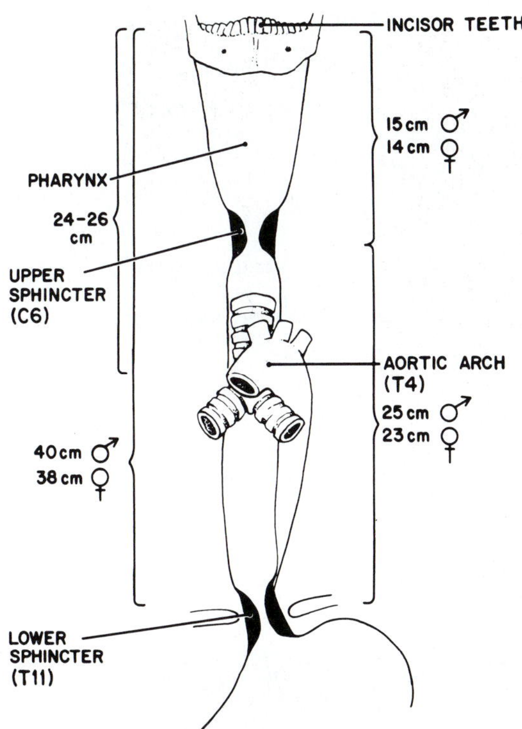


**Figure 39–3.** Important clinical endoscopic measurements of the esophagus in adults.

from the incisor teeth to the cricopharyngeus is 15 cm in men and 14 cm in women. The bifurcation of the trachea and the indentation of the aortic arch ranges between 24 and 26 cm from the incisor teeth. It is helpful to locate intraluminal lesions in reference to this landmark to decide on a left or right thoracotomy approach and avoid interference with the aortic arch.

## Anatomic Relations of the Esophagus

The cervical portion of the esophagus is approximately 5 cm long and descends between the trachea and the vertebral column from the level of the sixth cervical vertebra to the level of the interspace between the first and second thoracic vertebrae posteriorly, or the suprasternal notch anteriorly. The recurrent laryngeal nerves lie in the right and left grooves between the trachea and the esophagus. The left recurrent nerve lies somewhat closer to the esophagus than the right nerve owing to the slight deviation of the esophagus to the left and the more lateral course of the right recurrent nerve around the right subclavian artery. On the left and right sides of the esophagus are the carotid sheaths and the lobes of the thyroid gland.

From the thoracic inlet to the tracheal bifurcation the thoracic esophagus remains in intimate relation with the posterior wall of the trachea and the prevertebral fascia. Just above the tracheal bifurcation, the esophagus passes to the right of the aorta. This anatomic positioning can cause a notch indentation in the left lateral wall of the esophagus at barium swallow radiographic examination. Immediately below this notch, the esophagus crosses both the bifurcation of the trachea and the left main stem bronchus, because of the slight deviation of the terminal portion of the trachea to the right by the aorta (Fig. 39–4).

The right lateral surface of the thoracic esophagus is completely covered by the parietal pleura, except at the level of the fourth thoracic vertebra, where the azygos vein turns anteriorly over the esophagus to join the superior vena cava. The left lateral surface of the upper portion of the thoracic esophagus is covered anterolaterally by the left subclavian artery and posterolaterally by the parietal pleura. The distal portion of the esophagus, from the aortic arch down, lies to the right of the descending thoracic aorta. At the level of the eighth thoracic vertebra, the aorta disappears behind the esophagus, and its left lateral wall is covered only with the parietal pleura of the mediastinum and is the common site of perforation in Boerhaave's syndrome. From the bifurcation of the trachea downward, both the vagal nerves and the esophageal nerve plexus lie on the muscular wall of the esophagus.

As the esophagus passes through the diaphragmatic hiatus, it is surrounded by the phrenoesophageal membrane, a fibroelastic ligament that arises from the subdiaphragmatic fascia as a continuation of the transversalis fascia which lines the abdomen (Fig. 39–5). The phrenoesophageal membrane divides at the lower margin of the esophageal hiatus into a stout elongated ascending leaf that surrounds the terminal segment of the esophagus in a tent-like manner and into a shorter, thin, descending leaf, which merges as the visceral peritoneal covering of the stomach. The upper leaf of the membrane attaches itself in a circumferential manner around the esophagus 1–2 cm above the level of the hiatus. Between the upper leaf of the membrane and the cardia is a ring of fatty tissue interspersed with fibers from the lower leaf of the membrane. These fibers blend in with elastic-containing adventitia of the distal 2 cm of esophagus and the cardia of the stomach. This makes up the abdominal portion of the esophagus, which is subjected to the positive pressure environment of the abdomen.

The thoracic duct passes through the hiatus of the diaphragm on the anterior surface of the vertebral column behind the aorta and under the right crus. In the thorax it lies dorsal to the esophagus between the azygos vein on the right and the descending thoracic aorta on the left. From the level of the fifth thoracic vertebra upward, the thoracic duct gradually moves to the left and settles between the esophagus and the left parietal pleura, dorsal to the aortic arch and the intrathoracic part of the subclavian artery. In the neck the duct turns away from the esophagus and joins the venous system at the junction of the subclavian and internal jugular veins.

## Musculature of the Esophagus

The pharyngeal musculature consists of three overlapping, broad, flat, fan-shaped constrictors (Fig. 39–6). They are

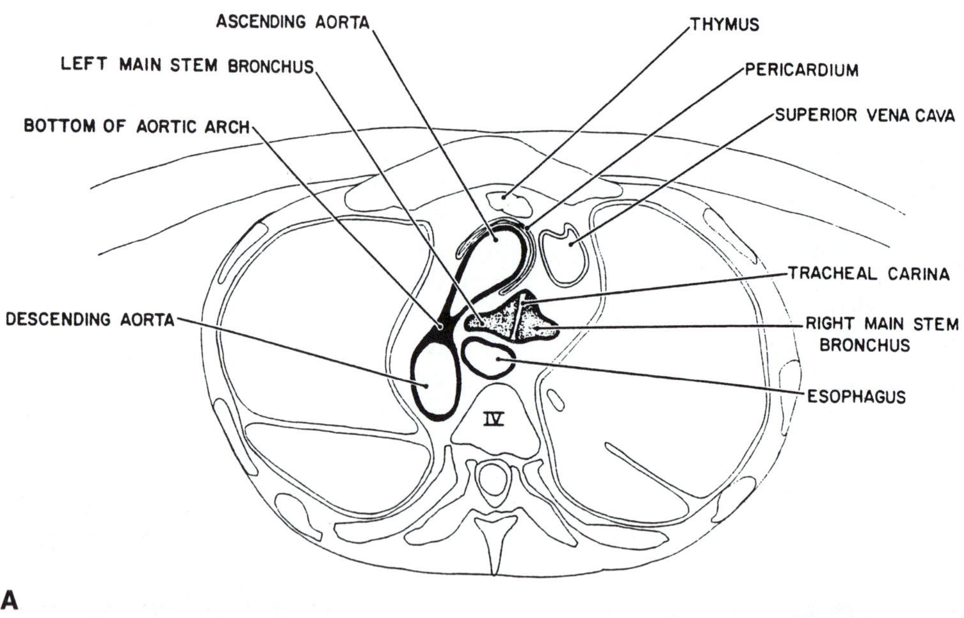


A

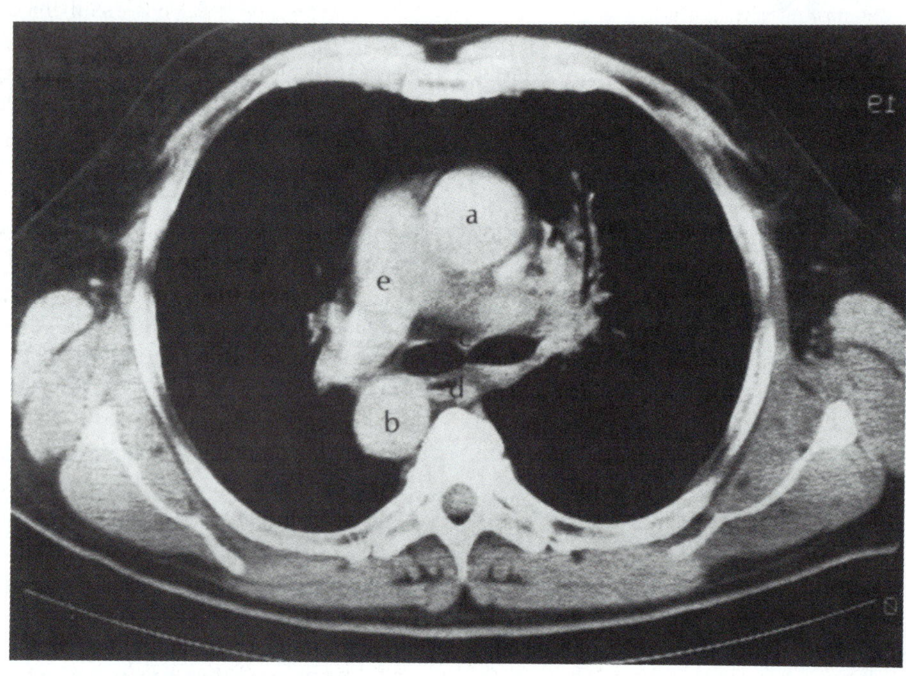


B

**Figure 39–4.** **A.** Cross-section of the thorax at the level of the tracheal bifurcation. **B.** CT scan at same level as **A** viewed from above. a = ascending aorta, b = descending aorta, c = tracheal carina, d = esophagus, e = pulmonary artery.

the superior constrictor, which originates mainly on the medial pterygoid plate; the middle constrictor, which originates on the hyoid bone; and the inferior constrictor, which originates on the thyroid and cricoid cartilages. These muscles insert with their corresponding muscle from the opposite side into a median posterior raphe.

The opening of the esophagus is collared by the cricopharyngeal muscle, which originates from both sides of the cricoid cartilage of the larynx and forms a continuous transverse muscle band without an interruption by a median raphe. The fibers of this muscle blend inseparably with those of the inferior pharyngeal constrictor above and the inner circular muscle fibers of the esophagus below. Some investigators believe that the cricopharyngeus is part of the inferior constrictor; that is, the inferior constrictor has two parts, an upper or retrothyroid portion that has diagonal fibers and a lower or retrocricoid portion that has transverse fibers. Keith[1] showed that these two parts of the same muscle serve different functions. The retrocricoid portion serves as the upper sphincter of the esophagus and relaxes when

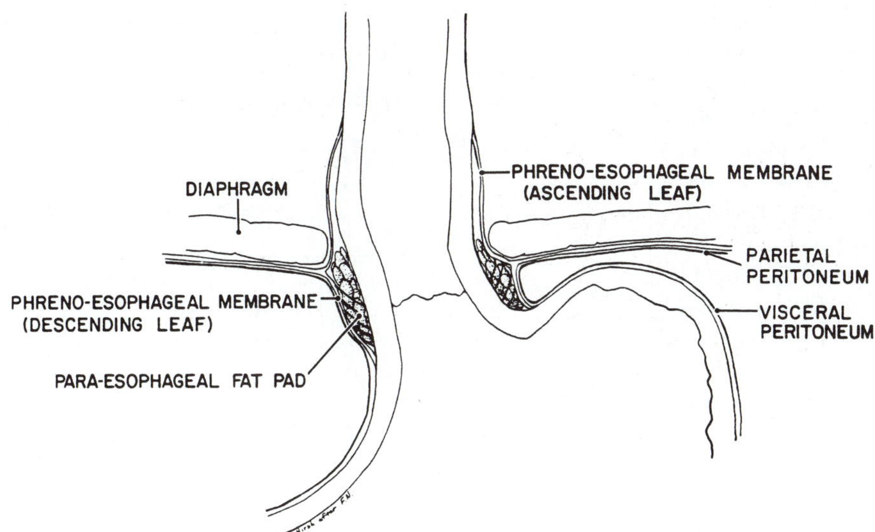


**Figure 39–5.** Attachments and structure of the phrenoesophageal membrane.

the retrothyroid portion contracts to force a swallowed bolus from the pharynx into the esophagus.

The musculature of the esophagus can be divided into an outer longitudinal and an inner circular layer. The upper 2–6 cm of the esophagus contains only striated muscle fibers. From there on smooth muscle fibers gradually become more abundant. At a distance of 4–8 cm from the superior end, or at the junction of the upper and middle thirds, the smooth musculature constitutes 50% of the esophageal muscle. The transition of striated to smooth muscle in the inner circular layer is at a higher level than in the outer longitudinal layer. Most of the clinically significant esophageal motility disorders involve only the smooth muscle in the lower two thirds of the esophagus. When a surgical esophageal myotomy is indicated, the incision usually needs only to extend this distance.

The circular muscle layer of the esophagus is thicker than the outer longitudinal layer. These fibers run horizontally only in the isolated and retracted esophagus. In situ, their course is elliptic and spiral with an inclination that varies according to the level of the esophagus: in the cervical portion the ellipse is dorsal, in the upper thoracic portion the highest point is right lateral, behind the heart ventral, and in the abdomen the fibers are horizontal. The arrangement of both the longitudinal and circular muscle fibers makes the peristalsis of the esophagus assume a worm-like drive as opposed to segmental and sequential squeezing. As a consequence, severe motor abnormalities of the esophagus assume a corkscrew-like pattern on a barium swallow radiograph.

## Vasculature of the Esophagus

The cervical esophagus receives its main arterial inflow from the inferior thyroid artery with smaller accessory

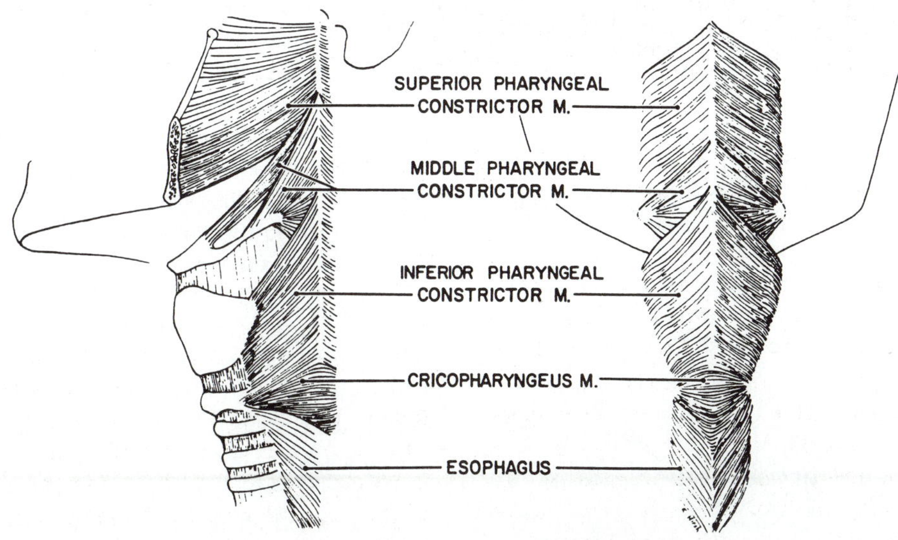


**Figure 39–6.** External muscles of the pharynx.

branches from the common carotid, subclavian, and superficial cervical arteries. The thoracic portion receives its blood supply from the bronchial arteries, 75% of individuals having one right-sided and one or two left-sided branches. Two esophageal branches originate directly from the aorta. The abdominal portion of the esophagus receives its blood supply mainly from esophageal branches of the left gastric and inferior phrenic arteries (Fig. 39–7). Upon penetrating the esophageal wall, the arteries assume a T-shaped division to form longitudinal anastomoses that give rise to an intramural vascular network in the muscular and submucosal layers. As a consequence the esophagus can be mobilized from the stomach to the level of the aortic arch without fear of devascularization and ischemic necrosis. Caution should be exercised, however, in patients who have had a previous thyroidectomy and ligation of the inferior thyroid arteries proximal to the origin of the esophageal branches.

Blood from the capillaries of the esophagus flows into a submucosal venous plexus and then into a periesophageal venous plexus from which the esophageal veins originate. In the cervical region, the esophageal veins empty into the inferior thyroid vein; in the thoracic region into the bronchial, azygos, or hemiazygous veins; and in the abdominal region into the coronary vein (Fig. 39–8). The submucosal venous networks of the esophagus and stomach freely communicate. In patients with portal venous obstruction, the networks function as a collateral pathway for portal blood to enter the superior vena cava through the azygos vein.

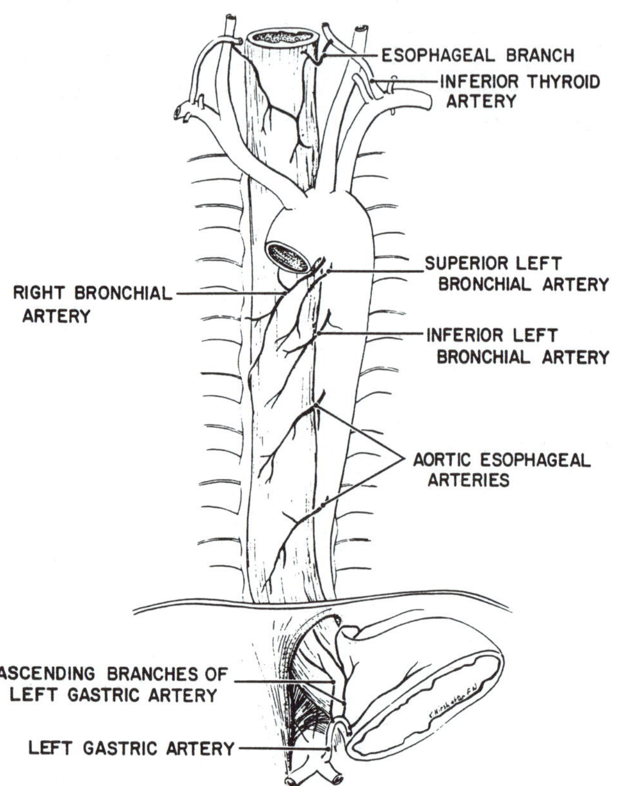


**Figure 39–7.** Arterial blood supply of the esophagus.

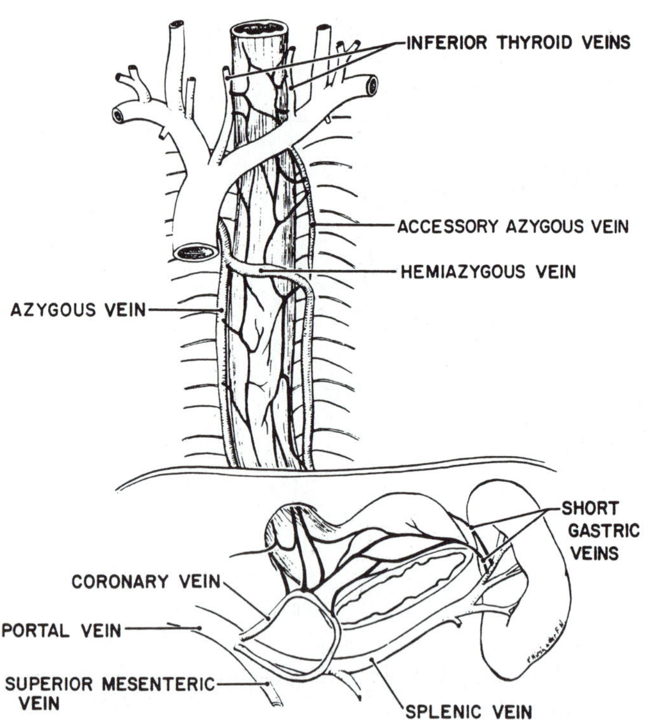


**Figure 39–8.** Venous drainage of the esophagus.

## Innervation of the Esophagus

The complete parasympathetic innervation of the esophagus is provided by the vagus nerves (Fig. 39–9). The cricopharyngeal sphincter and the cervical portion of the esophagus receive branches from both recurrent laryngeal nerves, which originate from the vagus nerves—the right recurrent nerve at the lower margin of the subclavian artery, the left at the lower margin of the aortic arch. The nerves are slung dorsally around these vessels and ascend in the groove between the esophagus and trachea, giving branches to each. Damage to these nerves not only interferes with the function of the vocal cords but also interferes with the function of the cricopharyngeal sphincter and the motility of the cervical esophagus, causing a predisposition to pulmonary aspiration on swallowing.

The upper thoracic esophagus receives branches from the left recurrent laryngeal nerve and directly from both vagus nerves as they descend through the superior mediastinum. The lower thoracic esophagus is innervated by the esophageal plexus located directly on both the anterior and posterior esophageal wall and formed by both vagal nerves after they pass behind the hilum of the lung and turn medially to reach the esophagus. The esophageal plexus also receives fibers from the thoracic sympathetic chain. The left vagus nerve splits before the esophageal plexus to form two branches. The first branch runs through the ventral esophageal plexus and constitutes the main element of the anterior or left abdominal vagal trunk. The second branch runs around the left esophageal wall, to join the dorsal esophageal plexus, and contributes to the formation of the

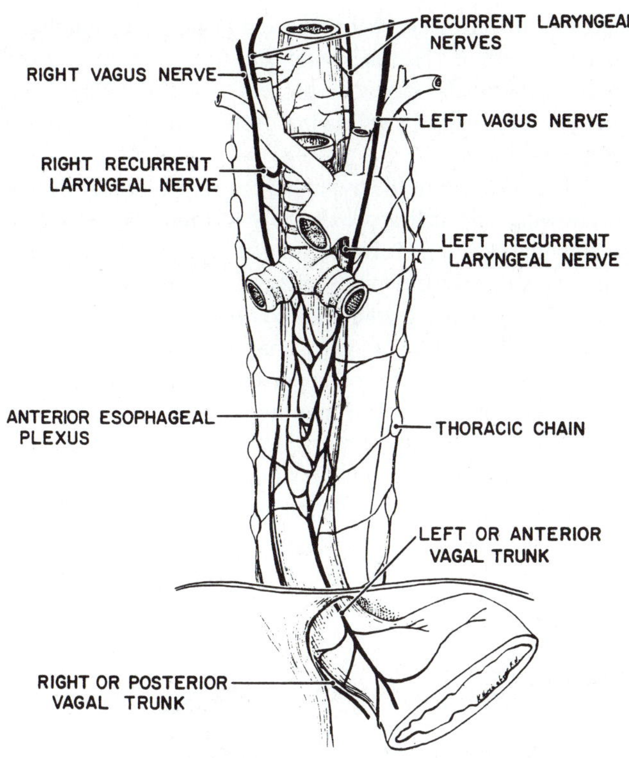


**Figure 39–9.** Innervation of the esophagus.

posterior or right abdominal vagal trunk. As a result of the intertwining of fibers from both the left and right vagus nerves in the esophageal plexus, both the left or anterior and the right or posterior abdominal vagal trunks contain fibers of the original left and right vagus nerves. The average distance above the diaphragm at which the left or anterior vagal trunk becomes a single nerve is 5.13 cm; the distance for the right or posterior vagal trunk is 3.7 cm.

Afferent visceral sensory pain fibers from the esophagus end without synapse in the first four segments of the thoracic spinal cord by means of a combination of sympathetic and vagal pathways. These pathways are also occupied by afferent visceral sensory fibers from the heart; hence, disorders of the esophagus and of the heart have similar symptoms.

## Lymphatic Drainage of the Esophagus

The lymph vessels in the submucosa of the esophagus are so dense and interconnected that they constitute a single plexus (Fig. 39–10). There are more lymph vessels than blood capillaries in the submucosa. Lymph flow in the submucosal plexus runs in a longitudinal direction. On injection of contrast medium, the longitudinal spread is seen to be about six times that of the transverse spread. In the upper two thirds of the esophagus the lymphatic flow is primarily cephalad; in the lower third it is caudad. In the thoracic portion of the esophagus the submucosal lymph plexus extends over a long distance in a longitudinal direction before penetrating the muscle layer to join the lymph vessels in the adventitia. As a consequence of this nonsegmental lymphatic drainage, a primary tumor can extend for a considerable length superiorly or inferiorly in the submucosal plexus, and free tumor cells can follow the submucosal lymphatic plexus in either direction for a long distance before they pass through the muscularis and on into the regional lymph nodes. On the contrary, the cervical esophagus has more direct segmental lymphatic drainage into the regional nodes. As a result, lesions in this portion of the esophagus have less submucosal extension and a more regionalized lymphatic spread.

The efferent lymphatics from the cervical esophagus

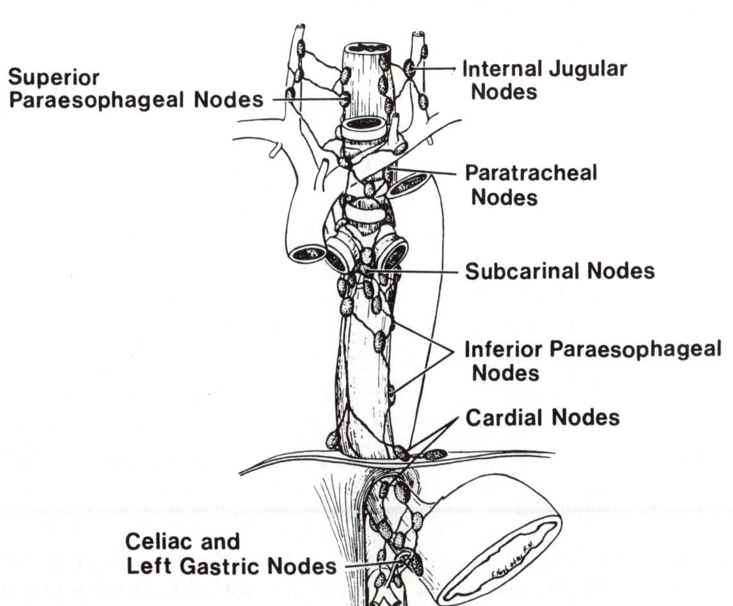


**Figure 39–10.** Lymphatic drainage of the esophagus.

drain into the paratracheal and deep cervical lymph nodes; those from the upper thoracic esophagus empty mainly into the paratracheal lymph nodes. Efferent lymphatics from the lower thoracic esophagus drain into the subcarinal nodes and into nodes in the inferior pulmonary ligaments. The superior gastric nodes receive lymph not only from the abdominal portion of the esophagus but also from the adjacent lower thoracic segment.

## NORMAL STRUCTURE AND FUNCTION

A thorough knowledge of the normal anatomy and physiology of the foregut is necessary to understand its pathophysiology and to treat its disorders.[2–5] Visualizing the pharynx, esophagus, and stomach as a series of mechanical pumps allows one to comprehend more clearly their integrated function. The tongue works with the pharynx as a piston works in a cylinder with its valves. The two valves of the pharyngeal cylinder are the soft palate and the cricopharyngeus muscle. The body of the esophagus works with the cardia as a propulsive pump with its valve. The terminal valve of the esophageal pump is the lower esophageal sphincter (LES). The fundus of the stomach works as a constant pressure reservoir that fills the antral pump. The pylorus works with the antral pump as a sizer that restricts the passage of larger particles, forcing them to return to the fundic reservoir for further digestion. Failure of these components individually or in combination leads to abnormalities, such as difficulties in food propulsion from mouth to stomach or regurgitation of gastric contents back into the esophagus and pharynx.

Food is taken into the mouth in portions of varying size. There it is broken up, mixed with saliva, and lubricated. The act of chewing is partly reflex and partly voluntary. Swallowing, once initiated, is entirely reflex. The degree to which a mouthful of food is chewed depends on the nature of the food, the quality of dentition, individual habit, and training. The amount of chewing has a negligible effect on digestion and usually proceeds unnoticed, unless there is dysphagia, which forces the person to chew his or her food particles until they are small enough to pass through the narrowed or dysfunctional zone.

When food is ready for swallowing, the tongue, acting like a piston, moves the bolus into the posterior oropharynx and forces it into the hypopharynx. Immobility of the tongue, such as from scarring secondary to irradiation or chemical burns, can produce great difficulty in the transoral movement of ingested food. Simultaneous with the posterior movement of the tongue, the soft palate is elevated, closing the passage between the oro- and nasopharynx. This separation prevents pressure generated in the oropharynx from being dissipated through the nose. When the soft palate is paralyzed, as after a cerebrovascular accident, food is commonly regurgitated into the nasopharynx. During swallowing, the larynx is elevated and pulled forward, opening the retrolaryngeal space and bringing the epiglottis under the tongue. The backward tilt of the epiglottis covers the opening of the larynx to prevent aspiration. The entire pharyngeal phase of swallowing occurs within 1.5 seconds (Fig. 39–11).

The pressure in the hypopharynx rises abruptly during swallowing to reach approximately 45 mm Hg. A sizable differential develops between the positive pharyngeal pressure and the negative midesophageal or intrathoracic pressure. This pressure gradient speeds the movement of food from the hypopharynx into the esophagus when the cricopharyngeus muscle or upper esophageal sphincter relaxes. The bolus is sucked into the thoracic esophagus and propelled by sequential contractions of the posterior pharyngeal constrictor muscles. It is important that the upper or striated portion of the esophagus be relaxed and compliant during this phase of the pharyngeal swallow so that it is prepared to accept the bolus when the cricopharyngeal sphincter relaxes. The upper esophageal sphincter closes within

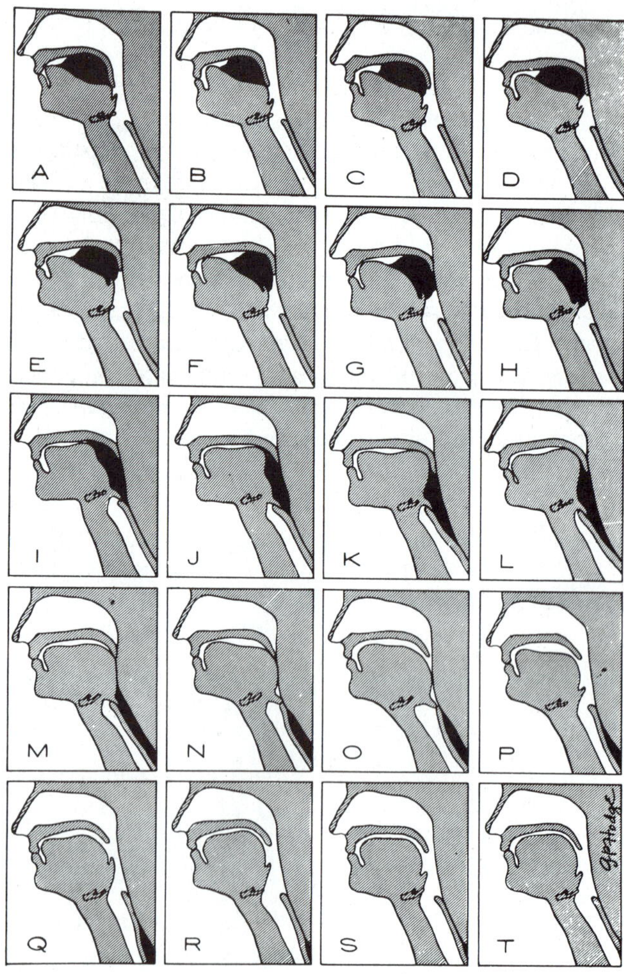


**Figure 39–11.** The sequence of events during the pharyngeal phase of swallowing. The piston-like action of the tongue coordinates with the valvular action of the soft palate, epiglottis, and cricopharyngeus muscle. The entire sequence takes 1.5 sec. **J.** Period of maximum compression in the pharyngeal cylinder.

another 0.5 seconds, the immediate closing pressure reaching approximately twice the resting level of 30 mm Hg. When the maximal cricopharyngeal pressure is reached, a peristaltic wave begins in the upper esophagus, which generates a pressure of approximately 30 mm Hg. The higher tone in the sphincter prevents reflux of the bolus from the esophagus into the pharynx. After the peristaltic wave has passed farther down the esophagus, the pressure in the upper esophageal sphincter returns to its resting level.

Swallowing can be started voluntarily or can be reflexly elicited by the stimulation of certain areas in the mouth and pharynx, among them the anterior and posterior tonsillar pillars and the posterolateral walls of the hypopharynx. The afferent nerves of the pharynx are the glossopharyngeal and superior laryngeal branch of the vagus. Once aroused by stimuli via these nerves, the swallowing center in the medulla coordinates the complete act of swallowing by discharging impulses through the fifth, seventh, tenth, eleventh, and twelfth cranial nerves as well as through the motor neurons of cervical nerves C1–C3. Discharges through these nerves occur in a specific pattern and last for approximately 0.5 sec. Little is known about the organization of the swallowing center except that it can trigger swallowing after a variety of different stimuli, but the response is always the same highly ordered pattern of outflow. After a cerebrovascular accident, this coordinated outflow may be altered, causing mild abnormalities in muscle coordination during swallowing. In severe injury, swallowing can be grossly disrupted, leading to repetitive aspiration. The latter is particularly apt to occur if the striated portion of the esophagus becomes spastic or loses its compliance as a result of deinnervation injury. The integrity of the swallowing center is required for the cricopharyngeus muscle to relax precisely at the moment of pharyngeal contraction and resume its resting tone once a bolus has entered the upper esophagus. Motor disorders of the pharyngeal phase of swallowing are characterized by abnormalities of incomplete upper sphincter relaxation, i.e., incomplete relaxation, premature closure after premature relaxation, and delayed relaxation, and, more important, the loss of compliance of skeletal portion of the cervical esophagus.

The pharyngeal phase of swallowing is followed by the esophageal phase. Once the swallowed bolus of food reaches the esophagus, orderly primary peristalsis propels the material into the stomach over a pressure gradient from –6 mm Hg intrathoracic pressure to an average of +6 mm Hg of intra-abdominal pressure (Fig. 39–12). The smooth muscle action in the lower third of the esophagus is most important in pumping the food across this barrier. The peristaltic wave generates an occlusive pressure that varies from 30 to 120 mm Hg. The wave rises to a peak in 1 sec, lasts at the peak for about 0.5 sec, and then subsides in about 1.5 sec. The whole course of rise and fall may occupy one point in the esophagus for 3–7 sec. The contraction wave, when measured from peak to peak, moves down the esophagus at 2–4 cm/sec and reaches the distal esophagus about 9 sec after swallowing starts (Fig. 39–13). Consecutive swallows produce similar primary peristaltic waves.

When the act of swallowing is rapidly repeated, the esophagus remains relaxed and the peristaltic wave occurs only after the last pharyngeal swallow. Progression of the wave in the esophagus is caused by sequential activation of its muscles modulated by efferent vagal nerve fibers discharging in a pattern determined by the swallowing center. Continuity of the esophageal muscle is not necessary if the nerves are intact. If the muscles are transected, but not the nerves, the pressure wave begins distally below the cut as it dies out at the proximal end above the cut. This allows a sleeve resection of the esophagus to be done without disruption of normal function. Vagal stimulation of the smooth-muscle portion of the esophagus does not appear to be necessary for a coordinated peristaltic wave. If the smooth-muscle portion of the esophagus is distended at any point, it initiates relaxation of the LES and propagation of a contractile wave that sweeps down the esophagus (Fig. 39–14). This secondary contraction occurs without any movement of the mouth or pharynx. This secondary wave may be helpful in clearing the esophagus of a large bolus

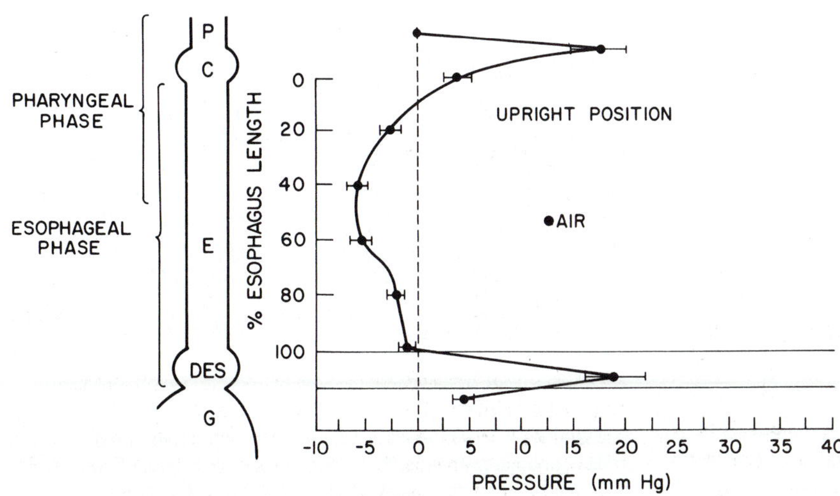


**Figure 39–12.** Resting pressure profile of the foregut showing the pressure differential between the atmospheric pharyngeal pressure (P) and the less-than-atmospheric midesophageal pressure (E) and the greater-than-atmospheric intragastric pressure (G), with the interposed high pressure zones of the cricopharyngeus muscle (C) and distal (lower) esophageal sphincter (DES). The necessity for the cricopharyngeus muscle to relax and DES pressure to decrease to move a bolus into the stomach is apparent. Esophageal work occurs when a bolus is pushed from the midesophageal area (E) with a pressure less than atmospheric into the stomach, which has a pressure greater than atmospheric (G).

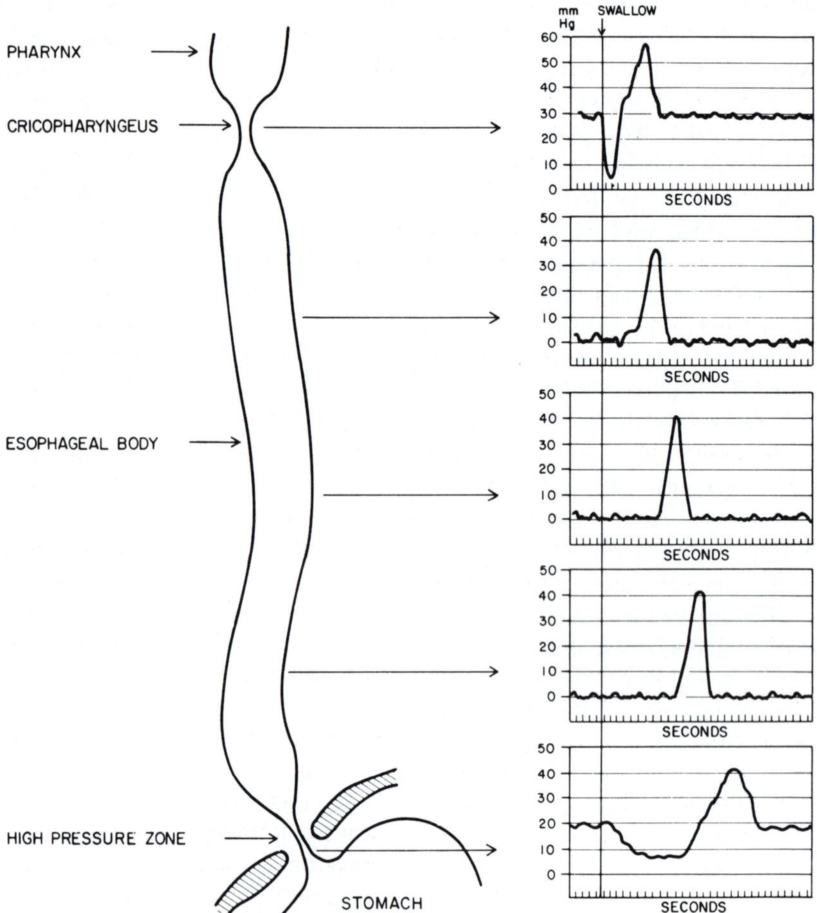


**Figure 39–13.** Intraluminal esophageal pressures in response to swallowing.

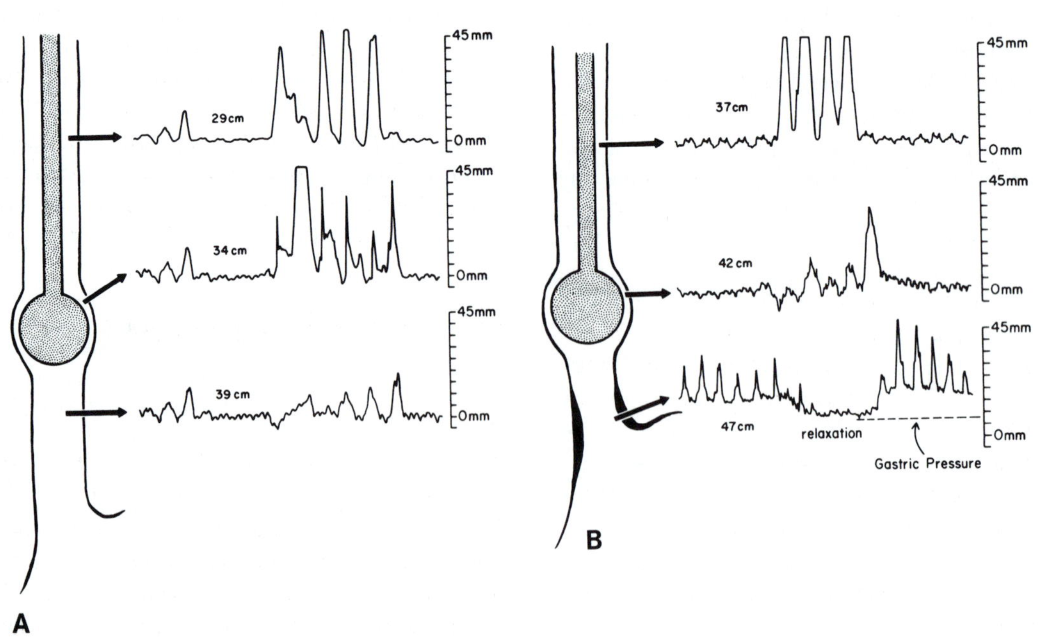


**Figure 39–14.** Intraluminal esophageal pressures in response to balloon distention. **A.** Forceful contraction of the esophageal body proximal to the balloon with no contraction of the body distal to the balloon. **B.** Concomitant relaxation of the lower esophageal sphincter.

that failed to be pushed through by the primary wave. The importance of the secondary wave has been questioned because it makes up only 2% of all esophageal waves.

The smooth muscle of the lower esophagus is supplied by the vagal preganglionic fibers, which end at synapses with ganglion cells in the myenteric plexi. The smooth-muscle cells receive motor innervation from the postganglionic fibers. Both the preganglionic and postganglionic fibers respond to a variety of neurotransmitters, the effects of which are not completely understood. There is no known sympathetic innervation of the esophagus.

Despite the rather powerful occlusive pressure, the propulsive force of the esophagus is relatively feeble. If a man attempts to swallow a bolus attached by a string to a counterweight, the maximum weight he can overcome is 5–10 g. The actual movement of a bolus of food through the body of the esophagus depends on the food's consistency and the position of the person. When water is swallowed by an upright person, it is propelled rapidly into the esophagus by the pharyngeal piston action and traverses the esophagus to reach the gastroesophageal junction within 1 sec. The water is sometimes held up briefly at the LES until the sphincter has time to relax. Usually, all the water flows into the stomach before the initial peristaltic wave is completed.

If water is swallowed repeatedly with the person upside-down, the esophagus fills progressively with liquid after each swallow. The column of water is supported by the closed cricopharyngeal sphincter. The weak propulsive force of the esophagus is incapable of raising the column of fluid into the stomach. On further swallowing, more water is forced into the esophagus by the piston action of the pharynx until the whole esophagus is filled with water. An equal volume at the top of the column is then delivered into the stomach with each successive swallow. With the person in any position, a semisolid mass moves more slowly than liquids through the pharynx and esophagus, the bolus splitting. The first portion reaches the stomach in 11 sec, and the second portion is usually cleared within three successive swallows. Solids move even more slowly and require pharynx-induced primary peristaltic waves for transit. Only occasionally are solids propelled to the stomach by a secondary wave initiated by local distention.

The pressure barrier between the esophagus and stomach is obliterated with pharyngeal swallowing and remains as such until the propulsive wave passes through the length of the esophagus (Fig. 39–13). The distal segment closes as the wave passes through, after which the LES returns to its resting pressure. In dogs, bilateral cervical vagotomy abolishes all the lower esophageal responses to pharyngeal swallowing or distention of the esophagus at any level, indicating the importance of vagal function in coordinating the relaxation of the LES.[6] Whether a similar response occurs in humans is unknown.

Disruption of the normal peristaltic pattern results in the specific and nonspecific esophageal motor disorders seen in clinical practice. Replacement of primary or secondary peristalsis by a simultaneous contraction over a large segment of the body of the esophagus is seen in diffuse esophageal spasm.

Loss of peristalsis throughout the body of the esophagus and failure of the LES to relax on swallowing are characteristic of the disorder called *achalasia.* In contrast, *scleroderma* results in the loss of contraction of the smooth-muscle portion of the esophagus and is primarily myogenic in etiology. The absence of distal esophageal contractions and LES tone is diagnostic of this condition. The absence of contractions in the proximal striated muscle portion of the esophagus occurs with inflammatory conditions that affect skeletal muscles, such as dermatomyositis.

Various disorders of esophageal motility and peristalsis may occur in association with reflux esophagitis. A normally functioning esophageal body is an important component of the antireflux mechanism. Even physiologic reflux episodes may result in prolonged acid exposure, leading to reflux esophagitis, if the ability of the esophageal body to clear refluxed material is impaired. If pathologic reflux is present, impaired esophageal clearance results in prolonged exposure, often contributing to a more severe degree of esophagitis, with complications such as stricture or Barrett's columnar-lined esophagus. Studies suggest that there are two components to the motility disorders associated with reflux esophagitis. One is proportional to, and the other independent of, the degree of esophagitis.[7] Some of these motility disturbances are reversible after an antireflux operation and others are not. These facts suggest that in some patients a preexisting motor disorder contributes to the pathogenesis of reflux esophagitis, whereas in others the esophagitis itself may result in disordered motility.

It has been suggested that the esophagus must be anchored both proximally and distally for it to clear refluxed material by a stripping peristaltic wave. The normal attachment of the distal esophagus is attenuated in patients with hiatal hernia, which can lead to inefficient clearance. The anchoring of the distal esophagus and consequent augmentation of esophageal clearance may be important components of antireflux procedures and may be responsible for the reversal of motility abnormalities in some patients.[8]

## THE ANTIREFLUX MECHANISM

### LES

The resting pressure of the LES is one of the primary components of the antireflux mechanism. The demonstration by Fyke et al[9] in 1956 of a functional lower esophageal high-pressure zone that possessed intrinsic tone and relaxed on swallowing set the scene for detailed investigation into the antireflux mechanism. A distinct anatomic sphincter muscle has been observed in some species, such as the dog and opossum, but the demonstration of its counterpart in primates, particularly humans, has been elusive. Microdissection studies by Liebermann-Meffert et al[10] did not show circumferential sphincter muscle fibers or uniform thickening of the distal esophagus. They did suggest, however, that the sphincter-like function in humans may be related to the muscular architecture of the cardia (Fig. 39–15). At the junction of the esophageal tube with the gastric pouch, there is an oblique muscular ring composed of an increased muscle mass inside the inner muscular layer. On the lesser-curve side of the cardia, the muscle fibers of the inner layer are oriented transversely and form semicircular muscle clasps, which insert into the submucosal connective tissues of the stomach. On the greater-curve side of the cardia, these muscle fibers form long, oblique loops, which run parallel to the lesser curve of the stomach and encircle the distal end of the cardia and gastric fundus. Both the semicircular muscle clasps and the oblique fibers of the fundus contract in a circular manner to close the cardia. This suggests that changes in gastric muscle tone may influence lower esophageal function. Diamant and Akin[11] showed that in dogs increases in LES pressure occurred simultaneously with gastric contractions. The studies by Petterson et al[12] confirmed this in humans and emphasized the importance of the proximal gastric sling fibers. The distal esophageal segment and the gastric fundus have been shown to relax simultaneously on swallowing.[13] These factors suggest that the distal esophageal segment and gastric fundus function as a single unit and have a common mural or myogenic control mechanism, which may be separate from the rest of the esophageal or gastric musculature.

A statistical correlation is seen between resting LES pressure and the incidence of gastroesophageal reflux disease (GERD) when large populations are examined.[14,15] A large number of studies have been performed in an attempt to identify the factors that influence resting LES pressure and account for its variation among individuals. Many factors, including neural, hormonal, myogenic, and mechanical factors, have been suggested. No neuroexcitatory mechanism for the maintenance of basal sphincter tone has been demonstrated in humans, since truncal vagotomy has no effect on resting LES pressure.[16] Furthermore, studies of isolated muscle strips from the distal esophageal muscle in animals and humans show a quantitatively different response to stimulation from that recorded in muscle fibers from the esophageal body.[17,18] Pharmacologic doses of cholinergic agents result in an increase in LES pressure; anticholinergic agents reduce it.[19] The relevance of these observations to normal physiologic function is unknown, particularly because the administration of atropine, while reducing LES tone, does not cause gastroesophageal reflux.[20]

The influences of many hormones on the LES have been investigated, but the effects noted are associated with pharmacologic doses and probably do not reflect the true physiologic situation.[19] Pharmacologic doses of secretin, cholecystokinin, glucagon, and prostaglandins reduce LES pressure. Exogenous gastrin, bombesin, and motilin augment it, but the influence of physiologic levels of these hormones is uncertain. Progesterones and estrogen decrease LES pressure and are thought to be relevant to the hypotensive LES seen in pregnancy.

It can currently be concluded that under normal physiologic circumstances, local, neural, or hormonal factors are not responsible for maintaining resting sphincter tone. The

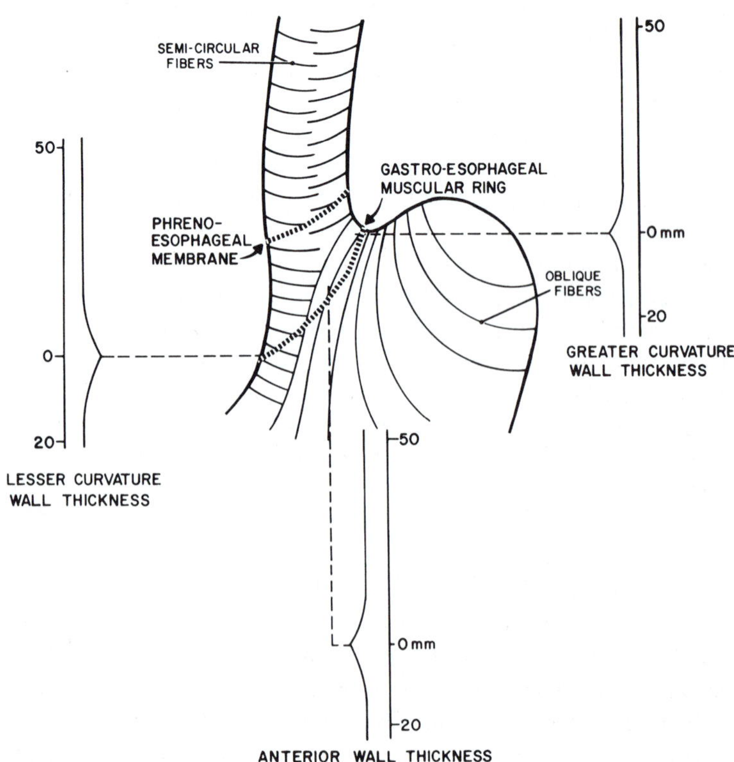


**Figure 39–15.** Wall thickness and orientation of muscle fibers at microdissection of the cardia.

cause of low LES pressure in patients with GERD is probably an abnormality of myogenic function. In support of this hypothesis, Biancani et al[21] showed that the LES pressure response to stretching is reduced in patients with an incompetent cardia, suggesting that sphincter pressure depends on the length-tension properties of the muscle.

Despite the statistical correlation between the amplitude of LES pressure and the presence of GERD in a population, considerable evidence exists that other factors are important in the antireflux mechanism. For example, there is considerable overlap in resting levels of LES pressure between people serving as controls and patients with GERD, and the results of antireflux operations are independent of changes in resting LES pressure.[22,23] Furthermore, myotomy can be performed along the length of the LES without resulting in reflux,[24] and competence can be maintained in the absence of the myogenic influence of the LES.[25,26] These observations suggest that intrinsic LES tone is but one of a complex of factors that maintain competence. For this reason, considerable attention has been focused on alternative mechanisms.

## Phrenoesophageal Ligament

Since the observations of Bombeck et al[27], who described a close relation between the insertion of the phrenoesophageal ligament into the esophageal wall and the incidence of GERD, considerable attention has been focused on the length of the intra-abdominal segment of the esophagus. The effect of this may be purely a mechanical one, in which Laplace's law operates. This physical law, which governs the behavior of soft tubes, states that the pressure required to distend a tube is inversely proportional to its diameter, provided that extrinsic pressure on the tube is constant. When an intra-abdominal segment of esophagus exists, both the esophagus and stomach are exposed to a positive intra-abdominal pressure, and the small-diameter esophagus opens into the large-diameter gastric pouch. Consequently, a very high intragastric pressure is necessary to overcome intraesophageal pressure, and hence allow reflux. This effective barrier is enhanced by the pressure differential between the intrathoracic esophagus, exposed to negative intrathoracic pressure, and the abdominal segment, exposed to positive intra-abdominal pressure, which results in apposition of the distal esophageal walls in a valve-like action, much like sucking on a softened soda straw causes it to collapse. In the absence of an intra-abdominal segment of esophagus, both these factors that promote competence are lost.

## Intra-abdominal Segment of Esophagus

Many experimental observations have supported the importance of the intra-abdominal segment of esophagus. Henderson[28] resected the distal esophagus, including the region of the LES, in dogs and replaced this segment with a tube constructed from the lesser curve of the stomach. When 6 cm of the gastric tube lay within the abdominal cavity, animals with histamine-induced gastric hypersecretion showed no esophagitis. Those in which the gastric tube opened into the stomach at the level of the hiatus, thereby eliminating the intra-abdominal segment, had esophagitis. When a similar experiment was conducted in monkeys, a high-pressure zone comparable with the LES existed in the intra-abdominal segment, and reflux, as detected by a modified standard acid reflux test, did not occur.[29] Furthermore, the high-pressure zone relaxed on swallowing, and the responses to infusions of gastrin, secretin and cholecystokinin were similar to those of the lower esophageal segment in healthy monkeys.

The in vitro model developed by DeMeester et al[30] demonstrated the close relation between competence and the length of esophagus exposed to positive intra-abdominal pressure. Various lengths of fresh cadaveric esophagi were exposed to intrathoracic, intra-abdominal, and intragastric pressure, and competence was found to be directly proportional to the length of the intra-abdominal segment. As this segment shortened, the intrinsic pressure of the LES had to increase exponentially to maintain reflux control. A minimum length of intra-abdominal esophagus was required to protect against changes in intra-abdominal pressure (Fig.

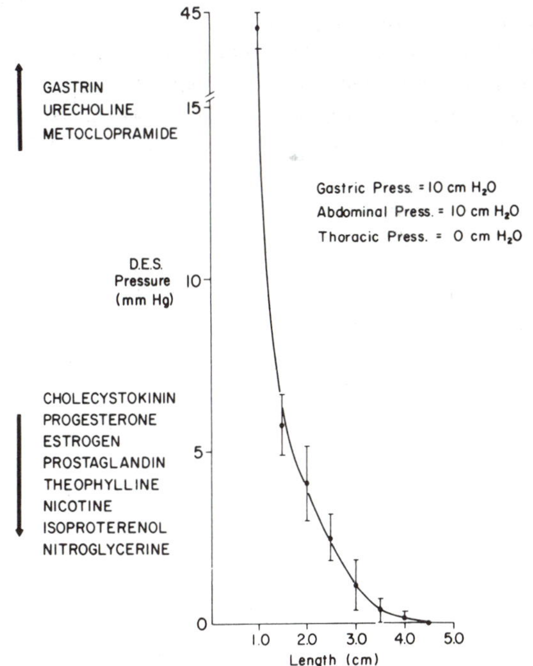


**Figure 39–16.** The plotted line shows the distal (lower) esophageal sphincter (DES) pressure necessary for competency of the cardia against challenges in intra-abdominal pressures for different lengths of DES exposed to the positive-pressure environment of the abdomen. Notice that an abdominal length of less than 1 cm requires an extraordinary amount of sphincter pressure to remain competent. The length of abdominal DES remains constant, but DES pressure can vary with pharmacologic and hormonal agents. Because one of these variables remains fixed (length of intra-abdominal esophagus), results differ among patients who undergo medical therapy.

39–16), and a minimum sphincter pressure was necessary to protect against the independent changes in intragastric pressure (Fig. 39–17). An intra-abdominal length of 4.5 cm, however, could in itself achieve total competence.

## GERD

The importance of intra-abdominal length of the LES, as well as resting LES pressure, was confirmed in a clinical study of 393 patients with symptoms.[15] Reflux resulted from a reduction in LES pressure, a shortening of the intra-abdominal esophagus, or both. Conversely, competence of the cardia required adequate LES pressure and intra-abdominal length. The probability of GERD was 80% when the LES pressure was less than 5 mm Hg, irrespective of the length of abdominal esophagus, and 80% when the abdominal segment was less than 1 cm, irrespective of the resting pressure. In contrast, the combination of a pressure greater than 20 mm Hg and length of abdominal esophagus greater than 2 cm was associated with a low incidence of GERD.

The fact that some GERD occurred in the presence of adequate resting LES pressure and length indicates that other mechanisms may be relevant to the antireflux barrier. The observed correlation between delayed gastric emptying and GERD, particularly in the supine posture,[31] suggests that gastric factors may be relevant. Despite Laplace's law, intragastric pressure may exceed intraesophageal pressure. Certain disorders, such as gastric outlet obstruction or gastroparesis secondary to diabetes or neuromuscular disease, may lead to gastric distention and increased intragastric pressure. Indeed, such distention arises early in the postprandial period, when physiologic reflux is known to occur in healthy people. The effect of elevated intragastric pressure and gastric dilatation is to shorten the length of the LES and, more important, the length of the intra-abdominal segment, just as inflation of a balloon shortens the length of its neck. Clinical and experimental observations have suggested that the critical overall length of LES at which reflux is likely to occur is 2 cm. Patients with shorter lengths at fasting manometric studies are prone to reflux.[32] The finding of a short LES in patients with GERD is not restricted to those with impaired gastric emptying. Thus, a third quality of the LES, its overall length, is a necessary component of competence, along with resting tone and intra-abdominal length.[34] The frequent association of gastric disorders, including duodenogastric bile reflux,[34,35] with GERD supports the early observations that the lower esophagus and gastric fundus function as a single unit. GERD is likely a manifestation of a diffuse motility disorder of the foregut.

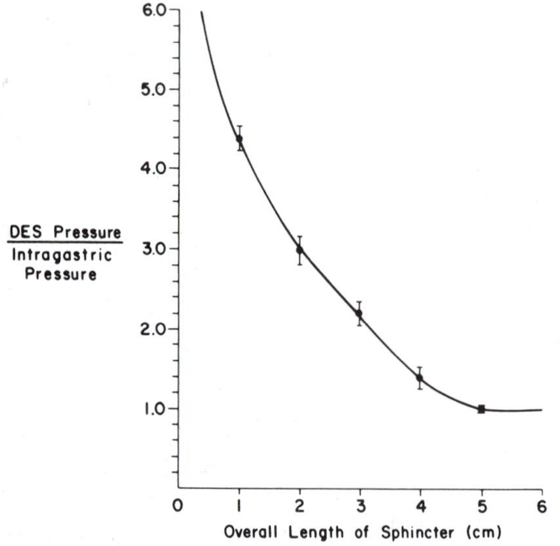


**Figure 39–17.** Plotted line shows the ratio of distal (lower) esophageal sphincter (DES) pressure to intragastric pressure necessary for competency of the cardia against challenges in intragastric pressure, independent of intra-abdominal pressures, for different overall lengths of the DES (intra-abdominal plus intrathoracic length). The overall DES length shortens with gastric distention—as the neck of the balloon shortens on inflation—requiring a higher ratio for competency. This explains the tendency of postprandial reflux to occur after a large meal.

The concept of the existence of a diffuse foregut motility disturbance is supported by the observation that many patients with GERD have motility changes in the esophageal body, resulting in impaired clearance.[7,36] The contribution of the esophageal body to clearance is highlighted by observations documenting a higher proportion of weak-amplitude contractions and simultaneous contractions, with resultant poor clearance, in patients with complications of GERD, namely stricture and Barrett's metaplasia.

In the physiologic situation, gravity, salivation, and swallowing all contribute to esophageal clearance and are important to the antireflux mechanism. Gravity aids clearance in the upright posture. Swallowed saliva has an important neutralizing effect on refluxed acid, as demonstrated by Helm et al.[37,38] Small amounts of refluxed gastric contents, occurring sporadically or in the postprandial period, are usually cleared rapidly by a primary peristaltic wave or even by saliva after a pharyngeal swallow that is not transmitted.

Bremner et al,[39] in a study utilizing 24-hour ambulatory esophageal pH monitoring combined with simultaneous monitoring of pharyngeal pressure and esophageal motility, studied the clearance of naturally occurring reflux episodes in healthy people and those with GERD. Esophageal clearance of acid, defined as a return of pH to greater than 4 after a reflux episode, occurred after primary peristalsis in 83% of such episodes (Fig. 39–18). Acid was cleared by pharyngeal swallows without an esophageal body response, a phenomenon that can be explained by the neutralizing properties of saliva aided by gravity, in an additional 11%. These findings are in accordance with a report that patients with xerostomia experience longer reflux episodes and more severe esophagitis than patients with normal salivation.[40] Secondary peristalsis only rarely was responsible for the clearance of a reflux episode. Patients and healthy subjects cleared reflux episodes similarly. The baseline swallowing frequency was 0.87 times per minute during the day, increasing to 2.59 times per minute during

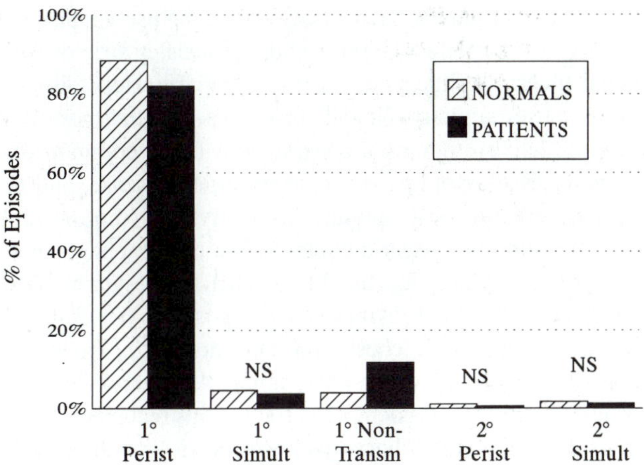


**Figure 39–18.** The types of contractions resulting in acid clearance from the esophagus. Most reflux episodes were cleared with a pharyngeal swallow followed by a primary peristaltic wave (1° Perist). 1° Simult = primary simultaneous wave, 1° Nontransm = primary nontransmittal wave, 2° Perist = secondary peristaltic wave, 2° Simult = secondary simultaneous wave.

daytime reflux episodes, but reaching only 1.42 times per minute during nighttime reflux episodes (Fig. 39–19). Thus, during sleep, the mechanisms of esophageal clearance are depressed; sleeping may dull the response of the esophagus to acidification.

The study gave support to the concept that pharyngeal swallowing, usually followed by primary peristalsis, is the most important mechanism for esophageal acid clearance in both healthy people and those with GERD. It also explains the air-swallowing behavior commonly observed in patients with pathologic gastroesophageal reflux. It is unlikely that medical therapy, aimed at improving contraction amplitude and frequency, will improve this protective mechanism. This is probably why prokinetic agents have been a disappointment in the treatment of patients with gastroesophageal reflux. Any impairment in esophageal motility may, therefore, predispose to abnormal exposure time, even in the presence of a mechanically competent cardia. The combination of a primary motility disturbance and one secondary to reflux esophagitis is likely to be present in patients with a mechanically incompetent cardia. It results in a severe form of reflux disease that may lead to further complications, such as stricture, Barrett's esophagus, or chronic aspiration.

Intrinsic sphincter tone, sphincter length, intra-abdominal length, gastric function, and esophageal pump function are the important factors determining competence against reflux in most patients. Prolonged manometric studies by Dodds et al,[41] however, have shown that spontaneous transient episodes of LES relaxation may allow abnormal esophageal exposure to gastric juice, even when the foregoing characteristics are normal. The LES may relax spontaneously, unrelated to swallowing, with a drop in pressure to gastric baseline, allowing reflux episodes to occur. Although the cause of these spontaneous relaxations is unknown, it probably is related to a gastric function, such as a belch. This mechanism may explain the increased esophageal acid exposure in patients whose antireflux mechanism appears intact. Prolonged manometry with a sleeve catheter is necessary to diagnose this abnormality. Studies have indicated that the transient relaxation episodes may be an artifact caused by catheter-induced nontransmitted pharyngeal swallows, because they were not recorded when the motility catheter was passed retrograde into the LES through a gastrostomy tube.

Primary sphincter failure, gastric abnormalities, impaired esophageal pump function, and inappropriate LES relaxation can result in pathologic GERD in the absence of a hiatal hernia. Statistics show, however, that more patients with troublesome reflux have a coexisting hiatal hernia, which undoubtedly has its own influence on the antireflux

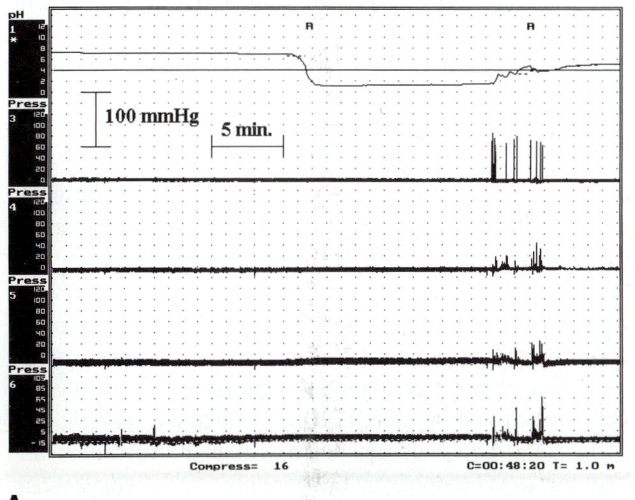


A

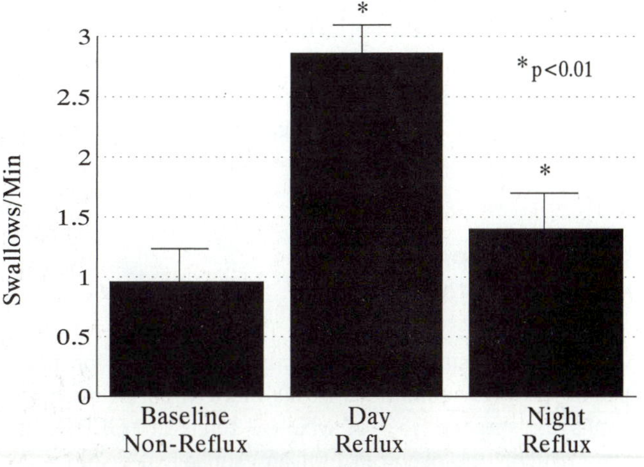


B

**Figure 39–19.** **A.** an example of a simultaneous recording of pharyngoesophageal motility and esophageal pH showing a reflux episode occurring at night. The swallowing response to reflux is delayed, resulting in a prolonged reflux episode. **B.** Swallowing frequency in patients during the baseline period and during daytime and nighttime reflux.

mechanism. A snug hiatal opening around the abdominal segment of esophagus, with a normally inserted phrenoesophageal ligament, limits distention of the abdominal esophagus and maintains the insertion of the narrow abdominal esophageal segment into the larger-caliber stomach, enabling Laplace's law to operate. In the presence of a hiatal hernia, however, these functions are lost. The acute angle of implantation is replaced by an inverted funnel shape, and the sharp gradient between the narrow esophagus and larger stomach disappears as they become a common channel. This may negate the effect of the "mucosal rosette," which serves as a mucosal plug when normal anatomic relations are present, particularly during gastric distention.[42]

While the role of the angle of His has been somewhat controversial, experience has shown that anatomical angles, in other situations such as at the neck of the bladder and the anorectum, are important factors in continence, although their relevance may be in enabling Laplace's law to operate. The autopsy studies of Butterfield,[43] in which appropriate anatomic relations enabled a water-filled stomach to be held upside down without leakage into the esophagus, demonstrated the importance of structurally related mechanical factors. The presence of a hiatal hernia may also result in an esophageal propulsive defect and inadequate esophageal acid clearance.[44,45] Our observations have shown that the presence of a hiatal hernia is associated with a greater proportion of supine reflux.

The antireflux mechanism, therefore, represents a complex of factors, some of which are easily amenable to measurement and others of which are not. Primary is the mechanical function of the LES, which depends on sphincter pressure, overall length, and intra-abdominal length.[33] Mechanical failure of one of these components can be compensated by an effective esophageal pump, but failure of all three invariably results in increased esophageal exposure to gastric juice. Antireflux operations effectively control reflux by restoring to normal the failed components of a mechanically defective sphincter.[33] The procedures vary mainly in the components they can correct. Some restore normal sphincter pressure, and others rely on accentuation of the intra-abdominal length and overall sphincter length.[46] Some operations restore all three components.[47] All reduce a hiatal hernia and appear to reconstruct the normal anatomic relation between stomach and esophagus.

## DIAGNOSTIC PROBLEMS IN ESOPHAGEAL DISEASE

A correct diagnosis provides the only rational basis for therapy. In few other conditions is this more important than in esophageal surgery, 75% of which is related to GERD. In many patients the occurrence of an esophageal disorder is indicated by typical symptoms of heartburn, regurgitation, and dysphagia. Ascribing these symptoms to reflux in the absence of esophagitis, however, may be misleading, because other diseases, such as achalasia, diffuse esophageal spasm, esophageal carcinoma, cholelithiasis, gastric or duodenal ulcer, alkaline gastritis, and coronary artery disease, may cause similar clinical problems. Furthermore, an esophageal disorder may coexist with other common alimentary tract disorders, or coronary artery disease, and result in a mixture of symptoms. Alternatively, symptoms due to regurgitation of gastric contents into the esophagus may be atypical and not attributable to GERD on symptomatic analysis alone. Such symptoms are postprandial fullness, belching, angina-like chest pain, chronic cough, wheezing, hoarseness and recurrent pneumonia. A common clinical problem is the assessment of patients with recurrent symptoms after previous biliary, gastroduodenal, hiatal, or coronary artery bypass operations. In some of these patients the underlying problem is an esophageal disorder. In all of these circumstances, objective methods are required to determine if an esophageal abnormality is present, and if so, to differentiate it from other conditions.

## OBJECTIVE ASSESSMENT OF ESOPHAGEAL DISORDERS

A number of tests are available for the diagnosis of esophageal disease; they vary greatly in reliability and appropriate application.[48] Commonly used investigative methods include radiographic barium studies, endoscopy, esophageal manometry, pH reflux tests, radionuclide studies, and the fiberoptic bile probe.

### Esophageal and Upper Gastrointestinal Radiographic Barium Studies

In a patient in whom esophageal disease is suspected, one of the simplest diagnostic tests is a barium swallow radiographic examination followed by a full assessment of the stomach and duodenum. The radiologist should be forewarned that esophageal disease is suspected, so that careful attention is paid to visualization and recording of all levels of swallowing from the pharynx to the stomach. Increased accuracy of analysis is achieved by cine or videotape recordings of the barium swallow and the use of both a liquid and a solid bolus. The studies are usually performed with the patient in the upright and supine positions and in several body rotations.

Barium studies may demonstrate a hiatal hernia, large mucosal ulceration, mucosal erosions, stricture, spastic contractions, rings, webs, diverticula, or neoplasm of the esophagus. Esophageal landmarks such as the cricopharyngeus muscle, aortic arch, tracheal bifurcation, phrenic ampulla, LES, and mucosal junction may be identified and help locate the esophageal abnormality. An esophageal narrowing or stricture should be reported without an attempt to make a definitive diagnosis (e.g., achalasia or neoplasia), because the overlap of radiographic findings among the several structural and motility disorders of the esophagus is too great for an imaging diagnosis to be considered definitive. Attempts to make a precise diagnosis by radiographic examination are a frequent cause of inappropriate management and therapy for esophageal disorders.

GERD is difficult for radiologists to demonstrate. In only about 40% of our patients who had documented reflux is spontaneous reflux observed by the radiologist. In most patients in whom free spontaneous reflux is seen on radiographs, the diagnosis of abnormal reflux is confirmed by pH studies. The radiographic demonstration of spontaneous reflux in the upright position, therefore, is a reliable indicator that reflux is present. A normal study, however, does not exclude GERD. Some authors have advocated observing for reflux while the patient is sipping water and pressure is simultaneously applied to the abdomen. This so-called water-sipping test is not an accurate assessment of pathologic reflux, because healthy people frequently demonstrate reflux of barium under these circumstances. The swallowing during sipping causes relaxation of the distal esophageal segment, and compression of the stomach encourages the reflux of barium to occur.

Mucosal disease, such as esophagitis or ulceration, can be detected by a careful double-contrast technique. The radiographic assessment of esophageal disease is not complete until the entire stomach and duodenum have been examined. A gastric or duodenal ulcer, a partially obstructing gastric neoplasm, or scarring of the duodenum or pylorus may contribute to GERD or symptoms otherwise attributable to esophageal disease.

When patient reports dysphagia, and no obstructing lesion is seen on the liquid barium swallow examination, it is useful to have the patient swallow a barium-impregnated marshmallow, a barium-soaked piece of bread, or a hamburger mixed with barium. This test may bring out a functional disturbance in esophageal transit that may be missed when liquid barium is used.

## Esophagoscopy

In any patient who reports dysphagia, esophagoscopy is indicated even in the presence of a normal barium swallow examination. Abnormal findings at barium swallow examination direct the endoscopist's attention to locations of subtle change and reduce the risk of endoscopy by making the operator aware of such dangers as a cervical vertebral osteophyte, an esophageal diverticulum, a deeply penetrating ulcer, or carcinoma. Regardless of the radiologist's interpretation of an abnormal finding, each structural abnormality of the esophagus should be confirmed with a biopsy, with the exception of a smooth extramucosal mass. Such masses are usually caused by a leiomyoma, a duplication cyst, or extrinsic compression, the management of which would be complicated by penetration through the mucosa in a biopsy. Esophagoscopy and biopsy may diagnose early esophagitis, mucosal abnormalities such as moniliasis, or small carcinomas not visible on radiographs. Advanced reflux esophagitis is graded by the visual appearance of the esophagus, but biopsy is necessary to exclude carcinoma and Barrett's metaplasia.

For the initial endoscopic assessment, a flexible fiberoptic esophagoscope is the instrument of choice, because it allows simultaneous assessment of the stomach and duodenum. This procedure is almost always performed with sedation with diazepam and meperidine and with a topical spray or viscous-liquid anesthesia of the pharynx. Under these circumstances, a continuous electrocardiogram (ECG) should be performed and cutaneous oxygen saturation should be monitored during the procedure. A flexible endoscopic evaluation is performed with the patient lying in the left lateral decubitus position, with knees, spine, and neck flexed. A useful maneuver is for the operator to pass an index finger alongside the bite block, guide the tip of the esophagoscope around the posterior pharyngeal curvature, and maintain the scope in the midline while the tip is advanced into the upper esophagus.

Every endoscopist should know how to use and have access to a rigid esophagoscope, because it may be essential when deep biopsies are required. Abnormalities of the pharynx, cricopharyngeus muscle, and upper esophagus may be more readily assessed with a rigid instrument, such as a direct laryngeal scope or a short esophagoscope. Rigid instruments allow more accurate biopsies and are easier to maintain in position at the midportion of the sphincter zone, or at the orifice of a high stricture, than are the flexible scopes. Rigid esophagoscopy in our clinic is almost always performed with general anesthesia or a block of the ninth cranial nerves.[49]

When GERD is the suspected diagnosis, the endoscopist pays particular attention to score the degree of esophagitis, look for the level of the squamocolumnar junction, and assess the presence of Barrett's columnar-lined esophagus. The endoscopic confirmation of a hiatal hernia is determined by the presence of a pouch lined with gastric rugal folds lying 2 cm or more above the indentation of the diaphragmatic crura; it is identified by having the patient sniff. When a hiatal hernia pouch is observed, particular attention is paid to exclude a gastric ulcer or gastritis within the pouch. An intragastric retroflex, or J maneuver, is important to evaluate the hernial pouch and the mucosal surface of the gastric fundus.

When esophagitis is present, its length and severity should be recorded. The most common grading system subdivides esophagitis into four grades.[50] Grade I is characterized by reddening of the mucosa without ulceration. Grade II is characterized by erosive and exudative mucosal lesions, usually in a linear arrangement, but not involving the entire circumference. Grade III is characterized by extensive mucosal involvement with confluence of erosions, leaving islands of edematous squamous mucosa, forming the so-called cobblestone esophagus. The mucosa is friable, but stricturing is absent. Grade IV is the presence of complications such as large ulcers, circumferential strictures, shortening of the esophagus, or the presence of columnar metaplasia. The specific grade of esophagitis present with the complication should be recorded.

When a stricture is present, the esophagoscope frequent does not pass. The benign nature of the stricture must be confirmed by multiple biopsies and brush cytologic sampling within the lumen of the stricture. The stricture may then be dilated and a fiberoptic esophagoscope of narrow caliber used, if necessary, to examine the length of the stricture and the upper gastrointestinal tract beyond.

Barrett's esophagus is suspected when there is difficulty visualizing the squamocolumnar junction at the normal location and there is a redder mucosa more luxuriant than is normally seen in the lower esophagus. The presence of Barrett's metaplasia should be confirmed with multiple biopsies. Dysplasia and neoplasia in Barrett's epithelium have a patchy distribution, so at least five biopsy specimens should be obtained from the Barrett's-lined portion of the esophagus. Further biopsy specimens should be obtained cephalad to ascertain the precise level at which the junction of Barrett's epithelium with normal squamous epithelium occurs. When a patient with Barrett's metaplasia undergoes endoscopic surveillance for the development of dysplasia, four circumferential biopsy specimens should be obtained at 2-cm intervals over the whole length of metaplastic mucosa.

When an esophageal diverticulum is seen, it should be carefully explored with a flexible esophagoscope to exclude ulceration or neoplasia within the pouch. When a submucosal mass is seen, biopsies are usually not performed. A submucosal leiomyoma or duplication cyst may be easily dissected away from the intact mucosa. If a biopsy specimen is taken, the mucosa may become fixed to the underlying abnormality so that a breach in the mucosa is caused during the surgical dissection, which complicates operative management and increases the risk of a subsequent infection.

### The Acid Perfusion Test

The acid perfusion test, introduced by Bernstein in 1958, determines the sensitivity of the esophageal mucosa to acid.[51] The test is performed with a catheter, often a manometry infusion catheter, with a port positioned 15 cm above the LES. The port is alternately infused with normal saline solution and 0.1N HCl. Both bottles of solution, preferably unmarked, are hung on an IV stand behind the patient's back and attached to a three-way stopcock. Ideally, the person performing the test should not know which solution is in which bottle. One solution is perfused through the catheter for 10 min or until symptoms are noted. The other solution is then perfused for an identical length of time or until symptoms change. The process may be repeated to establish consistency. The patient's symptoms are recorded in relation to whether solution A or solution B is being perfused at the time. Later, an assessment of the symptoms in relation to whether the infusion was acid or saline solution is made. A positive test is scored when the patient spontaneously reports symptoms during infusion of acid and relief during infusion of saline solution. The elicitation of symptoms other than the patient's spontaneous reports does not represent a positive test but may indicate acid sensitivity of the esophagus. Because people without GERD may have an acid-sensitive esophagus, the elicitation of chest pain or heartburn with infusion of acid does not diagnose GERD, nor does the absence of symptoms during an infusion exclude reflux. The test simply relates whether the patient's spontaneous symptoms can be reproduced by infusion of acid and not by saline solution. False-positive tests may occur in patients with gastric or duodenal ulcers, because the acid solution may stimulate these raw areas.

Applications, in our laboratory, of the acid perfusion test to patients with reflux-induced stricture and Barrett's esophagus have demonstrated considerably reduced sensitivity to acid perfusion in these patients, which may explain why these complications can develop in with mild symptoms.

### Manometry

Esophageal manometry is indicated whenever a motor abnormality of the esophagus is suspected or the patient reports dysphagia or odynophagia and the barium swallow examination does not show a clear structural abnormality. Manometry is indicated particularly to confirm the diagnoses of achalasia, scleroderma, and esophageal spasm. In patients with symptomatic GERD, the esophageal clearance mechanism should be assessed, because the outcome of antireflux surgery depends partly on the adequacy of esophageal motor function. In the past, many investigators studied the pressure of the distal esophageal segment as an indicator of reflux. This is, at best, an indirect assessment of competence of the cardia. Although patients with abnormal reflux have an average LES pressure that is considerably lower than normal, there is too much overlap between patients with and those without reflux in the amplitude of the high-pressure zone to make measurement of LES pressures alone reliable. When pressure measurements are coupled with the measurement of the overall sphincter length and the length exposed to the positive-pressure environment of the abdomen, manometry can be used to identify a mechanically defective sphincter as the cause of increased esophageal exposure to gastric juice.[33]

Manometry may be performed with pressure-sensitive transducers or water-perfused catheters with side hole ports attached to transducers outside the body. Usually a train of three to five pressure-sensing stations are bound together at 5-cm intervals. They are passed like a nasogastric tube into the stomach, and the gastric pressure pattern is confirmed. The catheters are then withdrawn across the cardia. Although some authors advocate steady, rapid withdrawal, we have found that a stepwise pull-through withdrawal of the catheter at 0.5-cm intervals provides reproducible and more quantitative information. When open-port catheters are used, a slow infusion of water is essential to obtain reproducible tracings. This is best achieved by using a low-compliance pneumohydraulic capillary infusion system (Arndorfer) that can perfuse as slowly as 0.6 mL/min.

As the pressure recorders are brought across the gastroesophageal junction, the high-pressure zone is entered. During this time, the patient is asked to swallow so that the relaxation of the distal esophagus can be assessed. Normally, the esophageal pressure should drop to the level of gastric pressure during a swallow. The location of the respiratory inversion point is noted between the upward deflection of abdominal pressure and the downward deflection of thoracic pressure on inspiration. The respiratory inversion point serves as a reference with which to measure the amplitude of the LES pressure (Fig. 39–20). It is also used to measure the length of the intra-abdominal portion of the LES, which is normally about 2 cm. As the pressure-sensitive stations are withdrawn into the body of the esophagus, the upper border of the LES is identified by the drop in pressure to the esophageal baseline. Using this measurement, the overall length of the sphincter can be determined.

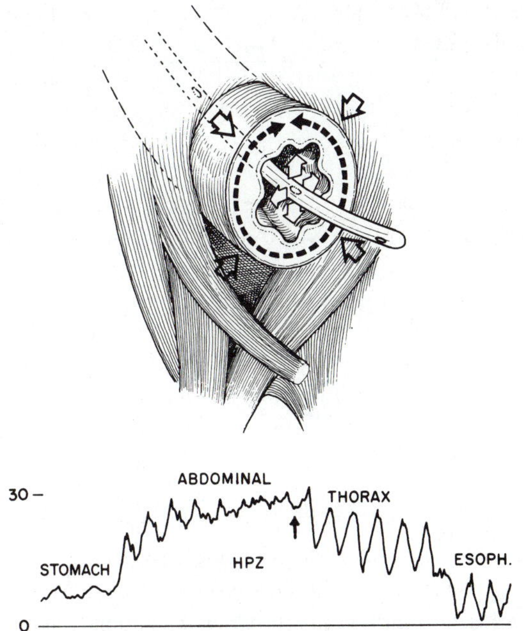


**Figure 39–20.** Measurement of LES pressure with the perfused catheter system. The outflow of the perfused fluid (*white arrows*) is retarded by the circular muscle tone of the cardia (*broken arrow*) and the external applied intra-abdominal pressure (*black-outlined arrows*). The abdominal and thoracic portions of the LES (HPZ) can be measured on the pressure recording by identification of the positive or negative effect of respiration on the tracing. The resting pressure of the LES (HPZ) is measured at the point where the abdominal and thoracic portions meet, or at the respiratory inversion point (*black arrowheads*).

Within the body of the esophagus, the response to 10 pharyngeal swallows is noted by assessing the amplitude of the contraction and the velocity of the wave, to determine whether it is peristaltic or synchronous. The swallow should be induced by 5-mL boluses of water, because wet swallows are often more sensitive in demonstrating motor abnormalities. As the pressure devices pass the cricopharyngeal area, recordings are taken at high chart speed to assess the timing of relaxation of the cricopharyngeus muscle in synchrony with the hypopharyngeal contraction.

Motor disorders of the esophagus can be classified according to motility findings. In classic achalasia, the LES does not fully reflux with swallowing, and all waves observed in the body of the esophagus are simultaneous; no primary peristaltic waves are seen. The resting pressure of the body of the esophagus is usually elevated (Fig. 39–21). In scleroderma, all muscular function of the distal esophagus is obliterated. There are no high-pressure zone and no contractions of the body for the skeletal portions (Fig. 39–22). The observation of simultaneous, repetitive, or broad-based powerful contractions may lead to a variety of diagnostic possibilities, including partial obstruction, presbyesophagus, and symptomatic esophageal spasm (Fig. 39–23). The proportion of simultaneous waves and length of esophagus involved are helpful in assessing the presence of esophageal spasm (Fig. 39–24).

It is becoming increasingly recognized that many nonspecific motor abnormalities, particularly those accounting for obscure chest pain of noncardiac origin, may be only transient phenomena and not be detected with conventional manometry. Portable systems are now available to record esophageal motility on an ambulatory basis over a prolonged time period, either with continuous sampling throughout a 24-hour interval or at the patient's command when symptoms occur.

## 24-Hour Esophageal Motility Monitoring

The diagnosis and classification of esophageal motor disorders and the proof of a causal relation between an abnormality and a symptom has been difficult in the past. The following reasons account for this:

1. There usually is no reliable mucosal lesion that can be observed at endoscopy to indicate the presence of an esophageal motor disorder.
2. Radiographic signs of esophageal motor disorders occur only in advanced disease.
3. The current standard of reference for the diagnosis of esophageal motor disorders, that is, stationary esophageal manometry, has several shortcomings. First, it is performed in a laboratory environment with the patient in a supine position. Second, the analysis is usually based solely on the motor response to 10 swallows; consequently, intermittent motor abnormalities may be missed.

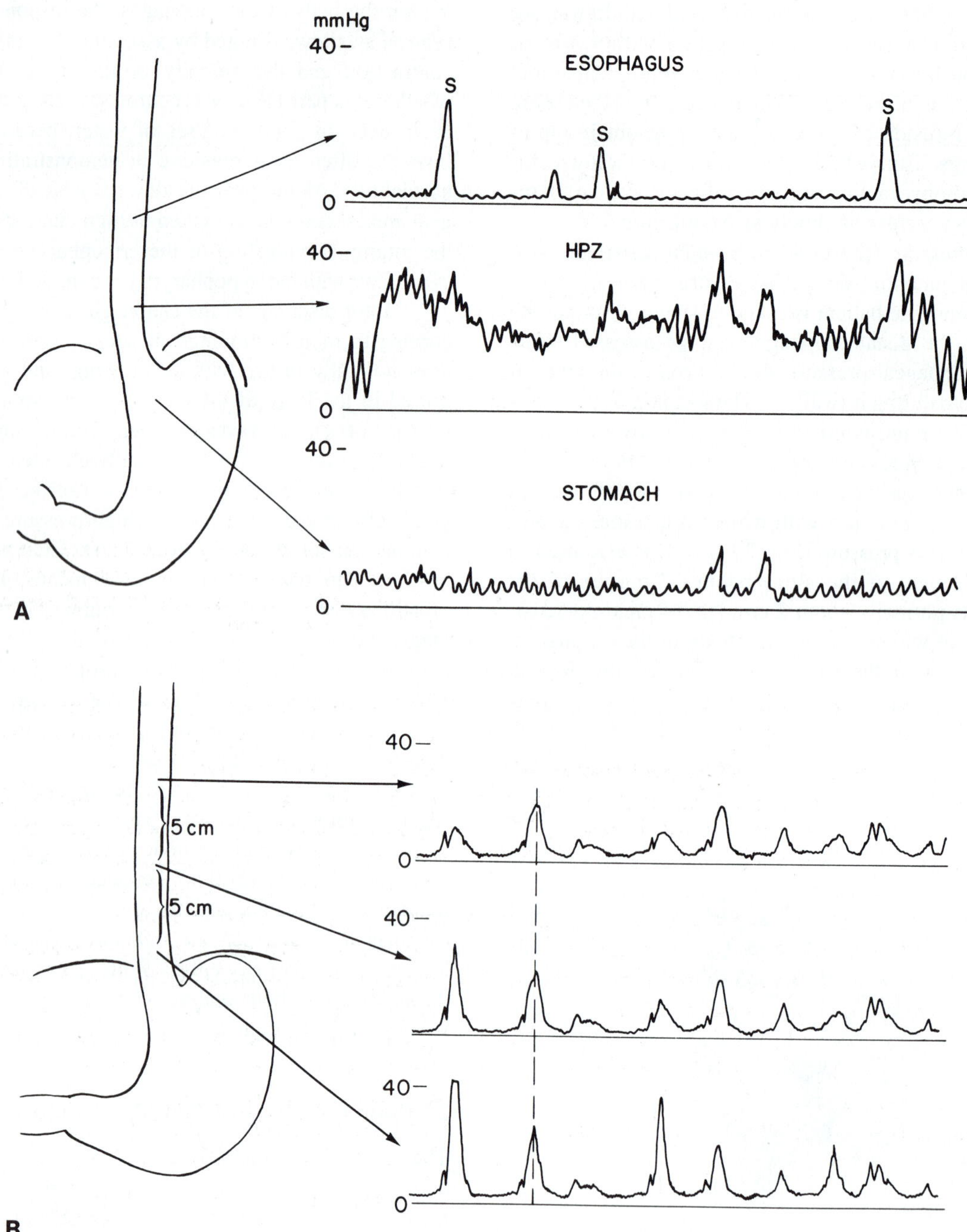


**Figure 39–21.** Motility record from a patient with achalasia. **A.** Failure of the LES (HPZ) to relax on swallowing (S). **B.** Aperistalsis in the body of the esophagus with only simultaneous contraction occurring on swallowing.

4. The current classification of motor disorders is controversial and does not allow for the quantitation of the severity of the abnormality.
5. Spontaneous symptoms rarely occur during a conventional motility study, and the finding of an esophageal motility disorder with conventional manometry in the absence of symptoms does not prove a causal relation between the abnormality and the reported symptoms.
6. The use of provocative studies, such as acid perfusion, administration of Tensilon (edrophonium chloride) or balloon distention, to reproduce the patient's symptoms is not helpful because most of these tests have a low yield, symptoms are reproduced with unphysiologic stimuli, the endpoint is based on the patient's symptom perception, and the results do not correlate with motility abnormalities associated with spontaneously occurring symptoms.[52]

Consequently, the current diagnosis of esophageal motility abnormalities is inexact. This may account for some of the

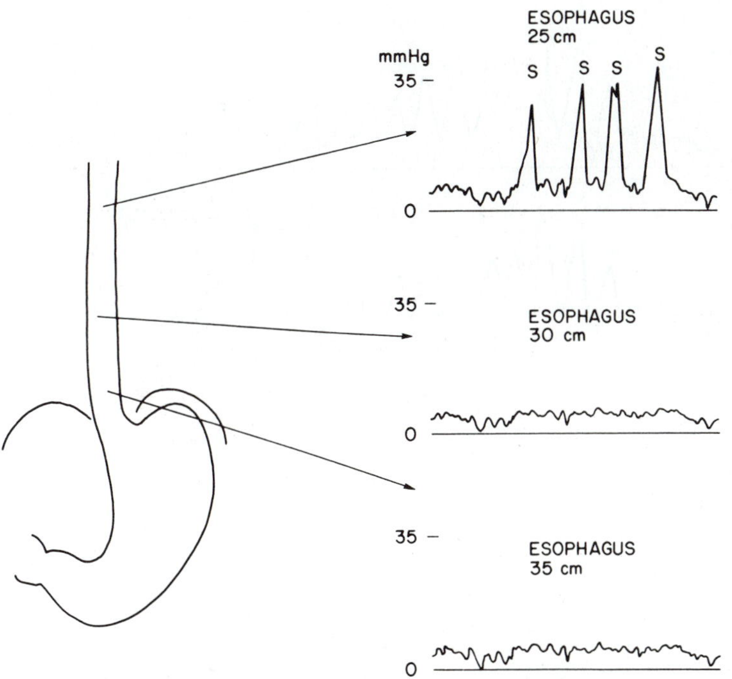


**Figure 39–22.** Motility record from a patient with scleroderma showing lack of muscle contraction in the distal two thirds of the esophageal body and contraction on swallowing (S) in the proximal third.

disappointing results of both pharmacologic and surgical therapy for these abnormalities.[52,53]

The recently introduced technique of ambulatory 24-hour esophageal motility monitoring overcomes the pitfalls of conventional manometry and provocative testing.[54,55] Ambulatory motility allows monitoring of esophageal motor activity over an entire circadian cycle and under a variety of physiologic conditions. This multiplies the amount of data on which a diagnosis can be based, increases the probability of documenting an intermittent abnormality, and allows correlation of spontaneously occurring symptoms with abnormal esophageal motor function, provided the symptom occurs during the 24-hour period. Furthermore, the combination of this technique with esophageal and gastric pH monitoring allows integrated evaluation of esophageal body function, gastroesophageal reflux, and gastric secretory and motor function in a physiologic environment within one circadian cycle.[56,57]

The technique of 24-hour ambulatory pH monitoring requires a portable digital data recorder, miniaturized electronic pressure transducers, and a personal computer (Fig. 39–25). Pressure data are sampled at a rate of 0.25 Hz and stored digitally on the data recorder.

All drugs that interfere with foregut function are discontinued for at least 48 hours before the study. The patient usually comes to the laboratory after an overnight fast. The LES is localized with manometry, and the electronic pressure transducers are placed transnasally into the distal esophagus. In most institutions, ambulatory esophageal manometry is performed with three transducers located 5,

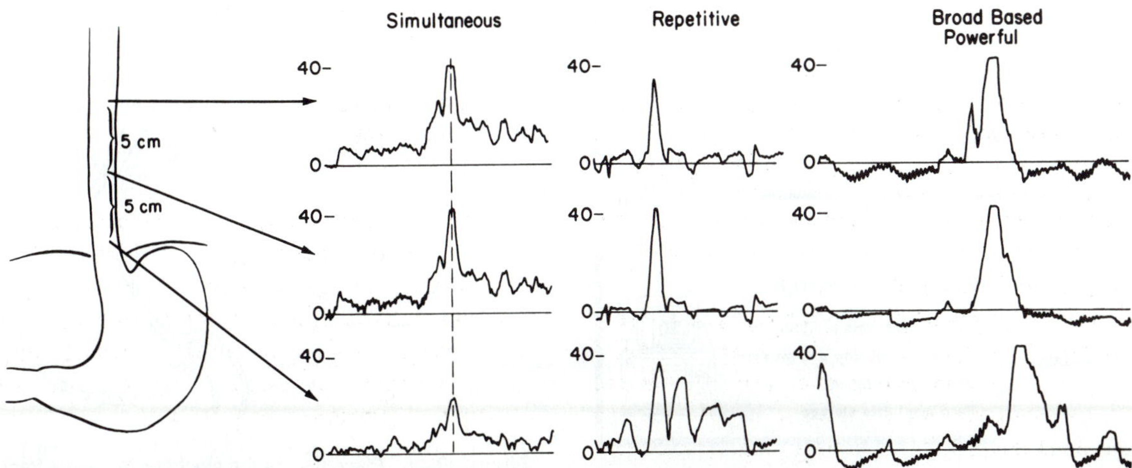


**Figure 39–23.** Examples of nonspecific motility disorders of the esophageal body. These are associated with a variety of abnormalities.

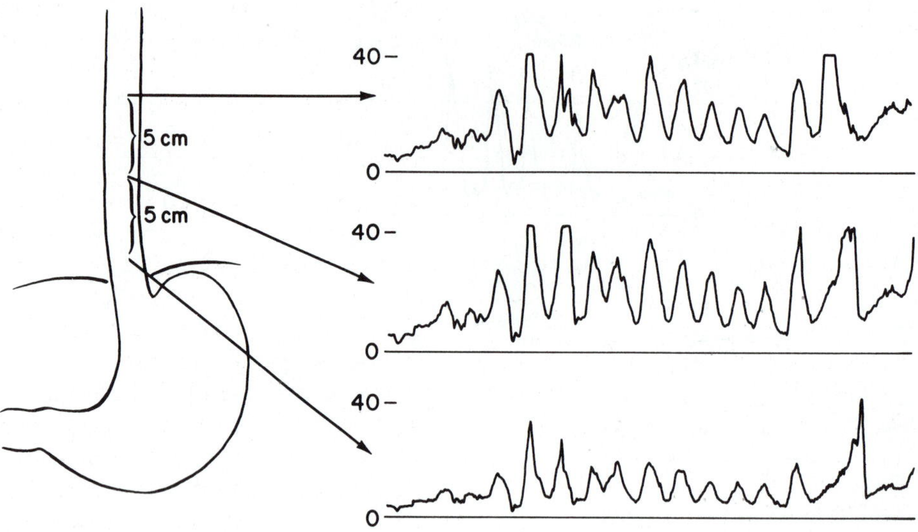


**Figure 39–24.** Motility record from a patient with diffuse esophageal spasm showing repetitive, broad-based, simultaneous contraction in the body of the esophagus over a length of 10 cm.

10, and 15 cm above the upper border of the LES (Fig. 39–26). After placement of the transducers, the patients are sent home and encouraged to perform normal daily activities. They are instructed to keep a diary for the next 24 hours that indicates the time of meals, when they assume the supine position in preparation for sleep, when they arise in the morning, and when symptoms occur.

With continuous monitoring, approximately 1000–1400 contractions are recorded by each pressure transducer over a 24-hour period. The contractions can be reviewed on the computer screen and a printout of the entire recording or of selected intervals can be obtained. The large amount of recorded data makes computerized evaluation essential. Dedicated software that allows for display, fully automatic analysis, and generation of a summary report for any recording interval has been developed and validated by several groups and is now commercially available.[55]

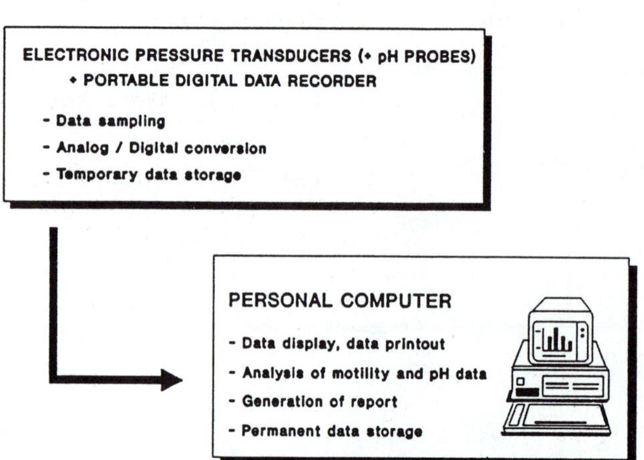


**Figure 39–25.** System for 24-hour ambulatory esophageal motility monitoring.

Table 39–1 gives the mean values for various parameters of the ambulatory motility recording during the supine, upright, and meal periods in 25 healthy volunteers without foregut symptoms or evidence of a foregut disorder on barium swallow examination and 24-hour esophageal pH monitoring.[58] The large standard errors indicate variability between subjects. Within the same person, however, the

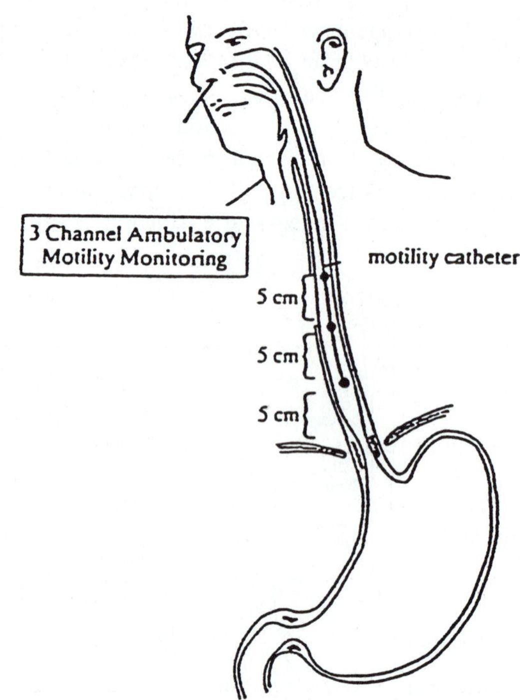


**Figure 39–26.** Placement of the electronic pressure transducers for ambulatory esophageal manometry 5, 10, and 15 cm above the LES.

**TABLE 39–1. NORMAL VALUES OF 24-HOUR AMBULATORY MOTILITY MONITORING (OBSERVED IN 25 HEALTHY VOLUNTEERS)[a]**

| Value | Supine | Upright | Meals |
|---|---|---|---|
| **Contractions per minute** | 0.5±0.1 | 1.2±0.2 | 2.6±0.3 |
| % peristaltic | 54.5±6.0 | 73.1±2.8 | 75.3±4.2 |
| % simultaneous | 43.3±6.0 | 23.7±3.0 | 21.4±3.6 |
| % isolated | 2.2±0.7 | 3.2±1.0 | 3.3±1.1 |
| % double peaked | 14.2±2.3 | 7.6±2.0 | 10.5±1.4 |
| % multiple peaked | 2.3±0.9 | 1.0±0.4 | 1.4±0.4 |
| % <30 mm Hg | 10.8±1.7 | 20.6±3.9 | 17.9±2.9 |
| % >180 mm Hg | 0.3±0.2 | 0.3±0.2 | 0.5±0.3 |
| % >7 sec | 12.0±2.6 | 2.8±1.4 | 4.8±1.4 |
| **Mean Contraction Amplitude (mm Hg)** | | | |
| 10 cm above LES | 49.3±3.5 | 39.5±3.9 | 42.2±4.0 |
| 5 cm above LES | 59.1±4.1 | 46.6±3.1 | 47.4±3.1 |
| **Mean Duration of Contractions (sec)** | | | |
| 10 cm above LES | 3.9±0.3 | 2.9±0.1 | 2.9±0.1 |
| 5 cm above LES | 4.2±0.3 | 3.4±0.2 | 3.6±0.1 |
| **Mean Area Under the Curve (mm Hg • sec)** | | | |
| 10 cm above LES | 112.2 ±14.1 | 62.1 ±8.1 | 68.8±8.4 |
| 5 cm above LES | 141.2 ±15.2 | 92.8 ±10.9 | 96.1±10.3 |

[a]Numbers are mean ± SEM.
LES = lower esophageal sphincter.

circadian esophageal motor pattern is highly reproducible.[59]

The classic criteria and thresholds for the diagnosis and classification of esophageal motility disorders based on stationary manometry and the corresponding thresholds for ambulatory esophageal motility monitoring are shown in Table 39–2. When the diagnoses obtained with both tests with these criteria were compared in a large series of consecutive patients there was surprisingly little agreement between the two tests (Fig. 39–27).[60–62] Ambulatory manometry frequently documented a more severe motility abnormality in patients thought to have normal esophageal motor function, a nonspecific motor disorder, or nutcracker esophagus on conventional manometry, suggesting that these findings with conventional manometry do not exclude the presence of a more severe disorder such as diffuse esophageal spasm. This finding appears to be due to the intermittent expression of esophageal motor abnormalities, which can be missed easily on conventional manometry but are detected when motor activity is monitored over an entire circadian cycle. Conversely, ambulatory manometry also frequently showed normal or only mildly disordered circadian motor function in patients thought to have a nonspecific disorder or nutcracker esophagus with conventional manometry, suggesting that the unphysiologic conditions under which conventional manometry is performed may trigger these abnormalities in patients known to have a low anxiety threshold.[63] A change in diagnosis was less prevalent in patients who met the criteria for diffuse esophageal spasm or achalasia with conventional manometry. This would indicate that a failure of peristalsis detected with conventional manometry is a reliable indicator of the presence of a severe motor disorder. These observations suggest that the current classification of esophageal motor disorders on the basis of conventional manometric findings may not be a reliable guide for the treatment of patients symptomatic with disease.[60,61]

Dysphagia in the absence of esophageal obstruction is a frequent symptom in patients with esophageal motor disorders. The underlying pathophysiologic abnormality responsible for the symptom, however, frequently cannot be determined with stationary manometry.[52,64] When 24-hour esophageal manometry is used, the circadian esophageal motility pattern in patients with dysphagia is characterized by an inability to organize the motor activity into peristaltic contractions during meals. Less than 60% of peristaltic contractions during meals were associated with a 92% prevalence of dysphagia.[65] When the percentage dropped below 30, dysphagia became so severe that it began to interfere with adequate nutrition, and a surgical myotomy was indicated. If myotomy is performed for dysphagia when a high per-

**TABLE 39–2. DIAGNOSTIC CRITERIA FOR THE CLASSIFICATION OF PRIMARY ESOPHAGEAL MOTOR DISORDERS BASED ON ESOPHAGEAL BODY FUNCTION**

| Disorder | Conventional Manometry | Ambulatory 24-Hour Manometry |
|---|---|---|
| Achalasia | Complete absence of peristalsis | Complete absence of peristalsis |
| Diffuse esophageal spasm | > 20% simultaneous contractions[a] | >55% simultaneous contractions upright, or >80% simultaneous contractions night[b] |
| Nutcracker esophagus | Mean amplitude >180 mm Hg[a] | Mean amplitude >105 mm Hg[b] |
| Nonspecific motor disorder | >20% multipeaked contractions,[a] or >20% interrupted contractions,[a] or >20% dropped contractions,[a] or >20% not transmitted contractions,[a] or Mean amplitude <30 mm Hg[c] | >20% multipeaked contractions,[b] or >20% isolated contractions,[b] or Mean amplitude <25 mm Hg[d] |

[a]> mean + 2 SD of 50 healthy volunteers.
[b]> mean + 2 SD of 25 healthy volunteers.
[c]< mean − 2 SD of 50 healthy volunteers.
[d]< mean − 2 SD of 25 healthy volunteers.

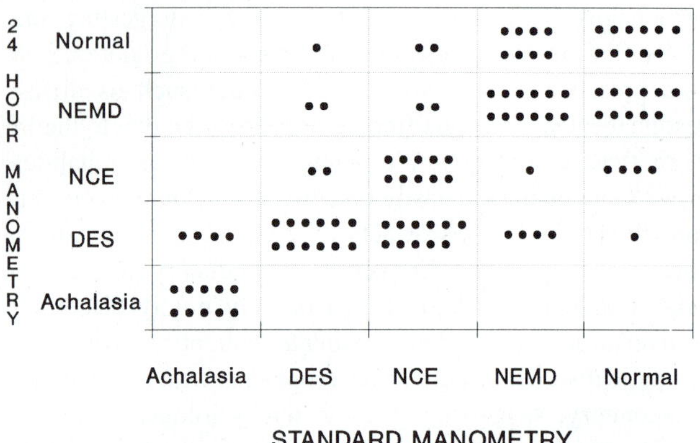


**Figure 39–27.** Classification of esophageal motor disorders in 108 patients with dysphagia or noncardiac chest pain according to the findings at conventional or ambulatory 24-hour manometry. Each dot represents one patient with his or her diagnosis from conventional manometry on the x axis and the diagnosis from 24-hour manometry on the y axis. DES = diffuse esophageal spasm, NCE = nutcracker esophagus, NEMD = nonspecific esophageal motor disorder.

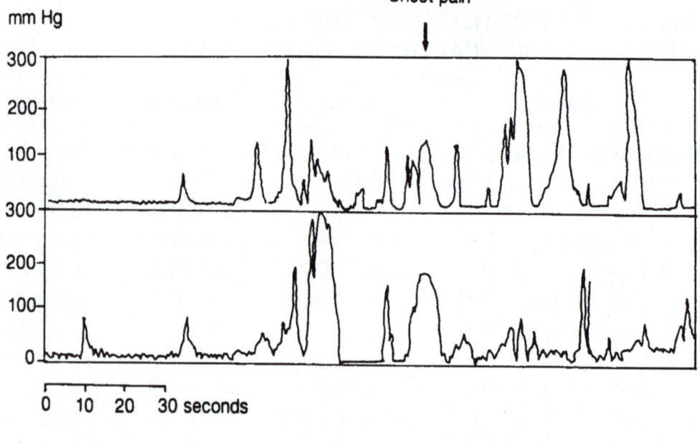


**Figure 39–28.** Section of an ambulatory esophageal motility record of a patient with nutcracker esophagus. In this patient esophageal motor function was monitored with two pressure transducers located 5 (bottom tracing) and 10 cm above (top tracing) the LES. The patient pressed the event button (*arrow*) at the onset of chest pain.

centage of waves are still peristaltic, then the loss of these peristaltic waves by the myotomy may add to the dysphagia.

Since its introduction in 1985, ambulatory esophageal manometry has been used primarily to identify esophageal motility abnormalities as the cause of noncardiac chest pain. Esophageal contractions of high amplitude or long duration have been suggested to be responsible for esophageal chest pain.[66–68] Contrary to this belief, ambulatory motility monitoring shows that the amplitude and duration of esophageal contractions associated with chest pain are similar to contractions during the asymptomatic recording periods.[61] Rather, the abnormal motor activity associated with the pain is characterized by an increased frequency of contractions immediately before and during the symptom. These contractions are mainly simultaneous, double and triple-peaked, and have a high amplitude, or they are of long duration (Figs. 39–28 and 39–29). These observations suggest that, similar to the heart, esophageal blood supply may be interrupted during bursts of abnormal esophageal contractions. This may become critical in situations in which the resting blood flow to the esophagus is already compromised, as has been shown for the hypertrophic esophageal muscle in patients with severe esophageal motor disorders.[69] A burst of disorganized motor activity in this situation may give rise to ischemic pain. Consequently, chest pain caused by a burst of uncoordinated esophageal motor activity under ischemic conditions has been termed *esophageal claudication.*[61,70] This theory has been supported by results of cold perfusion studies. Compared with healthy people, patients with esophageal motor disorders and chest pain have slower rewarming of the esophagus after an exposure to cold liquid, reflecting a reduction in blood flow or mild ischemia. The ability of the esophagus to produce these bursts of abnormal activity can be eliminated by a long esophageal myotomy (Fig. 39–30).[61,71]

For patients with symptoms and objective evidence of gastroesophageal reflux, 24-hour esophageal motility monitoring has several important applications. Esophageal clearance function can be assessed by the prevalence of efficient esophageal contractions, that is, peristaltic contractions with an amplitude greater than 30 mm Hg,[72] over an entire circadian period. Twenty-four-hour monitoring also has shown that esophageal contractility deteriorates with increasing severity of esophageal mucosal injury (Fig. 39–31).[73] The compromised clearance activity in this situation prolongs esophageal exposure to refluxed gastric juice, as indicated by the increased frequency of reflux episodes that last longer than 5 minutes in these patients.[74] Thus, a vicious circle is established. Because deteriorated contraction may not recover even after a successful antireflux operation,[75] an operation to correct the mechanically defective LES should be performed early in the course of the disease and before the development of organ failure. Once effective contractility has been lost, the surgical approach may have to be altered by the use of a repair with less outflow resistance, that is, a partial fundoplication. Assessment of esophageal clearance function by ambulatory motility monitoring in patients with GERD helps identify these patients.

Ambulatory esophageal motility monitoring allows for more precise classification of esophageal motility disorders than does conventional manometry and can help identify abnormal esophageal motor patterns associated with nonobstructive dysphagia, noncardiac chest pain, or gastroesophageal reflux. Ambulatory esophageal manometry, therefore, should replace stationary manometry in the assessment of esophageal body function. It also has the poten-

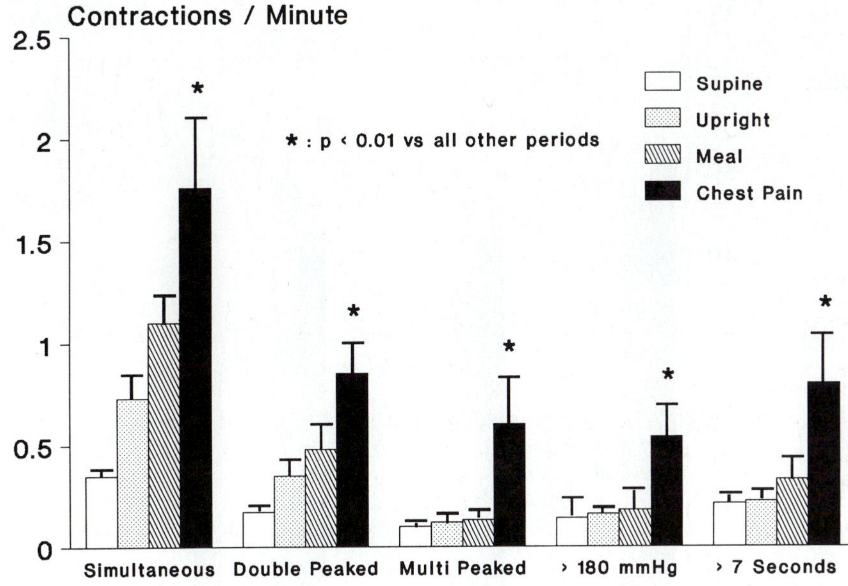


**Figure 39–29.** Frequency of simultaneous, double-peaked, multipeaked, high amplitude (>180 mm Hg), and long duration (>7 sec) contractions during the supine, upright, meal, and chest pain episodes. **P* < .01 vs all other periods.

tial to improve the diagnosis and treatment of patients with esophageal motor abnormalities.

## Three-Dimensional Imaging of the Lower Esophageal Sphincter

As previously discussed, manometric evaluation of the high-pressure zone at the gastroesophageal junction is usually performed by means of measuring the peak resting pressure or the pressure at the respiratory inversion point. Several studies have confirmed that this single pressure measurement is lower in patients with increased esophageal exposure to gastric juice than in healthy people and decreases with increasing severity of mucosal injury.[30,76] Despite this correlation, the method has been shown to be inadequate in identifying individual patients with mechanically defective sphincters because of the large overlap with healthy people.[33] A large number of patients with an adequate sphincter pressure at stationary manometry have increased esophageal acid exposure at 24-hour pH monitoring.

Studies have shown that the overall sphincter length and the length of the abdominal component are important in determining overall sphincter resistance, in that an overall length or abdominal length below the fifth percentile of normal can nullify a normal sphincter pressure.[15,32] Patients with low-normal values of each of these components, however, still can have an incompetent sphincter.[33] Consequently, simple measurement of the resting pressure, overall length, and abdominal length of the sphincter is insufficient to identify subtle mechanical defects in the sphincter that may result in increased esophageal acid exposure.

From a mechanical standpoint, the pressures exerted at each point over the entire length and around the circumference of the sphincter must be considered as contributing to the overall sphincter resistance. Bombeck et al[77] were the first to report on the use of radially measured sphincter pressures in the assessment of patients with GERD. Applying sophisticated computer technology, they analyzed the three-dimensional sphincter pressure profile obtained by a rapid pullback of a catheter with four to six radial side holes located at the same level. The concept of sphincter pressure vector volume was introduced as a parameter that integrates sphincter pressures exerted around the circumference and along the entire length of the sphincter into one value that represents LES resistance. Studies in our laboratory subsequently revealed that four radially oriented side holes are

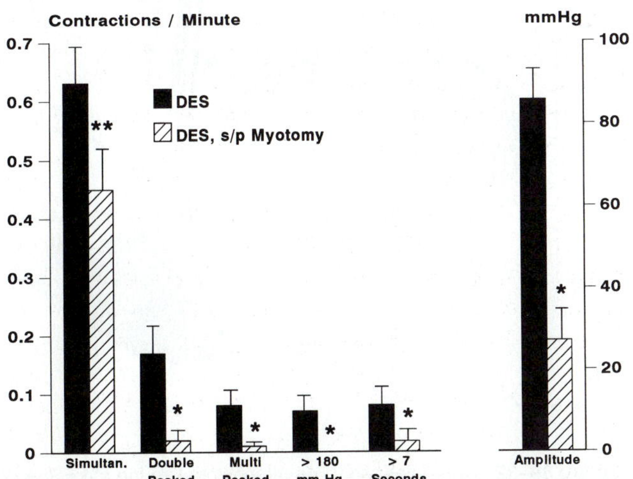


**Figure 39–30.** Frequency of simultaneous, double-peaked, multipeaked, high amplitude (>180 mm Hg), and long duration (>7 sec) contractions and mean contraction amplitude in patients with untreated diffuse esophageal spasm (DES) and patients who had undergone a long esophageal myotomy. **P* < .01 vs untreated DES.

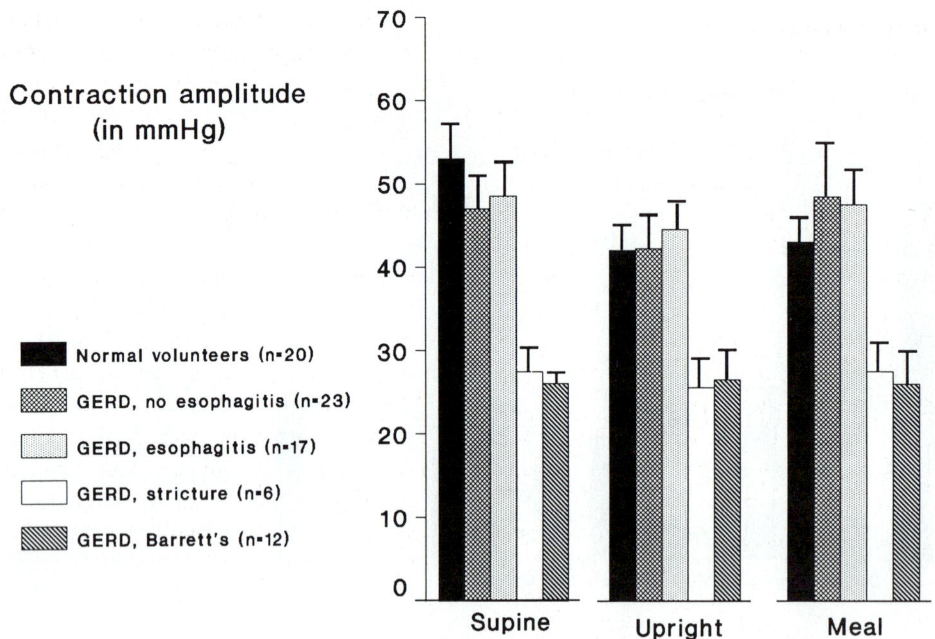


**Figure 39–31.** Mean amplitude of contractions and frequency of ineffective contractions, i.e., contractions with an amplitude less than 30 mm Hg, during the upright, supine, and meal periods in healthy volunteers and patients with gastroesophageal reflux disease (GERD) and various degrees of esophageal mucosal injury at endoscopy.

sufficient for reliable evaluation of sphincter pressure vector volume and that a stepwise pullback technique with a catheter containing radial side holes at the same level, or placed sequentially at 5 cm intervals, is superior to a rapid pullback in differentiating patients with GERD from healthy people.[78] A catheter with four sequential radial side holes used in a stepwise pullback allows evaluation of esophageal body function in the same setting and is, thus, the method of choice (Fig. 39–32). In addition, calculation of the sphincter pressure vector volume by this technique is not complex and does not require sophisticated computerized data acquisition and analysis systems.

Evaluation of the three-dimensional sphincter pressure profile in a large population of patients with increased esophageal acid exposure showed that both total and abdominal sphincter pressure vector volumes were markedly lower than in 50 healthy volunteers and decreased with increasing severity of mucosal injury (Fig. 39–33). Although it is tempting to ascribe the loss of sphincter function to inflammation or tissue damage, the observation of a low sphincter pressure vector volume in the absence of mucosal damage suggests that the loss of sphincter resistance is primary and probably due to smooth muscle abnormalities.[21]

Calculation of sphincter pressure vector volume did not provide an advantage over conventional manometric techniques in detecting a defective sphincter in patients with advanced complications of GERD, but did increase the sensitivity of manometry in identifying a mechanically defective sphincter in patients with increased esophageal acid exposure but no mucosal damage (Fig. 39–34). This indicates that conventional manometric techniques, that is, measurement of sphincter pressure, overall length, and abdominal length, can reliably identify gross sphincter defects but are insufficient to detect subtle sphincter abnormalities.

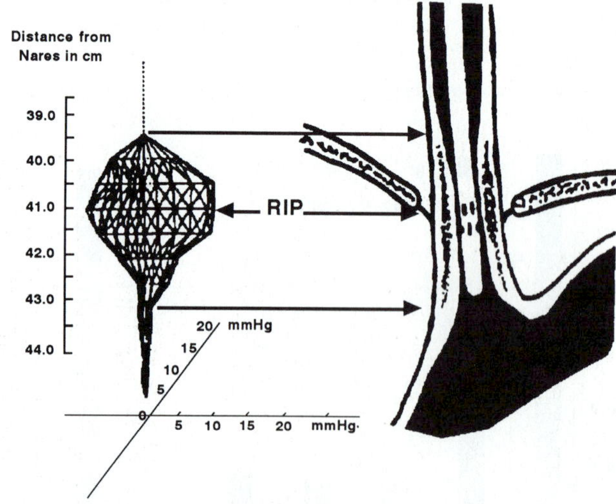


**Figure 39–32.** Computerized three-dimensional image of LES. A catheter with four to eight radial side holes is withdrawn through the gastroesophageal junction. For each level of the pullback, the radially measured pressures are plotted around an axis that represents gastric baseline pressure. When a stepwise pullback technique is used, the respiratory inversion point (RIP) can be identified.

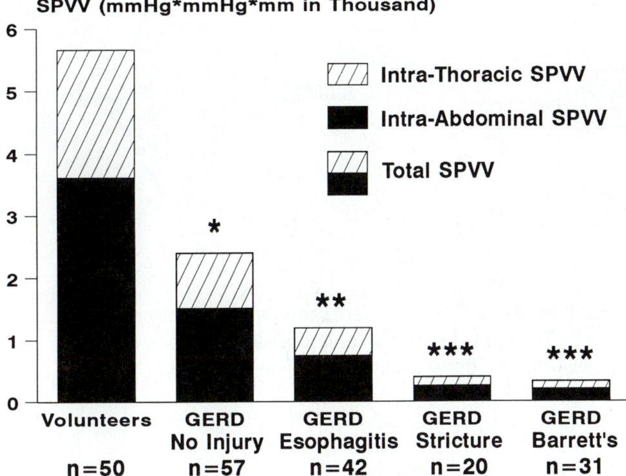


**Figure 39–33.** Mean total and intra-abdominal sphincter pressure vector volume (SPVV) in 50 healthy volunteers and 150 patients with gastroesophageal reflux disease (GERD) and various degrees of mucosal damage. *P* values are given for total and intra-abdominal SPVV. $^*P < .01$ vs volunteers, $^{**}P < .01$ vs volunteers and GERD patients with no mucosal injury, $^{***}P < .01$ vs all other groups.

Despite three-dimensional sphincter imaging in assessing sphincter resistance, a number of patients still have increased esophageal acid exposure and an apparently normal LES. Marked asymmetry of the sphincter, which is not taken into account when calculating the sphincter pressure vector volume, may be responsible for reflux in some of these patients.[79] In the other patients, other causes of increased esophageal exposure to gastric juice are likely to be present. In such patients, a careful evaluation of esophageal body function, gastric emptying, gastric acid secretion, and duodenogastric reflux should be performed.[80]

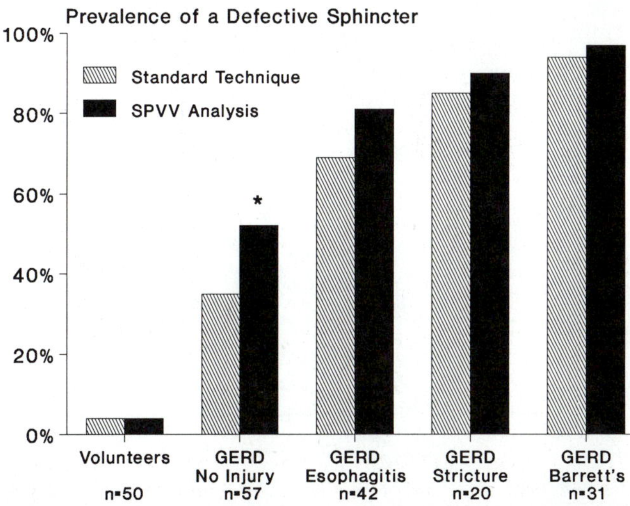


**Figure 39–34.** Comparison of standard manometric techniques and sphincter pressure vector volume (SPVV) analysis in the identification of a mechanically defective LES. $^*P < .05$ vs conventional manometry.

In patients with increased esophageal acid exposure due to abnormality of the LES, reconstruction of a functional sphincter with an antireflux procedure effectively abolishes reflux more than 90% of the time.[47] Our studies demonstrated that this result is achieved by increasing the total and abdominal sphincter pressure vector volume to normal after either a Nissen or a Belsey fundoplication (Figs. 39–35 and 39–36).[78] Failure to return this sphincter pressure profile to normal is associated with persistent or recurrent reflux (Fig. 39–37).

In summary, calculation of the sphincter pressure vector volume increases the sensitivity of manometry in identifying a mechanically defective LES, allowing identification of patients who would benefit from an antireflux procedure before the development of mucosal injury and loss of esophageal body function. This manometric technique should become the standard for the evaluation of the LES in patients with GERD.

## ESOPHAGEAL PH TESTS

### The pH Electrode Withdrawal Test

The gastric pH electrode was developed by Tuttle and Grossman in collaboration with the Beckman Instrument Company and was introduced for assessment of the cardia in 1958.[81] In this test, a pH electrode is passed into the stomach and then slowly withdrawn in a stepwise manner across the distal esophageal segment into the midesophagus. Healthy people demonstrate a sharp rise in pH from intragastric acid levels to a pH of 5–7 in the esophagus. Usually this rise occurs over a short 1- to 2-cm distance. Patients with a severely incompetent cardia may have no rise in pH across the distal esophageal segment, or a gradual slope in the elevation of the pH tracing. This procedure was the original esophageal pH test. Unfortunately, subsequent analysis showed that the test has a false-positive rate of approximately 20%, presumably because of adherence of acid mucus to the glass electrode, and a similarly high false-negative rate. As a result, this simple test of the cardia has been abandoned in favor of more quantitative methods of measuring reflux with the pH electrode.

### Standard Acid Reflux Test

In the standard acid reflux test (SART), after esophageal manometry, a pH electrode is introduced to a position 5 cm above the top of the LES. A manometric catheter is then placed temporarily in the stomach, and a load of 300 mL of 0.1N HCl is introduced, for an average-sized adult. The acid load is reduced accordingly in small people. The manometric catheter is flushed and then pulled back into the body of the esophagus. The patient is asked to perform a series of respiratory maneuvers (deep breathing, Valsalva

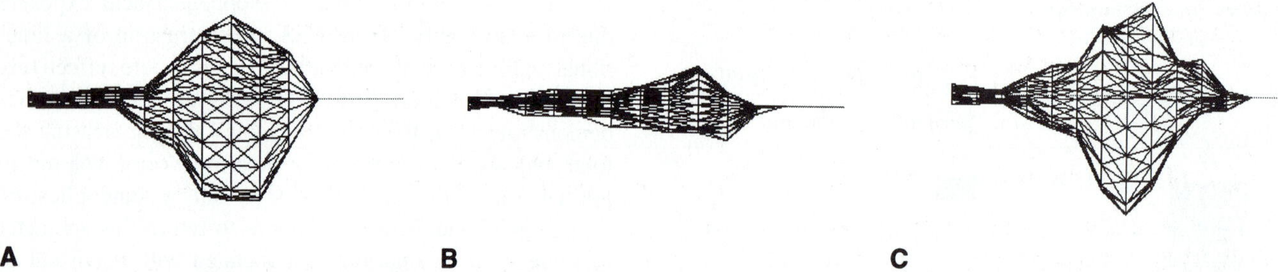


**Figure 39–35. A.** Three-dimensional LES pressure profile in a healthy volunteer. **B.** Profile in a patient with a mechanically defective sphincter. **C.** Profile in same patient as in **B** 1 year after Nissen fundoplication. The pressure profile was obtained by means of a stepwise pullback of eight radially oriented pressure transducers. Radial pressures along the gastroesophageal junction are plotted around an axis that represents the gastric baseline pressure.

and Muller maneuvers, and coughing) in four different body positions (supine, right and left lateral decubitus, and 20° head-down), providing 16 different challenge positions for the cardia. Among 90 healthy young volunteers, more than two reflux episodes in this study occurred in only two volunteers. Accordingly, one or two drops in pH during these challenges to the cardia are considered normal, and three or more drops in pH are taken as evidence of incompetence of the cardia. Patients with severe reflux may be unable to clear acid from the esophagus after reflux has been documented. If reflux of acid occurs and cannot be cleared, a maximal score is recorded. Although approximately 20% of patients who have abnormal reflux documented by other tests, particularly prolonged pH monitoring, may have a normal SART, 80% have an abnormal SART. Consequently, false-positives of three or more reflux episodes are sufficiently infrequent to make this test valuable in clinical practice. The test is simple to interpret and can be readily performed in an outpatient setting.[14]

## Acid Clearance Test

For penetration of the esophageal mucosa by acid to occur and cause esophagitis, both reflux and the persistent contact of gastric contents with the esophageal mucosa are required. The acid clearance test is a method to assess the ability of the esophagus to remove regurgitated gastric contents. The test is performed immediately after esophageal manometry and SART, at the same sitting. The pH electrode is left in position 5 cm above the LES, and 15 mL of 0.1N HCl is instilled through the proximal manometric catheter, 10 cm above the tip of the probe. The patient is asked to swallow at 30-sec intervals. Healthy young volunteers normally clear the bolus of acid from the esophagus back to a pH greater than 5 with fewer than 10 swallows. Abnormal acid clearance is identified when a large number of swallows are required or when the acid cannot be cleared at all. The results of the acid clearance test show a statistically significant correlation with the presence of proved

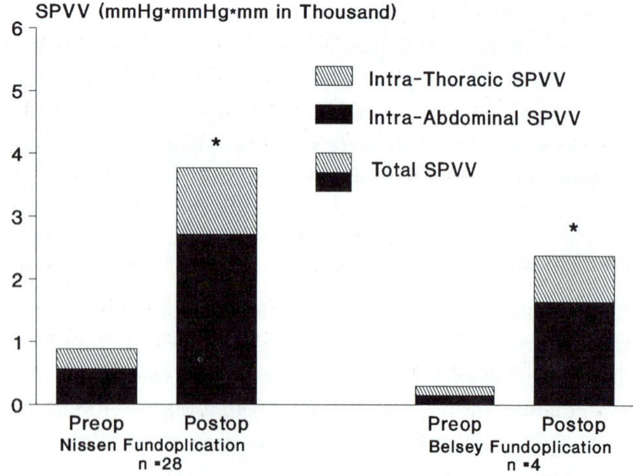


**Figure 39–36.** Effect of the Nissen (N = 28) and Belsey (N = 4) fundoplication on the sphincter pressure vector volume (SPVV). *$P < .001$ vs preoperative values.

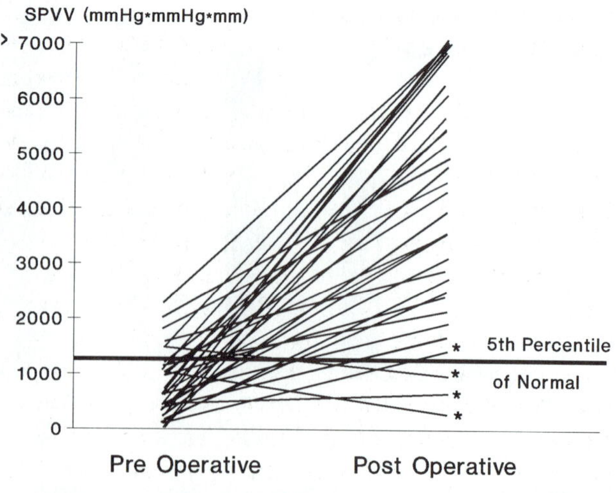


**Figure 39–37.** Individual pre- and postoperative sphincter pressure vector volumes (SPVV) in 32 patients who underwent antireflux operations. *Patients with persistent or recurrent reflux.

esophagitis and with the duration of reflux episodes observed during overnight pH monitoring. This test, in essence, evaluates esophageal motor function and should not be confused with a test for reflux.[82]

### 24-hour pH Monitoring

Prolonged recording of pH in the distal esophagus with an ambulatory recorder provides the most sensitive method of analyzing complicated esophageal problems thought to be associated with reflux.[83,84] The pH electrode is left in position 5 cm above the manometrically demonstrated LES. A variety of arrangements for a reference electrode have been used. We have found that the use of the combined probe and reference electrode provides a reliable and dependable method of completing the circuit. Esophageal pH is monitored continuously while the patient goes through a 24-hour cycle, in the hospital or at home, eating, sleeping, walking, sitting, and following a normal routine. An acid reflux episode is scored when the pH drops below 4, and alkaline reflux is determined when the pH rises above 7. The patient's intake is restricted to foods with a pH between 5 and 6; the use of a standardized diet to minimize variables is helpful.[85] The patient is asked to record the duration of meals, various body positions assumed, and the occurrence of symptoms of any type, so that reflux episodes can be related to such events. Computer analysis of the completed tracing allows determination of the cumulative acid or alkaline exposure in both the upright and supine positions, the frequency of reflux episodes per 24 hours, the number of episodes that last 5 minutes or longer, and the duration of the longest episode (Fig. 39–38). The relation of symptoms such as chest pain, heartburn, cough, wheezing, and regurgitation to reflux episodes is determined from observation of their relative timing (Fig. 39–39).

A quantitative scoring system has been developed on the basis of studies in healthy volunteers. To simplify data presentation, the following three units are used: cumulative time the pH is less than 4 expressed as the percentage of total, upright, and supine times; the frequency of a pH drop below 4 expressed as the number of episodes per 24 hours; and the duration the pH stayed below 4 expressed as the number of episodes lasting longer than 5 minutes and the duration in minutes of the longest episode. This gives six components to express the 24-hour pH record (Fig. 39–40).

The value of 24-hour pH monitoring has been enhanced considerably by the availability of portable microprocessor data recorders, which allow monitoring on an ambulatory basis, including the patient's normal range of activities. The test has proved to be extremely accurate and reproducible, with surprisingly little variation between inpatient and outpatient studies. Another advancement of this test has been the ability to simultaneously monitor intraesophageal and intragastric pH levels with separate electrodes placed above and below the LES. Such an arrangement allows documentation of alkaline reflux episodes, which can then be compared with data obtained from healthy people who serve as controls.[34] This technique, which recognizes the interactions between various foregut abnormalities, is beginning to be used routinely in specialized units. It enables the correlation of GERD with disorders of antroduodenal motility (Fig. 39–41).

### Application of Manometry and pH Testing

For a patient whose symptoms suggest GERD and in whom endoscopy has shown unequivocal evidence of reflux or esophagitis, manometry and pH recording are clearly not necessary to establish a diagnosis. These studies should be performed, however, before any surgical antireflux procedure is done. They provide useful information in quantifying and categorizing the pattern of reflux and coexisting motility disorders, and they identify a mechanically defective sphincter.[33] A group at risk can be identified, such as people with predominantly supine reflux, high acid scores, mechanically defective sphincters and associated motility problems, in whom aggressive treatment is needed and who are likely to require surgical correction to prevent permanent esophageal damage. Furthermore, the identification of very high acid scores or a predominantly alkaline refluxate may indicate the need to modify the antireflux operation to incorporate either proximal gastric vagotomy or a bile diversion procedure as a necessary adjunct. When symptoms are atypical, or when findings at endoscopy are equivocal, manometry and pH recording are essential to differentiate the symptoms from those of other foregut disorders such as esophageal dysmotility, peptic ulceration, bile reflux gastritis, and biliary tract disease.

It is our opinion that 24-hour ambulatory pH monitoring is indicated for (1) all patients with typical symptoms of GERD in whom the diagnosis is in question on the basis of other diagnostic tests; (2) all patients who fulfill the other criteria for needing an antireflux operation, so objective evidence of a mechanically defective cardia can be obtained and incompetence confirmed as responsible for the patient's symptoms; (3) patients with unexplained laryngeal symptoms or atypical symptoms of GERD, such as nonanginal chest pain, unexplained cough, or wheezing; (4) patients in whom gastric hypersecretion or bile reflux gastritis is suspected; (5) patients with dysphagia and an esophageal motor disorder that might be secondary to GERD; (6) pediatric or other patients who are unable to communicate their symptoms and in whom a diagnosis of GERD is suspected; and (7) all patients who have undergone esophageal or gastric operations who present with recurrent symptoms.

### Radionuclide Studies

The use of radioisotopes in the investigation of esophageal disease has the attraction that the tests are relatively nonin-

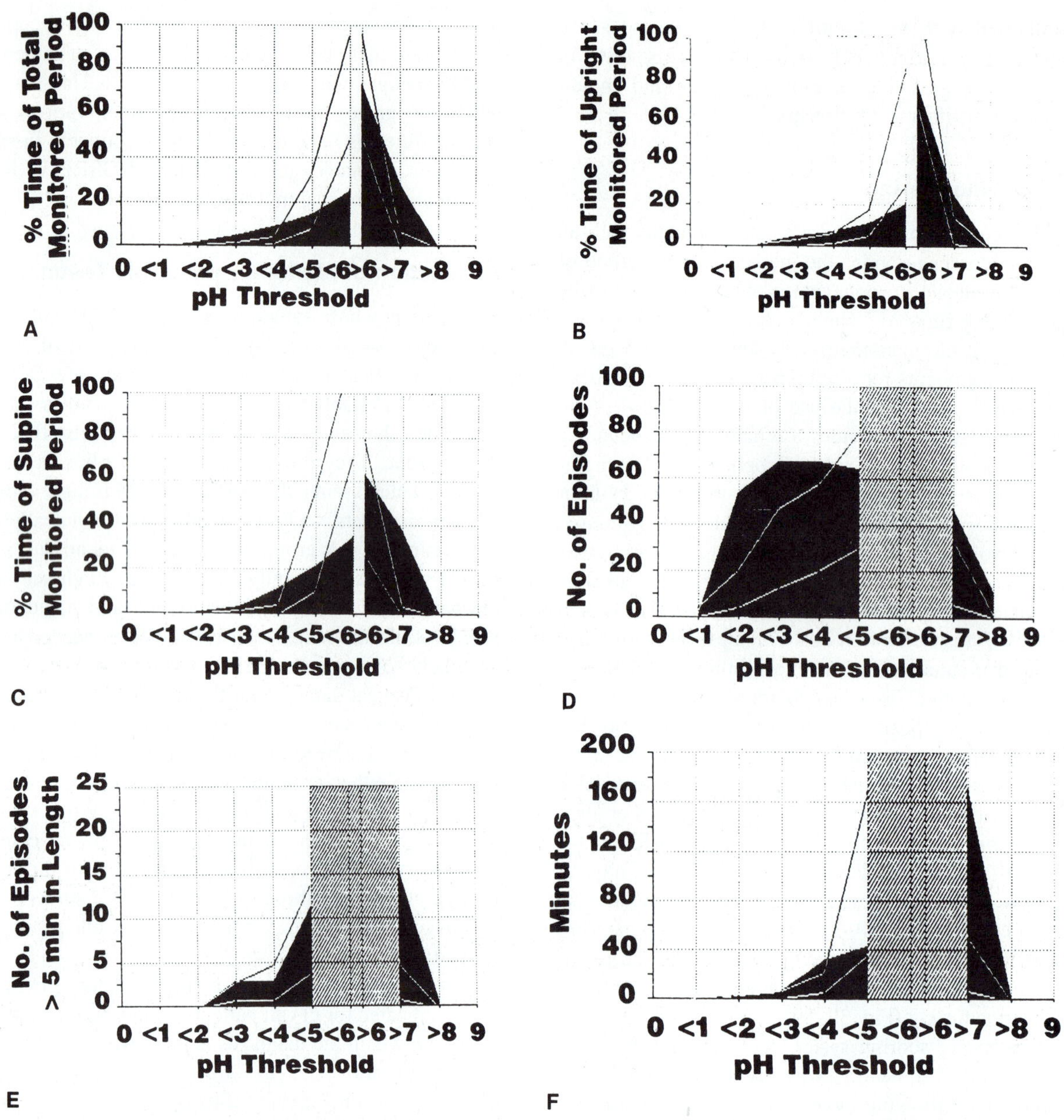


**Figure 39–38.** Graphic display of ESOpHOGRAM (24-hour pH monitoring software package) for whole pH threshold values. Graphs show median and 95th percentile levels in 50 healthy volunteers. Gray area in D, E, F represents the normal pH environment of the esophagus with exposure to pH outside of gray area representing reflux episodes. The *black area* represents measurements made in a patient. When the black area exceeds the 95th percentile line for a given pH threshold, the patient is considered to have an abnormal value for the component measured. **A.** Percentage cumulative exposure for total time less than 1–6 and greater than 6–8. **B.** Percentage cumulative exposure for upright time less than 1–6 and greater than 6–8. **C.** Percentage cumulative exposure for supine time less than 1–6 and greater than 6–8. **D.** Number of episodes. **E.** Number of episodes lasting longer than 5 minutes. **F.** Length of longest reflux episode.

vasive. Radioisotopes have been used in the following situations relevant to esophageal disease:

1. Localization of Barrett's columnar-lined esophagus.
2. Diagnosis and quantitation of GERD.
3. Measurement of esophageal transit.
4. Detection of duodenogastric bile reflux.
5. Measurement of gastric emptying.

## Localization of Barrett's Columnar-lined Esophagus

Berquist et al[86] described a small series in which intravenous $^{99m}$Tc pertechnetates were used to localize gastric mucosa in Barrett's columnar-lined esophagus. The number of patients with and those without Barrett's esophagus was too small to draw meaningful conclusions, and there is no evidence to suggest that the more clinically significant in-

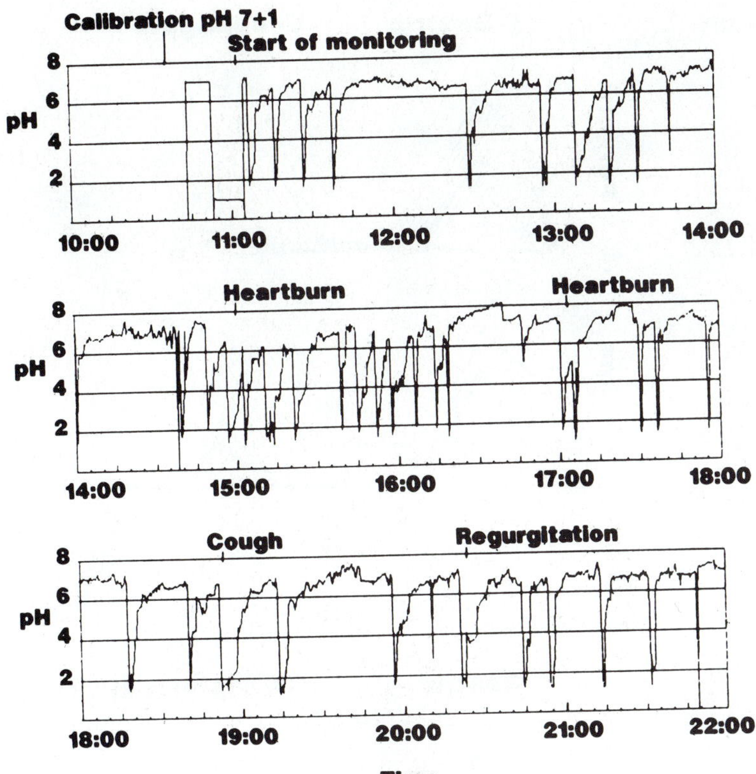


**Figure 39–39.** Plotting of pH values over time, with times at which symptoms occurred. Plotting allows correlation of symptoms with changes in pH to determine if the changes are reflux-induced.

testinal metaplasia can be detected. In any event, endoscopic and histologic diagnosis must remain the standard of reference. The use of radionuclide studies in this area has not been widely applied.

## Diagnosis and Quantitation of GERD

The attractive concept of detecting gastroesophageal reflux with scintigraphy was investigated by Fisher et al[87] using

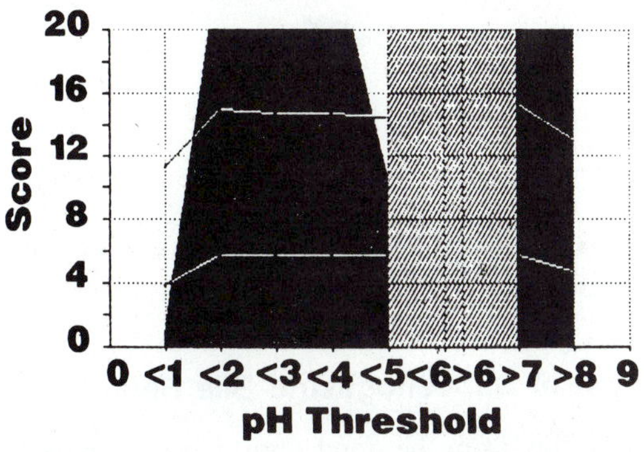


**Figure 39–40.** Composite score used to express the overall pH result. The *white lines* represent the median score and the 97.5 percentile of 50 healthy volunteers. *Gray area* represents normal pH environment of the esophagus. The *black area* represents the score of a patient at various pH thresholds. If the black area surpasses the 97.5 percentile time at a specific pH, the patient has excessive esophageal exposure at that pH. A pH level of 4 has been the standard.

$^{99m}$Tc sulfur colloid. The isotope, diluted with isotonic saline solution, was instilled into the stomach via a nasogastric tube. Serial gastroesophageal scans were performed as abdominal pressure was progressively increased by means of a pneumatic abdominal binder. Quantitation of reflux was attempted by calculating a reflux index that related counts of isotope activity in the esophagus to those in the stomach. A subsequent study[88] reported statistically significant correlation between the reflux index, symptom scores, and degree of endoscopic esophagitis.

Although high sensitivity is reported for the scintigraphic detection of GERD, the test is not physiologic, because of the necessity to use abdominal compression, and because the test is conducted over a relatively short period of time. There is a paucity of studies using the technique in healthy volunteers and comparing the results with those of 24-hour ambulatory pH monitoring. Thus, the true predictive value is difficult to assess.

## Measurement of Esophageal Transit

Radioisotopes have been used in the measurement of esophageal transit and the detection of motility disorders. Most studies involved an isotopically labelled liquid bolus of $^{99m}$Tc sulfur colloid in 10 mL of water instilled into the mouth and subsequently swallowed.[89,90] Computer images are made at areas of interest and processed to produce a clearance curve. Healthy people require 4–15 seconds to achieve 90% clearance of the esophagus. Prolonged clear-

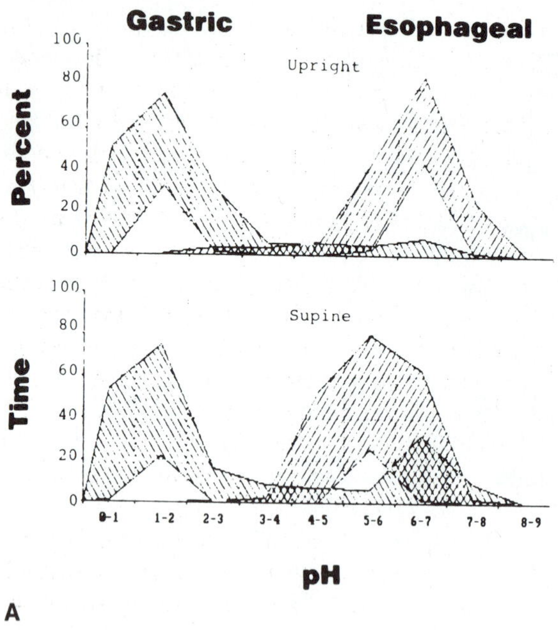


B

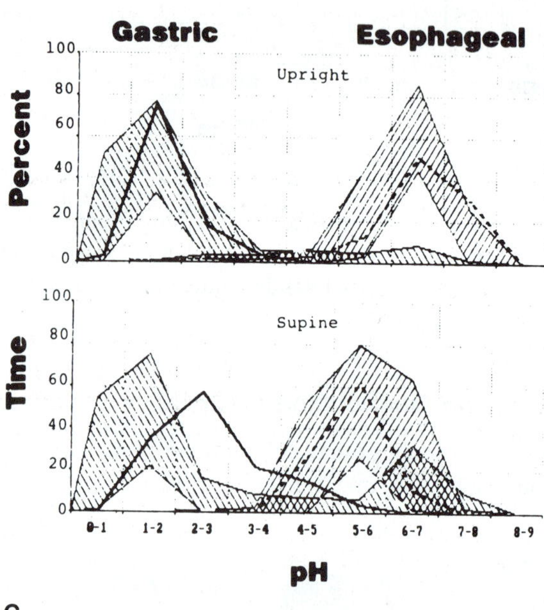


**Figure 39–41.** Computer graphic display showing simultaneous pH exposure of the esophagus and stomach as percentage of time for which the pH level was in a given range (1–2, 2–3, 3–4, etc.) during the upright and supine portions of the monitored period. **A.** The *hatched area* shows the normal pH exposure of the stomach (left) and esophagus (right). **B.** The *solid black line* is the gastric pH exposure of a patient plotted against a background of normal gastric exposure. The *dashed line* is the esophageal pH exposure plotted against a background of normal esophageal exposure. Note that the esophageal exposure has shifted to the left, indicating a loss of separation between the stomach and esophageal compartment because of gastroesophageal reflux. **C.** A study obtained in a patient with duodenogastric reflux, which has caused a shift of the patient's supine gastric pH to the right *(solid black line)* while esophageal pH exposure remains normal *(dashed line).* This represents duodenal gastric reflux which alkalizes the gastric pH environment. This type of analysis is very helpful in sorting out complex abnormalities of the foregut.

ance times are demonstrated in achalasia, scleroderma, diffuse esophageal spasm, and nonspecific motility disorders. The technique has been compared with manometry and found to have an overall sensitivity of 75%, compared with 83% for manometry and 30% for conventional barium radiography. Radionuclide transit is less reliable than manometry in detecting nutcracker esophagus and hypertensive LES. In some patients, abnormalities detected in scintigraphic transit were not confirmed with manometry.[91]

Although radionuclide transit undoubtedly provides useful information noninvasively, it has limitations as a screening test for motility disorders, for the aforementioned reasons. The limitations also may be due to the use of a liquid bolus in most studies. Encouraging results are emerging with the use of an isotopically labelled solid bolus.[92,96]

### Detection of Duodenogastric Bile Reflux

Alkaline reflux from the duodenum into the stomach, and into the esophagus, can be detected by $^{99m}$Tc HIDA dynamic biliary imaging.[93] The isotope is injected IV, is excreted by the hepatocytes into the biliary system, and is then passed into the duodenum. Sequential computer images can be produced, with the stomach and esophagus as areas of interest, to detect alkaline duodenogastric reflux and gastroesophageal reflux. False-positive and false-negative results are not uncommon, a situation not helped by the fact that duodenogastric reflux may be an intermittent phenomenon and, indeed, occasionally occurs physiologically. The use of this method will likely diminish with the increasing availability of simultaneous esophageal and gastric pH monitoring and the fiberoptic bile probe, discussed later, which appear to be more accurate tests of alkaline reflux.

## Measurement of Gastric Emptying

Delayed gastric emptying may be of considerable relevance to the pathogenesis of GERD in some patients. Conventional barium radiography is relatively inaccurate, except in gross disturbances. Radioisotopic clearance studies, however, using $^{113}$In for liquids and $^{99m}$Tc sulfur colloid-labeled egg or chicken liver for solids, have been much more accurate. Labeled oatmeal appears to be the best compromise, being easily available and providing curves very similar to those obtained with labeled chicken liver. Several studies have shown impaired gastric emptying in as many as 40% of patients with GERD,[46,94,95] predominantly those with supine reflux.[32] This phenomenon presumably is related to the frequent coexistence of delayed esophageal transit and delayed gastric emptying in patients with GERD,[47] reinforcing the viewpoint that GERD may be a component of a diffuse foregut motility disorder.

## Bilirubin Monitoring in the Esophagus with a Fiberoptic Probe

Reflux of alkaline duodenal contents into the stomach and esophagus is being increasingly recognized as an important physiologic factor in GERD. About 25% of patients with gastroesophageal reflux have recurrent, progressive disease, while undergoing medical therapy.[96] The disease is manifested by erosive esophagitis that advances to complications such as stricture, ulceration or Barrett's esophagus. Evidence is accumulating that the composition of the refluxed gastric juice plays an important role in the development of this progressive mucosal injury.[97,98] Studies in animals have shown marked augmentation of the acid-induced mucosal injury by the presence of components of duodenal juice.[99,100] Clinical observations have shown that the prevalence of complications such as esophagitis, stricture, and Barrett's esophagus in patients with GERD is related to an increased esophageal exposure to both acid and alkali, and the severity of these complications is greater in patients with acid-alkaline reflux as compared with acid reflux alone.[101] Prolonged ambulatory esophageal aspiration studies of the refluxate in the esophagus have shown an increase in bile acids in patients with severe esophagitis and Barrett's esophagus.[102] These observations strongly suggest a noxious and synergistic role of components of duodenal juice in the refluxed gastric juice.

An ambulatory monitoring system has been developed[103,104] that allows spectrophotometric measurement of luminal bilirubin concentration over a long time. Bilirubin is used as a marker for measurement of the time of esophageal exposure to duodenal contents while the patient is going about normal daily activities, eating, and sleeping. The apparatus consists of a portable optoelectronic data logger that can be passed transnasally and positioned 5 cm above the manometrically determined upper border of the LES (Bilitec 2000, by SRL, Florence, Italy, and Prodotec, by Synectics, Dallas, Texas). The tip of the probe contains a 2-mm space for sampling. Fluids and blenderized solids can easily flow through the space and their bilirubin concentration can be measured (Fig. 39–42). The probes are flexible, durable, reusable, and easy to sterilize. For a detailed discussion of the manner in which these probes function, see the excellent review by Kauer et al.[105]

The optimal absorbance range for the Bilitec 2000 is 0.14–0.5.[103] When combined with a strictly controlled diet, the absorbance threshold of 0.2 in healthy volunteers shows minimal esophageal exposure to bilirubin while still allowing a large range above this level to detect increased esophageal exposure to duodenal juice in patients.[105]

According to this absorbance threshold of 0.14, patients with GERD have elevated esophageal exposure to bilirubin. No difference is observed in bilirubin exposure between patients with reflux without mucosal injury and healthy controls. Patients with GERD and erosive esophagitis or Barrett's esophagus, however, have increased esophageal bilirubin exposure, indicating that the gastric content refluxed is a mixture of gastric and duodenal juice (Fig. 39–43). The highest bilirubin exposure occurs in patients with Barrett's esophagus. Attwood et al in 1989[106] and Stein in 1992[101] demonstrated the importance of mixed acid and alkaline reflux in causing mucosal injury. By performing simultaneous bilirubin and pH monitoring, Kauer et al were able to show exposure to bilirubin occurring when the esophageal pH was below 4 or between 4 and 7, when reflux of duodenal contents is undetectable with the

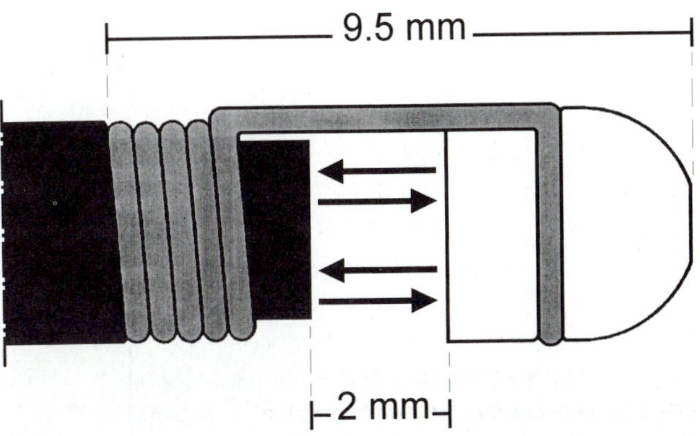


**Figure 39–42.** The tip of the fiberoptic probe with a 2-mm space for sampling. Fluid can easily move into and out of the space, and the presence of bilirubin can be detected because of its particular absorbance.

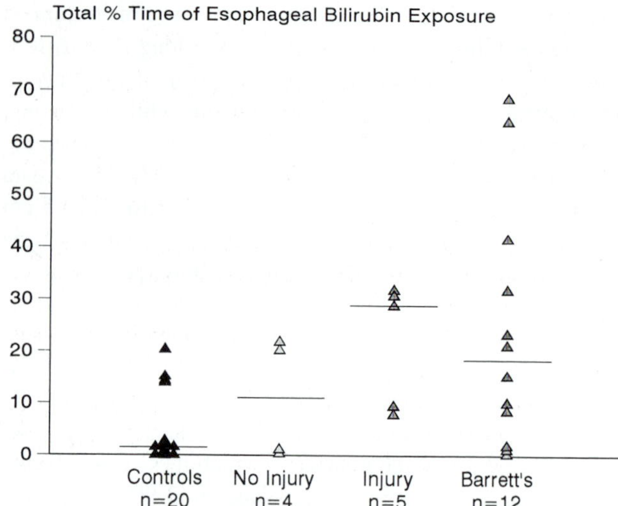


**Figure 39–43.** Percentage of total study period during which the esophageal mucosa of each subject was exposed to bilirubin (ie, above an absorbance of 0.2). Values for each subject are plotted and the median of each group is denoted by the *horizontal line*. Patients with mucosal injury and Barrett's esophagus had a significantly higher bilirubin absorbance compared with controls ($P < .004$, Mann-Whitney).

pH probe (Fig. 39–44).[105] Patients with Barrett's esophagus had a significantly higher bilirubin exposure than controls when the pH was less than 4 or between 4 and 7. The results of these studies suggest that the reflux of mixed gastric and duodenal juice into the esophagus may cause esophageal mucosal injury and that these reflux events may be asymptomatic because the esophageal pH remains within its normal range.

These findings may be a particularly important factor in the medical treatment of reflux esophagitis. Overall medical treatment is effective in the healing of 75% of patients with reflux esophagitis. In the other patients, reflux persists despite prolonged treatment with standard doses of acid suppression.[106] These patients are likely to have a mechanically defective LES and duodenogastroesophageal reflux. Under these conditions, acid suppression therapy reduces acid exposure and relieves heartburn while exposure to duodenal juice and neutralized gastric juice continues unabated. The resulting esophageal pH of 4–7 may provide the environment for continued mucosal damage from components in the neutralized refluxed gastric juice while the patient is experiencing symptomatic relief. An antireflux procedure prevents both acid and alkaline reflux and should, in these situations, be the treatment of choice.

The flexible photometric bile probe is a very useful and reliable complementary tool to esophageal pH monitoring in the examination of patients with foregut symptoms. Results from our laboratory show that reflux of duodenal juice, in addition to gastric juice, does occur in patients with severe GERD and that gastroesophageal reflux can occur at normal esophageal pH levels and go unnoticed when esophageal pH monitoring is performed in isolation. The combination of pH and bilirubin esophageal monitoring will further our understanding and improve our care of patients with GERD.

## CONCLUSION

The diversity of disease processes related to the esophagus and foregut poses challenges to clinicians. Only with a thorough understanding of both normal anatomy and physiology and the usual deviations from normal can a surgeon begin to approach the evaluation of these maladies in a systematic manner. Through a variety of diagnostic modalities much as been learned in recent years about the nature of benign esophageal disease. Ambulatory probes for measuring esophageal and gastric pH motility and bile reflux over prolonged periods has added to the information gained from stationary studies. Radiographic, endoscopic, and scintigraphic techniques have become more refined as well.

Although our understanding of basic esophageal and foregut pathophysiology has been expanded by these newer techniques, much remains to be learned, and the potential

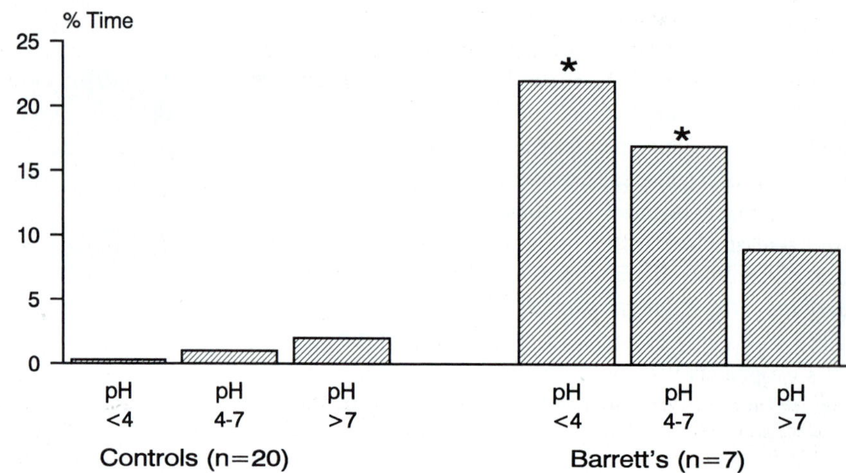


**Figure 39–44.** Percentage of time in the indicated pH intervals that the esophagus was exposed to bilirubin in controls and patients with Barrett's esophagus. Values are represented as medians. *Patients with Barrett's esophagus vs controls ($P < .01$, Mann-Whitney).

avenues for investigative research are numerous. Surgeons have led the way in many of these advances and will continue to do so. Only surgical specialists can offer a full array of diagnostic and therapeutic techniques and provide the care essential to the optimal well-being of patients with disorders of the foregut.

## REFERENCES


1. Keith A: A demonstration on diverticula of the alimentary tract of congenital or of obscure origin. *Br Med J* **1:**376, 1910
2. Davenport H: Motility. *Physiology of the Digestive Tract,* Part 1. Chicago, Year Book, 1962, pp 1–69
3. Dent J: What's new in the esophagus? *Dig Dis Sci* **26:**161–172, 1981
4. Cade CF, Creamer B, Schlegel JF: *An Atlas of Esophageal Motility in Health and Disease.* Springfield, Illinois, Thomas, 1981
5. Bosma JF: Deglutition: Pharyngeal stage. *Physiol Rev* **37:**275–300, 1957
6. Price LM, El-Sharkawy TY, Mui HY, Diamant NE: Effects of bilateral cervical vagotomy on balloon-induced lower esophageal sphincter relaxation in the dog. *Gastroenterology* **77:**324, 1979
7. Jenkinson LR, Norris TL, Watson A: Manometric function of the lower oesophageal sphincter and oesophageal body in reflux oesophagitis. *Br J Surg* **74:**323, 1987
8. Watson A, Jenkinson LR, Norris TL: Lower oesophageal sphincter characteristics after a simplified antireflux procedure. In Siewert JR, Hölscher AH (eds): *Diseases of the Esophagus.* New York, Springer-Verlag, 1987, pp 1180–1187
9. Fyke FE, Code DF, Schlegel JF: The gastroesophageal sphincter in healthy human beings. *Gastroenterologia (Basle)* **86:**135, 1956
10. Liebermann-Meffert D, Allgöwer M, Schneid P, Blum A: Muscular equivalent of the esophageal sphincter. *Gastroenterology* **76:**31–38, 1979
11. Diamant NE, Akin AW: Effect of gastric contractions on the lower esophageal sphincter. *Gastroenterology* **63:**38–44, 1982
12. Pettersson GB, Bombeck CT, Nyhus LM: The lower esophageal sphincter: Mechanisms of opening and closure. *Surgery* **88:** 307–314, 1980
13. Lind JF, Duthie HL, Schlegel JF, Code CF: Motility of the gastric fundus. *Am J Physiol* **201:**197–202, 1961
14. Skinner DB, Booth DJ: Assessment of distal esophageal function in patients with hiatal and/or gastroesophageal reflux. *Ann Surg* **172:**627, 1970
15. O'Sullivan GC, DeMeester TR, Joelsson BE, et al: Interaction of lower esophageal sphincter pressure and length of sphincter in the abdomen as determinants of gastroesophageal competence. *Am J Surg* **143:**40–47, 1982
16. Mazur JM, Skinner DB, Jones EL, Zuidema GD: Effect of transabdominal vagotomy on the human gastroesophageal high pressure zone. *Surgery* **73:**818–822, 1973
17. Goyal RK, Ratten S: Nature of the vagal inhibiting innervation to the lower esophageal sphincter. *J Clin Invest* **55:**1119–1126, 1975
18. Christensen J: Innervation and function of the esophagus. In Stipa S, Belsey RHR, Moraldi A (eds): *Medical and Surgical Problems of the Esophagus.* New York, Academic Press, 1981, pp 12–17
19. Castell DO: The lower esophageal sphincter: Physiologic and clinical aspects. *Ann Intern Med* **83:**290–401, 1975
20. Skinner DB, Camp TF: Relation of esophageal reflux to lower esophageal sphincter pressures decreased by atropine. *Gastroenterology* **54:**543, 1968
21. Biancani P, Zabinski MP, Behar J: Pressure, tension and force of closure of the human lower esophageal sphincter and esophagus. *J Clin Invest* **56:**476–483, 1975
22. Hope CE, Micyer GW, Castell DO: Is measurement of lower esophageal sphincter pressure clinically useful? *Dig Dis Sci* **26:** 1025–1030, 1981
23. Fisher RS, Malmud LS, Lobis IF: Antireflux surgery for symptomatic gastroesophageal reflux: Mechanism of action. *Dig Dis Sci* **23:**152–160, 1978
24. Ellis FH, Crozier RE, Watkins E: Operation for esophageal achalasia: Results of esophagomyotomy without an antireflux operation. *J Thorac Cardiovasc Surg* **88:**345–351, 1984
25. Higgs RH, Castell DO, Farrell RL: Evaluation of the effect of fundoplication on the incompetent lower esophageal sphincter. *Surg Gynecol Obstet* **141:**571–575, 1975
26. Bombeck TC, Coelho RGP, Nyhus LM: Prevention of gastroesophageal reflux after resection of the lower esophagus. *Surg Gynecol Obstet* **136:**1035–1043, 1970
27. Bombeck CT, Dillard DH, Nyhus LM: Muscular anatomy of the gastroesophageal junction and role of phrenoesophageal ligament: Autopsy study of sphincter mechanism. *Ann Surg* **164:**643–654, 1966
28. Henderson RD: Gastroesophageal junction in hiatus hernia. *Can J Surg* **15:**63, 1972
29. Moossa AR, Hall AW, Hughes RG, et al: Effect of gastrointestinal hormone infusions on lower esophageal competence of rhesus monkeys. *Br J Surg* **65:**499–504, 1978
30. DeMeester TR, Wernly JA, Bryant GH, et al: Clinical and in vitro determinants of gastroesophageal competence: A study of the principles of antireflux surgery. *Am J Surg* **137:**39–46, 1979
31. Little AG, DeMeester TR, Kirchner PT, et al: Pathogenesis of esophagitis in patients with gastroesophageal reflux. *Surgery* **88**(1):101–107, 1980
32. Bonavina L, Evander A, DeMeester TR, et al: Length of the distal esophageal sphincter and competency of the cardia. *Am J Surg* **151:**25–34, 1986
33. Zaninotto G, DeMeester TR, Schwizer W, et al: The lower esophageal sphincter in health and disease. *Am J Surg* **155:**104–111, 1988
34. Fuchs KH, DeMeester TR, Schwizer W, Albertucci M: Concomitant duodenogastric and gastroesophageal reflux: The role of twenty-four-hour gastric pH monitoring. In Siewert JR, Hölscher AH (eds): *Diseases of the Esophagus.* New York, Springer-Verlag, 1987, pp 1073–1076
35. Ball CS, Norris TL, Watson A: Clinical applications of simultaneous 24 hour ambulatory gastric and oesophageal pH monitoring. *Gut* **38:**1377, 1987
36. Joelsson BE, DeMeester TR, Skinner DB, et al: The role of the esophageal body in the antireflux mechanism. *Surgery* **92:**417–424, 1982
37. Helm JF, Dodds WK, Hogan WS, et al: Acid neutralizing capacity of human saliva. *Gastroenterology* **83:**75–80, 1982
38. Helm JF, Dodds WL, Pelc LR, et al: Effect of esophageal emptying and saliva on clearance of acid from the esophagus. *N Engl J Med* **310:**284–288, 1984
39. Bremner RM, Hoeft SF, Costantini M, et al: Pharyngeal swallowing: The major factor in clearance of esophageal reflux episodes. *Ann Surg* **218:**364–370, 1993
40. Madsen T, Wallin L, Boesby S, et al: Oesophageal peristalsis in normal subjects: Influence of pH and volume during imitated gastro-oesophageal reflux. *Scand J Gastroenterol* **18:**13–18, 1983
41. Dodds WJ, Dent J, Frugen WJ, et al: Mechanisms of gastroesophageal reflux in patients with reflux esophagitis. *N Engl J Med* **307:**1547–1552, 1982
42. Botha GSM: Mucosal folds at the cardia as a component of the gastro-oesophageal closing mechanism. *Br J Surg* **45:**569–580, 1958
43. Butterfield WC: Current hiatal hernia repairs: Similarities, mechanisms and extended indications—An autopsy study. *Surgery* **69:**910–916, 1971
44. DeMeester TR, Lafontaine E, Joelsson BE, et al: The relationship of

a hiatal hernia to the function of the body of the esophagus and the gastroesophageal function. *J Thorac Cardiovasc Surg* **82:**547–558, 1981
45. Jenkinson LR, Norris TL, Watson A: The influence of hiatal hernia on oesophageal function. *Gut* **28:**1377, 1987
46. Maddern GJ, Chatterton BE, Collin PJ, et al: Solid and liquid gastric emptying in patients with gastroesophageal reflux. *Br J Surg* **72:**344–348, 1985
47. DeMeester TR, Bonavina L, Albertucci M: Nissen fundoplication for gastroesophageal reflux disease. *Ann Surg* **204:**9–20, 1986
48. DeMeester TR, Johnson LF: The evaluation of objective measurements of gastroesophageal reflux and their contribution to patient management. *Surg Clin North Am* **56:**39–53, 1976
49. DeMeester TR, Skinner DB, Evans RH, Benson DW: Local nerve block anesthesia for peroral endoscopy. *Ann Thorac Surg* **24**(3):278–283, 1977
50. Tytgat GNJ: Non-radiological investigation of the oesophagus. In Watson A, Celestin LR (eds): *Disorders of the Oesophagus.* London, Pitman, 1984, pp 24–36
51. Bernstein LM, Baker LA: A clinical test for esophagitis. *Gastroenterology* **34:**760–781, 1958
52. Stein HJ, DeMeester TR, Hinder RA: Outpatient physiological testing and surgical management of foregut motor disorders. *Curr Probl Surg* **24:**418–555, 1992
53. DeMeester TR: Surgery for esophageal motor disorders. *Ann Thorac Surg* **34:**225–229, 1982
54. Peters L, Maas L, Petty D: Spontaneous non-cardiac chest pain: Evaluation by 24-hour ambulatory esophageal motility and pH monitoring. *Gastroenterology* **94:**878–886, 1988
55. Eypasch EP, Stein HJ, DeMeester TR, et al: A new technique to define and clarify esophageal motor disorders. *Am J Surg* **159:**144–151, 1990
56. Smout AJPM, Breediyk M, van der Zouw C, et al: Physiological gastroesophageal reflux and esophageal motor activity studied with a new system for 24-hour reading and automated analysis. *Dig Dis Sci* **34:**372–378, 1989
57. Stein HJ, DeMeester TR, Eypasch EP: A new modality for integrated outpatient evaluation of foregut disorders. *Gastroenterology* **98:**131, 1990
58. Stein HS, DeMeester TR: Indications, technique, and clinical use of ambulatory 24-hour esophageal motility monitoring in a surgical practice. *Ann Surg* **217:**128–137, 1993
59. Emde C, Ciluffo T, Castiglione F: Digital ambulatory long-term manometry: Low intraindividual and high interindividual variability impede the determination of generally applicable "normal values." *Gastroenterology* **96:**139, 1989
60. Stein HJ, DeMeester TR: Evaluation of esophageal motor disorders: 24-hour ambulatory esophageal motility monitoring. *Gastroenterol Int* **4:**60–64, 1991
61. Stein HJ, DeMeester TR, Eypasch EP, Klingman RP: Ambulatory 24-hour esophageal manometry in the evaluation of esophageal motor disorders and non-cardiac chest pain. *Surgery* **110:**753–763, 1991
62. Stein HJ, Eypasch EP, DeMeester TR: Circadian esophageal motility pattern in patients with classic diffuse esophageal spasm and nutcracker esophagus. *Gastroenterology* **96:**491, 1989
63. Clouse RE, Lustman JJ. Psychiatric illness and contraction abnormalities of the esophagus. *N Engl J Med* **309:**1337–1342, 1983
64. Katz PO, Dalton CB, Richter JE, et al: Esophageal testing of patients with non cardiac chest pain or dysphagia. *Ann Intern Med* **106:**593–597, 1987
65. Stein HJ, DeMeester TR, Singh S: Circadian esophageal motor function in patients with non-obstructive dysphagia and normal esophageal acid exposure. *Gastroenterology* **100:**168, 1991
66. Hennington JP, Burns TW, Balart LA: Chest pain and dysphagia in patients with prolonged peristaltic contractile duration of the esophagus. *Dig Dis Sci* **29:**134–140, 1984
67. Brand DL, Martin D, Pope CE: Esophageal manometrics in patients with angina type chest pain. *Am J Dig Dis* **23:**300–304, 1977
68. Ferguson ME, Little AG: Angina-like chest pain associated with high amplitude peristaltic contractions of the esophagus. *Surgery* **104:**713–719, 1988
69. MacKenzie J, Belch J, Land D, et al: Oesophageal ischaemia in motility disorders associated with chest pain. *Lancet* **2:**592–595, 1988
70. Stein HJ, Eypasch EP, DeMeester TR: "Esophageal claudication" as the cause of chest pain in diffuse spasm and nutcracker esophagus? *Gastroenterology* **96:**491, 1989
71. Eypasch EP, DeMeester TR, Klingman RR, Stein HJ: Physiologic assessment and surgical management of patients with diffuse esophageal spasm. *J Thorac Cardiovasc Surg* **104:**859–869, 1991
72. Kahrilas PJ, Dodds WJ, Hogan WJ: Effect of peristaltic dysfunction on esophageal volume clearance. *Gastroenterology* **94:**73–80, 1988
73. Stein HJ, DeMeester TR, Eypasch EP: Circadian esophageal motor function in patients with gastroesophageal reflux disease. *Surgery* **108:**769–778, 1990
74. Stein HJ, DeMeester TR: Barrett's esophagus: An esophageal motility disorder? *Gastroenterology* **100:**168(A), 1991
75. Stein HJ, Bremner RM, Jamieson J, DeMeester TR: Effect of Nissen fundoplication on esophageal function. *Arch Surg* **127:**788–791, 1992
76. Haddad JE: Relation of gastroesophageal reflux to yield sphincter pressures. *Gastroenterology* **58:**175–184, 1970
77. Bombeck CT, Vaz O, DeSalvo J, et al: Computerized axial manometry of the esophagus. *Ann Surg* **206:**465–472, 1987
78. Stein HJ, DeMeester TR, Naspetti R, et al: Three-dimensional imaging of the lower esophageal sphincter in gastroesophageal reflux disease. *Ann Surg* **214:**374–384, 1991
79. Crookes PF, Kaul BK, DeMeester TR, et al: Manometry of individual segments of the distal esophageal sphincter: Its relation to functional incompetence. *Arch Surg* **128:**411–415, 1993
80. DeMeester TR, Stein HJ. Gastroesophageal reflux disease. In Moody FG, Carey LC, Jones RC, et al (eds): *Surgical Treatment of Digestive Disease,* 2nd ed. Chicago: Year Book, 1989, pp 65–108
81. Tuttle SC, Grossman MI: Detection of gastroesophageal reflux by simultaneous measurements of intraluminal pressures and pH. *Proc Soc Exp Biol Med* **98:**225–227, 1958
82. Booth DJ, Kemmerer WT, Skinner DB: Acid clearing from the distal esophagus. *Arch Surg* **96:**731–734, 1968
83. DeMeester TR, Wang CI, Wernly JA, et al: Technique, indications and clinical use of 24-hour esophageal pH monitoring. *J Thorac Cardiovasc Surg* **79**(5):565–667, 1980
84. Branicki FJ, Evans DF, Ogilvie AL, et al: Ambulatory monitoring of oesophageal pH in reflux oesophagitis using a portable radio telemetry system. *Gut* **23:**992–998, 1982
85. Jenkinson LR, Norris TL, Watson A: Dietary guidelines for ambulatory pH recording. *Gut* **27:**549–550, 1986
86. Berquist TH, Nolan NG, Stephens DH, et al: Radioisotope scintigraphy in diagnosis of Barrett's esophagus. *Surg Gynecol Obstet* **123:**401–411, 1975
87. Fisher RT, Malmud LS, Roberts GS, et al: Gastroesophageal (GE) scintiscanning to detect and quantitate GE reflux. *Gastroenterology* **70:**301–308, 1976
88. Menin RA, Malmud LS, Petersen RP, et al: Gastroesophageal scintigraphy to assess the severity of gastroesophageal reflux disease. *Ann Surg* **191:**66–71, 1980
89. Tolin RD, Malmud LS, Reilley G, et al: Esophageal scintigraphy to quantitate esophageal transit (quantitation of esophageal transit). *Gastroenterology* **76:**1402–1408, 1979
90. Russell CO, Hill LD, Holmes ER III, et al: Radionuclide transit: A sensitive screening test for esophageal dysfunction. *Gastroenterology* **80:**887–892, 1981
91. De Caestecker JS, Blackwell JN, Adam RD, et al: Clinical value of radionuclide oesophageal transit measurement. *Gut* **27:**659–666, 1986

92. Eriksen CA, Holdsworth RJ, Sutton D, et al: The solid bolus oesophageal egg transit test: Its manometric interpretation and usefulness as a screening test. *Br J Surg* **74:**1130–1133, 1987
93. Shaffer EA, McOrmond P, Duggan H: Quantitation cholescintigraphy: Assessment of gall bladder filling and duodenogastric reflux. *Gastroenterology* **79:**899–906, 1980
94. Velasco N, Hill LD, Gannan RM, et al: Gastric emptying and gastroesophageal reflux: Effects of surgery and correlation with esophageal motor function. *Am J Surg* **144:**58–62, 1982
95. McCallum R, Berkowitz D, Lerner E: Gastric emptying in patients with gastroesophageal reflux. *Gastroenterology* **80:**285–291, 1981
96. Ollyo JB, Monnier P, Fontolliet C, Savary M: The natural history and incidence of reflux oesophagitis. *Gullet* **3:**3–10, 1993
97. Iascone C, DeMeester TR, Little AG, Skinner DB: Barrett's esophagus: Functional assessment, proposed pathogenesis and surgical therapy. *Arch Surg* **118:**543–549, 1983
98. Gillen P, Keeling P, Bryne PJ, Hennessy TPJ. Barrett's oesophagus: pH profile. *Br J Surg* **74:**774–776, 1987
99. Attwood SEA, Smyrk TC, DeMeester TR, et al: Duodenoesophageal reflux and development of esophageal adenocarcinoma in rats. *Surgery* **111:**503–10, 1992
100. Clark GWB, Smyrk TC, Mirvish SS, et al: Effect of gastroduodenal juice and dietary fat on the development of Barrett's esophagus and esophageal neoplasia: An experimental rat model. *Ann Surg Oncol* **1**(3):252–261, 1994
101. Stein HJ, Barlow AP, DeMeester TR, Hinder RA: Complications of gastroesophageal reflux disease: The role of the lower esophageal sphincter, esophageal acid/alkaline exposure, and duodenogastric reflex. *Ann Surg* **216:**35–43, 1992
102. Stein HJ, Feussner H, Kauer W, et al: "Alkaline" gastroesophageal reflux: Assessment by ambulatory esophageal aspiration and pH monitoring. *Am J Surg* **167:**163–168, 1994
103. Bechi P, Falciai R, Baldini F, et al: A new fiber optic sensor for ambulatory entero-gastric reflux detection. In Katzir A (ed): *Fiber Optic Medical and Fluorescent Sensors and Applications.* Proceedings of SPIE 1648. Bellingham, Washington, SPIE, 130–135, 1992
104. Bechi P, Pucciani F, Baldini F et al: Long-term ambulatory enterogastric reflux monitoring: Validation of a new fiberoptic technique. *Dig Dis Sci* **38:**1297–1306, 1993
105. Kauer KH, Burdiles P, Ireland AP, et al: Does duodenal juice reflux into the esophagus of patients with complicated GERD? Evaluation of a fiberoptic sensor for bilirubin. *Am J Surg* **169:**98–104, 1995
106. Attwood SE, DeMeester TR, Bremner CG, et al: Alkaline gastroesophageal reflux: Implications in the development of complications in Barrett's columnar-lined lower esophagus. *Surgery* **106:**763–70, 1989

CHAPTER

40

# Childhood Esophageal Abnormalities and Their Management

James A. O'Neill, Jr.

This chapter describes the most commonly encountered congenital disorders of the esophagus. The most important and most common of these, esophageal atresia, is discussed in detail because the principles of care of this anomaly and its variants are applicable to many other esophageal disorders in childhood. It was this entity that led surgeons to tackle other difficult neonatal anomalies and provided a strong stimulus for the development of the field of pediatric surgery.

The first anatomic description of esophageal atresia was presented by Durston[1] in 1670. He described the condition in one member of a pair of conjoined twins. In 1697, Gibson[2] presented the first clinical description of an infant with esophageal atresia and tracheoesophageal fistula. For the next 250 years, all attempts at surgical repair failed.

The development of successful surgical management of esophageal atresia paralleled the development of pediatric surgery itself. Before 1939, not one patient with esophageal atresia and tracheoesophageal fistula survived despite a variety of surgical approaches to this anomaly. A number of staged corrections were attempted over the years, but it was not until Lanman analyzed a series of 32 consecutive failures that changes in management were suggested.[3] The first two survivors of staged correction were described by Ladd in 1944[4] and Levin[5] in 1940. In 1943, Haight and Towsley described 14 patients with esophageal atresia and tracheoesophageal fistula, including the first successful primary repair performed years previously.[6]

## ESOPHAGEAL ATRESIA

Experimental embryologic studies in various species indicate that the esophagus appears as a short tube extending from pharynx to stomach at about 4 weeks of gestation. At this time, the esophagus is developing in conjunction with the trachea; both are entodermal in origin. The laryngotracheal groove, which runs lengthwise in the floor of the primitive gut and eventually separates the latter two structures, begins to develop at about 3 weeks of gestation. The trachea and the esophagus are separate structures by 4–5 weeks. By 8 weeks, the lungs are recognizable structures adjacent to the trachea and the esophagus on each side of the mediastinum. Thus, esophageal atresia probably develops somewhere between the third and sixth weeks of gestation. The influences responsible for incomplete separation of the early laryngotracheal groove from the gut are unknown, since the anomaly has not been reproduced experimentally. There is reason to speculate, however, that vascular accidents in utero may be responsible, much as is the case with the production of intestinal atresia. Because the epithelial lining of the esophagus develops later, probably around the fifth month of gestation, stenosis of the esophagus is an anomaly that probably has its origin then. Numerous classifications of the various types of esophageal atresia resulting from embryologic maldevelopment were suggested by Gross[7] and Vogt[8], but it is more useful to use a descriptive classification instead.

The common forms of esophageal atresia are shown in Figure 40–1. Esophageal atresia with tracheoesophageal fistula (Vogt type I) constitutes 85–90% of the variants of esophageal atresia; isolated esophageal atresia (type III) 5–8%, and H-type tracheoesophageal atresia (type IV) the rest. The extremely rare type II with a fistula to the trachea from the proximal esophageal pouch and the distal esophagus is not shown. Esophageal atresia with fistula is estimated to occur in approximately 1 in every 8000 births. The incidence of associated anomalies, as reported by Holder et al,[9] is about 50%. The most frequent associated anomalies are gastrointestinal, cardiac, and genitourinary, in that order. Cardiac malformations are particularly important to identify preoperatively because they have a profound effect on survival, as described by Hartenberg et al.[10] Chiba et al[11] described associated pulmonary and foregut anomalies. The VATER association is common, particularly if one considers this to be a spectrum including any three or more of the following: vertebral defects, anal atresia, tracheoesophageal fistula with esophageal atresia, and radial and renal dysplasia, as described by Quan and Smith in 1973.[12] Lim[13] described a number of cases of so-called CHARGE association: choanal atresia, heart anomalies, esophageal atresia, and gastrointestinal anomalies.

## ESOPHAGEAL ATRESIA WITH TRACHEOESOPHAGEAL FISTULA

### Signs and Symptoms

The presenting clinical signs of esophageal atresia and tracheoesophageal fistula are related to esophageal obstruction and respiratory complications resulting from reflux of acid-peptic juice into the lungs. Such infants have copious salivary secretions because the proximal part of the esophagus is obstructed; if fed, these infants tend to choke while feeding. As time progresses, gastroesophageal reflux causes aspiration pneumonia and atelectasis in a diffuse manner, and gas exchange becomes inadequate. This results in tachypnea and respiratory distress. As pulmonary resistance increases, air is forced through the tracheoesophageal fistula into the stomach causing progressive abdominal distention. A particular problem in this regard occurs in low-birth-weight infants with esophageal atresia and tracheoesophageal fistula who present with severe respiratory distress syndrome and increased pulmonary resistance necessitating assisted ventilation. Maternal polyhydramnios occurs in approximately one fourth of infants with this anomaly and in virtually all of those who have associated duodenal atresia.

### Diagnosis

Some cases of esophageal atresia and tracheoesophageal fistula are diagnosed with prenatal ultrasonography, but most cases are not suspected until symptoms occur after birth. Once the diagnosis of esophageal atresia and tracheoesophageal fistula in a neonate is suspected because of copious oral secretions, a relatively stiff nasogastric feeding tube should be passed. (Too pliable a tube might coil in the upper esophageal pouch and give the false impression that it was passing into the stomach.) If the tube does not pass beyond the upper thorax, the diagnosis should be strongly suspected. A chest radiograph confirms the thoracic position of the tube. Air in the intestinal tract indicates the presence of a distal tracheoesophageal fistula. Although some authors consider this sufficient for diagnosis, I prefer injec-

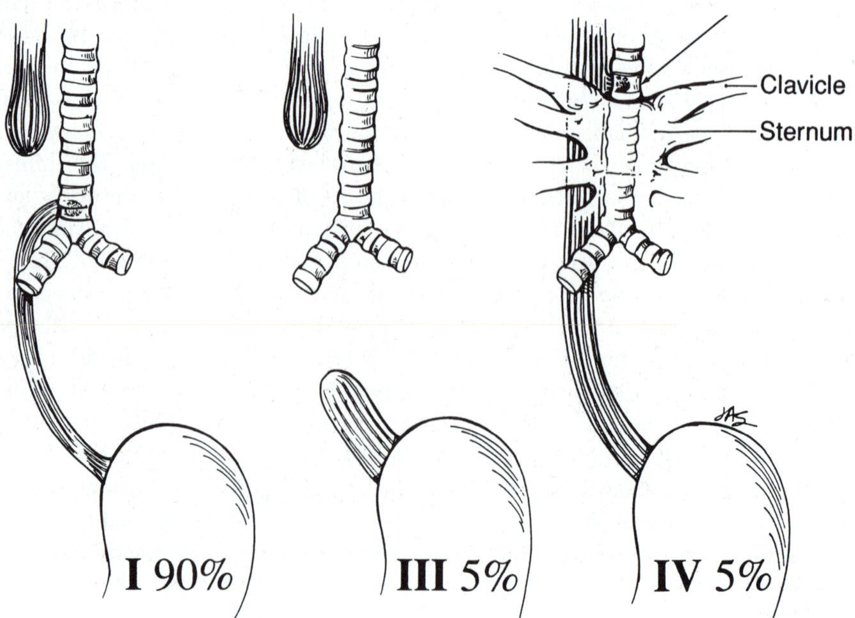


**Figure 40–1.** The common variants of esophageal atresia and their relative frequency. Esophageal atresia with tracheoesophageal fistula (**left**), isolated esophageal atresia (**center**), and H-type fistula (**right**). Variations of these forms occur but are quite rare.

tion of 0.5 mL of soluble contrast material into the upper pouch while anteroposterior and lateral radiographs are obtained with the infant in the upright position (Fig. 40–2). This technique clearly demonstrates the length of the upper pouch and rules out the presence of the occasional fistula from the upper pouch into the trachea (Type II), as suggested by Yun et al.[14] Furthermore, it rules out the possibility of a pseudodiverticulum resulting from pharyngeal perforation associated with traumatic intubation efforts in infants with respiratory distress syndrome[15] (Fig. 40–3).

If a right aortic arch is suspected because the upper esophageal pouch appears to be deviated toward the left, or if congenital heart disease is present, it is helpful to determine this with echocardiography before the operation.

The appearance of the abdominal portion of the radiograph may be helpful in making a diagnosis of associated gastrointestinal malformations such as duodenal atresia. The presence of pneumonia, atelectasis, and characteristic patterns of congenital cardiac disease also may be demonstrated. In the postoperative period, ultrasound examination of the genitourinary tract should be performed on all infants because of the high incidence of associated genitourinary malformations, particularly when anorectal malformations are present.

Preoperative bronchoscopy may be helpful to premature infants with a short upper pouch demonstrated on chest radiographs because bronchoscopy may help identify carinal insertion of the distal pouch and a long gap, which may require staged management.

## Treatment

### *Preoperative Management*

Although operative management of esophageal atresia in its various forms is a relative surgical emergency, there is always time for thorough evaluation and improvement of the patient's preoperative status. The preoperative considerations are the same for all forms of esophageal atresia.

In instances of esophageal atresia with tracheoesophageal fistula, the infant should be placed in the semisitting position, since reflux of acid-gastric contents is the prime danger. Replogle[16] and Ohkawa et al[17] described methods of sump tube drainage to clear the upper pouch of saliva.

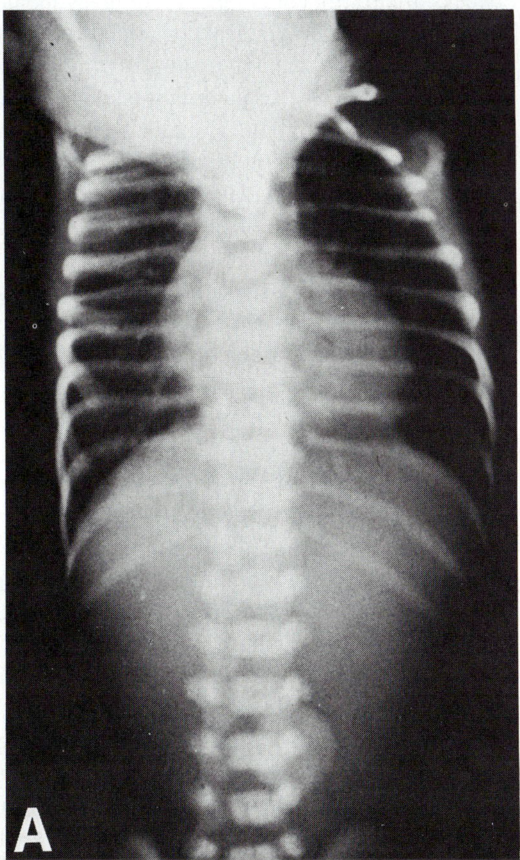


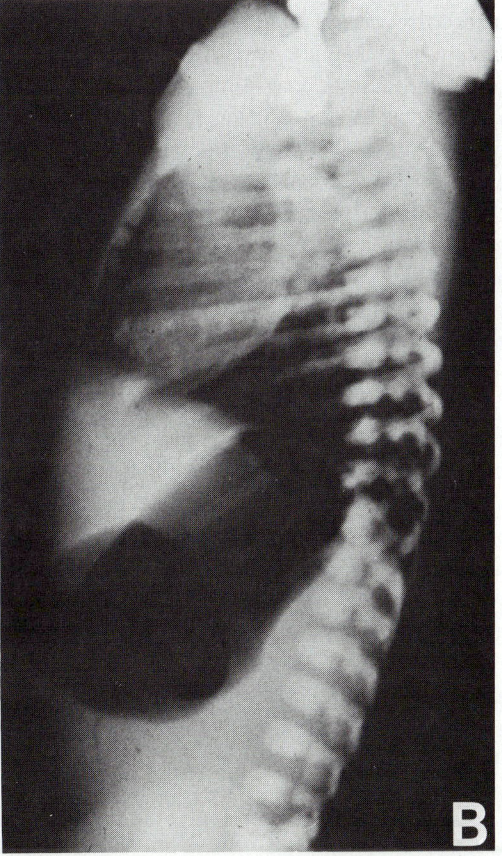


**Figure 40–2. A.** Radiograph showing typical findings of isolated esophageal atresia—a blind upper pouch and a flat, airless abdomen. **B.** Lateral view of an infant with proximal esophageal atresia, tracheoesophageal fistula, and the "double-bubble" sign of duodenal atresia.

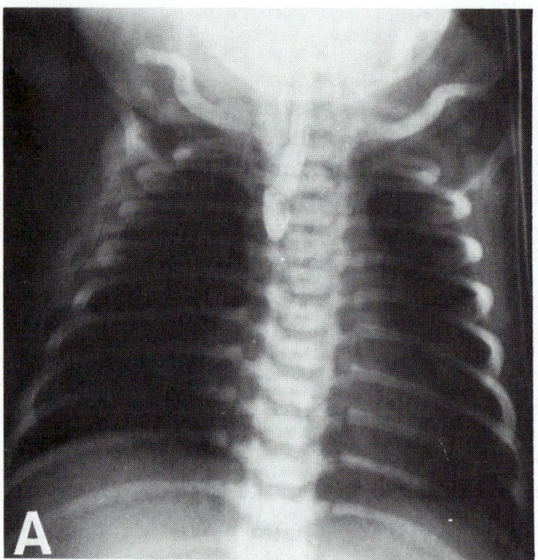


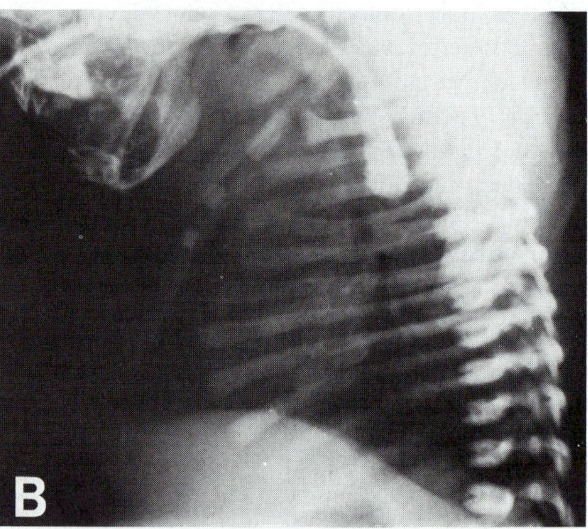


**Figure 40–3.** Posteroanterior (**A**) and lateral (**B**) radiographs obtained with injection of contrast material through a nasogastric tube demonstrate typical finding of a traumatic pseudodiverticulum—an irregular, eccentric pouch that is different from that seen in esophageal atresia. *(From Heller RM, et al: AJR 129:336, 1977, with permission.)*

However, because these patients require frequent suctioning anyway, I prefer to have the nurse suction the baby every 30 min to avoid the use of drainage tubes that occlude the nares and stimulate the production of even more secretions. Bar-Maor et al[18] described the use of cimetidine to reduce the risk of acid reflux into the lungs. This therapy may be useful in infants who must undergo delayed or staged operative management because of poor clinical condition.

Infants should be cared for in an intensive care unit with attention paid to maintenance of normal body temperature, evaluation of coagulation, and correction of hypoglycemia, hyperbilirubinemia, and acid-base and mineral disturbances. Antibiotics should always be administered. If an infant appears to be in respiratory distress or if there is radiographic evidence of pneumonitis or atelectasis, an endotracheal tube should be passed and the infant provided with assisted ventilation at the lowest effective pressures and with aggressive tracheobronchial toilet. In patients with increased pulmonary resistance, high-frequency ventilation with low mean airway pressure may be more effective than conventional ventilation, as shown by Bloom et al.[19] Often, as little as 8 hours of aggressive respiratory care can make the operation safe.

Infants with isolated esophageal atresia should be cared for preoperatively in much the same manner as those who have a tracheoesophageal fistula, except that they are probably best placed in the horizontal prone position because aspiration of saliva is the only real consideration. Infants with H-type fistula without esophageal atresia should be cared for exactly as are infants with esophageal atresia and tracheoesophageal fistula.

### *Surgical Treatment*

The choice of surgical approach and the timing of operation are directly related to the size and condition of the infant (Fig. 40–4). Primary repair is preferable for almost all infants. Extreme prematurity (less than 1500 g in weight), especially when associated with severe respiratory distress syndrome, may dictate delayed primary or staged repair 1–8 weeks after birth. Other reasons for delay include severe aspiration pneumonia, critical congenital cardiac disease, and any other life-threatening conditions that indicate to an experienced surgeon that the infant could not tolerate a complex thoracic operation. I, and others, no longer use the Waterston classification of risk as a guide to choosing primary or staged repair. I choose the operation on the basis of physiologic status, even in patients as small as 1200 g.[20] Just as an infant requires a good surgeon, an experienced anesthesiologist is also necessary. The operating room environment must be capable of providing warmth to the infant to prevent metabolic deterioration. Careful monitoring of all physiologic values, including volume status and pH and blood gases, during the operation helps maintain the infant in ideal condition.

Most infants with esophageal atresia and tracheoesophageal fistula do not require a preliminary gastrostomy before thoracotomy, as thought in the past, unless staging is required.[21] Gastrostomy may be helpful postoperatively if an anastomotic stricture occurs, because it facilitates dilation procedures. Louhimo,[22] Bishop,[23] and my group have successfully treated infants with this anomaly without gastrostomy. Furthermore, we have identified a high-risk group of infants with severe respiratory distress syndrome in whom preliminary gastrostomy may be dangerous.[24] In the latter instance, infants with severe respiratory distress syndrome may require such high ventilatory pressures for physiologic support that gastrostomy allows escape of ventilatory flow though the tracheoesophageal fistula to such a degree that acute deterioration occurs. Filston et al[25] and Reichenbacher and Ballantine[26] described use of a Fogarty

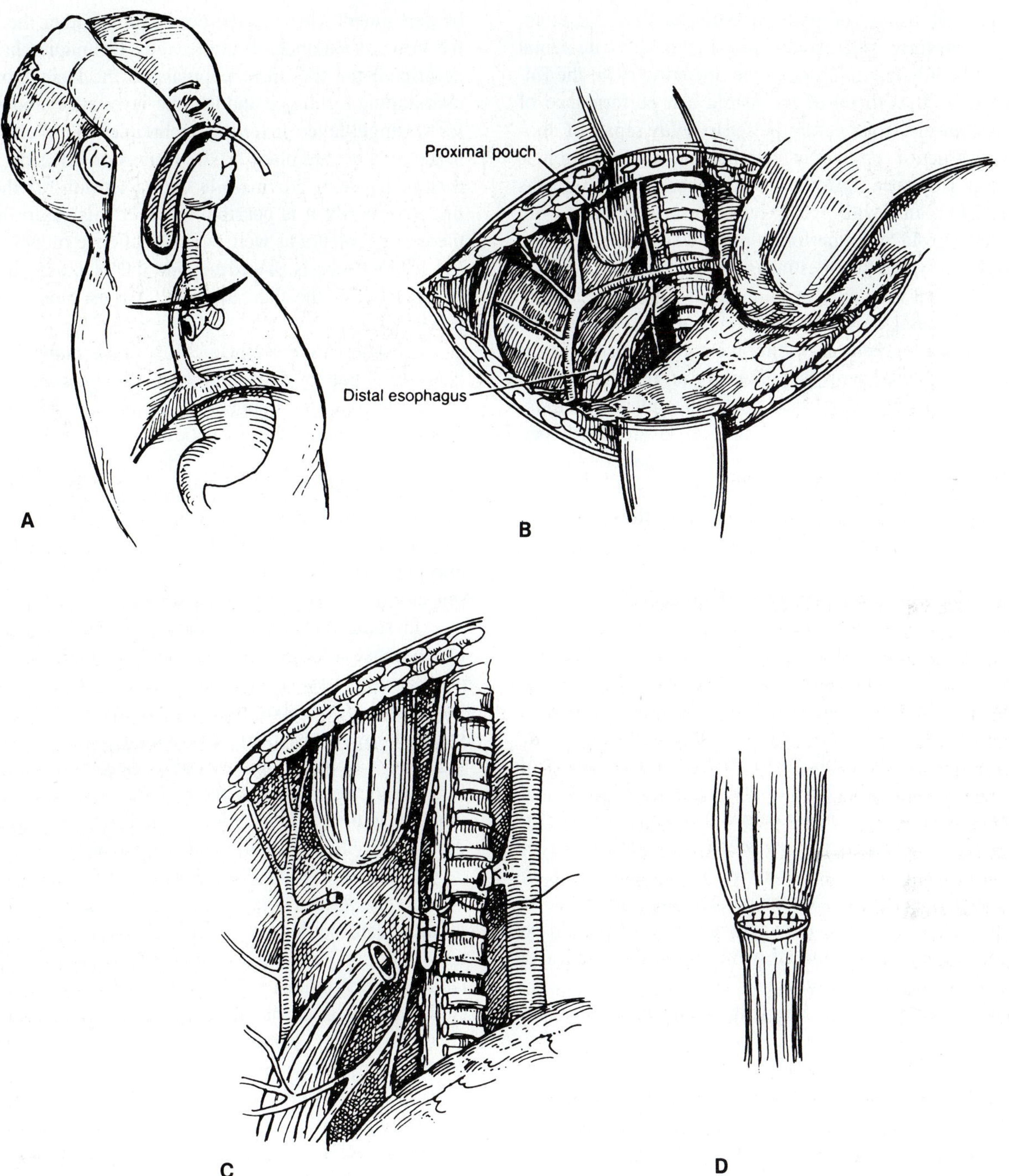


**Figure 40–4.** Surgical repair of type I esophageal atresia. **A.** Right thoracotomy. **B.** Exposure of proximal pouch and distal esophagus. **C.** Division and closure of tracheoesophageal fistula. **D.** Single-layer interrupted esophageal anastomosis. *(From O'Neill JA: Operative Surgery, Principles and Techniques, 3rd ed. Philadelphia, Saunders, 1990, p 1072.)*

balloon catheter as an aid to management of such infants before fistula ligation.

In the occasional instances in which gastrostomy is performed as the first step of the operation, the infant is positioned supine with the head of the table elevated. Ordinarily, the infant is intubated while awake and anesthetized gently with careful ventilation to avoid inducing reflux from passage of air through the fistula into the stomach. The stomach is approached through a left rectus muscle–splitting incision, and a No. 12 or No. 14 de Pezzer catheter is placed in the fundus through a double purse-string suture of 5-0 silk. The stomach may then be fixed to the posterior rectus sheath and the remainder of the closure performed in the routine way.

Special mention should be made of infants who have associated duodenal atresia or imperforate anus. I correct the duodenal atresia or perform colostomy, if indicated, first and perform gastrostomy in patients with duodenal atresia. The infant is returned to the operating room the following day for division of the fistula and performance of the anastomosis. Spitz et al[27] prefer to delay repair of duodenal obstruction until after the thoracic malformation is corrected. However, at my institution, there were no deaths among 24 infants with esophageal atresia combined with duodenal atresia or imperforate anus who underwent the procedure in which the intestine is repaired first.

The infant is usually positioned for right thoracotomy in the left lateral decubitus position with the head of the table elevated to avoid gastric reflux until the fistula is divided. Left thoracotomy is preferred for patients with a right aortic arch. A horizontal posterolateral thoracotomy incision is made and a retropleural exposure developed through the fourth intercostal space. Some surgeons prefer to use the transpleural approach, and current evidence suggests that the results are no different from those with the retropleural approach even when an anastomotic leak occurs.

The key to locating the site of the fistula is division of the azygos vein and identification of the vagus nerve. The upper blind pouch should not be mobilized until the exact positions of the distal pouch and fistula have been determined. The distal esophagus is then dissected just inferior to the entry of the fistula into the trachea, and gentle traction placed on it with a silicone rubber loop. Stay sutures of 5-0 nonabsorbable material are placed at the superior and inferior borders of the fistula before it is divided, and closure is performed with running technique. During dissection of the lower esophagus, every effort should be made to preserve the mediastinal vascular connections with the aorta and all small branches of the vagus nerve. Care should be taken to leave a small amount of tissue on the trachea to avoid narrowing that structure. It is usually possible to cover the tracheal suture line with a flap of mediastinal pleura.

After testing the integrity of the tracheal closure by having the anesthesiologist inflate the lungs with saline solution placed over the suture line, the surgeon may proceed with esophageal anastomosis. If the anastomosis is to be performed in a different operation, the distal pouch is simply closed and fixed as high as possible along the vertebral column, and the area is marked with a silver clip. Low birth weight is not a contraindication to esophageal anastomosis provided the infant's physiologic condition is satisfactory. The upper pouch is easily identified by having the anesthesiologist push a small catheter downward within it. The upper pouch receives its blood supply longitudinally from above, so it may be mobilized extensively. It is important to close the fistula from the proximal pouch to the trachea if such a fistula (type II) is present. At times the gap between the two ends of esophagus is long, particularly in low-birth-weight infants. If 1–3 cm of additional length is needed, either a circular myotomy as described by Livaditis[28] or multiple longitudinal incisions as described by Lindell[29] may be performed. This may be done within either the chest or the neck. A number of anastomotic techniques have been described; the two most popular are the Haight two-layer overlapping technique and the one-layer anastomosis. I prefer a single-layer inverting technique. With either technique, it is best to place all the sutures on one side first and then to tie them down while taking tension off the suture line. Ordinarily it is possible to cover this suture line with mediastinal pleura as well. A small silicone rubber nasogastric feeding tube is placed beyond the anastomosis into the stomach before the chest is closed. A chest tube is left in the retropleural space.

An alternative method of operative management has been described by Duhamel[30] and Sulamaa et al.[31] They found that the blood supply of the distal segment is more easily preserved if the tracheoesophageal fistula is ligated with two heavy silk sutures. Then an anastomosis is performed between the end of the upper pouch and the side of the distal pouch just beyond the two ligatures. Pietsch et al[32] and Touloukian[33] reported good results with this procedure, but they and others also reported the frequent occurrence of recanalization of the fistula.

In some instances, primary anastomosis is not possible, because a long gap exists between the ends even if a circular myotomy is performed, or not desirable after division of the fistula, because of the critical condition of the infant. In these instances, staged anastomosis is performed 2–8 weeks later. An uncommonly used method of staging for complicated cases is banding of the gastroesophageal junction with a silicone rubber band with gastrostomy, as described by Bloom et al[19] and Todd et al.[34]

Postoperatively the infant is cared for exactly as preoperatively. Assisted ventilation is used as indicated by the infant's cardiopulmonary status. Nasogastric or gastrostomy feedings may be started whenever the infant has established gastrointestinal function and passed transitional stools. If the infant has no evidence of esophageal leak, a contrast-swallow radiographic examination is performed on the seventh postoperative day. If the anastomosis is found to be intact, the chest tube may be removed and oral feedings begun. About 3 weeks after the operation, I calibrate the anastomosis using Tucker dilators passed through the infant's mouth. Ordinarily, when 24 F size is reached, the esophagus dilates in response to the normal swallowing mechanism, and stricture is not anticipated. On the other hand, a tight anastomosis is better dilated early if a rigid stricture is to be prevented.

## Complications

Serious congenital heart disease frequently complicates the pre- and intraoperative management of esophageal atresia when multiple anomalies coexist. Greenwood and Rosenthal[35] reviewed a series of 326 infants with esophageal atresia and tracheoesophageal fistula and noted the frequency of associated congenital heart disease to be 15%; but in 30–50% of infants it was associated with other gastrointestinal problems and various genetic syndromes. This has been the experience at my institution. At times, systemic–to–pulmonary artery shunting may be indicated in association with transpleural repair of the atresia. Right aortic arch is particularly common in these instances. Cardiac catheterization is probably best used in the preoperative phase of management when severe, symptomatic, complex congenital heart disease coexists with esophageal atresia and tracheoesophageal fistula.

The various complications encountered after surgical repair of esophageal atresia and tracheoesophageal fistula are related primarily to the size and condition of the patient, associated malformations, or tension at the suture line.[20,36,37] The most common complications are pneumonia and atelectasis, which may require replacement of an endotracheal tube with assisted ventilation and frequent suctioning. Another common problem is anastomotic leak, particularly when the anastomosis has been performed under tension. Most of these leaks become apparent from the drainage of saliva through the chest tube or occurrence of pneumothorax anytime from the first to the seventh postoperative day. Often a late leak is localized around the esophagus and appears only as a small diverticulum adjacent to the suture line on an esophogram. Unfortunately, strictures develop in most patients who have anastomotic leakage, but most of these strictures can be dilated over a period of weeks to months. If tapered dilators cannot be passed easily, gastrostomy, placement of a string, and guided dilation should be performed. Sometimes, even when every precaution has been taken, perforation of the esophagus occurs. If this is limited, the patient may be treated with antibiotics, and feedings may be withheld with the expectation that a small tear will seal. Sometimes the rupture is so extensive that operative closure and drainage, with or without a pericardial or other patch, are needed.

Some patients have periodic apneic spells. Many have this problem because of gastroesophageal reflux and associated laryngospasm. It has been theorized that this problem may be due to distention of the upper esophageal pouch with vagal stimulation. Schwartz and Filler[38] emphasized that the innominate artery may cause tracheal obstruction if the esophagus is dilated posteriorly and compresses the trachea against this artery. They described a series of patients treated with aortopexy with good results. Kimura et al[39] described the use of dynamic studies of the trachea with cine CT to demonstrate tracheal compression by the aortic arch in patients such as this; they also reported good results with aortosternopexy. Spitz[40] described a method of Dacron-patch aortopexy for this problem. Good results have been reported with this approach in approximately 70% of patients, whereas the others require tracheostomy and long-term ventilatory management.

All patients with esophageal atresia have disordered motility postoperatively, probably because of abnormal innervation, as described by Nakazato et al.[41] However, Shono et al[42] reported results of studies of patients before and after they underwent esophageal anastomosis that indicated that abnormal postoperative peristalsis is the result of operative damage. Although peristalsis is usually normal in the upper pouch, it is disordered in the lower segment of the esophagus, as manifested by slow contractions, poor wave transmissions, and to-and-fro movement. The lower esophageal sphincter (LES) is frequently incompetent as well. In some patients this is severe enough to be associated with esophageal obstruction and aspiration. Although these and other theories have been offered to explain the phenomenon of postoperative apnea, no ready explanation is apparent in most cases. Manifestations of postoperative apnea usually resolve by 2 years of age.[43] Chronic abnormalities in respiratory function following repair of esophageal atresia were analyzed by LeSouef et al,[44] whose studies indicated that recurrent pneumonia is probably related to lung damage from chronic gastroesophageal reflux and diminished LES pressures.

In patients in whom leak has occurred at the suture line or who required prolonged repeated dilations for resistant stricture, a recurrent tracheoesophageal fistula may form. The symptoms are generally those of repeated aspiration during feedings. Endoscopy is the best method of establishing this diagnosis. At the same time, endoscopic electrosurgical obliteration of the fistula may be attempted, as reported by Rangecroft et al.[45] If that is not successful, recurrent fistula must be closed surgically, usually in association with anastomotic revision.

Mention has already been made of gastroesophageal reflux as a postoperative complication in most patients. Fonkalsrud[46] described the need to perform Nissen fundoplication in more than half of a small series of patients. Only about 10% of patients at my institution[47] and patients described by Spitz et al[48] and Touloukian[33] required this procedure because of continuing severe reflux, recurrent pneumonia, or esophageal stricture.

## Results

The standard for comparison of operative results for patients with esophageal atresia and tracheoesophageal fistula has been the risk classification of Waterston et al.[49] I no longer use it as a guide to selection of operative approach. The categorization is as follows: group A, infants who present in good condition with birth weights in excess of 2.5 kg; group B, infants with birth weights between 1.8 and 2.5 kg or with higher birth weight but with mild pneumonia or an additional congenital abnormality that is not potentially lethal; and group C, infants with birth weights less than 1.8 kg or with a higher birth weight but with severe pneumonia or life-threatening congenital malformations. In my series of more than 100 patients with esophageal atresia and distal tracheoesophageal fistula, group A and group B patients had no early mortality, but there was a 15% early mortality among group C patients, giving an overall mortality of 4.6%. Late mortality in this series of patients, seen over a 10-year period, raised the overall mortality to 10%. Most good medical centers are achieving results of this sort.[20,21,33,36,37] The early deaths among the group C patients with esophageal atresia and tracheoesophageal fistula all were related to either serious cardiac disease or respiratory distress syndrome. The late deaths encountered were due to cardiac disease primarily, and to trauma in one instance. Spitz et al[48] described a 5-year experience with 148 patients, with 100% survival among Waterston group A patients and 85.1% survival overall. Louhimo[22] reported on 500 consecutive patients with an 85% survival rate. He indicated and I agree that because of the marked increase in the numbers of group C patients that most medical centers are seeing today, mortality may not improve further from this point on.

In general, the long-term outlook for patients with esophageal atresia and tracheoesophageal fistula is excellent. Motility disturbances seem to become less symptomatic in time as the size of the esophagus and the maturity of the child progress. Studies by Duranceau et al,[50] Orringer et al,[51] Parker et al,[52] and Putnam et al[53] documented long-term problems with disordered peristalsis and particularly gastroesophageal reflux with varying degrees of symptoms. Barium swallow radiographic examination is inadequate for complete examination of such patients and should be supplemented with pH monitoring and gastroesophageal radionuclide scans. I do not usually use esophageal manometry in small patients. As increasing numbers of patients are surviving and the follow-up period lengthens, it is likely that more patients will require antireflux surgery to prevent the complications of recurrent pneumonia and stricture, particularly those with long-gap atresias.

## ISOLATED ESOPHAGEAL ATRESIA

### Signs and Symptoms

Infants with isolated esophageal atresia present in much the same manner as those with an associated tracheoesophageal fistula—namely, copious oral secretions related to an obstructed blind upper esophageal pouch. Most infants with isolated esophageal atresia weigh less than 2.5 kg, and virtually all have associated maternal polyhydramnios. A scaphoid abdomen is the rule; chest radiographs demonstrate an airless abdomen. Pneumonia and atelectasis are less common in patients with solitary esophageal atresia than in patients with a fistula, probably because aspiration of mucus and saliva, although undesirable, is less damaging than reflux of gastric secretions.

### Surgical Treatment

In infants with isolated esophageal atresia, the lower esophageal segment is short, although intrathoracic lower esophagus is present. Because primary esophageal anastomosis is usually not possible, gastrostomy should be performed initially in all infants with this anomaly. Once the gastrostomy has healed completely, in 3 weeks or so, I initiate daily lengthening of the upper esophageal pouch by means of gentle pressure applied with a stiff orogastric tube, as described by Howard and Myers.[54] This procedure also promotes distal esophageal distention from gastroesophageal reflux associated with the gag reflux. Some authors believe that lengthening of both the upper and lower esophageal pouches will occur naturally, by means of the infant's swallowing and gastroesophageal reflux. Kleinman et al[55] described a method of daily dilation of the distal esophageal pouch using a balloon catheter passed through a gastrostomy with hydrostatic distention while the gastroesophageal junction is occluded by the balloon. After 6 weeks to 3 months, each end of the esophagus may be demonstrated at radiograph to be sufficiently close to allow anastomosis. In the interim, frequent suctioning is required.

As soon as the ends of the esophagus appear sufficiently lengthened to allow anastomosis, right thoracotomy is performed—unless a right aortic arch is present, which is rare. It is usually necessary to perform one or more myotomies as described by Livaditis[28] or Lindell.[29] An alternative approach to stretching has been described by Bar-Maor et al.[56] Their procedure involves lengthening the upper pouch by development of a mucomuscular flap that is rolled into a tube and anastomosed to the lower segment. Whenever possible, I prefer use of the patient's own esophagus to esophageal replacement.

### Esophageal Replacement

Esophageal replacement is described in detail in Chapters 52–54. However, it is worthwhile to emphasize certain considerations in the pediatric age group. When delayed primary esophageal anastomosis either is not possible or is thought to be undesirable because of critical associated disease, gastrostomy and cervical esophagostomy are in order. Cervical esophagostomy may be performed through either the right or the left side of the neck, by means of a short transverse supraclavicular incision. After lateral retraction of the carotid sheath structures and sternocleidomastoid muscle, the esophagus can easily be palpated behind the trachea if a catheter is placed in the esophagus preoperatively. The end of the esophagus is brought to the surface and sutured to the skin and subcutaneous tissue. These patients are then treated, until the age of 1 year or more, by means of gastrostomy feedings.

A variety of methods of esophageal replacement are available. Ordinarily, jejunal interposition is no longer used because it is relatively difficult to perform, unless, for some reason, none of the other forms of replacement is possible. Colonic interposition with either the right or the left colon as described by Dale and Sherman[57] and by Longino et al[58] provides satisfactory results. I prefer either substernal right colonic interposition or the intrathoracic use of left or left transverse colon as described by Waterston.[59] The latter procedure allows use of the native upper and lower esophagus and maintains the LES in use. I have also used the reversed gastric tube described by Gavrilu[60] for esophageal replacement. Finally, Valente et al[61] and Spitz[62] described esophageal replacement with the whole stomach in infants and children with isolated esophageal atresia. Valente et al used the transthoracic approach in 10 patients with no operative deaths. Spitz prefers gastric transposition via the mediastinal route, but the long-term results are no better than with the reversed gastric tube or the colon. Lindahl et al[63] analyzed a group of 34 patients who underwent either colonic interposition or gastric tube replacement of the esophagus for isolated esophageal atresia. Follow-up studies of this group of patients indicated that colonic replacement with either right or left colon and gastric tube replacement had identical long-term results, although the gastric tube procedure was considered easier to perform and was associated with fewer long-term complications.

The most serious complication of colonic interposition is gangrene due to congestion. If this occurs, the segment must be removed, and definitive replacement should be performed at a later date. The most common complication of colonic replacement, however, is leak of the coloesophageal anastomosis. Ordinarily this situation is easily handled by simple drainage, although subsequent stricture is common. If stricture does occur, operative revision ordinarily is required. Late complications of colonic interposition are uncommon. However, duodenal obstruction can occur if the colon is initially brought anterior to the stomach. If the colon has been placed in the right intrathoracic position, tortuosity may develop, necessitating surgical shortening. This problem is less common when the colon is placed substernally or when the Waterston left transverse colon technique is used, because the colon segment usually remains straight under these circumstances. Finally, peptic ulceration at the cologastrostomy site has occasionally been reported, suggesting that vagotomy and pyloroplasty should be added to the original operative procedure. I prefer this procedure. Late ulceration can occur within gastric tubes, usually resulting in loss of the tube. If esophageal replacement is undertaken before the infant is 1 year of age or before the patient is upright, most of the time reflux too frequently results in troublesome pulmonary aspiration.

### Results

My associates and I have operated on 30 patients with isolated esophageal atresia without mortality. Twelve patients underwent esophageal lengthening, myotomy, and delayed primary anastomosis with success, although stricture occurred in 10 of these patients. Nine of 10 responded to dilation, and one required surgical revision. Three patients underwent successful gastric tube replacement, and the other 15 underwent colonic interposition. Of the 15 patients who underwent colon interposition in the past 10 years, one suffered loss of a colonic segment but subsequently underwent successful repeat colonic interposition.

## H-TYPE FISTULA

### Signs and Symptoms

In cases of tracheoesophageal fistula with an intact esophagus—so-called H-type fistula—symptoms suggestive of aspiration during feeding are characteristic, although usually intermittent. Depending on the size of the communication, patients may present as neonates or even at the age of 1 or 2 years. Aspiration pneumonia is usually evident. In addition, if the infants are given thin feedings, they tend to cough and demonstrate signs of aspiration. The prime differential in this regard is whether the infant has dysfunctional swallowing or is actually swallowing correctly but aspirating during the act of swallowing. It is usually possible to make this distinction by means of careful observation.

### Diagnosis

Patients with H-type fistula and an intact esophagus present a diagnostic problem. Although some authors continue to advocate radiographic demonstration of a tracheoesophageal fistula using a contrast-material swallow, I find contrast esophagography to be both unreliable and unsafe. It is far preferable to perform endoscopy, which is the most definitive diagnostic maneuver available. Bronchoscopy also allows one to pass a small Fogarty balloon catheter into the esophagus through the fistula so that the exact level of the fistula may be determined (Fig. 40–5). Most of these fistulas are located low in the neck, although I encountered two within the thorax in a series of 24 patients. Direct observation is also the best method of diagnosis and evaluation for infants with laryngoesophageal clefts. I also have used analysis of gastric air for oxygen content in infants breathing 100% oxygen.[47] High levels of gastric oxygen indicate a tracheoesophageal fistula under these circumstances. This test may occasionally be useful preliminary to bronchoscopy for definitive diagnosis.

### Treatment

Infants with an H-type fistula and an intact esophagus frequently present with such severe pneumonia that they should be treated vigorously with tracheobronchial toilet, systemic antibiotics, and IV nutrition until their condition is satisfactory for operation. There usually is no need to perform an emergency operation under these circumstances.

Preliminary gastrostomy is not necessary in the most infants with an H-type fistula. Isolated tracheoesophageal fistulas usually occur at the level of the sternal notch, so most can be approached through the neck—unless endoscopy has demonstrated the fistula to be within the tho-

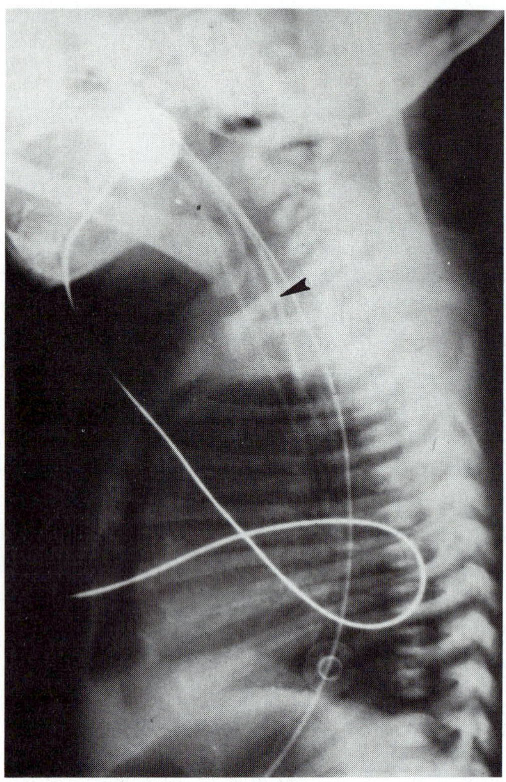

**Figure 40–5.** At the time of endoscopy a catheter (arrow) was passed from the esophagus into the trachea in this patient with an H-type fistula. This is the most reliable approach to diagnosis.

rax, in which case right thoracotomy is in order. I have encountered a single bronchoesophageal fistula. The operative approach is the same as that used for right cervical esophagostomy (Fig. 40–6). Preoperative placement of a Fogarty catheter through the fistula enhances identification and dissection. After identifying the recurrent laryngeal nerve, the surgeon dissects the esophagus away from the posterior wall of the trachea, mobilizing as little of each structure as possible. With gentle traction on the esophagus, it is possible to dissect, divide, and suture both sides of the fistula. Two-layer closure is usually possible on the esophageal side but not on the tracheal side. A small amount of paraspinal muscle is interposed between the two sides of the closure, and a small drain is left in the depths of the incision for a few days.

Respiratory complications related to aspiration of mucus are common. Vocal cord paralysis sometimes occurs. The rare esophageal leak ordinarily heals rapidly if no oral feedings are given.

### Results

Twenty-four patients with isolated H-type tracheoesophageal fistula were treated surgically. There was no mortality and only one temporary esophageal leak. There were no long-term problems in this group of patients. Further, there were no instances of phrenic nerve palsy, pneumothorax, tracheal obstruction, or mediastinitis. Myers and Egami's series of 28 patients with isolated congenital tracheoesophageal fistula had similarly good results, although there were two deaths.[64]

## ESOPHAGEAL STENOSIS

Although esophageal stenosis is ordinarily acquired from gastroesophageal reflux or caustic ingestion, congenital esophageal stenosis occasionally occurs. The diagnosis usually is not suspected until solid food is introduced into the diet, at which point dysphagia may occur. Two of our patients with esophageal atresia and tracheoesophageal fistula had congenital stenosis of the lower esophagus detected at the time of the initial operation. Stenoses that present as a web or diaphragm may be amenable to endoscopic dilation. Numerous cases of esophageal stenosis associated with tracheobronchial remnants have been reported (Fig. 40–7). Nishima et al[65] reviewed their series and demonstrated that 17% of patients had associated anomalies, esophageal atresia and anorectal malformations being the most common. Fekete et al[66] reviewed the cases of 20 patients with congenital esophageal stenosis, four of whom had tracheobronchial remnants; six of whom had membranous diaphragms; and 10 of whom had fibromuscular stenoses. All stenoses were responsive to bougienage except those with cartilaginous tracheobronchial remnants. Seven of this series of 20 patients (35%) had other associated anomalies, particularly esophageal atresia. Most webs occur in the upper and middle esophagus; those associated with esophageal atresia tend to be lower, and stenoses due to retrained cartilaginous tracheobronchial remnants occur in the lower third of the esophagus. The long-term results of treatment of congenital esophageal stenosis, whether by dilation or resection, are excellent. This was the case at my institution.

## ESOPHAGEAL DUPLICATIONS

Duplications of the esophagus generally lie within the posterior mediastinum; symptoms are related either to esophageal obstruction or to impingement on available thoracic space. Most of these lesions are asymptomatic and are discovered when chest radiographs are taken for other reasons. Approximately 30% of the mediastinal masses encountered in infants and children are of foregut origin. It is likely that these congenital cystic masses are of similar origin, whether they be esophageal, bronchogenic, neurenteric, or isolated. The lesions have similar histologic features and may or may not have a muscle all but are usually lined by ciliated epithelium. Sometimes the lining is gastric in nature; ulceration and bleeding may be a problem in these instances. Almost none of these lesions communicate with the lumen of the esophagus, although occasionally there is an

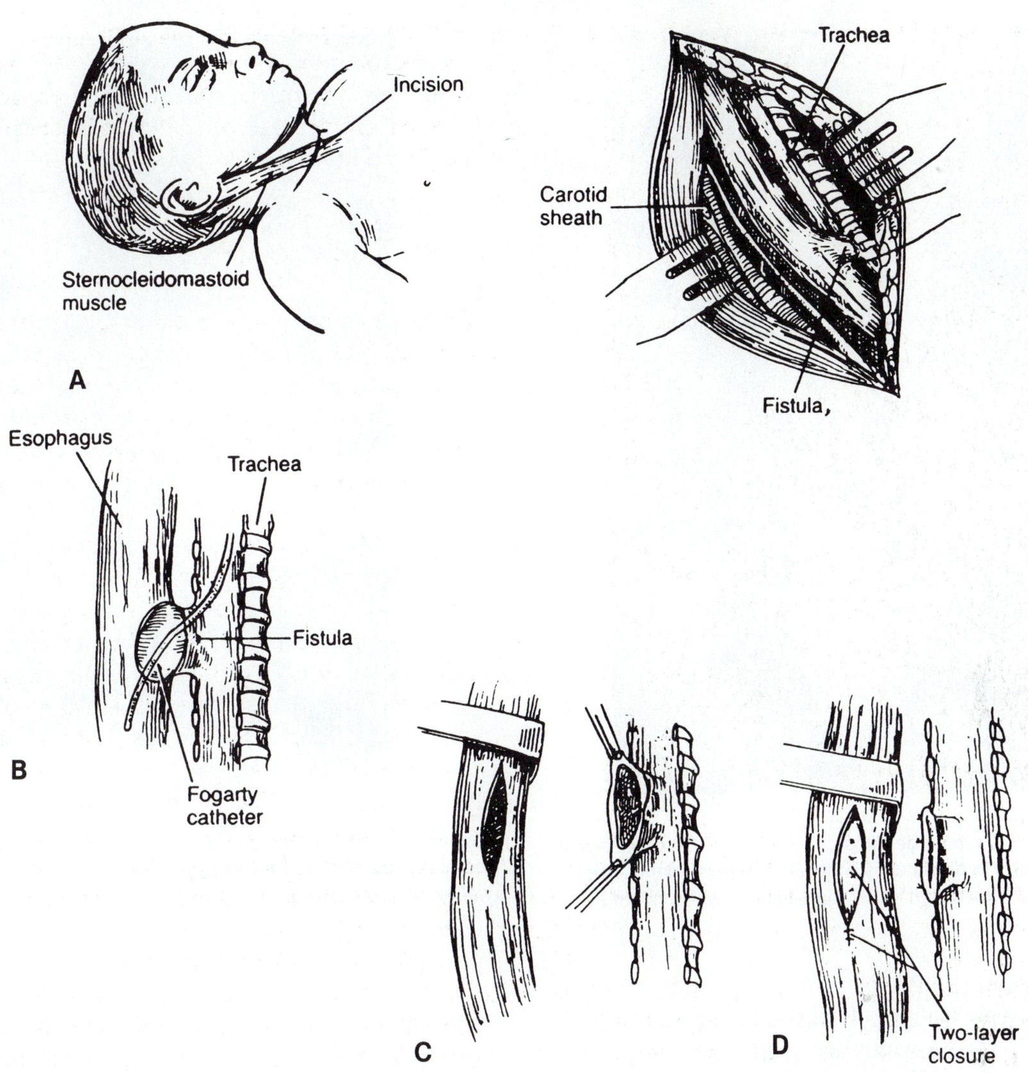


**Figure 40–6.** Repair of type IV H-type tracheoesophageal fistula. **A.** Cervical exposure of tracheoesophageal fistula. **B.** Endoscopic localization of fistula before operation with placement of Fogarty balloon catheter to assist identification of the fistula. **C.** Division of the H-type fistula avoiding injury to the recurrent laryngeal nerve. **D.** Closure of the tracheal and esophageal sides of the fistula. *(From O'Neill JA: Operative Surgery, Principles and Techniques, 3rd ed. Philadelphia, Saunders, 1990, p 1073.)*

attachment to the dura through a cervical vertebral defect. These are called neurenteric cysts.[67] On occasion, large paraesophageal cysts communicate through the diaphragm to a visceral structure below, usually the stomach. The pattern of blood supply is related to the anatomic location and extension of the lesion. In a large series of patients with mediastinal masses described by Haller et al,[68] 12% had duplications. In a series of enteric duplications reported by Grosfeld et al,[69] approximately 18% of patients had lesions related to the esophagus.

## Diagnosis

Because enteric duplications that involve the thorax do not usually communicate with the lumen of the esophagus, precise diagnosis may be difficult unless the characteristic features of a neurenteric duplication are seen—namely, bifid vertebrae in the lower cervical or upper thoracic region.[69] A barium esophogram is capable of demonstrating a smooth filling defect in the continuity of the esophagus (Fig. 40–8). I prefer to use computed tomography (CT) with esophageal contrast enhancement because this modality demonstrates the spatial relation within the mediastinum more accurately than any other study (Fig. 40–9). It is worthwhile to perform an ultrasound examination of the abdomen as well. I have encountered patients with coexisting duplication cysts within the mediastinum and along the abdominal gastrointestinal tract.[69] When a neurenteric cyst is suspected because of the presence of bifid vertebrae, technetium radionuclide scanning is in order, since many such patients have gastric mucosa present. Magnetic resonance imaging (MRI) of the vertebral column is in order to rule out an intraspinal component of the neurenteric cyst, as described by Superina et al.[70]

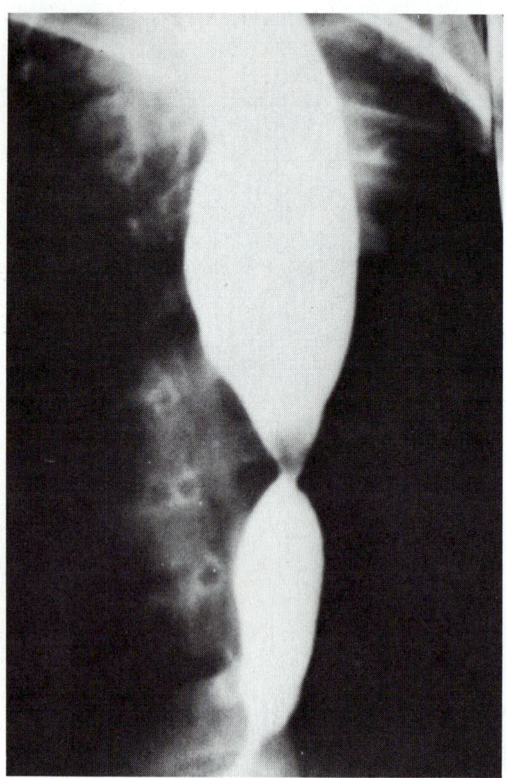

Figure 40–7. Esophogram demonstrating a congenital esophageal stenosis secondary to persistent tracheobronchial remnants. The lesion necessitates resection rather than dilation, which might be used to treat webs.

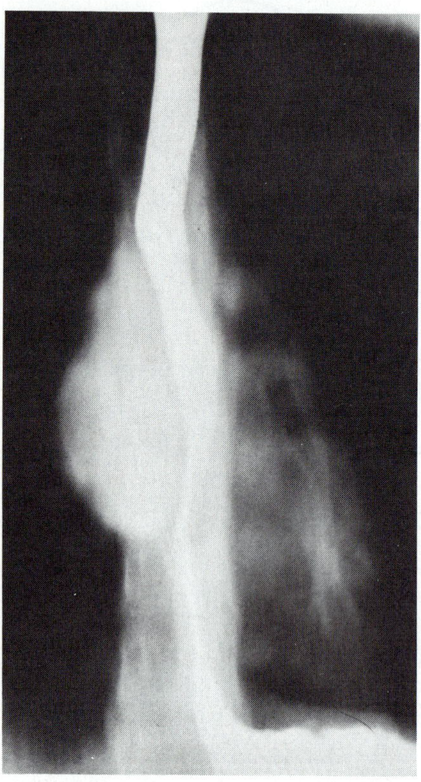

Figure 40–8. Tomographic cut of an esophogram demonstrating the typical deformity of a duplication cyst that shares a common wall with the esophagus but does not communicate with the lumen.

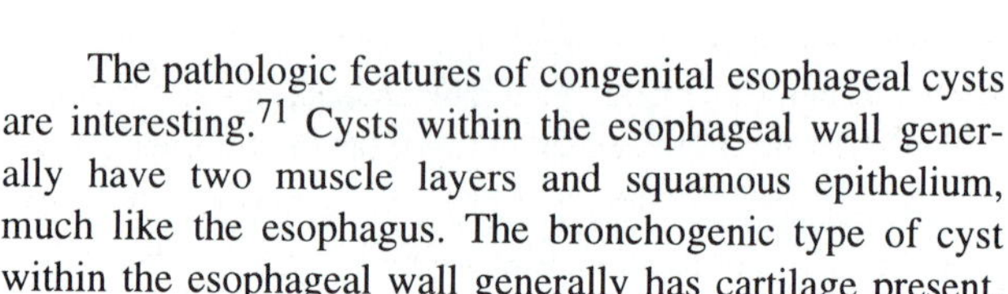

The pathologic features of congenital esophageal cysts are interesting.[71] Cysts within the esophageal wall generally have two muscle layers and squamous epithelium, much like the esophagus. The bronchogenic type of cyst within the esophageal wall generally has cartilage present. Neurenteric cysts in the posterior mediastinum tend to be covered by well-developed muscular walls; gastric or other intestinal mucosa is often present. At times esophageal atresia may be associated with esophageal duplication cysts, as reported by Hamalatha et al.[72]

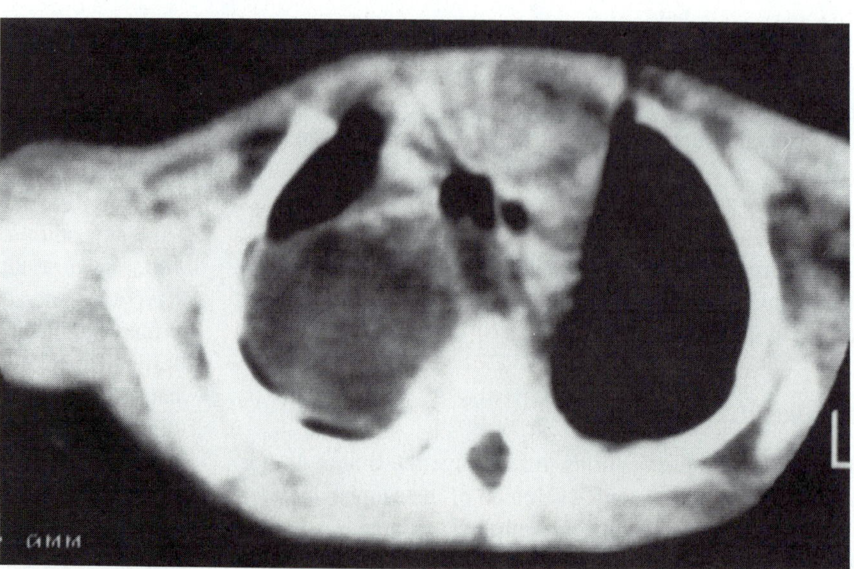

Figure 40–9. CT scan demonstrating an esophageal duplication cyst and all its relations with the mediastinum. This is the preferred diagnostic tool for the evaluation of esophageal duplication cysts.

### Treatment

At one time the preferred treatment of esophageal duplications was partial resection, mucosal stripping, and marsupialization.[73] However, the preferred approach now is complete resection with repair of the esophageal wall. We have not encountered any duplications of the esophagus that could not be completely resected. When esophageal duplications have been thoracoabdominal, complete resection has occasionally necessitated division of the diaphragm at its periphery, abdominal extension of the thoracic incision, or separate abdominal and thoracic incisions, depending on the length and nature of the attachments. Careful attention must be paid to the blood supply of large duplications, particularly when they extend below the diaphragm. When the mucosa of the esophagus is violated during the course of resection or when the esophageal lumen has been narrowed, gastrostomy has been used to protect the esophagus during healing or dilation, respectively.

### Results

In instances in which complete resection of esophageal duplications has been performed (this category includes most patients) no long-term sequelae have been encountered. When it has been necessary to reconstruct long segments of the esophageal wall, temporary motility disturbances have been noted, but they all have corrected within several months. There were no deaths or serious complications in a series of 21 patients with esophageal duplications treated at my institution.

## ESOPHAGEAL DIVERTICULA

Esophageal diverticula are extremely rare, and very few have been reported. The typical Zenker's diverticulum seen in adults is not a true diverticulum. The rare congenital diverticulum seen in infants and children tends to have a complete muscular wall.[74] In newborns, the usual symptom is excessive mucous secretions that simulate esophageal atresia. If a tube has been passed into the esophagus and happens to enter the diverticulum, esophageal atresia is suspected. If the diverticulum is large enough and fills on feeding, it may cause respiratory obstruction. The real danger of large diverticula filled with food is sudden spillover and aspiration. Resection is the treatment of choice.

Reference was made in the section on esophageal atresia with tracheoesophageal fistula to traumatic pseudodiverticulum of the pharynx. In four patients treated at my institution, nothing more than antibiotic therapy and tube feedings were required. Healing was complete within 10 days. Initial diagnosis and observation of healing are best accomplished with endoscopy.

Diverticula of the esophagus that occur within the thorax are generally associated with some variation of esophageal atresia and tracheoesophageal fistula. They may or may not be symptomatic, depending on their size.

## GASTROESOPHAGEAL REFLUX

A thorough discussion of gastroesophageal reflux, including the various surgical procedures applicable to this problem, is presented in Chapters 42–46. However, the presentation of gastroesophageal reflux in infants and children is somewhat different from that in adults and is worthy of further mention here. In patients with an intact esophagus and no other esophageal anomaly, the most likely cause of gastroesophageal reflux is failure of maturation of the LES sphincter. Boix-Ochoa and Canales[75] reported on manometric studies that confirmed the original studies of Carre.[76] In studies by the Boix-Ochoa and Canales, an effective LES mechanism was generally present by 6–7 weeks of life, although it took longer is some infants. This observation has some implications for the timing of surgical intervention in infants with gastroesophageal reflux.

Another potential cause of gastroesophageal reflux in infants is abnormal innervation of the esophagus. This is believed to be responsible for the high incidence of gastroesophageal reflux in patients with esophageal atresia and its variants.[53] Psychomotor retardation also has been shown to predispose to gastroesophageal reflux.[77]

### Signs and Symptoms

The most common presenting symptom of gastroesophageal reflux is frequent regurgitation; upper gastrointestinal bleeding, apneic spells, chronic intermittent pneumonia, and even sudden death occasionally may be encountered. Chronicity of these findings, particularly after 6 months of age, generally indicates that surgical intervention is in order. Infants who experience minor but persistent spitting up into late childhood are prone to strictures, so close long-term follow-up study is important.[76]

### Diagnosis

The diagnosis of pathologic gastroesophageal reflux is outlined in Chapter 42. The two methods I prefer are 24-hour pH monitoring, noting the number of reflux episodes and the rate of esophageal clearing, and technetium milk scans looking for reflux, esophageal clearing, episodes of aspiration, and rate of gastric emptying. I have not used esophageal manometry routinely in recent years. Although an upper gastrointestinal radiographic series has usually been performed, the study is probably no more than 50% accurate in verifying the presence of gastroesophageal reflux, so it is not considered a primary diagnostic tool. I have used esophagoscopy routinely to determine the presence of both esophagitis and Barrett's esophagus. The latter is a consideration in children older than 8 years.

## Treatment

Most infants who present with gastroesophageal reflux do not have a congenital hiatal hernia and respond to nonoperative therapy if it is aggressive enough. I use either elevated prone positioning or upright positioning, in a special seating device, in association with thickened feedings for infants. For the past 10 years, I have used Urecholine (bethanechol) 0.6 mg/kg every 24 hours, in three divided doses, with an 80% success rate in terms of permanent resolution of gastroesophageal reflux in infants. In older children, I have not found Urecholine to be beneficial, but I have found cimetidine to be extremely helpful in patients who have associated peptic esophagitis. I also have used metoclopramide routinely because many patients have delayed gastric emptying. Infants with chronic gastroesophageal reflux unresponsive to therapy, or with life-threatening symptoms, infants with congenital hiatal hernias, and older children with clinically significant gastroesophageal reflux, esophagitis, or other problems undergo surgical fundoplication (Table 40–1). Two primary approaches have been used. I prefer, as do most authors, the Nissen fundoplication. The other approach, promoted by Ashcraft et al,[78] is modified Thal fundoplication. The reported results are somewhat superior with the Nissen technique.

Nissen fundoplication (Chap. 44) is performed in infants and children according to the same basic principles as in adults, but the procedure is modified according to the size of the patient. I mobilize a sufficient length of esophagus to allow the entire wrap to be positioned within the abdominal cavity. A 1.5–2.0 cm wrap around the intra-abdominal esophagus is used in infants, and a 3.0 cm wrap in older patients. The wrap is usually made to be loose so that food of a consistency appropriate for the patient's age will easily pass into the stomach. As a guide, a nasogastric tube and esophageal dilator are placed within the esophagus into the stomach before the sutures used for construction of the wrap are tied. The size of the dilator ranges from 24 F in infants to 40 F in children. The complications seen in children are the same as those seen in adults, but gas bloat syndrome is of particular concern in small infants, whose feeding routine usually involves the need to burp. For this reason, I usually perform temporary gastrostomy in infants younger than 6 months who require fundoplication for intractable gastroesophageal reflux.

**TABLE 40–1. INDICATIONS FOR SURGERY FOR GASTROESOPHAGEAL REFLUX**

**Infants**
- Chronic regurgitation despite treatment
- Failure to thrive
- Chronic or recurrent pneumonia associated with reflux
- Recurrent apneic spells following initial nonsurgical treatment

**Children**
- Chronic esophagitis
- Recurrent pulmonary aspiration
- Severe neurologic impairment associated with reflux
- Esophageal stricture

The special group of patients with gastroesophageal reflux evident after repair of esophageal atresia and tracheoesophageal fistula requires careful continued follow-up, because persistent reflux may result in stricture at the level of the esophageal anastomosis. Should this or other serious complications occur, fundoplication is in order.

Another group who requires special consideration are older children with esophageal strictures associated with chronic gastroesophageal reflux. In a follow-up study of 18 consecutive children who underwent correction of peptic esophageal strictures, long-term follow-up findings indicated that preoperative dilation or direct surgical management before correction of reflux was ineffective.[79] The most effective approach was intraoperative dilation, Nissen fundoplication, and guided dilation after the operation. In only one patient with Barrett's esophagus was esophageal replacement required for a reflux stricture that was persistent despite successful Nissen fundoplication.

Patients in whom there was evidence of delayed gastric emptying and, occasionally, esophageal motor dysfunction underwent follow-up studies. Gastric emptying routinely returned to normal after successful fundoplication, but patients with esophageal motor dysfunction had continuing dysfunction.[79] The recurrence rate after Nissen fundoplication has been 10% at my institution; patients who had recurrences almost exclusively also had neurologic impairment.

## ACHALASIA

Much less common than reflux is achalasia or cardiospasm. This disorder of motility is of unknown causation and is common in adults. It is distinctly uncommon in childhood; only about 5% of all patients who present with this disorder are in the early years of life. Rare patients present with this disorder in infancy, but most young patients appear in the early teenage years with poor nutrition and chronic vomiting.

The diagnosis of achalasia at the gastroesophageal junction may be suspected on the basis of symptoms alone, but verification depends on careful performance of a barium esophogram and esophageal motility (manometry) studies. These details are described in Chapter 49. Differentiation of achalasia from stricture due to reflux depends on performance of esophagoscopy. At the time of esophagoscopy, no esophagitis and no permanent narrowing are noted. (Interestingly, this procedure alone may be therapeutic in infants.) In no patient have I found pharmacologic approaches to achalasia to be successful.

Achalasia may also rarely present in the region of the cricopharyngeus muscle. Cricopharyngeal achalasia is a disorder most frequently encountered in elderly patients who have sustained severe strokes, but it may be seen in in-

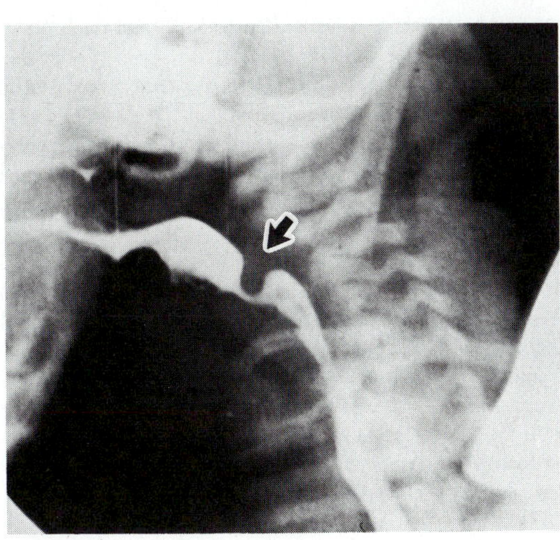

**Figure 40–10.** View of the pharynx and upper esophagus at the time of barium swallow demonstrating the persistent posterior impression of the cricopharyngeus muscle (arrow) associated with cricopharyngeal achalasia.

fants as well. It is likely that these patients have suffered some imbalance of cricopharyngeal innervation resulting in chronic constriction. The symptoms in infants up to several weeks of age are severe dysphagia, inability to control secretions, and aspiration pneumonia. Barium esophogram is generally diagnostic, demonstrating the characteristic features of persistent posterior obstruction of the esophagus at the level of the crichopharyngeas muscle (Fig. 40–10).

Nakayama et al[80] reported on a series of 19 patients with achalasia. Fifteen patients underwent pneumatic balloon dilation first, with four failures. These four patients and an additional four patients underwent left thoracic esophagocardiomyotomy with reconstitution of the hiatus, as described by Ellis et al.[81] Fundoplication was not used in association with esophagocardiomyotomy, and all patients were well at follow-up. I propose, on the basis of experience at my institution, that children with cardiospasm undergo pneumatic balloon dilation first and that surgical intervention be used only if there is rapid recurrence of symptoms. The long-term functional results are generally good in more than 90% of patients. Esophagocardiomyotomy is also being done via laparoscopy and thoracoscopy (see Chap. 50A).

Infants with cricopharyngeal achalasia have undergone myotomy performed through a left lateral cervical approach. Even after myotomy, relief is not immediate, and swallowing tends to remain uncoordinated for 7–10 days. After that time, patients are able to control their secretions, and swallowing progresses well, with no likelihood or recurrence of symptoms.

## REFERENCES


1. Durston W: A narrative of monstrous birth in Plymouth October 22, 1670; together with the anatomical observations taken thereupon by William Durston, Doctor of Physic and communication to Dr. Tim Clerk. *Philos Trans R Soc* **5:**2096, 1670
2. Gibson T: *The Anatomy of Humane Bodies Epitomized,* 6th ed. London, Awnsham & Churchill, 1703
3. Lanman TH: Congenital atresia of the esophagus: A study of thirty-two cases. *Arch Surg* **41:**1060, 1940
4. Ladd WE: The surgical treatment of esophageal atresia with tracheoesophageal fistulas. *N Engl J Med* **230:**625, 1944
5. Levin NL: Congenital atresia of the esophagus with tracheoesophageal fistula: Report of successful extrapleural ligation of fistulous communication and cervical esophagostomy. *J Thorac Surg* **10:**648, 1940
6. Haight C, Towsley HA: Congenital atresia of the esophagus with tracheoesophageal fistula: Extrapleural ligation of fistula and end-to-end anastomosis of esophageal segments. *Surg Gynecol Obstet* **76:**672, 1943
7. Gross RE: *The Surgery of Infancy and Childhood.* Philadelphia, Saunders, 1953, p 76
8. Vogt EC: Congenital esophageal atresia. *AJR* **22:**463, 1929
9. Holder TM, Cloud DT, Lewis JE, Pilling GP: Esophageal atresia and tracheoesophageal fistula: A survey of its members by the Surgical Section of the American Academy of Pediatrics. *Pediatrics* **34:**542, 1964
10. Hartenberg MA, Salzberg AM, Krummel TM, Bush JJ: Double aortic arch associated with esophageal atresia and tracheoesophageal fistula. *J Pediatr Surg* **24:**488, 1989
11. Chiba T, Ohi R, Hayashi Y, Uchida T: Bronchopulmonary foregut malformation in 3 infants: With special references to cases in childhood. *Z Kinderchir* **44:**105, 1989
12. Quan L, Smith DW: The VATER association. Vertebral defects, and atresia, T-E fistula with esophageal atresia, T-E fistula with esophageal atresia, radial and renal dysplasia: A spectrum of associated defects. *J Pediatr* **82:**104, 1973
13. Lim SY: CHARGE association: A case report and short annotation. *J Singapore Paediatr Soc* **32:**46, 1990
14. Yun K-L, Hartman GE, Schochat SJ: Esophageal atresia with triple congenital tracheoesophageal fistulae. *J Pediatr Surg* **27:**1527, 1992
15. Heller RM, Kirchner SG, O'Neill JA: Perforation of the pharynx in the newborn: A near look-alike for esophageal atresia. *AJR* **129:**335, 1977
16. Replogle RL: Esophageal atresia: Plastic sump catheter for drainage of the proximal pouch. *Surgery* **54:**296, 1963
17. Ohkawa H, Ochi G, Yamazaki Y, Sawaguchi S: Clinical experience with a sucking sump catheter in the treatment of esophageal atresia. *J Pediatr Surg* **24:**333, 1989
18. Bar-Maor JA, Shoshany G, Monies-Chass I: Use of cimetidine in esophageal atresia with lower tracheoesophageal fistula. *J Pediatr Surg* **16:**8, 1981
19. Bloom BT, Delmore P, Park YI, Nelson RA: Respiratory distress syndrome and tracheoesophageal fistula: Management with high frequency ventilation. *Crit Care Med* **18:**447, 1990
20. Randolph JG, Newman KD, Anderson KD: Current results in repair of esophageal atresia: Review of 16 years' experience. *J Pediatr Surg* **23:**805, 1988
21. Shaul DB, Schwartz MZ, Marr CC, Tyson RR: Primary repair without gastrostomy is the treatment of choice for neonate with esophageal atresia and tracheoesophageal fistula. *Arch Surg* **124:**1188, 1989
22. Louhimo I: Esophageal atresia: Primary result of 500 consecutively treated patients. *J Pediatr Surg* **18:**217, 1983
23. Bishop PJ, Klein MD, Phillipart AJ, et al: Transpleural repair of esophageal atresia without primary gastrostomy: 240 patients treated between 1951–1983. *J Pediatr Surg* **20:**823, 1985
24. Templeton JM, Templeton JJ, Schnaufer L, et al: Management of esophageal atresia and tracheoesophageal fistula in the neonate with severe respiratory distress syndrome. *J Pediatr Surg* **20:**394, 1985
25. Filston HC, Chitwood WR, Schkolne B, et al: The Fogarty balloon

catheter as an aid to management of the infant with esophageal atresia and tracheoesophageal fistula complicated by severe RDS or pneumonia. *J Pediatr Surg* **17:**149, 1982
26. Reichenbacher WE, Ballantine TV: Esophageal atresia, distal tracheoesophageal fistula, and an air shunt that compromised mechanical ventilation. *J Pediatr Surg* **25:**1216, 1990
27. Spitz L, Ali M, Brereton RJ: Combined esophageal and duodenal atresia: Experience of 18 patients. *J Pediatr Surg* **17:**149, 1982
28. Livaditis A: Esophageal atresia: A method of overbridging large segmental gaps. *Z Kinderchir* **13:**298, 1973
29. Lindell IL: Modification of Livadits' myotomy for long gap esophageal atresia. *Ann Chir Gynaecol* **79:**101, 1990
30. Duhamel B: *Technique Chirurgicale Infantale.* Paris, Masson, 1957, p 87
31. Sulamaa M, Gripenberg L, Ahvenainen EK: Prognosis and treatment of congenital atresia of the esophagus. *Acta Chir Scand* **102:**141, 1951
32. Pietsch JB, Stokes KB, Beardmore HE: Esophageal atresia with tracheoesophageal fistula: End-to-end versus end-to-side repair. *J Pediatr Surg* **13:**677, 1978
33. Touloukian RJ: Reassessment of the end-to-side operation for esophageal atresia and distal tracheoesophageal fistula: 22 year experience with 68 cases. *J Pediatr Surg* **27:**562, 1992
34. Todd DW, Shoemaker CT, Agarwal I, Browdie DA: Temporary banding of the gastroesophageal juncture in a very small neonate with esophageal atresia and tracheoesophageal fistula. *Minn Med* **73:**30, 1990
35. Greenwood RD, Rosenthal A: Cardiovascular malformations associated with tracheosophageal fistula and esophageal atresia. *Pediatrics* **57:**87, 1976
36. McKinnon LJ, Kosloski AM: Prediction and prevention of anastamotic complications of esophageal atresia and tracheoesophageal fistula. *J Pediatr Surg* **25:**778, 1990
37. Sillen U, Hagberg S, Rubenson A, Werkmaster K: Management of esophageal atresia: Review of 16 years' experience. *J Pediatr Surg* **23:**805, 1988
38. Schwartz MZ, Filler RM: Tracheal compression as a cause of apnea following repair of tracheoesophageal fistula: Treatment by aortopexy. *J Pediatr Surg* **15:**842, 1980
39. Kimura K, Soper RT, Kao SC, et al: Aortosternopexy for tracheomalacia following repair of esophageal atresia: Evaluation by cine-CT and technical refinement. *J Pediatr Surg* **25:**769, 1990
40. Spitz L: Dacron-patch aortopexy. *Prog Pediatr Surg* **19:**117, 1986
41. Nakazato Y, Wells TR, Landing BH: Abnormal tracheal innervation in patients with esophageal atresia and tracheoesophageal fistula: Study of the intrinsic tracheal nerve plexuses by a microdissection technique. *J Pediatr Surg* **21:**838, 1986
42. Shono T, Suita S, Arima T, et al: Motility function of the esophagus before primary anastomosis in esophageal atresia. *J Pediatr Surg* **28:**673, 1993
43. Cozzi F, Myers NA, Madonna L, et al: Esophageal atresia, choanal atresia, and dysantonomia. *J Pediatr Surg* **26:**548, 1991
44. LeSouef PN, Myers NA, Landau LI: Etiologic factors in long-term respiratory function abnormalities following esophageal atresia repair. *J Pediatr Surg* **22:**918, 1987
45. Rangecroft L, Bush GH, Lister J, et al: Endoscopic diathermy obliteration of recurrent TEF. *J Pediatr Surg* **19:**41, 1984
46. Fonkalsrud EW: Gastroesophageal fundoplication for reflux following repair of esophageal atresia: Experience with nine patients. *Arch Surg* **114:**48, 1979
47. O'Neill JA, Holcomb GW, Neblett WW: Recent experience with esophageal atresia. *Ann Surg* **114:**48, 1979
48. Spitz L, Kiely E, Brereton RJ: Esophageal atresia: Five year experience with 148 cases. *J Pediatr Surg* **22:**103, 1987
49. Waterston DJ, Bonham-Carter RE, Aberdeen E: Oesophageal atresia: Tracheoesophageal fistula—A study of survival in 218 infants. *Lancet* **1:**819, 1962
50. Duranceau A, Fisher SR, Flye MW, et al: Motor function of the esophagus after repair of esophageal atresia and tracheoesophageal fistula. *Surgery* **82:**116, 1977
51. Orringer MB, Kirsh MM, Sloan H: Long-term esophageal function following repair of esophageal atresia. *Ann Surg* **186:**436, 1977
52. Parker AF, Christie DL, Cahill JL: Incidence and significance of gastroesophageal reflux following repair of esophageal atresia and tracheoesophageal fistula and the need for anti-reflux procedures. *J Pediatr Surg* **14:**5, 1979
53. Putnam TC, Lawrence RA, Wood BP, et al: Esophageal function after repair of esophageal atresia. *Surg Gynecol Obstet* **158:**344, 1984
54. Howard R, Myers NA: Esophageal atresia. A technique for elongating the upper pouch. *Surgery* **58:**725, 1965
55. Kleinman PK, Waite RJ, Cohen IT, et al: Atretic esophagus: transgastric balloon-assisted hydrostatic dilation. *Radiology* **171:**831, 1989
56. Bar-Maor JA, Shoshany G, Sweed Y: Wide gap esophageal atresia: a new method to elongate the upper pouch. *J Pediatr Surg* **24:**882, 1989
57. Dale WA, Sherman CD: Late reconstruction of congenital esophageal atresia by intrathoracic colon transplant. *J Thorac Cardiovasc Surg* **40:**507, 1960
58. Longino L, Woolley MM, Gross RE: Esophageal replacement in infants and children with use of a segment of colon. *JAMA* **171:**1187, 1959
59. Waterston D: Colonic replacement of esophagus (intrathoracic). *Surg Clin North Am* **44:**1441, 1964
60. Gavriliu D: Aspects of esophageal surgery. *Curr Probl Surg* Oct., 1975
61. Valente A, Brereton RJ, Mackersie A: Esophageal replacement with whole stomach in infants and children. *J Pediatr Surg* **22:**913, 1987
62. Spitz L: Gastric transposition via the mediastinal route for infants with long-gap esophageal atresia. *J Pediatr Surg* **19:**149, 1984
63. Lindahl H, Louhimo I, Virkola K: Colon interposition or gastric tube? Follow-up study of colon-esophagus and gastric tube-esophagus patients. *J Pediatr Surg* **18:**58, 1983
64. Myers NA, Egami K: Congenital tracheo-esophageal fistula: "H" or "N" fistula. *Pediatr Surg* **22:**986, 1987
65. Nishima T, Tsuchida Y, Saito S: Congenital esophageal stenosis due to tracheobronchial remnants and its associated anomalies. *J Pediatr Surg* **16:**190, 1981
66. Fekete C, DeBacker A, Lortat-Jacob S, et al: Congenital esophageal stenosis: A review of 20 cases. *Pediatr Surg Int* **2:**86, 1987
67. Holcomb GW, Gheissari A, O'Neill JA, et al: Surgical management of alimentary tract duplications. *Ann Surg* **209:**167, 1989
68. Haller JA, Mazur DO, Morgan WW: Diagnosis and management of mediastinal masses in children. *J Thorac Cardiovasc Surg* **58:**385, 1969
69. Grosfeld JL, O'Neill JA, Clatworthy HW: Enteric duplications in infancy and childhood: An 18-year review. *Ann Surg* **172:**83, 1970
70. Superina RA, Ein SH, Humphreys RP: Cystic duplications of the esophagus and neurenteric cysts. *J Pediatr Surg* **19:**527, 1984
71. Arbona JL, Figueroa JG, Mayoral J: Congenital esophageal cysts: Case report and review of the literature. *Am J Gastroenterol* **79:**177, 1984
72. Hemalatha V, Batcup G, Brereton RJ, et al: Esophageal atresia associated with esophageal duplication cyst. *J Pediatr Surg* **22:**984, 1987
73. Ladd WE, Scott HW: Esophageal duplications or mediastinal cysts of enteric origin. *Surgery* **16:**815, 1944
74. Brintnall ES, Kridelbaugh WW: Congenital diverticulum of posterior hypopharynx simulating atresia or esophagus. *Ann Surg* **131:**564, 1950
75. Boix-Ochoa J, Canales J: Maturation of the lower esophageal sphincter. *J Pediatr Surg* **11:**749, 1976
76. Carre IT: The natural history of the partial thoracic stomach (hiatus hernia) in children. *Arch Dis Child* **34:**344, 1959
77. Staiano A, Cucchiara S, DelGiudice E, et al: Disorders of oesophageal motility in children with psychomotor retardation and gastroesophageal reflux. *Eur J Pediatr* **150:**638, 1991
78. Ashcraft KW, Holder TM, Amoury RA: Treatment of gastro-

esophageal reflux in children by Thal fundoplication. *J Thorac Cardiovasc Surg* **82:**706, 1981

79. O'Neill JA, Betts JM, Ziegler MM, et al: Surgical management of reflux strictures of the esophagus in childhood. *Ann Surg* **196:**453, 1982
80. Nakayama DK, Shorter NA, Boyle JT, et al: Pneumatic dilation and operative treatment of achalasia in children. *J Pediatr Surg* **22:**619, 1987
81. Ellis FH, Kister JC, Schlegel JF, et al: Esophagomyotomy for esophageal atresia: Experimental, clinical and manometric aspects. *Ann Surg* **166:**640, 1967

CHAPTER

# 41

# Esophageal Injury

## *Perforation, Chemical Burns, Foreign Bodies, and Bleeding*

John R. Handy, Jr., and Carolyn E. Reed

## ESOPHAGEAL INJURY

Esophageal injury is an infrequent component in the practice of thoracic surgery, but one that is dramatic in presentation. The successful management of such infrequently encountered clinical entities is challenging, and the consequences of incorrect decisions are devastating. The care of these often critically ill patients with unusual injuries requires an understanding of esophageal pathophysiology, a knowledge of the literature, and a good deal of common sense combined with patience.

### Esophageal Perforation

Esophageal perforation is an unusual but catastrophic event. The mortality for perforated esophagus has declined somewhat in recent history but still is about 20%.[1] A thorough understanding of the treatment options is required to successfully manage such a devastating injury.

#### *History*

The earliest reference to esophageal perforation is in the Edwin Smith Papyrus (2500 BC) which describes a complication thereof—a cervical esophagocutaneous fistula. In 1724, Boerhaave[2] described the clinical course and subsequent autopsy of a barogenic esophageal rupture in the High Admiral of the Dutch Navy, the Baron van Wessenaer, after the Baron had feasted and induced vomiting. Thus, barogenic esophageal rupture is named Boerhaave's syndrome. Meyer[3] made the first clinical diagnosis in 1858. Frink[4] described the first surgical drainage of an esophageal perforation. In 1944, Collins et al[5] made the first attempt at surgical repair, but the patient died. In 1947, Barrett[6] and Olsen with Claggett[7] described successful surgical repairs. Brewer and Burford[8] in 1947 described the successful repair of a traumatic perforation. In 1952, Satinsky and Kron[9] successfully performed esophagectomy for perforation.

Esophageal perforation once was a lesion of barogenic or traumatic causation, but now it is usually iatrogenic. Over the last 40 years, invasive techniques for the diagnosis of and therapy for gastrointestinal disease have been developed and disseminated. At the same time, the incidence of esophageal perforation has increased markedly.

#### *Pathophysiology*

Perforation of the esophagus exposes the involved body cavity to leakage of ingested material and gastrointestinal secretions. This results in a chemical insult to the surrounding tissues, which leads to chemical mediastinitis or peritonitis. Superimposed on this chemical burn is a bath of oral bacterial flora involving aerobic and anaerobic organisms. These organisms cause a mixed necrotizing superinfection in a closed space adjacent to vital organs of the mediastinum and upper abdomen. This combination of insults leads rapidly to severe systemic sepsis and capillary leak. Even today with sophistication of diagnostic and operative techniques and anesthetic and critical care, the mortality for perforated esophagus is high.

### Etiology

A comprehensive review article by Jones and Ginsberg[1] indicated that iatrogenic causes accounted for 51% of esophageal perforations (Fig. 41–1). Types of instrumentation that frequently cause perforation included esophagoscopy, pneumatic dilation, bougienage, and sclerotherapy, accounting for 43% of perforations. Esophageal perforation also has been described with placement of nasogastric tubes,[10] endotracheal tubes,[11] endoesophageal prostheses,[12,13] endoesophageal tamponading tubes,[14] and transesophageal echocardiography.[15] An additional 8% of iatrogenic perforations involved operative injury incurred during mediastinoscopy, thyroidectomy, leiomyoma enucleation, proximal gastric vagotomy, gastric reflux procedures, and even spinal operations.[16] Other rare iatrogenic causes of esophageal perforation have been described, such as transcatheter ablation of accessory cardiac conduction pathways.[17]

The actual risk of perforation during instrumentation of the esophagus is quite low. A review[18] of 211,410 flexible esophagogastroduodenoscopies revealed a rate of perforation of 0.03%. The rate of perforation for 13,139 mercury bougienages was 0.09%, 9431 metal olive dilations was 0.35%, and for 1,224 pneumatic dilations was 1.14%.

Areas at risk for instrumental esophageal perforation are inherently weak regions or sites of anatomic or pathologic narrowing. The cervical and thoracic portions of the esophagus are the areas most frequently perforated with instrumentation.[1] The area primarily jeopardized by weakness is Lannier's triangle. This triangle is bordered by the pharyngeal inferior constrictor and the cricopharyngeus muscles, leaving an area of esophageal mucosa without muscularis and directly abutting the prevertebral fascia. This region of anatomic weakness is brought prominently anterior by cervical osteophytic spurs, kyphosis or by maneuvers such as neck hyperextension, exposing the area to injury by tubes or scopes being passed. Anatomic areas of narrowing include not only the physiologic sphincters but also the esophagus adjacent to the aortic arch and the left main stem bronchus. Finally, benign or malignant strictures can occur at any site within the esophagus, putting it at risk for perforation.

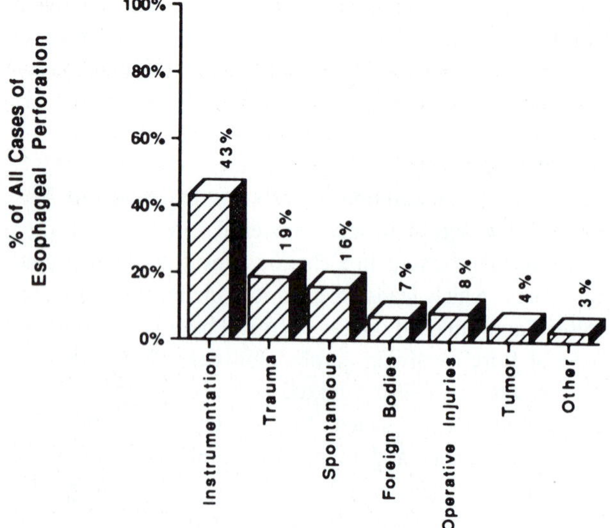


**Figure 41–1.** Causes of esophageal perforation. *(From Jones WG, Ginsberg RJ: Ann Thorac Surg 1992; 53:534–43, with permission.)*

Trauma accounts for about 20% of esophageal perforations. Traumatic causes are almost always secondary to penetrating injury and involve the cervical esophagus. Thus penetrating injury to the neck or thorax must always evoke the diagnostic consideration of esophageal perforation. Blunt trauma is a rare cause of perforation. Cervical esophageal perforation has been diagnosed after boxing[19] and forcible neck hyperextension.[20] Thoracic esophageal disruption has been described with motor vehicle collisions.[21,22] Unusual traumatic causes include perforation secondary to blast effect[23] or compressed air.[24]

Barogenic rupture is the cause of about 15% of esophageal perforations. Barogenic disruption virtually always follows vomiting or, much less frequently, a maneuver that suddenly and drastically increases intra-abdominal pressure, such as weight lifting, child birth, seizures, or even a paroxysm of laughter.[25] The disruption involves the left wall of the supradiaphragmatic esophagus, and 80% of the time drains into the left pleura or peritoneum.

The mechanism of barogenic rupture has been studied with experiments. In 1884, MacKenzie[26] determined the bursting point of the esophagus by filling 18 specimens with water. He found an average of 7 lb (3.15 kg) disrupted the esophagus, always along the lower esophagus in a longitudinal manner. He also noted the mucosa was more resistant to rupture than was the muscularis. In 1967, Tidman and John,[27] in studies of intact cadavers, found the esophagus ruptured at 4.6 psi (5 psi = 259 mm Hg). Intragastric pressures as high as 850 mm Hg have been measured during vomiting. These pressures easily exceed that needed to disrupt the esophagus if transmitted intraesophageally and contained within the organ by a closed upper esophageal sphincter or spasm.

Other rare causes of esophageal perforation include tumor erosion and cavitation, Barrett's ulcer,[28] and viral infections.[29]

Because instrumentation, trauma and barogenic mechanisms figure so prominently in the etiology of esophageal perforation, it is understandable that approximately 50% of perforations occur in an otherwise normal esophagus. The abnormalities present in the remaining half include benign stricture (25% of perforations), diverticula (15%), carcinoma (10%), and achalasia (5%).[1,30]

### Clinical Manifestations

The symptoms of esophageal perforation depend on the cause, the location, and the duration since perforation. Pain, dyspnea, and dysphagia are found to varying degrees.[31] A patient who reports chest pain or manifests fever after instrumentation of the upper aerodigestive tract should be considered to have a perforation until proved otherwise. The symptoms of trauma-induced perforations usually are overshadowed by symptoms of associated injuries.

The symptoms of barogenic perforation are usually nonspecific and catastrophic. Chest pain, abdominal pain, dyspnea, dysphagia, and fever are found in various combinations or all together. Barogenic perforations classically show Mackler's triad: vomiting, lower thoracic pain, and subcutaneous emphysema.[32] However, because of the nonspecific nature of the symptoms, the diagnosis is often confused with other life-threatening illnesses. Disorders commonly confused with barogenic esophageal rupture include myocardial infarction, acute aortic dissection, pancreatitis, perforated peptic ulcer, spontaneous pneumothorax, and pneumonia.[31]

The physical findings also depend on the cause, location, and duration of perforation. Fever and tachypnea are found in most patients irrespective of location. Crepitus is most frequently noted in cervical and less commonly in thoracic perforation. Mediastinal emphysema may be evident as a Hammon's crunch. Rales, tubular breath sounds, dullness to percussion, and egophony are manifestations of pleural effusion found with thoracic and abdominal perforation. Abdominal perforation can present as acute abdomen. If capillary leak syndrome from chemical burn and sepsis is well established from a misdiagnosed or ignored perforation, the patient has hypoperfusion manifested by hypotension, tachycardia, and cyanosis.

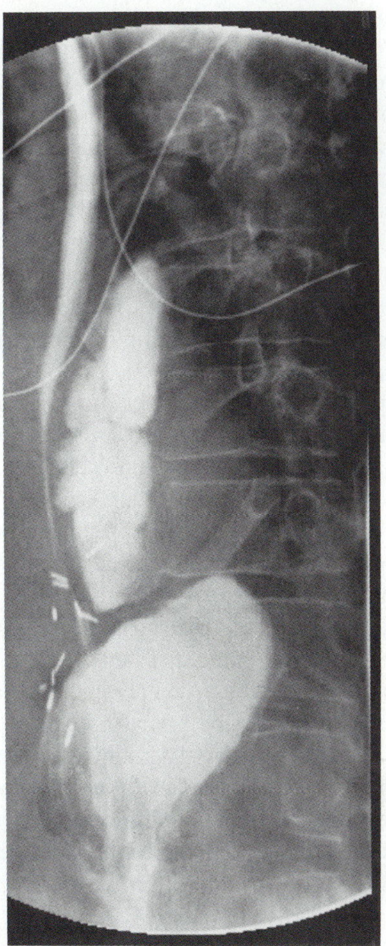

**Figure 41–2.** Contrast-enhanced radiograph illustrating perforations of the thoracic esophagus.

## *Diagnosis*

The diagnosis of esophageal perforation should be considered with the development of any suspicious symptoms after endoscopy. Complications and mortality increase with duration until initiation of therapy.[33,34]

A plain chest radiograph has been found to suggest esophageal perforation in 90% of patients but is diagnostic in association with history and physical examination in only approximately 15% of patients.[35] Pleural effusion, pneumothorax, pneumomediastinum, atelectasis, and soft-tissue emphysema are the most common findings.[36] Chest radiographs are normal in approximately 10% of patients.[35]

Contrast studies continue to be the standard in the diagnosis and determination of site of esophageal perforation (Fig. 41–2). Debate continues about the use of water-soluble contrast material as opposed to barium sulfate.[35,36] The argument for water-soluble contrast material is based on the known adverse effect of barium leakage into a contaminated peritoneal cavity. Experiments have shown no detrimental effect of bacterially contaminated barium placed into the mediastinum.[37] This finding has been confirmed clinically.[35] The superior mucosal coating of barium and the ability of barium to stain the tissues and demonstrate not only the primary leak at exploration but also the rare unsuspected additional esophageal perforation lead us to recommend using dilute barium sulfate to diagnose and localize esophageal perforation. Nonetheless, contrast studies continue to have approximately a 10% rate of false-negative diagnoses.[35,36]

Esophagogastroduodenoscopy and (CT) are adjunct measures in the diagnosis of esophageal perforation. The primary role of each is in the diagnosis of chronic perforation when other studies have not allowed diagnosis.[38] CT findings suggestive of esophageal perforation include mediastinal fluid and air.[39]

## *Therapy*

Treatment goals in the management of esophageal perforation are prevention of further contamination, elimination of infection, restoration of gastrointestinal integrity, and provision of nutritional support.[40,41] Thus, the treatment principles are debridement of infected and necrotic tissue, elimination of distal obstruction, secure closure of the perforation, drainage, and establishment of enteral access and antibiotic therapy.[1] Factors that affect the outcome of treatment include patient age and condition, clinical response to the incident, associated esophageal disease, the cause, site, and size of the perforation, the space into which the perforation drains, and the time to initiation of treatment.

Treatment options are operative or nonoperative. Absolute indications for operation are pneumothorax, pneumoperitoneum, extensive mediastinal emphysema, sepsis, shock, respiratory failure, or nonoperative therapy resulting in abscess or empyema.[31] Operative options include reinforced primary closure, continuous irrigation and drainage of the perforation, drainage alone, T-tube drainage, resection, exclusion and diversion, and placement of an intraluminal stent.

The operative approach depends on accurate determination of the site of perforation. A cervical esophageal perforation is approached through the left neck anterior to the sternocleidomastoid muscle and carotid sheath but lateral to the thyroid and trachea. The upper two thirds of the thoracic esophagus is approached through a right thoracotomy entering the sixth intercostal space. The lower third of the thoracic esophagus is exposed by means of a left thoracotomy through the seventh intercostal space. The abdominal esophagus is reached through an upper midline laparotomy.

Collins et al introduced primary repair of esophageal perforation.[5] The components of a primary repair include debridement of necrotic tissue, myotomy to expose the full extent of mucosal disruption, secure mucosal closure, and drainage of the area of contamination. Reinforcement of a primary repair is always necessary. Primary repair has been shown to have a mortality of 25% and a 39% rate of fistula formation versus a morality of 6% and a rate of fistula formation of 13% for reinforced primary repair.[42] Reinforcement of the site of repair requires secure anastomotic suturing of the flap around the repair, not simple tacking of the pedicle in the vicinity of the perforation. Repairs of cervical perforation are best reinforced with mobilized strap muscle. Figure 41–3 indicates the various buttressing flaps and tissues that have been described for thoracic perforation. Our preference is the intercostal muscle flap, which is most easily harvested immediately from the intercostal space used for thoracotomy, before placement of the rib spreader. This pedicle reaches easily to any thoracic esophageal site and does not open any previously uncontaminated spaces. The success of reinforced primary repair relies on the ability of the esophageal tissue to hold sutures; therefore, tissue edema, necrosis, and infection cannot be too extensive. Reinforced primary repair is doomed to failure and leads to death if performed on an organ with unaddressed distal obstruction.[43] Contrast-enhanced esophagraphy is performed approximately 7 days after repair. If no leak exists, oral intake is resumed and the drains are removed.

Irrigation and drainage of perforations diagnosed late and thus not amenable to reinforced primary closure was introduced in 1986 by Santos and Frater.[44] The method is demonstrated in Figure 41–4. Precise chest tube drainage at

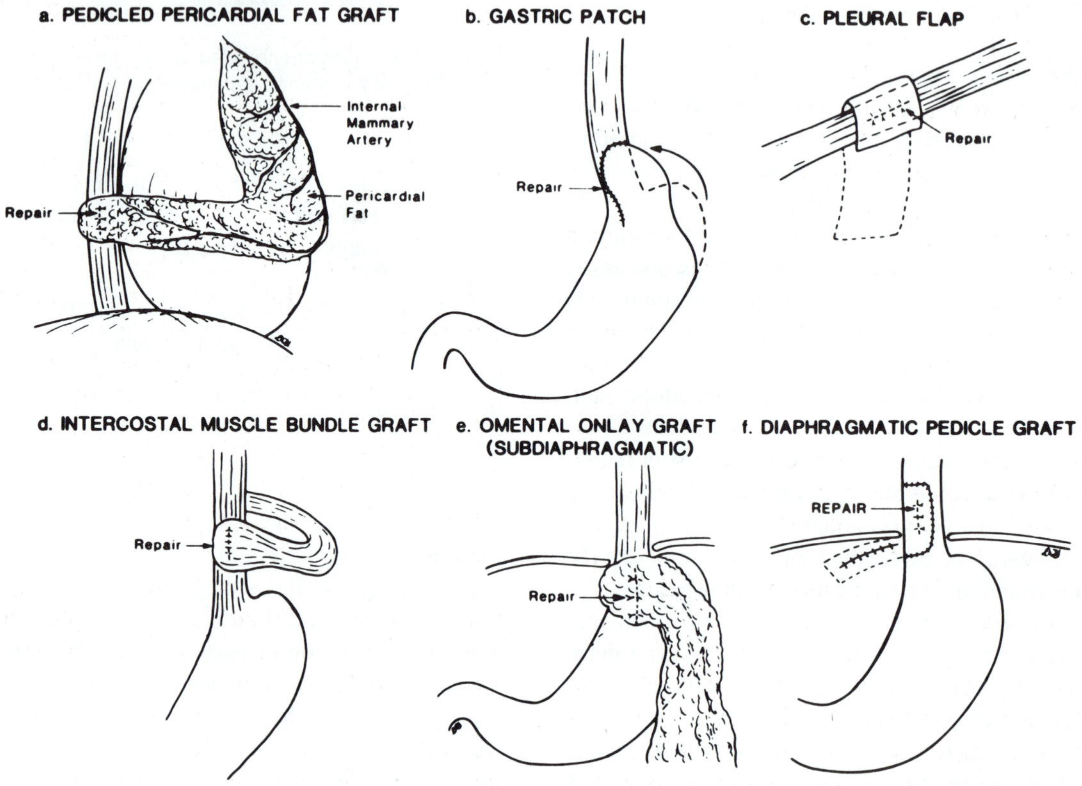


**Figure 41–3.** Techniques of buttressing the primary repair of esophageal perforation. *(From Brewer LA, et al: Am J Surg 1986; 152:62–69, with permission.)*

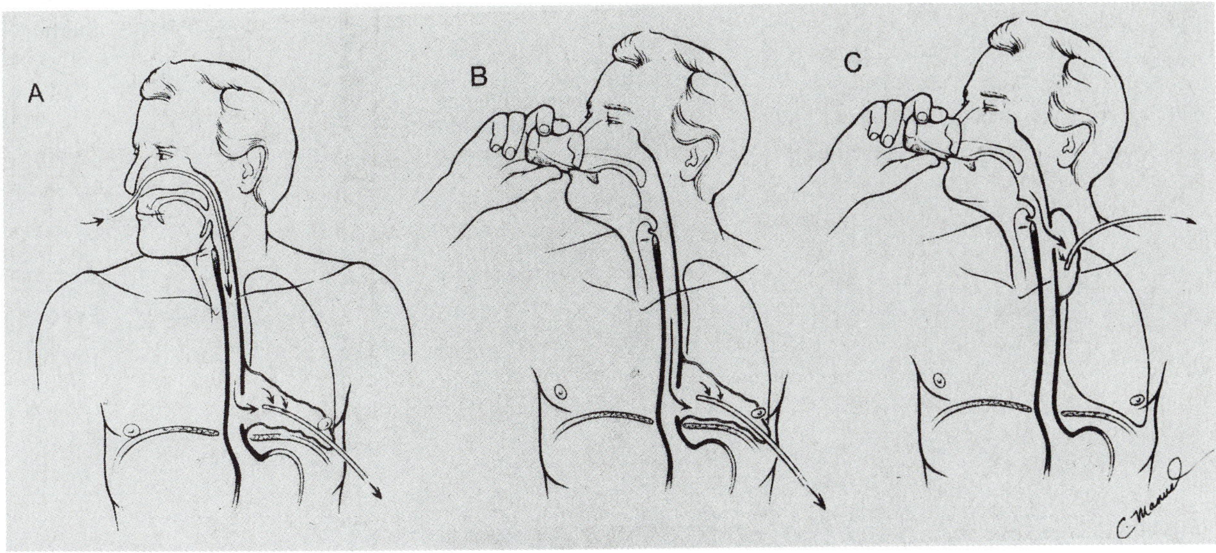


**Figure 41–4.** Technique of irrigation and drainage for late esophageal perforations. **A.** Irrigant is introduced through nasogastric tube positioned proximal to perforation. **B,C.** Patient drinks irrigant *(From Santos GH, Frater RWM: J Thorac Cardiovasc Surg 1986; 91:57–62, with permission.)*

the perforation site is established at operation after debridement. In the rare case of inoperability, drain placement is performed under CT guidance. The perforation is irrigated with saline solution either continuously through nasogastric tube or by frequent oral saline intake. As the chest tube output diminishes and finally ceases, the chest tubes are advanced. Serial esophagraphy or esophagoscopy helps establish the continued adequacy of drainage.

Distal esophageal obstruction requires concomitant treatment. Perforated carcinoma necessitates resection[45] or placement of an intraluminal stent if the tumor is unresectable.[13] If achalasia was unrelieved by the perforating procedure, treatment should be myotomy opposite the site of perforation repair. If severe gastroesophageal reflux is present, an antireflux procedure should accompany and buttress the esophageal repair. A Belsey repair is preferred for thoracic perforation and a Nissen fundoplication for abdominal perforation.

Drainage alone is reserved for small cervical perforations. Drainage alone is unacceptable in thoracic perforations because continued soilage is not prevented, and the hemithorax cannot be as effectively drained as the neck. Late diagnosis of thoracic perforation led to the development of T-tube drainage of the perforation. This allows for a controlled esophagocutaneous fistula.[46]

Resection is reserved for massive necrosis or malignant obstruction. Resection eliminates the perforation as the source of sepsis as well as the underlying esophageal disease, providing alimentary continuity. Transhiatal esophagectomy has been convincingly argued as the technique of choice.[45] Transhiatal esophagectomy has the advantage of performing the anastomosis in the neck distant from the area of contamination, thus avoiding edematous tissues and perianastomotic infection.

Multiple exclusion and diversion techniques have been described to deal with late diagnosis of perforation in a moribund patient. These techniques are illustrated in Figure 41–5. The treatment principles are the same regardless of the technique chosen. These principles include the best possible closure of the perforation, wide drainage, and proximal and distal diversion of the gastrointestinal tract excluding the involved esophagus to prevent further contamination. All exclusion and diversion techniques require a second operation to restore alimentary continuity. Techniques have been described wherein esophageal ligation has been performed with absorbable material, negating the necessity for a second restorative operation.[47]

Nonoperative therapy for esophageal perforation evolved because of recent developments. Instrumentation, the most common cause of perforation, usually results in limited injury and prompt diagnosis. Effective, broad-spectrum antibiotics have been developed and continually improved. CT allows adequate drainage and monitoring of the effectiveness of therapy. Finally, nutritional support has been exquisitely refined. Cameron et al[48] defined the four criteria for nonoperative treatment as (1) confinement of the perforation within the mediastinum, (2) the perforation well-drained back into the esophagus, (3) minimal symptoms, and (4) minimal sepsis. Nonoperative therapy involves keeping the patient fasting, administration of broad-spectrum antibiotics for 7–14 days, drainage of pleural effusions, total parenteral nutrition, and possibly placement of a nasogastric tube. If the patient's condition does not improve within 24 hours, surgical intervention should be strongly considered.

### Results

Outcome is affected by the cause and location of the perforation, the delay to treatment, the method of treatment, and the underlying esophageal disease.[30,49,50] An excellent

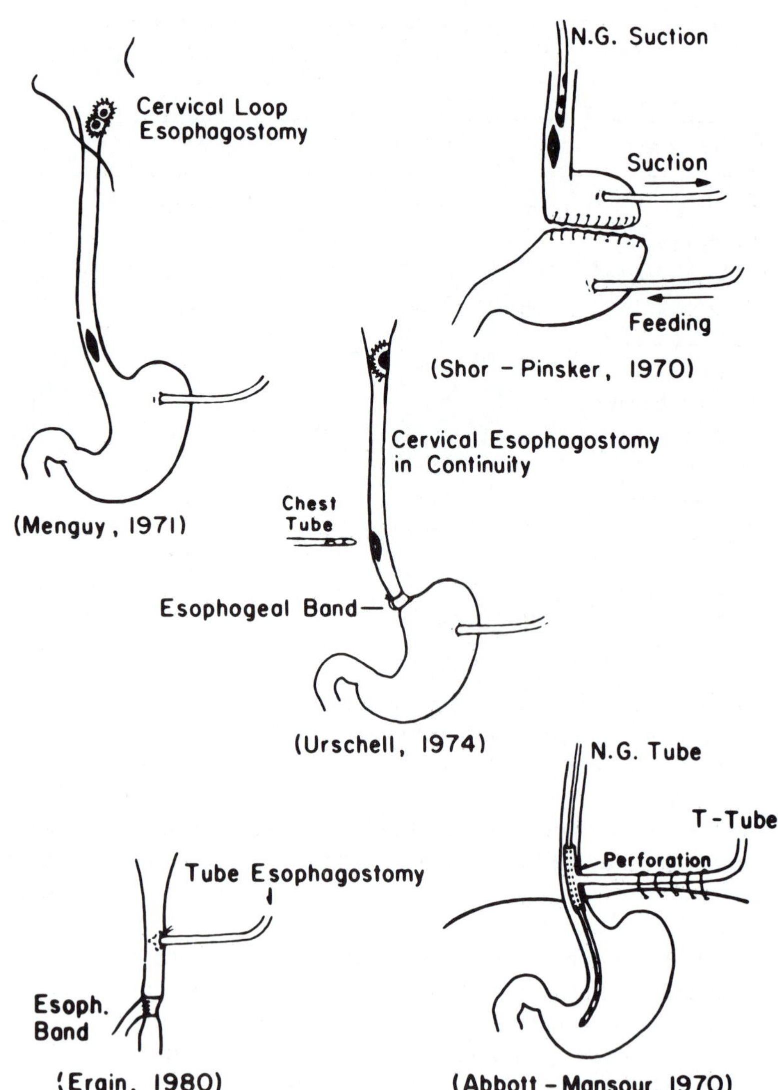


**Figure 41–5.** Exclusion and diversion techniques. *(From Goldstein LA, Thompson WR: Am J Surg 1982; 143:495–503, with permission.)*

summary of the results of treatment in this modern era of antibiotics and nutritional support was provided by Jones and Ginsberg.[1] As noted in accumulated clinical series from 1980 to 1990, instrumentation as the cause of perforation has a mortality of 19%; barogenic rupture, 39%; and trauma, 9%. Barogenic rupture is typically the most confusing diagnostic problem. Barogenic rupture, therefore, is generally treated later in the course of the disease, making its increased mortality understandable.

If the site of perforation is cervical, the mortality is 6%; thoracic, 34%; and abdominal, 29%. Perforation in the neck is usually well contained by fascial compartments, and reflux of gastric content is unlikely through a cervical rent, accounting for the decreased mortality at this location.

Delay to treatment has figured prominently in the risk of complications and death.[51,52] In a series from Duke University,[30] treatment within 24 hours had a mortality of 15%; treatment more than 24 hours after injury had a 33% mortality. Clearly, a gravely ill patient with well-established sepsis fares worse no matter what the treatment. Because of the condition of the esophagus in patients in whom treatment is delayed, more extensive procedures are often used, such as exclusion and diversion or resection. These procedures impose more physiologic demand on an already highly strained system. However, the increased sophistication of modern critical and anesthetic care has made delay to treatment less a factor than it formerly was.[31]

Table 41–1 lists the outcome of the different methods of treatment of esophageal perforation. Primary repair, which is performed on the patients in best condition, has the best results. Patients who cannot undergo primary repair undergo drainage, resection, or exclusion and diversion with a correspondingly higher mortality. Nonoperative treatment has a mortality of approximately 20%, although this figure includes patients who are not operative candi-

**TABLE 41–1. OUTCOME AFTER TREATMENT OF ESOPHAGEAL PERFORATION IN SERIES PUBLISHED BETWEEN 1980 AND 1990[a]**

| Reference | Year | Primary Repair | Drainage | Resection | Exclusion and Diversion | Nonoperative | Overall Mortality[b] |
|---|---|---|---|---|---|---|---|
| Skinner et al[34] | 1980 | 0/15 | 4/8 | 3/9 | 2/11 | — | 9/43 (21) |
| Goldstein and Thompson[35] | 1982 | 4/23 | — | — | 6/9 | 4/12 | 14/44 (32) |
| Sarr et al[53] | 1982 | 0/15[c] | 0/13 | 3/8 | 0/3 | 1/8 | 4/47 (9) |
| Larsen et al[14] | 1983 | 10/47 | 4/8 | — | — | 0/2 | 14/57 (25) |
| Ajalat and Mulder[54] | 1984 | 0/12 | 1/5 | 0/1 | 1/2 | 3/13 | 5/33 (15) |
| Borjeskov et al[55] | 1984 | 9/22 | 3/7 | 2/2 | — | 5/8 | 19/39 (49) |
| Radmark et al[56] | 1986 | 1/17[d] | — | 0/2 | 1/2 | 5/17 | 7/38 (18) |
| Brewer et al[41] | 1986 | 9/53 | 0/6 | 0/2 | 0/2 | 0/15 | 9/78 (12) |
| Nesbitt and Sawyers[31] | 1987 | 3/20 | 3/4 | — | 1/8 | 1/2 | 8/34 (24) |
| Moghissi and Pender[43] | 1988 | 7/13[e] | 4/5 | 2/11 | — | — | 13/29 (45) |
| Flynn et al[57] | 1989 | 1/44 | 2/9 | 1/4 | 1/2 | 0/8 | 5/67 (7) |
| Gouge et al[42] | 1989 | 0/14 | 0/1 | 1/1 | 2/2 | — | 3/18 (17) |
| Attar et al[50] | 1990 | 5/30 | 7/17 | 2/9 | 4/5 | — | 18/61 (30) |
| Total | | 49/325 | 28/83 | 14/49 | 18/46 | 19/85 | 128/588 |
| Mortality (%) | | 15.1 | 34 | 29 | 39 | 22 | 22 |

[a]Data are presented as number of deaths per number of patients undergoing procedure.
[b]Numbers in parentheses are percentages.
[c]This includes two patients who also underwent an antireflux procedure.
[d]This includes two patients who also underwent myotomy.
[e]This includes five patients who also underwent fundoplication.
*(From Jones WG, et al: Ann Thorac Surg 1992;53:534–543, with permission.)*

dates because of other medical conditions. Nonetheless, this mortality is higher than that of primary repair.

### *Conclusion*

Early diagnosis and intervention lead to the best results in esophageal perforation. Our preference in the treatment of esophageal perforation is reinforced primary repair if periesophageal inflammation is not severe and the esophagus is nonedematous. If the diagnosis is made late, we debride the periesophageal tissue and institute continuous irrigation with precisely placed chest tubes immediately at the perforation site. Over the last 4 years, we have used this method preferentially and successfully, including use in a delayed diagnosis of Boerhaave's syndrome in a recipient of a renal transplant. Distal obstruction must be eliminated. Nonoperative therapy is occasionally appropriate. One must be knowledgeable in all therapeutic options. No single approach is always correct in dealing with this devastating injury.

## Chemical Burns

Chemical burns of the upper gastrointestinal tract are infrequently encountered and are potentially catastrophic. Chemical burns need to be approached systematically in diagnosis and treatment.

### *Epidemiology*

In western society, 65% of chemical ingestion is alkali, 16% acid, and the rest is bleach.[58] The composition of ingested materials depends on the chemicals available in a particular society.[59] Approximately 50% of ingestion in adults and almost all ingestion in children is accidental.[60] The remainder of the adult chemical ingestion is suicidal. Adult accidental and suicidal ingestion is frequently associated with inebriation.[61]

### *Pathophysiology*

The degree of enteric injury depends on the character, concentration, and pH of the corrosive material as well as the duration of contact with the mucosa. Liquid alkali is tasteless and odorless, making accidental or suicidal ingestion of a large amount feasible. Granular caustics stick to the oral mucosa and burn, hindering voluminous ingestion. Alkali causes liquefactive necrosis and therefore penetrates deeply into the surrounding tissue.[60]

Acid has a severely unpleasant taste, causing choking and gagging. This leads to epiglottic burns, threatening airway patency. Acid produces coagulation necrosis and less penetration.[62] The esophageal squamous epithelium is somewhat resistant to acid. Intraesophageal acid has a short transit time. This tends to spare the esophagus but produce coagulation necrosis of the stomach.[59]

Bleaches have a neutral pH and are esophageal irritants. Clinical series of bleach ingestion have shown no serious complications or mortality. Extensive evaluation of patients with bleach ingestion is not indicated.[62]

Upper gastrointestinal chemical burns have a necrotic followed by a healing phase. The healing phase depends on the extent of injury. Mucosal injury requires 20–30 days to heal. Submucosal involvement heals in 90–120 days. Deep injury is associated with edema and local infection with resultant fibrosis. Strictures develop in 20% of patients and are usually extensive.[58]

### Diagnosis

Assessment of corrosive ingestion starts with an accurate history of the nature and concentration of the agent, time of ingestion, and the circumstances. No correlation exists between the presence of oropharyngeal burns at physical examination and upper gastrointestinal burns.[61] Therefore, a complete flexible endoscopic examination must be performed. This should be carried out within 24 hours to allow the injury to be visually manifest but before the walls of the organ are weakened. Complete examination is required. The risk of perforation has been overemphasized.[61] Therapy and prognosis depend on accurate staging of the extent of injury.

### Staging

Stage 1 is mucosal inflammation manifested by edema and hyperemia. Stage 2A is characterized by superficial ulcers, blisters, and white membranes. Stage 2B has deep or circumferential ulcers and necrosis. There is little hemorrhage. Stage 3 is defined by extensive necrosis involving the entire organ and massive hemorrhage. Stage 4 has the same endoscopic findings as stage 3 with the presence of systemic metabolic derangements, such as metabolic acidosis or disseminated intravascular coagulation.

### Therapy

The patient is resuscitated. Broad-spectrum IV antibiotics are begun and oral intake is prohibited. Emergency surgical exploration is indicated depending on the nature and quantity of chemical ingested, voluminous bloody emesis, endoscopic determination of burn extending beyond the pylorus, signs of peritonitis, and the presence of shock. Stage 3 or 4 injury requires operation. Exploratory laparotomy should assess the damage to the anterior and posterior stomach. If the stomach is viable, a feeding jejunostomy is placed. If partial or total gastric necrosis exists, transhiatal esophagogastrectomy is performed with feeding jejunostomy, establishment of an end cervical esophagostomy, and drainage of the posterior mediastinal and submesenteric spaces. Transhiatal resection is facilitated by thrombosis of periesophageal vessels and lack of mediastinal adhesion.[59] Gastrointestinal continuity is restored with a colonic interposition performed 2–3 months after resection.

Alimentation is provided parenterally or through a nasoduodenal tube or feeding jejunostomy. Oral intake resumes depending on the stage of injury. Patients with stage 1 injury can eat immediately. Patients with stage 2A injury can eat in 25 days; stage 2B, 35 days; and stage 3, 43 days.[61] The patient undergoes serial esophagogastroduodenoscopies to assess healing. The role of early dilation, steroids, and stents is controversial. Steroids provided no benefit in a prospective study in children.[63] The degree of burn, not the use of controversial treatment modalities,[60] is the main determinant of risk of stricture.

If no resection has been required, the esophagus is dilated by the fourth week after injury. The character of the dilation allows division into three groups. The first group dilates easily with little risk. This group is cured by bougienage. The second group dilates with moderate difficulty and little risk. Approximately 50% of these patients require esophageal surgery, usually within 1 year. The last group dilates with great difficulty and risk. This group requires esophageal replacement. Six to eight weeks should elapse before an operation is performed to allow scar maturation and identification of possible gastric outlet obstruction. If gastric and esophageal injury coexist, the gastric emptying disturbance is addressed first, usually with gastric resection. A second operation consisting of thoracotomy and esophageal resection is then performed. Thoracotomy is chosen because of extensive periesophageal scarring. Colonic interposition is the method of reconstruction.[64]

### Results

Complications are not encountered in stage 1 injury. Complications are rare in stage 2A. Fifty percent of stage 2B injuries produce strictures in the esophagus, stomach, or duodenum. Bleeding is encountered in less than 10% of stage 2B injuries. In stage 3, 70% of injuries produce strictures of the esophagus or stomach. In one series, bleeding developed in 15% of patients and perforation in 20% with 15% mortality.[61] When an emergency operation is required, operative mortality ranges from 30% to 100% depending on the acute illness of the patients undergoing operation.[58,59,61,64]

If a functional esophagus with fibrosis can be achieved, the patient requires surveillance endoscopy. The risk of carcinoma in a fibrosed esophagus is 5–7.2% over 10–15 years.[58,64]

## Foreign Body Ingestion

Seventy-five percent of ingested foreign bodies enter the gastrointestinal tract and about 15% the tracheobronchial tree. Most ingested foreign bodies pass spontaneously. Approximately 10–20% require endoscopic removal, and 1% require surgical treatment.[65]

### Pathophysiology

Ingested foreign bodies entering the gastrointestinal tract impact at areas of anatomic, physiologic, or pathologic narrowing. Esophageal anatomic and physiologic sites of narrowing include the cricopharyngeus muscle, crossing of the aortic arch, crossing of the left main stem bronchus, and the lower esophageal sphincter. Once a site is impacted, esophageal damage can occur because of direct penetration, which leads to perforation or submucosal tear and bleeding.

Perforation may lead to mediastinitis or injury of the periesophageal structures such as the great vessels.[66] Pressure necrosis or simply luminal compromise and obstruction may occur.

### Epidemiology

Eighty percent of foreign body ingestion occurs in the pediatric population. Toddlers 2–4 years of age are most commonly involved. The ingestion generally occurs during an unsupervised period, making diagnosis difficult because no clear history is obtainable.[62] One review noted only 41% of children were seen by a physician on the first day after the initial episode.[67] The most common esophageal foreign body readily seen on radiographs is a coin. The foreign body that causes death most often is an unchewed hot dog lodged in the esophagus, impacting in the child's airway and causing obstruction.[62]

In the adult population, non-food foreign bodies are involved if the person is younger than 40 years. In this population, 30% of patients are noted to be alcoholics; 38% are prison inmates; 25% have a history of suicide attempts; and 50% have a history of psychiatric illness.[68] A new population has joined this mechanism of esophageal injury: drug smugglers. Esophageal obstruction and perforation occur with ingestion of condoms filled with cocaine or marijuana.[69]

Among people older than 60 years, foreign bodies that cause difficulty are usually food. In food impaction, more than 95% of patients have underlying esophageal disease. Denture use is associated with food impaction because decreased palatal sensitivity allows swallowing of poorly chewed food. Esophageal tears due to swallowed tortilla chips or even dentures have been described.[70,71]

Drug-induced esophageal injury due to intentional ingestion of commercially available medications being used therapeutically is being increasingly reported. This injury combines esophageal chemical burn and foreign body ingestion.[72] Antibiotic or nonsteroidal anti-inflammatory medications are the most common culprits. More than 80% of patients have normal deglutition. Improper ingestion of tablets, such as not drinking enough water with them and lying down too soon after taking them, may predispose to esophageal injury. Drug characteristics such as size, shape, and coating are important. Esophageal injury includes ulceration, stricture, perforation, and fistula. This condition carries a mortality of 3.5%.[73]

### Clinical Manifestations

Symptoms of foreign body ingestion in children include coughing or wheezing because of airway compromise.[62] The diagnosis of retained foreign body should be entertained in any child with unexplained prolonged respiratory problems.[62] Otherwise, the symptoms are similar to those in adults and include odynophagia, dysphagia, and drooling with obstruction. Esophageal mucosal tears are manifested by bleeding, and perforation has the symptoms previously described.

### Diagnosis

Diagnosis should begin with routine radiographs. If the foreign body is radiolucent, thin barium is used to outline the object. If no foreign body is identified but the patient continues to have symptoms, flexible endoscopy is performed.[65]

### Treatment and Results

The method of removal varies according to the sharpness of the foreign body. One can remove blunt objects by passing a Foley catheter distal to the object under fluoroscopic guidance, inflating the balloon, and withdrawing the balloon and object. A steep Trendelenburg position is used for withdrawal to keep the object posterior to the larynx. This method has been criticized for lack of control and the risk of airway obstruction.[61] However, it has a reported success rate of 85% with only minor complications.[74] Blunt objects can be removed with esophagoscopy. Polypectomy snares or alligator forceps are used to grasp and remove the object under direct visualization. We prefer to use flexible esophagoscopy. Rigid esophagoscopy is used for objects that require large alligator forceps or direct manipulation. Impacted food can be pushed into the stomach or removed piecemeal at endoscopy.

The Heimlich maneuver has been used successfully to eject blunt esophageal foreign bodies. Complications of the Heimlich maneuver include vomiting and aspiration, visceral perforation, cardiac valve rupture, great vessel trauma, diaphragmatic rupture, and pneumomediastinum. These risks are warranted in the case of acute airway obstruction, which is a life-threatening emergency. Esophageal obstruction is dangerous but not immediately life-threatening; therefore the risks of the Heimlich maneuver are not justified.[75]

Sharp foreign bodies should be removed. Fifteen to 30 percent of sharp objects that pass through the gastrointestinal tract cause perforation, usually at the ileocecal valve. When dealing with pins, the adage "advancing points puncture, trailing points do not" dictates the method of endoscopic removal. Intraesophageal pins pointing toward the stomach can be grasped and withdrawn. Pins pointing cephalad should be pushed into the stomach and then withdrawn, point trailing. Razor blades are engaged, an overtube is maneuvered over the blade, and the conglomerate removed. If removal has been difficult, esophageal perforation is ruled out with a barium swallow radiograph.

Surgical removal is indicated if a sharp object is not removable with endoscopy or a blunt object has not advanced for 3 days. Drug-filled condoms should be removed surgically to avoid the risk of rupture.

### Conclusion

Esophageal injury is expertly handled by surgeons with a knowledge of esophageal anatomy, pathophysiology, and the various treatment modalities. This method of treatment assures the best results possible with these devastating injuries, which not only threaten life in the acute phase but also profoundly affect the quality of life afterward.

## ESOPHAGEAL BLEEDING

Although gastroenterologists usually manage acute esophageal bleeding, a thoracic surgeon may be called for the initial consult. The surgeon must be familiar with the different causes, diagnostic procedures, and management options because esophageal bleeding may be life-threatening, and early intervention is mandatory.

### Bleeding Esophageal Varices

The most frequent and devastating source of esophageal bleeding is variceal. Esophageal varices result from portal hypertension, which has a number of possible causes. In the United States, progressive fibrosis of the hepatic sinusoids most frequently results from alcoholic cirrhosis. As fibrosis occurs, portal venous flow decreases, and portal collateral flow increases, primarily via the coronary and short gastric veins. These venous complexes connect with the azygos and hemiazygos systems via the esophagogastric variceal plexus. Varices do not bleed until corrected portal pressure exceeds 12 mm Hg.[76] Current therapy suggests that bleeding results from the internal disruption or explosion of varices because of increased pressure or thinning of overlying supportive structures.[77] Bleeding usually occurs from vessels in the lower 5 cm of the esophagus.

All patients with suspected bleeding from esophageal varices require hospitalization. After appropriate resuscitation maneuvers, immediate endoscopy is essential. The number, size, length, and distribution of varices can be determined and active bleeding sites visualized. As many as 20% of patients with varices have nonvariceal causes of upper gastrointestinal hemorrhage (e.g., gastritis, bleeding ulcer).[78] Once variceal bleeding is confirmed, immediate therapy is instituted. Options include endoscopic sclerotherapy, endoscopic ligation, pharmacologic control, and balloon-tube tamponade.

Sclerotherapy can be performed at the time of initial endoscopy or be delayed until after variceal hemorrhage has been controlled with more conservative measures. Emergency sclerotherapy is the treatment of choice if the bleeding site can be visualized. Bleeding is halted in more than 90% of patients.[76,79] The procedure is relatively simple and inexpensive. The sclerosant material, frequency of repeat endoscopies, and technique (intravariceal versus paravariceal) are debatable issues. Side effects of sclerotherapy include esophageal ulceration, stricture, perforation, and pleural effusions. Endoscopic ligation of varices is an alternative to sclerotherapy and has been shown to be equally effective.[80]

Substances that reduce portal pressure are often used in the initial management of variceal bleeding. Vasopressin, a powerful splanchnic vasoconstrictor, is the most frequently used agent in the United States. Other commonly used drugs include terlipressin and somatostatin.[79,81] The addition of nitroglycerin to vasopressin has ben shown to decrease the side effects of vasopressin alone (cardiac and mesenteric ischemic effects), but controlled studies have not definitely shown improved efficacy.[82–84] Pharmacologic treatment yields an early bleeding control of 50%.[79]

Balloon tamponade, when properly performed, temporarily controls ongoing variceal bleeding in 80–90% of patients.[77,79] However, the rate of serious complications is high (10–17% in controlled trials), tube-related mortality is 3–5%, and the tube is difficult for nonexperts to place.[79] A high rebleeding rate of 30–60% is to be expected at removal.[85,86] At present, balloon tamponade is reserved most often for 5–10% of patients in whom bleeding is relentless despite sclerotherapy and IV vasoconstrictor therapy.

For patients who experience rebleeding within 48 hours of initial therapy and who do not respond to a second injection of sclerosant, mortality approaches 90%.[87] Such patients are examined for either a portosystemic shunt or esophageal transection with a staple gun. For Child's class C patients, a new alternative is placement of a transjugular intrahepatic protosystemic shunt (TIPS) with expandable metallic stents.[88–90] Portal decompression is achieved through a percutaneously established shunt between the hepatic and portal veins within the liver. TIPS is an attractive nonoperative therapeutic maneuver for patients who are potential candidates for liver transplantation.

Recurrence of variceal bleeding is high (48% of Child's class B, 68% of Child's class C patients).[76] The most common long-term treatment after variceal bleeding is continued sclerotherapy. Varices can be eradicated with this technique. Controlled clinical trials have shown that the incidence of recurrent variceal bleeding is markedly reduced, but the beneficial effect on survival remains in question.[91–95] Trials that compared sclerotherapy with the use of a selective distal splenorenal shunt showed that recurrent hemorrhage is more frequent with sclerotherapy.[96–98] An alternative long-term approach is an elective devascularization-and-transection operation.[99] The best approach in a patient with alcoholic cirrhosis remains to be determined. Risk of rebleeding must be weighed against technically demanding operations with high associated morbidity and mortality and risks of encephalopathy and accelerated liver damage. The only curative therapy for bleeding esophageal varices and associated underlying hepatic dysfunction is liver transplantation. However, for a variety of reasons, this alternative is a limited one for many patients with alcoholic cirrhosis.

### Mallory-Weiss Syndrome

Bleeding due to the Mallory-Weiss syndrome comes from mucosal tears or lacerations of the gastroesophageal junction caused by vomiting. Typically, these patients have a hiatal hernia with or without symptoms of gastroesophageal reflux. The lacerations cross the gastroesophageal junction but are predominantly gastric in location. Although these lesions may be responsible for considerable blood loss, at least 90% of the lesions can be managed nonsurgically.[100] Early endoscopy is required for a prompt and definitive diagnosis. Systemic vasopressin has been shown to have some effect against continued bleeding. Approximately 10% of patients do not respond to conservative therapy and require surgical intervention. These patients are approached through a high, midline abdominal incision, and the mucosal tear is oversewn through a high gastrotomy.

## Unusual Causes of Esophageal Bleeding

Esophageal carcinoma infrequently presents with bleeding (4–7% of patients). Reflux esophagitis is also an unusual cause of esophageal bleeding. On occasion a patient presents with anemia that is the result of chronic bleeding from esophagitis, but clinically significant hemorrhage is rare. Esophageal ulcers may be associated with the usage of nonsteroidal anti-inflammatory drugs.[101] Barrett's ulcers have been reported in 10–15% of cases of Barrett's esophagus and are characteristically deep.[102] Occult bleeding may lead to chronic anemia, and massive hemorrhage occurs in a few patients. Medical management is initiated in cases of bleeding secondary to reflux. The success of medical therapy for Barrett's ulcer has been variable.[103,104]

## REFERENCES


1. Jones WG, Ginsberg RJ: Esophageal perforation: A continuing challenge. *Ann Thorac Surg* **53**:534–543, 1992
2. Derbes VJ, Mitchell RE: Hermann Boerhaave's (1) Atrocis, nec Descripti Prius, Morbi Historia (2). *Bull Med Libr Assoc* **43**:217–240, 1955
3. Meyer J: Ueber Zemeissung der Speierohre. *Med Zeitung* **1**:189–195, 1858
4. Frink NW: Spontaneous rupture of the esophagus: Report of a case with recovery. *J Thorac Surg* **16**:291–292, 1941
5. Collins JL, Humphreys DR, Bond WH: Spontaneous rupture of the oesophagus. *Lancet* **2**:179, 1944
6. Barrett NR: Report of a case of spontaneous perforation of the esophagus successfully treated by operation. *Br J Surg* **35**:216–219, 1947
7. Olson AM, Claggett OT: Spontaneous rupture of the esophagus: Report of a case with immediate diagnosis and successful surgical repair. *Postgrad Med* **2**:417–421, 1947
8. Brewer LA, Burford TH: Special types of thoracic wounds. In *Medical Department: US Army Surgery in World War II, Thoracic Surgery,* 38th ed. Washington: US Government Printing Office, 1965, p 269
9. Satinsky VP, Kron SD: One-stage esophagectomy in the presence of mediastinitis. *Arch Surg* **64**:124–127, 1952
10. Jackson RH, Payne DK, Bacon BR: Esophageal perforation due to nasogastric intubation. *Am J Gastroenterol* **85**:439–442, 1990
11. Johnson KG, Hood DD: Esophageal perforation associated with endotracheal intubation. *Anesthesiology* **64**:281–283, 1986
12. Reed CR, Marsh WH, Carlson LS, et al: Prospective, randomized trial of palliative treatment for unresectable cancer of the esophagus. *Ann Thorac Surg* **51**:552–556, 1991
13. Kratz JM, Reed CE: A comparison of endoesophageal tubes: Improved results with the Atkinson tube. *J Thorac Cardiovasc Surg* **97**:19–23, 1989
14. Larsen K, Skov JB, Axelsen F: Perforation and rupture of the esophagus. *Scand J Thorac Cardiovasc Surg* **17**:311–316, 1983
15. Urbanowicz JH, Kernoff RS, Oppenheim G, et al: Transesophageal echocardiography and its potential for esophageal damage. *Anesthesiology* **72**:40–43, 1990
16. Kelly MF, Rizzo KA, Spiegle J, Zwillenberg D: Delayed pharyngoesophageal perforation: A complication of anterior spinal surgery. *Ann Otol Rhinol Laryngol* **100**:201–205, 1991
17. Sebag C, Lavergne T, Millat B, et al: Rupture of the stomach and the esophagus after attempted transcatheter ablation of an accessory pathway by direct current shock. *Am J Cardiol* **63**:890–891, 1989
18. Silvis SE, Nebel O, Rogers G: Endoscopic complications: Results of the 1974 American Society of Gastrointestinal Endoscopy Survey. *JAMA* **235**:928–930, 1976
19. Niezgoda JA, McMenamin P, Graeber GM: Pharyngoesophageal perforation after blunt neck trauma. *Ann Thorac Surg* **50**:615–617, 1990
20. Latimer EA, Clevenger FW, Osler TM: Tear of the cervical esophagus following hyperextension from manual traction: Case report. *J Trauma* **31**:1448–1449, 1991
21. Micon L, Geis L, Sidreys H, et al: Rupture of the distal thoracic esophagus following blunt trauma: Case report. *J Trauma* **30**:214–217, 1990
22. Carter MP, Long RF, Pellegrini RA, Wynn RA: Traumatic esophageal rupture: Unusual cause of acute mediastinal widening. *South Med J* **84**:767–769, 1991
23. Guth AA, Gouge TH, Depan HJ: Blast injury to the thoracic esophagus. *Ann Thorac Surg* **51**:837–839, 1991
24. Curci MR, Dibbins AW, Grimes CK: Compressed air injury to the esophagus: Case report. *J Trauma* **29**:1713–1715, 1989
25. Henderson JA, Peloquin AJM: Boerhaave revisited: Spontaneous esophageal perforation as a diagnostic masquerader. *Am J Med* **86**:559–567, 1989
26. Mackenzie M: *Diseases of the Nose and Throat,* 2nd ed. New York, William Wood, 1885, pp 111–125
27. Tidman MK, John HT: Spontaneous rupture of the oesophagus. *Br J Surg* **54**:286–292, 1967
28. Limburg AJ, Hesselink EJ, Kleibeuker JH: Barrett's ulcer: Cause of spontaneous oesophageal perforation. *Gut* **30**:404–405, 1989
29. Cronstedt JL, Bouchama A, Hainau B, et al: Spontaneous esophageal perforation in herpes simplex esophagitis. *Am J Gastroenterol* **87**:124–127, 1992
30. Bladergroen MR, Lowe JE, Postlethwait RW: Diagnosis and recommended management of esophageal perforation and rupture. *Ann Thorac Surg* **42**:235–239, 1986
31. Nesbitt JC, Sawyers JL: Surgical management of esophageal perforation. *Am Surg* **53**:183–191, 1987
32. Mackler SA: Spontaneous rupture of the esophagus: An experimental and clinical study. *Surg Gynecol Obstet* **95**:345–356, 1952
33. Grillo HC, Wilkins EW: Esophageal repair following late diagnosis of intrathoracic perforation. *Ann Thorac Surg* **20**:387–399, 1975
34. Skinner DB, Little AG, DeMeester TR: Management of esophageal perforation. *Am J Surg* **139**:760–764, 1980
35. Goldstein LA, Thompson WR: Esophageal perforation: A 15 year experience. *Am J Surg* **143**:495–503, 1982
36. White RW, Morris DM: Diagnosis and management of esophageal perforations. *Am Surg* **58**:112–119, 1992
37. James AE, Montali RJ, Chaffee V, et al: Barium or Gastrografin: Which contrast media for diagnosis of esophageal tears? *Gastroenterology* **68**:1103–1113, 1975
38. Kim-Deobald J, Kozarek RA: Esophageal perforation: An 8 year review of a multispeciality clinic's experience. *Am J Gastroenterol* **87**:1112–1119, 1992
39. Backer CL, LoCicero J, Hartz RS, et al: Computed tomography in patients with esophageal perforation. *Chest* **98**:1078–1080, 1990

40. Michel L, Grillo HC, Malt RA: Operative and nonoperative management of esophageal perforations. *Ann Surg* **194:**57–63, 1981
41. Brewer LA, Carter R, Mulder GA, Stiles QR: Options in the management of perforations of the esophagus. *Am J Surg* **152:**62–69, 1986
42. Gouge TH, Depan HJ, Spencer FC: Experience with the Grillo pleural wrap procedure in 18 patients with perforation of the thoracic esophagus. *Ann Surg* **209:**612–617, 1989
43. Moghissi K, Pender D: Instrumental perforations of the oesophagus and their management. *Thorax* **43:**642–646, 1988
44. Santos GH, Frater RWM: Transesophageal irrigation for the treatment of mediastinitis produced by esophageal rupture. *J Thorac Cardiovasc Surg* **91:**57–62, 1986
45. Orringer MB, Stirling MC: Esophagectomy for esophageal disruption. *Ann Thorac Surg* **49:**35–43, 1990
46. Abbott OA, Mansour KA, Logan WD, et al: Atraumatic so-called "spontaneous" rupture of the esophagus. *J Thorac Cardiovasc Surg* **59:**67–83, 1970
47. Lee YC, Lee ST, Chu SH: New technique of esophageal exclusion for chronic esophageal perforation. *Ann Thorac Surg* **51:**1020–1022, 1991
48. Cameron JL, Kieffer RF, Hendrix TR, et al: Selective nonoperative management of contained intrathoracic esophageal disruption. *Ann Thorac Surg* **27:**404–408, 1979
49. Michel L, Grillo HC, Malt RA: Esophageal perforation. *Ann Thorac Surg* **33:**203–210, 1982
50. Attar S, Hankins JR, Suter CM, et al: Esophageal perforation: A therapeutic challenge. *Ann Thorac Surg* **50:**45–51, 1990
51. Ohri SK, Kiakakos TA, Pathi V, et al: Primary repair of iatrogenic thoracic esophageal perforation and Boerhaave's syndrome. *Ann Thorac Surg* **55:**603–606, 1993
52. Cohn HE, Hubbard A, Patton G: Management of esophageal injuries. *Ann Thorac Surg* **48:**309–314, 1989
53. Sarr HG, Pemberton JH, Payne WS: Management of instrumental perforations of the esophagus. *J Thorac Cardiovasc Surg* **84:**211–218, 1982
54. Ajalat GM, Mulder DG: Esophageal perforations: the need for an individualized approach. *Arch Surg* **119:**1318–1320, 1984
55. Borgeskov S, Brynitz S, Siemenssen O: Perforation of the esophagus: Experience from a department of thoracic surgery. *Scand J Thorac Cardiovasc Surg* **18:**93–96, 1984
56. Radmark T, Sandberg N, Pettersson G: Instrumental perforation of the esophagus: A ten year study from two ENT clinics. *J Laryngol Otol* **100:**461–465, 1986
57. Flynn AE, Verrier ED, Way LW, et al: Esophageal perforation. *Arch Surg* **124:**1211–1214, 1989
58. Noirclerc MJ, Di Costanzo J, Sastre B, et al: Surgical management of caustic injuries to the upper gastrointestinal tract. In DeMeester TR, Matthews HR (eds): *International Trends in General Thoracic Surgery,* vol 3. St. Louis: Mosby, 1987, 261–268
59. Horvath OP, Olah T, Zentai G: Emergency esophagogastrectomy for treatment of hydrochloric acid injury. *Ann Thorac Surg* **52:**98–101, 1991
60. Spitz L, Lokhoo K: Caustic ingestion. *Arch Dis Child* **68:**157–158, 1993
61. Zargar SA, Kochhar R, Nagi B, et al: Ingestion of strong corrosive alkalis: Spectrum of injury to upper gastrointestinal tract and natural history. *Am J Gastroenterol* **87:**337–341, 1992
62. Friedman EM: Caustic ingestions and foreign bodies in the aerodigestive tract of children. *Recent Adv Pediatr Otolaryngol* **36:**1403–1410, 1989
63. Anderson KD, Rouse TM, Randolph JG: A controlled trial of corticosteroids in children with corrosive injury of the esophagus. *N Engl J Med* **323:**637–640, 1990
64. Horvath OP: Surgical management of caustic injuries to the upper gastrointestinal tract: discussion. In DeMeester TR, Matthews HR (eds): *International Trends in General Thoracic Surgery,* vol 3. St. Louis: Mosby, 1987, 266–268
65. Webb WA: Management of foreign bodies of the upper gastrointestinal tract. *Gastroenterology* **94:**204–216, 1988
66. Scher RL, Tegtmeyer CJ, McLean WC: Vascular injury following foreign body perforation of the esophagus. *Ann Otol Rhinol Laryngol* **99:**698–702, 1990
67. Cohen SR, Lewis FH: The emergency management of caustic ingestions. *Emerg Med Clin North Am* **2:**77–86, 1984
68. Taylor RB: Esophageal foreign bodies. *Emerg Med Clin North Am* **5:**301–309, 1987
69. Johnson JA, Landreneau RJ: Esophageal obstruction and mediastinitis: A hard pill to swallow for drug smugglers. *Am Surg* **57:**723–726, 1991
70. Longstreth GF: Esophageal tear caused by a tortilla chip. *N Engl J Med* **322:**1399–1400, 1992
71. Treska T, Smith CC: Swallowed partial denture. *Oral Surg Oral Med Oral Pathol* **72:**756–757, 1991
72. Nwakama PE, Jenkins HJ, Bailey RT, et al: Drug-induced esophageal injury: A case report of Percogesic. *Ann Pharmacother* **23:**227–229, 1989
73. Oakes DD, Sherck JP: Drug-induced esophageal injuries. In: DeMeester TR, Matthews HR (eds): *International Trends in General Thoracic Surgery,* vol 3. St. Louis: Mosby, 1987, 269–279
74. Mariani PJ, Wagner DK: Foley catheter extraction of blunt esophageal foreign bodies. *J Emerg Med* **4:**301–306, 1986
75. Sams JS: Dangers of the Heimlich maneuver for esophageal obstruction. *N Engl J Med* **321:**980–981, 1989
76. Johansen K, Helton WS: Portal hypertension and bleeding esophageal varices. *Vasc Surg* **6:**553–561, 1992
77. Terblanche J, Burroughs AK, Hobbs KEF: Controversies in the management of bleeding esophageal varices. I. *N Engl J Med* **320:**1393–1398, 1989
78. Sutton FM: Upper gastrointestinal bleeding in patients with esophageal varices: What is the most common source? *Am J Med* **83:**273–275, 1987
79. Söderlund C, Eriksson LS: Medical and surgical treatment of acute bleeding from esophageal varices in patients with cirrhosis. *Scand J Gastroenterol* **26:**897–908, 1991
80. Stiegmann GV, Goff JS, Michaletz-Onody PA, et al: Endoscopic sclerotherapy as compared with endoscopic ligation for bleeding esophageal varices. *N Engl J Med* **326:**1527–1532, 1992
81. Walker S: Vasoconstrictor therapy in bleeding esophageal varices. *Hepatogastroenterology* **37:**538–543, 1990
82. Gimson AES, Westaby D, Hegarty J, et al: A randomized trial of vasopressin and vasopressin plus nitroglycerin in the control of acute variceal hemorrhage. *Hepatology* **6:**410–413, 1986
83. Tsai YT, Lay CS, Lai KH, et al: Controlled trial of vasopressin plus nitroglycerin vs. vasopressin alone in the treatment of bleeding esophageal varices. *Hepatology* **6:**404–409, 1986
84. Bosch J, Groszmann RJ, Garcia-Pagan JC, et al: Association of transdermal nitroglycerin to vasopressin infusion in the treatment of variceal hemorrhage: A placebo-controlled clinical trial. *Hepatology* **10:**962–968, 1989
85. Novis BH, Duys P, Barbezat GO, et al: Fiberoptic endoscopy and the use of the Senkstaken tube in acute gastrointestinal hemorrhage in patients with portal hypertension and varices. *Gut* **17:**258–263, 1976
86. Panes J, Teres J, Bosch J, Rhodes J: Efficacy of balloon tamponade in treatment of bleeding gastric and esophageal varices: Results in 151 consecutive episodes. *Dig Dis Sci* **33:**454–459, 1988
87. Paquet KJ, Mercado MA, Aichner W, et al: Conservative and semi-invasive modalities for treating bleeding esophageal varices. *Hepatogastroenterology* **37:**561–564, 1990
88. Rin EJ, Lake JR, Roberts JP, et al: Using transjugular intrahepatic portosystemic shunts to control variceal bleeding before liver transplantation. *Ann Intern Med* **116:**304–309, 1992
89. LaBerge JM, Ring EJ, Lake JR, et al: Transjugular intrahepatic portosystemic shunts: Preliminary results in 25 patients. *J Vasc Surg* **16:**258–267, 1994

90. Conn HO: Transjugular intrahepatic portal-systemic shunts: The state of the art. *Hepatology* **17**:148–158, 1993
91. Copenhagen Esophageal Varices Sclerotherapy Project: Sclerotherapy after first variceal hemorrhage in cirrhosis. *N Engl J Med* **311**:1594–1600, 1984
92. Soederlund C, Ihre T: Endoscopic sclerotherapy vs. conservative management of bleeding oesophageal varices. *Acta Chir Scand* **151**:449–456, 1985
93. Terblanche JP, Bornman PC, Kahn D, et al: The failure of long-term injection sclerotherapy after variceal bleeding to improve survival. *Lancet* **2**:1328–1332, 1983
94. Westaby D, MacDougall BRD, Williams R: Improves survival following injection sclerotherapy for esophageal varices: Final analysis of a controlled trial. *Hepatology* **5**:627–631, 1985
95. Korula J, Balart A, Radvan G, et al: Prospective randomized controlled trial of chronic oesophageal variceal sclerotherapy. *Hepatology* **5**:584–589, 1984
96. Warren WD, Henderson JM, Millikan WJ, et al: Distal splenorenal shunt versus endoscopic sclerotherapy for long-term management of variceal bleeding: Preliminary report of a prospective, randomized trial. *Ann Surg* **203**:454–462, 1986
97. Rikkers LF, Burnett DA, Volentine GD, et al: Shunt surgery versus endoscopic sclerotherapy for long-term treatment of variceal bleeding: Early results of a randomized trial. *Ann Surg* **206**:261–271, 1987
98. Teres J, Bordas JM, Bravo D, et al: Sclerotherapy vs distal splenorenal shunt in the elective treatment of variceal hemorrhage: A randomized controlled trial. *Hepatology* **7**:430–436, 1987
99. Terblanche J, Burroughs AK, Hobbs KEF: Controversies in the management of bleeding esophageal varices. II. *N Engl J Med* **320**:1469–1475, 1989
100. Kanuer CN: Mallory-Weiss syndrome. *Gastroenterology* **71**:5–8, 1976
101. Wolfesen HC, Wang KK: Etiology and course of acute bleeding esophageal ulcers. *J Clin Gastroenterol* **14**:342–346, 1992
102. Ellis FH: Barrett's esophagus. *Postgrad Med* **90**:135–146, 1991
103. Williamson WA, Ellis FH, Gibb SP, Aretz HT: Barrett's ulcer: A surgical disease? *J Thorac Cardiovasc Surg* **103**:2–7, 1992
104. Pearson FG, Cooper JD, Patterson GA, Praskash D: Peptic ulcer in acquired columnar-lined esophagus: Results of surgical treatment. *Ann Thorac Surg* **43**:241–244, 1987

CHAPTER

# 42

# Medical and Surgical Treatment of Hiatal Hernia and Gastroesophageal Reflux

Keith S. Naunheim and Arthur E. Baue

## HISTORY

Herniation of abdominal contents through the diaphragm into the thoracic cavity has been recognized for several centuries. Bowditch credited Ambroise Paré with a description of a patient with herniation of the stomach through the esophageal hiatus in 1610.[1] The first description of a hiatal hernia in the English literature was probably Bright's in 1836.[2] In 1884, Potempski performed a successful repair of a diaphragmatic hernia and in 1889 he reported on six cases.[3] Early writings on this subject in the 20th century all focused on the anatomic problems of the herniated stomach into the chest, and most reports were on herniation due to trauma. In 1935, Winklestein was the first to call attention to the occurrence of peptic esophagitis, which was secondary to reflux.[4] The anatomic characteristics of the esophagogastric junction emphasized as important factors in preventing reflux included an abdominal segment of esophagus, the esophagogastric angle, the pinchcock effect of the right crus of the diaphragm, and the rosette of mucosal folds at the esophagogastric junction. Although a lower esophageal sphincter (LES) mechanism had been suggested by the work of Kronecker and Meltzer in the 19th century, this was largely ignored until recently.[5] Their manometric investigations of esophageal motility led to the studies by Code and Ingelfinger and their associates that demonstrated a zone of pressure elevation 2–5 cm long on the lower portion of the esophagus.[6,7] Since that time, a large body of sophisticated work has been performed to investigate the pathophysiology of gastroesophageal reflux (GER) (see Chapter 39). Although GER does occur in the absence of a hiatal hernia, most patients with reflux do have such a hernia. It is apparent that the normal anatomic relations in this region maintain and support the protective function of the gastroesophageal junction.

## ANATOMY OF THE ESOPHAGOGASTRIC JUNCTION

A detailed review of esophageal anatomy may be found in Chapter 39; however, a brief review is pertinent here. The tubular esophagus extends for a variable distance below the level of the diaphragm before merging with the saccular stomach. In its distal portion the esophagus is enclosed by the right crus of the muscular diaphragm that arises from the lumbar vertebrae (Fig. 42–1). The most important supporting structure is the phrenoesophageal membrane, first described by Laimer in 1883.[8] This membrane consists of fascial attachments of the distal esophagus to the diaphragm (Fig. 42–2). This structure is a continuation of the transversalis fascia on the inferior aspect of the diaphragm. It behaves as a fibroelastic sleeve enclosing the lower portion of the esophagus within the confines of the esophageal hiatus. The phrenoesophageal membrane is attached to the muscular wall of the esophagus several centimeters above the junction. The membrane is designed to distribute tension over a wide area of the esophageal wall and thus maintain the esophagogastric junction in its intra-abdominal location. When it fails to do so and the junction moves up through the hiatus, a hiatal hernia results.

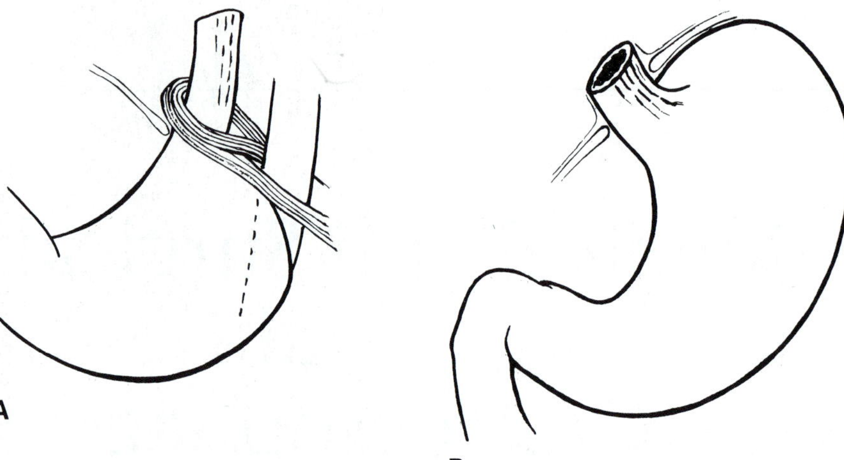


**Figure 42–1. A.** This diagram of the esophageal hiatus shows that it is made up of fibers of the right crus, which decussate and form both sides of the esophageal hiatus. There is little contribution from the left crus. **B.** The normal esophagogastric junction.

## CLASSIFICATION

Hiatal hernias are classified as Type I, II, or III depending on the specific abnormality present.

- Type I, also known as a sliding hiatal hernia. The phrenoesophageal ligament is weakened or stretched so that the esophagogastric junction can migrate through the hiatus into the posterior mediastinum to occupy an intrathoracic position. In this type, the esophagogastric junction remains cephalad to the stomach (Fig. 42–3). This hernia is usually reducible. However, in cases of chronic esophagitis and advanced stricturing, the esophagus may be foreshortened, and the gastroesophageal junction remains fixed in the thoracic cavity.
- Type II, known as paraesophageal hiatal hernia. In this

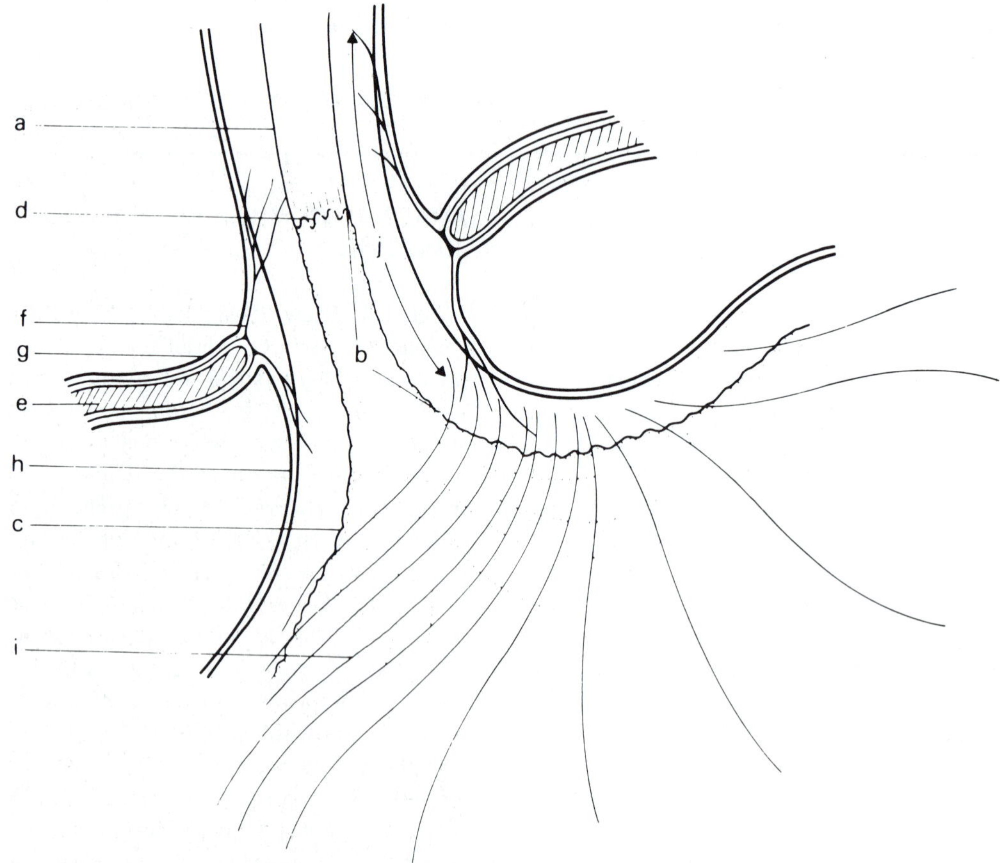


**Figure 42–2.** Anatomy of the gastroesophageal junction. **a.** Esophageal mucosa. **b.** Junctional mucosa. **c.** Gastric mucosa. **d.** "Z" line. **e.** Diaphragm. **f.** Phrenoesophageal membrane. **g.** Pleura. **h.** Peritoneum. **i.** Gastric hiatal sling fibers. **j.** High-pressure zone area. *(Courtesy of John Clark, Glan Clwyd Hospital, Rhyl, Wales.)*

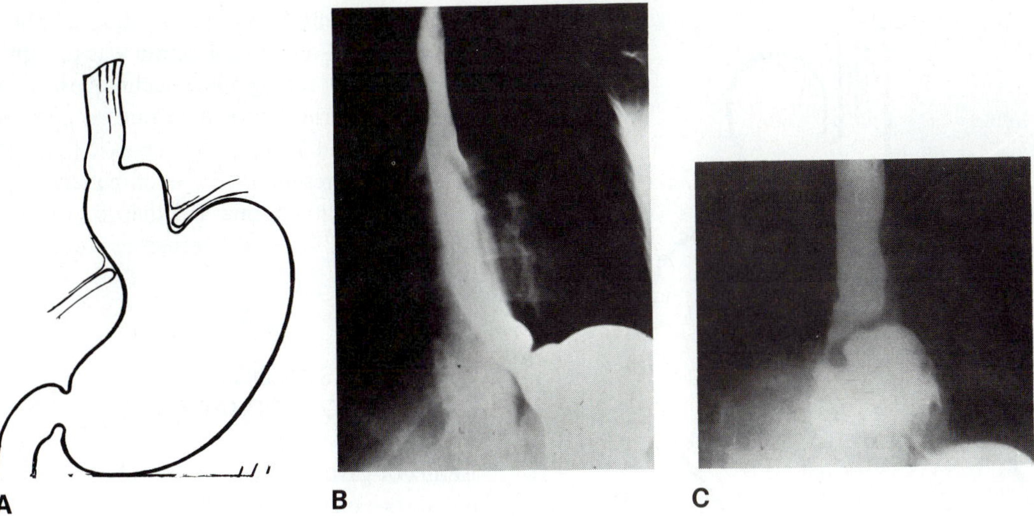

**Figure 42–3. A.** This diagram shows the protrusion of the esophagogastric junction and proximal stomach through the hiatus in a siding hiatal hernia. **B.** Barium swallow demonstrates small sliding hiatal hernia. **C.** Barium swallow demonstrates a large sliding hiatal hernia in which the fundus of the stomach is also pushing into the chest.

type of hernia, the phrenoesophageal ligament remains firm and binds the distal esophagus to the preaortic fascia and the median arcuate ligament. Therefore the gastroesophageal junction lies at or near its normal location near the hiatus. However, the fundus and body of the stomach roll up into the chest alongside the esophagus (Fig. 42–4). This entity is fully covered in Chapter 48.

- Type III, also known as sliding-and-rolling hernia. The esophagogastric junction herniates into the chest along with most of the greater curvature and body of the stomach (Fig. 42–5).

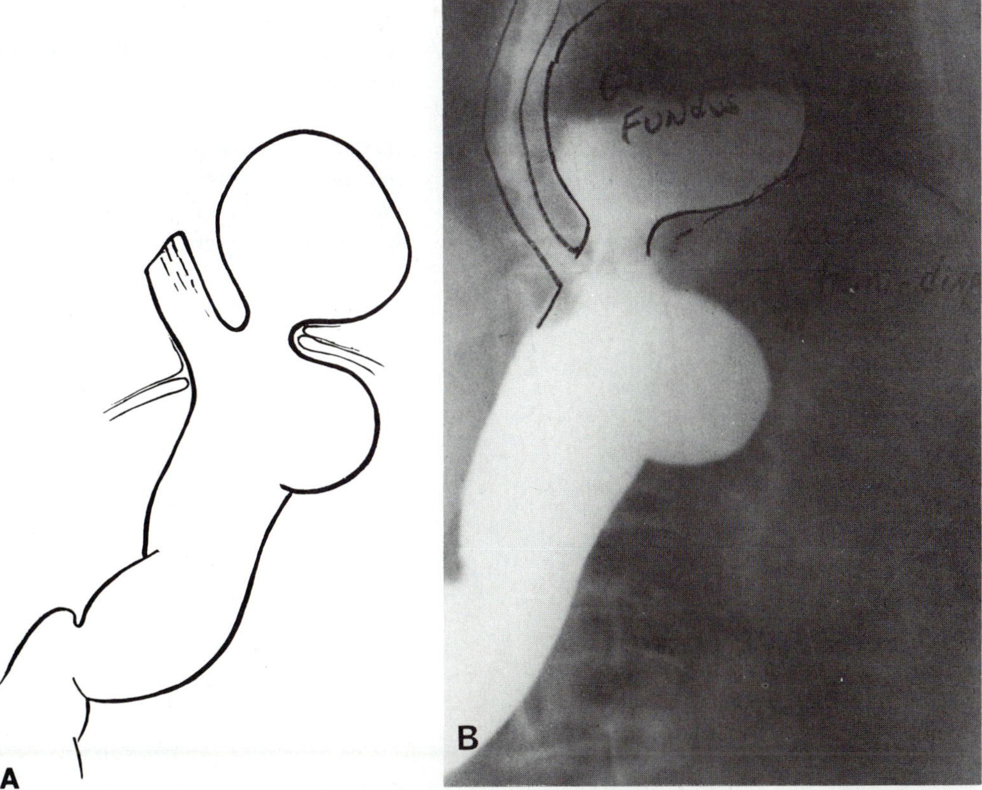


**Figure 42–4. A.** This diagram depicts a paraesophageal hernia. The esophagogastric junction is in the normal location, and the fundus of the stomach is protruding alongside the esophagogastric junction into the chest. **B.** Barium swallow shows this abnormality.

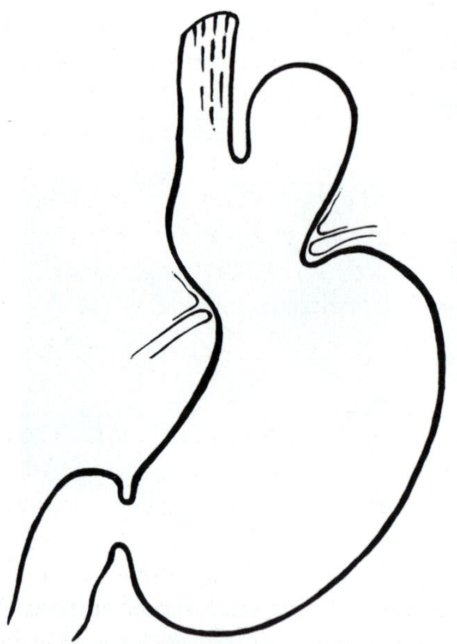

**Figure 42–5.** This diagram depicts the combined type of hernia, in which there are both sliding and rolling components, with the esophagogastric junction and part of the fundus of the stomach above the diaphragm.

Although there are undoubtedly occasional instances of congenital esophageal hiatal hernia,[2] most of these hernias occur later in life, and the cause has yet to be clearly determined. Obesity and pregnancy are important factors; the increased intra-abdominal pressure in these conditions causes stretching and weakening of the diaphragmatic attachments of the esophagus, setting the stage for herniation. However, hiatal hernias occur in many people in the absence of obvious anatomic causes, probably because of intrinsic weakness of muscular or fascial tissue in the hiatal region, either congenital or acquired.

Hiatal hernia is a relatively common problem encountered at the time of upper gastrointestinal radiographic examination. Special diagnostic maneuvers may disclose such a hernia in as many as 30% of patients.[9] The predominance of Type I or sliding hiatal hernia was recognized soon after the advent of radiographic techniques. Type II or paraesophageal hernia is far more rare, as confirmed by the report of Hill and Tobias, who reported that a paraesophageal hernia was present in 3.5% of patients operated on for esophageal hiatal hernia and that these patients accounted for less than 2% of all herniations through the esophageal hiatus.[10]

## PATHOPHYSIOLOGY OF GASTROESOPHAGEAL REFLUX

Reflux of gastric contents and acid into the esophagus is not an all-or-none phenomenon, as anyone who has overindulged will recognize. Most healthy people have occasional bouts of reflux and infrequently experience mild esophagitis. In most people even those with a sliding hiatal hernia, this process subsides with reasonable eating habits or with the taking of antacids. Thus many patients with a small sliding hiatal hernia have few or no symptoms. When reflux is a continuing or persistent problem, the patient has sufficient symptoms to require investigation and therapy.

Several factors may play a role in the pathologic development of severe GER and the resultant esophageal mucosal inflammation (Fig. 42–6 and Table 42–1). These include the following

1. Lower esophageal sphincter. The greatest emphasis has been placed on the LES. This functional sphincter resides at the gastroesophageal junction. When competent, the LES helps prevent pathologic reflux of gastric contents into the esophagus. Using esophageal manometry, one can measure the resting pressure, length, and site (intra-abdominal or intrathoracic) of this sphincter. A decreased pressure or length of the LES may facilitate reflux of gastric fluid into the esophagus.
2. Esophageal clearance. In a normal esophagus, reflux of

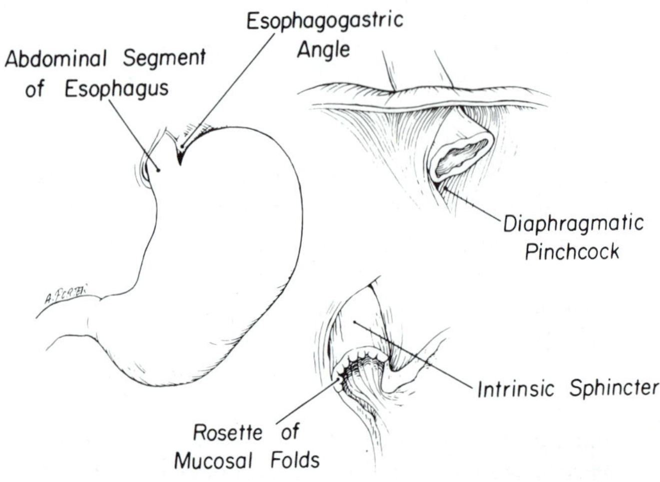


**Figure 42–6.** Anatomic characteristics that are features of the esophagogastric junction. They serve to support the intrinsic sphincter in a position of maximum effectiveness.

**TABLE 42–1. GASTRIC AND ESOPHAGEAL FACTORS INVOLVED IN THE PATHOPHYSIOLOGY OF GASTROESOPHAGEAL REFLUX**

| |
|---|
| Lower esophageal sphincter |
| Esophageal clearance |
| Mucosal resistance |
| Salivary neutralization |
| Gastric secretion |

gastric contents is be cleared by a combination of gravity (in the upright position) and reactive esophageal peristalsis. Normal esophageal motor activity and postural changes therefore play a critical role in preventing esophageal injury by effecting rapid clearance of the inflammatory material from the esophagus. This minimizes the time of mucosal exposure to the refluxate. If esophageal clearance is impaired, stasis of reflux material occurs, and damage may result. Patients with primary motor disorders are therefore predisposed to more severe esophagitis because of impaired motor function. Similarly, in nocturnal reflux, gravity can no longer play a role because of the supine position, and persistent mucosal inflammation results.

3. Mucosal resistance. The resistance to injury of the esophageal mucosa may differ from person to person. Some patients with documented reflux have no visible or histologic evidence for mucosal injury, but others suffer severe, diffuse esophagitis with the same degree of reflux. Mucosal resistance factors are poorly understood, although it is generally held that secretions from glands within the mucosa form a coating that protects the esophageal lining from chemical injury during reflux. This protective coating may be eroded by combinations of acid, pepsin, and bile. To date, no cellular or histochemical characteristics can be used to identify patients particularly susceptible to reflux damage and esophagitis. Histopathologic and ultrastructural facets of reflux esophagitis have been reviewed but are beyond the scope of this chapter.[11]
4. Salivary neutralization. The importance of saliva in protection of the esophageal mucosa has only recently come to light. Both the composition and the amount of swallowed saliva are important factors in dilution and neutralization of refluxed acid material. They represent an important mechanism for esophageal protection.[12]
5. Gastric secretion. Several aspects of gastric physiology may play a critical role, including the nature and volume of gastric secretion. The sensitivity of esophageal mucosa to gastric acid and pepsin has been documented by numerous investigators using models that include pyloric obstruction, destruction of the gastroesophageal sphincter, and chronic perfusion of esophageal mucosa with acid.[13] The reflux of alkaline bilous material has long been known clinically to result in severe esophagitis,[14] and this has been demonstrated experimentally.[15] However, the combination of acid, pepsin, and bile in gastric refluxate leads to a more erosive esophagitis than any of the three components alone. The volume of gastric secretion can also play a critical role. Delayed emptying secondary either to gastric stasis or pyloric obstruction may lead to high retained gastric volumes, which can exacerbate or cause reflux. Indeed, gastric emptying has been shown to be slower than normal in patients with reflux[16] and may play a role in as many as 40% of patients with reflux esophagitis.[17]

When clinically significant defects arise in these physiologic mechanisms, pathologic GER occurs, and peptic esophagitis often follows. Potential complications of severe GER include anemia due to chronic blood loss, esophageal strictures (see Chapter 47), and Barrett's esophagus. Specific complications for Barrett's esophagus (see Chapter 43) include the abovementioned problems in addition to severe erosive Barrett's ulceration and the tendency for malignant degeneration in the columnar-lined esophagus.

It is important to realize that just as not every patient with a hiatal hernia suffers from esophagitis, not every patient with GER has a concomitant hiatal hernia. Primary incompetence of the LES is an uncommon but well-recognized abnormality first described by Hiebert and Belsey in 1961.[18] It was dubbed by them to be "the patulous cardia." Clinical confirmation was forthcoming from Olsen et al[19] and Cohen and Harris[20] (Fig. 42–7). The pathophysiology of this entity is covered in detail in Chapters 39 and 40. Lack of radiologic evidence for such a hernia may sometimes delay the diagnosis. However, patients with primary incompetence of the gastroesophageal junction should be treated in the same manner as those with concomitant hiatal hernia.

## SYMPTOMS AND DIAGNOSIS

Most patients in whom a sliding hiatal hernia is demonstrated are free of any clinically significant or continuing symptoms. This hernia is one of the most common abnormalities of the esophagus and stomach in patients between the ages of 40 and 70 years. Excellent documentation of the epidemiology of this disease has been published.[21] Because involvement of viscera other than the esophagus and stomach in sliding hiatal hernia is extremely rare, such a hernia is not ordinarily associated with a risk of incarceration, obstruction, or strangulation of the intestine. The severity of symptoms of GER may be highly subjective and vary widely from one person to the next. One patient may describe extreme heartburn yet have no demonstrable esophagitis, and another may have little or no heartburn, yet present with an established stricture. Thus, symptoms are not necessarily a reliable indicator of the extent of organic disease. The typical symptoms of retrosternal or epigastric

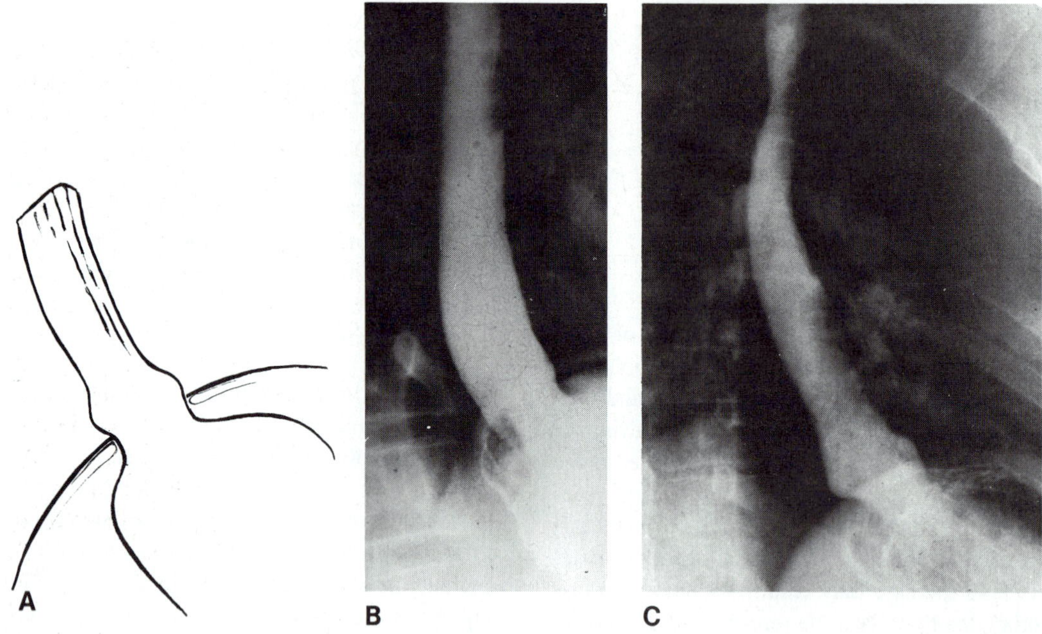


**Figure 42–7. A.** This diagram depicts a patulous cardia, or primary incompetence of the gastroesophageal junction, with free reflux but no hiatal hernia. **B.** A barium swallow showing primary gastroesophageal incompetence. **C.** A barium swallow showing another example in a patient with primary gastroesophageal incompetence and reflux without a sliding hiatal hernia. The bulges just above the diaphragm represent the phrenic ampulla and not a hiatal hernia.

heartburn, postural regurgitation, gaseous eructation, and intermittent dysphagia are manifestations of incompetence of the cardia with varying degrees of esophagitis. The symptoms are often worse after meals and aggravated by postural changes (lying down, stooping, bending over, or straining). Relief may occur with sitting or standing. Regurgitation of fluid into the mouth may produce a sour, hot, or bitter taste (waterbrash). In some patients, symptoms occur only at night, waking the patient from sleep with cough, pain, bitter taste, or fluid in the mouth. Heartburn or pyrosis may be mild and occur occasionally with overindulgence in food or drink or may be so severe as to be constant and interfere seriously with daily life. The pain may be only substernal or may be referred to the neck, ears, jaw, or arms.

Bleeding and anemia due to esophagitis may occur but are not frequent. Erosion of the esophagus may be so severe as to produce a protein-losing enteropathy. The greatest threat to the patient is the development of a stricture due to prolonged esophagitis. Other complications of reflux that have not been generally appreciated are those that involve the respiratory tract. Respiratory involvement occurs in 20% of patients and may be the dominant or sole symptom in some patients.[22,23] Aspiration of regurgitated gastric contents may occur, particularly during sleep, resulting in recurrent bouts of pneumonia or persistent cough. These may be the only indications of reflux. Some research suggests there may be a second mechanism producing pulmonary symptoms that is neurogenic. Intraesophageal instillation of dilute hydrochloric acid in patients with both reflux and asthma has produced reactive bronchoconstriction, probably by vagally mediated reflexes.[24,25]

A membrane or diaphragm may be seen on radiolographs of the esophagogastric mucosal junction as a ring and may become thickened or fibrotic, producing intermittent or persistent dysphagia. This has been called a Schatzki ring and is always associated with a hiatal hernia.[26] The ring is composed of esophageal squamous mucosa on the top and gastric mucosa on the bottom with a variable degree of fibrous tissue, smooth muscle, and scarring in between. Although this abnormality is usually seen only as a slight indentation at the esophagogastric junction on barium swallow examination, it may be so severe as to produce a diaphragm with only a small hole at the esophagogastric junction (Fig. 42–8). The most common problem caused by such a ring is intermittent dysphagia, particularly for solid foods. Most of these rings produce few, if any, symptoms and serve only to indicate the location of the gastroesophageal junction and the presence of a hiatal hernia. If symptoms of dysphagia occur, dilation with a balloon or a bougie is indicated. If the concomitant hiatal hernia is symptomatic, operative hiatal hernia repair with dilation of the ring may be undertaken. Although operative excision of the ring with gastrostomy has been performed in the past, virtually all true Schatzki rings may be managed with dilation alone.

Prolonged reflux may lead to variable reactive and inflammatory changes in the squamous epithelium of the lower esophagus and metaplasia of the columnar epithelium

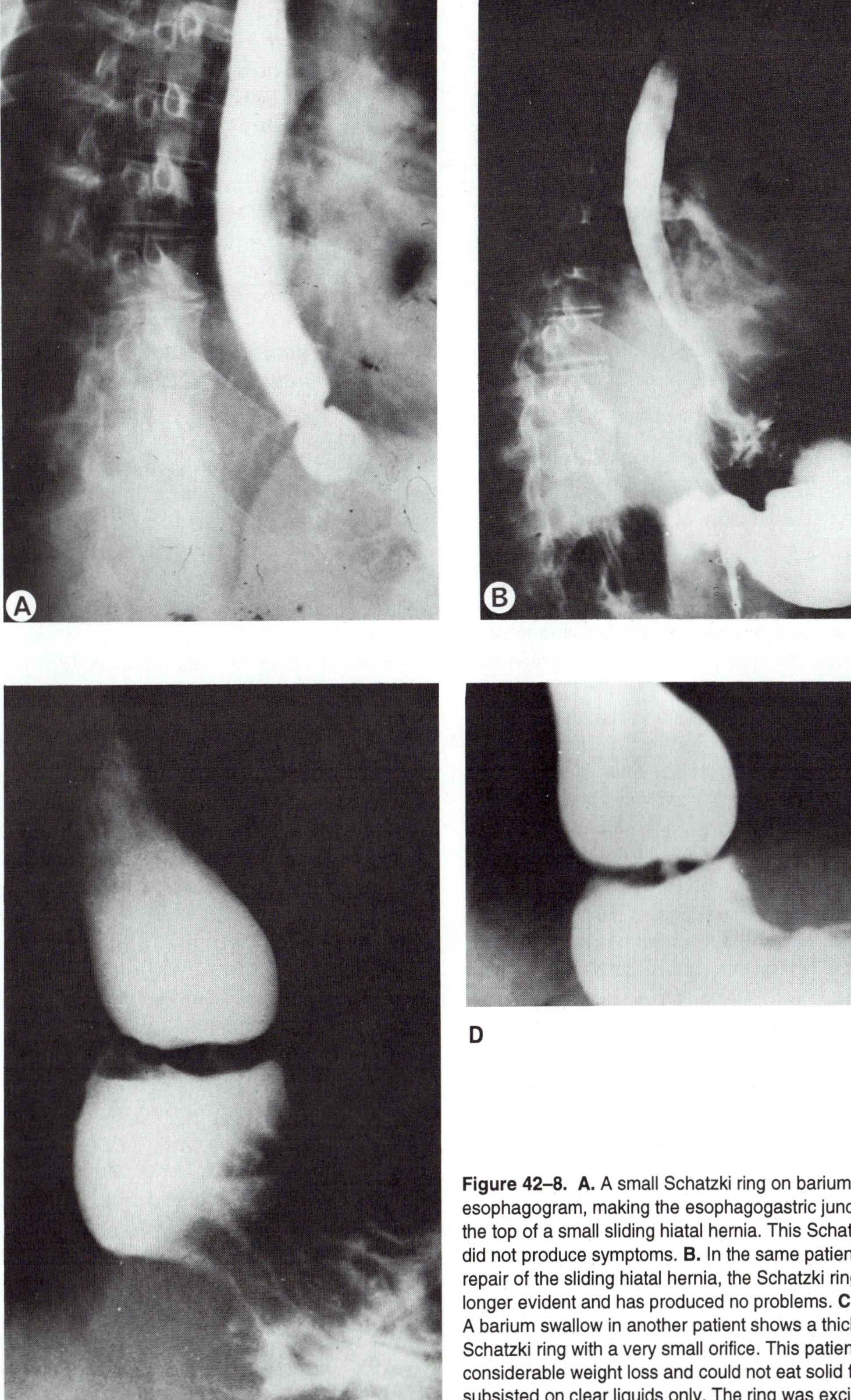

**Figure 42–8.** **A.** A small Schatzki ring on barium esophagogram, making the esophagogastric junction at the top of a small sliding hiatal hernia. This Schatzki ring did not produce symptoms. **B.** In the same patient, after a repair of the sliding hiatal hernia, the Schatzki ring is no longer evident and has produced no problems. **C and D.** A barium swallow in another patient shows a thickened Schatzki ring with a very small orifice. This patient had considerable weight loss and could not eat solid food but subsisted on clear liquids only. The ring was excised through a gastrotomy incision with reapproximation of the esophagogastric mucosal junction, and the sliding hiatal hernia was repaired with complete relief of symptoms and restoration of normal swallowing.

lining this portion. Ulceration or fibrous stricture may then occur high in the esophagus, often in the region of the aortic arch. The entire esophagus below the stricture is usually lined with columnar epithelium. This is invariably associated with a sliding hiatal hernia and clinically significant reflux. This condition is commonly known as Barrett's esophagus (see Chapter 43).

The diagnosis of a sliding hiatal hernia with reflux is usually made by radiographic means, which may include barium swallow examination along with special maneuvers to assess reflux. Esophagoscopy should be performed in all patients with symptoms of GER or with unexplained respiratory symptoms. The endoscopic findings of reflux vary from normal mucosa to slight erythema, severe hyperemia, irregular mucosa, linear or punctate ulcerations, and frank ulceration with mucosal destruction. The pliability of the esophageal wall can be assessed as can fixation of the esophagogastric junction above the diaphragm, the status of the fundus of the stomach, and the possibility of coincidental malignant disease. The severity of symptoms is not always related to the degree of esophagitis. For this reason, biopsy of the mucosa, even though the mucosa appears normal, may be helpful in evaluating the extent of esophageal inflammation. A detailed review of the technique of esophagoscopy and the findings in reflux can be found in Chapter 9.

Formal testing of esophageal function is not necessary for all patients with classic symptoms of GER. Medical therapy can be instituted without detailed analysis of esophageal function. However, before surgical intervention, formal testing should be undertaken and include both esophageal manometry and 24-hour pH testing. Esophageal manometry testing assesses not only the upper and lower esophageal sphincters but also the motility of the body of the esophagus. The standard for diagnosis of GER is 24-hour esophageal pH monitoring. These and other esophageal function tests are covered in Chapter 40.

Differential diagnosis is particularly important because the clinical features of esophageal disease can mimic other conditions, and vice versa. Chest pain may be due to angina pectoris, duodenal ulceration, cholecystitis, colonic disease, and diffuse spasm of the esophagus, among other problems. Similarly, these problems may present with epigastric or chest discomfort that is burning in nature and may mimic heartburn.

## MEDICAL TREATMENT

As noted, the pathophysiology of GER is multifactorial (Fig. 42–6 and Table 42–1). The different nodes of medical management are designed to address the individual factors in the hope of preventing or minimizing the severity of GER. Modes of medical therapy include lifestyle changes and pharmacologic agents.

### Lifestyle Modification

#### *Elevation of the Head of the Bed*

Gravity may be used to advantage in the treatment of symptoms of GER. The head of the bed should be elevated 6–10 inches (15–25 cm) by means of blocks under the feet of the bed or a foam wedge under the mattress. These maneuvers take advantage of gravity to decrease the number of reflux episodes and increase the rate of refluxate clearance.[27] This helps to prevent sustained nocturnal acid exposure of the esophagus, which occurs in many patients with GER who have supine reflux.[28]

#### *Weight Reduction*

Although no certain correlation between obesity and decreased LES pressure has been documented, some studies have demonstrated a correlation between reflux and morbid obesity.[29] The increased intra-abdominal pressure present in such patients may result in an increased transsphincteric gradient, which may cause any reflux episode to be more severe. It has been demonstrated that weight loss can lead to marked improvement of symptoms of GER.[30]

#### *Smoking*

Cigarette smoking can both decrease LES pressure and increase the frequency of episodes of GER.[31,32] It can also impair attempts at pharmacologic management of reflux symptoms.[33] Although cessation of smoking decreases the frequency of reflux episodes, the total time of acid exposure has not been shown to be greatly altered.[34] There are conflicting data on the rate of healing of esophagitis with cessation of smoking,[35,36] but most clinicians suggest this course of action to their patients with GER who smoke.

#### *Alcohol*

Ethanol has been demonstrated to lower LES pressure and to impair esophageal peristalsis.[37,38] These effects tend to increase the rate of reflux and slow normal esophageal clearance, both of which can lead to an increased risk of esophagitis.

#### *Diet Modification*

Several foods have been recognized to cause a decrease in LES pressure. These include coffee,[39] chocolate,[40] peppermint,[41] and rich fatty foods.[42] Although some authors have implicated coffee in lowering LES pressure,[39] others have suggested there is no direct effect on sphincter pressure[43] but that there is a stimulatory effect on gastric acid production.[44] Some foods (cola beverages, milk products) are also known to exacerbate GER because of their stimulatory effects on gastric acid secretion.[44] Other insults to the esophagus include direct mucosal irritation, which can occur with acidic beverages such as citrus or tomato juice.[45] The food that incite symptoms of GER often vary from patient to patient. The avoidance of such foods should be encouraged during medical management and may ameliorate symptoms. The timing of meals is also important; patients should avoid meals or snacks just before bedtime and avoid recumbency within 2–3 hours after any meal.

### *Medications*

A number of medications utilized for concomitant medical problems may produce exacerbation of symptoms of GER. The best example is theophylline, which has been shown both to decrease LES pressure and increase baseline acid secretion.[46] Other medicines with a potential detrimental effect on sphincter pressure include dopamine, nitrates, opiates, diazepam, and calcium channel blockers.[47] Although many of these medications cannot be avoided entirely, attempts at lowering the dose or substitution of different forms of medication (i.e., inhaled bronchodilators for people with asthma) may be beneficial in the management of GER.

## Pharmacologic Therapy

Pharmacologic therapy is aimed at achieving several physiologic goals that help minimize GER (Table 42–2). Commonly used agents can be categorized into four general classifications: cytoprotective regimens, antacids, acid suppressors, and prokinetic agents.

### *Cytoprotective Agents*

The most commonly used mucosal coating agent is sucralfate, which is a polysulfated aluminum salt of sucrose purported to have a cytoprotective effect. Sucralfate has no known effect on gastric or esophageal motility, sphincter pressure, or gastric secretion. This aluminum salt both coats damaged mucosal surfaces and binds potentially noxious agents such as bile acids and pepsin. However, despite the theoretic therapeutic advantages of the drug, the literature regarding efficacy is somewhat uncertain. Several studies assessing clinical benefit suggest sucralfate is superior to placebo[48] and as effective as $H_2$-blockers[49] for the treatment of reflux esophagitis. Other studies, however, show no significant difference between sucralfate and placebo.[50] At present, sucralfate is used primarily for adjunctive therapy in combination with acid suppressive medications rather than as a primary stand alone therapy.

**TABLE 42–2. DRUGS USED TO TREAT GASTROESOPHAGEAL REFLUX**

| Drug | Action |
|---|---|
| Cytoprotective agents | Improve mucosal resistance |
| Antacids | Neutralize gastric contents |
| Acid suppressors | Minimize secretion |
| Prokinetic agents | Strengthen LES<br>Enhance esophageal clearance<br>Accelerate gastric emptying<br>Minimize gastroduodenal reflux |

### *Antacids*

Antacids alkalinize the gastric pH and have been demonstrated to yield an increase in LES pressure.[51] Although these agents provide excellent relief of mild reflux symptoms,[52] large volumes are required to obtain an effect similar to that of $H_2$-blockers, and improvement of esophagitis is not easily demonstrated.

### *Acid Suppression*

The acid suppressive agents are of two types: $H_2$-receptor antagonists and proton pump inhibitors. The most commonly prescribed agents for GER are histamine receptor antagonists, otherwise known as $H_2$-blockers. Their mechanism or action is a blockade of the $H_2$-receptors on the gastric parietal cell, which decreases the volume and concentration of gastric acid available for reflux. These drugs have no primary effect on LES pressure, gastric motility, or esophageal clearance. Cimetidine and ranitidine have been clinically available for the longest time and thus the greatest number of studies have been performed on these two agents. The other $H_2$-blockers (famotidine, nizatidine, ethintidine, and roxatidine) appear comparable, but fewer studies have documented their efficacy. Unfortunately, the $H_2$-blockers have been found to be somewhat less effective for GER than they are for peptic ulcer disease. Prospective randomized trials have demonstrated improvement in reflux symptoms when cimetidine and ranitidine are compared with placebo.[53] However, the rate of healing documented at endoscopy is less than that found in peptic ulcer disease. Pooled data from several studies suggest that an aggressive cimetidine regimen yields a 50–60% rate of healing in patients with moderate (grade II–III) esophagitis.[54] This compares favorably with a 30% rate of healing in placebo controls. However, such healing occurs slowly, thus, $H_2$-blocker administration should be continued for a prolonged course of at least 3–6 months. Pooled data on ranitidine shows similar endoscopic healing rates as seen with cimetidine.[54] Patients with symptoms of GER and esophagitis refractory to standard dosages have been shown to respond to higher doses of up to 1800 mg per day.

The newest and most exciting agent to be developed for the treatment of GER is the proton pump inhibitor omeprazole. This class of acid suppressant agent has proved to be one of the most effective weapons to date in the treatment of reflux. Omeprazole suppresses both basal and stimulated gastric acid production[55] and results in a 95% inhibition of overall acid secretion.[56] This drug has no known effect on LES pressure, gastric motility, or esophageal clearance. It acts by blocking the $H^+$-$K^+$-ATPase pump on the surface of gastric parietal cells. Dosages range from 20–60 mg daily. This drug has been found superior to placebo,[57] ranitidine and cimetidine in the treatment of gastroesophageal reflux.[58,59] Omeprazole is found to be highly effective in patients with severe erosive esophagitis refractory to $H_2$-blockers with or without the use of prokinetic agents.[60]

There are, however, concerns regarding prolonged treatment with omeprazole because of chronic gastric acid suppression. This suppression causes hypergastrinemia, and the elevated gastrin levels have been associated with hyperplasia of enterochromaffin-like cells in experimental animals. This has raised the worry that there might be a predisposition toward development of carcinoid tumors in the setting of chronic omeprazole therapy. Thus current recommendation suggests cessation of proton pump blockers after 2-months of continuous usage.

### *Prokinetic Agents*

Prokinetic agents affect GER by means of a modulating effect on the motility of the upper digestive tract. The desired effect of such motility agents in an increase in resting LES pressure, improved esophageal peristalsis and clearance, and an increase in gastric motility with resultant acceleration of gastric emptying. The latter effect may also minimize the incidence of bile reflux from the duodenum into the stomach. Metoclopramide acts as a dopamine antagonist and was the first prokinetic agent widely used; it has proved somewhat disappointing. Although symptomatic relief was superior to placebo, improvement in endoscopic healing could not be reliably demonstrated.[61–63] Domperidone, another dopamine antagonist, proved to be similarly disappointing; the rate of endoscopic healing was poor when the drug was used as a single agent.[64] The main role for these medications has proved to be one in which they are used in combination with an $H_2$-blocker.[65]

Cisapride is a new prokinetic agent that increases contractility by enhancing acetylcholine release from the myenteric plexus of intestinal smooth muscle. It has been shown to increase LES pressure and accelerate gastric emptying. Studies suggest that when used as a single agent, cisapride is superior to placebo in the relief of reflux symptoms and the healing of esophagitis.[66,67] Cisapride in doses of 10 mg qid has been demonstrated to yield results similar to those of ranitidine with regard to control of symptoms and resolution of esophagitis.[68] The combination of cisapride and cimetidine has been demonstrated to be superior to cimetidine alone in the treatment of GER.[69]

## Strategy of Medical Therapy

The treatment of GER begins with conservative therapy consisting mainly of lifestyle modifications. Elevation of the head of the bed 6–10 inches (15–25 cm) helps prevent and minimize nocturnal reflux episodes. A sensible weight reduction regimen is encouraged by many physicians to minimize the transdiaphragmatic pressure gradient, which may promote reflux episodes. Cessation of smoking and limitation of alcohol consumption also may ameliorate mild to moderate GER symptoms. Finally, avoidance of foods and medications known to exacerbate GER is advisable. A large number of patients with mild GER symptoms can add over-the-counter antacids (taken after meals and at bedtime) to these lifestyle modifications and require no further therapy.

The second phase of treatment involves pharmacologic management and should begin only if the aforementioned measures fail an adequate trial. Patients with moderate to severe reflux symptoms or endoscopic evidence of esophagitis often require the institution of such measures. It is important to recognize that administration of medication should be undertaken in addition to and not in place of the lifestyle changes. Initial therapy usually involves use of $H_2$-receptor antagonists such as cimetidine or ranitidine. The latter medication is preferred by many physicians because it can be given twice a day, increasing the chance of patient compliance. It must be remembered that there is a wide therapeutic range for $H_2$-blockers, and the initial dose can usually be doubled for symptoms refractory to the starting dosage. If the single medication fails to prove effective or if the presenting symptoms are severe, a prokinetic agent may be added. Cisapride is most commonly used for two reasons. Its efficacy in combination with $H_2$-blockers has been very encouraging in early studies, and it appears to have a lower incidence of side effects (lethargy, fatigue, extrapyramidal symptoms) than metoclopramide.

Persistent reflux or unhealed esophagitis in the face of two-drug therapy may warrant the addition of a mucosal protective agent such as sucralfate. As an alternative, sucralfate can be used in place of a motility agent as the second drug.

Failure of the combinations of medications signals the need for use of a proton pump blocker. Currently, omeprazole is substituted for the $H_2$-blocker. Because of its remarkable efficacy, omeprazole alone may be sufficient therapy, and prokinetic agents and mucosal protectants can be withdrawn. Unfortunately, the official recommendation for omeprazole limits use to a 2-month period, although many clinicians persist with a longer course. The incidence of long-term side effects is as yet unknown, so committing a patient to chronic therapy with a proton pump blocker cannot as yet be approved.

Patients successfully treated with the foregoing regimen should continue treatment for 3–6 months before discontinuing pharmacologic therapy. Unfortunately, studies suggest that most patients note recurrence of symptoms in 6 months and as many as 90% have relapses within 1 year after withdrawal of medication.[70,71] Although therapy can be reinstituted for such patients, frequent relapses occur despite continued pharmacologic therapy.[72] Increasing $H_2$-blocker dosage may be beneficial in the short run, but in many patients relapses persist. Maintenance therapy with omeprazole, although logical, cannot yet be recommended.

It is for just such people that the last phase of therapy is appropriate—surgical intervention. Current indications for surgical treatment include symptoms refractory to medical management and complications of reflux disease, such as stricture, bleeding, and severe ulceration. Patients who present at a young age with clinically significant GER that is difficult to control should also be considered with the hope of obviating the need for a long-term and expensive medication regimen.

## SURGICAL TREATMENT

### Indications

The indications for surgical correction of GER vary from specialist to specialist and institution to institution. Surgeons usually recommend an antireflux operation to all patients who have complications of reflux, such as stricture, bleeding, or recurrent respiratory symptoms due to regurgitation. The indications for surgical repair in uncomplicated disease include symptoms refractory to medical therapy, failure of patient compliance, and presence of clinically significant symptoms and esophagitis in young patients.[73]

However, most patients with GER are treated not by surgeons but by medical specialists. Many such patients are treated only with conservative medical therapy despite the presence of the aforementioned complications. Often it appears as if gastroenterologists wish to "protect" their patients from surgical intervention at all costs. This bias is exemplified by a recent report from the Veterans Gastroesophageal Reflux Disease Study group.[74] In a randomized trial of men with complicated GER, patients were assigned randomly to receive continuous medical therapy, intermittent medical therapy for symptoms, or surgical therapy. There were frequent side effects in both medical therapy groups, and over a 2-year follow-up period the surgical cohort demonstrated decreased severity of reflux symptoms, esophagitis, and acid reflux. In addition, the patient satisfaction was greater with surgical therapy than with either of the two medical regimens. The conclusion, however, suggested only that surgical treatment was a valid alternative as opposed to being a preferential method of treatment.

### Operative Approach

The ideal surgical procedure for and approach to the treatment of GER has yet to be defined. There has long been a controversy regarding the route by which an antireflux procedure should be undertaken. General surgeons have insisted that virtually all cases of GER can be approached via the transabdominal route, whereas many cardiothoracic surgeons have insisted that a transthoracic approach be used for all patients. Several procedures can be performed only via an abdominal or a thoracic approach, whereas others, such as the Nissen fundoplication, can be undertaken from either side of the diaphragm. The answer to which route is appropriate lies in the physiologic principles underlying an antireflux repair. One of the goals of almost every antireflux operation is to restore a 4- to 6-cm length of esophagus within the abdominal cavity. The LES and distal esophagus are normally in an intra-abdominal location, and even in patients with small to moderate reducible hiatal hernias these structures can be approached via the abdominal approach. Although a procedure can also be accomplished via the transthoracic approach, there are several disadvantages to operations on the chest. First is the occurrence of postthoracotomy pain, which lasts longer than that following laparotomy and which can become chronic and disabling in 5–10% of patients. In addition, patients with underlying pulmonary disease have less respiratory compromise after an abdominal operation. Finally, it is quite easy to address any concomitant abdominal diseases when a laparotomy is performed.

Most patients with uncomplicated reflux esophagitis can be adequately treated with an abdominal incision and operation. There are, however, several strong indications for a transthoracic approach. Patients with considerable shortening of the esophagus often require a thoracic approach so the esophagus can be dissected up to the aortic arch to free enough length of esophagus to return the LES to the abdomen. Similarly, when patients have undergone a prior esophageal procedure, the circumferential dissection of the body of the esophagus is often best undertaken under direct vision through the chest, as opposed to use of a transhiatal approach. Esophageal dysmotility that necessitates a concomitant esophageal myotomy (achalasia or diffuse spasm) can also best be approached via the thoracic route. Finally, patients with associated pulmonary disease that can be addressed through a left thoracotomy should undergo a transthoracic approach so that both procedures can be done simultaneously.

One of the most recent advances in antireflux surgery is the introduction of laparoscopic repair. Repairs described include the Nissen,[75,76] Rossetti–Nissen,[77] Troupet[77] and Hill repair.[78] The advantages of the laparoscopic technique are decreased postoperative pain and a shorter postoperative hospital stay. Early results have been promising. Patients have had excellent symptomatic results and improvement in objective measurements such as LES tone and 24-hour pH monitoring.[76] Details of technique and results can be found in Chapter 50. However, it must be emphasized that it is still early in the experience, and it is unknown what the incidence of clinically significant perioperative complications will be. Also, there is still question as to the durability of a laparoscopic antireflux repair. It would behoove the surgeon to remember the history of laparoscopic inguinal hernia repair and colectomy. Both initially enjoyed a great surge of activity and a great deal of operator enthusiasm; however, significant drawbacks have been reported with both procedures and they are now being performed less frequently. Laparoscopic antireflux repairs should not be considered the standard of care until such time as the durability of the repairs have been confirmed.

## Operative Procedures

Since Allison's first report of hiatal hernia repair in 1951,[79] multiple procedures have been devised for anatomic repair of the hiatal hernia and for prevention of reflux of gastric contents. Although many authors have proposed multiple physiologic mechanisms purported to decrease the incidence and severity of reflux, the exact mechanism that makes the repairs effective is not well understood.[80] Suggested mechanisms include surgical manipulation of the LES with regard to pressure, length and location, accentuation of the angle of His to strengthen the mucosal flap valve at the gastroesophageal junction, and an increase in the opening pressure of the cardia. To date, it is uncertain which factor or combination of factors comes into play for any given repair.

The operations for GER can be divided into four basic classifications: complete fundoplication; partial fundoplication; lesser gastric curve plication; and prosthetic implant. It is difficult to directly compare results and therefore evaluate the relative merits of these procedures for a number of reasons. First, the patient populations differ from study to study with regard to how reflux was diagnosed and the severity of the reflux. Many of the newer procedures appear promising but lack the long-term follow-up results available for some of the more established operations. Finally, the series differ with regard to the level of objective documentation of results (systematic evaluation of symptoms, endoscopic findings, and esophageal function). It is therefore difficult for the individual practitioner to determine the best operation for GER.

### *Complete Fundoplication*

Although the Nissen fundoplication is the best known and most widely used 360° fundic wrap, it should be realized that the term *Nissen* is now used somewhat loosely. A detailed analysis of this procedure is provided in Chapter 44 and specifics of the procedure are not presented here. However, multiple modifications of the Nissen fundoplication have been described since the operation was developed, and they deserve mention. One of the earliest was the Nissen–Rossetti modification, which changed the technique of fundic wrapping (Fig. 42–9). The esophagus is dissected circumferentially, and the anterior wall of the fundus is brought posteriorly behind the esophagus and stitched to the anterior wall of the body of the stomach. Short gastric vessels are not routinely ligated and the fundoplication stitches are placed through the walls of the gastric wrap but are not passed through the esophagus. A long-term follow-up study of 590 such patients documented that 87% were free of reflux symptoms.[81] The rationale for the modification was its simplicity and the reduced need for dissection. A low incidence of bothersome postoperative symptoms (4%) was reported when a 3-cm loose Nissen–Rossetti fundoplication was performed.[82] However, not all investigators have reported excellent results. Failure to anchor the fundic wrap to the esophagus with the plication sutures has been reported to lead to a 22% failure rate with this technique.[83]

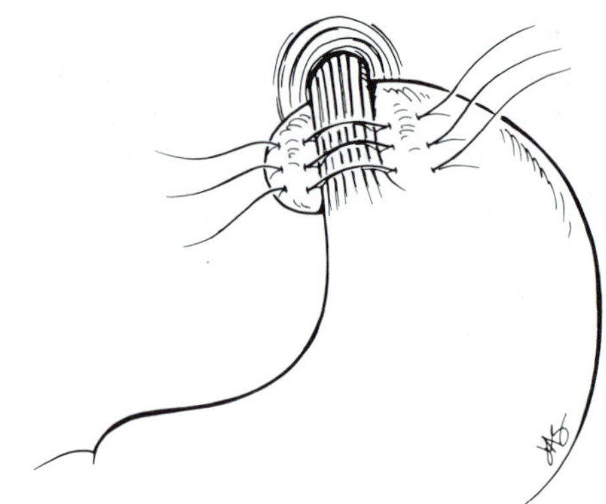

**Figure 42–9.** The Rosetti modification of the Nissen procedure consists of a three- or four-suture complete fundoplication. However, in the Rosetti repair, the short gastric vessels are left intact, the fundoplication sutures do not include the esophagus, and the wrap is performed using the anterior (not posterior) wall of gastric fundus, which is sutured to itself after being wrapped around the esophagus.

Another commonly used modification of the Nissen fundoplication is the floppy repair championed by Donahue et al.[84] In their report, the authors emphasized the importance of loosely wrapping the esophagus to lessen the tendency of the gastric wrap to act as a one-way valve, which can lead to symptoms of gas bloat and dysphagia. The key points of modification were the production of a short wrap (2–3 cm) around an intraluminal dilator that would easily allow passage of the finger in the space between the wrap and the esophagus, ensuring the wrap was not too tight. Many surgeons believe this type of repair is associated with less gas bloat after the operation.

Nearly every component of the original Nissen procedure has been altered by one investigator or another. Success has been reported despite variations in the length of the wrap, the number of sutures used, the presence or absence (and size) of an indwelling dilator, the performance of crural closure, and whether or not short gastric vessels are divided. A loose or floppy fundoplication appears to be the most common procedure undertaken and has generally met with good results and low operative morbidity.

### *Partial Fundoplication*

The frequent occurrence of clinically significant symptoms after Nissen fundoplication has prompted many surgeons to undertake a partial rather than a complete fundoplication. The best known partial wrap is the Belsey Mark IV, which was initially performed in 1952. The technical details and outcome with this procedure are provided in Chapter 46 by its inventor and his disciple.

A number of other partial fundoplication procedures have been designed and performed since the conception of the Belsey Mark IV procedure. One of these is the Lind transabdominal partial fundoplication procedure, first described in 1965.[85] The repair consists of a partial fundoplication that encompasses 300° the esophagus in the lateral and posterior aspects and leaves a 60° bare area anteriorly (Fig. 42–10). This fundoplication is made with three rows of sutures that attach the gastric fundus to the esophagus in the left lateral and right lateral positions and a fourth row more anteriorly. A recent prospective randomized trial compared the Lind procedure with a floppy Nissen with 26 patients in each group.[86] Repeat esophageal manometry, pH monitoring, and endoscopy were performed a mean of 13 months after the operation and revealed no significant difference between the two groups with regard to resolution of symptoms or objective findings of reflux. Interestingly, 10 patients (38%) in each group reported symptoms of gas bloat soon after the operation. Although the Lind procedure appears to be a satisfactory fundoplication in the short run, there is no apparent advantage over a Nissen fundoplication, which has a longer record of success.

In 1963, Toupet first reported his partial fundoplication procedure, which has since become widely used in Europe.[87] It is a 180° posterior fundoplication constructed after division of short gastric vessels. It imbricates the distal 2–3 cm of esophagus and usually involves four sets of sutures (Fig. 42–11). The medial aspects of the left and right portions of the fundoplication are sutured directly to the esophagus to prevent slippage of the fundus away from the esophagus. In addition, the lateral aspect of the left and right portions of the gastric wrap are sutured to their respective limbs of the crus to prevent the fundoplication from migrating out of the abdomen. Two prospective randomized studies were performed to compare the Toupet procedure with a Rossetti modification of the Nissen fundoplication. Lundell et al reported that both procedures nearly abolished both reflux symptoms and objective evidence of reflux as documented with 24-hour pH monitoring 6 months after the operation.[88] Manometry revealed the LES had a significantly increased resting pressure in both groups but was higher in the Rossetti–Nissen group. Thor and Silander found similar improvement of reflux with an approximate 90% improvement in esophagitis in both the Toupet and Rossetti–Nissen groups at 5 years.[89] However, the overall success rate was lower for the Nissen group, because three patients in this group had a slipped Nissen, which necessitated reoperation. It should be noted that in this study the investigators used the Rossetti modification in which the short gastric vessels were not divided to relieve tension on the wrap. It has been suggested that failure to perform this maneuver may result in a higher incidence of wrap dehiscence. Also, the complete fundoplication was 4 cm long, perhaps increasing the risk for dysphagia and gas bloat. These reports suggest that the Toupet procedure as widely practiced in Europe can be an effective and long-lasting antireflux repair.

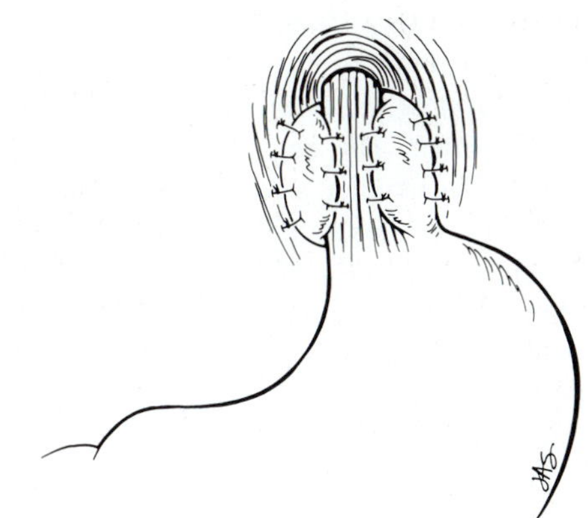

**Figure 42–11.** The Toupet partial fundoplication. The fundus is fixed in a posterior position with two rows of interrupted sutures 180° degrees apart.

Yet another partial fundoplication procedure was devised by Watson et al.[90] The repair is performed transabdominally in all patients except those with severe shortening of the esophagus, for whom a left thoracoabdominal approach is used (Fig. 42–12). The distal esophagus is mobilized, and the crura are closed with interrupted silk su-

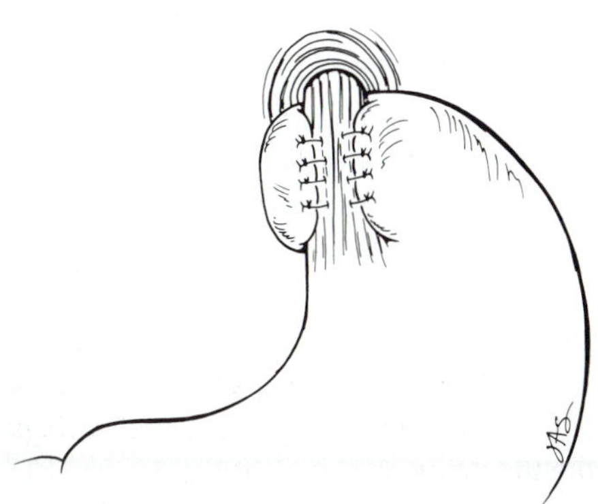

**Figure 42–10.** The Lind partial fundoplication. The third and most posterior row of interrupted sutures is not depicted in this view.

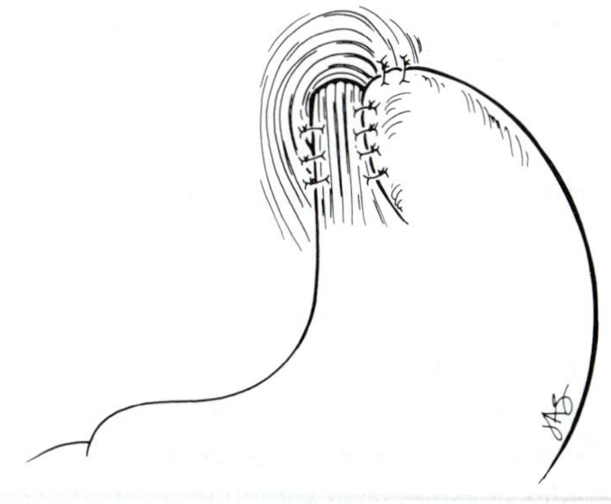

**Figure 42–12.** The Watson partial fundoplication. The right medial row of interrupted sutures is placed to both close the crura and fix the right aspect of the esophagus within the abdominal cavity.

tures. The needles are retained on the crural closure stitches and are then passed through the right posterolateral aspect of the muscular layer of the esophagus to fix 4–6 cm of the organ in the abdomen. The angle of His is reconstituted with placement of interrupted silk sutures from the superomedial aspect of the fundus to the inferior surface of the diaphragm just anterior to the hiatus. In addition, a 120° anterolateral fundoplication is performed with folding the gastric fundus over the anterior aspect of the esophagus and suturing the anterior wall of the fundus to the anterior aspect of the esophagus. The principles behind the operation are fixation of the distal esophagus below the diaphragm, production of an effective flap valve, and augmentation of the LES by means of intragastric pressure changes. Follow-up study of 100 consecutive patients revealed improvement of symptoms in 94% and total abolishment of symptoms in 82%. Transient dysphagia in 13% resolved spontaneously in all but two patients (2%) who had underlying motility disturbances and required endoscopic dilation. Improvement in esophagitis as assessed with endoscopy occurred in 91% of patients, with complete healing in 75%. Prolonged pH monitoring revealed reflux control in 84% of patients. These data suggest that the Watson procedure, at least in the hands of its inventor, provides good to excellent control of reflux during a short follow-up period. Whether these good results will persist and can be achieved by other practitioners will only be answered with time.

### The Hill Repair

In 1959 Hill devised a posterior gastropexy designed to accomplish three goals: restoration of an intra-abdominal segment of esophagus; accentuation of the esophagogastric angle; and tightening of the cardiac sling musculature at the LES to increase the resting tone of the high pressure zone.[91] Details of the procedure and recent modifications are provided by its originator in Chapter 45.

### Angelchik Prosthesis

In 1979, Angelchik and Cohen first described implantation of a prosthetic device for the treatment of GER.[92] The device consists of an annular silicone-filled implant somewhat resembling a horse collar. The prosthesis has an inner diameter of 2.5 cm and an outer diameter of 7 cm. A circumferential Dacron polyester tape is incorporated into the waist of the device to allow closure of the silicone ring around the LES. Insertion of the device can easily be accomplished after minimal mobilization of a tunnel around the gastroesophageal junction. The annulus is placed around the gastroesophageal junction, the tapes are tied, and in some patients the tapes themselves are fixed to the diaphragm with a suture to prevent rotation of the ring. Some authors have suggested simultaneous crural closure.

Few topics in esophageal surgery have incited as much controversy as the Angelchik prosthesis. There have been anecdotal reports of prosthetic migration into the chest or onto the fundus to obstruct the stomach. Erosion of the prosthesis into the gastrointestinal lumen also has been described, and a high incidence of postoperative dysphagia has been reported. Despite these negative events, several reports have documented the short-term efficacy of the prosthesis.[93–95] There have also been three prospective randomized trials comparing the Angelchik prosthesis to Nissen fundoplication in adults.[96–98] In none of the prospective randomized trials were there statistically significant differences between the Nissen fundoplication and the Angelchik prosthesis with regard to short-term efficacy of reflux control. However, Kmiot et al abandoned the use of the prosthesis because of what they deemed inferior results secondary to complications.[97] Twenty percent of the patients with Angelchik devices had persistent dysphagia compared with none of the patients who underwent Nissen fundoplication. Three prostheses were removed because of severe dysphagia, and a good or excellent result was obtained in only 60% of the Angelchik group versus 88% of the Nissen cohort. Although there was no statistically significant difference between the results of the two patient cohorts, Kmiot et al believed the lack of statistical significance was the result of small sample size. The authors considered the differences between the two groups to be clinically significant, and thus in good conscience declined to randomize patients to receive the Angelchik prosthesis.

Long-term results for the Angelchik device have been reported. Evans et al followed 42 patients for a median of 4.5 years and found that in six patients the prosthesis had to be removed. Four of these patients underwent removal because of persistent dysphagia, and in two the ring migrated into the chest, leading to failure with recurrent reflux.[96] Eleven of the 36 patients who could be contacted continued to have mild to moderate dysphagia because of the presence of the ring. Interestingly, esophageal manometry and 24-hour pH monitoring revealed that although the prosthesis was effective in the early postoperative period, there appeared to be a gradual deterioration of the artificially augmented LES and gradual recurrence of mild GER in many patients. Evans et al, however, also cited the known complications of the Nissen fundoplication, including gas-bloat syndrome, persistent dysphagia, and the need for a second operation because of recurrence. They concluded that the Angelchik prosthesis is an alternative to fundoplication for the control of reflux. Similar conclusions were reached by Eyre-Brook et al during a review of long-term (4–6 years) follow-up in a series of 119 patients who underwent insertion of the Angelchik prosthesis.[98]

Proponents on each side continue to argue strongly for their respective positions. Although it is true that a glass is both half empty and half full, recent medicolegal issues dealing with silicone breast implants may render moot this controversy regarding an esophageal prosthesis manufactured from silicone.

## SUMMARY

It appears clear from the literature that several different antireflux procedures yield good to excellent results when undertaken by skilled and experienced practitioners. However, even a good operation provides poor results when performed by untrained hands. The choice of operation for the treatment of uncomplicated GER should be based on the training and experience of the surgeon.

## REFERENCES

1. Bowditch HI: Peculiar case of diaphragmatic hernia. *Buffalo Med J Monthly Rev* **91:**(1)65, 1853
2. Tarnay TJ: Diaphragmatic hernia. *Ann Thorac Surg* **5:**66, 1968
3. Potempski P: Nuovo processo operativo per la riduzione cruenta della ernie diaframmatiche de trauma e per la sutura delle ferite del diaframma. *Bull Reale Accad Med Roma* **15:**191, 1889
4. Winklestein A: Peptic esophagitis (a new clinical entity). *JAMA* **104:**906, 1935
5. Kronecker H, Meltzer S: Der Schluckmechanismus, seine Erregung and seine Hemmung. *Arch Anat Physiol Suppl,* p 328, 1883
6. Fyke FE Jr, Code CF, Schlegel JF: The gastroesophageal sphincter in healthy human beings. *Gastroenterologia* **86:**135, 1956
7. Ingelfinger RJ, Kramer P, Sanchez GC: Gastroesophageal vestibule: Its normal function and its role in cardiospasm and gastroesophageal reflux. *Am J Med Sci* **228:**417, 1954
8. Laimer E: Beitrag zur Anatomie des Oesophagus. *Med Jahrb Wien* p 333, 1883
9. Clagett OT: Present concepts regarding the surgical treatment of oesophageal hiatal hernia. *Ann Royal Coll Surg* **38:**195, 1966
10. Hill LD, Tobias JA: Paraesophageal hernia. *Arch Surg* **96:**735, 1968
11. Hopwood D, Ross PE, Bouchier IA: Reflux esophagitis. *Clin Gastroenterol* **10:**505–520, 1981
12. Helm JF, Dodds WJ, Riedel DR, et al: Determinants of esophageal acid clearance in normal subjects. *Gastroenterology* **85:**607–610, 1983
13. Salo J, Kivilaakso E: Role of luminal hydrogen ions in the pathogenesis of experimental esophagitis. *Surgery* **92:**61–67, 1982
14. Gillison EW, Kusakari K, Bombeck CT, Nyhus LM: Importance of bile in reflux esophagitis and the success in its prevention by surgical means. *Br J Surg* **59:**794–797, 1972
15. Bateson MC, Hopwood D, Milne G, Bouchier IA: Oesophageal epithelial ultrastructure after incubation with gastrointestinal fluids and their components. *J Pathol* **133:**33–51, 1981
16. Little AG, DeMeester TR, Kirchner PT, et al: Pathogenesis of esophagitis in patients with gastroesophageal reflux. *Surgery* **88:**101–107, 1980
17. McCallum RW, Berkowitz DM, Learner E: Gastric emptying in patients with gastroesophageal reflux. *Gastroenterology* **80:**285–287, 1981
18. Hiebert CA, Belsey R: Incompetency of the gastric cardia without radiologic evidence of hiatal hernia. *J Thorac Cardiovasc Surg* **42:**352, 1961
19. Olsen AM, Schlegel JF, Payne WP: The hypotensive gastroesophageal sphincter. *Mayo Clin Proc* **48:**165, 1973
20. Cohen S, Harris LD: Does hiatus hernia affect competence of the gastroesophageal sphincter? *N Engl J Med* **284:**1053, 1971
21. Mobley JE, Christensen NA: Esophageal hiatal hernia: Prevalence, diagnosis and treatment in an American city of 30,000. *Gastroenterology* **30:**1, 1956
22. Barish CF, Wu WC, Castell DO: Respiratory complications of gastroesophageal reflux. *Arch Intern Med* **145:**1882, 1985
23. Pelligrini CA, DeMeester TR, Johnson LF, et al: Gastroesophageal reflux and pulmonary aspiration: Incidence, functional abnormality, and results of surgical therapy. *Surgery* **86:**110, 1979
24. Mansfield LE, Hameister HH, Spaulding HS, et al: The role of the vagus nerve in airway narrowing caused by intraesophageal hydrochloric acid provocation and esophageal distension. *Ann Allergy* **47:**431, 1981
25. Schan CA, Harding S, Haile JM, et al: Gastroesophageal reflux induced bronchoconstriction. *Chest* **106:**731–737, 1994
26. Schatzki R, Gary JE: Dysphagia due to diaphragmatic localized narrowing in the esophagus ("lower esophageal ring"). *Am J Roentgenol* **70:**911, 1953
27. Johnson LF, DeMeester TR: Evaluation of elevation of the head of the bed, bethanechol, and antacid foam tablets on gastroesophageal reflux. *Dig Dis Sci* **26:**673–680, 1981
28. Stanciu C, Bennett JR: Effects of posture on gastro-oesophageal reflux. *Digestion* **15:**104–109, 1977
29. O'Brien TF: Lower esophageal sphincter pressure and esophageal function in obese humans. *J Clin Gastroenterol* **2:**145–148, 1980
30. O'Hanrahan T, Marples M. Blount A, et al: Weight reduction and gastroesophageal reflux. *Gut* **30:**1491A, 1989
31. Dennish GW, Castell DO: Inhibitory effect of smoking on the lower esophageal sphincter. *N Engl J Med* **284:**1136–1137, 1971
32. Kahrilas PJ, Gupta RR: Mechanisms of acid reflux associated with cigarette smoking. *Gut* **31:**4–10, 1990
33. Schürer-Maly C-C, Varga L, Koelz HR, Halter F: Smoking and pH response to $H_2$-receptor antagonists. *Scand J Gastroenterol* **24:**1172–1178, 1989
34. Schindlbeck NE, Heinrich C, Dendorfer A, et al: Influence of smoking and esophageal intubation on esophageal pH-metry. *Gastroenterology* **92:**1994–1997, 1987
35. Koelz HR, Birchler R, Bretholz A, et al: Healing and relapse of reflux esophagitis during treatment with ranitidine. *Gastroenterology* **91:**1198–1205, 1986
36. Berenson MM, Sontag S, Robinson MG, et al: Effect of smoking in a controlled study of ranitidine treatment in gastroesophageal reflux disease. *J Clin Gastroenterol* **9:**499–503, 1987
37. Hogan WJ, Viegas de Andrade SR, Winship DH: Ethanol-induced acute esophageal motor dysfunction. *J Appl Physiol* **32:**755–760, 1972
38. Vitale G, Cheadle WG, Patel B, et al: The effect of alcohol on nocturnal gastroesophageal reflux. *JAMA* **258:**2077–2079, 1987
39. Thomas FB, Steinbaugh JT, Fromkes JJ, et al: Inhibitory effect of coffee on lower esophageal sphincter pressure. *Gastroenterology* **79:**1262–1266, 1980
40. Murphy DW, Castell DO: Chocolate and heartburn: Evidence of increased esophageal acid exposure after chocolate ingestion. *Am J Gastroenterol* **83:**633–636, 1988
41. Sigmund CJ, McNally EF: The action of a carminative on the lower esophageal sphincter. *Gastroenterology* **56:**13–18, 1969
42. Becker DJ, Sinclair J, Castell DO, Wu WC: A comparison of high and low fat meals on postprandial esophageal acid exposure. *Am J Gastroenterol* **84:**782–786, 1989
43. Salmon PR, Fedail SS, Wurzner HP, et al: Effect of coffee on human lower oesophageal function. *Digestion* **21:**69–73, 1981
44. McArthur K, Hogan D, Isenberg JI: Relative stimulatory effects of commonly ingested beverage on gastric acid secretion in humans. *Gastroenterology* **83:**199–203, 1982
45. Price SF, Smithson KW, Castell DO: Food sensitivity in reflux esophagitis. *Gastroenterology* **75:**240–243, 1978
46. Foster LJ, Trudeau WL, Goldman AL: Bronchodilator effects on gastric acid secretion. *JAMA* **241:**2613–2615, 1979
47. Castell DO: The lower esophageal sphincter: Physiologic and clinical aspects. *Ann Intern Med* **83:**390–401, 1975
48. Carling L, Cronstedt J, Engqvist A, et al: Sucralfate versus placebo in reflux esophagitis. *Scand J Gastroenterol* **23:**1117–1124, 1988

49. Hameeteman W, Van Den Boomgaard DM, Dekker W, et al: Sucralfate versus cimetidine in reflux esophagitis: A single blind multicentre study. *J Clin Gastroenterol* **9:**390–394, 1987
50. Williams RM, Orlando RC, Bozymski EM, et al: Multicenter trial of sucralfate suspension for the treatment of reflux esophagitis. *Am J Med* **83**(Suppl 3B):61–66, 1987
51. Higgs RH, Smith RD, Castell DO: Gastric alkalinization: Effect on lower esophageal sphincter pressure and serum gastrin. *N Engl J Med* **291:**486–488, 1974
52. Weberg R, Berstad A: Symptomatic effect of a low-dose antacid regimen in reflux oesophagitis. *Scand J Gastroenterol* **24:**401–406, 1989
53. Colin-Jones DG: Histamine-2-receptor antagonists in gastro-oesophageal reflux. *Gut* **30:**1305–1308, 1989
54. Katz PO: Pathogenesis and management of gastroesophageal reflux disease. *J Clin Gastroenterol* **13**(Suppl 2):S6–S15, 1991
55. Lind T, Cederberg C, Ekenved G, Olbe L: Inhibition of basal and betazole and sham-feeding–induced acid secretion by omeprazole in man. *Scand J Gastroenterol* **21:**1004–1010, 1986
56. Herrera JL, Shay SS, McCabe M, et al: Combined sucralfate suspension (SS) and cimetidine therapy vs cimetidine alone in patients with severe erosive esophagitis: A randomized double-blind trial. *Dig Dis Sci* **9:**1143, 1989 (abstr)
57. Hetzel DJ, Dent J, Reed WD, et al: Healing and relapse of severe peptic esophagitis after treatment with omeprazole. *Gastroenterology* **95:**903–912, 1988
58. Klinkenberg-Knol EC, Jansen JMBJ, Festen HPM, et al: Double-blind multicentre comparison of omeprazole and ranitidine in the treatment of reflux oesophagitis. *Lancet* **1:**349–351, 1987
59. Havelund T, Laursen LS, Skoubo-Kristensen E, et al: Omeprazole and ranitidine in treatment of reflux oesophagitis: Double blind comparative trial. *Br Med J* **296:**89–92, 1988
60. Lee FI, Isaacs PET: Barrett's ulcer: Response to standard dose ranitidine, high dose ranitidine, and omeprazole. *Am J Gastroenterol* **83:**914–917, 1988
61. Bright-Asare P, El-Bassoussi M: Cimetidine, metoclopramide, or placebo in the treatment of symptomatic gastroesophageal reflux. *J Clin Gastroenterol* **2:**149–156, 1980
62. McCallum RW, Fink DM, Winnan GR, et al: Metoclopramide in gastroesophageal reflux disease: Rationale for its use and results of a double-blind trial. *Am J Gastroenterol* **79:**165–172, 1984
63. Venable CW, Bill D, Echolston D: A double-blind study of metoclopramide in symptomatic peptic esophagitis. *Postgrad Med J* (Suppl):**49:**73, 1973
64. Masci E, Testoni PA, Passaretti S, et al: Comparison of ranitidine, domperidone maleate and ranitidine + domperidone maleate in the short-term treatment of reflux oesophagitis. *Drugs Exp Clin Res* **11:**687–692, 1985
65. Liebermann DA, Keefe DB: Treatment of severe reflux esophagitis with cimetidine and metoclopramide. *Ann Intern Med* **104:**21–26, 1986
66. Creytens G: Effects of cisapride on gastro-oesophageal reflux symptoms in hiatal-hernia patients. *Digestion* **34:**145, 1986
67. Baldi F, Bianchi-Orro G, Dobrilla G, et al: Cisapride versus placebo in reflux esophagitis: A multicenter double-blind trial. *J Clin Gastroenterol* **10:**614–618, 1988
68. Janisch HD, Hüttemann W, Bouzo MH: Cisapride versus ranitidine in the treatment of reflux esophagitis. *Hepatogastroenterology* **35:**125–127, 1988
69. Galmiche JP, Brandstatter G, Evreux M, et al: Combined therapy with cisapride and cimetidine in severe reflux oesophagitis: A double-blind controlled trial. *Gut* **29:**675–681, 1988
70. Liebermann DA: Medical therapy for chronic reflux esophagitis. *Arch Intern Med* **147:**1717–1721, 1987
71. Glise H: Healing, relapse rates and prophylaxis of reflux esophagitis. *Scand J Gastroenterol* **24**(Suppl 156):57–64, 1989
72. Castell DO: Long-term therapy for chronic gastro-esophageal reflux. *Arch Intern Med* **147:**1701–1702, 1987
73. Coley CM, Barry MJ, Mulley AG, et al: Medical vs. surgical therapy for gastroesophageal reflux disease: A decision analysis. *Gastroenterology* **89:**32A, 1990
74. Spechler SJ and the Department of Veterans Affairs Gastroesophageal Reflux Disease Study Group: Comparison of medical-surgical therapy for complicated gastroesophageal reflux disease in veterans. *N Engl J Med* **326:**786–92, 1992
75. Weerts JM, Dallemagne B, Hamoir E, et al: Laparoscopic Nissen fundoplication: Detailed analysis of 132 patients. *Surg Laparosc Endosc* **3:**359–364, 1993
76. Hinder RA, Filipi CJ, Neary PF, Wetscher GH: Laparoscopic Nissen fundoplication is an effective treatment for gastroesophageal reflux disease. *Ann Surg* **220:**472–481, 1994
77. Cuschieri AE: Hiatal hernia and reflux esophagitis. In Hunter JG, Sachia JM (eds): *Minimally Invasive Surgery*. New York, McGraw Hill, 1993, pp 87–111
78. Hill LD, Kraemer SJ, Aye RW, et al: Laparoscopic Hill repair. *Contemp Surg* **44:**13–20, 1994
79. Allison PR: Reflux esophagitis, sliding hiatal hernia and anatomy of repair. *Surg Gynecol Obstet* **92:**419–423, 1951
80. Little AG: Mechanisms of action of antireflux surgery: Theory and fact. *World J Surg* **16:**320–325, 1992
81. Rosetti M, Hill K: Fundoplication for the treatment of gastroesophageal reflux in hiatal hernia. *World J Surg* **1:**439–446, 1977
82. Bjerkeset T, Edna TH, Fjosne U: Long-term results after floppy Nissen/Rossetti fundoplication for gastroesophageal reflux disease. *Scand J Gastroenterol* **27:**707–710, 1992
83. Luostarinen M: Nissen fundoplication for reflux esophagitis: long-term clinical and endoscopic results in 109 of 127 consecutive patients. *Ann Surg* **217:**329–337, 1993
84. Donahue PE, Samelson S, Nyhus LM, Bombeck CT: The floppy Nissen fundoplication: Effective long-term control of pathologic reflux. *Arch Surg* **120:**663–669, 1985
85. Lind JF, Burns CM, MacDougall JT: "Physiological" repair for hiatus hernia: Manometric study. *Arch Surg* **91:**233–237, 1965
86. Walker SJ, Holt S, Sanderson CJ, Stoddard CJ: Comparison of Nissen total and Lind partial fundoplication in the treatment of gastroesophageal reflux. *Br J Surg* **79:**410–414, 1992
87. Toupet MA: Technique D'oesophago-gastroplastie avec phrenogastropexie applique dans la cure radicale des hernies hiatales et comme complement de l'operation de heuer dans les cardiospasmes. *Acad Chir* **89:**394–397, 1963
88. Lundell L, Abrahamsson H, Ruth M, et al: Lower esophageal sphincter characteristics and esophageal and exposure following partial or 360° fundoplication: Results of a prospective randomized trial. *World J Surg* **15:**115–21, 1991
89. Thor KBA, Silander T: Long-term randomized prospective trial of the Nissen procedure versus a modified Toupet technique. *Ann Surg* **210:**719–724, 1989
90. Watson A, Jenkinson LR, Ball CS, et al: A more physiologic alternative to total fundoplication for the surgical correction of resistant gastroesophageal reflux. *Br J Surg* **78:**1088–1094, 1991
91. Hill LD: An effective operation for hiatal hernia: An eight year appraisal. *Ann Surg* **166:**681–684, 1967
92. Angelchik JP, Cohen R: A new surgical procedure for the treatment of gastroesophageal reflux and hiatal hernia. *Surg Gynecol Obstet* **148:**246–248, 1979
93. Gear MWL, Gillison EW, Dowling BL: Randomised prospective trial of the Angelchik anti-reflux prosthesis. *Br J Surg* **71:**681, 1985
94. Stuart RC, Dawson K, Keeling P, et al: A prospective randomised trial of the Angelchik prosthesis versus Nissen fundoplication. *Br J Surg* **76:**87–89, 1989
95. Deakin M, Mayer D, Temple JG: Surgery for gastro-oesophageal reflux: The Angelchik prosthesis compared to the Nissen fundoplication—Two-year follow-up and five-year evaluation. *Ann R Coll Surg* **71:**249–251, 1989
96. Evans DF, Ledingham SJ, Robertson CF, et al: An objective long-

term evaluation of the Angelchik antireflux prosthesis. *Ann Royal Coll Surg* **73:**355–360, 1991

97. Kmiot WA, Kirby RM, Akinola D, Temple JG: Prospective randomized trial of Nissen fundoplication and Angelchik prothesis in the surgical treatment of medically refractory gastro-oesophageal reflux disease. *Br J Surg* **78:**1181–1184, 1991

98. Eyre-Brook IA, Codling BW, Gear MWL: Results of a prospective randomized trial of the Angelchik prosthesis and of a consecutive series of 199 patients. *Br J Surg* **80:**602–604, 1993

CHAPTER

# 43

# Barrett's Esophagus

Mark K. Ferguson

## HISTORY

Barrett's esophagus is a condition in which portions of the squamous epithelium of the lower esophagus are replaced by glandular epithelium. Although this entity was recognized many years ago, interest in it has increased since the 1980s because of its association with gastroesophageal acid reflux and adenocarcinoma of the esophagus. Peptic ulceration of the columnar-lined esophagus was noted as early as 1925 by Chevalier Jackson,[1,2] and its eponymous description was reported by Barrett in 1950. Barrett stated that foreshortening of the esophagus developed secondary to peptic ulceration, with subsequent migration of the gastric fundus into the thorax.[3] He asserted that such patients had actual gastric, rather than esophageal, ulceration. Bosher and Taylor were the first to accurately describe the circumferential extension of gastric mucosa into the esophagus.[4] The term *Barrett's ulcer* was coined by Allison and Johnstone in 1953[5]; they were the first to propose that these histologic changes were acquired rather than congenital, and resulted from gastroesophageal acid reflux. In a second report in 1957, Barrett adopted the view that columnar mucosa could line the esophagus.[6] He described numerous cases in which the existence of such epithelium within the esophagus was associated with inflammation and ulceration; he also reported the development of adenocarcinoma in this mucosa.

These publications generated little immediate interest in Barrett's esophagus. Adler described clinical complications, including malignancy, associated with Barrett's esophagus in 1963.[7] Mossberg and de la Pava et al contributed evidence supporting the acquired nature of this condition.[8,9] Interest in Barrett's esophagus was reawakened in the mid-1970s by reports of Naef et al on the association of this condition and adenocarcinoma.[10]

## ANATOMY AND PHYSIOLOGY

Congenital rests of columnar epithelium similar to gastric mucosa are sometimes found in the esophagus. The original description of columnar mucosa within the esophagus is attributed to Schridde,[11] who found microscopic foci typically lying just distal to the cricopharyngeus muscle but also in other portions of the esophageal body. Islands of columnar epithelium entirely surrounded by squamous epithelium and unrelated to the mucosa of the gastric cardia are referred to as ectopic or heterotopic.[12] In contrast, the condition known as Barrett's esophagus (endobrachyesophagus) exists when the columnar lining extends continuously from the gastric cardia proximally into the esophagus over distances ranging from a few centimeters to the entire esophageal length.

The normal squamocolumnar junction in adults may be found over a wide range of levels in the distal esophagus. Columnar mucosa often extends proximally over the entire length of the lower esophageal sphincter (LES) and can commonly occupy 2 cm of distal esophagus. Barrett's esophagus is defined as the condition in which the esophagus is lined with columnar mucosa more than 3 cm proximal to the distal end of the muscular esophageal tube. If metaplastic epithelium exists in columnar mucosa within 3 cm of the gastroesophageal junction, this must also be considered Barrett's esophagus.

The columnar epithelium found in Barrett's esophagus may be of three types: gastric fundic, junctional, and specialized columnar.[13] Gastric fundic epithelium has a surface layer containing foveoli but not goblet cells, whereas the glandular layer contains mucous glands, parietal cells, and chief cells (Fig. 43–1). Gastric fundic epithelium is atrophic compared with the epithelium in the body and fundus of the stomach. Junctional epithelium contains mucous glands but

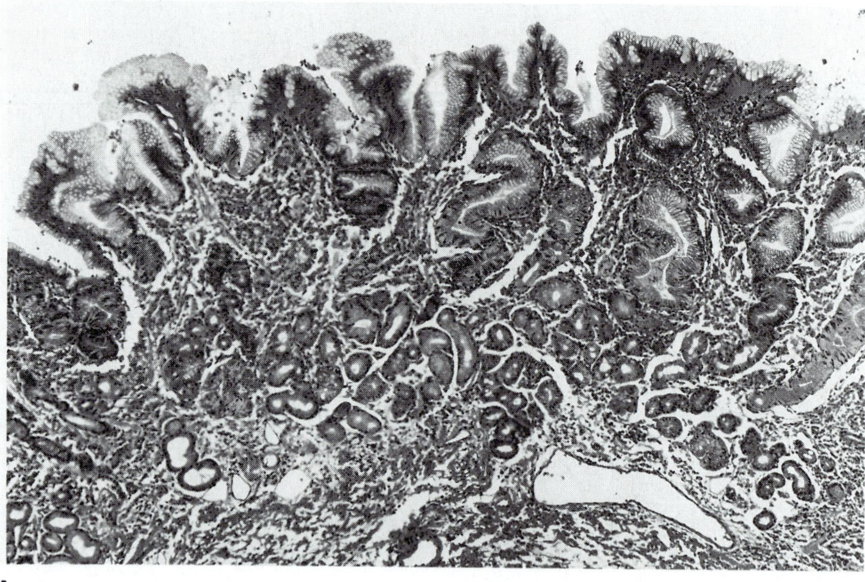

A

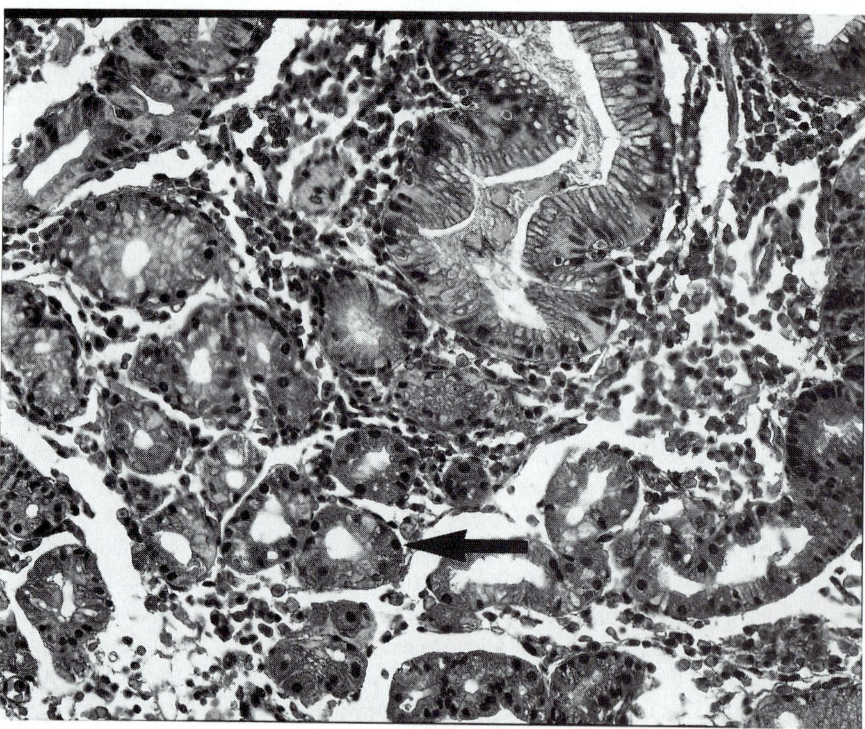

B

**Figure 43–1. A.** Fundic type of gastric epithelium, demonstrating foveolar cells lining the surface (hematoxylin and eosin stain, original magnification × 25). **B.** Atrophic glands beneath the gastric epithelium contain parietal cells (arrow; hematoxylin and eosin stain, original magnification × 40).

no parietal cells and closely resembles the epithelium of the normal gastric cardia (Fig. 43–2). Specialized columnar epithelium occurs in 80% of patients, closely resembling intestinal mucosa with a villiform surface and crypts (Fig. 43–3). The villi contain both columnar and goblet cells. This epithelium appears to be a type of incomplete intestinal metaplasia, lacking intestinal absorptive cells and appearing functionally immature.

The functional characteristics of Barrett's epithelium have been investigated intensively because of the high incidence of peptic stricture and esophageal ulceration in this condition. Although acid is produced by Barrett's mucosa, the amount is insufficient to make it a significant factor in the development of peptic complications of Barrett's esophagus.[14,15] Barrett's mucosa also contains pepsinogens and has the ability to secrete pepsin and gastrin, although the amount of the latter is insignificant relative to that produced in the gastric antrum and duodenum.[16–19] Barrett's epithe-

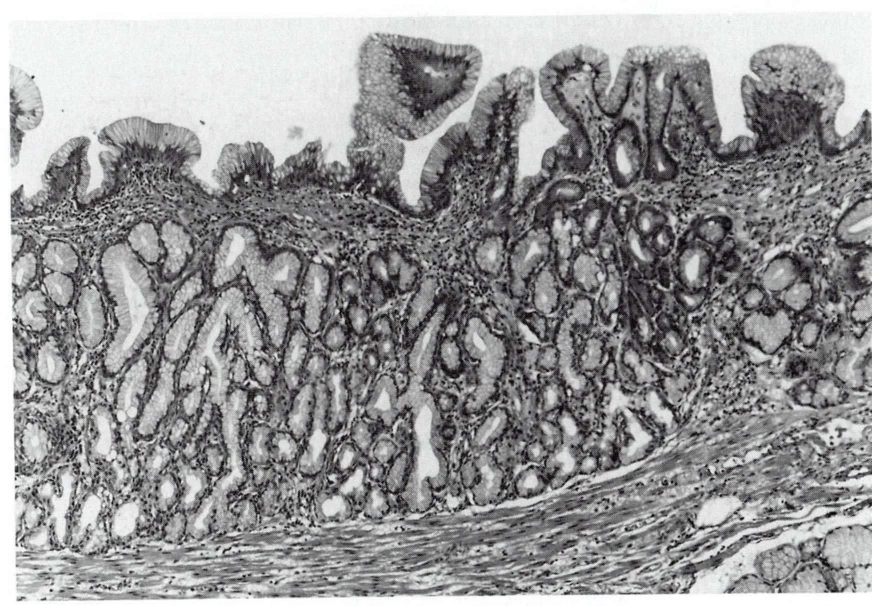

**Figure 43–2.** Junctional type of gastric epithelium. Simplified foveolar cells overlie submucosal esophageal glands (hematoxylin and eosin stain, original magnification × 25).

lium also contains serotonin, somatostatin, secretin, and pancreatic polypeptide.[20]

## PATHOGENESIS

Barrett himself originally ascribed an acquired causation to the condition that now bears his name.[3] Allison and Johnstone first proposed that Barrett's mucosa is due to chronic gastroesophageal acid reflux, and many subsequent reports support that contention.[21,22] Patients with reflux esophagitis examined over time with repeat esophagoscopy show development of progressively higher levels of Barrett's mucosa.[23] Nearly every patient with documented Barrett's esophagus has pathologic gastroesophageal acid reflux. Although many children and even some infants are reported to have this condition, it has never been described in a newborn. It is most likely that Barrett's esophagus is acquired and in most cases is related to chronic gastroesophageal acid reflux or other processes that damage the esophageal mucosa, such as alkaline reflux.[24–26]

The source of the columnar epithelium that replaces damaged squamous epithelium in the distal esophagus was once thought to be the gastric mucosa. It now appears that the orad migration of gastric mucosa is an insufficient explanation for all cases of Barrett's esophagus. For example, Barrett's mucosa is known to arise in patients who have undergone total gastrectomy and in whom the columnar epithelium is found adjacent to an esophagojejunostomy or

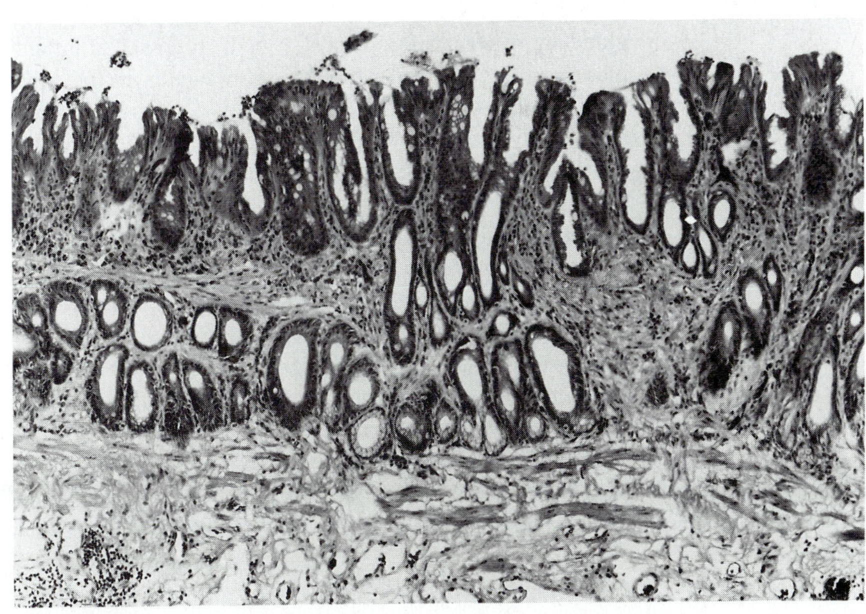

**Figure 43–3.** Specialized columnar epithelium with many goblet cells lining the villiform surface (hematoxylin and eosin stain, original magnification × 25).

esophagocolostomy.[27,28] It is currently believed that Barrett's esophagus arises through a process of metaplasia of pleuripotential cells found in the submucosal esophageal glands. Attempts to validate this theory using laboratory animal models have met with varied success, because the production of esophageal injuries similar to those seen in the clinical setting is difficult. Some investigators have managed to combine trauma and iatrogenic gastroesophageal reflux (GER) to produce mucosal changes similar to those found in human Barrett's esophagus. The healing in these animal models supports the theory that replacement cells migrate from the submucosal glands of the esophagus and not from the gastric cardia.[29,30]

## EPIDEMIOLOGY

The epidemiologic features of Barrett's esophagus are difficult to describe because of variations in the definition of Barrett's esophagus and in techniques used to document its existence. For example, reliance on blind suction biopsies raises the problem of identifying the relation of the biopsy site to the gastroesophageal junction. This is particularly troublesome in patients with sliding hiatal hernias, among whom the distance of the junction from the incisors varies constantly. In one autopsy series, 12% of bodies were said to have a columnar-lined esophagus.[9] The prevalence of Barrett's esophagus in patients without symptoms who undergo endoscopy is 1%, whereas Barrett's mucosa is observed in 10–20% of patients with symptoms of reflux.[10,31–33] Barrett's esophagus is found in 34% of patients with chronic peptic strictures of the esophagus.[32–34]

The average patient is 50–60 years of age at the time of diagnosis; the age range varies from 1 month to 90 years. Men are three times more likely than women to receive a diagnosis of Barrett's esophagus.[33] There is a relative lack of Barrett's esophagus among the black population, for reasons that are unknown. Familial occurrences have been reported, but are rare.[35–38] Barrett's esophagus in children is similar to the condition found in adults in most respects. It is usually associated with pathologic acid reflux and is thought to be an acquired disorder. Barrett's mucosa is found in 8–13% of children who undergo endoscopy for evaluation of suspected reflux.[39–41]

## DIAGNOSIS

Barrett's esophagus may be associated with a variety of nonspecific symptoms that arise from gastroesophageal acid reflux and its complications or from the development of an adenocarcinoma. As a result, the most common symptoms accompanying Barrett's esophagus are heartburn and regurgitation, dysphagia, chest pain, and bleeding (Table 43–1).[21,35,42–46] Patients with pathologic reflux may experience diminishing heartburn as Barrett's mucosa develops, presumably because of the relative resistance of the columnar epithelium to the damaging effects of acid.

**TABLE 43–1. INCIDENCE OF SYMPTOMS IN PATIENTS WITH BARRETT'S ESOPHAGUS AND BARRETT'S ADENOCARCINOMA**

| Symptom | Barrett's Esophagus (%) | Barrett's Adenocarcinoma (%) |
|---|---|---|
| Heartburn | 56 | 61 |
| Dysphagia | 73 | 77 |
| Bleeding | 24 | 15 |

*(Data from references 21,35,42–46.)*

Contrast-enhanced radiography is relatively insensitive in diagnosing Barrett's esophagus. The motility pattern is usually normal, and the columnar-lined portion of the esophagus can be slightly dilated. The use of double-contrast studies provides increased sensitivity, sometimes revealing mucosal thickening or irregularities that suggest reflux-associated inflammation in the squamous-lined esophagus. A reticular mucosal pattern also is described that is relatively specific for Barrett's mucosa if located adjacent to a stricture.[47,48] Although 10–15% of patients have no identifiable abnormalities, a hiatal hernia is present in more than 80%, a stricture in 75%, and a superficial or penetrating esophageal ulcer in nearly 50%.[41,42]

Endoscopy is the primary technique with which Barrett's esophagus is diagnosed. The squamous esophageal mucosa is pale and transparent with a subepithelial vascular network. The normal squamocolumnar junction is usually circumferential, slightly irregular (z-line), and horizontal with respect to the esophageal axis. The presence of Barrett's esophagus is suggested when the squamocolumnar junction is very irregular, with tongues of columnar epithelium extending orad. Barrett's epithelium is red, smooth, and feathery when benign (Fig. 43–4, see Color Plates following page 608) but may be thickened or polypoid when glandular hyperplasia is present or in the presence of inflammation or a malignant neoplasm. Esophagitis in the squamous-lined segment in common. Strictures frequently accompany Barrett's esophagus and normally involve the squamocolumnar junction or lie within the squamous epithelium. The columnar-lined esophagus may contain ulcers that are usually superficial and longitudinal, although deep ulcers do occur that are similar to gastric ulcers in appearance and behavior and occasionally resemble malignant ulcers.

The endoscopic recognition of Barrett's epithelium is not always reliable.[49] The diagnosis should not be made without histologic confirmation from endoscopic biopsies, which should be performed at multiple levels within the esophagus, care taken to note both the distance from the incisors and the circumferential location. Biopsies above the squamocolumnar junction provide evidence of the proximal extent of the columnar epithelium, since squamous mucosa can overgrow columnar epithelium, giving an inaccurate impression of its true margin.[21] Biopsies may be directed with the use of vital stains, because the application of Lugol's solution results in uptake by squamous mucosa without discoloration of columnar mucosa, whereas toluidine blue stains columnar mucosa dark blue and leaves normal squamous mucosa unstained.[50]

Motility studies in patients with Barrett's esophagus demonstrate only moderate manometric disorders. Because the LES is of critical importance in limiting gastroesophageal acid reflux, particular attention has been paid to this region. LES pressure is lower in patients with Barrett's esophagus compared with healthy people and patients with pathologic reflux but without Barrett's esophagus.[24–26,51] LES pressure is also lower in patients with Barrett's esophagus and complications of reflux (ulcers, stricture, or esophagitis) than in those with Barrett's esophagus unaccompanied by such complications. Relaxation of the LES in response to swallowing is normal. Most patients exhibit peristaltic contractions in the body of the esophagus that are normally coordinated, although the amplitude is often low and contraction duration is prolonged.[52]

## BENIGN COMPLICATIONS

Benign complications of Barrett's esophagus are similar to those of pathologic GER. They include stricture, mucosal ulceration, and bleeding (Table 43–2).[21,35,42–44] Strictures occur in as many as 75% of patients, developing in the distal segment of the squamous-lined esophagus or at the squamocolumnar junction (Fig. 43–5). The level of the squamocolumnar junction in Barrett's esophagus is quite variable, and these strictures may sometimes be found proximal to the aortic arch. Although they frequently cause dysphagia, these strictures rarely result in odynophagia. Although severe gastrointestinal hemorrhage and chronic gastrointestinal blood loss are infrequent complications of acid reflux, they occur in more than 25% of patients with Barrett's esophagus. Penetrating ulcers, also known as Barrett's ulcers, may arise within the columnar-lined esophagus in as many as 10% of patients. They are associated with a high morbidity and mortality, including fatal perforation into the mediastinum (Fig. 43–6).[53–55] Many ulcers are successfully treated with intensive acid suppression therapy requiring high-dose $H_2$-receptor blockers or omeprazole.[56] In some instances control of reflux by fundoplication is necessary; resection is required for ulcers that have penetrated into the mediastinum.

**TABLE 43–2. CLINICAL FEATURES OF BENIGN BARRETT'S ESOPHAGUS**

| Feature | Incidence (%) |
|---|---|
| Stricture | 75 |
| Ulcer | 23 |
| Reflux | 84 |

*(Data from references 21,35,42–44.)*

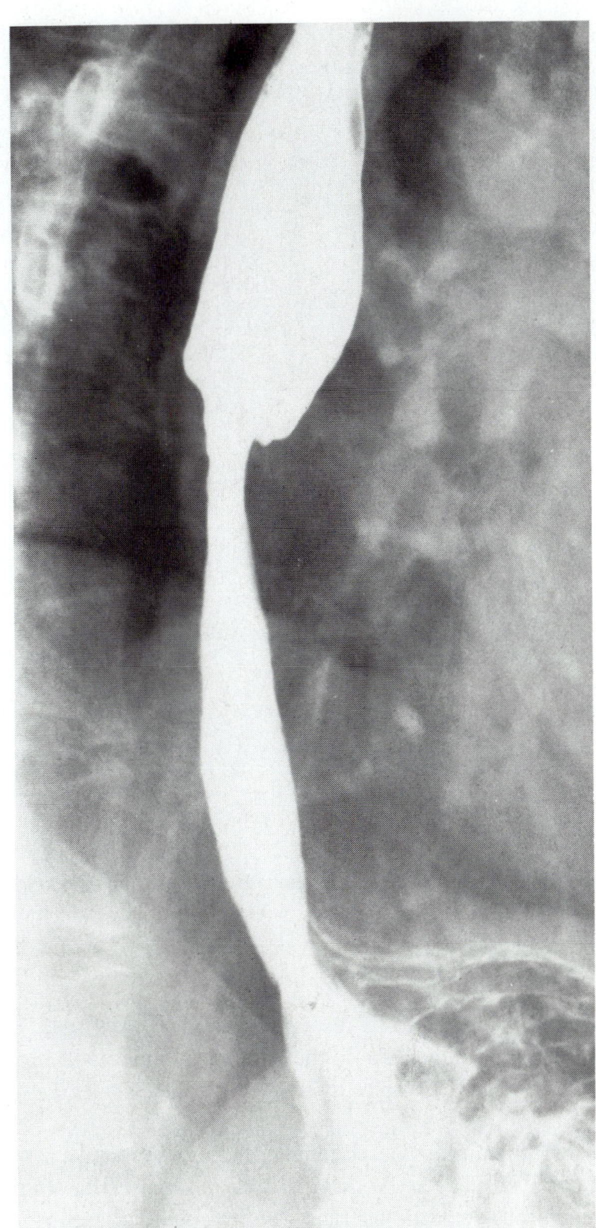

**Figure 43–5.** Benign stricture in the midesophagus at the squamocolumnar junction atop a long segment of Barrett's mucosa.

## DYSPLASIA AND ADENOCARCINOMA

Naef et al first suggested that the columnar-lined esophagus represents a premalignant condition in an irreversible transition state to adenocarcinoma.[10] Numerous subsequent publications reported experiences detailing the prevalence and incidence of dysplasia and adenocarcinoma in conjunction with Barrett's esophagus. The general concept now exists that persistent pathologic gastroesophageal acid reflux,

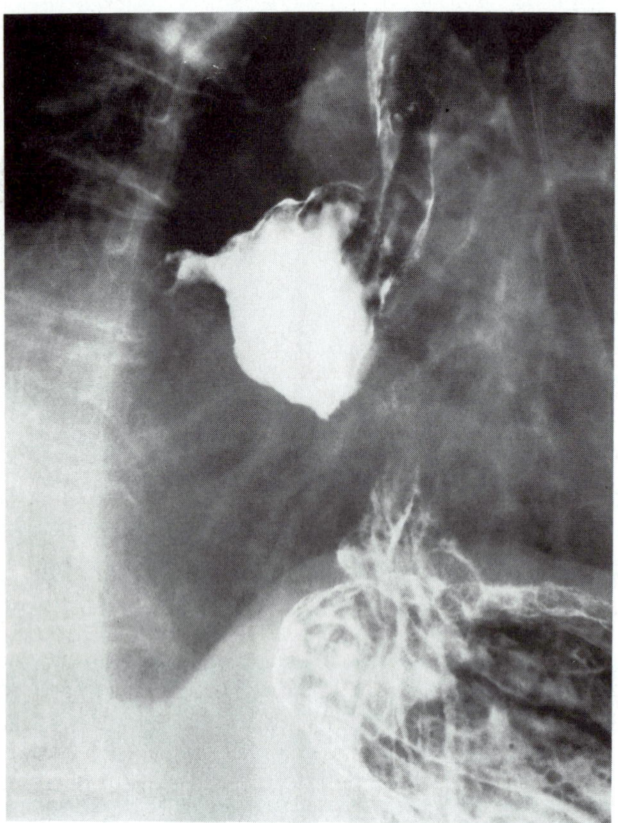

**Figure 43–6.** A benign Barrett's ulcer that has penetrated into the mediastinum.

which is believed to be responsible for the metaplastic development of Barrett's epithelium, is also involved in the development of dysplastic and malignant changes in this mucosa.

The definitions used in determining the relative severity of dysplasia vary widely. Dysplasia is defined as an unequivocal neoplastic alteration in the columnar esophageal mucosa.[57] No dysplasia is present when the nuclei of the metaplastic epithelium are similar to those found in similar epithelium in its normal anatomic location. Low-grade dysplasia is characterized by dysplastic nuclei confined to basal parts of the cells. High-grade dysplasia exists when nuclear changes are more severe and are found in the upper polar regions of the cells. Dysplasia is sometimes difficult to differentiate from inflammation due to reflux. Most pathologists agree that high-grade dysplasia and carcinoma in situ are distinct histologic entities, but it is often a difficult task to reliably differentiate between the two, particularly on the basis of small endoscopic biopsy specimens.

It has been suggested that dysplasia is a necessary precursor to malignant degeneration in Barrett's epithelium,[58] indicating that surveillance of patients with dysplasia may allow the diagnosis of cancer at an early stage. In addition to the use of dysplasia as a marker for patients at risk for cancer, other methods of assessing the potential for later development of invasive carcinoma include DNA flow cytometry and the detection of oncogenes and tumor suppressor genes. DNA aneuploidy and an increase in $G_2$-tetraploid fractions with flow cytometry have been shown to correlate with the severity of dysplasia and the likelihood of malignant degeneration,[59–61] although the degree of correlation is not universally accepted as being high,[62] and the use of this modality for assessing risk is considered experimental. Mutations in the three *ras* oncogenes (H-*ras,* K-*ras,* N-*ras*) that frequently are reported in other malignant gastrointestinal tumors have not been identified in patients with Barrett's dysplasia or adenocarcinoma. Preliminary data suggest that p17 allelic deletions, which include the region of the tumor suppressor gene p53, are found with increased frequency in patients with Barrett's adenocarcinoma, and are associated with overexpression of p53 protein.[63,64]

The risk of malignant degeneration in Barrett's epithelium is related clinically to the duration and severity of GER, tobacco use, and the overall extent of columnar mucosal spread.[23,65] Most Barrett's adenocarcinomas occur in the lower third of the esophagus; 15% are located in the middle third. These cancers develop almost exclusively in specialized columnar epithelium. Most tumors at the time of diagnosis have transmural extension with associated lymph node involvement. Differentiation between Barrett's adenocarcinoma and a tumor of the gastric cardia may be difficult. True gastric cancers are usually ulcerating, whereas Barrett's adenocarcinomas are often nodular or polypoid.

Estimates of the risk that a cancer will develop in Barrett's epithelium are exaggerated by many factors, including the increased incidence of invasive examinations in such patients because of symptoms and an uneven distribution in the incidence of autopsies performed on patients with Barrett's esophagus complicated by stricture or adenocarcinoma. Early studies focused on the high prevalence of carcinoma in Barrett's esophagus, initially reported in a range of 0–46%,[45,65,66] which were interpreted by some authors as showing a high incidence of the problem. Long-term studies have shown that the incidence of esophageal cancer in a Barrett's esophagus is about 1 per 140 patient years, or 40 times the usual rate among the North American population (Table 43–3).[65–70] This accounts for 10–20% of all esophageal cancers.

## MEDICAL MANAGEMENT OF BARRETT'S ESOPHAGUS

Because Barrett's esophagus is usually the result of GER, its medical management is similar to that of reflux itself. The aims of therapy are to improve esophageal clearance, optimize the function of the LES, and minimize the contributions of abnormal gastric function. Elevating the head of the bed 6 inches (15 cm) above the foot limits reflux and promotes clearance from the lower esophagus. A number of

**TABLE 43–3. INCIDENCE OF ADENOCARCINOMA IN BARRETT'S ESOPHAGUS**

| Reference | Year | No. of Patients | Mean Follow-up (y) | No. of Cancers Detected | Incidence per Patient-Year of Follow-up |
|---|---|---|---|---|---|
| Spechler et al[65] | 1984 | 105 | 3.3 | 2 | 1/175 |
| Cameron et al[66] | 1985 | 122 | 8.5 | 2 | 1/441 |
| Robertson et al[67] | 1988 | 56 | 3.0 | 4 | 1/56 |
| Van der Veen et al[68] | 1989 | 155 | 4.4 | 4 | 1/170 |
| Hameeteman et al[69] | 1989 | 50 | 5.2 | 5 | 1/52 |
| Williamson et al[70] | 1990 | 176 | 1.7 | 3 | 1/99 |
| Total | | 664 | 4.2 | 20 | 1/140 |

substances reduce LES pressure and adversely affect reflux management. Elimination of these substances, which include caffeine, nicotine, fats, chocolate, alcohol, peppermint, theophylline, anticholinergic agents, diazepam, opiates, and calcium channel blocking agents, can promote a higher resting LES pressure. The gastric contribution to reflux may be limited by weight reduction, refraining from eating before sleeping, and abstinence from very acidic foods, such as citrus juices and tomato products. Gastric acid neutralization can also control mild symptoms of reflux disease. Initial therapy for patients with mild symptoms and no stricture includes use of an $H_2$-receptor blocker; omeprazole is indicated for patients with severe symptoms or a peptic stricture. LES tone and gastric emptying may be improved with use of a prokinetic agent such as cisapride. Medical management reduces symptoms of gastroesophageal acid reflux in patients with Barrett's esophagus, and intensive therapy sometimes is effective in healing Barrett's ulcers and in preventing recurrence of peptic strictures.[56,71,72] Elimination of symptoms does not correlate with regression of Barrett's epithelium,[51,73] suggesting that the risk for dysplasia or adenocarcinoma is unaffected by medical management.

## SURVEILLANCE

The appropriate interval for follow-up examinations of patients with Barrett's epithelium is unknown. Because earlier reports were interpreted as showing a high incidence of adenocarcinoma in such patients, initial recommendations were that endoscopy be performed every 3–6 months accompanied by multiple biopsies throughout the region of columnar epithelium. Estimates of the costs of endoscopy and biopsy every 6 months with an accompanying barium swallow radiographic examination once a year range as high as $54,000 and nearly 80 lost work days[46] for detecting one asymptomatic adenocarcinoma in a patient with Barrett's epithelium. Additional information provided by more recent epidemiologic studies has tempered the initial recommendations regarding surveillance. Although no definite interval can be suggested, some means of surveillance should be performed at least once a year because of the increased incidence of adenocarcinoma among these patients (Fig. 43–7). Cytologic screening of the esophagus has been employed for a number of years. It is similar to screening methods used in geographic areas in which esophageal cancer is endemic.[74] Cytologic specimens may be obtained with a conventional gastroscopy brush, a mesh-covered intraesophageal balloon, or an encapsulated sponge. Both dysplastic and malignant changes may be detected, providing indications for follow-up endoscopy and barium swallow with an overall accuracy similar to that of histologic diagnosis.[75–77] Surveillance endoscopy allows detection of Barrett's adenocarcinoma at an early stage and improves long-term survival after resection compared with survival of patients who do not undergo surveillance endoscopy.[78]

## SURGICAL TREATMENT OF BENIGN DISEASE

Operative treatment of GER is indicated when medical management of reflux fails or when complications of reflux arise. Although symptomatic improvement occurs in patients with Barrett's esophagus after a period of medical management, it is unknown whether regression of Barrett's epithelium or reversion of dysplasia can be expected. Because dysplasia and adenocarcinoma are linked to the severity and duration of reflux, optimal control of reflux is important in these patients. Either a partial or a total fundoplication may be used. I select the transthoracic route because of features common among these patients, including hiatal hernias and strictures. A thorough mobilization of the intrathoracic esophagus is necessary to achieve a tension-free anastomosis. When a Barrett's ulcer is present, the depth of penetration can be evaluated by direct inspection before an antireflux procedure is chosen as sufficient treatment. A careful inspection of the esophagus and surrounding lymph nodes for evidence of carcinoma is also possible when the transthoracic route is used. Because of uncertainty whether the level of Barrett's epithelium or the degree of dysplasia regresses after adequate surgical treatment, the usual indications for an antireflux operation should be present before such an operation is performed, specifically fail-

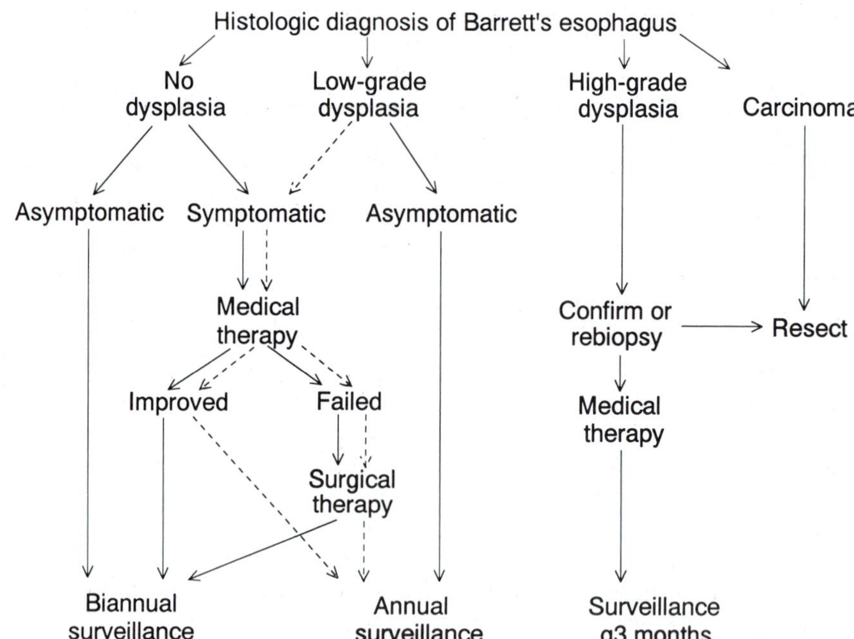


**Figure 43–7.** Flow diagram for managing Barrett's esophagus.

ure of medical management or complications of reflux. In addition to fundoplication, resection is sometimes necessary, especially in patients with penetrating ulcers or nondilatable strictures.[79] All Barrett's mucosa is removed, and reconstruction is performed by means of interposition of a segment of intestine or by means of cervical esophagogastrostomy. Performance of an intrathoracic esophagogastrostomy carries a high risk of recurrent Barrett's esophagus, particularly in patients with benign disease.

## SURGICAL MANAGEMENT OF DYSPLASIA AND ADENOCARCINOMA

The appropriate management of patients with high-grade dysplasia is controversial. Early reports suggested that high-grade dysplasia and carcinoma in situ were synonymous and that esophagectomy should be performed routinely in such patients because of the high likelihood of identifying invasive adenocarcinoma in the resected specimen. A summary of current information indicates that insufficient data are available to make a firm recommendation for appropriate therapy of high-grade dysplasia (Table 43–4).[80–87] When high-grade dysplasia is diagnosed in an endoscopic biopsy specimen, the reading should be corroborated by an independent and expert pathologist. Repeat biopsy for confirmation of the diagnosis is often useful. Current management options are intensive medical therapy with rebiopsy at 3-month intervals or resection. In patients who can tolerate an esophagectomy, resection should be seriously considered because of the moderate risk that an invasive carcinoma is present. The optimal technique for resection in patients with a preoperative diagnosis of high-grade dysplasia is not generally agreed on. Nearly 70% of operated patients have high-grade dysplasia or intramucosal carcinoma in the resected specimen,[81,82,84–86] and a limited resection including all Barrett's mucosa is sufficient therapy in such instances. This can be accomplished by either a

**TABLE 43–4. INCIDENCE OF ADENOCARCINOMA IN PATIENTS WITH BARRETT'S ESOPHAGUS AND HIGH-GRADE DYSPLASIA**

| Reference | Year | No. of Patients | No. of Cancers Identified | Percentage Affected |
|---|---|---|---|---|
| Lee[80] | 1985 | 2 | 1 | 50 |
| Hamilton and Smith[81] | 1987 | 4 | 2 | 50 |
| Reid et al[82] | 1988 | 4 | 0 | 0 |
| DeMeester et al[83] | 1990 | 2 | 1 | 50 |
| Altorki et al[84] | 1991 | 8 | 3 | 37.5 |
| Pera et al[85] | 1992 | 18 | 9 | 50 |
| Rice et al[86] | 1993 | 16 | 6 | 37.5 |
| Levine et al[87] | 1993 | 7 | 0 | 0 |
| Total | | 61 | 22 | 36 |

transhiatal approach or a conventional transthoracic excision. Unfortunately, it usually is impossible to predict preoperatively which patients are likely to require a more extensive esophagectomy and lymph node dissection, making selection of therapy a continuing challenge.

In patients with adenocarcinoma documented preoperatively, an esophagectomy is performed as part of the primary therapy. It is important to excise all the columnar epithelium, whether by a radical en bloc esophagectomy or conventional esophagectomy, to limit the risk of development of new Barrett's adenocarcinoma. Reconstruction is performed with interposition of a segment of colon or small intestine after limited resections. A long segment of colon or stomach pull-up with cervical esophagogastrostomy is used for patients who undergo subtotal esophagectomy. As is the case with other esophageal cancers, prognosis depends on the depth of penetration of the primary tumor, involvement of regional lymph nodes, and the presence of distant metastatic disease. A general algorithm for the care of patients with Barrett's esophagus is presented in Figure 43–7.

## REFERENCES


1. Jackson C: Carcinoma and sarcoma of the esophagus: A plea for early diagnosis. *Am J Med Sci* **169:**625, 1925
2. Jackson C: Peptic ulcer of the esophagus. *JAMA* **92:**369, 1929
3. Barrett NR: Chronic peptic ulcer of the oesophagus and "oesophagitis." *Br J Surg* **38:**175, 1950
4. Bosher LH, Taylor FH: Heterotopic gastric mucosa in the esophagus with ulcerations and stricture formation. *J Thorac Surg* **21:**306, 1951
5. Allison PR, Johnstone AS: The oesophagus lined with gastric mucous membrane. *Thorax* **8:**87, 1953
6. Barrett NR: The lower esophagus lined by columnar epithelium. *Surgery* **41:**881, 1957
7. Adler RH: The lower esophagus lined by columnar epithelium. *J Thorac Cardiovasc Surg* **45:**13, 1963
8. Mossberg SM: The columnar-lined esophagus (Barrett syndrome): An acquired condition? *Gastroenterology* **50:**671, 1966
9. de la Pava S, Pickren JW, Adler RH: Ectopic gastric mucosa of the esophagus: A study on histogenesis. *NY State J Med* **65:**1831, 1964
10. Naef AP, Savary M, Ozzello L: Columnar-lined lower esophagus: An acquired lesion with malignant predisposition. *J Thorac Cardiovasc Surg* **70:**826, 1975
11. Schridde H: Uber Magenschleimhaut-Inseln vom bauder Cardiadrusenzone und fundusdrusen Region und den unteren, oesophagealen Cardialdrusen gleichende drusen in obersten Cardialdrusen gleichende drusen in obersten Oesophagusabschnitt. *Virchows Arch Pathol Anat* **175:**1, 1904
12. Rector LE, Connerley ML: Aberrant mucosa in the esophagus in infants and children. *Arch Pathol* **31:**285, 1941
13. Paull A, Trier JS, Dalton MD, et al: The histologic spectrum of Barrett's esophagus. *N Engl J Med* **295:**476, 1976
14. Hershfield NB, Lind JF, Hildes JA, et al: Secretory function of Barrett's epithelium. *Gut* **6:**535, 1965
15. Ustach TJ, Tobon F, Schuster MM: Demonstration of acid secretion from esophageal mucosa in Barrett's ulcer. *Gastrointest Endosc* **16:**98, 1969
16. Mangla JC, Kim Y, Guarasci G, et al: Pepsinogens in epithelium of Barrett's esophagus. *Gastroenterology* **65:**949, 1973
17. Mangla JC, Schenk EA, Desbaillets L, et al: Pepsin secretion, pepsinogen, and gastrin in "Barrett's esophagus." *Gastroenterology* **70:**669, 1976
18. Dayal Y, Wolfe HG: Gastrin-producing cells in ectopic gastric mucosa of developmental and metaplastic origins. *Gastroenterology* **75:**655, 1978
19. Dalton MD, McGuigan JE, Camp RC, et al: Gastric content of columnar mucosa lining the lower (Barrett's) esophagus. *Am J Dig Dis* **22:**970, 1977
20. Griffin M, Sweeney EC: The relationship of endocrine cells, dysplasia and carcinoembryonic antigen in Barrett's mucosa to adenocarcinoma of the oesophagus. *Histopathology* **11:**53, 1987
21. Skinner DB, Walther BC, Riddell, RH, et al: Barrett's esophagus: Comparison of benign and malignant cases. *Ann Surg* **198:**554, 1983
22. Iascone C, DeMeester TR, Little AG, et al: Barrett's esophagus: Functional assessment, proposed pathogenesis, and surgical therapy. *Arch Surg* **118:**543, 1983
23. Iftikhar SY, James PD, Steele RJC, et al: Length of Barrett's oesophagus: An important factor in the development of dysplasia and adenocarcinoma. *Gut* **33:**1155, 1992
24. Attwood SEA, DeMeester TR, Bremner CG, et al: Alkaline gastroesophageal reflux: Implications in the development of complications in Barrett's columnar-lined lower esophagus. *Surgery* **106:**764, 1989
25. Stein HJ, Hoeft S, DeMeester TR: Reflux and motility pattern in Barrett's esophagus. *Dis Esoph* **5:**21, 1992
26. Stein HJ, Hoeft S, DeMeester TR: Functional foregut abnormalities in Barrett's esophagus. *J Thorac Cardiovasc Surg* **105:**107, 1993
27. Meyer W, Vollmar F, Bar W: Barrett-esophagus following total gastrectomy. *Endoscopy* **2:**121, 1979
28. Horvath OP, Csanadi J, Szendrenyi V: Adenocarcinoma arising in Barrett's esophagus after esophageal resection and jejunal interposition. In Nabeya K, Hanaoka T, Nogami H (eds): *Recent Advances in Diseases of the Esophagus.* Tokyo, Springer-Verlag, 1993, pp 150–155
29. Li H, Walsh TN, O'Dowd G, et al: Mechanisms of columnar metaplasia and squamous regeneration in experimental Barrett's esophagus. *Surgery* **115:**176, 1994
30. Gillen P, West AB, Keeling P, et al: Barrett's oesophagus: A pathophysiological study. In Siewert JR, Hölscher AH (eds): *Diseases of the Esophagus.* Berlin, Springer-Verlag, 1988, pp 540–541
31. Herlihy KH, Orlando RC, Bryson JC, et al: Barrett's esophagus: Clinical endoscopic, histologic, manometric, and electrical potential difference characteristics. *Gastroenterology* **86:**436, 1984
32. Savary M, Ollyo JB, Monnier P: Frequency and importance of Barrett's esophagus in reflux disease. In Siewert JR, Hölscher AH (eds): *Diseases of the Esophagus.* Berlin, Springer-Verlag, 1988
33. Gruppo Operativo per lo Studio delle Precancerosi dell 'Esofago(GOSPE): Barrett's esophagus: Epidemiological and clinical results of a multicentric survey. *Int J Cancer* **48:**364, 1991
34. Spechler SJ, Sperber H, Doos WG, et al: The prevalence of Barrett's esophagus in patients with chronic peptic esophageal strictures. *Dig Dis Sci* **28:**769, 1983
35. Borrie J, Goldwater L: Columnar cell-lined esophagus: Assessment of etiology and treatment. *J Thorac Cardiovasc Surg* **71:**825, 1976
36. Gelfand MD: Barrett esophagus in sexagenarian identical twins. *J Clin Gastroenterol* **5:**251, 1983
37. Everhart CW Jr, Holtzapple PG, Humphries TJ, et al: Barrett's esophagus: Inherited epithelium or inherited reflux? *J Clin Gastroenterol* **5:**357, 1983
38. Fahmy N, King JF: Barrett's esophagus: An acquired condition with genetic predisposition. *Am J Gastroenterol* **88:**1262, 1993
39. Hassall E, Weinstein WM, Ament ME: Barrett's esophagus in childhood. *Gastroenterology* **89:**1331, 1985
40. Dahms BB, Rothstein FC: Barrett's esophagus in children: A consequence of chronic gastroesophageal reflux. *Gastroenterology* **86:**318, 1984
41. Hassall E: Barrett's esophagus: Congenital or acquired? *Am J Gastroenterol* **88:**819, 1993

42. Ransom JM, Patel GK, Clift SA, et al: Extended and limited types of Barrett's esophagus in the adult. *Ann Thorac Surg* **33:**19, 1982
43. Radigan LR, Glover JL, Shipley FE, et al: Barrett esophagus. *Arch Surg* **112:**486, 1977
44. Robbins AH, Hermos JA, Schimmel EM, et al: The columnar-lined esophagus: Analysis of 26 cases. *Radiology* **123:**1, 1977
45. Saubier EC, Gouillat C, Samaniego C, et al: Adenocarcinoma in columnar-lined Barrett's esophagus. *Am J Surg* **150:**365, 1985
46. Achkar E, Carey W, Hall G, et al: The clinical features and biological behaviour of adenocarcinoma of the esophagus complicating Barrett's esophagus. In Siewert JR, Hölscher AH (eds): *Diseases of the Esophagus.* Berlin, Springer-Verlag, 1988, pp 562–565
47. Levine MS, Kressel HY, Caroline DF, et al: Barrett esophagus: Reticular pattern of the mucosa. *Radiology* **147:**663, 1983
48. Vincent RE, Robbins AH, Spechler SJ, et al: The reticular pattern as a radiographic sign of the Barrett esophagus: An assessment. *Radiology* **153:**33, 1984
49. Woolf GM, Riddell RH, Irvine EJ, Hunt RH: A study to examine agreement between endoscopy and histology for the diagnosis of columnar lined (Barrett's) esophagus. *Gastrointest Endosc* **35:**541, 1989
50. Chobanian SJ, Cattay EL Jr, Winters C Jr, et al: In vivo staining with toluidine blue as an adjunct to the endoscopic detection of Barrett's esophagus. *Gastrointest Endosc* **33:**99, 1987
51. Mann NS, Tsai MF, Nair PK: Barrett's esophagus in patients with symptomatic reflux esophagitis. *Am J Gastroenterol* **84:**1494, 1989
52. Mason RJ, Bremner CG: Motility differences between long-segment and short-segment Barrett's esophagus. *Am J Surg* **165:**686, 1993
53. Ferguson MK, Little AG, Skinner DB: The clinical spectrum of benign penetrating Barrett's ulcers. In Siewert JR, Hölscher AH (eds): *Diseases of the Esophagus.* Berlin, Springer-Verlag, 1988, pp 542–544
54. Andersson R, Nilsson S: Perforated Barrett's ulcer with esophagopleural fistula. *Acta Chir Scand* **151:**495, 1985
55. Pearson FG, Cooper JD, Patterson GA, Prakash D: Peptic ulcer in acquired columnar-lined esophagus: Results of surgical treatment. *Ann Thorac Surg* **43:**241, 1987
56. Lee FI, Isaacs PET: Barrett's ulcer: Response to standard dose ranitidine, high dose ranitidine, and omeprazole. *Am J Gastroenterol* **83:**914, 1988
57. Riddell RH: Dysplasia and regression in Barrett's epithelium. In Spechler SJ, Goyal RK (eds): *Barrett's Esophagus: Pathophysiology, Diagnosis and Management.* New York, Elsevier, 1985, pp 143–152
58. Miros M, Kerlin P, Walker N: Only patients with dysplasia progress to adenocarcinoma in Barrett's oesophagus. *Gut* **32:**1441, 1991
59. Reid BJ, Haggitt RC, Rubin CE, Rabinovitch PS: Barrett's esophagus. Correlation between flow cytometry and histology in detection of patients at risk for adenocarcinoma. *Gastroenterology* **93:**1, 1987
60. Reid BJ, Blount PL, Rubin CE, et al: Flow-cytometric and histological progression to malignancy in Barrett's esophagus: Prospective endoscopic surveillance of a cohort. *Gastroenterology* **102:**1212, 1992
61. Rabinovitch PS, Reid BJ, Haggitt RC, et al: Progression to cancer in Barrett's esophagus is associated with genomic instability. *Lab Invest* **60:**65, 1988
62. Fennerty MB, Sampliner RE, Way D, et al: Discordance between flow cytometric abnormalities and dysplasia in Barrett's esophagus. *Gastroenterology* **97:**815, 1989
63. Blount PL, Ramel S, Raskind WH, et al: 17p Allelic deletions and p53 protein overexpression in Barrett's adenocarcinoma. *Cancer Res* **51:**5482, 1991
64. Ramel S, Reid BJ, Sanchez CA, et al: Evaluation of p53 protein expression in Barrett's esophagus by two-parameter flow cytometry. *Gastroenterology* **102:**1220, 1992
65. Spechler SJ, Robbins AH, Rubins HB, et al: Adenocarcinoma and Barrett's esophagus: An overrated risk? *Gastroenterology* **87:**927, 1984
66. Cameron AJ, Ott BJ, Payne WS: The incidence of adenocarcinoma in columnar-lined (Barrett's) esophagus. *N Engl J Med* **313:**857, 1985
67. Robertson CS, Mayberry JF, Nicholson DA, et al: Value of endoscopic surveillance in the detection of neoplastic changes in Barrett's oesophagus. *Br J Surg* **75:**760, 1988
68. Van der Veen AH, Dees J, Blankenstein JD, Van Blankenstein M: Adenocarcinoma in Barrett's oesophagus: An overrated risk. *Gut* **30:**14, 1989
69. Hameeteman W, Tytgat GNJ, Houthoff HJ, van den Tweel JG: Barrett's esophagus: Development of dysplasia and adenocarcinoma. *Gastroenterology* **96:**1249, 1989
70. Williamson WA, Ellis FH Jr, Gibb SP, et al: Effect of antireflux operation on Barrett's mucosa. *Ann Thorac Surg* **49:**537, 1990
71. Atkinson M, Robertson CS: Benign oesophageal stricture in Barrett's columnar epithelialised oesophagus and its responsiveness to conservative management. *Gut* **29:**1721, 1988
72. Lundell L: Acid suppression in the long-term treatment of peptic stricture and Barrett's oesophagus. *Digestion* **51:**(Suppl I) 49, 1992
73. Attwood SEA, Barlow AP, Norris TL, Watson A: Therapy in Barrett's esophagus: Medical treatment versus antireflux surgery. In Nabeya K, Hanaoka T, Nogami H (eds): *Recent Advances in Diseases of the Esophagus.* Tokyo, Springer-Verlag, 1993, pp 156–161
74. Skinner DB, Dowlatshahi KD, DeMeester TR: Potentially curable cancer of the esophagus. *Cancer* **50:**2571, 1982
75. Robey SS, Hamilton SR, Gupta PK, Erozan YS: Diagnostic value of cytopathology in Barrett esophagus and associated carcinoma. *Am J Clin Pathol* **89:**493, 1988
76. Wang HH, Doria MI Jr, Purohit-Buch S, et al: Barrett's esophagus. The cytology of dysplasia in comparison to benign and malignant lesions. *Acta Cytol* **36:**60, 1992
77. Geisinger KR, Teot LA, Richter JE: A comparative cytopathologic and histologic study of atypia, dysplasia and adenocarcinoma in Barrett's esophagus. *Cancer* **69:**8, 1992
78. Streitz JM Jr, Andrews CW Jr, Ellis FH Jr: Endoscopic surveillance of Barrett's esophagus. *J Thorac Cardiovasc Surg* **105:**383, 1993
79. Altorki NK, Skinner DB, Segalin A, et al: Indications for esophagectomy in nonmalignant Barrett's esophagus: A 10-year experience. *Ann Thorac Surg* **49:**724, 1990
80. Lee RG: Dysplasia in Barrett's esophagus. *Am J Surg Pathol* **9:**845, 1985
81. Hamilton SR, Smith RRL: The relationship between columnar epithelial dysplasia and invasive adenocarcinoma arising in Barrett's esophagus. *Am J Clin Pathol* **87:**301, 1987
82. Reid BJ, Weinstein WM, Lewin KJ, et al: Endoscopic biopsy can detect high-grade dysplasia or early adenocarcinoma in Barrett's esophagus without grossly recognizable neoplastic lesions. *Gastroenterology* **94:**81, 1988
83. DeMeester TR, Attwood SEA, Smyrk TC, et al: Surgical therapy in Barrett's esophagus. *Ann Surg* **212:**528, 1990
84. Altorki NK, Sunagawa M, Little AG, Skinner DB: High-grade dysplasia in the columnar-lined esophagus. *Am J Surg* **161:**97, 1991
85. Pera M, Trastek VF, Carpenter HA, et al: Barrett's esophagus with high-grade dysplasia: An indication for esophagectomy? *Ann Thorac Surg* **54:**199, 1992
86. Rice TW, Falk GW, Achkar E, Petras RE: Surgical management of high-grade dysplasia in Barrett's esophagus. *Am J Gastroenterol* **88:**1832, 1993
87. Levine DS, Haggitt RC, Blount PL, et al: An endoscopic biopsy protocol can differentiate high-grade dysplasia from early adenocarcinoma in Barrett's esophagus. *Gastroenterology* **105:**40, 1993

CHAPTER

44

# Nissen Fundoplication

F. Henry Ellis, Jr.

The modern era of hiatal hernia repair has been profoundly influenced by increasing awareness that gastroesophageal reflux (GER) is the result of a physiologic abnormality, not an anatomic abnormality. Careful analysis of the long-term results of anatomically designed operations revealed a high percentage of unsatisfactory results,[1] and it became clear that restoration of normal function of the antireflux mechanism was a prerequisite of a successful antireflux procedure. This mechanism is complex and controversial and is addressed elsewhere in this book. Suffice it to say that the amplitude and length of the lower esophageal sphincter (LES) pressure play an important role and that hypotension of the LES is commonly encountered in patients with GER. It has become increasingly evident that hypotension of the LES can occur under a variety of circumstances not only in association with a sliding esophageal hiatal hernia. Many physicians, including me, believe that the Nissen fundoplication best restores the competence mechanism, and the operation has been performed throughout the world with great success. However, before detailing the technical aspects of the procedure and its results, a preliminary discussion of historical and experimental aspects will provide a better understanding of the operation.

## HISTORICAL ASPECTS

In December 1955, Professor Rudolph Nissen of Basel, Switzerland, operated on a 49-year-old woman with a long history of GER without radiographic evidence of a hiatal hernia.[2] He used a technique he had used nearly 20 years before to minimize postoperative reflux after resection of a peptic ulcer in the region of the cardia.[3] This involved enveloping the lower esophagus with gastric fundus by suture approximation of anterior and posterior fundal folds anterior to the esophagus within which a large intraesophageal bougie had been positioned.

Since the original description, the Nissen fundoplication has undergone a variety of modifications designed to minimize complications and poor results. Nissen[4] himself combined the operation with anterior gastropexy only to discontinue that modification. Later, with Rossetti, Nissen suggested that only the anterior wall of the stomach be wrapped around the lower esophagus.[5] In neither of these techniques did Nissen recommend division of the short gastric vessels. Most surgeons currently performing the Nissen operation recommend this maneuver to facilitate the procedure. In fact, in a comparative study by Luostarinen et al, better results were achieved when complete mobilization of the fundus was accomplished.[6] Other modifications of the original Nissen operation have been proposed, including closure of the esophageal hiatus,[7] anchoring of the plication to the preaortic fascia,[8,9] and the addition of highly selective vagotomy to the plication.[10,11] The degree of fundal wrap has been varied to encircle less than 360° of the esophageal tube to avoid the "gas bloat" syndrome.[12–14] For a similar reason, construction of a loose (floppy) wrap has been described.[15] Whereas the wrap initially performed by Nissen extended over 4–6 cm of the esophagus, a shorter wrap is now preferred.[16,17] Modifications, such as the cut and uncut Collis–Nissen procedures, are usually reserved for patients with a shortened esophagus with or without stricture; they are not considered here. Thus, the term *Nissen fundoplication,* while perhaps adhering to the basic principles originally proposed by Nissen, is a relatively imprecise term. The exact technique used must be elucidated for one to understand what is meant when the term is used.

## EXPERIMENTAL BACKGROUND

Considerable experimental evidence indicates that the Nissen fundoplication with a 360° wrap is more effective in preventing reflux than other antireflux procedures.

Bombeck et al,[18] working with dogs, and Butterfield,[19] working with cadaveric specimens, support this view. In vitro studies by Alday and Goldsmith[20] showed that a wrap greater than 270° best fulfilled the criteria of establishing competence, and the cadaveric studies of Lortat-Jacob et al[21] pointed out that at least 4 cm of esophagus must be wrapped to achieve competence. More pertinent is the report of Leonardi et al,[22] who performed in vivo studies on cats, whose esophagus is similar to that of humans. When the effectiveness of the Nissen, Hill, and Belsey procedures as measured with postoperative manometry and pH testing was compared, the Nissen fundoplication proved superior to the others in raising LES pressures and in preventing GER. Leonardi et al[23] also showed that a complete wrap was preferable to a partial wrap in restoring normal LES function.

The precise mechanism by which these procedures prevent reflux is debatable. Condon et al[24] explained the results purely on the basis of mechanical factors. However, Siewert et al[25] demonstrated with in vitro studies that excised strips of smooth muscle from the LES and adjacent gastric fundus exhibit similar responses to such stimuli as pentagastrin (Peptavlon), suggesting that the physiologic response of the newly created high-pressure zone is restored to normal after fundoplication because the smooth muscle of the gastric fundus that composes the wrap acts in a manner similar to the smooth muscle of the normal LES. The anatomic studies by Libermann-Meffert[26] support this concept. Alterations in the length and tension characteristics of the LES muscle produced by surgical repair were suggested by Lipshutz et al[27] as being important. They hypothesized that the LES muscle is placed at its optimal degree of stretch by antireflux procedures, enabling it to respond normally to both neural and hormonal stimulation. It has also been suggested that antireflux operations may interrupt distracting forces of the LES by limiting tension at the gastroesophageal junction.[28] Incomplete abolition of the high-pressure zone during LES relaxation also has been suggested as a possible mechanism.[29] A variety of factors are no doubt involved in the success of fundoplication in preventing reflux; most postoperative manometric studies identify an increase in amplitude and length of LES pressure.

## PATIENT SELECTION

Proper patient selection is essential for good results to be achieved with the Nissen fundoplication. Because medical treatment of GER controls the symptoms in most patients, operation should be undertaken only when symptoms persist after a prolonged period (3–6 mo) of intensive medical therapy or when endoscopic evidence of esophageal ulceration persists despite some alleviation of symptoms. Some surgeons have adopted a more aggressive approach in the presence of Barrett's esophagus. However, I use the same indications for operation in patients with Barrett's esophagus as in other patients with GER because antireflux operations fail to achieve predictable regression of the abnormal mucosa and do not protect against malignant degeneration.[30] The exception is a patient with high-grade dysplasia, who should be treated with resection.[31]

Lack of success after fundoplication encircling a distal esophageal stricture has discouraged application of this technique to patients with panmural fibrotic strictures. In such circumstances, an esophageal lengthening procedure (Collis gastroplasty) with a Nissen wrap performed over the newly formed gastric tube rather than around the strictured area of the distal esophagus is preferred. This modification is also preferable in the presence of esophageal shortening to avoid leaving the wrap in the thorax, a potentially dangerous maneuver.[32,33] The Nissen total wrap should be avoided in patients with poor peristaltic activity of the esophagus, particularly those with achalasia or scleroderma, because it usually leads to obstructive symptoms postoperatively. Preoperative manometry can differentiate such patients definitively. Lesser wraps of the Belsey, Dor, or Toupet variety are appropriate for patients who do not have normal esophageal peristalsis. Although some surgeons have advocated performing an antireflux procedure in every patient who undergoes an operation for paraesophageal hiatal hernia,[34] this is not necessary. To be sure, mixed varieties of sliding and paraesophageal hernias exist, but the symptoms are usually the result of mechanical factors related to the paraesophageal element, and only rarely is LES hypotension present, thus necessitating an antireflux maneuver.[35]

## TECHNIQUE OF FUNDOPLICATION

An abdominal approach is preferred except in patients who have had a previous thoracotomy and in those believed to have anatomic shortening of the esophagus. In such patients, thoracotomy provides optimal exposure for the performance of the procedure. An upper midline incision that skirts to the left of the umbilicus is used. The left lobe of the liver is mobilized to allow exposure of the esophagogastric junctional area. Several centimeters of intra-abdominal esophagus are developed by dividing the peritoneum and phrenoesophageal membrane overlying this organ. The short gastric vessels are ligated and divided as is the posterior gastric artery arising from the splenic artery and a branch of the left inferior phrenic artery, if present. These vessels are rarely illustrated in anatomy texts and, with few exceptions,[36,37] are not described in surgical articles that deal with the technical aspects of fundoplication.

The mobilized esophagus is encircled with a Penrose drain, care being taken to protect the vagus nerves (Fig. 44–1). A 46–50 F Maloney dilator is passed transorally across the esophagogastric junction, and the gastric fundus is then passed behind the mobilized esophagus from left to

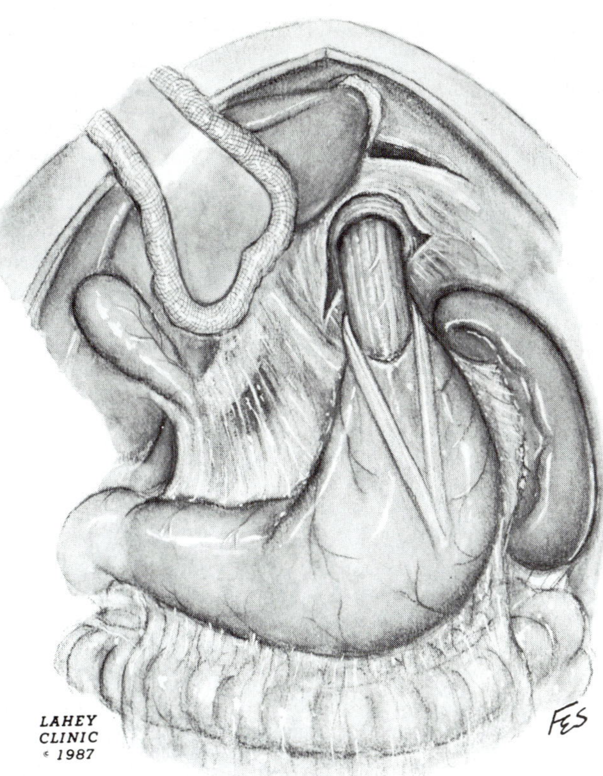


**Figure 44–1.** After mobilization, the intrathoracic esophagus is partially delivered into the abdomen and encircled with a Penrose drain. *(Reprinted with permission of the Lahey Clinic.)*

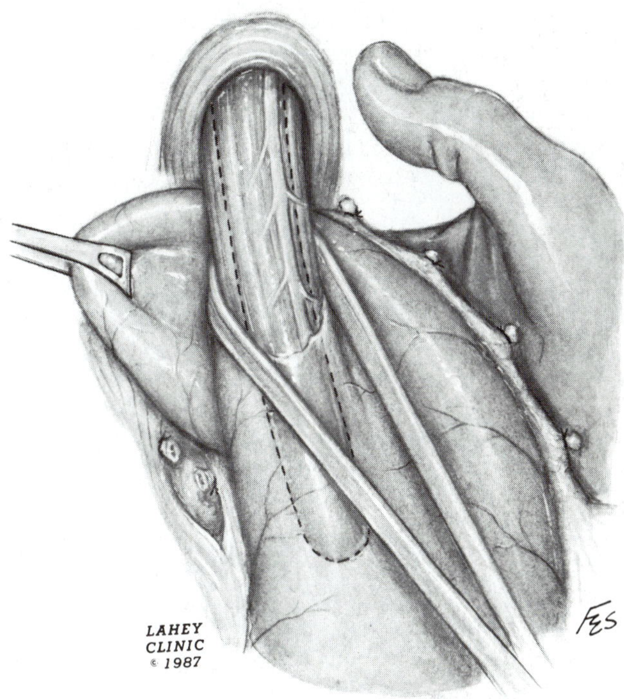


**Figure 44–2.** After the short gastric vessels are divided, the mobilized gastric fundus is passed behind the esophagus and grasped with a Babcock clamp. *(Reprinted with permission of the Lahey Clinic.)*

right and grasped with a Babcock clamp (Fig. 44–2). Adjacent folds of anterior and posterior gastric fundus are approximated anterior to the esophagus with two No. 0 nonabsorbable interrupted sutures that incorporate a small portion of anterior esophageal wall. Care is taken to avoid the vagus nerves (Fig. 44–3). I currently envelop a shorter segment of esophagus than in past years, 1.5–2.5cm long, to minimize the risk of postoperative dysphagia. Additional sutures of finer material (3-0 silk) are placed between these sutures to ensure security of the wrap, and the position of the collar of the wrap around the esophagus is secured with placement of several fine interrupted sutures between the seromusculature wall of the gastric fundus and the esophageal wall (Fig. 44–4). The esophagus, now wrapped with gastric fundus, is elevated with an appropriate retractor, and the esophageal hiatus is narrowed posterior to the wrap with two or three nonabsorbable heavy (No. 0) sutures in the diaphragmatic crura. Only then is the large-bore indwelling stent removed.

Postoperative care is usually straightforward. A nasogastric tube is used only in a reoperative procedure. If both vagi have been damaged, pyloromyotomy should be performed concomitantly. In the uncomplicated situation, oral feedings are allowed when bowel sounds return to normal. Early ambulation is encouraged, and patients are usually ready for discharge within a week of the operation. Some patients may notice transient dysphagia a week to 10 days after the operation, but rarely is bougienage required. If splenic injury occurs during the procedure and necessitates splenectomy, the postoperative complication rate is said to be tripled.[38]

## RESULTS OF OPERATION

Opinions differ regarding the relative merits of the various antireflux procedures currently available to the surgeon. Criticisms of the Nissen fundoplication are numerous, and a number of complications associated with the operation may require reoperation. Recurrent reflux, postoperative dysphagia, and the gas-bloat syndrome predominate among the criticisms of the procedure. On the other hand, the hospital mortality is low, approaching 0%, and overall clinical results are good in 80–90% of patients.

Favorable reports of the results of the operation are numerous. Several studies have compared results of different antireflux operations performed in the same hospital and with few exceptions have documented the superiority of the Nissen fundoplication.[39–47] DeMeester et al[42] evaluated results after Nissen, Belsey, and Hill procedures and found the Nissen fundoplication to be superior to the other operations in restoring LES function and preventing GER. Nicholson and Nohl-Oser[43] confirmed the superiority of the Nissen procedure over the Belsey Mark IV operation in pre-

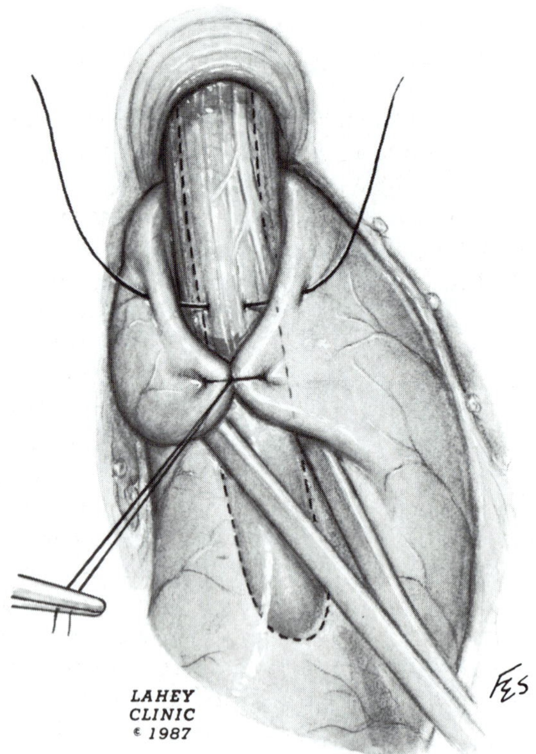


Figure 44–3. The adjacent seromuscular layers of gastric fundus are approximated with two heavy nonabsorbable sutures incorporating some of the anterior wall of the esophagus. Note indwelling large-bore (42 to 46 French) bougie. *(Reprinted with permission of the Lahey Clinic.)*

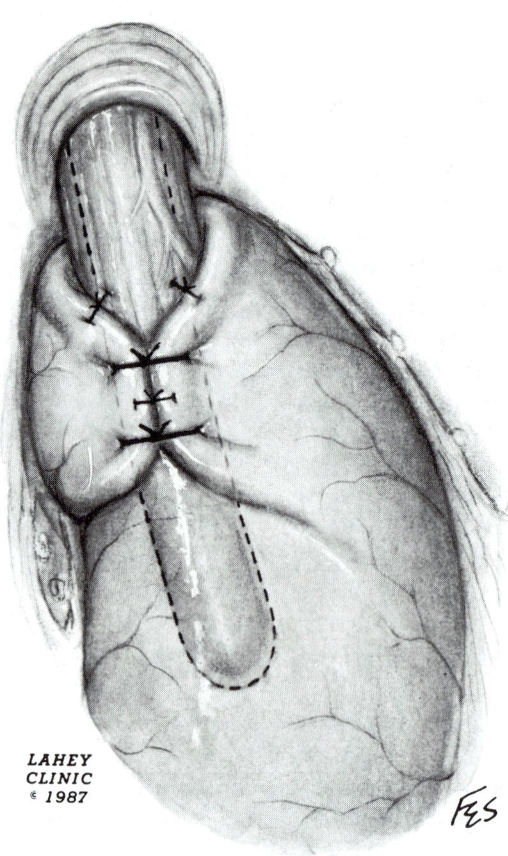


Figure 44–4. Completed fundoplication with reinforcing fine sutures of nonabsorbable material anchoring the collar of the wrap to the esophagus, being careful to preserve the vagus nerve. *(Reprinted with permission of the Lahey Clinic.)*

venting GER, as did Dilling et al.[44] Sillin and et al,[45] in a comparative study of 207 patients undergoing antireflux operations, found the failure rate with the Belsey Mark IV to be 18% and with the Hill posterior gastropexy to be 13%, but the failure rate was only 8% with the Nissen fundoplication. In a similar study of 101 patients, Ferraris and Sube[39] compared results after the Belsey, Hill, and Nissen procedures and found the lowest recurrence rate to be associated with the Nissen operation combined with posterior gastropexy. The superiority of the Nissen procedure over the teres cardiopexy[46] and the Angelchick prosthesis[47] has also been documented.

Undoubtedly, the largest reported series of Nissen fundoplications is that of Rossetti and Hell,[48] who performed operations over a 20-year period on 1400 patients at the University of Basel, where the procedure originated. Patients operated on during the latter part of this period underwent the modified procedure, in which only the anterior wall of the fundus was used for the wrap. A long-term follow-up study of 590 patients with uncomplicated reflux esophagitis showed that 87.5% were free of symptoms. Four hundred patients reported on by Polk[49] had a failure rate of only 4.5%. DeMeester and Bonavina[16] reviewed results for 100 consecutive patients with GER without stricture or motility abnormality treated by a different version of the Nissen fundoplication, modified in recent years with complete mobilization of the gastric fundus and shortening of the length of the wrap to 1.5 cm. The operation was 91% effective in controlling symptoms of reflux over a follow-up period of up to 10 years. Of 241 fundoplication procedures performed at the Lahey Clinic between 1970 and 1987, 157 were of the Nissen type; 121 of these procedures were performed as described in this chapter on patients with GER without stricture, the wrap being left within the abdomen. One fourth of the procedures were reoperations. The results disclosed that reflux symptoms were permanently relieved in more than 90% of patients, and 80% of the patients were able to belch postoperatively.[50] Results of primary operations were better than those after reoperations, and postoperative dysphagia and recurrent reflux have been minimized since use of a large-bore indwelling stent during performance of the fundoplication was introduced. Most of these reports involved relatively short postoperative intervals. More recent long-term (5–10 years) studies revealed that the early good results persist.[51–53] Even more important is a study involving a long-term randomized comparison of the results of medical therapy with those of Nissen fundoplication for patients with complicated GER disease. The conclusion was that operation was statistically significantly more effective than medical therapy in relieving symptoms and endoscopic signs of esophagitis.[54]

In addition to these excellent clinical results, ample objective documentation of the effect of the Nissen fundoplication on LES function can be found. Not only does the operation triple the amplitude of LES pressure and the length of the high-pressure zone, but also the neurohumoral responsiveness of the LES is restored. Twenty-four-hour pH monitoring provides objective confirmation of restoration of the competence mechanism.[50,52,55–57] In addition to these favorable effects of the Nissen fundoplication on LES function, the operation also increases the amplitude of esophageal deglutitory contractions[58] and enhances gastric emptying.[59] Nonetheless, not all surgeons agree that these favorable changes in LES function are responsible for restoration of gastroesophageal competence.[60,61]

## COMPLICATIONS

As already stated, the causes of poor results after the Nissen fundoplication are recurrent reflux, dysphagia, and the gas-bloat syndrome. In the opinion of Negre,[62] the postoperative complications of inability to belch and vomit are so severe as to compromise the overall success of the operation. The Mayo Clinic group[63] abandoned the Nissen fundoplication in preference for the uncut Collis-Nissen operation because of failure of the Nissen repair to prevent telescoping of the esophagogastric junction out of the wrap. These complications can be avoided or minimized by using a floppy wrap facilitated with placement of a large-bore indwelling stent at the time of fundoplication and with suture fixation of the wrap to the esophagus. It should be emphasized that the gas-bloat syndrome is now rare. However, many patients notice increased flatus after the Nissen procedure.

In addition to these postoperative problems, a number of other less frequently observed phenomena have been reported, including paraesophageal hernia,[64] gastric ulceration,[65–67] gastric obstruction caused by a slipped Nissen fundoplication,[68] and perforation of the wrap with fistula formation.[69] That these complications are rare if the operation is properly applied is evident from the results detailed earlier.

A number of reports of reoperations for failed Nissen fundoplication deserve comment. Hill et al[70] reported on 25 reoperations, the most common cause of failure being recurrent reflux resulting from incomplete repair or disruption of the wrap. Obstruction secondary to a slipped Nissen or too tight a wrap was the next most common cause of reoperation. Little et al[71] reported on 61 reoperations for failed antireflux procedures, most of which were transabdominal Nissen fundoplications. Recurrent reflux or failure of esophageal clearance or both were the most common causes of failure of the original procedure. Various reoperative procedures were used, most commonly a transthoracic Nissen or Belsey procedure. Excellent or good results were achieved in 42–85% of patients, depending on how many previous operative procedures each patient had undergone.

Ninety-eight patients on my service required reoperation from January 1970 to January 1994 for failure of a previous antireflux procedure; I performed seven of these operations (unpublished data, 1994). These 98 patients had undergone 153 previous upper gastrointestinal tract operations, the most common of which was a Nissen fundoplication (84 patients). The most common symptom necessitating reoperation was dysphagia (58 patients) caused by either an incorrect original diagnosis in approximately one third of the patients or a wrap performed inappropriately in a patient without esophageal peristalsis. Persistent or recurrent reflux was the next most common symptom that necessitated reoperation (23 patients). Twelve patients required reoperation because of a postoperative paraesophageal hiatal hernia, and only four required reoperation because of the gas-bloat syndrome. Perforation of a fundoplication necessitated reoperation in one patient. It was estimated that faulty technique accounted for failure of the antireflux procedure in nearly two thirds of the patients. Poor patient selection was the next most common reason for failure.

It is difficult to determine the overall incidence of reoperation after a failed antireflux procedure. On the basis of a literature review, Jamieson stated that it is probably on the order of 4–6%.[72] Although the operative mortality after reoperation is higher than after a primary procedure, the clinical results are not very different from those following primary operations. However, clinical results vary depending on the number of previous operations. They are twice as good in patients who had undergone only one previous operation, compared with those who had undergone three or more previous procedures.[71] Although complications may occur after the Nissen procedure, it is important to emphasize that excellent results can be obtained if the operation is used appropriately.

For good results, patients should be selected carefully and certain technical aspects of the operation must be observed. When these recommendations are followed, satisfactory and permanent relief of symptoms of GER can be achieved in more than 90% of patients.[73] Postoperative symptoms of persistent or recurrent reflux, dysphagia, and gas bloat are extremely rare and few patients require reoperation.

## REFERENCES

1. Allison, PR: Hiatus hernia: A 20-year retrospective study. *Ann Surg* **178**:273, 1973
2. Nissen R: Eine einfache Operation zur Beeinflussung der Reluxoesophagitis. *Schweiz Med Wochenschr* **86**(Suppl):590, 1956

3. Nissen R: Die transpleurale Resektion der Kardia. *Deutsche Ztschr Chir* **249:**311, 1937
4. Nissen R: Gastropexy and "fundoplication" in surgical treatment of hiatal hernia. *Am J Dig Dis* **6:**954, 1961
5. Nissen R, Rossetti M: Surgery of hiatal and other diaphragmatic hernias. *J Int Coll Surg* **43:**663, 1965
6. Luostarinen M, Koskinen M, Karronen J: Nissen fundoplication for gastroesophageal reflux disease: Effect of fundic mobilization on belching ability and abdominal gas volume. *Scand J Gastroenterol* **28:**31, 1993 (abstr)
7. Ellis FH Jr: Techniques of fundoplication. In Stipa S, Belsey RHR, Moraldi A (eds): *Medical and Surgical Problems of the Esophagus.* New York, Academic Press, 1981, pp 61–65
8. Cordiano C. Rovere GQD, Agugiaro S, Mazzilli G: Technical modification of the Nissen fundoplication procedure. *Surg Gynecol Obstet* **143:**977, 1976
9. Kaminski DL, Codd JE, Sigmund CJ: Evaluation of the use of the median arcuate ligament in fundoplication for reflux esophagitis. *Am J Surg* **134:**724, 1977
10. Jordan PH Jr: Parietal cell vagotomy facilitates fundoplication in the treatment of reflux esophagitis. *Surg Gynecol Obstet* **147:**593, 1978
11. Jones NA, Anders CJ: A new approach to the surgical treatment of reflux oesophagitis. *Ann R Coll Surg* **61:**48, 1979
12. Guarner V, Martinez N, Gavino JF: Ten year evaluation of posterior fundoplasty in the treatment of gastroesophageal reflux: Long-term and comparative study of 135 patients. *Am J Surg* **139:**200, 1980
13. Dor J, Humbert P, Dor V, Figarella J: L'intérêt de la technique de Nissen modifiée la prevention du reflux après cardiomyotomie extra muqueuse de Heller. *Mem Acad Chir* **88:**877, 1962
14. Toupet A: Technique d'oesophagogastroplastie avec phrenogastropexie applikquée dans la cure radicale des hernia hiatales et comme completment de l'operation de Heller dans les cardiospasmus. *Mem Acad Chir* **89:**374, 1963
15. Donahue PE, Samelson S, Nyhus LM, Bombeck CT: The floppy Nissen fundoplication: Effective long-term control of pathologic reflux. *Arch Surg* **120:**663, 1985
16. DeMeester TR, Bonavina L, Albertucci M: Nissen fundoplication for gastroesophageal reflux disease: Evaluation of primary repair in 100 consecutive patients. *Ann Surg* **204:**9, 1986
17. Henderson RD: Dysphagia complicating hiatal hernia repair. *J Thorac Cardiovasc Surg* **88:**922, 1984
18. Bombeck CT, Coelho RG, Castro VA, et al: An experimental comparison of procedures for the operative correction of gastroesophageal reflux. *Bull Soc Int Chir* **30:**435, 1971
19. Butterfield WC: Current hiatal hernia repairs: Similarities, mechanisms and extended indications—An autopsy study. *Surgery* **69:**910, 1971
20. Alday ES, Goldsmith HS: Efficacy of fundoplication in preventing gastric reflux. *Am J Surg* **126:**322, 1973
21. Lortat-Jacob JL, Maillard JN, Fékété F: A procedure to prevent reflux after esophagogastric resection: Experience with 17 patients. *Surgery* **50:**600, 1961
22. Leonardi HK, Lee ME, El-Kurd MF, Ellis FH Jr: An experimental study of the effectiveness of various antireflux operations. *Ann Thorac Surg* **24:**215, 1977
23. Leonardi HK, Ellis FH Jr, Cormack J, Gorrilla M: Experimental fundoplication: Comparison of results of different techniques. *Surgery* **82:**514, 1977
24. Condon RE, Kraus MA, Wolheim D: Cause of increase in "lower esophageal sphincter" pressure after fundoplication. *J Surg Res* **20:**445, 1976
25. Siewert R, Jennewein HM, Waldock F, et al: Experimentelle und klinische Untersuchungen zum Wirkungsmechanismus der Fundoplication. *Langenbecks Arch Chir* **333:**519, 1973
26. Libermann-Meffert D: Architecture of the musculature at the gastroesophageal junction and in the fundus. *Chir Gastroenterol* **9:**425, 1975
27. Lipshutz WH, Eckert RJ, Gaskins RD, et al: Normal lower-esophageal-sphincter function after surgical treatment of gastroesophageal reflux. *N Engl J Med* **291:**1107, 1974
28. Anderson KW, Bombeck CT: Why antireflux surgery works. *Surg Rounds* **11:**49, 1987
29. Ireland AC, Holloway RH, Joouli J, Dent J: Mechanisms underlying antireflux actions of fundoplication. *Gut* **34:**303, 1993
30. Williamson WA, Ellis FH Jr, Gibb SP, et al: Effect of antireflux operation on Barrett's mucosa. *Ann Thorac Surg* **49:**537, 1990
31. Streitz JM Jr, Andrews CW Jr, Ellis FH Jr: Endoscopic surveillance of Barrett's esophagus: Does it help? *J Thoracic Cardiovasc Surg* **105:**383, 1993
32. Mansour KA, Burton HG, Miller JI Jr, Hatcher CR Jr: Complications of intrathoracic Nissen fundoplication. *Ann Thorac Surg* **32:**173, 1981
33. Richardson JD, Larson GM, Polk HC Jr: Intrathoracic fundoplication for shortened esophagus: Treacherous solution to a challenging problem. *Am J Surg* **143:**29, 1982
34. Pearson FG, Cooper JD, Ilves R, et al: Massive hiatal hernia with incarceration: A report of 53 cases. *Ann Thorac Surg* **35:**45, 1983
35. Williamson WA, Ellis FH Jr, Streitz JM Jr, Shahian DM: Paraesophageal hiatal hernia: Is an antireflux procedure necessary? *Ann Thorac Surg* **56:**447, 1993
36. Suzuki K, Prates JC, Liberato JA, Didio JA: Incidence and surgical importance of the posterior gastric artery. *Ann Surg* **187:**134, 1978
37. Wald H, Polk HC Jr: Anatomical variations in hiatal and upper gastric areas and their relationship to difficulties experienced in operation. *Ann Surg* **197:**389, 1983
38. Rogers DM, Herrington JL Jr, Morton C: Incidental splenectomy associated with Nissen fundoplication. *Ann Surg* **191:**153, 1980
39. Ferraris VA, Sube J: Retrospective study of the surgical management of reflux esophagitis. *Surg Gynecol Obstet* **152:**17, 1981
40. Thor KBA, Selander T: A long term randomized prospective trial of the Nissen procedure versus a modified Toupet technique. *Ann Surg* **210:**719, 1989
41. Stipa S, Fegiz G, Iascone C, et al: Belsey and Nissen operations for gastroesophageal reflux. *Ann Surg* **210:**583, 1989
42. DeMeester TR, Johnson LF, Kent AH: Evaluation of current operations for the prevention of gastroesophageal reflux. *Ann Surg* **180:**511, 1974
43. Nicholson DA, Nohl-Oser HC: Hiatus hernia: A comparison between two methods of fundoplication by evaluation of the long-term results. *J Thorac Cardiovasc Surg* **72:**938, 1976
44. Dilling EW, Peyton MD, Cannon SP, et al: Comparison of Nissen fundoplication and Belsey Mark IV in the management of gastroesophageal reflux. *Am J Surg* **134:**730, 1977
45. Sillin LF, Condon RE, Wilson SD, Worman LW: Effective surgical therapy of gastroesophagitis: Experience with Belsey, Hill, and Nissen operations. *Arch Surg* **114:**536, 1979
46. Janssen IMB, Gouma DJ, Klementschitsk P, et al: Prospective randomized comparison of teres cardiopexy and Nissen fundoplication in the surgical therapy of gastroesophageal reflux disease. *Br J Surg* **80:**875, 1993
47. Kimot WA, Kirby DA, Temple JG: Prospective randomized trial of Nissen fundoplication and Angelchik prosthesis in the surgical management of gastroesophageal reflux disease. *Br J Surg* **78:**1181, 1991
48. Rossetti M, Hell K: Fundoplication for the treatment of gastroesophageal reflux in hiatal hernia. *World J Surg* **1:**439, 1977
49. Polk HC Jr: Indications for, technique of, and results of fundoplication for complicated reflux esophagitis. *Am Surg* **44:**620, 1978
50. Ellis FH Jr, Crozier RE: Reflux control by fundoplication: A clinical and manometric assessment of the Nissen operation. *Ann Thorac Surg* **38:**387, 1984
51. MacIntyre IMC, Goulbourne IA: Long term results after Nissen fundoplication: A 5–15 year review. *J R Coll Surg Edinb* **35:**159, 1990
52. Martinez de Haro LF, Ortiz A, Parrilla P, et al: Long term results of Nissen fundoplication in reflux esophagitis without strictures:

Clinical, endoscopic and pH metric evaluation. *Dig Dis Sci* **37:**523, 1992

53. Loustarinen M: Fate of Nissen fundoplication after 20 years: A clinical, endoscopical and functional analysis. *Gut* **34:**1015, 1993
54. Spechler SJ: Comparison of medical and surgical therapy for complicated gastroesophageal reflux disease with veterans. *N Engl J Med* **326:**786, 1992
55. DeMeester TR, Johnson LF: Evaluation of the Nissen procedure by esophageal manometry and twenty-four hour pH monitoring. *Am J Surg* **129:**94, 1975
56. Johnson F, Joelson B, Gudmundson K, et al: Effects of fundoplication on the antireflux mechanism. *Br J Surg* **74:**1111, 1987
57. Breumenholf R, Smout ASPM, Schyns MWRJ, et al: Prospective evaluation of the effect of Nissen fundoplication. *Surg Gynecol Obstet* **171:**115, 1990
58. Stein HJ, Bremner RM, Jamieson J, DeMeester TR: Effects of Nissen fundoplication on esophageal motor function. *Arch Surg* **127:**788, 1992
59. Maddern GJ, Chatterton BE, Collins PJ, et al: Solid and gastric emptying in patients with gastro-oesophageal reflux. *Br J Surg* **72:**344, 1985
60. Fisher RS, Malmud LS, Lobis IF, Maier WP: Antireflux surgery for symptomatic gastroesophageal reflux: Mechanisms of action. *Am J Dig Dis* **23:**152, 1978
61. Bancewicz J, Mughal M, Marples M: The lower oesophageal sphincter after floppy Nissen fundoplication. *Br J Surg* **74:**162, 1987
62. Negre JB: Post-fundoplication symptoms: Do they restrict the success of Nissen fundoplication? *Ann Surg* **198:**698, 1983
63. Piehler JM, Payne WS, Cameron AJ, Pairolero PC: The uncut Collis-Nissen procedure for esophageal hiatal hernia and its complications. *Probl Gen Surg* **1:**1, 1984
64. Balison JR, Macgregor AM, Woodward ER: Postoperative diaphragmatic herniation following transthoracic fundoplication: A note of warning. *Arch Surg* **106:**164, 1973
65. Bremner CG: Gastric ulceration after a fundoplication operation for gastroesophageal reflux. *Surg Gynecol Obstet* **148:**62, 1979
66. Herrington JL Jr, Meacham PW, Hunter RM: Gastric ulceration after fundic wrapping: Vagal nerve entrapment, a possible factor. *Ann Surg* **195:**574, 1982
67. Campbell R, Kennedy T, Johnston GW: Gastric ulceration after Nissen fundoplication. *Br J Surg* **70:**406, 1903
68. Mattox HE III, Albertson DA, Castell DO, Richter JE: Dysphagia following fundoplication: "Slipped" fundoplication versus achalasia complicated by fundoplication. *Am J Gastroenterol* **857:**1468, 1991
69. Burnett HF, Read RC, Morris WD, Campbell GS: Management of complications of fundoplication and Barrett's esophagus. *Surgery* **82:**521, 1977
70. Hill LD, Ilves R, Stevenson JK, Pearson JM: Reoperation for disruption and recurrence after Nissen fundoplication. *Arch Surg* **114:**542, 1979
71. Little AG, Ferguson MK, Skinner DB: Reoperation for failed antireflux operations. *J Thorac Cardiovasc Surg* **91:**511, 1986
72. Jamieson GB: The results of antireflux surgery and reoperative antireflux surgery. *Gullet* **3:**41, 1993
73. Dunnington GL, DeMeester TR: Outcome effect of adherence to operative principles of Nissen fundoplication by multiple surgeons. *Am J Surg* **166:**654, 1993

CHAPTER

45

# The Hill Procedure

Lucius D. Hill

Gastroesophageal reflux disease (GERD) with its complications of heartburn, esophagitis, and pneumonia is the most common abnormality of the upper gastrointestinal tract. Despite the high incidence of GERD, the pathophysiology of this disorder has been poorly understood until recently. Basically, reflux occurs when the antireflux barrier fails. To understand the disorder and the principles of surgical correction, it is essential to understand the components of the antireflux barrier.

## ANTIREFLUX BARRIER

The antireflux barrier consists of the gastroesophageal valve (GEV), the lower esophageal sphincter (LES), the diaphragm, the posterior fixation of the gastroesophageal (GE) junction, and esophageal clearance. In 1956, Fyke et al produced manometric evidence of a LES.[1] Attention was then focused on the LES as the sole barrier to reflux. The GEV is made by the angle of entry of the esophagus into the stomach. It was described 100 years ago and was noted by Allison[2] and Barrett[3] and many others, but these descriptions were ignored. With the ability to view the GE junction with a retroflexed fiberoptic esophagoscope, it became clear that the GEV is an important component of the antireflux barrier. The LES generates a pressure of 15–18 mm Hg in the resting state and can generate pressures of 100 mg Hg or more. However, a weak sphincter alone cannot withstand the high pressures exerted against the GE junction with heavy lifting, straining, and trauma.

In 33 cadavers, with no premorbid evidence of hiatal hernia or esophageal disease, my colleagues and I[4] showed that a measurable gradient of approximately 15 cm of water exists across the GE junction. This gradient can be eliminated by depressing the fundus of the stomach 45°. This maneuver causes the angle of His to become obtuse, eliminates the GE flap valve, converts the osteum of the esophagus into a funnel, and results in free reflux. Because there is no LES function in cadavers, the presence of a gradient across the GE junction and the maneuver of depressing the cardia to eliminate the gradient helped to confirm the importance of this valve.

The appearance of the valve was studied through a retroflexed endoscope in 20 healthy volunteers without reflux to determine how the normal valve appears. The valve opened only with swallowing, belching, and vomiting and closed promptly and adhered to the scope at all times.

Thirty-two patients with and without reflux were examined with a retroflexed endoscope, and the valves were graded by gastroenterologists blinded to the clinical status of the patient. From this and other studies, we developed a grading system of the valve (Fig. 45–1). No patient with grade I or II GEV showed reflux, whereas all patients with grade III and IV valves showed reflux. In 33 other patients seen in the gastric laboratory who had both standard acid reflux tests and grading of the valve, the results were shown in terms of prediction of the clinical status of the patient (Fig. 45–2). Grading of the GEV more accurately predicted clinical status in 32 of 33 patients, whereas measurement of the LES correlated with clinical status in only 17 patients.[5] A grade I valve is a normal valve (Fig. 45–3, see Color Plates following page 608) that consists of a musculomucosal fold that adheres to the endoscope through all phases of respiration, opens for swallowing and belching and closes promptly.[5,6] We have also viewed the valve through a gastrostomy during a surgical procedure, in patients with a gastrostomy, and in cadavers. It has the same structural appearance as that seen through a retroflexed endoscope.[4]

A grade II GEV is only slightly less well-defined and shorter than a normal valve. It opens but closes promptly

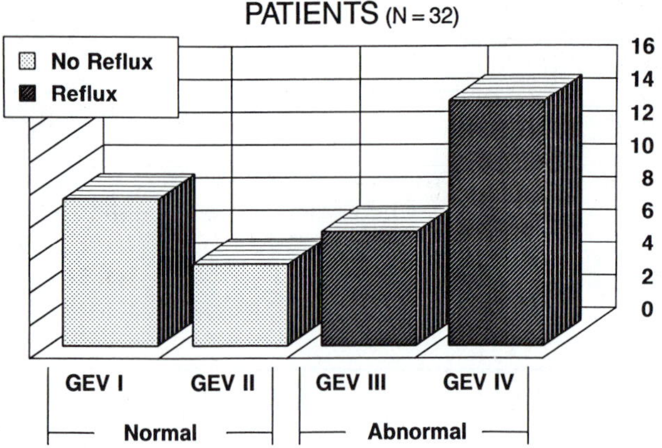


**Figure 45–1.** Grading system of the GEV developed with the aid of retroflexed endoscopy in 32 patients with and without GERD. GEV = gastroesophageal valve.

(Fig. 45–4, see Color Plates following page 608). A grade III valve opens frequently, remains open for varying periods of time, is poorly defined, and is often associated with a hiatal hernia (Fig. 45–5, see Color Plates following page 608). The grade IV valve shows no well-defined musculomucosal fold. The esophageal orifice is wide open, and it is invariably accompanied by a hiatal hernia (Fig. 45–6, see Color Plates following page 608).

These studies show clearly that the GEV is an important component of the antireflux barrier.

## PRINCIPLES OF OPERATIVE TREATMENT

The role of surgical therapy is to re-establish the function of the antireflux barrier with a normal, grade I, 180° valve.

In addition to reconstructing the valve, calibrating the LES is important and can be performed by means of intraoperative measurement of sphincter pressure. A computer-generated view shows that the sphincter resides inside the valve and aids the valve in discriminating among gas, liquids, and solids while the valve does the heavy work in terms of preventing reflux (Fig. 45–7). Increased intragastric pressure serves to close the valve against the lesser curve.

Posterior fixation of the GE junction is essential. This is lost when a hiatal hernia develops and the GE junction ascends into the posterior mediastinum. The esophagus can no longer generate propulsive waves that are necessary for esophageal clearance, because the esophagus no longer has a fulcrum or point of fixation from which to work. The entire gastrointestinal tract, including the hollow and solid viscera in humans and most vertebrate animals, is suspended by the dorsal mesentery to the posterior body wall. The esophagus is no exception to this rule. Extensive cadaveric dissections demonstrate that the esophagus is primarily fixed posteriorly by a dense plate of fibroareolar tissue that extends from the median arcuate ligament to the aortic arch. The posterior attachment of the GE junction by

| Measurement of LESP | Grading of Esophageal Value |
|---|---|

33 Patients

Correlation with Clinical Picture of GERD

| LESP | Grading of GEV |
|---|---|
| 17 of 33 | 32 of 33 |

Endoscopist Blinded to Clinical Picture

**Figure 45–2.** Results of correlation with clinical status of patients seen in the gastroenterology laboratory. Grading of the GEV correlated more closely with clinical status than the measurement of LES pressure (LESP).

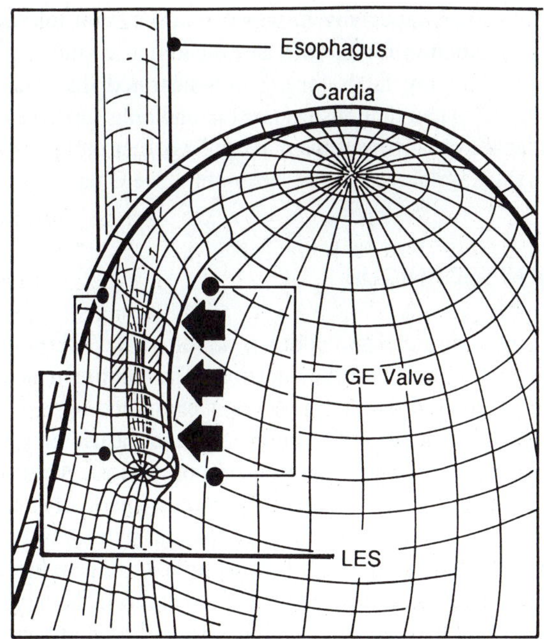


**Figure 45–7.** Computer-generated view shows the relation between the sphincter and the GEV. The sphincter resides inside the valve and aids the valve in discriminating among gas, liquid, and solids and aids in the prevention of reflux. The arrows are pressure vectors demonstrating that increased intragastric pressure closes the valve.

the dorsal mesentery to the preaortic fascia is key to the entire barrier to reflux. In cadavers, division of the posterior attachment allows the GE junction to slide into the chest, and the effect of the GEV is lost. As the GE junction ascends into the posterior mediastinum, the valve is lost, and the sphincter is distracted.

Closure of the enlarged diaphragmatic opening is important to prevent recurrence of hiatal hernia.[7] The diaphragm should be closed loosely about the esophagus, so that at least one finger can be placed alongside the esophagus with a nasogastric tube in the lumen. Fixation of the cardia to the rim of the diaphragm is also important to accentuate the valve and to close the opening into the posterior mediastinum, to prevent herniation of the cardia into the posterior mediastinum.

To summarize, the goals of surgery are restoration of the GEV, calibration of the LES to the proper range, posterior fixation of the GE junction to restore esophageal peristalsis and clearance, reduction of hiatal hernia, and partial closure of the enlarged hiatus.

## INDICATIONS FOR OPERATION

Because the symptoms of esophagitis, including heartburn and dysphagia, are so common, it is important that the indications for surgical intervention remain strict. The important indications for operation are as follows.

### Intractability

Medical management should be carried out by a gastroenterologist or internist interested in gastrointestinal disorders.[8,9] If medical treatment fails under the guidance of a competent physician, the patient should be considered for surgical treatment.[10]

### Esophagitis

Esophagitis may vary from edema and erythema of the mucosa accompanied by spasm to severe forms of ulcerative esophagitis with stricture.

### Stricture and Ulceration

Approximately 14% of patients at my institution underwent operations for stricture; 2.5% had discrete ulceration with or without stricture. A stricture usually indicates that esophagitis has been allowed to proceed too long.[11,12] Perforations into the mediastinum and even into the pericardium occur but are rare. Large hernias may produce pressure on the heart and lungs, produce chest discomfort, and limit reserve.

### Bleeding

Bleeding is usually chronic and low grade, producing persistent anemia. Sometimes a tear or penetrating ulceration with mucosal bleeding may lead to acute, serious bleeding. About 10% of the patients in our series had chronic anemia.

### Respiratory Complications

Larrain and Pope reviewed the pulmonary complications of GE reflux that are often overlooked by physicians.[13] A number of patients in our series underwent long-term treatment of what was considered asthma. Careful questioning revealed that the so-called asthma occurred when the patient lay down or after an episode of reflux. Even with acid neutralization with proton pump inhibitors like omeprazole, the refluxed material damages the tracheobronchial tree and the vocal cords. Surgical treatment is rewarding in such patients, because it eliminates reflux and aspiration.

### Large Hernias

In a small group of patients operation is required because the hernia is large enough to produce pressure symptoms in the chest with cardiorespiratory embarrassment (see Chap. 48). Episodes of incarceration may cause pain so severe, it is interpreted as a myocardial infarction. Trauma to the stomach, at the point where the diaphragm impinges on the displaced viscus, can lead to what is called a callus ulceration of the gastric mucosa, which may bleed.

### Barrett's Esophagus

Patients with documented Barrett's esophagus who have progressive and increasing dysplastic changes in the Barrett's epithelium while undergoing intensive medical treatment are candidates for operation.[14] Studies by Reid et al, who used flow cytometry to correlate genomic instability (diploidy and aneuploidy), provided additional data to identify patients with Barrett's epithelium who are at increased risk for esophageal cancer.[15,16] Esophageal reflux is currently the primary factor investigated in the evolution of Barrett's epithelium. Some patients who have undergone successful antireflux operations have been shown to have regression of Barrett's esophagus after control of reflux. Brand et al found that four of 10 patients with Barrett's esophagus had reversion to squamous epithelium after an antireflux procedure.[17] This is a controversial point, however. Patients with severe dysplasia may well have carcinoma in situ and should be considered for resection (see Chap. 43).

## PREOPERATIVE EVALUATION

Preoperative evaluation should identify the presence and severity of reflux and its complications while excluding or documenting co-existent problems (see Chap. 39). Upper gastrointestinal radiographs are somewhat insensitive to reflux. They demonstrate the level and length of stenosis and ulceration and the type of hiatal hernia. More objective tests include esophageal manometry with pH studies to establish the level of acid in the stomach, the volume of acid that is refluxing, and the pressure of the LES. These studies can be used postoperatively to test the success of the operation. A sphincter pressure less than 10 mm Hg raises the question of sphincter incompetence. A sphincter pressure 30 mm Hg or more raises the possibility of a hypertensive sphincter, or so-called super squeeze. The standard acid reflux text can demonstrate the motility of the esophagus and the presence of high-pressure, simultaneous waves, which suggest diffuse spasm.[18]

Twenty-four-hour pH monitoring is reserved for patients in whom endoscopy and standard acid reflux testing have not clarified the problem. It can indicate the frequency and severity of reflux. This has helped us identify patients with reflux in the upright position but little or no reflux in the supine position.

Preoperative endoscopy, with or without biopsy, provides valuable information regarding the presence of esophagitis, ulceration, and Barrett's esophagus and helps rule out carcinoma.

Radionuclide studies are a valuable test for the detection of reflux, especially in patients who cannot tolerate or refuse intubation for the pH and manometric studies. Russell et al, in my laboratory,[19] demonstrated that radionuclide studies can demonstrate reflux and help separate early achalasia from diffuse spasm as well as other motility disorders, such as delayed gastric emptying (see Chap. 49).

## OPEN TECHNIQUE

The open surgical procedure is accomplished through an upper abdominal midline incision. The abdomen is thoroughly explored, and the pylorus is examined for evidence of pyloric stenosis, which might impede gastric emptying. Preoperative endoscopy should rule out pyloric stenosis or duodenal ulcer. Only if the duodenum is markedly scarred or if there is active ulceration, should pyloroplasty and vagotomy be performed. It is imperative to relieve any gastric outlet obstruction to obtain a good result from an antireflux procedure. On the other hand, to add a vagotomy to a routine hiatal hernia repair is unwise. This has led to complications of vagotomy without benefit to the patient.

The triangular ligament of the left lobe of the liver is divided so that the left lobe can be retracted to the patient's right. This exposes the esophageal hiatus with its covering phrenoesophageal membrane. An upper-hand retractor with two blades facilitates exposure of the upper abdomen. The phrenoesophageal membrane is divided on the diaphragm (Fig. 45–8). As much of the fibroareolar tissue that makes up the phrenoesophageal bundles as possible is kept with the GE junction. These bundles normally hold the GE junction in place in the diaphragm and are used to anchor the

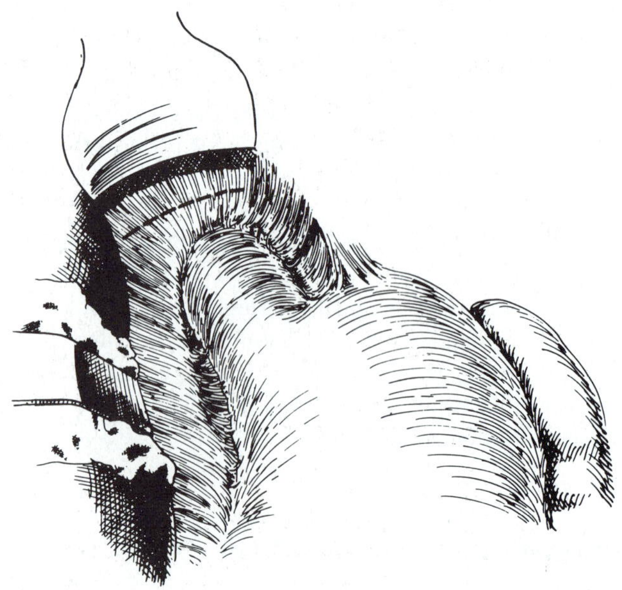

**Figure 45–8.** The phrenoesophageal membrane is divided on the diaphragm to retain the fibroareolar tissue on the stomach to be used in the repair.

GE junction to the preaortic fascia. The lesser omentum is divided, and the esophageal hiatus is exposed. The esophagus is gently diverted to the patient's left, and the attachment of the cardia to the diaphragm is divided. Only rarely must we divide the short gastric vessels. Such dissection must be done with care so as not to damage the spleen. Capsular tears of the spleen may be repaired with cauterization, suturing, or application of a topical hemostat such as Avitene.

Division of the phrenogastric and superior portions of the gastrosplenic ligament mobilizes the upper part of the gastric fundus. The fundus can then be rotated so that the posterior part of the stomach can be visualized. This allows the GE junction to be retracted down and the hiatal hernia reduced. The bundles of tissue that constitute the anterior and posterior attachments of the GE junction to the diaphragm, the anterior and posterior phrenoesophageal bundles, can then be displayed. With caudal retraction of these bundles, an intraabdominal segment of the esophagus becomes visible. The anterior and posterior vagus nerves are visualized and kept in view so as not to be damaged.

Retracting the stomach to the patient's left exposes the preaortic fascia. The aorta and celiac axis are easily felt. The median arcuate ligament lies immediately above the celiac trunk. It can be exposed with careful blunt dissection at this point over the midpoint of the aorta. The celiac artery usually arises cephalad to the median arcuate ligament. When the free edge of the median arcuate ligament has been exposed, the celiac artery can be compressed into the aorta, and the fibroareolar tissue overlying the artery can be carefully divided. An instrument such as a Goodell dilator is then passed beneath the median arcuate ligament. If the instrument is in the correct plane, it should simply float beneath the preaortic fascia. If the instrument meets an obstruction, there may be a branch of the celiac artery in the midline. The branch may be damaged if force is used at insertion. Dissection of the celiac axis has been the deterrent to performing this operation, in the opinion of other surgeons. If it is difficult to locate the median arcuate ligament and if the surgeon is not familiar with vascular surgery and is uncomfortable dissecting out the celiac axis, a safer alternative procedure is recommended.

The fibroareolar tissue overlying the aorta and the esophageal hiatus can be divided with sharp dissection, exposing the aorta. A finger placed gently beneath the preaortic fascia down to the celiac artery lifts the preaortic fascia off the aorta. The fascia can be grasped with a Babcock clamp and sutures placed through the preaortic fascia. This is a safer approach than dissecting out the celiac artery. This technique was described by Van Sant (Fig. 45–9) and is used by us quite frequently. In passing the finger behind the fascia, care is taken not to damage short branches that pass from the aorta to the crura. If dissection is kept in the midline, these branches are avoided. We find that this approach is preferable, and we now rarely dissect the median arcuate ligament.

The crura of the esophageal hiatus are loosely approximated behind the esophagus with nonabsorbable sutures. The crura are closed so that a finger can be placed alongside the esophagus, making certain the closure is not too tight.

The stomach is rotated to expose the anterior and posterior phrenoesophageal bundles. The bundles are grasped with Babcock clamps well above the left gastric artery, care taken not to traumatize the vagal nerves. Strong, nonabsorbable sutures are taken through the anterior and posterior phrenoesophageal bundles. These are then passed through the preaortic fascia, which is lifted well off the aorta with a Babcock clamp. Usually five sutures are placed in the anterior and posterior phrenoesophageal bundles and carried through the preaortic fascia (Fig. 45–10). These sutures are placed with the vagus nerves in full view in order not to damage the nerves. A single knot is then placed in the top three sutures, which are then clamped with long hemostats. One measures the barrier pressure by passing the side hole

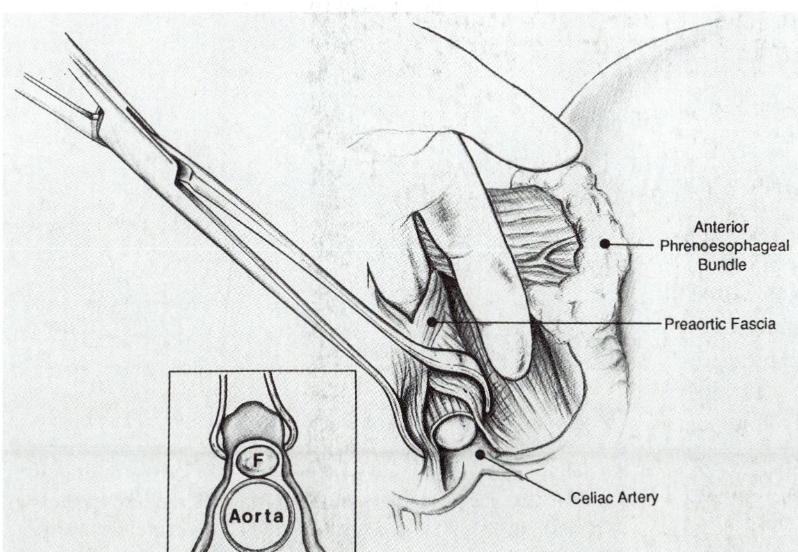


**Figure 45–9.** The fibroareolar tissue in the esophageal hiatus is divided, and a finger (F) is passed down posterior to the preaortic fascia. Sutures may then be placed in the preaortic fascia without dissecting out the median arcuate ligament. The preaortic fascia is lifted off the aorta with a Babcock or stay suture.

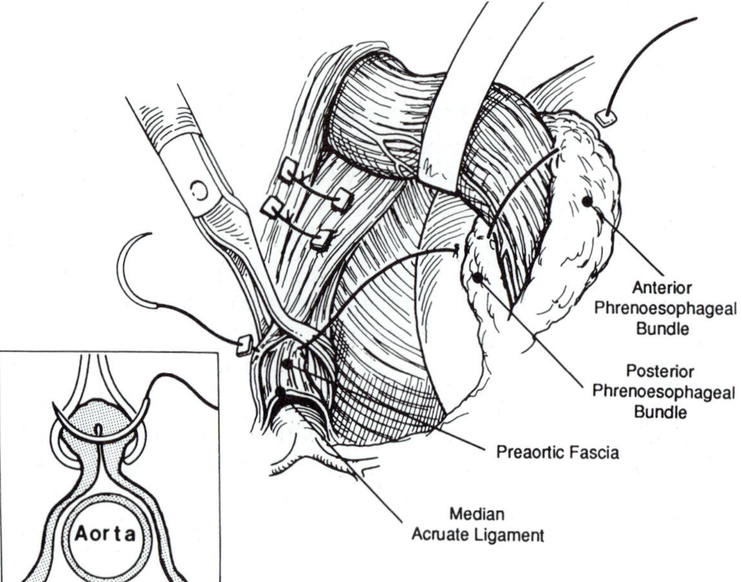


**Figure 45–10.** The hiatus is closed loosely about the esophagus, and suturing is begun in the anterior and posterior phrenoesophageal bundles and carried through the preaortic fascia. The median arcuate ligament is not dissected out. Four such sutures are placed, and the top suture is tied with a single throw and a knot tied to allow for pressure measurements and alteration of the sutures according to the pressure obtained.

of the modified nasogastric tube attached to a monitor through the GE junction. If the pressure is greater than 40 mm Hg, the sutures are loosened. If it is less than 25 mm Hg, the sutures are tightened, depending on the problem at hand. After the proper pressure of 25–35 mm Hg is obtained, all five sutures are tied, and the surgeon takes a final pressure measurement by pulling the tube out at a steady rate. The barrier is usually 3–4 cm long. Additional cardiodiaphragmatic sutures are placed. The final appearance of the repair is shown in Figure 45–11. In addition to restoration of the sphincter, the GEV is accentuated and can be readily palpated through the wall of the stomach. The valve measures 3–4 cm along the lesser curve and is important in the prevention of reflux. In patients who have had previous operations with scarring and destruction of the GE junction, the valve may be destroyed or inadequate. In these patients, a gastrostomy is performed and the valve is secured with sutures in the anterior and posterior edges of the valve, lengthening the valve to 3–4 cm. Attempts to calibrate the cardia with a bougie are unsatisfactory. It is impossible to determine whether the wrap around the bougie is too tight or too loose.

## LAPAROSCOPIC TECHNIQUE

The laparoscopic technique is basically the same as the open technique. It is performed through six 10-mm ports with a pneumoperitoneum with carbon dioxide to a pressure of 14–15 mm Hg. A 30°, 10 mm laparoscope (forward oblique) and video camera are used. Trocars and retractors are introduced under direct vision (Fig. 45–12). The phrenoesophageal membrane is incised, and the phrenoesophageal bundles are retained on the stomach as described earlier. The diaphragm and preaortic fascia are exposed, and the crura are then closed loosely about the esophagus. Four repair sutures are placed through the anterior and posterior phrenoesophageal bundles and the preaortic fascia and tied with a single throw in the knot with a knot pusher. This maneuver approximates the phrenoesophageal bundles to the preaortic fascia and places tension on the cardia.

Intraoperative pressure measurements are then performed by adjusting suture tension, and an intraluminal

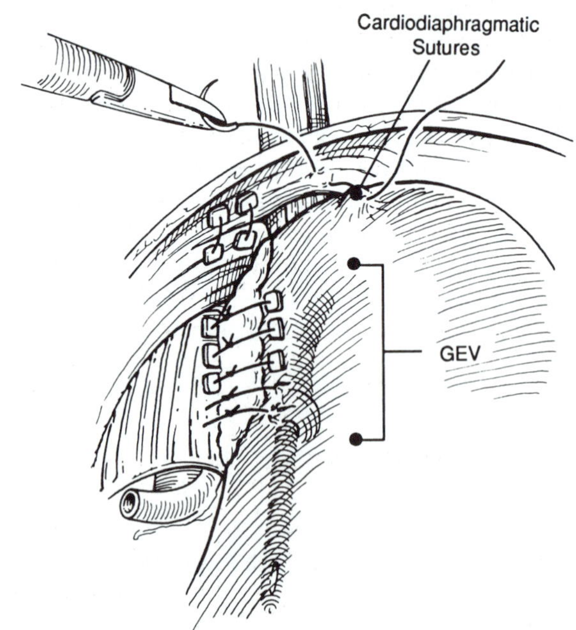


**Figure 45–11.** The final appearance of the repair. All four to five sutures are tied, anchoring the GE junction to the preaortic fascia. If the procedure is open, the GEV can be palpated. If it is done closed, endoscopy is done to check the valve. Cardiodiaphragmatic sutures are placed in to prevent herniation back into the posterior mediastinum.

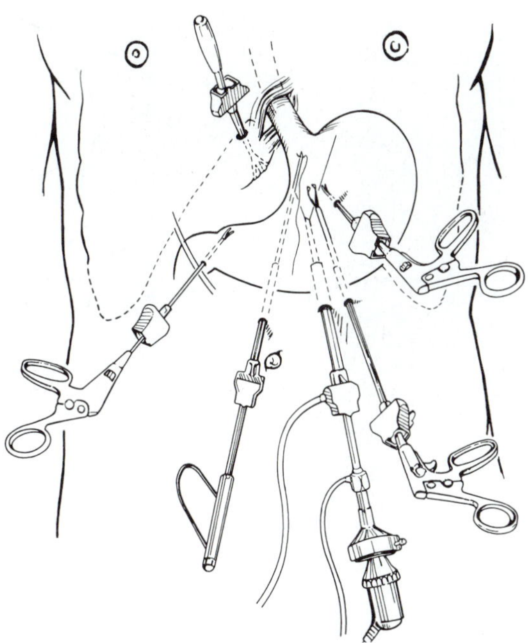

Figure 45–12. For the laparoscopic repair, six trocars are placed as shown. Five of these are 10-mm trocars and one is a 5-mm trocar.

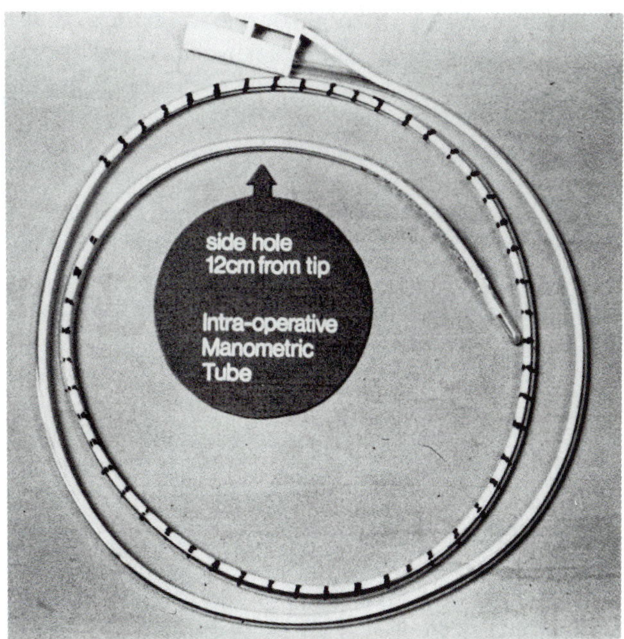


Figure 45–13. Modified nasogastric tube with a side hole, which can be passed back and forth across the LES during the operation to determine the appropriate barrier pressures.

pressure of 25–30 mm Hg is developed. The 15-mm pressure of the pneumoperitoneum should be added to the intraluminal pressure. This produces a postoperative pressure of 18–25 mm Hg, which is ideal. An intraoperative pressure less than 12 mm Hg may not prevent reflux. Intraoperative endoscopy is then performed to ensure that a grade I GEV has been constructed. The musculomucosal fold is tightly apposed to the endoscope through all phases of respiration; it is 3–4 cm long. When the desired suture tension is reached and GEV grade I has been achieved, all sutures are tied. The GEV is further accentuated with placement of three or more additional sutures from the seromuscular layer of the gastric fundus to the edge of the crura of the esophageal hiatus. After final inspection, a second reading of the barrier pressure is obtained. This usually is very close to the first reading. The trocars are removed, and the wounds are closed.

## INTRAOPERATIVE MANOMETRY

In 1978 we reported a simple method of measuring the pressure in the antireflux barrier during operation to give an objective determination of the pressure created.[20] The tip of the smaller polymeric silicone sump portion of a nasogastric tube is sealed, and a 1-cm side hole is cut 18 cm from the tip of the tube (Fig. 45–13). This small tube is attached to a strain gauge and manometer that produces a digital reading. If this manometer is not available, the pressure tube can simply be attached to the arterial line that the anesthesiologist has available. The tube is constantly perfused at a slow rate (0.7 mL/min). This apparatus is identical to the one used in the gastric laboratory and has been thoroughly standardized and used in more than 19,000 patients at our institution. The side hole is passed across the GE junction at operation, and a baseline pressure is obtained before repair. Most often, there is no pressure whatever in the GE junction. As the side hole passes through the junction, both a tracing and a digital readout are obtained. After the repair, pressures are measured and adjustments made as described earlier.

Intraoperative pressure measurements could avoid complications of the Nissen procedure when the wrap is too lose or too tight. The measurement technique described herein is safe and simple and requires only a few minutes to obtain valuable information. An antireflux operation depends on the construction of an adequate barrier. This intraoperative assessment of the barrier should be a standard part of any technique.

The Hill repair is not a fundoplication. The phrenoesophageal bundles are imbricated together with no wrap around the lower esophagus. Often this operation is erroneously described as a partial fundoplication or a wrap. A blind wrap-around of the stomach is not performed but rather careful calibration of the antireflux barrier, restoration of the GEV, and posterior fixation of the GE junction. There is no wrap to slip. The differences between this GE restoration repair and the Nissen repair are as follows.[21]

1. The Hill procedure depends on augmentation of the intrinsic pressure and its special features. By placing tension on the collar-sling musculature, the repair restores

the GEV, which has been shown to be important in the prevention of reflux. The Nissen repair depends on extrinsic pressure of a wrap around the lower esophagus, with indirect pressure on the lower esophagus.[21]

2. The Hill procedure anchors the GE junction posteriorly to its normal primary attachment, the preaortic fascia. The Nissen repair is allowed to float freely, and the GE junction is not anchored. The unanchored esophagus has no fulcrum from which to operate and almost always develops dysmotility, since the esophagus cannot generate propulsive waves.
3. In the Hill procedure, no sutures are used in the esophagus. The esophagus has no serosa and no strength. The Nissen procedure uses esophageal sutures to hold the wrap in place. The weakness of these sutures accounts for the frequency of the slipped Nissen.[22,23] If these sutures are taken deeply, there is a risk of fistula formation from the esophagus.
4. In the Hill procedure, intraoperative pressure measurements calibrate the barrier constructed, giving an objective assessment of the competence of the reflux barrier. This measurement should be used in all repairs, whether the Hill, the Belsey, or the Nissen. In the Nissen procedure, the surgeon relies on a bougie or a finger placed into the esophageal lumen. We have seen a number of patients in whom a large bougie was used, only to find that as soon as the bougie was removed from a wrap that was made too tight, the repair simply closed down. After the bougie was removed from a wrap that was made too loose, the wrap remained open.

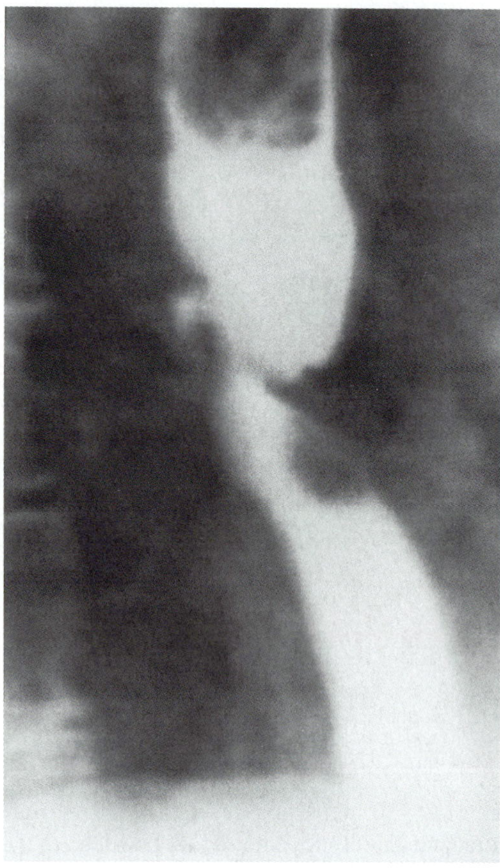

**Figure 45–14.** Stricture with a very narrow lumen and a deep penetrating ulcer. This was considered an undilatable stricture in a short esophagus. The patient was treated with a simplified antireflux procedure.

## PEPTIC ESOPHAGEAL STRICTURE

Surgical management of peptic strictures was controversial because Barrett[3] said in 1950, "Any portion of the gullet lined by columnar epithelium must be stomach." Thus columnar epithelium above the diaphragm was believed to represent congenital shortening of the esophagus, with an intrathoracic stomach. This concept persisted despite the fact that Allison and Johnstone[2] described the columnar epithelium-lined esophagus and stated that the tubular portion of the gullet, even though lined with columnar epithelium above the diaphragm, was indeed esophagus. In 1970 we reported on our experience with 37 patients with advanced stricture, treated with a simplified antireflux procedure.[24] After successful antireflux procedures, these strictures and ulcers opened up with surprising rapidity. Dilation was performed during a surgical procedure and was required in less than half of the patients postoperatively. A representative patient in the reported series had a stricture of the midesophagus with a deep penetrating ulcer (Fig. 45–14). She had been unable to swallow solid food for 3 years and had been told she had an undilatable stricture with a short esophagus. At operation, the esophagus was straightened and the tortuosity eliminated, whereupon bougies could be passed and the stricture dilated. An antireflux gastrointestinal radiograph showed the stricture to be open (Fig. 45–15). This patient underwent surgical treatment in 1970. At last follow-up examination she was well, swallowed all solid food, and had normal upper GI radiographs. Mercer and I reviewed a 20-year experience involving 160 patients undergoing antireflux operations with dilation for peptic esophageal stricture.[25] The mean follow-up period was 47 mo (range 6–240 mo). One hundred seven patients operated on early in the course of the disease had the best results (90% good, 9% fair, 1% poor). Thirty-one patients after a previous failed operation had 52% good, 23% fair, and 26% poor results. Twenty-two patients had multiple dilations. Antireflux procedures in these patients yielded 45% good, 23% fair, and 32% poor results. The postoperative LES pressure in patients without reflux was 17.7±1.3 mm Hg. This was higher than the pressure in patients with reflux (8.9±0.8 mm Hg). Thus a conservative antireflux operation with dilation is the treatment of choice for peptic esophageal strictures. The series has now been expanded to more than 200 patients, which has further confirmed these observations. In patients with multiple previous operations

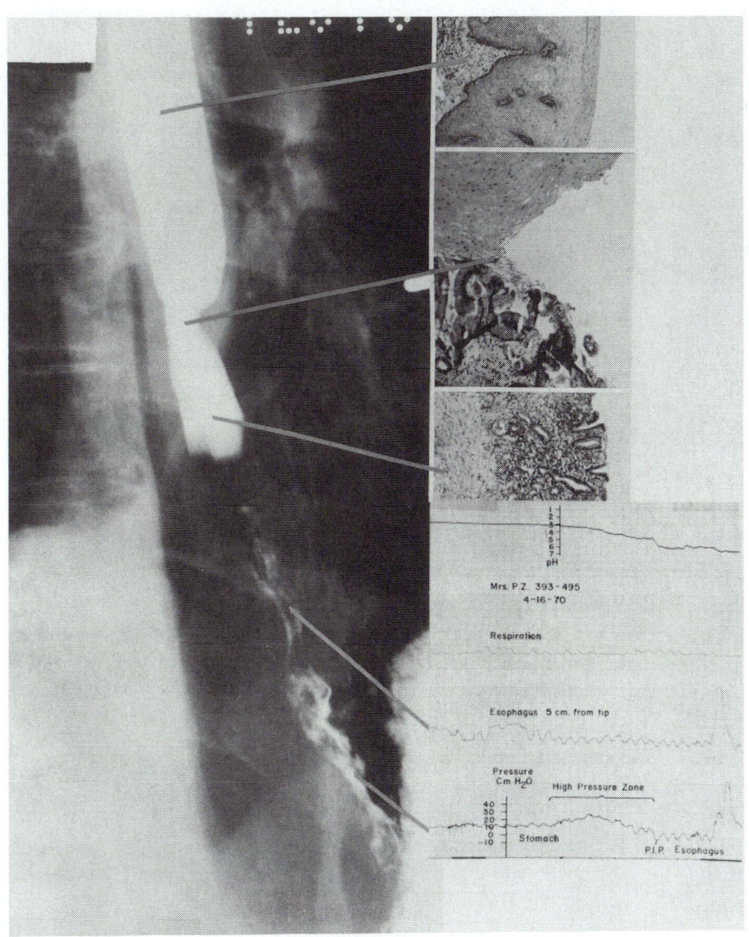


**Figure 45–15.** A composite postoperative study in patient in Figure 45–14 3 weeks after the operation. The stricture has been dilated and an antireflux procedure done. Reflux has been corrected as evidenced by the pH and pressure study, and the stricture has opened. The patient was well 18 years after the operation.

or multiple dilations, in whom transmural damage and fibrosis has destroyed the function of the esophagus, resection with either gastric or colonic interposition is the only choice (see Chap. 47).

## RESULTS

The most important criterion of success is patient satisfaction. If a patient is free of heartburn, can eat a full meal, can resume normal activity, and be productive, then the operation should be considered a success. We have added to this a meticulous follow-up program using pH and pressure studies 2–3 months after the operation, whenever possible.[26]

Numerous series examined the relatively short-term success of currently popular antireflux operations, the Nissen and the Belsey.[27–29] My colleagues and I have performed three retrospective studies of the long-term effect of surgical treatment with the Hill repair. More than 2000 patients have undergone operations over a 25-year-period.[30] The results are excellent or good in more than 94%, with a recurrence rate of about 5%. The complication and mortality rates have been very low at 2.5%, with one death in the last 600 operations for primary repair.

A 15–20 year (mean, 17.8 years) follow-up study of 167 patients is the only study that includes evaluation at an early stage and then a general reassessment of the same population over a 20-year-period.[31] This study showed good to excellent results in 88% of patients. These patients underwent surgical treatment before intraoperative manometrics was introduced into practice. A more recent study of 115 patients who participated in a follow-up study for as long as 8 years after intraoperative pressure measurements and other technologic advances became available showed good to excellent results in 96% of patients. This study was conducted by an ophthalmologist who was far removed from the field of gastrointestinal surgery so that the study might be unbiased.[31]

The main complication in the last 500 patients was dysphagia that necessitated esophageal dilation. Adjustments in intraoperative manometrics and, more recently, raising the level of the intraoperative pressure in the antireflux barrier to only 25–35 mm Hg has nearly eliminated the need for postoperative dilation. Early in our experience, four fistulas resulted from deep biopsy in the esophagus before surgical intervention. If a biopsy of the lower esophagus is required to rule out carcinoma or Barrett's esophagus, we wait at least 2 weeks to allow for the biopsy site to heal before performing an antireflux operation. Only one fistula occurred in a primary repair. The others were in patients who had had previous operations. We have not encountered the devastating fistulas and the severe gas bloat and other complications that have been seen with a slipped Nissen procedure.

## REPRODUCIBILITY

For an operation to be of value, it should be reproducible, with good results, when performed by many surgeons. The Hill repair has been performed and reported by a number of surgeons around the world. Csendes and Larrain in Chile achieved 93% good results and no radiologic recurrence in 29 patients followed as long as 16 months.[32,33] Hermreck and Coates reported success in the United States.[34] Mercer performed the Hill procedure on 110 patients with 95% good results (written communication, 1994). Van Sant et al reported treating 400 patients with about 90% good results over the long term without the complications reported with the Nissen procedure.[35]

## SUMMARY

The Hill procedure includes reconstruction of the normal GE junction, restoration of the GEV, and restoration of the esophagus to its normal point of attachment or fulcrum, which allows it to generate forceful peristaltic waves to propel food into the stomach. Thus esophageal motility is restored. The sphincter is calibrated, and the pressure is measured to produce pressure that is high enough to prevent reflux but not so high as to produce dysphagia. The GEV is restored, and the diaphragm is closed loosely around the esophagus. With careful selection of patients and careful performance of the procedure, good results can be obtained over the long term.

## ACKNOWLEDGMENT

This work was supported in part by the Ryan Hill Research Foundation.

## REFERENCES

1. Fyke RE, Code CF, Schleggel JF: The GE sphincter in healthy human beings. *Gastroenterology* **86:**135–150, 1956
2. Allison PR, Johnstone AS: The oesophagus lined with gastric mucous membrane. *Thorax* **8:**87–101, 1953
3. Barrett NR: The lower esophagus lined by columnar epithelium. *Surgery* **41:**881–894, 1957
4. Thor KBA, Hill LD, Mercer CD, Kozarek RA: Reappraisal of the flap valve mechanism: A study of a new valvuloplasty procedure in cadavers. *Acta Chir Scand* **153:**25–28, 1987
5. Morgan EH, Hill LD, Siemsen JK, et al: Studies of intraluminal esophageal and gastric pressure and pH. *Bull Mason Clin* **14:**53–89, 1960
6. Hill LD, Morgan EH, Kellogg HB: Experimentation as an aid in management of esophageal disorders. *Am J Surg* **102:**240–253, 1961
7. Mittal RK, Dudley F, Rochester DF, McCallum R: Sphincteric action of the diaphragm during a relaxed lower esophageal sphincter in humans. *J Am Physiol Soc* G139, 1989
8. Havelund T, Laursen LS, Skubo-Kristensen E, et al: Omeprazole and ranitidine in treatment of reflux oesophagitis: Double blind comparative trial. *Br Med J* **296:**89–92, 1988
9. Klinkenberg-Knol EC, Jansen JMB, Festen HPM, et al: Double-blind multicenter comparison of omeprazole and ranitidine in the treatment of reflux oesophagitis. *Lancet* **1:**349–351, 1987
10. Spechler SJ and the VA GERD Study Group, Department of Veteran's Affairs: Comparison of medical and surgical therapy for complicated gastroesophageal reflux disease in veterans. *N Engl J Med* **362:**786–792, 1992
11. Patterson DJ, Graham DY, Smith JL, et al: Natural history of benign esophageal stricture treated by dilatation. *Gastroenterology* **85:**346–350, 1983
12. Watson A: The role of antireflux surgery combined with fiberoptic endoscopic dilatation in peptic esophageal stricture. *Am J Surg* **148:**346–349, 1984
13. Larrain A, Pope CE: Respiratory complications of gastroesophageal reflux. In Hill LD, Kozarek R, McCallum R, Mercer CD (eds): *The Esophagus: Medical and Surgical Management.* Philadelphia, Saunders, 1988, pp 70–77
14. Cameron AJ, Ott BJ, Payne WS: The incidence of adenocarcinoma in columnar-lined (Barrett's) esophagus. *N Engl J Med* **313:**857–859, 1985
15. Reid BJ, Weinstein WM, Lewin KJ, et al: Endoscopic biopsy can detect high-grade dysplasia or early adenocarcinoma in Barrett's esophagus without grossly recognizable neoplastic lesions. *Gastroenterology* **94:**81–90, 1988
16. Reid BJ, Haggitt RC, Rubin CE, Rabinovitch PS: Barrett's esophagus: Correlation between flow cytometry and histology in detection of patients at risk for adenocarcinoma. *Gastroenterology* **93:**1–11, 1987
17. Brand DL, Vivisaker JT, Gelfard M, Pope CE II: Regression of columnar esophageal (Barrett's) epithelium after anti-reflux surgery. *N Engl J Med* **302:**844–848, 1980
18. Brand DL, Eastwood IR, Martin D, et al: Esophageal symptoms, manometry and histology before and after antireflux surgery: A long-term follow-up study. *Gastroenterology* **76:**1393–1401, 1979
19. Russell COH, Hill LD, Holmes ER III, et al: Radionuclide transit: A sensitive screening test for esophageal dysfunction. *Gastroenterology* **80:**887–892, 1981
20. Hill LD: Intraoperative measurement of lower esophageal sphincter pressure. *J Thorac Cardiovasc Surg* **75:**378–382, 1978
21. Nissen R: Eine einfache operation zur beeinflussung der refluxoesophagitis. *Schweiz Med Wochenschr* **86:**590, 1956
22. Leonardi HK, Crozier RE, Ellis FH: Reoperation for complications of the Nissen fundoplication. *J Thorac Cardiovasc Surg* **81:**50–56, 1981
23. Negre JB: Post fundoplication symptoms: Do they restrict the success of Nissen fundoplication? *Ann Surg* **198:**698–700, 1983
24. Hill LD, Gelfland M, Bauermeister D: Simplified management of reflux esophagitis with stricture. *Ann Surg* **172:**639–651, 1970
25. Mercer CD, Hill LD: Surgical management of peptic esophageal stricture. *J Thorac Cardiovasc Surg* **91:**371–378, 1986
26. Hill LD, Chapman KW, Morgan EH: Objective evaluation of surgery for hiatus hernia and esophagitis. *J Thorac Cardiovasc Surg* **41:**60, 1961
27. Little AG, Ferguson MK, Skinner DB: Reoperation for failed antireflux operations. *Surgery* **91:**511–517, 1986
28. Rossetti M, Hell K: Fundoplication for the treatment of gastroesophageal reflux in hiatal hernia. *World J Surg* **1:**439–444, 1977
29. Low DE, Mercer CD, James EC, Hill LD: Post Nissen syndrome. *Surg Gynecol Obstet* **167:**1–5, 1988

30. Hill LD, Aye RW, Ramel SO: Antireflux surgery: A surgeon's look. *Gastroenterol Clin North Am* **19:**745–775, 1990
31. Low DE, Anderson RP, Ilves R, et al: Fifteen to twenty year results after the Hill antireflux operation. *J Thorac Cardiovasc Surg* **98:**444–450, 1989
32. Csendes A, Braghetto I: Highly selective vagotomy, posterior gastropexy and calibration of the cardia for reflux esophagitis. In Hill LD, Kozarek R, McCallum R, Mercer CD (eds): *The Esophagus: Medical and Surgical Management.* Philadelphia: Saunders, 1988, Chap 9, pp 129–135
33. Larrain A, Carrasco J, Galleguillos P, Pope CE II: Reflux treatment improves lung function by patients with intrinsic asthma. *Gastroenterology* **80**(5, Part 2):1204, 1978
34. Hermreck AS, Coates NR: Results of the Hill antireflux operation. *Am J Surg* **140:**764–767, 1980
35. Van Sant JH, Baker JW, Ross DG: Modification of the Hill technique for repair of hiatal hernia. *Surg Gynecol Obstet* **143:**637–642, 1976

CHAPTER

# 46

# The Belsey Mark IV Procedure

Ronald H.R. Belsey and Arthur E. Baue

The surgical management of gastroesophageal reflux and hiatal hernia remains controversial. There is a lack of agreement on the indications for surgical treatment. A variety of antireflux procedures currently are used with little objective information about the merits and lack of merit of each technique in relation to the patient's condition or the underlying disease. Because of the lack of intensive long-term follow-up studies based on personal interview and laboratory investigation, obscurity shrouds the late results of various operations. Surgeons and gastroenterologists disagree on the criteria for assessing the long-term results of treatment. Many surgeons in this field do not comprehend the basic pathophysiology of reflux and the logical approach to the technical problems involved in the restoration of a permanent and competent antireflux mechanism to the gastroesophageal junction. The solution is further obscured by uncertainty regarding the contribution of various physiologic factors to the maintenance of gastroesophageal competence in healthy people. The development of new and powerful acid-reducing agents has controlled symptoms in many patients, allowed esophagitis to heal, and decreased the need for operative treatment.

Comparison of the results of various techniques and clarification of the special indications for these techniques in different clinical circumstances demand the general acceptance and application of the following rigid criteria for assessing late results: (1) complete and permanent relief of all symptoms and complications, (2) the ability to belch and relieve gas distention of the stomach (the gas-bloat syndrome) voluntarily when necessary, (3) the ability to vomit when necessary, (4) objective proof of the control of reflux with 24-hour pH studies, (5) the ability to communicate the technique to the resident or trainee surgeon of average competence, and (6) restoration of the patient's ability to lead a normal, full life with no further medical, postural, or dietetic treatment. The satisfaction of these criteria should be the minimum requirement for any method of treatment to be regarded as adequate.

## MARK IV REPAIR

### Advantages of the Thoracic Approach

1. If retention of the lower esophageal sphincter, the distal 4–5 cm of esophagus in the high-pressure region below the diaphragm, is the essential feature of a satisfactory antireflux procedure, extensive mobilization of the esophagus is necessary. This can be achieved only by the thoracic route. The laboratory studies of DeMeester et al have confirmed this operative concept as the basis of antireflux surgery.[1]
2. Adequate access to the upper abdomen for attention to coexisting abnormalities is afforded by an extended left sixth interspace thoracotomy or by taking the diaphragm down from the chest wall.
3. For recurrent gastroesophageal reflux and especially after multiple previous surgical interventions, the thoracic route is mandatory.
4. The thoracic route is the mandatory approach in the treatment of reflux complicated by chronic fibrosing esophagitis with shortening and stenosis when resection and reconstruction or a Collis gastroplasty may be necessary.
5. The Mark IV repair is effective when an antireflux procedure is a necessary adjunct to a long myotomy for various functional disorders of the esophagus, such as achalasia of the cardia and diffuse esophageal spasm. A Nissen fundoplication following a myotomy can result in intractable dysphagia.
6. The long-term results of the Mark IV repair have been well documented. The recurrence rate is 6% or less

when the operation is performed by a trained surgeon as opposed to 14.6% when performed by residents or interns at an early stage of training.[2,3]

### Disadvantages of the Thoracic Route

1. Most surgeons confronted with the problem of gastroesophageal reflux are oriented toward the abdomen and less familiar with thoracotomy techniques and management of postthoracotomy complications.
2. It is claimed that the abdominal approach facilitates the correction of coexisting upper abdominal disease, a claim unsubstantiated in fact and outweighed by the other advantages of the thoracic approach.
3. Postthoracotomy discomfort is the main disadvantage but can be controlled or eliminated by attention to details of thoracotomy technique.
4. The abdominal approach can be justified in cases of reflux complicated by severe pulmonary fibrosis due to recurring aspiration pneumonitis in the absence of chronic fibrosing esophagitis.

## TECHNIQUE OF THE MARK IV REPAIR

### Preoperative Treatment

A course of thoracic physiotherapy to control aspiration pneumonitis and maintain pulmonary function in the immediately postoperative period is necessary.

### Thoracotomy Technique

Access is through an oblique posterolateral thoracotomy incision over the sixth left interspace. The latissimus dorsi and serratus anterior muscles are divided as low as possible or dissected from their costal origins to maintain maximum function. The intercostal tissues are dissected from the upper border of the seventh rib, and the left pleura is entered through the periosteal bed of this rib. The intercostal incision is carried forward to the costal margin. Posteriorly, the sacrospinalis muscle is retracted backward, and 1 cm of the posterior end of the seventh rib is resected subperiosteally beneath the muscle, which stabilizes the cut ends of the seventh rib when restored to its normal position. The seventh intercostal bundle is ligated and divided before the ribs are distracted to prevent traction injuries to the posterior nerve root. Most postthoracotomy discomfort is situated in the cord or posterior roots rather than lateral chest wall. In children it is not necessary to divide a rib. The sixth and seventh ribs should be separated gently and only sufficiently to achieve manual access to the hiatus. Aggressive distraction by mechanical rib spreaders, such as the Finocietto, inevitably increases postoperative discomfort.

The technique of closure is important. The sixth and seventh ribs should be restored to their normal relations with loosely tied pericostal sutures. Tight approximation of these ribs causes pain. Airtight closure of the intercostal incision is unnecessary with correctly placed catheter drainage of the pleura, and no surgical emphysema results. The chest wall is repaired in three layers with continuous monafilament stainless steel wire suture material, which causes no tissue reaction and, in the event of superficial wound infection, does not retard healing or cause stitch sinuses. The thoracotomy technique has been described in some detail, because attention to these points reduces or eliminates postoperative discomfort.

### The Extended Left Thoracotomy

When access to the upper abdomen is necessary to allow treatment of additional disease such as cholecystitis or peptic ulceration of the stomach or duodenum, the incision is extended forward and downward to the margin of the rectus sheath, the costal margin is divided at the anterior extremity of the sixth interspace, and the oblique muscles are divided for 1–2 inches (2.5–5.0 cm). The diaphragm is then separated from its costal origin anteriorly for a distance of approximately 15 cm, leaving a 2-cm fringe on the chest wall for subsequent reattachment, and retracted upward with its nerve supply intact. An excellent exposure of the upper abdomen is thus presented. During closure a short segment of the costal margin can be resected to prevent any unsightly overlap of the cut ends, but these ends should not be wired together, since a painful chondritis may ensue and necessitate a later resection of the inflamed cartilage.

Peritoneal cavity exposure can also be obtained with an intact costochondral arch. Should it be necessary to gain access to the peritoneal cavity through a left thoracotomy, this can be done by incising the diaphragm about 2 cm from its insertion into the chest wall from the substernal region to the lateral chest wall (Fig. 46–1). The costochondral arch is intact, and the problems of postoperative pain are avoided. Such an approach could be required to mobilize the stomach with a recurrent hernia, to do a pylorotomy, or for other problems. The diaphragm can then be closed with interrupted mattress sutures. The diaphragm and its phrenic nerve innervation are intact and fully functional.

### Objective of the Mark IV Repair

The basic principle of the Mark IV procedure is restoration of the lower esophageal sphincter zone to the high-pressure region below the diaphragm and its permanent maintenance in that situation. The exact position and extent of the sphincter cannot be determined accurately at external examination of the lower esophagus during the dissection. In a series of more than 2000 procedures according to this principle, however, it was observed by trial and error that restoration of a length of 4–5 cm of lower esophagus to the high-pressure region resulted in an effective antireflux mechanism. The repair is physiologic in objective and de-

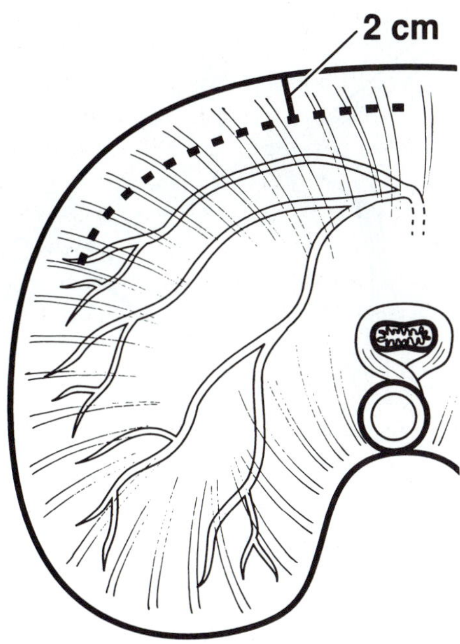


**Figure 46–1.** The peritoneal cavity can be entered by way of an incision in the diaphragm close to the costal insertion. This preserves the costochondral junction and the diaphragm.

signed to restore all the normal functions of a competent cardia, including the ability to belch and vomit when necessary. Mechanical obstruction plays no part in the completed repair. The purpose of the 240° fundoplication involved in the procedure is to enable the fundus of the stomach to embrace the lower sphincter zone with sufficient determination to retain it permanently in the high-pressure region when restored to the abdomen.

A posterior buttress is made by means of approximation of the two halves of the right crus to afford counterpressure against which the lower sphincter zone can be compressed by the positive intraabdominal and intragastric pressures. Narrowing the hiatus plays no part in the control of reflux. Technical errors perpetrated by surgeons not intimately acquainted with the subtlety of the Mark IV technique arise chiefly from failure to appreciate these basic principles.[4,5]

## Details of Operative Technique

1. Mobilization of the esophagus and cardia.
2. Construction of the posterior buttress.
3. 240° fundoplication.
4. Reduction of the hernia and restoration of the lower sphincter zone to the abdomen.

### *Mobilization*

Adequate exposure through a left sixth interspace thoracotomy incision is essential. The esophagus is mobilized up to the point where the vagus nerves pass from the hila of the lungs to the middle third of the esophagus, close to the aortic arch. This mobilization involves division of the middle esophageal artery, the large vessel running from the descending aorta to the junction of the middle and lower thirds of the organ and frequently the inferior bronchial artery (Fig. 46–2). It may be necessary to mobilize the esophagus up to and under the aortic arch. Provided that the ascending or esophageal branch of the left gastric artery is preserved, no risk to the viability of the lower half of the esophagus is involved in this degree of mobilization.

Mobilization of the cardia is equally important. After opening the peritoneal cavity through the hiatus, four or five of the uppermost short gastric arteries are divided. An important limitation for the novice in performing this operation is inadequate mobilization of the greater curve of the stomach for the wrap around the esophagus. Sufficient free greater curve allows a loose partial wrap around the esophagus. The finger is passed medially and posteriorly through the upper portion of the gastrohepatic omentum into the lesser sac. The finger is passed between the left gastric artery and a band of tissue at the upper limit of the gastrohepatic omentum that contains an important vessel known as Belsey's artery. This artery is a communicating vessel between the esophageal branch of the left gastric artery and the inferior phrenic artery. The artery and the surrounding band of tissue must be divided before complete mobilization of the cardia can be achieved. The proximal end of the artery is doubly ligated, because on division it retracts into the abdominal cavity, and any subsequent hemorrhage due to slipping of the ligatures will be difficult to control. A common error is failure to identify and to divide this vessel and failure to mobilize the cardia adequately. The entire esophagogastric junction must be free from the hiatus of the diaphragm. If the stomach is attached to the hiatus, it cannot be placed down far enough into the peritoneal cavity to have 4–5 cm of intraperitoneal esophagus.

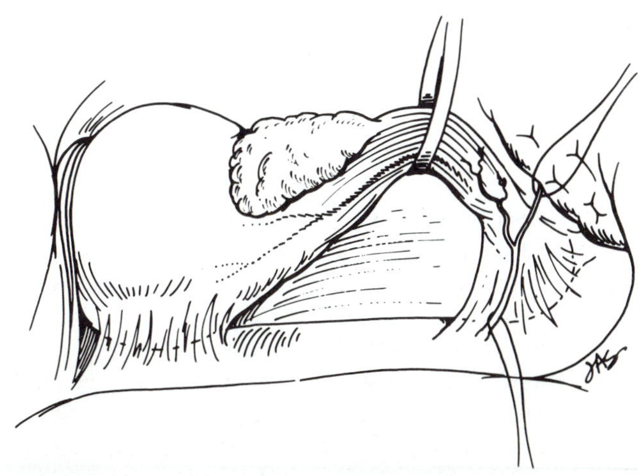

**Figure 46–2.** The esophagus is mobilized from the hiatus to the aortic arch with division of the esophageal vessels. A tape around the esophagus facilitates exposure.

### *Preparation of the Posterior Buttress*

Stout sutures are passed through the two halves of the right crus posteriorly (Fig. 46–3). It is essential that these sutures include the dense fibrous core of the inner half of the right crus. This is facilitated by putting tension on the crus with traction forceps applied to the central tendon of the diaphragm. The sutures do not pass through the weak intercrural muscle fibers. Failure to place the buttressing sutures correctly may lead to a posterior recurrence of the hernia. Three to five sutures are usually required, depending on the size of the hiatus. They are not tied until a later stage in the operation.

### *The Fundoplication*

Before the fundoplication is performed, the fat pad lying in front of the cardia and esophagus must be completely removed, because its retention results in an oily bursa lying between the fundus of the stomach and the esophagus, which prevents the necessary adhesion between these organs (Fig. 46–4). As the fat paid is resected, the vagus nerves are mobilized and allowed to fall posteriorly behind the esophagus. The integrity of the vagi must be preserved. Mobilization of the vagi does not interfere with esophageal peristalsis. If the vagi are damaged during this maneuver, the thoracotomy is extended anteriorly, the diaphragm is detached, and a pyloromyotomy is performed to prevent gastric stasis. A pyloromyotomy involves less risk of duodenal reflux than a formal pyloroplasty.

A 240° anterior fundoplication is performed with two rows of mattress sutures of nonabsorbable suture, three sutures to a row, to embrace the lower 4–5 cm of esophagus. Silk should not be used, because it will fragment later. These mattress sutures are designed to obtain an adequate grip of both the circular and longitudinal muscle fibers of the esophagus. The esophageal and gastric mucosae must not be penetrated by these sutures. Each suture is passed vertically, first with a bite of the seromuscular layer of the stomach 2–3 cm below the apparent esophageal junction, then through the muscle layer of the esophagus 2 cm above the junction. Manual shortening of the esophagus elevates the muscle layer off the underlying mucosa and protects the latter from perforation during the passage of the suture. The suture is then reversed and re-entered to the muscle layer 5 mm nearer the midline of the organ. The suture now descends through this layer, again attaining an adequate bite of both longitudinal and circular muscle layers. It then picks up a similar bite of the seromuscular layer of the stomach wall 2 cm below the junction, emerging 5 mm lateral to the original point of entry. Three mattress sutures are inserted in the first row to embrace 240° of the anterior circumference of the organ. These sutures are now tied very gently to achieve tissue apposition without tissue strangulation. Only living tissue heals (Fig. 46–5). Aggressive suturing in this situation damages the esophageal muscle layer and leads to breakdown of the repair.

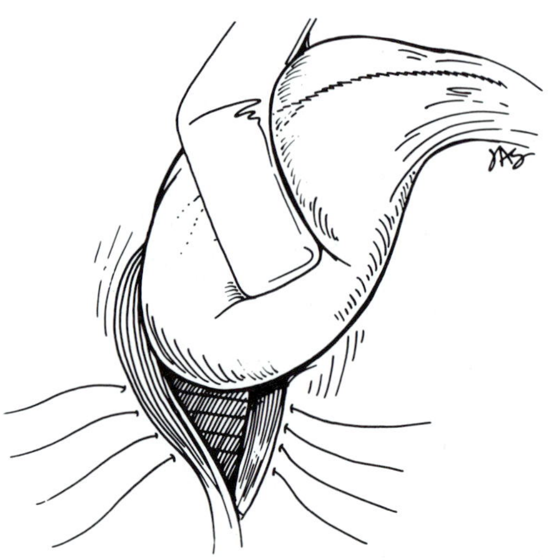

Figure 46–3. Sutures are placed with large bites through each side of the right crus of the diaphragm. These are tied later, approximating the right crus of the diaphragm behind the esophagus to form a buttress and also to narrow the hiatus.

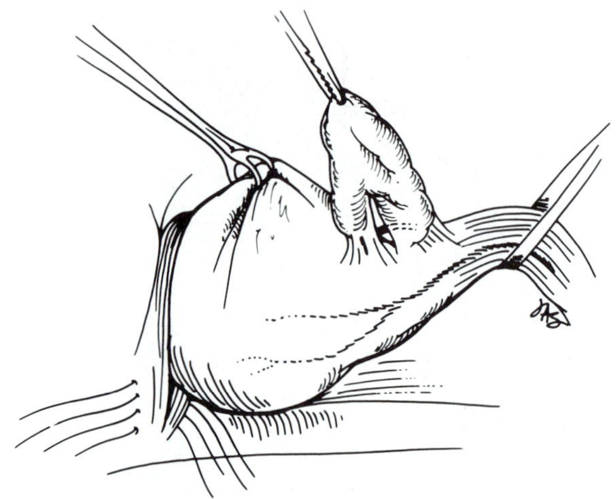

Figure 46–4. The fat pad at the esophagastric junction is removed.

A second row of three mattress sutures is inserted. These sutures are passed down through the diaphragm, first at the point where the muscular margin of the hiatus meets the central tendon, then through the muscular layers of the stomach and of the esophagus as in the initial row but at a higher level in the esophagus. They return in the opposite direction and up through the diaphragm in the reverse direction (Fig. 46–6). The placement of these sutures through the diaphragm is facilitated by a spoon-shaped retractor passed through the hiatus to prevent inclusion of any abdominal viscera in the sutures. The necessity for gentle tying of the second row of fundoplicating sutures, to preserve the integrity of the fragile muscle layer, must again be emphasized.

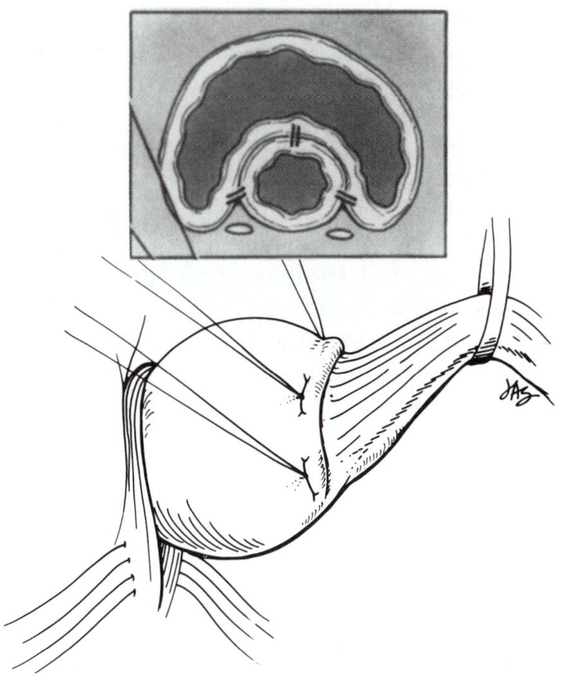

Figure 46–5. The first row of three mattress sutures is in place and tied, plicating the stomach around the esophagus through 240° from just above one vagus nerve to the other.

### Reduction of the Hernia

The reduction must be achieved manually to avoid damage to the esophagus by traction on the mattress sutures. If adequate mobilization has been achieved initially, there will be no tendency for the lower segment of esophagus to return to the pleural cavity. The stomach and esophagus are gently pushed below the diaphragm. As this is done the mattress sutures are gently pulled up to take out the slack. The hernia must not be reduced by pulling up on the mattress sutures, or the sutures will pull out. After the complete manual reduction has been effected, the second row of mattress sutures is again tied very gently to preserve the integrity of the esophageal muscle layer. The object of these sutures is merely to maintain the reduction achieved manually. If the mattress sutures have been correctly placed, 4–5 cm of esophagus lie in the high-pressure region below the diaphragm embraced by a 240° wrap of gastric fundus. Finally, the posterior buttress is made by tying the intercrural sutures, previously placed, from behind forward. Before the last stitch is tied, a finger must be passed through the hiatus posteriorly to ascertain that there is no aggressive reduction in the size of the hiatus, since this plays no part in the antireflux mechanism (Fig. 46–7). If there is doubt it is better to leave the hiatus too loose than too tight, and it may be necessary to remove the last buttress suture. The object of the buttress is to produce counterpressure against which the lower esophagus can be compressed by the positive intragastric pressure. Mild dysphagia in the immediately postoperative period due to edema of the tissue is acceptable, but persisting dysphagia should never occur if the posterior buttress is correctly established.

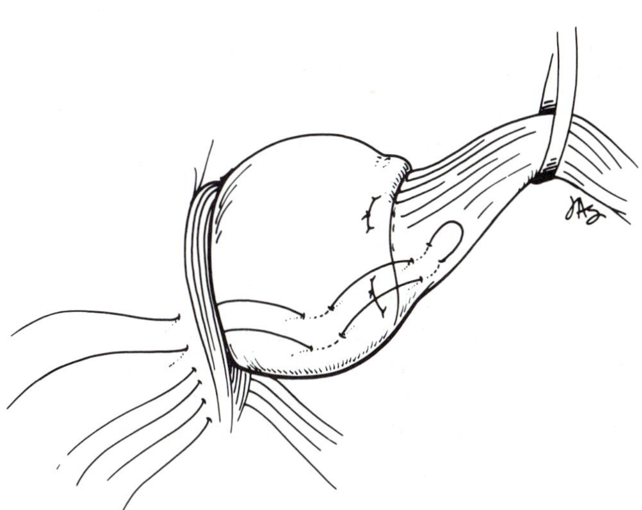

Figure 46–6. The second row of mattress sutures is being placed from the esophagus to the stomach and then through the hiatus and out through the diaphragm on the pleural surface. When the hernia is reduced and these sutures are tied, further stomach is imbricated around the esophagus, and this entire repair is held firmly beneath the diaphragm.

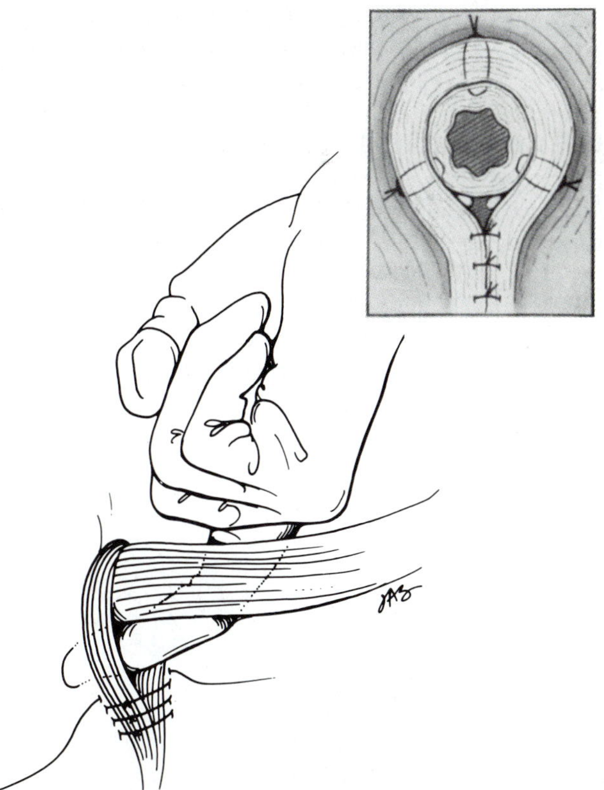

Figure 46–7. The second row of sutures has been tied after reduction of the hernia. A finger has been inserted posteriorly. The posterior sutures in the right crus of the diaphragm have been tied, approximating it, and the finger tests the size of the lumen. An index finger should be able to pass easily through the hiatus posterior to the repair. This completes the repair and the plication.

### The Belsey Mark V Operation

The senior author (R.H.R.B.) predicted that someone, sometime would modify the Mark IV operation to try to improve on it. The junior author (A.E.B.) treated two young male patients who had recurrences a few years after a Mark IV operation. Both patients had very physical occupations, climbing telephone poles and carrying hods. Both had first one row and then later the second row of sutures pull out of the esophagus during vigorous exertion. These patients were unlike the housewives and pubkeepers of Bristol, England, whom Belsey had treated when he developed the operation. A modification was in order. Sutures in the muscle layer of the esophagus were similar to sewing closed an incision in the muscle of the left ventricle of the heart. Pledgets were required to buttress the mattress sutures in the heart. Muscle repairs of inguinal hernias are known to be inadequate. Thus for the sutures on the esophagus, small pledgets of Teflon (polytetrafluoroethylene) felt was used (Fig. 46–8). Pledgets also were used on the stomach for the first row of three stitches and on the esophagus and diaphragm for the second row (Fig. 46–9). This procedure has been used routinely since 1964 by the junior author. There have been no complications from these pledgets. They have not eroded into the esophagus or stomach. There have been no fistulas and no recurrences. This modification was called the Belsey Mark V.[6] It has been roundly condemned by some Mark IV zealots on the basis of inadequate evidence.

## POSTOPERATIVE CARE

Thoracic physiotherapy is resumed immediately after the patient emerges from anesthesia. The intercostal catheter is removed as soon as the left lung is fully expanded, and any drainage of serum is reduced to a trickle, usually at the end of 24–48 hours. A nasogastric tube is not inserted routinely at the end of the operation, because of the tendency of the tube to cause reflux and to increase the risk of postoperative pulmonary complications. In the event of gastric distention in the postoperative period, a nasogastric tube can be passed temporarily to relieve the distention. Some surgeons use a nasogastric tube routinely for 1–2 days. Almost all patients can be extubated at the end of the procedure and returned to their rooms. Of the more than 2000 patients who underwent this procedure in the Bristol unit and in the Bristol Children's Hospital, in not one instance was there any necessity for positive-pressure pulmonary support in the postoperative period. Routine use of an epidural catheter is helpful for pain control and may require admission to an intensive care unit for 24 hours.

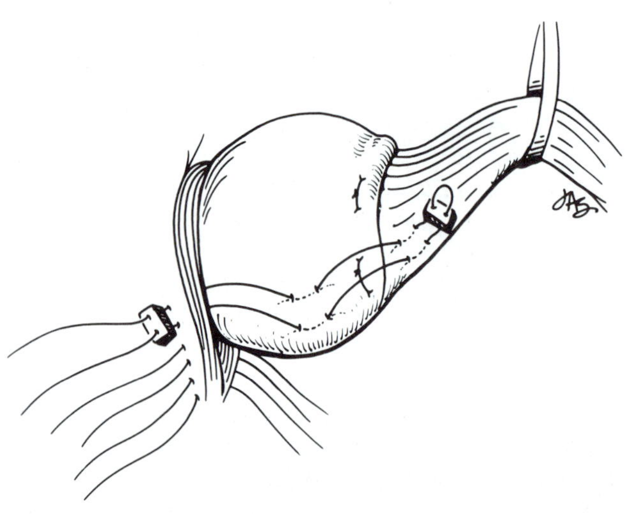

Figure 46–8. The Belsey Mark V adds Teflon felt pledgets to buttress the sutures in muscle.

## POSTOPERATIVE COMPLICATIONS

Apart from the complications that can follow any mismanaged thoracotomy incision, such as inadequate pleural drainage, there are no specific complications attendant upon the technique. Intraperitoneal hemorrhage may follow failure to identify and secure Belsey's artery during mobilization of the cardia. Postoperative dysphagia may result from unnecessary narrowing of the hiatus during construction of the posterior buttress, but the gas-bloat syndrome has not been encountered. Mechanical obstruction plays no part in the control of reflux with this technique. Gastric stasis may rarely follow unrecognized damage to the vagus nerves during mobilization of the esophagus. The only late complication recorded has been recurrent reflux due to technical errors perpetrated by residents and surgeons unfamiliar with the subtleties of the technique. An important advantage has been elimination of dramatic late complications, occasionally lethal, that have been reported after alternative techniques.

The mortality in a series of more than 2500 operations performed by us or by residents and assistants has been less than 1%; the deaths were usually due to cerebrovascular or cardiac complications.

## ERRORS IN TECHNIQUE

1. Inadequate exposure.
2. Inadequate mobilization of the esophagus and the cardia of the stomach.
3. Faulty placement of the posterior buttressing sutures.
4. Overaggressive suturing in creating the 240° fundoplication.

## CONTRAINDICATIONS TO THE MARK IV ANTIREFLUX PROCEDURE

1. Lack of familiarity with the technique.
2. Inadequate training in thoracotomy technique and postthoracotomy management.

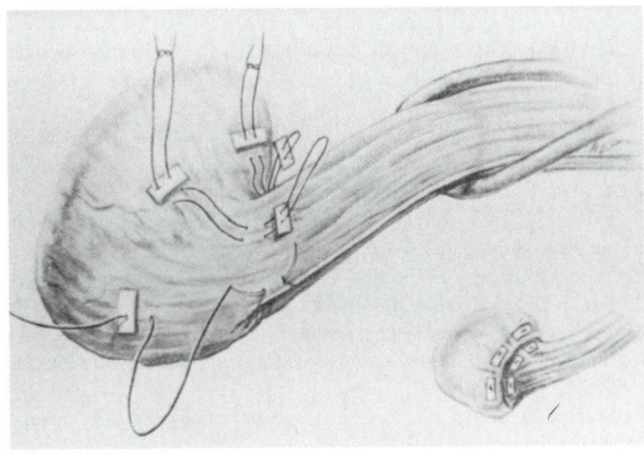

A

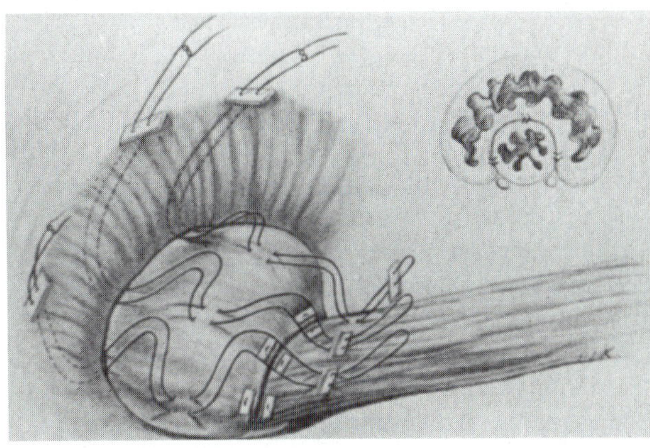

B

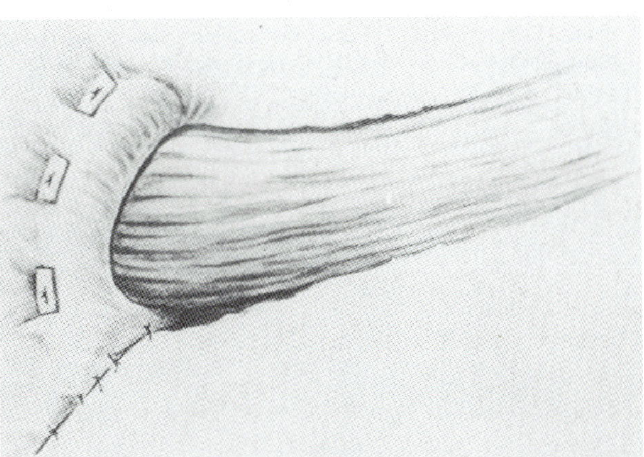

C

**Figure 46–9.** Details of the Belsey Mark V. **A.** First row **B.** Second row **C.** Completed repair.

3. Extensive acquired shortening of the organ from chronic esophagitis, preventing the restoration of the lower sphincter segment to the high-pressure infradiaphragmatic region. A modified Collis gastroplasty or resection and replacement of the stenosed segment by means of interposition of an isoperistaltic segment of left colon or jejunum may be indicated in this situation.[7]
4. Pulmonary insufficiency due to recurring aspiration pneumonitis, which may indicate an abdominal rather than a thoracic approach.

## LONG-TERM RESULTS

In a series of 892 consecutive patients in the Bristol series whose records were reviewed by Orringer et al, 680 of whom were followed for 5 years or longer, the recurrence rate following procedures performed by faculty members was 5.9%. After procedures performed by residents and interns in a resident training program the recurrence rate was 14.6%. (The overall recurrence rate was 12%).[2] Few recorded results indicate the influence of operator experience. The late results were documented as satisfactory only when all the criteria for an acceptable antireflux procedure had been fully met. The causes of recurrence were attempts to perform a physiologic repair in unsuitable cases of chronic peptic esophagitis with stenosis and acquired shortening of the organ due to mural fibrosis, attempts to control reflux in infants and young children, and the technical errors inevitable in any resident training program.

It is not possible to compare the long-term results of various surgical antireflux procedures because there is no general agreement as to the indications for operation and the criteria for assessing late results. No survey has so far been encountered reporting the late results of other techniques, on the basis of the criteria outlined, in a series of 500 patients or more followed by personal interview for a minimum period of 5 years or longer after the operation.

The frequent claims on behalf of many techniques for an initial success rate of 95–100% must be assessed against a background of an increasing tide of patients with recurrent reflux being referred back for further surgical correction, medical treatment having failed to provide symptomatic relief. In a series of cases of recurrent reflux reported by Little et al from the University of Chicago, the Mark IV antireflux procedure was the technique of choice after failure of other techniques, both abdominal and thoracic.[8] This may ultimately prove a major role for the Mark IV technique when all else has failed to control reflux.

## SUMMARY

As confirmed by the experimental work of DeMeester[1] (see Chap. 39) in addition to extensive clinical evidence, the Mark IV operation is a physiologic procedure that fulfills the six criteria discussed earlier.[9] The main disadvantage of this procedure appears to be that its success depends on certain technical subtleties and that, therefore, it is more difficult to perform. The Mark V modification may help with some of these problems. However, as recorded in a series of cases described in 1972, the fact that residents could be trained in 6 months to achieve an 85% success rate with this operation suggests that the technical difficulties are not insuperable.[2]

## REFERENCES

1. DeMeester TR, Wernly JA, Bryant GE, et al: Clinical and in vitro analysis of determinates of gastroesophageal competence: A study of the principles of antireflux surgery. *Am J Surg* **137**:39, 1979
2. Orringer M, Skinner D, Belsey R: Long-term results of the Mark IV operation for hiatal hernia and analyses of recurrences and their treatment. *J Thorac Cardiovasc Surg* **63**:25, 1972
3. Skinner D, Belsey R: Surgical management of oesophageal reflux and hiatus hernia. *J Thorac Cardiovasc Surg* **53**:33, 1972
4. Skinner D, Belsey R, Hendrix T, Zuidema G: *Gastroesophageal Reflux and Hiatal Hernia.* Boston, Little, Brown, 1972
5. Belsey RHR: Gastroesophageal reflux. *Am J Surg* **139**:775, 1980
6. Baue AE: The Belsey Mark V procedure. *Ann Thorac Surg* **29**:265, 1980
7. Pearson FG: Surgical treatment of peptic esophagitis and stricture. *World J Surg* **1**:463, 1977
8. Little AG, Ferguson MK, Skinner DB: Reoperation for failed antireflux operations. *J Thorac Cardiovasc Surg* **91**:511, 1986
9. Baue AE, Belsey RHR: The treatment of sliding hiatus hernia and reflux esophagitis by the Mark IV technique. *Surgery* **62**:396, 1967

CHAPTER

# 47

# Benign Strictures of the Esophagus

Alex G. Little

A stricture is simply a narrowing. A stricture of the esophagus can be due to either benign or malignant causes. This chapter focuses on benign causes, but an astute clinician is always mindful that esophageal cancer must always be considered. That diagnosis should be excluded before one proceeds on the assumption that any stricture is benign. Otherwise, hope of curative intervention is diminished proportional to the duration of time lost in establishing the true, malignant, diagnosis. All patients with strictures identified by radiologic means must be examined with endoscopy. Both brushings and biopsy specimens of the affected area have to be obtained before therapy is initiated on the basis of an assumption of benign stricture.

## HISTORICAL PERSPECTIVE

Before the advent of radiologic and endoscopic methods of imaging or viewing the esophagus, identifying an esophageal stricture as a cause of dysphagia was not possible. Esophageal stricture, or esophageal fibrosis, was identified as an anatomic and pathologic entity as early as 1933.[1] The cause of these strictures was unclear. An infectious process was frequently assumed although gastroesophageal reflux was properly identified as the correct cause in 1935 by Winkelstein.[2] In spite of the uncertainty regarding the pathogenesis of esophageal strictures, empiric treatment with various types of esophageal dilators was introduced into clinical practice with reasonable outcomes.[3]

Surgical treatment was first described in the 1940s and 1950s by such thoracic surgery pioneers as Belsey and Allison. Their approach included esophagogastric resection and reconstruction with repositioned stomach or interposed colon or jejunum.[4,5] These surgeons were obviously dealing with chronic and advanced fibrotic disease that was not amenable to more conservative measures. Their use of these relatively morbid procedures was, therefore, justified. Thal et al developed a procedure to open the stricture and repair the esophagus with stomach.[6] In 1957, Collis described a gastroplasty that involved formation of a tube of lesser curve of the stomach followed by hernia repair.[7] In 1971, Pearson et al combined the Collis gastroplasty with a Belsey hiatal hernia repair to allow a dilatable stricture to heal.[8] Since these early experiences, two surgical goals have evolved. The first goal is early intervention in patients with reflux esophagitis to prevent progression of esophagitis to a fibrous stricture. The second goal, when the first is not achieved, is to develop esophagus-sparing operative alternatives to resection in patients with fully developed fibrous strictures. This chapter describes the current status of the surgical movement toward these goals.

## PATHOGENESIS

### Gastroesophageal Reflux Disease

By far the most common cause of esophageal stricture is gastroesophageal reflux disease (GERD). The pathophysiologic mechanism involves reflux of gastric contents through an ineffective lower esophageal sphincter with subsequent exposure of the squamous esophageal mucosa to these injurious materials. The overwhelming evidence suggests that when reflux damages the epithelium and causes esophagitis, the precursor of a stricture, the most devastating agents are acid and pepsin in combination. This is the reason that reflux strictures are often called peptic strictures. Although bile, trypsin, and other pancreatic enzymes have been implicated as contributing to or exacerbating acid and peptic injury, the effect of these biliary and pancreatic substances appears to be much less important in pathogenesis than the acid-pepsin combination.[9–11]

It has been shown in several studies that the combination of acid and pepsin is more injurious to the squamous epithelium than any other combination of upper gastrointestinal secretions.[12,13] In one study, an incompetent gastroesophageal junction was surgically constructed in dogs, and the esophagus was subsequently exposed to reflux under varying conditions.[14] These experimental groups included dogs with reflux and no gastric stimulation, maximal gastric stimulation, and biliary diversion into the stomach. Only the combination of an incompetent cardia and maximal stimulation of gastric output with pentagastrin resulted in erosive esophagitis. This is not surprising when one considers the physical chemistry of the involved enzymes. When duodenal contents mix with gastric contents, the relative number of hydrogen ions is diminished because of neutralization by duodenal bicarbonate. The resulting pH is one at which all enzymes are relatively ineffective. This theoretic reasoning and experimental findings were corroborated by a clinical study. The study showed that patients with GERD with an increased amount of alkaline duodenal gastric reflux actually had a lower incidence of esophagitis and stricture formation than patients with less duodenogastric reflux, presumably because of buffering of gastric acid by duodenal bicarbonate.[15]

It has been estimated that 40–65% of patients who undergo endoscopy for reflux symptoms have erosive or ulcerative esophagitis.[12] Why all patients with reflux do not have esophagitis or strictures is not entirely clear. The inherent injuriousness of the gastric contents, including considerations such as pH and the presence of various upper gastrointestinal enzymes, is an important factor.[15] In addition, in some patients the natural esophageal defenses prevent reflux contents from breaking down the esophageal mucosal barrier. These esophageal protective mechanisms include secondary peristalsis, which returns refluxed materials to the stomach,[16] and the protective action of swallowed saliva, which is rich in bicarbonate and neutralizes acid.[17] Other important protective factors are the inherent properties of the esophageal mucosa, such as the richness of its blood supply and the ability of mucosal flow to increase in response to injury. This process removes hydrogen ions that diffuse from the esophageal lumen into the mucosal cells.[18] When the reflux contents are sufficient to overcome these defense mechanisms, esophagitis is produced. Figure 47–1 shows that at this stage the mucosa is thinned and in some areas even denuded.

One possible resolution of mild esophagitis is healing. This has been shown to occur in approximately 50% of patients with esophagitis when appropriate medical management is used.[19] The introduction of the proton pump inhibitor omeprazole has increased the acute rate of healing of esophagitis, although long-term results are not improved when patients must return to standard medical management. The corollary to this observation is that esophagitis in approximately 50% of patients does not heal or resolve, and fibrous scar tissue develops, which constitutes the final stricture. At this stage the esophagus is shortened as a consequence of inflammation, and normal tissue is replaced by fibrous tissue. This fibrotic stricture is permanent and does not change. Figure 47–2 shows the radiographic appearance of a typical reflux stricture, and Figure 47–3 (see Color Plates, following page 608) shows the endoscopic appear-

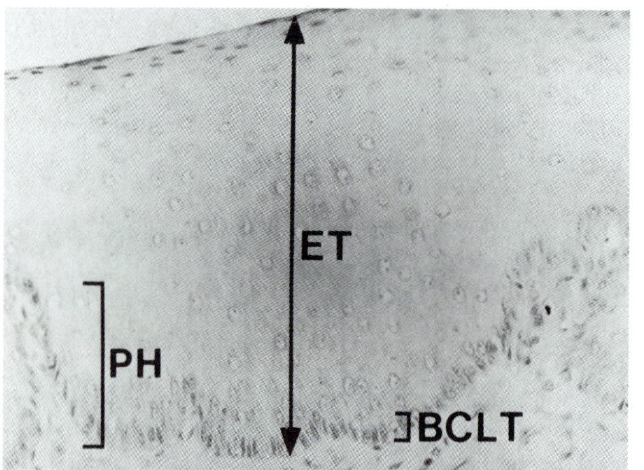


A

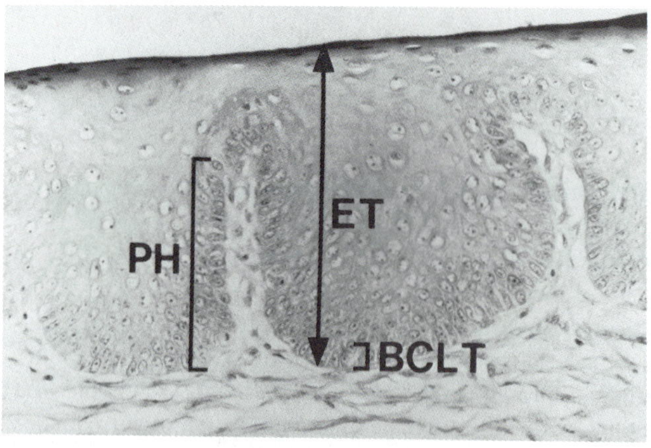


B

**Figure 47–1. A.** Micrograph of the normal histologic appearance of the distal esophageal mucosa. **B.** Micrograph of the histologic appearance of the distal esophagus of a patient with reflux esophagitis. The squamous epithelial thickness is diminished so that the relative magnitude of the basal cell layer and the submucosal papillae are increased. ET = epithelial thickness of the squamous epithelium, BCLT = basal cell layer thickness, PH = height of the submucosal papilla (hemotoxolin and eosin stain, original magnification × 35).

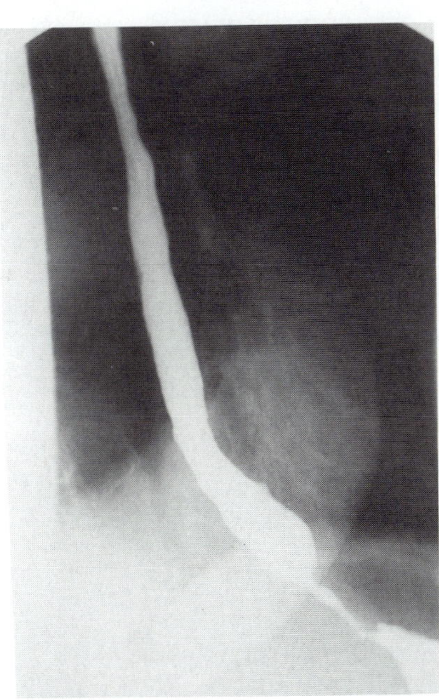

**Figure 47–2.** Barium swallow radiograph shows the typical appearance of a distal esophageal reflux stricture.

ance. Although these appearances suggest a benign condition, appearances can be deceiving, and obtaining brushings and biopsy specimens of the stricture is mandatory. Figure 47–4 presents the gross appearance of a resected specimen.

Depicted in Figure 47–5 is the radiographic appearance of a Schatzki's ring. This lower esophageal ring is a diaphragm-like structure that is constituted of reactive mucosal hyperplasia at the squamocolumnar junction. This is thought to be an acquired, rather than congenital, abnormality that is a complication of GERD.[20–22] A Schatzki's ring is not a fibrous structure but is an esophageal narrowing caused by reflux. It can, therefore, be thought of as a forme fruste of a true stricture.

## Barrett's Esophagus

Barrett's esophagus, or a columnar epithelium-lined esophagus, is associated with gastroesophageal reflux. All patients with Barrett's esophagus have an incompetent cardia and, regardless of symptoms, can be shown with esophageal pH monitoring to have pathologic reflux.[23] Whether reflux actually causes the abnormal epithelium or the two phenomena are developmentally but not causally linked is suggested but not firmly established.[24] Strictures at the squamocolumnar junction are a common feature of this disorder. Figure 47–6 shows the usual radiographic appearance of a midesophageal stricture in a patient with a Barrett's esophagus. Because the squamocolumnar junction and the stricture are typically 5 cm or more above the true gastroesophageal junction, it is not certain whether these strictures are actually due to the reflux. The stricture may also represent part of the developmental abnormality of the upper gastrointestinal tract seen in Barrett's esophagus. These strictures are usually both shorter and associated with less overall fibrous tissue formation than are distal esophageal strictures of the normal peptic variety.

## Drugs

It is well known that some orally administered drugs contain substances that injure the gastrointestinal mucosa, including the esophageal epithelium. Table 47–1 identifies some of these substances. It is unlikely that drugs are a primary cause of strictures in many patients. A review of drug-induced esophageal injuries between 1970 and 1985 could identify only 251 reported cases, and 49% of them were due to one agent, tetracycline.[25] There is no question, however, that drugs can be the primary cause of stricture in some patients and can exacerbate development of strictures in patients with abnormal esophageal motility or underlying

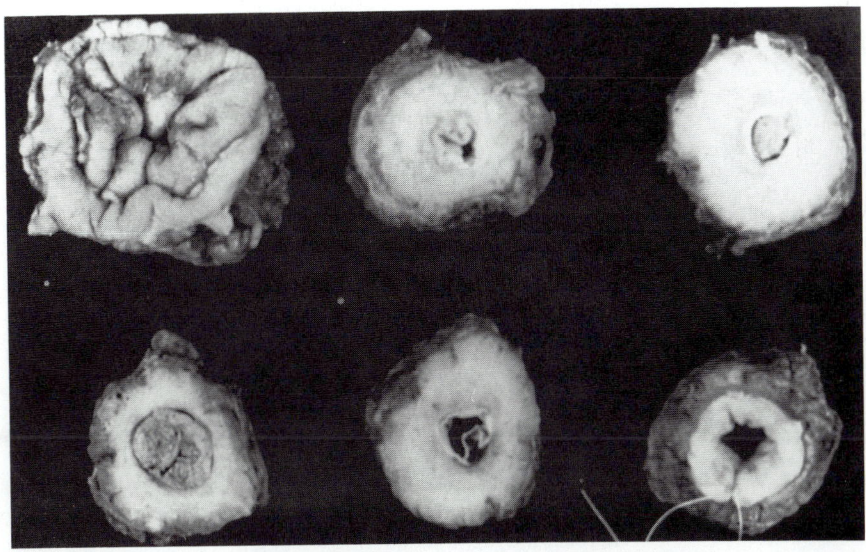

**Figure 47–4.** A resected esophageal stricture has been sliced open to demonstrate the extreme narrowing of the esophageal lumen and the degree to which the normal esophageal tissue has been replaced by dense fibrous tissue. *(From Postlethwait RW: Complications of gastroesophageal reflux. In Posttelthwait RW (ed): Surgery of the Esophagus, 2nd ed. Norwalk, Connecticut, Appleton-Century-Crofts, 1986, with permission.)*

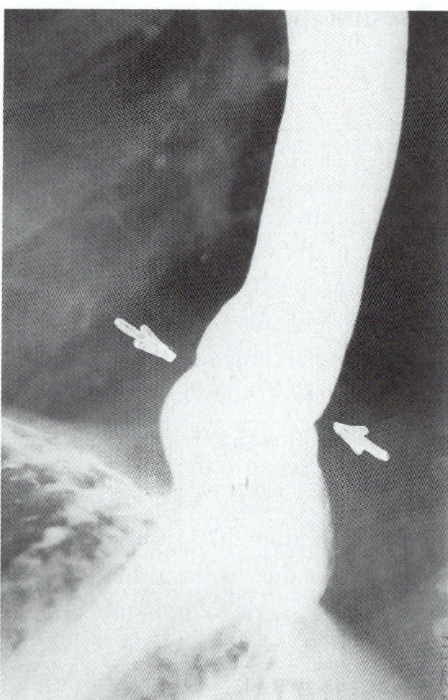

**Figure 47–5.** Barium swallow radiograph shows a Schatzki's ring (arrow) at the level of the squamocolumnar junction.

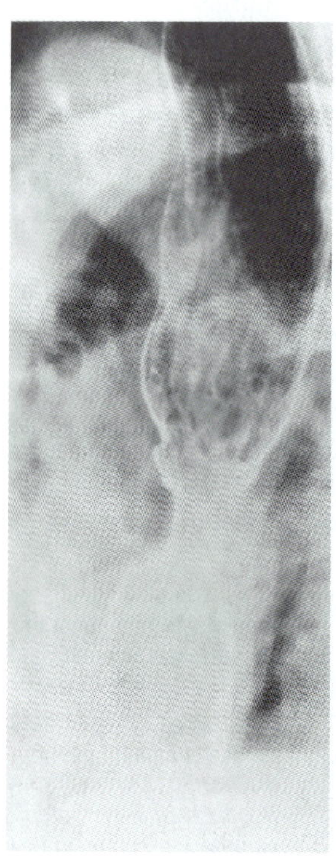

**Figure 47–6.** A midesophageal stricture of the squamocolumnar junction is demonstrated in a patient with Barrett's esophagus.

**TABLE 47–1. ETIOLOGY OF BENIGN ESOPHAGEAL STRICTURES**

| |
|---|
| **Nonreflux Related** |
| Congenital |
| Infectious |
| *Candida albicans* infection |
| Mucormycosis |
| Syphilis |
| Tuberculosis |
| Herpes |
| Traumatic |
| Caustic ingestion |
| Prolonged nasogastric drainage |
| Irradiation |
| Foreign body impaction |
| Iatrogenic (perforation or anastomotic leak) |
| Medication |
| Tetracycline |
| Doxycycline |
| Aspirin |
| Nonsteroidal anti-inflammatory drugs |
| Theophylline and derivatives |
| Miscellaneous |
| Cutaneous diseases (pemphigus, toxic epidermal necrolysis) |
| Behçet's syndrome |
| Crohn's disease |
| Cricopharyngeal web |
| Schatzki's ring |
| **Reflux Related** |
| Reflux esophagitis |
| Barrett's esophagitis |
| Primary motor disorders |

GERD when the duration of contact between the offending drug and the esophageal mucosa is prolonged.

### Caustic Ingestion

Ingestion of acid or, more commonly, alkaline caustic materials can produce esophageal damage that results in strictures. This entity is addressed thoroughly in Chapter 41.

## CLINICAL FEATURES

### Gastroesophageal Reflux Disease

Although some patients present with a peptic stricture without any prior symptoms, most patients with reflux or peptic strictures have an antecedent history of heartburn and perhaps other symptoms of GERD such as regurgitation. The symptom associated with stricture is, of course, dysphagia or difficulty swallowing. The degree of difficulty swallowing is variable and depends on both the length and degree of esophageal narrowing. A minimum esophageal diameter of 1.2 cm is necessary for unimpeded swallowing. As the lumen progressively narrows or as the length of narrowing increases, dysphagia becomes worse.

Because of impairment of the quality of life associated with stricture formation and because an appropriately timed operation can prevent development of a fibrous stricture, all patients with symptoms of GERD sufficient to occasion a visit with a physician should be examined with endoscopy to detect and determine the severity of esophagitis. Patients with esophagitis should be carefully monitored while being treated with medical management. When esophagitis fails to resolve during treatment or recurs after a course of medical therapy, the patients should be treated with an elective antireflux operation to prevent the development of a fibrous stricture. If this opportunity is missed and dysphagia has developed and a stricture is found, endoscopic examination is of extreme importance to look for the presence of Barrett's esophagus and to rule out the possibility of a malignant neoplasm. This requires both brushings and biopsy specimens from the area of the stricture. Brushing and biopsy may have to be repeated after dilation to give the endoscopist access to the full length of the strictured esophagus. At this point, documentation of reflux with esophageal pH monitoring is a bit academic. If there is any doubt about the cause then complete esophageal function tests are warranted. Manometry rules out the possibility of a primary motility disorder if that is a clinically significant possibility. After a stricture has been dilated, pH monitoring can document the presence or absence of acid reflux if that is an open clinical question.

### Barrett's Esophagus

Barrett's esophagus, despite the presence of reflux in essentially every patient, may be surprisingly asymptomatic. Many patients with very profound acid reflux are completely without any history of heartburn or regurgitation.[23] However, when Barrett's esophagus is identified in the diagnostic evaluation of reflux symptoms or in the investigation of a stricture, it is mandatory that the endoscopist obtain multiple biopsy specimens of the columnar epithelium to look for an early, occult carcinoma. Typically the stricture in these patients is in the middle esophagus at the squamocolumnar junction rather than at the gastroesophageal junction, as is the case for reflux-peptic strictures. In fact, an astute clinician suspects Barrett's esophagus when a barium swallow documents stricture in the middle esophagus.

## TREATMENT AND RESULTS

### Medical Therapy

Patients with GERD and a distal stricture require simultaneous esophageal dilation and gastric acid suppression and neutralization. Dilation is usually performed with tapered dilators of either the Maloney type, which do not require endoscopy, or guided dilators, such as the Savary dilator, which do require endoscopic control. Balloon dilation is also an alternative, but excessive, sudden stretching of a fibrous stricture can result in esophageal disruption. Simultaneous suppression of gastric acid output with either $H_2$-blockers or omeprazole and acid neutralization with antacid preparations prevents further reflux damage to the esophagus as the stricture is opened. In addition to stretching the fibrous tissue, some resolution of peristricture edema and inflammation occurs during this process of medical management. This facilitates surgical correction, if it becomes necessary, by restoring some degree of esophageal pliability.

Medical treatment of strictures can be successful. Several reports of dilational therapy combined with medical treatment of reflux suggest that dysphagia is relieved or improved in 50–88% of patients.[26–29] However, over time these results deteriorate because of persisting reflux symptoms and recurrence of the stricture, which necessitates repeat esophageal dilation. One recent report of 106 consecutive patients with reflux strictures is particularly helpful.[30] All strictures were dilated with a Savary-Gilliard bougie system. Dilation failed in 20 patients (19%) within 1 month of treatment. Of the remaining 86 patients, who also received standard medical reflux therapy, only 16 (19%) remained free of dysphagia after the initial dilation sessions. Fifty-seven (66%) patients required multiple dilations after the initial sessions, and 22 patients ultimately underwent surgical treatment. This experience also found that dilation was more likely to be successful for strictures shorter than 2 cm and with a diameter in excess of 9 mm. The dilators are shown in Figure 47–7.

Both the gastroenterologist and physician should be willing to acknowledge that frequent and repetitive esophageal dilations and rigid medical management of reflux do not constitute the ideal lifestyle over an extended period of time. Occasional dilation in combination with tolerable medical management and lifestyle modification is entirely reasonable and may be elected by the patient and gastroenterologist. However, when the stricture is persistent, and multiple or frequent dilations are required, exposing the patient both to the risk of perforation, which is usually less than 1%,[26–30] and to the inconvenience and unpleasantness of frequent dilation sessions, surgical correction becomes a reasonable consideration.

Patients with a Schatzki's ring require no treatment unless they have dysphagia, which is usually present when the internal diameter is less than 13 mm. In that case, simple dilation with a Maloney or Savary dilator system is curative. Typical symptoms of GERD such as heartburn, however, may appear when the ring has been obliterated as underlying reflux is unmasked and gastric contents gain access to the esophageal epithelium above the site of the ring. Patients should then receive symptom-based medical therapy for GERD.

Treatment of patients with Barrett's esophagus is determined by symptoms, complications of the primary dis-

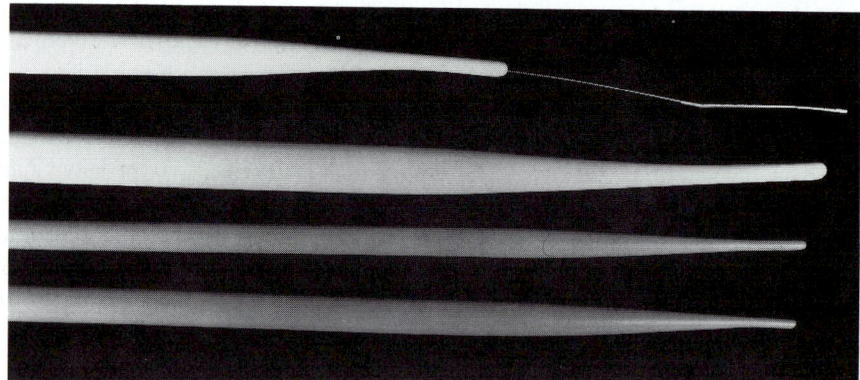

**Figure 47–7.** Comparison of the Maloney and wire-guided Savary dilators. Note the tapered tips on both dilators. The Savary dilator contains a central channel that facilitates passage over the guide wire.

ease, and endoscopic findings. Patients without symptoms and no evidence of dysplasia in biopsy specimens need only surveillance. Patients with reflux symptoms and no dysplasia should receive symptomatic GERD treatment and also undergo endoscopy on a regular basis. Finally, patients with stricture should receive simultaneous gastric acid suppression-based medical therapy and esophageal dilation. Unfortunately, this conservative approach frequently fails, and complete reflux control with an antireflux operation is required. Only then does the dilated stricture remain open.

## Surgical Therapy

Despite any conclusive proof that strictures in patients with Barrett's esophagus are truly related to reflux, experience shows that persistence of the reflux is associated with persistence of the stricture.[31] Accordingly, these patients can be considered therapeutically exactly as patients with primary GERD. In other words, resection of the abnormally epithelized esophagus is not indicated unless severe dysplasia or carcinoma is identified. There is the caveat that routine endoscopic surveillance is necessary even after an antireflux operation, because curtailment of reflux does not appear to reduce the premalignant potential of the Barrett's epithelium.

When an esophageal stricture can be dilated to a lumen size adequate to relieve dysphagia, usually requiring a bougie size greater than 13–15 mm (40–45 F), multiple options exist. By far the ideal is performing a standard antireflux procedure such as a Nissen fundoplication. This possibility can be anticipated when the stricture is relatively short and dilation results in a nearly normally anatomically located gastroesophageal junction, suggesting only a modest amount of inflammation and esophageal foreshortening. Some surgeons would operate on this sort of patient through the abdomen. This approach has been shown to be successful when performed by experienced surgeons, and the siren song of laparoscopy can be heard. For example, one report documented that 90% of 107 patients with strictures had good results (defined as no or minimal dysphagia) after one dilation session and a transabdominal Hill antireflux procedure.[32] Results deteriorated if multiple preoperative dilations were required.

I believe it is safer to approach this type of patient through a left thoracotomy than through an abdominal incision. Left thoracotomy allows extensive esophageal mobilization, which should be carried out to the level of the aortic arch. Depending on training and experience, the surgeon can perform either a Nissen or a Belsey type of antireflux procedure as a primary repair.[33] It is absolutely essential that as the final step the fundoplication and gastroesophageal junction be able to lie without any vertical tension beneath the closed hiatus. If this is not the situation, the fundoplication will tend to be distracted and ultimately disrupted by being retracted into the mediastinum as the inflamed and somewhat shortened esophagus produces vertical tension after the operation. My experience with 32 patients with dilatable strictures treated with a transthoracic antireflux procedure documents an excellent (no dysphagia) or good (minimal dysphagia) outcome in 88% of the patients.[33] These results were obtained with no perioperative deaths. Of note, two additional patients treated with a transabdominal Nissen fundoplication had poor results, which eventually necessitated a reoperation through the chest, which was successful in both instances.

The thoracic approach also allows options that are not available with a laparotomy. When the final repair, typically a Nissen fundoplication, cannot be reduced without tension beneath the diaphragm, the surgeon has two alternatives. One option is positioning the antireflux procedure in the chest. This procedure is competent to prevent reflux; however, it is also associated with quite serious complications. Compression of the stomach at the hiatus can produce gastric obstruction and sequelae related to the intrathoracic pouch of stomach, which is essentially a closed loop.[34,35] These sequelae range from postprandial bloating to actual gastric perforation. Widening of the hiatus with incisions in the limiting diaphragmatic muscle eliminates gastric narrowing and obstruction and thereby greatly reduces the incidence of complications.[36]

A more attractive option when the esophagus or fundoplication cannot be reduced beneath the diaphragm without tension is lengthening of the esophagus with a Collis gastroplasty. As illustrated in Figure 47–8, this technique effectively lengthens the foreshortened esophagus with construction of a gastric tube from the lesser curve. It is extremely important that the GIA stapler be pressed firmly against the internal bougie so that the gastric tube, i.e., the neoesophagus, is the same diameter as the true esophagus. Either a Nissen or Belsey type antireflux procedure can be combined with the Collis lengthening procedure to construct an antireflux fundoplication that is based on the neoesophagus and lies tension-free beneath the approximated hiatus.

Patients who require this approach have more periesophagitis, fibrosis, and esophageal shortening than patients with easily dilatable strictures and a relatively normal esophageal length. Even so, the combined Collis plus Nissen or Belsey approach has been shown to be effective. Stirling and Orringer[37] achieved control of GERD symptoms in 81% of 59 patients and eliminated dysphagia in 71% by combining dilation with the Collis–Nissen procedure. Pearson et al[38] reported on their experience with the Collis–Belsey technique in 138 patients with peptic stricture and a short esophagus. They obtained good results in 93% of patients with an operative mortality of only 0.5%.

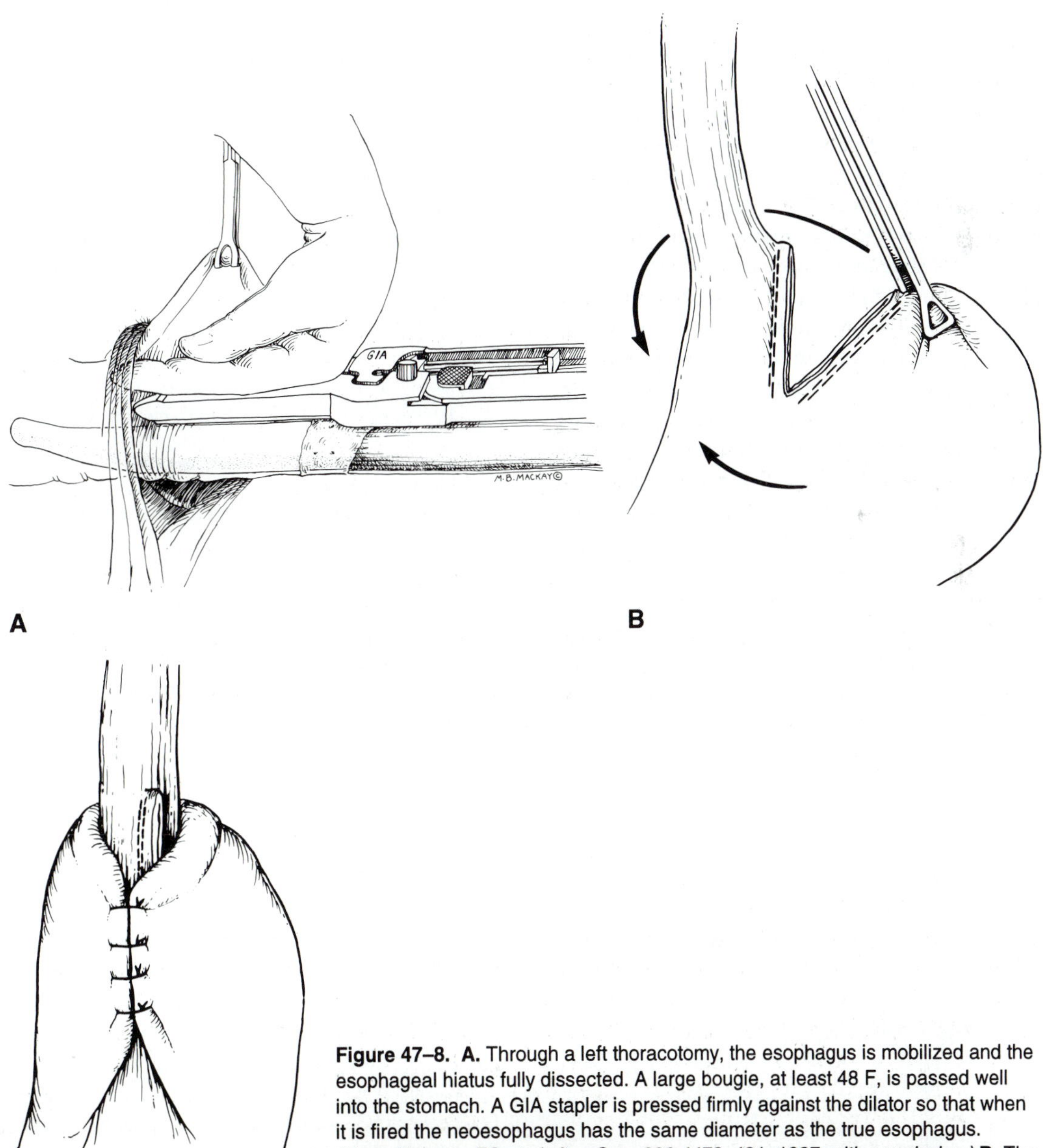


**Figure 47–8.** **A.** Through a left thoracotomy, the esophagus is mobilized and the esophageal hiatus fully dissected. A large bougie, at least 48 F, is passed well into the stomach. A GIA stapler is pressed firmly against the dilator so that when it is fired the neoesophagus has the same diameter as the true esophagus. *(From Pearson FG et al: Ann Surg 206:4473–481, 1987, with permission.)* **B.** The schematic appearance of the lengthened esophagus after the GIA stapler has been fired. **C.** After the gastroplasty tube has been constructed, either a Belsey or, as depicted in these figures, a Nissen fundoplication can be performed.

A surgical alternative that is not frequently used at present is a Thal patch.[6,39] As illustrated in Figure 47–9, in this operation a longitudinal incision is made in the stricture. An appropriately sized skin graft is laid on the gastric fundus, and the skin graft–fundus complex is sutured to the esophagotomy. This enlarges the stricture and provides a squamous epithelium lining. The procedure is completed by construction of a full gastric wrap for a Nissen fundoplication.

The final consideration is strictures that cannot be dilated. These uncommon strictures must be resected and continuity of the gastrointestinal tract restored. This undertaking is associated with considerably more morbidity and mortality than antireflux operations performed in the absence of clinically significant esophagitis, again emphasizing the benefits of early surgical intervention. However, resection is the only option when dilation is unsuccessful. In this case, options include a transhiatal resection with a cervical esophagogastrostomy or a left thoracotomy with reconstruction using stomach, colon, or jejunum. The only completely unacceptable alternative is an intrathoracic reconstruction using stomach. This anatomy, with resection of any remnant of a native antireflux mechanism at the gastroesophageal junction and placement of the anastomosis in the negative pressure environment of the thorax, results in unrelenting reflux with heartburn and regurgitation and eventual stricture recurrence.[40] Both colon and jejunum provide satisfactory postreconstruction function. I prefer using an isoperistaltic segment of the splenic flexure of the left colon because of the reliability of its blood supply and the ability to obtain a relatively straight colonic segment.[33,41]

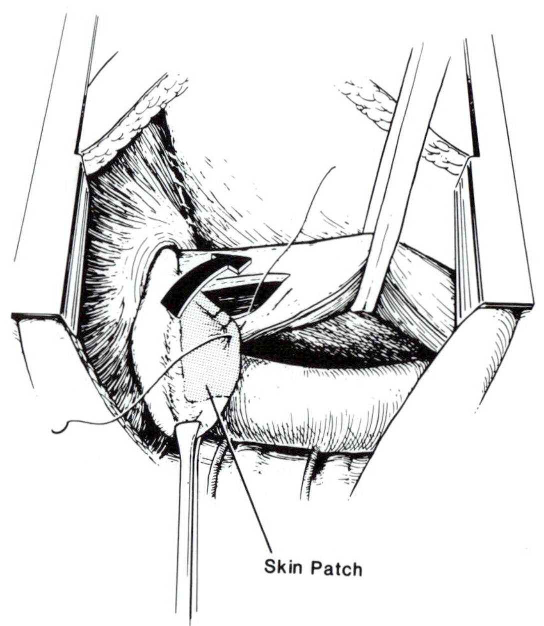


**Figure 47–9.** A Thal patch. A Nissen fundoplication is added to provide reflux control.

When resection is required for an undilatable stricture in a patient with a Barrett's esophagus, the resection should include all the abnormal epithelium. If a remnant is retained, the patient remains at risk for development of an adenocarcinoma in the residual columnar epithelium, even though there is no further provocation by acid reflux.[42]

An uncommon but occasionally encountered scenario is a stricture that the surgeon is loath to approach directly. This may be because the patient is considered to be at too high an operative risk, because the hiatal tissues are considered too inflamed to allow safe dissection, or because there are contradictions to use of stomach, colon, or jejunum for reconstruction. In this setting, antrectomy with Roux-en-Y gastrojejunostomy is a reasonable compromise. Some reflux persists, but the combination of reduction in gastric output and diversion of pancreatobiliary secretions diminishes both the volume and harmfulness of the reflux.[43]

## REFERENCES


1. Mosher HP: Involvement of the esophagus in acute and chronic infections. *Arch Otolaryngol* **18:**563–572, 1993
2. Winkelstein A: Peptic esophagitis: A new clinical entity. *JAMA* **104:**906–9, 1935
3. Jackson C, Jackson CJ: *Bronchoesophagology.* Philadelphia, Saunders, 1950, pp 267–77
4. Belsey R: Diaphragmatic hernia. In: *Modern Trends in Gastroenterology.* New York, Hoeber, 1952, pp 128–78
5. Allison PR: Peptic ulcer of the oesophagus. *Thorax* **3:**20–9, 1948
6. Thal AP, Hatafuku T, Kurtzman R: New operation for distal esophageal stricture. *Arch Surg* **90:**464–472, 1965
7. Collis JL: An operation for hiatus hernia with short esophagus. *J Thorac Cardiovasc Surg* **34:**768, 1957
8. Pearson FG, Langer B, Henderson RD: Gastroplasty and Belsey hiatus hernia repair. *J Thorac Cardiovasc Surg* **61:**50–61, 1971
9. Lillemoe KD, Johnson LF, Harmon JW: Taurodeoxycholate modulates the effects of pepsin and trypsin in experimental esophagitis. *Surgery* **97:**622–7, 1985
10. Gotley DC, Morgan AP, Cooper MJ: Bile acid concentrations in the refluxate of patients with reflux oesophagitis. *Br J Surg* **75:**587–90, 1988
11. Salo JA, Myllarniemi H, Kivilaakso E: Morphology of lysolecithin-induced damage on esophageal mucosa. *J Surg Res* **42:**290–7, 1987
12. Little AG, DeMeester TR, Kirchner PT, et al: Pathogenesis of esophagitis in patients with gastroesophageal reflux. *Surgery* **88:**101–7, 1980
13. Goldberg HI, Dodds WJ, Gee S, et al: Role of acid and pepsin in acute experimental esophagitis. *Gastroenterology* **56:**223–30, 1969
14. Evander A, Little AG, Riddell RH, et al: Composition of the refluxed material determines the degree of reflux esophagitis in the dog. *Gastroenterology* **93:**280–86, 1987
15. Little AG, Martinez EI, DeMeester TR, et al: Duodenogastric reflux and reflux esophagitis. *Surgery* **96:**447–54, 1984
16. Kahrilas PJ, Dodds WJ, Hogan WJ, et al: Esophageal peristaltic dysfunction in peptic esophagitis. *Gastroenterology* **91:**897–904, 1986
17. Ferguson MK, Ryan JW, Little AG, Skinner DB: Esophageal emptying and acid neutralization in patients with symptoms of gastroesophageal reflux. *Ann Surg* **201:**728–35, 1985
18. Bass BL, Schweitzer EJ, Harmon JW, Kraimer J: $H^+$ back diffusion interferes with intrinsic reactive regulation of esophageal mucosal blood flow. *Surgery* **96:**404–13, 1984
19. Koelz HR, Birchler R, Bretholz A, et al: Healing and relapse of reflux

esophagitis during treatment with ranitidine. *Gastroenterology* **91:**1198–1203, 1986

20. Eastridge CE, Pate JW, Mann JA: Lower esophageal ring: Experiences in treatment of 88 patients. *Ann Thorac Surg* **37**(2):103–107, 1984
21. Wilkins EW Jr: The lower esophageal ring: How unique? *Ann Thorac Surg* **37**(2):101–102, 1984
22. Scharschmidt BF, Watts HD: The lower esophageal ring and esophageal reflux. *Am J Gastroenterol* **69**(5):544–549, 1978
23. Iascone C, DeMeester TR, Little AG, Skinner DB: Barrett's esophagus: Functional assessment, proposed pathogenesis and surgical therapy. *Arch Surg* **118:**543–9, 1983
24. Little AG: Barrett's esophagus: Another esophageal Sphinx. *Ann Thorac Surg* **55:**1359–60, 1993 (editorial)
25. Oakes DD, Sherck JP: Drug-induced esophageal injuries. In DeMeester TR, Matthews HR (eds): *International Trends in General Thoracic Surgery.* St. Louis, Mosby, 1987, pp 269–77
26. Shemesh E, Czerniak A: Comparison between Savary-Gilliard and balloon dilation of benign esophageal strictures. *World J Surg* **14:**518–22, 1990
27. Tytgat GN: Dilation therapy of benign esophageal stenoses. *World J Surg* **13:**142–8, 1989
28. Kozarek RA: Hydrostatic balloon dilation of gastrointestinal stenoses: A national survey. *Gastrointest Endosc* **32:**15–20, 1986
29. Patterson DJ, Graham DY, Smith JL: Natural history of benign esophageal stricture treated by dilation. *Gastroenterology* **85:**346–51, 1983
30. Bonavina L, Norberto L, Cusumano A, et al: Reflux-induced esophageal strictures: Factors influencing long-term results of dilation. In: Little AG, Ferguson MK, Skinner DB (eds): *Diseases of the Esophagus, Vol 2, Benign Diseases.* Mount Kisco, New York, Futura, 1990, pp 247–54
31. Lundell L: Acid suppression in the long-term treatment of peptic stricture and Barrett's oesophagus. *Digestion* **51:**49–58, 1992
32. Mercer CD, Hill LD: Surgical management of peptic esophageal stricture. *J Thorac Cardiovasc Surg* **91:**371–8, 1986
33. Little AG, Naunheim KS, Ferguson MK, Skinner DB: Surgical management of esophageal strictures. *Ann Thorac Surg* **45:**144–7, 1988
34. Pennell TC: Supradiaphragmatic correction of esophageal reflux strictures. *Ann Surg* **193:**655–65, 1981
35. Richardson JD, Larson GM, Polk HC: Intrathoracic fundoplication for shortened esophagus: Treacherous solution to a challenging problem. *Am J Surg* **143:**29–35, 1982
36. Maher JW, Hocking MP, Woodward ER: Supradiaphragmatic fundoplication: Long-term follow-up and analysis of complications. *Am J Surg* **147:**181–6, 1984
37. Stirling MC, Orringer MV: The combined Collis-Nissen operation for esophageal reflux strictures. *Ann Thorac Surg* **45:**148–57, 1988
38. Pearson FG, Cooper JD, Patterson GA, et al: Gastroplasty and fundoplication for complex reflux problems: Long-term results. *Ann Surg* **206:**433–441, 1987
39. Maher JW, Hocking MP, Woodward ER: Long-term follow-up of the combined fundic patch fundoplication for treatment of longitudinal peptic strictures of the esophagus. *Ann Surg* **194:**64–9, 1981
40. Bender EM, Walbaum PR: Esophagogastrectomy for benign esophageal stricture: Fate of the esophagogastric anastomosis. *Ann Surg* **205:**385–8, 1987
41. Curet-Scott MJ, Ferguson MJ, Little AG, Skinner DB: Colon interposition for benign esophageal disease. *Surgery* **102:**568–74, 1987
42. Hamilton SR, Hutcheon DF, Ravich WJ, et al: Adenocarcinoma in Barrett's esophagus after elimination of gastroesophageal reflux. *Gastroenterology* **86:**356–60, 1984
43. Fekete F, Pateron D: What is the place of antrectomy with Roux-en-Y in the treatment of reflux disease? Experience with 83 total duodenal diversions. *World J Surg* **16:**349–53, 1992

CHAPTER

# 48

# Paraesophageal Hiatal Hernia

Arthur E. Baue and Keith S. Naunheim

Paraesophageal hiatal hernias have also been called intrathoracic stomachs, "upside-down stomachs," massive hiatal hernias, parahiatal hernias, and rolling hiatal hernias. They are much less common than and different from sliding hiatal hernias. In sliding hernias (type I), the phrenoesophageal ligament fails to keep the esophagogastric junction below the diaphragm and within the abdomen. This type of hernia is commonly associated with inadequacy of the lower esophageal sphincter mechanism, which allows the development of reflux and esophagitis. In paraesophageal hernias (type II), the esophagogastric junction is often in or near its normal position below the diaphragm. The greater curve of the stomach is often the leading point for this rotational herniation, and the fundus or body of the stomach is rotated into the chest. As a rule, these patients suffer not from reflux but from symptoms of bleeding, fullness after eating, or obstruction as a complication of the hernial defect. Paraesophageal hiatal hernias account for only 3–6% of operations for hiatal hernias.[1–3] When the gastroesophageal junction moves upward and lies within the chest along with herniation of the fundus or body of the stomach into the chest, it is called a combined or type III hernia and is more commonly associated with reflux esophagitis in addition to the symptoms of partial obstruction due to rotation of the stomach.

## HISTORICAL NOTE

Recognition of different kinds of hiatal hernias has been a recent development. Originally, they were all categorized together. The early history of diagnosis and treatment of hiatal hernias is found in Chapter 42, as is the classification of hernias through the hiatus of the diaphragm.

Early in thoracic surgical history, hernias through the hiatus of the diaphragm or close to it were thought to be either congenital problems of a short esophagus or parahiatal herniation through a defect through the diaphragm alongside the hiatus.[4] It is now known that congenital short esophagus does not occur. It is an acquired abnormality of a sliding hiatal hernia or reflux esophagitis, producing a Barrett's esophagus. Parahiatal hernia also was described as one in which muscle fibers of the diaphragm were said to be present alongside the esophagus on the left with a defect in the diaphragm lateral to the hiatus. No one has ever seen such an entity. Thus, there is no such thing as a parahiatal hernia. Some authors who do not want to take a stand on this issue and who also have never seen a parahiatal hernia suggest that perhaps it is an extremely rare variant. We question how in the world a defect would develop in the muscle of the hiatus of the diaphragm lateral to the hiatus. It may well be in the past that posttraumatic hernias that were close to the hiatus were interpreted to be parahiatal hernias. A recent case report describes a strangulated parahiatal hernia through a small (1–2 cm) diaphragmatic defect that was separate from and 4 cm lateral to the esophageal hiatus.[5] The patient had no history of previous trauma. The only other case cited was in a woman 5 years after a Belsey repair; the hernia was probably produced by the sutures pulling through the diaphragm.[6] Ellis cited that a parahiatal hernia is extraordinarily rare.[7] Ellis recalls seeing one such hernia over a 40-year-period (written communication, 1994). Certainly there are traumatic ruptures of the diaphragm with herniation, but a paraesophageal hernia is not one of them.

All herniations of the fundus or body of the stomach into the chest anterior or lateral to the esophagus are paraesophageal hernias. Some authors have maintained that all paraesophageal hernias began as sliding hernias and enlarged to allow a paraesophageal component.[8] This has not been our experience, nor that of many of our colleagues. Many patients have a pure massive paraesophageal hernia with the esophagogastric junction lying posterior along the aorta but in a position where the intrinsic sphincter of the esophagus and the valve mechanism at the gastroesophageal junction are sufficient to decrease or prevent reflux and esophagitis.

Borchardt in 1904 described a triad of chest pain with retching but inability to vomit and inability to pass a nasogastric tube, which he called volvulus of the stomach.[9] Volvulus of the stomach occurs with a huge rotated paraesophageal hernia.

## ANATOMY

The esophageal hiatus is formed by muscle fibers of the right crus of the diaphragm with little or no contribution from the left crus. These fibers overlap inferiorly where they attach over and along the right side of the median arcuate ligament, which is securely attached to the lateral aspects of the vertebral bodies. The orifice is thus teardrop-shaped with the point to the right of the aorta. The rounded portion is in the midline close to the connecting portion of the central tendon of the diaphragm. Thus, the crural fibers enclose the esophagus in a tunnel. The phrenoesophageal ligament that holds the distal esophagus in place is formed by fusion of the endothoracic and endoabdominal fascia at the diaphragmatic hiatus. It is not a very strong ligament, which is why sliding hiatal hernias are so common. Ronald Belsey once described the phrenoesophageal ligament as a figment of Philip Allison's imagination.

The initial abnormality of a paraesophageal hernia is a protrusion of the fundus or body of the stomach alongside or anterior to the esophagogastric junction and into the chest (Fig. 48–1). As the defect enlarges anterior to the esophagus and with positive intra-abdominal and negative intrathoracic pressures, the most mobile portion of the stomach tends to move up through the defect and into the chest. The gastric cardia is fixed in place by the left gastric vessels and by the gastrosplenic and gastrohepatic ligaments. In a similar manner, the pylorus and first portion of the duodenum are fixed by the short attachments of the lesser omentum and the retroperitoneal position of the duodenum. Although the greater curve of the stomach is attached to the transverse colon by the greater omentum, the latter structures are quite mobile. Thus it is the greater curve and body of the stomach that migrate through the defect initially.

As the hernia progresses, the stomach rotates upward, utilizing the fixed lesser curve as an axis of rotation, thus the term *organoaxial rotation.* The greater curvature of the stomach eventually rotates up and over into the chest toward the right shoulder. Organoaxial rotation of the stomach is most commonly upward into the chest and to the

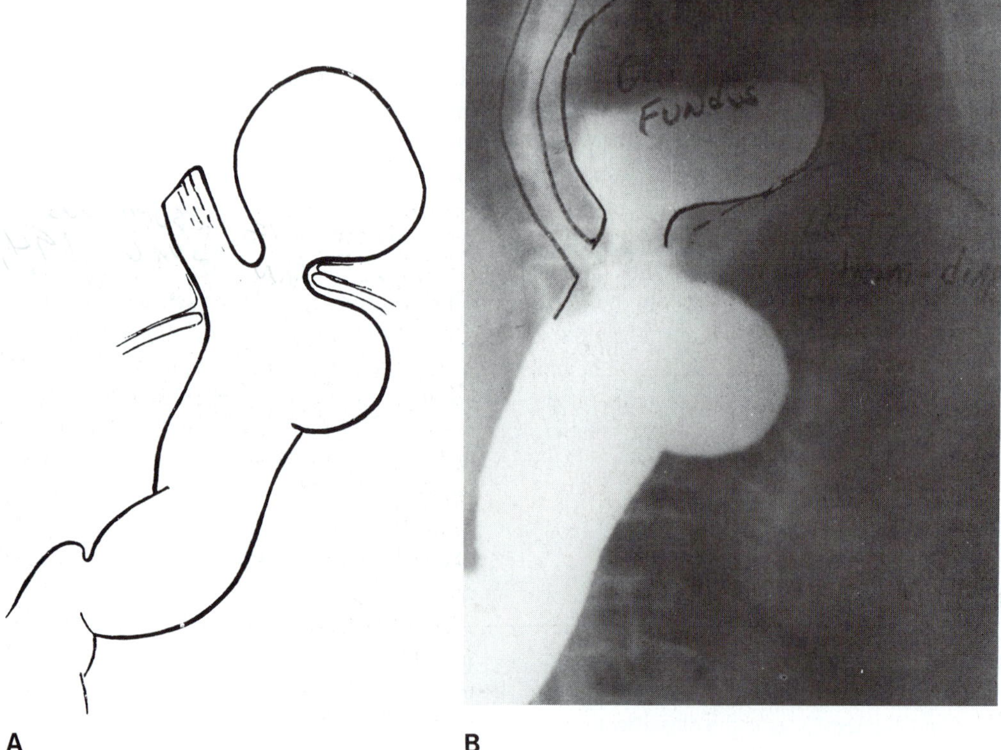


**Figure 48–1.** **A.** The diagram depicts a paraesophageal hernia. The esophagogastric junction remains in the normal location and the fundus protrudes alongside the junction up into the chest. **B.** Barium swallow depicting this abnormality.

right. This is the path of least resistance because of the aorta to the left and the heart to the left and anterior. On occasion, however, the stomach may rotate superiorly and not to the right so that the greater curve lies transversely behind the heart. As this process continues, the tension on the pylorus and lesser curve results in increased mobility of these areas with their migration toward the thorax. The greater curve, gastric body, and antrum eventually rotate upward through the defect, giving the radiographic picture of an "upside-down stomach." If the hernia is allowed to progress, the greater omentum and transverse colon may also be drawn into the defect, producing a giant paraesophageal hernia lying within the right chest.[10] On rare occasions, small intestine and spleen may herniate as well (Fig. 48–2). As the hiatus enlarges and more stomach herniates, the esophagogastric junction is placed under tension and may eventually migrate up into the chest. This produces the combined hernia (type III). Some physicians believe these are not true paraesophageal hernias but rather combinations of the sliding and rolling abnormalities.[8]

The variations and progression of paraesophageal herniation (Fig. 48–3) include protrusion of a portion of fundus of the stomach alone (Fig. 48–1), rotation of the fundus and greater curve into the chest, the entire stomach upside down in the chest (Fig. 48–2), and organoaxial rotation of the body of the stomach into the chest, with the fundus prolapsing back below the diaphragm (Fig. 48–3) or the obstructed fundus staying below the diaphragm.

Thus, a paraesophageal hernia may vary from a portion of gastric fundus protruding through the hiatus to a large hernial defect containing the entire stomach, omentum, and transverse colon.

## SYMPTOMS AND PATHOPHYSIOLOGY

Paraesophageal hernias produce few symptoms when they are small. This is the reason why so few small hernias are discovered. If left unchecked, however, most hernias enlarge until most of the stomach lies within the thorax, at which time clinically significant symptoms often develop and draw attention to the condition. Most of these hernias are very large when the diagnosis is made. It may be that the symptoms are so mild or nonspecific when the hernia is small that the patients do not seek medical attention. It may also be that once this type of hernia begins to develop it progresses rapidly to a large size because of negative intrathoracic and positive intra-abdominal pressures.

The essential anatomic difference between paraesophageal and sliding hernias—the intact posterior fixation of the esophagus to the preaortic fascia and the median arcuate ligament—is responsible for the differences in pathophysio-

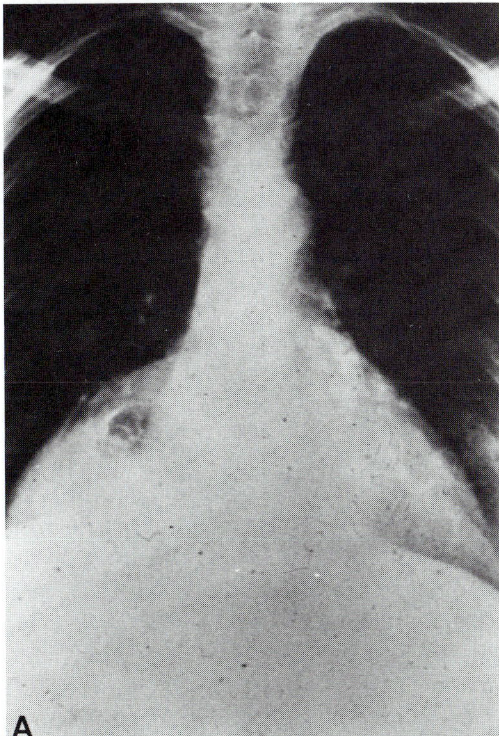


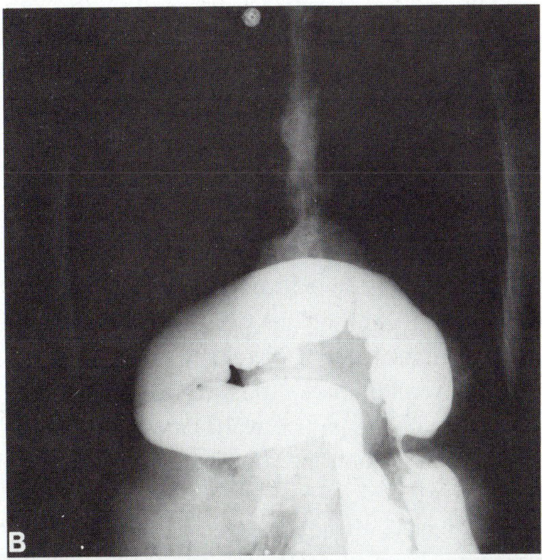


**Figure 48–2. A.** A chest radiograph in a patient with a giant paraesophageal hernia (Type III) shows a mass containing air density in the right lower chest. **B.** Barium enema in the same patient demonstrates the transverse colon drawn up into the intrathoracic hernia sac.

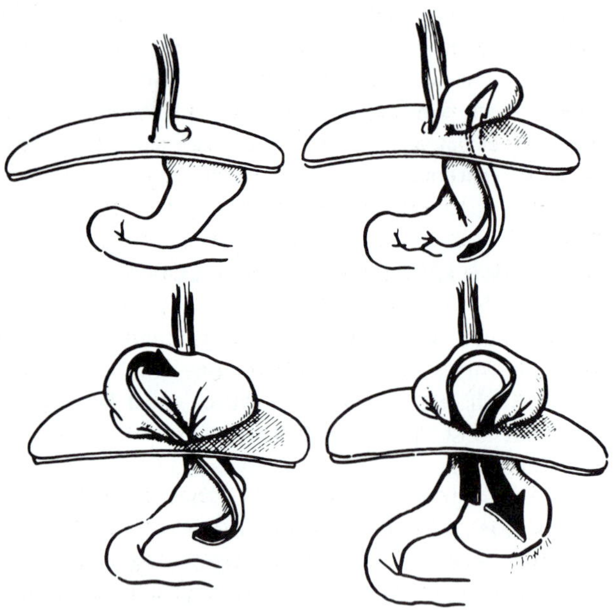

**Figure 48–3.** Mechanics of incarceration and strangulation with paraesophageal hernia. Note the fundus prolapsing back into the abdomen, producing a trapped intrathoracic gastric segment. *(Reprinted with permission from Postlethwait RW: Surgery of the Esophagus, 2nd ed, Appleton-Century Crofts, 1986, p 256.)*

logic features and clinical manifestations. Patients with a type II hernia may have a long history of postprandial distress and discomfort accompanied by occasional wretching and the sensation of nausea after eating. Severe substernal fullness and belching are usually present. True dysphagia is uncommon, and there is a striking absence of heartburn and other symptoms of esophagitis in most patients. The patient often learns to live with a sense of substernal discomfort until a complication occurs. Pulmonary complications, which vary from dyspnea to recurrent pneumonia, are common in paraesophageal hernias. The dyspnea characteristically follows ingestion of a heavy meal and results from compression of one or both pleural spaces by a huge hernial sac. Such compression may cause chronic atelectasis that may progress to pneumonia in some cases. The combination of dyspnea and the sensation of substernal fullness after meals can occasionally be misdiagnosed as postprandial angina. Spillover into the tracheobronchial tree can also occur from the partially obstructed stomach.

A frequent complication of this disorder is ulceration of the herniated stomach with resultant bleeding and chronic anemia. This condition is produced by poor gastric emptying and torsion of the gastric wall, particularly after repeated incarcerations, which interfere with blood supply and lymphatic drainage.

The type II defect is a true anatomic hernia in which the physical contents are completely surrounded by a peritoneal hernial sac. A paraesophageal hiatal hernia is prone to the same complications as herniation of a viscus elsewhere in the body. These complications include incarceration, obstruction, torsion, gangrene, and perforation. The most feared and lethal complication of this defect is gastric volvulus with subsequent strangulation obstruction. Volvulus usually occurs after a meal when the fundus, filled with food, descends from its intrathoracic position into the abdomen (Fig. 48–3). This causes the stomach to become twisted and angulated in its midportion just proximal to the antrum, resulting in partial or complete obstruction. Distention of the intrathoracic stomach and further rotation of the intra-abdominal fundus may result in obstruction at the gastroesophageal junction. Further twisting may lead to complete pyloric obstruction, resulting in an incarcerated gastric segment and a closed loop obstruction. If neglected, this obstruction leads to strangulation, necrosis, and perforation.[11,12] Unless the problem is recognized and corrected, gastric gangrene leads to leakage of gastric contents with resulting mediastinitis and shock, which is fatal in a high percentage of patients.

Patients present in extreme distress. The symptoms are those of a high obstruction with inability to swallow. Severe substernal and epigastric pain or pressure is often the chief symptom and may be accompanied by nausea. Sometimes this condition is misdiagnosed as myocardial infarction. Vomiting can occur, but more frequently the complete inability to swallow or regurgitate is the most prominent manifestation. Approximately 30% of paraesophageal hernias present with this problem. Borchardt's triad of chest pain—retching but inability to vomit and inability to pass a nasogastric tube—indicates volvulus of the stomach. It was found in three patients reported by Allen et al from the Mayo Clinic.[13] They had five patients who required emergency operations for suspected strangulation, three of whom had gastric necrosis and one of whom died.

Although symptoms of gastroesophageal reflux can occur in patients with paraesophageal hernias, most authors note that this is an uncommon occurrence. However, Pearson reported that most of his patients with massive hiatal hernias had clinically significant reflux. This may be due to the high percentage of combined type III hernias in their population.[8]

## DIAGNOSIS

Whether or not symptoms are present, the diagnosis of paraesophageal hiatal hernia is often first suspected because of an abnormal chest radiograph. The most frequent finding is a retrocardiac mass filled with air or an air–fluid level (Fig. 48–4). In a giant type II hernia, this may present as a posterior mediastinal mass that extends into the lower right thoracic cavity. The differential diagnosis includes a cyst or abscess in the lung, mediastinum, or pericardium. The diagnostic test of choice is a barium study of the upper gastrointestinal tract. The pathognomonic finding is that of an upside-down stomach within the thoracic cavity (Fig. 48–5). Another example of a variation on the theme is that of rota-

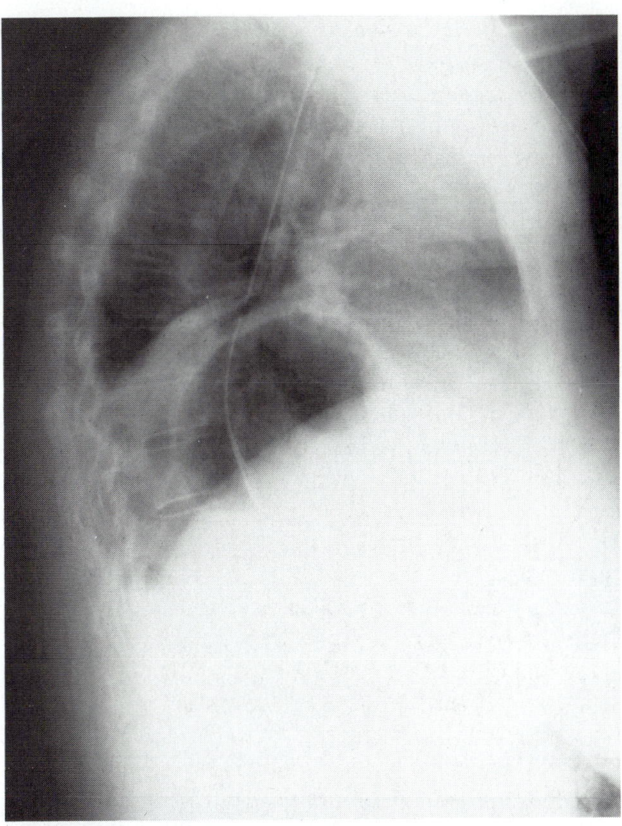

**Figure 48–4.** Chest radiograph of patient with paraesophageal hernia demonstrating retrocardiac air bubble.

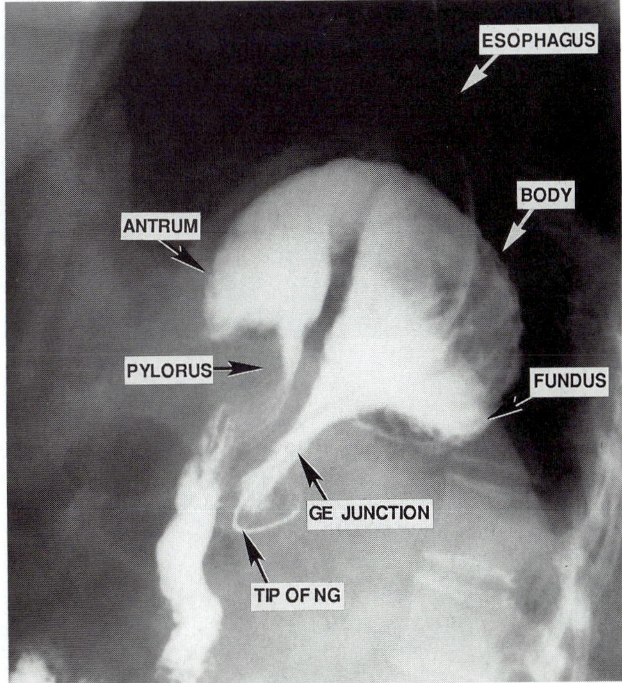


**Figure 48–5.** Barium swallow depicting "upside-down stomach." It is important to note the course of the nasogastric catheter (NG). The catheter tip lies in the esophagogastric junction, which is located well below the hiatus.

tion of the anterior wall and greater curve of the body of the stomach into the chest (Fig. 48–6). The fundus of the stomach may remain in the abdomen. A barium swallow radiograph is virtually diagnostic unless there is acute obstruction by volvulus and incarceration at the esophagogastric junction. Occasionally such a hernia can be found on a barium swallow radiograph obtained during a routine investigation for anemia. It is important that the radiologist pay strict attention to the position of the gastroesophageal junction. This sign not only confirms the diagnosis of a type II defect but also may be helpful in determining whether or not an antireflux procedure is needed at the time of repair. A barium enema may also be helpful in delineating the presence of part or all of the transverse colon in the hernial sac (Fig. 48–2).

Once the presence of the type II defect has been established radiologically, it is important to determine whether it has had a functional effect on lower esophageal sphincter competence. Symptoms of gastroesophageal reflux are rare in paraesophageal hernias, but their presence may indicate the existence of peptic esophagitis. Unfortunately, a lack of symptoms is no guarantee there is no gastroesophageal reflux. Preoperative esophageal testing should be undertaken to confirm or refute the suspicion of reflux. Ambulatory 24-hour esophageal pH testing can help determine whether reflux is present and whether a fundoplication is indicated at the time of surgical correction. Walther et al found evidence of clinically significant gastroesophageal reflux in nine of 15 (60%) of their patients with paraesophageal hernias who underwent 24-hour esophageal pH testing.[14] Of interest is the fact that one third of the patients with reflux had no symptoms of esophagitis.

Upper gastrointestinal endoscopy may play an important role in the diagnostic evaluation of hemorrhage. Reports from the literature citing endoscopic results are conflicting. Pearson et al[8] performed endoscopy on all 51 patients with primary incarcerated giant hiatal hernias and found that 30% had grade I esophagitis and an additional 30% had grade II–IV esophagitis. However, in most series the incidence of esophagitis is considerably lower. Walther et al[14] noted that only two of 15 patients (13%) had mild grade I esophagitis, figures identical to those quoted by Ellis et al (13%, five of 39 patients) in their series of type II hiatal hernia defects.[15] It must be remembered that in this disorder, esophagoscopy can be fraught with hazard. The instrument may fail to gain access to the stomach because of acute angulation, and vigorous efforts to pass the instrument despite resistance can cause perforation.

Although the literature is controversial, it appears that preoperative esophageal testing may yield important information with regard to the presence or absence of gastroesophageal reflux. Although patients with gastric volvulus and obstruction would not be candidates, it seems reasonable to perform these tests before all elective paraesophageal hernia repairs, and we recommend it. The results of the tests help the surgeon determine whether a fundoplica-

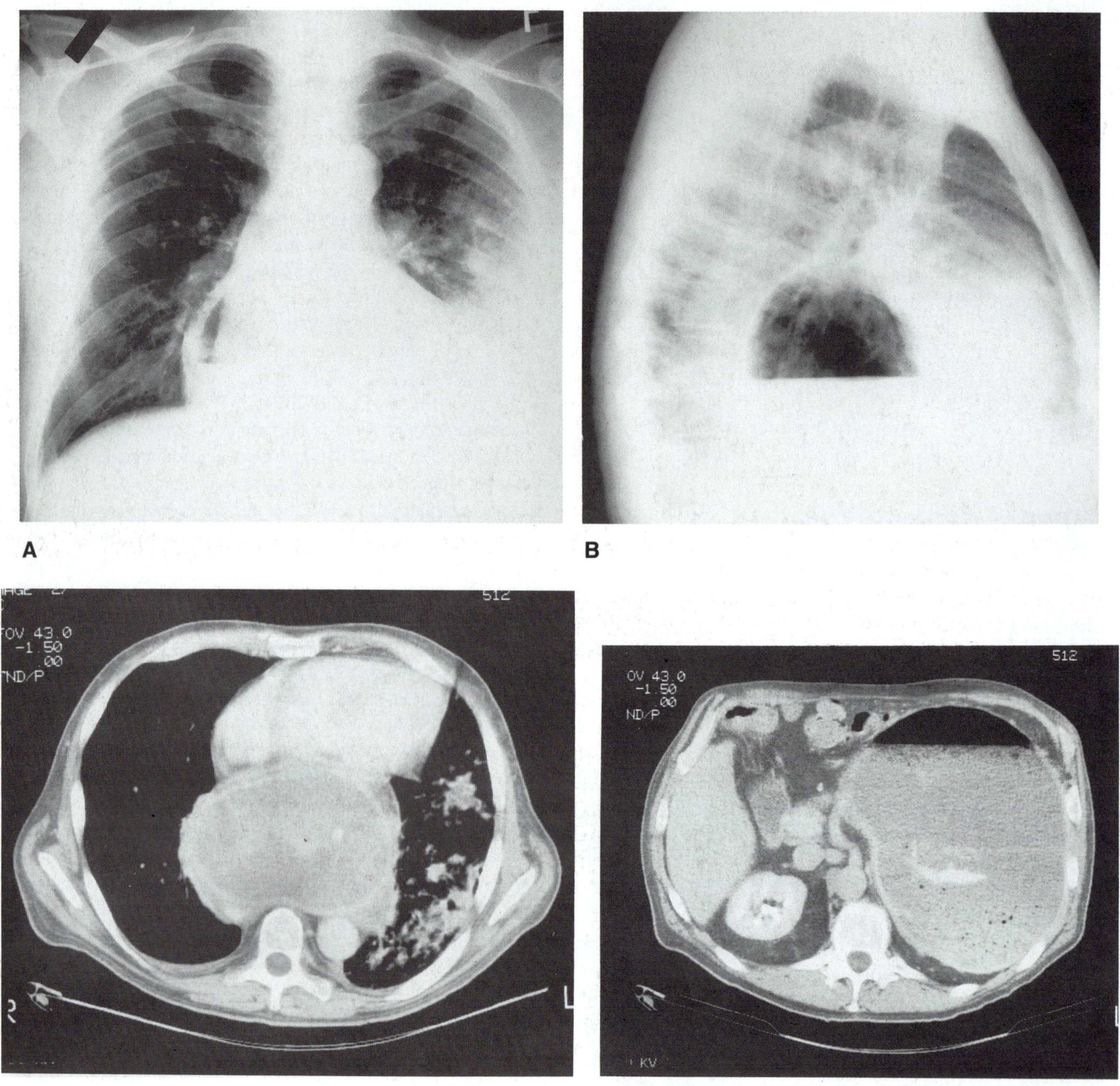


**Figure 48–6. A.** Posteroanterior chest radiograph shows the large air–fluid level protruding into the right chest with chronic destruction of the left lower lobe from aspiration. **B.** A lateral chest radiograph shows the large retrocardiac air–fluid level indicating a giant paraesophageal hiatal hernia. These radiographs are pathognomonic of this abnormality. There is almost nothing else that can simulate it. **C.** CT scan shows the large thick-walled fluid filled stomach in the posterior mediastinum within a hernial sac. There is also chronic change in the left lower lobe of the lung. **D.** CT scan of the abdomen shows the distended, thick-walled, partially obstructed fundus of the stomach, which is pushing the kidney and the spleen downward. *(Continued.)*

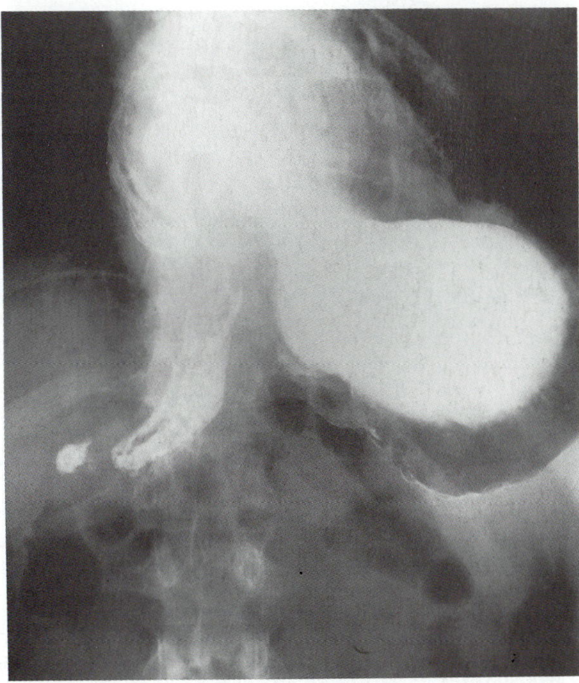

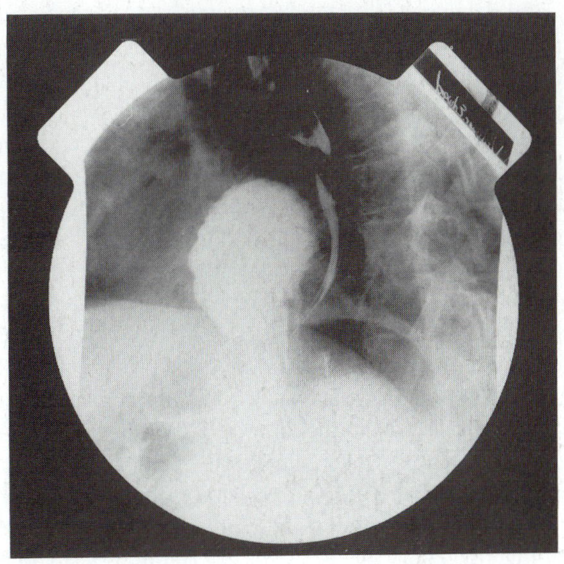

E F

**Figure 48–6.** *(Continued.)* **E.** Barium swallow radiograph shows the body of the stomach in the mediastinum with a partially obstructed antrum beneath the diaphragm on the right side and the antrum of the stomach pulled up into the chest. The esophagogastric junction can be seen in its usual position with some difficulty. **F.** The esophagus can be seen easily and the esophagogastric junction at or below the diaphragm leading into the partially obstructed fundus with the greater curve of the body of the stomach protruding into the chest.

tion is required at the time of correction of the paraesophageal hernia.

## THERAPY

There is no acceptable medical treatment for patients with paraesophageal hiatal hernias. Neutralization of gastric acid does not correct the interference with gastric drainage, nor does it prevent trauma to the gastric wall. Patients followed expectantly are at high risk, as evidence in the study of Skinner and Belsey,[16] who noted that of 21 patients treated medically because of minimal symptoms, six (29%) died of complications of strangulation, perforation, exsanguinating hemorrhage, or acute gastric dilatation within the thorax. The presence of a paraesophageal hernia, no matter the size or symptoms, is sufficient indication for operation. This is a mechanical anatomic defect that will progress and cause life-threatening problems in the future.

Gastric volvulus and obstruction are surgical emergencies. Decompression should be attempted with nasogastric tube or endoscopy. If decompression is promptly performed and there are no signs of toxicity, an operation can be scheduled at the earliest convenience. Inability to decompress the volvulus constitutes a surgical emergency and mandates immediate operative intervention, whether or not signs of toxicity exist.

Although the necessity for surgical repair is widely recognized, two controversies regarding management still exist among surgeons: (1) Should a fundoplication be performed routinely at the time of repair? (2) What is the optimal approach—transthoracic or transabdominal?

Many authors, including Pearson et al,[8] Ozdemir et al,[2] and Postlethwait,[17] routinely perform an antireflux procedure on all patients regardless of the presence or absence of reflux symptoms. Hill and Tobias[1] espouse a simple anatomic repair alone and have had excellent results with no recurrences and no postoperative reflux in 19 patients. Perhaps the most enlightened approach is that of Williamson et al,[18] who suggested that patients with type II hiatal herniation undergo preoperative endoscopy, manometry, and pH testing. Only patients with symptoms or objective evidence for gastroesophageal reflux should have an antireflux repair, such as a loose Nissen fundoplication.

Both the transthoracic and transabdominal approach have been advocated. Surgeons who endorse the thoracic approach emphasize the ease of intrathoracic dissection of the hernial contents and sac.[8,16] In a type III defect, the thoracic approach allows thorough dissection and mobilization of the esophagus in cases of moderate to severe esophageal shortening. This may allow reduction of a fundoplication beneath the hiatus without the need for a lengthening procedure such as a Collis gastroplasty. However, the proponents of a transthoracic repair often neglect to note the increased morbidity or discomfort attendant to a thoracotomy. In addition, a transthoracic repair may allow the stomach to rotate again in an organoaxial manner after it is pushed back into the peritoneal cavity. This may produce volvulus of the body of the stomach in which the greater curve becomes adherent to the liver. We are aware of two patients in whom this occurred. A laparotomy was required in the postoperative period to correct the volvulus in both patients.

Surgeons who suggest an abdominal approach point out that the procedure is easily performed through the abdomen and that concomitant abdominal procedures can be undertaken simultaneously.[19] In addition, it allows placement of a gastrostomy tube, which obviates the need for a nasogastric tube and may also decrease the risk of recurrent volvulus postoperatively. The only patient in whom this approach might prove difficult is one with a proved type III, or combined, hernia with known reflux and a foreshortened esophagus. In this patient the thoracic approach would be a better alternative. However, familiarity with dissection of the esophagus done with a transhiatal esophagectomy allows mobilization of most of the esophagus through an enlarged diaphragmatic hiatus. Also, the addition of a Collis gastroplasty allows lengthening, if necessary, to reduce the tube and perform a fundoplication around the gastric tube below the diaphragmatic hiatus.

## OPERATIVE TECHNIQUE

The principles of repair are reduction of the hernia with return of its contents to the peritoneal cavity and repair of the hiatal defect to prevent recurrence of the hernia. We prefer and recommend the abdominal approach through an upper midline incision. The left lobe of the liver is mobilized from the diaphragm and retracted to the right. The contents of the hernial sac are reduced back into the peritoneal cavity with gentle traction. If resistance is encountered while the contents are reduced into the abdomen, a small rubber catheter inserted into the hernial sac allows entry of air as the contents of the hernia are reduced and decreases the suction effect holding them inside the thorax. Sometimes in cases of tight incarceration, the hiatal ring itself may have to be incised to allow return of the organs to the abdominal cavity.

In some patients dense adhesions of the stomach to the sac require careful dissection. If possible, the hernial sac is dissected free from the thoracic cavity and resected. The dead space in the mediastinum disappears as the lungs reexpand, and routine drainage of this space is not necessary. The usual finding is a grossly enlarged hiatus with the esophagogastric junction forming the posterior aspect of the defect. It is often easier to mobilize the esophagus, free it circumferentially from the hiatus, and narrow the hiatus beginning at the posterior aspect. Sutures that narrow the hiatus anterior to the esophagus distort the normal anatomy. Moving the esophagus anteriorly restores it to its normal

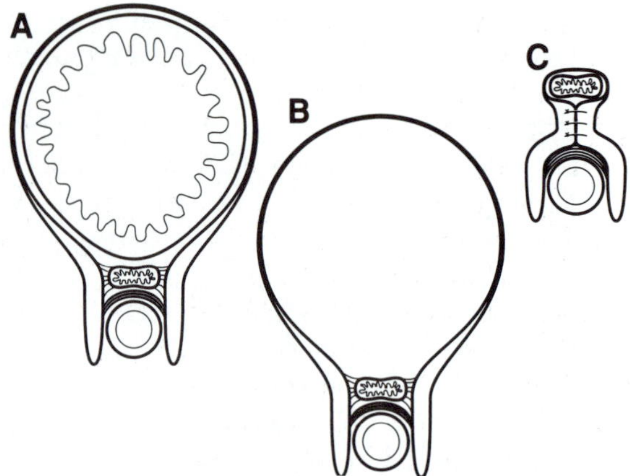


**Figure 48–7.** Diagram shows the large anterior defect in the hiatus containing stomach with the esophagus pushed posteriorly (**A**). After the stomach is freed and brought back into the peritoneal cavity and after the hernial sac is resected (**B**), the esophagus is mobilized and the crus of the diaphragm repaired posteriorly, restoring the esophagus to its normal anterior position (**C**).

position (Fig. 48–7). In a lateral view, the esophagus is normally seen to move anteriorly as it goes through the diaphragm.

Often when the esophagus and esophagogastric junction are mobilized, sufficient length of esophagus lies easily below the diaphragm. This gives the intrinsic esophageal sphincter a mechanical advantage, which should maintain competence. The hiatal defect is rarely larger than the size of a fist and is closed with stout (No. 0) nonabsorbable sutures in an interrupted manner. The surgeon must be certain to take large bites at the right and left sides of the defect, lest the sutures tear out postoperatively. The closure is continued until the hiatus just admits the tip of the index finger when placed beside the esophagus with a nasogastric tube in place. To prevent recurrent hernia, the stomach should be fixed below the diaphragm. This can be accomplished most expeditiously by a Hill type of suture.[1] A series of three or four sutures placed from the posterior to the anterior aspect of the lesser curve of the stomach are affixed to the median arcuate ligament. This series of sutures holds the lesser curve of the stomach, the esophagogastric junction, and 2–4 cm of the distal esophagus well below the diaphragm.

If the patient has objective evidence of reflux or esophagitis at preoperative studies or if the posterior attachments of the lower esophagus were taken down during dissection, it is likely that the lower esophageal sphincter is incompetent, and a fundoplication should be performed at the time of surgical correction. In such patients, our procedure of choice is a loose Nissen fundoplication constructed over a No. 50 Maloney dilator. If the esophagus has been mobilized and its posterior attachments divided, the hiatus can be narrowed with posterior sutures. The esophagus is held up and the left and right sides of the crus of the diaphragm approximated, beginning over the aorta and moving anteriorly. In this way the esophagus is returned to a more normal anterior position. If there is a question about reflux and the location of the gastroesophageal junction, it is safer to do a fundoplication and have a more assured repair.

Last, we fix the stomach within the peritoneal cavity with a Stamm gastrostomy. This discourages recurrent rotation and herniation of the stomach by fixing it to the anterior abdominal wall and removes the need for a nasogastric tube. Many patients with incarcerated type II hernias have a prolonged period of postoperative gastric stasis. A gastrostomy allows continued drainage without the discomfort or complications of an in-dwelling nasogastric catheter. The gastrostomy can be routinely removed 10 days after the operation.

In the patients in whom gangrene or perforation is found at the time of operation, resection of all devascularized tissue must be done in combination with debridement of the infected tissue. Broad-spectrum antibiotics that include anaerobic coverage are strongly advised in this setting because of the possibility of perforation and mediastinal contamination by salivary leakage. Recently a few paraesophageal hernias have been repaired transabdominally by laparoscopic techniques. Laparoscopic repair of type I hernias with fundoplication has been reported by Cuschieri and is being performed frequently by other surgeons.[20] Probably because of the relative rarity of paraesophageal hernia, laparoscopic repair has been reported only once, by Congreve in 1992.[21] Recent experiences and details of the technique are described in Chapter 50A.

## RESULTS

Elective repair of paraesophageal hernias is a very safe procedure. In 300 patients the operative mortality was 0.3%, a figure similar to that quoted for repair of sliding hiatal hernias (Table 48–1). Emergency procedures for gastric volvulus have a much higher mortality, about 14%. The 30-fold increase in operative risk underscores the need for elective repair at the time of initial diagnosis. Complications are the same as for any reflux procedure, with two additions. In patients with gastric volvulus and obstruction, there appears to be an increase in pulmonary complications, probably because of episodes of regurgitation and aspiration. Also, prolonged gastric stasis may persist 7–10 days after operative repair because of the lingering inflammation and edema in the released gastric segment.

Long-term results are generally excellent, whether or not an antireflux procedure is performed in addition to simple repair. Hill and Tobias[1] performed simple repair and saw no hernia recur or reflux develop in 22 patients over a 15-year follow-up period. Identical results were noted by Wichterman et al,[10] who routinely performed concomitant antireflux procedures. However, recurrent sliding (type I) hernias with reflux were reported by Ozdemir et al[2] (10%),

**TABLE 48–1. OPERATIVE MORTALITY FOR PARAESOPHAGEAL HERNIA REPAIR**

| Reference | Year | Elective (%) | Emergency (%) |
|---|---|---|---|
| Beardsly and Thompson[11] | 1964 | — | 3/10 (30) |
| Sanderud[3] | 1967 | 0/14 (0) | 1/7 (14) |
| Hill and Tobias[1] | 1968 | 0/19 (0) | 2/10 (20) |
| Ozdemir et al[2] | 1973 | 0/19 (0) | 2/12 (17) |
| Wichterman et al[10] | 1979 | 0/16 (0) | 1/6 (17) |
| Carter et al[12] | 1980 | — | 1/14 (7) |
| Pearson et al[8] | 1983 | 0/47 (0) | 1/4 (25) |
| Walther et al[14] | 1984 | 0/15 (0) | — |
| Ellis et al[15] | 1986 | 1/39 (2.6) | — |
| Landreneau et al[22] | 1992 | 0/12 (0) | 0/5 (0) |
| Allen et al[13] | 1993 | 0/119 (0) | 1/5 (20) |
| Williamson et al[18] | 1994 | 1/119 (0.84) | 1/7 (14) |
| Total | | 2/419 (0.48) | 13/80 (16) |

Operative mortality reported as number of deaths divided by number of patients operated on. Emergency defined as gastric volvulus.

Pearson et al,[8] (8%), and Sanderud[3] (8%) as late complications of paraesophageal hernial repair despite fundoplication at the time of initial operation. Therefore, it does not appear that simultaneous fundoplication is completely effective prophylaxis against recurrent herniation. Fundoplication could be more appropriately performed on a selective basis in those patients with documented reflux.[22]

Williamson et al reviewed the records of 117 patients with paraesophageal hiatal hernias.[18] The most common presenting symptom was epigastric or substernal pain in 76% of patients. Only 17 patients underwent antireflux procedures in addition to anatomic repair of the hernia. The antireflux procedures were performed for esophagitis determined by symptoms and at esophagoscopy, which showed a hypotensive lower esophageal sphincter ($\leq$ 10 mm Hg) or abnormal findings of 24-hour pH monitoring. However, after the operation two patients had severe reflux symptoms and findings (1.7%) and 17 others (14.5%) had mild and controllable symptoms. The authors reported the development of a recurrent hernia in 10 of 117 patients who underwent operations with good to excellent results in 86% of patients. Allen et al[13] in their review reported that 111 (93.3%) patients had a transthoracic repair with the addition of an uncut Collis–Nissen fundoplication, a Belsey Mark IV fundoplication, or a Nissen fundoplication. Eight patients (6.7%) underwent an abdominal repair with an antireflux procedure. Thus the authors routinely performed an antireflux procedure in spite of the fact that only 15% of their patients had esophagitis. They reported excellent results in 60% of their patients, good in 33%, fair in 5.2%, and poor in 1.7%. The results were similar with all types of repair. Twenty-three patients were followed without an operation. Four of these patients had progressive symptoms and one died of aspiration.

## REFERENCES


1. Hill LD, Tobias JA: Paraesophageal hernia. *Arch Surg* **96:**735, 1968
2. Ozdemir IA, Burke WA, Ikins PM: Paraesophageal hernia: a life-threatening disease. *Ann Thorac Surg* **16:**547, 1973
3. Sanderud A: Surgical treatment for the complications of hiatal hernia. *Acta Chir Scand* **133:**223, 1967
4. Sauerbruch F, O'Shaughnessy L: *Thoracic Surgery,* a revised and abridged edition of Sauerbruch's *Die Chirurgie der Brustorgane.* London, Edward Arnold, 1937, pp 348–382
5. Demmy TL, Boley TM, Curtis JJ: Strangulated parahiatal hernia: Not just another paraesophageal hernia. *Ann Thorac Surg* **58:**227–229, 1994
6. Vallieres E, Waters PF: Incarcerated parahiatal hernia with gastric necrosis. *Ann Thorac Surg* **44:**82, 1987
7. Ellis FH Jr: Diaphragmatic hiatal hernias: Recognizing and treating the major types. *Postgrad Med* **88:**113–124, 1990
8. Pearson FG, Cooper JD, Ilves R: Massive hiatal hernia with incarceration: A report of 53 cases. *Ann Thorac Surg* **35:**45, 1983
9. Borchardt M.: Zur Pathologie and Therapie des magen Volvulus. *Arch Klin Chir* **74:**243, 1984
10. Wichterman K, Geha AS, Cahow CE, Baue AE: Giant para-esophageal hiatal hernia with intra-thoracic stomach and colon: The case for early repair. *Surgery* **86:**497, 1979
11. Beardsley JM, Thompson WR: Acutely obstructed hiatal hernia. *Ann Surg* **159:**49, 1964
12. Carter R, Brewer LA, Hinshaw DB: Acute gastric volvulus: A study of 25 cases. *Am J Surg* **140:**99, 1980
13. Allen MS, Trastek VF, Deschamp C, Pairolero PC: Intrathoracic stomach: Presentation and results of operation. *Ann Thorac Surg* (in press)
14. Walther B, DeMeester RR, Lafontaire E: Effect of paraesophageal hernia on sphincter function and its implication on surgical therapy. *Am J Surg* **147:** 111, 1984
15. Ellis FH, Crozier RE, Shea JA: Paraesophageal hiatus hernia. *Arch Surg* **121:**416, 1986
16. Skinner DB, Belsey RHR: Surgical management of esophageal reflux and hiatus hernia: Long-term results with 1030 patients. *J Thorac Cardiovasc Surg* **53:**33, 1967
17. Postlethwait RW: *Surgery of the Esophagus.* Norwalk, Connecticut, Appleton-Century-Crofts, 1986, p 257
18. Williamson WA, Ellis FH Jr, Shahian DM, Streitz JM Jr: Para-esophageal hiatal hernia: Is an anti-reflux procedure necessary? *Ann Thorac Surg* (in press)
19. Naunehim KS, Baue AE: Paraesophageal hiatal hernia. In Baue AE et al (eds): *Glenn's Thoracic and Cardiovascular Surgery.* Norwalk, Connecticut, Appleton & Lange, 1990, pp 741–746
20. Cuschieri A, Shim S, Nathanson LK: Laparoscopic reduction, crural repair and fundoplication of large hiatal hernia. *Am J Surg* **163:**425, 1992
21. Congreve DP: Laparoscopic paraesophageal hernia repair. *J Laparoendosc Surg* **2:**45, 1992
22. Landreneau RJ, Johnson JA, Marshall JB, et al: Clinical spectrum of paraesophageal herniation. *Dig Dis Sci* **37:**537, 1992

CHAPTER

# 49

# Esophageal Dysmotility

André Duranceau

The esophagus is a hollow muscular tube the function of which is to transport swallowed material from the pharynx to the stomach. Performance of this function depends on coordinated muscular activity. Disorders of motility may be classified into those involving the upper esophageal sphincter (UES) and swallowing mechanism (oropharyngeal dysphagia), those involving the body of the esophagus (transport dysphagia), and those dealing with the lower esophageal sphincter (LES) (esophagogastric dysphagia). They may also be classified into abnormalities of hyperactivity, hypoactivity, and incoordination. These may occur separately or in combination and usually produce swallowing difficulty manifested clinically by the symptoms described herein. In addition, these disorders may contribute to the formation of pulsion diverticula, which can occur in a cervical location proximal to the UES (Zenker's) or within the thoracic cavity in the mid or distal esophagus (epiphrenic).

Any disorder that disrupts normal esophageal motility impairs the ability of the esophagus to transport swallowed material. Symptoms reflect either this disturbance in function or the motor abnormality itself. Dysphagia is the most common symptom of esophageal motor disease. It is typically intermittent and may occur with both solids and liquids, although many patients have specific difficulty with the latter. Cold liquids are commonly more of a problem than are warm. Dysphagia is often poorly localized, being perceived retrosternally or at the level of the sternal notch. Various maneuvers such as the Valsalva maneuver and repeated swallowing may help to relieve dysphagia. In severe cases, dysphagia may be associated with regurgitation of swallowed nondigested food.

Normal esophageal contractions are not noticed by most people; however, high-pressure esophageal contractions may be perceived as chest pain. This pain is typically retrosternal, sometimes radiating to the back, to the interscapular area, or to the jaw or arms. It may be severe and mimic the pain of coronary insufficiency. Episodes can last from a few minutes to several hours and may occur spontaneously or be precipitated by swallowing. The pain is sometimes associated with dysphagia.

Aspiration of swallowed material may be another symptom of motility disorders. Malfunction of the hypopharynx and UES can lead to aspiration during deglutition. Functional obstruction of the distal esophagus from poor peristalsis or failure of the LES to relax may cause accumulation of material within the esophagus. Postural maneuvers (lying down) or acts that increase intrathoracic pressure (coughing, bending over) may lead to regurgitation of this material into the pharynx with resultant aspiration.

## NORMAL DEGLUTITION

The act of swallowing requires the coordinated interaction of the tongue, soft palate, pharyngeal musculature, larynx, and faucial pillars. Deglutition can be divided into four separate phases. In the oral preparatory phase, food is chewed and mixed with saliva, during which time the soft palate is pulled anteriorly up against the back of the tongue, maintaining the food bolus within the mouth. In the orovoluntary phase of swallowing, the tongue is displaced upward against the hard palate. This milks the food bolus posteriorly. When the bolus strikes and stimulates the anterior faucial arch, the pharyngeal phase of swallowing is initiated reflexively. The remainder of deglutition is an involuntary process. The soft palate elevates to close off the nasopharynx and prevent oronasal regurgitation. The pharyngeal constrictors are stimulated and squeeze the food bolus through the pharynx to the level of the cricopharyngeus muscle. During this time, the laryngeal musculature has elevated the larynx up against the epiglottis to cover the laryngeal opening and prevent tracheal aspiration. The cricopharyngeus muscle relaxes and allows passage of the bolus into the upper esophagus. These three phases of deglutition are a smooth, unbroken process that lasts approximately 1 second.

Both gravity and active esophageal peristalsis milk the bolus through the body of the esophagus to a level above the LES. Once the peristaltic wave has propelled the food to this level, the LES relaxes in a coordinated manner and allows passage of the food into the stomach. This last stage of swallowing is called the esophageal phase.

## OROPHARYNGEAL DYSPHAGIA AND DISORDERS OF THE UPPER ESOPHAGEAL SPHINCTER

Oropharyngeal dysphagia refers to a symptom complex characterized by difficulty propelling food or liquid from the oral cavity into the cervical esophagus. The etiology of the special category or dysphagia is summarized in Table 49–1.

### Symptoms

Three categories of symptoms result from misdirection of the swallowed bolus: pharyngonasal and pharyngo-oral regurgitation and laryngotracheal aspiration. Discomfort during meals and bronchopulmonary complications from aspiration are the main presenting patterns for oropharyngeal dysphagia, and the pattern of symptoms varies with cause.

#### *Neurologic Disease*

Symptoms in patients with neurologic disease and proximal dysphagia are often difficult to assess and to treat. This type of dysphagia is most often secondary to cerebrovascular disease with concomitant difficulties with speech and expression. Dysarthria is accompanied by poor control and coordination of pharynx and larynx. UES dysfunction may also be present. Patients who have had cerebrovascular accidents often reveal difficulties in bolus formation and propulsion. In patients with Parkinson's disease, hesitancy in bolus preparation and in the initiation of swallows may be observed. In diseases like amyotrophic lateral sclerosis, dysarthria and the absence of voluntary deglutition may result in repetitive aspiration.

**TABLE 49–1. ETIOLOGY OF OROPHARYNGEAL DYSPHAGIA**

| |
|---|
| **Neurogenic** |
| Central |
| Peripheral |
| **Myogenic** |
| End-plate disease |
| Muscle disease |
| **Structural** |
| Idiopathic UES dysfunction |
| Without pharyngoesophageal diverticulum |
| With pharyngoesophageal diverticulum |
| **Iatrogenic** |
| After surgery, radiation therapy |
| **Distal esophageal disease** |
| Motor disorders |
| Reflux disease |
| **Mechanical** |

#### *Muscular Disease*

Muscular disease that causes oropharyngeal dysphagia is often associated with bilateral palpebral ptosis and muscular weakness in both upper and lower limbs. In this category of patient, oropharyngeal dysphagia results from the same weakness that affects all striated muscles. In such cases the UES becomes a functional obstacle to the powerless pharynx, and pharyngo-oral regurgitation results. When the velopharyngeal muscles are too weak to effectively close the nasopharynx, pharyngonasal regurgitation is reported by patients. Repetitive tracheal aspiration results from hypopharyngeal pooling with poor control of the laryngeal additus.

#### *Iatrogenic Dysphagia*

Scarring from neck incisions is inevitable after tracheostomy, thyroidectomy, or pharyngolaryngectomy. Limitations to the normal excursion of the larynx cause oropharyngeal dysphagia. When more extensive ablative or explorative operations have been performed in the neck, poor pharyngeal and UES function may result. Similar symptoms may appear with the dense ischemic fibrosis of irradiation at the pharyngoesophageal junction.

#### *Distal Esophageal Disease*

Dysfunction in the esophageal body and at the LES level may cause referred symptoms at the pharyngoesophageal junction level. Both reflux disease and idiopathic motor disorders have been known to present as oropharyngeal dysphagia.

### Diagnosis

The assessment of oropharyngeal dysphagia includes videoradiologic evaluation, pharyngoesophageal radionuclide scintigrams, endoscopic assessment, and motility studies.

#### *Radiology*

Precise evaluation of oropharyngeal dysphagia requires multiphasic multipositional studies with modern video recording equipment.[1,2] Because of the rapidity of events during the act of swallowing, dysfunction of the pharynx, larynx, and UES can be accurately recorded only when these techniques are used. They allow observation of the movements of the tongue and soft palate, the symmetry of the pharyngeal contraction, the organization and activity of the laryngeal excursion, and the activity of the UES at rest and during swallowing. Even minute abnormalities in the function of these muscle groups can be documented with these techniques. Hypopharyngeal pooling and stasis as well as pooling in the pyriform sinuses and in the valleculae are the most frequent observations that suggest abnormal emptying (Figs. 49–1 and 49–2).

### *Radionuclide Emptying Studies*

The capability of the oropharynx and hypopharynx to empty can be quantified with pharyngoesophageal radionuclide transit studies. In all categories of oropharyngeal dysphagia these studies provide more objective documentation of emptying problems with either a liquid or a solid bolus. Although this method depends on and is limited by the ability of the patient to cooperate, this quantification allows objective assessment of results after either medical or surgical management of dysphagia (Figs. 49–3 and 49–4).[3]

### *Endoscopy*

After clinical and radiologic assessment of the oropharyngeal dysphagia, endoscopy is used to rule out an endoluminal lesion. I prefer direct laryngoscopy and use of a short rigid esophagoscope to obtain a detailed evaluation of larynx, pharynx, hypopharynx, and UES. A flexible endoscope is used to complete the assessment of the esophageal body and of the esophagogastric junction. If a pharyngoesophageal diverticulum is present, endoscopy is not considered necessary unless an underlying malignant neoplasm is suspected in the diverticulum. In the presence of a diverticulum, endoscopic assessment of the rest of the esophagus is delayed until the oropharyngeal problem has been completely corrected.

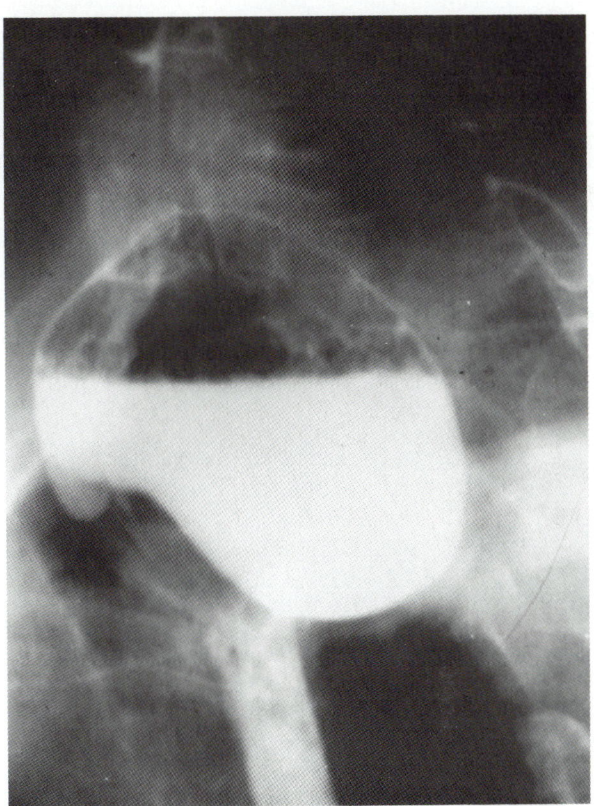

**Figure 49–2.** Large Zenker's diverticulum with liquid and food retention responsible for aspiration symptoms.

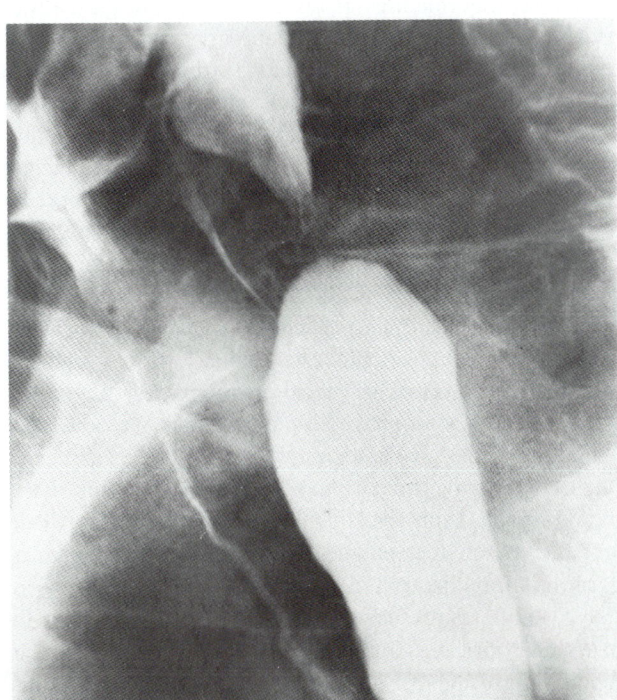

**Figure 49–1.** Pseudotumor effect and laryngeotracheal aspiration in a patient with oropharyngeal dysphagia from muscular dystrophy.

### *Motility Studies*

Manometric evaluation of the whole esophagus and both its sphincters is essential to document distal esophageal func-

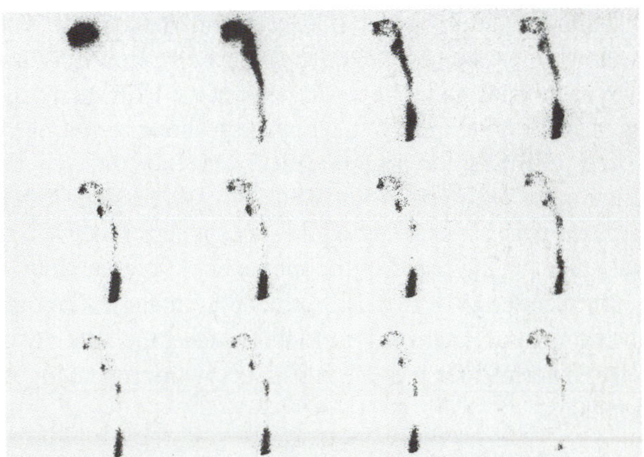

**Figure 49–3.** Pharyngoesophageal emptying scintigram demonstrating retention in valleculae and pyriform sinuses.

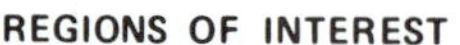


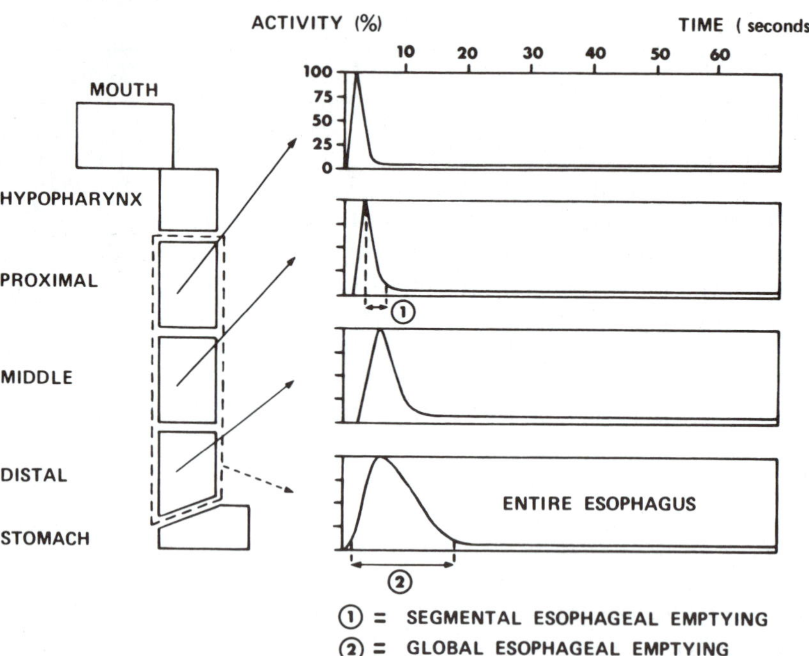


**Figure 49–4.** Scintigrams can help assess segmental or global esophageal emptying capacity.

tion and the physiologic abnormalities of the pharyngoesophageal junction. Precise and meticulous evaluation of the UES is difficult to perform. Current manometric techniques must take into consideration two factors: the radial and axial asymmetry of the sphincter and the upward and anterior excursion of the sphincter during every swallow. Single-port recording catheters are notably inaccurate in assessing UES resting pressures. A study by Winans documented that when UES resting pressures are recorded at the same level with a multilumen recording catheter, pressures in the anterior and posterior axis are twice as high as pressures in the lateral axis.[4] A circumferential pressure transducer, as used by Castell et al, provides the most accurate pressure recordings.[5,6] The Dent sleeve catheter provides the advantage of recording sphincter pressures at any level along the sleeve membrane, allowing accurate measurement even during the sphincter displacement that occurs with swallowing.[7] A composite probe using a microtransducer at pharyngeal level and a sleeve catheter at the UES can be assembled. Despite improvement in the accurate recording of resting pressures, the assessment of relaxation and coordination in the UES remains difficult. For that reason, Castell proposed positioning the recording sensor above the UES to study the opening phase of the sphincter. At present, manometric recordings of the UES provide accurate resting and closing pressure values but underestimate the true functional abnormalities present in patients with oropharyngeal dysphagia.

## Treatment and Results

Simple cricopharyngeal myotomy is performed for oropharyngeal dysphagia and UES dysfunction resulting from various causes. When a pharyngoesophageal diverticulum is present, cricopharyngeal myotomy is accompanied by either diverticulum suspension or diverticulum resection.

### *Neurologic Dysphagia*

Patients with dysphagia of pure neurologic origin reveal functional abnormalities of resting pressure in the UES as well as incoordination and relaxation defects. UES hypertension was described by Ellis and Crozier.[8] Bonavina et al described incoordination and poor relaxation of the sphincter during contraction.[9] My associates and I observed normal resting pressures in the UES, but relaxation was incomplete in seven of 20 patients who underwent studies because of dysphagia secondary to neurologic disease. Poor coordination of sphincter opening during pharyngeal contraction was observed in 80% of all patients. Only patients with neurologic oropharyngeal dysphagia showed complete absence of relaxation or achalasia of their UES (Fig. 49–5). The results of cricopharyngeal myotomy for neurologic dysphagia (Fig. 49–6) have been reported for more than 200 patients.[10] Although the underlying motor abnormalities remain unchanged, patients may be expected to improve if they present with intact voluntary deglutition, normal movements of the tongue, normal phonation, and no dysarthria from the central disease.

Overall results have been mixed and vary with the neurologic disease. Approximately 50% of treated patients report improvement. The other patients may show initial improvement but with subsequent deterioration. Poor results are seen when the prognostic factors mentioned cannot be met. The mortality following this operation for a neurologic condition may be as high as 12–20%. This morbidity

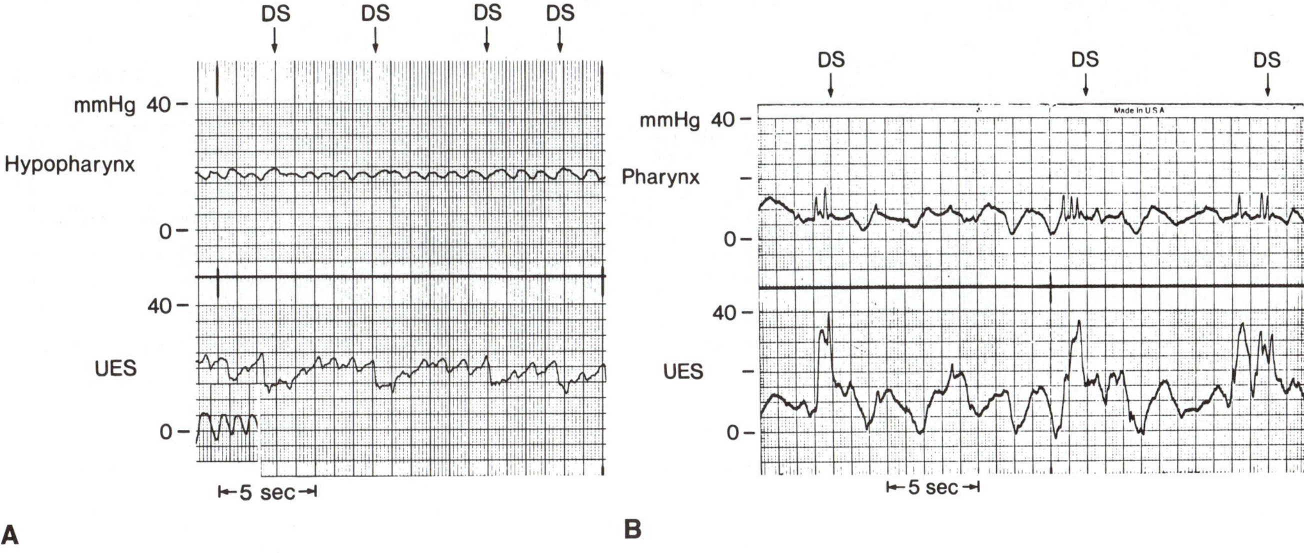


**Figure 49–5. A.** Absent pharyngeal contractions and unrelaxing UES in patient with neurologic dysphagia. **B.** Uncoordinated pharyngeal contraction with active contractions at UES.

and mortality result from persistent aspiration with subsequent pulmonary and cardiovascular complications.

### *Muscular Dysphagia*

Weaker and longer contractions in the pharynx of patients with muscular disease do not produce enough power to propel the bolus past the cricopharyngeus muscle (Fig. 49–7A). The UES is thus a functional obstacle to bolus transit. Just as for patients with neurologic disorders, the intent of cricopharyngeal myotomy is to abolish the resistance of the pharyngoesophageal junction (Fig. 49–7B). The operation follows the same technique as described in Figure 49–6.

Although patients with muscular disease have a weakened pharynx, improvement in oropharyngeal dysphagia is observed in more than 75% of patients who undergo operations.[3,10] These patients retain adequate voluntary deglutition. If the patients have appropriate muscular control of their laryngeal structure, comfortable swallowing is afforded after cricopharyngeal myotomy. Symptoms are decreased by the operation, and improvement in pharyngeal emptying is usually observed. Progression of the disease over time is the main factor that determines the evolution of symptoms after myotomy. Appearance of dysphagia and hoarseness suggest deterioration of muscular function with the potential for increased aspiration episodes. In these patients, laryngeal exclusion or excision becomes necessary to stop the repetitive aspirations.

### *Idiopathic Dysfunction of the UES*

More than 80 patients have undergone a cricopharyngeal myotomy for exclusive dysfunction of the UES. Seven of eight patients are reported to show excellent improvement after the operation.

When a pharyngoesophageal diverticulum was present, Cook et al[11] and Jamieson et al[12] used a sleeve sensor to assess sphincter function and documented high intrabolus pressures in the hypopharynx during swallows (Fig. 49–8). At the same time this occurs, a restricted opening area occurs in the UES. This decreased opening of the sphincter was caused by histologically documented fibrosis and inflammation that produced a restrictive myopathy of the UES. Both decreased sphincter compliance and high hypopharyngeal intrabolus pressures lead to diverticulum formation. Cricopharyngeal myotomy (Fig. 49–6) with either a diverticulum suspension or a diverticulum resection (Fig. 49–9) brings uniformly good results in the management of this type of oropharyngeal dysphagia.

### *Iatrogenic and Distal Esophageal Dysfunction*

Functional abnormalities of the UES are most commonly seen after extensive cervical operations such as laryngectomy. In this situation, recurrent malignant disease must be ruled out before the standardized cricopharyngeal myotomy is performed.

## IDIOPATHIC MOTOR DISORDERS OF THE ESOPHAGUS

### Hypomotility and Achalasia

Achalasia of the esophagus is the best described idiopathic motor disorder of the esophagus. It is a rare condition with an incidence described in many countries as approximately one case per 100,000 population.

### *Etiology*

The exact mechanism that leads to achalasia as a motor disorder remains unknown. The basic defect seems to be a

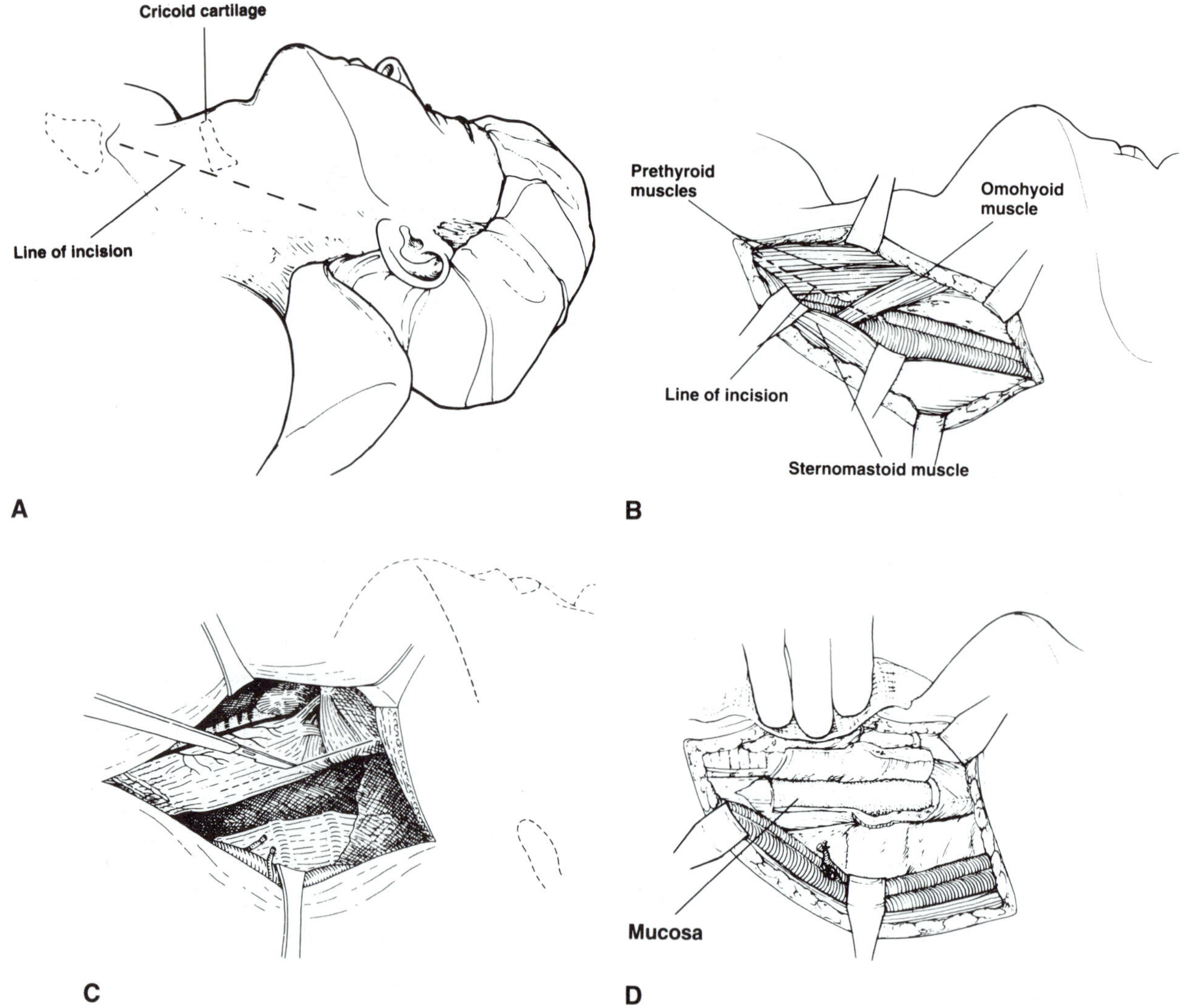


**Figure 49–6. A.** The approach to a cricopharyngeal myotomy is through incision along the anterior border of the sternomastoid muscle. **B.** With the sternothyroid muscle retracted laterally, the omohyoid and prethyroid muscles are transected along the line of incision. **C.** The middle thyroid vein and inferior thyroid artery are ligated and divided to expose the cricopharyngeal area. The pharyngoesophageal junction is further exposed by medial extraction and everting pressure on the right side of the neck. A 6-cm cricopharyngeal myotomy extends from the hypopharynx to the cervical esophagus. **D.** A flap of muscularis is dissected from the mucosa and resected, leaving the pharyngoesophageal junction without posterior muscle. *(From Duranceau A, Jamieson GG, Beauchamp G: Surg Clin North Am 1983;63:833–839.)*

neuromuscular disorder resulting from a loss of control at the postganglionic level of nonadrenergic and noncholinergic inhibitory nerves. These abnormalities explain the loss of peristalsis in the esophageal body and the absent relaxation in the LES with lesions of the intramural nerve plexus, which become more severe with progression of the disease. The intrinsic motor neurons of the plexus between the inner circular and outer longitudinal muscular layers are either reduced in number or entirely absent. These abnormalities are seen at all levels of both striated and smooth muscle in the esophagus but are more prominent in the distal portion and the LES. Histopathologic changes also exist in the preganglionic nerve axons and in the brain stem nuclei.[13] The smooth muscle itself shows variable and nonspecific changes, including sclerosis of the muscle and loss of intermuscular connection. These findings suggest denervation atrophy and are presumptive evidence of a neurogenic pathogenesis of achalasia.

Chagas disease produces a motor disturbance quite similar to classic achalasia. This condition is seen mostly in South America and is caused by a parasitic infection with *Trypanosoma cruzi.* This disease is responsible for a systemic type of disorder that affects both the digestive tract and the cardiopulmonary system.

### *Clinical Presentation*

Achalasia is seen most commonly in young adults; patients commonly present between 35 and 45 years of age. This motor disorder also may be seen in the very young and in the elderly.[14] Dysphagia is the earliest symptom of achala-

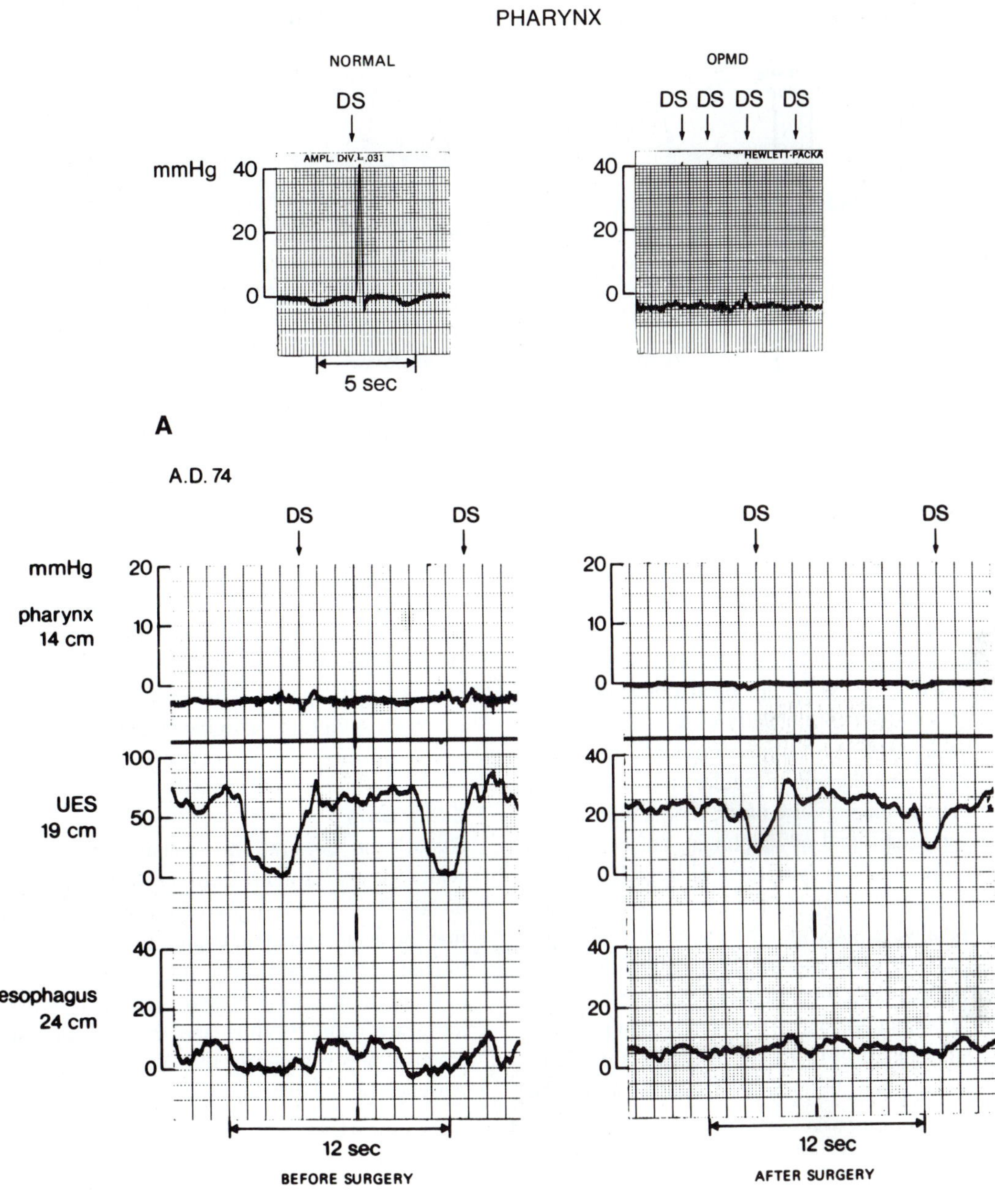


**Figure 49–7. A.** Manometry reveals a normal pharyngeal contraction (left) with powerless pharyngeal contractions (right) in a patient with muscular dystrophy. **B.** Cricopharyngeal myotomy in a patient with muscular dystrophy. Resting pressures are decreased at the UES. The duration of UES opening during pharyngeal contraction is decreased as well. DS = dry swallow.

sia and is described in nearly all patients as a sticking sensation in the substernal area. Occasionally, the symptoms are referred to the pharyngoesophagel junction as oropharyngeal dysphagia. The dysphagia may be influenced by tension or anxiety; regurgitation is present in more than 70% of patients. The regurgitated food is not sour, regurgitation tends to occur immediately after a meal. In later stages it occurs during sleep, occasionally manifesting as tracheobronchial aspiration. Odynophagia is recorded in approximately 30% of patients, usually in the early phase of the condition, when the dysfunction is recorded as vigorous. The pain is usually substernal and constrictive, radiating to the midback or toward the neck and the jaw. Pain may be precipitated by drinking of cold liquids. The pulmonary complications seen in achalasia are usually associated with the late phase of the disease. Tracheobronchopulmonary soilage occurs secondary to regurgitation and aspiration of esophageal contents. Recurrent bouts of bronchitis and pneumonia usually dominate the clinical situation. The incidence of pulmonary complications in patients with achalasia is approximately 10%.

The evolution of achalasia may be divided into three

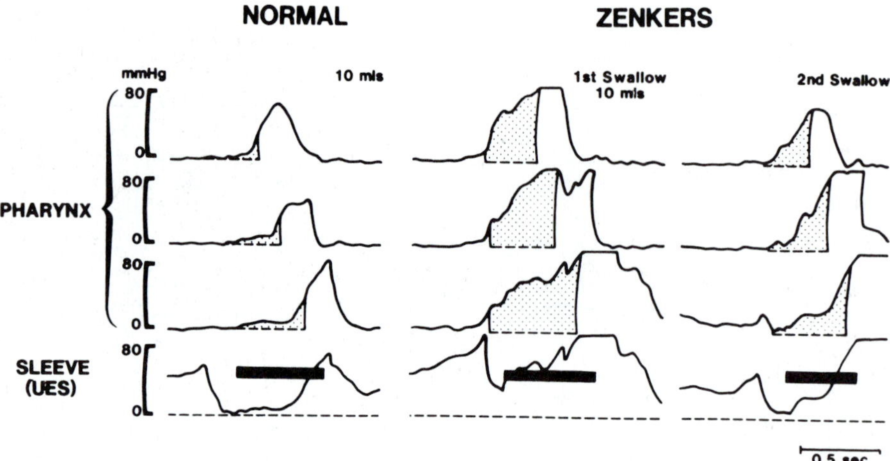


Figure 49–8. Normal intrabolus pressure (left) in the hypopharynx. Increased intrabolus pressures in the hypopharynx of patients with Zenker's diverticulum (right). *(From Cook IJ, et al: Gastroenterology 1992;103:1229–1235.)*

clinical stages. Stage I disease exists in patients with an esophagus less than 4 cm in diameter. Dysphagia, odynophagia, and regurgitation result in weight loss in this early stage. In stage II disease, the esophageal diameter varies from 4 to 7 cm, and patients usually note a decrease in symptoms (Fig. 49–10A). Dysphagia persists,but the esophagus becomes more dilated, and muscular resistance at the cardia is overcome by the pressure of the food column. This results in less dysphagia and odynophagia, but occasional regurgitation still occurs. The symptoms of stage III disease are those of a nonfunctioning esophagus—dysphagia and regurgitation are always present. The esophagus is larger than 7 cm in diameter and remains chronically filled with ingested material that does not progress into the stomach (Fig. 49–10B). Frequent episodes of nocturnal regurgitation and aspiration may result in recurrent pneumonia and pulmonary abscess. This late stage of the disease is now seen infrequently and may be accompanied by symptoms of compression with substernal discomfort. Although it is practical to divide the clinical evolution into these three stages for the purpose of reporting, it remains difficult to correlate symptoms with the size of the esophagus.

### *Diagnosis*

**Radiologic Evaluation.** A chest radiograph may show a widened mediastinum from a dilated esophagus containing an air–fluid level. Signs of chronic pulmonary aspiration may be seen. Dynamic evaluation of the esophagus with a videoesophagogram may demonstrate various stages of esophageal dilatation. Spastic contractions may be seen, but these are nonperistaltic, and there is retention of contrast material above a poorly relaxing esophagogastric junction. Absence of a gastric air bubble is noted in at least 50% of

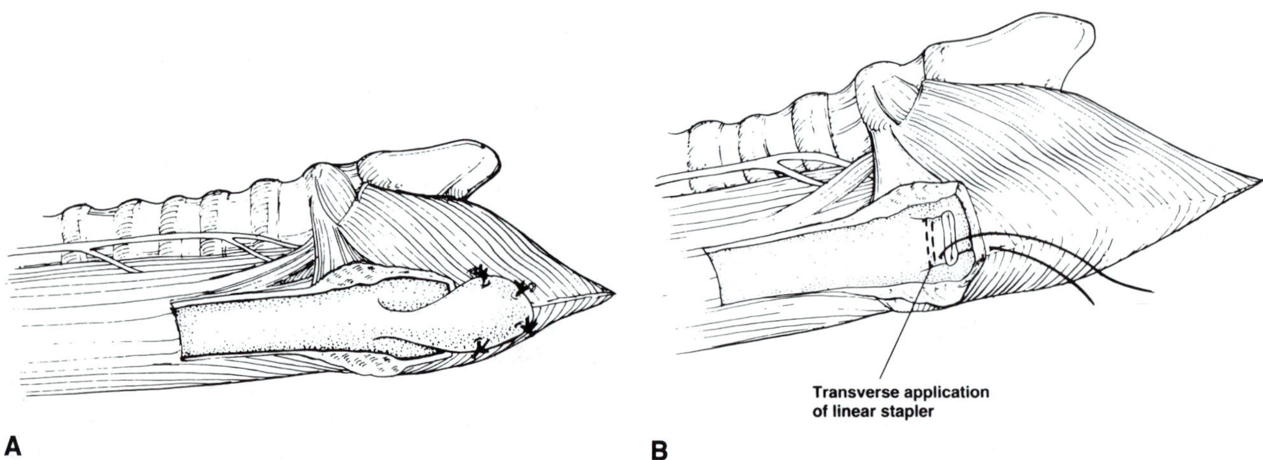


**Figure 49–9. A.** Cricopharyngeal myotomy is the most important part of the operation. It extends from hypopharynx to cervical esophagus. When the diverticulum is small, it is suspended and tied to the posterior pharyngeal wall. **B.** When the diverticulum is large (usually when greater than 4 cm), it should be resected.

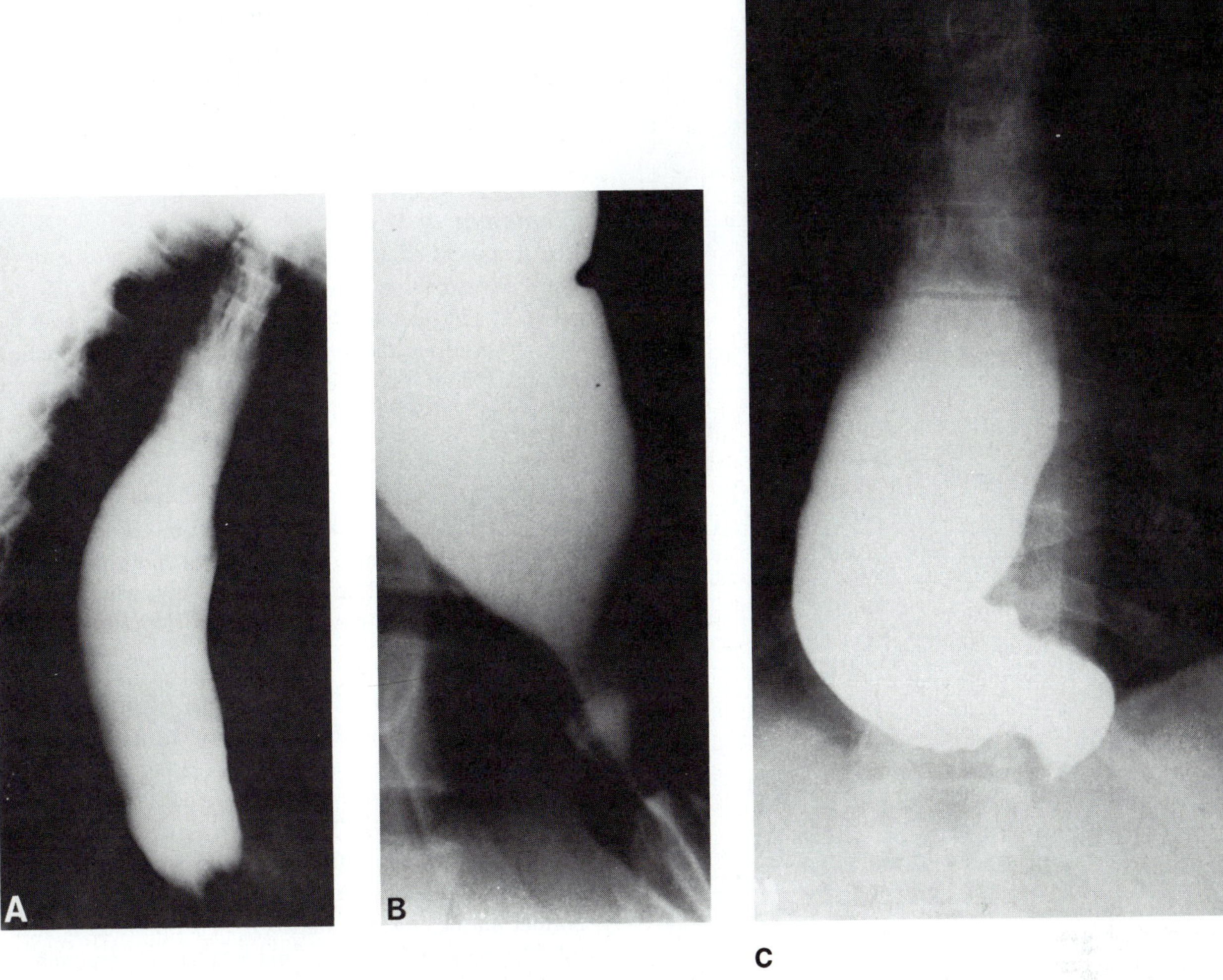


**Figure 49–10.** **A.** A barium swallow radiograph in a 17-year-old with achalasia shows a large dilated esophagus, which, however, is still smooth and has not acquired the sigmoid shape. The esophageal wall is also smooth. **B.** The distal esophagus and area of the LES in this patient are smooth with normal mucosa and unrelaxed LES. **C.** The barium swallow shows a dilated sigmoid-shaped esophagus with failure of relaxation of the LES at the point of narrowing with the beak-like appearance of the distal esophagus.

patients with achalasia. The end-stage esophagus is larger than 7 cm and demonstrates food retention and has a sigmoid-like appearance of the esophageal body (Fig. 49–10C).

**Endoscopy.** The endoscopic features of achalasia show indirect evidence of a malfunctioning esophagus with stasis. The dilated esophageal body may show retained food and liquid or saliva. Inflammation in the areas of stasis as well as thickened mucosa may be observed. The LES area may offer resistance to the passage of the instrument, but it is essential to rule out an esophageal cancer, which may mimic achalasia in all its aspects. Other causes of organic strictures also must be ruled out.

**Manometric Evaluation.** The motor abnormalities seen in achalasia are diagnostic. They reveal normotensive or hypertensive LES resting pressures, incomplete or absent relaxation of the LES with swallows, increased resting pressure in the esophageal body, and absence of normal peristalsis in the esophageal body. During the early stages of the disease, the simultaneous contraction pattern may show a higher-amplitude contraction. All swallows are replaced by simultaneous, low-amplitude, mirror-like activity at all recording levels. This is the sine qua non for the diagnosis of achalasia. The UES functions normally (Figs. 49–11 and 49–12).

Because of ganglionic denervation of the esophageal body and LES, denervation hypersensitivity has been reported in achalasia. When a cholinergic stimulus is given to the patient as with the administration of Urecholine (bethanechol chloride), the esophageal body demonstrates an increase in baseline pressure, an increase in spontaneous activity, and more frequent and stronger contractions. Chest

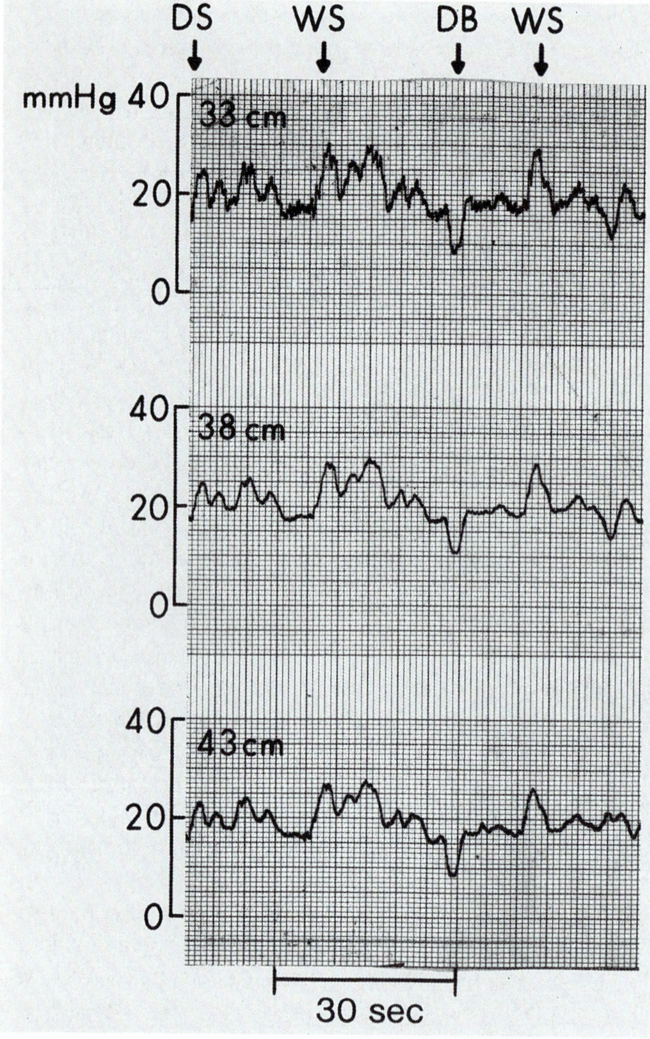


Figure 49–11. Esophageal motor dysfunction in achalasia. Resting pressure is elevated. All swallows are followed by weak and simultaneous waves. DB = deep breath, DS = dry swallow, WS = wet swallow.

pain usually occurs with esophageal spasm, and this is relieved by the administration of IV atropine.

**Radionuclide Emptying Studies.** Liquid and solid radionuclide emptying studies have been used to quantify the emptying capacity of the achalasic esophagus. Whereas a normal esophagus clears an ingested bolus within 15 seconds, in achalasia the esophagus always shows retention 2 minutes after ingestion of the bolus (Fig. 49–13). Isotope-labeled liquid, semiliquid, and solid boluses do not allow diagnosis of the motor disorder. However, they help quantitate improvement in emptying capacity after medical or surgical management.

### Treatment

The treatment of achalasia involves relieving the obstruction caused by the hypertensive, nonrelaxing LES to improve dysphagia and esophageal emptying. Whatever methods are used for therapy, the abnormal motor function of achalasia does not return to normal. All treatments are strictly palliative.

**Medication.** Traube et al showed a decrease in LES pressure with the use of calcium channel blocking agents.[15,16] Esophageal emptying, however, was not improved and there was no clinical improvement in dysphagia or regurgitation in a comparison with placebo.

**Pneumatic Dilation.** The functional obstruction of the nonrelaxing LES may be improved by the progressive inflation of a dilator bag to a pressure of 300–500 mm Hg. The balloon of the dilator is positioned under endoscopic or fluoroscopic monitoring. The dilation is accomplished while the bag is centered on the esophagogastric junction. Single or multiple dilations aim at stretching or rupturing the abnormal musculature of the LES. When dilation is successful, LES pressure decreases and esophageal emptying is improved on scintograms (Figs. 49–14 and 49–15).

Good to excellent results are reported in approximately 65% of patients. The main complication of pneumatic dilation for achalasia is perforation. This complication occurs in 0–15% of patients and averages a rate of 4.5% in large series. The incidence of perforation is believed to be inversely proportional to the experience of the dilating team. When perforation is suspected, immediate documentation should be obtained with a Gastrogafin (meglumine diatrizoate) swallow radiograph. Urgent surgical intervention should be planned, both to repair the disruption and to un-

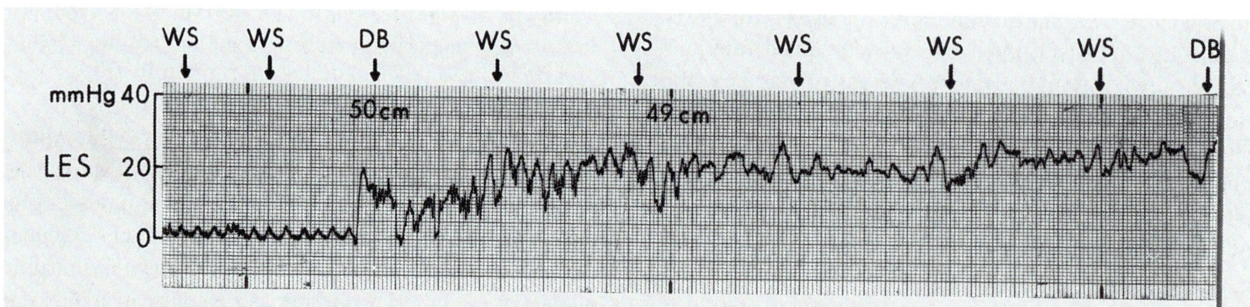


Figure 49–12. The LES in achalasia. Resting pressures are normotensive or hypertensive. Incomplete or absent relaxation is observed with swallows. WS = wet swallow, DB = deep breath.

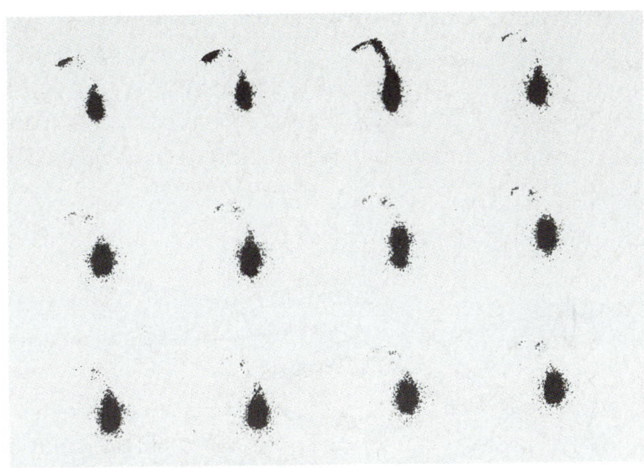

**Figure 49–13.** Radionuclide transit study in patient with achalasia before treatment. Considerable radioactivity is present in the esophagus 24 seconds after ingestion of a single bolus.

dertake definitive treatment by performing an esophageal myotomy 180° away from the site of perforation.

Another potential complication is symptomatic gastroesophageal reflux, which is rarely mentioned as following forceful dilation. Although the true incidence of reflux disease is undocumented, Yon and Christensen[17] reported a 7% incidence, whereas Bennett and Hendrix[18] observed clinical and radiologic signs of reflux in 17% of their patients who underwent dilation. In two prospective studies, Csendes et al detected acid reflux in 8% of their patients who underwent dilation.[19,20] Smart et al used ambulatory 24-hour pH measurement to document acid reflux in 12% of their patients after dilation.[21] Anecdotal evidence of increased inflammation and fibrosis in the esophageal submucosa has been reported at operations following hydrostatic dilation. No clear correlation can be established between such damage and the number of dilation episodes.

**Surgical Treatment.** The surgical alternative for the management of achalasia is esophageal myotomy of the esophagogastric junction (Fig. 49–14). This operation can be performed through a left thoracotomy, by means of laparotomy, or by a thoracoscopic technique.[22] The operation is described as offering a more precise technical approach to the dysfunction of the LES and is considered to improve obstructive symptoms more effectively than dilation.[19,20] Short- and long-term results of this operation reveal absent dysphagia in more than 90% of patients who undergo surgical intervention. This is accompanied by a decrease in resting pressure at the LES, but the functional abnormalities remain unchanged. Some return of propulsive activity has been documented in the proximal esophagus after surgical treatment of achalasia.[23]

The complications of esophageal myotomy for achalasia were reviewed by Andreollo and Earlam,[24] Moreno-Gonzales et al,[25] and by my associates and me.[26] Early complications may occur during operation and include perforation of the mucosa. Perforation occurs in 1.1% of myotomies reported and may lead to esophageal fistula formation and empyema in 0.4% of patients. If mucosal perforation occurs, it is closed with interrupted sutures and buttressed with healthy tissue for added protection. The fundus of the stomach (partial fundoplication) or a pleural flap is usually preferred. Dissection of the esophageal supporting structure in the diaphragmatic hiatus carries the risk of postoperative hernia. Other complications involve early or late recurrence of dysphagia related to the motor disorder. Although it may be difficult to differentiate between incomplete myotomy and healing of the myotomy edges, gradual reappearance of symptoms with return of manometric findings of achalasia suggests rehealing of the myotomy. Reflux esophagitis and stricture are considered the primary late complications of esophageal myotomy for achalasia. The reported incidence of reflux following this operation ranges from 0 to 52%. The reviews by Andreollo and Earlam[24] and by Moreno-Gonzalez et al[25] suggested that the incidence of reflux is higher (13%) in patients operated on with laparotomy as opposed to patients operated on through a thoracotomy (7%). Jara et al observed an increasing incidence of reflux complications with the passage of time: 24% at 1 year, 48% at 10 years, and a stabilization of the complication rate at 52% 13 years after the myotomy.[27] Overall, 19% of these patients had a stricture at long-term follow-up studies. With the increasing objectivity and accuracy of evaluation methods during follow-up care, damage to the esophagus by reflux disease becomes more evident. Thus the 3% incidence of reflux disease following myotomy reported by Ellis and Olsen based on clinical and radiologic observations needs to be reassessed using more accurate methods.[14] Peptic esophagitis accounts for most of the poor results following any procedure for achalasia. Long-term complications of reflux after myotomy also include the appearance of a Barrett's mucosa with ulceration, fistula, bleeding, and malignant transformation.

The length of the myotomy is still vigorously debated, in regard to both its proximal extension and its distal extension onto the gastric wall. The addition of a concomitant antireflux operation following myotomy to prevent the complications of reflux disease also remains controversial. Ellis and Olsen consider this added procedure unnecessary; however, many surgeons now add some form of antireflux operation to protect against this eventuality.[14] Adding an antireflux operation at the end of a nonperistaltic esophagus adds the risk of producing an impediment to emptying. Total fundoplication after myotomy, despite being used by a number of authors, has been documented to result in poor emptying. Progressive dilation of the esophagus and recurrent obstructive symptoms develop in these patients. Myotomy with partial fundoplication has brought uniformly good results without undue dysphagia and with satisfactory control of reflux.[28] This technique seems to offer excellent, symptomatic results by allowing esophageal emptying while protecting against reflux.

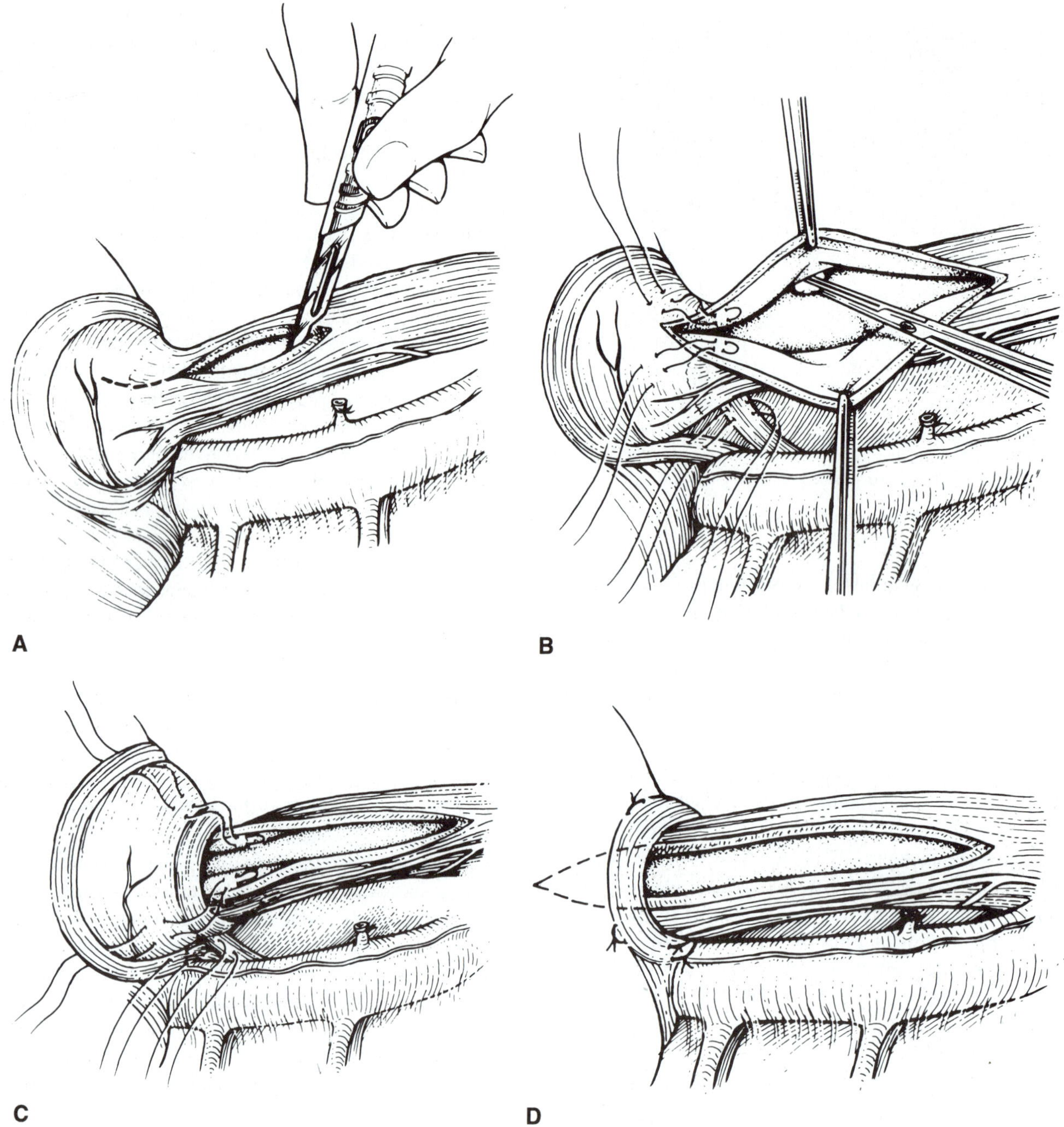


**Figure 49–14. A.** Esophageal body myotomy extends from the inferior pulmonary vein to include the LES and 1–1.5 cm of the gastric wall muscle. **B.** The mucosa is freed over 50% of the esophageal circumference to allow pouting of the mucosa between the transected pieces of muscle. A partial fundoplication is added to protect the esophagus from reflux disease. Two stitches approximate the esophageal muscle layer and the gastric fundus. This modified Belsey fundoplication omits the third suture, which normally would lie at the site of the myotomy. **C.** A second row of sutures approximate esophageal muscle and gastric fundus. These same sutures are then passed through the diaphragm and tied on the thoracic side of the hiatus. This maneuver both reduces the repair into the abdomen and anchors it there. **D.** Operative appearance after repair.

## Hypermotility Disorders

Over the last two decades, meticulous assessment of hypermotility disorders led Castell to propose a reclassification of these conditions.[29] Hypermotility disorders are subdivided into idiopathic diffuse esophageal spasm, hyperperistalsis, and the hypertensive LES. The diagnosis is based on the objective information made available by means of motility recordings. Nonspecific esophageal motor disorders represent a group of unclassified functional abnormalities.

### *Diffuse Esophageal Spasm*

Symptomatic idiopathic esophageal spasm is a motor dysfunction that affects the smooth muscle of the esophagus.

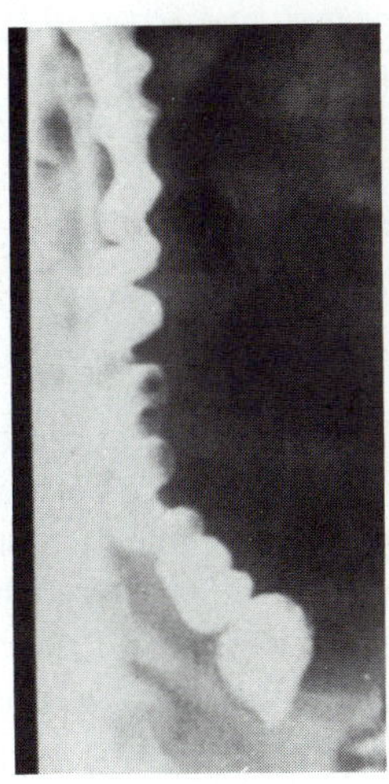
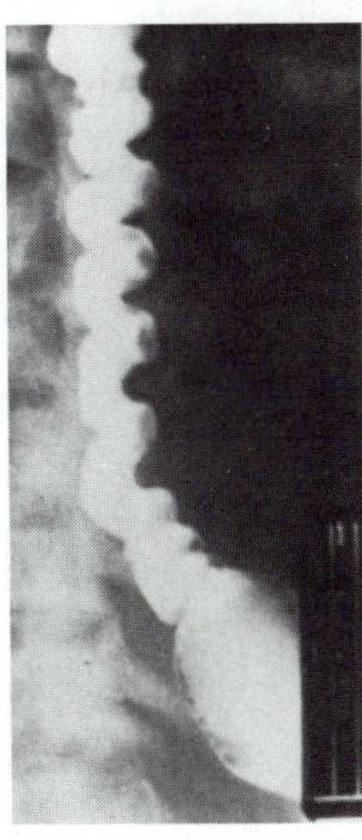

**Figure 49–15.** Barium swallow radiograph indicates diffuse esophageal spasm. The scalloped appearance of uncoordinated contractions occurring throughout the body of the esophagus is seen with a small sliding hiatal hernia.

The diagnostic criteria for diffuse esophageal spasm have been modified in a number of publications but are not yet quite as uniform and precise as for achalasia.[29] Chest pain and dysphagia are often present, but regurgitation is not as frequently reported as in achalasia. The typical patient is anxious and reports symptoms exacerbated during periods of emotional stress. The pain may mimic angina pectoris or myocardial infarction, and these patients are frequently referred to a thoracic surgeon after a normal cardiac assessment. A combination of atypical chest pain associated with dysphagia should suggest this diagnosis. This is a rare condition; only 4% of all patients who undergo tests in an esophageal function laboratory are considered to have true idiopathic diffuse esophageal spasm.[30]

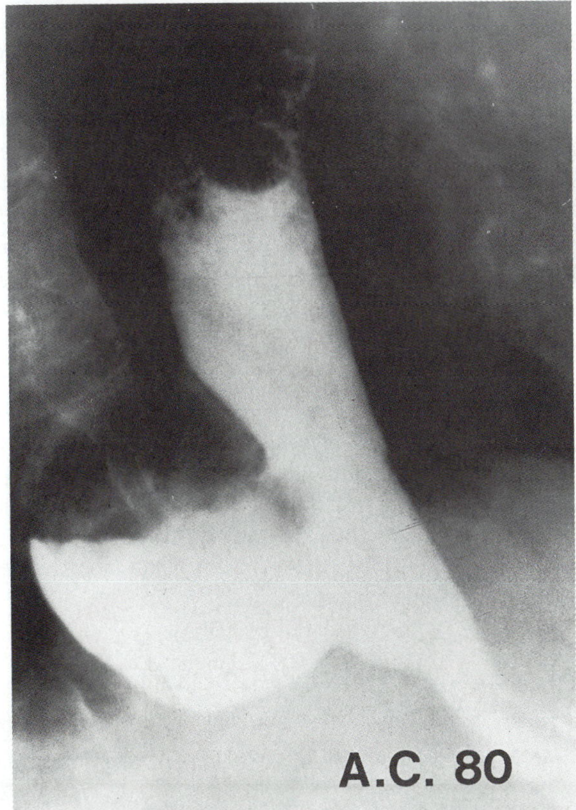


**Figure 49–16.** Large epiphrenic diverticulum in an 80-year-old patient with dysphagia.

**Etiology.** The pathogenesis of diffuse esophageal spasm is unknown. The esophageal musculature may show an increased thickness in both its longitudinal and circular layers.[31] The innervation of the esophageal wall has normal histologic features, in contrast to the pathologic findings of achalasia. Some focal infiltration by chronic inflammatory cells may be observed. Although hypertrophied, the esophageal muscle cells do not show appreciable ultrastructural changes.

**Diagnosis.** The correlation of symptoms, radiologic abnormalities, and manometric abnormalities is considered essential before a diagnosis of diffuse esophageal spasm is confirmed.

***Radiology.*** Most patients with diffuse esophageal spasm do not experience chest pain during their barium evaluation, and often the results appear completely normal. When abnormal contractions appear during radiologic assessment, they suggest a disorder affecting the smooth muscle portion of the esophagus. Abnormal radiographic findings include segmental contractions resulting in the appearance of a corkscrew or rosary beads over the distal two thirds of the esophagus (Fig. 49–15). The esophagus may show dilatation proximal to the dysfunctional segment. Frequently, transient or persistent diverticula have been observed in association with these contractions (Fig. 49–16). Because of the intermittent nature of this disorder, Stein and DeMeester suggested using ambulatory esophageal manometry as a more accurate way to diagnose and classify motor disorders of this type.[32]

### *Endoscopy*

Endoscopy is indicated to exclude any esophageal lesion that might explain abnormal contractions. Segmental contraction may occasionally cause resistance to the passage of the endoscope, but otherwise the mucosa is usually normal, and no intraluminal lesions are visualized.

***Manometry.*** The manometric criteria for diffuse esophageal spasm have been described and modified repeatedly, and they remain the subject of considerable discussion.[29] The functional abnormalities usually affect the distal two thirds of the esophagus. Repetitive tertiary contractions (triphasic or more) are observed in response to at least 30% of deglutitions, with normal peristaltic contractions seen between the episodes of spasm. The frequency of nonperistaltic activity may vary from 30% to 80% but is less than 100%. Whereas originally the diagnosis of diffuse esophageal spasm required the presence of high-amplitude repetitive and nonpropulsive activity,[31] it has since been recognized that patients may show abnormal contractions of normal amplitude.[30,33] The LES is usually reported as functioning normally[34]; however, it may be hypertensive and its relaxation may be recorded as incomplete.[35]

The duration of esophageal contraction is increased over two standard deviations above that of healthy people. Repetitive contractions (triphasic) are considered the most typical feature of diffuse spasm. Cholinergic stimulation of the esophagus may increase the contractions considerably. However, the relevance of this stimulation remains unclear. In the LES, incomplete or absent relaxation has been observed with premature sphincter closure. The differential diagnosis includes motor disorders associated with diabetes, scleroderma, alcoholism, or gastroesophageal reflux disease.[36]

**Treatment.** Treatment is aimed at controlling chest pain and dysphagia. Psychologic assessment of patients with these contraction abnormalities is mandatory, because it may play a role in pathogenesis.[37] These patients frequently are very tense and often have an unusually strong desire for medical attention. Control of anxiety with sedatives may decrease symptoms. Medication known to decrease esophageal contraction pressures such as sublingual nitroglycerin or calcium channel blocking agents may be taken before meals to control symptoms. Blackwell et al recorded decreased amplitude in contractions and lower LES pressures when utilizing this therapy.[38] Pneumatic dilation of the LES area may be suggested if the sphincter is considered abnormal.

Surgical intervention for diffuse esophageal spasm is offered only after a prolonged period of medical therapy and follow-up care. Full reassessment of esophageal function is indicated before a decision is made regarding therapy. The surgical treatment of choice is a long esophageal myotomy similar to that performed for achalasia (Fig. 49–14). However, the operative results are not as good as those reported for achalasia. The overall improvement observed in the Mayo Clinic experience was 67%.[14] In more recent reports Ellis et al described experience with 42 patients with chest pain due to diffuse esophageal spasm and related disorders.[39,40] When possible, Ellis et al restricted the myotomy to the diseased portion of the esophagus as demonstrated with manometry. This required extension of the myotomy to include the LES in more than 50% of patients. The overall results were excellent in 70% of patients with a median follow-up period of 5 years. The functional effects of long myotomy have been reported by Paris et al,[41] Leonardi et al,[42] and Ellis.[40] There is a statistically significant decrease in peak contraction pressures in the esophageal body. The LES high pressure zone remains intact when left untouched. When the LES is transected, a hypotensive sphincter must be expected, and a partial fundoplication of the Belsey type is added to protect against reflux. The same treatment philosophy must be followed in the treatment of patients with a pulsion diverticulum of the distal esophagus.

## Epiphrenic Diverticulum

The origin of an epiphrenic or lower esophageal diverticulum is less well understood than that of Zenker's diverticulum. It seems to be associated with intermittent spasm or failure of complete relaxation of the LES. There may be an associated small sliding hiatal hernia with or without reflux. Most patients have an associated motility disorder such as achalasia, diffuse esophageal spasm, or a hypercontracting LES. Symptoms are pain, regurgitation, and dysphagia. Most commonly, symptoms are not due to the diverticulum but to the associated esophageal disorder. Because of the frequent occurrence of these other lesions, it is important that the patient undergo a careful and complete esophageal evaluation, including cine esophagography, barium swallow radiography, esophageal motility study, pH study, and esophagoscopy. Carcinoma can be present in such a diverticulum, but it is a rare occurrence. If the patient has clinically significant symptoms, operative repair is recommended and entails both diverticulectomy and a distal myotomy. A left thoracotomy is the best approach, even for diverticula that protrude on the right. The diverticulum is excised with a careful two-layer interrupted suture closure (Fig. 49–17A–D). Care must be taken not to narrow the esophagus. An alternative to diverticulectomy espoused by Belsey is the suspension of the diverticulum similar to that performed with a Zenker's abnormality. Whichever alternative is chosen, it must be followed in all cases by a long modified Heller myotomy, which is best performed 180° away from the site of the diverticulum. Controversy exists whether the myotomy should end at the gastroesophageal junction or be carried onto the stomach and combined with an antireflux procedure. I prefer the latter approach, and our repair of choice is a modified Belsey Mark IV fundoplication that omits the middle mattress suture over the myotomy (Fig. 49–14A,D). With this approach, results are excellent with a low (1–5%) mortality and a recurrence rate of approximately 5%. If a myotomy is not simultaneously performed, the diverticulum is likely to recur, and an esophageal leak at the site of the diverticulectomy can occur, usually with disastrous results.[43]

## Hyperperistalsis (Nutcracker or Super Squeeze Esophagus)

The most common symptom in hyperperistalsis is substernal chest pain. Coronary disease must be ruled out by appropriate investigation. Patients with hyperperistalsis often show a strong emotional influence on their symptoms. They tend to be hypochondriacal, seeking early and frequent medical attention for their symptoms.[44] Radiologic and en-

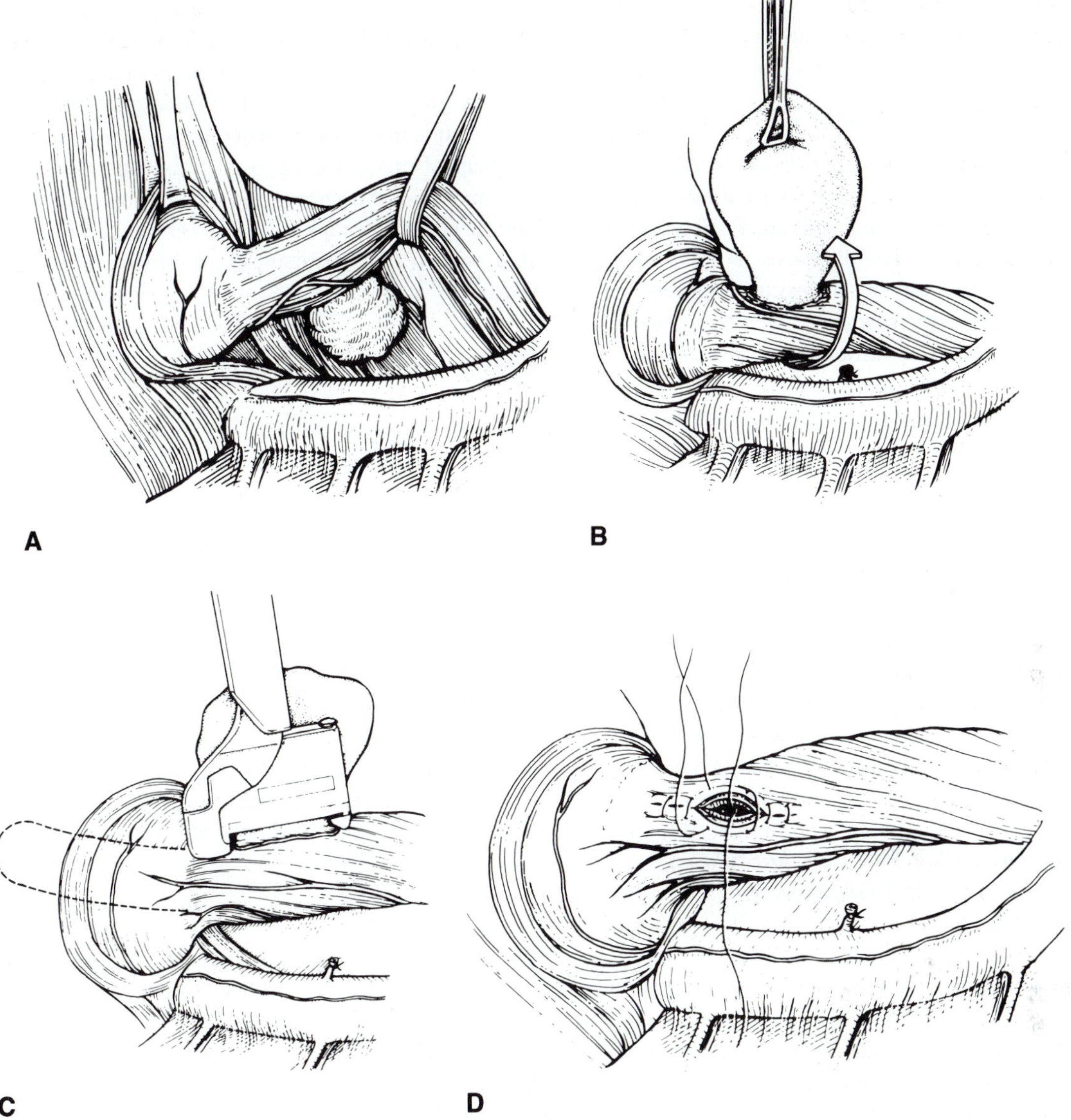


**Figure 49–17. A.** The esophagus is mobilized to the aortic arch. When a diverticulum is present, it usually protrudes toward the right chest. **B.** Full mobilization of the esophagogastric junction is necessary to twist the esophagus and rotate the diverticulum into the left chest. **C.** A large mercury-filled bougie is passed into the esophagus and stomach to protect the integrity of the esophageal lumen during dissection of the collar of the diverticulum. With the bougie still in place, the collar of the diverticulum is closed with a linear stapler. **D.** The muscularis is closed, including the transected neck of the diverticulum.

doscopic examinations are usually normal. Although radionuclide transit studies revealed poor bolus transit in most of the patients studied by Benjamin,[45] Richter[46] observed abnormal transit only in patients with nonperistaltic contractions and low-amplitude waves. In the latter study, transit times were not affected by the amplitude or duration of esophageal contraction. The intermittent simultaneous contractions occasionally present in these patients may account for some of the abnormal transit observed.

### *Manometry*

Patients with hyperstalsis show normal peristaltic progression but achieve a contraction amplitude greater than two standard deviations above normal. The mean amplitude in the distal esophagus is usually greater than 180 mm Hg, and the esophageal contraction duration is increased to more than 6 sec. The LES resting pressure may be elevated and exhibit an occasional incomplete relaxation.

### *Treatment*

Psychologic assessment and treatment are essential in these patients as with other patients suffering from hypermotility disorders. Nifedipine[36] and diltiazem[33] have been shown to decrease both the symptoms of chest pain and the amplitude and duration of distal esophageal contraction. These medications also decrease LES resting pressures. Hydrostatic dilation and bougienage do not seem to offer appreciable benefit.[47] Surgical myotomy has now been reported in 10 patients with documented hyperperistalsis. In eight of these 10 operations, the myotomy extended onto the stomach and was accompanied by a Belsey fundoplication. Results were reported to be good to excellent in all patients.[48–50]

### Hypertensive Lower Esophageal Sphincter

Hypertension of the LES is a resting pressure greater than 45 mm Hg. LES relaxation is usually normal with occasional incomplete opening of the sphincter. Esophageal body peristalsis is normal.[51] The diagnosis is documented with manometric studies, and the therapeutic approach is similar to that for other hyperdynamic disorders. Psychologic assessment, anxiety medication, and smooth muscle relaxants are used. Periodic reassessment of esophageal function is recommended to rule out deterioration of function over time.

### Nonspecific Esophageal Motor Abnormalities

Peristalsis, spontaneous tertiary activity, and occasional prolonged or repetitive contractions are considered abnormal but may not be part of a fixed pattern of contractions. These recorded motor dysfunctions are not typical of a given condition and cannot be classified into a specific disease category. Symptomatic treatment is recommended because surgical treatment is of no benefit to these patients.

## MOTOR DISORDERS OF REFLUX DISEASE, IDIOPATHIC GASTROESOPHAGEAL REFLUX DISEASE

Atkinson et al documented the weakness of the LES when gastroesophageal reflux was present.[52] It was subsequently clarified that if the LES remains constantly hypotensive, reflux episodes occur more often. In contrast, normal resting pressure in the LES is rarely associated with abnormal reflux episodes.[53,54] Dent et al described physiologic reflux episodes occurring in healthy people in association with transient LES relaxations.[55] Dodds et al observed that in patients with esophagitis most of the reflux episodes initially occurred in the presence of a normal LES.[56] LES tone becomes weaker with an increase in severity of the esophagitis. In experiments, LES pressures return to normal values with the healing of esophagitis.[57]

When disappearance of LES tone leads to increased reflux episodes and mucosal damage, disordered motility results. Kahrilas et al studied noninflammatory reflux and mild and severe esophagitis.[58] They reported an increased incidence of failed peristalsis and decreased contraction pressures that were more severe with increasing mucosal damage and circumferential columnar esophagus. Contraction abnormalities are usually worst with poor amplitude and aperistalsis accompanied by a weak or virtually absent LES.[59,60] Stein et al suggested a correlation between the severity of LES hypotension and the extent of functional abnormalities in the esophageal body.[61]

When reflux disease occurs in an esophagus rendered atonic by disease, the usual defense mechanisms that afford protection are absent. Scleroderma, which causes smooth muscle atrophy and collagen infiltration of the esophageal wall, results in one of the worst forms of reflux disease. The esophageal mucosa is exposed frequently to a refluxate of bile and acid. Absence of an LES, poor contractions, and loss of peristalsis rapidly lead to prolonged mucosal exposure with a high percentage of severe reflux complications.[62–64]

## REFERENCES

1. Curtis DJ, Hudson T: Laryngotracheal aspiration: Analysis of specific neuromuscular factors. *Radiology* **149:**517–522, 1983
2. Curtis DJ, Cruess DF, Berg T: The cricopharyngeal muscle: A video-recording review. *Am J Radiol* **142:**497–500, 1984
3. Taillefer R, Duranceau A: Manometric and radionuclide assessment of pharyngeal emptying before and after cricopharyngeal myotomy in patients with oculopharyngeal muscular dystrophy. *J Thorac Cardiovasc Surg* **95:**868–875, 1988
4. Winans CS: The pharyngoesophageal closure mechanism: A manometric study. *Gastroenterology* **63:**768–777, 1972
5. Castell JA, Dalton CB, Castell DO: Pharyngeal and upper esophageal sphincter manometry in humans. *Am J Physiol* **258:**173–178, 1990
6. Castell JA, Dalton CB: Esophageal manometry. In Castell DO (ed): *The Esophagus.* Boston, Little, Brown, 1992, pp 143–160
7. Kahrilas PJ, Dodds WJ, Dodds WJ, et al: A method for continuous monitoring of upper esophageal sphincter pressure. *Dig Dis Sci* **32:**121–128, 1987
8. Ellis FH, Crozier RE: Cervical esophageal dysphagia: Indications for and results of cricopharyngeal myotomy. *Ann Surg* **194:**279–289, 1981
9. Bonavina L, Khan HA, DeMeester TR: Pharyngoesophageal dysfunctions: The role of cricopharyngeal myotomy. *Arch Surg* **120:**541–549, 1985
10. Duranceau A, Lafontaine E, Taillefer R: Oropharyngeal dysphagia. In Jamieson GG (ed.): *Jamieson's Surgery of the Oesophagus.* London, Churchill Livingston, 1988 pp 413–434
11. Cook IJ, Gabb M, Panagopoulos V, et al: Pharyngeal (Zenker's) diverticulum is a disorder of upper esophageal sphincter opening. *Gastroenterology* **103:**1229–1335, 1992
12. Jamieson GG, Cook IJ, Shaw D: The pathogenesis of Zenker's diverticulum and its normalization by cricopharyngeal myotomy. *International Society for Diseases of the Esophagus Meeting Report,* Kyoto, 1993
13. Cassella RR, Brown AL Jr, Sayre GP, Ellis FH Jr: Achalasia of the esophagus: Pathologic and cytologic considerations. *Ann Surg* **60:**474–486, 1964
14. Ellis FH, Olsen AM: Achalasia of the esophagus. *Major Problems in Clinical Surgery,* Vol 9. Philadelphia, Saunders, 1969
15. Traube M, Hongo M, Magyar L, McCallus RW: Effects of nifedipine in achalasia and in patients with high amplitude peristaltic esophageal contractions. *JAMA* **252:**1733–1736, 1984
16. Traube M, Dubovik S, Lange RC, McCallus RW: The role of nifedipine therapy in achalasia: Results of a randomized, double-blind, placebo controlled study. *Am J Gastroenterol* **84:**1259, 1989
17. Yon J, Christensen J: An uncontrolled comparison or treatments for achalasia. *Ann Surg* **182:**672–676, 1975
18. Bennett JR, Hendrix TR: Treatment of achalasia with pneumatic dilatation. *Mod Treat* **7:**1217–1228, 1970
19. Csendes A, Braghetto I, Henriquez A, et al: Late results of a prospective randomized study comparing forceful dilatation and esophagomyotomy in patients with achalasia. *Gut* **30:**299–305, 1989

20. Csendes A, Velasco N, Braghetto I, Henriquez A: A prospective randomized study comparing forceful dilatation and esophagomyotomy in patients with achalasia of the esophagus. *Gastroenterology* **80:**789–795, 1981
21. Smart HL, Foster PN, Evans DF, et al: Twenty-four hour esophageal acidity in achalasia before and after pneumatic dilatation. *Gut* **28:**883–887, 1987
22. Pellegrini C, Wetter A, Patti M, et al: Thoracoscopic esophagomyotomy: Initial experience with a new approach for treatment of achalasia. *Ann Surg* **216:**291–299, 1992
23. Topart P, Deschamps C, Taillefer R, Duranceau A: Long-term effect of total fundoplication on the myotomized esophagus. *Ann Thorac Surg* **54:**1046–1052, 1992
24. Andreollo NA, Earlam RJ: Heller's myotomy for achalasia: Is an added antireflux procedure necessary? *Br J Surg* **74:**765–769, 1987
25. Moreno-Gonzales E, Garcia AA, Garcia LI, et al: Results of surgical treatment of esophageal achalasia: Multicenter retrospective study of 1850 cases. *Int Surg* **73:**69–77, 1988
26. Duranceau A, Lafontaine E, Deschamps C: Complications of operations for esophageal motor disorders. In Waldhausen JA, Orringer MB (eds): *Complications in Cardiothoracic Surgery.* St. Louis, Mosby Year Book, 1991, p 397
27. Jara FM, Toledo PLH, Lewis JW, Magilligan DJ Jr: Long term results of esophagomyotomy for achalasia of the esophagus. *Arch Surg* **115:**935–936, 1979
28. Little AG, Soriano A, Ferguson MK, et al: Surgical treatment of achalasia: Results of esophagomyotomy and Belsey repair. *Ann Thorac Surg* **45:**489, 1988
29. Castell DO: Achalasia and diffuse esophageal spasm. *Arch Intern Med* **136:**571–579, 1976
30. Boag DC, Castell DO, Hewson EG, et al: Diffuse esophageal spasm: A rare motility disorder not characterized by high amplitude contractions. *Dig Dis Sci* **36:**1025–1028, 1991
31. Ellis FH, Olsen AM, Schlegel JF, Code CF: Surgical treatment of esophageal hypermotility disturbances. *JAMA* **188:**862–866, 1964
32. Stein HJ, DeMeester TR: Indications, technique and clinical use of ambulatory 24-hour esophageal motility monitoring in a surgical practice. *Ann Surg* **217:**128–137, 1993
33. Richter JE, Spurling TJ, Cordova CM, Castell DO: Effects of oral calcium blocker diltiazem on esophageal contractions. *Dig Dis Sci* **29:**646–656, 1984
34. DiMarino AJ, Cohen S: Characteristics of lower esophageal sphincter function in symptomatic diffuse esophageal spasm. *Gastroenterology* **66:**1–6, 1974
35. Campo S, Traube M: Lower esophageal sphincter dysfunction in diffuse esophageal spasm. *Am J Gastroenterol* **84:**928–932, 1989
36. Richter JE, Dalton CB, Bradley LA, Castell DO: Oral nifedipine in the treatment of non-cardiac chest pain in patients with nutcracker esophagus. *Gastroenterology* **93:**21–28, 1987
37. Clouse RE, Lusman PJ: Psychiatric illness and contraction abnormalities of the esophagus. *N Engl J Med* **309:**1337–1342, 1983
38. Blackwell JN, Holt S, Heading RC: Effect of nifedipine on oesophageal motility and gastric emptying. *Digestion* **21:**50–56, 1981
39. Ellis FH, Crozier RE, Shea JA: Long esophagomyotomy for diffuse esophageal spasm and related disorders. In Siewert JR, Hölscher AH: *Diseases of the Esophagus.* Berlin, Springer-Verlag, 1988, pp 913–917
40. Ellis FH: Esophagomyotomy for noncardiac chest pain resulting from diffuse esophageal spasm and related disorder. *Am J Med* **92(5A):**129S–131S, 1992
41. Paris F, Benages A, Berenguer J, et al: Pre and postoperative manometric studies in diffuse esophageal spasm. *J Thorac Cardiovasc Surg* **70:**126–132, 1975
42. Leonardi HK, Shea JA, Crozier RE, Ellis FH Jr: Diffuse spasm of the esophagus: Clinical, manometric and surgical considerations. *J Thorac Cardiovasc Surg* **74:**736–743, 1977
43. Allen TH, Claggett OT: Changing concepts in the surgical treatment of pulsion diverticula of the lower esophagus. *J Thorac Cardiovasc Surg* **40:**455, 1965
44. Richter JE, Obrecht WF, Bradley LA, et al: Psychological comparison of patients with nutcracker esophagus and irritable bowel syndrome. *Dig Dis Sci* **31:**131–138, 1986
45. Benjamin SB, O'Donnell JK, Hancock J, et al: Prolonged radionuclide transit in nutcracker esophagus. *Dig Dis Sci* **278:**775–779, 1983
46. Richter JE: Diffuse esophageal spasm. In Castell DO, Richter JE, Boag DC (eds): *Esophageal Motility Testing.* New York, Elsevier, 1987
47. Winters C, Artnak EJ, Benjamin SB, Castell DO: Esophageal bougienage in symptomatic patients with nutcracker esophagus. *JAMA* **252:**363–366, 1984
48. Brown M, Taxier MS, May ES: Esophageal myotomy and treatment of nutcracker esophagus. *Am J Gastroenterol* **82:**1331–1333, 1987
49. Traube M, Tummala V, Baue AE, McCallum RW: Surgical myotomy in patients with high amplitude peristaltic esophageal contractions: Manometric and clinical effects. *Dig Dis Sci* **32:**16–21, 1987
50. Shimi SM, Nathanson LK, Cushieri A: Thoracoscopic long oesophageal myotomy for nutcracker oesophagus: Initial experience of a new surgical approach. *Br J Surg* **79:**533–536, 1992
51. McCallum RW: The hypertensive LES has quite special features: In Giuli R, McCallum RW, Skinner DB (eds): *Primary Motility Disorders of the Esophagus.* London, Libbey Eurotext, 1991, pp 825–829
52. Atkinson M, Edwards DAW, Honour AJ, Rowlands EN: The oesophagogastric sphincter in hiatus hernia. *Lancet* **2:**1138–1142, 1957
53. Haddad JK: Relation of gastroesophageal reflux to yield sphincter pressures. *Gastroenterology* **58:**175–184, 1970
54. Ahtarides G, Snape WJ, Cohen S: Lower esophageal sphincter as an index of gastroesophageal acid reflux. *Dig Dis Sci* **26:**993–998, 1981
55. Dent J, Dodds WJ, Friedman RH, et al: Mechanism of gastroesophageal reflux in recumbent asymptomatic subjects. *J Clin Invest* **65:**245–247, 1980
56. Dodds WJ, Dent J, Hogan WJ, et al: Mechanisms of gastroesophageal reflux in patients with reflux esophagitis. *N Engl J Med* **307:**1547–1552, 1982
57. Eastwood GL, Castell DO, Higgs RH: Experimental esophagitis in cats impairs lower esophageal sphincter pressure. *Gastroenterology* **69:**146–153, 1975
58. Kahrilas PJ, Dodds WJ, Hogan WJ, et al: Esophageal peristaltic dysfunction in peptic esophagitis. *Gastroenterology* **91:**897–904, 1986
59. Ransom JM, Patel GK, Clift SA, et al: Extended and limited types of Barrett's esophagus in the adult. *Ann Thorac Surg* **33:**19–27, 1982
60. Iascone C, DeMeester TR, Little AG, Skinner DB: Barrett's esophagus functional assessment, proposed pathogenesis and surgical therapy. *Arch Surg* **118:**543–549, 1983
61. Stein HJ, Hoeft S, DeMeester TR: Reflux and monthly pattern in Barrett's esophagus. *Dis Esoph* **5:**21, 1992
62. Henderson RD, Pearson FG: Surgical measurement of esophageal scleroderma. *J Thorac Cardiovasc Surg* **66:**686–692, 1973
63. Orringer MB: Surgical management of scleroderma reflux esophagitis. *Surg Clin North Am* **63:**859–867, 1983
64. Poirer NC, Taillefer R, Topart P, Duranceau A: Gastroesophageal reflux control in operated scleroderma patients. *Ann Thorac Surg* **58:**66–73, 1994

CHAPTER

# 50A

# The Treatment of Achalasia and Gastroesophageal Reflux by Minimally Invasive Techniques

Mika Sinanan and Carlos A. Pellegrini

## ACHALASIA

Achalasia, from the Greek meaning *lack of relaxation,* is a motility disorder of the esophagus characterized by the lack of peristalsis, inadequate or incomplete lower esophageal sphincter (LES) relaxation, and the presence of a high resting pressure at the lower end of the esophagus.[1–4] Because there is no way to improve the peristaltic activity of the esophagus in these patients, therapy is directed to decreasing resistance to flow through the sphincter. Both pneumatic dilation and Heller myotomy can achieve this effect, which facilitates emptying in most patients.

### Historical Aspects

Thomas Willis provided the first clinical description of achalasia in 1674[2] and introduced passage of an esophageal dilator as treatment. The first effective method to lower resistance through the sphincter in a reliable manner was described in 1913 by Heller.[5,6] It entailed an extramucosal cardiomyotomy performed through either a left thoracic or an abdominal approach. For many years it proved the treatment of choice for patients with achalasia. The procedure was successful in relieving dysphagia in more than 90% of patients with negligible morbidity and mortality.[7,8] Nevertheless, because of the pain and convalescence associated with both thoracocotomy and laparotomy, a less invasive alternative was sought. When balloon dilation was developed[9] it soon replaced myotomy as the initial approach to the treatment of achalasia. Balloon dilation is often performed on an outpatient basis and is generally not associated with substantial pain. However, balloon dilation does not appear to be as effective as myotomy. In the series of 537 patients reported on by Vantrappen and Janssen,[10] 37.5% of patients had excellent results (no dysphagia) and 39.5% of patients had good results (occasional dysphagia of short duration), a 77% success rate. Perforation of the esophagus occurred in 2.6% of patients with a 0.2% mortality. Ferguson reviewed the results of pneumatic dilation in many centers in the United States, Europe, and South America between 1980 and 1990[4] and confirmed Vantrappen's data. In almost 900 patients treated with different types of dilators, the overall improvement rate was 71%. Gastroesophageal reflux disease (GERD) occurred in 27% of patients. More than 16% of patients required further dilations, and 8% eventually required a Heller myotomy. The overall mortality was 0.3%. Ferguson also analyzed the results of esophagomyotomy for achalasia performed in centers in the United States and abroad during the same decade. The overall success rate among 1199 patients was 89%. Less than 3% of patients required a second operation, and the incidence of GERD was 10%. The mortality was 0.3%.

Only one prospective study[11] compared the results of myotomy with those of pneumatic dilation. In 1989, Csendes et al published the late results of their trial (mean follow-up period, 62 months), which included 81 patients, 39 treated with dilation with a pneumatic balloon and 42 with surgical intervention. Overall results were good in 65% of patients after one or more dilations. By contrast, good results were observed in 95% of patients who underwent myotomy. Although the results of this study supported surgical intervention as the initial treatment, this remains a subject of vigorous debate.[10,12–14]

We believe that surgical treatment is the superior alternative. A myotomy performed under direct vision can relieve the obstruction more precisely and reliably (and with fewer complications) than the blind rupture of the muscle fibers that occurs with dilation. In 1991, stimulated by the excellent results of laparoscopic cholecystectomy, we applied minimally invasive techniques to the treatment of achalasia and started performing the Heller myotomy by means of thoracoscopy. We subsequently found that laparoscopic techniques also are possible. This section describes the indications for, techniques of, and results of extramucosal esophagomyotomy performed via laparoscopic and thoracoscopic approaches.

## Indications and Preoperative Planning

Most patients report a long history of dysphagia with regurgitation of undigested food. Some suffer from chronic malnutrition, recurrent pneumonia, or other complications. Patients with symptomatic achalasia confirmed with radiographic, endoscopic, and manometric studies[15–19] may be considered for thoracoscopic or laparoscopic treatment. A thorough functional and morphologic evaluation of the esophagus must be done in all patients to diagnose and characterize the disease. An upper gastrointestinal radiographic series usually shows a dilated esophagus with bird-beak appearance at the distal end (Fig. 50A–1). This provides invaluable information about location, shape (particularly useful in patients with sigmoid deformities of the esophagus), and relations of the distal esophagus. Endoscopy is important to rule out a tumor. Esophageal manometry typically demonstrates diminished or absent peristalsis in the esophageal body and a high LES pressure with defective relaxation. Pulmonary function should be evaluated in older patients or those with evidence of associated chronic obstructive lung disease.

Patients must be at reasonable risk for undergoing anesthesia and have no uncorrectable coagulopathy. Prior extensive upper abdominal operations or portal hypertension increases the risk of a transabdominal approach. A prior left thoracotomy or poor pulmonary function may hinder transpleural access and single-lung ventilation. Prior balloon dilation or surgical myotomy does not preclude myotomy via the videoendoscopic approach. A history of such treatment certainly influences the endoscopic approach. If a patient has had a previous operation through the left chest we prefer to perform a laparoscopic myotomy; otherwise the thoracoscopic route remains our choice. Should patients with a large sigmoid esophagus be excluded? Our experience suggests that myotomy may be ineffective in these patients; however some patients have experienced improvement. Because there is little to lose, we undertake myotomy for most patients regardless of esophageal shape or caliber.

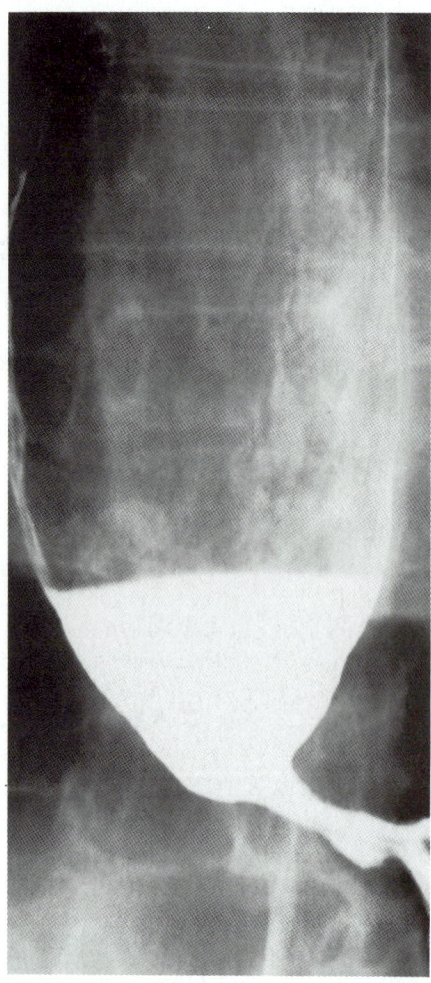

**Figure 50A–1.** Esophagogram shows a dilated esophagus, an air-fluid level, and a bird-beak appearance typical of achalasia.

## Operative Management

### *General Considerations*

Patients should take nothing by mouth for at least 24 hours before the procedure lest they retain food in the esophagus, which may be aspirated during induction of anesthesia. Prophylactic antibiotics are routinely administered. Patients are advised that a thoracotomy or a laparotomy may be required to complete the procedure safely.

### *Thoracoscopic Myotomy*

Anesthesia is induced in a conventional manner, and single-lung ventilation is made possible by placement of a double-lumen endotracheal tube. The patient is positioned in an extended right lateral decubitus position, and dual video monitors are positioned off the right and left sides of the table. The surgeon and one assistant are positioned at the patient's back, and a second assistant is positioned at the patient's front. A fiberoptic endoscope is positioned in the esophagus transorally. This instrument plays a key role during thoracoscopic Heller myotomy. At the beginning of the procedure it facilitates identification of the esophagus with transillumination; subsequently it helps gauge depth of penetration of instruments and provides invaluable assistance in exposure as well as helping gauge the extent of the myotomy.[20,21]

The left pleural space is accessed with five transthoracic ports placed in a diamond-shaped pattern (Fig. 50A–2). Before the parts are inserted, all sites are locally infiltrated with 0.5% bupivicaine as a local anesthetic agent. The first port (A) is inserted after blunt dissection through the pleura anterior to the posterior axillary line in the fourth intercostal space. The scope is inserted to assess the degree of lung collapse and to examine the pleura and mediastinal structures. Three additional 10-mm ports are placed. One telescope port (B) is inserted through the sixth intercostal space 5 cm behind the posterior axillary line, and two operative ports are placed at the posterior axillary line one or two intercostal spaces above (E) and below (C) the telescope port. These ports are used to pass the instruments held in the surgeon's right hand (E) and left hand (C). The telescope enters between these ports and 5 cm behind, establishing a triangle that helps orient the surgeon. The fifth port (D, retraction-separation port) is placed through the sixth intercostal space in the anterior axillary line. Additional ports may be necessary for retraction of the lung or diaphragm and should be placed to provide appropriate access while avoiding conflict with other instruments.

Initially, the posterior mediastinal pleura is obscured by overlying lung and diaphragm, which must be retracted to gain access to the esophagus. A grasping forceps introduced through the D port is used to depress the dome of the diaphragm inferiorly while the collapsed lung is retracted superiorly with an articulated fan-type retractor passed through the superior port (A). The inferior pulmonary ligament is thus placed under tension and can be divided with scissors or cautery. Care is taken to avoid injury to the inferior pulmonary vein. Pleura overlying the groove between the pericardium and the aorta is incised sharply, and the lateral margin of the esophagus is pushed up into the field with the tip of the fiberoptic endoscope (Fig. 50A–3).

After exposure of the muscular wall of the esophagus, the myotomy is begun midway between the esophageal hiatus and the inferior pulmonary vein. With a 90° hook and a blended coagulation current (25–30 W), the longitudinal and circular layers of the esophagus are progressively elevated and divided while the underlying mucosa is protected. Transillumination with a fiberoptic endoscope may be helpful in identifying the layers of the esophagus, especially in patients with previous pneumatic disruption of the muscle or a failed myotomy. The myotomy is extended distally under endoscopic guidance with the hook cautery or bipolar cautery scissors until the endoscopically visible constriction at the LES is completely divided. This part of the dissection is facilitated with cephalad retraction on the esophagus and depression of the diaphragm. Gastric distention from the endoscopic insufflation may have to be intermittently relieved with aspiration of the stomach with the endoscope, especially if the left hemidiaphragm starts to encroach into the operative field. After complete division of the LES, gastric muscle fibers with a different orientation and increased vascularity are encountered. In most patients the myotomy is extended only a short distance (0.5 cm) onto the gastric cardia to reduce the risk of bleeding and postoperative reflux. Patients with "vigorous achalasia" are identified by a history of chest pain associated with diffuse, nonperistaltic contractions of the esophagus demonstrated manometrically. Such patients may achieve additional pain relief if the myotomy is extended proximally to the inferior pulmonary vein.

After longitudinal completion of the myotomy, the submucosal plane is dissected along each muscle edge. A third or more of the mucosa may be mobilized circumferentially by this technique, which allows the mucosa to pouch out through the myotomy and prevents reapproximation of the muscle margins. Thoracoscopic and endoscopic inspection ensures that there is no bleeding and that the mucosa has not been injured. A straight chest tube (22F) connected to a water-seal apparatus is passed through the lowest trocar site and positioned posteriorly. The lung is re-expanded and all ports are removed under direct vision. Trocar wounds are closed superficially and dressed.

Postoperatively the patient can eat a soft diet as soon

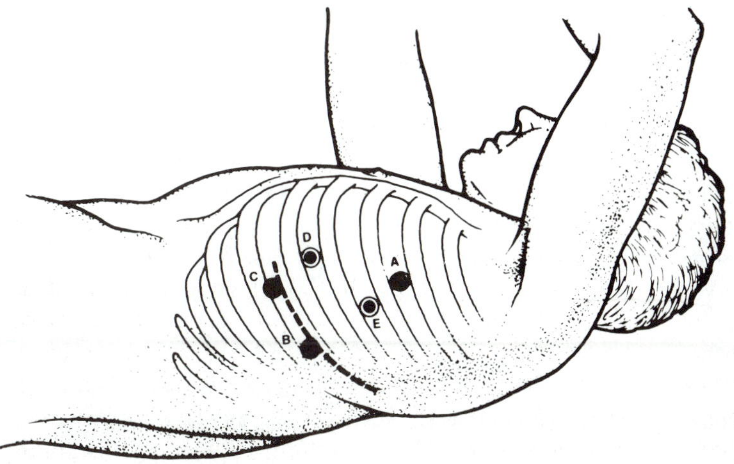


**Figure 50A–2.** Placement of ports for thoracoscopic myotomy.

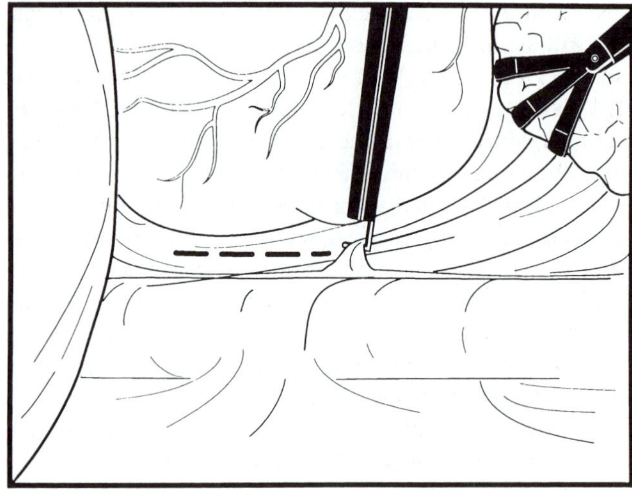

Figure 50A–3. The lung is retracted upward for exposure of the pleura overlying the esophagus in the groove between the aorta and the pericardium.

as he or she is comfortable enough and willing to do so. The chest tube is removed if there is no evidence of an air leak. Most patients are discharged eating a normal diet on the third postoperative day.

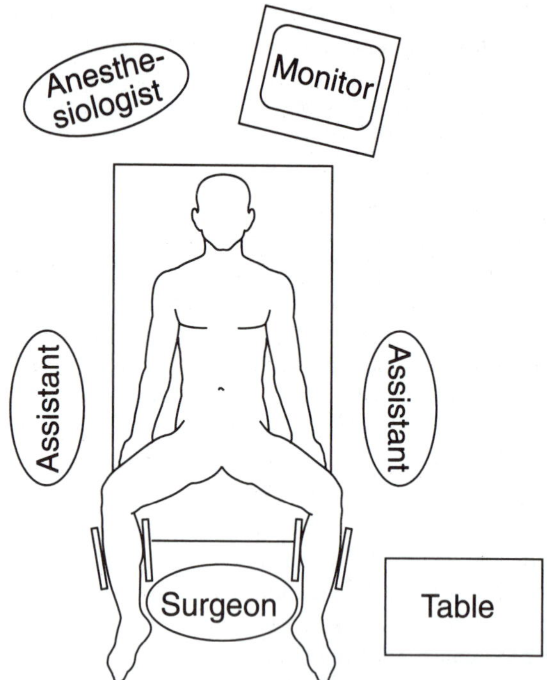


Figure 50A–4. The position of the patient, the surgeon, anesthesiologists, table, assistants, and monitor.

### *Laparoscopic Myotomy*

The patient is positioned in low lithotomy with steep Trendelenberg. The monitor is placed on either side of the patient's head, and the surgeon stands between the patient's legs with an assistant on each side (Fig. 50A–4). Pneumoperitoneum is achieved, and 10- to 11-mm laparoscopic ports are placed as follows: 5 cm above the umbilicus and 2 cm to the left of the midline (telescope port), half way between the xiphoid and the right costal margin (surgeon's left-hand instrument), in the upper left abdomen (surgeon's right-hand instrument), and at the right (liver retractor) and left costal margins in the midclavicular line (gastric retractor) (Fig. 50A–5). This pattern of port placement is the same for most procedures performed at or around the gastroesophageal junction. During the procedure, the 30° telescope is placed through the supraumbilical port between and below the surgeon's two instrument ports. After exploration of the abdomen, the left lobe of the liver is elevated superiorly and the stomach retracted inferiorly with instruments inserted through the right and left subcostal ports. After passage of the endoscope to verify the location of the esophagus, the anterior portion of the phrenoesophageal ligament is divided. This exposes the esophagus anteriorly, after which its anterior wall is cleared for a distance of 5 cm from hiatus to cardia, preserving the anterior vagus nerve. The division of the phrenoesophageal ligament during laparoscopic myotomy does increase the risk of postoperative reflux compared with that of thoracoscopic myotomy. For this reason, we believe that the procedure should be completed with the addition of a partial fundoplication. Therefore, the posterior attachments of the esophagus are divided and the fundus is freed in preparation for the Toupet procedure that will be done later. This allows the placement of a variable-shape memory retractor around the lower esophagus, which better defines the site for the myotomy. The endoscope is then used to locate the narrowed section of lumen and to elevate the esophagus for initiation of the myotomy (Fig. 50A–6). Using the hook cautery technique previously described, longitudinal and circular muscle layers are divided beginning in the middle third of the exposed esophagus to the left of the vagus. It is usually necessary to

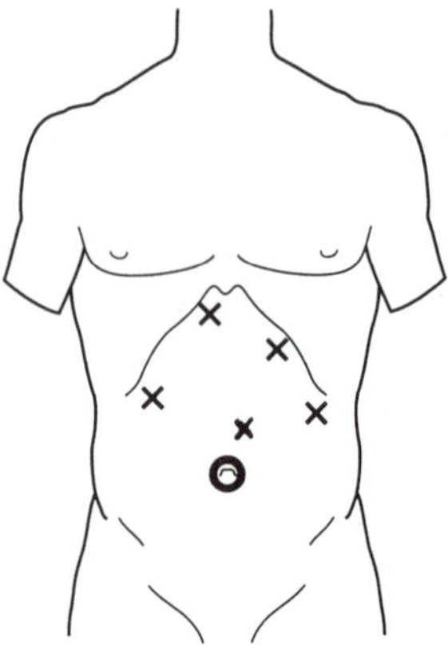

Figure 50A–5. The position of the ports for operations on the cardia.

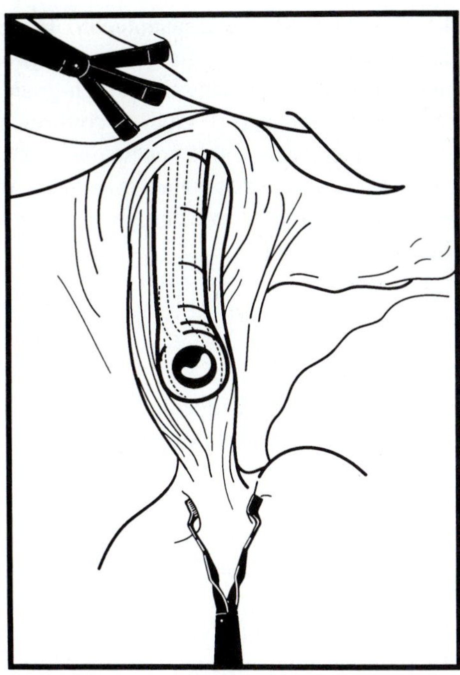

**Figure 50A–6.** An endoscope in the esophagus helps identify the anterior wall of the organ.

carry the myotomy onto the stomach for a distance of up to 1 cm to relieve all endoscopically visible constriction. Postoperatively patients are offered a full-liquid diet on the evening of the operation (unless nausea is present). The next day they eat a regular diet as tolerated. Discharge occurs on the second or third day.

### Results of Esophageal Myotomy

Laparoscopic and thoracoscopic management of achalasia are new procedures with limited published experience. Thoracoscopic myotomy is preferred in patients with vigorous achalasia[22] because of limited proximal extent of the myotomy at laparoscopy. In the largest reported series,[21] we found excellent or good relief of dysphagia in 21 of 24 (88%) patients who underwent esophagomyotomy with a median follow-up period of 12 months, though the first three patients required a second procedure to complete the myotomy. As of May 1994, 36 patients had undergone myotomy with this approach. Excellent (no dysphagia at all) and good relief (occasional dysphagia, less than once a week) was observed in 92% of patients, with a median follow-up period of 16 months. LES pressures declined from a mean of 33.5 ± 7 mm Hg before the operation to 14 ± 5 mm Hg after the operation. No severe morbidity or mortality was recorded in this series. Heartburn was seen in about 25% of the patients in the first postoperative week. Treatment for 4 weeks with $H_2$-blockers was successful in all patients. Despite the substantial reduction in LES pressure, no patient reported heartburn at the time of follow-up examination. Twenty-four-hour pH monitoring in 16 patients, however, showed mild abnormal reflux limited to the distal esophagus in eight patients.

Several reports have indicated that laparoscopy provides reasonable access to the distal esophagus. Shimi et al[23] described a laparoscopic approach to cardiomyotomy that leaves esophageal attachments intact posteriorly. Jorgensen et al[24] included a laparoscopic Nissen fundoplication for treatment of reflux because their procedure included circumferential mobilization of the esophagus. Most patients in these series achieved improvement or relief of symptoms. Experience with open Heller myotomy suggests that the transabdominal approach results in a greater degree of reflux than procedures performed through the chest.[25–27] Although this remains unproved for laparoscopic esophagomyotomy,[27] these considerations are another reason for recommending thoracoscopic over laparoscopic myotomy.

### Complications of Esophageal Myotomy

Potential complications of thoracoscopic myotomy include those associated with anesthesia and single-lung ventilation as well as cardiac arrhythmias from instrument contact or electrocautery near the pericardium. Excessive traction on the lung or too extensive a dissection of the inferior pulmonary ligament can tear the inferior pulmonary vein and cause bleeding. For both thoracoscopic and laparoscopic procedures, care must be taken when manipulating the endoscope to avoid mucosal perforation, especially after the mucosa has been exposed during myotomy. Unrecognized cautery burns to the mucosa may lead to delayed esophageal perforation. The risk of this complication is small when proper procedures are followed during the myotomy. Any question of a postoperative esophageal leak must be evaluated to minimize the severe morbidity of this complication. Mucosal perforation recognized during the procedure may be treated effectively with intracorporeal suture closure of the perforation and muscularis propria. Because almost all perforations occur in the lowest portion of the myotomy (i.e., at the cardia) the area can easily be buttressed with stomach. An additional myotomy is usually not necessary. Intraoperative endoscopy also confirms the completeness of the myotomy as the last constricting fiber is cut, assuring relief of obstruction. Controlling the extent of the myotomy prevents excessive mobilization of the hiatus or unnecessary extension onto the stomach, which may contribute to postoperative gastroesophageal reflux,[26] especially when the procedure is performed through the abdomen.

## ANTIREFLUX PROCEDURES

Abnormal gastroesophageal reflux frequently is associated with a mechanically defective cardia. The defect consists of an abnormally low LES pressure (4–8 mm Hg), an abnormally short sphincter, and an increase in the number of spontaneous episodes of sphincter relaxation. Many patients have an associated hiatal hernia and a low insertion of the phrenoesophageal ligament. Restoration of cardioesophageal competency is the goal of an antireflux procedure.

## Historical Aspects

Because the defect appears to be a mechanical one, numerous operations were described over the years to deal with abnormal reflux. Originally, the focus was the associated hiatal hernia, and attention centered on correction of the anatomic defect. Later, both Allison[28] and Russell and Hill[29] emphasized the role of the angle of His and the importance of reconstruction of the flap valve in the restoration of competency. Skinner and Belsey[30] and Nissen[31] emphasized construction of a long segment of intra-abdominal esophagus and designed a partial or a total wrap of fundus to anchor the esophagus in place. Zaninotto et al[32] defined the physiologic basis of antireflux surgery and identified the relative importance of the intra-abdominal length of esophagus as well as LES length and pressure in determining competency of the cardia.[33]

Today, the principles of surgical treatment of GERD include rebuilding the LES, constructing a passive valve at the gastroesophageal junction, and raising the opening pressure of the cardia. Currently, encircling the esophagus partially or completely with a fundic wrap is the most reliable technique for attaining these goals.[34,35] Until recently, the morbidity of an upper abdominal laparotomy or thoracotomy has been an important deterrent to surgical treatment of reflux. Experience with laparoscopic treatment of reflux suggests that control of reflux can be achieved with little morbidity and a rapid return to normal activities.[36] Although preliminary reports of a laparoscopically placed prosthesis (Angelchik),[37] ligamentum teres cardiopexy,[38,39] and Hill repair[40] have appeared, fundoplication is the most widely practiced laparoscopic antireflux procedure. When guided by an adequate preoperative evaluation and specific technical principles,[41] fundoplication holds promise for effective relief of symptoms in 90% or more of patients.[42]

## Indications and Preoperative Planning

Surgical treatment should be considered for patients with refractory symptoms, frequent recurrences after medical therapy, or complications from reflux. Relative contraindications include obesity, prior upper abdominal operations, or a coagulopathy. Reflux disease with a peptic esophageal stricture can be treated laparoscopically if dilation of the stricture is possible. However, clinically significant shortening of the esophagus cannot be managed effectively with laparoscopic techniques, at least at present.[36]

Preoperative evaluation of patients considering a laparoscopic antireflux operation includes endoscopy with appropriate biopsies, an upper gastrointestinal radiographic series, 24-hour pH testing,[43] and manometry. These studies confirm the presence of pathologic reflux and exclude severe strictures, Barrett's esophagus with high-grade dysplasia, and cancer. Manometry is vital to confirm adequate esophageal body peristalsis with a concomitant loss of pressure in the LES, a pattern not found in patients with secondary reflux disease due to poor esophageal clearance or abnormal gastric emptying.[44]

## Operative Management

Antibiotics are administered to cover common orogastric flora. The patient's position is illustrated in Figure 50A–4 and the position of the trocars in Figure 50A–5. An additional 10- to 11-mm port at the xiphoid process is occasionally useful when passing the variable-curvature shape-memory dissector (EndoRetract; US Surgical Corporation, Norwalk, Connecticut). The procedure is carried out with the 30° laparoscope passed through the upper midline port positioned between the surgeon's operating ports. The length of the operation and the difficulty of the procedure are directly related to the degree of obesity, the ease with which the fundus can be mobilized, and the extent of periesophagitis present.

After inspection of the peritoneal cavity, an articulated fan retractor is passed from the right lateral port to elevate the lateral segment of the liver. The triangular ligament of the liver is not divided because it anchors the liver margin. The stomach is retracted inferiorly with a Babcock retractor placed through the left lateral port. The stomach is decompressed with an orogastric tube, which is then replaced with a 50–52 F bougie to facilitate localization and dissection of the esophagus. This is withdrawn into the upper esophagus during dissection of the posterior esophageal attachments and then readvanced for suturing of the wrap.

The area of the hiatus is examined. When present, a hiatal hernia can usually be reduced using the Babcock retractor and atraumatic forceps. Next, the peritoneum overlying the hiatus is divided. During this step, care must be taken not to divide the gastrohepatic ligament too far to the right because this maneuver can injure the nerve of Latarjet and may encourage displacement or slippage of the wrap onto the stomach. Therefore, we favor dissecting the left crus of the diaphragm first, exposing and dividing the gastrophrenic attachments early in the operation. Although some authors claim that a loose fundoplication can be constructed with the anterior wall of the fundus without dividing the short gastric vessels,[45,46] we believe that dividing the short gastric vessels allows easier and complete mobilization of the top of the fundus and left side of the posterior wall of the esophagus. We divide these vessels early during the operation. We perform this step as a natural extension of division of the phrenogastric ligament. Once four or five short gastric vessels have been divided to achieve ample mobility of the fundus, we open the remaining part of the phrenoesophageal membrane and expose and dissect the right crus. The inner aspect of each crural tendon is separated from the esophagus, and any remaining phrenoesophageal membrane or attachments of a hernial sac to the cardia are divided. This maneuver is done with the bougie in the body of the esophagus to facilitate identification of the esophagus and decrease the risk of esophageal perforation.

Once the crura are exposed, the abdominal portion of the esophagus must be dissected free. The anterior wall of the esophagus is identified with the help of the bougie, and periesophageal tissues are separated from the esophagus with a combination of blunt and sharp dissection. This maneuver can be difficult or not, depending on the vascularity of the tissue and the degree of periesophagitis present. The anterior vagus nerve is eventually identified on the anterior aspect of the esophagus, where it is usually tightly adherent, running either parallel to the esophagus or angling to the right. Dissection is continued down along either side of the esophagus. For this dissection a combination hook/electrocautery/irrigation/suction device is particularly useful. The posterior vagus nerve is found between the right crus of the diaphragm and the esophagus, commonly quite separate from the esophagus. In most patients, the posterior vagus is mobilized laterally away from the esophagus to form the window through which the wrap is placed, between the vagus nerve and the esophagus (Fig. 50A–7).

Dissection of the posterior attachments of the esophagus is one of the more difficult portions of the operation. In preparation, the bougie is withdrawn into the upper esophagus and the 30° scope is angled to provide a view of the right posterior esophagus, where most of the dissection is performed. Rotating and displacing the esophagus to the left exposes these attachments in a progressive manner. Esophageal branches from the aorta and left gastric artery must be identified and controlled with clips or cautery. Posterior dissection is facilitated with a periodic return to the anterior and left sides of the esophagus. Eventually, a window is achieved posteriorly and the esophagus is ready to be retracted anteriorly. The variable shape-memory dissecting-retracting instrument is inserted through the surgeon's right-hand port or a separate xiphoid port, and the esophagus (without bougie) is hooked and retracted anteriorly. Posterior and intercrural dissection is completed. The fundus must be now assessed for mobility and laxity. We prefer to test this by wrapping the fundus around the esophagus to see if there is any tension once the bougie is brought back into the stomach. If the wrap retracts spontaneously behind the esophagus when released, excessive tension is present. Additional short gastric blood vessels must then be divided until the wrap no longer retracts when released.

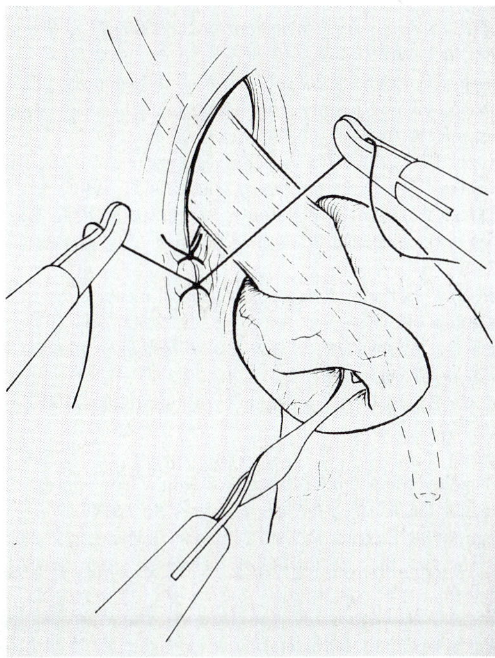

**Figure 50A–7.** The posterior window through which the wrap will be passed.

The surgeon brings the wrap through the retroesophageal window by moving the liver retractor to another port and bringing a Babcock retractor through the right flank port. The Babcock retractor is advanced from right to left behind the esophagus (and anterior to the posterior vagus nerve). The fundus is then grasped, usually by bringing it to the Babcock retractor with a grasper positioned through the left flank port. Anterior retraction of the esophagus with the variable shape-memory dissecting instrument also facilitates this maneuver. Once a satisfactory portion of fundus has been brought through for the wrap, the bougie is advanced once again to avoid excessive narrowing of the hiatus, and the crura are closed. With the wrap and esophagus retracted to the left, one or two sutures of 2–0 silk are individually placed by means of standard endoscopic suturing techniques. Total fundoplication is then completed in a floppy manner with individual 3–0 silk sutures that approximate the wrap to the anterior stomach and incorporate the esophagus. Care is taken not to injure the anterior vagus nerve. Finally, the wrap is anchored superiorly on both the left and right sides to the esophagus in with one 2-0 silk suture (coronal or crowning) in each side to prevent slippage. In patients with severely compromised esophageal body peristalsis, the procedure may be modified to construct a partial wrap in the manner of Toupet[46,47] to reduce the risk for postoperative dysphagia. Similarly, in patients undergoing a laparoscopic myotomy, a Toupet or Dor (anterior partial fundoplication) should be performed (see Chapter 42).

Nasogastric suction is not necessary in the postoperative period. The patient usually eats a soft diet on the first postoperative day and is discharged by the second or third day.

## Results

A prospective randomized trial comparing medical therapy with open surgical therapy for complicated GERD demonstrated that Nissen fundoplication, when performed in an open manner, effectively improved the symptoms and endoscopic signs of complicated esophagitis for as long as 2 years.[42] Few reports of laparoscopic fundoplication have been published since 1991.[36,48–50] These served to indicate the feasibility of the procedure during a process of refinement. Cuschieri et al reported on a multicenter experience[51] with 116 patients who underwent laparoscopic antireflux operations, most treated with an operation similar to that described herein. The median duration for the procedure was 2.5 hours, and the median hospital stay was 2 days. At endoscopy, esophagitis was completely healed in 71% and partially healed in 21% of the patients 3 months after the operation. Twenty-four-hour pH monitoring was initially abnormal in 93% of patients and corrected to normal in 95% after the procedure. With a median follow-up period of 13 months, the authors documented symptomatic improvement in 106 (91%) of their patients, including 96 (83%) who were free of symptoms. In the study, only 10 patients had persistent troublesome reflux, which was considered evidence that the treatment was effective. Studies by Hutson and Hunter[52] and by Bittner et al[53] confirmed these results. In our experience with 63 patients between July 1991 and March 1994, we saw substantial relief in 60 patients and moderate improvement of symptoms in three patients. Postoperative dysphagia was seen in about one third of the patients; it usually lasted less than 1 week and resolving in most patients without the need for dilation.

## Complications

Intraoperative complications specific to fundoplication include perforation of the esophagus or stomach, bleeding, splenic injury, and pneumothorax. Cuschieri et al[51] reported one or more of these complications in 10% of patients, but serious complications were rare and most could be treated with laparoscopy. In their series, only one patient with both perforation and bleeding had to undergo an open operation, and there were no deaths. One of our patients had perforation of the fundus of the stomach, which was discovered within 24 hours of the operation. The patient was successfully treated with an open operation. In retrospect we realized that, this perforation occurred at the time of the operation while the surgeon was trying to bring the wrap around the esophagus with an instrument that had teeth. At the time of reoperation, the sharp imprints of the instrument were visible in the minute gastric perforation that the patient sustained.

Postoperative complications include wound infections, dysphagia, or complete obstruction of the esophagus, gas-bloat syndrome, injury to the vagi with gastroparesis or diarrhea, and recurrence of reflux symptoms. Cuschieri et al[51] found that minor wound infections are uncommon; appropriate care to make a loose wrap results in late dysphagia or gas-bloat in less than 10% of patients. However, early during the postoperative period dysphagia is much more common after laparoscopic than after open Nissen fundoplication. The reason is not apparent.

Although long-term follow-up data are not available, it appears that the laparoscopic approach is rapidly becoming the choice for patients who require reconstruction of the gastric cardia.

## REFERENCES


1. Reynolds JD, Parkman HP. Achalasia. *Gastroenterol Clin North Am* **18**:223–255, 1993
2. Mayberry JF, Probert CSJ, Sher KS, et al: Some epidemiological and aetiological aspects of achalasia. *Dig Dis;* **9**:1–8, 1991
3. Feldman M: Esophageal achalasia syndromes. *Am J Med Sci* **295**:60–81, 1988
4. Ferguson MK: Achalasia: Current evaluation and therapy. *Ann Thorac Surg* **52**:336–342, 1991
5. Payne W: Heller's contribution to the surgical treatment of achalasia of the esophagus. *Ann Thorac Surg* **48**:876–881, 1989
6. Heller E: Extramukose cardioplastik bein chronischen cardiospasmus mit dilatation des oesophagus. *Mitt Grenzgeb Med Chir* **27**:141, 1913
7. Csendes A: Results of surgical treatment of achalasia of the esophagus. *Hepatogastroenterology* **38**:474–480, 1991
8. Sauer L, Pellegrini CA, Way LW: The treatment of achalasia: A current perspective. *Arch Surg* **124**:929–932, 1989
9. Kurlander DJ, Raskin HF, Kirsner JB, et al: Therapeutic value of the pneumatic dilator in achalasia of the esophagus: Long term results in sixty-two living patients. *Gastroenterology,* **45**:604–613, 1963
10. Vantrappen G, Janssens J: To dilate or to operate? That is the question. *Gut* **24**:1013–1019, 1983
11. Csendes A, Braghetto I, Henriquez A, Cortes C: Late results of a prospective randomized study comparing forceful dilatation and oesophagomyotomy in patients with achalasia. *Gut* **30**:299–304, 1989
12. Richter JE: Surgery or pneumatic dilatation for achalasia: A head-to-head comparison—Now are all the questions answered? *Gastroenterology* **97**:1340–1341, 1989
13. Temple J: Achalasia: Dilatation or operation? *J R Soc Med* **79**:695–969, 1986
14. Parkman HP, Reynolds JC, Ouyang A et al: Pneumatic dilatation or esophagomyotomy treatment for idiopathic achalasia: Clinical outcomes and cost analysis. *Dig Dis Sci* **38**:75–85, 1993
15. Couturier D, Samama J: Clinical aspects and manometric criteria in achalasia. *Hepatogastroenterology* **338**:481–487, 1991
16. Blackwell JN, Hannan WJ, Adam RD, et al: Radionuclide transit studies in the detection of esophageal dysmotility. *Gut* **24**:421–426, 1983
17. Brand DL, Martin D, Pope CE: Esophageal manometrics in patients with angina-like chest pain. *Am J Dig Dis* **22**:300–304, 1977
18. Castell DO, Richter JO, Dalton CB: *Esophageal Motility Testing.* New York, Elsevier, 1987.
19. Katz PO, Castell DO: Esophageal motility disorders. *Am J Med Sci* **290**:61–69, 1985
20. Pellegrini CA, Wetter LA, Patti M, et al: Thoracoscopic esophagomyotomy: Initial experience with a new approach for the treatment of achalasia. *Ann Surg* **216**:291–296, 1992
21. Pellegrini CA, Leichter R, Patti M, et al: Thoracoscopic esophageal myotomy in the treatment of achalasia. *Ann Thorac Surg* **56**:680–682, 1993
22. Shimi SM, Nathanson LK, Cuschieri A: Thoracoscopic long oesophageal myotomy for nutcracker oesophagus: Initial experience of a new surgical approach. *Br J Surg* **79**:533–536, 1992
23. Shimi S, Nathanson LK, Cuschieri A: Laparoscopic cardiomyotomy for achalasia. *J R Coll Surg Edinb* **36**:152–154, 1991

24. Jorgensen JO, Hunt DR: Laparoscopic management of pneumatic dilatation resistant achalasia. *Aust N Z J Surg* **63:**386–388, 1993
25. Ellis FHJ: Oesophagomyotomy for achalasia: A 22-year experience. *Br J Surg* **80:**882–885, 1993
26. Andreollo NA, Earlam RJ: Heller's myotomy for achalasia: Is an added anti-reflux procedure necessary? *Br J Surg* **74:**765–769, 1987
27. Jaakkola A, Ovaski J, Isolauri J: Esophagocardiomyotomy for achalasia: Long term clinical and endoscopic evaluation of transabdominal vs. transthoracic approach. *Eur J Surg* **157:**407–410, 1991
28. Allison PR: Reflux esophagitis, sliding hiatal hernia, and the anatomy of repair. *Surg Gynecol Obstet* **92:**419–423, 1951
29. Russell CO, Hill LD: Gastroesophageal reflux. *Curr Probl Surg* **20:**205–278, 1983
30. Skinner DB, Belsey RH: Surgical management of esophageal reflux and hiatus hernia: Long-term results with 1030 patients. *J Thorac Cardiovasc Surg* **53:**33–38, 1967
31. Nissen R: Eine einface operation zur beeinflussung der refluxosophagitis. *Schweiz Med Wochenschr* **86:**590–595, 1956
32. Zaninotto G, DeMeester TR, Schwizer W, et al: The lower esophageal sphincter in health and disease. *Am J Surg* **155:**104–109, 1988
33. Sivri B, McCallum RW: What has the surgeon to know about pathophysiology of reflux disease. *World J Surg* **16:**294–299, 1992
34. Little AG: Mechanisms of action of antireflux surgery: Theory and fact. *World J Surg* **16:**320–325, 1992
35. Siewert JR, Feussner H, Walker SJ: Fundoplication: How to do it? Peri-esophageal wrapping as a therapeutic principle in gastroesophageal reflux prevention. *World J Surg* **16:**326–334, 1992
36. Cuschieri A: Laparoscopic antireflux surgery and repair of hiatal hernia. *World J Surg* **17:**40–45, 1993
37. Berguer R, Stiegmann GV, Yamamoto M, et al: Minimal access surgery for gastroesophageal reflux: Laparoscopic placement of the Angelchik prosthesis in pigs. *Surg Endosc* **5:**123–126, 1991
38. Nathanson LD, Shimi S, Cuschieri A: Laparoscopic ligamentum teres (round ligament) cardiopexy. *Br J Surg* **78:**947–951, 1991
39. Janssen IM, Gouma DJ, Klementschitsch P, et al: Prospective randomized comparison of teres cardiopexy and Nissen fundoplication in the surgical therapy of gastro-oesophageal reflux disease. *Br J Surg* **80:**875–878, 1993
40. Hill LD, Kraemer SJM, Aye RW, et al: Laparoscopic Hill repair. *Contemp Surg* **44:**13–20, 1994
41. Dunnington GL, DeMeester TR, Department of Veterans Affairs Gastroesophageal Reflux Disease Study Group: Outcome effect of adherence to operative principles of Nissen fundoplication by multiple surgeons. *Am J Surg* **166:**654–658, 1993
42. Spechler SJ, VA Gastroesophageal Reflux Disease Study Group: Comparison of medical and surgical therapy for complicated gastrooesophageal reflux disease in veterans. *N Engl J Med* **326:**786–792, 1992
43. DeMeester TR, Wang C-I, Wernly JA, et al: Technique, indications, and clinical use of 24 hour esophageal pH monitoring. *World J Surg* **79:**656–670, 1980
44. Stein HJ, DeMeester TR: Who benefits from antireflux surgery? *World J Surg* **16:**313–319, 1992
45. Rosetti M, Hell K: Fundoplication for the treatment of gastroesophageal reflux in hiatal hernia. *World J Surg* **1:**439–443, 1977
46. Boutelier P, Jonsell G: An alternative fundoplicative manoeuver for gastroesophageal reflux. *Am J Surg* **143:**260–264, 1982
47. Toupet A: Technique d'oesophago-gastroplastie avec phrenogastopexie appliquee dans la cure radicale des hernies hiatales et comme complement de l'operation d'Heller dans les cardiospasmes. *Mem Acad Chir* **89:**394–397, 1963
48. Cuschieri A, Shimi S, Nathanson LK: Laparoscopic reduction, crural repair, and fundoplication of large hiatal hernia. *Am J Surg* **163:**425–430, 1992
49. Geagea T: Laparoscopic Nissen's fundoplication: Preliminary report on ten cases. *Surg Endosc* **5:**170–173, 1991
50. Falk GL, Brancatisano RP, Hollinshead J, et al: Laparoscopic fundoplication: A preliminary report of the technique and postoperative care. *Aust N Z J Surg* **62:**969–972, 1992
51. Cuschieri A, Hunter J, Wolfe B, et al: Multicenter prospective evaluation of laparoscopic antireflux surgery: Preliminary report. *Surg Endosc* **7:**505–510, 1993
52. Hutson WR, Hunter JG: Manometric and 24 hour esophageal pH findings following laparoscopic Nissen or Toupet procedures for gastroesophageal reflux disease (GERD). *Gastroenterology* **104:**107, 1993
53. Bittner HB, Meyers WC, Brazer SR, et al: Laparoscopic Nissen fundoplication: Operative results and short-term follow-up. *Am J Surg* **167:**193–200, 1994

CHAPTER

# 50B

# Thoracoscopic Esophageal Surgery

Toni Lerut

Recent developments in video-assisted and minimally invasive technology have opened a new dimension to surgeons. This has been demonstrated by the rapid standardization of laparoscopic cholecystectomy. Although a prospective, randomized trial has not been performed, this procedure is now accepted as the standard procedure for symptomatic cholelithiasis.[1]

Video-assisted thoracic surgery (VATS) has been introduced.[2] VATS results in less morbidity than open operations, resulting in quicker recovery and return to normal activity. Recent data from international meetings and the literature show that VATS addresses a wide variety of complex problems. The thoracic cavity is particularly suited to endoscopic procedures.[3] The rigid thoracic wall and collapsible lung allow a sufficiently large working space. Minimally invasive procedures are therefore replacing a number of operations classically performed through an open thoracotomy, including some esophageal procedures.[4] The purpose of this chapter is to describe some of the technical aspects of thoracoscopic treatment of esophageal disease and to comment on indications and results for this new type of approach.

## STANDARD TECHNIQUE OF THORACOSCOPY IN ESOPHAGEAL DISEASE

Although the essentials of thoracoscopy are explained in Chapter 12, a brief description of a standard VATS approach to esophageal disease is described in this chapter. Most procedures that involve the esophagus are performed through a right-sided approach, but procedures on the gastroesophageal junction are undertaken from the left side. In both instances the patients are placed in the lateral decubitus position, and the corresponding lung is collapsed to obtain necessary exposure and working space. It is important to have the patient's upper arm appropriately positioned to provide adequate exposure, especially when procedures are performed on the upper half of the esophagus. Usually, five thoracoports are used (Fig. 50B–1): one for the camera and four working channels. Two of these channels are used by the surgeon and two by the assistant who is responsible for keeping the lung retracted. An initial port is inserted just below and anterior to the tip of the scapula in the midaxillary line to introduce the thoracoscope. A 10-mm 0° thoracoscope is most frequently used.

After introducing the scope, the surgeon can inspect the pleural cavity for adhesions. Dense adhesions may preclude thoracoscopy and necessitate conversion to open thoracotomy. If no dense adhesions are present, four additional 10-mm ports are made under direct vision, two ports in the anterior axillary line and two in the posterior axillary line.

Once the lung has been deflated, the mediastinal pleura over the esophagus is opened to allow mobilization of the esophagus. For disease of the upper half of the esophagus or when full mobilization of the esophagus is required, the azygos vein is divided with a linear vascular endostapler (Fig. 50B–2). The exposure of the lateral aspect of the esophagus is achieved with anterior and medial distraction of the esophagus, which allows exposure and clipping of the arteries from the aorta. When the esophagus is deflected posterolaterally, a dissection plane can be developed between the esophagus and both the pericardium and the posterior membranous trachea.

After this maneuver, the attachments to the posterior mediastinum are divided so that a sling or Penrose drain

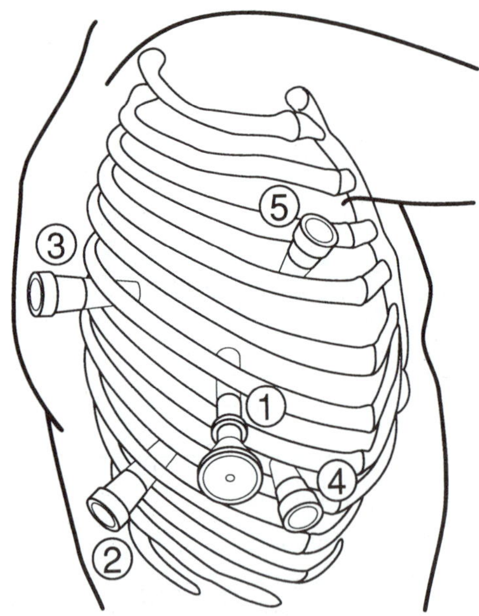


Figure 50B–1. Placement of thoracoports with the patient in the left lateral decubitus position. Port 1 is used for the telescope. Port 2 is the main operating port for the right hand of the surgeon. Port 3 is for the left hand. The esophagus can be transected through this port with a 30-mm linear stapler. Port 4 is used for suction probes and dissecting forceps. Port 5 is used for the retractor for the lung.

may be passed around the esophagus, usually from medial to lateral (Fig. 50B–3). The sling is brought out of the chest alongside one of the thoracoports and is used to exert traction on the esophagus when necessary.

Instruments used for dissection are endograsps, endodissectors, an electrosurgical hook knife or endoshears attached to the electrocautery. A wide variety of disposable and reusable endoinstruments are available. A number of reusable coaxial distal curved instruments that are introduced through a reusable metal flexible cannula have proved useful for dissection at sharp angles. In addition, thoracoports can be removed and conventional long instruments can be introduced to facilitate some parts of the dissection.

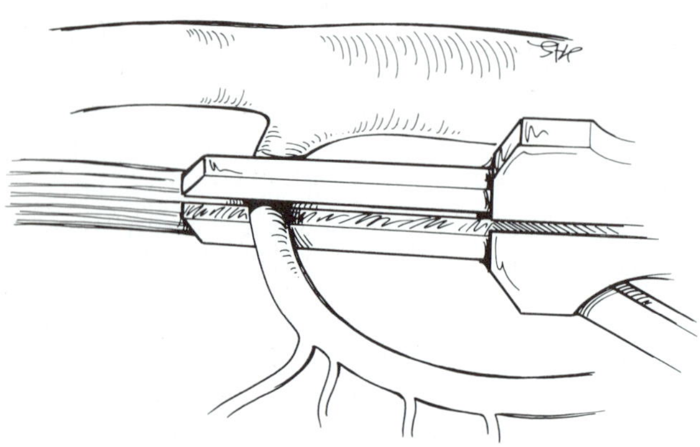

Figure 50B–2. Section and stapling of the azygos vein.

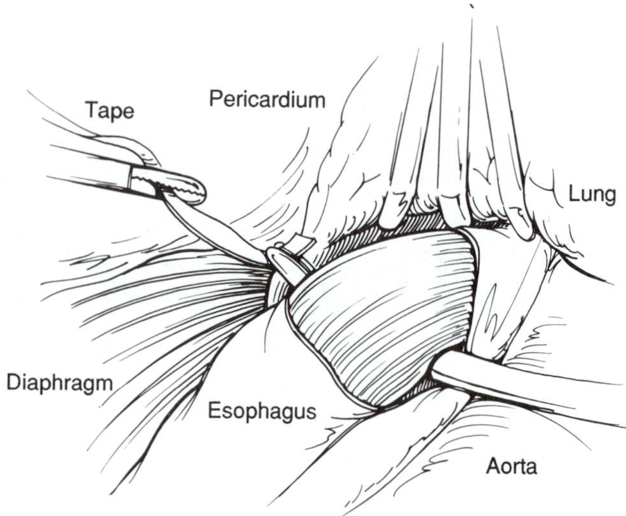


Figure 50B–3. Mobilization of the esophagus and insertion of a sling brought around the esophagus.

It is essential that an open thoracotomy instrument tray be available during all thoracoscopic procedures in the event that urgent thoracotomy is required.

A number of variations in gaining access to the esophagus have been described by several authors. The most relevant of these procedures are presented in discussions of the esophageal conditions in which these methods may be used.

## BENIGN TUMORS

A symptomatic leiomyoma of the esophagus is the most common benign esophageal tumor and is an ideal lesion to approach with thoracoscopy. Complete excision of this lesion results in definitive cure. Because most of these lesions are located in the middle third of the esophagus, the chest is entered from the right side.[5] At operation the tumor usually can be easily located because of its extrinsic appearance.

After the overlying pleura is incised and the leiomyoma is located, the muscular wall covering the lesion is divided, usually with an electrosurgical hook knife (Fig. 50B–4A). Once the whitish hard surface of the tumor is encountered, a plane of cleavage between muscle and tumor is easily made (Fig. 50B–4B). At this point, a stitch may be placed through the tumor (Fig. 50B–4C), which allows one to lift and manipulate the mass to facilitate dissection and separation from the mucosa (Fig. 50B–4D). This enucleation can usually be done without difficulty, but one should be particularly cautious when previous endoscopic biopsies have been performed. In such a case adhesions between mucosa and tumor may jeopardize easy dissection and cause unintentional entry into the esophageal lumen. When the tumor is small and protrudes to the right, the whole procedure can be performed without formal mobilization of the esophagus. Once the tumor is completely dissected, it is placed in a plastic bag and removed through one of the tho-

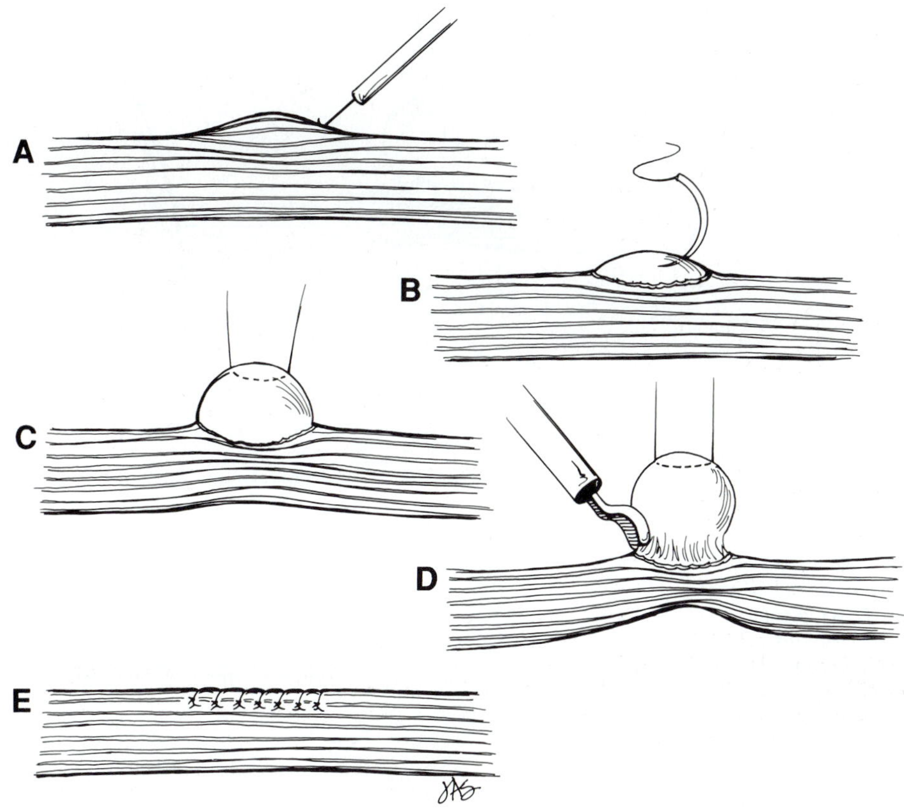


**Figure 50B–4.** Operation for leiomyoma of the esophagus. **A.** Incision of the muscular wall. **B.** Dissection of the muscular wall. **C.** A traction stitch placed through the tumor. **D.** Separation of the tumor from the mucosa. **E.** Closure of the myotomy.

racoports. Removing larger tumors requires conversion of one of the thoracoports into a minithoracotomy. Morcellation of the tumor into smaller fragments is not recommended.

If the tumor protrudes to the left or is horseshoe-shaped, full mobilization of the esophagus is essential to allow rotation of the esophagus.

After enucleation, insufflation of the esophagus is performed with a nasogastric tube to confirm that the mucosa is intact. The edges of the muscle are approximated with placement of two or more sutures (Fig. 50B–4E). This approximation avoids a pseudodiverticulum of the mucosa, which may result in swallowing difficulties. Some surgeons use a flexible esophagoscope to monitor the depth of dissection and mucosal integrity during this procedure.[6] The operation is finished with introduction of a chest tube through the lowest posterior thoracoport and re-expansion of the lung.

## DIVERTICULA

Pulsion diverticula of the thoracic esophagus are part of a more complex underlying motor disorder of the esophagus. The principle of treatment consists in a diverticulectomy associated with an extramucosal myotomy of the esophageal body. The extent of this myotomy is determined on the basis of manometric findings but usually extends from a level just proximal to the neck of the diverticulum down to the gastroesophageal junction in cases of diffuse spasm and across the gastroesophageal junction in cases of achalasia. The approach is left-sided for distal diverticula and right-sided for more proximal diverticula.

A diverticulum is usually easy to identify and is grasped by an endoscopic Babcock retractor or an endograsp (Fig. 50B–5A). With upward traction the sac can be freed from surrounding structures circumferentially. At the level of the neck, the surrounding muscle fibers are gently pushed away to free the entire base of the neck. The diverticulectomy can be removed with either a standard linear stapler introduced through a widened intercostal port or with a linear endostapler. Use of a linear endostapler requires the introduction of the instrument through the lowest posterior thoracoport in such a way that the stapler is parallel to the neck of the diverticulum. This maneuver can be cumbersome and difficult to perform.

When the neck of the diverticulum is small, the application of one 35-mm stapler suffices. If the diverticulum has a broad base, two or more applications or the use of a 60-mm endostapler are needed. The disadvantage of use of a 60-mm endostapler, however, is its large diameter of 18 mm, which makes the instrument difficult to manipulate.

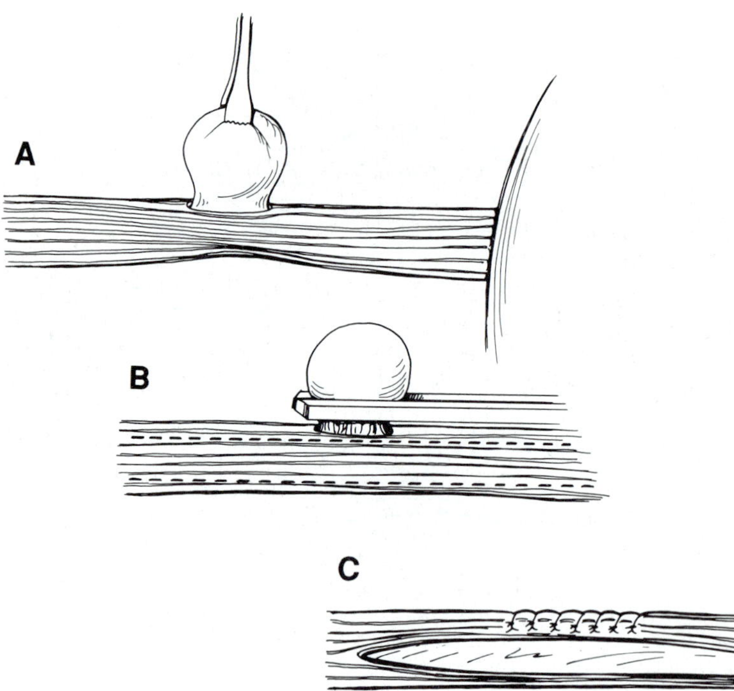


**Figure 50B–5.** Operation for diverticulum of the thoracic esophagus. **A.** Diverticulum is identified and grasped. **B.** A Maloney bougie is passed endoluminally. Resection of the diverticulum with the endostapler. **C.** Closure of the myotomy above the resected diverticulum and contralateral myotomy of the esophageal body.

Moreover, the port of entry in the thorax has to be located well away from the neck of the diverticulum because the instrument is introduced into the chest at least 8 cm before the jaws can be opened. To avoid narrowing of the esophageal lumen, it is advisable to introduce either an esophagoscope or a 50 F Maloney bougie into the esophagus before the diverticulum is stapled (Fig. 50B–5B).

After the diverticulum is resected, the surgeon begins the myotomy by marking the area of the muscle to be divided with an electrocautery (Fig. 50B–5C). The longitudinal fibers are incised in an area at least 90° away from the diverticular staple line. The underlying circular muscle layer is incised with the electrocautery hook. Great care is taken to lift the fibers during coagulation to avoid injury to the mucosa.

Once a small length of the circular layer is divided, it becomes easy to find a dissection plane between submucosa and muscle fibers. The myotomy is then continued cauded to or across the gastroesophageal junction according to the manometric findings. The myotomy is taken cephalad to a level proximal to the neck of the diverticulum. After an adequate myotomy, the mucosa should bulge fully between the cut edges of the muscular wall. Insufflation of air through a nasogastric tube rules out mucosal perforation. The procedure ends with approximation of the two edges of the muscular wall to cover the diverticular staple line. In the event of mucosal perforation, the defect usually can be closed with a simple fine-needle suture.

My experience with benign tumors and diverticula includes 10 patients: six with leiomyoma, one with an enterogenic cyst, one with a benign inflammatory tumor, and two with diverticula. In all patients with leiomyoma, the tumor was enucleated without great difficulty even when it was large. The patient with the inflammatory tumor had adhesions between the tumor mass and the mucosa that necessitated use of a linear endostapler to resect the adherent mucosa with the tumor (Fig. 50B–6). In the patient with the enterogenic cyst it was possible to dissect and remove the entire wall of the cyst without difficulty. The two patients with diverticula had manometric tests strongly suggestive of diffuse spasm. In both, the diverticulum was resected, and a long myotomy was performed down to but not across the gastroesophageal junction. There was no operative mortality, and all patients were discharged by the fifth postoperative day. After discharge a large but localized hemothorax developed in one patient who had undergone enucleation of a leiomyoma. This complication necessitated chest tube drainage. No patient suffered persistent postthoractomy pain.

Although VATS appears ideal for the treatment of benign tumors and diverticula of the esophagus, several caveats seem in order. Only symptomatic leiomyomas require surgical treatment because these tumors are benign and can be monitored with endoscopic ultrasonography. When a leiomyoma is in the distal third of the esophagus, associated gastroesophageal reflux must be considered. If present the reflux is treated with a concomitant antireflux procedure after enucleation of the leiomyoma.[5]

There is continuing debate regarding the need to perform a concomitant antireflux procedure after a combined

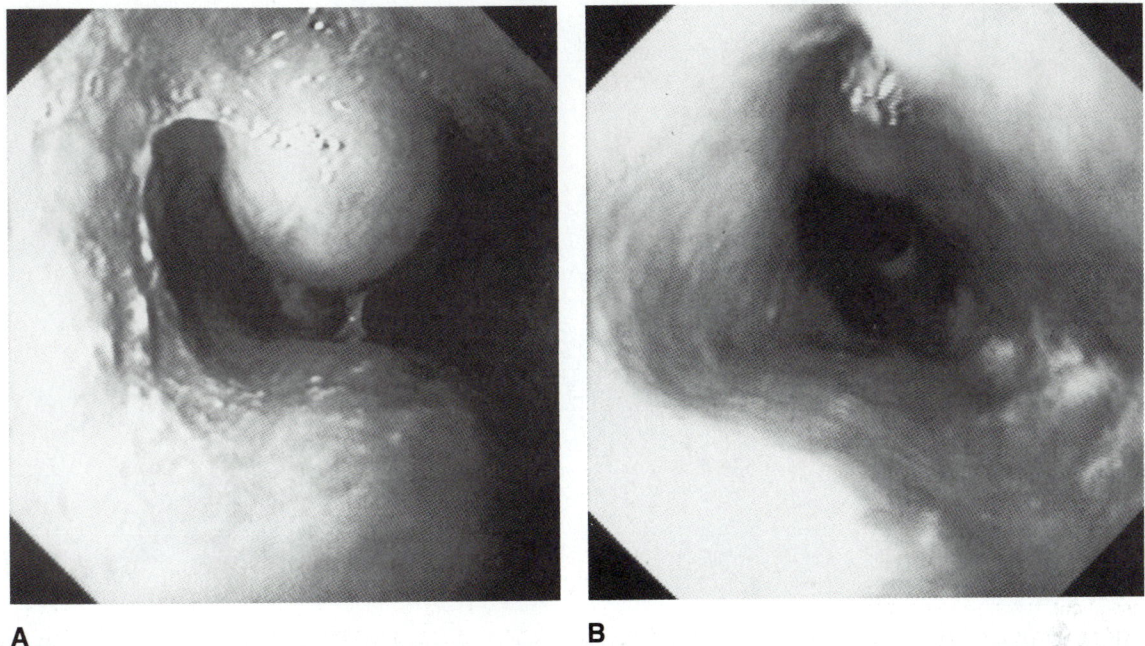


**Figure 50B–6.** Endoscopic views of inflammatory benign tumor of the esophagus. **A.** Preoperative view. **B.** Postoperative view in which the staples are clearly visible.

diverticulectomy and Heller myotomy in patients with achalasia.[7–12] The desire to use a minimally invasive approach is not ample justification for avoiding an antireflux procedure in these patients. Each patient should undergo careful preoperative analysis, and surgical decisions should be made only after thoughtful consideration of the manometric and 24-hour pH results. Occurrence of pathologic acid reflux during a 24-hour pH study has already been reported after VATS Heller myotomy. Further long-term follow-up study is needed to determine whether this reflux results in symptomatic esophagitis.[13]

Finally, one must be aware of the possibility of a leak from the closure at the site of diverticulectomy (Gayet B, personal communication, 1994). This complication is due to technical difficulties in the application of a linear endostapler. Illustrates the need for extreme caution during this operation.

## MOBILIZATION AND DISSECTION OF THE ESOPHAGUS FOR A BENIGN OR MALIGNANT CONDITION

The simple vascular supply and the tubular structure of the esophagus allow for easy thoracoscopic mobilization for both benign and malignant conditions. Today en bloc resection of the esophagus combined with extensive mediastinal or abdominal lymphadenectomy is the technique of choice for many surgeons who treat carcinoma of the thoracic esophagus and cardia.[14–16] Transhiatal esophagectomy is preferred by other surgeons, who believe that a radical operation is of secondary importance in the field of cancer surgery.[17] A videoscopic procedure can be performed for each of these approaches.

## TRANSMEDIASTINAL ENDOSCOPIC ESOPHAGEAL DISSECTION

Endoscopic mediastinal dissection of the esophagus was developed by Buess between 1986 and 1989.[18] A specially designed rigid mediastinoscope with a rotating conical overtube is used for dissection (Fig. 50B–7A). The front of the cone is circular and the lower third is concave, enabling the instrument to ride on the esophagus. The scope contains both fiberoptic channels and a large working channel through which a number of specially adapted instruments are passed to allow dissection of the esophagus under direct vision within the mediastinum.

Through a left cervical incision, the esophagus is approached medial to the sternocleidomastoid muscle and carotid sheath. The cervical esophagus is freed from the membranous wall of the trachea and encircled carefully; trauma to the recurrent nerves is avoided. The mediastinoscope is then inserted between the esophagus and vertebral fascia so that the posterior esophageal wall comes into view. With blunt dissection, electrocautery, and sharp dissection with scissors, the esophagus is carefully separated from the trachea and mediastinal tissues. Progress is easy as long as only soft tissue, including some smaller vessels, is dissected (Fig. 50B–7B). Vagal branches that join

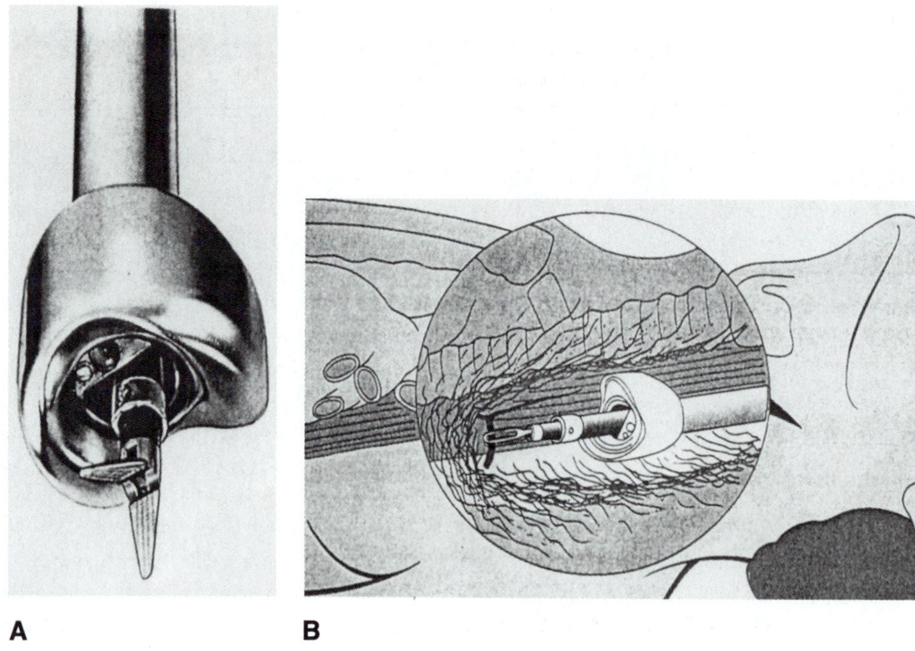


**Figure 50B–7. A.** Instrument used in transmediastinal endoscopic esophageal dissection. **B.** Smaller vessels are grasped, coagulated, and divided.

the esophagus are identified and divided. It is essential to remain in the appropriate dissection plane at the level of the tumor to prevent perforation of the esophagus.

During mediastinal dissection, a second team of surgeons performs a laparotomy and dissects and mobilizes the stomach. After a gastric tube has been constructed and hemostasis has been achieved in the mediastinum, the gastric tube is advanced into the neck by way of the posterior mediastinal route. Advantages of this technique over the conventional transhiatal approach include reduced pain, bleeding, pulmonary complications, and fewer injuries to the recurrent laryngeal nerves. Disadvantages are the limited endoscopic field and the inability to perform lymphadenectomy.[19] Furthermore, this method requires great care in manipulation of instruments because of the minimal degree of freedom and because movements are possible only in the line of vision. Loss of orientation, avulsion of esophageal muscle wall, arterial bleeding, and bronchial or tracheal damage can result. One randomized, prospective study of conventional transhiatal esophagectomy and endoscopic mediastinal dissection for carcinoma has been performed.[19] There was no difference in terms of mortality, blood loss, sepsis, or anastomotic leak. The only statistically significant difference was a decrease in pulmonary complications in the endoscopic dissection group. The most important disadvantage of this method may be the long-term outcome when dealing with carcinoma. In the series of Mannoke et al only patients with a T1 tumor survived long term. Patients with T2 tumors had a survival of 30 months, those with a T3 tumor survived 18 months, and all those with T4 tumors died within 1 year.[20] This poor outcome may be related to the limited dissection in the area surrounding the tumor and inability to perform adequate lymphadenectomies. This method may be most appropriate in patients at high risk with a clinical T1N0 lesions.

## TRANSTHORACIC THORACOSCOPIC OR VIDEO-ASSISTED ESOPHAGECTOMY

Thoracoscopic esophagectomy is best accomplished with the patient in the left lateral position. Placement of a large nasogastric tube or introduction of a flexible endoscope stents the esophagus and facilitates the dissection. It is important to establish a plane of dissection well away from the tumor. A flexible endoscope can be of great help in lifting the esophagus out of its mediastinal bed. A dry field with meticulous hemostasis is essential, and frequent irrigation and suction are needed to remove blood clots, which both absorb light and obscure the field. The right vagus nerve is identified before the takeoff of its pulmonary branches and is divided below the origin of the right recurrent laryngeal nerve. A dissection plane between the esophagus, the posterior wall of the trachea, and the superior vena cava can easily be identified, allowing dissection well up in the neck. Electrocoagulation must be avoided in this region because of the risk of damage to the recurrent laryngeal nerves.

As one dissects caudad, separation of the esophagus from the tracheal bifurcation and pericardium is usually performed without great difficulty. Subcarinal lymph nodes and periesophageal lymph nodes can be dissected and removed en bloc with the esophagus or separately. Electrocoagulation on the pericardium must be used sparingly because of the risk of cardiac arrhythmias. In the distal portion of its course, the esophagus is mobilized without opening of the opposite pleura unless the pleura adheres to the tumor. The inferior pulmonary ligament is divided, and surrounding periesophageal lymph nodes are included in the dissection, which is continued until the esophagus is identified. At this point, the mobilization of the esophagus is completed, and after insertion of a chest tube, the trocar sites are closed. The patient is then reprepared and draped in the supine position. Further steps consist of a left cervical incision and a laparotomy. After mobilization and dissection of the stomach, a gastric tube is constructed. The mobilized esophagus is delivered from the neck incision, and the gastric tube is brought up through the posterior mediastinum. A cervical esophagogastrostomy completes the operation.

This technique of thoracoscopic dissection and mobilization of the esophagus is technically feasible with acceptable morbidity.[21] Other variations of this thoracoscopic dissection vary with regard to number and size of chest wall opening. Some surgeons use a minithoracotomy, which allows easy introduction of conventional instruments, facilitating dissection (so-called thoracoscopic surgery without thoracoports).[22] The operation can also be performed with a limited 5- to 10-cm skin and muscle incision that is enlarged between the ribs so that a Finochietto retractor can be introduced. In these situations the camera operates merely to illuminate the operative field (Giudicelli R, personal communication, 1993). Some groups use a more radical dissection for esophageal carcinoma. They perform an en bloc resection that includes resection of the azygos vein and the thoracic duct[23] (Fig. 50B–8).

My colleagues and I attempted mobilization of the esophagus for carcinoma in seven patients. All patients had an early stage of carcinoma—T1 tumor and no evidence of lymph node involvement. In two patients, the procedure had to be converted to an open procedure because of dense lung adhesions; in the other five patients, the procedure was completed without difficulty. In one patient, we evaluated the possibility of extended lymphadenectomy. In this patient, it was possible to remove all subcarinal lymph nodes as well as the lymph nodes in the aortopulmonary window and in the posterior mediastinum below the aortic arch, including the thoracic duct. Removal of the paratracheal lymph nodes, however, was judged technically too difficult and too time-consuming. After mobilization of the esophagus, the patient was turned to the supine position, and the procedure was continued with a gastric pull-up with a cervical esophagogastrostomy. Pathologic examination confirmed that all patients had a T1 carcinoma and no lymph node involvement. One patient with a T1 tumor and liver cirrhosis died 32 days after the operation of liver failure and hepatic coma. The postoperative course in the other patients was similar to that of patients operated on through the transthoracic approach.

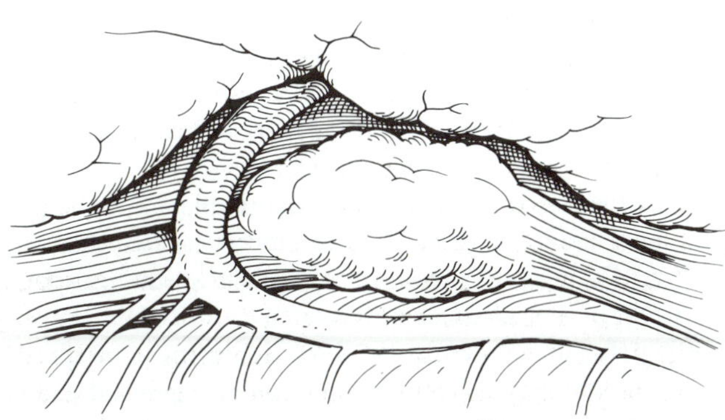

**Figure 50B–8.** Thoracoscopic en bloc esophagectomy.

Only a few centers have reported preliminary experiences in small numbers of patients[4,21,23–25] (Table 50B–1). From these data it becomes clear that thoracoscopic mobilization of the esophagus carries a mortality risk equivalent to that reported for open transthoracic operations. The operative morbidity and postoperative hospital course also appear similar to that seen after an open operation. The expected decrease in pulmonary complications was not realized, probably because of the need for prolonged one-lung ventilation. In an attempt to obviate the requirement for prolonged one-lung ventilation, Cuschieri is placing the patient in the prone posterior jack-knife position. This maneuver is said to result in excellent access to the mediastinum and intrathoracic esophagus without one-lung ventilation because the right lung drops away from the operative field because of gravity.[25] At this time I believe a VATS esophageal mobilization should not be performed in patients who are at high risk.

Of more concern, however, is the long-term outcome from the cancer. Peracchia reported on a patient in whom an early mediastinal recurrence developed and another who had tumor at a trocar site 6 months after VATS esophagectomy.[24]

Additional concerns are the difficulty in obtaining a complete dissection of the lymph nodes in the paratracheal region especially along the left recurrent laryngeal nerve and the aortopulmonary window. I consider these steps to be an essential part of the operation, especially for carcinomas of the middle and upper thirds of the esophagus. Many lymph nodes may be removed in fragments, which may partially account for the unusually high number of lymph nodes reported to be removed.[23] Even if this kind of lymphadenectomy could be performed, it is likely to be at the price of considerable prolongation of the time of the operation. I therefore believe that the open transthoracic approach is superior because it offers several advantages. Accurate staging is assured because of radical dissection and extensive lymphadenectomy in the paratracheal, posterior mediastinal, celiac, and cervical regions. There is increasing evidence that radical dissection and extensive lymphadenectomies result in better 5-year survival rates for pa-

**TABLE 50B–1. THORACOSCOPIC ESOPHAGEAL DISSECTION**

| Reference | Feasibility[a] | Blood Loss | Duration | Mortality (no. of pts/ no. of operations) | Mobidity[b] |
|---|---|---|---|---|---|
| Cuschieri[25] | 19/27 | Not measured; 1 pt required 7L | 5.5 h (4.5–7 h) | 0 | 44 |
| Gossot et al[21] | 12/15 | 200 mL mean | 125 min | 0 | 3 |
| Collard et al[23] | 9/12 | 2 of 9 pts required transfusions | 150–390 min | 1/9 | 2 |
| Coosemans et al[4] | 5/7 | 200–400 mL | — | 1/5 | 1 |
| Peracchia[24] | — | — | 125 min | 0 | 1 |

[a]Number of patients who underwent procedure/number of patients who required surgical treatment.
[b]Number of pulmonary complications.

tients in whom the operation is performed with curative intent.[14,16]

This impression was confirmed in my associates' and my retrospective review in which we compared radical with nonradical transthoracic esophagectomy in patients with potentially curable esophageal carcinoma. We noted a statistically significantly better 5-year survival rate in favor of radical resection with extensive lymphadenectomy.[15] Hagen et al prospectively compared transhiatal versus transthoracic resections and found a highly significant difference in 5-year survival rate favoring patients who underwent radical, en bloc transthoracic esophagectomy[26] for early disease. At present, transthoracic esophagectomy can be performed by experienced surgeons with a mortality rate of 1–2%. Until there is further refinement in both equipment and technique, there will be very few indications for VATS esophagectomy in the treatment of esophageal carcinoma.

## THORACOSCOPIC STAGING PROCEDURES

Survival after resection of esophageal carcinoma is strongly related to the presence or absence of lymph node involvement. Lymph node status has for many years fueled the debate between the "nihilists," who advocate simple esophagectomy, and the "radicalists," who advocate en bloc resection combined with two- or even three-field lymphadenectomy.

Besides the potential improvement in cure rate, an argument favoring extensive lymph node dissection is improvement in the accuracy of staging. Accurate pathologic staging may prove to be critical in the near future because of mounting evidence that suggests preoperative induction therapies are beneficial in improving resectability and survival rates. The important disadvantage, however, of these preoperative regimens is the lack of accuracy in clinical staging, which makes it difficult to stratify patients according to stage. Such stratification is vital if one is to identify which patients will benefit from such a regimen. Even with sophisticated imaging techniques such as endoscopic ultrasonography, there is still a margin of error of approximately 30% in clinical staging.[15] Currently, the only way to improve these figures is with open lymph node biopsy, which requires large incisions with the attendant morbidity.

Thoracoscopic surgery provides more accurate staging of the intrathoracic lymph nodes associated with the primary tumor and metastatic pleural implants or pulmonary lesions. Such an exploration, when combined with laparoscopic staging of the abdominal compartment, could improve staging accuracy with minimal morbidity and discomfort for the patient. However, there are several disadvantages:

1. The mediastinal pleura must be opened and the esophagus partially dissected to obtain accurate tumor staging and lymph node sampling, which may make subsequent resection difficult.
2. Adequate laparoscopic exploration requires introduction of several trocars and instruments with full mobilization along the lesser curvature to obtain the necessary exposure at the level of the celiac trunk and its branches. This is time-consuming and is not a minor procedure.
3. Manipulation of tumor masses or nodes may result in dispersion of cancer cells in the abdominal cavity enhanced by the continuous flow of carbon dioxide. Inoculation of trocar sites has been reported after laparoscopic operations for carcinoma.[27,28]

At this time we perform thoracoscopic or laparoscopic staging procedures on patients with very large and long tumors in whom the probability of extensive lymph node involvement is high and when clinical staging suggests suspicious abnormalities.

## THORACOSCOPIC ANTIREFLUX PROCEDURE

Today there is great interest in laparoscopic antireflux procedures, and large series of these procedures have been reported. Postoperative recovery and return to activity appear to occur more quickly than with an open procedure, and excellent functional results are claimed in most patients.[29] The antireflux procedure itself, however, requires the same surgical skills and expertise as an open operation. Even when performed by the most experienced surgeons and despite refinements such as the floppy Nissen, the morbidity is as high as 50% in late follow-up studies after open operations.[30,31] Potent medications such as omeprazole have decreased the need for surgical treatment. Thus the indications for surgery are restricted to more complex or complicated, drug-resistant reflux problems. The feasibility of the videoscopic approach in these patients is in question.

Complicated reflux disease can be difficult to treat even with an open thoracotomy. Therefore, the surgeon should be careful in deciding whether to perform an antireflux procedure and whether to perform it with a videoscopic approach. Randomized studies comparing open with videoscopic antireflux procedures are mandatory.

Besides the Nissen fundoplication, the Belsey Mark IV antireflux procedure is one of the more common procedures used in the last three decades. My associates and I used the Belsey Mark IV in open operations on more than 250 patients and had excellent to very good overall results in 70% and reflux control in 92% of the patients.[32] We believe patients eat and drink more comfortably after a Belsey repair than after a Nissen fundoplication. We became interested in performing the Belsey repair using VATS hoping that this approach might decrease morbidity, especially the incidence of postthoracotomy pain (the most important disadvantage related to this operation). In six patients, we tried to perform a Belsey antireflux procedure using VATS. In two patients, the operation was converted to an open procedure because it became too technically difficult. In the other four patients the Belsey procedure was performed without great difficulty. To perform the operation, two small utility thoracotomies are located on the anterior and posterior sides of the sixth interspace. These incisions allow the surgeon to introduce not only the typical endoscopic equipment but also routine instruments, making the operation easier. The camera is introduced through a separate thoracoport in the sixth interspace on the midaxillary line (Fig. 50B–9).

The first step of the operation is to mobilize the esophagus up to the aortic arch. The cardial dissection is begun with an incision in the structures that give access to the peritoneal cavity: the overlying pleura, the phrenoesophageal ligament, and the peritoneum. Once the peritoneum is incised, one can enter the greater sac. From the greater sac, the surgeon gains access to the lesser sac by going through the top of the hepatogastric ligament and tying off the connecting vessel, which runs from the phrenic artery to the branches of the left gastric artery (Belsey's artery). See Chapter 46 for details of the Belsey procedure. It is performed in exactly the same way whether it is done as an open operation or with thoracoscopic assistance.

The next step is to dissect the gastroesophageal fat pad from the distal esophagus and to dissect both vagus nerves so that they might be positioned posteriorly. The two halves of the right crus are prepared for approximation by placement of as many stitches as necessary to narrow the hiatus. These sutures are not tied until the end of the procedure.

The fundoplication is begun with placement of a stitch in the lateral gastric fundus 2 cm below the gastroesophageal junction and taking of a bite in the esophagus approximately 2 cm above the junction.

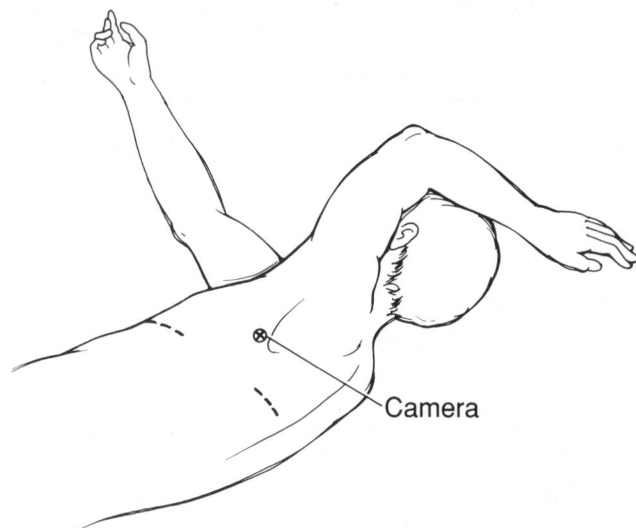


**Figure 50B–9.** Position of the patient, camera, and two minithoracotomies in the thoracoscopic Belsey Mark IV procedure.

The stitch is reversed and passed back to form a U-shaped mattress suture. Two more such sutures are placed in such a way that approximately 240°–270° of the esophagus is enfolded by the gastric fundus with both vagal nerves lying posteriorly on the uncovered portion of the esophagus. A second row of three mattress stitches is placed. Each begins by passing through the diaphragm at about the junction of the muscular and tendinous part of the diaphragm. They are then placed through the stomach, into the esophagus, and back again through esophagus, stomach, and diaphragm. This second row of sutures is placed to invaginate another 2 cm of esophagus over a circumference of 240°–270°.

Once the second row of sutures is tied, the distal 4 cm of esophagus is plicated by the gastric fundus and fixed in a subdiaphragmatic position. The stitches in the crura are tied after it is assured that the hiatal closure is not too tight. The postoperative course was uneventful in all four patients who underwent this operation, but it was not appreciably different from that of an open approach in terms of respiratory comfort or hospital stay. None of the patients reported postthoracotomy pain. All were eating and drinking well without clinical evidence of reflux. One patient, however, suffered from flatulence, episodes of diarrhea, and shortness of breath when performing physical effort.

## ZENKER'S DIVERTICULUM

Although the treatment of pharyngoesophageal diverticulum or Zenker's diverticulum is not a thoracic condition, it is a part of the spectrum of esophageal disease that can be addressed with videoscopic technology (Fig. 50B–10A).

The development of endostaplers has provided an opportunity for treating Zenker's diverticulum with endoscopic assistance. The introduction into the pharynx of a Weerda diverticuloscope (Storz; Karl Storz, Tuttlingen, Germany) offers good visualization of the mouth of the diverticulum, the esophageal orifice, and the cricopharyngeal bar, which separates them (Fig. 50B–10B). The endostapler is applied by insertion of one limb, or jaw, of the stapler into the diverticulum while the second limb is passed into the esophageal lumen. When closed, the jaws of the stapler compress the wall of the esophagus and the wall of the diverticular sac for a distance of 3 cm (Fig. 50B–10C). When the stapler is fired, this wall, which includes the cricopharyngus muscle, is divided between two rows of sta-

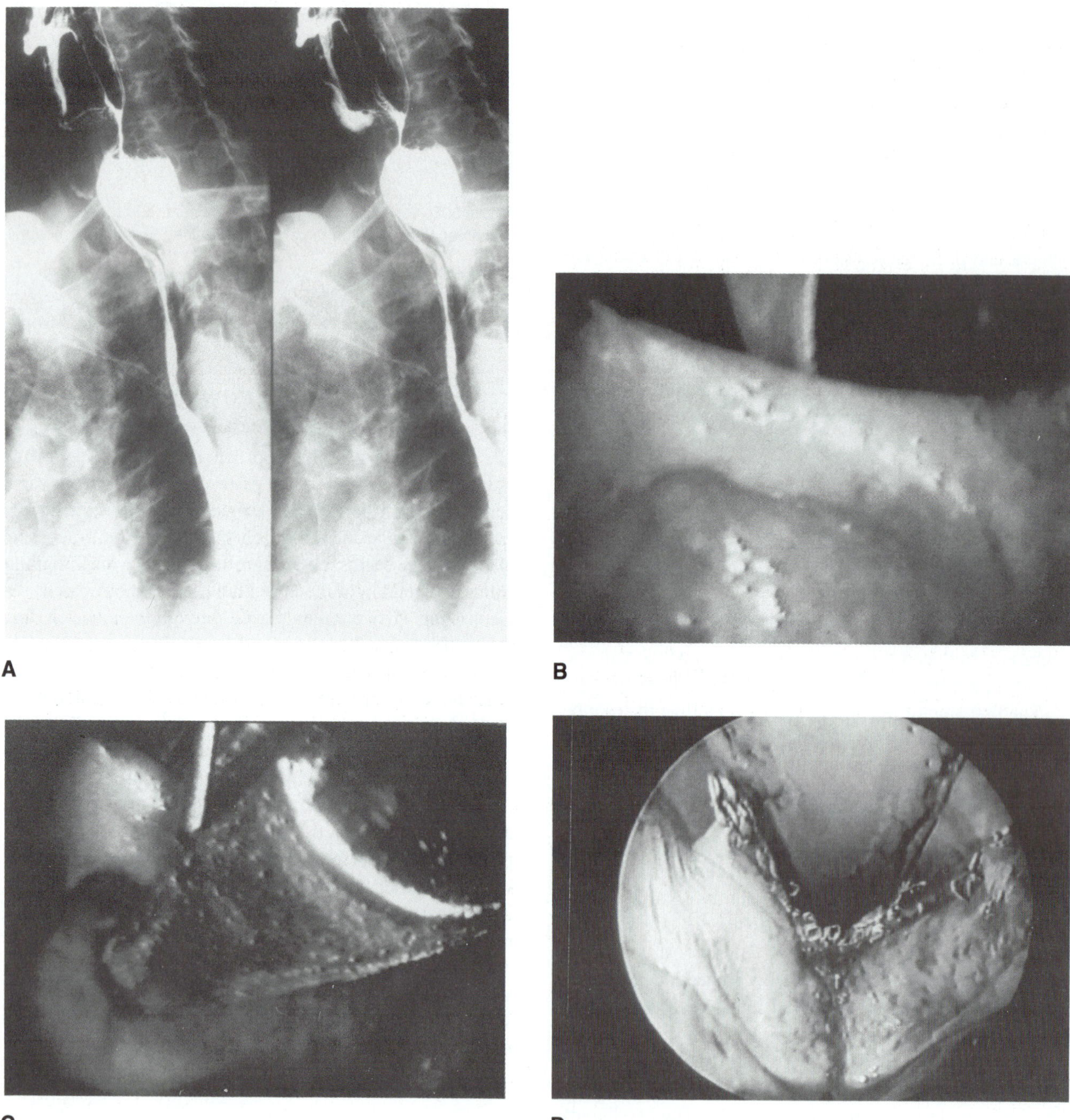

**Figure 50B–10.** Treatment of Zenker's diverticulum. **A.** Preoperative barium swallow radiograph. **B.** Preoperative view through the diverticuloscope showing the cricopharyngeal bar. The nasogastric tube is in the esophageal lumen. **C.** Application of the endostapler. **D.** Postoperative view after firing of the endostapler. *(Continued.)*

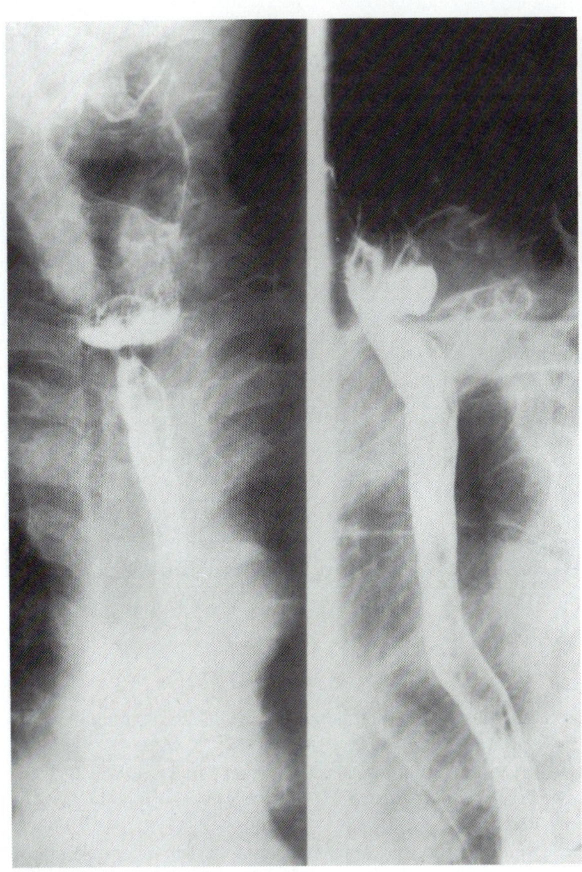

E

**Figure 50B–10.** *(Continued.)* **E.** Postoperative barium swallow radiograph shows filling of the cul-de-sac of the diverticulum.

ples. This division results in a myotomy and forms a common space between the sac and the esophageal lumen, which allows easy passage of swallowed food. With endoscopy, one can visualize the retracted, stapled edges of the cricopharyngus muscle and the common opening of diverticulum and esophagus (Fig. 50B–10D). This procedure is quick and simple and allows the patient to eat and drink on the first postoperative day (Fig. 50B–10E).[33]

A prospective study was undertaken to evaluate endoscopic diverticuloesophagostomy. Twenty patients (mean age 64 years) with symptomatic Zenker's diverticulum (Table 50B–2) underwent either endoscopic treatment (n = 11) or a standard cervical approach with a diverticulopexy and extramucosal myotomy (n = 9). There are two perioperative complications in the endoscopic treatment group, including one case of subcutaneous emphysema (but no leak on contrast study) and one case of temporary vocal cord paralysis. In the open myotomy group, one patient with a history of having undergone an operation on the carotid artery had an incisional hematoma that required drainage. The long-term follow-up period ranged from 1 to 16 months. No patient in the open myotomy group had new symptoms, and all had excellent functional results.

In the endoscopy group, one patient had an episode of unexplained hematemesis. Another patient experienced slight dysphagia after eating dry meat and reported vocal weakness. Two patients experienced return of moderate dysphagia after an initial period of excellent functional recovery. At endoscopy it seemed that the U-shaped suture line had been transformed into a web-like ridge of scar tissue that impaired passage of a solid bolus of contrast material (Fig. 50B–11). In both patients, endostapler application was repeated, and the patients had an excellent early outcome.[34]

**TABLE 50B–2. ZENKER'S DIVERTICULUM**

| Type of Procedure | No. of Preoperative Complications | No. of Postoperative Complications | Late Complications | | Final Outcome | |
|---|---|---|---|---|---|---|
| Open (n = 9) | — | (Hematoma) | — | | Excellent | 9 |
| Endoscope (n = 11) | (Subcutaneous emphysema) | (Left vocal cord paresis) | Hematemesis | 1 | Excellent | 4 |
| | | | Dysphagia | | | |
| | | | Slight | 1 | Good | 5 |
| | | | Moderate | 2 | Fair | 2 |

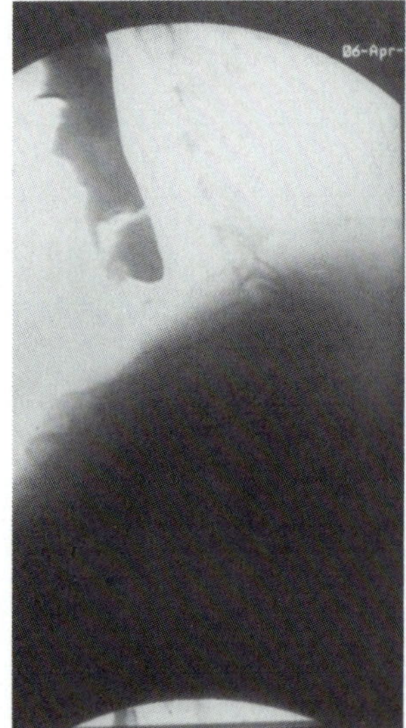
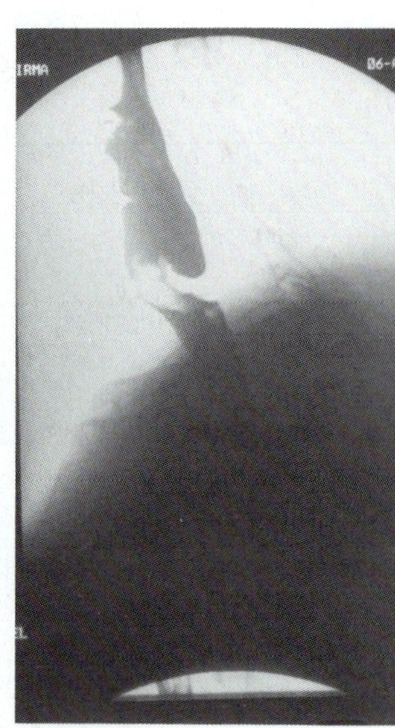

**Figure 50B–11.** Recurrent dysphagia in Zenker's diverticulum. Difficult passage of a solid bolus if barium over the remaining cricopharyngeal ridge is shown.

Although endoscopic therapy for Zenker's diverticulum is technically feasible, the long-term follow-up results suggest that symptoms persist or recur in as many as 30% of patients. The recurrence rate for open myotomy and diverticulopexy is less than 10%, so at present this must be considered the treatment of choice.

## REFERENCES


1. Cuschieri A, Dubois F, Mouiel J, et al: The European experience with laparoscopic cholecystectomy. *Am J Surg* **161**:385–387, 1991
2. Torre M, Pierangelo Belloni P: Nd: YAG laser pleurodesis through thoracoscopy: New curative therapy in spontaneous pneumothorax. *Ann Thorac Surg* **47**:887–889, 1989
3. Landreneau RJ, Mack MJ, Hazelrigg SR, et al: Video-assisted thoracic surgery: Basic technical concepts and intercostal approach strategies. *Ann Thorac Surg* **54**:800–807, 1992
4. Coosemans W, Lerut TE, Van Raemdonck DE: Thoracoscopic surgery: The Belgian experience. *Ann Thorac Surg* **56**:721–730, 1993
5. Lerut T, Coosemans W, Gruwez JA, Geboes K: Leiomyoma and leiomyosarcoma of the oesophagus. *Dis Esoph* **3**:37–42, 1991
6. Bardini R, Segalin A, Ruol A, et al: Videothoracoscopic enucleation of esophageal leiomyoma. *Ann Thorac Surg* **54**:576–577, 1992
7. Black J, Vorbach AN, Collis JL: Results of Heller's operation for achalasia of the esophagus: The importance of hiatal repair. *Br J Surg* **63**:949–953, 1976
8. Okike N, Payne WS, Neufeld DM, et al: Esophagomyotomy versus forceful dilatation of achalasia of the esophagus: Results in 899 patients. *Ann Thorac Surg* **28**:119–125, 1979
9. Jara FM, Toledoo-Pereyra LH, Lewis JW, Magilligan DJ Jr: Long term results of esophagotomy for achalasia of the esophagus. *Arch Surg* **114**:935–936, 1979
10. Pai GP, Ellison RG, Rubin JW, et al: Two decades of experience with modified Heller's myotomy for achalasia. *Ann Thorac Surg* **38**:201–210, 1984
11. Ellis FH Jr, Crozier RE, Watkins E Jr: Operation for esophageal achalasia: Results of esophagomyotomy without an antireflux operation. *J Thorac Cardiovasc Surg* **88**:344–351, 1984
12. Ellis FH Jr: Surgery for achalasia: How do I do it? In Wu YK, Peters RM: *International Practice in Cardiothoracic Surgery* Beijing, Science Press, 1985, pp 524–529
13. Pellegrini CA: Thoracoscopic myotomy for achalasia or motor disorder of the esophageal body. *Dis Esoph* **7**:14–16, 1994
14. Altorki NK, Skinner DB: En bloc oesophagectomy: The first 100 patients. *Hepatogastroenterology* **37**:360–363, 1990
15. Lerut T, deLeyn P, Coosemans W, et al: Surgical strategies in esophageal carcinoma with emphasis on radical lymphadenectomy. *Ann Surg* **216**:583–590, 1992
16. Akiyama H, Tsurumaru M, Kawanura T, Ono Y: Principles of surgical treatment for carcinoma of the esophagus: Analysis of lymph node involvement. *Ann Surg* **194**:435–446, 1981
17. Orringer MB, Marshall B, Stirling MC: Transhiatal esophagectomy for benign and malignant disease. *J Thorac Cardiovasc Surg* **2**:265–277, 1993
18. Buess G, Beker HD, Mentges B, et al: Die endoskopischemikrochirurgische Dissektion der Speiseröhre. *Chirurg* **61**:308–311, 1990
19. Bumm R, Hoelscher AH, Fuessner H, et al: Endodissection of the thoracic oesophagus: Technique and clinical results in transhiatal esophagectomy. *Ann Surg* **218**:97–104, 1993
20. Manncke K, Raestrup H, Walter D, et al: Technique of endoscopic mediastinal dissection of the oesophagus. *Endosc Surg 2*:21–25, 1994
21. Gossot D, Fourquier P, Celerier M: Thoracoscopic esophagectomy: Technique and initial results. *Ann Thorac Surg* **56**:667–670, 1993
22. Roviaro GC, Rebuffat C, Varioli F, et al: Videoendoscopic thoracic surgery. *Int Surg* **78**:4–9, 1993
23. Collard JM, Lengele B, Otte JB, Kestens PJ: En bloc and standard esophagectomies by thoracoscopy. *Ann Thorac Surg* **56**:675–679, 1993
24. Peracchia A, Bonavina L, Segalin A, et al: Esophagectomy without thoracotomy or transmediastinal endodissection for esophageal carcinoma. *Dis Esoph* **7**:36–38, 1993
25. Cuschieri A: Endoscopic subtotal oesophagectomy for cancer using the right thoracoscopic approach. *Surg Oncol* **2**:(Suppl 1) 3–12, 1993
26. Hagen JA, Peters H, DeMeester TR: Superiority of extended en bloc

oesophagogastrectomy for carcinoma of the lower esophagus and cardia. *J Thorac Cardiovasc Surg* **106:**850–858, 1993

27. Cava A, Ronian J, Gonzalez Quintala A, et al: Subcutaneous metastasis following laparoscopy in gastric adenocarcinoma. *Eur J Surg Oncol* **16:**63–67, 1990
28. Guillou PJ, Darzi A, Monson JR: Experience with laparoscopic colorectal surgery for malignant disease. *Surg Oncol* **2**(Suppl 1):43–49, 1993
29. Dallemagne B, Weerts JM, Jehaes C, et al: Laparoscopic Nissen fundoplication: Preliminary report. *Surg Laparosc Endosc* **1:**138–143, 1991
30. Luostarinen M: Nissen fundoplication for reflux esophagitis: Long term clinical and endoscopic results in 109 of 127 consecutive patients. *Ann Surg* **217:**329–337, 1993
31. Jamieson GG, Maddern GJ, Myers JC: Gastric emptying after fundoplications with and without proximal gastric vagotomy. *Arch Surg* **126:**1414–1417, 1991
32. Lerut T, Coosemans W, Christiaens R, Gruwez JA: The Belsey MIV antireflux procedure: Indications and long-term results. *Acta Gastroenterol Belg* **3:**585–590, 1990
33. Lerut T, Van Raemdonck D, Guelinckx P, et al: Zenker's diverticulum: Is a myotomy of the cricopharyngeus useful? How long should it be? *Hepatogastroenterology* **39:**127–131, 1992
34. Collard JP, Kestens PJ: Endoscopic suture of the hypopharyngeal diverticulum: A new technique. *Abstracts of the Fifth World Congress of the International Society for Diseases of the Esophagus,* August 1992, Kyoto, p 238

# CHAPTER 51

# Carcinoma of the Esophagus

Nasser K. Altorki, David B. Skinner,
Bruce D. Minsky, and David P. Kelsen

The earliest historical records describing syndromes of dysphagia date back almost 2000 years. The "hard of swallowing disease" was apparently endemic in northern China and instilled a profound fear among the population. Almost 20 centuries later, carcinoma of the esophagus remains a dreaded neoplasm with dismal survival rates. Fortunately, squamous cell carcinoma is uncommon in the United States and accounts for fewer than 10,000 new cases per year. However, a recent alarming increase in the incidence of esophageal adenocarcinoma has been reported, especially among white men.[1] The increase in incidence remains poorly understood in epidemiologic terms and has spurred renewed interest in research efforts directed at both the basic and clinical aspects of esophageal carcinoma.

## INCIDENCE

### Squamous Cell Carcinoma

Squamous cell carcinoma of the esophagus demonstrates a remarkable variability in prevalence worldwide. Whereas the disease is relatively uncommon outside Asia, it is among the leading causes of cancer deaths in large areas of central and southeast Asia. A high-incidence esophageal cancer belt seems to extend from the Caspian littoral region of northern Iran, across the southern republics of the former Soviet Union and into northern China; the highest incidence rates are reported in Iran and northern China.[2] The national mortality for esophageal cancer in the Peoples Republic of China is 19.6 per 100,000 for men and 9.8 per 100,000 for women. The disease accounts for 23% of all deaths from cancer.[3] Some of the areas of highest incidence are in the three northern Chinese provinces of Hunan, Shanxi, and Hebei, where the average incidence exceeds 100 per 100,000 population per year. Variability in incidence is encountered within various counties of these provinces. The influence of local dietary habits and environmental factors on these widely disparate incidences have been the subject of extensive epidemiologic studies. Within the Asian continent, carcinoma of the esophagus also is common in Sri Lanka,[4] the Indian subcontinent,[5] and among people of Chinese descent in Singapore.[6] In the African continent, an area of high incidence is found among the Zulu and Bantu tribes of the Cape Province and the Transkei regions of South Africa.[7]

Squamous esophageal cancer is relatively uncommon in most of Europe and the Americas. The average incidence in the western hemisphere is 5–10 per 100,000 population. High-incidence areas are nestled in northwestern France, namely Brittany and Normandy[8] as well as the northeastern regions of the Italian peninsula. Within the continental United States, the national incidence of squamous cell carcinoma is approximately six cases per 100,000 people per year and has remained stable since the mid 1980s.[9] Squamous cell carcinoma of the esophagus accounts for 70% of all esophageal tumors in the United States primarily because of a dramatic increase in the prevalence of esophageal adenocarcinoma.[1] High incidence rates are observed in the low country of the Carolinas and in major metropolitan centers such as Los Angeles, New York, Detroit, and Washington, DC, where the incidence approaches 28 cases per 100,000 population.[10] The incidence of esophageal cancer has remained relatively stable among white men older than 30 years but has nearly tripled over the same period among black men. Esophageal cancer is now the second leading cause of death from cancer among black men younger than 55 years.[11]

### Adenocarcinoma

Adenocarcinoma of the esophagus is no longer a medical rarity. These tumors accounted for at least 30% of all esophageal tumors by the mid 1980s and increased in incidence by approximately 10% per year over the 1980s.[1] Esophageal adenocarcinoma currently accounts for 50% of esophageal tumors in white men.[12] A similar increase in incidence of esophageal adenocarcinoma has been observed in the United Kingdom and various regions of northern and western Europe.[13] The epidemiologic reasons for this quasiepidemic increase in incidence remain unknown. An increase in the incidence of Barrett's metaplasia, a known premalignant condition, also was observed over the same time period.[14] The reported incidence of malignant degeneration in patients with Barrett's' esophagus is variable but is estimated at 1 in 200 persons per year of follow-up study.[15] Those estimates are 30–40 fold higher than the expected incidence of esophageal cancer among Caucasian men in North America. However, the true incidence of esophageal adenocarcinoma may be underestimated because tumors of the gastric cardia are often dismissed as being gastric in origin. Remarkably, careful pathologic examination of specimens resected for carcinoma of the cardia reveals evidence of residual benign Barrett's epithelium in 70% of patients.[16] It is quite likely that most tumors of the gastric cardia originate within the specialized intestinal epithelium of Barrett's esophagus, the remnant of which may on occasion be entirely overgrown with tumor. Clinicopathologic studies have shown the remarkable epidemiologic, clinical, and morphologic similarities between carcinoma of the gastric cardia and Barrett's adenocarcinoma.[17] The combined incidence of adenocarcinoma of the cardia and esophagus in white men is currently estimated at 5.8 per 100,000 population ranking this tumor among the top 15 cancers of white men in the United States.[12]

## EPIDEMIOLOGY

### Squamous Cell Cancer

In the western hemisphere, epidemiologic evidence has strongly implicated alcohol and tobacco consumption as predisposing factors for squamous cell carcinoma of the esophagus. Tobacco is one of the important sources of nitrosamines, by-products of which are known potent esophageal carcinogens.[18] Cohort and case-control studies in the United States, western Europe, and South America show that smokers are at high risk for squamous cell carcinoma of the esophagus.[19–21] The risk is strongly dose-related. Ex-smokers show a reduced risk relative to current smokers; the highest risk occurs among those who smoke two or more packs a day. The hazard from smoking is not confined to cigarettes alone; cigar and pipe smokers exhibit high risk relative to nonsmokers. Paradoxically, smoking does not seem to play an important role in the pathogenesis of esophageal cancer in the high-risk areas of the world. Smoking of locally grown tobacco in China has not been correlated with esophageal cancer, and smoking is quite uncommon among the inhabitants of the Caspian littoral region. Chewing of opium, a commonly practiced habit in northern Iran, has been suggested as a risk factor because of the known mutagenicity of some opiate residues.[22]

Consumption of alcohol has been strongly associated with esophageal squamous cell carcinoma in the Americas and Europe. Case-control studies conducted in Los Angeles,[23] New York,[24] Washington, DC,[25] Uruguay,[21] and France[26] confirmed a strong association between alcohol intake and the development of esophageal cancer. Relative to nondrinkers, regular drinkers displayed a dose-related hazard for esophageal carcinoma. The risk was highest among consumers of hard liquor and lowest with beer drinkers; wine drinkers occupied an intermediate position. The combination of smoking and drinking exerted a multiplicative rather than an additive effect. The synergy between alcohol and tobacco consumption may be due to facilitation of diffusion of tobacco-related carcinogens through the esophageal wall by alcoholic beverages or due to the generally poor nutritional status of most alcoholics. Once again, alcohol consumption does not appear to be an important risk factor in the high-incidence areas of northern China and the Moslem population of northern Iran.

Environmental and dietary factors are heavily implicated in the etiology of esophageal cancer in most of the high-incidence areas. Considerably higher levels of nitrates are detected in the drinking water in the northern provinces of the Chinese mainland. Furthermore, the consumption of pickled vegetables is positively correlated with esophageal cancer mortality within those provinces.[27] The mutagenicity of extracts of pickled vegetables has been documented in rats.[28] A higher level of secondary amines is also noted in food material commonly consumed in these areas, such as fermented fish, fungal infested corn, or sweet potatoes.[29] Although dietary habits are substantially different in various geographic areas along the esophageal cancer belt, the population in general seems to manifest poor nutritional status. Studies among black Americans have confirmed that poor nutritional status is an important contributing factor. Along with alcohol and tobacco consumption poor nutrition may be responsible for the almost three-fold increase in the incidence of esophageal cancer in that racial group.[23]

Environmental factors believed to predispose to esophageal carcinoma include asbestos or radiation exposure and ingestion of silica fragments, but the evidence so far remains sparse. A possible viral cause was suggested when papilloma virus particles were found within esophageal cancer cells.[30]

### Adenocarcinoma

Among all adenocarcinomas of the cardia and esophagus seen at our institution, almost 50% are associated with residual benign columnar metaplasia. In the other patients, benign mucosa may have been completely overgrown by the tumor. Careful histologic examination of specimens resected for Barrett's adenocarcinoma often reveals multiple dysplastic lesions associated with an invasive carcinoma and thus strongly suggests that the entire mucosal lining is exposed to a carcinogen that drives the cells toward the malignant phenotype.[31] Evidence derived from flow cytometric analysis shows that most patients with Barrett's adenocarcinoma have a multiple aneuploid population that often overlaps the site of invasive cancer.[32]

Strong evidence implicates gastroesophageal reflux as the culprit in the pathogenesis of adenocarcinoma of the esophagus and cardia. Clinical studies have shown that approximately 60–70% of patients with confirmed Barrett's adenocarcinoma have a long-standing history of gastroesophageal reflux.[33,34] The lack of similar history in the other remaining 30–40% of patients may be attributable to the known acid insensitivity of the metaplastic mucosa in some patients. The exact component of the refluxate contributing to the malignant phenotype is unknown. Recent clinical evidence suggest that patients with combined increased acid and alkaline esophageal exposure are more prone to complications of Barrett's esophagus, including dysplasia, than those with isolated acid reflux.[35] This clinical evidence remains preliminary and certainly lacks a correlation with malignant degeneration.

Neither alcohol consumption nor smoking of tobacco is positively correlated with esophageal adenocarcinoma.

## PREMALIGNANT LESIONS

### Barrett's Esophagus

The premalignant nature of Barrett's esophagus has been confirmed by various studies since Morson and Belcher's original report of an esophageal adenocarcinoma that arose in a columnar-lined esophagus.[36] The incidence of malignant degeneration and its pathogenesis are discussed earlier in this chapter. The frequency and tempo of progression from metaplasia to dysplasia and finally carcinoma remain largely unknown. Patients with Barrett's esophagus should be included in a surveillance program aimed at early detection of high-grade dysplasia and early adenocarcinoma.

### Achalasia

The first report of esophageal carcinoma associated with achalasia of the cardia was by Fagge in 1872.[37] Several authors have since confirmed that association, and prevalence rates vary between 0–20% per year. This wide range is probably due to confusion over *incidence* and *prevalence* figures and the variability in the length of follow-up periods reported in each study. Incidence is the number of new cases that occur over a specified time, whereas prevalence is the number of cases that exist at any one time. Ellis reported an "incidence" of 24% among 24 patients seen at the Mayo Clinic between 1944 and 1952,[38] whereas Chuong did not observe a single case of esophageal cancer among 91 patients followed for a period of 6 years.[39] A retrospective analysis reported that over a 23-year follow-up period carcinoma of the esophagus developed in 10 of 147 patients who underwent esophagomyotomy (7% prevalence).[40] In one of the few prospective studies, 195 patients with confirmed achalasia treated with pneumatic dilation underwent esophagoscopy and biopsy on a biannual basis.[41] Carcinoma of the esophagus developed in three patients an average of 5.8 years since the diagnosis of achalasia and 17 years since the onset of symptoms. The observed incidence was 33-fold higher than that expected in the general population. Two of the three patients had early tumors that were successfully resected, leading to long-term disease-free survival.

Squamous cell carcinoma is the predominant cell type and is mostly located in the middle third of the esophagus. The tumors are quite advanced in most patients primarily because of the insidious nature of the symptoms that are often indistinguishable from the pre-existing symptoms of achalasia. In addition, the dilated esophagus allows the tumor to grow to a substantial size before producing appreciable luminal obstruction. Approximately 80% of tumors are thus unresectable at the time of diagnosis, leading to a dismal survival rate.

### Chronic Esophagitis

The high prevalence of chronic esophagitis among the population in areas of high risk for esophageal cancer strongly suggests that esophagitis is a precursor lesion for squamous cell carcinoma of the esophagus. In the high-risk area of Huixian in northern China, the prevalence of esophagitis approaches 50% in adults older than 35 years and 40% in younger people.[42] In neighboring areas with a lower incidence of esophageal cancer, the incidence of chronic esophagitis is only 17%. In general, the presence of chronic esophagitis is positively correlated with the intake of burning hot beverages and low consumption of fresh fruit and vegetables. An epidemiologic study conducted in France[43] suggested that esophagitis was positively correlated with cigarette smoking and frequent consumption of butter. Studies from South America also associated the presence of esophagitis or dysplasia with cigarette smoking, alcohol consumption, and maté drinking.[44] It appears that whatever the noxious agent, the esophageal response to injury is an inflammatory reaction that may progress to various degrees of dysplasia and eventual carcinoma. The concept of a dysplasia–carcinoma sequence in squamous cell carcinoma of the esophagus is supported by indirect and direct clinicopathologic evidence. Careful examination of esophagi resected for squamous cell carcinoma reveals at least one focus of carcinoma in situ closely associated with the invasive lesion in most cases. In 14% of cases various degrees of dysplasia are noted throughout the resected specimen.[45]

## Tylosis

Tylosis (keratopalmar keratosis) is an autosomal dominant inherited defect of keratinization associated with a very high risk for squamous cell carcinoma of the esophagus. Howell-Evans, in the first detailed description of the disease, estimated the risk of malignant degeneration at 95% by the age of 65.[46] Although hyperkeratosis of the palms and soles is a clinical characteristic of the disease, the esophageal epithelium does not manifest clinically significant abnormalities of keratinization.

## Plummer Vinson Syndrome

Also known as the Patterson-Kelly syndrome, Plummer Vinson syndrome is rare except in northern Scandinavia, where it appears predominately in women. The syndrome is characterized by webs of the cervical esophagus, iron deficiency anemia, stomatitis, pharyngitis, and dystrophic changes in the nail beds.[47] An increased incidence of cervical esophageal cancer has been observed and is possibly linked to the various nutritional deficiencies implicated in the pathogenesis of the disorder.

## Caustic Strictures

The propensity of caustic strictures to undergo malignant degeneration is well recognized. Tumors tend to develop within the esophagus at the site of the bronchial bifurcation and are usually of the squamous cell type. A latent period as long as 40 years occurs between lye ingestion and the development of carcinoma.[48] All patients with lye strictures should undergo endoscopic or cytologic surveillance to detect early tumors. When surgical intervention is required for palliation of dysphagia in patients without associated carcinoma, serious consideration should be given to resection of the esophagus and reconstruction rather than simple bypass because a carcinoma can still develop in the excluded portion of the gullet.[49]

## Miscellaneous Disorders

A variety of disorders have been associated with carcinoma of the esophagus. The spectrum of radiation injury to the esophagus following mediastinal or breast irradiation varies between an acute, self-limiting esophagitis and important complications such as stricture, perforation, and occasionally carcinoma.[50] Carcinoma has been found in association with epiphrenic and pharyngoesophageal diverticula, but a cause-and-effect relation is hard to establish.

# PATHOLOGY

## Squamous Cell Carcinoma

Squamous cell carcinoma accounts for 50–60% of esophageal cancers. Squamous cell carcinoma is predominantly located in the middle third (50%) followed by the distal third (30%) and finally the proximal third of the intrathoracic esophagus. Squamous cell carcinoma of the cervical esophagus occurs in 10% of patients. The tumors are usually moderately differentiated, displaying sheets of polygonal and polyhedral cells with keratin pearls. Spread along submucosal lymphatic vessels occurs both proximal and distal to the primary tumor. Synchronous noncontiguous foci of carcinoma are seen 2–10 cm away from the primary lesion in 14% of patients. These findings suggest the need for subtotal esophagectomy in most patients as well as frozen-section examination of the proximal resected margin at operation.

## Squamous Cell Variants

Two unusual variants of squamous cell carcinoma are occasionally seen. Verrucous carcinoma presents as a papillary intraluminal exophytic growth with low metastatic potential. The surface of the tumor is composed of well-differentiated squamous epithelium, and thus only deep biopsies that demonstrate submucosal invasion prove its malignant nature. Another variant is carcinosarcoma of the esophagus, in which, in addition to the epithelial component, there is a prominent spindle-cell component with interlacing spindle-shaped cells that demonstrate pleomorphism, hyperchromatism, and frequent mitoses. Misconceptions regarding the metastatic potential of the sarcomatous elements resulted in the misnomer *pseudosarcoma.* At gross inspection, the tumor presents predominantly intraluminal growth with a wide or narrow pedicle and little propensity toward full-wall penetration of the esophagus.

## Adenocarcinoma

Adenocarcinomas commonly arise from an associated Barrett's mucosa and rarely from the submucosal esophageal glands or islands of heterotropic columnar epithelium. Tumors in the distal third of the esophagus are usually fungating or polypoid in appearance, although stenotic variants are not uncommon. Most tumors are well differentiated, and 80–100% are associated with intraepithelial neoplasia. Other tumors included with adenocarcinoma are adenoid cystic and mucoepidermoid carcinomas. These rare tumors are morphologically similar to their salivary gland counterparts but are indistinguishable clinically and prognostically from the more common type of esophageal cancer.

## Small Cell Carcinoma

Small cell carcinoma accounts for less than 2% of all esophageal tumors. The tumor arises from the APUD (amine precursor uptake and decarboxylation) cell system present in the basal part of the lower esophageal epithelium. The tumors are composed of small round or fusiform cells with high nuclear-cytoplasmic ratios and hyperchromatic nuclei. Neurosecretory granules are seen in a large number of patients.

### Malignant Melanoma

Malignant melanoma, which is exceedingly rare in the esophagus, is more common in men than in women. It presents a bulky, polyploid intraesophageal mass that varies in color according to its melanin content. Sheets of spindle or polygonal cells are seen at histologic examination with abundant eosinophillic cytoplasm that stains positively for melanin granules. The prognosis is uniformly poor even after surgical resection.

### Esophageal Sarcoma

Among all esophageal tumors of mesenchymal origin, leiomyosarcoma is probably the most common, yet it accounts for only 1% of all esophageal tumors. The tumors often present as a bulky, intraluminal mass that displays hemorrhage and necrosis on cut section. The presence of frequent mitotic figures is said to differentiate the tumor from its benign counterpart. The absence of intracellular organelles characteristic of smooth muscle and detected with electron microscopy is proving to be a more reliable marker for malignancy. Eventually it is the biologic behavior of the tumor as detected intraoperatively that determines its malignant nature. Leiomyosarcomas are large tumors that usually ulcerate through the mucosa or are firmly attached to it, precluding the easy enucleation that is possible with esophageal leiomyoma.

## EARLY DETECTION

Most patients with esophageal carcinoma present with locally advanced or metastatic disease—their survival rates are dismal. Cure, however, is possible when early lesions are detected in patients with no or minimal symptoms. Five-year survival rates higher than 90% have been reported from mass screening programs in Asia.[51] Similar results after resection of stage I esophageal carcinoma have been reported by investigators in Europe.[52] Mass screening programs are not economically feasible in North and South America because of the relatively low incidence of esophageal carcinoma. Screening is more reasonably directed toward groups of patients at high risk for esophageal carcinoma. There is consensus that cytologic screening is both reliable and cost effective. Abrasive balloon cytology has been widely used in China and the sponge and capsule method has been used in Japan with good results.[53] We prefer a modification of an abrasive brush technique developed in northern Iran.[54] The frequency of surveillance is debatable. Data from some studies suggest that esophageal cancer has a prolonged preclinical latency period, which allows surveillance of groups at high risk as infrequently as once a year.

## CLINICAL PRESENTATION

Dysphagia is the presenting symptom in most patients with esophageal carcinoma. Unfortunately dysphagia occurs late in the natural history of the disease. The lack of a serosal coat allows the esophagus to distend and accommodate an intraluminal growth without noticeably impeding deglutition. Dysphagia occurs when the tumor encroaches on 60–80% of the esophageal circumference. Solid-food dysphagia may rapidly progress to total dysphagia. Although some patients may be able to point to the site of obstruction, this does not always correlate with the actual location of the tumor in the esophagus. Odynophagia is experienced by 20% of patients and is occasionally the only symptom. Persistent chest pain or discomfort unrelated to meals is an ominous sign that may indicate mediastinal penetration. Weight loss occurs in most patients, but cachexia is rarely seen.

A variety of symptoms indicate extraesophageal spread, including hoarseness secondary to recurrent nerve invasion, aspiration resulting from esophagobronchial fistula, and massive hematemesis from major vessel invasion. Approximately half the patients have locally unresectable disease or distant metastases at presentation.

## DIAGNOSIS

### Contrast Studies

A barium esophagram is usually the initial study performed in the examination of patients with dysphagia. It is essential that the study include the cervical esophagus as well as the stomach and duodenum. A single-contrast study readily reveals structural abnormalities, such as masses, ulcerations, or strictures. Double-contrast studies provide precise definition of the mucosal pattern, allowing detection of early lesions.

### Esophagoscopy

Esophagoscopy is an essential diagnostic modality that not only allows a tissue diagnosis but also allows the surgeon to map out the extent of the lesion. The choice of side of the planned thoracotomy is partly determined by the location of the tumor and its relation to the indentation of the aortic arch as noted at endoscopy. An abnormally placed squamous columnar j-junction, as in associated Barrett's metaplasia, or the presence of satellite lesions is carefully sought. The surgeon should be familiar with the appearance of an early malignant lesion—mild erythema, induration, and small ulcerations. Vital stains such as Lugol's iodine or toluidine blue should be used when findings are equivocal to guide endoscopic biopsies. The esophagus is initially washed with 1% acetic acid followed by the stain and then decolorized by a second application of acetic acid. Malignant lesions retain the dye with toluidine blue but remain unstained with Lugol's iodine. In each case staining allows directed biopsies.

Strictures when encountered are dilated to allow passage of an endoscope. Multiple biopsy specimens are obtained because a positive yield increases with the number of biopsy specimens. Direct brush cytologic examination is performed because on occasion a diagnosis is established with this technique in the face of a normal biopsy. The combined diagnostic accuracy of brushings and biopsies exceeds 90%. Rarely an undilatable stricture is encountered, and a diagnosis of malignancy is difficult to establish. Rigid esophagoscopy is performed under general anesthesia with another attempt at dilation and four-quadrant biopsies. If a diagnosis cannot be established the patients are treated as if they had a presumptive diagnosis of esophageal cancer.

### Staging

The staging system adopted by the American Joint Committee on Cancer and the Union Internationale Contre le Cancer (Table 51–1) represents a definite improvement over previous staging systems. The degree of tumor penetration through the esophageal wall emerged as a more important determinant of survival than tumor length or degree of obstruction. Staging of nodal disease remains fairly nebulous. A single N1 descriptor encompasses all possible sites of nodal spread. An emerging body of evidence from European and Japanese investigators indicates that survival rates are negatively correlated with the number of involved nodes as well as the location of the metastatic nodes. The current tumor stages are shown in Table 51–2.

## STAGING MODALITIES

### Bronchoscopy

Bronchoscopy is always done in patients with carcinoma of the cervical as well as the upper and middle thoracic esophagus. Mobility of the vocal cords is carefully evaluated. A mere bulge into the membranous trachea or main stem bronchi does not necessarily indicate malignant invasion. However, erythema and edema are ominous signs of airway invasion, and biopsy specimens and cytologic samples are retrieved from suspicious areas. An esophagorespiratory fistula is present in 5% of patients and usually requires emergency intervention.

**TABEL 51–1. TNM SYSTEM**

| | |
|---|---|
| **Primary Tumor** | |
| TX | Primary tumor cannot be assessed |
| T0 | No evidence of primary tumor |
| Tis | Carcinoma in situ |
| T1 | Tumor invades lamina propria or submucosa |
| T2 | Tumor invades muscularis propria |
| T3 | Tumor invades adventitia |
| T4 | Tumor invades adjacent structures |
| **Lymph Node** | |
| NX | Regional nodes cannot be assessed |
| N0 | No regional lymph node metastasis |
| N1 | Regional lymph node metastasis |
| **Distant Metastasis** | |
| M0 | No distant metastasis |
| M1 | Distant metastasis (including positive celiac nodes) |

**TABLE 51–2. TUMOR STAGES**

| | | | |
|---|---|---|---|
| Stage 0 | Tis | N0 | M0 |
| Stage I | T1 | N0 | M0 |
| Stage IIA | T2 | N0 | M0 |
| | T3 | N0 | M0 |
| Stage IIB | T1 | N1 | M0 |
| | T2 | N1 | M0 |
| Stage III | T3 | N1 | M0 |
| | T4 | Any N | M0 |
| Stage IV | Any T | Any N | M1 |

### Computed Tomography

Computed tomography (CT) of the chest and upper abdomen is routinely performed. The primary tumor is usually marked by thickening of the esophageal wall. A blurring of the contour of the esophagus in the region of the tumor indicates full-thickness penetration of the wall. Using this criterion for the T descriptor, we were able to predict wall penetration with a 75% accuracy. Prediction of nodal involvement is less reliable, however. Diagnostic accuracy is only 50% because of false-negative rates with small nodes. The criteria that determine invasion of adjacent structures are not well defined. Aortic invasion is predictable when the tumor encroaches on more than 90° of the aortic circumference, but the diagnostic accuracy of this sign is poor with lesser degrees of encroachment. CT criteria for gross airway invasion include distortion of airway anatomy or an obvious endoluminal extension of the tumor. Nonetheless, CT signs of early invasion of the airway are not uniformly reliable and should not prevent exploration in an otherwise favorable case. Evidence of hepatic or adrenal metastases should be diligently sought. CT has largely supplanted liver scintigraphy for detection of liver metastases. However, metastatic lesions from adenocarcinoma of the gastric cardia or esophagus on occasion may be isodense with the liver parenchyma and hence only detectable with radionuclide scintigraphy.

### Endoscopic Ultrasonography

Endoscopic ultrasonography has emerged over the past decade as a useful modality in the clinical staging of esophageal cancer.[55] The topic is covered in Chapter 8.

### Miscellaneous

Invasive measures such as mediastinoscopy, cervical node biopsy, thoracoscopy, laparoscopy, and occasionally laparotomy should be used liberally when suggested by abnormal CT findings. Histologic documentation of metastatic disease should be obtained whenever possible, specifically for isolated metastatic lesions.

## SURGICAL THERAPY

Czerny performed the first resection for carcinoma of the cervical esophagus in 1877.[56] Attempts at resection of the intrathoracic esophagus were stymied by the inevitable catastrophic pneumothorax and mediastinal tamponade before the introduction of positive pressure ventilation. Nonetheless the first successful transthoracic esophagectomy was performed in New York by Franz Torek (1913) before the advent of intratracheal ventilation and ether anesthesia.[57] The intraoperative survival of Torek's patient was no doubt due to the dense pleural adhesions that fixed the mediastinum. The procedure was done through a left thoracotomy and was completed in a little less than 2 hours of operating time. The patient survived for 13 years with a cervical esophagostomy and a gastrostomy connected by an extracorporeal tube. Subsequent attempts by other surgeons met with catastrophic consequences for a variety of reasons, including severe intrathoracic anastomotic dehiscences. The first successful resection of the thoracic esophagus with immediate reconstruction was accomplished by Oshawa in 1933.[58] The procedure was later popularized by Adams and Phemister in 1938.[59] In the ensuing decades, advances in the evolution of esophageal resection and reconstruction were made by pioneering thoracic surgeons such as Sweet[60] and Belsey.[61] In 1978 Orringer and Sloan reported their experience with transhiatal blunt esophagectomy for carcinoma of the thoracic esophagus.[62] Despite the uproar incited by this blind technique, enucleation of the intrathoracic esophagus had been proposed and performed by Denk in 1913.[63] Several other esophageal surgeons, such as Akiyama et al, had also used transhiatal resection of the thoracic esophagus as an adjunct to resection of cancer of the cervical esophagus and postcricoid region.[64] However, it was Orringer who popularized this technique for resection of tumors of the thoracic esophagus. To date he remains a proponent of this approach (see Chap. 52).

Despite substantial advances in surgical and anesthetic techniques, a report published in 1980 analyzed the world literature on esophagectomy for carcinoma of the esophagus between 1953 and 1978.[65] The cumulative resectability rate was 22% with a 3% 5-year survival rate and an operative mortality in excess of 25%. This report is clearly no longer representative of the current state of the art. A review of the world literature published in 1990 showed that hospital mortality worldwide was 11% and indeed in many centers that specialize in esophageal surgery less than 5%.[66] Nonetheless, substantial improvement in survival rates remains elusive. The dismal survival rates are mainly due to the advanced stage of the tumor at the time of presentation.

Surgical procedures vary between limited resection and extended resection depending primarily on the expertise and preference of the surgeon. Unfortunately, limited resection techniques do not allow for full staging of the extent of nodal disease. Therefore, understaging may be a common problem that precludes a stage-for-stage comparison of survival between various procedures. Also, terms such as *curative* or *palliative* add to the confusion because palliation of dysphagia is almost universally accomplished regardless of the curative nature of the resection. The International Society of Diseases of the Esophagus proposed the following classification of resections:

- R0 No residual gross or microscopic disease
- R1 Residual microscopic disease
- R2 Residual gross disease

The use of the R descriptor in staging may partly resolve some of the confusion in analysis of various reports. The controversy surrounding the extent of resection is unlikely to be resolved in the near future.

## SURGICAL APPROACH

Resection of the thoracic esophagus can be accomplished with a variety of surgical approaches. The most commonly used approach worldwide is a right thoracotomy and laparotomy as initially proposed by Lewis.[67] A modification was proposed by McKeown whereby an additional cervical incision allows the anastomosis to be performed in the neck, thus avoiding the potential hazards of an intrathoracic anastomosis.[68] A less commonly used incision for esophageal resection is left thoracotomy. This approach, preferred by Sweet and others, was gradually abandoned because of the significant increase in pulmonary morbidity incurred with the radial incision of the diaphragm required for exposure of the upper abdomen. Belsey modified the technique by adopting a peripheral semilunar incision located approximately 1 1/2 inches from the chest wall and thus preserving diaphramatic innervation. This exposure is popular in China and in a few centers in the United States and Europe.

Resections of the intrathoracic esophagus may be accomplished through a transhiatal approach with an upper abdominal and cervical incision. Special retractors allow adequate exposure of the hiatal tunnel and the lower mediastinum up to the tracheal bifurcation. Surgeons who use this approach should be both willing and capable of performing a thoracotomy to deal with the potential but rare intrathoracic vascular or tracheal injuries that might occur during esophageal resection.

Tumors of the cervical esophagus are exposed through a generous collar or U-shaped incision. Additional exposure can be obtained through an upper sternal split, a technique that is potentially useful in exposing tumors that extend into the thoracic inlet. A laryngectomy and a terminal tracheostomy are also performed. Reconstruction is achieved by advancing the stomach or an isoperistaltic segment of colon. A free jejunal graft may also be used for reconstruction.

Our approach to tumors of the thoracic esophagus is dictated by the distance between the proximal end of the tumor and the aortic pulsation noted at endoscopy. Tumors of the cardia or those situated 10 cm distal to the aortic arch are approached through a left thoracotomy. This approach provides excellent exposure of the lower mediastinum, hiatal tunnel, and left upper quadrant. Reconstruction may be performed either in the mediastinum or, preferably, in the neck after mobilization of the rest of the intrathoracic esophagus. Tumors whose proximal extent is within 10 cm of the aortic arch and those of the upper thoracic esophagus are approached through a right posterorlateral thoracotomy. The stomach is prepared through a separate laparotomy or occasionally mobilized through the hiatus without a laparotomy, as proposed by Belsey and Hiebert.[61] Transhiatal resection is best reserved for patients in whom palliation is clearly the objective of treatment because of the advanced stage of the disease or the presence of serious co-morbidity.

## Transhiatal Esophagectomy

Transhiatal esophagectomy is best suited for resection of carcinoma of the cardia but is also used for resection of carcinoma of the intrathoracic esophagus. A description of the technical aspects of transhiatal esophagectomy is provided in Chapter 52. Perhaps the largest single experience with transhiatal esophagectomy is that of Orringer et al. They reported on 417 patients with carcinoma of the esophagus and cardia resected with this technique over a 15-year period.[69] The overall hospital mortality was low (5%), and complications were no more clinically significant than those encountered with standard transthoracic resections. The overall 5-year actuarial survival rate was 27% and did not vary greatly with cell type or tumor location. Tumor stage was the only statistically significant determinant of survival (Table 51–3). Paradoxically the survival rate among patients with stage IIA disease was worse than that among patients with stage IIB tumors. This peculiarity may be caused at least in part by understaging of mediastinal lymph nodes with transhiatal esophagectomy. Gelfand et al reported on 160 patients who underwent transhiatal esophagectomy for carcinoma of the lower esophagus and cardia.[70] Most tumors were adenocarcinomas and most presented in earlier stages. Survival rates at 1, 2 and 5 years were 62%, 40% and 21%. Vigenswaran et al reported on 131 patients who underwent transhiatal resection with an operative mortality of 2%.[71] The overall 5-year survival rate was 21%. Five-year survival rates for stages I, II, and III disease were 47.5%, 37.7% and 5.8%. In the latter study, the 5-year survival rate for adenocarcinoma was 27%; none of the patients with squamous cell carcinoma were alive at 5-year follow-up study.

**TABLE 51–3. SURVIVAL RATES AFTER TRANSHIATAL ESOPHAGECTOMY**

| Stage | Survival Rate (%) |
|---|---|
| Stage 0 | 59 |
| Stage I | 63 |
| Stage IIA | 24 |
| Stage IIB | 38 |
| Stage III | 12 |
| Stage IV | 16 |

*(Data from Orringer MB, Marshall B, Stirling MC: Transhiatal esophagectomy for benign and malignant disease. J Thorac Cardiovasc Surg 105(2):265–277, 1993.)*

Proponents of transhiatal esophagectomy maintain that overall survival rates are not significantly different with standard transthoracic or even extended resections and that occasional cures are possible only in the few patients with superficial tumors and without nodal metastases (T1–T2N0). Critics of transhiatal esophagectomy, however, argue that a complete lymphadenectomy is a necessary component of resection for carcinoma, primarily for staging and possibly for curative purposes, at least in some patients with limited nodal metastases. A large body of data indicating the presence of nodal metastases in 30–50% of patients in whom the tumor is limited to the submucosa lends support to the latter argument, particularly because more extensive resections result in 50–60% 5-year survival rates among patients with T1–T2N1 disease.[72] The controversy is likely to continue until a well-designed, random-assignment study produces a direct comparison of survival rates.

## Standard Transthoracic Esophagectomy

Standard transthoracic esophagectomy is performed through either a right or left thoracotomy depending on the location of the tumor. When a right thoracotomy is chosen, the chest is entered through the fifth interspace. Because this approach is often used for midesophageal tumors that abut the aortic arch or tracheal bifurcation, the fifth interspace provides excellent exposure of these structures. Single-lung ventilation greatly enhances the exposure. The arch of the azygos vein is divided, and the esophagus is mobilized from its mediastinal bed. Particular care is exercised to avoid injuries to the recurrent nerves. Mobilization of the esophagus is carried distally to the hiatus and proximally into the prevertebral cervical space. The right lung is reinflated, and the thoracotomy is closed. The stomach is then mobilized through an upper abdominal incision while the previously mobilized cervical esophagus is exposed through a cervical collar incision. The esophagus is divided at a suitable site in the neck, and the specimen is retrieved through the abdominal incision. Distal transection of the specimen is performed to include the initial four branches of the left gastric artery along the lesser curvature. The resultant gastric tube is advanced to the neck through the posterior mediastinum, and a hand-sewn, end-to-side esophagogastric anastomosis is performed. A frozen section of the proximal margin is always obtained before the anastomosis is performed.

Some surgeons advocate that the operation begin with abdominal exploration and gastric mobilization followed by a thoracotomy with an eventual intrathoracic esophagogastrostomy. We believe that an initial thoracotomy allows for early assessment of resectability and that the longer operative time with a cervical incision is a reasonable price to pay for the relative safety of a cervical anastomosis.

When the procedure is performed through a left thoracotomy, the chest is entered through the sixth interspace. Access to the left upper quadrant is obtained through a semilunar diaphragmatic incision 1 inch (2.5 cm) away from the chest wall. Extending the incision across the costal margin into the abdomen adds little to the exposure and is not advisable. After mobilization and resection of the proximal stomach and lower half of the thoracic esophagus, reconstruction is performed in the mediastinum or, preferably, in the neck. If the latter is chosen, the esophagus is mobilized from under the aortic arch and along its course in the supra aortic posterior mediastinum and freed well into the neck. The gastric tube is then passed under the aortic arch and attached to the esophageal stump; both are loosely tucked in the prevertebral cervical space. The diaphragm is reattached and the thoracotomy closed. With the patient in the supine position, a small cervical incision is performed and dissection is carried to the prevertebral space, where the esophageal stump and gastric tube are encountered and easily delivered into neck for a cervical anastomosis.

Several studies have shown little difference in operative mortality or morbidity between transthoracic and transhiatal esophagectomy.[73,74] Survival rates reported with this technique are essentially identical to those reported after transhiatal resection.

## En Bloc Resection

En bloc resection of carcinoma of the cardia and lower esophagus was originally proposed by Logan in 1962.[75] He reported on 250 patients who underwent resection with the en bloc technique with an impressive 16% 5-year survival rate but a formidable 21% operative mortality. The technique was modified in 1969 and later extended to resection of carcinoma of the thoracic and cervical esophagus.[76] Skinner described his initial experience with en bloc resection for neoplasms of the esophagus and cardia performed in 80 patients with an 11% operative mortality and 18% survival rate at 5 years.[76] In a subsequent detailed analysis of 58 specimens resected with the en bloc technique, a staging system was based on the degree of wall penetration (W) and the number of involved nodes (N0, N1, N2) (Table 51–4).[77] A subgroup of patients with potentially curable carcinoma was defined as those with less than full-wall penetration (W1) and a limited number of positive nodes (N1) or those in whom full-wall penetration occurred but without nodal metastases. Both groups had a 50% long-term survival rate without tumor recurrence after en bloc resection. Those survival rates have since been reported by other investigators. Lerut et al reported on 257 patients with an overall 5-year survival rate of 30%.[78] The 5-year survival rate was significantly better among patients with comparable stages who underwent curative (M0) radical resections (48%) as opposed to curative (M0) nonradical resections. Hagen et al reported a 5-year survival rate of 41% after en bloc resection versus a 21% 5-year survival rate among patients who underwent resection with the transhiatal technique.[79] The survival benefit was even more apparent in patients with early lesions (W1N0, W1N1) after en bloc resection compared with transhiatal resections (75% vs 21%). Despite what appears to be an important survival advantage produced by en bloc esophagectomy, the operation has not been widely adopted and is performed in only a limited number of centers in Europe and the United States. The procedure is technically demanding and is associated with a considerable learning curve. The high operative mortalities initially reported have now decreased to the 5–10% range.

The basic principle of en bloc resection is the extirpation of the esophagus within an envelope of adjoining normal tissue. This includes the posterior pericardium and both pleural surfaces where they abut on the tumor-bearing esophagus as well as the lymphovascular tissue (thoracic duct, azygos veins and their tributaries) wedged dorsally between the esophagus and the spine. This "mesoesophagus" is probably with remnant of the embryonic esophageal mesentery that determines the pathways of vascular supply and lymphatic drainage.[80] Because the esophagus lacks a defined serosal coat, both pleural surfaces and the pericardium are construed as the serosal counterpart, especially because the lower esophageal longitudinal muscle layer is partly attached to the subpleural and pericardial fibrous lay-

**TABLE 51–4. WNM SYSTEM**

| | |
|---|---|
| **Primary tumor** | |
| W0 | Tumor into but not through submucosa |
| W1 | Tumor into muscularis propria |
| W2 | Tumor transmural |
| **Nodal metastasis** | |
| N0 | No nodal metastasis |
| N1 | 1–4 nodal metastases |
| N2 | 5 or more positive nodes |
| **Distant metastasis** | |
| M0 | No distant metastasis |
| M1 | Distant metastasis |

ers. For tumors of the cardia and intra-abdominal esophagus, a 1-inch (2.5 cm) cuff of diaphragm is resected en bloc with the specimen. Upper abdominal and mediastinal lymphadenectomy completes the procedure. The gastrointestinal tract is divided approximately 10 cm on either side of the tumor, and gastrointestinal continuity is established with the esophageal substitute of choice. Because of the extensive nature of the resection, the procedure is performed only when preoperative and intraoperative staging maneuvers indicate a potentially favorable situation. At the time of operation, evidence of occult hematogenous metastases is diligently sought. Frozen-section evaluation of celiac nodal biopsies and biopsies of lymph nodes located 10 cm on either side of the tumor are performed. The presence of celiac nodal metastasis or positive nodes beyond the limits of the proposed resection signals incurability, and the operation is converted to a more conventional resection.

### Three-field Lymphadenectomy

The Japanese concept of the surgical treatment of carcinoma of the esophagus has always emphasized the need for a subtotal esophagectomy with resection of the thoracic duct and an extensive mediastinal and upper abdominal lymphadenectomy (two-field lymphadenectomy). Despite the salutary survival rates reported by Japanese investigators (and unmatched in the West), large follow-up studies indicate that as many as 30–40% of patients have recurrences in the cervical nodes.[81] This has prompted several esophageal centers in Japan to adopt an extended lymphadenectomy, which includes dissection of the cervical, mediastinal, and abdominal nodes for patients with carcinoma of the thoracic esophagus. Isono et al reported the results of a study performed at 35 institutions in Japan between 1983 and 1989 that dealt with three-field lymph node dissection for carcinoma of the esophagus.[82] Despite the enormity of the data generated by this large study, several important points emerged that provide insight into the patterns of nodal spread of squamous cell carcinoma of the esophagus. These points are as follows:

1. Metastases to the cervical nodes occurred in almost one third of the 1791 patients treated with three-field lymphadenectomy. Although the incidence of nodal metastases was highest when the tumor was located in the upper third of the thoracic esophagus (42%), almost 20% of patients with cancer of the lower third had cervical nodal metastases.
2. The frequency of nodal metastases increased with the depth of tumor penetration through the esophageal wall. Although none of the patients with carcinoma in situ (intramucosal carcinoma) had positive nodes, tumor invasion into the submucosa (T1) signaled a 50% probability of nodal metastases. Patients with a T2 or T3 tumor had a 60–80% probability of nodal involvement. These multi-institutional data have since been substantiated by subsequent reports and cast doubt on the efficacy of limited resection for the treatment of patients with Stage I disease.
3. The cervical nodes most frequently involved with metastatic carcinoma included the chain of nodes along the right and left recurrent nerves as well as the deep cervical nodes along the posterior aspect of the proximal extent of the internal jugular vein. Involvement of the supraclavicular nodes was infrequent and often associated with extensive nodal disease.
4. In the mediastinum, the location of nodal metastases from carcinoma of the thoracic esophagus varied with the location of the tumor. Nonetheless, the most commonly involved nodes were those along the right recurrent nerve, which represented a continuum of nodes into the neck. The left paratracheal, periesophageal, subcarinal, and right paratracheal nodes were involved in approximately 20% of patients.
5. Within the abdomen, nodal metastasis was predominantly located along the cardia, the lesser curvature, the left gastric trunk, and the celiac axis—a pattern defined by Akiyama in the early 1980s.[83]

There is little doubt that the results of three-field lymph node dissection have contributed considerably to our understanding of the pathways and patterns of lymphatic spread in thoracic esophageal cancer. It is also clear that a large number of tumors will be inaccurately staged after isolated mediastinal and abdominal lymphadenectomy. Most studies of three-field lymph node dissection have shown a consistent improvement in survival rates beyond those obtained with two-field lymphadenectomy in patients without nodal metastasis. In the study by Isono et al that compared two- and three-field lymph node dissection, the 5-year survival rate was significantly better in patients without nodal metastases after three-field lymph node dissection (56% vs 45%). This finding suggested the presence of occult cervical nodal metastases in patients who underwent two-field lymphadenectomy.[82] The effect of extended lymphadenectomy on survival once nodal metastases has occurred has been contested in the west. Nonetheless, the results from the extensive data generated in Japan since the mid 1980s are compelling. Kato et al reported on 79 patients who underwent transthoracic esophagectomy with mediastinal, abdominal, and bilateral cervical lymphadenectomy with an operative mortality of 3.8%. The overall survival rate for 57 patients with positive nodes was an impressive 33.6%.[84] Patients with cervical nodal metastasis had a 30% 5-year survival rate, suggesting that the cervical nodal basin should be considered a regional (N1) rather than a distant (M1) site of spread. Akiyama et al reported on 538 patients with comparable stages of disease treated with either two- or three-field lymphadenectomy over a 20-year period.[85] The 5-year survival for patients with positive nodes was 42% after three-field dissection compared with 28% after two-field lymphadenectomy.

Matsuhara et al reported similar survival data and confirmed previous Japanese and western data that correlated survival with the number of positive nodes.[86] A 5-year survival rate of 40–50% for patients with fewer than seven positive nodes reported by both Akiyama et al and Matsuhara et al is in agreement with similar data reported in the early 1980s. Although the survival advantage for a three-field lymphadenectomy has not been confirmed in the western literature, these recent reports serve to highlight the importance of this issue.

## RADIATION THERAPY

### Radiation Therapy as Primary Modality

#### *External Beam*

Many authors have reported results of external beam radiation therapy alone for esophageal carcinoma. Most series include patients with unfavorable features such as clinical T4 lesions, positive lymph nodes, and unresectable disease. For example, in the series treated by De-Ren, 184 of the 678 patients had stage IV disease.[87]

The use of radiation therapy in the potentially curative setting requires doses of at least 5000 cGy at 180–200 cGy per fraction. Given the large size of many unresectable esophageal cancers, doses of 6000 cGy or greater are probably required. The results of selected series of radiation therapy alone are presented in Table 51–5.[87–89] The overall 5-year survival rate for patients with carcinoma of the esophagus treated with radiation therapy alone is approximately 10%.

#### *External Beam and Intraluminal Brachytherapy*

Intraluminal brachytherapy has been used in a variety of settings for esophageal cancer. It can be delivered with a high dose rate or a low dose rate.[90,91] Although there are technical differences between the two dose rates, there are no clear therapeutic advantages. Briefly, the technique involves placement of a radioactive source intraluminally by means of esophagoscopy or a nasogastric tube.

The most important limitation of brachytherapy is the effective treatment distance. The primary isotope is $^{192}$Ir, which can effectively treat to a distance of 1 cm from the source. Therefore, any portion of the tumor farther than 1 cm from the source receives a suboptimal radiation dose.

In the curative setting, the best approach is to add brachytherapy as a boost after external beam irradiation. The dose of brachytherapy in this setting is commonly 1000–2000 cGy. The limited nonrandomized data suggest that outcome may be improved when brachytherapy is added to external beam irradiation. This approach is being examined in a prospective study by the Radiation Therapy Oncology Group (RTOG 92-07). In the palliative setting, intraluminal brachytherapy is used to improve dysphagia due to obstruction by tumor. The effectiveness of brachytherapy in this setting is unclear.

### Adjuvant Radiation Therapy

The rationale for adjuvant therapy in clinically resectable esophageal cancer is based on the patterns of failure after potentially curative operations. Unfortunately, few surgical series report patterns-of-failure data. The incidences of local-regional failure in the surgical control arms of the preoperative radiation therapy randomized trials performed by Mei et al[92] and by Gignoux et al[93] were 12% and 67%. The local-regional failure rate in the surgical control arm of the postoperative radiation therapy randomized trial performed by Teniere et al[94] was 35% for patients with negative local-

**TABLE 51–5. RADIATION THERAPY ALONE FOR ESOPHAGEAL CANCER—SELECTED SERIES**

| Reference | Histology | Stage | No. of Pts | 5-Year Survival Rate (%) |
|---|---|---|---|---|
| De-Ren[87] | Various | II | 177 | 22 |
| | | III | 501 | 28 |
| | | <5 cm | 59 | 25 |
| | | 5 cm | 115 | 25 |
| | | >5 cm | 504 | 6 |
| | | Total[a] | 678 | 8 |
| Newaishy et al[88] | Squamous "Inoperable" | | 444 | 9 |
| Okawa et al[89] | Squamous I | | 43 | 20 |
| | | II | 130 | 10 |
| | | III | 92 | 3 |
| | | IV | 23 | 0 |
| | | T1 | 47 | 18 |
| | | T2 | 147 | 10 |
| | | T3 | 94 | 3 |
| | | Total | 288 | 9 |

[a]Includes 184 patients with stage IV diseases.

regional lymph nodes and 38% for patients with positive local-regional lymph nodes. Therefore, although most patients with esophageal cancer die of distant metastasis, the incidence of local-regional failure following surgical excision alone in patients with clinically resectable disease is high enough to support the use of adjuvant radiation therapy.

### Preoperative Radiation Therapy

Theoretically, preoperative radiation therapy in the treatment of esophageal cancer yields biologic (decreased tumor seeding and increased radiosensitivity due to more oxygenated cells), physical (increased resectability), and dosimetric (patients who undergo a gastric pull-up or intestinal interposition are not limited to the postoperative dose of 4500–5000 cGy) advantages.

Six randomized trials of preoperative radiation therapy for esophageal cancer have been performed (Table 51–6).[92,93,95–98] Overall, there were no differences in resectability rates between patients who underwent preoperative radiation therapy and those who underwent surgical excision alone. Local-regional failure rates were reported in only two of the six series. Mei et al[92] reported no difference in local-regional failure rates; however, Gignoux et al[93] reported a statistically significant decrease in local-regional failure rate (46% vs 67%) among patients who underwent preoperative radiation therapy compared with patients who underwent surgical excision alone.

Two of the six studies reported an improvement in survival with preoperative radiation therapy. Nygaard et al performed a four-arm trial in which patients were randomized preoperatively to undergo chemotherapy (cisplatin and bleomycin for two cycles), radiation therapy, combined modality therapy, or surgical therapy alone.[98] Patients who received preoperative radiation therapy (with or without chemotherapy) had a significant improvement in overall 3-year survival rate (18% versus 5%, $P = .009$). The 48 patients who received preoperative radiation therapy alone had a 20% 3-year survival rate that was not statistically significant. A similar improvement in survival rate was reported by Huang et al (46% versus 25%).[97]

In summary, because only two of the six studies reported local-regional failure rates, it is difficult to draw firm conclusions regarding the influence of preoperative radiation therapy on the incidence of local-regional failure. Regarding the impact on survival, two studies reported an improvement (one in which 50% of the patients received chemotherapy). However, four of the six studies reported no advantage in overall survival rate. Nonrandomized trials from Yadava et al[99] and Sugimachi et al[100] also reported no survival benefit. According to the results of the foregoing randomized, albeit poorly designed trials, adjuvant preoperative radiation therapy does not appear to improve local-regional control or survival.

### Postoperative Radiation Therapy

The primary advantage of adjuvant postoperative radiation therapy is accurate patient selection. Patients with T1–2N0M0 tumors on the basis of pathologic results and those with metastatic disease can be excluded from treatment. The disadvantage is dosimetric; patients who undergo a gastric pull-up or intestinal interposition are limited to 4500–5000 cGy.

There are many encouraging reports of nonrandomized studies of postoperative radiation therapy in the treatment of esophageal cancer. For example, Kasai et al reported an 88% 5-year survival rate among patients with node-negative disease who received postoperative radiation therapy.[101] Only two randomized trials have been performed. This discussion is limited to patients treated in the adjuvant setting (complete resection and negative margins with or without local-regional lymph nodes).

Teniere et al[94] reported results of the treatment of 221 patients with squamous cell carcinoma randomized to sur-

**TABLE 51–6. RANDOMIZED TRIALS OF PREOPERATIVE RADIATION THERAPY FOR ESOPHAGEAL CANCER**

| | | | | | Percentage of Tumors Resectable | | Local Failure Rate (%) | | 5-Year Survival Rate (%) | |
|---|---|---|---|---|---|---|---|---|---|---|
| Reference | Type | No. of Pts | Total Dose (cGy) | Fraction Size (cGy) | *Surgery* | *Radiation Therapy* | *Surgery* | *Radiation Therapy* | *Surgery* | *Radiation Therapy* |
| Arnott et al[96] | Squamous and adeno | 176 | 2000 | 200 | N/A[a] | N/A | N/A | N/A | 17 | 9 |
| Launois et al[95] | Squamous | 109 | 4000 | N/A | 70 | 76 | N/A | N/A | 10 | 10 |
| Huang et al[97] | N/A | 160 | 4000 | 200 | 90 | 92 | N/A | N/A | 25 | 46[b] |
| Mei et al[92] | N/A | 206 | 4000 | N/A | 85 | 93 | 12 | 13 | 30 | 35 |
| Gignoux et al[93] | Squamous | 229 | 3300 | 330 | 58 | 47 | 67 | 46[c] | 8 | 10 |
| Nygaard et al[98] | Squamous | 186 | 3500[d] | 175 | N/A | N/A | N/A | N/A | 5 | 18 (3-yr)[c] |

[a]N/A = Information not available in article.
[b]Statistical analysis not performed.
[c]($P = .009$)
[d]With or without chemotherapy.

gical excision alone or postoperative radiation therapy (4500–5500 cGy at 180 cGy per fraction). The minimum follow-up period was 3 years. For the total patient group, the addition of postoperative radiation therapy had no statistically significant impact on survival rate.

The study by Fok et al[102] included patients with both squamous cell carcinoma and adenocarcinoma. There was no statistically significant improvement in median survival rate, local failure rate, or distant failure rate with the addition of postoperative radiation therapy.

Postoperative radiation therapy is commonly recommended for patients with positive local-regional lymph nodes. Although the data from Teniere et al[94] support the use of postoperative radiation therapy for local-regional control, the benefit was limited to patients with negative lymph nodes (10% local failure rate for postoperative radiation therapy versus 35% local failure rate for surgery alone. There was no significant benefit for patients with positive nodes.

In summary, although adjuvant postoperative radiation therapy may improve local-regional control in patients with node-negative disease, it has no impact on overall survival rate.

## CHEMOTHERAPY

### Rationale

The failure of surgical or radiation therapy to cure clinically localized esophageal cancer is due to the inability to eradicate residual disease at the primary site and to early systemic dissemination of disease. Autopsy studies confirm the frequent systemic nature of the disease, even at or soon after initial presentation.[103,104] In these autopsies performed soon after diagnosis (median, 6 months), most patients were found to have evidence of distant metastatic disease whether or not residual local disease was present. The ability to treat metastatic disease with systemic treatment early in the disease has led to the incorporation of chemotherapy into combined-modality therapy that also use surgical excision and radiation therapy.

The role of chemotherapy as a single modality in the treatment of esophageal cancer has undergone considerable change over the last 15–20 years. Before 1976, few studies had been performed in patients with esophageal cancer. By 1994, although many single agents still had to be tested, a number of multidrug combinations had at least preliminary evaluation. Chemotherapy is used as palliative therapy for patients with advanced incurable cancer. In addition, however, the poor outcome among patients with local-regional tumors treated with the conventional treatment of surgical excision or radiation therapy has led to numerous studies of neoadjuvant chemotherapy or chemotherapy plus radiation therapy for local-regional tumors.

### Assessment of Response

Evaluating response to chemotherapy in patients with advanced metastatic disease is usually not difficult. These patients generally have measurable disease at physical or radiographic examination, and the standard criteria of response outlined by Miller et al[105] can be easily used. However, in patients with local-regional disease in which only the primary esophageal tumor is available for assessment of response to treatment, evaluating tumor regression can be quite difficult. A number of early studies used improvement in dysphagia as a criterion of tumor regression. Careful assessment of this criterion has shown it to be a misleading indicator of response, because minimal tumor shrinkage can lead to marked improvement in swallowing. This effect may be a reflection of a decrease in the resistance to flow, as described in Laplace's law, whereby small changes in radius have a large effect on resistance. On the other hand, several studies have demonstrated that objective assessment of response in patients with local-regional disease can be based on repeat barium esophagograms and the following criteria: (1) complete radiologic response—no tumor seen after repeat barium esophagram; (2) partial radiographic response—more than 50% reduction in tumor bulk but residual disease still evident; and (3) minor radiologic regression—tumor reduction clearly evident but less than 50% shrinkage.[106] The final assessment of effectiveness of chemotherapy requires endoscopic or surgical confirmation. Complete pathologic remission requires histologic confirmation in addition to a normal esophagram. The use of endoscopic ultrasonography may allow a more precise assessment of response in local-regional esophageal cancer.

### Single Agent Chemotherapy—Primary Modality

Sixteen chemotherapeutic agents have undergone adequate trials to allow at least preliminary analysis of their efficacy at the 15% level.[107–109] A serious disadvantages of many of the earlier studies is the absence of strict response criteria, and the small numbers of patients entered into these trials, which necessitated pooling of data from several studies.

Bleomycin was one of the earliest single agents to be studied in esophageal cancer. Initial studies were performed in the late 1960s and early 1970s. Bleomycin had a response rate of 15% among 80 patients in whom efficacy could be evaluated. The median duration of response was brief, 2–3 months. Because of potential pulmonary toxicity (making use of the drug in combined modality programs difficult), bleomycin is rarely used in current studies.

Mitomycin C has been tested as a single agent in three phase II trials. Overall, 15 of 58 patients (26%) in whom efficacy could be evaluated had major tumor regression with mitomycin C. However, most of these remissions occurred with a dose schedule of mitomycin that was very toxic. In addition, mitomycin has potential pulmonary toxicity.

Cisplatin is a common component of combination

chemotherapy for esophageal cancer. In all, 53 of 167 patients treated with cisplatin as a single agent had a response; the overall response rate was 32.4%. It should be noted, however, that in a random-assignment trial in patients with advanced disease, the response rate to single-agent cisplatin was quite low (11%).[110] Toxicity has generally been tolerable; it includes nausea, vomiting, nephrotoxicity, and ototoxicity.

Vindesine has undergone extensive trials in patients with esophageal cancer. The overall cumulative response rate in 86 patients in whom efficacy could be evaluated was 22%. In all the trials the worst side effects of vindesine were peripheral neuropathy and myelosuppression. However, the drug was, in general, well tolerated.

In two trials 5-fluorouracil (5-FU) was studied as a single agent. The cumulative response rate was 42% among 36 patients in whom efficacy could be evaluated.

Paclitaxel (Taxol) is a taxane derivative that has been extensively studied for breast and ovarian carcinomas. Investigators from Memorial Sloan-Kettering Cancer Center and The M.D. Anderson Cancer Center performed a joint phase II trial of treatment of patients with adenocarcinoma and epidermoid cancers of the esophagus.[111] All patients had advanced disease. Taxol was well tolerated; the worst toxicity was neutropenia. Substantial antitumor activity was demonstrated with this new agent. A 32% response rate including one complete remission, was seen in a group of 51 patients in whom efficacy could be evaluated. Equal activity was seen for patients with adenocarcinoma and those with epidermoid cancer. The number of patients who responded to treatment was not significantly different in this noncomparative trial from that seen when cisplatin-based combination therapy was used for advanced disease.

### Combination Chemotherapy—Primary Modality

The demonstration of modest antitumor activity for several single agents and the knowledge that combination chemotherapy seemed to be more effective than single-agent therapy in the treatment of a number of solid tumors led to the study of combination chemotherapy for epidermoid esophageal cancer. Many phase II single-arm trials of combination chemotherapy have been conducted in the last few years. The common denominator in most combination chemotherapy trials was cisplatin.

The combinations studied were cisplatin with a Vinca alkaloid plus or minus other agents and cisplatin-fluorouracil–based treatment. Kelsen et al treated 71 patients using the three-drug combination of cisplatin, vindesine, and bleomycin.[112] The overall response rate was 53%. Twenty-eight of 44 patients with local-regional disease achieved a partial response (64%) compared with eight of 24 extensive disease (33%). The dose-limiting toxicity of the regimen was myelosuppression.

Kies et al initially identified cisplatin–5-FU as an active combination for esophageal cancer.[113] In all, the combination of cisplatin and 5-FU has been used in 134 patients with advanced esophageal cancer, with a cumulative response rate of 49%. This regimen has mostly been used as part of multimodality treatment of esophageal cancer.

Several other combinations of the aforementioned agents as well as other drugs such as methotrexate, vincristine, Adriamycin (doxorubicin) and mitoguazone have been studied with variable response rates in small series. To date there have been no prospective, randomized studies comparing one combination regimen with another. The toxic effects of most of these regimens are tolerable but clinically significant.

Whenever reported, the response rate for local-regional disease has been significantly higher than that for metastatic disease (approximately 45–55% vs 25–30%). This may be related to the patient's performance status and tumor burden. Clearly chemotherapy can result in palliation of symptoms in a moderate but reproducible number of patients with advanced disease. However, the duration of response continues to be brief, and none of the chemotherapy regimens developed so far have induced complete remissions in a substantial percentage of patients. There is evidence that adenocarcinomas of the esophagus and the gastroesophageal junction respond to regimens similar to those used for epidermoid carcinoma.

### Combined Modality Therapy

The laboratory and clinical rationale for neoadjuvant chemotherapy was reviewed by Harris and Mastrangelo.[114] Resection can be difficult because the esophagus lies in close apposition to and may involve adjoining structures (spine, aorta, heart), many of which cannot be excised. Thus, one advantage of preoperative chemotherapy for esophageal cancer is the possibility of down-staging the primary tumor, which may enhance resectability and allow a more conservative surgical approach. This may also potentially improve local control. Another advantage is the ability to assess response of the primary tumor to preoperative chemotherapy. One can then identify the patients who respond to chemotherapy and who might therefore benefit from postoperative chemotherapy. Finally, and most important, administering chemotherapy early in the course of the disease has the advantage of treating subclinical metastatic cancer at a time when chemotherapy is likely to have its greatest impact. Neoadjuvant treatment is also delivered when the patient is usually best able to tolerate potential toxicities.

There are potential disadvantages to early use of systemic therapy. These include the possibility that chemotherapy-resistant tumor cells will emerge or that there may be a delay in achieving effective local tumor control. If these events occur, there is a risk of tumor spread from the primary lesion during the period of preoperative chemotherapy. There is also the possibility that patients who respond to chemotherapy might refuse the standard local measures of surgical or radiation-based therapy.

The rationale for concurrent chemotherapy and radiation therapy was reviewed by Vokes and Weichselbaum.[115] In essence, concurrent chemo- and radiation therapy may yield enhanced local control by several theoretic mechanisms, including radiosensitizing effects, while simultaneously treating potential systemic micrometastases.

Extensive laboratory studies involving a variety of models have been undertaken to evaluate the effect on survival of the timing of chemotherapy in relation to surgical intervention. Gunduz et al found in mice that resection of the primary tumor caused a marked increase in the labeling index of metastasis in comparison with leaving the primary tumor in place.[116] Survival was also shorter in the group that had the primary tumor resected. In a second study, Fisher et al administered chemotherapy either before or after resection.[117] The longest survival time was recorded when chemotherapy was given before operation, mimicking the neoadjuvant approach. Similar results have been reported by other investigators.[118–120]

Three neoadjuvant approaches involving chemotherapy have been studied in patients with apparently localized esophageal cancers: preoperative chemotherapy followed by an operation, a combination of chemotherapy and concurrent radiation followed by an operation, or chemotherapy with radiation and no operative procedure. Pilot trials involving a small number of patients and larger random assignment trials have suggested potential advantages for all of these approaches.

## Preoperative Chemotherapy

The use of preoperative chemotherapy in esophageal carcinoma has been studied in many phase II trials, involving more than 700 patients. In these studies, preoperative chemotherapy was given for one to six cycles and followed by a definitive surgical procedure. Patients received postoperative radiation therapy. In more recent trials, chemotherapy was used both before and after an operation. Results of selected phase II and the few phase III preoperative studies are outlined in Table 51–7.

Preoperative cisplatin-based combination chemotherapy achieves a major response in 17–66% of patients with pathologic complete responses in 3–10% of patients. Except for cisplatin–bleomycin, most regimens yield responses of 40–60%. Operability after chemotherapy has ranged from 50–100%, and resectability of tumors in patients who have undergone operations has ranged from 40% to 90% with no increase in operative mortality. Phase II studies supported the concept of preoperative chemotherapy as having no adverse affect on surgical outcome. An im-

**TABLE 51–7. ESOPHAGEAL CANCER PREOPERATIVE CHEMOTHERAPY PHASE II/III TRIALS**

| Reference[109] | Regimen | No. of Pts. | Percentage of Tumors Operable | Percentage of Tumors Resectable | Operative Mortality (%) | Major Response Rate (%) /Pathologic Complete Response (%) | Median Survival Period (mo) | 5-Year Survival Rate (%) |
|---|---|---|---|---|---|---|---|---|
| **Phase II Trials** | | | | | | | | |
| Coonley | CDDP-BL | 34 | 100 | 76 | 11 | 17/0 | 10 | 6 |
| Kelsen | CDDP-BL-VDS | 34 | 100 | 82 | 5.6 | 53/3 | 16 | 17.5 |
| Kelsen | CDDP-M-VDS | 14 | 93 | 86 | 7 | NS/7 | 8 | NS |
| Forastiere | CCDP-M-VLB | 27[a] | 86 | 86 | 0 | 44/3[a] | 14 | 21[b] |
| Kies | CDDP-FU | 25 | 54 | 38 | 0 | 42/0 | 17.8 | 17 |
| Hilgenberg | CDDP-FU | 35 | 89 | 77 | 4 | 57/7 | NS | 54[c] |
| **Phase III Trials** | | | | | | | | |
| Roth | CDDP-BL-VDS | 17 | 89 | 35[d] | 12 | 47/6 | 9 | 25[b,e] |
| | Surgery | 19 | 95 | 21[d] | 0 | — | 9 | 5[b,e] |
| Schlag | CDDP-FU | 29 | 83 | 71 | 21 | 47/NS | 8 | NS |
| | Surgery | 40 | 100 | 77 | 12 | — | 9 | NS |
| Nygaard | CDDP-BL | 50 | 82 | 58 | 15 | NS | NS | 3[b] |
| | Surgery | 41 | 93 | 69 | 13 | — | NS | 9[b] |
| | Radiation therapy 3500 cGy | 48 | 75 | 54 | 11 | NS | NS | 21[b] |
| | Radiation therapy CDDP-BL | 47 | 72 | 66 | 24 | NS | NS | 17[b] |

CDDP = cisplatin, BL = bleomycin, VDS = vindesine, M = mitoguazone, VLB = vinblastine, FU = 5-fluorouracil, NS = not stated.
[a]Trial treated adenocarcinoma and epidermoid carcinoma. Response proportion represents pooled adenocarcinoma and epidermoid carcinoma patients.
[b]Three-year actuarial survival rate.
[c]Actuarial survival rate at 3.5 years.
[d]Curative resection.
[e]Not statistically significant.
*(From Ilson DH, Kelsen DP: Combined Modality Therapy in the Treatment of Esophageal Cancer, Semin Oncol 21:493–507, 1994)*

provement in the percentage of patients achieving long-term survival has been suggested in preoperative chemotherapy trials. There was a clear trend toward improved survival among patients who manifested a major objective response to chemotherapy. However, it is not known if response to chemotherapy is independent of other favorable prognostic factors.

The role of preoperative chemotherapy in the treatment of local-regional esophageal carcinoma can only be clearly defined by means of random-assignment trials with a surgery-only control arm. Three small, randomized trials compared surgical treatment alone with preoperative chemotherapy followed by surgical intervention. With small numbers, the power of these trials to identify small to moderate (but clinically significant) differences was very weak. In fact, none of them demonstrated an appreciable overall survival advantage for preoperative chemotherapy. In one trial the subgroup of patients who responded to chemotherapy showed a trend toward improved survival compared with surgical controls.[108] Schlag et al in Ilson[109] reported no difference between survival rate among patients who received 5-FU and cisplatin and survival rate among patients who underwent surgical treatment alone. Although the same result was found by Nygaard et al, the use of a suboptimal chemotherapy regimen in the latter study may have diminished the effect of chemotherapy.[98]

### Preoperative Chemoradiation

Most preoperative chemoradiation therapy trials have used cisplatin or mitomycin-C in combination with 5-FU given by continuous infusion. On the basis of the initially encouraging results with 5-FU, cisplatin, and irradiation, both the Southwestern Oncology Group (SWOG) and the RTOG jointly conducted a large-scale phase II trial of treatment of epidermoid carcinoma in this way. The SWOG trial evaluated treatment of 106 patients and found the operability rate was only 63% (all tumors were initially operable). Only 49% of patients underwent resection and the operative mortality was 11%.[121] Pathologic complete responses were seen in 17% of patients and the median survival time of all patients was only 12 months. The RTOG study of treatment of 41 patients had similar results.[122] Two treatment-related deaths occurred. Toxicity was tolerable; it included mucositis, diarrhea, myelosuppression, and, rarely, neurotoxicity and nephrotoxicity.

Naunheim et al reported the results of treatment of 47 patients who received preoperative radiation therapy (3000–3600 cGy) and concurrent 5-FU–cisplatin followed by esophagectomy.[123] Of the 47 patients, 39 underwent surgical excision; the pathologic complete response rate was 21%. The overall treatment mortality was 5% with a median survival of 23 months and a 3-year actuarial survival rate of 40%. Using a different surgical technique, Forastiere et al at the University of Michigan studied an intensive 21-day preoperative trial of 5-FU and cisplatin given by continuous IV infusion in combination with vinblastine and radiation therapy delivered concurrently.[124] After preoperative therapy, patients underwent transhiatal esophagectomy. Forty-three patients were treated, 22 with epidermoid carcinoma and 21 with adenocarcinoma. The operability rate was 95%, and 91% of tumors were resectable; 84% were resected for potential cure. There was only one postoperative death. As in other trials, major responses were seen in 42% of patients and the pathologic complete response rate was 24%. Survival was longer than previously reported. The median survival period was 29 months, and the 5-year actuarial survival rate was 34% (34% for adenocarcinoma and 30% for epidermoid carcinoma).

Because of the encouraging survival results in this phase II study, a random-assignment trial comparing surgical treatment alone with preoperative chemoradiation therapy followed by surgical treatment is underway at the University of Michigan.

### Chemotherapy and Radiation

Radiation therapy with concurrent chemotherapy as definitive nonoperative therapy has been the subject of many single-arm phase II studies. Phase III trials also have been reported. Coia et al reviewed their experience over a 10-year period in 57 patients treated with continuous infusion 5-FU and mitomycin given for two cycles concurrently with high-dose radiation therapy (6000 cGy over 6–7 weeks).[125] The median survival time was 18 months, and 18% of patients survived 5 years. Eventually, local failure occurred in 48% of patients, and 72% had some component of distant failure. Severe toxicities were uncommon in this series, but there were two treatment-related deaths.

An important phase III random-assignment trial comparing radiation therapy alone (60 patients) with radiation given with concurrent 5-FU and cisplatin (61 patients) was reported by the RTOG.[126] In an update, 31% of patients treated with chemoradiation therapy were alive 3 years after treatment compared with no patients alive 3 years after treatment with radiation therapy alone.[127] Recurrence was decreased at both local and distant sites for those receiving both chemotherapy and radiation therapy. Still, 44% of patient treated with combined chemotherapy and radiation had either persistence or recurrence of local disease. Toxicity for chemoradiation therapy was greater than that seen with radiation therapy alone. Sixty-four percent of patients treated with chemoradiation therapy experienced severe or life-threatening toxicity as opposed to 28% of patients treated with radiation therapy alone. However, only one patient treated with chemoradiation therapy died of treatment-related toxicity (1.6%).

At present, chemotherapy (alone or with concurrent radiation therapy) before a planned operation is an investigational approach, and surgical treatment alone is standard treatment. The RTOG study strongly indicates that concurrent chemotherapy and radiation therapy are superior to radiation therapy alone for locally advanced epidermoid esophageal carcinoma.

## REFERENCES


1. Blot WJ, Devesa SS, Kneller RW, et al: Rising incidence of adenocarcinoma of the esophagus and gastric cardia. *JAMA* **265**(10):1287–1289, 1991
2. Waterhouse J, Muir C, Shammugaratnan K, et al: Cancer incidence in five continents. *International Agency for Research on Cancer,* Vol 4, Lyon, France, 1974
3. Office of Research on Cancer Prevention and Treatment of the Ministry of Health: *Atlas of Cancer Mortality of the Peoples Republic of China.* Beijing, China, Ministry of Health, 1980
4. Stephen SJ, Uragoda CG: Some observations on oesophageal cancer in Ceylon, including its relation to betel chewing. *Br J Cancer* **24:**11–15, 1970
5. Jussawalla DJ: Esophageal cancer in India. *J Cancer Res Clin Oncol* **99:**29–33, 1981
6. DeJong UW, Breslow N, Hong JG, et al: Aetiological factors in oesophageal cancer in Singapore Chinese. *Int J Cancer* **13:**291–303, 1974
7. Rose EF, McGlashan ND: The spatial distribution of oesophageal cancer in Transkei, South Africa. *Br J Cancer* **31:**197–206, 1979
8. Tuyns AJ, Masse G: Cancer of the esophagus: An incidence study in Ille-et-Vilaine. *Int J Epidemiol* **4:**55–59, 1975
9. Blot WJ, Fraumeni JF: Geographic epidemiology of cancer in the United States. In Schotterfeld D, Fraumeni J (eds): *Cancer Epidemiology and Prevention.* Philadelphia, Saunders, 1982, p 179
10. Fraumeni JF, Blot WJ: Geographic variation in esophageal cancer mortality in the United States. *J Chron Dis* **30:**759–767, 1977
11. Blot WJ, Fraumeni JF Jr: Trends in esophageal cancer mortality among U.S. blacks and whites. *Am J Public Health* **77:**296–298, 1987
12. Blot WJ, Devesa SS, Fraumeni JF Jr: Continuing climb in rates of esophageal adenocarcinoma: An update. *JAMA* **270**(11):1320, 1993
13. Johnston BJ, Reed PI. Changing pattern of oesophageal cancer in a general hospital in the UK. *Eur J Cancer Prev* **1**(1):23–25, 1991
14. Cameron AJ, Zinsmeister AR, Ballard DJ, et al: Prevalence of columnar-lined (Barrett's) esophagus. *Gastroenterology* **99:** 918–922, 1990
15. Spechler JS, Robbins AH, Rubbins HB, et al: Adenocarcinoma and Barrett's esophagus: An overrated risk? *Gastroenterology* **87:**927–933, 1984
16. Hamilton S, Smith R, Cameron J, et al: Prevalence and characteristics of Barrett's esophagus in patients with adenocarcinoma of the esophagus or the esophagogastric junction. *Hum Pathol* **19:**942–948, 1988
17. Kalish RJ, Clancy PE, Orringer MB, et al: Clinical, epidemiological and morphologic comparison between adenocarcinomas arising in Barrett's esophageal mucosa and in the gastric cardia. *Gastroenterology* **86:**461–467, 1984
18. Bartsch J, Montesano R: Relevance of nitrosamines to human cancer. *Carcinogenesis* **5:**1381–1391, 1984
19. Hammond EC: Smoking in relation to death rates of one million men and women. *Natl Cancer Inst Mongor* **19:**127–204, 1966
20. Rogot E, Murray JL: Smoking and causes of death among U.S. veterans: 16 years of observation. *Publ Health Rep* **95:**213–222, 1980
21. De Stefani E, Muno N, Esteve J, et al: Mate drinking, alcohol, tobacco, diet, and esophageal cancer in Uruguay. *Cancer Res* **50:**426–431, 1990
22. Chadirian P, Stein GF, Gorodetsky C, et al: Oesophageal cancer studies in the Caspian littoral of Iran: Some residual results, including opium as a risk factor. *Int J Cancer* **35:**593–597, 1985
23. Mimic Y, Garabrant DH, Peters JM, et al: Tobacco, alcohol, diet, occupation and cancer of the esophagus. *Cancer Res* **48:**3843–3848, 1988
24. Wynder EL, Bross IJ: A study of etiological factors in cancer of the esophagus. *Cancer* **14:**389–413, 1961
25. Pottern LM, Morris LE, Blot WJ, et al: Esophageal cancer among black men in Washington DC. I. Alcohol, tobacco and other risk factors. *JNCI* **67:**777–783, 1981
26. Tuyns AJ, Pequignot G, Jensen OM: Le cancer de l'oesophage en Ille-et-Vilaine en fonction des niveaux de consommation d'alcohol et de tabac: des risques qui se multiplient. *Bull Cancer* **64:**63–65, 1977
27. Yang J, Chen ML, Hu GG, et al: Preliminary studies on the etiology and conditions of carcinogenesis of the esophagus in Linxian. In Yang J, Gao J (eds): *Experimental Research on Esophageal Cancer.* Beijing, Renmin Weisheng, 1980
28. Department of Chemical Etiology of CICAMS and LRTPTEC: Preliminary investigation on the carcinogenicity of extracts of pickles in Linxian. *Res Cancer Prev Treatment* **2:**46–49, 1977
29. Lu SH, Ohshima H, Fu HM, et al: Urinary excretion on N-nitrosamino acids and nitrate by high and low esophageal risk populations in northern China: Endogenous formation of N-nitrosproline and its inhibition by vitamin C. *Cancer Res* **46:**1485–1491, 1986
30. Hille JJ, Markowitz S, Margoliusk A, et al: Human papillomavirus and carcinoma of the esophagus. *N Engl J Med* **213:**1707, 1985
31. Schmidt HG, Riddell RH, Walter B, et al: Dysplasia in Barrett's esophagus. *Cancer Res Clin Oncol* **110:**145–152, 1985
32. Rabinovitch PS, Reid BJ, Haggitt RC, et al: Progression to cancer in Barrett's esophagus in associated with genomic instability. *Lab Invest* **60:**65–71, 1988
33. Sanfey H, Hamilton SR, Smith RR, et al: Carcinoma arising in Barrett's esophagus. *Surg Gynecol Obstet* **161:**570–574, 1985
34. Harle IA, Finley RJ, Belsheim M, et al: Management of adenocarcinoma in columnar-lined esophagus. *Ann Thorac Surg* **40:**330–336, 1985
35. DeMeester TR, Attwood SE, Smyrk TC, et al: Surgical therapy in Barrett's esophagus. *Ann Surg* **212**(4):528–542, 1990
36. Morson BC, Belcher JR: Adenocarcinoma of the oesophagus and ectopic gastric mucosa. *Br J Cancer* **6:**127–130, 1953
37. Fagge CH: A case of simple stenosis of the oesophagus followed by epithelioma. *Guy's Hosp Rep* **17:**413–421, 1872
38. Ellis FG: The natural history of achalasia of the cardia. *Proc R Soc Med* **53:**663–66, 1960
39. Chuong JJ, DuBovik S, McCallum RW: Achalasia as a risk factor for esophageal carcinoma. A reappraisal. *Dig Dis Sci* **29**(12):1105–1108, 1984
40. Aggestrup S, Holm JC, Sorenson HR: Does achalasia predispose to cancer of the esophagus? *Chest* **102**(4):1013–1016, 1992
41. Meijssen MAC, Tilanus HW, van Blankenstein M, et al: Achalasia complicated by oesophageal squamous cell carcinoma: a prospective study in 195 patients. *Gut* **33**(2):155–158, 1992
42. Chang-Claude JC, Wahrendorf J, Liang QS, et al: An epidemiological study of precursor lesions of esophageal cancer among young persons in a high-risk population in Huixian, China. *Cancer Res* **50:**2268–2274, 1990
43. Jacob JH, Riviere A, Mandard AM, et al: Prevalence survey of precancerous lesions of the oesophagus in a high-risk population for oesophagus in a high-risk population for oesophageal cancer in France. *Eur J Cancer Prev* **2**(1):53–59, 1993
44. Castelletto R, Munoz N, Landoni N, et al: Pre-cancerous lesions of the oesophagus in Argentina: Prevalence and association with tobacco and alcohol. *Int J Cancer* **51:**34–37, 1992
45. Mandard AM, Marnay J, Gignoux M, et al: Cancer of the esophagus and associated lesions: detailed pathologic study of 100 esophagectomy specimens. *Hum Pathol* **15:**660–669, 1984
46. Howell-Evans W, McConnel RB, Clarke CA, et al: Carcinoma of the oesophagus with keratosis palmaris et plantaris (tylosis): A study of two families. *Q J Med* **27:**413–429, 1958
47. Vinson PP: Hysterical dysphagia. *Minn Med* **5:**107–108, 1992

48. Csikos M, Horvath O, Petri A, et al: Late malignant transformation of chronic corrosive oesophageal strictures. *Langenbecks Arch Chir* **365**(4):231–238, 1985
49. Imre J, Kopp M: Argument against long-term conservative treatment of oesophageal strictures due to corrosive burns. *Thorax* **27**:594–598, 1972
50. Goffman TE, McKeen EA, Curtis RE, et al: Esophageal carcinoma following irradiation for breast cancer. *Cancer* **52**(10):1808–1809, 1983
51. Shao LF, Hunag GJ, Zhang DW, et al: Detection and surgical treatment of early esophageal carcinoma. In *Proceedings of the Beijing Symposium on Cardiothoracic Surgery, Beijing.* New York, John Wiley, 1981, p 168
52. Moghissi K: Surgical resection for stage I cancer of the oesophagus and cardia. *Br J Surg* **79**(9):935–937, 1992
53. Nabeya K, Hanoaka T, Onozawa K, et al: New measures for early detection of carcinoma of the esophagus. In Siewert Jr, Hölscher AH (eds): *Diseases of the Esophagus.* Berlin, Springer-Verlag, 1988, p. 105
54. Dowlatshahi K, Skinner DB, DeMeester TR, et al: Evaluation of brush cytology as an independent technique for detection of esophageal carcinoma. *J Thorac Cardiovasc Surg* **89**:848–851, 1985
55. Tio TL, Cohen P, Coene P, et al: Endosonography and computed tomography of esophageal carcinoma. *Gastroenterology* **96**: 1478–1486, 1989
56. Czerny V: Neue operationen. *Zentralbl Chir* **4**:443–434, 1877
57. Torek F: The first successful case of resection of the thoracic portion of the oesophagus for carcinoma. *Surg Gynecol Obstet* **166**:614–617, 1913
58. Oshsawa T: Surgery of the esophagus. *Arch Jpn Surg* **10**:605–695, 1933
59. Adams W, Phemister DB: Carcioma of the lower thoracic esophagus: Report of a successful resection and esphagogastrostomy. *J Thorac Surg* **7**:621–632, 1938
60. Sweet RH: Surgical management of carcinoma of the mid thoracic esophagus. *N Engl J Med* **233**:1–7, 1945
61. Belsey R, Hiebert CA: An exclusive right thoracic approach for cancer of the middle third of the esophagus. *Ann Thorac Surg* **18**:1–5, 1974
62. Orringer MB, Sloan H: Esophagectomy without thoracotomy. *J Thorac Cardiovasc Surg* **76**:643–654, 1978
63. Denk, W: Zur Radikaloperation des oesophaguskarzinoms (Vorlaufige Mitteilung). *Zentralbl Chir* **40**(2):1065–1068, 1913
64. Akiyama H, Hiyama M, Miyazono H: Total esophageal reconstruction after extraction of the esophagus. *Ann Surg* **182**:547–552, 1975
65. Earlam R, Cunha-Melo JR: Oesophageal squamous cell carcinoma. I. A critical review of surgery. *Br J Surg* **67**:381, 1980
66. Muller JM, Erasmi H, Stelzner M, et al: Surgical therapy of oesophageal carcinoma. *Br J Surg* **77**:845–857, 1990
67. Lewis I: The surgical treatment of carcinoma of the oesophagus with special reference to a new operation for growths in the middle third. *Br J Surg* **34**:18–31, 1946
68. McKeown KC: Total three-stage oesophagectomy for cancer of the oesophagus. *Br J Surg* **63**:259, 1976
69. Orringer MB, Marshall B, Stirling MC: Transhiatal esophagectomy for benign and malignant disease. *J Thorac Cardiovasc Surg* **105**(2):265–277, 1993
70. Gelfand GA, Finley RJ, Nelems B, et al: Transhiatal esophagectomy for carcinoma of the esophagus and cardia: Experience with 160 cases. *Arch Surg* **127**(10):1164–1167, 1992
71. Vigneswaran WT, Trastek VF, Pairolero PC, et al: Transhiatal esophagectomy for carcinoma of the esophagus. *Ann Thorac Surg* **56**(4):838–844, 1993
72. Isono K, Ochiai T, Okuyama K, et al: The treatment of lymph node metastasis from esophageal cancer by extensive lymphadenectomy. *Jpn J Surg* **20**(2):151–157, 1990
73. Tilanus HW, Hop WC, Langenhorst BL, et al: Esophagectomy with or without thoracotomy: Is there any difference? *J Thorac Cardiovasc Surg* **105**(5):898–903, 1993
74. Goldminc M, Maddern G, Le Prise E, et al: Oesophagectomy by a transhiatal approach or thoracotomy: A prospective randomized trial. *Br J Surg* **80**(3):367–370, 1993
75. Logan A: The surgical treatment of carcinoma of the esophagus and cardia. *J Thorac Cardiovasc Surg* **46**:150–161, 1963
76. Skinner DB: En-bloc resection for neoplasms of the esophagus and cardia. *J Thorac Cardiovasc Surg* **85**:59–69, 1983
77. Skinner DB, Dowalatshahi KD, DeMeester TR: Potentially curable cancer of the esophagus. *Cancer* **50**:2571–2575, 1982
78. Lerut T, De Leyn P, Coosemans W, et al: Surgical strategies in esophageal carcinoma with emphasis on radical lymphadenectomy. *Ann Surg* **216**(5):583–590, 1992
79. Hagen JA, Peters JH, DeMeester TR: Superiority of extended en bloc esophagogastrectomy for carcinoma of the lower esophagus and cardia. *J Thorac Cardiovasc Surg* **106**(5):850–858, 1993
80. Arey LB: *Development Anatomy: A Textbook and Laboratory Manual of Embryology.* Philadelphia, Saunders, 1954
81. Isono K, Onoda S, Okuyama K, et al: Recurrence of intrathoracic esophageal cancer. *Jpn J Clin Oncol* **15**:49–60, 1985
82. Isono K, Sato H, K, Nakayama K: Results of nationwide study on the three-field lymph node dissection of esophageal cancer. *Oncology* **48**:411–420, 1991
83. Akiyama H: Surgery of the esophagus. *Curr Probl Surg* **17**:55–120, 1980
84. Kato H, Tachimori Y, Watanabe H, et al: Lymph node metastasis in thoracic esophageal carcinoma. *J Surg Oncol* **48**:106–111, 1991
85. Akiyama H, Tasurumaru M, Udagawa Y, et al: Systematic lymph node dissection for esophageal cancer-effective or not? *Dis Esoph* **7**(1):1–12, 1994
86. Matsubara T, Mamoru U, Yanagida O, et al: How extensive should lymph node dissection be for cancer of the thoracic esophagus? *J Thorac Cardiovasc Surg* **107**(4):1073–1078, 1994
87. De-Ren S: Ten-year follow-up of esophageal cancer treated by radical radiation therapy: Analysis of 869 patients. *Int J Radiat Oncol Biol Phys* **16**:329–334, 1989
88. Newaishy GA, Read GA, Duncan W, et al: Results of radical radiotherapy of squamous cell carcinoma of the esophagus. *Clin Radiol* **33**:347–352, 1982
89. Okawa T, Kita M, Tanaka M, et al: Results of radiotherapy for inoperable locally advanced esophageal cancer. *Int J Radiation Oncol Biol Phys* **17**:49–54, 1989
90. Armstrong JG: High dose rate remote afterloading brachytherapy for lung and esophageal cancer. *Semin Radiat Oncol* **4**:270–277, 1993
91. Caspers RJL, Zwinderman AH, Griffioen G, et al: Combined external beam and low dose rate intraluminal radiotherapy in oesophageal cancer. *Radiother Oncol* **27**:7–12, 1993
92. Mei W, Xian-Zhi G, Weibo Y, et al: Randomized clinical trial on the combination of preoperative irradiation and surgery in the treatment of esophageal carcinoma: Report on 206 patients. *Int J Radiat Oncol Biol Phys* **16**:325–327, 1989
93. Gignoux M, Roussel A, Paillot B, et al: The value of preoperative radiotherapy in esophageal cancer: Results of a study of the E.O.R.T.C. *World J Surg* **11**:426–432, 1987
94. Teniere P, Hay J, Fingerhut A, et al: Postoperative radiation therapy does not increase survival after curative resection for squamous cell carcinoma of the middle and lower esophagus as shown by a multicenter controlled trial. *Surg Gynecol Obstet* **173**:123–130, 1991
95. Launois B, Delarue D, Campion JP, et al: Preoperative radiotherapy for carcinoma of the esophagus. *Surg Gynecol Obstet* **153**:690–692, 1981
96. Arnott SJ, Duncan W, Kerr GR, et al: Low dose preoperative radiotherapy for carcinoma of the oesophagus: Results of a randomized clinical trial. *Radiother Oncol* **24**:108–113, 1993

97. Huant GJ, Gu XZ, Wang LJ, et al: Combined preoperative irradiation and surgery for esophageal carcinoma. In *International Trends in General Thoracic Surgery,* St. Louis, Mosby, 1988, pp 315–318
98. Nygaard K. Hagen S, Hansen HS, et al: Pre-operative radiotherapy prolongs survival in operable esophageal carcinoma: A randomized, multicenter study of pre-operative radiotherapy and chemotherapy—The second Scandinavian trial in esophageal cancer. *World J Surg* **16:**1104–1110, 1992
99. Yadava OP, Hodge AJ, Matz LR, et al: Esophageal malignancies: Is preoperative radiotherapy the way to go? *Ann Thorac Surg* **51:**189–193, 1991
100. Sugimachi K, Matsufuji H, Kai H, et al: Preoperative irradiation for carcinoma of the esophagus. *Surg Gynecol Obstet* **162:**174–176, 1986
101. Kasai M, Mori S, Watanabe T: Follow-up results after resection of thoracic esophageal carcinoma. *World J Surg* **2:**543–551, 1978
102. Fok M, Sham JST, Choy D, et al: Postoperative radiotherapy for carcinoma of the esophagus: A prospective, randomized controlled trial. *Surgery* **113:**138–147, 1993
103. Anderson I, Ladd T: Autopsy findings in squamous cell carcinoma of the esophagus. *Cancer* **50:**1587, 1982
104. Bosch A, Frias Z, Caldwell W, et al: Autopsy findings in carcinoma of the esophagus. *Acta Radiol Oncol* **18:**103, 1979
105. Miller AB, Hoogstrated B, Staquet M, Winkler A: Reporting results of cancer treatment. *Cancer* **47:**207–214, 1981
106. Kelsen DP, Heelan R, Coonley C, et al: Clinical and pathological evaluation of response to chemotherapy in patients with esophageal carcinoma. *Am J Clin Oncol* **6:**539–546, 1983
107. Kelsen D, Atiq, O.T. Therapy of upper gastrointestinal tract cancers. In: Current Problems in Cancer, edited by Haskell, C.M. St. Louis, Mosby Year Book, 1991 p 239–294
108. Roth JA, Putnam JB Jr, Lichter AS, Forastiere AA: Cancer of the esophagus. In DeVita VT Jr, Hellman S, Rosenberg SA (eds): *Cancer: Principles & Practice of Oncology,* Philadelphia: Lippincott, 1993, p 776–817
109. Ilson DH, Kelsen DP: Combined modality therapy in the treatment of esophageal cancer. *Semin Oncol* **21:**493–507, 1994
110. Bleiberg H: Management of esophageal gastric, pancreatic and hepatobiliary neoplasms. *Curr Opin Oncol* **3:**737–744, 1991
111. Ajani J, Ilson DH, Daughert K, et al: Activity of taxol on patients with squamous cell carcinoma and adenocarcinoma of the esophagus. *J Natl Cancer Inst* **86**(14):1086–1091, 1994
112. Kelsen D, Hilaris B, Coonley C, et al: Cisplatin, vindesine, and bleomycin chemotherapy of local-regional and advanced esophageal carcinoma. *Am J Med* **75:**645–652, 1983
113. Kies MS, Rosen ST, Tsang TK, et al: Cisplatin and 5-fluorouracil in the primary management of squamous esophageal cancer. *Cancer* **60:**2156–2160, 1987
114. Harris DT, Mastrangelo MJ: Theory and application of early systemic therapy. *Semin Oncol* **18:**493–503, 1991
115. Vokes EE, Weichselbaum RR: Concomitant chemoradiotherapy: Rationale and clinical experience in patients with solid tumors. *J Clin Oncol* **8:**911–934, 1990
116. Gunduz N, Fisher B, Saffer E: Effect of surgical removal on the growth and kinetics of residual tumor. *Cancer Res* **39:**3861–3865, 1979
117. Fisher B, Gunduz N, Saffer EA: Influence of the interval between primary tumor removal and chemotherapy on kinetics and growth of metastases. *Cancer Res* **43:**1488–1492, 1983
118. Schatten WE: An experimental study of postoperative tumor metastases. I. Growth of pulmonary metastases following total removal of primary leg tumor. *Cancer* **11:**455–459, 1958
119. Simpson-Herren L, Sanford AH, Holmquist JP: Effects of surgery on the cell kinetics of residual tumor. *Cancer Treat Rep* **60:**1749–1760, 1976
120. Pendegrast WJ Jr, Drake WP, Mardiney MR Jr: A proper sequence for the treatment of B16 melanoma: Chemotherapy, surgery and immunotherapy. *J Natl Cancer Inst* **57:**539–544, 1976
121. Poplin E, Fleming T, Leichman L, et al: Combined therapies for squamous-cell carcinoma of the esophagus, a Southwest Oncology Group Study (SWOG-8037). *J Clin Oncol* **5:**622–628, 1987
122. Seydel HG, Leichman L, Byhardt R, et al: Preoperative radiation and chemotherapy for localized squamous cell carcinoma of the esophagus: A RTOG Study. *Int J Radiat Oncol Biol Phys* **14:**33–35, 1988
123. Naunheim KS, Petruska PJ, Roy TS, et al: Preoperative chemotherapy and radiotherapy for esophageal carcinoma. *J Thorac Cardiovasc Surg* **5:**887–895, 1992
124. Forastiere AA, Orringer MB, Perez-Tamayo C, et al: Preoperative chemoradiation followed by transhiatal esophagectomy for carcinoma of the esophagus: Final report. *J Clin Oncol* **11:**1118–1123, 1993
125. Coia LR, Engstrom PF, Paul AR, et al: Long-term results of infusional 5-FU, mitomycin-C and radiation as primary management of esophageal carcinoma. *Int J Radiat Oncol Biol Phys* **20:**29–36, 1991
126. Herskovic A, Martz K, Al-Sarraf M, et al: Combined chemotherapy and radiotherapy compared with radiotherapy alone in patients with cancer of the esophagus. *N Engl J Med* **326:**1593–1598, 1992
127. Al-Sarraf M, Pajak T, Herskovic A, et al: Progress report of combined chemo-radiotherapy (CT-RT) vs. radiotherapy (RT) alone in patients with esophageal cancer: An intergroup study. *Proc Am Soc Clin Oncol* **12:**197, 1993

CHAPTER

# 52

# Surgical Options for Esophageal Resection and Reconstruction with Stomach

Mark B. Orringer

The first reports of successful transthoracic esophagectomy and intrathoracic esophagogastric anastomosis appeared in 1938.[1,2] Since that time, this operation has become the most common surgical procedure for malignant tumors of the esophagus. During the past 55 years, there have been substantial advances in preoperative assessment, nutritional support, anesthetic and operative techniques, and postoperative care of patients undergoing esophageal resection and reconstruction. Unfortunately, although several modern series report a hospital mortality lower than 5%,[3–5] esophageal resection and reconstruction for carcinoma is still performed with substantial risk to patients, the mortality ranging from 15% to 40%[6,7] and averaging 33%[8,9] in many parts of the world. Disruption of an intrathoracic esophagogastric anastomosis with secondary mediastinitis and sepsis continues to be the most dreaded complication of esophageal surgery and is a leading cause of postoperative morbidity and mortality in virtually every large reported series of esophageal resection and reconstruction. Postoperative pulmonary complications are also common in these often debilitated patients, who have esophageal obstruction that requires combined thoracic and abdominal operations.

In an effort to reduce the physiologic insult of conventional transthoracic esophagectomy and esophageal reconstruction while still providing efficient surgical palliation of dysphagia in patients with esophageal carcinoma, the technique of transhiatal esophagectomy without thoracotomy has been rediscovered, refined, popularized, and debated in the past decade.[10–20] Performed through an upper midline incision and a cervical incision, transhiatal esophagectomy avoids a thoracotomy and is therefore more readily tolerated by the patient. The cervical esophagogastric anastomosis used routinely to re-establish alimentary continuity virtually eliminates mediastinitis and sepsis as a cause of postoperative death. Despite these advantages, considerable controversy surrounds the use of transhiatal esophagectomy. The procedure has been criticized as a dangerous operation that violates the basic surgical principles of adequate exposure and hemostasis.[21,22] Some surgeons disapprove of the use of transhiatal esophagectomy in patients with esophageal carcinoma because it precludes an en bloc regional mediastinal lymph node dissection and is therefore not a traditional cancer operation. In this regard, transhiatal esophagectomy contrasts sharply with the concept of radical en bloc esophagectomy, another procedure first described years ago[23] and recently rediscovered and advocated by Skinner.[24] This chapter reviews the surgical options available to patients who require esophageal resection and reconstruction with stomach as well as the advantages and disadvantages of each technique.

## ESOPHAGEAL REPLACEMENT WITH STOMACH

The stomach is the best organ with which to replace the entire thoracic esophagus. Its advantages over other segments of the alimentary tract are its extraordinarily rich blood supply and submucosal collateral circulation, its thick resilient muscular wall, and its ability to reach superiorly to any level of the chest or neck for esophageal substitution.

## Blood Supply of the Mobilized Stomach

Mobilization of the stomach for esophageal replacement requires division of the left gastroepiploic and short gastric vessels along the high greater curve of the stomach as well as division of the left gastric artery and vein. Even with these two sources of blood supply divided, the stomach is still nourished by two vessels, the right gastric and the more substantial right gastroepiploic artery along the low greater curve. The latter vessel alone can support the entire stomach in the rare situation in which the right gastric artery is unavailable or is unintentionally divided. When the short gastric vessels are divided, care should be taken not to ligate them so near the gastric wall that subsequent necrosis occurs. Similarly, as the greater omentum is separated from the stomach, it must be divided at least 1–2 cm inferior to the right gastroepiploic arcade to prevent injury to this vessel.

The esophagus and stomach, upper alimentary tract organs, have thick muscular walls that facilitate the passage of chewed, semisolid food. The relatively tough, resilient gastric wall is a considerable contrast to the thin, flaccid wall of the large and small intestines and explains why late redundancy and tortuosity, so common after colonic interposition, are not seen when stomach is used to replace the esophagus.

## Gastroesophageal Reflux after Esophagogastric Anastomosis

A concern with esophagogastric anastomosis is the subsequent development of gastroesophageal reflux and esophagitis in a patient whose lower esophageal sphincter has been resected and an "iatrogenic hiatal hernia" produced. The inverse relation between the height of the esophagogastric anastomosis and the degree of subsequent gastroesophageal reflux is well established. That is, a low intrathoracic esophagogastric anastomosis is almost invariably associated with marked reflux esophagitis, whereas with high intrathoracic or cervical esophagogastric anastomoses, considerable gastroesophageal reflux is uncommon. This complication of esophageal resection is less important in patients with esophageal carcinoma and limited longevity. However, in patients undergoing distal esophagectomy for benign disease, a low intrathoracic esophagogastric anastomosis should never be performed lest subsequent development of a stricture from reflux esophagitis leave the patient with recurrent dysphagia and a problem as bad as that for which he or she originally underwent operation. If only the distal esophagus is to be resected for benign disease, it is best to perform a reconstruction with either a jejunal or short-segment colonic interposition (see Chapters 53 and 54), which provide somewhat of a barrier for the remaining esophagus against regurgitated gastric contents.

Although it has been taught that a patient who undergoes esophagogastric anastomosis for carcinoma seldom lives long enough for reflux esophagitis to develop, I have examined a number of patients in whom severe low intrathoracic esophagogastric anastomotic strictures developed within 6–12 months of a resection for carcinoma. The differentiation between a benign reflux stricture and a malignant stricture due to recurrent tumor may be extremely difficult in these patients. This is one important reason that I prefer total thoracic esophagectomy and cervical esophagogastric anastomosis whenever an esophageal resection is required for either benign or malignant disease regardless of the level of the esophageal disease. An even more compelling reason for avoiding an intrathoracic esophagogastric anastomosis is the striking difference between the consequences of a cervical and those of an intrathoracic anastomotic leak. A cervical leak is most often nothing more than a transient cervical salivary fistula that is virtually never associated with systemic sepsis, mediastinitis, or death.

## Mobilization of the Stomach for Cervical Esophagogastric Anastomosis

A relatively few years ago, before cervical esophagogastric anastomosis was used commonly in the United States, there was a widely held belief that the North American Caucasian stomach would seldom reach to the neck, in contrast to the longer Asian stomach. It has in fact been shown by means of careful postmortem measurements that the average Japanese stomach is 5 cm longer than the North American Caucasian stomach.[25] However, with adequate mobilization, as evidenced by my experience with more than 800 cervical esophagogastric anastomoses, a normal stomach virtually always reaches to the neck. Certain key technical maneuvers facilitate the upward reach of the stomach. A generous Kocher maneuver is routine. It separates the duodenocolic attachments and sweeps the second portion of the duodenum and pancreas medially, away from the inferior vena cava, until the pylorus is relocated from its usual position in the right upper quadrant of the abdomen to the level of the xiphoid process in the midline.

Dividing the lesser curve of the stomach sequentially with a GIA stapler, beginning at the midportion of the lesser curve and proceeding toward the fundus, eliminates the natural curve of the mobilized stomach toward the right and allows "straightening" of the stomach for its upward reach. In patients with carcinomas localized to the cardia, this maneuver, carried out 4–6 cm distal to gross tumor, also allows preservation of the high greater curve of the stomach so that a cervical anastomosis is still possible.[10,26]

## Need for Gastric Drainage Procedure

In most patients, the vagus nerves are divided in the process of esophagectomy. Because of concern about impaired gastric emptying owing to gastric atony or pylorospasm most esophageal surgeons recommend some type of gastric drainage procedure after esophagectomy. A pyloroplasty is the most commonly performed drainage procedure. Some surgeons simply dilate the pylorus vigorously between their fingers. I prefer an extramucosal pyloromyotomy of the Ramstadt type beginning 1.5 cm on the stomach and extending through the pylorus and onto the duodenum for another 0.5–1 cm. This is carried out with a microvascular mosquito clamp, which is used to elevate the muscle fibers of the stomach, pylorus, and duodenum and divide them with a needle-tip electrocautery. A pyloromyotomy has the advantage of eliminating an intra-abdominal gastric suture-line at right angles to the long axis of the stomach, which is pulled upward into the chest. The pyloromyotomy may be covered with omentum before the abdomen is closed. I have seen one postoperative pyloromyotomy site leak in more than 800 patients who underwent this method of gastric drainage after esophageal resection. Two patients required late (at 2 and 4 years) reoperations for gastric outlet obstruction that developed after a pyloromyotomy. Several authors have indicated that in most patients who undergo esophagectomy a gastric drainage procedure is unnecessary.[27,28] However, in one prospective randomized trial, gastric emptying was four times longer in patients who did not undergo pyloroplasty after an esophageal resection and esophagogastric anastomosis than in those who did, and the patients who did not undergo pyloroplasty had more adverse symptoms after eating.[29] The consequences of impaired emptying of the intrathoracic stomach in these patients may be so devastating that disruption of the pyloric sphincter, by whatever technique preferred, is a mandatory component of esophagectomy.

## Position of the Intrathoracic Stomach

After a standard transthoracic subtotal esophageal resection, the mobilized stomach is positioned in the posterior mediastinum in the original esophageal bed, and an intrathoracic esophagogastric anastomosis is performed. When a cervical esophagogastric anastomosis is to be performed, the surgeon has the option of positioning the stomach either in the usual posterior mediastinal location or retrosternally in the anterior mediastinum. The posterior mediastinum is the preferred position for the esophageal substitute in both benign and malignant disease. It is the shortest and most direct route between the neck and abdominal cavity, and if subsequent anastomotic dilation is required, it is relatively easy to carry out endoscopy and dilation when the usual anastomotic course of the swallowing passage has been preserved. Under certain circumstances, however, it may be preferable to use the retrosternal route for esophageal replacement. In some patients with carcinoma that cannot be totally resected, residual tumor in the posterior mediastinum may cause late obstruction of the intrathoracic stomach. In addition, in some patients who have undergone radiation therapy or have other causes of previous mediastinal inflammation (e.g., multiple past esophageal operations or a remote perforation), the posterior mediastinum may be so fibrotic and contracted that it does not comfortably accommodate the stomach. In these situations, the anterior mediastinum provides an acceptable, although second best, alternative route for the intrathoracic stomach. When the stomach is positioned in the anterior mediastinum, routine resection of the medial clavicle and adjacent manubrium is recommended to enlarge the superior opening of the anterior thoracic inlet and to prevent compression of the retrosternal stomach by the posterior prominence of the head of the clavicle[30] (Fig. 52–1).

The cervical esophagus normally lies posterior to and slightly to the left of the trachea. Therefore the left neck is always the preferred side from which to approach the cervical esophagus. When the organ being used to replace the esophagus must be positioned retrosternally, the cervical esophagus is elevated away from the prevertebral fascia and angles anteriorly for the anastomosis with the anterior mediastinal stomach or colon. This angulation, although necessary, makes subsequent endoscopy or dilations, if required, difficult. The anterior mediastinal route also requires that the intrathoracic stomach reach approximately 2 cm more cephalad than when the stomach is positioned in the posterior mediastinum in the original esophageal bed. Another disadvantage of the anterior mediastinum for esophageal substitution is the increased incidence of early cervical anastomotic disruption that occurs when this route is used. When the cervical esophagus is anastomosed to the stomach, which has been positioned in the posterior mediastinum in the normal esophageal bed, the anastomosis is supported by the spine posteriorly, the trachea medially, the carotid sheath and its contents laterally, and the strap muscles of the neck anteriorly. In contrast, a cervical esophageal anastomosis to the retrosternal stomach is relatively unsupported in its essentially subcutaneous position. Any subsequent increase in intrathoracic pressure, as occurs with coughing or a Valsalva maneuver, is transmitted cephalad inside the stomach. If the upper esophageal sphincter is closed, stress on the anastomosis may result in disruption during the critical first 10 postoperative days of anastomotic wound healing. Use of a nasogastric tube for at least 7 days after construction of a cervical esophagogastric anastomosis is indicated when the stomach has been positioned retrosternally, primarily to keep the upper esophageal sphincter incompetent and to minimize the chance of early anastomotic disruption. This is in distinct contrast to a cervical esophageal anastomosis with the posterior mediastinal stomach, where a nasogastric tube is seldom required beyond 2–3 days, and the leak rate is quite low.

Although historically the antethoracic (presternal or subcutaneous) route was used for visceral esophageal substitution before endotracheal anesthesia made transthoracic esophageal operations possible, it is mentioned here only for the sake of completeness and to condemn it. Subcutaneous placement of an esophageal substitute is cosmetically

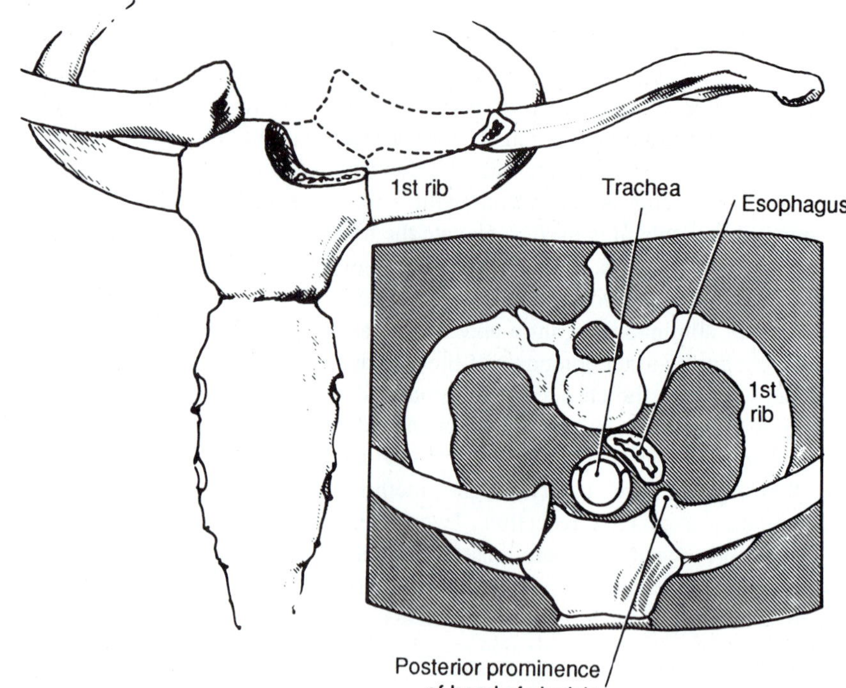


**Figure 52–1.** Resection of the medial clavicle, sternoclavicular joint, and upper corner of manubrium (dotted lines) performed to enlarge the anterior thoracic inlet when the retrosternal route is used for esophageal replacement. This achieves removal of the posterior prominence of the clavicular head, thereby widening the superior opening of the anterior mediastinum and allowing more room for the transposed substernal stomach (or colon) at the anterior thoracic inlet. *(Reproduced with permission from Orringer MB, Sloan H: Substernal gastric bypass of the excluded thoracic esophagus for palliation of esophageal carcinoma. J Thorac Cardiovasc Surg 70:836, 1975.)*

unacceptable—swallowed food can be seen moving through the intestine along the anterior chest wall. In addition, late fibrosis within the subcutaneous tunnel may produce intestinal obstruction and a poor functional result. There is little if any indication to use this route for esophageal substitution.

### Use of a Jejunostomy Feeding Tube

I advocate routine placement of a jejunostomy feeding tube in every patient undergoing esophageal resection and reconstruction.[31] Despite the recently popularized needle-catheter jejunostomy, a 14 F rubber tube secured in place with a Weitzel maneuver is more reliable. The relatively few potential complications of a feeding tube are far outweighed by its advantages: facilitation of early ambulation, supplemental nutritional support, and the best means of providing calories in the event of an anastomotic disruption. IV hyperalimentation, with its potential metabolic and septic complications, is seldom as valuable as enteral feedings either pre- or postoperatively in a patient with esophageal obstruction. Because esophageal replacement with stomach is essentially an upper abdominal operation that requires minimal manipulation of the intestines, postoperative ileus for more than 48–72 hours is unusual. It is therefore possible to benign jejunostomy tube feedings with dextrose and water within 2–3 days of the operation and advance to full-strength tube feedings soon thereafter, allowing discontinuation of IV fluids and greater ease of ambulation for the patient as oral intake is being increased. After discharge from the hospital, for the first several weeks after the operation, supplementation of calorie intake with 8 oz (240 mL) of tube feeding at night can provide an additional 500–600 calories until the patient's appetite and general sense of well-being are restored, but this is not routine.

## ESOPHAGEAL RESECTION THROUGH THE LEFT CHEST

Historically, lesions of the distal esophagus and gastric cardia have been approached through a variety of left chest incisions, which vary in the degree to which they extend into the abdomen (Fig. 52–2). The most commonly used is a left posterolateral thoracotomy in the seventh or eighth intercostal space. Division of the costal arch is not absolutely essential for a distal esophagectomy and esophagogastrostomy through the left chest. However, by extending the thoracotomy incision forward through the costal arch, oblique abdominal muscles, and the left rectus muscle and dividing the diaphragm, one can assess the upper abdomen and mobilize either the stomach, left colon, or jejunum for esophageal replacement. In addition, duodenal mobilization and performance of a gastric drainage procedure, not normally possible through a thoracic incision alone, are readily achieved through a left thoracoabdominal incision. Division of the costal arch and the anterior abdominal extension of the incision usually allow ample exposure of the low mediastinum and upper abdomen without as long an incision as the conventional posterolateral thoracotomy. Division of the diaphragm should always be performed with a circumferential peripheral incision 3–5 cm from the chest wall to

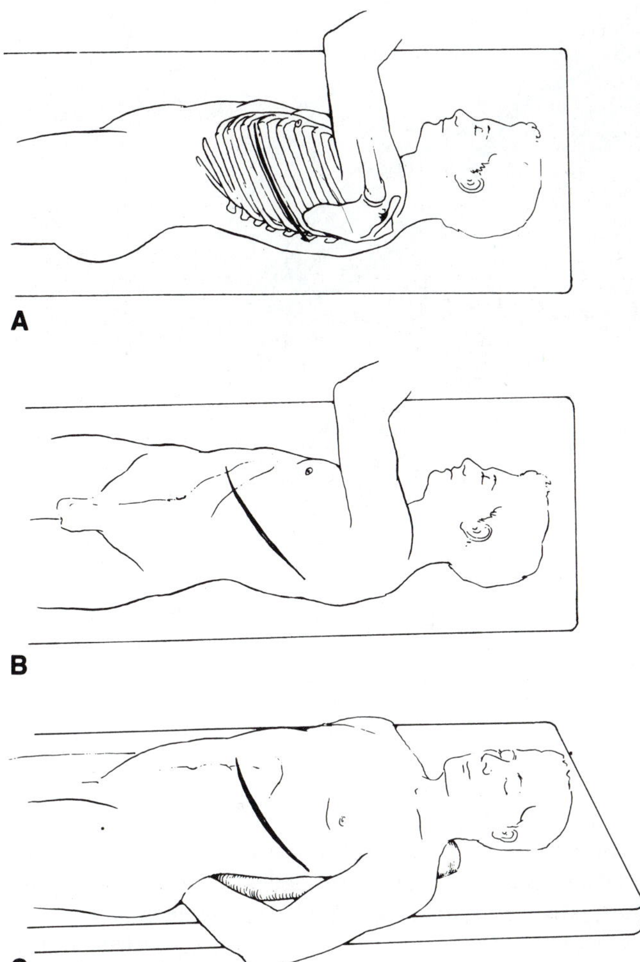


**Figure 52–2.** Left thoracic approaches to the esophagus. **A.** Posterolateral thoracotomy. **B.** Thoracoabdominal incision. **C.** Abdominothoracic incision. The abdominothoracic incision provides only marginal exposure of the distal esophagus and makes construction of an esophagogastric anastomosis very difficult.

facilitate subsequent closure rather than a radial incision through the hiatus. This minimizes injury to the phrenic nerve branches and postoperative diaphragmatic dysfunction.

Once the mediastinal pleura has been opened, the esophagus is mobilized, and the local extent of the tumor is assessed. Involvement of the cardia is evaluated from above the diaphragm as well as from below through the counterincision (Fig. 52–3). At times, a rim of diaphragmatic hiatal muscle must be resected with the tumor. Although some authors advocate inclusion of the greater omentum with the specimen, this is not routine, and most often the greater omentum is separated from the stomach by means of division of the short gastric and left gastroepiploic vessels and careful preservation of the right gastroepiploic arcade. I do not perform routine splenectomy on these patients, although this has been advocated by some surgeons to remove splenic hilar lymph nodes, which may contain metastatic disease.

Along the lesser curve of the stomach, the gastrohepatic omentum is divided, and the origin of the left gastric artery from the celiac axis is identified. This vessel is doubly ligated and divided near its origin; involved lymph nodes are taken with the stomach (Fig. 52–4). Transection of the stomach is facilitated with use of a TA-90 surgical stapler (Fig. 52–5). The stapled suture line is inverted with a running polypropylene Lembert stitch. The stomach is then mobilized into the chest, and the most superior edge is sutured to the prevertebral fascia with seromuscular sutures. The esophagus is transected at a sufficient distance cephalad to the tumor, and an end-to-side esophagogastrostomy is performed (Fig. 52–6). Considerable individual variation exists in the method of constructing the anastomosis. Some surgeons use an EEA stapling device to join the stomach and esophagus. Others use two layers of either silk and catgut or silk, and still others use a single layer of running 5-0 wire. I prefer a single layer of interrupted absorbable 4-0 polyglycolic acid suture for construction of all esophagogastric anastomoses. If possible, the anastomosis is supported with greater omentum. Some surgeons advocate an ink well technique of inversion of the anastomosis into the stomach, but I have found there is usually insufficient remaining stomach for this procedure. It is preferable to minimize the number and rows of esophageal sutures and potential anastomotic ischemia. Attempts to prevent gastroesophageal reflux with construction of an intrathoracic fundoplication around the esophagogastric anastomosis are seldom successful, and I do not use them.

The edges of the diaphragmatic counterincision must be carefully reapproximated to prevent subsequent disruption and herniation of abdominal viscera into the chest. I use everting interrupted nonabsorbable 2-0 or 1-0 horizontal mattress sutures, each one penetrating pleura, diaphragmatic muscle, and then peritoneum and placed 1 cm from the edge of the incision, reinforced by a running 2-0 whipstitch. After closure of the counterincision, the diaphragmatic hiatus is inspected. It should comfortably admit three fingers alongside the stomach, which has been drawn into the chest. The edge of the hiatus should be tacked gently to the stomach with seromuscular sutures to prevent subsequent herniation of intestine.

I deplore distal esophagectomy with a proximal gastrectomy and intrathoracic esophagogastrostomy for benign esophageal disease for the reasons cited earlier. However, this is still a commonly used operative approach worldwide in patients with carcinoma of the gastric cardia or lower third of the esophagus. There are several important and unresolved technical issues here: the need to divide the costal arch; the appropriate length of the proximal esophageal margin of resection; the amount of stomach distal to the tumor that should be resected; and the necessity for a splenectomy as part of the "cancer operation." Division of the costal arch may have tremendous morbidity, particularly in patients with marginal respiratory reserve. Movement of the two edges of the divided cartilage against one

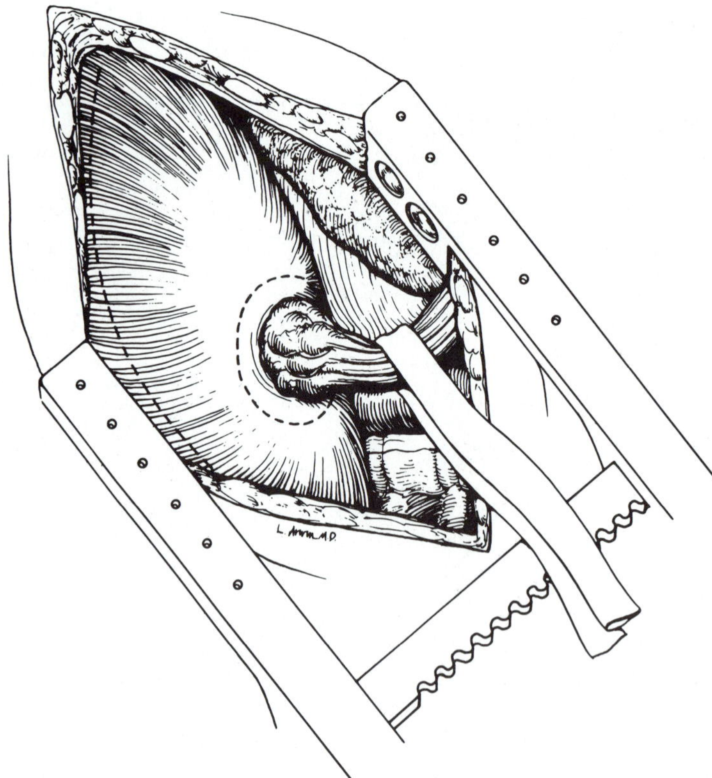

Figure 52–3. Left thoracoabdominal exposure of a carcinoma of the cardia through the seventh or eighth intercostal space. With division of the costal arch and opening of the diaphragm, exposure of the upper abdomen and low mediastinum is optimal. The peripheral, not radial, diaphragmatic incision is shown. A cuff of diaphragmatic hiatus (*dotted line*) adjacent to the tumor may be resected with the specimen.

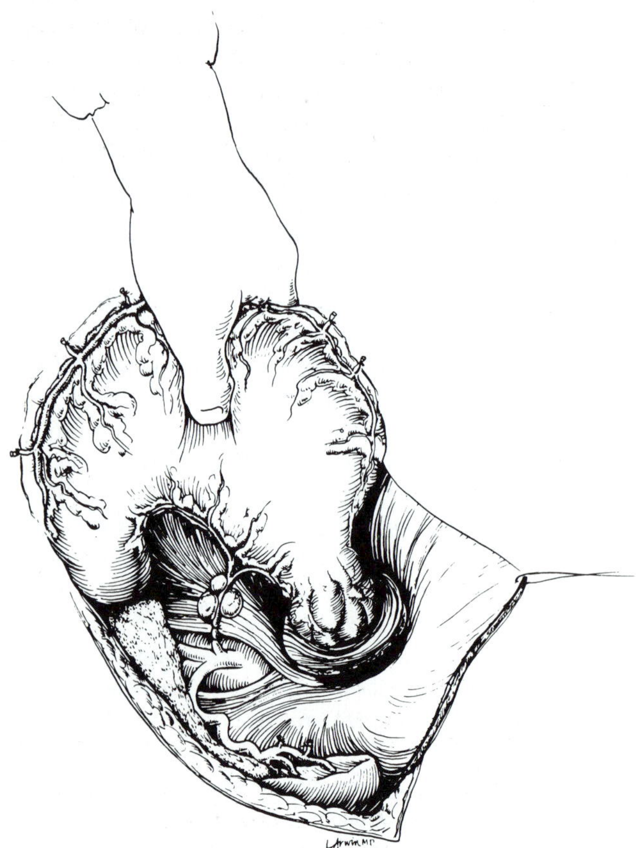

Figure 52–4. The left gastric artery is exposed, doubly ligated, and divided at its origin by means of retraction of the stomach upward through the diaphragmatic incision. Readily accessible lymph nodes along the left gastric artery are resected with the specimen.

another can be quite painful and result in secondary splinting and atelectasis. If the costal arch must be divided, careful reapproximation and stabilization of the cartilage during closure of the wound, or resection of several centimeters of cartilage so that the two edges cannot make contact, is essential.

The notorious submucosal lymphatic spread of esophageal carcinoma has prompted the recommendation that a 10-cm margin proximal and distal to gross tumor be obtained. If, however, the gastric extension of the tumor necessitates resection of a considerable portion of the stomach, there may be an insufficient length of remaining stomach to allow an esophagogastric anastomosis. Some surgeons advocate as limited an esophageal and gastric resection as possible to allow a palliative esophagogastrostomy. Others recommend total thoracic esophagectomy and total gastrectomy, which re-establishes alimentary continuity with a long-segment colonic interposition. I believe a malignant tumor of the cardia that is so extensive as to require total esophagectomy and gastrectomy for gross removal is almost certainly incurable, and the added morbidity of colonic interposition in such a patient is not justified. Another option when considerable stomach must be resected is reconstruction with an esophagojejunal anastomosis to a Roux-en-Y limb, but again, this is seldom necessary.

## ESOPHAGEAL RESECTION THROUGH THE RIGHT CHEST

The upper two thirds of the esophagus are most directly approached through a right thoracotomy, usually in the fifth

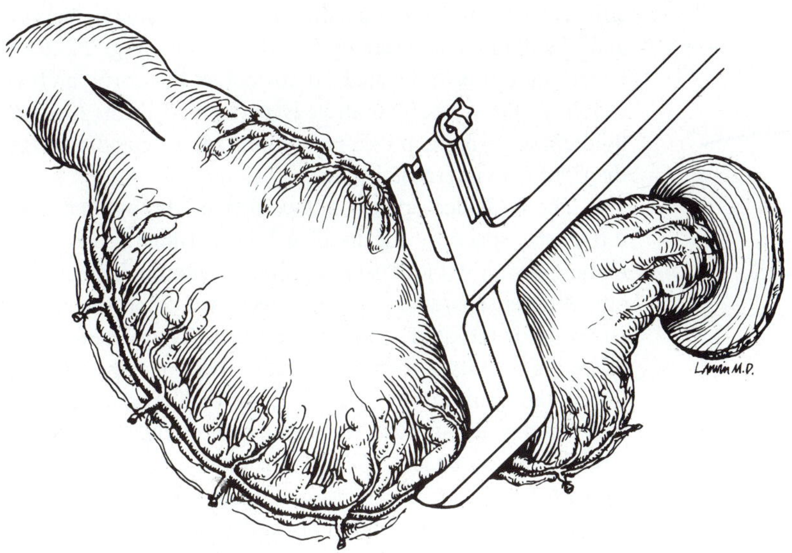

**Figure 52–5.** Transection of the stomach with a TA-90 surgical stapler. The staple suture line should always be oversewn for additional support.

interspace (Fig. 52–7A). On this side, the aortic arch is not an obstacle to exposure, and the azygos vein is relatively easily controlled and divided to provide visualization of almost the entire length of the thoracic esophagus. It is possible to mobilize the stomach through an abdominal incision and to perform a right thoracotomy for the esophagectomy without the necessity of repositioning the patient (Fig. 52–7B). Most surgeons, however, prefer to perform an initial exploratory laparotomy, mobilize the stomach, and then close the abdomen and reposition the patient in a true left lateral decubitus position for a full right posterolateral thoracotomy (Fig. 52–8). Most often, a high intrathoracic anastomosis is performed at the apex of the right chest (Fig. 52–8B). An alternative is to drape the arm into the field, so that exposure to the neck can be achieved by lowering the arm to the patient's side once the thoracic phase of the operation is completed (Fig. 52–7B). A cervical esophagogastric anastomosis can then be performed.

Another variation of the three-incision procedure involves positioning the patient supine with the right anterior chest elevated on a rolled blanket beneath the right posterior thorax. The right arm is bent, the elbow well padded, and the hand placed in the small of the back. When the operating table is rolled toward the right, the patient is flattened so that a standard laparotomy with the patient supine may be performed. The table is rotated toward the left for the thoracic portion of the operation. Use of a double-lumen endotracheal tube allows collapse of the right lung, which is

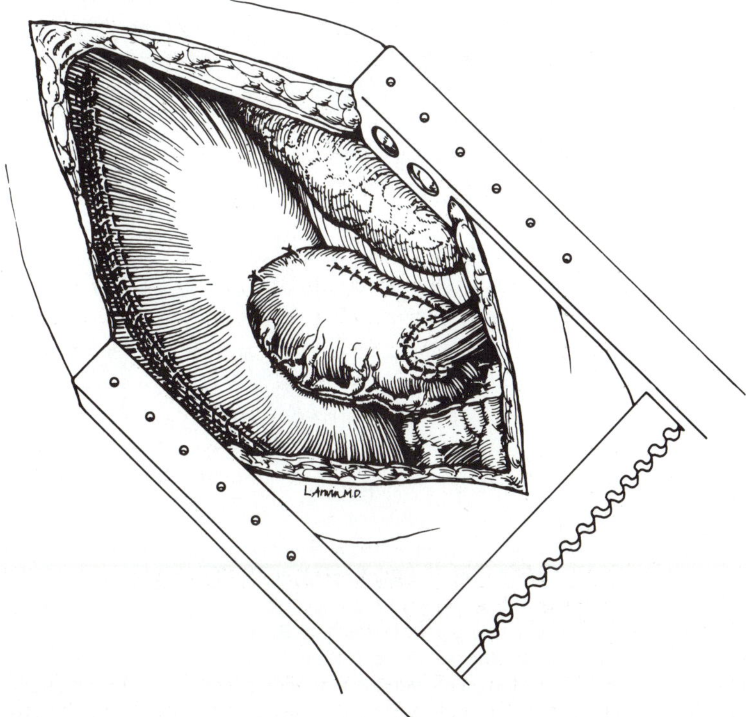

**Figure 52–6.** The remaining distal stomach has been mobilized into the chest through the diaphragmatic hiatus. After the stomach is suspended from the prevertebral fascia with several sutures, the esophagogastric anastomosis is constructed away from the suture line of the gastric transection. The edge of the diaphragmatic hiatus is sutured to the stomach to prevent subsequent herniation of abdominal viscera into the chest. The diaphragmatic incision is closed carefully with interrupted, everting horizontal mattress sutures followed by a running whip-stitch of nonabsorbable suture.

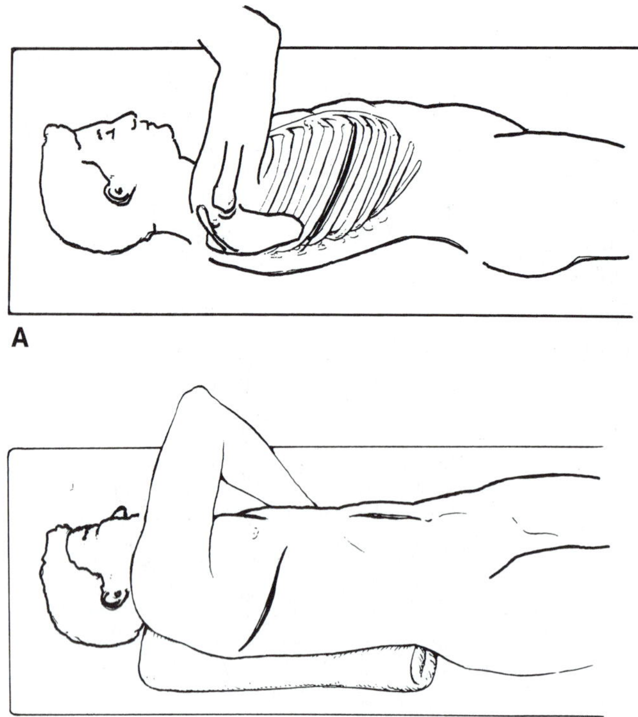


Figure 52–7. Positions used for right transthoracic approaches to the esophagus. A. Standard posterolateral thoracotomy through the fifth intercostal space. B. With the right side elevated 30° by rolled blankets placed beneath the right shoulder and hip and the right arm suspended, simultaneous performance of an anterolateral thoracotomy for esophageal exposure and a laparotomy is possible. If the right arm is prepared and draped into the field, once the thoracic and abdominal phases of the operation are completed, the arm can be lowered to the patient's side, allowing exposure of the neck for construction of a cervical anastomosis.

retracted anteriorly through a right anterolateral thoracotomy. The azygos vein can be visualized and divided and a cervical incision performed for anastomosis above the clavicles without having to reposition the patient. This three-incision operation without repositioning the patient is best suited for very thin patients in whom visualization within the chest is facilitated by the patient's small size. Belsey and Hiebert described an exclusive right-sided thoracic approach for cancer of the middle third of the esophagus.[32] This procedure involves a standard transthoracic esophagectomy and then progressive mobilization of the stomach into the chest by means of division of the short gastric vessels through the hiatus without repositioning the patient. This is a difficult operation that may unnecessarily traumatize the stomach; for this reason I do not advocate its use.

## RADICAL EN BLOC ESOPHAGECTOMY FOR ESOPHAGEAL CARCINOMA

As defined by Skinner,[24] the objective of en bloc resection is complete removal of the esophagus 10 cm above and 10 cm below the tumor whenever possible and total excision of adjacent tissues, including the arterial and venous supply and the lymphatic drainage of the tumor (Fig. 52–9A). When the tumor is located 10 cm below the aortic arch at esophagoscopy, the operation is performed through a left thoracotomy; more proximal tumors are resected through the right fifth intercostal space.

The left-sided operation is performed through the sixth intercostal space by means of a long peripheral diaphragmatic incision without dividing the costal arch. The greater omentum is separated from the transverse colon and mesocolon but is left attached to the stomach. The spleen is mobilized from its subdiaphragmatic location, the splenic artery and vein are divided at the tip of the pancreas, and the spleen is left attached to the stomach by the short gastric vessels. The stomach, spleen, and omentum are retracted forward to provide access to the celiac axis and retroperitoneum. Retroperitoneal lymph nodes and fat superior to the pancreas are reflected toward the diaphragmatic hiatus. The left gastric artery and vein are divided at the origin of the artery from the celiac axis. Tissue anterior to the left adrenal gland is reflected toward the hiatus, and the left gastric artery and vein are divided and ligated where they pass from behind the adrenal gland toward the diaphrag-

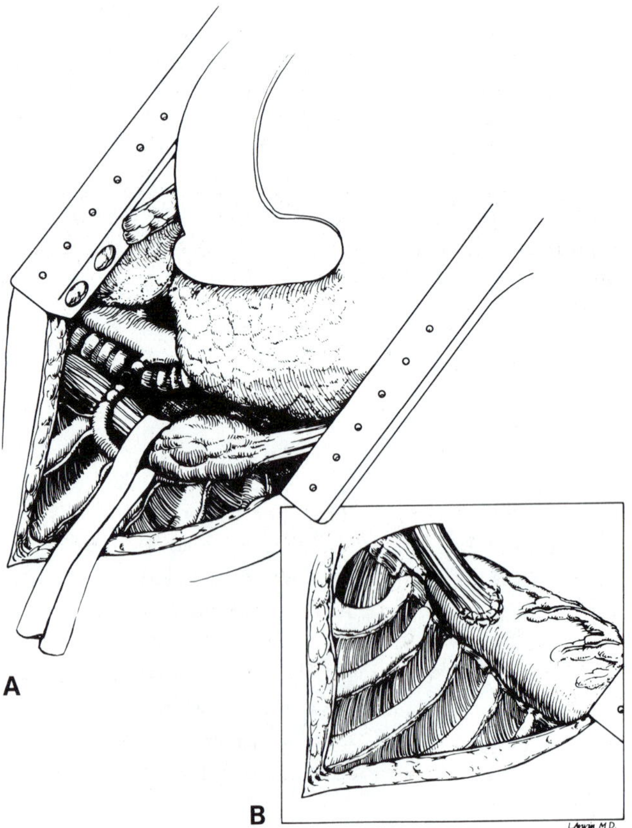


Figure 52–8. A. Mobilization of a midesophageal carcinoma through a right posterolateral thoracotomy. The azygos vein is divided and the esophagus is encircled and dissected away from the posterior membranous trachea. B. High intrathoracic esophagogastric anastomosis performed at the apex of the right chest after the gastric fundus is suspended from the prevertebral fascia.

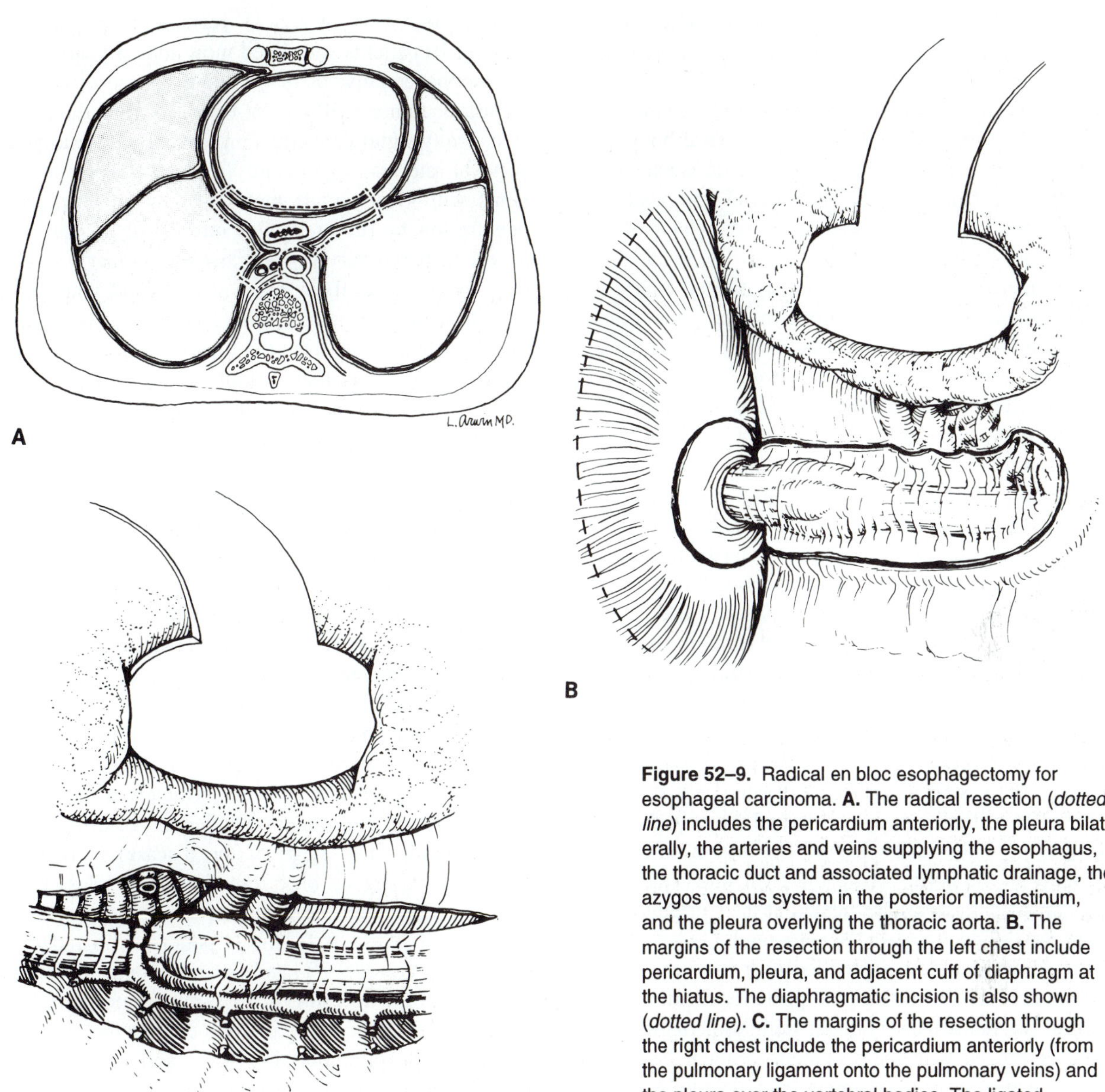


**Figure 52–9.** Radical en bloc esophagectomy for esophageal carcinoma. **A.** The radical resection (*dotted line*) includes the pericardium anteriorly, the pleura bilaterally, the arteries and veins supplying the esophagus, the thoracic duct and associated lymphatic drainage, the azygos venous system in the posterior mediastinum, and the pleura overlying the thoracic aorta. **B.** The margins of the resection through the left chest include pericardium, pleura, and adjacent cuff of diaphragm at the hiatus. The diaphragmatic incision is also shown (*dotted line*). **C.** The margins of the resection through the right chest include the pericardium anteriorly (from the pulmonary ligament onto the pulmonary veins) and the pleura over the vertebral bodies. The ligated intercostal vessels and azygos vein are shown.

matic hiatus. A rim of diaphragm is resected with the esophagus at the hiatus, thereby minimizing contact with the tumor. Visualization of the thoracic aorta to the level of the aortic hiatus is readily achieved once the esophageal hiatus has been enlarged. The thoracic duct is identified and divided in the aortic hiatus. The ascending lumbar veins at the level of the hiatus and several intercostal arteries and veins are ligated and divided behind the esophagus as the dissection up the anterior surface of the thoracic vertebrae proceeds.

The intrathoracic portion of the operation is begun with an incision in the pleura over the aorta from the diaphragm to the aortic arch (Fig. 52–9B). The pleura is dissected medially off the anterior surface of the aorta, and the exposed esophageal and bronchoesophageal arteries arising from the aorta are ligated and divided. With the lateral prevertebral dissection completed, the medial dissection is begun back at the level of the diaphragmatic hiatus. The right side of the prevertebral soft tissue is progressively elevated and the lymphatics entering the thoracic duct and the intercostal vessels are sequentially identified, ligated, and divided. The azygos vein and thoracic duct remain in continuity within the mediastinal fat and pleura surrounding the esophagus. The dissection proceeds superiorly to 10 cm above the tumor, where the thoracic duct and azygos vein are ligated again. The esophagus is encircled beneath the aortic arch.

After the pulmonary ligament is divided to the level of the inferior pulmonary vein, the pericardium is opened along the inferior pulmonary vein and is incised distally to the diaphragm along the pleuropericardial junction. The pericardial incision proceeds along the posterior surface of the heart to the right pulmonary veins. The subcarinal lymph nodes and those adjacent to both main stem bronchi are dissected with the specimen. Any bronchial arteries encountered are ligated. The right pleura and pericardium are incised anterior to the esophagus, and the incision is carried inferiorly to the diaphragm anterior to the right pulmonary ligament. The pleural reflection off the vertebral bodies is incised distally, and the posterior right incision is extended upward on the vertebral bodies. The anterior and posterior right pleural incisions are joined by means of division of the right pulmonary ligament against the lung. The distal ends of the right intercostal vessels, previously ligated lateral to the esophagus, are divided again along the vertebral bodies as they pass toward the right intercostal spaces, completing the en bloc posterior mediastinal dissection.

The stomach is divided 10 cm distal to the tumor; the right gastroepiploic arcade is preserved. If the tumor is squamous carcinoma, Skinner[24] resects the entire thoracic esophagus and performs a cervical esophagogastric anastomosis. For most adenocarcinomas, once a 10-cm margin is obtained, an intrathoracic anastomosis beneath the aortic arch or occasionally a left colonic interposition based on the ascending branch of the left colic artery is performed.

Middle-third tumors are approached through the fifth right intercostal space, and the pleura over the right side of the vertebral bodies is incised from the diaphragm to the clavicles, aiming for a 10-cm margin, if possible, proximal and distal to palpable tumor (Fig. 52–9C). The intercostal vessels along the vertebral bodies are divided, and all anterior soft tissue, including azygos vein and thoracic duct, is mobilized along with the esophagus. The dissection is carried medially to the aorta, where the right intercostal and bronchoesophageal arteries are ligated at their origins. The vagus nerve is divided beneath the aortic arch.

After the azygos vein is divided near the vena cava, the esophagus is separated from the posterior membranous trachea, and the subcarinal and main stem bronchial lymph nodes are mobilized with the specimen; bronchial vessels are divided as necessary. A segment of pericardium is excised from the level of the pulmonary veins to the diaphragm. On the left, the pericardium is incised anteriorly along the pulmonary veins and posteriorly at the pleural reflection off the aorta. As described for left thoracic dissection, a mediastinal envelope surrounding the esophagus is resected. Skinner[24] proceeds with esophageal replacement either by mobilizing the stomach into the chest through the diaphragmatic hiatus as advocated by Belsey and Hiebert[32] or using a long-segment left colonic interposition through an abdominal incision.

### Results of Radical en Bloc Esophagectomy for Esophageal Carcinoma

In his initial review of en bloc resection for carcinoma of the esophagus and cardia, Skinner reported on 80 patients who underwent this operation.[24] Nine (11%) died within 30 days of the operation, and another 11 died within 1–6 months of the operation, four of pneumonia. The actuarial survival rate was 24% at 3 years and 18% at 5 years. Among 10 patients who lived more than 3 years after radical esophagectomy, there was no evidence of recurrent or metastatic tumor. Cell type or tumor location did not have a statistically significant effect on survival rate, but the 2-year survival rate was significantly ($P < .01$) worse among patients with lymph node metastases or full-thickness wall penetration by tumor. It was interesting to note that the 3-year actuarial survival rate among Skinner's 29 patients with midesophageal tumors was 14% and that among 37 patients with lower-third tumors, the rate was 33%. These results differed little from the reported 3-year actuarial survival rate after transhiatal esophagectomy for middle-third tumors (17%) and for distal-third tumors (31%).[15]

The most recent follow-up report of en bloc esophagectomy performed by Skinner et al emphasized a more selected application of the operation in patients with potentially "curable" tumors considered at preoperative assessment not to be transmurally invasive or to involve more than five lymph nodes.[33] Among 31 patients fulfilling these criteria at preoperative staging and who underwent en bloc resection, nine (29%) were found at pathologic examination to have more extensive disease than anticipated. Compared with 21 patients treated with conventional esophagectomy, those treated with en bloc esophagectomy had a statistically significantly greater survival rate at all time intervals after 6 months. However, one must ask critically if this difference in survival rate is not more a reflection of different pathologic findings (i.e., stage of the disease) in two groups, those undergoing en bloc resection having less extensive disease, rather than the extent of the resection performed. The hospital mortality for the 31 patients who underwent en bloc resection was 9.7%, and five other patients died within 6 months of the operation (26% 6-month mortality). The 21 patients who underwent palliative conventional esophagectomy had a hospital mortality of 5% and a 6-month mortality of 33%. The average blood loss at en bloc resection was 2.4 L compared with 1.5 L for conventional esophagectomy. Patients who underwent en bloc resection spent an average of 5 days in the intensive care unit postoperatively compared with 3 days, and average hospitalization was 17 days as opposed to 13 days. En bloc resection resulted in an average of eight more lymph nodes per specimen at pathologic examination than conventional esophagectomy. Another, more recent nonrandomized series suggested the superiority of extended en bloc resection over transhiatal esophagectomy without thoracotomy for carcinoma of the lower esophagus and cardia.[34]

## TRANSHIATAL ESOPHAGECTOMY WITHOUT THORACOTOMY

In my experience with more than 800 transhiatal esophagectomies without thoracotomy, the technique has been applicable in virtually every patient requiring esophagectomy for either benign or malignant disease. Concern about untoward bleeding with this method of esophagectomy is based on long-held misconceptions about the blood supply of the esophagus. The main arteries supplying the esophagus are the superior thyroid, bronchial, left gastric, and splenic. Three-dimensional anatomic investigations of the esophageal blood supply with injection techniques in autopsy specimens refute the notion that the major esophageal arteries arise directly from the intercostal or phrenic arteries or the aorta.[35] Rather, it has been shown that most arteries that nourish the esophagus divide into fine branches several centimeters from the esophagus and form an extensive interconnecting submucosal network. When these small vessels are torn, contractive hemostasis, not massive hemorrhage, occurs. Thus, unless a great vessel is torn during an inappropriate attempt at transhiatal esophagectomy, blood loss is normally not in excess of 1000 mL and now averages around 500 mL.

Patients with benign esophageal disease, particularly those who have undergone one or more previous esophagomyotomies for neuromotor dysfunction, may have extensive periesophageal mediastinal adhesions that prevent transhiatal mobilization of the esophagus. This, however, is determined at operation by palpation through the hiatus, and if necessary, a transthoracic approach is undertaken. For esophageal carcinoma, I regard every patient who is deemed a candidate for esophageal resection a candidate for transhiatal esophagectomy. All patients with upper or middle thoracic esophageal tumors undergo preoperative bronchoscopic assessment. If tracheobronchial invasion (not contiguity) is documented, transhiatal esophagectomy without thoracotomy is absolutely contraindicated. Patients with intrathoracic esophageal carcinoma and distant metastatic disease (e.g., biopsy proved metastasis to the liver, a supraclavicular lymph node) are not regarded as candidates for esophagectomy. The expected survival time with these stage IV tumors is approximately 6 months, and the risk of a complex operative undertaking generally outweighs the short-term benefits. Although a computed tomographic (CT) scan of the chest and upper abdomen is useful in determining the presence or extent of metastatic disease, I find this diagnostic modality not to be a reliable indicator of resectability of esophageal carcinoma.[36] The CT finding of contiguity of an esophageal tumor with the aorta, for example, does not prove that invasion is present and that the tumor is unresectable. When undertaking a transhiatal esophagectomy, whether for benign or malignant disease, the surgeon must be prepared to open the thorax to resect the esophagus if local invasion by the tumor or periesophageal adhesions prevent transhiatal resection or if untoward bleeding occurs.

## Anesthetic Management

During transhiatal esophagectomy, when the surgeon's hand is inserted into the posterior mediastinum, cardiac displacement may interfere with filling of the heart. To avoid prolonged hypotension during this dissection, continuous monitoring of intra-arterial pressure is routine. This is achieved with a radial artery catheter, which is sutured in place and well protected by padding, since the patient's arms are placed at the sides during the operation so that the surgeon has access to the neck, the chest, and the abdomen without the interference of arm boards. Although intraoperative blood loss now averages 500 mL, two large-bore IV catheters are inserted for rapid volume replacement. Central venous pressure usually is not monitored, but if required, monitoring should be done through a right neck vein, away from the operative field in the left neck.

An unshortened standard endotracheal tube is most commonly used. In the event that a membranous tracheal tear occurs during the transhiatal dissection, it is possible to advance this longer tube into the distal trachea so that the balloon is beyond the tear and direct repair can be carried out. I avoid use of a double-lumen endotracheal tube, which is larger than a standard endotracheal tube and may complicate transhiatal dissection of the esophagus away from the airway. During the actual transhiatal dissection, inhalation anesthetic agents are temporarily discontinued and inspired oxygen concentration is increased to minimize the adverse affects of transient hypotension that may occur when the surgeon's hand inserted into the posterior mediastinum through the diaphragmatic hiatus displaces the heart. The anesthetist and surgeon must work closely together to minimize severe or prolonged hypotension.

## Operative Technique

The patient is supine with the head turned toward the right and stabilized with a head ring beneath the occiput. A small folded sheet is placed beneath the scapulae to extend the neck. The skin is prepared and draped from the mandibles to the pubis and anterior to both midaxillary lines. The padded arms are placed at the patient's side. A table-mounted, self-retaining (upper hand) retractor facilitates the entire abdominal operation. Transhiatal esophagectomy is carried out in three separate phases: the abdominal, the mediastinal, and the cervical.

## Abdominal Phase

A supraumbilical upper midline incision is usually adequate (Fig. 52–10). The triangular ligament of the liver is divided, and the left hepatic lobe is retracted to the right. The stomach is inspected to be certain that there is no gastric scarring or shortening from prior disease that precludes its use as an esophageal substitute. The right gastroepiploic artery is carefully identified and the presence of its pulse confirmed, particularly in patients who have undergone prior abdominal operations.

The lesser sac behind the greater omentum is entered through an avascular area where the right gastroepiploic

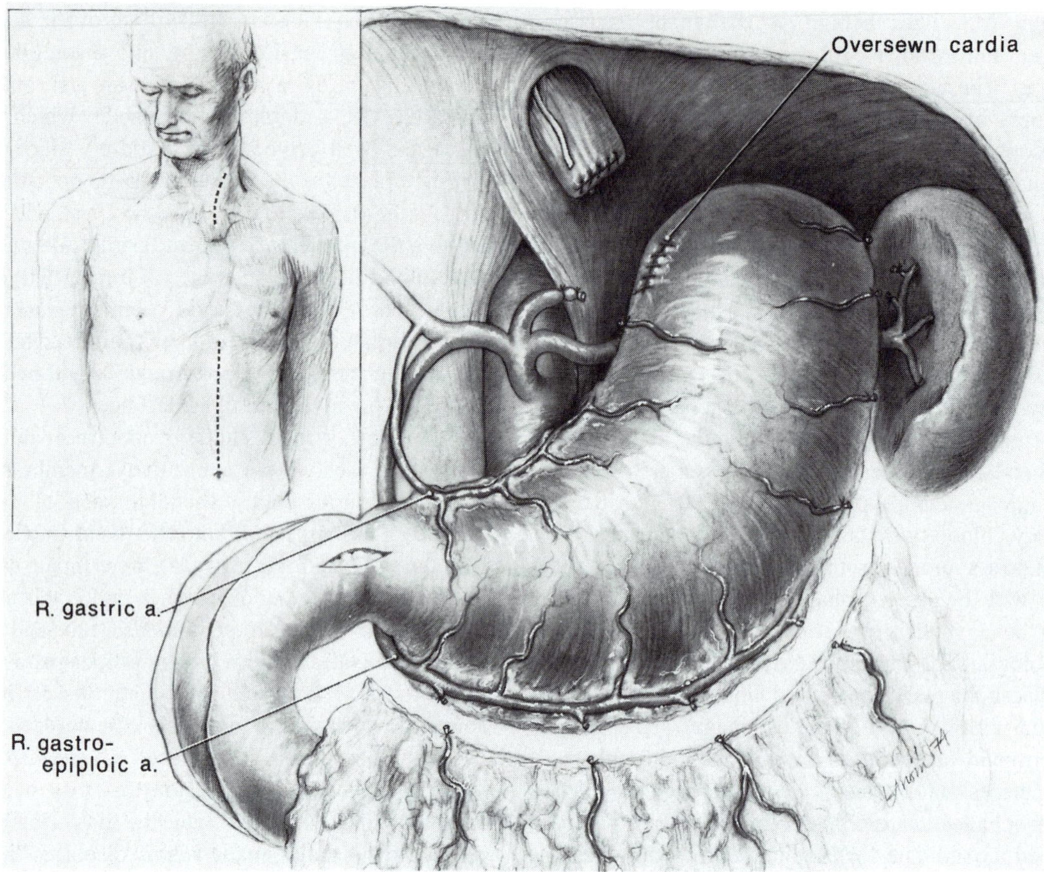


**Figure 52–10.** Mobilization of the stomach for esophageal replacement following transhiatal esophagectomy. Inset shows the standard left anterior cervical and supraumbilical midline abdominal incisions used. *(Reproduced with permission from Orringer MB, Sloan H: Substernal gastric bypass of the excluded thoracic esophagus for palliation of esophageal carcinoma. J Thorac Cardiovasc Surg 70:836, 1975.)*

artery terminates as it enters the stomach or anastomoses with small branches of the left gastroepiploic artery. The omentum is separated from the right gastroepiploic artery at least 1.5–2 cm below the vessel to minimize the chance of injury to this artery. The greater omentum is separated from the stomach to the level of the pylorus and the origin of the right gastroepiploic artery from the gastroduodenal artery. The left gastroepiploic and short gastric arteries are divided along the high greater curve of the stomach, carefully avoiding injury to the spleen as well as gastric necrosis from ligation of these vessels too near the wall of the stomach. Once the entire greater curve of the stomach is mobilized, the peritoneum overlying the esophageal hiatus is incised. The gastrohepatic omentum along the lesser curve of the stomach is incised, and the left gastric artery is isolated, ligated, and divided. If possible, celiac axis lymph nodes containing metastatic carcinoma are resected with the specimen by dividing the left gastric artery near its origin from the celiac axis. If there is a large celiac axis lymph node mass containing metastatic tumor, however, cure is not possible. Unless these lymph nodes are relatively easily removed, they need not be resected because there is little logic in risking uncontrolled hemorrhage for incurable disease. The right gastric artery is protected throughout the gastric mobilization. Because of concern about the possibility of delayed gastric emptying after the vagotomy that accompanies the esophagectomy, a gastric drainage procedure is performed routinely. I prefer a pyloromyotomy that extends from 1.5 cm on the stomach through the pylorus and onto the duodenum for 0.5–1.0 cm. This is performed with the cutting current of a needle-tipped electrocautery and a fine-tipped mosquito clamp to dissect the gastric and duodenal muscle away from the underlying submucosa. Silver clip markers are placed at the level of the pyloromyotomy for future radiographic evaluation of gastric emptying. A generous Kocher maneuver is performed to ensure maximum upward reach of the stomach. When adequate pyloroduodenal mobilization has been carried out, the pylorus can be displaced from its usual position in the right upper quadrant of the abdomen almost to the level of the xiphoid process in the midline.

Gentle mobilization of the distal 5–10 cm of esophagus from the mediastinum is carried out with retraction of the esophagogastric junction downward with a Penrose drain encircling it while dissection is carried upward into the mediastinum with the opposite hand (Fig. 52–11). Divi-

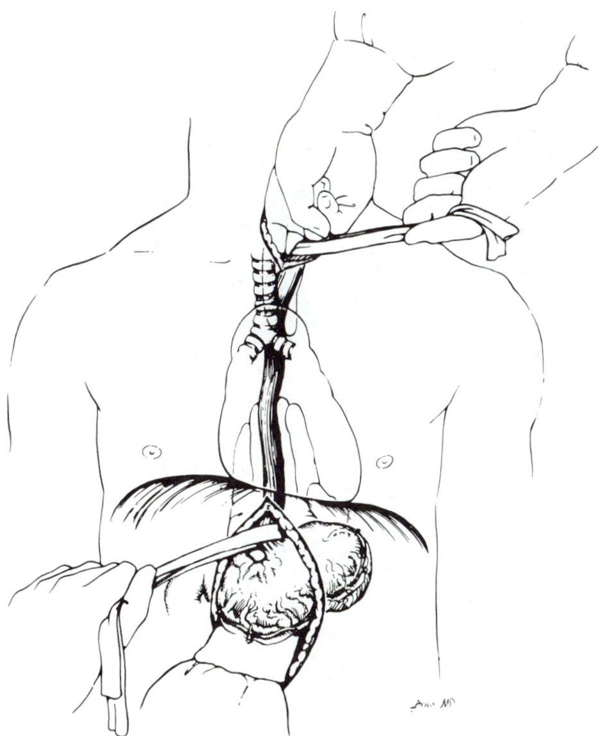

**Figure 52–11.** Transhiatal esophagectomy is performed as a midline dissection with the volar aspects of the fingers against the esophagus. Penrose drains encircling the cervical esophagus and esophagogastric junction are used to provide countertraction. *(Modified from Orringer MB, Sloan H: Esophagectomy without thoracotomy. J Thorac Cardiovasc Surg 76:643, 1978.)*

sion and ligation of the lateral esophageal vascular attachments under direct vision are facilitated with use of deep narrow retractors in the diaphragmatic hiatus and long 13-inch right-angle clamps. Mobility of the esophagus within the posterior mediastinum can be assessed at this time. If no contraindication to transhiatal esophagectomy is encountered at this point, the mediastinal dissection is discontinued and the abdominal phase of the operation completed. A 14 F rubber jejunostomy tube is inserted and secured with a Weitzel maneuver. Until the mediastinal dissection has been completed, however, the jejunostomy is not brought out through the abdominal wall.

## Mediastinal Phase

The cervical esophagus is approached through an oblique incision that parallels the anterior border of the left sternocleidomastoid muscle. The incision extends from the level of the cricoid cartilage toward the suprasternal notch and is approximately 5–7 cm long. An extensive cervical incision is unnecessary because the cervical esophagus begins at the level of the cricoid cartilage, and exposure much superior to this point offers little advantage. After the platysma and omohyoid fascial layers are incised, the sternocleidomastoid muscle and carotid sheath and its contents are retracted laterally, and the larynx and trachea medially. *It is imperative that no retractor be placed against the recurrent laryngeal nerve in the tracheoesophageal groove during this portion of the operation or the subsequent esophagogastric anastomosis.* The inferior thyroid artery and middle thyroid vein are generally but not always ligated and divided.

Dissection is carried medially to the carotid sheath and proceeds directly posteriorly to allow identification of the prevertebral fascia. Blunt finger dissection is carried into the superior mediastinum. The tracheoesophageal groove is developed with sharp dissection; the recurrent laryngeal nerve is kept in constant view (but not dissected) and protected. The cervical esophagus is encircled with a Penrose drain; care is taken not to tear the posterior membranous trachea. The drain around the cervical esophagus is retracted upward as blunt dissection of the upper thoracic esophagus from the superior mediastinum is carried out; the volar aspects of the fingers are constantly kept against the esophagus in the midline (Fig. 52–11). In this way, the upper thoracic esophagus may be mobilized almost to the level of the carina through the neck incision.

The transhiatal esophageal mobilization is not a random wrenching of the esophagus from the posterior mediastinum, but rather is performed in an orderly, sequential manner. The surgeon determines the resectability of thoracic esophageal tumors with this technique by grasping the tumor-containing portion of the esophagus through the diaphragmatic hiatus and rocking the mass to determine if there is fixation to the prevertebral fascia or adjacent, pericardium, aorta, or tracheobronchial tree. If the esophagus feels mobile enough to be resected through the hiatus, one hand is inserted through the diaphragmatic hiatus posterior to the esophagus as the other hand is inserted through the neck incision along the prevertebral fascia and proceeds downward. The dissection may be facilitated with a half-sponge on a stick inserted into the superior mediastinum through the cervical incision (Fig. 52–12). The esophagus is swept away from the prevertebral fascia from above until the sponge stick makes contact with the hand inserted through the diaphragmatic hiatus. This completes the posterior mobilization of the esophagus from the prevertebral fascia. A 28 F Argyle Saratoga sump catheter is inserted from the cervical incision downward into the mediastinum and is connected to suction to facilitate accurate assessment of intraoperative blood loss. Intra-arterial blood pressure is carefully monitored by both the surgeon and the anesthetist during the transhiatal dissection to minimize prolonged hypotension resulting from cardiac displacement as the surgeon's hand is inserted into the posterior mediastinum. A surgeon whose glove size is larger than 7 may have difficulty with the transhiatal dissection because of unacceptable cardiac displacement.

The anterior esophageal dissection is carried out as a mirror image of the posterior mobilization. The esophagogastric junction is retracted downward as the surgeon's hand is inserted palm down through the diaphragmatic hiatus with the volar aspect of the fingers against the anterior

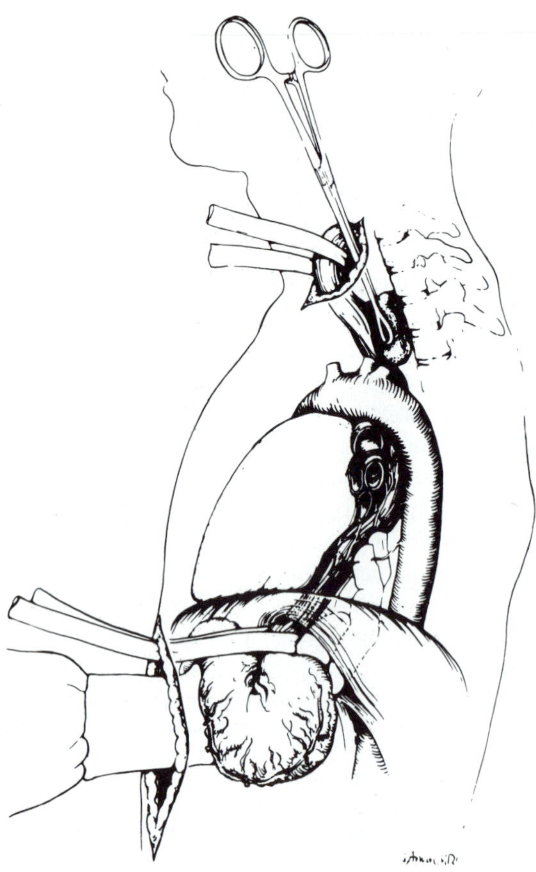

**Figure 52–12.** A "half-sponge-on-a-stick" inserted through the cervical incision into the posterior mediastinum facilitates mobilization of the esophagus away from the prevertebral fascia. *(Modified from Orringer MB, Sloan H: Esophagectomy without thoracotomy. J Thorac Cardiovasc Surg 76:643, 1978.)*

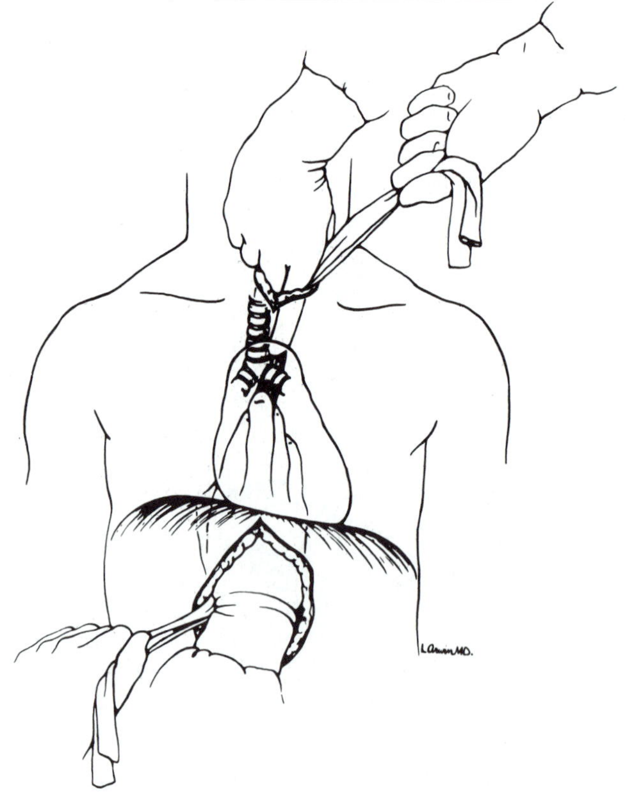

**Figure 52–13.** Mobilization of the anterior aspect of the thoracic esophagus during transhiatal esophagectomy is a mirror image of the posterior dissection, with the volar aspects of the fingers against the esophagus to avoid injury to the posterior membranous trachea. *(Modified from Orringer MB: Transhiatal blunt esophagectomy without thoracocomy. In Cohn LH (ed): Modern Technics in Surgery—Cardiothoracic Surgery. New York, Futura Publishing Co., 1983.)*

esophagus (Fig. 52–13). The esophagus is swept posteriorly away from the pericardium and carina. Mobile subcarinal lymph nodes may be identified and resected through the diaphragmatic hiatus. Simultaneously, through the neck incision, fingers placed against the anterior wall of the esophagus and behind the trachea gently dissect the esophagus away from the posterior membranous trachea (Fig. 52–14). A sponge-on-a-stick may be passed anterior to the esophagus to facilitate its dissection away from the posterior membranous trachea. It is particularly important during this dissection along the posterior wall of the esophagus to keep the fingers and palm of the hand flattened against the esophagus and to apply constant posterior pressure to minimize anterior cardiac displacement and hypotension.

As the cervical esophagus is retracted superiorly by its encircling Penrose drain, lateral attachments delivered into the neck wound are progressively dissected away bluntly until 5–8 cm of upper esophagus has been circumferentially mobilized. The right hand inserted through the diaphragmatic hiatus anterior to the esophagus and advanced into the superior mediastinum behind the trachea can identify the circumferentially mobilized upper esophagus and its intact lateral attachments (Fig. 52–15). With the esophagus trapped against the prevertebral fascia between the index and middle fingers, a downward gentle raking motion of the hand avulses the remaining periesophageal attachments (Fig. 52–16). Occasionally, denser fibrotic adhesions between the esophagus and periesophageal tissues make transhiatal resection difficult. One may find that the entire intrathoracic esophagus has been mobilized except for a 1–2 cm segment in the subcarinal or subaortic area. This tissue may be fractured by firm pressure between the index finger and thumb. As an alternative, an upper partial sternal split may provide access to the upper thoracic esophagus to the level of the carina so that the remaining adhesions can be divided under direct vision (Fig. 52–17).

Once the entire intrathoracic esophagus is mobile, several inches of esophagus are delivered into the cervical wound, and the esophagus is divided with the GIA surgical stapler. A Penrose drain is sutured to the distal end before the stapler is removed. Downward traction on the stomach through the abdominal incision draws the thoracic esopha-

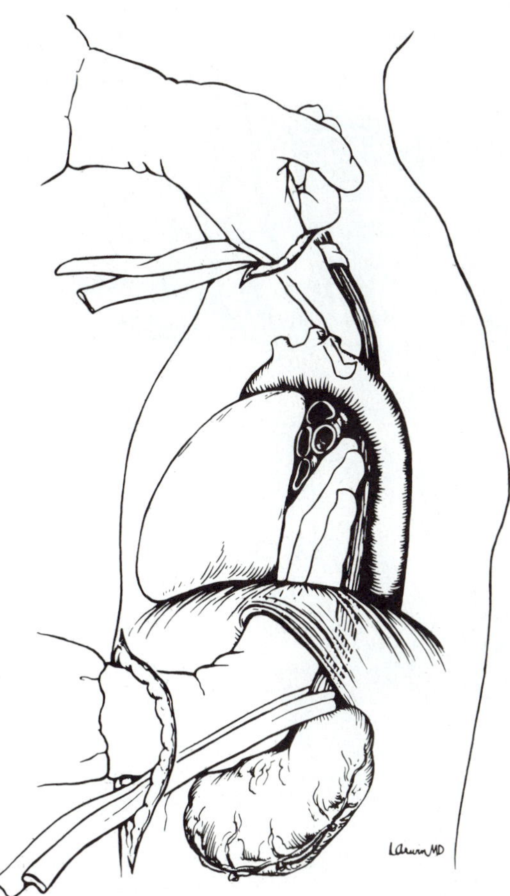

**Figure 52–14.** During the anterior esophageal dissection, constant posterior pressure is exerted against the esophagus to minimize cardiac displacement and secondary hypotension. *(Modified from Orringer MB: Transhiatal blunt esophagectomy without thoracotomy. In Cohn LH (ed): Modern Technics in Surgery—Cardiothoracic Surgery. New York, Futura Publishing Co., 1983.)*

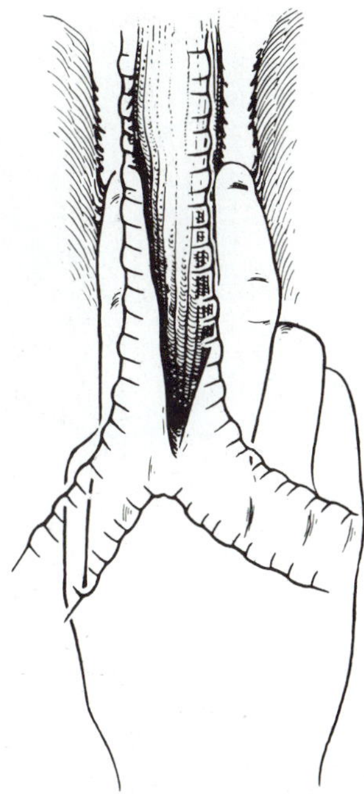

**Figure 52–15.** The right hand inserted through the diaphragmatic hiatus reaches up into the superior mediastinum until the undivided lateral esophageal attachments can be felt. *(Reproduced with permission from Orringer MB: Transhiatal esophagectomy. In Dudley H, Pories WJ, Carter D (eds): Rob and Smith's Operative Surgery (4th ed). London, England, Butterworths, 1983.)*

gus out of the posterior mediastinum through the diaphragmatic hiatus. The Penrose drain attached to the divided upper esophagus is also pulled downward through the posterior mediastinum. The cervical end of the Penrose drain is clamped with a hemostat. Once the entire thoracic esophagus has been delivered out of the posterior mediastinum along with its attached Penrose drain, the distal end of the drain is clamped with a hemostat and divided from the specimen. The Penrose drain now traverses the mediastinum and is held in place by a hemostat at either end. An Argyle Saratoga sump catheter is again used to evacuate the posterior mediastinum and to assess bleeding. With the esophagus removed, narrow retractors are placed in the diaphragmatic hiatus to facilitate both visual and manual inspection of the mediastinal pleura. Abdominal packs are gently placed into the posterior mediastinum through the hiatus to help tamponade only small vessels and achieve hemostasis. If either chest cavity has been entered because of a pleural tear, a 32 F chest tube is inserted in the appropriate midaxillary line and connected to underwater chest-tube suction. The stomach and attached esophagus are placed on

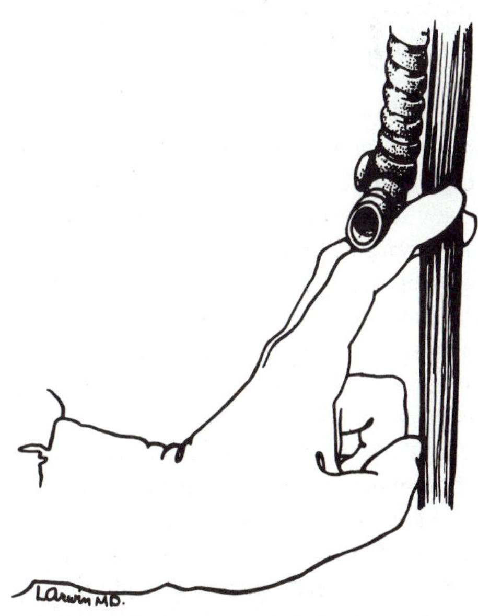

**Figure 52–16.** A gentle downward raking motion, with the esophagus trapped between the index and middle fingers, avulses the remaining periesophageal attachments. *(Reproduced with permission from Orringer MB: Transhiatal blunt esophagectomy without thoracotomy. In Cohn LH (ed): Modern Technics in Surgery—Cardiothoracic Surgery. New York, Futura Publishing Co., 1983.)*

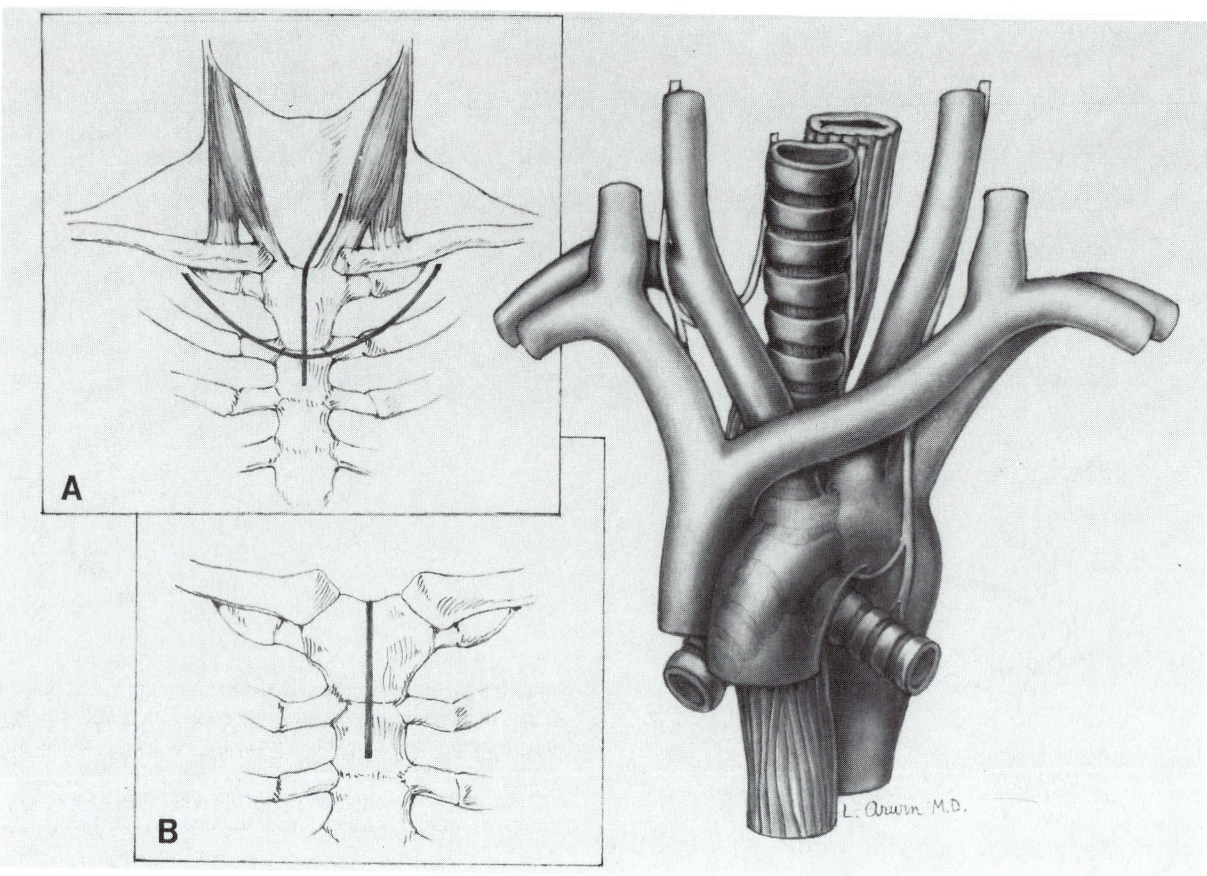


**Figure 52–17.** Exposure of the upper thoracic esophagus through a partial upper sternal split (main illustration). The course of the left recurrent laryngeal nerve beneath the aortic arch and then in the tracheoesophageal groove is demonstrated. Inset **A** shows the usual left cervical incision extended onto the anterior chest in the midline and the alternative curved anterior thoracic skin incision, which avoids a scar on the lower anterior neck. Inset **B** shows the sternotomy incision, which extends from the suprasternal notch through the manubrium and across the angle of Louis. *(Reproduced with permission from Orringer MB: Partial median sternotomy: Anterior approach to the upper thoracic esophagus. J Thorac Cardiovasc Surg 87:124, 1984.)*

the anterior abdominal wall. The gastric fundus is grasped and retracted superiorly as the lesser curve of the stomach is progressively divided with a GIA stapler beginning at approximately the second vascular arcade from the cardia (see Fig. 52–23). When the partial proximal gastrectomy is completed, the esophagus is removed from the field. The gastric stapled suture line is oversewn with a running 4-0 polypropylene Lembert stitch; care is taken not to pursestring the lesser curve and thereby hinder its upward reach.

The point along the greater curve of the stomach that reaches most superiorly to the neck is identified, and the distal end of the transmediastinal Penrose drain is sutured to the gastric fundus at this site with two interrupted 3-0 silk sutures (Fig. 52–18). The posterior mediastinal packs are removed through the hiatus, and hemostasis is ensured with one last inspection of the mediastinum assisted by the narrow retractors again placed in the hiatus. The stomach is then positioned into the posterior mediastinum more with gentle manipulation and pushing through the diaphragmatic hiatus than with traction on the cervical end of the rubber drain. When the fundus appears in the cervical wound above the level of the clavicles, it is gently grasped and pulled upward while the other hand inserted into the mediastinum from the abdomen continually pushes the stomach upward. The stomach should be carefully palpated along its anterior surface from above and below to be certain that it has not been twisted during its positioning in the chest. When the gastric fundus is properly located so that several centimeters are superior to the level of the clavicles, the pylorus comes to rest within 1–3 cm of the diaphragmatic hiatus in the abdomen. The gastric fundus is suspended from the cervical prevertebral fascia with two interrupted 4-0 absorbable sutures (Fig. 52–19B). This avoids subsequent suspension of the stomach from the anastomosis. The prevertebral fascia overlying in the longus coli muscles laterally rather than that immediately over the disk spaces should be used for the suspension sutures to prevent potential bacterial seeding of the intervertebral disks and vertebral osteomyelitis.

Before the cervical anastomosis is performed, the abdominal portion of the operation is completed to avoid contamination by oral bacteria, which might occur once the

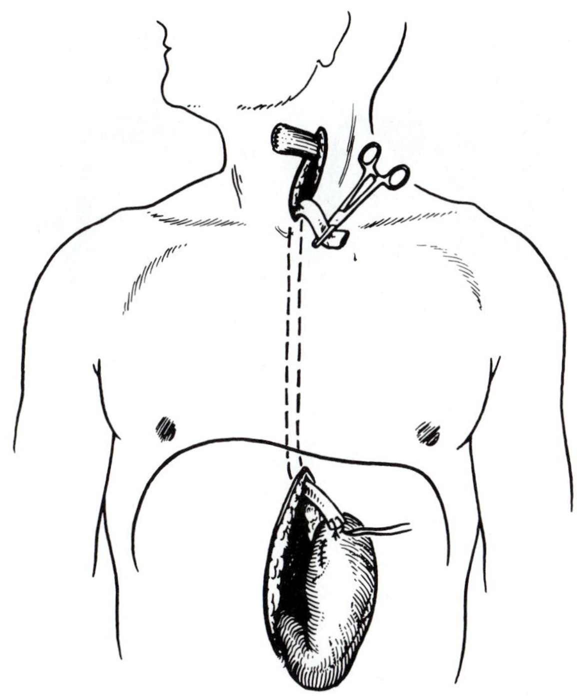

**Figure 52–18.** Gastric fundus sutured to transmediastinal rubber drain before stomach is positioned in posterior mediastinum. *(Reproduced with permission from Orringer MB: Transmediastinal esophagectomy. In Dudley H, Pories WJ, Carter D (eds): Rob and Smith's Operative Surgery, 4th ed. London, England, Butterworths, 1983.)*

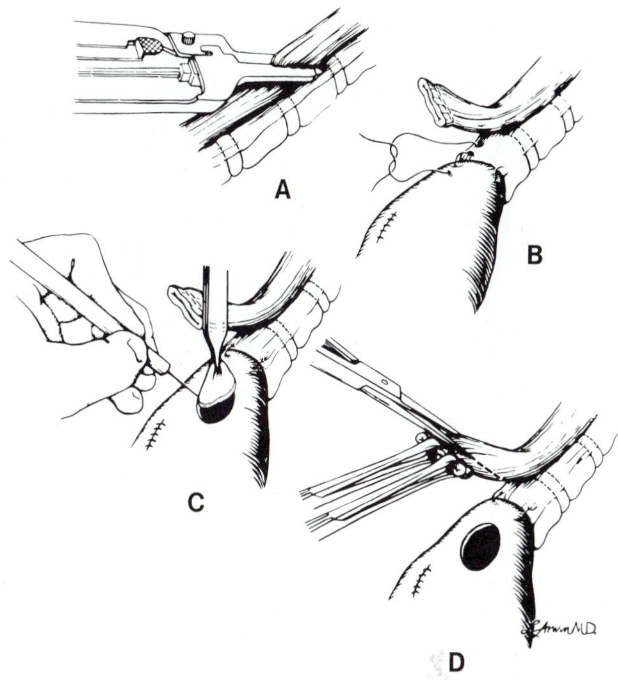


**Figure 52–19.** **A.** Division of cervical esophagus with GIA stapler. **B.** Suspension of gastric fundus from cervical prevertebral fascia. **C.** Removal of a 2-cm "button" of stomach with needle-tip electrocautery in preparation for the anastomosis. **D.** Oblique amputation of cervical esophagus leaving the anterior wall longer than the posterior wall. *(Modified from Orringer MB: Esophageal replacement after blunt esophagectomy. In Nyhus LM, Baker RJ (eds): Mastery of Surgery. Boston, Little, Brown & Co., 1984.)*

cervical esophagus is opened. The inevitably enlarged diaphragmatic esophageal hiatus is narrowed with several nonabsorbable sutures of No. 1–gauge material placed to the left of the stomach; care is taken to avoid injury to the right gastroepiploic vessels. The hiatus should easily admit three fingers alongside the stomach. The anterior gastric wall is sutured at several points to the edge of the diaphragmatic hiatus to prevent intrathoracic herniation of abdominal viscera. The pyloromyotomy is covered with adjacent omentum, and the previously retracted left hepatic lobe is restored to its normal location, further buttressing the pyloromyotomy. The feeding jejunostomy tube is brought out through a left upper quadrant stab wound, and the jejunum is fixed to the anterior abdominal wall with several interrupted sutures. The abdominal incision is closed without the routine use of abdominal or mediastinal drains.

## Cervical Phase

The last portion of the operation consists of a single-layered cervical esophagogastric anastomosis performed with absorbable 4-0 polyglycolic acid sutures (Figs. 52–19 and 20). Once the posterior half of the anastomosis is completed, a 46 F Maloney esophageal dilator is passed orally by the anesthetist across the anastomosis, and the anterior half of the anastomosis is completed with this dilator in place to ensue an adequate lumen. The dilator is removed and replaced with a nasogastric tube. Silver clip markers are placed on either side of the anastomosis for future radiographic assessment. When the operation is completed, the cervical anastomosis is 4–5 cm distal to the upper esophageal sphincter (approximately 19–20 cm from the incisors at endoscopy), and the pyloromyotomy is 2–3 cm below the diaphragmatic hiatus (Fig. 52–21). The cervical wound is closed loosely over a rubber drain. A chest radiograph is obtained in the operating room at the end of the operation to be certain that there is no unrecognized pneumo- or hemothorax that requires chest-tube drainage and that the nasogastric tube is in proper position within the intrathoracic stomach. Mechanical ventilation is generally continued the night of operation, and the endotracheal tube is removed and the patient transferred out of the intensive care unit the next morning.

## Transhiatal Esophagectomy and Proximal Partial Gastrectomy for Carcinoma of the Esophagogastric Junction

The technique of transhiatal esophagectomy is applicable in many patients with carcinoma of the cardia and proximal

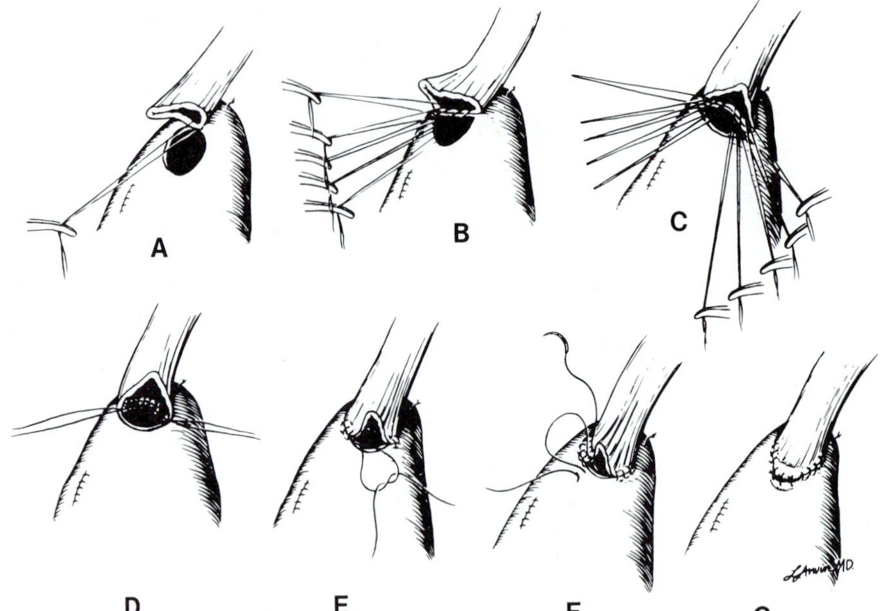


**Figure 52–20.** Construction of the cervical esophagogastric anastomosis. **A–D.** The two posterior quadrants are completed with the knots tied on the inside of the lumen. **E–G.** The anterior two quadrants of the anastomosis are completed with a 46 bougie (not shown) within the esophagus to prevent narrowing. *(Modified from Orringer MB: Esophageal replacement after blunt esophagectomy. In Nyhus LM, Baker RJ (eds): Mastery of Surgery. Boston, Little, Brown & Co., 1984.)*

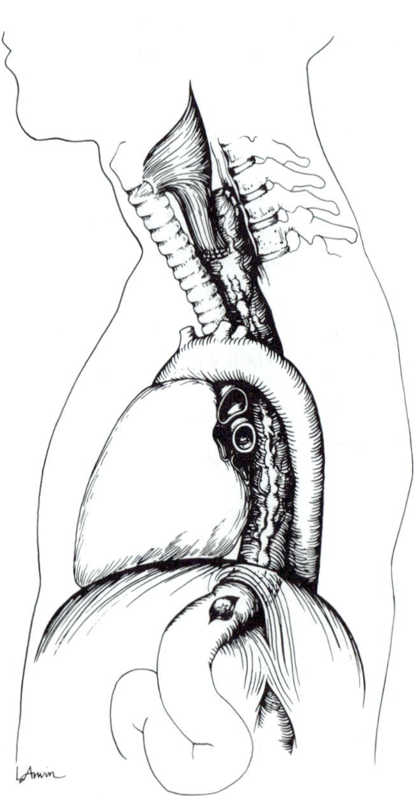

**Figure 52–21.** Final position of the intrathoracic stomach after transhiatal esophagectomy. The gastric fundus is suspended from the prevertebral fascia several centimeters above the cervical anastomosis, and the pyloromyotomy is located 2-3 cm below the diaphragmatic hiatus. *(Reproduced with permission of the C.V. Mosby Co. from Orringer MB, Sloan H: Esophagectomy without thoracotomy. J Thorac Cardiovasc Surg 76:643, 1978.)*

stomach. As long as the entire greater curve of the gastric fundus can be preserved, including the point that reaches most cephalad to the neck (Fig. 52–22), esophageal resection and reconstruction can still be performed without opening of the thorax, and a reasonable gross distal margin beyond the tumor can be obtained. In most of these patients, associated celiac axis lymph node spread precludes a curative resection, and a traditional proximal hemigastrectomy for the sake of performing a better "cancer operation" wastes valuable stomach that can be used for esophageal replacement, contributes little to the patient's longevity, and commits the surgeon to an intrathoracic esophageal anastomosis.

When the technique of transhiatal esophagectomy is used for tumors at the esophagogastric junction, the cervical esophagus must not be divided until the surgeon is satisfied that there is adequate remaining stomach to reach to the neck. If the thoracic esophagus is removed after the cervical end is divided and then the esophagogastric junction tumor is found to involve so much stomach that a proximal hemigastrectomy is required to remove it, there will be insufficient gastric length to reach to the neck. The patient will be left with a cervical esophagostomy and feeding tube—a disastrous result from an esophageal operation performed to restore the enjoyment of eating.

Once the mobilized thoracic esophagus and stomach have been placed on the anterior abdominal wall, the stomach may be divided with a GIA stapler 4–6 cm from gross palpable tumor (Fig. 52–23). The remaining greater curve gastric tube is then sutured to the transmediastinal Penrose drain as described earlier. After the stomach is positioned in the posterior mediastinum in the original esophageal bed and suspended stomach from the prevertebral fascia, the cervical esophagogastric anastomosis is performed on the

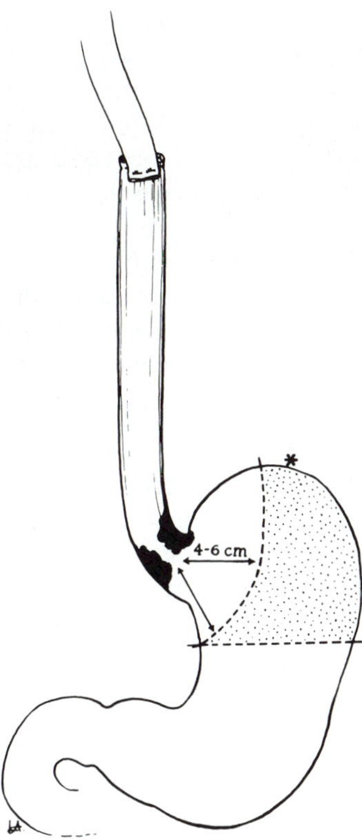


**Figure 52–22.** Transhiatal esophagectomy may be combined with a partial proximal gastrectomy for lesions of the cardia and distal esophagus. A 4-6 cm gastric margin is obtained while preserving the entire greater curvature and that point (*) that reaches most cephalad. (Stippled area shows that portion of stomach that is typically resected in a standard hemigastrectomy, thereby eliminating the possibility of a cervical esophagogastric anastomosis.) *(Reproduced with permission from Orringer MB, Sloan H: Esophagectomy without thoracotomy. J Thorac Cardiovasc Surg 76:643, 1978.)*

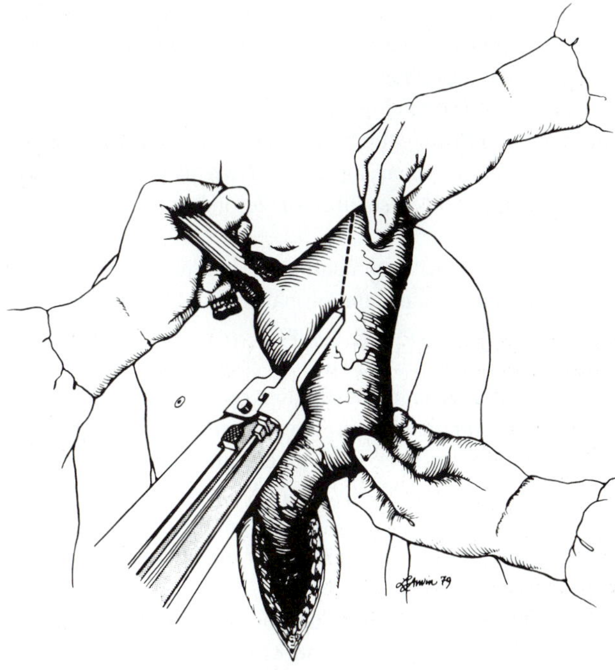

**Figure 52–23.** After transhiatal resection, the proximal partial gastrectomy is performed using the GIA surgical stapler applied to the stomach 4-6 cm distal to palpable tumor. *(Reproduced with permission from Orringer MB, Sloan H: Esophageal replacement after blunt esophagectomy. In Nyhus LM, Baker RJ (eds): Mastery of Surgery, Boston, Little, Brown & Co., 1984, pp 426-439, Chap 52.)*

anterior gastric wall, away from the gastric staple suture line as described earlier.

## Results of Transhiatal Esophagectomy for Benign and Malignant Disease

My colleagues and I reported results with transhiatal esophagectomy without thoracotomy[10,11] in 583 patients with diseases of the intrathoracic esophagus.[37] One hundred sixty-six patients (28.5%) had benign disease that necessitated esophageal replacement, and 417 (71.5%) had carcinoma (Table 52–1). The ages of the patients with benign disease ranged from 14 to 88 years (average, 48 years), whereas the ages of those with carcinoma ranged from 29 to 92 years (average, 63 years). Ninety-five (22.8%) patients with carcinoma were 70 years of age or older. Among the patients with carcinoma, 148 (35.5%) had squamous cell carcinoma (18 upper, 85 middle, and 45 lower third), and 258 (61.9%) had adenocarcinoma (two upper third, 28 middle third, 228 lower third of cardia). Barrett's mucosa was associated with 136 (32.6%) of these carcinomas. Seven patients had adenosquamous carcinoma, two had anaplastic, and two had poorly differentiated carcinomas.

Mediastinal inflammation from prior operations, perforations, or radiation therapy has not precluded transhiatal esophagectomy. One hundred (60.2%) of the patients with

**TABLE 52–1. INDICATIONS FOR TRANSHIATAL ESOPHAGECTOMY (583 PATIENTS)**

| Condition | No. (%) |
|---|---|
| **Benign Conditions** | **166 (28.5%)** |
| Stricture | 67 (40.4) |
| Gastroesophageal reflux esophagitis | 51 |
| Caustic ingestion | 13 |
| Other | 3 |
| Neuromotor dysfunction | 54 (32.5) |
| Achalasia | 40 |
| Spasm | 14 |
| Recurrent gastroesophageal reflux | 27 (16.3) |
| Acute perforation | 9 (5.4) |
| Acute caustic injury | 4 (2.4) |
| Other | 5 (3.0) |
| **Carcinoma of Intrathoracic Esophagus** | **417 (71.5%)** |
| Upper third | 23 (5.5) |
| Middle third | 115 (27.6) |
| Lower third thoracic, cardia, or both | 279 (66.9) |

*(Reproduced with permission from Orringer MB, Marshall B, Stirling MC: Transhiatal esophagectomy for benign and malignant disease. J Thorac Cardiovasc Surg 105:265–277, 1993.)*

benign disease had undergone one or more prior esophageal or periesophageal operations, including antireflux repairs (64 patients); esophagomyotomy (42 patients); vagotomy (13 patients); esophagogastrostomy (five patients); colonic interposition (four patients); repair of perforation, esophagoplasty, laryngopharyngectomy (two patients each); and sclerotherapy and resection of leiomyoma (one patient each).

Three patients with acute caustic injuries were treated with emergency transhiatal esophagectomy, cervical esophagostomy, and feeding jejunostomy followed by delayed esophageal reconstruction 2–8 weeks later. Esophageal resection and reconstruction were performed at the same operation in all but five patients, four with acute caustic injuries and one with severe mental retardation and recurrent aspiration due to a reflux stricture. The stomach was used as the visceral esophageal substitute in 553 (94.8%) of these patients who underwent immediate esophageal replacement (Table 52–2). Four of the 17 patients with acute or chronic caustic injuries required either partial or total gastric resection. Colon was used to replace the esophagus in the four patients with caustic injuries. In the patients with carcinoma colon was used only when prior gastric resection for peptic ulcer disease precluded use of the stomach as an esophageal substitute. The posterior mediastinum was used for the esophageal substitute in all but nine patients in whom either residual posterior mediastinal tumor or fibrosis and narrowing prevented adequate positioning of the stomach for a tension-free cervical anastomosis. The retrosternal route was used in these nine patients. In patients with carcinoma, accessible subcarinal, paraesophageal, and celiac axis lymph nodes were routinely sampled, but no attempt was made to perform en bloc wide resection of the esophagus and its continuous lymph node–bearing tissues. Postsurgical tumor-node-metastasis (TNM) staging of these carcinomas indicated that 200 (48%) were either transmurally invasive or metastatic beyond regional lymph nodes (stage III or IV tumors) (Table 52–3). Thirty-five (8.4%) were staged as T0, having no residual tumor after preoperative chemotherapy or radiation therapy or both.

There was one intraoperative death in this series. It was caused by hemothorax that occurred during esophageal mobilization. Measured intraoperative blood loss averaged 817 mL in patients with carcinoma and 1035 mL in patients with benign disease (Table 52–4).

### Intraoperative Complications

Entry into one or both pleural cavities during transhiatal esophagectomy is quite common; 74% of our patients required a chest tube. There were four intraoperative membranous tracheal lacerations. Three involved the high membranous trachea and were repaired through a partial upper sternal split. The other tear involving the membranous carina required a right thoracotomy for repair. Twenty-four patients (4.1%) required a splenectomy because of intraoperative injury.

### Postoperative Complications

Three patients required a thoracotomy for control of mediastinal bleeding within 24 hours of transhiatal esophagectomy, two with a megaesophagus of achalasia and one after inappropriate pharmacologic hypotensive anesthesia was used intraoperatively. Early in our experience, left recurrent laryngeal nerve paresis was common. This complication was initially believed to be an unavoidable consequence of blunt dissection in the subaortic area along the course of the

**TABLE 52–2. ESOPHAGEAL RECONSTRUCTION AFTER TRANSHIATAL ESOPHAGECTOMY (583 PATIENTS)**

| Timing of Reconstruction | Benign (No.) | Carcinoma (No.) | Total [No. (%)] |
|---|---|---|---|
| Immediate | | | |
| Cervical Esophago-gastrostomy | 145 | 408 | 553 (94.8) |
| Posterior Mediastinal | 143 | 402 | |
| Retrosternal | 2 | 6 | |
| Cervical Esophago-colostomy | 16 | 9 | 25 (4.3%) |
| Posterior Mediastinal | 9 | 9 | |
| Retrosternal | 7 | — | |
| Delayed (2–8 weeks) | | | |
| Retrosternal | 3 | | 3 (0.5%) |
| None (Esophagostomy, Tube) | 2 | | 2 (0.3%) |
| Total | 166 | 417 | 583 |

*(Reproduced with permission from Orringer MB, Marshall B, Stirling MC: Transhiatal esophagectomy for benign and malignant disease. J Thorac Cardiovasc Surg 105:265–277, 1993.)*

**TABLE 52–3. POSTSURGICAL RESECTION STAGING OF 417 INTRATHORACIC ESOPHAGEAL CARCINOMAS**

| | Tumor Site | | | |
|---|---|---|---|---|
| Stage | *Upper* | *Middle* | *Lower* | Total [No. (%)] |
| 0[a] | 3 | 11 | 21 | 35 (8.4) |
| I | 1 | 14 | 27 | 42 (10.1) |
| IIA | 6 | 29 | 64 | 99 (23.7) |
| IIB | 2 | 7 | 30 | 39 (9.4) |
| III | 7 | 39 | 111 | 157 (37.6) |
| IV | 4 | 14 | 25 | 43 (10.3) |
| Unstaged[b] | — | 1 | 1 | 2 (0.5) |
| TOTAL | 23 | 115 | 279 | 417 |

[a]Includes seven Tis and 28 T0 after prior chemotherapy or radiation therapy or both

[b]Includes one patient who died of intraoperative bleeding before esophagectomy could be completed and one patient whose pathology report could not be located.

*(Reproduced with permission from Orringer MB, Marshall B, Stirling MC: Transhiatal esophagectomy for benign and malignant disease. J Thorac Cardiovasc Surg 105:265–277, 1993.)*

**TABLE 52–4. MEASURED INTRAOPERATIVE BLOOD LOSS WITH TRANSHIATAL ESOPHAGECTOMY**

| Type of Disease | No. | Range (mL) | Average (mL) |
|---|---|---|---|
| Benign Disease | 164[a] | 100–4000 | 1023 |
| Carcinoma | 415[a] | 125–4360 | 817 |
| Upper third | 23 | 125–3000 | 988 |
| Middle third | 114 | 125–3700 | 861 |
| Lower third | 278 | 125–4360 | 784 |
| TOTAL | 579 | 100–4360 | 875 |

[a]Excludes two patients with benign disease and two patients with carcinoma who experienced inordinate intraoperative blood loss ranging from 6600 to 18,000 mL.

*(Reproduced with permission from Orringer MB, Marshall B, Stirling MC: Transhiatal esophagectomy for benign and malignant disease. J Thorac Cardiovasc Surg 105:265–277, 1993.)*

left recurrent laryngeal nerve. However, after we began compulsively avoiding placement of any retractor against the tracheoesophageal groove during the cervical portion of the operation, the incidence of postoperative hoarseness has fallen to less than 4% in the past 4 years. The total incidence of postoperative hoarseness in patients undergoing a cervical anastomosis was 9% (59 patients), but in 40 patients, this resolved spontaneously within 2–12 weeks. Chylothorax due to injury to the thoracic duct occurred in 13 patients (2.2%), eight with carcinoma and five with benign disease. In each case, this complication was treated aggressively with transthoracic ligation of the intrathoracic duct within 7–10 days of the operation, and the patients recovered uneventfully.[38] The overall anastomotic leak rate following cervical esophagogastric anastomosis with the stomach positioned in the posterior mediastinum in the original esophageal bed was 7.9% (46 patients) as compared with 63% (five patients) among the eight patients with retrosternal placement of the stomach. All but three of these 51 anastomotic leaks were successfully treated with opening of the cervical wound at the bedside and local packing until spontaneous healing occurred. Necrosis of the tip of the stomach necessitated takedown of the intrathoracic stomach and a cervical esophagostomy in three patients.

### *Mortality*

Among these 583 patients who underwent transhiatal esophagectomy, the overall hospital mortality was 4.6% (27 deaths), the same for patients with both benign and malignant disease. No patient in this series died of sepsis due to an anastomotic leak, and there were only two deaths of respiratory insufficiency.

### *Hospitalization*

Overall, 235 (42%) of the 556 patients who survived transhiatal esophagectomy were discharged within 10 days of the operation, 181 (32%) within 11–14 days, and 67 (12%) by 3 weeks after the operation.

### *Functional Results*

The functional results of esophageal substitution with stomach were assessed by means of a careful evaluation of symptoms of dysphagia, regurgitation, and postvagotomy dumping as well as weight compared with preoperative status.[37] The 138 patients with benign disease for whom follow-up information was available (average follow-up period, 47 months) best reflect the results of esophageal substitution with stomach. At the time of their most recent follow-up examination, 42 patients (31.1%) had excellent results (completely asymptomatic); 50 (37.0%), good results (mild symptoms requiring no treatment); 39 (28.9%), fair results (symptoms necessitating occasional treatment such as a dilation or antidiarrheal medication; and four patients (3.0%) had poor results (symptoms necessitating ongoing treatment, such as regular anastomotic dilations or an intensive anti-dumping regimen). One hundred five patients (77.8%) of patients had either good or excellent ability to swallow; 26 (19.2%) required an occasional anastomotic dilation; and four patients (3.0%) required regular dilation for severe stricture. Three anastomoses were revised because of severe stenosis. Eighty-nine patients (65.9%) reported no regurgitation; 39 (28.9%) had intermittent, nontroublesome nocturnal reflux that was easily controlled with proper posturing; and seven (5.2%) had regular and severe nocturnal regurgitation. None of our patients, however, experienced pulmonary complications due to aspiration after a cervical esophagogastric anastomosis. Regarding weight after transhiatal esophagectomy for benign disease, at the time of latest follow-up examination, 55 (40.7%) of the patients weighed 1–54 pounds (0.45–24.3 kg) (average 11 pounds [4.95 kg]) more than they did before the operation; 66 (48.9%) weighed 1–20 pounds (0.45–54 kg) (average, 18 pounds [8.1 kg]) less, and 12 (8.9%) weighed the same as they did before the operation. A perceived decrease in gastric capacity is common after esophageal substitution with stomach, not unlike that experienced years ago when resection was commonly performed for peptic ulcer disease.

### *Survival of Patients with Carcinoma*

The overall Kaplan-Meier actuarial survival rate after transhiatal esophagectomy for carcinoma of the intrathoracic esophagus and cardia in our 417 patients was 41% at 2 years and 27% at 5 years (Fig. 52–24). The 5-year survival rate after treatment of lower-third tumors was 32% compared with 18% after treatment of middle-third and 22% after treatment of upper-third carcinomas. The survival rate was not statistically significantly different among patients with adenocarcinoma as opposed to those with squamous cell carcinoma. As expected, the most important determinant of survival after transhiatal esophagectomy is tumor stage. Patients with stage 0 and I tumors live considerably longer than those with more advanced disease (Fig. 52–25).

One interesting subgroup of our patients is a group of 43 with locoregional esophageal cancer (adenocarcinoma in 21, squamous cell carcinoma in 22) who received preopera-

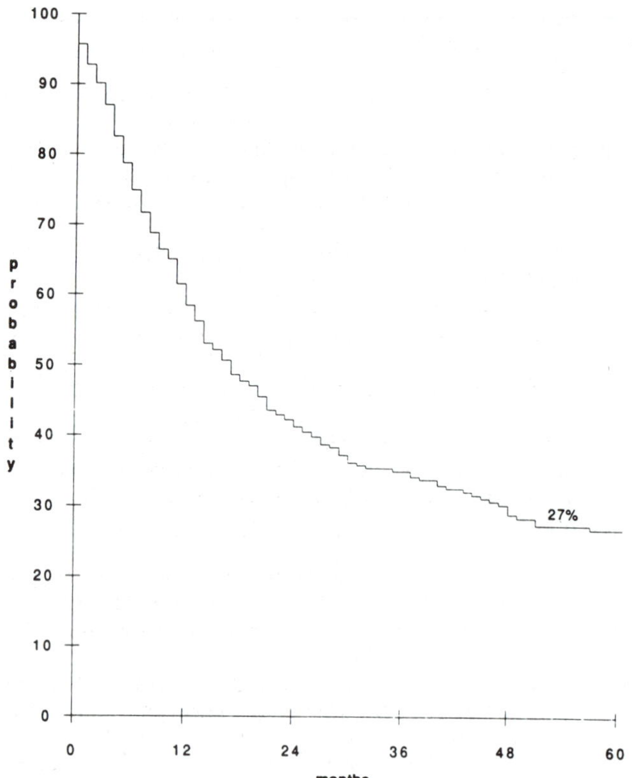


**Figure 52–24.** Kaplan-Meier actuarial survival curve of 417 patients who underwent transhiatal esophagectomy for carcinoma of the intrathoracic esophagus and cardia. *(Reproduced with permission from Orringer MB, Marshal B, Stirling MC: Transhiatal esophagectomy for benign and malignant disease. J Thorac Cardiovasc Surg 105:265–277, 1993.)*

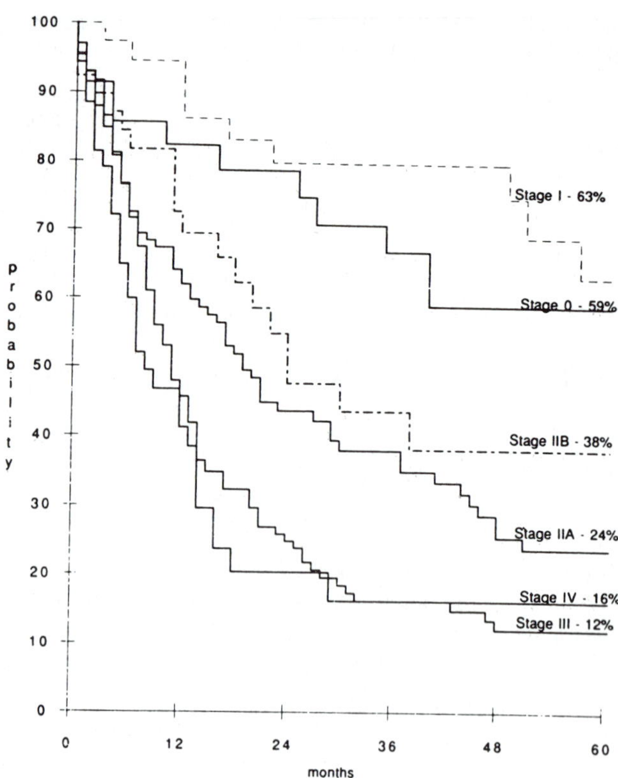


| | No. | No. Patients Followed Through Interval | | | | |
|---|---|---|---|---|---|---|
| Stage 0 | 35 | 26 | 21 | 18 | 12 | 9 |
| Stage I | 42 | 31 | 25 | 22 | 17 | 11 |
| Stage IIA | 99 | 58 | 34 | 26 | 16 | 13 |
| Stage IIB | 39 | 22 | 14 | 9 | 7 | 7 |
| Stage III | 157 | 61 | 25 | 14 | 10 | 8 |
| Stage IV | 43 | 16 | 6 | 5 | 2 | 1 |

**Figure 52–25.** Stage-dependent Kaplan-Meier actuarial survial curves for patients who underwent transhiatal esophagectomy for carcinoma of the intrathoracic esophagus and cardia. *(Reproduced with permission from Orringer MB, Marshall B, Stirling MC: Transhiatal esophagectomy for benign and malignant disease. J Thorac Cardiovasc Surg 105:265–277, 1993.)*

tive chemotherapy (cisplatin, vinblastine, and 5-fluorouracil) concurrent with 4500-cGy radiation therapy as part of a phase II trial for 21 days before planned transhiatal esophagectomy.[39] Transhiatal resections were performed in 39 patients (91% resectability rate). Of the 41 patients who underwent operations 10 (24%) had no tumor in the resected esophagus or lymph nodes (T0N0). The median survival duration of the 43 patients was 20 months, and 17 patients (34%) were alive at 5 years. Survival rate was not statistically significantly different among patients with adenocarcinoma as opposed to those with squamous cell carcinoma. Among these patients with no residual tumor (T0N0), the 5-year survival was 60%.[40] Among patients with residual disease, the 5-year survival was 32%. This study suggested that survival after transhiatal esophagectomy for carcinoma is significantly improved with preoperative radiation and chemotherapy. A phase III trial to validate these encouraging results is now in progress.

## SUMMARY

Each of the alternative techniques for resecting the thoracic esophagus has its proponents, who can provide strong arguments about the merits of their preferred approaches. Objective assessment of available data indicates that the operative mortality for any of these operations, when performed by skilled surgeons, can be held below 5%. Controversy centers on the adequacy of the type of esophagectomy as a "cancer operation." Proponents of the long-respected Halstedian principles of en bloc cancer resection object to transhiatal esophagectomy for carcinoma because it precludes a mediastinal lymphadenectomy. They argue for radical resection as a patient's best chance for survival.[34] They are in a distinct minority, however, because, unfortunately, except in countries where mass-screening techniques provide a large population of patients with early esophageal carcinoma, this tumor is rarely encountered in a localized, surgically curable form. Nodal metastases and transmural tumor invasion characterize most esophageal cancers in western countries. In approximately 80% of patients, the tumor is advanced (NM stage III or IV). Such "systemic" disease is unlikely to be cured by any operation.

The era of radical operations to cure cancer is coming to an end as objective comparison with less radical methods of therapy is made. For example, en bloc dissection of regional lymph nodes in continuity with a primary lesion of the breast at the time of mastectomy for breast carcinoma offers no better survival than simple mastectomy followed by postoperative radiation therapy.[41–43] Similarly, survival statistics after transhiatal esophagectomy for carcinoma are similar to those reported in most modern western series of standard transthoracic esophagectomies[44,45] and to those reported after so-called radical en bloc esophagectomy and mediastinal lymphadenectomy. In most patients I encounter, esophageal carcinoma is a systemic disease, and systemic therapy (e.g., chemotherapy or immunotherapy) is ultimately required to control it. Stage 0 (TisN0M0) and I (T1N0M0) carcinomas confined to the esophageal mucosa are curable by any type of esophagectomy. Thus I prefer to avoid a thoracotomy and its attendant morbidity if possible when treating such tumors. In the occasional patient whose esophageal cancer is associated only with regional lymph node spread, a more radical technique of esophagectomy may have benefit.

The argument which technique of esophagectomy is best for esophageal carcinoma is fast becoming passé. Developments in thoracic oncology have begun to demonstrate improved survival with combinations of systemic chemotherapy, radiation therapy, and surgical therapy. Additional practical questions for the future concern the best method of esophagectomy and esophageal replacement for benign disease, in which long-term functional results are far more critical. Long-term follow-up findings are beginning to validate my belief that a total thoracic esophagectomy with a cervical esophagogastric anastomosis is preferable in patients who require esophageal resection for benign disease as well as in patients with carcinoma.[37] When the stomach is used to replace the entire thoracic esophagus, placement in the posterior mediastinum is the preferred route, and a gastric drainage procedure is indicated to avoid the potential adverse effects of gastric outlet obstruction associated with vagotomy.

## REFERENCES


1. Ohsawa T: The surgery of the oesophagus. *Jpn Chir* **10:**604, 1933
2. Adams WE, Phemister DB: Carcinoma of the lower thoracic esophagus: Report of a successful resection and esophagogastrostomy. *J Thorac Surg* **7:**621, 1938
3. Akiyama H, Tsurumaru M, Kawamura T, Ono Y: Principles of surgical treatment for carcinoma of the esophagus: Analysis of lymph node involvement. *Ann Surg* **194:**438, 1981
4. Mitchell RL: Abdominal and right thoracotomy approach as standard procedure for esophagogastrectomy with low morbidity. *J Thorac Cardiovasc Surg* **93:**205, 1987
5. Mathisen DJ, Grillo HC, Wilkins EW Jr, et al: Transthoracic esophagectomy: A safe approach to carcinoma of the esophagus. *Ann Thorac Surg* **45:**137, 1988
6. Ellis FH Jr: Carcinoma of the esophagus. *Cancer* **33:**264, 1983
7. Postlethwait RW: Complications and deaths after operations for esophageal carcinoma. *J Thorac Cardiovasc Surg* **85:**827, 1983
8. Giuli R, Gignoix M: Treatment of carcinoma of the esophagus: Retrospective study of 2400 patients. *Ann Surg* **192:**44, 1980
9. Earlam R, Cunha-Melo JR: Oesophageal squamous cell carcinoma. I. A critical review of surgery. *Br J Surg* **67:**381, 1980
10. Orringer MB, Sloan H: Esophagectomy without thoracotomy. *J Thorac Cardiovasc Surg* **76:**643, 1978
11. Szentpetery S, Wolfgrant T, Lower RR: Pull-through esophagectomy without thoracotomy for esophageal carcinoma. *Ann Thorac Surg* **27:**399, 1979
12. Garvin PJ, Kaminski DL: Extrathoracic esophagectomy in the treatment of esophageal cancer. *Am J Surg* **140:**772, 1980
13. Steiger Z, Wilson RF: Comparison of results of esophagectomy with and without a thoracotomy. *Surg Gynecol Obstet* **153:**653, 1981
14. Orringer MB, Orringer JS: Transhiatal esophagectomy without thoracotomy a dangerous operation? *J Thorac Cardiovasc Surg* **85:**72, 1983
15. Orringer MB: Transhiatal esophagectomy without thoracotomy for carcinoma of the thoracic esophagus. *Ann Surg* **200:**282, 1984
16. Orringer MB: Transhiatal esophagectomy for benign disease. *J Thorac Cardiovasc Surg* **90:**649, 1985
17. Stewart JR, Sarr MG, Sharp KW, et al: Transhiatal (blunt) esophagectomy for malignant and benign esophageal disease: Clinical experience and technique. *Ann Thorac Surg* **40:**343, 1985
18. Baker JW, Schechter GL: Management of panesophageal cancer by blunt resection without thoracotomy and reconstruction with stomach. *Ann Surg* **203:**491, 1986
19. Shahian DM, Neptune WB, Ellis FH Jr, Watkins E Jr: Transthoracic versus extrathoracic esophagectomy: Mortality, morbidity and long-term survival. *Ann Thorac Surg* **41:**237, 1986
20. Hankins JR, Miller JE, Attar S, McLaughlin JS: Transhiatal esophagectomy for carcinoma of the esophagus: Experience with 26 patients. *Ann Thorac Surg* **44:**123, 1987
21. Belsey R: Discussion of Orringer MB, Sloan H: Esophagectomy without thoracotomy. *J Thorac Cardiovasc Surg* **76:**652, 1978
22. Skinner DB: Discussion of Orringer MB, Sloan H: Esophagectomy without thoracotomy. *J Thorac Cardiovasc Surg* **76:**652, 1978
23. Logan A: The surgical treatment of carcinoma of the esophagus and cardia. *J Thoracic Cardiovasc Surg* **46:**150, 1963
24. Skinner DB: En bloc resection for neoplasms of the esophagus and cardia. *J Thorac Cardiovasc Surg* **85:**59, 1983
25. Goldsmith HS, Akiyama H: A comparative study of Japanese and American gastric dimensions. *Ann Surg* **190:**690, 1979
26. Goldfaden D, Orringer MB, Appleman H, Kalish R: Adenocarcinoma of the distal esophagus and gastric cardia. *J Thorac Cardiovasc Surg* **91:**242, 1986
27. Angorn IB: Esophagogastrostomy without a drainage procedure in esophageal carcinoma. *Br J Surg* **62:**601, 1975
28. Huant GJ, Zhang DC, Zhang DW: A comparative study of resection of carcinoma of the esophagus with and without pyloroplasty. In TR DeMeester, DB Skinner (eds): *Esophageal Disorders: Pathophysiology and Therapy.* New York, Raven Press, 1985, pp 383–388
29. Fok M, Cheng WK, Wong J: Pyloroplasty versus no drainage in gastric replacement of the esophagus. *Am J Surg* **162:**447, 1991
30. Orringer MB, Sloan H: Substernal gastric bypass of the excluded thoracic esophagus for palliation for esophageal carcinoma. *J Thorac Cardiovasc Surg* **70:**836, 1975
31. Gerndt S, Orringer MB: Tube jejunostomy as an adjunct to esophagectomy. *Surgery* **115:**164, 1994
32. Belsey R, Hiebert CA: An exclusive right thoracic approach for cancer of the middle third of the esophagus. *Ann Thorac Surg* **18:**1, 1974
33. Skinner DB, Ferguson MK, Soriano A, et al: Selection of operation for esophageal cancer based on staging. *Ann Surg* **204:**391, 1986

34. Hagen JA, Peters JH, DeMeester TR. Superiority of extended en bloc esophagogastrectomy for carcinoma of the lower esophagus and cardia. *J Thorac Cardiovasc Surg* **106:**850, 1993
35. Liebermann-Meffert DMI, Luescher U, Neff U, et al: Esophagectomy without thoracotomy: Is there a risk of intramediastinal bleeding? *Ann Surg* **206:**184, 1987
36. Quint LE, Glazer GM, Orringer MB, Gross BH: Esophageal carcinoma: CT findings. *Radiology* **155:**171, 1985
37. Orringer MB, Marshall B, Stirling MC. Transhiatal esophagectomy for benign and malignant esophagel disease. *J Thorac Cardiovasc Surg* **105:**265, 1993
38. Orringer MB, Bluett M, Deeb GM: Aggressive treatment chylothorax complicating transhiatal esophagectomy without thoracotomy. *Surgery* **104:**720, 1988
39. Orringer MB, Forastiere AA, Perez-Tamayo C, et al: Chemotherapy and radiation therapy before transhiatal esophagectomy for esophageal carcinoma. *Ann Thorac Surg* **49:**348, 1990
40. Forastiere AA, Orringer MB, Perez-Tamayo C, et al: Preoperative chemoradiation followed by transhiatal esophagectomy for carcinoma of the esophagus: Final report. *J Clin Oncol* **11:**1118, 1993
41. Donegan WL: Surgical clinical trends. *Cancer* **53:**691, 1984
42. Veronesi V, Saccozi R, DelVecchio M, et al: Comparing radical mastectomy with quandrantectomy, axillary dissection, and radiotherapy in patients with small cancers of the breast. *N Engl J Med* **306:**6, 1981
43. Fisher B, et al: 10-year results of a randomized clinical trial comparing radical mastectomy and total mastectomy with or without radiation. *N Engl J Med* **312**(11):674, 1985
44. Pac M, Gasoglu A, Kocal H, et al: Transhiatal versus transthoracic esophagectomy for esophageal cancer. *J Thorac Cardiovasc Surg* **106:**205, 1993
45. Tilanus HW, Hop WCJ, Langenhorst BLAM, vanLanschot JJB. Esophagectomy without thoracotomy: Is there any difference. *J Thorac Cardiovasc Surg* **105:**898, 1993

CHAPTER

53

# Surgical Options for Esophageal Excision Replacement

## *Colonic Interposition*

Clement A. Hiebert

Stomach, small intestine, and colon as well as free revascularized grafts have been substituted for excised esophagus (Table 53–1). Of these stomach is unquestionably the most convenient and widely used.[1] Stomach was the replacement organ used by Huang[2] in 98.2% of 1874 patients who required esophagectomy for either benign or malignant disease. The stomach, however, is occasionally disqualified by caustic burn, scar, ulceration, or previous operation. Under these circumstances the colon becomes a Cinderella.

### HISTORY

Kelling, in 1911, is credited with first using transverse colon to replace the esophagus.[3] Von Hacker employed the right colon in 1914[4] and, 7 years later, Lundblad followed by using colon in the total replacement of a segment of esophagus damaged by a lye stricture in a 3-year-old child.[5] For two decades the operation remained something of a feat; in 1934 Ochsner and Owens were able to find only 20 cases of colonic interposition.[6] Dale and Sherman[7] identified and used the substernal route in 1955, and Waterston[8] and Belsey[9] pioneered the transthoracic route for the left colon in the 1950s and 1960s. Many surgeons attempted these procedures and eventually abandoned them because of frequent complications and high mortalities. Good results were possible, however, as noted by Wilkins and Burke in 1975, when they reported on 30 patients with no colonic necrosis, a single anastomotic leak, and a 6.6% mortality.[10] By 1980, Belsey was able to report 360 reconstructions using the left colon based on the blood supply of the left colic artery.[11] In 1988, DeMeester et al[12] reported on a series of 80 patients with colonic interposition or bypass. The 30-day surgical mortality was 3%. Seventy-six percent of the group were entirely relieved of preoperative symptoms, and the remainder were improved.

### RATIONALE AND INDICATIONS

Champions of colonic substitution have used the organ for virtually every kind of esophageal malady, including, for example, long segment esophageal atresia, malignant tracheoesophageal fistula, esophageal varices, esophagitis with or without stricture, lye burns, esophageal perforation, and failed gastric pull-up or failed operations for achalasia. I reserve the technique for adults with nonmalignant conditions or whose stomach is diseased or has been removed. A three-anastomosis operation for cancer in a cachectic patient may be feasible but is not ordinarily justified. In children, colonic substitution is especially useful for caustic burns or for long-segment esophageal atresias.[13] A special benefit of using the colon is that the surgically displaced colon remembers, albeit variably,[14] its commitment to peristalsis. An interposed colonic segment flushed with a bolus of 0.1 N HCl[15] clears promptly, a worthy trait for an organ recruited to serve both as a conduit and a barrier to reflux. Finally, the left colon has approximately the same caliber as

**TABLE 53–1. REPLACEMENT ORGANS COMPARED**

| Organ | Best Level of Usefulness | Type of Esophageal Lesion | No. of Anastomoses | Inherent Morbidity and Difficulty |
|---|---|---|---|---|
| Stomach | Midesophagus to pharynx | Any lesion amenable to a high anastomosis | 1 | + |
| Small intestine | Lower third | Peptic stricture | 3 | ++ |
| Colon | All | Failed operations at hiatus, lye stricture, childhood stricture or atresia | 3 | +++ |
| Free revascularized graft | Cervical esophagus | Cancer | 5 (including 2 microvascular) | ++++ |

+ = low, ++ = moderate, +++ = high, ++++ = extremely high.

the esophagus, sufficient length, and a generally reliable blood supply.

## ASSESSMENT AND PREPARATION

As with any procedure, the surgeon must assess the patient's general risk factors and the modifiable hazards peculiar to the proposed operation.

Two specific areas of concern are the vascular supply of the intestine and the absence of intrinsic disease. The vascular supply to the intestine can be assessed with a selective transfemoral arteriogram of the superior and inferior mesenteric arteries. Attention should be paid to the size of the parent vessel, the integrity of the arcades close to the colon, and variant anatomy. Angiography must, of course, be performed with an intestine free of contrast material.

There should be little or no intrinsic disease in the portion of colon to be used for substitution. The presence of diverticulitis, polyps, stricture, or a malignant tumor is a contraindication. Although the reassuring confirmation of normal colon with a barium enema radiograph in a child or young adult may not be necessary, a patient older than 40 years should undergo the examination. Ideally, this investigation should take place before the patient is admitted to the hospital but, in any event, at least 5 days before the operation to avoid the presence of retained barium in the perioperative period.

In the preparation of the patient, four major areas need attention:

1. Pulmonary. A regimen of chest percussion and postural drainage is helpful to achieve optimal pulmonary toilet. Esophageal disorders go hand in hand with chronic aspiration. After a transthoracic colonic substitution, furthermore, the patient experiences impairment of the abdominal, diaphragmatic, and intercostal muscles because of pain. An experienced physiotherapist can do much to improve breathing mechanics and prepare the patient for postoperative treatment.
2. Dental. Postoperative pulmonary and mediastinal infection is likely to occur in the presence of oral sepsis. Periodontal infection must be treated and carious teeth removed. It is preferable that the dental work be done before endoscopy.
3. Nutrition. It should be assumed that the patient is malnourished. Measurements of total protein, skin-fold thickness, and tests of anergy are not substitutes for daily weight measurements and common sense. A full discussion of supplementary oral or tube feedings and total parenteral nutrition is beyond the scope of this chapter. It should be emphasized, however, that enteral or parenteral alimentation should begin 5 days before the operation for two reasons. First, the patient has fasted for the radiologic studies and endoscopy; the less starvation the better. Second, although the expectation is that the patient will be swallowing normally by the fifth or sixth postoperative day, this may not be the case. It is wise to be ahead nutritionally.
4. Antibiotic prophylaxis. Given the magnitude of the proposed procedure and the probability of at least microscopic soilage, antibiotic prophylaxis is appropriate. I use an oral antibiotic regimen starting the day before the operation, e.g., erythromycin 1 g and neomycin 1 g given at 1:00 PM, 2:00 PM, and 11 PM. In addition, a cephalosporin, cefoxitin 2 g IV, is administered 1–2 hours before the operation and subsequently every 6 hours for 24 hours.
5. Intestinal preparation. A patient with an obstructive swallowing disorder has been eating a self-determined low-residue diet, leaving the colon with little bulk. A clear liquid diet is given for the 2 days before the operation. If the barium enema radiograph is obtained within a few days of the operation, evacuation of the material must be a high priority. Bowel movement can be promoted with oral bisacodyl 10 mg; cathartics whose action depends on expanding the colon with fluid are apt to lead to liquid spillage and contamination during the operation. For the same reason preoperative enemas are avoided.

## TECHNICAL CONSIDERATIONS

### Preparing the Team

Two teams are ideal in this procedure, one working in the abdomen preparing the intestine and the other working in a semi-isolated manner in the neck.[10] The anesthesiologist, in addition to routine considerations, must comprehend the operative plan so that the surgeon is spared the irritation of working around a jugular vein line or wishing belatedly, in the instance of a thoracotomy, for one-lung ventilation. Finally, placing an epidural catheter to control postoperative pain is helpful, and time for its insertion must be allowed.

## GOALS, STRATEGIES, AND DECISIONS

### Palliation or Cure?

In an operation for cancer, it is useful to know if the extent of disease makes removal of the growth feasible. The goal should determine the surgical approach. For example, substernal bypass of a lesion not to be resected requires the supine position, but the presence of a curable condition in a youth argues for a left thoracotomy and short-segment transplant.

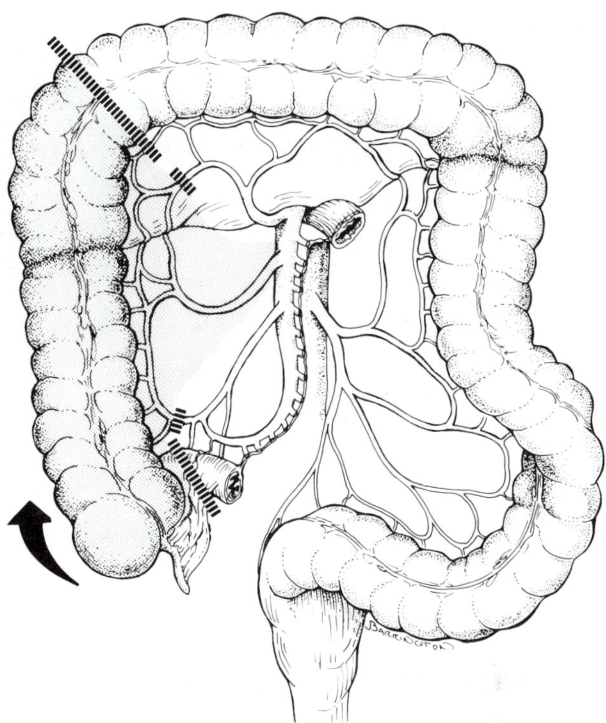

**Figure 53–1.** Right colonic mobilization is easy, but the short vascular pedicle limits its usefulness; the rotated cecum seldom reaches higher than the suprasternal notch.

### Right or Left Colon?

The *right colon* (Fig. 53–1) is the easiest to mobilize and works well enough. Neville and Najem reported satisfactory results in 84% of patients with a 28-year follow-up period.[16] Owing to its variable blood supply, shorter vascular pedicle, and disparate size, however, the right colon is used less commonly now as a replacement segment.

The *left colon* has better caliber, is thicker, and is therefore easier to suture. It can readily span defects from stomach to pharynx because of a straight and usually adequate mesenteric arterial arcade.[10] Belsey noted that the left colon, in contrast to the right, is "trained for a solid bolus."[11] It can be mobilized through the abdomen, transdiaphragmatically through the chest, or through a thoracoabdominal incision. Irrespective of whether right or left colon is used, wide mobilization is done as for a colectomy. The critical difference is avoiding trauma to the vessels in the mesentery and to the intestine itself. Until the graft segment is actually isolated, no clamps are placed and manual traction of intestine and mesentery is kept to a minimum.

### Isoperistaltic or Antiperistaltic?

In its natural location, the colon is committed to unidirectional pulsion. Clinical observation as well as fluoroscopic and manometric studies attest to this.[17] Others reckon the principal thrust to be gravity.[18] Late follow-up contrast studies in some patients do show barium cascading from haustra without discernible peristalsis.[19]

I place the organ in an isoperistaltic direction whenever possible to avoid even the small chance of functional obstruction or reflux and aspiration.

### Route of the Colon

Five routes are possible: subcutaneous, retrosternal, transpleural, posterior mediastinal, and endoesophageal (Fig. 53–2).[20] The latter operation is the brainchild of Saidi,[21] who stripped the mucosa of the esophagus to form a dilatable muscular sleeve through which colon or stomach may be passed to the neck. Ostensible advantages include a short straight lie of the substitute esophagus, prevention of redundancy, minimal blood loss, and elimination of injury to the airway or thoracic duct. Saidi used the endoesophageal pull-through operation in 136 esophageal resections, including 34 in which colon was the transposed organ.[22]

### Free Transplant or Pedicled Graft?

For a cervical lesion, a revascularized free transplant spares excision of a normal thoracic esophagus.[18] This theoretic advantage, however, is more than offset by the necessity for a longer operation with two microvascular and three intestinal anastomoses (see Chap. 54).

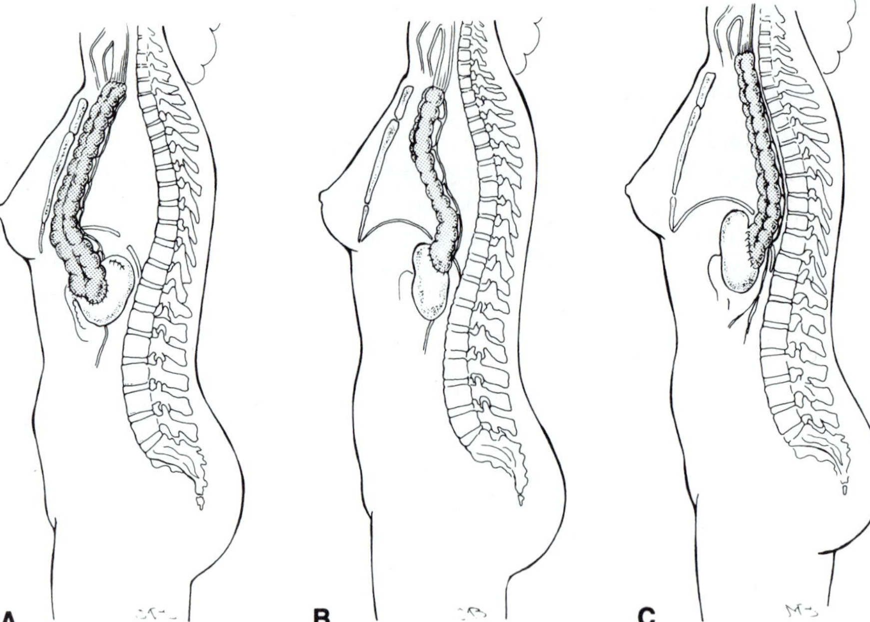


**Figure 53–2.** Three of the five possible routes of explanted colon. **A.** Substernal route. **B.** Transpleural route. **C.** Posterior mediastinal route. If the *substernal route* is used, closure of the peritoneum is begun just caudal to the point where the explant emerges from the abdomen and enters the retrosternal space. *Transpleural* positioning of the graft may be either anterior or posterior to the hilum of the lung.

### Colon or Jejunum?

Jejunum is handy and does not require intestinal preparation, useful characteristics for an ad hoc interposition when stomach or colon is unavailable. Placed in an isoperistaltic position, jejunum is both a reliable transporter of food and a barrier to refluxed acid. Like colon, jejunum is agreeable to suturing because both its wall thickness and diameter approximate those of the esophagus. Jejunum, however, is doomed by vascular arcades that make a long and straight lie next to impossible. It is occasionally useful in reoperations for complicated strictures,[23] failed hiatal reconstruction, or as the Roux-en-Y component of an acid-suppression and alkaline diversion procedure for gastroesophageal reflux disease.[24–26]

### Concomitant Esophagectomy or Not?

Should the diseased esophagus be removed? Omitting removal of a lye stricture, for example, poses the risk of a mucocele, carcinoma, or reflux esophagitis. The true incidence of these lesions is unknown but appears to be low. The risk of excision must be weighed against the more extensive dissection of the mediastinum that may be required to remove the esophagus. I ordinarily perform an excision but not when the patient is extremely old or debilitated or when there is mediastinal fibrosis. In the instance of cancer, a case has been made for bypass followed by radiation and chemotherapy followed by extirpation. The problem with this approach is that too much of the patient's remaining life is consumed with treatment. I prefer a single-stage operation followed by radiation treatment of residual disease.

The approach may be midline abdominal, left thoracic, left thoracoabdominal, or a combination of abdominal and thoracic or cervical depending on the level of the upper anastomosis. Irrespective of the approach, the first step is to determine the suitability of the colon.

### Mobilization of the Colon

The segment of colon to be used is freed to gauge both the health of the organ and the status of the blood supply. Transillumination of the mesentery helps define the vascular anatomy. To accomplish this, the surgeon's headlamp is extinguished temporarily and the operating room light adjusted for back lighting.

### Selection of the Graft

The transverse colon and splenic flexure usually contain the optimal segment with blood supply derived from the left colic artery (Fig. 53–3). Should a long segment be required, the midcolic vessels are divided and ligated close to their origin to preserve collateral circulation.[9] A short-segment colonic graft (for lower esophageal reconstruction) allows the proximal division line to be to the left of the midcolic artery (see Fig. 53–3A). Measurements of the graft reassure the operator that a sufficient length is available *before* the second team transects the upper esophagus. The colon can then be divided, leaving the graft segment tethered by its vascular pedicle. Pulsatile bleeding at the site of the division is a favorable sign, as is pink mucosa and absence of venous congestion. If these portents are less than ideal, a warm moist pack is placed on the graft, the blood supply is straightened, and the operating team waits and watches.

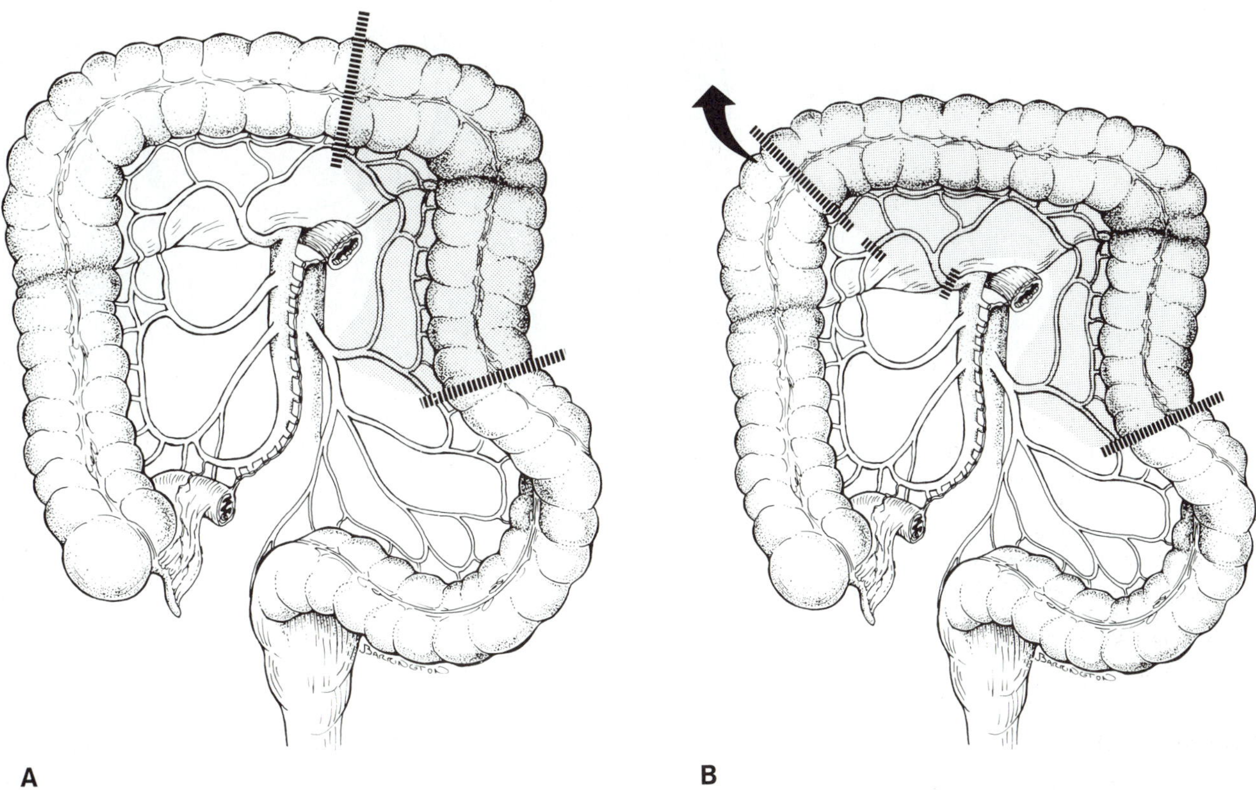


**Figure 53–3.** Left colonic mobilization. The left colon can be used to span either a short (**A**) or a long (**B**) esophageal defect. The ascending limb of the left colic artery is the critical vessel.

## Exposure of the Cervical Esophagus

Incision is made along the anterior border of either sternocleidomastoid muscle extending from the suprasternal notch to the thyroid cartilage. If one is right-handed, it is easier to work from the right. Division of the omohyoid muscle, branches of the ansa hypoglossal nerve, and middle thyroid veins allows retraction of the carotid sheath laterally and the thyroid and trachea medially. The ipsilateral recurrent laryngeal nerve lies between esophagus and trachea at the level of the inferior thyroid artery; traction or retraction must be avoided. The contralateral nerve is spared if the operator hugs the esophagus with the encircling instruments and tape.

## Route Development

An extrapleural retrosternal tunnel is developed with blunt finger dissection. It is usually possible to pass one's hand from below upward into the cervical wound. Irrespective of the thoracic route of the colon, the segment selected is passed posterior to the stomach to provide the most direct path for its vascular pedicle. The colonic segment is covered with a plastic bag the surface of which is moistened with saline solution. The plastic bag helps to prevent soilage and the saline solution affords lubrication. The upper end of the graft is inspected for venous engorgement. If there is any doubt, the graft is withdrawn and passed again to be certain there is no twisting or kinking of the vessels. If the substernal route has been chosen, excision of the manubrium and medial head of the clavicle may be required to avoid crowding at the thoracic inlet.

## Anastomoses

The abdominal team completes the colocolic and cologastric anastomoses while the thoracic team performs the esophagocolic approximation. Conventional two-layer technique is used for anastomosing the colon to the anterior aspect of the mid stomach if the substernal route is used or to the posterior aspect if the transthoracic approach is used. The colonic segment should drain through a straight line (Fig. 53–4). We agree with DeMeester et al[12] that in tailoring the distal end of the transplant the mesentery should be left untrimmed. The cervical anastomosis is performed with interrupted 4-0 silk for the seromuscular layer and chromic catgut or polyglactin 910 for the mucosal layer. Repeated grabbing with forceps causes trauma to the mucosa and should be avoided. Sutures are taken approximately 4 mm back from the edge and about the same interval apart so as not to compromise the blood supply. Before the cervical wound is closed, a $\frac{3}{8}$-inch Penrose drain is inserted both as an indicator wick and as a vent for fluid.

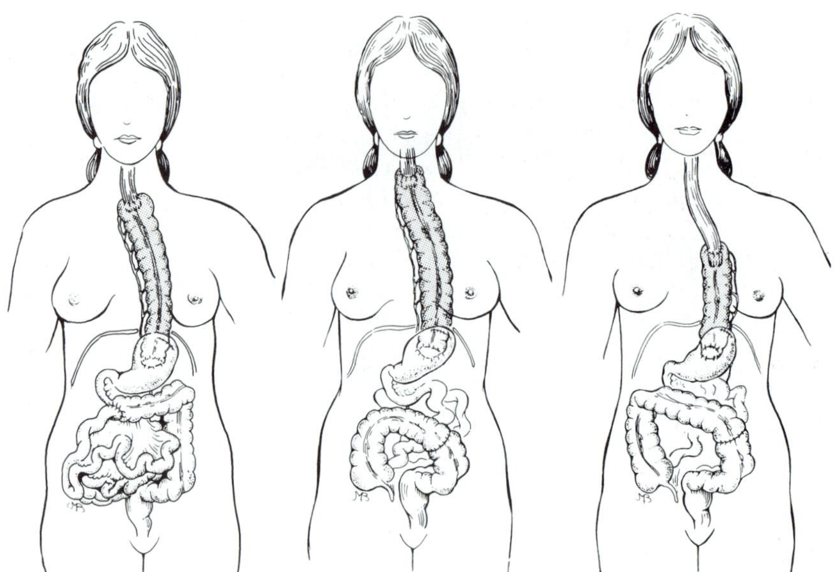

**Figure 53–4.** Completed appearance of several options. A straight line without tension is the essential feature.

### Pyloroplasty, Gastrostomy, Jejunostomy

Pyloroplasty is not invariably essential to gastric emptying. Besides, it may be followed by dumping symptoms. If the patient is operated on through the abdomen and if the patient has a history of duodenal ulcer, however, a pyloroplasty is done. It is not possible to perform a pyloroplasty through the left transthoracic transdiaphragmatic approach; therefore, this route is not chosen if there is a history of gastric outlet obstruction. A Witzel gastrostomy affords a vent pending return of peristalsis. Jejunostomy is done using the needle-catheter technique. Temporary decompression of the colonic segment can be achieved with a Levine tube.

## POSTOPERATIVE CARE

Pulse, temperature, blood pressure, central venous pressure, pulmonary capillary wedge pressure, ECG, and arterial blood gases are usually monitored. A chest radiograph is taken on arrival to the intensive care unit and repeated at least once daily for 3 days and again before discharge. Measurements of hemoglobin and hematocrit are determined in the recovery area and repeated daily for 3 days and again before discharge. Measurements of urine output, BUN, and creatinine are checked as indicated by history and postoperative course. A discussion of monitoring for parenteral nutrition is beyond the scope of this chapter.

Fluid requirements in the first 24 hours may be considerable both because of the patient's depleted state and because of the large internal wound occasioned by the dissection of intestine, retroperitoneum, and mediastinum.

### Drains and Tubes

Early weaning from the respirator in the recovery room is recommended. The gastrostomy tube is irrigated with water or saline solution every 2 hours and is placed on gentle suction the remainder of the time. I have identified venous infarction on the night of operation by profuse bloody drainage from the drain site. A chest tube is used in every thoracotomy, but if the substernal route has been used, a thoracotomy catheter is placed only if the chest radiograph shows a pneumothorax or fluid collection.

### Nutrition

Elemental feedings through the jejunostomy tube are started on the first or second day. Oral fare is withheld until flatus is passed and there is evidence that the graft segment is emptying well. A Gastrografin (meglumine diatrizoate) swallow is useful in determining the latter. The weight of swallowed fluid in the colonic segment must be considered a distracting force on the upper anastomosis, and feeding the patient too soon or too much may be a factor in anastomotic dehiscence.

### Pain Control

A thoughtful discussion with the patient before the operation does much to allay anxiety afterward. Beyond this, the use of an epidural catheter for narcotic analgesia, patient-controlled analgesia, and avoidance of opening the chest retractor more than 3 inches (7.5 cm) during the operation constitute the principal components of pain control.

## COMPLICATIONS

### Anastomotic Leak

Cervical esophageal anastomotic leak used to occur in as many as one fourth of patients; stricture developed in about half of these patients.[26] Leakage is treated with drainage, and stricture with endoscopic dilation or eventual revision of the anastomosis. Colonic ischemia occurs in 3–8%[10,26] of patients and is fatal unless the dead graft is promptly removed. Venous infarction, secondary to kinking and stretching or compression of the veins draining the colonic segment, is a second important cause of graft failure. The remedy is prevention. Antibiotics can obscure symptoms and thereby delay diagnosis. Although dead intestine may present on the third or fourth postoperative day, the critical vascular event doubtless occurs during or immediately after the operation.

## SUMMARY

A pedicled isoperistaltic segment of colon, especially left colon, is a useful substitute for excised esophagus. Although it becomes indispensable when the stomach is diseased or unavailable, a surgeon may elect to use colon routinely for reasons of personal preference. Versatility. Competence. These are the right stuff in esophageal surgery.

## REFERENCES

1. Akiyama H, Miyazono H, Tsurumaru M, et al: Use of the stomach as an esophageal substitute. *Ann Surg* **188**:606–610, 1978
2. Huang GJ: Replacement of the esophagus with stomach. In Shields TW: *General Thoracic Surgery,* 3rd ed., Philadelphia, Lea & Febiger, 1989, Chap 39, p 433
3. Kelling GE: Esophagoplasty with the aid of the transverse colon (Oesophagoplastik mit Hilfe der Querkolon). *Zentralbl Chir* **38**:1209, 1911
4. Von Hacker V: On esophagoplasty in general and on the repair of the esophagus by the antethoracic construction of a skin-colon tube in particular (Ueber Oesophagoplastik in allgemeinen under über den Ersatz der Speiserohre durch Antethorakale Haut Dickdarmschlauchbildung im besonderen). *Arch Klin Chir* **105**:973, 1914 (Cited by Saint: *Arch Surg* **19**:53, 1929)
5. Lundblad O: Ueber antethorakale oesophagoplastik. *Acta Chir Scand* **53**:535, 1921
6. Ochsner A, Owens N: Anterothoracic oesophagoplasty for impermeable stricture of the esophagus. *Ann Surg* **100**:1055, 1934
7. Dale WA, Sherman CD Jr: Late reconstruction of congenital esophageal atresia by intrathoracic colon transplantation. *J Thorac Surg* **29**:344, 1955
8. Waterston D: Colonic replacement of esophagus (intrathoracic). *Surg Clin North Am* **44**:1441, 1964
9. Belsey R: Reconstruction of the esophagus with left colon. *J Thorac Cardiovasc Surg* **49**:33, 1965
10. Wilkins EW Jr, Burke JF: Colon esophageal carcinoma. *Am J Surg* **129**:394, 1975
11. Belsey R: Palliative management of esophageal carcinoma. *Am J Surg* **139**:789, 1980
12. DeMeester TR, Johansson K, Franze I, et al: Indications, surgical technique, and long-term functional results of colon interposition or bypass. *Ann Surg* **208**:460, 1988
13. Kelly JP, Shackelford GD, Roper CL: Esophageal replacement with colon in children: Functional results and long-term growth. *Ann Thorac Surg* **36**:634, 1983
14. Moreno-Osset E, Tomas-Tidocci M, Paris F, et al: Motor activity of esophageal substitute (stomach, jejunal, and colonic segments). *Ann Thorac Surg* **41**:515, 1986
15. Jones EL, Skinner DB, DeMeester TR, et al: Response of the interposed human colonic segment to an acid challenge. *Ann Surg* **177**:75, 1973
16. Neville WE, Najem AZ: Colon replacement of the esophagus for congenital and benign disease. *Ann Thorac Surg* **3**:636, 1983
17. Postlethwait RW: Colonic interposition for esophageal substitution. *Surg Gynecol Obstet* **156**:377, 1983
18. Sieber AM, Sieber WK: Colon transplants as esophageal replacement: Cineradiographic and manometric evaluation in children. *Ann Surg* **168**:116, 1968
19. Matthews HR: Colon replacement of the oesophagus. In Jackson JW, Cooper DKC (eds): *Rob and Smith's Operative Surgery (Thoracic Surgery),* 4th ed. London, Butterworths, 1983, pp 357–362
20. Postlethwait RW, *Surgery of the Esophagus* 2nd ed., Norwalk, Appleton-Century-Crofts, 1986, pp 469–524
21. Saidi F: Endoesophageal pull through. *Ann Surg* **207**:446, 1988
22. Saidi F: Transhiatal endoesophageal pullthrough operation. In Pearson FG, Deslauriers J, Ginsberg RJ, et al (eds): *Thoracic Surgery/Esophageal Surgery,* New York, Churchill Livingstone, 1995, Chap 46, pp 719–728
23. Polk HC Jr, Richardson JD: Non-functional esophagogastric junction: Treatment by jejunal interposition. *Serono Symposia,* **43**: 188, 1981
24. Ellis FH Jr, Anderson HA, Clagett OT: Treatment of short esophagus with stricture by esophagogastrectomy and antral exclusion. *Ann Surg* **148**:526, 1958
25. Fekete F, Pateron D: What is the place of antrectomy with Roux-en-Y in the treatment of reflux disease? Experience with 83 total duodenal diversions. *World J Surg* **16**:349, 1992
26. Shackelford RT: *Surgery of the Alimentary Tract,* Philadelphia, Saunders, 1978, Vol 1, 2nd ed

CHAPTER

# 54

# Esophageal Replacement

## *Microvascular Jejunal Transplantation*

Christian E. Paletta and M. J. Jurkiewicz

### HISTORY

Many techniques have been used through the years to reconstruct the cervical esophagus. The simplest technique is application of a split-thickness skin graft within a tube developed from the adjacent pharynx and esophagus. This method is rarely applicable in large resections and has a high rate of stricture with contracture of the skin graft.

Wookey in 1942 described a second method for cervical esophageal reconstruction using lateral neck flaps.[1] These flaps were initially designed as a tube, leaving a lateral cervical sinus. Several weeks later, the sinus track was closed and the skin-tube for swallowing established. In 1965, Bakamjian introduced the deltopectoral flap in head and neck reconstruction. This flap, based on medial perforators from the internal mammary artery,[2] is transposed to the neck and a tube made for esophageal replacement. It is also a two-stage procedure with initial division of the base of the flap and later insertion into the esophageal remnant.

Myocutaneous flaps were developed in the 1970s.[3] The pectoralis major muscle can be transposed to the neck with an overlying skin island, deriving its blood supply from the thoracoacromial vessels. The skin island can then be made into a tube for esophageal replacement. However, this flap is not the first choice in cervical esophageal replacement because of its bulk.

A third method mobilizes the stomach or colon to the neck in a single stage as an interpositional graft. With adequate mobilization, the stomach or colon can adequately reach the middle or lower neck region. However, there may be excessive tension when these organs are mobilized to the base of the tongue (see Chapters 52 and 53).

A fourth method is microvascular transfer of a jejunal segment to the neck. Alexis Carrel first described this technique in 1907 when he successfully transplanted the small intestine into the neck of a dog.[4] In 1946, Longmire and Ravitch described a technique of augmenting the blood supply to a transferred loop of jejunum in esophageal reconstruction for lye stricture.[5] Using loupe magnification, they performed an end-to-end anastomosis of the primary mesenteric vessel of an ischemic jejunal segment to the internal mammary vessels. In 1959, Seidenberg et al performed the first free jejunal transplantation in a patient.[6] During the 1960s, there were multiple case reports of cervical esophageal replacement with a revascularized segment of jejunum.[7]

Free tissue transfer emerged from the domain of experimental surgery during the 1970s with the development of microsurgical techniques and instrumentation. A variety of tissues were suitable for distant transfer, including muscle (latissimus dorsi, gracilis, rectus abdominis), cutaneous flaps (groin, scapular), osteal flaps (iliac crest and fibula), and intestine (jejunum, ileum, and colon).

As the success of microvascular free tissue transfer reached 90–95%, the use of the free jejunal graft was established.[8] The primary advantage of the free jejunal transfer is that it can be used as a one-stage procedure without disrupting the continuity of the gastroesophageal junction and pylorus.

### ANATOMY

The blood supply of the jejunum and the ileum comes from the superior mesenteric artery, which originates from the anterior wall of the abdominal aorta just below the celiac axis. It courses behind the neck of the pancreas and anterior to the third portion of the duodenum. Its first major branch is the middle colic artery. It also gives rise to the right colic artery, the ileocolic artery, and multiple segmental jejunal and ileal arterial branches.

There are normally 12–15 intestinal arterial branches from the superior mesenteric artery to the jejunum and ileum. Each intestinal artery divides into branches, which unite to form an arcade within the mesentery of the jejunum and ileum. In the proximal jejunum the intestinal arteries are long and straight, with a single arcade pattern near the mesenteric wall of the small intestine. As one progresses distally in the jejunum and ileum, the intestinal arteries become shorter. A series of arcades develop to the point where in the terminal ileum the intestinal arteries are quite short and there is a multitude of arcades within the mesentery. For this reason, the ideal segment of small intestine for microvascular transfer is the proximal jejunum, because one can obtain a long vascular pedicle and avoid interpositional vein grafts.

The length of the vascular pedicle ranges between 8 and 12 cm. The lumen of the artery and vein is between 1.5 and 3.0 mm. In the proximal jejunum, a segment of intestine up to 22 cm long can be transferred on a single vascular pedicle.

## INDICATIONS AND CONTRAINDICATIONS

Indications for jejunal transplantation are listed in Table 54–1. The primary indication is for reconstruction of the cervical esophagus after radical resection. Most patients have undergone a partial or complete pharyngolaryngectomy for squamous cell carcinoma in the supraglottic, glottic, or subglottic region. For smaller tumors in this region, a partial pharyngectomy allows an adequate amount of pharyngeal tissue to be preserved for closure. Many of these patients receive either preoperative or postoperative irradiation. Some then experience a stricture with or without an accompanying fistula. This can be very difficult to alleviate with dilation alone, and it is usually best to resect the irradiated and scarred tissue and perform free jejunal replacement.

This technique can also be used for the treatment of benign, isolated, cervical esophageal strictures that have not responded to dilation. If a stricture due to caustic ingestion is limited to the upper portion of the esophagus, a free jejunal graft can adequately replace the diseased segment. If, on the other hand, caustic ingestion has produced a diffuse stricture involving more than a 25-cm length of the esophagus, the stomach or colon should be used.

There are several contraindications to microvascular free jejunal esophageal reconstruction (Table 54–2). If the patient is in too poor a condition to undergo a 6-hour operation, a jejunal reconstruction should not be performed. The procedure is a highly technical one. Although blood loss is usually minimal, technical difficulties can arise and prolong the procedure. In addition, thrombosis may occur in either the arterial or venous anastomosis, necessitating re-exploration soon after the operation. Patients should have adequate cardiopulmonary reserve.

Either the transverse cervical artery or a branch of the external carotid artery can serve for inflow to the free jejunal transplant. Severe atherosclerosis involving the carotid vessels should be evaluated before the free jejunal transplant. If the patient has had a previous carotid endarterectomy, finding appropriate recipient vessels may be difficult. An end-to-side anastomosis to the external carotid or the use of the thyrocervical trunk is an option.

Another contraindication is patient age less than 3 years, because the jejunal vessels are too small for safe transfer. The youngest patient upon whom we performed a transplant was 3 years of age. A history of intestinal adhesions from peritonitis or multiple previous abdominal operations is a relative contraindication. Intestine with inflammatory or benign lesions in the proximal portion is not used for microvascular transfer.

**TABLE 54–1. INDICATIONS FOR FREE JEJUNAL TRANSPLANTATION**

1. Pharyngeal and cervical esophageal replacement following:
   (a) extensive resection of neoplasms of the oropharynx, hypopharynx, larynx, or cervical esophagus
   (b) extensive trauma to the pharynx or cervical esophagus (e.g., motor vehicle collision, gun-shot wound to the neck)
   (c) caustic ingestion refractory to repeat dilation
2. Recurrent pharyngeal or cervical esophageal stricture
3. Persistent pharyngeal or cervical esophageal fistula after tumor resection or trauma
4. Cervical esophageal replacement when a gastric pull-up or colonic interposition is not possible because of previous gastric or colon operation
5. Replacement of intraoral lining after oropharyngeal tumor resection or trauma

## SURGICAL TECHNIQUE

The operative approach depends on whether the reconstruction is done immediately following pharyngolaryngo-

**TABLE 54–2. CONTRAINDICATIONS TO FREE JEJUNAL TRANSPLANTATION**

1. Patient's condition not stable enough for prolonged operation
2. Age less than 3 years, because the vessels are too small for microvascular anatomosis
3. Extensive carotid atherosclerotic disease
4. Extensive intestinal adhesions
5. Inflammatory bowel disease
6. Benign tumors of the small intestine (eg, Gardner's syndrome)

esophagectomy or several months to years later for a complication of a resection and irradiation (stricture or fistula). If reconstruction is immediate, the jejunal dissection should be delayed until an adequate tumor resection has been performed and instruments and drapes have been changed.

Following tumor resection, a two-team approach minimizes operative time. One surgical team dissects the appropriate recipient cervical artery and vein while a second team performs a laparotomy to obtain the jejunal segment. When done as an immediate procedure, dissection in the neck usually goes rapidly, because the tissue planes have already been dissected and the recipient artery is not bound in scarred, irradiated tissue. If, during the dissection of the recipient artery, an appropriate artery cannot be isolated, one should go to the opposite side of the neck to find a suitable artery. Fortunately, this is made possible by the adequate length of the intestinal arterial donor vessel. If the esophageal reconstruction is done as an immediate procedure, the transverse cervical artery and vein are excellent recipient vessels, because they are normally outside the field of resection. If the transverse cervical vessels are not available, one can dissect the various branches of the external carotid artery and choose the one best suited (eg, the lingual artery, occipital artery, or superior thyroid artery). The draining vein is often more of a problem than the recipient artery. The internal jugular vein is usually resected with the tumor and neck dissection. If one can preserve the external jugular vein during resection, this can provide an excellent source of venous drainage. If the internal jugular vein is not available, one should turn to the transverse cervical vein or use a vein graft to the opposite neck for venous drainage.

Once the recipient vessels have been isolated, the margins of the pharyngeal and esophageal lumens are identified and adequately mobilized. The neck is then ready for the jejunal transplant.

The donor site dissection begins with exploration of the abdominal cavity. Palpation of the liver is performed routinely to assess intrinsic liver disease (cirrhosis) and to rule out the uncommon but real possibility of metastatic disease. In addition, manual exploration of the spleen, colon, small intestine, and para-aortic region is accomplished.

The ligament of Treitz is identified. A segment of jejunum is chosen approximately 15–30 cm distal to the ligament of Treitz. The primary determining factor for the segment of jejunum chosen for transplantation is the length of the mesentery along the transplanted portion. Once an appropriate segment has been identified, 3-0 silk sutures are placed along the serosa of the jejunum, both proximally and distally, to mark the segment to be dissected. The mesenteric arcade of this segment is evaluated with transillumination. Usually, there are two intestinal arteries to this segment. In most patients, 10–15 cm of jejunum is required for cervical esophageal replacement. After identification of the arteries to the segment of jejunum, an incision is made into the mesentery past the arterial arcade. A parallel incision is made in the mesentery on the opposite side as well. The vascular interconnections with the adjacent proximal and distal arcades are carefully dissected, clamped, and tied with 3-0 silk suture. Once a pedicle length of approximately 10 cm has been obtained, the intestinal artery is carefully separated from the intestinal vein. These vessels are fragile and must be handled with utmost care.

Intestinal clamps are placed both proximally and distally on the jejunum segment. This segment is then divided but is still attached to its vascular pedicle. The segment for transplantation is placed on a moist towel while intestinal continuity is re-established with either a one- or two-layer technique (Fig. 54–1).

Following completion of the anastomosis, the segment of jejunum to be transferred is carefully inspected for viability. One usually has dissected several extra centimeters of jejunum. This can be discarded if its viability is in question.

The jejunal segment is ready for transfer to the neck. The radial intestinal artery is clamped first to prevent engorgement of the jejunal segment. The vein is clamped, and the intestinal vessels are transected and ligated with 3-0 silk suture. The ends of the intestinal artery and vein are carefully irrigated with a heparin solution before anastomosis in the neck.

It is essential that the intestinal vessels not be ligated until the neck dissection is completed and the recipient vessels appropriately prepared. With this technique, the ischemia time of the jejunal transplant is kept to a minimum. In most cases, ischemia time is less than 60 min. Thus, we have not found it necessary to cool the transplanted segment to prevent ischemic damage to the mucosa.

With the transplant in the neck, a posterior row of sutures is placed both proximally in the pharynx and distally in the esophagus. This secures the jejunum in place and helps determine the length of its vascular pedicle to prevent kinking. The intestine is normally placed in an isoperistaltic manner.

The operating microscope is brought into the field. The more difficult or deeper anastomosis is performed first. The microvascular anastomosis is performed usually in an end-to-end manner with interrupted 9-0 or 10-0 nylon or polypropylene.

Once the microvascular anastomoses have been accomplished and there are no leaks, the microvascular clamps are removed. Immediately, one should see pulsations in the mesenteric arcade and peristalsis in the jejunum. Careful inspection ensures that there is no kink or twist in the intestinal vessels. The mesentery is usually bulky and can be used to cover an adjacent exposed carotid artery (Fig. 54–2).

A No. 16 or No. 18 F red rubber catheter is passed into the nose through the jejunal segment and into the upper esophagus. The purpose of the catheter is to provide adequate drainage for saliva and intestinal secretions through the jejunal transplant during its collapsed state in the early

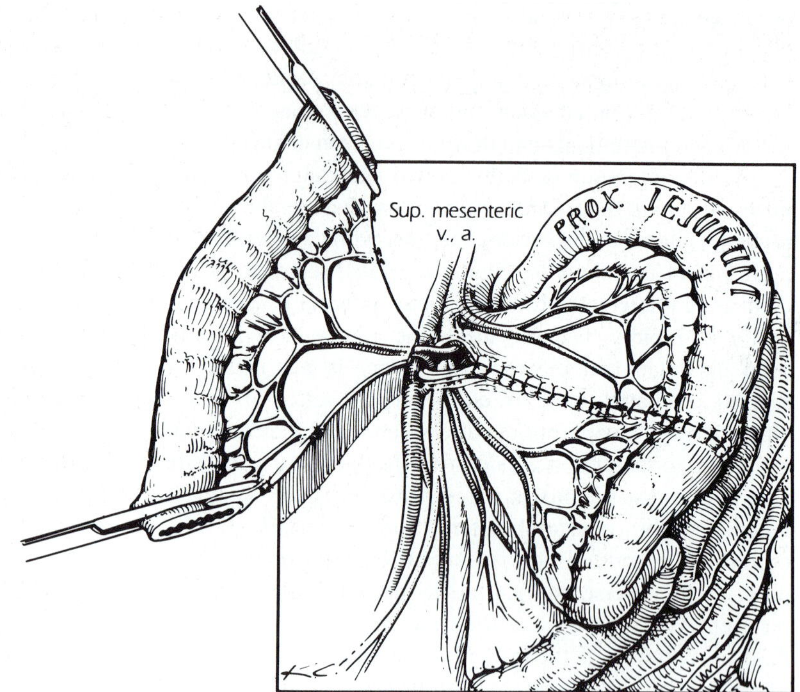


**Figure 54–1.** A segment of proximal jejunum has been dissected with its vascular pedicle. The proximal intestinal continuity has been re-established and the mesenteric defect closed. *(From Jurkiewicz MJ, Paletta CE: Free jejunal graft. In Grillo HC, Austen WG, Wilkins EW, Mathisen DJ, Vlahakes GJ (eds): Current Therapy in Cardiothoracic Surgery, Philadelphia, B.C. Decker, Inc., 1989.)*

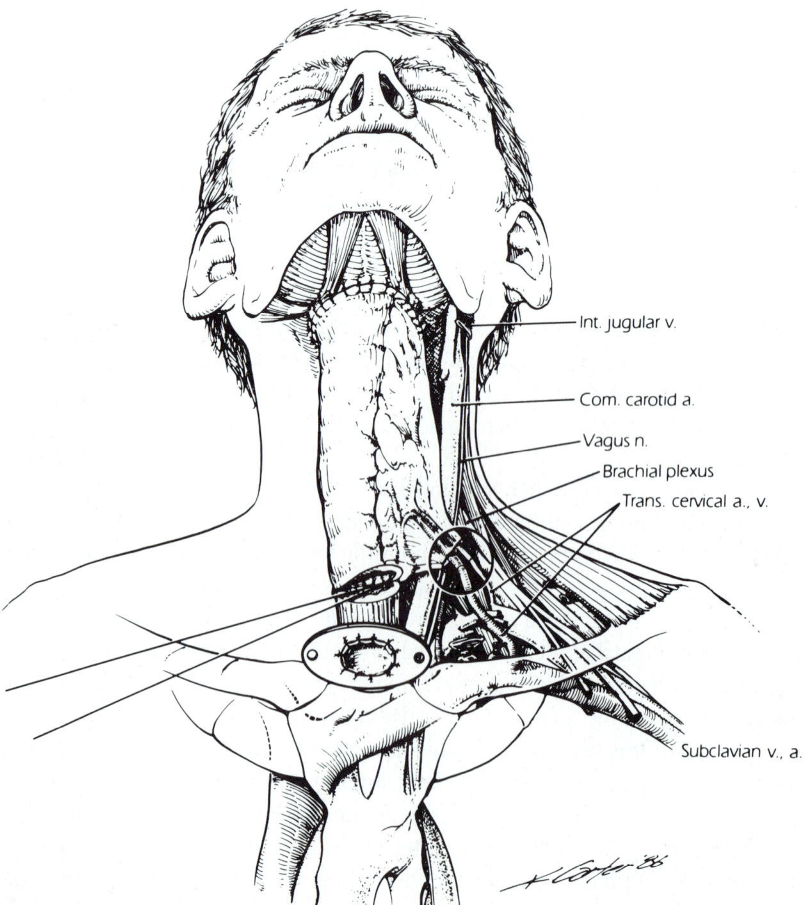


**Figure 54–2.** The jejunal segment has been transplanted to the neck. The proximal suture line has been completed. The jejunal vascular pedicle has been anastomosed to adjacent neck vessels. *(From Jurkiewicz MJ, Paletta CE: Free jejunal graft. In Grillo HC, Austen WG, Wilkins EW, Mathisen DJ, Vlahakes GJ (eds): Current Therapy in Cardiothoracic Surgery. Philadelphia, B.C. Decker, Inc., 1989.)*

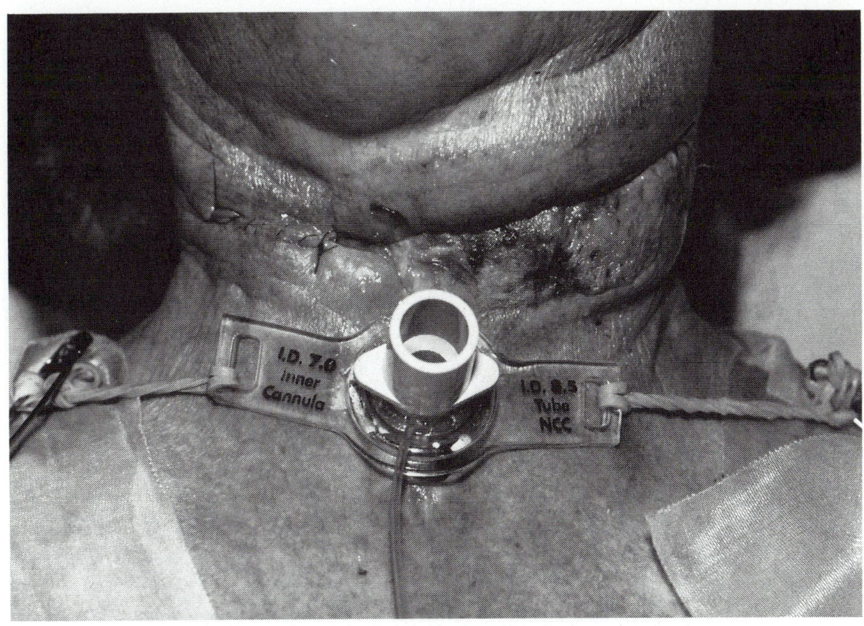


**Figure 54–3.** This patient underwent laryngopharyngectomy and irradiation for squamous cell carcinoma of the larynx. The pharyngoesophageal suture line broke down, and the patient presented with a chronic fistula in her neck.

postoperative period. The anterior wall of the transplanted jejunum is then sutured. Saline solution is introduced into the posterior pharynx through the mouth to determine the presence of any anastomotic leak.

After completion of the microvascular anastomosis, low-molecular-weight dextran is given IV and continued for 5 days. The neck wound is closed with skin flaps. A portion of the jejunum is covered with a meshed skin graft. Both the color and peristalsis of the jejunum can be observed and monitored carefully through this "window" postoperatively (Figs. 54–3 to 54–6).

Following removal of the jejunal segment from the abdomen, the abdominal closure is performed in a routine manner. A feeding jejunostomy is normally placed distal to the jejunal anastomosis for early postoperative feeding. The feeding jejunostomy can be very useful if complications arise in the neck. In addition, a gastrostomy is placed both to prevent the necessity of a nasogastric tube through the jejunal transplant in the neck and for adequate gastric decompression.

The patient begins jejunal tube feedings on the second or third postoperative day. A barium swallow radiograph is obtained on the seventh postoperative day to determine the integrity of the proximal and distal jejunal anastomoses. If a leak is not demonstrated, the patient begins ingesting clear liquids. Oral feedings are then advanced as tolerated. Most

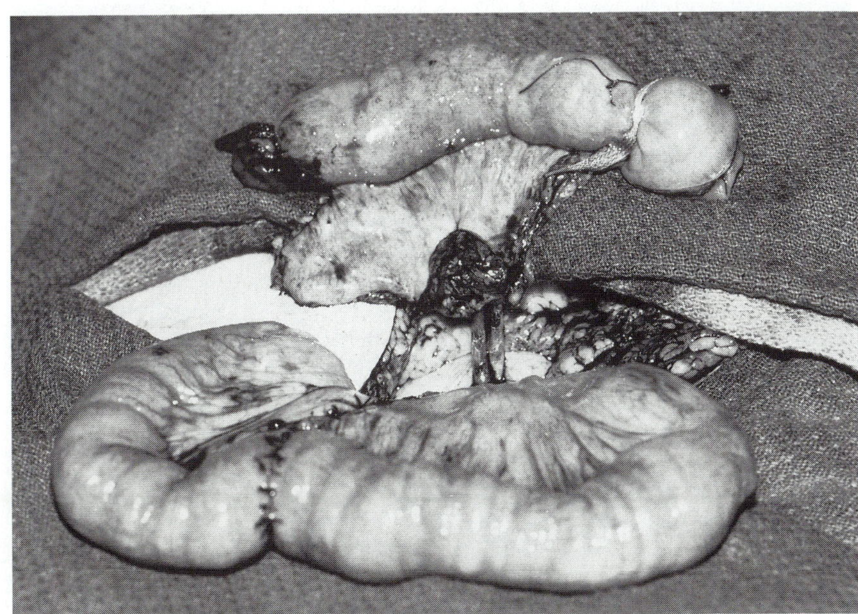

**Figure 54–4.** An 18-cm portion of proximal jejunum has been dissected on its vascular pedicle. The jejunal continuity has been reestablished.

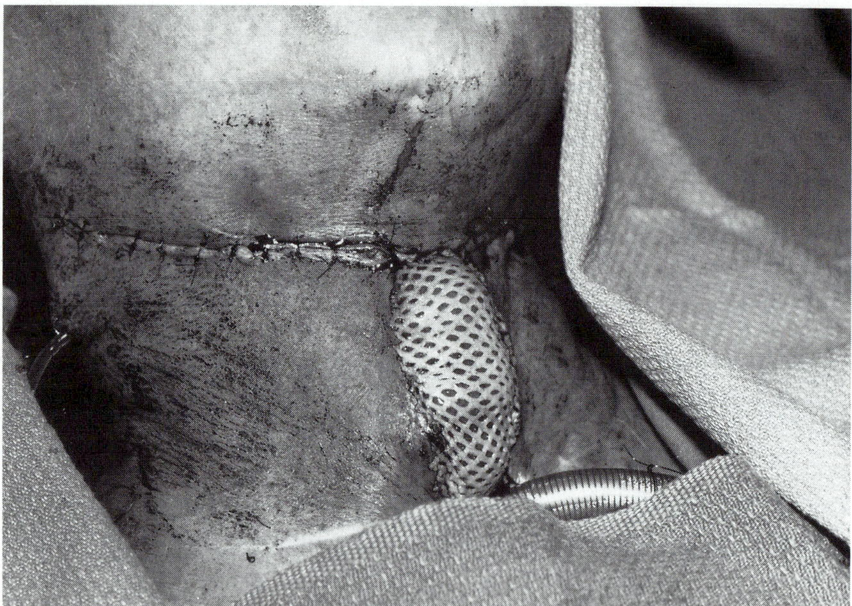

**Figure 54–5.** The segment of jejunum has been transplanted to the neck. Vascular anastomoses have been accomplished with the transverse cervical artery and vein. A meshed, split-thickness skin graft has been placed over the jejunal transplant. Intestinal viability and peristalsis can be monitored through this graft.

patients can resume essentially normal oral intake within 2 weeks of the transplant. The feeding jejunostomy is left intact in the event of any late postoperative complications. It is removed 6–8 weeks after the operation. The gastrostomy tube is clamped and removed after discharge.

## RESULTS

There are now more than 500 reported cases of jejunal autotransplantation in cervical esophageal reconstruction. The graft survival rate ranges between 85% and 95% (Table 54–3). In the Emory University series, there were 111 grafts with 96 graft survivals (86.5% graft survival rate).[9–13] Harashina reported 40 small-intestine transplants, with only one case of partial graft necrosis.[14] In a retrospective review Schusterman et al compared different methods of total reconstruction of the hypopharynx and cervical esophagus. Based on return of oral alimentation and shortened length of hospitalization, free jejunal transfer has become their preference for pharyngoesophageal reconstruction.[12]

The perioperative mortality in the Emory series was 5%. This compares favorably with a 19% mortality reported by Ujiki et al in a series of 42 patients who underwent a gastric pull-up for pharyngoesophageal reconstruction.[15] The mortality for free jejunal transplantation also compares favorably with that in Postlethwait's series. Postlethwait reported a 25% postoperative mortality using colonic interpo-

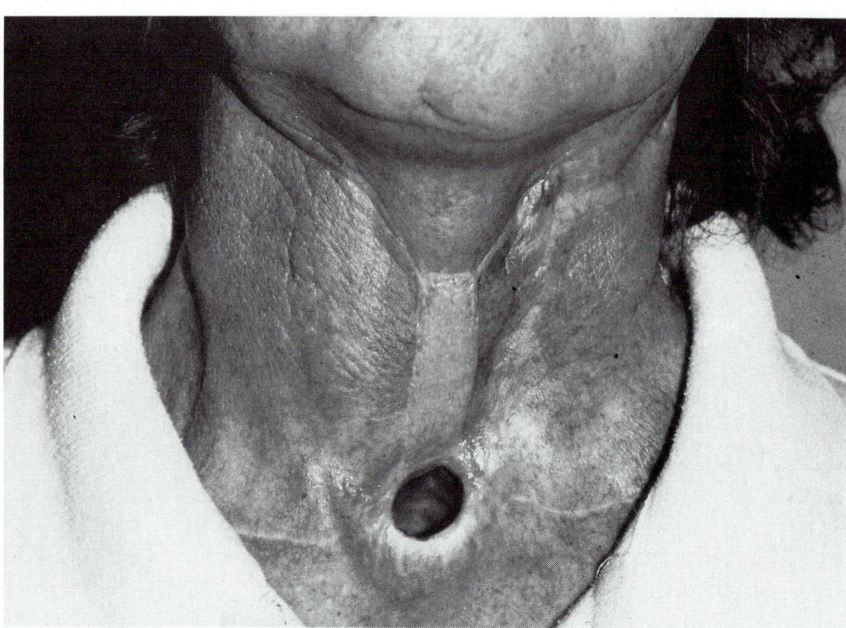

**Figure 54–6.** Two months postoperatively, the jejunal transplant is functioning well as a conduit. The graft has healed and the patient is swallowing without difficulty.

**TABLE 54–3. RESULTS OF JEJUNAL TRANSPLANTATION**

| Study (No. of Grafts) | Graft Survival Rate (%) | Perioperative Mortality (%) | Successful Swallowing Rate (%) |
|---|---|---|---|
| Emory[9] (n = 111) | 86 | 5 | 83 |
| MD Anderson[10] (n = 50) | 94 | 2 | 88 |
| Duke[11] (n = 47) | 89 | 8 | 92 |

sition and a 28% mortality using an isoperistaltic gastric tube for esophageal bypass.[16,17] Because the technique of free jejunal transplantation avoids mediastinal dissection and gastric mobilization, many of the complications associated with these procedures in patients at high risk are avoided. These include postoperative gastroesophageal reflux, mediastinitis, empyema, and abdominal abscesses.

Adequate postoperative swallowing can be achieved in 80–90% of patients with free jejunal transplantation. Although there is no evidence that jejunal transplantation prolongs survival after resection for malignant disease, it does provide palliation, with improved nutrition and oral satisfaction for the patient. Because transplantation can be achieved in one stage with a relatively short hospital stay, the benefit of palliation is maximized. The patient can assume a normal eating pattern for the remainder of his or her life without having to spend a prolonged period of time in a hospital undergoing multiple staged procedures. In addition, because mediastinal dissection and gastric mobilization are unnecessary, complications associated with these procedures and prolonged hospitalization are avoided.

Postoperative function of the jejunal transplant was evaluated by Meyers et al.[18] They used cinefluoroscopy, manometry, and electrical studies to examine nine patients who underwent jejunal autotransplantation for replacement of the pharyngoesophagus. They demonstrated free passage of liquid through the grafts. Solid materials exhibited some delay in passage, but there was no clinically significant functional obstruction at radiographic analysis. A variety of esophageal contractile patterns were noted. However, these did not correlate with any symptoms of dysphagia. Interestingly, the authors found an increase in the electrical activity in the transplanted jejunal segment after instillation of food into the stomach. They suggested a hormonal mechanism separate from any neural pathway, because the nerve fibers are transected during jejunal transplantation.

McConnel et al used manofluorography to evaluate deglutition in patients who underwent total laryngopharyngectomy.[19] They compared swallowing in patients who had undergone reconstruction with either a gastric pull-up or a jejunal graft. In a series of 10 patients, the authors found prolonged swallowing in all patients. They correlated the presence of jejunal contractions with symptoms of dysphagia. They concluded that the most important determinant of swallowing was a widely patent and nonmotile graft segment.

**TABLE 54–4. COMPLICATIONS OF FREE JEJUNAL TRANSPLANTATIONS**

**Donor Site**
- Breakdown of jejunal anastomosis
- Small-intestinal obstruction
- Abdominal wall dehiscence
- Prolonged postoperative ileus

**Recipient Site**
- Infection
- Microvascular thrombosis leading to partial or complete graft loss
- Anastomotic stricture or stenosis
- Pharyngocutaneous fistula
- Pseudoaneurysm at arterial anastomosis
- Dysphagia

**TABLE 54–5. ADVANTAGES OF FREE JEJUNAL TRANSPLANTATION**

1. The jejunal free graft is easy to harvest.
2. The intestinal jejunal vessels are well suited for microvascular anastomosis.
3. The diameter of the lumen in the jejunum is similar to that of the cervical esohagus.
4. The size and consistency of the jejunal segment best match the cervical esophagus compared with regional skin flaps, muscle flaps, or colon.
5. The jejunal transplant is a one-stage procedure that can be performed either for immediate reconstruction after resection or as a delayed reconstruction after the development of a stricture or fistula.
6. Rate of successful microvascular transfer is 90–95%.
7. Adequate swallowing is obtained in most patients usually within 7–10 days of the operation, thereby achieving effective palliation of the patient's preoperative dysphagia.
8. The functional integrity of the upper gastrointestinal tract is preserved (i.e., the gastroesophageal junction and the pylorus).
9. Mortality is low: <5%.
10. If the initial transfer fails, another jejunal graft can be harvested.
11. Incidence of postoperative stricture and fistula is low.
12. The proximal and distal anastomoses are tension-free, even when the graft is sutured to the base of the tongue.
13. The jejunal graft can be used to replace a portion of the cervical esophagus (6–8 cm) or the entire pharynx and cervical esophagus (up to 25 cm).
14. If only a portion of the pharyngeal wall or cervical esophagus needs replacement, the jejunal segment can be split open and used as a patch graft.
15. The mesentery of the jejunum can be used as a protective cover for the exposed carotid vessels.
16. Complications of mediastinal dissection and gastric mobilization are avoided.
17. Hospital stay is short compared with more traditional, multistaged procedures.
18. A thoracotomy is avoided.

## COMPLICATIONS

As expected with this group of patients with complex problems, a variety of complications can be encountered with esophageal replacement using a free jejunal autograft. The complications can be divided into those at the abdominal donor site and those at the recipient site in the neck (Table 54–4).

The primary complications of harvesting the jejunal graft include breakdown of the jejunal anastomosis, small-intestine obstruction, abdominal wall dihiscence, and prolonged ileus. These complications can be kept to a minimum with meticulous technique and preoperative nutritional supplementation in depleted patients.

Many complications have been encountered at the recipient site. The neck wound is heavily contaminated, because it is exposed to the aerodigestive system. In addition, this region may have been heavily irradiated. Complications include infection, microvascular thrombosis, anastomotic stricture, pharyngocutaneous fistula, pseudoaneurysm at the arterial anastomosis, and dysphagia.

Most of the neck-wound complications can be handled with local care because the transplanted intestine is well vascularized. Thirty percent of the patients in the Emory series experienced postoperative fistulas in the neck. More than half of these fistulas healed without intervention. This compares favorably with other methods of cervical esophageal replacement, including colonic interposition and gastric transposition.

## SUMMARY

Free jejunal transplantation using microvascular technique offers an ideal method for reconstruction of the cervical esophagus and pharynx with many advantages over traditional local flap techniques. Because the jejunal transplant is well vascularized with a tension-free anastomosis, there are many advantages over gastric transposition and colonic interposition. (Table 54–5). Although there are several disadvantages to free jejunal transplantation (Table 54–6), these are shared with the other techniques and are not a major consequence.

**TABLE 54–6. DISADVANTAGES OF FREE JEJUNAL TRANSPLANTATION**

1. It is a technically demanding procedure with a long operative time of 6–10 hours.
2. Flap viability is all or none.
3. Jejunal graft peristalsis may not coordinate well with the swallowing mechanism, leading to delayed transit time.
4. Esophageal speech is not usually achieved after jejunal grafting.

## REFERENCES


1. Wookey H: The surgical treatment of carcinoma of the pharynx and upper esophagus. *Surg Gynecol Obstet* **75:**499, 1942
2. Bakamjian VY: A two-stage method for pharyngeosophageal reconstruction of the cervical esophagus and pharynx. *Plast Reconstr Surg* **36:**509, 1965
3. Ariyan S, Cuono CB: Myocutaneous flaps in head and neck reconstruction. *Head Neck Surg* **2:**321, 1980
4. Carrel A: The surgery of blood vessels, etc. *Johns Hopkins Hosp Bull* **190:**18, 1907
5. Longmire WP Jr, Ravitch MM: A new method for constructing an artificial esophagus. *Ann Surg* **123:**819, 1946
6. Seidenberg B, Rosenak SS, Hurwitt ES, Som ML: Immediate reconstruction of the cervical esophagus by a revascularized isolated jejunal segment. *Ann Surg* **149:**162, 1959
7. Jurkiewicz MJ: Vascularized intestinal graft for reconstruction of the cervical esophagus and pharynx. *Plast Reconstr Surg* **35:**509, 1965
8. Hester TR, McConnell F, Nahai F, et al: Pharyngoesophageal stricture and fistula: Treatment by free jejunal graft. *Ann Surg* **199:**762, 1984
9. Coleman JJ III, Tan K, Searles JM Jr, et al: Jejunal free autograft: Analysis of complications and their resolution. *Plast Reconstr Surg* **84:**589, 1989
10. Carlson GW, Schusterman MA, Guillamondegui OM: Total reconstruction of the hypopharynx and cervical esophagus: A 20 year experience. *Ann Plast Surg* **29:**408, 1992
11. Fisher S, Cameron R, Hoyt D, et al: Free jejunal interposition graft for reconstruction of the esophagus. *Head Neck* **12:**126, 1990
12. Schusterman MA, Shestak K, de Vries E, et al: Reconstruction of the cervical esophagus: Free jejunal transfer versus gastric pull-up. *Plast Reconstr Surg* **85:**16, 1990
13. Coleman JJ III, Searles JM Jr, Hester TR, et al: Ten years experience with the free jejunal autograft. *Am J Surg* **154:**394, 1987
14. Harashina T: Analysis of 200 free flaps. *Br J Plast Surg* **41:**33, 1988
15. Ujiki GT, Pearl GJ, Poticha S, et al: Mortality and morbidity of gastric "pull-up" for replacement of the pharyngoesophagus. *Arch Surg* **122:**644, 1987
16. Postlethwait RW: Technique for isoperistaltic gastric tube for esophageal bypass. *Ann Surg* **189:**673, 1979
17. Postlethwait RW, Sealy WC, Dillon ML, Young WG: Colon interposition for esophageal substitution. *Ann Thorac Surg* **12:**89, 1971
18. Meyers WC, Seigler HF, Hanks JB, et al: Postoperative function of "free" jejunal transplants for replacement of the cervical esophagus. *Ann Surg* **192:**439, 1980
19. McConnel FMS, Hester TR, Mendelsohn MS, Logemann JA: Manofluorography of deglutition after total laryngopharyngectomy. *Plast Reconstr Surg* **81:**346, 1988

CHAPTER

# 55

# Palliative Treatment of Carcinoma of the Esophagus

Donald E. Low and K. Michael Pagliero

In our generally aging population the incidence of esophageal carcinoma is on the increase.[1–3] Unfortunately, screening programs are generally ineffectual. Presentation is usually late, because the earliest symptoms of dysphagia do not arise until 50% of the circumference of the esophagus has become involved with tumor. Survival of patients who do not receive effective treatment is less than 10 months from the onset of symptoms.[4] Of the patients amenable to resection, 72% have lymph node metastasis,[5] and only 25% undergo potentially curative surgical treatment.[6]

Belsey described surgical cure of esophageal cancer as a fortunate accident[7]; with modern surgical and intensive care and diagnostic approaches, patients with early, especially those with node-negative, disease can be offered cure rates as high as 25–50%. When the operation is performed by an experienced surgeon, the mortality among these patients should be less than 5%. Thus, we believe that all patients with localized disease who are medically able to tolerate an operation should be offered a potential curative resection.

However, for the large percentage of patients who, on the grounds of extent of disease or medical condition, are not surgical candidates, methods of medical, surgical, and endoscopic palliation of dysphagia, chest pain, malnutrition, aspiration, anemia, and esophagorespiratory fistulas are required.

With increased use of flexible endoscopy, a wide variety of new palliative techniques have been introduced. Ideal palliative treatment should be safe, efficacious, well tolerated, easy to learn and apply, cost effective, and adaptable to a variety of clinical applications. The goal in patients with malignant dysphagia should be successful restoration of the patient's ability to take adequate oral nutrition while spending as little time in the hospital as possible. Newer techniques over the past decade, used alone or in combination with other palliative methods, are moving us closer to these goals.

## THE OPTIONS

1. Palliative resection or bypass.
2. Esophageal dilation.
3. Prosthetic intubation or stenting.
4. Antineoplastic chemotherapy.
5. Brachytherapy (intracavitary irradiation).
6. Laser photoablation.
7. Photodynamic therapy.

### Palliative Resection or Bypass

Historically, patients who could not undergo curative surgical treatment were offered palliative operations to decrease local recurrence. Palliative resection or bypass can offer good symptomatic results but at a cost of high morbidity and mortality.[8–11] The mortality for bypass operations is 20–40%. Nonfatal complications occur in 25% of patients.[12] These figures are unacceptably high for patients with stage III and IV esophageal cancer, whose survival is usually measured in months.

As a result, it is our policy to consider palliative operations in only two circumstances. The first is esophagorespiratory fistulas in young, fit patients, and the second is disease that is unresectable for cure at operation in a patient in whom partial resection or bypass would add only a small part to an already complex operation.

Palliative operations with resection of the primary tumor follow the same techniques as curative resections. When the primary tumor is left in situ, either because of involvement of structures in the thorax or because of a fistula, an alternative route for the reconstructed gullet is chosen (Fig. 55–1). If the primary tumor is left in situ, the retrosternal route offers the best direct conduit to the neck.[13] This route reduces the possibility of recurrent malignant dysphagia or malignant fistulization and allows portals for palliative radiation therapy to be planned specifically to avoid the neoesophagus (Fig. 55–2). The presternal route has been advocated by Mannel,[14] but we believe it should be reserved for rare situations in which the retrosternal route is unavailable because of a previous cardiac or mediastinal operation. The retrosternal option is safer and easier to use, although Orringer observed a higher incidence of anastomotic leak when extra-anatomic bypasses are performed.[11] Stricture and anastomotic leak can be decreased in retrosternal bypasses if the thoracic inlet is enlarged by means of removal of the upper manubrium and adjacent clavicular heads before a cervical anastomosis is performed.[9] In conventional esophagectomies, when the stomach is used to construct the neoesophagus, we do not routinely perform a pyloromyotomy or pyloroplasty when the graft is placed in the bed of the resected esophagus. We do recommend a gastric emptying procedure with extra-anatomic bypasses.

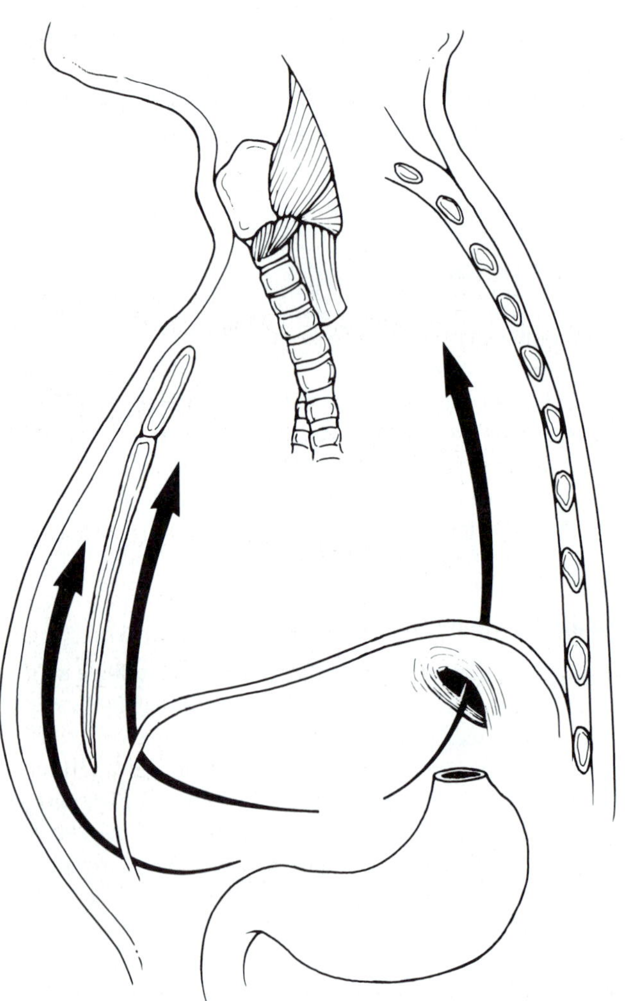

**Figure 55–1.** The three potential routes for passage of the neoesophagus during esophageal bypass operations.

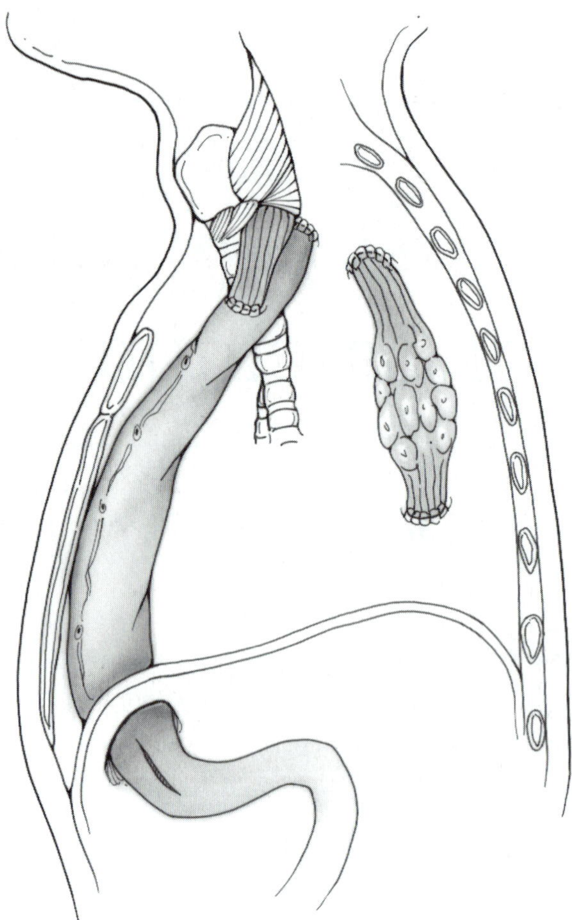

**Figure 55–2.** Example of retrosternal bypass that leaves the primary tumor in situ.

Kirschner advocated bypass and then drainage of the unresected esophageal remnant with a Roux-en-Y segment of small intestine[15] (Fig. 55–3). However, we agree with other authors[16,17] that unresected tumor and a short isolated segment of esophagus can be left in situ and undrained (Fig. 55–2) without worry about an esophagocele due to the paucity of esophageal glands.

Patients with tracheoesophageal fistulas have had survival periods of weeks. Palliation and survival can be improved in young, otherwise fit patients by use of esophageal exclusion and extra-anatomic bypass.[18–20] Surgical therapy also avoids a particularly unpalatable death due to constant aspiration of food and saliva. The only other reasonable op-

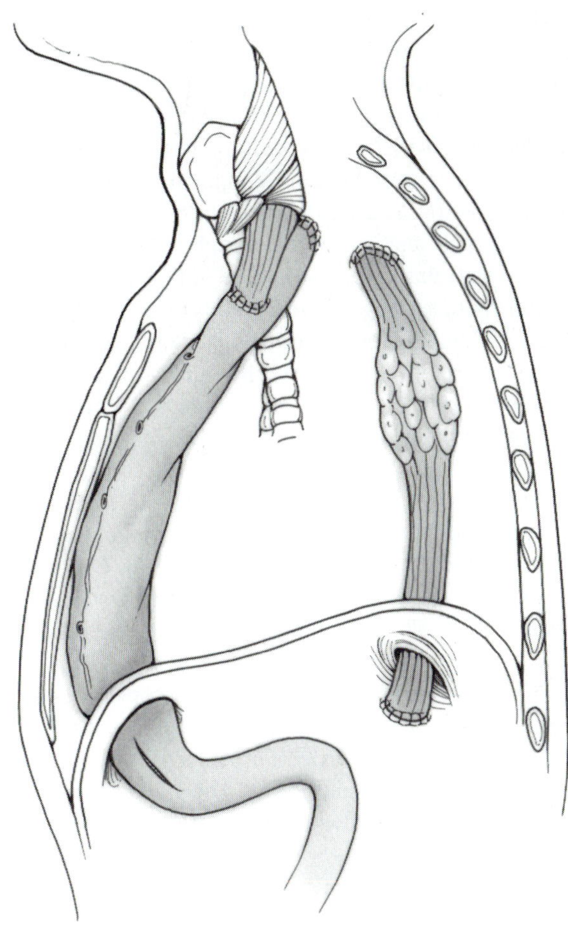

**Figure 55–3.** Kirschner operation featuring retrosternal gastric bypass with Roux-en-Y drainage of the esophageal remnant.

tion for managing esophageal fistulas is esophageal intubation.

## Esophageal Dilation

Esophageal dilation is the oldest palliative treatment of malignant tumors of the esophagus. It can often rapidly restore esophageal patency in patients who cannot take an adequate diet or control their production of saliva. A small group of patients with only a short time to live can undergo palliation dilation alone.[21–23] In most patients dilation has a supportive role in conjunction with other treatment modalities to make those modalities safe and efficient.[24–26] The experience of Heit et al is representative of that of other authors. It showed that multiple dilations and return trips to hospital are necessary for patients with esophageal cancer.[25,27–31] Long-term and repeated commitment to hospital treatment is unacceptable for patients with a very limited life expectancy.

The techniques of esophageal dilation have improved dramatically over the last 20 years. Mercury-filled red rubber (Maloney or Hurst) bougies are still the most commonly used dilators (Fig. 55–4). However, various wire-directed systems, such as the Puestow system of directed, graded, metal olive dilators have evolved since the 1950s (Fig. 55–5).[32] The wire-directed systems evolved into the stepped, high-density polymer dilators, variable-diameter polyethylene balloons, and hollow-core polyvinyl dilators. Short tumors with an easily visible lumen can usually be safely dilated with Maloney mercury-filled dilators. Fluoroscopy increases safety and accuracy by ensuring that the dilator is not curling above the stricture. Long, angulated, or eccentric strictures are best dilated with guide-wire systems under fluoroscopic control.[33]

The Puestow dilating system (either single-olive or tridil) has been used widely but has been supplanted by the hollow-core polyvinyl dilating systems,[34,35] such as the American (C.R. Bard; Belmont, Massachusetts) or Savary-Gillard (Wilson Cook; Winston-Salem, North Carolina) systems (Fig. 55–4). These systems require fluoroscopic or endoscopic placement of a guide wire into the stomach. Care must be taken not to attempt too aggressive a program of dilation based on the ease with which these dilators can be passed through even the tightest malignant strictures.

Other reports advocate variable-sized polyethylene Gruntzig balloons to dilate malignant strictures (Fig. 55–4).[31] This system has the advantage of allowing the dilating balloon to be placed either over a guide wire or under

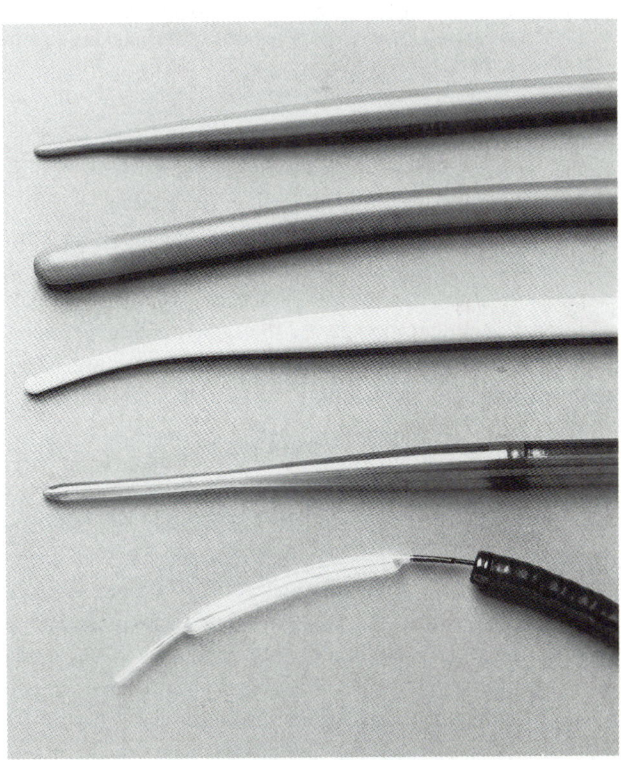

**Figure 55–4.** Selection of dilation systems from top to bottom: Maloney and Hurst mercury-filled red rubber dilators; American and Savary wire-directed dilators; and a 12-mm through-the-scope dilator.

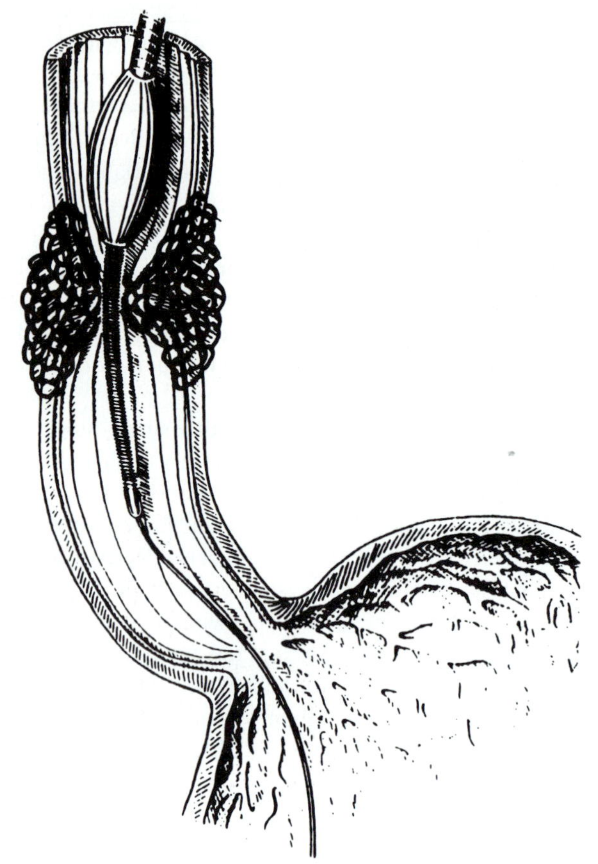

**Figure 55–5.** Eder-Puestow wire-directed dilation system, which works on the basis of interchangeable metal olives used to sequentially dilate tumors.

direct vision with endoscopy. Dilation is performed by means of application of radial rather than vector forces, which potentially decreases the risk of perforation.

We do not take primary dilations of malignant strictures higher than No. 45 F gauge. If histologic confirmation is available at the time of initial dilation, we often apply an additional treatment modality at the same treatment session. If the patients are not surgical candidates, we use either stent placement, brachytherapy, or laser photoablation.

## Esophageal Intubation

Insertion of stents to relieve the obstruction in malignant disease of the esophagus was first reported by Sir Charles Symonds in 1885.[36] The Souttar tube is a tightly coiled wire stent that is inserted through a rigid esophagoscope. It was the first widely applied esophageal stent.[37] A vast array of intubation methods and devices have been developed.[38,39] Most are constructed with a proximal funnel for easy collection of food and liquids, and many of the newer stents also have a distal flange to help prevent displacement. Most stents have an internal diameter of at least 10 mm, which should routinely allow passage of well-masticated food.

Historically, there have been two general approaches to esophageal stenting. The traction method requires a surgical procedure and general anesthesia. The pulsion method involves insertion with IV sedation and endoscopic methods. The most widely used traction stent is the Celestin tube,[40] which is introduced in conjunction with a limited upper laparotomy. A pilot bougie is introduced through the patient's mouth and retrieved through a gastrotomy (Fig. 55–6A). The Celestin tube is sutured to the proximal end of the pilot bougie (Fig. 55–6B) and then gently pulled through the malignant stricture. Once the cup abuts the proximal aspect of the tumor, the cup is stitched to the lesser curve of the stomach over a buttress of Teflon (polytetrafluoroethylene) felt (Fig. 55–6C). The tube is then trimmed to length and the gastrotomy closed. Oral passage of the pilot bougie sometimes is not possible because of complete obstruction or tortuosity of the malignant stricture. In this circumstance, the obstruction can often be negotiated with passage of a fine bougie retrograde through the gastrotomy. This can then be used to guide the pilot bougie into the stomach.

Pulsion intubation involves the endoscopic insertion of a tube over a guidewire under fluoroscopic control. This process can be usually carried out under IV sedation without the need for general anesthesia. The guidewire is passed through the tumor, and the malignant stricture is initially dilated to not greater than 45 F with a wire-directed dilating system. It is important not to dilate the tumor too aggressively before tube insertion to avoid early displacement. The tumor is inspected with endoscopy. The length of the tumor is measured, and fluoroscopy is used to mark the proximal and distal extents of the tumor by means of metal markers on the anterior chest wall.

The most commonly used pulsion stents are the Celestin tube, the Atkinson tube, and the Wilson Cook polyvinyl wire-reinforced esophageal stents (Fig. 55–7). The Atkinson tube comes in three lengths and two diameters. The tube is inserted over a guide wire with a Nottingham introducer, which holds the prosthesis in place with an expandable metal olive at its tip. The prosthesis is positioned with fluoroscopy with the funnel proximal to the tumor and the flange distal to the tumor. The metal olive is then released and the introducer withdrawn while a pushing tube is used to stabilize the prosthesis. This system offers the advantage of allowing repositioning of the prosthesis by means of reinsertion of the introducer and re-expansion of the olive.

The Savary system (Wilson Cook; Winston-Salem, North Carolina) uses a guide wire, pusher tube, and 33 F polyvinyl dilator as an introducer. These polyvinyl wire–reinforced tubes are resistant to compression, but if removal or position readjustment is required, the tube must be pushed into the stomach or pulled back with a forceps or a balloon dilator inflated within the tube.

We compared the pulsion and traction methods of esophageal intubation[41] (Table 55–1) and found that hospi-

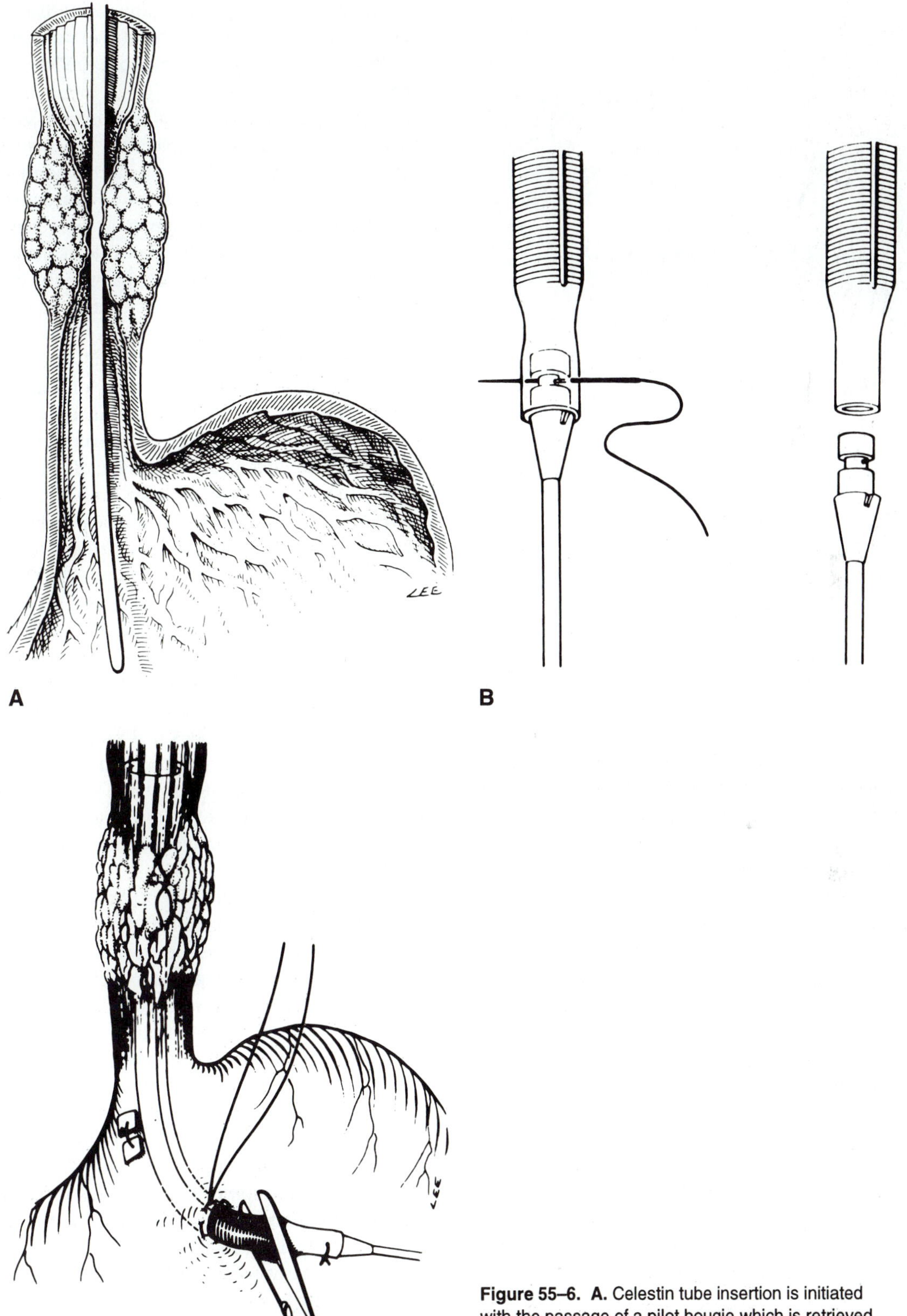


**Figure 55–6. A.** Celestin tube insertion is initiated with the passage of a pilot bougie which is retrieved through a small gastrotomy. **B.** The Celestin tube is sutured to the proximal end of the pilot bougie. **C.** The bougie is guided into place through the tumor. The Celestin tube is trimmed to size and fixed to the lesser curve with a pledgeted suture.

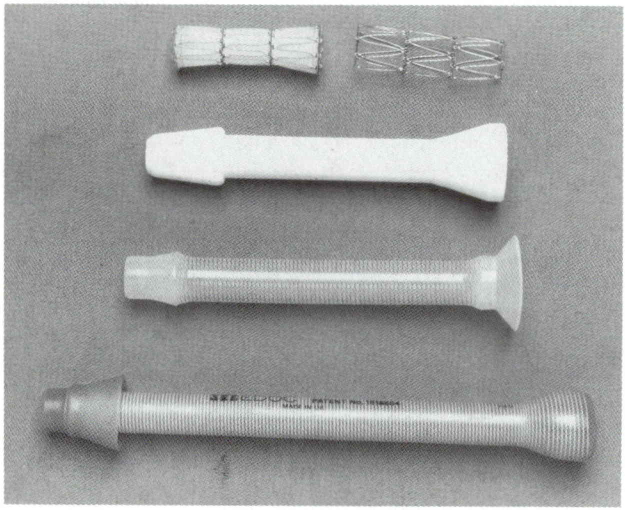

**Figure 55–7.** Various pulsion stents and endoscopically placed wire mesh stents. From top to bottom are examples of covered and uncovered expandable metal Z stents and the Atkinson, Wilson-Cook, and Celestin pulsion stents.

tal stay was shorter in the pulsion group (8.4 vs 18.6 days). Our findings agree with other reports[42] that demonstrated decreased hospital mortality with the pulsion method (14% vs 23%). Wound infection and dehiscence occur in as many as one fourth of patients who undergo traction intubation, but tube displacement is seen much more frequently with pulsion tubes (17.4% vs 0%). We reserve traction insertion of Celestin tubes for patients who have severe dysphagia and are found to have inoperable tumors at surgical exploration and for the rare patients in whom we cannot pass a guide wire. When performed by an experienced surgeon, pulsion tube insertion can be successful and improved swallowing can be achieved by more than 90% of patients.[43–45] However, even after successful stent placement, 40–50% of patients are limited to a predominantly pureed diet.

**TABLE 55–1. PULSION VS TRACTION INTUBATION**

| Variable | Pulsion Intubation Group | Traction Intubation Group |
|---|---|---|
| Number of patients | 49 | 39 |
| Mean age (y) | 77.3 | 70.5 |
| Sex—Male | 24 | 31 |
| Female | 25 | 8 |
| Hospital stay (d) | 8.4 | 18.6 |
| Hospital mortality [no. of deaths (%)] | 7 (14) | 9 (23) |
| Failed insertions (no. pts.) | 3 (9) | 1 (3) |
| Perforations (no. pts.) | 4 | 2 |
| Nonfatal | 3 | 0 |
| Fatal | 1 | 1 |
| Wound problems (no. pts.) | 0 | 7 |
| Aspiration pneumonia [no. pts. (%)] | 3 (9) | 1 (3) |
| Tube bolus obstruction [no. pts. (%)] | 3 (9) | 2 (5) |
| Tube displacement [no. pts (%)] | 6 (17) | 0 |
| No symptomatic improvement (no. pts.) | 2 | 1 |

Common complications of endoscopic stent placement are reflux esophagitis with bleeding or stricture formation, perforation, tube dislocation, tumor overgrowth, pressure necrosis, and secondary airway compression. Reflux esophagitis and aspiration are most prevalent in patients with lower-third carcinomas whose stents cross the gastroesophageal junction. These patients should be advised to sleep with the head of the bed elevated. Routine treatment with omeprazole and gastric motility agents such as cisapride can also be helpful.

Perforation occurs in 4–12% of patients[18,41,42,46]; 4–9% of patients die.[45,47] Surgical management after perforation is usually contraindicated. Treatment includes nothing by mouth, intercostal drainage of any contaminated pleural space, IV broad-spectrum antibiotics, and adequate nutritional support. This approach helps some of these patients when the perforation is localized and noted at an early stage.[48]

Tube displacement occurs in 10–20% of patients.[18,46,47] Proximally displaced tubes either are regurgitated or require endoscopic removal. Distal displacement is rarely a problem in that the tube either remains in the stomach or is passed. Food bolus obstruction is variable and can be managed with techniques that range from drinking carbonated beverages, endoscopic removal of the bolus, or substituting a larger-diameter stent. Tumor overgrowth can be corrected with the insertion of a longer prosthesis or with neodymium: yttrium-aluminum-garnet (Nd:YAG) laser photoablation.

Pressure necrosis usually occurs at the edge of the funnel. It is usually seen in patients with associated kyphoscoliosis, large hiatal hernias, or previous radiation therapy. It can lead to pain, bleeding, and mediastinal contamination. The tube should be removed and replaced with a longer or different model. Intubation of bulky tumors adjacent to airways can result in severe respiratory embarrassment. When this occurs, the tube must be removed and a smaller diameter tube inserted or alternative palliation applied.

External compression of the esophagus is a difficult problem that is resistant to many palliative measures.[49–51] Endoscopic intubation in these patients offers an excellent method of relieving dysphagia before the application of radiation therapy or chemotherapy.

An important recent advance in esophageal stenting is the availability and use of expandable metal wire stents for esophageal cancers and esophagorespiratory fistulas (Fig. 55–7). These stents can be inserted with greater ease and safety than the other pulsion stents because most of these devices are introduced with a 34 F introducer. This often eliminates the need to dilate tumors before stent insertion. These stents can be placed with local anesthesia under fluoroscopic control. When open they produce funnel-shaped dilation both proximal and distal to the tumor. These stents routinely become imbedded within the tumor and esophageal mucosa within several days, decreasing the chance of displacement. Knyrim et al showed a decrease in hospital stay, serious complications, and mortality with the use of expansile metal stents as opposed to conventional pulsion stents.[52] The disadvantages of the metal stents are increased cost (metal stents are up to ten times more expensive than conventional stents), and if the stents are placed incorrectly, they are extremely difficult to remove or dislocate. The tumor can also grow through the wire mesh.[52,53] Coating the wire framework with silicone may minimize this complication.[54]

We have found expandable metal stents particularly helpful in patients with esophagorespiratory fistulas who are not good candidates for bypass operations. Figure 55–8 shows the result obtained in a patient who presented with a large fistula and was able to resume a semisoft diet immediately after insertion of an expandable wire stent.

With increased application of brachytherapy and laser photoablation, we have seen a decrease in need for esophageal stents. We recommend primary intubation only for patients with malignant external compression of the esophagus and for patients with esophagorespiratory fistulas who are not surgical candidates. Continued improvement in expandable metal stents may result in resurgence of that treatment approach.

## Chemotherapy

The relatively low long-term survival rates among patients with seemingly curable esophageal cancer is explained by the high incidence of unrecognized metastatic disease at the time of diagnosis.[55,56] Improvement in results therefore requires methods of detecting esophageal cancer at an earlier stage or the successful application of antineoplastic drugs in addition to surgical therapy. Since the mid 1980s, a large number of trials used single- and multiple-drug chemotherapeutic regimens with or without radiation therapy. The single agents with the highest response rates were continuous infusion of 5-fluorouracil (5-FU)[57] and cisplatin,[58] but they were effective in only 15–20% of patients.[59,60]

Better results have been seen with multidrug trials, predominantly with cisplatin with a variety of other agents.[61–64] These trials involved treatment of incurable or recurrent disease rather than primary treatment of early cancer. Nevertheless, response rates were 33–50%. Other trials using combinations of chemo- and radiation therapy for stage III and IV disease showed that 77% of patients were free of dysphagia after treatment and that 60% could swallow normally at the time of death.[65] Median survival times as long as 12.5 months with regimens of 5-FU, cisplatin, and radiation therapy has been reported. It should be noted, however, that this trial reported a rate of severe life-threatening side effects of 44%.[66] (See Chapter 51).

## Brachytherapy

Brachytherapy is a technique whereby a radioactive source is afterloaded into a closed tube, which is placed adjacent to a malignant esophageal tumor with endoscopy and fluoroscopy. Under fluoroscopic guidance, the upper and lower extent of the tumor can be precisely located by means of external metal markers on the skin. The guide wire is then passed through the tumor and into the stomach and an 8-mm (23 F) polyvinylchloride catheter (Fig. 55–9A) is passed over the wire to straddle the esophageal tumor (Fig. 55–9B). The catheter has radiopaque markers so that during insertion, the 13 cm that constitute the active treatment zone can be visualized with fluoroscopy. If the clinical situation warrants, two catheters can be inserted so that 26 cm (which usually embraces the entire esophagus) can undergo treatment. Once positioned, the catheter is fixed at the level of the mouth or nose, and the patient is transferred to the brachytherapy suite for treatment. The radioactive sources are automatically loaded to provide a single, high-dose fraction of 3500 cGy at the surface of the catheter. The fraction is diminished to 1500 cGy 1cm from the central axis of the catheter.

Brachytherapy has made the delivery of radiation to a malignant growth more exact because of two factors. The first involves use of cesium-137 and iridium-192, which produces less scatter within tissues and allows increased accuracy of dose calculation and shorter treatment intervals than radium or cobalt sources. The second factor is that the radioactive source is directly adjacent to the malignant tissue, minimizing the need to irradiate through normal thoracic viscera.

Since our original report,[67] we have reviewed the results in 72 patients with a median age of 76 years who underwent treatment with a single-dose high-fraction technique.[68] Indications for brachytherapy were evidence of distant metastases in 36% of the patients, anastomotic recurrence after esophagogastrectomy in 4%, and medical contraindications to surgical treatment in 60%. Hospital stay was less than 3 days for 70% of the patients. Three patients were unable to tolerate having the brachytherapy catheter in place for the 1 hour required for treatment. Seven patients (10%) required re-treatment for recurrent dysphagia, and 15 patients (21%) underwent esophageal intubation because of treatment failure or early symptom recurrence.

It became apparent during this study that patients with dysphagia secondary to extrinsic malignant compression were more likely to have treatment failure and require intubation. Overall, 75% of patients had an improvement in dysphagia score as graded by an independent observer. The 1-year survival rate was 10% in patients with squamous cell carcinoma and 20% in those with adenocarcinoma.

Complications in the 69 patients who completed treatment included sore throat (two patients), mild esophagitis (two patients), epigastric pain (five patients), and nausea

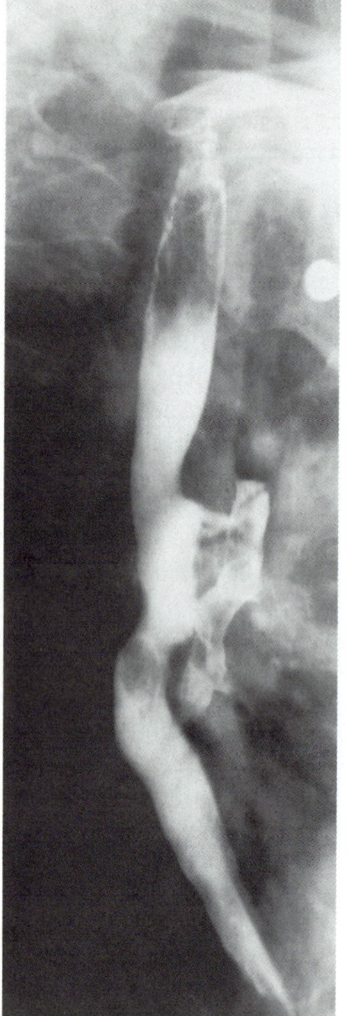

**Figure 55–8.** **A.** Barium radiograph showing a large esophagorespiratory fistula in a patient with esophageal cancer. **B.** Endoscopic photograph of an expandable metal stent bridging the fistula. **C.** Barium radiograph showing passage of barium through the stent without any evidence of residual communication with the airway. **D.** Lateral chest radiograph showing the stent in situ.

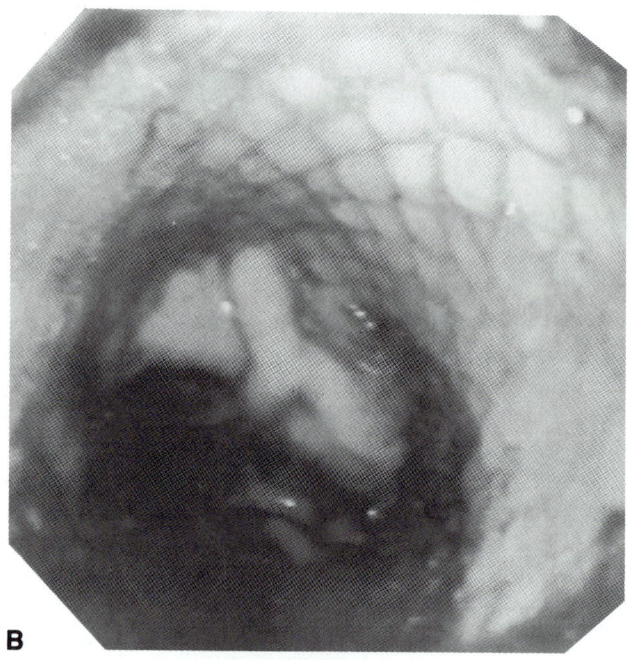

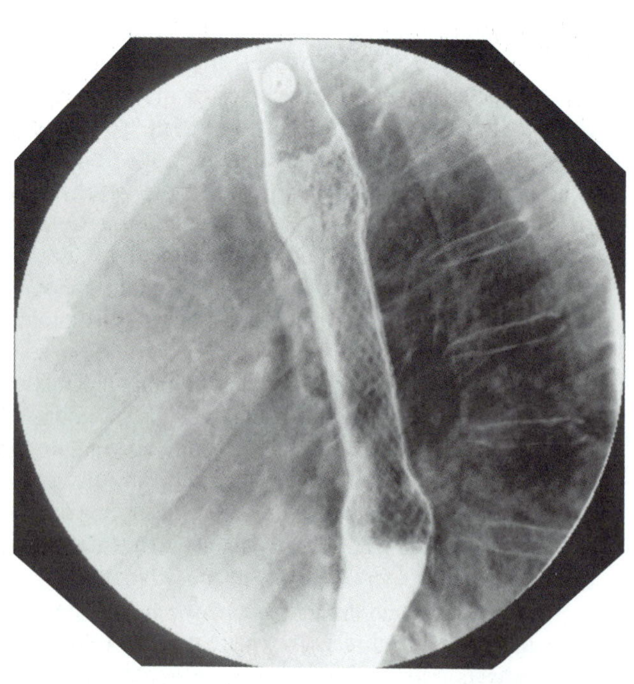

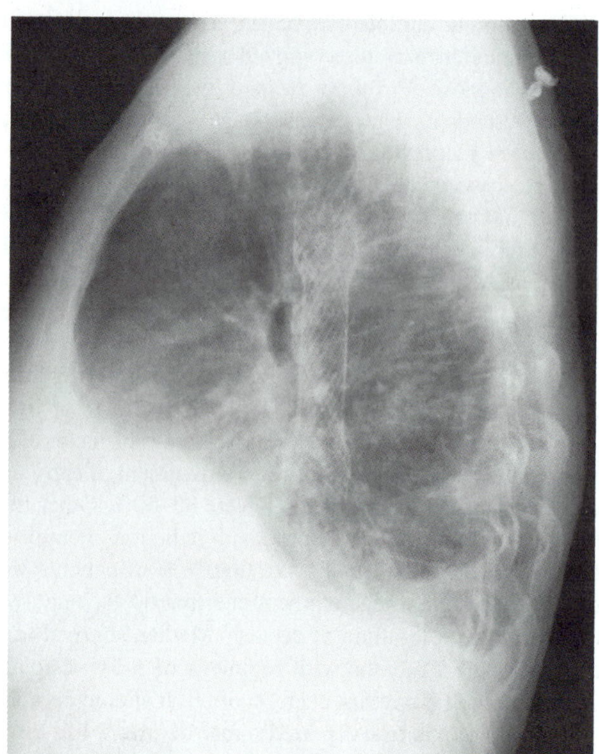

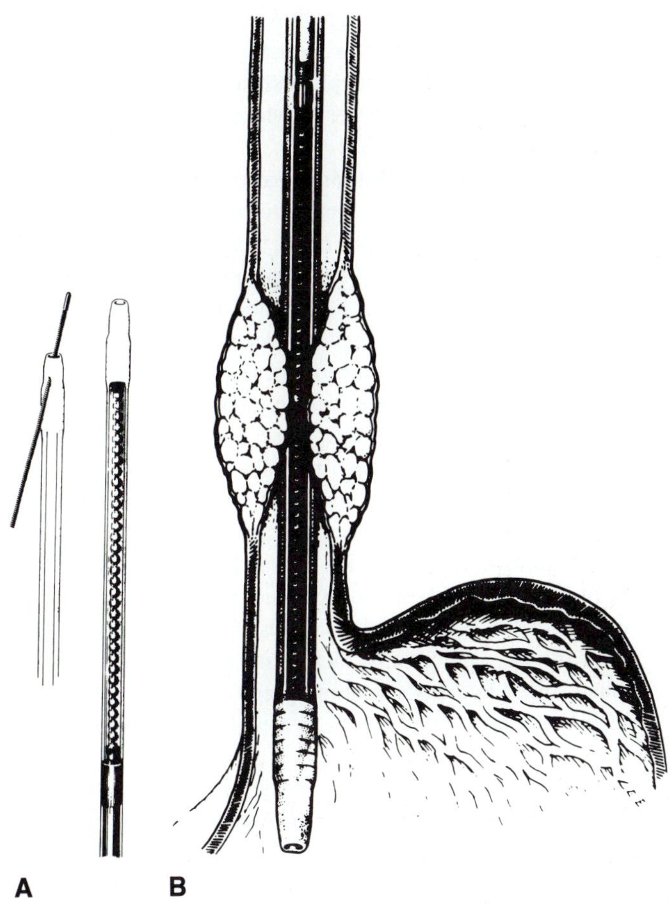


**Figure 55–9. A.** Brachytherapy catheter and the method by which it is placed over a guide-wire. **B.** Brachytherapy catheter in situ bridging the esophageal tumor.

and diarrhea (one patient). One patient had a fibrous radiation stricture that responded to a single dilation. There was no direct procedure-related mortality; however, one patient was later admitted with an esophagorespiratory fistula of which he died. Flores et al reported using brachytherapy in combination with external beam radiation.[69] They reported complete restoration of swallowing in 62% of patients. Dilation was required in 7% of patients immediately after treatment and in 30% of patients at some point after treatment. One patient died of radiation pneumonitis 3 months after treatment; however, radiation esophagitis was extremely common (92% mild, 8% severe). Bader et al reported that the application of brachytherapy after laser photoablation reduces the requirement for repeat laser treatments.[70]

We performed a prospective, randomized trial that compared the effectiveness of brachytherapy with that of laser treatment in 23 consecutive patients.[51] Brachytherapy required shorter hospitalization time and was less likely to require re-treatments. Both treatments were equally effective in allowing the patients to eat a relatively normal diet until death and allowing patients to die without readmission to tertiary referral centers. The only serious complication was a nonfatal perforation that occurred in a patient who underwent laser therapy. One-third of the patients who underwent brachytherapy showed a tendency toward post-treatment dysphagia, which resolved spontaneously in 48–72 hours. Although the numbers were small, there was a suggestion of increased survival time in patients who underwent laser therapy.

## Laser Photoablation

The most common laser used in palliation of malignant esophageal tumors is the Nd:YAG (wavelength 1,060 nm) because it can be delivered through a quartz fiber and has greater tissue penetration than other lasers. Laser treatment works on the principle of tissue vaporization and thermal necrosis of surrounding tissue. At high power settings, temperatures as high as 100°C are generated in the tissue directly adjacent to the treatment areas.[71,72] It has also been suggested that laser treatment may produce secondary fibrosis, which can limit the subsequent rate of tumor growth.[73]

When performed by an experienced practitioner, individual laser treatments should take 20–40 min. If the endoscope cannot go through the tumor stenosis, a guide wire should be passed under fluoroscopic control and the tumor dilated.

We believe that immediate efficiency and long-term efficacy can be improved with snare cautery debridement of all exophytic tumor before laser treatment.[73] We also recommend routine laser re-treatment 2–4 days after the initial session. This provides time for treated tissue to slough, allowing treatment of the secondary layer with additional snare debridement and laser photoablation.

Laser treatment is effective irrespective of tumor type[74] and can be applied to tumors located at any position within the esophagus. It is generally accepted, however, that exophytic, noncircumferential tumors are more successfully treated than submucosal tumors or obstruction due to extrinsic malignant compression.[50,74–77] Cervical tumors and growths with a substantial gastric component, as well as excessively long tumors (greater than 8 cm), also lead to poor clinical results.[75,77,78] Multiple studies have demonstrated that laser palliation is relatively safe, efficacious, well-tolerated, cost-effective, and requires only a minimal amount of time in the hospital.[24,49,50,74,76,79] Studies also have demonstrated that laser therapy can improve quality of life.[80,81] The incidence of serious complications is highly dependent on the skill and experience of the operator.[24,39,49,79] Minor complications occur in 10–50% of patients. The most serious complications are bleeding and perforation. When an experienced practitioner performs the ablation, the perforation rate should be less than 5%.[77] Posttreatment bleeding has been reported in as many as 4% of patients, but, paradoxically, is best treated with additional laser treatment. Ell et al conducted a survey of 20 laser units combining the results for a total of 1184 patients.[84] They found an overall complication rate of 4.1%. Laser-related mortality is most commonly associated with perforation and occurs in 1–2.7% of patients.[79,82]

The success rate of laser photoablation is usually reported to be about 80%.[50,74,76,83,84] It is important, however, to differentiate between the technical success of achieving luminal patency and the functional success of restoring the ability to eat a normal diet. Laser treatment does not cure malignant anorexia, which occurs in 25–30% of patients.[72,74] One group who has been particularly resistant to laser treatment are patients with obstruction due to malignant extrinsic compression.[21,50] These patients rarely have good functional results with laser therapy alone and are usually best treated with esophageal intubation.

### Photodynamic Therapy

Photodynamic therapy uses IV photosensitizing agents to inactivate biologic systems and an energy transfer process that causes irreversible oxidation of essential cellular components.[85] The most commonly used photosensitizing agents are hematoporphyrin derivatives and phthallocyanines. When given IV, these compounds disseminate widely to malignant and normal tissues, but clearance occurs more rapidly from normal tissue. After 48–72 hours, there is a differential concentration of photosensitizing agent between tumor cells and adjacent normal tissues. Dye lasers can be tuned to the precise wavelength required to activate the sensitizing agent. The effect of photodynamic therapy is achieved through tumor necrosis secondary to vascular occlusion and laser hyperthermia.[81] Photodynamic therapy is a photochemical process rather than a thermal reaction or coagulative necrosis, which occurs with the Nd:YAG laser.

McAughan and Williams have the largest series of photodynamic therapy for palliation of inoperable esophageal cancer.[86] In 25 patients, the mean survival time was 6.8 months. Eighty-eight percent of these patients could consume at least a liquid diet at the time of death. Complications occurred in only three patients, who required posttreatment dilation. One of these patients had a sterile pleural effusion, and there was no treatment-related mortality.

Photodynamic therapy produces considerable tumor necrosis without accompanying fibrosis. Theoretically the therapy may result in increased risk of perforation or esophagorespiratory fistula. In addition, photochemical necrosis produced by photodynamic therapy does not result in the coagulation of blood vessels that takes place during laser therapy, potentially increasing the chance of subsequent bleeding. It is encouraging that McAughan and Williams's series did not have a high rate of bleeding or perforation.

The injection of hematoporphyrins produces cutaneous photosensitivity, which can lead to severe burns when patients are exposed to sunlight. Problems can be avoided with sunscreen, protective clothing, and a nocturnal lifestyle. Some patients find these sunlight restrictions difficult over the 6–8 weeks they are necessary. The restrictions are especially troublesome to patients whose treatment has to be repeated and whose survival is measured in months.

Photodynamic therapy has the advantage that treatment is aimed directly and potentially exclusively at malignant tissue. The treatment is unsuitable for large, bulky tumors and has little effect on extraluminal tumor. The best application may be in conjunction with preliminary tumor debulking with snare cautery with or without laser photoablation.

## SUMMARY

With so many options for palliative treatment the decision should be based on the expertise and equipment available, patient factors favoring one technique over another, financial considerations, experience, and equipment adaptability. All of these methods require a degree of confidence with basic endoscopic techniques—no method is safe and easy if one is not comfortable with the delivery system.

Fundamentally, "cure" should always be the goal in all patients who present with localized and apparently resectable malignant esophageal tumors. Palliation should therefore be reserved for four groups of patients: (1) those who cannot undergo a major operation because they are not fit enough; (2) those whose preoperative assessment demonstrates incurable disease; (3) those whose operative findings demonstrate unresectability; and (4) those who decline surgical treatment.

Ideally, several palliative methods should be available so that treatment can be tailored to each patient. Fluoroscopically wire-directed dilation systems play a role in palliation in most patients, but only in combination with other treatment. Esophageal stents are of greater interest because of new expandable metal stents. Stents remain the primary treatment for patients with dysphagia secondary to external malignant compression and malignant esophagorespiratory fistula. Brachytherapy is performed in many radiation therapy units because of its wide use in the treatment of other malignant tumors. It can be performed with extremely low morbidity and mortality, few side effects, and is highly efficacious in a large percentage of patients after only a single treatment.

Laser therapy has a prominent learning curve and a high potential for complications but is now widely used and adaptable for primary palliation or in conjunction with other treatments. It has an immediate effect and is of proved efficacy when administered by an experienced practitioner. Photodynamic therapy has been reported to be safe, efficacious, and easily applied; however, the long period of cutaneous photosensitivity can be troublesome for patients with a limited life expectancy.

Prospective randomized trials from units experienced with different techniques are required to compare single and combination treatment. It is our expectation that brachytherapy or photodynamic therapy extends the initial effect of laser treatment so that most patients can be offered safe and efficacious treatment with a minimum time in the hospital.

## REFERENCES


1. Matthews HR, Waterhouse JAH, Powell J, et al: Epidemiology: demographic aspects. In: Matthews HR, Waterhouse JAH, Powell J (eds): *Cancer of the Oesophagus,* Vol 1, 1st ed. Southampton, England, Macmillan, 1987, pp 11–39
2. Earlam RJ, Cunha-Melo Jr, Donnon SPB, Evans SJW: The epidemiology of oesophageal cancer with special reference to England and Wales. *Ital J Gastroenterol* **14**:244–249, 1982
3. Blot WJ, Devesa SS, Kneller RW, Fraumeni JF: Rising incidence of adenocarcinoma of the esophagus and gastric cardia. *JAMA* **265**:1287–1289, 1991
4. Pei VH, Zhang YD, Hou J: Natural evolution and follow-up study of early esophageal carcinomas in 23 patients. *Cancer Res Prevent Treat* **9**:75–79, 1982
5. Watson D: A study of the quality and duration of survival following resection, endoscopic intubation and surgical intubation in oesophageal carcinoma. *Br J Surg* **69**:585–590, 1982
6. Orringer MB: Palliative procedures for esophageal cancer. *Surg Clin North Am* **63**:941–950, 1983
7. Belsey R: Is it possible to talk of cure of carcinoma of the esophagus? In Maloine SA (ed): *Cancer of the Oesophagus in 1984: 135 Questions.* Paris, Presses Palais-Royal, p 382
8. Earlam R, Cunha-Melo JR: Oesophageal squamous cell carcinoma: A critical review of surgery. *Br J Surg* **67**:381, 1980
9. Conlan AA, Nicolaou N, Hammond CA, et al: Retrosternal bypass for inoperable esophageal cancer: Report of 71 patients. *Ann Thorac Surg* **36**:396, 1983
10. Postlethwait RW: Carcinoma of the esophagus. *Curr Probl Cancer* **2**(8), 1978 (monograph)
11. Orringer MB: Esophageal carcinoma: What price palliation? *Ann Thorac Surg* **36**:377, 1983
12. Postlethwait RW: Complications and deaths after operations for esophageal carcinoma. *J Thorac Cardiovasc Surg* **85**:827–831, 1983
13. Kirk RM: A trial of total gastrectomy combined with total thoracic oesophagectomy without formal thoracotomy for carcinoma at or near the cardia of the stomach. *Br J Surg* **68**:577, 1981
14. Mannell A: Presternal gastric bypass for unresectable carcinoma of the thoracic oesophagus: A preliminary report. *Br J Surg* **67**:522, 1980
15. Kirschner MB: Ein neues Verfahren der oesophagoplastik. *Arch Klin Chir* **114**:606, 1920
16. Deaton WR, Bradshaw HH: The fate of an isolated segment of the oesophagus. *J Thorac Surg* **32**:827, 1956
17. Johnson J, Schwegman CW, Kirby CK: Esophageal exclusion for persistent fistula following spontaneous rupture of the esophagus. *J Thorac Surg* **32**:827, 1956
18. Segalin A, Little AG, Ruol A, et al: Surgical and endoscopic palliation of esophageal carcinoma. *Ann Thorac Surg* **48**:267–271, 1989
19. Weaver RM, Matthews HR: Palliation and survival in malignant oesophagorespiratory fistula. *Br J Surg* **67**:539–542, 1980
20. Burt M, Diehl W, Martini N, et al: Malignant esophagorespiratory fistula: Management options and survival. *Ann Thorac Surg* **52**:1222–1229, 1991
21. Cox J, Bennett JR: Light at the end of the tunnel? Palliation for oesophageal carcinoma. *Gut* **28**:781–785, 1987
22. Tytgat GM, Jager DH: To dilate or intubate. *Gastrointest Endosc* **29**:58–59, 1983
23. Heit HA, Johnson LF, Seiger SR, Boyce HW: Palliative dilation for dysphagia of esophageal carcinoma. *Ann Intern Med* **89**:629–631, 1978
24. Pietrafitta JJ, Dwyer RM: Endoscopic laser therapy of malignant esophageal obstruction. *Arch Surg* **121**(4):395–400, 1986
25. Riemann JF, Ell C, Lux G, Demling L: Combined therapy of malignant stenoses of the upper gastrointestinal tract by means of laser beam and bougienage. *Endoscopy* **17**:43–48, 1985
26. Lux G, Groitl H, Ell C: Tumour stenoses of the upper gastrointestinal tract: Therapeutic alternatives to laser therapy. *Endoscopy* **1**:21–26, 1986
27. Jensen DM: Palliation of esophagogastric cancer via endoscopy. *Gastroenterol Clin Biol* **11**:361–363, 1987
28. Moses FM, Peura DA, Wong R, Johnson LF: Palliative dilation of esophageal carcinoma. *Gastrointest Endosc* **31**:61–63, 1985
29. Cassidy DE, Nord HJ, Boyce HW: Management of malignant oesophageal strictures: Role of oesophageal dilation and peroral prosthesis. *Am J Gastroenterol* **76**:173, 1981
30. Watson D: Palliative therapy. In Hurt RL (ed): *Management of Oesophageal Carcinoma.* London, Springer, 1989, pp 211–222
31. Kozarek RA: Endoscopic Gruntzig balloon dilation of gastrointestinal stenoses. *J Clin Gastroenterol* **6**:401–407, 1984
32. Puestow KL: Conservative treatment of stenosing diseases of the esophagus. *Postgrad Med* **18**:6–14, 1955
33. Tulman AB, Boyce HW: Complications of esophageal dilation and guidelines for prevention. *Gastrointest Endosc* **27**:320–324, 1981
34. Aste H, Munizzi F, Martines H, Pugliese V: Esophageal dilation in malignant dysphagia. *Cancer* **56**:2413–2715, 1985
35. Celestin LR, Campbell WB: A new and safe system for oesophageal dilation. *Lancet* **1**:45–75, 1981
36. Symonds CJ: The treatment of malignant stricture of the esophagus by tubage or oral catheterization. *Br Med J* **1**:870–874, 1887
37. Souttar HS: A method of intubating the oesophagus for malignant stricture. *Br Med J* **1**:782–783, 1924

38. Dwyer RM: The technique of gastrointestinal laser endoscopy. In Goldman L (ed): *The Biomedical Laser: Technology and Clinical Application.* New York, Springer, 1981, pp 255–269
39. Kozarek RA. Neodymium–YAG laser application in the esophagus. In Hill LD, Kozarek RA, McCallum R, Mercer CD (eds): *The Esophagus: Medical and Surgical Management.* Philadelphia, Saunders, 1988, pp 295–301
40. Celestin LR: Permanent intubation in inoperable cancer of the esophagus and cardia. *Ann R Coll Surg Engl* **25:**165–170, 1959
41. Unruh HW, Pagliero KM: Pulsion intubation versus traction intubation for obstructing carcinomas of the esophagus. *Ann Thorac Surg* **40:**337–342, 1982
42. Lishman AH, Dellipiani AW, Devlin HB: The insertion of oesophagogastric tubes in malignant oesophageal strictures: Endoscopy or surgery? *Br J Surg* **67:**257–259, 1980
43. Angorn IB, Haffejee AA: Endoesophageal intubation for palliation in obstructing esophageal carcinoma. In Delaure NC, Wilkins EW, Wong J (eds): *International Trends in General Thoracic Surgery, Esophageal Cancer,* Vol. IV. St. Louis, Mosby, 1988, pp 410–419
44. Den Hartog Jager FC, Bartelsman JF, Tytgat GN: Palliative treatment of obstructing esophagogastric malignancy by endoscopic positioning of a plastic prosthesis. *Gastroenterology* **77:**1008–1014, 1979
45. Ogilvie AL, Dronfield MW, Ferguson R, Atkinson M: Palliative intubation of oesophagogastric neoplasms at fiberoptic endoscopy. *Gut* **23:**1060–1067, 1982
46. Tytgat GNJ, Den Hartog Jager FCA, Bartelman JF: Endoscopic prosthesis for advanced esophageal cancer. *Endoscopy* **18**(Suppl): 32–39, 1986
47. Jones DB, Davies PS, Smith PM: Endoscopic insertion of palliative oesophageal tubes in oesophagogastric neoplasms. *Br J Surg* **68:**197–198, 1981
48. Wesdrop IC, Bartelsman JF, Huibregtse K, et al: Treatment of instrumental oesophageal perforation. *Gut* **25:**398–401, 1984
49. Mellow MH, Pinkas H: Endoscopic laser therapy for malignancies affecting the esophagus and gastroesophageal junction. *Arch Intern Med* **145:**1443–1446, 1985
50. Krasner N, Barr H, Skidmore C, Morris AI: Palliative laser therapy for malignant dysphagia. *Gut* **23:**792–798, 1987
51. Low DE, Pagliero KM: Prospective randomized clinical trial comparing brachytherapy and laser photoablation for palliation of esophageal cancer. *J Thorac Cardiovasc Surg* **104:**173–179, 1992
52. Knyrim K, Wagner HJ, Bethge N, et al: A controlled trial of an expansible metal stent for palliation of esophageal obstruction due to inoperable cancer. *N Engl J Med* **329:**1302–1307, 1993
53. Boyce HW: Stents for palliation of dysphagia due to esophageal cancer. *N Engl J Med* **329:**1345–1346, 1993 (editorial)
54. Schaer J, Katom RM, Ivancer K, et al: Treatment of malignant esophageal obstruction with silicone coated metallic expanding stents. *Gastrointest Endosc* **38:**669–675, 1992
55. Anderson L, Lad T: Autopsy findings in squamous cell carcinoma of the oesophagus. *Cancer* **50:**1587, 1982
56. Bosch A, Friza Z, Caldwell WL, et al: Autopsy findings in carcinoma of the oesophagus. *Acta Radiol Oncol* **18:**103, 1979
57. Lokich J, Shea M, Chaffey J, et al: Sequential infusional 5-fluorouracil followed by concomitant radiation for tumors of the esophagus and the gastroesophageal junction. *Cancer* **60:**275–279, 1987
58. Miller JL, McIntyre MD, Hatcher CR: Combined treatment approach in surgical management of carcinoma of the esophagus: A preliminary report. *Ann Thorac Surg* **40**(3):289, 1985
59. Falkson G, Ckoetzer BJ, Jerblanch AP: Oesophageal cancer: Chemotherapy overview. *S Afr Med J* **71:**21, 1987
60. Leichman L, Berry BT: Experience with cisplatin in treatment regimens for esophageal cancer. *Semin Oncol* **18**(Suppl 3):64, 1991
61. Kelsen DP, Hilaris B, Coonley C, et al: Cisplatin, vindesine and bleomycin combination chemotherapy of local-regional and advanced esophageal carcinoma. *Am J Med* **75:**645, 1983
62. Vogl SE, Camacho F, Berenzweig M, et al: Chemotherapy for esophageal cancer with mitoguazone, methotrexate, bleomycin and cisplatin. *Cancer Treat Rep* **69:**21, 1985
63. De Basi P, Sileni VC, Salvagno L, et al: Phase II study of cisplatin, 5-FU, and allopurinol in advanced esophageal cancer. *Cancer Treat Rep* **70:**909–910, 1986
64. Iizuka T, Kakegawa T, Ide H, et al: Phase II study of CDDP + 5-FU for squamous esophageal carcinoma: JEOG Cooperative Study results. *Proc Am Soc Clin Oncol* **10:**157, 1991 (Abstract 496)
65. Coia LR, Engstrom PF, Paul AR, et al: Long-term results of infusional 5-FU, mitomycin-C, and radiation as primary management of esophageal carcinoma. *Int J Radiat Oncol Biol Phys* **20:**29–36, 1991
66. Herskovic A, Martz K, Al-Sarraf M, et al: Combined chemotherapy and radiotherapy compared with radiotherapy alone in patients with cancer of the esophagus. *N Engl J Med* **326:**1593–1598, 1992
67. Rowlands CG, Pagliero KM: Intracavitary irradiation in palliation of carcinoma of the oesophagus and cardia. *Lancet* **2:**981–982, 1985
68. Pagliero KM, Rowland CG: Brachytherapy for inoperable cancer of the oesophagus and cardia. In Delaure NC, Wilkins EW, Wong J (eds): *International Trends in General Thoracic Surgery, Esophageal Cancer,* Vol IV. St. Louis, Mosby, 1988, pp 361–367
69. Flores AD, Stoller JL, Nelems B, et al: Combined primary treatment of cancer of the esophagus and cardia by intracavitary and external irradiation. In Siewert JR, Hölscher AH (eds): *Diseases of the Esophagus.* Berlin, Springer-Verlag, 1988, pp 745–753
70. Bader M, Dittle HJ, Ultsch B, et al: Palliative treatment of malignant stenoses of the upper gastrointestinal tract using a combination of laser and afterloading therapy. *Endoscopy* **18:**27–31, 1986
71. Kelly DF, Bown SG, Calder BM, et al: Histological changes following Nd: YAG laser photocoagulation of canine gastric mucosa. *Gut* **24:**915–920, 1983
72. Fleischer D, Kessler F: Endoscopic ND-YAG laser therapy for carcinoma of the esophagus: A form of palliative treatment. *Gastroenterology* **85:**600–606, 1983
73. Low DE, Kozarek RA: Snare cautery debridement prior to Nd:YAG photoablation improves treatment efficiency of broad-based adenomas of the colorectum. *Gastrointest Endosc* **35**(4):288–291, 1989
74. Fleischer D, Sivak MV: Endoscopic Nd:YAG laser therapy as palliation for esophagogastric cancer: Parameters affecting initial outcome. *Gastroenterology* **89**(4):827–831, 1985
75. Maunoury V, Brunetaud JM, Cochelard D, et al: Palliative treatment of cancer of the esophagus and cardia by laser photoablation. *Gastroenterol Clin Biol* **11**(5):371–375, 1987
76. Naveau S, Zourabichvili O, Poitrine A, et al: Palliative treatment of cancers of the esophagus and cardia with Neodymium YAG laser: Short term results and multidimensional analysis of factors related to functional improvement and tumour destruction. *Gastroenterol Clin Biol* **11**(5):364–370, 1987
77. Fleischer D: The Washington Symposium on endoscopic laser therapy, April 18 and 19, 1985. *Gastrointest Endosc* **31**(6):397–400, 1985
78. Fleischer D, Sivak MV: Endoscopic Nd:YAG laser therapy as palliative treatment for advanced adenocarcinoma of the gastric cardia. *Gastroenterology* **87:**815–820, 1984
79. Matthewson K: Laser therapy. In Hurt RL (ed): *Management of Oesophageal Carcinoma.* London, Springer, 1989, pp 251–256
80. Loizou LA, Rampton D, Atkinson M, et al: A prospective assessment of quality of life after endoscopic intubation and laser therapy for malignant dysphagia. *Cancer* **70**(2):386–391, 1992
81. Barr H, Krasner N: Prospective quality-of-life analysis after palliative photoablation for the treatment of malignant dysphagia. *Cancer* **68**(7):1660–1664, 1991
82. Ell C, Rieman JF, Lux G, Demling L: Palliative laser treatment of malignant stenoses in the upper gastrointestinal tract. *Endoscopy* **18**(Suppl 1):21–26, 1986
83. Mathus Vliegen EM, Tytgat GN: Laser photocoagulation in the palliative treatment of upper digestive tract tumours. *Cancer* **57**(2):396–399, 1986

84. Moon BC, Woolfson IL, Mercer CD: Neodymium: yttrium aluminum garnet laser vaporization for palliation of obstructing esophageal carcinoma. *J Thorac Cardiovasc Surg* **98:**11–15, 1989
85. Dougherty TJ: Photodynamic therapy. *Clin Chest Med* **6**(2):219–236, 1985
86. McCaughan JS, Williams TE: Palliation of esophageal malignancy with photodynamic therapy. In Delaure NC, Wilkins EW, Wong J: *International Trends in General Thoracic Surgery, Esophageal Cancer,* Vol IV. St. Louis, Mosby, 1988, pp 402–409

# Index



Page numbers followed by *t* or *f* indicate tables or figures, respectively. *CP* indicates color plates, which follow page 608 in Vol I; page 2072 in Vol. II.

Page numbers followed by *t* or *f* indicate tables or figures, respectively. *CP* indicates color plates, which follow page 608 in Vol I; page 2072 in Vol. II.

Page numbers followed by *t* or *f* indicate tables or figures, respectively. *CP* indicates color plates, which follow page 608 in Vol I; page 2072 in Vol. II.

Page numbers followed by *t* or *f* indicate tables or figures, respectively. *CP* indicates color plates, which follow page 608 in Vol I; page 2072 in Vol. II.

Page numbers followed by *t* or *f* indicate tables or figures, respectively. *CP* indicates color plates, which follow page 608 in Vol I; page 2072 in Vol. II.

Page numbers followed by *t* or *f* indicate tables or figures, respectively. *CP* indicates color plates, which follow page 608 in Vol I; page 2072 in Vol. II.

Page numbers followed by *t* or *f* indicate tables or figures, respectively. *CP* indicates color plates, which follow page 608 in Vol I; page 2072 in Vol. II.

Page numbers followed by *t* or *f* indicate tables or figures, respectively. *CP* indicates color plates, which follow page 608 in Vol I; page 2072 in Vol. II.

Page numbers followed by *t* or *f* indicate tables or figures, respectively. *CP* indicates color plates, which follow page 608 in Vol I; page 2072 in Vol. II.

Page numbers followed by *t* or *f* indicate tables or figures, respectively. *CP* indicates color plates, which follow page 608 in Vol I; page 2072 in Vol. II.

Page numbers followed by *t* or *f* indicate tables or figures, respectively. *CP* indicates color plates, which follow page 608 in Vol I; page 2072 in Vol. II.

Page numbers followed by *t* or *f* indicate tables or figures, respectively. *CP* indicates color plates, which follow page 608 in Vol I; page 2072 in Vol. II.

Page numbers followed by *t* or *f* indicate tables or figures, respectively. *CP* indicates color plates, which follow page 608 in Vol I; page 2072 in Vol. II.

Page numbers followed by *t* or *f* indicate tables or figures, respectively. *CP* indicates color plates, which follow page 608 in Vol I; page 2072 in Vol. II.

Page numbers followed by *t* or *f* indicate tables or figures, respectively. *CP* indicates color plates, which follow page 608 in Vol I; page 2072 in Vol. II.

Page numbers followed by *t* or *f* indicate tables or figures, respectively. *CP* indicates color plates, which follow page 608 in Vol I; page 2072 in Vol. II.

Page numbers followed by *t* or *f* indicate tables or figures, respectively. *CP* indicates color plates, which follow page 608 in Vol I; page 2072 in Vol. II.

Page numbers followed by *t* or *f* indicate tables or figures, respectively. *CP* indicates color plates, which follow page 608 in Vol I; page 2072 in Vol. II.

Page numbers followed by *t* or *f* indicate tables or figures, respectively. *CP* indicates color plates, which follow page 608 in Vol I; page 2072 in Vol. II.

Page numbers followed by *t* or *f* indicate tables or figures, respectively. *CP* indicates color plates, which follow page 608 in Vol I; page 2072 in Vol. II.

Page numbers followed by *t* or *f* indicate tables or figures, respectively. *CP* indicates color plates, which follow page 608 in Vol I; page 2072 in Vol. II.

Page numbers followed by *t* or *f* indicate tables or figures, respectively. *CP* indicates color plates, which follow page 608 in Vol I; page 2072 in Vol. II.

---

Page numbers followed by *t* or *f* indicate tables or figures, respectively. *CP* indicates color plates, which follow page 608 in Vol I; page 2072 in Vol. II.

Page numbers followed by *t* or *f* indicate tables or figures, respectively. *CP* indicates color plates, which follow page 608 in Vol I; page 2072 in Vol. II.

Page numbers followed by *t* or *f* indicate tables or figures, respectively. *CP* indicates color plates, which follow page 608 in Vol I; page 2072 in Vol. II.

Page numbers followed by *t* or *f* indicate tables or figures, respectively. *CP* indicates color plates, which follow page 608 in Vol I; page 2072 in Vol. II.

Page numbers followed by *t* or *f* indicate tables or figures, respectively. *CP* indicates color plates, which follow page 608 in Vol I; page 2072 in Vol. II.

Page numbers followed by *t* or *f* indicate tables or figures, respectively. *CP* indicates color plates, which follow page 608 in Vol I; page 2072 in Vol. II.

Page numbers followed by *t* or *f* indicate tables or figures, respectively. *CP* indicates color plates, which follow page 608 in Vol I; page 2072 in Vol. II.

Page numbers followed by *t* or *f* indicate tables or figures, respectively. *CP* indicates color plates, which follow page 608 in Vol I; page 2072 in Vol. II.

Page numbers followed by *t* or *f* indicate tables or figures, respectively. *CP* indicates color plates, which follow page 608 in Vol I; page 2072 in Vol. II.

---

Page numbers followed by *t* or *f* indicate tables or figures, respectively. *CP* indicates color plates, which follow page 608 in Vol I; page 2072 in Vol. II.

Page numbers followed by *t* or *f* indicate tables or figures, respectively. *CP* indicates color plates, which follow page 608 in Vol I; page 2072 in Vol. II.

Page numbers followed by *t* or *f* indicate tables or figures, respectively. *CP* indicates color plates, which follow page 608 in Vol I; page 2072 in Vol. II.

Page numbers followed by *t* or *f* indicate tables or figures, respectively. *CP* indicates color plates, which follow page 608 in Vol I; page 2072 in Vol. II.

Page numbers followed by *t* or *f* indicate tables or figures, respectively. *CP* indicates color plates, which follow page 608 in Vol I; page 2072 in Vol. II.

Page numbers followed by *t* or *f* indicate tables or figures, respectively. *CP* indicates color plates, which follow page 608 in Vol I; page 2072 in Vol. II.

Page numbers followed by *t* or *f* indicate tables or figures, respectively. *CP* indicates color plates, which follow page 608 in Vol I; page 2072 in Vol. II.

Page numbers followed by *t* or *f* indicate tables or figures, respectively. *CP* indicates color plates, which follow page 608 in Vol I; page 2072 in Vol. II.

Page numbers followed by *t* or *f* indicate tables or figures, respectively. *CP* indicates color plates, which follow page 608 in Vol I; page 2072 in Vol. II.

Page numbers followed by *t* or *f* indicate tables or figures, respectively. *CP* indicates color plates, which follow page 608 in Vol I; page 2072 in Vol. II.

Page numbers followed by *t* or *f* indicate tables or figures, respectively. *CP* indicates color plates, which follow page 608 in Vol I; page 2072 in Vol. II.

Page numbers followed by *t* or *f* indicate tables or figures, respectively. *CP* indicates color plates, which follow page 608 in Vol I; page 2072 in Vol. II.

Page numbers followed by *t* or *f* indicate tables or figures, respectively. *CP* indicates color plates, which follow page 608 in Vol I; page 2072 in Vol. II.

Page numbers followed by *t* or *f* indicate tables or figures, respectively. *CP* indicates color plates, which follow page 608 in Vol I; page 2072 in Vol. II.

---

Page numbers followed by *t* or *f* indicate tables or figures, respectively. *CP* indicates color plates, which follow page 608 in Vol I; page 2072 in Vol. II.

Page numbers followed by *t* or *f* indicate tables or figures, respectively. *CP* indicates color plates, which follow page 608 in Vol I; page 2072 in Vol. II.

Page numbers followed by *t* or *f* indicate tables or figures, respectively. *CP* indicates color plates, which follow page 608 in Vol I; page 2072 in Vol. II.

Page numbers followed by *t* or *f* indicate tables or figures, respectively. *CP* indicates color plates, which follow page 608 in Vol I; page 2072 in Vol. II.

Page numbers followed by *t* or *f* indicate tables or figures, respectively. *CP* indicates color plates, which follow page 608 in Vol I; page 2072 in Vol. II.

Page numbers followed by *t* or *f* indicate tables or figures, respectively. *CP* indicates color plates, which follow page 608 in Vol I; page 2072 in Vol. II.

Page numbers followed by *t* or *f* indicate tables or figures, respectively. *CP* indicates color plates, which follow page 608 in Vol I; page 2072 in Vol. II.